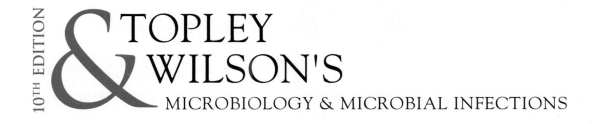

10TH EDITION

& TOPLEY WILSON'S

MICROBIOLOGY & MICROBIAL INFECTIONS

VIROLOGY

VOLUME 1

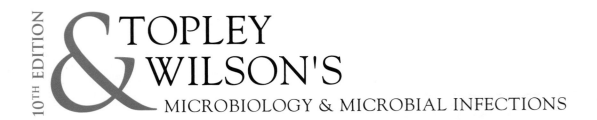

TOPLEY & WILSON'S
MICROBIOLOGY & MICROBIAL INFECTIONS

10TH EDITION

Topley & Wilson's Microbiology and Microbial Infections has grown from one to eight volumes since first published in 1929, reflecting the ever-increasing breadth and depth of knowledge in each of the areas covered. This tenth edition continues the tradition of providing the most comprehensive reference to microorganisms and the resulting infectious diseases currently available. It forms a unique resource, with each volume including examples of the best writing and research in the fields of virology, bacteriology, medical mycology, parasitology, and immunology from around the globe.

www.topleyandwilson.com

VIROLOGY Volumes 1 and 2

Edited by Brian W.J. Mahy and Volker ter Meulen
Volume 1 ISBN 0 340 88561 0; Volume 2 ISBN 0 340 88562 9; 2 volume set ISBN 0 340 88563 7

BACTERIOLOGY Volumes 1 and 2

Edited by S. Peter Borriello, Patrick R. Murray, and Guido Funke
Volume 1 ISBN 0 340 88564 5; Volume 2 ISBN 0 340 88565 3; 2 volume set ISBN 0 340 88566 1

MEDICAL MYCOLOGY

Edited by William G. Merz and Roderick J. Hay
ISBN 0 340 88567 X

PARASITOLOGY

Edited by F.E.G. Cox, Derek Wakelin, Stephen H. Gillespie, and Dickson D. Despommier
ISBN 0 340 88568 8

IMMUNOLOGY

Edited by Stephan H.E. Kaufmann and Michael W. Steward
ISBN 0 340 88569 6

Cumulative index

ISBN 0 340 88570 X

8 volume set plus CD-ROM

ISBN 0 340 80912 4

CD-ROM only

ISBN 0 340 88560 2

For a full list of contents, please see the *Complete table of contents* on page 945

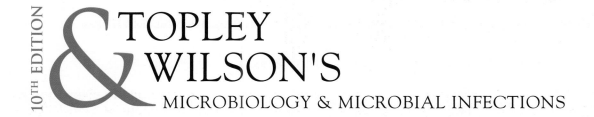

10TH EDITION

& TOPLEY & WILSON'S
MICROBIOLOGY & MICROBIAL INFECTIONS

VIROLOGY

VOLUME 1

EDITED BY

Brian W.J. Mahy MA PhD ScD DSc
Senior Scientific Research Advisor, National Center for Infectious Diseases
Centers for Disease Control and Prevention, Atlanta, GA, USA

Volker ter Meulen MD
Professor Emeritus of Clinical Virology and Immunology
Former Chairman of the Institute for Virology and Immunobiology
University of Würzburg, Würzburg, Germany

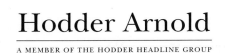 Hodder Arnold
A MEMBER OF THE HODDER HEADLINE GROUP

 ASM PRESS

First published in Great Britain in 1929
Second edition 1936; Third edition 1946
Fourth edition 1955; Fifth edition 1964; Sixth edition 1975
Seventh edition 1983 and 1984; Eighth edition 1990
Ninth edition 1998.
This tenth edition published in 2005 by
Hodder Arnold, an imprint of Hodder Education and a member of the Hodder Headline Group,
338 Euston Road, London NW1 3BH

http://www.hoddereducation.com

Distributed in the United States of America by ASM Press, the book publishing division of the American Society for Microbiology, 1752 N Street, N.W. Washington, D.C. 20036, USA

Hodder Headline's policy is to use papers that are natural, renewable and recyclable products and made from wood grown in sustainable forests. The logging and manufacturing processes are expected to conform to the environmental regulations of the country of origin.

Whilst the advice and information in this book are believed to be true and accurate at the date of going to press, neither the author[s] nor the publisher can accept any legal responsibility or liability for any errors or omissions that may be made. In particular (but without limiting the generality of the preceding disclaimer) every effort has been made to check drug dosages; however it is still possible that errors have been missed. Furthermore, dosage schedules are constantly being revised and new side-effects recognized. For these reasons the reader is strongly urged to consult the drug companies' printed instructions before administering any of the drugs recommended in this book.

British Library Cataloguing in Publication Data
A catalogue record for this book is available from the British Library

Library of Congress Cataloging-in-Publication Data
A catalog record for this book is available from the Library of Congress

Volume 1 ISBN-10   0 340 885 610   ISBN-13 978 0 340 88561 1
Volume 2 ISBN-10   0 340 885 629   ISBN-13 978 0 340 88562 8
Two volume set ISBN-10 0 340 885 637   ISBN-13 978 0 340 88563 5
Complete set and CD-ROM ISBN-10   0340 80912 4   ISBN-13   978 0 340 80912 9
Indian edtion ISBN-10   0 340 88559 9   ISBN-13   978 0 340 88559 8

1 2 3 4 5 6 7 8 9 10

Commissioning Editor: Serena Bureau / Joanna Koster
Development Editor: Layla Vandenberg
Project Editor: Zelah Pengilley
Production Controller: Deborah Smith
Cover Designer: Sarah Rees
Cover image: Herpes simplex virus, TEM. Dr. Linda Stannard, UCT / Science Photo Library

Typeset in 9/11 Times New Roman by Lucid Digital, Salisbury, UK
Printed and bound in Italy

What do you think about this book? Or any other Hodder Arnold title? Please send your comments to www.hoddereducation.com

Contents

Please note: Chapter names shown in gray can be found in Virology Volume 2

Contributors

Adriano Aguzzi MD PHD hcFRCP FRCPATH
Institute of Neuropathology
University Hospital of Zürich
Zürich, Switzerland

Antonio Alcami PHD
Department of Medicine
University of Cambridge
Addenbrooke's Hospital, Cambridge, UK; and
Centro Nacional de Biotecnologia (CSIC)
Campus Universidad Autónoma
Madrid, Spain

L. Andrew Ball DPHIL
Professor of Microbiology
University of Alabama at Birmingham
Birmingham, AL, USA

Jangu E. Banatvala CBE MA MD FRCP FRCPATH
FMEDSCI
Emeritus Professor of Clinical Virology
Guy's, King's and St Thomas' Medical
and Dental School
London, UK

Bettina Bankamp PHD
Measles, Mumps, Rubella and Herpes Team
Respiratory and Enteric Viruses Branch
Division of Viral and Rickettsial Diseases
National Center for Infectious Diseases
Centers for Disease Control and Prevention
Atlanta, GA, USA

Alan D.T. Barrett PHD
Department of Pathology
University of Texas Medical Branch
Galveston, TX, USA

Thomas Barrett PHD
Institue for Animal Health
Pirbright Laboratory
Pirbright, UK

William J. Bellini PHD
Chief, Measles, Mumps, Rubella and
Herpesviruses Team
Respiratory and Enteric Viruses Branch
Division of Viral and Rickettsial Diseases
National Center for Infectious Diseases
Centers for Disease Control and Prevention
Atlanta, GA, USA

Mauro Bendinelli MD PHD
Professor of Microbiology; and
Director of Virology and Retrovirus Center
Department of Experimental Pathology
Virology Section, University of Pisa
Pisa, Italy

Kenneth I. Berns MD PHD
Director, UF Genetics Institute; and
Professor, Molecular Genetics and Microbiology
College of Medicine
University of Florida
Gainesville, FL, USA

Jennifer M. Best PHD FRCPATH
Reader in Virology,
Department of Infectious Diseases
King's College London,
London, UK

Roumiana S. Boneva MD PHD
Medical Epidemiologist
National Center for Infectious Diseases
Centers for Disease Control and Prevention
Atlanta, GA, USA

Thomas Briese PHD
Jerome L. and Dawn Greene
Infectious Disease Laboratory
Mailman School of Public Health
Columbia University
New York, NY, USA

William J. Britt MD
Department of Pediatrics
University of Alabama at Birmingham
Birmingham, AL, USA

Jo Ellen Brunner PHD
Instructional Support Group
School of Biological Sciences
University of California
Irvine, CA, USA

Michael J. Carter BA PHD
School of Biomedical and Molecular Sciences
University of Surrey
Guildford, UK

Pierre-Emmanuel Ceccaldi PHD
Senior Scientist
Unit 'Epidémiologie et Physiopathologie
des Virus Oncogènes'
Institut Pasteur
Paris, France

Ian N. Clarke BSC PHD
Professor of Virology
Division of Infection, Inflammation and Repair
School of Medicine
University of Southampton
Southampton, UK

J. Barklie Clements FRSE FMEDSCI
Professor of Virology
Division of Virology
Institute of Biological and Life Sciences
University of Glasgow
Glasgow, UK

Leslie Collier MD DSC FRCP FRCPATH
Professor Emeritus of Virology
The London Hospital and Medical College, London;
Formerly Director, Vaccines and Sera Laboratories
The Lister Institute of Preventive Medicine
Elstree, Hertfordshire, UK

Richard C. Condit PHD
Department of Molecular Genetics and Microbiology
University of Florida College of Medicine
Gainesville, FL, USA

James F. Conway BSC PHD
Group Leader
Laboratoire de Microscopie Electronique Structurale
Institut de Biologie Structurale
Grenoble, France

Samantha Cooray MBIOCHEM PHD
Department of Virology
Wright Fleming Institute
Imperial College Faculty of Medicine
London, UK

Susan F. Cotmore PHD
Senior Research Scientist
Department of Laboratory Medicine
Yale University School of Medicine
New Haven, CT, USA

Nancy J. Cox PHD
Chief, Influenza Branch
Division of Viral and Rickettsial Diseases
Centers for Disease Control and Prevention
Atlanta, GA, USA

Dorothy H. Crawford MBBS PHD MD FRCP
DSC FRSE
Professor of Medical Microbiology
School of Biomedical & Clinical Laboratory Sciences
University of Edinburgh
Edinburgh, UK

Andrew J. Davison MA PHD
MRC Virology Unit
Institute of Virology
University of Glasgow
Glasgow, UK

Terence S. Dermody MD
Professor of Pediatrics and Microbiology
and Immunology
Elizabeth B. Lamb Center for Pediatric Research
Vanderbilt University School of Medicine
Nashville, TN, USA

Ulrich Desselberger MD FRCPATH FRCP
Clinical Microbiology and Public Health Laboratory
Addenbrooke's Hospital
Cambridge, UK (until July 2002)

Charlene S. Dezzutti PHD
HIV and Retrovirology Branch
Division of AIDS, STD, and TB Laboratory Research
National Center for HIV, STD, and TB Prevention
Centers for Disease Control and Prevention
Atlanta, GA, USA

Esteban Domingo PHD
Professor CSIC
Centro de Biología Molecular "Severo Ochoa"
CSIC-UAM, Universidad Autónoma de Madrid
Cantoblanco, Madrid, Spain

Ruben O. Donis DVM PhD
Chief, Molecular Genetics Section
Influenza Branch
Division of Viral and Rickettsial Diseases
National Centers for Infectious Diseases
Centers for Disease Control and Prevention
Atlanta, GA, USA

Bernadette M. Dutia BSc PhD
Senior Research Fellow
Laboratory for Clinical and Molecular Virology
Division of Veterinary Biomedical Sciences
University of Edinburgh
Edinburgh, UK

Andrew J. Easton BSc PhD
Professor of Virology
Department of Biological Sciences
University of Warwick
Coventry, UK

Richard M. Elliott BSc DPhil FRSE
Professor of Molecular Virology
Division of Virology
Institute of Biomedical and Life Sciences
University of Glasgow
Glasgow, UK

Gisela Enders MD
Professor of Virology
Head of the Institute of Virology
Infectiology and Epidemiology; and
Chief, Laboratory Prof. G. Enders and Partners
Stuttgart, Germany

M. Anthony Epstein MA MD DSc PhD FRS
Nuffield Department of Clinical Medicine
University of Oxford, John Radcliffe Hospital
Oxford, UK

Dean D. Erdman Dr PH
Team Leader
Respiratory Virus Diagnostics Section
Division of Viral and Rickettsial Diseases
National Center for Infectious Diseases
Centers for Disease Control and Prevention
Atlanta, GA, USA

Mary K. Estes PhD
Professor, Department of Molecular Virology
and Microbiology
Baylor College of Medicine
Houston, TX, USA

Heinz Feldmann MD
Chief, Special Pathogens Program
National Microbiology Laboratory

Public Health Agency of Canada; and
Associate Professor
Department of Medical Microbiology
University of Manitoba
Winnipeg, MB, Canada

Hugh J. Field ScD FRCPath
Reader in Comparative Virology
Centre for Veterinary Science
University of Cambridge
Cambridge, UK

Bernhard Fleckenstein MD
Professor and Chairman
Institute for Clinical and Molecular Virology
University of Erlangen-Nürnberg
Erlangen, Germany

Thomas M. Folks PhD
HIV and Retrovirology Branch
Division of AIDS, STD, and
TB Laboratory Research
National Center for HIV, STD, and TB Prevention
Centers for Disease Control and Prevention
Atlanta, GA, USA

Ilya V. Frolov PhD
Department of Microbiology and Immunology
University of Texas Medical Branch
Galveston, TX, USA

Yves Gaudin PhD
Director
Laboratoire de Virologie Moléculaire et Structurale
UMR-CNRS 2472; UMR-INRA 1157 CNRS
Gif-sur-Yvette, Cedex, France

Wolfram H. Gerlich PhD
Professor and Director
Institute of Medical Virology
Justus Liebig University Giessen
Giessen, Germany

Alexander E. Gorbalenya PhD DSci
Associate Professor
Department of Medical Microbiology
Leiden University Medical Center
Leiden, The Netherlands

Jim Gray FIBMS PhD FRCPath
Head, Enteric Virus Unit
Virus Reference Department
Health Protection Agency, Centre for Infections
London, UK

Duane J. Gubler ScD
Director of Asia-Pacific Institute for Tropical Medicine
and Infectious Diseases; and
Chair, Department of Medicine and
Medical Microbiology
John A. Burns School of Medicine
Honolulu, HI, USA

Stephen C. Hadler MD
Senior Advisor for Strengthening Childhood
Immunization, Global Immunization Division
National Immunization Program
Centers for Disease Control and Prevention
Atlanta, GA, USA

Walid Heneine PHD
HIV and Retrovirology Branch,
Division of AIDS, STD, and TB Laboratory Research
National Center for HIV, STD, and TB Prevention
Centers for Disease Control and Prevention
Atlanta, GA, USA

John J. Holland PHD
Emeritus Professor
Division of Biology and Institute of
Molecular Genetics, University of California
San Diego, La Jolla, CA, USA

Mady Hornig MA MD
Director of Translational Research
Jerome L. and Dawn Greene Infectious Disease
Laboratory; and
Associate Professor of Epidemiology
Mailman School of Public Health
Columbia University
New York, NY, USA

Li Jin MD PHD MRCPATH
Clinical Scientist, Enteric Virus Reference
Department, Health Protection Agency
Centre for Infections, London, UK

Michael Kann MD
Professor of Virology
Justus Liebig University Giessen
Giessen, Germany

Yoshihiro Kawaoka DVM PHD
Professor and Director
International Research Center for Infectious Diseases;
and Division of Virology
Department of Microbiology and Immunology
Institute of Medical Science
University of Tokyo, Tokyo, Japan; and
Professor, Department of Pathobiological Sciences
School of Veterinary Medicine

University of Wisconsin-Madison
Madison, WI, USA

Kamel Khalili PHD
Professor and Director
Center for Neurovirology and Cancer Biology
Temple University
Philadelphia, PA USA

Michael P. Kiley † PHD
Formerly USDA, Agricultural Research Service
Animal Production, Product Value
Beltsville, MD, USA

Hans-Dieter Klenk MD
Institute of Virology Medical School
Philipps-University
Marburg, Germany

Wendy A. Knowles BSC PHD MIBIOL
Clinical Scientist, Enteric, Respiratory and
Neurological Virus Laboratory
Specialist and Reference Microbiology Division
Health Protection Agency, Centre for Infections
London, UK

Myriam S. Künzi PHD
Postdoctoral Fellow, John Hopkins Oncology Center
Baltimore, MD, USA

Paul R. Lambden BSC PHD
Senior Research Fellow, Molecular Microbiology
University Medical School
Southampton General Hospital
Southampton, UK

R. Michael Linden PHD
Associate Professor
Department of Gene and Cell Medicine, and
Department of Microbiology
Mount Sinai School of Medicine
New York, NY, USA

W. Ian Lipkin MD
Jerome L. and Dawn Greene Infectious
Disease Laboratory
Mailman School of Public Health
Columbia University
New York, NY, USA

Graham Lloyd BSC MSC PHD FIBMS
Head, Special Pathogens Reference Unit
Health Protection Agency
Centre for Emergency, Preparedness and Response
Porton Down, Salisbury, UK

Fabrizio Maggi MD PhD
Assistant, Clinical Virology
Department of Experimental Pathology
Virology Section, University of Pisa
Pisa, Italy

Brian W.J. Mahy MA PhD ScD DSc
Senior Scientific Research Advisor
National Center for Infectious Diseases
Centers for Disease Control and Prevention
Atlanta, GA, USA

Myra McClure PhD DSc FRCPATH
Professor of Retrovirolgy and
Honorary Consultant in GU Medicine
Head of Section of Infectious Diseases
Jefferiss Research Trust Laboratories
Wright-Fleming Institute, Faculty of Medicine
Imperial College London
London, UK

Philip Minor BA PhD
National Institute for Biological Standards and
Control (NIBSC), Division of Virology
South Mimms, Potters Bar
Herts, UK

Anthony C. Minson BSc PhD
Professor of Virology, Virology Division
Department of Pathology, University of Cambridge
Cambridge, UK

Arnold S. Monto MD
Professor of Epidemiology, Director
The University of Michigan Bioterrorism
Preparedness Initiative
University of Michigan School of Public Health
Ann Arbor, MI, USA

Anne Moscona MD
Professor, Pediatrics and Microbiology/Immunology
Vice Chair of Pediatrics for Research
Weill Medical College
Cornell University
New York, NY, USA

Richard W. Moyer PhD
Senior Associate Dean for Research
Development; and
Professor, Department of Molecular Genetics
and Microbiology
University of Florida College of Medicine
Gainesville, FL, USA

Frederick A. Murphy DVM PhD
School of Veterinary Medicine
University of California Davis
Davis, CA, USA

David Mutimer MBBS MD FRACP FRCP
Reader in Hepatology, University of Birmingham; and
Consultant Hepatologist, Liver and Hepatobiliary Unit
Queen Elizabeth Hospital
Birmingham, UK

Anthony A. Nash PhD FRSE
Laboratory for Clinical and Molecular Virology
Centre for Infectious Diseases
University of Edinburgh
Edinburgh, UK

Neal Nathanson MD
Associate Dean, Global Health Programs
University of Pennsylvania School of Medicine
Philadelphia, PA, USA

James C. Neil BSc PhD FRSE
Professor of Virology and Molecular Oncology
Institute of Comparative Medicine
University of Glasgow Veterinary School
Glasgow, UK

Frank Neipel MD
Institute for Clinical and Molecular Virology
University of Erlangen-Nürnberg
Erlangen, Germany

Gabriele Neumann PhD
Department of Pathobiological Sciences
School of Veterinary Medicine
University of Wisconsin-Madison
Madison, WI, USA

Jessica Otte BS
Center for Neurovirology and Cancer Biology
Temple University
Philadelphia, PA, USA

Richard W. Peluso PhD
Vice President Process Sciences and
Manufacturing, Targeted Genetics
Seattle, WA, USA

Mark Pett MA PhD
Postdoctoral Research Associate
MRC Cancer Cell Unit
Hutchinson MRC Research Centre
Cambridge, UK

Paula M. Pitha MS PhD
Sidney Kimmel Comprehensive Cancer Centre
Johns Hopkins School of Medicine
Baltimore, MD, USA

Craig R. Pringle BSc PhD
Emeritus Professor, Biological Sciences Department
University of Warwick
Coventry, UK

Axel Rethwilm MD
Institut für Virologie und Immunbiologie
Universität Würzburg
Würzburg, Germany

Betty Robertson PhD
Division of Viral Hepatitis
Centers for Disease Control and Prevention
Division of Viral Hepatitis
Atlanta, GA, USA

Juan D. Rodas DVM MSc PhD
Assistant Professor
Facultad de Ciencias Agrarias y
Laboratorio de Immunovirologia
Universidad de Antioquia
Medellin, Columbia

John T. Roehrig PhD
Chief, Arbovirus Diseases Branch
Division of Vector-Borne Infectious Diseases
National Center for Infectious Diseases
Centers for Disease Control
and Prevention Public Health Service
Fort Collins, CO, USA

Paul A. Rota PhD
Measles, Mumps, Rubella and Herpesvirus Team
Respiratory and Enteric Viruses Branch
Division of Viral and Rickettsial Diseases
Centers for Disease Control and Prevention
Atlanta, GA, USA

David J. Rowlands PhD
School of Biochemistry and Microbiology
University of Leeds
Leeds, UK

Rob W.H. Ruigrok PhD
Laboratoire de Virologie Moléculaire et Structurale
FRE 2854 CNRS-Université Joseph Fourier
Grenoble, France

Willie Russell BSc PhD FRSE
Emeritus Research Professor
School of Biology
University of St Andrews
Fife, UK

Mahmut Safak PhD
Head, Laboratory of Molecular Virology
Center for Neurovirology and Cancer Biology
Temple University
Philadelphia, PA USA

Maria S. Salvato PhD
Professor, Institute of Human Virology
University of Maryland Biotechnology Institute
Baltimore, MD, USA

Jürgen Schneider-Schaulies PhD
Professor of Virology
Institute for Virology and Immunobiology
University of Würzburg, Würzburg, Germany

Sibylle Schneider-Schaulies PhD
Professor of Virology
Institute for Virology and Immunobiology
University of Würzburg
Würzburg, Germany

Guy Schoehn PhD
Laboratoire de Virologie Moléculaire et Structurale
FRE 2854 CNRS-Université Joseph Fourier
Grenoble, France

Ulrich Schubert PhD
Institute for Clinical and Molecular Virology
University of Erlangen-Nürnberg
Erlangen, Germany

Bert L. Semler PhD
Professor and Chair
Department of Microbiology and Molecular Genetics
University of California
Irvine, CA, USA

Jane F. Seward MBBS MPH
Chief, Viral Vaccine Preventable Diseases Branch
Epidemiology and Surveillance Division
National Immunization Program
Centers for Disease Control and Prevention
Atlanta, GA, USA

Robert E. Shope MD†
Formerly John S. Dunn Distinguished
Chair in Biodefense
Department of Pathology
University of Texas Medical Branch
Galveston, TX, USA

Stuart G. Siddell BSc PhD
Professor of Virology
Department of Pathology and Microbiology
University of Bristol
Bristol, UK

Peter Simmonds BM PhD MRCPath
Centre for Infectious Diseases
University of Edinburgh
Edinburgh, UK

Anthony Simmons MA MB BChir PhD
Professor, Pediatrics, Pathology, Microbiology
and Immunology, 2.330 Children's Hospital
University of Texas Medical Branch at Galveston
Galveston, TX, USA

Geoffrey L. Smith PhD FRS
Professor of Virology; and
Wellcome Trust Research Fellow
Department of Virology
Faculty of Medicine
Imperial College London
London, UK

Eric J. Snijder PhD
Associate Professor,
Department of Medical Microbiology
Leiden University Medical Center
Leiden, The Netherlands

Steven Specter PhD
Professor, Medical Microbiology and Immunology and
Associate Dean for Admissions and Student Affairs
University of South Florida College of Medicine
Tampa, FL, USA

Margaret Stanley PhD
Professor of Epithelial Biology
Department of Pathology
University of Cambridge, UK

Peter Tattersall PhD
Professor, Departments of Laboratory
Medicine and Genetics
Yale University School of Medicine
New Haven, CT, USA

John M. Taylor PhD
Senior Member
Fox Chase Cancer Center
Philadelphia, PA, USA

Volker ter Meulen MD
Professor Emeritus of Clinical Virology
and Immunology
Former Chairman of the Institute for Virology
and Immunbiology
University of Würzburg
Würzburg, Germany

Noël Tordo PhD
Chief of Laboratory; and
Head, Unit 'Stratégies Antivirales'
Virology Department, Institut Pasteur
Paris, France

Ralph A. Tripp PhD
Professor and GRA Chair, University of Georgia,
College of Veterinary Medicine
Department of Infectious Diseases
Athens, GA, USA

Kenneth L. Tyler MD
Reuler-Lewin Family Professor of Neurology and
Professor of Medicine
Microbiology and Immunology
University of Colorado Health Sciences
Center and Chief, Neurology Service
Denver Veterans Affairs Medical Center
Denver, CO, USA

Marc H.V. Van Regenmortel PhD
Emeritus Research Director, CNRS
Biotechnology School of the University of Strasbourg
Illkirch, France

Alex I. Wandeler PhD
Canadian Food Inspection Agency
Ontario Laboratory Fallowfield
Nepean, Ontario, Canada

Scott C. Weaver PhD
Director for Tropical and Emerging Infectious Diseases
UTMB Center for Biodefense and
Emerging Infectious Disease; and
Professor, Departments of Pathology
Microbiology & Immunology
University of Texas Medical Branch
Galveston, TX, USA

Sandra K. Weller PhD
Professor and Chair
Molecular, Microbial and Structural Biology
University of Connecticut Health Center
Farmington, CT, USA

Richard J. Whitley MD
Professor of Pediatrics, Microbiology,
Medicine and Neurosurgery
University of Alabama at Birmingham
Children's Hospital
Birmingham, AL, USA

Margaret M. Willcocks BSc PhD
School of Biomedical and Molecular Sciences
University of Surrey
Guildford, UK

John A. Wyke MA, VetMB, PhD, MRCVS, FRSE
Senior Research Fellow
Institute of Comparative Medicine
University of Glasgow Veterinary School
Glasgow, UK

John Ziebuhr MD
Associate Professor, Institute of Virology
and Immunology, University of Würzburg
Würzburg, Germany

Preface

The remarkable progress of research in virology has led to the expansion from 47 chapters in the 9th edition to 70 in this 10th edition. Since the preparation of the 9th edition we have seen the emergence of several hitherto unknown human viruses as well as some remarkable examples of viruses of animals or birds crossing the species barrier and infecting humans. So far as the latter phenomenon is concerned, two incidents occurred involving avian influenza viruses. In 1997, avian influenza subtype H5N1 was recovered for the first time from humans, when it caused 18 cases of severe influenza with six deaths in children and adults in Hong Kong. The slaughter of more than a million chickens in early 1998 ended this disease outbreak, but in 1999 another avian influenza subtype, H9N2, was recovered from two young children in Hong Kong. The H5N1 virus has continued to infect poultry and other birds in South East Asia, and to cause further morbidity and mortality in humans in 2005. In both these incidents the viruses which affected humans were found to have all gene segments derived from the avian virus, a situation never previously encountered in influenza virology.

A second example of crossing the species barrier occurred in 1999 and involved a newly recognized paramyxovirus, Nipah virus, which caused disease outbreaks with severe mortality in Malaysia and Singapore. The causative virus was acquired from infected pigs, and disease control measures included the slaughter of more than a million pigs in Malaysia. Nipah virus appears to have a wide host range including dogs and cats as well as pigs and humans, and will be an important new area for investigation over the next several years. The virus is now causing human disease outbreaks in Bangladesh, apparently without the involvement of pigs as an intermediate host.

New human viruses that have recently emerged include TT virus, originally thought to be associated with transfusion-acquired hepatitis in Japan, but now not thought to be a cause of hepatitis. TT virus has a small circular, single-stranded DNA genome, and appears to have a global distribution. There is evidence that infection is acquired at an early age in some parts of the world, but its disease significance remains unknown. TT virus thus joins GB virus C/Hepatitis G virus as a newly recognized human virus infection of unknown disease significance.

In 2003, a new disease was recognized in Asia which became known as severe acute respiratory syndrome (SARS). Unexpectedly, the causative agent of this disease was identified as a hitherto unknown coronavirus. A remarkable international collaboration led to rapid determination of the complete genome sequence of the SARS human coronavirus which showed that this virus had not previously been seen. The precise origin of this virus remains unknown. As outlined in the preface to the 9th edition, it is likely that the identification of new viruses by gene sequencing or other technologies will continue to raise questions for virologists, who need to investigate their relevance.

The chapters in this 10th edition are grouped into four parts.

Several new chapters are now included in Part I (General Characteristics of Viruses).

The changes in virus classification and nomenclature that were approved by the International Committee on Taxonomy of Viruses (ICTV) in August 1999 are outlined in Chapters 3 and 4. During this period three new Orders were established, and the characteristics of those infecting vertebrates are described in two new chapters on Mononegavirales and Nidovirales (Chapters 19 and 20). We have also included three new chapters on replication of negative strand RNA viruses, positive-strand RNA viruses, and DNA viruses (Chapters 8-10), and a new chapter on Viral evasion of the immune response (Chapter 16), an increasingly recognized component of viral pathogenesis.

In Part II, the number of chapters on specific viruses and viral infection has increased from 26 to 40 in this 10th edition. There are new chapters on Borna disease virus (Chapter 52), an increasingly studied member of the Mononegavirales that may be a cause of some human psychiatric disorders, and on TT virus and other members of the *Anellovirus* genus (Chapter 57).

Other new chapters deal with polyoma viruses (Chapter 24), human herpes virus 8 (Chapter 28), poxvirus replication (Chapter 31) paramyxoviruses (Chapters 34-38), rotaviruses (Chapter 44), foamy viruses (Chapter 59), human immunodeficiency virus

(Chapter 65), and viral vectors for gene therapy (Chapter 68).

Chapters from the 9th edition that have undergone substantial revision include those on Human enteric RNA viruses (Chapters 41 and 42); Retroviruses and associated diseases in humans (Chapter 58); Bunya-viruses (Chapter 48); Betaherpesviruses (Chapter 27); Orthomyxoviruses (Chapter 32); Prions of human and animals (Chapter 61); Coronaviruses, Toroviruses, and Arteriviruses (Chapter 39); Reoviruses (Chapter 43); Hepatitis C (Chapter 54); Parvoviruses (Chapter 21); Immunoprophylaxis of viral diseases (Chapter 67); and Antiviral Chemotherapy (Chapter 69).

We are extremely indebted to all the authors for their excellent contributions to this text, which now provides a realistic representation of the state of the art in understanding human viral infections. As in previous editions, little prominence has been given to infections of nonhuman species, except where they bear upon human infections as zoonoses, models of pathogenesis, or economic importance.

We wish to thank Penny Mahy for her excellent editorial work.

During the preparation of this text, we deeply regret that two of our authors passed away. Michael Kiley (Chapter 65), a world expert on biosafety, died on 24th January 2004 (Johnson 2004) and Robert Shope (Chapter 48), the world's most distinguished arbovirologist, died on 19th January 2004 (Murphy and Calisher 2004). Their obituaries can be found in Archives of Virology (see below), but we hope that this text will serve as a continuing tribute to their memory.

References

Johnson, K.M., 2004. In Memoriam Michael Patrick Kiley (1942–2004). *Arch Virol* **149**, 1467–8.

Murphy, F.A., Calisher, C.H. et al. 2004. In Memoriam Robert Ellis Shope (1929–2004). *Arch Virol* **149**, 1061–6.

Brian W.J. Mahy and Volker ter Meulen
Atlanta and Würzburg
May 2005

Abbreviations

aa	amino acid		**APD**	average pore diameter
AB	antibody		**APOBEC3G**	apolipoprotein B mRNA editing enzyme
AAFP	American Academy of Family Physicians		**APOIV**	Apoi virus
A+T	adenine and thymine		**APV**	avian pneumovirus
AAP	American Academy of Pediatrics		**Ara-A**	adenine arabinoside
AAV	adeno-associated virus		**Ara-C**	1-β-D-arabinofuranosylcytosine
ABLV	Australian bat lyssavirus		**Ara-MP**	adenine arabinoside-monophosphate
ABSV	Absettarov virus		**Ara-TP**	adenine arabinoside-triphosphate
ACE2	angiotensin-converting enzyme 2		**ARDS**	acute respiratory distress syndrome
ACIP	Advisory Committee on Immunization Practices (USA)		**ARIMA**	autoregressive integrated moving average
ACMHV-2	avian carcinoma virus Mill Hill virus 2		**AROAV**	Aroa virus
ACOG	American College of Obstetricians and Gynecologists		**ART**	antiretroviral therapy
			ARV	Adelaide river virus
ACTG	acquired immunodeficiency syndrome clinical trial group		**ASCUS**	atypical squamous cells of undetermined significance
ACV	aciclovir; or acyclovir		**ASFV**	African swine fever virus
ACV-MP	acyclovir monophosphate		**AST**	alkaline phosphatase
ACV-TP	acyclovir triphosphate		**As₂O₃**	arsenic trioxide
AD	autodisable		**ATCC**	American Type Culture Collection
ADC	acquired immunodeficiency syndrome dementia complex		**α-TIF**	α-*trans*-inducing factor
			ATL	acute T-cell leukemia; or adult T-cell leukemia
ADCC	antibody-dependent cell-mediated cytotoxicity		**AZT**	azidothymidine; or 3′-azido-3′-deoxythymidine
ADE	antibody-dependent enhancement		**AZT-DP**	azidothymidine diphosphate
Ad pol	adenovirus polymerase		**AZT-TP**	azidothymidine triphosphate
ADRP	adenosine diphosphate-ribose1′-phosphatase			
Ad35	adenovirus type 35		**BaEV**	baboon endogenous virus
AFP	α-fetoprotein		**BAGV**	Bagaza virus
AGMK	African green monkey kidney		**BAL**	bronchoalveolar lavage
AGUS	atypical glandular cells of undetermined significance		**BANV**	Banzi virus
			BAstV	bovine astrovirus
AHC	acute hemorrhagic conjunctivitis		**BBB**	blood–brain barrier
AHSV	African horse sickness virus		**BBV**	Bukalasa bat virus
AIDS	acquired immunodeficiency syndrome		**BCC**	basal cell carcinoma
ALFV	Alfuy virus		**BCoV**	bovine coronavirus
ALT	alanine amino transferase		**BCR**	B-cell receptor
ALV	avian leukosis virus		**BCRF**	B-cell regulatory factor
ALV-E	avian leukosis virus subgoup E		**BCV**	Batu Cave virus
AM	'aseptic' meningitis		**BD**	borna disease
AMDV	Aleutian mink disease virus		**bDNA**	branched DNA; or branched-chain DNA
AMP-RT	amplified reverse transcriptase		**BDPV**	Barbarie duck parvovirus
AMV	avian myeloblastosis virus		**BDV**	Border disease virus; or borna disease virus
ANP	acyclic nucleoside phosphonate		**BEFV**	bovine ephemeral fever virus
ANV	avian nephritis virus		**BFDV**	beak and feather disease virus
APC	antigen presenting cell		**BFPyV**	budgerigar fledgling polyomavirus
			BFU-E	burst-forming units erythroid

BFV	Barmah Forest virus; or bovine foamy virus
Bgp1	biliary glycoprotein 1
BH	black-hooded
BHK	baby hamster kidney
BIV	bovine immunodeficiency virus
BKPyV	BK polyomavirus
BKV	BK virus
BKVN	BKV-associated nephropathy
BL	Burkitt's lymphoma
BLV	bovine leukemia virus
BMI	body mass index
B19	human parvovirus B19
BOUV	Bouloui virus
BPL	β-propiolactone
BPV	bovine parvovirus; or bovine papillomavirus
BPV-1	bovine papillomavirus type 1
BPyV	bovine polyomavirus
BSE	bovine spongiform encephalopathy
BSL	biosafety level
BSQV	Bussuquara virus
BToV	bovine torovirus
BTV 10	bluetongue virus type 10
BVaraU	bromovinylarabinosyl-uracil
BVDU	bromovinyl deoxyuridine
BVDU-DP	bromovinyl deoxyuridine-diphosphate
BVDU-MP	bromovinyl deoxyuridine-monophosphate
BVDV	bovine viral diarrhea virus
BVU	bromovinylarabinosyl-uracil
C	cytosine
CA	capsid
CAdV	canine adenovirus
CAH	chronic active hepatitis
CAM	cell adhesion molecule; or chorioallantoic membrane
CAR	coxsackie adenovirus receptor
CART	combined antiretroviral therapy
CAT	chloramphenicol acetyl transferase
CAV	chicken anemia virus
CCA	chimpanzee coryza agent
cccDNA	covalently closed circular DNA
CCE	cornified cell envelope
CCHFV	Crimean–Congo hemorrhagic fever virus
CCPP	contagious caprine pleuropneumonia
CCoV	canine enteric coronavirus
CCV	channel catfish virus
CD	circular dichroism
CDC	Centers for Disease Control and Prevention (USA)
CDI	conformation-dependent immunoassay
CDKI	cyclin-dependent kinase inhibitor
CDV	canine distemper virus
CEA	carcinoembryonic antigen
CEE	central European encephalitis
CEV	cell-associated enveloped virus
CF	complement fixation; or cystic fibrosis
CFU-E	colony-forming units erythroid

CHIKV	Chikungunya virus
CHO	Chinese hamster ovary
CI	complementation index
CIC	circulating immune complex
CID	cytomegalic inclusion disease
CIEBOV	Côte d'Ivoire ebola virus
CIN	cervical intraepithelial neoplasia
CIV	Carey island virus
CJD	Creutzfeldt–Jakob disease
CK II	casein kinase II
CLP	core-like particle
CMI	cell-mediated immunity
CMV	cytomegalovirus
CnMV	canine minute virus
CNS	central nervous system
COPV	canine oral papillomavirus
cp	cytopathic
CPCV	Cacipacore virus
CPD	cyclic phosphodiesterase
CPE	cytopathic effect
CPH	chronic persistent hepatitis
CPMV	cowpea mosaic virus
CPSF	cleavage and polyadenylation specificity factor
CPT	cycling probe technology
CPV	canine parvovirus
CPXV	cowpox virus
CRE	*cis*-acting replication element
CREB	cyclic AMP-responsive element-binding protein
CRF	circulating recombinant forms
CRM	chromosome region maintenance
CrmA	cytokine response modifier A
CRPV	cottontail rabbit papillomavirus
CRS	congenital rubella syndrome
CRV	Cowbone Ridge virus
cryo-EM	cryo-electron microscopy
CsA	cyclosporin A
CSD	Cambridge Structural Database (UK)
CSE	conserved sequence element
CSF	cerebrospinal fluid; or colony stimulating factor
CSFV	classical swine fever virus
CT	computer tomography
CTE	constitutive RNA transport element
CTFV	Colorado tick fever virus
CTL	cytotoxic T-lymphocyte
CVB3	coxsackie virus B3
cVDPV	circulating vaccine-derived poliovirus
CVS	challenge virus standard; or chorionic villi sampling; or congenital varicella syndrome
CWD	chronic wasting disease
CypA	cyclophilin A
D	aspartate
DA	dopamine
DAF	decay accelerating factor
DANA	2,3-didehydro-2-deoxy-N-acetylneuraminic acid
DBP	DNA-binding protein
DBS	dried blood spots

DBV	Dakar bat virus
DC	dendritic cell
DD	death domains
DDA-TP	dideoxyadenosine 5′ triphosphate
DDC	dideoxycytidine
DDI	2′,3′-dideoxyinosine
DDI-MP	2′,3′-dideoxyinosine monophosphate
DED	death effector domain
DEET	diethylmethylbenzamide; or diethyltoluamide
DENV	dengue virus
D4T	2′,3′-didehydro-2′-deoxythymidine; or didehydrodeoxyuridine
D4T-DP	D4T diphosphate
D4T-TP	D4T triphosphate
DHBV	duck hepatitis B virus
DHF	dengue hemorrhagic fever
DHF/DDS	Dengue hemorrhagic fever/dengue shock syndrome
DI	defective interfering
DIC	disseminated intravascular coagulation
DMSO	dimethyl sulfoxide
DMV	dolphin morbillivirus; or double membrane vesicle
DNApol	DNA polymerase
DNCB	dinitrochlorobenzene
DR	direct repeat
DRADA	double-stranded RNA adenosine deaminase activity
DRM	detergent-resistant membrane
dsRNA	double-stranded RNA
DSS	dengue shock syndrome
DTaP	diphtheria and tetanus toxoids and acellular pertussis vaccine
DY	drowsy
E	glutamate
EA	early antigen
EAE	experimental allergic encephalomyelitis
EAV	equine arteritis virus; or endogenous avian virus
EBER	Epstein–Barr virus-encoded small RNA
EBHSV	European brown hare syndrome virus
EBLV	European bat lyssavirus
EBNA	Epstein–Barr virus nuclear antigen
EBOV	Ebola virus
EBV	Epstein–Barr virus
EC50	effective concentration
ECTV	ectromelia virus
EDTA	ethylenediaminetetraacetic acid
EEEV	eastern equine encephalomyelitis virus
EEV	extracellular enveloped virus
EF-1α	elongation factor 1 alpha
EFV	equine foamy virus
EGF	epidermal growth factor
EHDV	epizootic hemorrhagic disease virus
EHV	Edge hill virus
EHV-2	equine herpesvirus 2
EI	erythema infectiosum

EIA	enzyme immunoassay
EIAV	equine infectious anemia virus
eIF-2α	eukaryotic translation initiation factor 2α
eIF3	eukaryotic translation initiation factor 3
EIPV	enhanced potency inactivated poliovirus vaccine
ELISA	enzyme linked immunosorbent assay
ELVIS	enzyme-linked virus-inducible system
EM	electron microscopy
EMCV	encephalomyocarditis virus
ENTV	Entebbe bat virus
EP	early palindrome
EPI	expanded program on immunization
EPO	erythropoietin
ER	endoplasmic reticulum
ERGIC	endoplasmic reticulum–Golgi intermediate compartment
ES	embryonic stem
EToV	equine torovirus
EV	epidermodysplasia verruciformis
F	fusion; or phenylalanine
FADD	Fas-associated death domain
FasL	Fas ligand
FAstV	feline astrovirus
FAT	fluorescent antibody test
FCoV	feline coronavirus
FcR	Fc receptor
FCV	famciclovir; or feline calicivirus
FDA	Food and Drug Administration (USA)
FDC	follicular dendritic cell
FeLV	feline leukemia virus
FFI	fatal familial insomnia
ffu	focus-forming unit
FFV	feline foamy virus
4-GuDANA	4-guanidino-Neu5Ac2en
FI-RSV	formalin-inactivated respiratory syncytial virus
FIPV	feline infectious peritonitis virus
FIV	feline immunodeficiency virus
5HT	serotonin
FMDV	foot-and-mouth disease virus
FPV	feline panleukopenia virus; or fowlpox virus
FRET	fluorescence resonance energy transfer
FrMLV	Friend murine leukemia virus
FSE	feline spongiform encephalopathy
FTIR	Fourier-transformed infrared
FV	foamy virus
GABA	γ-amino butyric acid
GAG	glycosaminoglycans
GalC	galactosylceramide
G+C	guanosine and cytosine
GAPDH	glyceraldehyde-3-phosphate dehydrogenase
GAV	gill-associated virus
GAVI	Global Alliance for Vaccines and Immunization
gB	glycoprotein B
GBV-A	GB virus A
GBV-B	GB virus B

GBV-C	GB virus C
GCV	ganciclovir
GCV-MP	ganciclovir monophosphate
GCV-TP	ganciclovir triphosphate
GDD	glycine–aspartic acid–aspartic acid
GETV	Getah virus
gG	glycoprotein G
GGTP	γ-glutamyl transpeptidase
GGYV	Gadget's gully virus
GM	growth medium
GM-CSF	granulocyte/macrophage colony stimulation factor
GmDNV	*Galleria mellonella* densovirus
GP	glycoprotein
GPCR	G-protein-coupled receptor
GPI	glycophosphatidylinositol
GPV	Goose parvovirus
GR	glycine–arginine-rich
GRE	glucocorticoid-responsive element
GREP	Global Rinderpest Eradication Programme
GSHV	ground squirrel hepatitis virus
GSS	Gerstmann–Sträussler–Scheinker
H	hemagglutinin; or histidine
HA	hemagglutination; or hemagglutinin
HAA	human T-cell leukemia virus-associated arthropathy
HAART	highly active antiretroviral therapy
HAD	human immunodeficiency virus-associated dementia
HAI	hemagglutination inhibition
HAM	human T-cell leukemia virus-associated myelopathy
HAM/TSP	human T-cell leukemia virus-1-associated myelopathy/tropical spastic paraparesis
HANV	Hanzalova virus
HaPyV	hamster polyomavirus
HAstV	human astrovirus
HAV	hepatitis A virus
Hb	hemoglobin
HBeAg	hepatitis B e antigen
HBIG	hepatitis B immunoglobulin
HBcAg	hepatitis B virus core antigen
HBsAg	hepatitis B surface antigen
HBSP	hepatitis B spliced protein
HBSS	Hank's balanced salt solution
HBV	hepatitis B virus
HCC	hepatocellular carcinoma
hCG	human chorionic gonadotropin
HCMV	human cytomegalovirus
HCoV	human coronavirus OC43, 229E, or NL63
HCV	hepatitis C virus; or hog cholera virus
HD	helper dependent; or Hodgkin's disease
HDCS	human diploid cell strain
HDV	hepatitis delta virus
HE	hemagglutinin–esterase; or hematoxylin and eosin

HECoV	human enteric coronavirus
HEF	hemagglutinin–esterase fusion
HEK	human embryonic kidney
HEPA	high efficiency particulate air
HERV	human endogenous retroviruses
HEV	hepatitis E virus
HF	host factor; or hydrops fetalis
HFMD	hand-foot-and-mouth disease
HFRS	hemorrhagic fever with renal syndrome
HFV	human foamy virus
HGH	human grown hormone
HGSIL	high-grade squamous intraepithelial lesion
HGV	hepatitis G virus
HHBV	heron hepatitis B virus
HHV-1	human herpesvirus 1
HHV-6	human herpesvirus 6
HHV-7	human herpesvirus 7
HHV-8	human herpesvirus 8
HI	hemagglutination inhibition
Hib	*Haemophilus influenzae* type b
HIV	human immunodeficiency virus
HIV-1	human immunodeficiency virus type 1
HIV-2	human immunodeficiency virus type 2
HL	hemolysis
HMO	health maintenance organization
hMPV	human metapneumovirus
HN	hemagglutinin-neuraminidase
HNF	hepatonuclear factor
HNIG	human normal immunoglobulin
hnRNP	heterogeneous nuclear ribonucleoprotein
Hoc	highly antigenic outer capsid
HPIV-3	human parainfluenza virus type 3
HPLC	high performance liquid chromatography
HPMPC	hydroxyphonosphonylmethoxycytosine
HPV	human papilloma virus
HR	heptad repeat
HR-HPV	high-risk human papillomavirus
HRIG	human anti-rabies immunoglobulin
HRSV	human respiratory syncytial virus
HRV	human rhinovirus
HS	heparan sulfate
Hsc	heat-shock cognate
HSC	hematopoietic stem cell
HSK	herpes simplex virus-induced keratitis
HSV	herpes simplex virus; or herpesvirus saimiri
HSV-1	herpes simplex virus type 1
HSV-2	herpes simplex virus type 2
HTLV	human T-cell leukemia virus
HTLV-1	human T-cell leukemia virus-1
HTLV-2	human T-cell leukemia virus-2
HToV	human torovirus
HU	human T-cell leukemia virus-associated uveitis
Hu	human
huIgG	unspecific pooled human immunoglobulin
HuR	human RNA-binding protein
HVEM	herpesvirus entry mediator

HVR	hypervariable region
HVS	herpesvirus saimiri
HY	hyper
HYPRV	Hypr virus
I	isoleucine
IAA	infection-associated antigen
IAP	inhibitor of apoptosis protein
IATA	International Air Transport Association
IBV	infectious bronchitis virus
ICA	islet cell antibody
ICAM	intracellular adhesion molecule
ICAM-1	intercellular adhesion molecule 1
ICAO	International Civil Aviation Organization
ICE	interleukin-1β-converting enzyme
iCJD	iatrogenic Creutzfeldt–Jakob disease
ICNV	International Committee on Nomenclature of Viruses
ICTV	International Committee on Taxonomy of Viruses
ICTVdB	International Committee on Taxonomy of Viruses database
ID	immunodiffusion; or infective dermatitis
IDDM	insulin-dependent diabetes mellitus
IDU	idoxuridine; or injecting drug user
IDU-TP	idoxuridine triphosphate
IE	immediate–early
IEF	isoelectric focusing
IEM	immunoelectron microscopy
IEV	intracellular enveloped virus
IF	immunofluorescence; or intermediate filament
IFA	immunofluorescence assay
IFAT	indirect fluorescent antibody test
IFN	interferon
IFN-α	interferon-alpha
IFN-γ	interferon-gamma
IFT	immunofluorescence testing
Ig	immunoglobulin
IgA	immunoglobulin A
IgG	immunoglobulin G
IgM	immunoglobulin M
IHA	indirect hemagglutination
IL	interleukin
IL-6	interleukin-6
ILHV	Ilhéus virus
IM	infectious mononucleosis
IMP	inflammation modulatory protein
IMV	intracellular mature virus
IN	integrase
iNOS	inducible nitric oxide synthetase
Int	integrase
IOM	Institute of Medicine (USA)
IP	inflammatory protein; or internal promoter
IPA	immunoperoxidase assay
IPV	inactivated poliovirus vaccine
IR	inverted repeat
IRES	internal ribosomal entry site

IRF	interferon regulatory factor
IRF-3	interferon regulatory factor 3
IRF-7	interferon regulatory factor 7
ISAV	infectious salmon anemia virus
ISDR	interferon-sensitivity determining region
ISG	interferon-stimulated gene
ISRE	interferon-specific response element
ISVP	infectious subvirion particle
ITAM	immunoreceptor tyrosine-based activation motif
ITIM	immunoreceptor tyrosine-based inhibitory motif
ITR	inverted terminal repeat
ITV	Israel turkey meningo-encephalitis virus
IU	international unit
IUMS	International Union of Microbiological Societies
IV	immature virion
IVDU	intravenous drug user
IVF	in vitro fertilization
IVIG	intravenous immunoglobulin
IVN	nucleoid-containing IV
JAK	Janus kinase
JAM1	junctional adhesion molecule 1
JCPyV	JC polyoma virus
JCV	Jamestown Canyon virus
JEV	Japanese encephalitis virus
JLP	juvenile laryngeal papillomatosis
JSRV	jaagsiekte sheep retrovirus
JUGV	Jugra virus
JUTV	Jutiapa virus
JV	Jena virus
K	lysine
KADV	Kadam virus
KEDV	Kedougou virus
KFDV	Kyasanur Forest disease virus
KIR	killer cell immunoglobulin-like receptor; or killer inhibitory receptor
KOKV	Kokobera virus
KOUV	Koutango virus
KRV	Kilham rat virus
KS	Kaposi's sarcoma
KSHV	Kaposi's sarcoma herpesvirus
KSIV	Karshi virus
KUMV	Kumlinge virus
KUNV	Kunjin virus
L	large; or late; or leucine
LA	latex agglutination
LAIV	live-attenuated influenza vaccine
LAK	L-associated kinase
LAP	leukemia-associated protein
LAT	latency-associated transcript
LCL	lymphoblastoid cell line
LCMV	lymphocytic choriomeningitis virus
LCR	ligase chain reaction
LDL	low density lipoprotein

LDLR	low density lipoprotein-related		**MK**	monkey kidney
LDV	lactate dehydrogenase-elevating virus		**MLV**	murine leukemia virus
LGSIL	low-grade squamous intraepithelial lesion		**MM**	maintenance medium
LGTV	Langat virus		**MMLV**	Montana myotis leukoencephalitis virus
LIP	lymphoid interstitial pneumonitis		**MMP**	matrix metalloproteinase
LIV	Louping ill virus		**MMR**	measles, mumps, and rubella
LMP	last menstrual period; or latent membrane protein; or low-molecular-weight protein		**MMTV**	mouse mammary tumor virus
			MMV	mice minute virus
LMP1	latent membrane protein 1		**Mo**	mouse
LNYV	lettuce necrotic yellows virus		**MOCV**	molluscum contagiosum virus
LOD	logarithm of odds		**MODV**	Modoc virus
LP	leader protein		**MOI**	multiplicity of infection
LPD	lymphoproliferative disease		**MoMLV**	Moloney murine leukemia virus
LPMV	La-Piedad Michoacan-Mexico virus		**MPGN**	membranoproliferative glomerulonephritis
LPS	lipopolysaccharide		**MPMV**	Mason–Pfizer monkey virus
LPV	lymphotropic papovavirus		**MPV**	murine pneumonia virus
LR-HPV	low-risk human papillomavirus		**MPyV**	murine polyomavirus
LRSV	lychnis ringspot virus		**MRA**	microbiological risk assessment
LT	lymphotoxin		**MRI**	magnetic resonance imaging
LT-βR	LT-β receptor		**mRNA**	messenger RNA
LT-βR-IgFcγ	LT-βR-immunoglobulin fusion protein		**MS**	multiple sclerosis
LTR	long terminal repeat		**MSM**	men who have sex with men
			MST	mean survival time
			MT	methyltransferase
M	matrix; or methionine		**MuLV**	murine leukemia virus
MA	matrix; or membrane antigen		**MuV**	mumps virus
mAb	monoclonal antibody		**MV**	measles virus
MADT	morphological alteration and disintegration test		**MVA**	modified virus Ankara
MALT	mucosal-associated lymphoid system		**MVB**	multivesicular body
MAP	mitogen-activated protein		**MVEV**	Murray valley encephalitis virus
MAR	monoclonal antibody-resistant		**MVM**	minute virus of mice
MARV	Marburg virus		**MYXV**	myxoma virus
MAYV	Mayaro virus			
MBL	mannose-binding lectin			
MBM	meat and bone-meal		**N**	asparagine; or nucleocapsid; or nucleoprotein
MBP	myelin basic protein		**NA**	neuraminidase
MCA	middle cerebral artery		**nAChR**	nicotinic acetylcholine receptor
MCD	multifocal Castleman disease		**NACI**	National Advisory Committee on Immunization (Canada)
M cells	membranous epithelial cell			
MCMV	murine cytomegalovirus		**NANB**	non-A, non-B
MCP	membrane co-factor protein		**NANBH**	non-A, non-B hepatitis
MCV	molluscum contagiosum virus		**NaPTA**	sodium phosphotungstate
MDBK	Madin–Darby bovine kidney		**NAS**	nuclear addressing signal
MDCK	Madin–Darby canine kidney		**NASBA**	nucleic acid sequence-based amplification
MDPV	muscovy duck parvovirus		**NAT**	nucleic acid amplification technique
ME	myalgic encephalomyelitis		**NC**	nucleocapsid
MEAV	Meaban virus		**NCAM**	neuronal cell adhesion molecule
MEK	MAPK/ERK kinase		**NCCLS**	National Committee for Clinical Laboratory Standards (USA)
MeV	measles virus			
MEV	Meaban virus		**NCR**	noncoding region
MGF	myxoma growth factor		**NDUV**	Ndumu virus
MHC	major histocompatibility complex		**NDV**	Newcastle disease virus
MHV	murine hepatitis virus; or mouse hepatitis virus		**NE**	norepinephrine
MHV-68	murine gammaherpesvirus 68		**NEGV**	Negishi virus
MHVR	mouse hepatitis virus receptor		**NEP**	nuclear export protein
MIBE	measles inclusion body encephalitis		**NES**	nuclear export signal
MIDV	Middelburg virus		**NFAT**	nuclear factor activated T cell
MIP	macrophage inflammatory protein		**NF-κB**	nuclear factor-κB

NF1	nuclear factor I	**Pap**	papanicolaou
NFT	neurofibrillary tangles	**PAS**	periodic acid–Schiff
NGF	nerve growth factor	**PAstV**	porcine astrovirus
NHEJ	nonhomologous end joining	**PBL**	peripheral blood lymphocyte
NHP	nonhuman primate	**PBMC**	peripheral blood mononuclear cell
NID	national immunization days	**PBS**	phosphate-buffered saline; or primer binding site
NIH	National Institutes of Health (USA)	**PCBP**	poly(rC) binding protein
NIV	Nipah virus	**PCBP1**	poly(rC) binding protein 1
NJLV	Naranjal virus	**PCBP2**	poly(rC) binding protein 2
NK	natural killer	**PcG**	polycomb group
NLS	nuclear localization signal	**PCNA**	proliferating cell nuclear antigen
NLV	Norwalk-like viruses	**PCoV**	puffinosis coronavirus
NMSC	nonmelanoma skin cancer	**PCR**	polymerase chain reaction
NNRTI	nonnucleoside reverse transcriptase inhibitor	**PCV**	porcine circovirus; or penciclovir
NNS	nonsegmented negative-strand	**PCV-MP**	penciclovir-monophosphate
NO	nitric oxide	**PCV-TP**	penciclovir-triphosphate
noncp	noncytopathic	**PD**	prenatal diagnosis
NP	nucleocapsid-associated protein; or nucleo-protein	**PDB**	protein database
		PDGF	platelet derived growth factor
NPC	nasopharyngeal carcinoma; or nuclear pore complex	**PDR**	Physicians' Desk Reference (USA)
		PDV	phocine distemper virus
n-PCR	nested polymerase chain reaction	**PEDV**	porcine epidemic diarrhea virus
NPS	nasopharyngeal secretion	**PEG**	polyethylene glycol
NRE	negative regulatory element	**PEL**	primary effusion lymphoma
NRTI	nucleoside reverse transcriptase inhibitor	**PEMS**	poult enteritis mortality syndrome
nRT-PCR	nested reverse transcription-polymerase chain reaction	**PEP**	postexposure prophylaxis
		PFA	phosphonoformic acid
NS	nonstructural	**pfu**	plaque forming unit
NSP	nonstructural protein	**PFV**	prototype foamy virus
nt	nucleotide	**PHC**	primary hepatocellular carcinoma
NT	virus-neutralizing	**PHCoV**	pheasant coronavirus
NTAV	Ntaya virus	**PHEV**	porcine haemagglutinating encephalomyelitis virus
NTR	non-translated region; or noncoding region; or non-translated RNA	**PHLS**	Public Health Laboratory Service (UK)
		PI	protease inhibitor
NtRTI	nucleotide reverse transcriptase inhibitor	**PIC**	preintegration complex
NV	Nipah virus; or nonvirion	**PIE**	postinfectious encephalitis
nvCJD	new variant Creutzfeldt–Jakob disease	**PIF**	parvoviral initiation factor
		PIV2	parainfluenza virus 2
OAE	otoacoustic emission	**PKCε**	protein kinase Cε
OAS	2′,5′-oligoadenylate synthetase	**PKR**	protein kinase dsRNA
OAstV	ovine astrovirus	**PLpro**	papainlike cysteine proteinase
OHFV	Omsk hemorrhagic fever virus	**PMEA**	9-(2-phosphonylmethoxyethyl) adenine
OIE	World Organization for Animal Health	**PMKC**	primary cynomolgus or rhesus monkey kidney cell
ONNV	O'nyong-nyong virus		
OPV	oral poliovirus vaccine	**PML**	progressive multifocal leukoencephalopathy
ORF	open reading frame	**PMLP**	promyelocyte leukemia protein
ORI	origin of replication	**PMPA**	R-9-(2-phosphonylmethoxypropyl) adenine
ORS	oral rehydration solution	**PMTV**	potato mop-top virus
		PMV	porpoise morbillivirus
P	phosphoprotein; or pneumonia; or proline	**PoEV**	porcine endogenous retrovirus
PA	platelet-aggregating	**poly(A)**	polyadenylate
PABP	poly(A) binding protein	**POTV**	Potiskum virus
PABPII	poly(A) binding protein II	**POWV**	Powassan virus
PAGE	polyacrylamide gel electrophoresis	**PPBV**	Phnom Penh bat virus
PAHO	Pan American Health Organization	**PPD**	purified protein derivative
PAMP	pathogen-associated molecular pattern	**PPIase**	peptidyl-prolyl isomerase
P&I	pneumonia and influenza		

PPRV	peste des petits ruminants virus		**ROCV**	Rocio virus
PPS	postpolio syndrome		**RPA**	replication protein A
PPV	porcine parvovirus		**RPC**	replication protein C
PR	protease		**RPV**	rinderpest virus; or rabbitpox virus
PRCoV	porcine respiratory coronavirus		**RPXV**	rabbitpox virus
PRE	post-transcriptional regulatory element		**RR**	ribonucleotide reductase
PRN	plaque reduction neutralization		**RRE**	rev responsive element
PRNT	plaque reduction neutralization test		**RREID**	rapid rabies enzyme immunodiagnosis
PRR	pattern recognition receptor		**rRNA**	ribosomal RNA
PRRSV	porcine reproductive and respiratory syndrome virus		**RRP**	recurrent respiratory papillomatosis
PR-RT/RN	protease-reverse transcriptase/RNase H		**RRV**	rhesus monkey rhadinovirus; or Ross river virus
PSG	peripheral sensory ganglia		**RSP**	recombinant subviral particle
PSLV	poa semilatent virus		**RSSE**	Russian spring–summer encephalitis
PSV	peak systolic velocity		**RSV**	respiratory syncytial virus
PT/SAP	Pro–Thr/Ser–Ala–Pro		**RT**	reverse transcriptase
PTA	phosphotungstate		**RTA**	replication and transcription activator
PTB	polypyrimidine tract binding		**RTC**	reverse transcription complex
PTK	protein tyrosine kinase		**RtCoV**	rat coronavirus
PTLD	post-transplant lymphoproliferative disease		**RT-PCR**	reverse transcriptase polymerase chain reaction
PToV	porcine torovirus		**RUBV**	rubella virus
pTP	precursor of the terminal protein		**RV**	rabies virus
PV	papillomavirus; or polyomavirus		**RVV**	rhesus–human reassortant rotavirus
PVC	polvinylchloride			
PVR	poliovirus receptor		**S**	serine
PYV	polyomavirus		**SA**	sialic acid; or splice acceptor
			SA12	simian agent 12
Q	glutamine		**SABV**	Saboya virus
			SAC	Staphylococcus aureus Cowan strain I
R	arginine; or direct repeat		**SAF**	scrapie-associated fibril
RABV	rabies virus		**SAg**	superantigen
RANTES	regulated upon activation of normal T cell expressed and secreted		**SaHV-1**	herpes saimiri
RBC	red blood cell		**SAR**	secondary attack rate; or structure–activity relationship
RBS	rep binding site		**SARS**	severe acute respiratory syndrome
RBV	Rio Bravo virus; or ribavirin		**SARS-CoV**	severe acute respiratory syndrome coronavirus
rc	relaxed circular		**SCBV-IM**	sugarcane bacilliform virus-Ireng Maleng
RD	rhabdomyosarcoma cells		**SCC**	squamous cell carcinoma
RdRp	RNA-dependent RNA polymerase		**SCID**	severe combined immunodeficiency
REA	restriction enzyme analysis		**sCJD**	sporadic Creutzfeldt–Jakob disease
REBOV	Reston ebola virus		**SCR**	short consensus repeat
RER	rough endoplasmic reticulum		**SD**	splice donor
RF	recombination frequency; or replicative form; or retroperitoneal fibromatosis; or rheumatoid factors		**SDA**	strand displacement amplification
			SDAV	sialodacryoadenitis virus
RF-C	replication factor C		**SDD**	serine–aspartic acid–aspartic acid
RFLP	restriction fragment length polymorphism		**SDS-PAGE**	sodium dodecyl sulfate polyacrylamide gel electrophoresis
RFV	Royal Farm virus		**SEBOV**	Sudan ebola virus
RHDV	rabbit hemorrhagic disease virus		**SELP**	simian virus 40 early leader protein
RHR	rolling hairpin replication		**SEPV**	Sepik virus
RI	replicative intermediate		**SFA**	sanglifehrin A
RIA	radioimmunoassay		**SFFV**	spleen focus-forming virus
RID	receptor internalization and degradation		**SFGF**	Shope fibroma growth factor
RKV	rabbit kidney vacuolating virus		**SFV**	Semliki Forest virus; or simian foamy virus
RML	Rocky Mountain Laboratory		**sg**	subgenomic
RNAi	RNA interference		**SH**	small hydrophobic
RNP	ribonucleocapsid particle; or ribonucleoprotein		**SHa**	Syrian hamster
			SHa/Mo	Syrian hamster/mouse

SHFV	simian haemorrhagic fever virus
SIL	squamous intraepithelial lesion
SIN	self-inactivating
SINV	Sindbis virus
SIV	simian immunodeficiency virus
SL	stem-loop
SLAM	signaling lymphocyte activation molecule
SLEV	St. Louis encephalitis virus
SLV	Sapporo-like viruses
SN	serum neutralization
SNHL	sensorineural hearing loss
SNS	segmented negative-stranded
Soc	small outer capsid
SOKV	Sokoluk virus
SP	structural protein
SPDV	salmon pancreas disease virus
SPIEM	solid-phase immunoelectron microscopy
SPOV	Spondweni virus
SPV	San Perlita virus
SREV	Saumarez Reef virus
SRF	serum-response factor
SRH	single radial hemolysis
SRP	signal recognition particle
SRSV	small round structured virus
SRV	Saumarez Reef virus; or simian type D virus; or small round virus
ssDNA	single-stranded DNA
SSPE	subacute sclerosing panencephalitis
ssRNA	single-stranded RNA
SST	sodium silicotungstate
STAT	signal transducers and activators of transcription
STD	sexually transmitted disease
STE	surface tubule element
STIKO	German Vaccinee Commission
STLV	simian T-lymphotropic virus
STMV	stump-tailed macaque virus
STORCH	syphilis, toxoplasma, other diseases, rubella, cytomegalovirus, herpes simplex virus
STRV	Stratford virus
SU	surface
SV	subvirion
SV-5	simian virus 5
SV40	simian vacuolating virus 40; or simian virus 40
SVDV	swine vesicular disease virus
SVP	subviral particle
SVV	Sal Vieja virus
T	thymine
TABV	Tamana bat virus
TAP	transporter associated with antigen processing
TAstV	turkey astrovirus
TBEV	tick-borne encephalitis virus
TBP	TATA-binding protein
3CLp	3C-like protease; or 3C-like proteinase
TCoV	turkey coronavirus
TCR	T-cell receptor
2D	two-dimensional

3D	three-dimensional
TF	transcription factor
TfR	transferrin receptor
TFT	trifluridine; or trifluorothymidine
Tg	transgenic
TGEV	transmissible gastroenteritis virus
TGF-β	transforming growth factor β
TGF-β1	tumor growth factor β1
Th	T helper
Th1	T-helper-1
Th2	T-helper-2
TH	tyrosine hydroxylase
TIBO	thiobenzimidazolone
TIR	terminal inverted sequence region; or Toll/interleukin-1 receptor
TK	thymidine kinase
TLMV	TTV-like minivirus
TLR	Toll-like receptor
TLR2	Toll-like receptor 2
TM	transmembrane
TMA	transcription-mediated amplification
TMEV	Theiler's murine encephalomyelitis virus
TMUV	Tembusu virus
TMV	tobacco mosaic virus
TNF	tumor necrosis factor
TNF-α	tumor necrosis factor α
TNFR	tumor necrosis factor receptor
T1L	type 1 Lang (virus)
TOP	termination of pregnancy
topo I	topoisomerase I
TORCH	toxoplasma gondii, other diseases, rubellavirus, cytomegalovirus, herpes simplex virus
TORCHES-CLAP	toxoplasma gondii, other diseases, rubellavirus, cytomegalovirus, herpes simplex virus, enterovirus, syphilis, chickenpox virus, Lyme disease, AIDs, parvovirus B19
TP	terminal protein
TPA	tetradecanoylphorbol acetate
TR	terminal repeat
TRAF	tumor necrosis factor receptor activating factor
TRBP	tat region binding protein
TRE-1	tax response element 1
TR-FIA	time-resolved fluoroimmunoassay
TRIS	tris(hydroxymethyl)amino-methane
tRNA	transfer RNA
TROCV	Trocara virus
TRS	terminal resolution sequence; or transcription-regulating sequence
ts	temperature-sensitive
TS	thymidylate synthase
TSE	transmissible spongiform encephalopathy
TSG	tumor suppressor gene
TSP	tropical spastic paraparesis
TSP/HAM	tropical spastic paraparesis/human T-cell leukemia virus-I associated myelopathy
3TC	2'-deoxy-3'-thiacytidine
T3D	type 3 Dearing (virus)

T2J	type 2 Jones (virus)		**VLP**	virus-like particle
TTMV	torque-teno-minivirus		**VLTF**	viral late transcription factor
TTP	thymidine triphosphate		**VMK**	vervet monkey kidney
TTV	torque-teno-virus		**VN**	virus neutralization
TUT	terminal uridylate transferase		**VNA**	virus-neutralizing antibody
TYUV	Tyuleniy virus		**Vpr**	viral protein R
			Vpu	viral protein U
UEV	ubiquitin E2 variant		**VSIV**	vesicular stomatitis Indiana virus
UGSV	Uganda S virus		**VSV**	vesicular stomatitis virus
ULBP	UL16 binding protein		**VTF**	viral termination factor
UNICEF	United Nations International Children's Emergency Fund		**VTM**	viral transport medium
			VZIG	varicella-zoster immune globulin
UPS	ubiquitin proteasome system		**VZV**	varicella zoster virus
UPU	Universal Postal Union			
URR	upstream regulatory region		**W**	Tryptophan
USUV	Usutu virus		**WB**	western blot
UTR	untranslated region		**WEEV**	western equine encephalomyelitis virus
UV	ultraviolet		**WESSV**	Wesselsbron virus
			WG	week of gestation
V	valine		**WHO**	World Health Organization
VA	virus-associated		**WHV**	woodchuck hepatitis virus
VACV	vaccinia virus; or valaciclovir		**WNV**	West Nile virus
VAERS	vaccine adverse events reporting system			
VAP	virus attachment protein		**X-SCID**	X-linked severe combined immunodeficiency
VAPP	vaccine-associated paralytic poliomyelitis		**XLA**	X-linked agammaglobulinemia
vCJD	variant Creutzfeldt–Jakob disease		**XLPS**	X-linked lymphoproliferative syndrome
vCKBP	viral chemokine binding protein			
vCKR	viral chemokine receptor		**Y**	tyrosine
VCP	viral complement control protein		**YAOV**	Yaounde virus
VEEV	Venezuelan equine encephalitis virus		**YFV**	yellow fever virus
VEGF	vascular endothelial growth factor		**YHV**	yellow head virus
VETF	viral early transcription factor		**YLDV**	yaba-like disease virus
vFLIP	viral FLICE inhibitory protein		**YMTV**	yaba monkey tumor virus
VHSV	viral hemorrhagic septicemia virus		**YOKV**	yokose virus
Vif	virus infectivity factor			
VIG	vaccinia immunoglobulin		**ZDV**	zidovudine
vIL-18BP	viral interleukin-18 binding protein		**ZEBOV**	Zaire ebola virus
vIL-1βR	viral interleukin-1β receptor		**ZF**	zinc-finger
VITF	viral intermediate transcription factor		**ZIG**	zoster immunoglobulin
VL	viral load		**ZIKV**	Zika virus
VLBW	very low birth weight			

PART I

GENERAL CHARACTERISTICS OF VIRUSES

A short history of research on viruses

LESLIE COLLIER

INTRODUCTION

Virus (Latin, from Greek φιοσ): a poisonous or slimy fluid. I have not called this chapter 'The history of virology' because it pertains almost entirely to viruses themselves, and not to the whole subject, which includes epidemiology, immune responses, pathogenicity, and many other topics. Such extended coverage would have demanded a chapter of inappropriate length. The survey deals mainly with the period from the end of the nineteenth century to about the end of the twentieth, and includes references to papers that are now seen to have provided points of departure for major advances.

THE FOUNDATIONS

The discovery of viruses

Bacteria were seen and cultivated before their association with disease was determined. By contrast, the nature of viruses was not elucidated until well after it was realized that certain diseases of plants and animals could be transmitted by an invisible infective principle that differed considerably from that of the known parasites. This discovery was made amid the ferment of ideas and experimentation on microbes that took place in the closing decades of the nineteenth century; the technical advance on which it was based was the invention by Charles Chamberland (1884), a colleague of Louis Pasteur, of a porcelain filter originally designed to sterilize drinking water. In 1892, Ivanowski in Russia showed that such a filter allowed passage of the agent that caused mosaic disease of tobacco. Somewhat diffidently, he suggested that the infective principle might be a toxin elaborated by bacteria, but did not pursue the matter. In 1898, Beijerinck independently made similar observations on this infection, but extended them much further (Beijerinck 1899, cited by Waterson and Wilkinson 1978: 27). To exclude the possibility that his porcelain filter was letting through a very small bacterium he used the then novel device of diffusing sap through agar gel, after which it still retained infectivity. He also observed that the agent multiplied only in dividing cells, and that it withstood desiccation but was inactivated by boiling. Having failed with the means at his disposal to demonstrate its particulate nature, he termed it a *contagium vivum fluidum*. In the same year, Loeffler and Frosch (1898), both associates of Robert Koch, reported passage of the agent of foot-and-mouth disease through a bacteria-retaining filter. They ruled out the idea of an inert toxin on the basis of the dilution factors involved, and concluded first, that the agent must be able to replicate, and second, that it must be smaller than the smallest bacterium then known, and thus beyond the resolving power of the best available microscopes. Although the great majority of viruses were beyond the bounds of resolution of the light microscope, Buist (1887) visualized one of the largest, vaccinia virus, after staining it with aniline methyl violet. He also assigned it the remarkably accurate measurement of 100–500 nm.

Propagation in tissue culture

By the end of the nineteenth century, viruses had been defined solely in terms of their infectivity, filterability, and, as a result of Beijerinck's percipience, their requirement for living cells as a substrate for growth. Hitherto, viruses had been propagated only in intact animals or plants. Further progress demanded a much more simple and controllable system, the foundation of which was laid by Harrison (1906–7), who devised the first tissue culture, not for propagating viruses but for studying the growth of frog nervous tissue in clotted lymph. Steinhardt et al. (1913) exploited Harrison's technique to grow vaccinia in fragments of guinea-pig cornea embedded in clotted plasma. They could not demonstrate the virus directly in these preparations, but concluded from the results of serial subcultures that replication had taken place.

In 1928, Maitland and Maitland propagated vaccinia in suspensions of minced hens' kidneys. Their method was not widely used and its potential was not fully realized until a quarter of a century later, when flask cultures of trypsinized fragments of monkey kidney were used to grow poliovirus on a large scale for vaccine production.

Quantification

Guérin (1905) found that the number of vesicles produced by a suspension of vaccinia inoculated into scarified rabbit skin was roughly proportional to its dilution. This method was used by Steinhardt et al. (1913) in their tissue culture experiments, and was the precursor of many later and more accurate methods of assaying viral infectivity.

Host range and pathogenicity: effects on cells

The discovery of animal and plant viruses was soon followed by the finding of others that affected insects and bacteria. Oncogenic viruses were discovered by Ellerman and Bang (1908) and by Rous (1911), who respectively showed that a leukemia and a sarcoma of fowls could be transmitted by filterable agents. Another category, bacterial viruses (Twort 1915; d'Herelle 1917), was also to prove of the first importance, particularly for the study of viral replication and bacterial genetics.

In the early years of this century various workers described intracellular inclusion bodies in the tissues of animals and humans infected with viruses (e.g. rabies, *Cytomegalovirus*, and vaccinia). As the only obvious manifestation of viral activity within cells, inclusions were long the objects of intense study and speculation; they were categorized in terms of staining properties (eosinophilic or basophilic), location (intranuclear or cytoplasmic), and morphology (Cowdry 1934). They are now largely of academic interest.

Immune responses

It was long ago appreciated that certain infectious illnesses were followed by resistance to a second attack.

This observation prompted the inoculation of material from cases of smallpox (variolation), which was for centuries practiced in eastern countries. The practice was associated with significant mortality (approximately 2 percent) and was eventually superseded by the use of cowpox as the result of astute observations in the eighteenth and early nineteenth centuries by Edward Jenner (1801) and by lesser-known figures such as Benjamin Jesty, a farmer in Dorset. The last two decades of the nineteenth century saw the pioneering work of Louis Pasteur and his associates on immunization against both bacterial and viral infections, the most dramatic example being rabies. Meanwhile, the mechanisms of immunity underlying these somewhat empirical observations were being unraveled in the laboratory. Elias Metchnikoff (1891) demonstrated the importance of phagocytes in combating certain bacterial infections, and thus founded the concept of cell-mediated immunity. This line of investigation was long overshadowed by work on humoral factors. Around the turn of the century, the quantitative and qualitative aspects of antigen–antibody reactions and their specificity were under intensive study by von Behring, Kitasato, Ehrlich, Landsteiner, and others; and Nuttall and Bordet discovered a heat-labile factor in blood, later to be designated complement, that was bactericidal in the presence of specific antibody. For a more detailed account of early research on immunology, see Chapter 2, History, in the Immunology volume of this series.

The end of the beginning

By the end of the First World War, therefore, the foundations of virology had been laid. It had been established that viruses are much smaller than bacteria, and appeared to be capable of growing only in living cells, sometimes leaving evidence of their presence in the form of inclusion bodies. The main categories of viruses affecting respectively vertebrates, invertebrates, bacteria, and plants had been identified, the existence of oncogenic viruses was established, and the outlines of the immune response to viruses and other microbes were beginning to take shape.

PROPAGATION OF VIRUSES IN THE LABORATORY

Before discussing work on the properties of viruses, mention must be made of their propagation outside the intact animal, because such techniques are essential for studying them and most other microorganisms.

Chick embryos

Before the advent of antibiotics, tissue culture methods depended mostly on the growth of explants in clotted plasma, and freedom from contamination was difficult to maintain. The removal of these constraints, which impeded both quantitative work and large-scale cultivation, was signaled in 1931 with the finding by Woodruff and Goodpasture that fowlpox virus inoculated on to the chorioallantoic membrane of 10–15-day-old embryos produced discrete lesions (pocks). Within the next few years other viruses, including herpes simplex, Newcastle disease virus of fowls, and louping ill virus, had been propagated in this way and infectivity titrations by the pock-counting method were being carried out (Burnet 1936). Later, the allantoic and amniotic routes of inoculation were used to grow a range of viruses (Beveridge and Burnet 1946), and some, notably yellow fever virus and influenza, were grown in large quantities for vaccine production.

Cell cultures

The tedious method of growing tissue fragments in plasma clot was quite unsuited to the propagation of viruses in any quantity. In the early 1950s, it was largely replaced by true cell cultures as a result of several technical advances, given impetus by the celebrated discovery of Enders et al. (1949) that poliomyelitis virus would grow in nonneural tissues. The technical advances were: (1) the introduction of antibiotics to control bacterial and fungal contamination; (2) the use of trypsin to obtain suspensions of single cells that could then be grown as monolayers on glass or plastic surfaces; and (3) the production of lines of cells that could be propagated by serial passage, which fell into two main groups. Some were derived either from malignant tumors, for example the HeLa line (Scherer et al. 1953), or from cells that had acquired malignant characteristics, including aneuploidy, during serial transfer, or after infection with certain viruses; these 'continuous' cell lines would grow indefinitely. Others were derived from normal tissues and retained their diploid karyotype for a limited number of transfers. Monolayer cultures had the great advantage that the effects of viruses in terms of cell destruction (cytopathic effect) could be readily observed by low-power microscopy.

Quantitative methods

The use of cell cultures greatly improved the accuracy of infectivity titrations, for which two principal methods were developed. The first was analogous to the counting of bacterial colonies obtained from a known dilution of suspension and, as we have seen, was applied to infectivity titrations of viruses that produced discrete lesions on the chick embryo chorioallantoic membrane. Suitably diluted suspensions of bacteriophage produced cleared areas ('plaques') in confluent lawns of bacteria on solid media, and, likewise, some animal viruses produced foci of destruction in cell monolayers overlaid with gel (Dulbecco and Vogt 1954). Because, in theory at least, each plaque resulted from the replication of one virus particle, the infectivity of the suspension could be accurately assayed as the mean of a number of replicate counts.

The second method was useful when plaque counting was impracticable. It depended on ascertaining the highest dilution of suspension producing a certain endpoint, for example the death of an animal or a cytopathic effect in a cell culture. The precision of the method was much enhanced by estimating the dilution producing the endpoint in 50 percent of the animals or cultures inoculated. The earliest and perhaps best known method for doing so was that of Reed and Muench (1938).

From about 1970 onwards, developments in rapid methods of nucleic acid and protein analysis contributed greatly to fundamental knowledge of the properties of viruses and to the diagnosis of viral infections. During the same period, the introduction of micromethods and automation made possible the use of techniques such as enzyme-linked immunosorbent assays (ELISA) for analyzing large numbers of specimens. Such methods progressively replaced the more cumbersome and less informative assays using, for example, complement fixation.

THE PROPERTIES OF VIRUSES

Physical characteristics

SIZE

Probably because of the difficulty of propagating them in the laboratory, research on the sizing of viruses by filtration and centrifugation was an important focus of attention until well into the 1940s.

In 1929, Elford described a method of making series of collodion membrane filters of known average pore diameter (APD); with the proviso that the conditions of filtration had to be carefully controlled, their availability greatly assisted the measurement of viruses. Thus, by 1940, the sizes of about 25 animal viruses, ranging from the enteroviruses (approximately 20 nm) to poxviruses (approximately 250 nm) had been measured with fair accuracy (see van Rooyen and Rhodes, 1940a). Such studies were further advanced by the use of high-speed centrifuges, notably of the Sharples and Svedberg varieties (reviewed by van Rooyen and Rhodes 1940b), to estimate size as a function of the sedimentation characteristics.

Centrifugation was also useful for purifying viruses and became more so with the introduction by Brakke (1953) of sucrose density gradients, in which particles within a mixture can be separated according to their sedimentation rates. Later, cesium chloride and other salts were used with great success in high-speed centrifuges to separate viruses from contaminating material on the basis of their differing buoyant densities.

MORPHOLOGY

Until 1939, next to nothing was known about the structure of viruses because of the constraints imposed by the limited resolving power of light, even of short wavelengths in the ultraviolet range. In that year Kausche, Pfannkuch, and Ruska visualized a virus with the newly invented electron microscope (EM), in which beams of electrons travelling in a vacuum are focused on the object with electromagnetic fields. Given the then current interest in crystalline tobacco mosaic virus (TMV) (see Chemical composition: the role of the nucleic acids), it is not surprising that this was the first virus to be examined. Kausche and his colleagues (Kausche et al. 1939) employed the technique of shadow-casting, whereby the objects on the specimen grid were coated with gold particles generated by heating the metal in a vacuum; they defined the size of the crystals as about 25×300 nm.

After the interruption of the Second World War, new techniques were introduced to exploit the potential of the EM; they are well reviewed by Almeida (1984). In brief, shadow-casting revealed important morphological features of viruses, including the fact that some have an icosahedral structure. Negative staining, in which the background, but not the virus, is stained with an electron-dense salt of tungsten, uranium, or osmium, found wide application, not least in the diagnostic laboratory, and demonstrated that the outer surfaces of virus particles are composed of subunits. Methods were developed for cutting ultrathin sections in the 2-nm range which, alone or treated with labeled antibodies, yielded much information about virus–host-cell relationships.

These techniques, together with X-ray diffraction studies, showed that most viruses fall into one of two groups: the icosahedral viruses with so-called cubic symmetry; and those with helical symmetry, in which the outer subunits are arranged like the treads in a spiral staircase.

Chemical composition: the role of the nucleic acids

The demonstration by Stanley (1935), that TMV could be obtained in an apparently crystalline form, further stimulated the active, but ultimately sterile, debate on whether viruses are living entities. More importantly, it prompted study of the chemical composition of such preparations; and in 1937, Bawden and Pirie showed that they were not, as Stanley at first thought, pure proteins but also contained a nucleic acid, probably

RNA. From this observation stemmed the realization that viruses consist of a nucleic acid contained within a protein coat; by the end of the decade, it was also clear that some viruses contain DNA rather than RNA. Following the demonstration by Avery et al. (1944) that the genetic information determining the type specificity of pneumococci resides in their DNA, Hershey and Chase (1952) confirmed the crucial role of nucleic acid in viral replication by showing that, after the attachment of bacteriophage T2, the DNA, but not the protein coat, enters the bacterial cell. A further major step was the demonstration by Gierer and Schramm (1956) and Fraenkel-Conrat (1956) that RNA in infective form could be extracted from TMV.

THE CONCEPT OF THE VIRION

Not long after Crick and Watson had solved the structure of DNA, they suggested that viral nucleic acid is protected by a shell of identical protein subunits (Crick and Watson 1956). This notion, based on the limited coding capacity of viral nucleic acid, proved essentially correct. All viruses were found to have this basic architecture (Klug and Caspar 1960; Caspar and Klug 1962), the nucleic acid being, with few exceptions, double-stranded DNA or single-stranded RNA. Caspar et al. (1962) proposed the following terminology: the complex of protein shell (capsid) and nucleic acid is the nucleocapsid; the mature nucleocapsid, surrounded in some viruses by an outer envelope, is referred to as the virion.

Replication

For well over half a century after their discovery, nothing was known of the way in which viruses reproduce themselves. From about 1940 onwards, however, research by Delbrück, Luria, Hershey, Lwoff, and many others elucidated the basic mechanisms. Much of the work was done with bacteriophages, which had the advantages over animal viruses of easy propagation in vitro, accurate quantification, and growth cycles measured in minutes rather than hours; considerable use was made of radiolabeling to trace the synthesis of nucleic acids and proteins. The mechanisms of viral attachment, penetration, and uncoating were defined, as was that of the coding of enzymic and structural proteins by messenger RNA.

By 1957, André Lwoff was able to crystallize the essential features that distinguish viruses from all other organisms: they are strictly intracellular and potentially pathogenic entities with an infectious phase, and (1) possess only one type of nucleic acid; (2) multiply in the form of their genetic material; (3) are unable to grow and undergo binary fission; and (4) are devoid of a Lipmann system of enzymes for energy production.

'Unconventional' viruses

Two groups of viruses or virus-like agents stand apart from the generality of animal viruses: these are the retroviruses and the prions.

RETROVIRUSES

The finding by Ellerman and Bang (1908) and Rous (1911) that certain malignancies of fowl are caused by a transmissible agent was followed by the observation that many others in birds and animals, both of the solid tissues and of blood, can be transmitted vertically, from parents to offspring, as well as horizontally. The oncogenic effects of the viruses concerned are characterized by unusually long incubation periods. Temin argued for many years that the persistence of these RNA-containing viruses was due to a DNA 'provirus' that had become integrated into infected cells. This was finally confirmed when it was discovered that their RNA is transcribed to a DNA copy by means of an enzyme, reverse transcriptase (Baltimore 1970; Temin and Mitu-zani 1970), so called because it reverses the usual flow of genetic information from DNA to RNA.

Fatal infections, also with long incubation periods but otherwise dissimilar, appeared among sheep in Iceland following the importation of Karakul sheep from Germany in 1933; known as maedi and visna, they respectively affected the lungs and central nervous system (Sigurdsson 1954a). Other viruses, the so-called 'foamy agents,' were first detected in monkey kidney cells used for polio vaccine production during the 1950s and later in the kidneys of other species, including humans; these agents appear not to cause disease.

The viruses concerned have now been grouped into the *Retroviridae* family. The insertion and integration of viral DNA (provirus) into the host-cell genome accounts both for the chronicity of these infections and for the oncogenic potential of many of the viruses in the family. Later, retroviruses were discovered that cause infections of humans, notably leukemias and acquired immunodeficiency syndrome, and viruses of other families, notably hepatitis B, were found to utilize reverse transcription during replication; but these developments are outside the scope of this chapter.

PRION DISEASES

For the past 200 years, a widespread disease of sheep and goats has been recognized that affects the central nervous system, has an incubation period of several years, and is always fatal; it is known as scrapie because the severe itching impels affected animals to rub against posts and fences. The disease could be transferred between sheep by injection of brain tissue (Cuillé and Chelle 1936); its transfer to mice (Chandler 1961) and hamsters, with an incubation period of less than a year, greatly facilitated experimental work. A similar disease, rida, was reported in sheep in Iceland (Sigurdsson 1954b), and such infections were later identified in other animals, notably cattle in the UK. All were characterized by, inter alia, severe neuronal degeneration and vacuolation (spongiform encephalopathy), and by the presence in the brain of tangles of fibrils (scrapie-associated fibrils (SAF)). Analogous infections were found in humans, in the form of Creutzfeldt–Jakob disease (Creutzfeldt, 1920; Jakob, 1921), Gerstmann–Sträussler–Scheinker syndrome, and kuru (Gajdusek and Zigas 1957), a now extinct disease of the Fore tribe in Papua New Guinea spread by endocannibalism.

The year 1986 saw the start of a major epizootic of bovine spongiform encephalopathy (BSE), first in the UK, and later in other countries, involving many thousands of cattle infected by meat and bone-meal (MBM) given as a dietary supplement; it was eventually brought under control by extensive slaughter and the banning of suspect foodstuffs. In 1995, two adolescents in the UK, and subsequently others, were diagnosed with a form of Creutzfeldt–Jakob disease whose agent was indistinguishable from that of BSE. These cases were characterized by their early onset, longer than usual time to death, amyloid plaques, and absence of the usual electroencephalographic changes. This syndrome is termed new variant CJD (nvCJD). The number of cases ran into three figures, but is now declining.

The causal agents of these infections differ in many respects from 'conventional' viruses and cannot be classified on similar criteria. They are very small and highly resistant to heat and ionizing radiation. Even so, they can reproduce themselves, and some, at least, can undergo genetic variation. Prusiner (1982) marshalled the evidence suggesting that these agents are protein and devoid of nucleic acid; he termed them prions (proteinaceous infectious particles). His view that they are an aberrant form (PrP^{Sc}) of a protein (PrP) normally found in the brain has now gained wide acceptance. The mode of reproduction is probably explained by repetitive conformational changes induced by PrP^{Sc} in the normal protein. (Weissmann 1991).

CLASSIFICATION OF VIRUSES

Now that the story of research on the properties of viruses has been described, it is appropriate to consider how they have been applied to viral classification. The early history of this topic was reviewed by Brown (1984); here, there is space to refer only to the main events.

The earliest attempts at grouping viruses were necessarily based on what they do rather than on what they are: the criteria included clinical effects, pathological changes, and tissue tropisms. The inadequacies of such systems were apparent, and in 1950 a Subcommittee on Virus Nomenclature under the chairmanship of C.H. Andrewes was set up at the International Congress of Microbiology held at Rio de Janeiro; it recommended use of a system based on the physical, chemical, and antigenic properties of the viruses themselves, and allotted names to some of the better known (e.g. poxvirus, herpesvirus, myxovirus). In 1961, Cooper proposed, inter alia, the fundamentally important grouping by type of nucleic acid. Soon afterwards, Lwoff et al. (1962) put forward a universal system that has contributed much to the modern classification. The criteria were:

1 the type of nucleic acid (DNA or RNA);
2 the symmetry of the virus;
3 the presence or absence of an envelope;
4 the diameter of the nucleocapsid for helical viruses or the number of capsomeres for cubic viruses.

On the basis of these and other criteria, viruses are assigned to families (and sometimes subfamilies), genera, and species. Baltimore (1971) provided a basis for further refining classification that takes into account genome conformation and strategies for mRNA synthesis, characteristics that are being used on an increasing scale (van Regenmortel et al. 2000.

IMMUNIZATION AND ANTIVIRAL THERAPY

At the beginning of this chapter, I stated that it would not be possible to cover applied virology. Nevertheless, at a time when major successes are being scored by both virus vaccines and antiviral drugs, it is only right to include mentions of these topics, brief though they must be.

Viral vaccines

Smallpox vaccine was the first to come into general use and the first to eradicate an infectious disease worldwide (Fenner and Henderson 1988), the last natural case having occurred in Somalia in 1977. The conquest of smallpox is set fair to be repeated with other vaccines, notably poliomyelitis and measles. The development of viral vaccines reflects the advances in virological techniques over the past two centuries, ranging successively from animal inoculation to the use of chick embryos, cell cultures, and finally recombinant DNA technology (Table 1.1).

Antiviral therapy

Because of the intimate association between viruses and their host cells, the development of antiviral agents lagged behind that of compounds active against other microbes. Because the replication of viruses was not well understood, its basis was at first purely empirical and depended largely on random screening of many potentially useful compounds; the devising of compounds directed against specific target activities, such as attachment to the host cell, nucleic acid synthesis, and the release of mature virus, is of more recent origin.

An early development in antiviral therapy was the discovery by Isaacs and Lindenmann (1957) of interferon (IFN), a low molecular weight protein produced by cells in response to infection with viruses, some bacteria, double-stranded nucleic acids, and other biological compounds (see also Isaacs et al. 1957). Three classes of IFN (α, β, and γ) with differing properties are now recognized. The early finding that IFN inhibited a

Table 1.1 *Vaccines for human use developed in the past two centuries*

Decade in which introduced	Vaccine	Live (L) or inactivated (I)	Derivation
1800–1809	Smallpox	L	Animals
1880–1889	Rabies	I	
1940–1949	Yellow fever	L	Chick embryos
	Influenza	I	
1950–1959	Polio (Salk type)	I	Cell cultures
1960–1969	Rabies	I	Cell cultures
	Polio (Sabin type)	L	
	Measles	L	
	Mumps	L	
	Rubella	L	
1980–1989	Hepatitis B	I	Human plasma
	Hepatitis B	I	Yeast[a]
	Japanese B encephalitis	I	Mice or cell cultures
	Varicella	L	Cell cultures
1990–1999	Hepatitis A	I	Cell cultures

a) Genetically engineered antigen.

Table 1.2 *Examples of antiviral compounds developed since 1960*

Year[a]	Compound	Target	Viruses inhibited
1960	Methisazone	Ribonucleoside reductase	Poxviruses
1963	Amantadine/Rimantadine	Inhibits virus uncoating	Influenza A
1972	Ribavirin	Not yet fully defined	Respiratory syncytial virus; Lassa fever
1978	Acyclovir	DNA synthesis	Some herpesviruses
1985	Azidothymidine	DNA synthesis	HIV
1990	Saquinavir	Protease inhibitor	HIV (and probably others)

a) Approximate only. Indicates an early description rather than when the compound was first licensed for clinical use.

wide range of viruses raised hopes that it would be in the nature of a universal panacea for viral infections. This expectation was not fulfilled, but more recently IFN have proved useful in treating some cases of chronic hepatitis B. The large doses required can be produced by recombinant DNA techniques.

The precursor of all synthetic antiviral compounds was *p*-amino-benzaldehyde, 3-thiosemicarbazone (Brownlee and Hamre 1951), which inhibited vaccinia virus. A related compound, methisazone, appeared to have a prophylactic effect in smallpox contacts, but was rendered superfluous by the success of the vaccine eradication campaign. However, a more profitable approach was becoming apparent. By 1955, Matthews and Smith were able to write: 'There is a growing body of evidence suggesting that the genetic properties of viruses may reside largely in their nucleic acids, and a number of recent observations show that virus multiplication can be delayed by compounds which interfere with nucleic acid metabolism. As a class, analogues of the purine and pyrimidine bases may inhibit growth by a variety of mechanisms' (Matthews and Smith 1955). This prediction was fulfilled; the greatest achievements have in fact been the therapy and prophylaxis of herpesvirus infections with nucleoside analogs, at first idoxuridine (5-iodo-2'-deoxyuridine) and latterly acyclovir (9-(2-hydroxyethoxymethyl) guanine) (Table 1.2). Another such compound, zidovudine, has had a limited measure of success against infection with human immunodeficiency virus. It is, however, clear that our successors will regard this era as still part of the early history of antiviral therapy. The benefits of molecules designed to block specific receptors, drugs accurately aimed at defined targets within the replication cycle, synthetic antigens, DNA vaccines, and novel delivery systems lie still in the future.

CONCLUSION

The virologist will readily appreciate how much has had to be omitted from this brief account, but I hope that it

will convey to the nonspecialist something of the many and complex strands that have combined to make the study of viruses such a leading influence in microbiology. From its beginnings, virology has provided a high degree of intellectual challenge that has attracted many leading minds, not least through its contributions to our knowledge of biological processes at the molecular level. The reader who wishes to study the fascinating story in more detail will find good accounts in the books by Lechevalier and Solotorovsky (1965) and Waterson and Wilkinson (1978).

REFERENCES

Almeida, J.D. 1984. Morphology: virus structure. In: Wilson, G.S., Miles, A.A. and Parker, M.T. (eds), *Topley and Wilson's Principles of bacteriology, virology and immunity*, 7th edn. London: Edward Arnold, 14–48.

Avery, O.T., MacLeod, C.M. and McCarty, M. 1944. Studies on the chemical nature of the substance inducing transformation of pneumococcal types. Induction of transformation by a desoxyribonucleic acid fraction isolated from *Pneumococcus* type III. *J Exp Med*, **79**, 137–57.

Baltimore, D. 1970. RNA-dependent DNA polymerase in virions of RNA tumour viruses. *Nature (Lond)*, **226**, 1209–11.

Baltimore, D. 1971. Expression of animal virus genomes. *Bacteriol Rev*, **35**, 235–41.

Bawden, F.C. and Pirie, N.W. 1937. The isolation and some properties of liquid crystalline substances from solanaceous plants infected with three strains of tobacco mosaic virus. *Proc Roy Soc Lond, B*, **123**, 274–320.

Beijerinck, M.W. 1899. Ueber ein Contagium vivum fluidum als Ursache der Fleckenkrankheit der Tabaksblätter. *Zentralbl Bakteriol Parasitenkd Infektionskr Hyg Abt 2*, **5**, 27–33, First published in Dutch in 1898.

Beveridge, W.I.B. and Burnet, F.M. 1946. *The cultivation of viruses and rickettsiae in the chick embryo. Special Report Series No. 256*. London: Medical Research Council/HMSO.

Brakke, M.L. 1953. Zonal separations by density-gradient filtration. *Arch Biochem Biophys*, **45**, 275–90.

Brown, F. 1984. Classification of viruses. In: Wilson, G.S., Miles, A.A. and Parker, M.T. (eds), *Topley and Wilson's Principles of bacteriology, virology and immunity*, 7th edn. London: Edward Arnold, 5–13.

Brownlee, K.A. and Hamre, D. 1951. Studies on chemotherapy of vaccinia virus. *J Bacteriol*, **61**, 127–34.

Buist, J.B. 1887. *Vaccinia and variola: a study of their life history*. London: Churchill.

Burnet, F.M. 1936. *The use of the developing egg in virus research.* *Special Report Series No. 220.* London: Medical Research Council/HMSO.

Caspar, D.L.D. and Klug, A. 1962. Physical principles in the construction of regular viruses. *Cold Spring Harbor Symp Quant Biol*, **27**, 1–24.

Caspar, D.L.D., Dulbecco, R., et al. 1962. Proposals. *Cold Spring Harbor Symp Quant Biol*, **27**, 49.

Chamberland, C. 1884. Sur un filtre donnant de l'eau physiologiquement pure. *CR Acad Sci*, **99**, 247–8.

Chandler, R.L. 1961. Encephalopathy in mice produced by inoculation with scrapie brain material. *Lancet*, **1**, 1378–9.

Cooper, P.D. 1961. A chemical basis for the classification of animal viruses. *Nature (Lond)*, **190**, 302–5.

Cowdry, E.V. 1934. The problem of intra-nuclear inclusions in virus diseases. *Arch Pathol*, **18**, 527–42.

Creutzfeldt, H.G. 1920. Über die eigenartige herdförmige Erkrankung des Zentralnervensystems. *Z ges Neurol Psychiatr*, **57**, 1–18.

Crick, F.H.C. and Watson, J.D. 1956. Structure of small viruses. *Nature (Lond)*, **177**, 473–5.

Cuillé, J. and Chelle, P.-L. 1936. La maladie dite tremblante du mouton est-elle inoculable? *CR Acad Sci*, **203**, 1552–4.

Dulbecco, R. and Vogt, M. 1954. Plaque formation and isolation of pure lines with poliomyelitis viruses. *J Exp Med*, **99**, 167–82.

Elford, W.J. 1929. Ultra-filtration methods and their application in bacteriological and pathological studies. *Br J Exp Pathol*, **10**, 126–44.

Ellerman, V. and Bang, O. 1908. Experimentelle leukämie bei Hühnerin. *Zentralbl Bakteriol Parasitenkd Infetktionskr Hyg Abt 1 Orig*, **46**, 595–609.

Enders, J.F., Weller, T.H. and Robbins, F.C. 1949. Cultivation of the Lansing strain of poliomyelitis virus in cultures of various human embryonic tissues. *Science*, **109**, 85–7.

Fenner, F. and Henderson, D.A. 1988. *Smallpox and its eradication.* Geneva: World Health Organization.

Fraenkel-Conrat, H. 1956. The role of the nucleic acid in the reconstitution of active tobacco mosaic virus. *J Am Chem Soc*, **78**, 882–3, Correspondence.

Gajdusek, D.C. and Zigas, V. 1957. Degenerative disease of the central nervous system in New Guinea: the endemic occurrence of 'kuru' in the native population. *N Engl J Med*, **257**, 974–8.

Gierer, A. and Schramm, G. 1956. Infectivity of ribonucleic acid from tobacco mosaic virus. *Nature (Lond)*, **177**, 702–3.

Guérin, M.C. 1905. Contrôle de la valeur des vaccins Jenneriens par la numération des éléments virulents. *Ann Inst Pasteur (Paris)*, **15**, 317–20.

Harrison, R.G. 1906-1907. Observations on the living developing nerve fibre. *Proc Soc Exp Biol Med*, **4**, 140–3.

d'Herelle, F. 1917. Sur un microbe invisible antagoniste des bacilles dysentériques. *CR Acad Sci*, **165**, 373–5.

Hershey, A.D. and Chase, M. 1952. Independent functions of viral protein and nucleic acid in growth of bacteriophage. *J Gen Physiol*, **36**, 39–56.

Isaacs, A. and Lindenmann, J. 1957. Virus interference. I. The interferon. *Proc Roy Soc Lond B*, **147**, 258–67.

Isaacs, A., Lindenmann, J. and Valentine, R.C. 1957. Virus interference. II. Some properties of interferon. *Proc Roy Soc Lond B*, **147**, 268–73.

Ivanowski, D.I. 1892. Ueber die Mosaikkrankheit der Tabakspflanze. *St Petersburg Acad Imp Sci Bull*, **35**, 67–70.

Jakob, A. 1921. Über eigenartigen Erkrankungen des Zentralnervensystems mit bermerkenswertem anatomische Befunde. *Z ges Neurol Psychiatr*, **64**, 147–228.

Jenner, E. 1801. *An inquiry into the causes and effects of the Variolae Vaccinae, a disease discovered in some of the western counties of England, particularly Gloucestershire, and known by the name of the Cow-pox.* London: Edward Jenner.

Kausche, G.A., Pfannkuch, E. and Ruska, H. 1939. Die Sichtbarmachung von pflanzlichem Virus im Übermikroskop. *Naturwissenschaften*, **27**, 292–9.

Klug, A. and Caspar, D.L.D. 1960. The structure of small viruses. *Adv Virus Res*, **7**, 225–325.

Lechevalier, H.A. and Solotorovsky, M. 1965. *Three centuries of microbiology.* New York: McGraw-Hill.

Loeffler, F. and Frosch, P. 1898. Berichte der Kommission zur Erforschung der Maul und Klauenseuche bei dem Institut für Infektionskrankheiten in Berlin. *Zentralbl Bakteriol Parasitenkd Infektionskr Hyg Abt Orig 1*, **23**, 371–91.

Lwoff, A. 1957. The concept of virus. *J Gen Microbiol*, **17**, 239–53.

Lwoff, A., Horne, R. and Tournier, P. 1962. A system of viruses. *Cold Spring Harbor Symp Quant Biol*, **27**, 51–5.

Maitland, H.B. and Maitland, M.C. 1928. Cultivation of vaccinia virus without tissue culture. *Lancet*, **2**, 596–7.

Matthews, R.E.F. and Smith, J.D. 1955. The chemotherapy of viruses. *Adv Virus Res*, **3**, 49–148.

Metchnikoff, E. 1891. Lecture on phagocytosis and immunity. *Br Med J*, **1**, 213–17.

Prusiner, S.B. 1982. Novel proteinaceous particles cause scrapie. *Science*, **216**, 136–44.

Reed, L.J. and Muench, H. 1938. A simple method of estimating fifty-percent end points. *Am J Hyg*, **27**, 493–7.

Rous, P. 1911. Transmission of a malignant new growth by means of a cell-free filtrate. *JAMA*, **56**, 198.

Scherer, W.F., Syverton, J.T. and Gey, G.O. 1953. Studies on the propagation in vitro of poliomyelitis viruses. IV. Viral multiplication in a stable strain of human malignant cells (strain HeLa) derived from an epidermoid carcinoma of the cervix. *J Exp Med*, **97**, 695–709.

Sigurdsson, B. 1954a. Maedi, a slow progressive pneumonia of sheep: an epizoological and a pathological study. *Br Vet J*, **110**, 255–70.

Sigurdsson, B. 1954b. Rida, a chronic encephalitis of sheep; with general remarks on infections which develop slowly and some of their special characteristics. *Br Vet J*, **110**, 341–54.

Stanley, W.M. 1935. Isolation of a crystalline protein possessing the properties of tobacco-mosaic virus. *Science*, **81**, 644–5.

Steinhardt, E., Israeli, C. and Lambert, R.A. 1913. Studies on the cultivation of the virus of vaccinia. *J Infect Dis*, **13**, 294–300.

Temin, H.M. and Mituzani, S. 1970. RNA-dependent DNA polymerase in virions of Rous sarcoma virus. *Nature (Lond)*, **226**, 1211–13.

Twort, F.W. 1915. An investigation on the nature of ultra-microscopic viruses. *Lancet*, **2**, 1241–3.

van Regenmortel, M.H.V., Fauquet, C.M., et al. 2000. *Virus taxonomy. Classification and nomenclature of viruses.* London: Academic Press.

van Rooyen, C.E. and Rhodes, A.J. 1940a. The particulate nature of viruses – a summary of results. In: van Rooyen, C.E. and Rhodes, A.J. (eds), *Virus diseases of Man.* London: Oxford University Press, 52–7.

van Rooyen, C.E. and Rhodes, A.J. 1940b. The centrifugalisation of elementary bodies. In: van Rooyen, C.E. and Rhodes, A.J. (eds), *Virus diseases of man.* London: Oxford University Press, 44–51.

Waterson, A.P. and Wilkinson, L. 1978. *An introduction to the history of virology.* Cambridge: Cambridge University Press.

Weissmann, C. 1991. A 'unified theory' of prime propagation. *Nature (Lond)*, **352**, 679–83.

Woodruff, M. and Goodpasture, E.W. 1931. The susceptibility of the chorio-allantoic membrane of chick embryos to infection with the fowl-pox virus. *Am J Pathol*, **7**, 209–22.

2

The origin and evolution of viruses

ESTEBAN DOMINGO AND JOHN J. HOLLAND

THEORIES ON THE ORIGIN OF VIRUSES

Some fundamental questions such as the origin of life or the origin of viruses cannot be answered with any precision because the critical events occurred eons ago, and the questions do not lend themselves to direct experimental studies. There is no fossil record of viral sequences and even if molecular techniques enabled recovery of putative viral sequences from well-preserved fossils, it is likely that such sequences would be cryptic and difficult to relate to modern viruses because of their rapid evolution. Thus questions such as if there were (and how they were) viruses during the Cambrian explosion (a critical period from around 550 until about 485 million years ago in which a relatively rapid diversification of animal life occurred) are unlikely ever to be answered.

There have been several theories of the origin of viruses (reviewed by Joklik 1974; Luria et al. 1978; Botstein 1981; Atkins 1993):

- Viruses may be the descendants of primitive, pre-cellular replicons that existed before the first cellular forms appeared on earth. These primitive replicons evolved to become dependent on cells for replication. Reverse transcription, which at some stage must have generated DNA from RNA, must have been active in producing primitive DNA viruses. According to this theory, the viruses we know today are the result of a long coevolutionary process of early viruses and cells which underwent a process of differentiation.

- In a completely different theory, viruses have never been descendants of simple replicons but, rather, they were the result of regressive evolution of complex microbial forms that displayed cellular organization and metabolism. A virus would be a parasitic, sub-genomic form of a formerly free-living organism.

- Viruses originated from cellular DNA or RNA, or from subcellular organelles (such as mitochondria or chloroplasts). Part of the DNA or RNA could evolve to become decreasingly dependent on the cell, and eventually could include an extracellular step in its replication cycle.

- Viruses are as ancient as early cellular forms with which they have shared functional modules. The growing list of complete genomic nucleotide sequences of viral genomes and many unicellular and differentiated organisms (Mount 2001; Bushman 2002) suggests that all life forms and subcellular replicons share some basic structural and functional motifs. There are similarities between viral and cellular RNA structures and proteins involved in genome replication, proteolytic enzymes, and general patterns of genome organization and expression. No viral functions outstandingly different from similar cellular functions have been characterized. These findings of molecular genetics support the view that exchanges of functional modules, mediated by several forms of genetic recombination, together with mutation, contributed to coevolution of cells and a number of autonomous replicons, including viruses (Botstein 1981; Zimmern 1988; Gorbalenya 1995; Holland and Domingo 1998; Baranowski et al. 2001; DeFilippis and Villarreal 2001; Brown 2003).

Regardless of the details of early evolution of life on earth, and of the earliest origins of viruses, it is clear that cellular nucleic acids interact with, exchange with, and coevolve with, the DNA and RNA of viruses, plasmids, transposons, retrotransposons, and other mobile genetic elements (Hayes 1968; Monroe and Schlesinger 1983; Boeke 1988; Berg and Howe 1989; Harrison et al. 1991; Coffin 1992; Doolittle and Feng 1992; Syvanen 1994; Lodish et al. 1995; Bushman 2002). Novel viruses are among the 'new' life forms that evolve from such interactions, and the 'origination' of viruses is therefore a never-ending process (van Regenmortel et al. 2000). Their ubiquity, mobility, and capacity to recombine with cellular and other viral genetic elements put viruses (and other mobile elements) in the mainstream of all evolution on earth.

DNA viruses and RNA viruses may have had different origins or even if they shared a common ancestor they may have coevolved with cells in substantially different patterns. Examination of some distinctive features of DNA and RNA viruses may provide some insight into their evolutionary origins.

DNA viruses

DNA viruses may have arisen from combinations of cellular genes or by reverse transcription of RNA molecules. It is not yet clear, for example, whether a hepadnavirus (such as hepatitis B virus) was formerly a DNA virus that acquired a reverse transcriptase to allow replication via RNA transcripts, or if it was a retrovirus that evolved to encapsidate DNA replication intermediates instead of the RNA 'genome' (Doolittle and Feng 1992). Regardless of ultimate origins, any DNA virus has the potential to capture useful genes from cell chromosomes via DNA recombination (Cooper 2000).

DNA viruses as mobile DNA replicons

The distinction between DNA viruses and other autonomously replicating DNA replicons is sometimes tenuous. Plasmids, insertion sequences, transposons, and retrotransposons are mobile autonomous DNA replicons (Boeke 1988; Berg and Howe 1989; Coffin 1992; Doolittle and Feng 1992; Syvanen 1994; Bushman 2002) that resemble viruses in many respects, but they lack the capsid protein coats (and lipid/glycoprotein envelopes) that package viral genomes, protect them, and deliver them to appropriate receptors on susceptible host cells. It is this extracellular infectious stage that distinguishes viruses from other mobile DNA elements. Bacteriophage Mu is an example of a virus that is also a transposon (Berg and Howe 1989; Bushman 2002). It is a temperate phage, which, unlike phage lambda, can insert its DNA into numerous sites in the host bacterial chromosome. Copies of Mu DNA then transpose to many thousands of other chromosomal sites, thereby causing an enormous increase in mutation frequency. Mu therefore differs from the more common transposons because it encodes phage coat proteins which enable efficient transfer as a virus. As first suggested by Botstein (1981), it is likely that virus genomes undergo 'modular evolution' in which 'new' viruses can be created by a combination of genes or gene clusters derived from multiple sources, including chromosomes, defective viruses, plasmids, and mobile elements (Zimmern 1988; Baranowski et al. 2001).

Viroids and circular satellite RNAs

Of all the infectious viruslike mobile genetic elements, the viroids and related circular satellite RNAs (Maramorosch 1991; Robertson 1992; Semancik and Duran-Vila 1999) are the most primitive, and the most likely to have descended directly from primordial RNAs during the early evolution of life on earth. The viroids are small, naked RNA molecules several hundred nucleotides in length. They are covalently closed circular strands of RNA with extensive secondary structure, which replicate autonomously when introduced into susceptible plants, frequently causing characteristic signs of disease. They have intrinsic ribozyme self-splicing activity related to group 1 introns, and apparently replicate via a rolling-circle mechanism by interaction with plant cell transcription components. They do not require a protein coat for transmission and do not encode capsid proteins, so genome transmission and disease progression can be very slow, but effective. However, there are related satellite viruses (sometimes termed 'virusoids') that depend on coinfection of plants with an infectious helper virus to provide them with capsid proteins for efficient transmission (Vogt and Jackson 1999).

As yet, there are no known viroids (or viroid diseases) of animals or humans. Robertson (1992) has, however, pointed out the close similarity between human hepatitis D virus (delta (δ) agent) and viroids. Delta agent contains a self-cleavage viroid domain joined to a protein-coding domain that encodes the δ antigen. Furthermore, the δ agent RNA is a defective circular 'satellite' RNA that depends on coinfection with hepatitis B virus as a helper virus to provide capsid protein. This striking similarity to viroids or circular satellite RNAs led Robertson (1992) to postulate mechanisms of evolution of early self-replicating RNA genomes to form various 'conjoined' RNA replicons that ultimately evolved into mosaic DNA systems. These plausible speculations envisage early RNA replicons as progenitors of both present-day viroids and the intricate DNA-based life forms which now predominate. It should be noted that naked viroid RNAs and circular satellite RNAs thereby bear a relationship to RNA viruses similar to that of naked DNA replicons, including plasmids and transposons, to DNA viruses. In both cases, viruses are distinguished as autonomously replicating nucleic acid mobile elements with the capacity to encode capsid proteins.

RNA viruses

RNA viruses are the most ubiquitous and diverse viruses, and they include two major groups, the riboviruses and the retroviruses. Both have very high mutation rates, and even clones (derived from a single parental genome) rapidly form diverse 'quasispecies' populations or 'mutant swarms.' The extreme mutability of RNA viruses and its biological consequences are discussed in detail in the sections on Mutation of virus genomes and Biological significance of virus quasi species.

RIBOVIRUSES

The ordinary non-retrovirus RNA viruses that replicate their RNA genomes entirely via RNA templates are called riboviruses. Their ultimate origins are uncertain, and are probably quite varied (see section on Theories on the origin of viruses). Some may be directly descended from early primordial RNA replicons, whereas others may have originated more recently by recombination, reassortment, or mutation of cellular RNAs. Regardless of their ultimate origins, it is likely that most riboviruses have exchanged RNA sequences with cellular RNAs (and other virus RNAs) and so their genomes are mosaics of sequences from multiple sources. 'New' riboviruses may frequently arise by recombination of genome segments from two or more different riboviruses. One example is western equine encephalomyelitis virus, which is a recombinant virus derived from parental genomes of eastern equine encephalomyelitis virus and from New World relatives of sindbis virus (Hahn et al. 1988; Weaver et al. 1994). Genetic recombination in all riboviruses may be common on evolutionary time scales (Strauss and Strauss 1988; Zimmern 1988). A striking laboratory example of the creation of a new virus by recombination of unrelated riboviruses was reported. Rolls et al. 1994, using recombinant DNA intermediates, created a remarkable infectious virus in which the surface glycoprotein of vesicular stomatitis virus (VSV) was expressed from a replicon of Semliki Forest virus (SFV). The SFV replicon encoded only the SFV replicase, and no structural proteins. When the VSV glycoprotein gene was inserted by molecular genetic techniques, infectious virus particles were formed by budding of plasma membrane vesicles containing the VSV glycoproteins enclosing RNA replicons. Because VSV is a negative-strand ribovirus and SFV is a positive-strand ribovirus, a highly unexpected 'hybrid virus' was created. This demonstrates not only that novel viral genome matings can be productive but also that enveloped infectious viruses can be much simpler than virologists had expected.

Chance may have played a role in the way functional modules have been linked together to form viable forms of viruses. Recently, G. Wertz and colleagues have altered the gene order of VSV and found that virtually all gene combinations tested yielded viable virus (Ball et al. 1999; Wertz et al. 2002). Therefore, founder events in processes of gene transfer and ligation may have exerted a definitive influence on the organization patterns of the viruses we see today.

RETROVIRUSES

Retroviruses, hepadnaviruses, and caulimoviruses share a unique capacity of their genomes to participate regularly as part of both the RNA and the DNA worlds. Although their ultimate origins are uncertain, it is probable that they have evolved from retroid transposable elements, as originally proposed in Temin's (1970) 'protovirus' hypothesis. There is a wide variety of 'viral' and 'nonviral' retrotransposons and related elements, including Gypsy, Copia, LINES and LINE-like elements, mitochondrial introns, mitochondrial retroplasmids, and bacterial reverse transcriptases (Boeke 1988; Temin 1989; Coffin 1992; Doolittle and Feng 1992; Bushman 2002; Brown 2003). The so-called 'viral' retrotransposons more closely resemble retrovirus genomes. All these elements have in common the presence of reverse transcriptase, but most lack envelope genes which allow cell-to-cell and organism-to-organism transmission as mature virus particles (virions). Other retroviral genes and domains such as long-terminal repeat (LTR), capsid protein, ribonuclease, integrase, and protease are variably present in various 'viral' and 'nonviral' retroid elements (Boeke 1988; Temin 1989; Coffin 1992; Doolittle and Feng 1992; Bushman 2002). Most of these retroid elements may represent little more than 'selfish' jumping genes which sometimes cause useful rearrangements of host cell DNA sequences and sometimes damage or kill their hosts via DNA alterations. At least some of them may, however, perform essential functions. For example, a LINE-like retrotransposon, TART in *Drosophila*, apparently preferentially retrotransposes to the termini of chromosomes in an essential process by which *Drosophila* telomeres are maintained (Sheen and Levis 1994). The telomerases involve reverse transcription to elongate chromosome termini (telomeres), a process required for indefinite periods of cell division in mammals (Kim et al. 1994; Cooper 2000).

Transposons have been found in the eukaryotic genomes sequenced to date such as the human genome, yeast, *Drosophila*, the worm *Caenorhabditis elegans*, mice, and several plant species (reviewed in Bushman 2002). Remarkably, 44 percent of the human genome is made up of transposons or transposonlike elements. It is suspected that much of the 50 percent of the human genome that has not been assigned to a function, was likely contributed by mobile elements.

These findings provide strong evidence that retroid elements have been around for eons, that they can acquire additional genes, and that they can become retroviruses only if they acquire envelope genes to confer infectivity. Even now, 'new' retroviruses are continuously born (or reborn) by recombinational acquisition of cellular genes (e.g. proto-oncogenes in the case of some transforming retroviruses). Another source is the acquisition of genes from other retroviruses (e.g. LTR sequences, or altered *env* genes from proviruses in the case of mouse lymphoma virus) (Coffin 1992).

The origin of viruses is likely to remain a mystery for a long time. New observations may suggest one of the proposed mechanisms (condensed in the section on Theories on the origin of viruses) over another. In fact, multiple mechanisms may have participated in several origins of viruses at different stages of the evolution of life on earth. While it is plausible that viroids and other simple RNA elements may have evolved from primitive replicons (Semancik and Duran-Vila 1999; Vogt and Jackson 1999) it is hard to conceive the origin of complex DNA viruses (such as poxviruses, iridoviruses or herpesviruses with genomes of 130 000 up to 370 000 bp) as not being related to cells or cell organelles, either as a source of functional modules or as the starting point of a degenerative process. An interesting outcome of the development of tools to probe cellular and viral genome structures and their replication strategies is that they offer a number of plausible mechanisms (based on gene transfers, recombination, and mutation) for virus origins. Remarkably, these same mechanisms are acting on present-day viruses, and they can be observed experimentally as affecting not only virus evolution but also disease manifestations on the hosts they parasitize.

VIRUS EVOLUTION AND MECHANISMS INVOLVED

Because they can replicate rapidly with high yields of progeny, and readily mutate, recombine, and reassort their genomes, most viruses can exhibit great genetic plasticity and adaptability. This provides the possibility for extremely rapid evolution, but does not dictate constant rapid genome evolution. Viruses, like other living things, can have periods of relative evolutionary stasis, punctuated by periods of evolutionary disequilibrium and rapid genetic change (Holland 1992).

Recombination

Recombination affords rapid, major rearrangements of viral genomes, and this mechanism for evolution is widespread among DNA viruses and RNA viruses. Both homologous and nonhomologous recombination are very common, and the latter has the potential to produce quite extensive genome alterations and bizarre phenotypes.

DNA VIRUS RECOMBINATION

Mechanisms of DNA recombination and transposition have been widely studied, are well characterized (Kucherlapati and Smith 1988; Cooper 2000; Bushman 2002) and will not be reviewed here. Recombination or transposition allows DNA viruses to acquire new genes from other viruses; to integrate into, and excise from, host-cell chromosomes; to generate defective virus genomes and to rescue genes from them; and to capture host-cell genes or to transfer them to new host cells. In short, DNA virus genomes have available to them all the recombinatorial mechanisms extant in the DNA-based world, and this gives them the potential for profound genome rearrangements and for extensive genetic interactions with DNA-based hosts. Many DNA virus genomes contain genes that have been captured (or rescued) from earlier hosts. For example, the thymidine kinase (TK) genes of herpesviruses exhibit broad substrate specificity, and have apparently evolved from cellular deoxycytidine kinase enzymes (Harrison et al. 1991), whereas poxvirus TK genes were apparently derived from cellular TK genes (Boyle et al. 1987). Defective viruses produced by recombination are ubiquitous among DNA viruses and may often help shape their evolution by maintaining functional (and rescuable) gene modules. Botstein (1981) suggested that the product of virus evolution 'is not a given virus but a family of interchangeable genetic elements (modules) each of which carries out a particular biological function. Each virus encountered in nature is a favorable combination of modules. . . .' Exchange of modules allows the evolution of viral genes to occur within differing viral genomes, host chromosomes, defective viruses, plasmids, transposons, etc. Viral genes can not only associate with plasmids and episomes and other replicons, but they can also become episomes or plasmids (autonomous, non-infectious replicons). Examples are bacteriophage F1 selected for 'benevolent' interactions with host *Escherichia coli* (Bull and Molineux 1992) and Epstein–Barr virus (EBV) virus 'episomal' circular genomes within transformed (immortalized) B lymphocytes (Lindahl et al. 1976; Lawrence et al. 1988; Middleton et al. 1991; Kirchmaier and Sugden 1995). The 'benevolent' F1 plasmids eventually lost viral genes and infectivity, but replicated efficiently within host bacteria, and the EBV episome genomes in EBV-immortalized B cell lines are generally non-infectious or poorly infectious unless 'induced' (Weigel and Miller 1983).

RETROVIRUS RECOMBINATION

Retroviruses, of course, have the potential to recombine at the proviral DNA level (as for any other DNA).

However, they have the additional capacity to undergo recombination as a result of the tendency for reverse transcriptases to switch from one template to another (copy choice) during DNA chain elongation. This occurs at an extremely high frequency, is responsible for most retrovirus recombination events, and can play a major role in retrovirus evolution (Coffin 1992). Recent quantifications have estimated a minimum rate of 2.8 crossovers per replication cycle of a HIV-1-based vector system (Zhuang et al. 2002).

One of the most striking developments during the acquired immunodeficiency syndrome (AIDS) epidemic has been the discovery of the contribution of recombination to generate new variant forms of HIV-1 (Thomson et al. 2002). An increase of the number of circulating HIV-1 recombinants is likely to be influenced by higher frequencies of re-infections with different HIV-1 viruses as the AIDS epidemic advances, and geographical boundaries for HIV-1 subtypes become gradually fuzzier. Also, HIV-1 evolution is associated with an expanded mutant repertoire which increases the probability of producing recombinants with sufficient relative fitness (a measure of the relative replication capacity of a virus; see section on Biological significance of virus quasi species) to become dominant in infected individuals and to be transmitted.

RIBOVIRUS RECOMBINATION

Riboviruses can also exhibit very high rates of genome recombination due to frequent copy choice switching from one template RNA strand to another by RNA replicase. The RNA replicase carries the growing RNA chain to another RNA template and can align it precisely by base pairing. Therefore, most recombination is homologous ('legitimate') for positive-strand RNA viruses, which replicate their genomes as naked RNA (King 1988; Lai 1992; Wimmer et al. 1993; Nagy and Simon 1997). Such homologous recombination is clearly important for RNA virus evolution. For example, recombinants between different serotypes of poliovirus vaccine strains occur frequently in vaccinated humans and can be rather strongly selected in their intestinal tract (Kew et al. 1981; Minor et al. 1986; Minor 1992; Agol 2002; Dahourou et al. 2002). During picornavirus infections, average recombination frequencies in cell culture using selectable markers have been estimated in 10–20 percent of the progeny; recombination frequencies tend to decrease with the genetic distance between the parental genomes (King 1988; Lai 1992). Frequent homologous recombination helps to shape the evolution of numerous riboviruses such as coronaviruses (Lai 1992) and brome mosaic virus of plants (Rao and Hall 1990; Nagy and Bujarski 1995; Nagy and Simon 1997). Even though copy choice recombination is much more common than non-homologous ('illegitimate') recombination among positive-strand riboviruses (and

retroviruses), non-homologous recombination can occasionally produce major genome changes of great evolutionary importance. For example, the coronavirus mouse hepatitis virus appears to have acquired its hemagglutinin-esterase gene by recombination with influenza C virus, a negative-strand virus (Luytjes et al. 1988). Mucosal disease variants of bovine viral diarrhea virus (BVDV), a positive-strand pestivirus, are cytopathogenic viruses often generated either by multiple mutations or by recombination of parental, nondefective, noncytopathogenic BVDV genomes with cellular mRNAs (Meyers et al. 1991; Tautz et al. 1994; Kummerer et al. 2000).

Negative-strand riboviruses, which replicate their genomes as ribonucleoprotein strands rather than naked RNAs, generally undergo homologous recombination much less frequently than positive-strand RNA viruses. Replicase template switching occurs frequently, but this nearly always produces nonhomologous recombination because the growing RNA strands, being ribonucleoprotein, are not able to anneal and align the growing RNA chain precisely on homologous segments of the new template (Barrett and Dimmock 1986; Roux et al. 1991). Recently, homologous recombination of the negative-strand RNA Tula virus has been described (Plyusnin et al. 2002). To what extent homologous recombination in nature occurs with negative-strand RNA viruses is not known, but the study by Plyusnin et al. (2002) has certainly opened prospects for interesting research. Recombination of negative-strand riboviruses regularly produces biologically important variant genomes, particularly defective interfering (DI) particles. These can exert significant modulatory effects on parental virus infections (Barrett and Dimmock 1986; Huang 1988; Roux et al. 1991). Occasionally, quite bizarre recombinants between cellular RNAs and viral RNA genomes arise. For example, when a 54 nucleotide segment of 28S ribosomal RNA was inserted into the hemagglutinin gene segment of influenza A virus (by recombination during growth in chick embryo cells), the resulting recombinant virus was much more virulent, causing systemic lethal infections in chickens (Khatchikian et al. 1989). Similarly, a number of isolates of potato leafroll virus have acquired a 119 nucleotide segment from plant chloroplast DNA (Mayo and Jolly 1991), and cell culture replication of well-characterized strains of poliovirus (Charini et al. 1994) and sindbis virus (Monroe and Schlesinger 1983) led to acquisition of a short ribosomal RNA segment and a tRNA, respectively. Thus, although major nonhomologous recombination events are generally infrequent in ribovirus evolution, they occur sufficiently often to have significant evolutionary effects. They might even influence the results of biotechnological manipulations in which resistance to virus is conferred on transgenic plants expressing viral mRNA segments. For example, recombination between a defective plant virus genome and a viral mRNA transcript expressed in transgenic plants restored infectivity to the defective viral genome (Greene and Allison 1994).

Recombination may have two disparate effects in evolution. It may produce entirely new genome combinations from distant parental molecules such as the heterologous recombination events that led to influenza viruses with a fragment of ribosomal RNA (Khatchikian et al. 1989). This is an exploratory activity that may produce novel genome combinations, and only an extremely small fraction out of many unsuccessful trials are likely to produce high fitness virus (see section on Biological significance of virus quasi species). For example, the influenza recombinant was very virulent for chickens, but did not survive to represent an epidemiologically relevant threat for other hosts. This unique recombinant probably occupied a very high fitness peak surrounded by deep, low fitness valleys in other environments (Wright 1982; Domingo et al. 2001a). Recombination may have an opposite effect in the rescuing of viable gene combinations from debilitated parents. This conservative activity will often be mediated by homologous recombination, and it is one of the possible mechanisms to counteract fitness loss in RNA virus due to Muller's ratchet (see section on Biological significance of virus quasi species).

Reassortment of ribovirus genome segments

A number of riboviruses have segmented genomes either of single-stranded RNA (influenza viruses, arenaviruses, bunyaviruses, several plant viruses) or double-stranded RNA (reoviruses, rotaviruses). Their genomes consist of a number of specific segments, each of which encodes one or more gene products. Each specific segment must be included in a virion together with all other segments in order for that virion to be infectious and to replicate infectious progeny. As expected, the various genomic segments from genetically different (but related) viruses can reassort to produce reassortant viruses, a process equivalent to the reassortment of maternal and paternal chromosomes that occurs during meiotic gametogenesis in diploid eukaryotic organisms. Ribovirus gene reassortment occurs when two distinct viruses simultaneously infect the same cell(s). Gene reassortment can cause major genome alterations during evolution of segmented riboviruses. The most striking examples are the influenza A viruses. Both the 1957 Asian and the 1968 Hong Kong influenza pandemics began in south China. These 'new' human viruses arose by reassortment of gene segments apparently derived from circulating avian viruses and from circulating human virus sources. Domestic pigs were suggested as the probable hosts in which the reassortment events took place ('mixing vessels') (Gorman et al. 1992; Webster et al. 1992; Webster 1999; Wuethrich 2003). It

is probable that the next major influenza A pandemic will emerge some time during the next few decades, and that it will be due to reassortment events occurring in swine or humans or another 'mixing vessel.' Influenza C viruses, which usually circulate as multiple, independently evolving lineages in humans, have also undergone gene reassortment in man (Peng et al. 1994).

Major gene reassortment events between avian and human influenza A viruses are rare. This is undoubtedly because the currently circulating gene segments are co-evolving (and selected) for optimal interactions with each other. Therefore, only rare events could create a new virus with optimally interacting gene segments derived from widely divergent sources. Reassortment is common; it is the low probability for efficient interactions among diversely derived gene segments that greatly restricts the emergence of new influenza A pandemics. Reoviruses and many other segmented riboviruses also readily undergo genetic reassortment of segments from related lineages, and similar principles apply (Ramig et al. 1983; Desselberger 1996). There is, for example, evidence for segment reassortment in nature among viruses related to hantavirus pulmonary syndrome (Li et al. 1995), and for interspecific segment reassortment in the evolution of cucumoviruses of plants (White et al. 1995).

Mutation of virus genomes

Mutation is the primary driving force for all evolution, and it occurs inevitably and inexorably in all life forms, including viruses. In the RNA viruses (both riboviruses and retroviruses), a combination of small genome size, high mutation rates, high virus yields and very rapid replication, can produce spectacular rates of evolution. DNA viruses apparently mutate and evolve at lower rates, but they can nevertheless be quite mutable and biologically adaptable.

MUTATION AND EVOLUTION OF DNA AND RNA VIRUSES

The mutation rates of DNA bacteriophages have been characterized much more thoroughly than have those of the DNA viruses of humans and animals. Drake 1969 estimated the mutation rate of E. coli bacteriophages λ and T4 to be about 2×10^{-8} substitutions per nucleotide, two orders of magnitude higher than that of the host bacterium. Although mutation rates vary widely at individual genome sites, Drake (1991) has shown that there is a rather constant rate of spontaneous mutations per genome per replication in DNA-based microbes (including bacteria, yeasts, molds, and three DNA bacteriophages). Their genomic mutation rates per replication varied only about 2.5-fold around an average value of 0.0033 mutations per genome per replication round. Because the genome sizes of these diverse

DNA-based microbes vary by thousands-fold, their average mutation rates per base pair also vary by thousands-fold. Drake (1993) later calculated the genomic rates of spontaneous mutation among RNA viruses (the only known life forms with RNA genomes) and found them to be consistently higher. Animal lytic viruses (riboviruses) and RNA bacteriophages have an average genomic mutation rate per replication in the neighborhood of one, and retroviruses average slightly (about ten-fold) lower genomic mutation rates (Drake 1993; Drake and Holland 1999). Over all, these calculations tell us that genomic mutation rates do not vary markedly. They are remarkably fixed for DNA-based organisms, and are also fairly constant, but higher for RNA-based life forms (riboviruses and retroviruses). Obviously, as Drake (1993) pointed out, evolutionary forces must be shaping genomic mutation rates.

Despite the quite constant nature of genomic mutation rates, there is enormous variation in the mutation rates per nucleotide, per genome replication. This difference arises from the huge variation in genome sizes among living cells and subcellular replicons (Drake 1991; Drake 1993). Complex DNA viruses such as the herpesviruses are replicated by a viral-coded DNA polymerase endowed with a $3' \rightarrow 5'$ exonuclease proofreading activity to increase DNA copying fidelity (Hwang et al. 1997). Proofreading and postreplicative misincorporation-correcting activities have evolved to ensure the copying fidelity needed for maintenance of genetic information of complex DNA genomes. By contrast, RNA replicases and reverse transcriptases lack exonuclease proofreading activities, as evidenced by biochemical tests (Steinhauer et al. 1992; Cameron et al. 2002). RNA viruses have mutation rates in the range of 10^{-3} to 10^{-5} substitutions per nucleotide copied, expected from their small genome size (Batschelet et al. 1976; Eigen and Biebricher 1988; Drake and Holland 1999). These values exceed by several million-fold the base misincorporations rates of their eukaryotic hosts. A clear example of this was given by Gojobori and Yokoyama (1985), who showed that the Moloney murine sarcoma virus, a retrovirus of mice, evolves at a rate a millionfold higher than the rate of its integrated cellular homologue, c-*mos*. This allows (but does not necessitate) rates of RNA virus evolution to proceed millions of times faster than that of their animal and human hosts (Holland et al. 1982; Smith and Inglis 1987; Domingo et al. 1988, 1992, 2001a; Eigen and Biebricher 1988; Domingo and Holland 1994; Duarte et al. 1994).

Extremely high mutation rates generate 'mutant swarms' or 'quasispecies' populations of RNA viruses, and can provide great adaptability. This factor must be balanced against the inevitable high levels of lethality when the rates are too high. Eigen and Biebricher (1988) have reviewed results that show by computer simulation that when mutation rates increase they suddenly exceed an 'error threshold' at which there is a 'melting' of genetic information or a transition into 'error catastrophe.' They have proposed that RNA virus quasispecies generally adapt to the error threshold at which the misincorporations rate per nucleotide per replication will be in the neighborhood of $1/v$ where v is the length (in bases) of the genome. This figure can vary somewhat, depending on a selectively factor for the most fit 'master' sequences within a quasispecies population (Eigen and Biebricher 1988). This threshold limit dictates that genomic mutation rates generally cannot exceed values of about one. Drake's (1993) calculations indicate that most RNA virus genomic mutation rates are in fact close to one. Strong chemical mutagenesis of RNA viruses (inducing high lethality in progeny) only slightly increases mutation rates in viable progeny (Holland et al. 1990). This indicates that RNA viruses are at or near their error threshold. As Eigen and Biebricher (1988) have pointed out, occasional, short duration violations of the error threshold can provide brief evolutionary advantages, but persistent violations are lethal for viral genomes.

One mechanism for radical mutational changes in RNA viruses is biased hypermutation (Cattaneo et al. 1988; Wain-Hobson 1992; Cattaneo 1994; Martínez et al. 1994; Meyerhans and Vartanian 1999). Biased hypermutation can produce long segments of viral genome in which certain bases are substituted in a regular, recurring pattern. There are two major mechanisms, one of which involves deamination mediated by cellular enzymes (Cattaneo 1994; Harris et al. 2003). The other mechanism involves reverse transcriptase errors in retrovirus replication due to biased deoxyribonucleotide triphosphate pool concentration (Wain-Hobson 1992; Martínez et al. 1994). Either can produce sudden, massive genome changes.

In general, most RNA viruses are life forms that replicate and evolve near the extreme limits of mutability and adaptability. Genomic mutation rates in the range around 0.1–1 dictate that even clones of riboviruses and retroviruses are quasispecies, or mutant swarms, rather than collections of identical virus genomes. This quasispecies nature of RNA virus populations has numerous biological consequences, some of which are outlined below.

BIOLOGICAL SIGNIFICANCE OF VIRUS QUASI SPECIES

First and foremost, quasispecies populations endow RNA viruses with enormous environmental adaptability and capacity for extremely rapid evolution (Holland et al. 1982, Holland et al. 1992; Domingo et al. 2001a). Mutations are immediately seen when an RNA virus starts replicating in a new host, as documented with recent emergences such as HIV-1 and the severe acute respiratory syndrome (SARS) coronavirus (Holmes and Enjuanes 2003; Marra et al. 2003; Rota et al. 2003).

Rates of evolution for RNA viruses are often in the range of 10^{-2}–10^{-4} substitutions per nucleotide site per year (Domingo and Holland 1994). During persistent infections of cattle with biological clones of foot-and-mouth disease virus (FMDV), rates of evolution approached 10^{-1} substitutions per site and year in the genomic region encoding capsid protein VP1. This is one of the largest evolutionary rates recorded and demonstrates the capacity for rapid genetic change of viral quasi species evolving in their natural hosts (Gebauer et al. 1988). In sharp contrast, rates of evolution for cellular genes have been estimated in 10^{-8}–10^{-9} substitutions per nucleotide and year (reviewed by Domingo and Holland 1994).

Certain regions of an RNA virus genome (and certain single-base sites) may be much less variable (more highly conserved) than others and therefore evolve at much slower rates. In any currently circulating human strain of influenza A virus, evolution is gradual, and virus surface antigens evolve much more rapidly than do internal proteins (Webster et al. 1992). Sequence comparisons among all influenza viruses, all rhabdoviruses or all viral reverse transcriptases show that, eventually, nearly all sites can undergo viable mutations. Influenza A virus strains apparently evolve much more slowly in birds than in humans, even though these human strains have been derived from avian sources (Webster et al. 1992). Similarly, many arthropod-borne RNA viruses such as alphaviruses evolve about an order of magnitude more slowly in nature than do most other RNA viruses (Weaver et al. 1992, 1994; Strauss and Strauss 1994). Presumably, adaptive constraints necessary for efficient replication in two quite different environments (animal and insect tissues) can limit the rate of arbovirus evolution. But it is the evolutionary adaptability of RNA viruses that allows insect vector–host transmission cycles to evolve in the first instance. With very few exceptions, viruses that infect both insects and animals (or insects and plants) are RNA viruses. Generally, only RNA virus quasi species have the diversity and adaptability to move readily back and forth between quite diverse selective environments. In a number of cases of evolutionary stasis of RNA viruses, evolutionary rates are in the range of 10^{-4} substitutions per nucleotide per year, still 10^{4}–10^{5}-fold more rapid than cellular genes (Domingo et al. 2001a). RNA virus populations can reach adaptive equilibrium with host species, and relative evolutionary stasis results, whereas the same virus genes and replication enzyme in a new host can be driven to disequilibrium and rapid evolution when introduced into different selective environments (Holland et al. 1982; Domingo et al. 1988, 2001a; Domingo and Holland 1994).

Wide variations in evolutionary rates (among different genomic regions or within the same region depending on epidemiologic features and time intervals between sequence determinations) are expected from quasi species dynamics. This is because perturbations of mutant spectra that lead to modifications of dominant sequences are unpredictable. Therefore, a 'molecular clock' will rarely operate during evolution of an RNA virus (Domingo et al. 2001a). Minimal requirements for the measurements of evolutionary rates are that a founder sequence and its time of appearance in nature be identified and that there is a proper reconstruction of the evolutionary pathways of its progeny (Hillis et al. 1996). But even these conditions will rarely yield a constant rate of RNA virus evolution in nature because the response of individual hosts to the infection will not be identical (Holland et al. 1992) and dominant sequences will not be renewed in a time-dependent manner but rather in an environment-dependent manner.

Quasi-species dynamics: fitness variations and molecular memory

Because of their rapid rate of replication, high mutation rates, frequently large population sizes, and their limited genome length, RNA viruses have a great capacity for exploration of sequence space. This refers to the total number of possible sequences theoretically available to a genome (Eigen and Biebricher 1988; Domingo et al. 2001a). A numerical approximation illustrates this point. A viral genome of 10 000 residues has a total of 3×10^4 possible single mutants, which is below the population size of many viral populations. By contrast, in a mammalian genome the number of possible single mutants is about 10^{10}, a value which is well above the population size of any mammalian species. An essential feature of sequence space is the high connectivity among its different points which facilitates 'walks' to high fitness points. Fitness is a measure of the relative replication capacity of a virus in a given environment. Fitness differences have been quantitated in vivo by infecting animals with two viruses which compete for replication (Carrillo et al. 1998) and ex vivo, by infection-competition experiments in cell culture using variant viruses from in vivo infections (Quiñones-Mateu and Arts 2002; Ball et al. 2003). Model studies in cell culture have shown that serial passages of large populations of viruses result in fitness gains when measured in that same environment (Novella et al. 1995a; Escarmís et al. 1999). By contrast, repeated plaque-to-plaque transfers (serial bottleneck events) of virus in cell culture result in fitness losses (Chao 1990; Duarte et al. 1992; Escarmís et al. 1996; Yuste et al. 1999). During large population passages, selection of the best adapted mutant distributions can occur, while upon plaque-to-plaque transfers genetic drift prevails with the random accumulation of mutations, and little opportunity for compensation of their deleterious effects. In this case Muller's ratchet operates (Muller 1964). However, the virus population size that leads to fitness gain or fitness loss depends on the initial fitness of the population. Low fitness virus tends to gain fitness upon passage of modest population numbers while for high fitness viruses the usual large population passages may not be sufficient for fitness gain (Novella et al. 1995b, 1999).

One of the consequences of quasispecies dynamics as it affects fitness variations is that viruses may maintain a memory of their past evolutionary history, as documented with independent evolutionary lineages and genetic markers of FMDV in cell culture (Ruíz-Jarabo et al. 2000, 2002; Arias et al. 2001). When FMDV genomes that were dominant in a population were outcompeted either by revertants or superior variants, the proportion of the outcompeted genomes did not return to a basal level dictated by mutational pressure but, instead, remained at a significantly higher level termed memory level. Memory levels were dependent on the initial fitness of the dominant genomes destined to become memory, and this is in agreement with theoretical predictions of quasispecies dynamics (Ruíz-Jarabo et al. 2002). Genetic bottlenecks erase memory as expected from memory being deposited in minority components of an evolving quasispecies. Memory reflects the behavior of viral quasispecies as complex adaptive systems (Frank 1996), and may allow viral quasispecies to respond more readily to a selective constraint that has been previously experienced by the same population, provided no genetic bottlenecks intervened. The presence of memory shows that mutant spectra of viral populations may not be only a random distribution of variants but may also be structured according to evolutionary history. This has a number of implications for viral diagnosis, now under investigation (Domingo et al. 2003).

EFFECT OF MUTATIONS ON VIRAL PHENOTYPES

Very often only one, or a few mutational changes can allow a virus to gain virulence, change its tissue tropism, or become resistant to an antiviral drug, or a monoclonal antibody, etc. (Holland et al. 1982; Smith and Inglis 1987; Domingo et al. 1988, 1992, 2001b; Domingo and Holland 1992, 1994; Duarte et al. 1994). Compared with the average (consensus) genome sequence, a large RNA virus quasispecies population will potentially contain almost every possible single-base change (see section on Quasi-species dynamics: fitness variations and molecular memory) and many double- and triple-base change combinations required for significant biological changes, so population selection rather than further mutation will often be sufficient. This is clearly illustrated by a study of HIV-infected individuals in whom antiretroviral inhibitor-resistant mutants were already present in the complete absence of current or prior drug treatment (Nájera et al. 1995). Following antiviral drug treatment of influenza-infected (Hayden and Hay 1992) or HIV-infected (Richman 1992) individuals, a

substantial proportion of drug-resistant variants can emerge within days or a few weeks. Use of additional antiretroviral inhibitors has not ceased to enlarge a list of single and multiple mutations in the reverse transcriptase and protease of HIV that confer various levels of resistance to one or several inhibitors due primarily to mutation but also to recombination. This manifestation of adaptability of HIV constitutes a major drawback for the control of AIDS (Coffin 1995; Cabana et al. 1999; Menéndez-Arias 2002). Inhibitor-resistant mutants of other RNA viruses are also readily selected, as expected from high mutation rates and quasispecies dynamics (Domingo et al. 2001b).

Mutations in structural and nonstructural viral proteins may alter host-cell tropism and host range, with implications for viral disease emergence and re-emergence (Baranowski et al. 2001). Because of a frequent overlap between receptor-recognition sites and antigenic sites located on the surface of viral capsids and envelopes, a coevolution of host-cell tropism and antigenicity can take place (Stewart and Nemerow 1997; Baranowski et al. 2001), a concept first described with influenza virus (review by Skehel and Wiley 2000).

Large population passages of FMDV in cell culture offer a striking example of phenotypic modification resulting in expansion of host-cell tropism, with the use of integrins, heparan sulfate, and a third unidentified entry pathway to infect even the same cell type (reviewed by Baranowski et al. 2001; Airaksinen et al. 2003). Recent evidence suggests that antigenic variation that affects integrin recognition may be operating in vivo, again a demonstration of the adaptive potential of viral quasispecies within natural hosts (Tami et al. 2003; Zhao et al. 2003).

VIRUS EVOLUTION AND NEW ANTIVIRAL STRATEGIES

The Darwinian principles of genetic variation, competition, and selection that dominate biological evolution underlie several problems of disease control (antibiotic resistance in bacteria, drug resistance in eukaryotic pathogens, heterogeneity of tumor cells and metastasis, etc.) (review by Domingo et al. 2001a). Difficulties are even greater for the control of diseases associated with some genetically and antigenically highly variable viruses, and no effective preventive vaccines or therapeutic designs have yet been developed for important diseases such as AIDS or hepatitis C infections.

A new antiviral design based on the concept of error catastrophe (Eigen and Biebricher 1988; Eigen 2002) is under intensive investigation. For any complexity (amount of genetic information) hereditarily transmitted, there is a maximum error rate compatible with the maintenance of genetic information. Experimental evidence for the existence of an error threshold has been obtained with a number of RNA viruses including poliovirus (Holland et al. 1990; Crotty et al. 2000, 2001), VSV (Holland et al. 1990; Lee et al. 1997), FMDV (Sierra et al. 2000; Pariente et al. 2001, 2003; Airaksinen et al. 2003), hepatitis GBV-B virus (Lanford et al. 2001), hantavirus (Severson et al. 2003), lymphocytic chorio-meningitis virus (LCMV) (Grande-Pérez et al. 2002; Ruiz-Jarabo et al. 2003; Baranowski et al. 2003), and HIV (Loeb et al. 1999; Loeb and Mullins 2000). Interestingly, the antiviral nucleoside analogue ribavirin (1-β-D-ribofuranosyl-1,2,4-triazole-3-carboxamide) has been shown to be mutagenic for a number of RNA viruses (Crotty et al. 2000, 2001; Lanford et al. 2001; Airaksinen et al. 2003; Severson et al. 2003). Its pharmacologically active ribavirin triphosphate form is a substrate for some viral RNA-dependent RNA polymerases (Crotty et al. 2000; Maag et al. 2001; Graci and Cameron 2002). Ribavirin is used clinically to treat some viral infections, including hepatitis C virus infections in combination with interferon. Therefore, it is possible that some of the antiviral effects already documented for ribavirin in clinical practice were exerted through the transition of viral replication into error catastrophe.

An encouraging result regarding the potential application of an error catastrophe-based antiviral approach has been obtained by de la Torre and his colleagues (Ruiz-Jarabo et al. 2003) by showing that administration of the mutagenic base analogue 5-fluorouracil to mice prevented the establishment of a persistent infection with LCMV in mice. This constitutes a proof of principle of the feasibility of an error catastrophe-based approach as an antiviral strategy.

This chapter has shown that in addition to the fascinations and mysteries of virus origins and their evolution that we can observe today, a knowledge of the mechanisms underlying virus evolution has important implications for the understanding of viral disease and for the design of better strategies for their control. This is an enlightening demonstration on how basic research may lead to practical applications in the most unexpected ways.

REFERENCES

Agol, V.I. 2002. Picornavirus genetics: an overview. In: Semler, B.L. and Wimmer, E (eds), *Molecular biology of picornaviruses*. Washington, DC: American Society for Microbiology, 269–85.

Airaksinen, A., Pariente, N., et al. 2003. Curing of foot-and-mouth disease virus from persistently infected cells by ribavirin involves enhanced mutagenesis. *Virology*, **311**, 339–49.

Arias, A., Lázaro, E., et al. 2001. Molecular intermediates of fitness gain of an RNA virus: characterization of a mutant spectrum by biological and molecular cloning. *J Gen Virol*, **82**, 1049–60.

Atkins, J.F. 1993. Contemporary RNA genomes. In: Gesteland, R.F. and Atkins, J.F. (eds), *The RNA world*. Cold Spring Harbor, NY: Cold Spring Harbor Laboratory Press, 535–56.

Ball, L.A., Pringle, C.R., et al. 1999. Phenotypic consequences of rearranging the P, M and G genes of vesicular stomatitis virus. *J Virol*, **73**, 4705–12.

Ball, S.C., Abraha, A., et al. 2003. Comparing the ex vivo fitness of CCR5-tropic human immunodeficiency virus type 1 isolates of subtypes B and C. *J Virol*, **77**, 1021–38.

Baranowski, E., Ruiz-Jarabo, C.M. and Domingo, E. 2001. Evolution of cell recognition by viruses. *Science*, **292**, 1102–5.

Baranowski, E., Ruíz-Jarabo, C.M., et al. 2003. Evolution of cell recognition by viruses: a source of biological novelty with medical implications. *Adv Virus Res*, **62**, 19–111.

Barrett, A.D. and Dimmock, N.J. 1986. Defective interfering viruses and infections of animals. *Curr Top Microbiol Immunol*, **128**, 55–84.

Batschelet, E., Domingo, E. and Weissmann, C. 1976. The proportion of revertant and mutant phage in a growing population, as a function of mutation and growth rate. *Gene*, **1**, 27–32.

Berg, D.E. and Howe, M.H. 1989. *Mobile DNA*. Washington, DC: American Society for Microbiology.

Boeke, J.D. 1988. Retrotransposons. In: Domingo, E., Holland, J.J. and Ahlquist, P. (eds), *RNA genetics*, vol. 2. Boca Raton, FL: CRC Press, 59–103.

Botstein, D. 1981. A modular theory of virus evolution. In: Fields, B.N., Jaenisch, R. and Fox, C.F. (eds), *Animal virus genetics*. New York: Academic Press, 363–84.

Boyle, D.B., Coupar, B.E., et al. 1987. Fowlpox virus thymidine kinase: nucleotide sequence and relationships to other thymidine kinases. *Virology*, **156**, 355–65.

Brown, J.R. 2003. Ancient horizontal gene transfer. *Nat Rev Genet*, **4**, 121–32.

Bull, J.J. and Molineux, I.J. 1992. Molecular genetics of adaptation in an experimental model of cooperation. *Evolution*, **46**, 882–3.

Bushman, F. 2002. *Lateral DNA transfer. Mechanisms and consequences*. Cold Spring Harbor, NY: Cold Spring Harbor Laboratory Press.

Cabana, M., Clotet, B. and Martinez, M.A. 1999. Emergence and genetic evolution of HIV-1 variants with mutations conferring resistance to multiple reverse transcriptase and protease inhibitors. *J Med Virol*, **59**, 480–90.

Cameron, C.E., Gohara, D.W. and Arnold, J.J. 2002. Poliovirus RNA-dependent RNA polymerase (3Dpol): structure, function and mechanisms. In: Semler, B.L. and Wimmer, E. (eds), *Molecular biology of picornaviruses*. Washington, DC: ASM Press, 255–67.

Carrillo, C., Borca, M., et al. 1998. In vivo analysis of the stability and fitness of variants recovered from foot-and-mouth disease virus quasispecies. *J Gen Virol*, **79**, 1699–706.

Cattaneo, R. 1994. Biased (A→I) hypermutation of animal RNA virus genomes. *Curr Opin Genet Dev*, **4**, 895–900.

Cattaneo, R., Schmid, A., et al. 1988. Biased hypermutation and other genetic changes in defective measles viruses in human brain infections. *Cell*, **55**, 255–65.

Chao, L. 1990. Fitness of RNA virus decreased by Muller's ratchet. *Nature*, **348**, 454–5.

Charini, W.A., Todd, S., et al. 1994. Transduction of a human RNA sequence by poliovirus. *J Virol*, **68**, 6547–52.

Coffin, J.M. 1992. Genetic diversity and evolution of retroviruses. *Curr Top Microb Immunol*, **176**, 143–64.

Coffin, J.M. 1995. HIV population dynamics in vivo: implications for genetic variation, pathogenesis, and therapy. *Science*, **267**, 483–9.

Cooper, G.M. 2000. *The cell. A molecular approach*. Washington, DC: ASM Press.

Crotty, S., Maag, D., et al. 2000. The broad-spectrum antiviral ribonucleotide, ribavirin, is an RNA virus mutagen. *Nat Med*, **6**, 1375–9.

Crotty, S., Cameron, C.E. and Andino, R. 2001. RNA virus error catastrophe: direct molecular test by using ribavirin. *Proc Natl Acad Sci USA*, **98**, 6895–900.

Dahourou, G., Guillot, S., et al. 2002. Genetic recombination in wild-type poliovirus. *J Gen Virol*, **83**, 3103–10.

DeFilippis, V.R. and Villarreal, L.P. 2001. Virus evolution. In: Knipes, D.M., Howley, P.M., et al. (eds), *Fields virology*. Philadelphia, PA: Lippincott-Raven, 353–70.

Desselberger, U. 1996. Genome rearrangements of rotaviruses. *Adv Virus Res*, **46**, 69–95.

Domingo, E. and Holland, J.J. 1992. Complications of RNA heterogeneity for the engineering of virus vaccines and antiviral agents.. *Genet Eng (NY)*, **14**, 13–31.

Domingo, E. and Holland, J.J. 1994. Mutation rates and rapid evolution of RNA viruses. In: Morse, S.S. (ed.), *Evolutionary biology of viruses*. New York: Raven Press, 161–84.

Domingo, E., Holland, J.J. and Ahlquist, P. 1988. *RNA genetics*. Boca Raton, FL: CRC Press.

Domingo, E., Escarmis, C., et al. 1992. Foot-and-mouth disease virus populations are quasispecies. *Curr Top Microbiol Immunol*, **176**, 33–47.

Domingo, E., Biebricher, C., et al. 2001a. *Quasispecies and RNA virus evolution: principles and consequences*. Austin, TX: Landes Bioscience.

Domingo, E., Mas, A., et al. 2001b. Virus population dynamics, fitness variations and the control of viral disease: an update. *Prog Drug Res*, **57**, 77–115.

Domingo, E., Ruíz-Jarabo, C.M., et al. 2003. Detection and biological implications of genetic memory in viral quasispecies. In Matsumori, A. (ed.), *Cardiomyopathies and heart failure: biomolecular, infectious and immune mechanisms*. London: Kluwer Academic Publishers, 259–76.

Doolittle, R.F. and Feng, D.F. 1992. Tracing the origin of retroviruses. *Curr Top Microbiol Immunol*, **176**, 195–211.

Drake, J.W. 1969. Comparative rates of spontaneous mutation. *Nature*, **221**, 1132.

Drake, J.W. 1991. A constant rate of spontaneous mutation in DNA-based microbes.. *Proc Natl Acad Sci USA*, **88**, 7160–4.

Drake, J.W. 1993. Rates of spontaneous mutation among RNA viruses. *Proc Natl Acad Sci USA*, **90**, 4171–5.

Drake, J.W. and Holland, J.J. 1999. Mutation rates among RNA viruses. *Proc Natl Acad Sci USA*, **96**, 13910–13.

Duarte, E., Clarke, D., et al. 1992. Rapid fitness losses in mammalian RNA virus clones due to Muller's ratchet. *Proc Natl Acad Sci USA*, **89**, 6015–19.

Duarte, E.A., Novella, I.S., et al. 1994. RNA virus quasispecies: significance for viral disease and epidemiology. *Infect Agents Dis*, **3**, 201–14.

Eigen, M. 2002. Error catastrophe and antiviral strategy. *Proc Natl Acad Sci USA*, **99**, 13374–6.

Eigen, M. and Biebricher, C.K. 1988. Sequence space and quasispecies distribution. In Domingo, E., Ahlquist, P. and Holland, J.J. (eds), *RNA genetics*, vol. 3. Boca Raton, FL: CRC Press, 211–45.

Escarmís, C., Dávila, M., et al. 1996. Genetic lesions associated with Muller's ratchet in an RNA virus. *J Mol Biol*, **264**, 255–67.

Escarmís, C., Dávila, M. and Domingo, E. 1999. Multiple molecular pathways for fitness recovery of an RNA virus debilitated by operation of Muller's ratchet. *J Mol Biol*, **285**, 495–505.

Frank, S.A. 1996. The design of natural and artificial adaptive systems. In: Rose, M.R. and Lauder, G.V. (eds), *Adaptation*. San Diego, CA: Academic Press, 451–505.

Gebauer, F., de la Torre, J.C., et al. 1988. Rapid selection of genetic and antigenic variants of foot-and-mouth disease virus during persistence in cattle. *J Virol*, **62**, 2041–9.

Gojobori, T. and Yokoyama, S. 1985. Rates of evolution of the retroviral oncogene of Moloney murine sarcoma virus and of its cellular homologues. *Proc Natl Acad Sci USA*, **82**, 4198–201.

Gorbalenya, A.E. 1995. Origin of RNA viral genomes; approaching the problem by comparative sequence analysis. In: Gibbs, A., Calisher, C.H. and Garcia-Arenal, F. (eds), *Molecular basis of virus evolution*. Cambridge, UK: Cambridge University Press, 49–66.

Gorman, O.T., Bean, W.J. and Webster, R.G. 1992. Evolutionary processes in influenza viruses: divergence, rapid evolution, and stasis. *Curr Top Microbiol Immunol*, **176**, 75–97.

Graci, J.D. and Cameron, C.E. 2002. Quasispecies, error catastrophe, and the antiviral activity of ribavirin. *Virology*, **298**, 175–80.

Grande-Pérez, A., Sierra, S., et al. 2002. Molecular indetermination in the transition to error catastrophe: systematic elimination of lymphocytic choriomeningitis virus through mutagenesis does not correlate linearly with large increases in mutant spectrum complexity. *Proc Natl Acad Sci USA*, **99**, 12938–43.

Greene, A.E. and Allison, R.F. 1994. Recombination between viral RNA and transgenic plant transcripts. *Science*, **263**, 1423–5.

Hahn, C.S., Lustig, S., et al. 1988. Western equine encephalitis virus is a recombinant virus. *Proc Natl Acad Sci USA*, **85**, 5997–6001.

Harris, R.S., Bishop, K.N., et al. 2003. DNA deamination mediates innate immunity to retroviral infection. *Cell*, **113**, 803–9.

Harrison, P.T., Thompson, R. and Davison, A.J. 1991. Evolution of herpesvirus thymidine kinases from cellular deoxycytidine kinase. *J Gen Virol*, **72**, 2583–6.

Hayden, F.G. and Hay, A.J. 1992. Emergence and transmission of influenza A viruses resistant to amantadine and rimantadine. *Curr Top Microbiol Immunol*, **176**, 119–30.

Hayes, W. 1968. *The genetics of bacteria and their viruses*. New York: John Wiley and Sons Inc.

Hillis, D.M., Mable, B.K. and Moritz, C. 1996. Applications of molecular systematics. In: Hillis, D.M., Moritz, C. and Mable, B.K. (eds), *Molecular systematics*. Sunderland, MA: Sinauer Associates, 515–43.

Holland, J. and Domingo, E. 1998. Origin and evolution of viruses. *Virus Genes*, **16**, 13–21.

Holland, J., Spindler, K., et al. 1982. Rapid evolution of RNA genomes. *Science*, **215**, 1577–85.

Holland, J.J. (ed.) 1992. *Genetic diversity of RNA viruses. , Current topics in microbiology and immunology*. Berlin: Springer-Verlag.

Holland, J.J., Domingo, E., et al. 1990. Mutation frequencies at defined single codon sites in vesicular stomatitis virus and poliovirus can be increased only slightly by chemical mutagenesis. *J Virol*, **64**, 3960–2.

Holland, J.J., de la Torre, J.C. and Steinhauer, D.A. 1992. RNA virus populations as quasispecies. *Curr Top Microbiol Immunol*, **176**, 1–20.

Holmes, K.V. and Enjuanes, L. 2003. Virology. The SARS coronavirus: a postgenomic era. *Science*, **300**, 1377–8.

Huang, A.S. 1988. Modulation of viral disease processes by defective interfering particles. In: Domingo, E., Holland, J.J. and Ahlquist, P. (eds), *RNA genetics*. Boca Raton, FL: CRC Press, 195–208.

Hwang, Y.T., Liu, B.Y., et al. 1997. Effects of mutations in the Exo III motif of the herpes simplex virus DNA polymerase gene on enzyme activities, viral replication, and replication fidelity. *J Virol*, **71**, 7791–8.

Joklik, W.K. 1974. Evolution in viruses. In: Carlile, M.J. and Skehel, J.J. (eds), *Evolution in the microbial world*. Cambridge: Cambridge University Press, 293–320.

Kew, O.M., Nottay, B.K., et al. 1981. Multiple genetic changes can occur in the oral poliovaccines upon replication in humans. *J Gen Virol*, **56**, 337–47.

Khatchikian, D., Orlich, M. and Rott, R. 1989. Increased viral pathogenicity after insertion of a 28S ribosomal RNA sequence into the hemagglutinin gene of an influenza virus. *Nature*, **340**, 156–7.

Kim, N.W., Piatyszek, M.A., et al. 1994. Specific association of human telomerase activity with immortal cells and cancer. *Science*, **266**, 2011–15.

King, A.M.Q. 1988. Genetic recombination in positive strand RNA viruses. In: Domingo, E., Holland, J.J. and Ahlquist, P. (eds), *RNA genetics*, vol. 2. . Boca Raton FL: CRC Press, 149–65.

Kirchmaier, A.L. and Sugden, B. 1995. Plasmid maintenance of derivatives of *oriP* of Epstein–Barr virus. *J Virol*, **69**, 1280–3.

Kucherlapati, R.S. and Smith, G.R. 1988. *Genetic recombination*. Washington, DC: American Society for Microbiology.

Kummerer, B.M., Tautz, N., et al. 2000. The genetic basis for cytopathogenicity of pestiviruses. *Vet Microbiol*, **77**, 117–28.

Lai, M.M.C. 1992. Genetic recombination in RNA viruses. *Curr Top Microbiol Immunol*, **176**, 21–32.

Lanford, R.E., Chavez, D., et al. 2001. Ribavirin induces error-prone replication of GB virus B in primary tamarin hepatocytes. *J Virol*, **75**, 8074–81.

Lawrence, J.B., Villnave, C.A. and Singer, R.H. 1988. Sensitive, high-resolution chromatin and chromosome mapping in situ: presence and orientation of two closely integrated copies of EBV in a lymphoma line. *Cell*, **52**, 51–61.

Lee, C.H., Gilbertson, D.L., et al. 1997. Negative effects of chemical mutagenesis on the adaptive behavior of vesicular stomatitis virus. *J Virol*, **71**, 3636–40.

Li, D., Schmaljohn, A.L., et al. 1995. Complete nucleotide sequences of the M and S segments of two hantavirus isolates from California: evidence for reassortment in nature among viruses related to hantavirus pulmonary syndrome. *Virology*, **206**, 973–83.

Lindahl, T., Adams, A., et al. 1976. Covalently closed circular duplex DNA of Epstein–Barr virus in a human lymphoid cell line. *J Mol Biol*, **102**, 511–30.

Lodish, H., Baltimore, D., et al. 1995. *Molecular cell biology.* New York: W.H. Freeman and Co, Scientific American Books.

Loeb, L.A., Essigmann, J.M., et al. 1999. Lethal mutagenesis of HIV with mutagenic nucleoside analogs. *Proc Natl Acad Sci USA*, **96**, 1492–7.

Loeb, L.A. and Mullins, J.I. 2000. Lethal mutagenesis of HIV by mutagenic ribonucleoside analogs. *AIDS Res Hum Retroviruses*, **13**, 1–3.

Luria, S.E., Darnell, J., et al. 1978. *General virology*, 2nd edn. New York: John Wiley and Sons.

Luytjes, W., Bredenbeek, P.J., et al. 1988. Sequence of mouse hepatitis virus A59 mRNA 2: indications for RNA recombination between coronaviruses and influenza C virus. *Virology*, **166**, 415–22.

Maag, D., Castro, C., et al. 2001. Hepatitis C virus RNA-dependent RNA polymerase (NS5B) as a mediator of the antiviral activity of ribavirin. *J Biol Chem*, **276**, 46094–8.

Maramorosch, K. 1991. *Viroids and satellites: molecular parasites at the frontier of life.* Boca Raton, FL: CRC Press.

Marra, M.A., Jones, S.J., et al. 2003. The genome sequence of the SARS-associated coronavirus. *Science*, **300**, 1399–404.

Martínez, M.A., Vartanian, J.P. and Wain-Hobson, S. 1994. Hypermutagenesis of RNA using human immunodeficiency virus type 1 reverse transcriptase and biased dNTP concentrations. *Proc Natl Acad Sci USA*, **91**, 11787–91.

Mayo, M.A. and Jolly, C.A. 1991. The 5′-terminal sequence of potato leafroll virus RNA: evidence of recombination between virus and host RNA. *J Gen Virol*, **72**, 2591–5.

Menéndez-Arias, L. 2002. Molecular basis of fidelity of DNA synthesis and nucleotide specificity of retroviral reverse transcriptases. *Prog Nucl Acid Res Mol Biol*, **71**, 91–147.

Meyerhans, A. and Vartanian, J.-P. 1999. The fidelity of cellular and viral polymerases and its manipulation for hypermutagenesis. In: Domingo, E., Webster, R.G. and Holland, J.J. (eds), *Origin and evolution of viruses.* San Diego, CA: Academic Press, 87–114.

Meyers, G., Tautz, N., et al. 1991. Viral cytopathogenicity correlated with integration of ubiquitin-coding sequences. *Virology*, **180**, 602–16.

Middleton, T., Gahn, T.A., et al. 1991. Immortalizing genes of Epstein–Barr virus. *Adv Virus Res*, **40**, 19–55.

Minor, P.D. 1992. The molecular biology of poliovaccines. *J Gen Virol*, **73**, 3065–77.

Minor, P.D., John, A., et al. 1986. Antigenic and molecular evolution of the vaccine strain of type 3 poliovirus during the period of excretion by a primary vaccinee. *J Gen Virol*, **67**, 693–706.

Monroe, S.S. and Schlesinger, S. 1983. RNAs from two independently isolated defective interfering particles of Sindbis virus contain a cellular tRNA sequence at their 5′ ends. *Proc Natl Acad Sci USA*, **80**, 3279–83.

Mount, D.W. 2001. *Bioinformatics. Sequence and genome analysis.* Cold Spring Harbor, NY: Cold Spring Harbor Laboratory Press.

Muller, H.J. 1964. The relation of recombination to mutational advance. *Mut Res*, **1**, 2–9.

Nagy, P.D. and Bujarski, J.J. 1995. Efficient system of homologous RNA recombination in brome mosaic virus: sequence and structure requirements and accuracy of crossovers. *J Virol*, **69**, 131–40.

Nagy, P.D. and Simon, A.E. 1997. New insights into the mechanisms of RNA recombination. *Virology*, **235**, 1–9.

Nájera, I., Holguín, A., et al. 1995. Pol gene quasispecies of human immunodeficiency virus: mutations associated with drug resistance in virus from patients undergoing no drug therapy. *J Virol*, **69**, 23–31.

Novella, I.S., Duarte, E.A., et al. 1995a. Exponential increases of RNA virus fitness during large population transmissions. *Proc Natl Acad Sci USA*, **92**, 5841–4.

Novella, I.S., Elena, S.F., et al. 1995b. Size of genetic bottlenecks leading to virus fitness loss is determined by mean initial population fitness. *J Virol*, **69**, 2869–72.

Novella, I.S., Quer, J., et al. 1999. Exponential fitness gains of RNA virus populations are limited by bottleneck effects. *J Virol*, **73**, 1668–1671.

Pariente, N., Sierra, S., et al. 2001. Efficient virus extinction by combinations of a mutagen and antiviral inhibitors. *J Virol*, **75**, 9723–30.

Pariente, N., Airaksinen, A. and Domingo, E. 2003. Mutagenesis versus inhibition in the efficiency of extinction of foot-and-mouth-disease virus. *J Virol*, **77**, 7131–8.

Peng, G., Hongo, S., et al. 1994. Genetic reassortment of influenza C viruses in man. *J Gen Virol*, **75**, Pt 12, 3619–22.

Plyusnin, A., Kukkonen, S.K., et al. 2002. Transfection-mediated generation of functionally competent Tula hantavirus with recombinant S RNA segment. *EMBO J*, **21**, 1497–503.

Quiñones-Mateu, M.E. and Arts, E.J. 2002. HIV-1 fitness: implications for drug resistance, disease progression, and global epidemic evolution. In: Kuiken, C., Foley, B., et al. (eds), *HIV-1 sequence compendium. Theoretical Biology and Biophysics Group.* Los Alamos, NM: Los Alamos National Laboratory, 134–70.

Ramig, R.F., Ahmed, R. and Fields, B.N. 1983. A genetic map of reovirus: assignment of the newly defined mutant groups H, I and J to genome segments. *Virology*, **125**, 299–313.

Rao, A.L. and Hall, T.C. 1990. Requirement for a viral trans-acting factor encoded by brome mosaic virus RNA-2 provides strong selection in vivo for functional recombinants. *J Virol*, **64**, 2437–41.

Richman, D.D. 1992. Selection of zidovudine-resistant variants of human immunodeficiency virus by therapy. *Curr Top Microbiol Immunol*, **176**, 131–42.

Robertson, H.D. 1992. Replication and evolution of viroid-like pathogens. *Curr Top Microbiol Immunol*, **176**, 213–19.

Rolls, M.M., Webster, P., et al. 1994. Novel infectious particles generated by expression of the vesicular stomatitis virus glycoprotein from a self-replicating RNA. *Cell*, **79**, 497–506.

Rota, P.A., Oberste, M.S., et al. 2003. Characterization of a novel coronavirus associated with severe acute respiratory syndrome. *Science*, **300**, 1394–9.

Roux, L., Simon, A.E. and Holland, J.J. 1991. Effects of defective interfering viruses on virus replication and pathogenesis in vitro and in vivo. *Adv Virus Res*, **40**, 181–211.

Ruíz-Jarabo, C.M., Arias, A., et al. 2000. Memory in viral quasispecies. *J Virol*, **74**, 3543–7.

Ruíz-Jarabo, C.M., Arias, A., et al. 2002. Duration and fitness dependence of quasispecies memory. *J Mol Biol*, **315**, 285–96.

Ruiz-Jarabo, C.M., Ly, C., et al. 2003. Lethal mutagenesis of the prototypic arenavirus lymphocytic choriomeningitis virus (LCMV). *Virology*, **308**, 37–47.

Semancik, J.S. and Duran-Vila, N. 1999. Viroids in plants: shadows and footprints of a primitive RNA. In: Domingo, E., Webster, J.P. and Holland, J.J. (eds), *Origin and evolution of viruses.* San Diego, CA: Academic Press, 37–64.

Severson, W.E., Schmaljohn, C.S., et al. 2003. Ribavirin causes error catastrophe during Hantaan virus replication. *J Virol*, **77**, 481–8.

Sheen, F.M. and Levis, R.W. 1994. Transposition of the LINE-like retrotransposon TART to *Drosophila* chromosome termini. *Proc Natl Acad Sci USA*, **91**, 12510–14.

Sierra, S., Dávila, M., et al. 2000. Response of foot-and-mouth disease virus to increased mutagenesis. Influence of viral load and fitness in loss of infectivity. *J Virol*, **74**, 8316–23.

Skehel, J.J. and Wiley, D.C. 2000. Receptor binding and membrane fusion in virus entry: the influenza hemagglutinin. *Annu Rev Biochem*, **69**, 531–69.

Smith, D.B. and Inglis, S.C. 1987. The mutation rate and variability of eukaryotic viruses: an analytical review. *J Gen Virol*, **68**, 2729–40.

Steinhauer, D.A., Domingo, E. and Holland, J.J. 1992. Lack of evidence for proofreading mechanisms associated with an RNA virus polymerase. *Gene*, **122**, 281–8.

Stewart, P.L. and Nemerow, G.R. 1997. Recent structural solutions for antibody neutralization of viruses. *Trends Microbiol*, **5**, 229–33.

Strauss, J.H. and Strauss, E.G. 1988. Evolution of RNA viruses. *Annu Rev Microbiol*, **42**, 657–83.

Strauss, J.H. and Strauss, E.G. 1994. The alphaviruses: gene expression, replication, and evolution. *Microbiol Rev*, **58**, 491–562.

Syvanen, M. 1994. Horizontal gene transfer: evidence and possible consequences. *Annu Rev Genet*, **28**, 237–61.

Tami, C., Taboga, O., et al. 2003. Evidence of the coevolution of antigenicity and host cell tropism of foot-and-mouth disease virus in vivo. *J Virol*, **77**, 1219–26.

Tautz, N., Thiel, H.J., et al. 1994. Pathogenesis of mucosal disease: a cytopathogenic pestivirus generated by an internal deletion. *J Virol*, **68**, 3289–97.

Temin, H.M. 1970. Malignant transformation of cells by viruses. *Perspect Biol Med*, **14**, 11–26.

Temin, H.M. 1989. Retrons in bacteria. *Nature (Lond)*, **339**, 254–5.

Thomson, M.M., Perez-Alvarez, L. and Najera, R. 2002. Molecular epidemiology of HIV-1 genetic forms and its significance for vaccine development and therapy. *Lancet Infect Dis*, **2**, 461–71.

van Regenmortel, M.H.V., Fauquet, C.M. et al. (eds) 2000. *Virus taxonomy. Seventh Report of the International Committee on Taxonomy of Viruses*. San Diego, CA: Academic Press.

Vogt, P.K. and Jackson, A.O. 1999. *Satellites and defective viral RNAs. Current Topics in Microbiology and Immunology*. Berlin: Springer-Verlag.

Wain-Hobson, S. 1992. Human immunodeficiency virus type 1 quasispecies in vivo and ex vivo. *Curr Top Microbiol Immunol*, **176**, 181–93.

Weaver, S.C., Rico-Hesse, R. and Scott, T.W. 1992. Genetic diversity and slow rates of evolution in New World alphaviruses. *Curr Top Microbiol Immunol*, **176**, 99–117.

Weaver, S.C., Hagenbaugh, A., et al. 1994. Evolution of alphaviruses in the eastern equine encephalomyelitis complex. *J Virol*, **68**, 158–169.

Webster, R.G. 1999. Antigenic variation in influenza viruses. In: Domingo, E., Webster, R.G. and Holland, J.J. (eds), *Origin and evolution of viruses*. San Diego: Academic Press, 377–90.

Webster, R.G., Bean, W.J., et al. 1992. Evolution and ecology of influenza A viruses. *Microbiol Rev*, **56**, 152–79.

Weigel, R. and Miller, G. 1983. Major EB virus-specific cytoplasmic transcripts in a cellular clone of the HR-1 Burkitt lymphoma line during latency and after induction of viral replicative cycle by phorbol esters. *Virology*, **125**, 287–98.

Wertz, G.W., Moudy, R. and Ball, L.A. 2002. Adding genes to the RNA genome of vesicular stomatitis virus: positional effects on stability of expression. *J Virol*, **76**, 7642–50.

White, P.S., Morales, F. and Roossinck, M.J. 1995. Interspecific reassortment of genomic segments in the evolution of cucumoviruses. *Virology*, **207**, 334–7.

Wimmer, E., Hellen, C.U. and Cao, X. 1993. Genetics of poliovirus. *Annu Rev Genet*, **27**, 353–436.

Wright, S. 1982. Character change, speciation, and the higher taxa. *Evolution*, **36**, 427–43.

Wuethrich, B. 2003. Chasing the fickle swine flu. *Science*, **299**, 1502–5.

Yuste, E., Sánchez-Palomino, S., et al. 1999. Drastic fitness loss in human immunodeficiency virus type 1 upon serial bottleneck events. *J Virol*, **73**, 2745–51.

Zhao, Q., Pacheco, J.M. and Mason, P.W. 2003. Evaluation of genetically engineered derivatives of a Chinese strain of foot-and-mouth disease virus reveals a novel cell-binding site which functions in cell culture and in animals. *J Virol*, **77**, 3269–80.

Zhuang, J., Jetzt, A.E., et al. 2002. Human immunodeficiency virus type 1 recombination: rate, fidelity, and putative hot spots. *J Virol*, **76**, 11273–82.

Zimmern, D. 1988. Evolution of RNA viruses. In: Domingo, E., Holland, J.J. and Ahlquist, P. (eds), *RNA genetics*, vol. 2. Boca Raton, FL: CRC Press, 211–40.

3

The nature and classification of viruses

MARC H.V. VAN REGENMORTEL

THE FILTERABILITY OF VIRUSES

The first evidence that viruses are infectious, disease-causing agents different from pathogenic bacteria was obtained by filtration experiments with Chamberland filters. These bacteria-retaining filters which had been used by Pasteur to remove pathogenic microorganisms from water were used by Dmitri Ivanovsky in his classical studies of tobacco mosaic disease published in 1892. Ivanovsky showed that when sap from a diseased tobacco plant was passed through the filter, the filtrate remained infectious and could be used to infect other plants. The same experiment was repeated in 1898 by Beijerinck who again showed that the filtered tobacco sap was still infectious. Beijerinck went further and established that the infectious agent was able to diffuse through several millimeters of an agar gel, from which he concluded that the infection was caused not by a microbe but by what he called a *contagium vivum fluidum* or contagious living liquid. He called the agent which reproduced itself in the plant, a virus. During the same year, Loeffler and Frosch who were investigating foot-and-mouth disease reported that although the causative agent passed through a Chamberland-type filter, it did not go through a Kitasato filter which had a finer grain than the Chamberland filter. From this result, Loeffler concluded that the virus was a corpuscular particle and not a soluble agent as claimed by Beijerinck.

Although all historical accounts of the beginnings of virology refer to the work of Ivanovsky, Beijerinck, and Loeffler, there is disagreement among various authors about who should be credited with the discovery that viruses were a new type of infectious agent (Lvov 1993; Bos 1995; Witz 1998). This is an interesting debate since it concerns the question of what is a scientific discovery. Although Ivanovsky was clearly the first one to show that the agent causing the tobacco mosaic disease passed through a bacteria-retaining filter, all his publications show that he did not grasp the significance of his observation. He actually believed that the filter he used might have had fine cracks and that small spores of a microbe might have passed through the filter. More than 10 years after his initial observations he remained convinced that he was dealing with a bacterium rather than with a new type of infectious agent (Bos 1995). Beijerinck on the other hand, realized he was dealing with something different from a microbe but he thought that the virus was an infectious liquid and not a corpuscular particle as claimed by Loeffler (Witz 1998). Only Loeffler correctly concluded that the virus causing foot-and-mouth disease was a small particle stopped by a fine-grain Kitasato filter. The debate about who should be considered the founder of virology may be settled only if it is accepted that, in order to make a discovery, it is not sufficient to make a novel observation (i.e. the filterability of an infectious agent) but that, in addition, it is also necessary to interpret the observation correctly (Root-Bernstein

1989). Good science does not consist only in making new observations or collecting new data but it requires also unbiased, imaginative thinking which enables the scientist to arrive at the correct interpretation of his experimental findings. Loeffler's interpretation of his filtration experiments came the closest to the modern concept of a virus. However, it was only the work of William Elford with graded collodion membranes, done more than 30 years later, which established that different viruses had particle diameters of 20–200 nm (Grafe, 1991). The actual morphology of virus particles was finally elucidated only when the particles could be visualized by electron microscopy.

THE NATURE OF VIRUSES

At the beginning of the last century, viruses were characterized only by negative features, i.e. they were not identifiable by light microscopy, they could not be cultured on conventional bacteriological media, and they were not retained by filters used for sterilization (Grafe 1991). The perception of what is a virus changed dramatically in 1935 when Wendel Stanley showed that tobacco mosaic virus could be crystallized. This seemed to indicate that an infectious virus was a chemical molecule rather than an organism and it stimulated an intense interest in viruses as entities at the borderline between chemistry and biology. Many scientists became fascinated with viruses 'as living molecules.' This led physicists like Max Delbrück to turn to the study of bacteriophages because these viruses were more suitable for the quantitative analysis of virus multiplication. A reductionist, chemical approach to the study of biology was also stimulated by Erwin Schrödinger's book *What is life* published in 1945. Viruses were increasingly studied by physicochemical techniques and these studies contributed significantly to the development of molecular biology (Grafe 1991).

As our knowledge of the biochemistry of virus multiplication increased, it became clear that viruses depended for their multiplication on the protein-synthesizing and energy-producing systems of the host cell. Viruses were recognized to be subcellular infectious agents that, at one stage of their growth cycle in the infected cell, were reduced to their nucleic acid component. The virus particle or virion appeared simply as one stage of the virus life cycle. The virion was seen to protect the viral genome from degradation by nucleases and ultraviolet radiation and to allow the infectious agent to be transferred to a new host.

Whether or not viruses should be regarded as living organisms was regarded by some to be only a matter of taste. The question was sidestepped by Lwoff (1957) who declared that 'viruses should be considered as viruses because viruses are viruses.' However, it was generally accepted that viruses belong to biology since they possessed some of the properties of living systems,

such as having a genome and being able to adapt to particular hosts and biotic habitats. On the other hand, viruses do not possess some of the essential attributes of living systems, such as the ability to capture and store free energy, and as a result they lack the characteristic autonomy that arises from the presence of a set of integrated, metabolic activities. Viruses are replicated through the metabolic activities of infected cells and they become part of a living system only after they have infected a host cell. The consensus among biologists at present is that the simplest system that can be said to be alive is a cell. The individual macromolecules and organelles found in a cell are not considered to be alive and there is indeed little justification for regarding viruses as living microorganisms. They are nonliving, infectious entities and they can be said, at best, to lead a kind of borrowed life (Van Regenmortel 2000a). According to D.J. McGeoch, viruses can be described as 'mistletoe on the Tree of Life' (Calisher et al. 1995).

The distinction between viruses and various types of organisms is highlighted when the functional roles of proteins present in viruses and in unicellular and multicellular organisms are compared. When proteins are classified in three broad, functional categories corresponding to energy utilization, carriers of information, and communication mediators, the proportion of each protein class found in viruses differs markedly from that found in living organisms (Tamames et al. 1996; Patthy 1999). Viruses have the highest proportion of proteins involved in information processes, i.e. in the control and expression of genetic information, and they have very few proteins of the energy and communication classes (Figure 3.1). This distribution obviously reflects the fact that viruses utilize the host cell's metabolic machinery and rely entirely on the energy supply system of the host they infect. By contrast, bacteria have the highest proportion of proteins of the energy

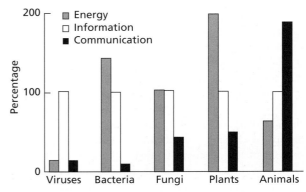

Figure 3.1 *The proteins of viruses, microorganisms, plants, and animals have different functional roles. The vertical bars represent the proportion of proteins in the categories of energy utilization and carrier of information relative to those in the category of mediator of information. Viruses have the highest proportion of proteins involved in information processes, i.e. in the control and expression of genetic information (from Patthy 1999).*

class involved in small molecule transformations whereas animals have a high proportion of proteins associated with intra- and intercellular communication (Figure 3.1).

VIRUSES SHOULD NOT BE CONFUSED WITH VIRUS PARTICLES OR VIRIONS

A virus is an elementary biosystem that replicates as an intracellular parasite in its host cell. During its multiplication cycle it takes on various forms and manifestations, for instance as a replicating nucleic acid in the host cell. One stage in the so-called 'life cycle' of a virus corresponds to the virus particle or virion which can be characterized by various intrinsic, structural, and chemical properties such as size, mass, chemical composition, etc. A virus, on the other hand, possesses, in addition, various relational properties that exist only by virtue of a relation with other objects such as a host or a vector. Some of these properties, for instance the replication cycle, are emergent properties that are possessed only by the system as a whole and are not present in its constituent parts. A virus should thus not be reduced to the physical constituents and chemical composition of a virion and it is necessary to include in its description also the functional activities that become actualized only inside the host as well as a variety of other biotic interactions (Van Regenmortel 2000a). Confusing the entity 'virus' with virion is similar to confusing the entity 'insect' with either a pupa, a caterpillar or a flying moth or butterfly. It is unfortunate that, in the scientific literature, virions are often referred to as the virus, for instance when one talks of 'the picture of the virus' or of 'the process of purifying the virus.'

VIRUS CLASSIFICATION AND NOMENCLATURE

The earliest attempts to classify viruses were based on the type of diseases they caused and the names given to the causative viruses were derived from the symptoms of the diseases and the hosts and organs that were infected. By the end of the 1950s, enough information on some types of virus particles had been gathered to allow the recognition of groups like the herpesviruses, the myxoviruses, and the poxviruses as well as several groups of elongated plant viruses. Following the development of the negative staining technique for observing virions in the electron microscope (Brenner and Horne 1959), it became relatively easy to establish the morphology of virus particles also in crude extracts. This in turn enabled the placement of viruses in genera and families according to virion morphology and stimulated the development of the Lwoff et al. (1962) scheme of virus classification. This hierarchical system was based on the assumption that the most important character-

istics for classifying viruses were nucleic acid type and virion morphology. Although this scheme was initially criticized because the choice of criteria was deemed to be arbitrary, the attempt to replace it by an Adansonian system that gives equal weight to a large number of different characteristics was short-lived (Matthews 1983). Properties such as the size of the genome and the strandedness and polarity of the nucleic acid are stable properties since they determine the viral genome expression strategy and cannot be altered without being lethal for the virus. Likewise, the structural elements that build up a virion cannot undergo major changes without resulting in lethal instability of the virion.

The 63 virus families recognized at present (Van Regenmortel et al. 2000b) were demarcated on the basis of the nature of the viral genome, the strategy of replication used by the virus, and the structure of the virion. The family level in the taxonomic hierarchy has changed very little over the years, the main changes being the addition of more families. As new types of viruses were discovered in the families *Poxviridae*, *Herpesviridae*, *Parvoviridae*, and *Paramyxoviridae*, subfamilies have been introduced that group genera possessing certain common features.

In recent years, three virus orders representing groupings of families of viruses that share common characteristics have been created (Fauquet 1999). The order *Mononegavirales* comprises the families *Bornaviridae*, *Filoviridae*, *Paraxymoviridae*, and *Rhabdoviridae* that contain viruses with similar replication strategy. The order *Caudovirales* comprises the families *Myoviridae*, *Podoviridae*, and *Siphoviridae*, consisting of tailed, double-stranded DNA bacteriophages. The third order *Nidovirales* comprises the families *Coronaviridae*, *Arteriviridae*, and *Roniviridae*.

Viral families are subdivided into genera on the basis of characteristics that differ from one family to another, for instance differences in genome size and organization, virus replication strategy, vector transmission, etc. In some cases, when it is not clear whether a group of viruses placed in a genus should be included in an existing family or not, the corresponding genus is given the status of unassigned or floating genus.

The names of orders, families, subfamilies, and genera are latinized and written in italics with a capital initial letter and with the endings – *virales* for orders, *viridae* for families, *virinae* for subfamilies and *virus* for genera.

The families and unassigned genera of viruses that have been recognized up to July 2002 are listed in Table 3.1.

THE INTERNATIONAL COMMITTEE ON TAXONOMY OF VIRUSES

The authority on matters concerning virus classification and nomenclature is the International Committee on Taxonomy of Viruses (ICTV), which is a Committee of

Table 3.1 *Families and unassigned genera of viruses[a]*

Family or unassigned genus	Morphology of virus particle	Host
The dsDNA viruses		
Myoviridae	Tailed phage	Bacteria
Siphoviridae	Tailed phage	Bacteria
Podoviridae	Tailed phage	Bacteria
Tectiviridae	Isometric	Bacteria
Corticoviridae	Isometric	Bacteria
Plasmaviridae	Pleomorphic	Mycoplasma
Lipothrixviridae	Rod-shaped	Archaea
Rudiviridae	Rod-shaped	Archaea
Fuselloviridae	Lemon-shaped	Archaea
'SNDV-like viruses'	Droplet-shaped	Archaea
Poxviridae	Pleomorphic	Vertebrates/Invertebrates
Asfarviridae	Spherical	Vertebrates
Iridoviridae	Isometric	Vertebrates/Invertebrates
Phycodnaviridae	Isometric	Algae
Baculoviridae	Bacilliform	Invertebrates
Nimaviridae	Rod-shaped	Invertebrates
Herpesviridae	Isometric	Vertebrates
Adenoviridae	Isometric	Vertebrates
Rhizidiovirus	Isometric	Fungi
Polyomaviridae	Isometric	Vertebrates
Papillomaviridae	Isometric	Vertebrates
Polydnaviridae	Rod, fusiform	Invertebrates
Ascoviridae	Reniform	Invertebrates
The ssDNA viruses		
Inoviridae	Filamentous	Bacteria
Microviridae	Isometric	Bacteria
Geminiviridae	Isometic	Plants
Circoviridae	Isometric	Vertebrates
Anellovirus	Spherical	Vertebrates
Nanoviridae	Isometric	Plants
Parvoviridae	Isometric	Vertebrates/invertebrates
The DNA and RNA reverse-transcribing viruses		
Hepadnaviridae	Spherical	Vertebrates
Caulimoviridae	Isometric, bacilliform	Plants
Pseudoviridae	Spherical	Fungi, plants, invertebrates
Metaviridae	Spherical	Fungi, plants, invertebrates
Retroviridae	Spherical	Vertebrates
The dsRNA viruses		
Cystoviridae	Spherical	Bacteria
Reoviridae	Isometric	Vertebrates/invertebrates, plants
Birnaviridae	Isometric	Vertebrates/invertebrates
Totiviridae	Isometric	Fungi, protozoa
Partitiviridae	Isometric	Fungi, plants
Chrysoviridae	Spherical	Fungi
Hypoviridae	Pleomorphic	Fungi
The negative-strand ssRNA viruses		
Bornaviridae	Spherical	Vertebrates
Filoviridae	Bacilliform	Vertebrates
Paramyxoviridae	Pleomorphic	Vertebrates
Rhabdoviridae	Bullet-shaped	Vertebrates/invertebrates, plants
Varicosavirus	Rod-shaped	Plants
Ophiovirus	Filamentous	Plants

(Continued over)

Table 3.1 *Families and unassigned genera of viruses[a] (Continued)*

Family or unassigned genus	Morphology of virus particle	Host
The negative-strand ssRNA viruses (continued)		
Orthomyxoviridae	Pleomorphic	Vertebrates
Bunyaviridae	Spherical	Vertebrates, invertebrates, plants
Tenuivirus	Filamentous	Plants
Arenaviridae	Spherical	Vertebrates
Deltavirus	Spherical	Vertebrates
The positive-strand ssRNA viruses		
Leviviridae	Isometric	Bacteria
Narnaviridae	Rnp complex	Fungi
Picornaviridae	Isometric	Vertebrates
Dicistroviridae	Spherical	Invertebrates
Sequiviridae	Isometric	Plants
Comoviridae	Isometric	Plants
Potyviridae	Filamentous	Plants
Caliciviridae	Isometric	Vertebrates
Astroviridae	Isometric	Vertebrates
Nodaviridae	Isometric	Vertebrates/invertebrates
Tetraviridae	Isometric	Invertebrates
Sobemovirus	Isometric	Plants
Luteoviridae	Isometric	Plants
Umbravirus	Rnp complex	Plants
Tombusviridae	Isometric	Plants
Coronaviridae	Isometric	Vertebrates
Arteriviridae	Isometric	Vertebrates
Roniviridae	Bacilliform	Invertebrates
Flaviviridae	Isometric	Vertebrates
Togaviridae	Isometric	Vertebrates
Tobamovirus	Rod-shaped	Plants
Tobravirus	Rod-shaped	Plants
Hordeivirus	Rod-shaped	Plants
Furovirus	Rod-shaped	Plants
Pomovirus	Rod-shaped	Plants
Pecluvirus	Rod-shaped	Plants
Benyvirus	Rod-shaped	Plants
Bromoviridae	Isometric	Plants
Ourmiavirus	Isometric	Plants
Idaeovirus	Isometric	Plants
Closteroviridae	Filamentous	Plants
Capillovirus	Filamentous	Plants
Tymoviridae	Isometric	Plants
Carlavirus	Filamentous	Plants
Potexvirus	Filamentous	Plants
Allexivirus	Filamentous	Plants
Foveavirus	Filamentous	Plants
Trichovirus	Filamentous	Plants
Vitivirus	Filamentous	Plants
Barnaviridae	Bacilliform	Fungi

a) Van Regenmortel et al. 2000a.

the Virology Division of the International Union of Microbiological Societies (IUMS). This Committee was established in 1966 at the International Congress for Microbiology held in Moscow and was initially called the International Committee on Nomenclature of Viruses. A few years later, the name of the Committee was changed to International Committee on Taxonomy of Viruses. The membership of ICTV comprises the 18 members of its Executive Committee, a number of Life members, over 40 National members and the members of its specialist subcommittees (Mayo and Fauquet 2000). The ICTV operates through six subcommittees responsible for Bacterial Viruses, Fungal Viruses, Invertebrate Viruses, Plant Viruses, Vertebrate Viruses, and an electronic Virus Database [the ICTV database (ICTVdB)]. The subcommittees coordinate the work of about 60 Study Groups comprising more than 500 virologists representing all areas of virology. The current membership of the ICTV is listed at the ICTV web site (www.ncbi.nlm.nih/ICTV).

The activities of ICTV are regulated by statutes approved by the Virology Division of IUMS and by an International Code of Virus Classification and Nomenclature (Mayo and Horzinek 1998). The International Code requires that virus classification and nomenclature must be international and uniformly applicable to all viruses infecting animals, plants, and microorganisms.

Although the virus classification system employs the hierarchical levels of order, family, subfamily, genus, and species, it is not obligatory to use all levels of the taxonomic hierarchy. Most virus species are classified into genera and most genera are classified into families. When it is uncertain to which genus a virus species should be allocated, even though its classification in a family is clear, the species is classified as an unassigned species of that family. If it is not clear to which family a genus belongs, it remains an unassigned genus. In its effort to develop an internationally agreed taxonomy for all viruses, the ICTV relies on guidance from individual Study Groups composed of recognized experts in each area of virology. However, any recommendations made by Study Groups are first evaluated by the subcommittees and Executive Committee of ICTV for their acceptability to the virological community in general. The ICTV Executive Committee then prepares taxonomic proposals for ratification by the full membership of the ICTV, either by post or at plenary sessions held during the triennial International Congresses of Virology. Recently the Executive Committee of ICTV has started to use the ICTVnet to allow more extensive consideration of proposals by Executive Committee members prior to an Executive Committee meeting. This procedure was extended to allow a wider consultation with the virological community than was possible previously. The new procedure goes through several stages of discussion, modifications, and public scrutiny and has been described in detail (Mayo et al. 2003).

At regular intervals, the ICTV publishes reports which represent the state of virus taxonomy and nomenclature at the time of publication. Seven reports have so far been published (Wildy 1971; Fenner 1976; Matthews 1979, 1982; Francki et al. 1991; Murphy et al. 1995; Van Regenmortel et al. 2000a). The 7th ICTV Report published in 2000 lists three orders, 63 families, 240 genera, and 1 550 viral species.

An important change in the 7th Report (Van Regenmortel et al. 2000a) was that the criteria used for demarcating species within many genera were defined for the first time. In the 6th Report, more than 3 600 viral 'entities' were listed, without, in many cases, a clear indication of their status as species, strains, serotypes, or isolates. In the 7th Report, only 1 550 viral species were officially recognized as distinct taxonomic entities. The major changes in the classification scheme introduced in the 7th Report have been summarized by Fauquet and Mayo (2001). The 7th ICTV Report needs to be consulted to ascertain the current status of virus taxonomy. This information is also available on the ICTVnet (www.danforthcenter.org/ITAB/ICTVnet). Subsequent changes introduced up to July 2002 and approved by the ICTV are listed in Mayo (2002). The 8th ICTV Report is currently under preparation and is likely to be published in 2005.

The activities of the ICTV are publicized in the 'Virology Division News' section of *Archives of Virology*, which is the official journal of the Virology Division of IUMS (Mayo and Van Regenmortel 2000).

THE SPECIES ISSUE IN VIROLOGY

All classifications are conceptual constructions made up of classes (hence their name) and the categories used for building them are not found in nature but arise in human minds. The categories of species, genus, family, and order are abstract concepts which, like all abstractions, have no location in space and time. The categories should therefore not be confused with groups of real objects or organisms which obviously are located in space and time. The distinction is readily accepted in the case of genera, families, and orders, and virologists have no difficulty in regarding these categories as abstract constructions that they will never physically encounter in their handling of viruses. It is indeed impossible to centrifuge a virus family, i.e. a concept, or to visualize it in an electron microscope. It is, therefore, rather odd that in the case of the species category, the distinction tends to be blurred with the result that species are often considered to have a real spatiotemporal existence. Part of the problem lies in the fact that the term species has been given different meanings. In addition to referring to a class or category, which is an abstract concept, the term species is sometimes used to refer to a collection of concrete objects, or real organisms localized in space and time (Ghiselin 1997). On the other hand, when a species is viewed, correctly, as an abstract class, it is impossible for concrete individuals to be part of such a species since the part–whole relationship does not apply to entities of different logical type. The entities or organisms belonging to such a species can only take part in a relation known as class membership (Mahner and Bunge 1997). An organism can only be a **member** of the species and not a **part** of it because it is logically impossible for a concrete object to be part of an abstract entity, i.e. of an entity of different logical type

(Van Regenmortel 2003). It is of course impossible for a virus species to cause a disease since abstractions do not cause diseases. On the other hand, a concrete virus entity that causes a disease can be a member of an abstract virus species. Unfortunately, many authors are inclined to use shorthand, sloppy expressions and will write that the species *Mus musculus* has been inoculated with one or other virus species, instead of saying correctly that a mouse (a member of the species *Mus musculus*) has been inoculated with a member of a certain virus species (i.e. with particles of an isolate of a certain species).

Another difficulty arises because classes like genera and families are so-called universal or Aristotelian classes, i.e. classes defined in terms of properties that are collectively necessary and sufficient for membership in the class. A virus family, for instance, is a universal class that consists of members, all of which share a number of defining properties that allow unambiguous identification of any member. For instance, all members of the family *Herpesviridae* are enveloped viruses that contain an icosahedral particle and double-stranded DNA and it is possible to allocate a virus to this family by considering only a few morphological and chemical features. By contrast, a virus species is not a universal class because its members undergo continual evolutionary changes and always show considerable variability. In practice, this means that it is not possible to rely on a single discriminating property for differentiating between two species. It is for this reason that although the species category is the most fundamental one in any biological classification, it has been the most difficult one to apply in virus classification.

Species are fuzzy sets

The difficulty of defining species is not a problem restricted to virus classification but is prevalent in all biological classifications. It often comes as a surprise that more than a century after the publication of Darwin's *On the origin of species* there is no general agreement about what constitutes a plant, animal, or microbial species. As many as 22 different species concepts have been used in various fields in biology (Mayden 1997).

The traditional view of species is that they correspond to groups of similar organisms that can breed among themselves and produce fertile offspring. A classical definition of biological species states that 'species are groups of interbreeding natural populations that are reproductively isolated from other such species' (Mayr 1963). One problem with this definition is that it can only be applied to organisms that reproduce sexually; furthermore, it also does not take into account the phenomenon of interspecies hybridization which is very common in the plant kingdom. In order to make it applicable to asexual organisms for which the criterion of interbreeding breaks down, Mayr (1982) modified his

definition to: 'a species is a reproductive community of populations, reproductively isolated from others, that occupies a specific niche in nature.' Another species concept is that of evolutionary species which has been defined as 'a single lineage of ancestor–descendant populations which maintains its identity from other such lineages and which has its own evolutionary tendencies and historical fate' (Wiley 1981). This concept emphasizes the historical dimension but does not provide any guidance on how far back in time a species can be traced. Life on earth is a biological and historical continuum and it is equally difficult to demarcate boundaries in time for identifying evolutionary species as it is to define clearcut breeding discontinuities in order to identify biological species. These difficulties led to the view that species are fuzzy sets with hazy boundaries and that it is not possible to draw sharp boundaries between them as is done with universal classes and classical sets. The use of fuzziness or vagueness for describing reality has a long history in Western thinking. Vagueness stems from the existence of a continuum with innumerable steps and is illustrated by the sorites paradox of the heap described by Greek philosophers. This paradox arises because it is impossible to say how many grains of sand can be removed from a heap before it stops being a heap. Clearly, the concept of a heap cannot be defined in a precise manner and it would be counterproductive to try to impose an artificial precision on such a term.

Fuzzy logic is a method that has been developed to handle concepts and entities that do not possess sharp boundaries (McNeill and Freiberger 1993). Fuzzy logic as a method for handling fuzzy sets accepts the inherent imprecision of terms and categories used in both ordinary language and in science. In ordinary language, a glass can be said to be full when it is only 95 or 98 percent full and the statement 100 percent full is rarely relevant. In classical logic, on the other hand, it will be maintained that a glass is necessarily either full or not full. In the real world of empirical and scientific observations this dichotomy is absent since fullness admits of degrees. Since fuzzy sets have no sharp boundaries, membership of a fuzzy set is not an all-or-nothing matter. This means that the two pillars of classical logic, the law of excluded middle (a swan is either white or nonwhite) and the law of noncontradiction (a swan cannot be both white and nonwhite) do not apply to fuzzy sets. Handling fuzzy sets falls outside the scope of classical, bivalent logic. When fuzziness is accepted as an unavoidable ingredient of the species concept, it becomes possible to describe species in terms of continuums devoid of artificial sharp edges (Van Regenmortel 1998). In a biological classification, it is often necessary to allocate an organism to a particular species purely as a matter of convenience and expediency rather than logical necessity. In a similar way, colors can be distinguished conceptually in spite of the continuous nature of the spectrum of electromagnetic waves and mountain peaks can be identified and are given names in spite of the absence of sharp boundaries in geological rock formations (Van Regenmortel 2000a).

What is a virus species?

The question of what is a virus species is related to the general problem of deciding if one virus is the same as another. This in turn requires that an answer be given to the identity question: how different must two virus isolates be in order to be considered different types of virus rather than the same virus? Although mutants or pathogenic variants may be clearly distinguishable from the wild-type virus, virologists usually have no difficulty in recognizing them as being the same type of virus. This ability to pass judgment on the significance of the extent of difference observed between individual objects is a typically human faculty that in turn gives rise to our urge to classify and order the world around us. In biology, the hierarchical categories of family, genus, and species are used to classify organisms, the species class being the most difficult one to define. Since viruses are biological entities, albeit not living organisms, the ICTV has attempted to use the same categories for classifying viruses. Whereas the categories of family and genus were readily accepted by most virologists, it took many years before the species category gained acceptance by the virological community as a whole. As recounted in detail elsewhere (Van Regenmortel 1989), there was considerable opposition among plant virologists to the idea that the concept of species could be applied to viruses (Milne 1984; Harrison 1985). The unwillingness of some plant virologists to accept the species category was due to two erroneous assumptions on their part (Milne 1984). They assumed that the only legitimate species concept was that of biological species defined by gene pools and reproductive isolation, thereby ignoring the many other definitions of species some of which may have been applicable to entities such as viruses (Ghiselin 1997; Mayden 1997). They also assumed that the acceptance of virus species would inevitably lead to the latinization of virus names which they strongly opposed (Matthews 1983; Van Regenmortel 1989).

The battle against the use of the species category in virology was very much an argument over semantics. For many years some of the plant virologists who objected strongly to the term species had been engaged in a most successful enterprise of delineating separate plant viruses known as the *CMI/AAB Descriptions of Plant Viruses* (Matthews 1985). These *Descriptions* of more than 300 plant viruses were widely accepted as the standard demarcation of separate viruses. Instead of calling them separate species, however, the editors of the *Descriptions* preferred to call them 'viruses' where the inverted commas were meant to convey the message

that these entities corresponded to a separate taxon and not merely to a particular viral strain or isolate. These 'viruses' really represented de facto species and plant virologists were in fact ahead of vertebrate virologists in delineating viral species, but without actually calling them species (for a review, see Van Regenmortel 1989).

The arguments against the use of the term species were also reinforced by the absence of an appropriate definition of the concept of virus species. In 1981, the ICTV had approved the following definition: 'A virus species is a concept that will normally be represented by a cluster of strains from a variety of sources, or a population of strains from a particular source, which have in common a set of correlating stable properties that separate the cluster from other clusters of strains' (Matthews 1982). Since this rather unhelpful definition did not explain what a strain was and did not indicate that viruses possess genes, Kingsbury (1985) suggested that it should be replaced by the following definition: 'A virus species is a population of viruses sharing a pool of genes that is normally maintained distinct from the gene pools of other viruses.' One difficulty with this definition is that many viruses reproduce entirely by clonal means and do not possess gene pools.

In order to emphasize the cohesive forces present in ancestral descendant clones that share a common biotic niche, the following definition was proposed in 1989: 'A virus species is a polythetic class of viruses that constitute a replicating lineage and occupy a particular ecological niche' (Van Regenmortel 1989). This is the definition which the ICTV endorsed in 1991 (Pringle 1991).

Virus species as polythetic classes

The concept of polythetic class was introduced in biology by Beckner (1959) who initially called this class polytypic to differentiate it from classical, universal classes defined by properties that are both necessary and sufficient for membership in the class. A polythetic class is characterized by a combination of properties, each of which might also occur outside the given class and could also be absent in a particular member of the class. Although the members of a polythetic class always have several properties in common, there is no single attribute absent in other classes which they all share (Figure 3.2). This means that no single property can be used as a defining property of a polythetic species on the basis that it is universally present in all the members of the species, and at the same time, always absent in the members of other species. It is for this reason that a single discriminating character, such as a certain percentage of genome sequence dissimilarity or a particular host reaction, cannot be used as a valid criterion for differentiating two virus species within the same genus. It is the inherent variability of the members of a species that prevents a single discriminating character from

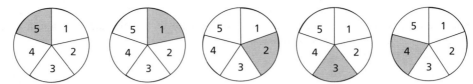

Figure 3.2 *Schematic representation of five members of a polythetic class characterized by five properties, 1–5. Each member possesses several of these properties, but no single property is present in all the members of the class. The missing property in each case is represented by the gray sector.*

being used for species differentiation (Van Regenmortel 2000a; 2003). It is always a combination of properties that must provide the justification for considering that two virus species are different.

The advantage of defining virus species as polythetic classes is that this makes it possible to accommodate individual viruses that lack one or other character that would normally be considered typical of the species. Polythetic classes are thus well-suited for dealing with biological entities like viruses which undergo continual evolutionary changes and show considerable variability.

Since there are mostly no sharp boundaries between different virus species, they are best treated as fuzzy sets (see section on Species are fuzzy sets). Species are thus very different from the other taxonomic categories used in virus classification, such as genera and families which can easily be defined in an unambiguous manner by a few morphological and chemical characteristics. The difficulties inherent in defining virus species are demonstrated by the fact that it was only in the 7th ICTV Report published in 2000 that the criteria used for differentiating many of the virus species were clearly stated for the first time.

Virus species as replicating lineages

The membership of a virus species varies over time and since all the members share descent from a common ancestor, they represent an evolving lineage. Since shared descent is a property that also links different species and genera, phylogeny is not a useful criterion for species demarcation. The same shortcoming applies to the evolutionary species concept since there are no clearcut criteria for deciding how far back in time a species can be traced (Wiley 1978; Lovtrup 1979). Virus species undergo continuous variation in time and transition from one species to another during evolution occurs within the continuity of gene duplication. As variations accumulate, a point will be reached where the importance of phenotypic and genotypic differences will lead an observer to conclude that he is dealing with a different virus species. Although increasing dissimilarity in genome sequence may provide some guidance, it must be stressed that there is no precise degree of genome difference which can be used as a cutoff point to differentiate between two species. The reason for this is that there is no direct quantitative relationship between the

extent of genome sequence similarity and the similarity in biological or phenotypic characteristics of a virus. Since the biological properties of viruses are the ultimate reason why virologists engage in species demarcation, it would be unrealistic to differentiate between viral species only on the basis of genome properties. Unfortunately, there is at present an increasing tendency to want to rely only on genomic data for virus classification (Calisher et al. 1995; Zanotto et al. 1996). It should be borne in mind that classifying viral genomes is not the same as classifying viruses (Van Regenmortel et al. 1997) and that a viral nucleic acid sequence is not the same as a virus (Drebot et al. 2002). Genome comparisons cannot by themselves justify taxonomic placements that would disregard the biotic and phenotypic characteristics of viruses which remain the most important justification for developing a practical viral taxonomy.

Ecological niche occupancy

The ecological niche refers to the biotic properties of members of a virus species such as the host range, tissue tropism, and vector. The ecological niche does not only refer to a location in space but is a functional concept based on the relational properties of the virus (see Viruses should not be confused with virus particles or virions) which involves aspects such as host responses, pathogenesis, and virulence. The niche is not a property of the environment but a property of the virus related to its biotic habitat. There are, therefore, no vacant or empty niches but only unoccupied habitats or geographic spaces. In the absence of the virus, its ecological niche property is also absent and the notion of a vacant niche is thus meaningless (Colwell 1992). A niche provides the needs that must be met for the virus to replicate and to survive.

What is a type species?

Although the term 'type species' appears in the *International Code of Virus Classification and Nomenclature* (Mayo and Horzinek 1998), a precise definition of the concept has been proposed only recently: 'A Type Species is a species whose name is linked to the use of a particular genus name. The genus so typified will always contain the Type Species' (Mayo et al. 2002).

A type species is thus a nomenclatural or name-bearing type corresponding to a class which itself is included in a particular genus class. A type species, therefore, only typifies the use of the genus name and is not typical in the sense of possessing the greatest number of characteristics of the genus. Some confusion may arise if the concept of virus species as an abstract class is not clearly differentiated from that of the concrete infectious entity called a virus. A virus species may have as one its members a reference type which could for instance be a culture collection isolate that can be exchanged between laboratories and is useful for making comparisons with any new isolate. Such a reference type is actually a type strain and should not be confused with a type species, which being a species, is an abstraction and not a virus culture (Mayo et al. 2002).

The quasi-species misnomer

In recent years it has become fashionable to refer to RNA viruses as quasi-species populations (Smith et al. 1997). RNA viruses have genomes that replicate in the absence of repair mechanisms and they possess a mutation frequency per nucleotide site of 10^{-3}–10^{-5}. A clone of an RNA virus will, therefore, always generate many thousands of different genomes, all of which compete during replication of the clone (Holland et al. 1992). This population consists of a master sequence corresponding to the most fit genome sequence with respect to a given environment, together with a very large number of competing virus mutants. Such a population is often referred to as a quasi species. This is an unfortunate term since it implies that the virus corresponds to some sort of imperfect species, as opposed to a true or genuine species that would possess a single, invariant genome sequence (Domingo et al. 1995). Such an idealized virus species consisting of members that all have the same sequence of course does not exist (Van Regenmortel et al. 1997). The confusion arises because a chemical concept, i.e. that of a molecular species consisting of molecules that are all identical, is applied to a biological entity that is not defined by chemical homogeneity but by its inherent variability. Like all biological entities that possess the ability to reproduce themselves or to replicate, viruses are endowed with an intrinsic variability that results from the error-prone process of nucleic acid duplication.

The term quasi species was introduced by Manfred Eigen and his colleagues to describe self-replicating RNA molecules which because of mutation do not consist of a unique molecular species (Eigen 1993). The members of a chemical species are all identical molecules whereas the members of a virus species are not. The biological and taxonomic concept of virus species, therefore, cannot be reduced to that of molecular or chemical species since it would amount to the reductionist fallacy of attempting to reduce biology to

chemistry. Taxonomic species are always quasi-species in the molecular sense and no additional clarification is provided by giving the label quasi species to viral species (Smith et al. 1997). It has been proposed that a 'virus quasi-species corresponds to a dynamic distribution of non-identical but closely related mutants and recombinant viral genomes subjected to a continuous process of genetic variation, competition and selection, and which act as a unit of selection' (Domingo 1999). However, such a definition reduces viruses to genome sequences. The term quasi species is, indeed, used appropriately for describing a population of genome sequences rather than a population of viruses since the implicit reference to a unique molecular species then applies to a chemical species consisting of a single nucleotide sequence.

Virus species demarcation

Although the acceptance of a definition of virus species by the virological community was an important step for establishing a virus classification based on traditional taxonomic categories, it should be stressed that such a definition did not solve the problem of demarcating individual virus species. Defining the virus species concept amounted to defining the category of species classes and it did not do away with the need to delineate individual virus species in the classification scheme.

Demarcating individual species is an attempt to introduce some order into the bewildering variety of viruses and this task requires the input of individuals with extensive experience and expertise with the viruses in a particular taxon (Van Regenmortel et al. 1997). This is the reason why the task of demarcating individual species was assigned to the ICTV Study Groups composed of virologists who possess in-depth knowledge of particular areas of virology. Only specialists are aware of the facts, issues, and nuances about viruses and their biotic interactions and of the importance of making certain distinctions, which may not be the same in all virus genera, for achieving a convenient and useful classification (Van Regenmortel et al. 1997).

In order to differentiate between individual species, it is necessary to rely on properties that are not present in all the members of a genus or family, since such properties obviously will not permit species demarcation. Characters such as virion morphology, genome organization, method of replication, and number and size of structural and non-structural proteins are properties that are shared by all the members of a genus or family and which, therefore, cannot be used for demarcating individual species within a genus. The properties that are useful for discriminating between individual virus species are characters that are not necessarily constant within the species and which can often change as a result of only few mutations. This situation is responsible for much of the difficulty of demarcating species. Another difficulty, discussed in the section Species are fuzzy sets is that species are fuzzy sets, which means that there is in most cases no logical necessity in any particular species demarcation. Taxonomy at the level of species tends to be mostly a matter of opinion. Properties that are useful for demarcating species are the natural host range, cell and tissue tropism, pathogenicity and cytopathology, mode of transmission, certain physicochemical properties, antigenic properties, and genome sequence similarities (Van Regenmortel et al. 1997). All these characters are not equally important for demarcating species in different viral genera and families. This is often deemed to be unsatisfactory, although there is really no need to harmonize discriminating criteria across all species, genera, and families. A classification scheme has to answer the practical needs of people who deal with viruses and these needs are not the same in all areas of virology. From a human perspective, all the organisms infected by viruses are not equally relevant and it is to be expected that human pathogens or pathogens that infect animals and plants of economic importance will be studied more intensely than, for example, the viruses that infect the myriad species of insects. Fine distinctions based on relatively minor differences in host range, pathogenicity, or antigenicity may thus seem to be more relevant for viruses that are of particular interest to humans (Van Regenmortel and Mahy 2004).

Since virus species are polythetic, the ICTV Study Groups, in order to demarcate the 1 550 species that are listed in the 7th ICTV Report, had to rely on a combination of properties rather than on the presence or absence of a single key feature. Once a species has been established in this manner it is possible, however, to identify a virus isolate as a member of that species by considering only a few of the properties of the species. For instance, if a virus isolate reacts with a panel of monoclonal antibodies in the same way as an established member of a given species, the virus will be considered a member of that species. This apparent contradiction between the need for many characters to define a virus species and the fact that a single property may suffice to identify a member of a species disappears when it is realized that species definition and demarcation is a different endeavor from virus identification (Van Regenmortel 2003).

VIRUS IDENTIFICATION

There is a common misconception that the existence of a definition of the concept of virus species should make it an easy matter to decide if a particular virus isolate is a member of an established virus species or not. One reason for this misconception is the failure to appreciate that it is only the abstract concept of species, as a class of classes, that can be defined by explaining the meaning of the concept. Individual viruses like any other concrete entities that are located in space and time cannot be

defined but can only be named (Kitts 1984; Van Regenmortel 1990) and identified by the use of so-called diagnostic properties (Ghiselin 1984). A definition only explains the meaning of a concept but it does not provide the means to decide which concrete entities are members of an abstract class. What is required is a set of characters and diagnostic properties that can be used for identifying individual members of a particular species. For different virus species, different types of properties may have to be used (Van Regenmortel et al. 1997).

The identification of a virus isolate is a comparative process based on a limited number of diagnostic properties which clarifies the extent of the relationship of the isolate with known members of an established species. Practical aspects of the virus identification process have been discussed by Murphy (1996). For unambiguous identification it is often convenient to compare new isolates with virus strains available in culture collections such as the American Type Culture Collection. These strains and reference types, which should not be confused with type species (see section on What is a type species?), are chosen and designated not by the ICTV but by international specialty groups, some of which operate under the auspices of the World Health Organization and other agencies. Levels of classification below the level of species, such as strain, serotype, and isolate, are not the remit of the ICTV, although such entities may be listed in ICTV Reports, admittedly without being defined (Drebot et al. 2002). A viral strain is a biological variant of a given virus that is recognizable because it possess some unique characteristics that remain stable under natural conditions. A viral serotype is a strain that is recognizable because it possess unique antigenic properties that remain constant under natural conditions. In the 7th ICTV Report, human polioviruses 1, 2, and 3 are considered serotypes of the species *Poliovirus* and they clearly constitute stable replicating lineages, a feature which allowed them to remain distinct over time (Drebot et al. 2002). The fact that these three serotypes do not cross-protect against each other is sufficient reason for epidemiologists to want to consider them as separate, clinically relevant entities. This important differentiation is clearly feasible even if the three serotypes are classified as members of the same virus species. In human and animal virology, individual viral serotypes are recognized only if they do not cross-protect against each other. In plant virology, the cross-protection criterion is not relevant and the label serotype is given to any antigenic variant that can be recognized as such. A viral isolate, on the other hand, is simply one particular virus culture that is being studied and it may correspond to a member of a species, a strain, or an entity of unknown taxonomic status.

Deciding whether viral isolates correspond to strains or serotypes of an established species or belong to separate species remains in many cases one of the most difficult challenges that virologists are faced with. The ICTV

Study Groups continue to address this issue by providing species demarcation criteria that can serve as guidelines for identifying which properties of viral isolates will be most useful for diagnostic purposes.

THE ICTV DATABASE (ICTVdB)

Although only about 1 600 virus species are currently recognized by the ICTV, it has been estimated that about 30 000 different viruses, strains, and subtypes are kept in specialized laboratories, reference centers, and culture collections. One of the aims of ICTV is to develop a universal virus database, the ICTVdB, which will store primary descriptive data of virus isolates formatted for the DELTA Computer System (DEscriptive Language for Taxonomy). The ICTVdB intends to be the main repository for descriptive information on viruses at the strain and isolate level and it will therefore be a valuable resource for virus researchers or anyone who needs information on currently known viruses (Büchen-Osmond et al. 2000). The ICTVdB uses a decimal numbering system similar to that used for enzymes (Büchen-Osmond and Dallwitz 1996). The database has been constructed using a descriptor list of several hundred characters which have been translated into single property statements which can be recognized by the search facilities of the database and can be used for virus identification. The ICTVdB also provides links with genome sequence and protein sequence databases (GenBank and SWISS-PROT).

Information on the ICTVdB is available from the US website www.ncbi.nlm.nih.gov/ICTVdb/ or the UK site www.ictvdb.iacr.ac.uk/

Information on individual viruses stored in the ICTVdB should in future be a useful tool for ICTV Study Groups when they need to make decisions regarding species demarcation and other taxonomic assignments.

NAMES AND TYPOGRAPHY OF VIRUS SPECIES

In the 6th ICTV report (Murphy et al. 1995), names of viral orders, families, subfamilies, and genera were written in italics with a capital initial letter. Following the 1998 revision of the International Code (Mayo and Horzinek 1998), the same typography was used for the names of virus species in the 7th Report. This typography provides a visible sign that species correspond to viral taxa, just like genera and families. For most viruses, the English common names of viruses became the species names and these were written in italics with the initial letter capitalized (Van Regenmortel 1999). This made it possible to differentiate virus species officially recognized by the ICTV from other viral entities such as tentative species, viral strains, and serotypes written in Roman characters. This new typography has met with some criticism (Bos 2000; Gibbs 2000) and

corresponding rebuttals (Van Regenmortel 2000b; Van Regenmortel et al. 2000b) and is now generally applied in most scientific publications (Mahy 2001). The use of italicized English names for virus species reflects the emergence of English as the international language of scientific communication and is in line with the general dislike of virologists for Latin virus names (Van Regenmortel 2000b; 2003).

It should be emphasized that italicized virus species names are not meant to replace existing vernacular or common names of viruses written in Roman characters (Van Regenmortel and Fauquet 2002). The viruses studied by virologists are concrete, disease-causing entities and not abstract classes and they should be referred to by their common, non-italicized names. It is only the names of viral taxonomic classes that are written in italics, not the names of viruses (Drebot et al. 2000). In a scientific paper it will be necessary to refer only once, for instance in the Materials and Methods section, to the official, taxonomic species name, while in the remainder of the text reference will be made to the virus as a physical entity, denoted by its common name written in Roman characters (Van Regenmortel and Mahy 2004).

The claim that common virus names can be used in an abstract, taxonomic sense (Bos 2002) is based on the erroneous assumption that a virus is an abstraction rather than a concrete entity. A virus name is a sign or label that designates a real, concrete object located in space and time, and the word virus corresponds to what logicians call a general term which denotes any number of concrete objects or entities. The word 'virus' itself as a term referring to an infectious entity and the picture of a 'virion' should not be confused with the real objects to which they refer and which are the entities studied by virologists. The painter Magritte reminded us of that distinction in his well-known painting of a pipe that included the caption 'this is not a pipe.' A pipe is a general term denoting concrete objects and is no more an abstraction than a virus or a virus-infected plant (Van Regenmortel 2003). Only confusion results if a virus is considered to be an abstraction (Bos 2000; Van Regenmortel 2000b). Abstractions are concepts that are not located in space and time; examples are concepts like beauty, generosity, disease, and class (Mahner and Bunge 1997). Taxonomic classes are abstractions and the use of italics for the names of viral classes is a useful reminder of their abstract nature. Common names of viruses actually refer to concrete objects and not to abstract taxonomic categories, and this distinction is a crucial one when constructing a virus classification.

A POSSIBLE FUTURE BINOMIAL NOMENCLATURE FOR VIRUS SPECIES

For many years, some plant virologists have been using an unofficial binomial system for referring to virus species. In this system, the word 'virus' appearing at the end of the current species name is replaced by the genus name, which also ends in 'virus;' *Tobacco mosaic virus* then becomes *Tobacco mosaic tobamovirus*, *Bluetongue virus* would become *Bluetongue orbivirus* and *Measles virus* would become *Measles morbillivirus*. The advantage of such as system is that inclusion of the genus name in the species name provides additional information about the properties of the viruses. To non-specialists, it would become immediately obvious that hepatitis A, B, and C viruses are very different entities belonging to separate genera if their species names would be *Hepatitis A hepatovirus*, *Hepatitis B orthohepadnavirus* and *Hepatitis C hepacivirus*. If such names became official names recognized by the ICTV, they should, of course, be written in italics, as they are in fact simply a contraction of the current species and genus names written in italics.

A binomial system for species names would have the additional advantage that there would then be a clear distinction between the species name written in italics (*Measles morbillivirus*) and the common non-italicized, virus name, measles virus. At present, the distinction between the name of the virus and that of the species relies in most cases only on typography (measles virus and *Measles virus*), which can lead to confusion (Van Regenmortel and Fauquet 2002).

The issue of whether nonlatinized binomial names should become the official species names of viruses has been hotly debated for many years (Bos 2000; Gibbs 2000; Van Regenmortel 2000b, 2001) and the ICTV has been criticized by some plant virologists for not making binomial names the official names of all virus species. However, the ICTV has moved cautiously since it was not clear whether a majority of virologists would be in favor of a binomial system that would lead to a change of all the current, official names of virus species. Efforts were made in 2002 to canvass the opinion of virologists regarding the acceptability of binomial names. The results of two ballots showed that a sizeable majority (80–85 percent) of the virologists (about 250) who expressed an opinion were in favor of a binomial system of species names (Mayo 2002; Van Regenmortel and Fauquet 2002; Van Regenmortel and Mahy 2004). This is the first time that the ICTV has obtained some indication about the way virologists feel about a particular taxonomic issue. Those who oppose a binomial system may still want to argue that the number of virologists who expressed an opinion is too small to justify a change in species names. Published taxonomic debates are usually conducted by a very small number of strongly opinionated individuals and the ICTV has always found it difficult to implement some sort of democratic decision-making since very few virologists bother to express their views on matters of taxonomy (Matthews 1983; Van Regenmortel 2000b; Van Regenmortel et al. 2000b). In the case of binomial species names there is now at least some indication on

how the virological community thinks about the issue. At present, it is not clear whether the ICTV will change the International Code of Virus Classification and Nomenclature and will introduce new binomial names for all virus species.

REFERENCES

Beckner, M. 1959. *The biological way of thought*. New York: Columbia University Press.

Bos, L. 1995. The embryonic beginning of virology: unbiased thinking and dogmatic stagnation. *Arch Virol*, **140**, 613–19.

Bos, L. 2000. Structure and typography of virus names. *Arch Virol*, **145**, 429–32.

Bos, L. 2002. International naming of viruses a digest of recent developments. *Arch Virol*, **147**, 1471–7.

Brenner, S. and Horne, R.W. 1959. A negative staining method for high resolution electron microscopy of viruses. *Biochim Biophys Acta*, **34**, 103–10.

Büchen-Osmond, C. and Dallwitz, M. 1996. Towards a universal virus database: progress in the ICTVdb. *Arch Virol*, **141**, 392–9.

Büchen-Osmond, C., Blaine, L. and Horzinek, M. 2000. The universal virus database of ICTV (ICTVdB). In: Van Regenmortel, M.H.V., Fauquet, C.M., et al. (eds), *7th ICTV Report*. San Diego, CA: Academic Press, 19–24.

Calisher, C.H., Horzinek, M.C., et al. 1995. Sequence analyses and a unifying system of virus taxonomy. *Arch Virol*, **140**, 2093–9.

Colwell, R.K. 1992. Niche: a bifurcation in the conceptual lineage of the term. In: Keller, E.F. and Lloyd, E.A. (eds), *Keywords in evolutionary biology*. Cambridge, MA: Harvard University Press, 241–8.

Domingo, E. 1999. Quasispecies. In: Granoff, A. and Webster, R.G. (eds), *Encyclopedia of virology*, 2nd edn. San Diego, CA: Academic Press, 1431–6.

Domingo, E., Holland, J.J., et al. 1995. Quasispecies: the concept and the word. In: Gibbs, A., Calisher, C.H. and Garcia-Arenal, F. (eds), *Molecular basis of virus evolution*. Cambridge, UK: Cambridge University Press, 171.

Drebot, M.A., Henchal, E., et al. 2002. Improved clarity of meaning from the use of both formal species names and common (vernacular) virus names in virological literature. *Arch Virol*, **147**, 2465–71.

Eigen, M. 1993. Viral quasispecies. *Sci Am*, **269**, 32–9.

Fauquet, C.M. 1999. Taxonomy, classification and nomenclature of viruses. In: Granoff, A. and Webster, R.G. (eds), *Encyclopedia of virology*, 2nd edn. San Diego, CA: Academic Press, 1730–56.

Fauquet, C.M. and Mayo, M.A. 2001. The 7th ICTV report. *Arch Virol*, **146**, 189–94.

Fenner, F. 1976. The classification and nomenclature of viruses. Second report of the International Committee on Taxonomy of Viruses. *Intervirology*, **7**, 1–115.

Francki, R.I.B., Fauquet, C.M., et al. 1991. *Classification and nomenclature of viruses. Fifth Report of the International Committee on Taxonomy of Viruses*. Wien/New York: Springer-Verlag.

Ghiselin, M.T. 1984. 'Definition', 'character' and other equivocal terms. *Syst Zool*, **33**, 104–10.

Ghiselin, M.T. 1997. *Metaphysics and the origin of species*. New York: New York State University of New York Press.

Gibbs, A. 2000. Virus nomenclature descending into chaos. *Arch Virol*, **145**, 1505–7.

Grafe, A. 1991. *A history of experimental virology*. Berlin: Springer-Verlag.

Harrison, B.D. 1985. Usefulness and limitations of the species concept for plant viruses. *Intervirology*, **24**, 71–8.

Holland, J.J., de la Torre, J.C. and Steinhauer, D.A. 1992. RNA virus populations as quasispecies. In: Holland, J.J. (ed.), *Genetic diversity of RNA viruses*. New York: Springer-Verlag.

Kingsbury, D.W. 1985. Species classification problems in virus taxonomy. *Intervirology*, **24**, 62–70.

Kitts, D.B. 1984. The names of species: a reply to Hull. *Syst Zool*, **33**, 112–15.

Lovtrup, S. 1979. The evolutionary species: fact or fiction? *Syst Zool*, **28**, 386–92.

Lvov, D.K. 1993. Centenary of virology. In: Mahy, B.W.J. and Lvov, D.K. (eds), *Concepts in virology. From Ivanovsky to the present*. Chur, Switzerland: Harwood Academic Publishers, 3–13.

Lwoff, A. 1957. The concept of virus. *J Gen Microbiol*, **17**, 239–53.

Lwoff, A., Horne, R.W. and Tournier, P. 1962. A system of viruses. *Cold Spring Harbor Symp Quant Biol*, **27**, 51–5.

Mahner, M. and Bunge, M. 1997. *Foundations of biophilosophy*. Berlin: Springer-Verlag.

Mahy, B.W.J. 2001. *A dictionary of virology*, 3rd edn. London: Academic Press.

Matthews, R.E.F. 1979. Classification and nomenclature of viruses. Third Report of the International Committee on Taxonomy of Viruses.. *Intervirology*, **12**, 132–296.

Matthews, R.E.F. 1982. Classification and nomenclature of viruses. Fourth Report of the International Committee on Taxonomy of Viruses. *Intervirology*, **17**, 1–200.

Matthews, R.E.F. 1983. The history of viral taxonomy. In: Matthews, R.E.F. (ed.), *A critical appraisal of viral taxonomy*. Boca Raton, FL: CRC Press, 1–35.

Matthews, R.E.F. 1985. Viral taxonomy for the nonvirologist. *Annu Rev Microbiol*, **39**, 451–74.

Mayden, R.L. 1997. A hierarchy of species concepts: the denouement in the saga of the species problem. In: Claridge, M.F., Dawah, H.A., et al. (eds), *Species, the units of biodiversity*. London: Chapman and Hall, 381–424.

Mayo, M.A. 2002. ICTV at the Paris ICV: results of the plenary session and the binomial ballot. *Arch Virol*, **147**, 2254–60.

Mayo, M.A. and Fauquet, C.M. 2000. The current composition of ICTV. *Arch Virol*, **145**, 1497–504.

Mayo, M.A. and Horzinek, M.C. 1998. A revised version of the International Code of Virus Classification and Nomenclature. *Arch Virol*, **143**, 1645–54.

Mayo, M.A. and Van Regenmortel, M.H.V. 2000. ICTV and the Virology Division News. *Arch Virol*, **145**, 1985–8.

Mayo, M.A., Maniloff, J., et al. 2002. The type species in virus taxonomy. *Arch Virol*, **147**, 1271–4.

Mayo, M.A., Fauquet, C.M. and Maniloff, J. 2003. Taxonomic proposals on the web: new ICTV consultative procedures. *Arch Virol*, **148**, 609–11.

Mayr, E. 1963. *Animal species and evolution*. Cambridge, MA: Harvard University Press.

Mayr, E. 1982. *The growth of biological thought; diversity, evolution and inheritance*. Cambridge, MA: Harvard University Press.

McNeill, D. and Freiberger, P. 1993. *Fuzzy logic*. New York: Simon and Schuster.

Milne, R.G. 1984. The species problem in plant virology. *Microbiol Sci*, **1**, 113–22.

Murphy, F.A. 1996. Viral taxonomy. In: Fields, B.N., Knipe, D.M., et al. (eds), *Fields virology*, 3rd edn. Philadelphia, PA: Lippincott-Raven, 15–57.

Murphy, F.A., Fauquet, C.M., et al. 1995. *Virus taxonomy. Sixth Report of the ICTV*. Vienna: Springer.

Patthy, L. 1999. *Protein evolution*. Oxford: Blackwell Science.

Pringle, C.R. 1991. The 20th Meeting of the Executive Committee of the ICTV. Virus species, higher taxa, a universal database and other matters. *Arch Virol*, **119**, 303–4.

Root-Bernstein, R.S. 1989. *Discovering, inventing and solving problems at the frontiers of scientific knowledge*. Cambridge, MA: Harvard University Press.

Smith, D.B., McAllister, J., et al. 1997. Virus 'quasispecies': making a mountain out of a molehill? *J Gen Virol*, **78**, 1511–19.

Tamames, J., Ouzounis, C., et al. 1996. Genomes with distinct function composition. *FEBS Lett*, **389**, 96–101.

Van Regenmortel, M.H.V. 1989. Applying the species concept to plant viruses. *Arch Virol*, **104**, 1–7.

Van Regenmortel, M.H.V. 1990. Virus species, a much overlooked but essential concept in virus classification. *Intervirology*, **31**, 241–54.

Van Regenmortel, M.H.V. 1998. From absolute to exquisite specificity. Reflections on the fuzzy nature of species, specificity and antigenic sites. *J Immunol Methods*, **216**, 37–48.

Van Regenmortel, M.H.V. 1999. How to write the names of virus species. *Arch Virol*, **144**, 1041–2.

Van Regenmortel, M.H.V. 2000a. Introduction to the species concept in virus taxonomy. In: Van Regenmortel, M.H.V., Fauquet, C.M., et al. (eds), *Seventh ICTV Report*. San Diego, CA: Academic Press, 3–16.

Van Regenmortel, M.H.V. 2000b. On the relative merits of italics, Latin and binomial nomenclature in virus taxonomy. *Arch Virol*, **145**, 433–41.

Van Regenmortel, M.H.V. 2001. Perspectives on binomial names of virus species. *Arch Virol*, **146**, 1637–40.

Van Regenmortel, M.H. 2003. Viruses are real, virus species are man-made taxonomic constructions. *Arch Virol*, **148**, 2483–90.

Van Regenmortel, M.H.V. and Fauquet, C.M. 2002. Only italicized species names of viruses have a taxonomic meaning. *Arch Virol*, **147**, 2247–50.

Van Regenmortel, M.H. and Mahy, B.W.J. 2004. Emerging issues in virus taxonomy. *Emerg Infect Dis*, **10**, 8–13.

Van Regenmortel, M.H.V., Bishop, D.H.L., et al. 1997. Guidelines to the demarcation of virus species. *Arch Virol*, **142**, 1505–18.

Van Regenmortel, M.H.V., Fauquet, C.M., et al. 2000a. *Seventh ICTV Report*. San Diego, CA: Academic Press.

Van Regenmortel, M.H.V., Mayo, M.A., et al. 2000b. Virus nomenclature: consensus versus chaos. *Arch Virol*, **145**, 2227–32.

Wildy, P. 1971. Classification and nomenclature of viruses. First Report of the International Committee on Taxonomy of Viruses. *Monogr Virol*, **5**, 1–65.

Wiley, E. 1978. The evolutionary species concept reconsidered. *Syst Zool*, **27**, 17–26.

Wiley, E.O. 1981. *Phylogenetics: the theory and practice of phylogenetic systematics*. New York: Wiley.

Witz, J. 1998. A reappraisal of the contribution of Friedrich Loeffler to the development of the modern concept of virus. *Arch Virol*, **143**, 2261–3.

Zanotto, P.M., Gibbs, M.J., et al. 1996. A reevaluation of the higher taxonomy of viruses based on RNA polymerases. *J Virol*, **70**, 6083–96.

4

The classification of vertebrate viruses

CRAIG R. PRINGLE

INTRODUCTION

A formal taxonomy of viruses, known now as The Universal System of Virus Taxonomy, has developed from the operational need for a uniform system of nomenclature of viruses to facilitate the accurate identification and control of nonbacterial disease-producing agents. The concept of virus originated from the discovery that tobacco mosaic disease of plants could be transmitted by sap that had been rendered free of bacteria by passage through a Chamberland filter. Subsequently, the particulate nature of viruses was established by Loeffler who observed that foot-and-mouth disease of cattle was transmitted by a nonbacterial agent that could pass through Kieselguhr filters, but was retained by finer-grained Kitasato filters (see Witz 1998). Following the discovery of these viruses at the turn of the century, several other diseases were recognized as virus-associated. The physical nature of viruses remained unknown for several decades, however, and viruses were named and grouped according to their biological attributes, for example, pathogenicity, host range, tissue and organ specificity, transmission routes, etc. As knowledge of the chemical and physical properties of viruses accrued, it became apparent that the disease-producing potential of viruses was an unsound basis for virus classification. With the rapid expansion of virology from the 1950s onwards, the requirement for a uniform system of nomenclature became compelling. Several competing classification schemes were proposed based on a variety of criteria, but none gained wide acceptance. Systems of nomenclature at the extremes ranged from a rigid hierarchical system embracing subphyla,

classes, orders, and families, based on an arbitrary set of characteristics (Lwoff et al. 1962), to a nonhierarchical system whereby any virus could be identified by a unique cryptogram defined by eight virus properties (Gibbs et al. 1966). To introduce order into this undertaking, an International Committee on Nomenclature of Viruses (ICNV) was established at the International Congress of Virology in Moscow in 1966. This committee was renamed the International Committee on Taxonomy of Viruses (ICTV) in 1973, and now operates under the auspices of the Virology Division of the International Union of Microbiological Societies (IUMS). The Universal System of Virus Taxonomy has been developed to its present state through a series of seven reports, the most recent of which was published in 2000 (Wildy 1971; Fenner 1976; Matthews 1979, 1982; Francki et al. 1991; Murphy et al. 1995; van Regenmortel et al. 2000). The classification presented in this chapter is a condensed version of the Universal System of Taxonomy (Pringle 1999), which was published in full as the Seventh Report of the ICTV in 2000 (van Regenmortel et al. 2000), and includes all revisions that have been approved by the ICTV up to the time of its plenary meeting in Paris in July 2002 (Mayo 2002). It is inherent in the design of the Universal Taxonomy that it can accommodate change in the nomenclature of viruses, as knowledge accrues, without obscuring previous usage. An Eighth Report is nearing completion and will be published under the title *Virus Taxonomy: VIIIth Report of the International Committee on Taxonomy of Viruses*, edited by C.M. Fauquet et al., London: Elsevier Academic Press. The overall structure of the higher level of the taxonomy remains largely unaltered, the principal difference being that the number of designated virus species has almost doubled, and is likely to continue to increase exponentially in future years.

The ICTV operates through six subcommittees, which coordinate the work of approximately 50 study groups, with a total involvement of some 450 virologists representing all areas of virology. Five of these six subcommittees have responsibility for bacterial viruses, fungal viruses, plant viruses, invertebrate viruses, and vertebrate viruses, while the sixth is concerned with the development of an electronic virus database (the ICTVdB). An executive committee oversees the activities of the subcommittees and their study groups, and prepares all taxonomic proposals for ratification by the full membership of the ICTV, which comprises the executive committee, the life members, and the national members (nominated by countries supporting a national microbiological society). Normally a new taxonomic proposal should be directed to the chair of the appropriate study group, who becomes responsible for its progress through the evaluation procedure. An updated list of the names and addresses of study group chairs and the membership of the ICTV can be accessed at the ICTV website (www.ncbi.nlm.nih.gov/ICTV). Taxonomic proposals under consideration can also be viewed at the ICTV website on an interactive basis.

The system of taxonomy adopted by the ICTV is sufficiently flexible to withstand the stress of the continual discovery of new viruses from an ever-increasing diversity of host organisms. A hierarchy of five taxa, ranked as orders, families, subfamilies, genera, and species, has been developed. Taxonomic categories below the species level, such as subspecies, strains, variants, genotypes, etc., are excluded from the taxonomy and are defined at the discretion of working virologists. The concept and definition of the category of virus species is central to the structure of the taxonomy, and the nature of the virus species is discussed separately under The concept of the virus species. Artificially constructed hybrid viruses, genetically engineered and re-engineered viruses, mutants, recombinants, and reassortants are not included in the Universal Taxonomy; their status is a matter for consideration by interested specialist groups. Satellite viruses, satellite genomes, viroids, and prions are included, but not dealt with in detail in this chapter.

DEFINITION OF TAXA

The order

The highest taxon, the order, comprises a group of families that have certain features in common. Currently only three orders are recognized. It is anticipated that the number of orders will increase in step with refinement of the methods of characterization of viruses. Orders are designated by names with the suffix -virales.

For example, the order embracing all the monopartite negative-sense single-stranded RNA viruses is the Mononegavirales.

The family

The taxon below the order is the family and 68 families are now recognized. Families consist of groups of genera exhibiting common properties not present in other genera, and they are identified by the ending -viridae, for example, Herpesviridae. In some instances subfamilies have been introduced to accommodate new knowledge regarding the relationships of genera within families. Subfamilies are indicated by the suffix -virinae, for example, Alphaherpesvirinae. In general, however, the policy is to avoid subdivision of primary taxa, except for reasons of expediency. The family is the bedrock of the universal taxonomy and most have been reinforced rather than undermined by the accumulation of knowledge. The members of the same family have similar morphology, genome organization, and replication strategy. However, since virology has no fossil record to fall back on, proof of common phylogeny is not a defining property. Of the 68 virus families currently recognized, only 28 (38 percent) contain viruses with vertebrate hosts.

The genus

Virus genera are assemblages of species of viruses that share common properties that distinguish them from the members of other genera. Genera are designated by the suffix -virus, for example, Simplexvirus. Currently 250 genera have been designated, 222 of which have been assigned to families. The remaining 28 genera, mostly positive-sense single-stranded RNA viruses of plants, are referred to as unassigned or 'floating' genera. There are 99 genera of viruses infecting vertebrates, four of which remain 'unassigned.' The genera occupy the most stable level of the hierarchy and establish the point of departure from which other taxa are defined. It is inherent in the taxonomy at its present stage of development that there is a lack of equivalence in different branches, and the criteria used for definition of genera differ from family to family. Evidence of common phylogeny is a desirable but not an exclusive criterion for definition of a genus. The horizontal transfer of genetic information during virus evolution and the occasional incorporation of host-derived genes can rapidly obscure or mimic phylogenetic relationship. It is implicit in the designation of a genus, however, that its constituent species will not exhibit conflicting phylogenetic relationships.

The species

The species is the most important category in any system of biological taxonomy. The concept of species in clonally related organisms is discussed under The concept of the virus species. The definition of virus species finally adopted by the ICTV is the one formulated by van Regenmortel (1990). This definition states that: 'A virus species is defined as a polythetic class of viruses that constitutes a replicating lineage and occupies a particular ecological niche.' A polythetic class is a class that is defined by more than one property, and no single property is necessary or sufficient to confer membership. The adjectival phrase 'ecological niche' refers to the total environment as distinct from its restrictive usage in contemporary environmental philosophies. The principal advantage of the van Regenmortel definition is that it takes account of the inherent variability of viruses and is not reliant on a single diagnostic characteristic. This definition is sufficiently elastic to accommodate the differing perceptions of virus species by virologists working in different fields of virology. One of the most difficult tasks facing virus taxonomists currently is to establish some uniformity in the nature of the phenotypic properties employed in the definition of species (van Regenmortel et al. 1997). The seventh report of the ICTV (van Regenmortel et al. 2000) should be consulted for detailed information concerning the criteria used for species designation in each family or floating genus.

The International Code of Virus Classification and Nomenclature

The naming of species has been codified (see Mayo and Horzinek 1998). A species name must be unambiguous and should consist of as few words as practicable, for example, *Human herpesvirus 1*. It must not consist solely of a host name with the word virus appended. A recent change in practice approved by the ICTV is that, in common with other biological taxonomies, virus species names will be rendered in italics with the initial letter capitalized. Tentative species, i.e. those with unconfirmed taxonomic status and awaiting approval are not italicized but do have the initial letter capitalized. Each species is also identifiable by a unique acronym (for example, see Fauquet and Martelli 1995; Fauquet and Pringle 1999a, b, 2000), which can be used unitalicized in text subsequent to the first mention of the species name, for example, ASFV is the approved acronym for *African swine fever virus*.

In future, all taxonomic categories from orders down to species should be rendered in italics with the initial letter capitalized. The name of the taxon should precede its actual name, for example, the genus *Simplexvirus*, rather than the *Simplexvirus* genus. This is the convention in the formal identification of a taxon, for example, in designation of the species *Tobacco mosaic virus*. In other circumstances, such as when used in an adjectival form, italicization and capitalization of the initial letter

are not required; e.g. in the adjectival statement, the tobacco mosaic virus polymerase.

The use of vernacular nomenclature can be a source of ambiguity where a common root name is employed in designation of both family and genus. A pertinent example is the confusion generated by the use of the vernacular term 'paramyxovirus.' This is ambiguous because the vernacular term could refer either to viruses belonging to the genus *Paramyxovirus,* or to constituent members of the family *Paramyxoviridae*. This usage lacks precision because the family *Paramyxoviridae* comprises five uniquely named genera. To deal with this problem the Paramyxovirus Study Group of the ICTV recently decided that the genus *Paramyxovirus* should be renamed the genus *Respirovirus*, notwithstanding the familiarity and historical associations of the original name. Although the International Code of Virus Classification and Nomenclature (see Mayo and Horzinek 1998) states that existing names should be retained wherever feasible, priority is not a factor that is given precedence. To increase precision and to avoid ambiguity it is the intention in the longer term to eliminate all vernacular names from the Universal Taxonomy and to replace them with international names, for example, the species formerly designated as lambda phage is now designated the species *Enterobacteria phage λ*.

The International Code also requires that the names of taxa should be easy to use, euphonious, and easy to remember. No person's name should be used in designation of a new taxon. Nor should subscripts, superscripts, hyphens, oblique bars, and Greek letters be used in the designation of a new taxon, notwithstanding the fact that examples of these remain in the existing taxonomy. Sigla may be accepted as names of taxa, provided that their meaning is obvious to the members of the relevant study group and to general virologists. For example, the name of the genus *Reovirus* is a siglum compounded from 'r' for 'respiratory', 'e' for 'enteric', and 'o' for 'orphan'.

THE UNIVERSAL SYSTEM OF VIRUS TAXONOMY

Strategy of the viral genome

The order of presentation of taxa adopted by the ICTV is based on the four criteria that define the strategy of the viral genome (see Chapter 11, The genetics of vertebrate viruses). The virus taxa are grouped according to (1) the nature of the viral genome; (2) the strandedness of the nucleic acid; (3) the facility for reverse transcription; and (4) the polarity of the genome. There are seven categories: single-stranded DNA viruses (Table 4.1), double-stranded DNA viruses (Table 4.2), reverse-transcribing viruses (Table 4.3), double-stranded RNA viruses (Table 4.4), negative-sense single-stranded RNA viruses (Table 4.5), positive-sense single-stranded

Table 4.1 *The taxonomy of single-stranded DNA viruses*

Order	Family [Subfamily]	Genus	Type species
–	*Inoviridae*	*Inovirus*	*Enterobacteria phage M13*
		Plectrovirus	*Acholeplasma phage MV-L51*
–	*Microviridae*	*Microvirus*	*Enterobacteria phage φX174*
		Spiromicrovirus	*Spiroplasma phage 4*
		Bdellomicrovirus	*Bdellovibrio phage MAC1*
		Chlamydiamicrovirus	*Chlamydia phage 1*
–	*Geminiviridae*	*Mastrevirus*	*Maize streak virus*
		Curtovirus	*Beet curly top virus*
		Topocuvirus	*Tomato pseudo curly top virus*
		Begomovirus	*Bean golden mosaic virus*
	Narnoviridae	*Nanovirus*	*Subterranean clover stunt virus*
		Babuvirus	*Banana bunchy top virus*
–	*Circoviridae*	*Circovirus*	*Porcine circovirus 1*
		Gyrovirus	*Chicken anaemia virus*
–	(Unassigned)	*Anellovirus*	*Torque teno virus*
–	*Parvoviridae [Parvovirinae]*	*Parvovirus*	*Murine minute virus*
		Erythrovirus	*B19 virus*
		Dependovirus	*Adeno-associated virus 2*
	[Densovirinae]	*Densovirus*	*Junonia coenia densovirus*
		Iteravirus	*Bombyx mori densovirus*
		Brevidensovirus	*Aedes aegypti densovirus*

Vertebrate virus taxa are indicated by absence of shading.
The dashes signify 'unassigned'.

RNA viruses (Table 4.6), and unconventional agents, comprising naked RNA viruses, viroids, and subviral agents (Table 4.7). The order of presentation does not imply hierarchical or phylogenetic relationship. In each table the viruses that infect vertebrates are indicated by the absence of shading. It will be obvious that no single strategy is typical of vertebrate viruses. The only unique strategy is exhibited by the wasp-infecting viruses of the family *Polydnaviridae*, which are the only viruses to possess segmented double-stranded DNA genomes. Otherwise segmentation is absent in DNA-containing viruses, although not uncommon among RNA-containing viruses, particularly those infecting plants. Segmentation of the genome may contribute to control of gene expression, but the consequences are different in the case of animal and plant viruses. The different segments of the genome of viruses infecting plants are encapsidated separately, possibly as an adaptation to movement within the host, and an infectious unit is a complement of particles. As far as is known in viruses infecting vertebrates the full complement of segments is encapsidated in each infectious particle.

The viruses infecting bacteria are predominantly DNA viruses, whereas the viruses infecting plants are either RNA viruses, viruses with a reverse-transcription stage in their multiplication cycle, or single-stranded DNA viruses. The viruses infecting fungi, invertebrates, and vertebrates may have either RNA or DNA genomes, and reverse-transcribing viruses infect all types of hosts except bacteria. The viruses of vertebrates and plants may also infect and multiply in invertebrates, but so far no virus is known that can infect all three types of host, and no vertebrate virus can multiply in plant hosts and vice versa.

The single-stranded DNA viruses

There are six families and one unassigned genus of viruses with single-stranded DNA genomes (Table 4.1). Viruses of two of the families and the unassigned genus infect vertebrates, and the remaining families embrace viruses found in bacteria, mycoplasmae, plants, and invertebrates.

THE FAMILY *CIRCOVIRIDAE*

The family *Circoviridae* comprises two genera, *Circovirus* and *Gyrovirus*, the type species of which are *Porcine circovirus 1* and *Chicken anemia virus*, respectively. The name of the family derives from the circular form of the approximately 2 kb genome. The vertebrate circoviruses resemble the plant nanoviruses, which have similar particle architecture and circular single-stranded DNA genomes. Indeed, the nanoviruses were initially classified as members of the family *Circoviridae* before achieving separate family status. *Porcine circovirus 1*, the type species of the genus *Circovirus*, resembles plant and bacterial viruses of the families *Geminiviridae* and *Microviridae* respectively, in terms of nucleic acid and protein homologies related to rolling circle DNA replication (Meehan et al. 1997).

The name *Anellovirus* has been proposed for an unassigned genus to include the recently discovered 'TT virus' and 'TT virus-like mini virus', which contain circular single-stranded DNA genomes of about 3.8 and 2.9 kb respectively. Despite their delayed recognition, these viruses are globally distributed in human and some nonhuman populations and may prove to be the most abundant of all viruses. The anelloviruses share similarities with the circoviruses regarding genome organization and expression, but all isolates possess negative sense genomes like chicken anemia virus (the sole member of the genus *Gyrovirus*) in contrast to the ambisense genomes of the circoviruses belonging to the genus *Circovirus*. The anelloviruses are unusual among DNA viruses in displaying extreme genetic heterogeneity.

THE FAMILY *PARVOVIRIDAE*

The family *Parvoviridae* comprises two subfamilies, the *Parvovirinae* comprising three genera of viruses infecting vertebrates and the *Densovirinae* comprising three genera of viruses infecting invertebrates. Viruses of both subfamilies possess linear single-stranded DNA genomes of 4–6 kb, unlike the other families of single-stranded DNA viruses where the DNA is circularized. The polarity of the single-stranded DNA encapsidated in virions varies according to species. *Murine minute virus* (genus *Parvovirus*) preferentially incorporates negative strands, whereas *Adeno-associated virus* (genus *Dependovirus*) incorporates strands of either polarity in quasi-equivalent amounts. The principal human pathogen in the single-stranded DNA virus category is *B19 virus*, which is classified as the type species of the third vertebrate-infecting genus, the genus *Erythrovirus*.

A feature distinguishing some viruses of the genus *Densovirus* from the vertebrate parvoviruses is encoding of the replicative function gene (REP) and the capsid protein gene (CP) on complementary strands. The processing of capsid proteins from the CP ORF involves splicing, which is mediated by an alternative splice donor in the case of viruses belonging to the genus *Parvovirus*, and an alternative splice acceptor in the case of viruses belonging to the genus *Densovirus*. Phylogenetic analyses support the formal taxonomy of the *Parvoviridae* (see *Virus Taxonomy, the Seventh Report of the ICTV*, van Regenmortel et al. 2000).

The double-stranded DNA viruses

There are 20 families and three unassigned genera of viruses with double-stranded DNA genomes (Table 4.2). Nine of the families and one of the unassigned genera contain viruses infecting bacteria, archaea or mycoplasmae, one family contains viruses infecting algae, four families contain viruses infecting invertebrates, and four families and one unassigned genus contain viruses infecting vertebrates. Two other families contain viruses with either vertebrate or invertebrate hosts. The unassigned fungal virus genus *Rhizidiovirus* was previously associated with the adenoviruses. There are no viruses infecting plants in this category.

The three families of bacterial viruses characterized by possession of complex contractile (*Myoviridae*) or noncontractile (*Siphoviridae* and *Podoviridae*) tail structures include 96 percent of the more than 4 500 bacterial viruses described in the literature. These three families are now grouped together as the order *Caudovirales* (Maniloff and Ackermann 1998). The species classified in these families infect hosts on most branches of the bacterial phylogenetic tree, and two of the three families include species infecting *Bacteria* and species infecting *Archaea*, suggesting that tailed viruses originated before the divergence of these hosts. The rationale for establishment of the order *Caudovirales* differs from that for the two orders of vertebrate viruses, *Mononegavirales* and *Nidovirales* (see The negative-sense single-stranded RNA viruses and The positive-sense single-stranded RNA viruses), where there is evidence of common phylogeny and genome organization. Evidence of common phylogeny of the constituent members of the order *Caudovirales* cannot be expected on account of the time scale of evolution, the enormous population sizes, and the ecological diversity of the tailed bacterial viruses. The occurrence of horizontal gene transfer is another complicating factor. The criteria for creation of the order *Caudovirales* are the following: a highly conserved complex morphology; a common replication pattern, involving injection of DNA, formation of concatamers and cleavage to unit length progeny genomes; the insertion of DNA into preformed proheads fabricated on scaffolding proteins; and the release of the tailed particle by virally encoded lytic enzymes. This example illustrates that a logical and useful taxonomy of viruses can be constructed in the absence of knowledge of phylogenetic relationships.

THE FAMILY *POXVIRIDAE*

The family *Poxviridae* comprises species of virus infecting either vertebrate or invertebrate hosts. The members of the family are distinguished from the other double-stranded DNA viruses by their cytoplasmic site of multiplication. The genome is a single, linear molecule of covalently closed double-stranded DNA, 139–375 kbp in size. The subfamily *Chordopoxvirinae* consists of eight genera of viruses infecting vertebrates generally with restricted host ranges. The subfamily *Entompoxvirinae* embraces three genera of viruses infecting distinct insect hosts. The two subfamilies are also distinguished by a different linear arrangement of core genes. Phylogenetic analyses of poxvirus DNA polymerases, NTPases, thymidine kinases, and DNA uracyl glycosulases support the formal taxonomy in

Table 4.2 *The taxonomy of double-stranded DNA viruses*

Order	Family [Subfamily]	Genus	Type species
Caudovirales	Myoviridae	'T4-like viruses'	Enterobacteria phage T4
		'P1-like viruses'	Enterobacteria phage P1
		'P2-like viruses'	Enterobacteria phage P2
		'Mu-like viruses'	Enterobacteria phage Mu
		'SPO1-like viruses'	Bacillus phage SPO1
		'ϕH-like viruses'	Halobacterium virus ϕH
	Siphoviridae	'λ-like viruses'	Enterobacteria phage λ
		'T1-like viruses'	Enterobacteria phage T1
		'T5-like viruses'	Enterobacteria phage T5
		'c2-like viruses'	Lactococcus phage c2
		'L5-like viruses'	Mycobacterium phage L5
		'ψM1- like viruses'	Methanobacterium ψM1
	Podoviridae	'T7-like viruses'	Enterobacteria phage T7
		'ψ29-like viruses'	Bacillus phage ψ29
		'P22-like viruses'	Enterobacteria phage P22
–	Rudiviridae	Rudivirus	Sulfolobus virus SIRV1
–	Tectiviridae	Tectivirus	Enterobacteria phage PRD1
–	Corticoviridae	Corticovirus	Alteromonas phage PM2
–	Lipothrixviridae	Lipothrixvirus	Thermoproteus virus 1
–	Plasmaviridae	Plasmavirus	Acholeplasma phage L2
–	Fuselloviridae	Fusellovirus	Sulfolobus virus SSV1
–	Phycodnaviridae	Chlorovirus	Paramecium bursaria Chlorella virus 1
		Prasinovirus	Micromonas pusilla virus SP1
		Prymnesiovirus	Chrysochromulina brevifilum virus PW1
		Phaeovirus	Ectocarpus siliculosis virus 1
–	–	'Sulfolobus SNDV-like viruses'	Sulfolobus virus SNDV
–	Poxviridae [Chordopoxvirinae]	Orthopoxvirus	Vaccinia virus
		Parapoxvirus	Orf virus
		Avipoxvirus	Fowlpox virus
		Capripoxvirus	Sheeppox virus
		Leporipoxvirus	Myxoma virus
		Suipoxvirus	Swinepox virus
		Molluscipoxvirus	Molluscum contagiosum virus
		Yatapoxvirus	Yaba monkey tumor virus
	[Entomopoxvirinae]	Entomopoxvirus A	Melolontha melolontha entomopoxvirus
		Entomopoxvirus B	Amsacta moorei entomopoxvirus
		Entomopoxvirus C	Chironomus luridus entomopoxvirus
–	Iridoviridae	Ranavirus	Frog virus 3
		Lymphocystivirus	Lymphocystis disease virus 1
		Itidovirus	Invertebrate iridescent virus 6
		Chloriridovirus	Invertebrate iridescent virus 3
–	Polydnaviridae	Ichnovirus	Campoletis sonorensis ichnovirus
		Bracovirus	Cotesia melanoscela bracovirus
–	Herpesviridae [Alphaherpesvirinae]	Simplexvirus	Human herpesvirus 1
		Varicellovirus	Human herpesvirus 3
		Mardivirus	Gallid herpesvirus 2
		Iltovirus	Gallid herpesvirus 1
	[Betaherpesvirinae]	Cytomegalovirus	Human herpesvirus 5
		Muromegalovirus	Murid herpesvirus 1
		Roseolovirus	Human herpesvirus 6

(Continued over)

Table 4.2 *The taxonomy of double-stranded DNA viruses (Continued)*

Order	Family [Subfamily]	Genus	Type species
	[*Gammaherpesvirinae*]	*Lymphocryptovirus*	*Human herpesvirus 4*
		Rhadinovirus	*Saimirine herpesvirus 2*
	(Unassigned)	*Ictalurivirus*	*Ictalurid herpesvirus 1*
–	*Polyomaviridae*	*Polyomavirus*	*Simian virus 40*
–	*Papillomaviridae*	*Papillomavirus*	*Cottontail rabbit papillomavirus*
–	*Adenoviridae*	*Mastadenovirus*	*Human adenovirus C*
		Atadenovirus	*Ovine adenovirus D*
		Aviadenovirus	*Fowl adenovirus A*
		Siadenovirus	*Frog adenovirus*
	(Unassigned)	*Rhizidiovirus*	*Rhyzidiomyces virus*
–	*Ascoviridae*	*Ascovirus*	*Spodoptera frugiperda ascovirus*
–	*Baculoviridae*	*Nucleopolyhedrovirus*	*Autographa californica nucleopolyhedrovirus*
		Granulovirus	*Cydia pomonella granulovirus*
–	*Asfarviridae*	*Asfivirus*	*African swine fever virus*
–	*Nimaviridae*	*Whispovirus*	*White spot syndrome virus 1*

Vertebrate virus taxa are indicated by absence of shading.
The dashes signify 'unassigned'.

Table 4.2. The major human pathogen, the species *Variola virus*, no longer exists in nature.

THE FAMILY *IRIDOVIRIDAE*

The family *Iridoviridae* comprises large enveloped icosahedral viruses with linear double-stranded DNA genomes of 140–300 kbp. Two of the four genera in the family are viruses with vertebrate hosts; that is, the genus *Ranavirus*, infecting amphibians, and the genus *Lymphocystivirus* infecting fish. The DNA of the vertebrate viruses is highly methylated, whereas the DNA of the invertebrate viruses is not. The vertebrate viruses possess an additional outer envelope derived by budding through the plasma membrane, which may also be present in invertebrate viruses grown in tissue culture, but this is not essential for infectivity. Phylogenetic analysis of major capsid protein sequences confirms the formal taxonomy, which is based on a variety of phenotypic properties.

The major capsid protein exhibits detectable amino acid sequence homology with the corresponding proteins of both *Paramecium bursaria Chlorella virus 1* of the family *Phycodnaviridae* and *African swine fever virus* of the family *Asfarviridae*. There are no recognized human pathogens in the famly *Iridoviridae*.

THE FAMILY *ASFARVIRIDAE*

The family *Asfarviridae* contains a single genus *Asfivirus*. The taxonomic position of the species *African swine fever virus* has been problematic in view of the distant homology with iridoviruses referred to above. Furthermore, there is resemblance to the *Poxviridae* in the intricate morphology, genome structure, and replication pattern of *African swine fever virus*. Originally this species was listed as a member of the family *Iridoviridae*, then later designated as the solitary member of an unassigned and unnamed genus. In the revised taxonomy of the seventh report it has been elevated to the status of type species of the genus *Asfivirus* of the family *Asfarviridae*. The name of the family is a siglum compounded from the phrase African swine fever and related viruses.

THE FAMILY *HERPESVIRIDAE*

The family *Herpesviridae* was one of the first taxonomic groups to be defined on the basis of virion properties rather than by disease association (Andrewes 1954). It now comprises three subfamilies and an unassigned genus. The order of the genes is largely conserved within subfamilies, but extensive gene rearrangement is observed between subfamilies. Each of the three subfamilies contains two or more genera, with important human pathogens in each subfamily. Related herpesviruses are classified as distinct species on the basis of quantifiable sequence differences across the whole genome and possession of distinct phenotypes with respect to host, epidemiology, or pathogenesis. For example the two serotypes of herpes simplex virus are now designated as the species *Human herpesvirus 1* and *Human herpesvirus 2* because these viruses exhibit sequence differences across the genome and infect different tissues with distinctive epidemiological consequences. The ability of these two species to undergo recombination in cultured cells is not considered relevant since no natural recombinants have been isolated despite the apparent parallel evolution of these viruses over millions of years.

The formal taxonomy of three subfamilies derived initially on the basis of phenotypic properties has been substantiated by phylogenetic analyses of eight well-conserved genes. The viral phylogenies fit well with the host phylogenies derived from the fossil record. On the assumption of the existence of a constant molecular clock and cospeciation of virus and host, the divergence of the three subfamilies is estimated to have occurred 180–220 million years ago. Major sublineages discernible within each subfamily were probably established before the radiation of the *Mammalia* 60 to 80 million years ago, with speculation within these sublineages occurring subsequently (McGeoch et al. 1995).

The fish herpesviruses are anomalous and have been consigned temporarily to the unassigned genus *Ictalurivirus*. The species *Ictalurid herpesvirus 1* (which includes channel catfish virus) is classified as a herpesvirus on the basis of virion morphology, and indeed this virus was instrumental initially in deriving the structure of the mammalian alphaherpesvirus genome. However, nucleotide sequence analysis has revealed no specific relationship with mammalian herpesviruses at the amino acid sequence level, other than with respect to ubiquitous enzymes not unique to mammalian herpesviruses (Davison 1998). Consequently the fish and mammalian herpesviruses may have arisen independently and may have acquired similar morphologies by convergent evolution. Alternatively they may have evolved by divergence from a common ancestral herpesvirus and their phylogenetic relationship has been obscured by 400 million years of progressive covariation with their hosts. These findings illustrate again that taxonomy cannot be reduced solely to the classification of viruses by extent of sequence homology. It has been suggested recently that two additional families should be created: one to accommodate the fish and amphibian herpesviruses and the other to embrace some recently discovered herpesviruses from molluscs. These viruses exhibit common structural and physical organization but appear to have separate evolutionary histories from the avian and mammalian herpesviruses. It was further suggested that to resolve the taxonomic difficulties the three families should together constitute a new virus order, the *Herpesvirales* (Davison 2002).

THE FAMILIES *POLYOMAVIRIDAE* AND *PAPILLOMAVIRIDAE*

As a result of continuing molecular and genetic characterization of the small oncogenic DNA viruses, the family *Papovaviridae* has disappeared to be replaced by two new families, the *Polyomaviridae* and the *Papillomaviridae*. Both families include human pathogens. *Simian virus 40* now becomes the type species of the single genus *Polyomavirus* of the family *Polyomaviridae*, and *Cottontail rabbit papilloma virus* becomes the type species of the single genus *Papillomavirus* of the family *Papillomaviridae*. This situation illustrates an unresolved problem in virus taxonomy. The assignment of taxonomic levels is peculiar to each group of viruses, and as yet there are no rules or criteria for achieving parallelism or equivalence between different taxonomic lineages. These two families of small oncogenic DNA viruses may be the next candidates for inclusion in an order.

THE FAMILY *ADENOVIRIDAE*

The taxonomy of the family *Adenoviridae* has been revised as a result of synthesis of the extensive literature on the molecular and genetic properties of these viruses. The serotypes of the traditional classification of adenoviruses have now been grouped into species. Species are designated on the basis of several properties in accordance with the van Regenmortel definition. For example, lack of cross-neutralization, phylogenetic difference exceeding 10 percent, etc. The criteria are flexible so that where phylogenetic distance is <1 percent, additional criteria may be used, such as ability to recombine, degree of oncogencity, GC content, etc. The type species of the genus *Mastadenovirus* is now designated *Human adenovirus C*, which includes human adenovirus types 1, 2, 5, and 6, bovine adenovirus type 9, and simian adenovirus types 13 and 26. As a consequence of this revision the diversity of mammalian adenoviruses has been reduced to about 20 species.

The avian adenoviruses are serologically distinct from the mammalian adenoviruses and are included in the genus *Aviadenovirus*. The type species is *Fowl adenovirus A*. The avian adenoviruses lack the genes of mammalian adenoviruses that encode proteins V and IX, and also lack homologues of early regions E1 and E3. The avian adenoviruses have been grouped into five species in the same manner as the mammalian adenoviruses.

Since publication of the seventh report, two new genera have been added to the *Adenoviridae* as a result of characterization of adenoviruses from nonhuman hosts. The genus *Siadenovirus* includes only two species: a virus isolated from a leopard frog and an avian virus distinguishable antigenically and genetically from the other avian adenoviruses. The genus *Atadenovirus* embraces a larger group of adenoviruses originating from several different hosts, and which includes several serotypes of bovine adenoviruses and adenoviruses from a wide range of reptiles.

The reverse-transcribing viruses

There are five families of viruses that have a reverse transcription stage in their replication cycle (Table 4.3). Reverse transcribing viruses have been isolated from fungi, plants, invertebrates, and vertebrates, but not from bacteria. The families differ with respect to the stage of the replication cycle sequestered in the extracellular particle. Consequently some viruses encapsidate DNA in the virion, whereas others encapsidate RNA. Remarkably all of the known double-stranded DNA-

Table 4.3 *The taxonomy of reverse-transcribing viruses*

Order	Family	Genus	Type species
–	Pseudoviridae	Pseudovirus	Saccharomyces cerevisiae Ty1 virus
		Hemivirus	Drosophila melanogaster copia virus
–	Metaviridae	Metavirus	Saccharomyces cerevisiae Ty3 virus
		Errantivirus	Drosophila melanogaster gypsy virus
–	Hepadnaviridae	Orthohepadnavirus	Hepatitis B virus
		Avihepadnavirus	Duck hepatitis B virus
–	Caulimoviridae	Badnavirus	Commelina yellow mottle virus
		Caulimovirus	Cauliflower mosaic virus
		Tungrovirus	Rice tungro bacilliform virus
		Soymovirus	Soybean chlorotic mottle virus
		Cavemovirus	Cassava vein mosaic virus
		Petuvirus	Petunia vein clearing virus
–	Retroviridae [Orthoretrovirinae]	Alpharetrovirus	Avian leukosis virus
		Betaretrovirus	Mouse mammary tumour virus
		Gammaretrovirus	Murine leukemia virus
		Deltaretrovirus	Bovine leukemia virus
		Epsilonretrovirus	Walleye dermal sarcoma virus
		Lentivirus	Human immunodeficiency virus 1
	[Spumaretrovirinae]	Spumavirus	Simian foamy virus

Vertebrate virus taxa are indicated by absence of shading.
The dashes signify 'unassigned'.

containing viruses of plants replicate via reverse transcription and have been grouped into the single family *Caulimoviridae*. Of the other four families, the *Hepadnaviridae* and the *Retroviridae* comprise viruses infecting vertebrate hosts only, and the *Metaviridae* and the *Pseudoviridae* contain viruses infecting either fungal or invertebrate hosts, according to genus.

THE FAMILY *RETROVIRIDAE*

The taxonomy of the retroviruses has been simplified in the latest revision, and there are now seven genera designated as *Alpharetrovirus, Betaretrovirus, Gammaretrovirus, Deltaretrovirus, Epsilonretrovirus, Lentivirus,* and *Spumavirus*. The genus *Alpharetrovirus* comprises the viruses previously designated as Avian type C retroviruses, and the genus *Betaretrovirus* embraces the viruses previously classified as the Mammalian type B retroviruses and the type D retroviruses. The genus *Gammaretrovirus* replaces the former Mammalian type C retroviruses and in addition includes the reptilian type C oncoviruses and the *Reticuloendotheliosis viruses*. The genus *Deltaretrovirus* includes the former 'BLV-HTLV-like retroviruses.' A new genus, *Epsilonretrovirus*, has been introduced to accommodate several complex retroviruses isolated from fish. The genus names *Lentivirus* and *Spumavirus* have been retained from earlier classifications on the principle inherent in the nomenclature code that 'existing names of taxa should be retained wherever feasible.'

The family *Retroviridae* embraces vertebrate viruses with genomes consisting of a dimer of linear positive-sense single-stranded RNA. The monomers range in size from 7 to 12.8 kb and are held together by hydrogen bonding. Purified virion RNA is not infectious. Each monomer is polyadenylated at the 3′ end, and has a type 1 cap structure at the 5′ end. A specific tRNA is base-paired to a primer-binding site near the 5′ end. Infectious virus has four major genes in the order 5′–gag–pro–pol–env–3′. The *pro* gene encodes a specific protease, and the *pol* gene encodes the reverse transcriptase and an integrase. Additional cell-derived genes may be present as additions or substitutions in retroviruses classified in the genera *Alpharetrovirus, Betaretrovirus,* and *Gammaretrovirus*, with important pathogenic consequences. Viruses may become helper-dependent as a result of gene substitution. Retroviruses classified in the genera *Deltaretrovirus, Epsilonretrovirus, Lentivirus,* and *Spumavirus* contain genes encoding additional nonstructural proteins, which play a role in control of gene expression and viral replication. Integration into cellular DNA is an obligatory stage in the multiplication cycle. As a consequence retroviruses exist as both exogenous infectious agents of vertebrates, and as endogenous proviruses inherited as Mendelian genes as a result of infection of germ line cells. The latter are not part of the universal taxonomy at present. Phylogenetic analysis of the pol genes of retroviruses produces trees consistent with the formal taxonomy (see *Virus Taxonomy, the Seventh Report of the ICTV*, van Regenmortel et al. 2000).

THE FAMILY *HEPADNAVIRIDAE*

The family *Hepadnaviridae* contains two genera of DNA viruses. The genome of hepadnaviruses consists of a single molecule of circular DNA, 3.0–3.3 kb in size, which is not covalently closed. The DNA may be partially single-stranded in the virion, the extent of this differing in the two genera. The reverse-transcription stage in the replication cycle occurs in the cytoplasm and consequently integration into cellular DNA is not an obligatory or usual part of the cycle. *Hepatitis B virus* is the type species of the genus *Orthohepadnavirus* and *Duck hepatitis B virus* is the type species of the genus *Avihepadnavirus*. Host range is the primary determinant of assignment of species to genus.

THE FAMILIES *CAULIMOVIRIDAE*, *METAVIRIDAE*, AND *PSEUDOVIRIDAE*, THE NONVERTEBRATE FAMILIES OF REVERSE-TRANSCRIBING VIRUSES

The family *Caulimoviridae* contains five genera of plant-infecting DNA viruses. The genome is a single molecule of circular DNA, 7.2–8.1 kbp in size. The genome contains between two and seven ORFs, depending on the genus. The organization of the genome is one of the principal distinguishing features of the individual genera. The functions of the virus-encoded proteins common to all genera are the following: the capsid protein gene, an aspartate protease, a reverse transcriptase, and ribonuclease H. Additional gene functions relate to movement in the plant host and vector transmissibility. The replica-

tion cycle is episomal and does not involve an integration phase.

The family *Metaviridae* includes species of retrotransposons infecting yeast (the genus *Metavirus*) or invertebrates (the genus *Errantivirus*), and the family *Pseudoviridae* includes the retroelements known as LTR-retrotransposons infecting yeast (the genus *Pseudovirus*) and invertebrates (the genus *Hemivirus*).

The double-stranded RNA viruses

Double-stranded RNA viruses have been isolated from bacteria, fungi, plants, invertebrates, and vertebrates (Table 4.4). These viruses are classified into six families and one unassigned genus. The double-stranded RNA viruses are predominantly segmented genome viruses. Four of the six families and the unassigned genus contain viruses with segmented genomes. Two of the families, the *Reoviridae* and the *Birnaviridae*, contain viruses infecting vertebrate hosts, although not exclusively.

THE FAMILY *REOVIRIDAE*

The family *Reoviridae* comprises ten genera: six (*Aquareovirus*, *Coltivirus*, *Orbivirus*, *Orthoreovirus*, *Rotavirus*, and *Seadornavirus*) contain vertebrate-infecting viruses, three (*Fijivirus*, *Phytoreovirus*, and *Oryzavirus*) plant-

Table 4.4 *The taxonomy of double-stranded RNA viruses*

Order	Family	Genus	Type species
–	Cystoviridae	Cystovirus	Pseudomonas phage (6
–	Reoviridae	Orthoreovirus	Mammalian orthoreovirus
		Orbivirus	Bluetongue virus
		Rotavirus	Rotavirus A
		Coltivirus	Colorado tick fever virus
		Seadornavirus	Kodipiro virus
		Aquareovirus	Aquareovirus A
		Cypovirus	Cypovirus 1
		Fijivirus	Fiji disease virus
		Phytoreovirus	Rice dwarf virus
		Oryzavirus	Rice ragged stunt virus
–	Birnaviridae	Aquabirnavirus	Infectious pancreatic necrosis virus
		Avibirnavirus	Infectious bursal disease virus
		Entomobirnavirus	Drosophila X virus
–	Totiviridae	Totivirus	Saccharomyces cerevisiae virus L-A
		Giardiavirus	Giardia lamblia virus
		Leishmaniavirus	Leishmania RNA virus 1-1
–	Partitiviridae	Partitivirus	Gaeumannomyces graminis virus 019/6-A
		Alphacryptovirus	White clover cryptic virus 1
		Betacryptovirus	White clover cryptic virus 2
–	Chrysoviridae	Chrysovirus	Penicillium chrysogenum virus
–	Hypoviridae	Hypovirus	Cryphonectria hypovirus 1-EP713
–	(Unassigned)	Varicosavirus	Lettuce big-vein virus

Vertebrate virus taxa are indicated by absence of shading.
The dashes signify 'unassigned.'

infecting viruses, and one (*Cypovirus*) invertebrate-infecting viruses. Reoviruses contain 10, 11, or 12 segments, depending on the genus, of linear double-stranded RNA. The cypoviruses share a property in common with the DNA-containing baculoviruses. Namely, possession of a gene encoding a polyhedrin protein which provides a protective matrix to enhance the survival of virus released into the environment after excretion from the gut or on death of the host.

In this family the prime determinant for classification of viruses into species is the Darwinian criterion of ability to exchange (reassort) genome segments. However, such information is rarely available and the genetic compatibility of isolates is estimated indirectly from serological, physical, and sequence data. The electropheretic migration patterns of the double-stranded RNA genome segments isolates (the electropherotype) may also be employed on account of their high resolution and reproducibility, particularly in the case of rotaviruses many of which cannot be propagated in vitro.

THE FAMILY *BIRNAVIRIDAE*

The family *Birnaviridae* comprises three genera of viruses with bisegmented linear double-stranded RNA genomes. The larger genome segment is variable around 3 kbp in size, and the smaller more homogeneous around 2.7 kbp. There are minor differences in the processing of the viral genes between genera, and the taxonomy is based on serology, host range, and pathology. Two of the three genera contain vertebrate-infecting viruses: species of the genus *Aquabirnavirus* are major pathogens of salmonid fish, and *Infectious bursal disease virus*, the type species of the genus *Avibirnavirus*, is an important pathogen in the poultry industry. The natural host of *Drosophila X virus*, the type species of the genus *Entomobirnavirus*, is probably *Culicoides* spp., with infection rendering the host sensitive to CO_2.

THE NONVERTEBRATE FAMILIES OF DOUBLE-STRANDED RNA VIRUSES

The bacterial viruses of the family *Cystoviridae* have tripartite genomes of some 13 kbp in total. The fungal and plant viruses of the family *Partitiviridae* have bipartite genomes of 2.8–6.0 kbp total. The unassigned genus *Varicosavirus* also has a bipartite linear genome of 13.5 kbp total. The *Totiviridae* and *Hypoviridae*, on the other hand, have nonsegmented linear double-stranded RNA genomes of some 4.6–7 kbp and 9–13 kbp total, respectively.

The negative-sense single-stranded RNA viruses

Vertebrate-infecting viruses are classified in all seven families of negative-sense single-stranded RNA viruses

(Table 4.5). Plant viruses are included in two of the seven families and are the sole representatives of the two unassigned genera, *Ophiovirus* and *Tenuivirus*. *Deltavirus* is formally included with the negative-sense RNA viruses as an unassigned genus, although the single species *Hepatitis D virus* exists only as a satellite of the species *Hepatitis B virus* (family *Hepadnaviridae*). At this time no negative-sense single-stranded RNA virus has been isolated from bacteria, fungi, or protozoa.

THE MONOPARTITE NEGATIVE-SENSE GENOME VIRUSES – THE ORDER *MONONEGAVIRALES*; COMPRISING THE FAMILIES *BORNAVIRIDAE*, *FILOVIRIDAE*, *PARAMYXOVIRIDAE*, AND *RHABDOVIRIDAE*

The first order in viral taxonomy was created to embrace the three families, *Filoviridae*, *Paramyxoviridae*, and *Rhabdoviridae*, on the basis of similar genome structure and individual gene functions, and the apparent absence of genetic recombination. The latter property suggests that evolutionary relationships are not obscured by horizontal transfer of genetic information. Phylogenetic analysis has supported the taxonomic association of these families (Pringle and Easton 1997; see Chapter 19, The order *Mononegavirales*). Subsequently the order *Mononegavirales* was extended to include the family *Bornaviridae* (see Chapter 52, Borna disease virus, and Pringle 1997). The bornaviruses are vertebrate viruses with monopartite negative-stranded RNA genomes, which have features in common with the other three families in the order. They are substantially different in other properties, however, such as their intracellular location and limited processing of mRNA by splicing. Some disputed evidence suggests that bornaviruses may be associated with human psychiatric disease.

The two genera of viruses, *Ebolavirus* and *Marburgvirus*, classified in the family *Filoviridae* are enigmatic human pathogens thought to be exclusively vertebrate viruses. The classification of these viruses remains in a fluid state due to the hazardous nature of these viruses, which restricts their characterization.

The viruses classified in the family *Paramyxoviridae* are predominantly associated with respiratory disease and childhood illnesses. Two subfamilies have been designated. The subfamily *Paramyxovirinae* comprises the three genera *Respirovirus*, *Morbillivirus*, and *Rubulavirus* described in the Seventh Report, and two newly designated genera; the genus *Avulavirus* accommodating *Newcastle disease virus*, a species now recognized to possess unique properties; and the genus *Henipavirus*, created to accommodate *Hendra virus* and *Nipah virus*, two recently discovered bat paramyxoviruses associated with outbreaks of life-threatening human disease. The subfamily *Pneumovirinae* contains the genera *Pneumovirus* and *Metapneumovirus*, both of which

Table 4.5 *The taxonomy of negative-sense single-stranded RNA viruses*

Order	Family [Subfamily]	Genus	Type species
Mononegavirales			
	Paramyxoviridae		
	[Paramyxovirinae]	*Respirovirus*	*Sendai virus 1*
		Morbillivirus	*Measles virus*
		Rubulavirus	*Mumps virus*
		Avulavirus	*Newcastle disease virus*
		Henipavirus	*Hendra virus*
	[Pneumovirinae]	*Pneumovirus*	*Human respiratory syncytial virus*
		Metapneumovirus	*Turkey rhinotracheitis virus*
	Rhabdoviridae	*Vesiculovirus*	*Vesicular stomatitis Indiana virus*
		Lyssavirus	*Rabies virus*
		Ephemerovirus	*Bovine ephemeral fever virus*
		Cytorhabdovirus	*Lettuce necrotic yellows virus*
		Nucleorhabdovirus	*Potato yellow dwarf virus*
		Novirhabdovirus	*Infectious hematopoietic necrosis virus*
	Filoviridae	*Marburgvirus*	*Lake Victoria marburgvirus*
		Ebolavirus	*Zaire ebolavirus*
	Bornaviridae	*Bornavirus*	*Borna disease virus*
–	*Orthomyxoviridae*	*Influenzavirus A*	*Influenza A virus*
		Influenzavirus B	*Influenza B virus*
		Influenzavirus C	*Influenza C virus*
		Thogotovirus	*Thogoto virus*
		Isavirus	*Infectious salmon anemia virus*
–	*Bunyaviridae*	*Orthobunyavirus*	*Bunyamwera virus*
		Hantavirus	*Hantaan virus*
		Nairovirus	*Dugbe virus*
		Phlebovirus	*Rift Valley fever virus*
		Tospovirus	*Tomato spotted wilt virus*
–	*Arenaviridae*	*Arenavirus*	*Lymphocytic choriomeningitis virus*
–	–	*Ophiovirus*	*Citrus psorosis virus*
–	–	*Tenuivirus*	*Rice stripe virus*
–	(Unassigned)	*Delta virus*	*Hepatitis delta virus*

Vertebrate virus taxa are indicated by absence of shading.
The dashes signify 'unassigned.'

contain viruses uniquely associated with respiratory disease of human infants. These two subfamilies are separated by differences in gene number, gene order, and gene size. Unexpected sequence homologies between pneumoviruses and members of the other families of monopartitite negative-sense RNA viruses was one of the initiating factors in the establishment of the taxon of order in virology.

The family *Rhabdoviridae* embraces one of the largest and most catholic of virus families. Four of the six genera include viruses infecting vertebrates. The hosts of rhabdoviruses include plants, invertebrates, and vertebrates, and different rhabdoviruses may multiply in invertebrates and plants, or invertebrates and vertebrates, but none is known which will multiply in vertebrates and plants. The plant rhabdoviruses classified in the genus *Nucleorhabdovirus* are exceptional, being located in the nuclei of infected cells. All other rhabdoviruses are cytoplasmic. Because of their distinctive

morphology many rhabdovirsues have been named on evidence from electron microscopy alone. The status of these viruses is unknown since they do not exist as isolates and as a consequence they are not considered in the current taxonomy.

THE SEGMENTED GENOME VIRUSES – THE FAMILIES *ORTHOMYXOVIRIDAE*, *BUNYAVIRIDAE*, AND *ARENAVIRIDAE*

Thee three families of segmented genome viruses have diverse properties and exhibit no common link other than segmentation of the genome. Consequently an order has not been created to embrace these three families. Reassortment of segments may occur among serologically related viruses, a property which can be employed in taxonomy at the species level. Reassortment of segments has been demonstrated in all three families, but in the absence of comprehensive genetic data, the definition of species within a genus is usually based on serological properties, host range, geographical distribution, and disease association.

The family *Orthomyxoviridae* includes three genera of vertebrate viruses (*Influenzavirus A*, *B*, and *C*) and the genus *Thogotovirus* containing a vertebrate-infecting species and an invertebrate-infecting species. The hemagglutinin-esterase (HE) protein of *Influenzavirus C* exhibits 30 percent amino acid identity with the HE protein of the positive-sense toroviruses, suggesting that genetic information may have passed horizontally by heterologous RNA recombination. Viruses in the genus *Thogotovirus* have six or seven segments and some of their genes exhibit homologies to influenza virus core protein genes. *Thogoto virus*, the type species of the genus *Thogotovirus*, is a biological enigma. The single glycoprotein gene has no homology with any influenza virus gene but does show similarity to the glycoprotein (*gp64*) gene of baculoviruses. The enigma is compounded by the fact that thogotoviruses are tick-borne viruses, whereas baculoviruses are DNA viruses predominantly para-sitizing lepidoptera. Since publication of the Seventh Report, a fifth genus, the genus *Isavirus*, has been added to accommodate *Infectious salmon anemia virus*, a pathogen of marine teleosts. Like the mammalian influenza viruses *Infectious salmon anemia virus* possesses an eight-segmented negative-sense single-stranded RNA genome of approximately 14.5 kb. Low sequence homology is exhibited at the amino acid level with the polymerase gene (*PB1*) of *Influenza C virus* (note: the type species of the genus *Influenzavirus C* is designated *Influenza C virus*, etc).

The family *Bunyaviridae* is possibly the most diverse of all the families of viruses, and many trisegmented bunya-like viruses have yet to be classified. Five genera are differentiated at present. Three of the genera, *Orthobunyavirus*, *Hantavirus*, and *Nairovirus*, are regular negative-sense RNA viruses, whereas the remaining two genera, *Phlebovirus* and *Tospovirus*, have one or more segments of ambisense RNA (see Chapter 27). The genera are defined on the basis of phylogenetic divergence, host range and transmission characteristics. Viruses of the genera *Orthobunyavirus*, *Nairovirus*, and *Phlebovirus* are arthropod-transmitted viruses of verte-brates. Viruses of the genus *Hantavirus* are vertebrate viruses with no known invertebrate hosts, and viruses of the genus *Tospovirus* are plant viruses transmitted by arthropods.

The family *Arenaviridae* comprises a single genus of vertebrate viruses with bipartite RNA genomes. Although included in the negative-sense RNA virus category, both segments of the genome have information encoded in an ambisense orientation. Variable amounts of viral complementary RNA, subgenomic mRNA, and cellular ribosomal RNA may be present in purified arenavirus particles.

The positive-sense single-stranded RNA viruses

These viruses have the most expansive taxonomy (Table 4.6). So far 22 families and 20 unassigned genera have been designated. Plant virus taxa are the most abundant with eight families and 18 unassigned genera, followed by vertebrate viruses with seven families and one unassigned genus. There are three families and one unassigned genus of invertebrate viruses, one family embracing both vertebrate and invertebrate viruses, two families of fungal viruses and one family of bacterial viruses. No positive-sense single-stranded RNA viruses have been isolated from protozoa.

The existence of three 'supergroups' of positive-sense single-stranded RNA viruses has been hypothesized on the basis of common features of genome organization and expression, reinforced by sequence analyses of conserved motifs within the replicase gene (Goldbach and de Haan 1994; Koonin and Dolja 1993; Ward 1993). Families have been clustered into supergroups of 'picorna-like viruses,' 'toga-like viruses' and 'flavi-like viruses,' and variously designated as higher taxa. The 'flavi-like' supergroup, however, is less homogeneous than the other two. None of these proposals has been ratified by the ICTV. The phylogenetic significance of these observations has been questioned recently and is discussed in the section Phylogenetic analysis and taxonomy.

THE FAMILY *PICORNAVIRIDAE*

The family *Picornaviridae* comprises nine genera of vertebrate viruses. The genome is a single molecule of positive-sense single-stranded RNA, 7.0–8.5 kb in size. The overall sequence identity between viruses of different genera is typically less than 40 percent. Most picornaviruses are specific for one or a few hosts, with the exception of the two species, *Foot-and-mouth disease virus* and *Encephalomyocarditis virus*.

The picornavirus species has been defined by the Picornavirus Study Group as a polythetic class of phylo-genetically related serotypes or strains which would normally be expected to share: (1) a limited range of hosts and cell receptors; (2) a significant degree of compatibility in proteolytic processing, replication, encapsidation, and genetic recombination; and (3) essen-tially identical genome maps (see, *Virus Taxonomy, the Seventh Report of the ICTV*, van Regenmortel et al. 2000). As a consequence, the familiar serotypes of picor-naviruses have been condensed into a limited number of species. For example, the type species *Poliovirus* of the genus *Enterovirus* includes serotypes 1, 2, and 3, and the type species *Foot-and-mouth disease virus* of the genus *Aphthovirus* includes the serotypes, A, C, O, SAT 1, SAT 2, SAT 3, and Asia 1. The genus *Parechovirus* has been created to accommodate two viruses formerly

Table 4.6 *The taxonomy of positive-sense single-stranded RNA viruses*

Order	Family [Subfamily]	Genus	Type species
–	Narnaviridae	Narnavirus	Saccharomyces cerevisiae namavirus 20S
		Mitovirus	Chryphonectria parasitica mitovirus 1-NB631
–	Leviviridae	Levivirus	Enterobacteria phage MS2
		Allolevivirus	Enterobacteria phage Qβ
–	Picornaviridae	Enterovirus	Poliovirus
		Rhinovirus	Human rhinovirus A
		Hepatovirus	Hepatitis A virus
		Cardiovirus	Encephalomyocarditis virus
		Aphthovirus	Foot-and-mouth disease virus
		Parechovirus	Human parechovirus
		Erbovirus	Equine rhinitis B virus
		Kobuvirus	Aichi virus
		Teschovirus	Porcine teschovirus
–	Dicistroviridae	Cripavirus	Cricket paralysis virus
	(Unclassified)	Iflavirus	Infectious flacherie virus
–	Sequiviridae	Sequivirus	Parsnip yellow fleck virus
		Waikavirus	Rice tungro spherical virus
–	Comoviridae	Comovirus	Cowpea mosaic virus
		Fabavirus	Broad bean wilt virus 1
		Nepovirus	Tobacco ringspot virus
–	Potyviridae	Potyvirus	Potato virus Y
		Rymovirus	Ryegrass mosaic virus
		Bymovirus	Barley yellow mosaic virus
		Macluravirus	Maclura mosaic virus
		Ipomovirus	Sweet potato mild mottle virus
		Tritimovirus	Wheat streak mosaic virus
–	Caliciviridae	Vesivirus	Vesicular exanthema of swine virus
		Lagovirus	Rabbit hemorrhagic disease virus
		Norovirus	Norwalk virus
		Sapovirus	Sapporo virus
		Hepevirus	Hepatitis E virus
–	Astroviridae	Astrovirus	Human astrovirus 1
		Avastrovirus	Turkey astrovirus
–	Nodaviridae	Alphanodavirus	Nodamura virus
		Betanodavirus	Striped jack nervous necrosis virus
–	Tetraviridae	Betatetravirus	Nudaurelia capensis β virus
		Omegatetravirus	Nudaurelia capensis ω virus
–	Tombusviridae	Tombusvirus	Tomato bushy stunt virus
		Carmovirus	Carnation mottle virus
		Necrovirus	Tobacco necrosis virus A
		Dianthovirus	Carnation ringspot virus
		Machlomovirus	Maize chlorotic mottle virus
		Avenavirus	Oat chlorotic stunt virus
		Aureusvirus	Pothos latent virus
		Panicovirus	Panicum mosaic virus
Nidovirales	Coronaviridae	Coronavirus	Infectious bronchitis virus
		Torovirus	Equine torovirus
	Arteriviridae	Arterivirus	Equine arteritis virus
	Roniviridae	Okavirus	Gill-associated virus
–	Togaviridae	Alphavirus	Sindbis virus
		Rubivirus	Rubella virus
–	Flaviviridae	Flavivirus	Yellow fever virus
		Pestivirus	Bovine viral diarrhea virus
		Hepacivirus	Hepatitis C virus

(Continued over)

Table 4.6 *The taxonomy of positive-sense single-stranded RNA viruses (Continued)*

Order	Family [Subfamily]	Genus	Type species
–	Bromoviridae	Alfamovirus	Alfalfa mosaic virus
		Ilarvirus	Tobacco streak virus
		Bromovirus	Brome mosaic virus
		Cucumovirus	Cucumber mosaic virus
		Oleavirus	Olive latent virus 2
–	Closteroviridae	Closterovirus	Beet yellows virus
		Crinivirus	Lettuce infectious yellows virus
		Ampelovirus	Grapevine leafroll associated virus 3
–	Barnaviridae	Barnavirus	Mushroom bacilliform virus
–	Luteoviridae	Luteovirus	Barley yellow dwarf virus-PAV
		Polerovirus	Potato leafroll virus
		Enamovirus	Pea enation mosaic virus-1
–	–	Tobamovirus	Tobacco mosaic virus
–	–	Tobravirus	Tobacco rattle virus
	–	Hordeivirus	Barley stripe mosaic virus
	–	Furovirus	Soil-borne wheat mosaic virus
–	–	Pomovirus	Potato mop-top virus
	–	Pecluvirus	Peanut clump virus
–	–	Benyvirus	Beet necrotic yellow vein virus
–	–	Idaeovirus	Raspberry bushy dwarf virus
–	–	Capillovirus	Apple stem grooving virus
–	–	Trichovirus	Apple chlorotic leaf spot virus
–	–	Sobemovirus	Southern bean mosaic virus
–	–	Umbravirus	Carrot mottle virus
–	Tymoviridae	Tymovirus	Turnip yellow mosaic virus
		Maculavirus	Grapevine fleck virus
		Marafivirus	Maize rayadofino virus
–	–	Carlavirus	Carnation latent virus
–	–	Potexvirus	Potato virus X
–	–	Allexivirus	Shallot virus X
–	–	Foveavirus	Apple stem pitting virus
–	–	Vitivirus	Grapevine virus A
–	–	Ourmiavirus	Ourmia melon virus

Vertebrate virus taxa are indicated by absence of shading.
The dashes signify 'unassigned.'

classified as enteroviruses and known as echovirus 22 and 23. These viruses have predicted protein sequences that have less than 30 percent identity with any other picornavirus. They are now ranked as members of the type species *Human parechovirus*. Since publication of the Seventh ICTV Report, three additional genera have been designated: the genus. *Erbovirus* to accommodate *Equine rhinitis B virus*, which is significantly different from the human rhinoviruses, the genus *Kobuvirus* to accommodate *Aichi virus*, which unlike other picornaviruses exhibits icosahedral surface structure by electron microscopy; and the genus *Teschovirus* to accommodate *Porcine teschovirus*.

The 'picornavirus supergroup' comprises the family *Picornaviridae* and the three families of plant viruses, *Comoviridae*, *Potyviridae*, and *Sequiviridae*. These families share common features of genetic organization (5'-VPg, 3'-polyA, post-translational cleavage of a polyprotein), similar capsid structure, and sequence similarity of the nonstructural proteins. However, there is no biological overlap and the apparent relationship of these families could equally be a consequence of convergent evolution, modular evolution, or divergence from a common ancestor.

THE FAMILY *CALICIVIRIDAE*

The family *Caliciviridae* includes four genera of vertebrate viruses. The assignment of genera is supported by phylogenetic analysis, and species are distinguished by differences in gene sequence, gene product sequences and serology. The caliciviruses have some properties in common with the vertebrate picornaviruses and the plant comoviruses and potyviruses, for example, a VPg at the 5' end and a poly(A) tract at the 3'end. The putative viral replicase of the caliciviruses shares sequence homology with that of picornaviruses.

THE UNASSIGNED GENUS *HEPEVIRUS*

Hepatitis E virus, which was loosely associated previously with the caliciviruses on morphological criteria, is now ranked as the type species of an unassigned genus. Phylogenetic analysis of polymerase and helicase regions justifies the separate status of the genus *Hepevirus*. Weak homology is evident with members of the *Togaviridae* (e.g. *Rubella virus*) and the plant furoviruses.

THE FAMILY *ASTROVIRIDAE*

The family *Astroviridae* comprises two genera: *Mamastrovirus* and *Avastrovirus*. The genus *Mamastrovirus* contains four species of viruses infecting mammals, and the genus *Avastrovirus* contains two species infecting avian hosts. Each species includes a range of serotypes; e.g. the seven serotypes of human astroviruses, as defined by immune electron microscopy and neutralization tests, are all included in the type species *Human astrovirus 1*.

THE FAMILY *NODAVIRIDAE*

The family *Nodaviridae* comprises two genera of viruses with bipartitite genomes; the *Alphanodavirus* infecting insects and the *Betanodavirus* infecting vertebrates. *Nodamura virus*, the type species of the genus *Alphanodavirus*, may occasionally infect vertebrates. Seven species are defined within this genus on the basis of a complex of molecular and biological characteristics. The genus *Betanodavirus* comprises seven species of viruses infecting different species of marine fish. There is 10 percent or less amino acid homology between the coat proteins of viruses in the two genera, whereas the level of identity is >80 percent within the genus *Betanodavirus*.

THE NESTED SET GENOME VIRUSES – THE ORDER *NIDOVIRALES*; COMPRISING THE FAMILIES *ARTERIVIRIDAE, CORONAVIRIDAE,* AND *RONIVIRIDAE*

The two families of vertebrate viruses, *Coronaviridae* and *Arteriviridae,* and the invertebrate (decapod crustacean) virus family *Roniviridae* are grouped as the order *Nidovirales* by virtue of their distinctive genome organization and similar morphology in the case of the vertebrate viruses (Cavanagh 1997; see Chapter 20, The order *Nidovirales*). The mRNAs are processed as a 3′ co-terminal (nested) set of subgenomic RNAs. Although the mRNAs are structurally polycistronic, translation is restricted with a few exceptions to the unique 5′ region, which is absent from the next smallest mRNA. Another unique feature of the order *Nidovirales* is the configuration of the replicase gene as two open reading frames with expression mediated by ribosomal frameshifting.

The viruses of the two families of vertebrate viruses are not serologically related, but sequence identity may reach 30 percent in selected regions.

The family *Coronaviridae* comprises two genera, *Coronavirus* and *Torovirus*, with little sequence similarity. There is a structural distinction also in that the coronaviruses have a helical nucleocapsid protected by a core shell, whereas the toroviruses have a tubular nucleocapsid. The coronavirus genome is the largest monopartite RNA genome at 27–31 kb in size. Species are distinguished on the basis of serology and sequence comparison. Phylogenetic analyses of gene sequences support the formal taxonomy, even though very high frequency recombination is an attribute of coronaviruses.

The family *Arteriviridae* comprises a single genus, *Arterivirus*. Macrophages are the primary target cells for all arteriviruses and the genus includes the type species *Equine arteritis virus*, and the species *Lactate dehydrogenase-elevating virus*, *Porcine respiratory and reproductive syndrome virus*, and *Simian hemorrhagic fever virus*. Genome strategy and replication pattern are similar to those of the *Coronaviridae*, but the genomes and virions of arteriviruses are about half the size of those of coronaviruses.

THE FAMILY *TOGAVIRIDAE*

The family *Togaviridae* comprises two disparate genera, *Alphavirus* and *Rubivirus*, associated by similar morphology and genome strategy. The species included in the genus *Alphavirus* are serologically related viruses infecting vertebrates and transmitted by mosquitoes. They exhibit a high level of sequence identity (>60 percent in the case of structural protein genes). The single species of the genus *Rubivirus* is a human pathogen with no arthropod vector and no sequence relationship with the alphaviruses.

The replicases of alphaviruses show some sequence homology with the nonstructural proteins of *Hepatitis E virus* and those of several groups of plant viruses, including the families *Bromoviridae* and *Closteroviridae*, and the unassigned genera *Hordeivirus*, *Tobamovirus*, and *Tobravirus*. These constitute the 'toga-like supergroup,' and transcription from genomic and subgenomic RNA is a feature of their multiplication cycle. The closteroviruses possess a toga-like polymerase, but their replication strategy more closely resembles that of the coronaviruses, although the latter have a picorna-like polymerase. These relationships may be a consequence of past recombination events and modular evolution, or merely fortuitous.

THE FAMILY *FLAVIVIRIDAE*

The family *Flaviviridae* comprises three biologically distinct genera. Most viruses of the genus *Flavivirus* are transmitted to vertebrate hosts by arthropod vectors. All flaviviruses are serologically related. The type species is *Yellow fever virus*. Species are defined on the basis of sequence data, antigenic characteristics, and various biological criteria, and more than 50 species have been designated. Viruses of the genus *Pestivirus* infect ruminants and pigs, have no arthropod vectors, and encode two gene products unique to this genus. Some cytopathogenic isolates of the type species, *Bovine viral diarrhea virus*, have a small insertion of host-derived nucleic acid integrated at a specific site, whereas others have gene duplications or deletions. The genus *Hepacivirus* contains a single species, *Hepatitis C virus*. This virus is transmitted between humans mainly by exposure to contaminated blood. No arthropod vectors are known. Three related viruses isolated from monkeys, *GB virus A*, *GB virus B*, and *GB virus C/Hepatitis G virus* are ranked for the present as unassigned species in the family. Only the latter is associated with hepatitis in humans.

Other categories

The Universal Taxonomy also covers several other agents (Table 4.7). The family *Narnaviridae* comprises two genera of mycoelements, which exist as ribonucleoprotein complexes but have no virion stage in their multiplication cycle. These have been listed here and also together with the positive-sense single-stranded RNA viruses, because some regard their status as viruses to be dubious. The viroids of plants are now classified as two families, using the suffix -*viroidae* to differentiate them from the true viruses. Finally, consistent nomenclatures for subviral satellites and prions are under consideration.

THE CONCEPT OF THE VIRUS SPECIES

The species is the basic taxonomic group in biological systematics, and because viruses are biological entities the species concept can be extended to virology. Viruses exhibit intrinsic genetic variability due to the error prone processes of nucleic acid duplication. Genetic variability enables biological systems to adapt and survive. As a consequence, unlike chemical compounds, viruses cannot be grouped into universal classes (e.g. species) defined by a single property or set of properties that are both necessary and sufficient for class membership (van Regenmortel et al. 1991). A virus with a positive-sense single-stranded RNA genome is per se a member of a class of positive-sense single-stranded RNA viruses. It could also be a member of several other universal classes defined by morphology, host, antigens, gene order, etc. It follows, therefore, that although viruses can be members of several universal classes, where each class is defined by a single property necessary and sufficient for class membership, the taxonomic grouping designated as a species is not a universal class definable by a single property. Members of a species can only be accommodated in a different type of class, the polythetic class, definable exclusively by several independent properties. In a polythetic class each member possesses most but not all of the properties of the set, and each property in the set is possessed by the majority but not all of the members. The polythetic class definition of a viral species implies that there can be no single defining property for class membership, and search for such a property is unrewarding. Such a property would have to differ from a common property defining a higher category in the taxonomic hierarchy. Common

Table 4.7 *Other categories*

Order	Family	Genus	Type species
Naked RNA viruses			
–	*Narnaviridae*	*Narnavirus*	*Saccharomyces cerevisiae 20SRNA narnavirus*
		Mitovirus	*Cryphonectria parasitica mitovirus 1-NB631*
Viroids			
–	*Pospiviroidae*	*Pospiviroid*	*Potato spindle tuber viroid*
		Hostuviroid	*Hop stunt viroid*
		Cocadviroid	*Coconut cadang-cadang viroid*
		Apscaviroid	*Apple scar skin viroid*
		Coleviroid	*Coleus blumei viroid 1*
–	*Avsunviroidae*	*Avsunviroid*	*Avocado sunblotch viroid*
		Pelamoviroid	*Peach latent mosaic viroid*
Subviral agents			
Agents	Genus		Example
Satellites	–		Tobacco necrosis virus satellite
Prions	–		Scrapie agent

Vertebrate virus taxa are indicated by absence of shading.
The dashes signify 'unassigned.'

properties shared by the members of different species, such as are used to designate higher tax (genera, families, and orders), cannot be species-defining properties.

The polythetic definition of virus species (see Definition of taxa) emphasizes the biological nature of viruses and has dispensed with the reference to 'gene pools', which featured in earlier definitions, because most viruses replicate clonally and do not share gene pools. The concept of the replicating lineage, which replaces it, indicates an inherited genealogy extending over many generations, unified by a common descent, and evolving in response to natural selection. The reference to ecological niche occupancy in the definition emphasizes the role of environmental factors (host, tissue tropism, vector specificity, etc.) in determining the identity of species.

This species definition establishes the meaning of the categories used in classification, but it does not provide rules for demarcating the boundaries between species. Nor does it establish equivalence between the diagnostic properties used for delineation of species in different parts of the taxonomy. The phenotypic properties available to define different polythetic classes of viral species are variable in quantity and quality, and progress towards equivalence will be a gradual process (see van Regenmortel et al. 1997).

The high mutability of replicating RNA viruses has led to the development of the 'quasi-species' concept. A quasi-species distribution is the result of self-replication and corresponds to a mutant distribution consisting of a master sequence and an attendant swarm of mutants derived from it. Implicit in the concept of quasi species, however, is the assumption that the species is a unique sequence. This is at variance with the polythetic species concept, which incorporates variability into the definition. Quasi-species distributions have been demonstrated in most RNA viruses at the genotypic level, but nonetheless many RNA viruses exhibit remarkable stability at the phenotypic level, reflecting the existence of powerful selective forces, which maintain an average sequence and genetic stability.

PHYLOGENETIC ANALYSIS AND TAXONOMY

The ascendancy of molecular virology has fostered the conception that viral taxonomy may eventually be reduced to a cataloging and ranking of genome sequences. This is a receding prospect (Mayo and Pringle 1998). Phylogenetic trees derived from nucleotide or inferred amino acid sequences are generally concordant with existing taxonomies over short ranges as noted throughout the section on The Universal System of Virus Taxonomy in this chapter. Furthermore, in monopartite negative-sense single-stranded RNA viruses, where horizontal transfer of genetic information by genetic recombination is rare or nonexistent,

sequence relationships can be used to substantiate taxonomic groups up to the level of the order. In particular situations useful inferences can be made about the evolution and origins of viruses (see Virus evolution below), and concerning the mechanics of epidemic diseases. Phylogenetic analysis is less successful in the analysis of more distantly related groups. Polymerase-based phylogenetic trees have suggested previously unsuspected putative links between the polymerases of plant and animal viruses (see The positive-sense single-stranded RNA viruses). However, such data establish relationships between individual genes only and should not be extrapolated to indicate phylogenetic relationships between complete genomes. The genomes of many viruses, particularly RNA viruses, often appear to have evolved in a 'modular' fashion acquiring genes or blocks of genes from the genomes of other viruses or even from their host (for examples, see Mayo and Pringle 1998).

More instructive is the statistical re-evaluation of the worth of RNA-dependent RNA polymerases of RNA viruses as a phylogenetic marker undertaken by Zanotto et al. (1996). The results of a Monte Carlo stimulation assay of sequence similarity among 40 RNA-dependent RNA polymerase and 40 RNA-dependent DNA polymerases were transformed to a gray scale density plot that allowed the significance of the 1 600 possible comparisons to be scanned visually and evaluated statistically by densometric scanning. The concentration of white and light gray squares along the diagonal in the density plots demonstrated that significant values were only obtained between viruses known to be similar on other criteria (i.e. within families). Overall the data do not provide statistical support for proposals for the existence of evolutionary groupings of RNA viruses above the family level (Ward 1993, Koonin and Dolja 1993, Goldbach and de Haan 1994), although they did not negate them. Similarly, this type of comprehensive analysis provided no statistical support for a presumptive common ancestry of viral RNA-dependent RNA polymerases and viral reverse transcriptases.

VIRUS EVOLUTION

The origin and evolution of viruses is too broad a question to consider here. The section on The Universal System of Virus Taxonomy in this chapter indicates that there is no genome strategy or molecular mechanism of processing genetic information that is peculiar to viruses infecting a specific type of host. Viruses leave no fossil record. Where there is evidence of co-speciation of virus and host, however, persuasive estimates of the origin and antiquity of particular viruses can be made (McGeoch and Cook 1994). In general, phylogenetic analysis is hampered by horizontal gene transfer and the absence of isolates from much before the present. The phylogenetic trees for some viruses are merely a reflection of isolate abundance rather than lineal descent. Where there are obvious relationships but no phylogenetic support, the direction of evolution may be difficult to discern, as for example in the case of the order *Caudovirales* cited in the section on The double-stranded DNA viruses, where convergent or divergent evolution cannot be distinguished (see also Chapter 11, Genetics of vertebrate viruses).

More problematic and challenging are the results of recent reverse genetic experiments involving the reengineering of viral genomes. Throughout the order *Mononegavirales* the order of genes is highly conserved. Nonetheless, several gene order variants of vesicular stomatitis virus have been produced by a reverse genetics. Surprisingly, most can be propagated in cultured cells and experimental animals without rearrangement or restoration of the wild-type conserved sequence (Wertz et al. 1997, 2002). Indeed several of the variants slightly exceed the wild-type virus in reproductive potential. It is clear that in the case of RNA viruses at least, strong selective forces maintain an average genome sequence. Until the nature of these selective forces is defined, it will be difficult to arrive at any sound conclusions regarding virus evolution.

REFERENCES

Andrewes, C.H. 1954. The nomenclature of viruses. *Nature*, **173**, 176–80.

Cavanagh, D. 1997. *Nidovirales*: a new order comprising *Coronaviridae* and *Arteriviridae*. *Arch Virol*, **142**, 629–33.

Davison, A.J. 1998. The genome of *Salmonid herpesvirus* 1. *J Virol*, **72**, 174–82.

Davison, A.J. 2002. Evolution of the herpesviruses. *Vet Microbiol*, **86**, 69–88.

Fauquet, C.M. and Pringle, C.R. 1999a. Abbreviations for vertebrate virus species names. *Arch Virol*, **144**, 1865–80.

Fauquet, C.M. and Pringle, C.R. 1999b. Abbreviations for invertebrate virus species names. *Arch Virol*, **144**, 2265–71.

Fauquet, C.M. and Pringle, C.R. 2000. Abbreviations for bacterial and fungal virus names. *Arch Virol*, **145**, 197–203.

Fauquet, C.M. and Martelli, G.P. 1995. Updated ICTV list of names and abbreviations of viruses, viroids and satellites infecting plants. *Arch Virol*, **140**, 393–413.

Fenner, F. 1976. The classification and nomenclature of viruses. Second Report of the International Committee on Taxonomy of Viruses. *Intervirology*, **7**, 1–115.

Francki, R.I.B., Fauquet, C.M., et al. 1991. *Classification and nomenclature of viruses. Fifth Report of the International Committee on Taxonomy of Viruses*. Wien, New York: Springer-Verlag.

Gibbs, A.J., Harrison, B.D., et al. 1966. What's in a virus name? *Nature*, **209**, 450–4.

Goldbach, R. and de Haan, P. 1994. RNA virus supergroups and evolution of RNA viruses. In: Morse, S.S. (ed.), *The evolutionary biology of viruses*. New York: Raven Press, 105–19.

Koonin, E.V. and Dolja, V.V. 1993. Evolution and taxonomy of positive strand RNA viruses: implications of comparative analysis of amino acid sequences. *Crit Rev Biochem Mol Biol*, **28**, 375–430.

Lwoff, A., Horne, R.W. and Tournier, P. 1962. A system of viruses. *Cold Spring Harb Ser Quant Biol*, **27**, 51–5.

McGeoch, D.J. and Cook, S. 1994. Molecular phylogeny of the *Alphaherpesvirinae* sub-family and a proposed evolutionary timescale. *J Mol Biol*, **238**, 9–22.

McGeoch, D.J., Cook, S., et al. 1995. Molecular phylogeny and evolutionary timescale for the family of mammalian herpesviruses. *J Mol Biol*, **247**, 443–58.

Maniloff, J. and Ackermann, H.-W. 1998. Taxonomy of bacterial viruses: establishment of tailed virus genera and the order *Caudovirales*. *Arch Virol*, **143**, 2051–63.

Matthews, R.E.F. 1979. Classification and nomenclature of viruses. Third Report of the International Committee on Taxonomy of Viruses. *Intervirology*, **12**, 132–296.

Matthews, R.E.F. 1982. Classification and nomenclature of viruses. Fourth Report of the International Committee on Taxonomy of Viruses. *Intervirology*, **17**, 1–199.

Mayo, M.A. 2002. ICTV at the Paris ICV: Results of the plenary session and the binomial ballot. *Arch Virol*, **147**, 2254–60.

Mayo, M.A. and Horzinek, M.C. 1998. A revised version of the International Code of Virus Classification and Nomenclature. *Arch Virol*, **143**, 1645–54.

Mayo, M.A. and Pringle, C.R. 1998. Virus taxonomy – 1997. *J Gen Virol*, **79**, 649–57.

Meehan, B.M., Creelan, J.L., et al. 1997. Sequence of porcine circovirus DNA: affinities with plant circoviruses. *J Gen Virol*, **78**, 221–7.

Murphy, F.A. and Fauquet, C.M. 1995. *Virus taxonomy: Sixth Report of the International Committee on Taxonomy of Viruses*. Wien, New York: Springer-Verlag, pp. 1–586.

Pringle, C.R. 1997. The order *Mononegavirales* – current status. *Arch Virol*, **142**, 2321–6.

Pringle, C.R. 1999. Virus taxonomy – 1999. *Arch Virol*, **144**, 421–9.

Pringle, C.R. and Easton, A.J. 1997. Monopartite negative strand RNA genomes. *Semin Virol*, **8**, 49–57.

van Regenmortel, M.H.V. 1990. Virus species, a much overlooked but essential concept in virus classification. *Intervirology*, **31**, 241–54.

van Regenmortel, M.H.V., Maniloff, J. and Calisher, C.H. 1991. The concept of virus species. *Arch Virol*, **120**, 313–14.

van Regenmortel, M.H.V., Bishop, D.H.L., et al. 1997. Guidelines to the demarcation of virus species. *Arch Virol*, **142**, 1506–18.

van Regenmortel, M.H.V., Fauquet, C.M., et al. 2000. *Virus taxonomy; 7th Report of the International Committee on Virus Taxonomy*. San Diego: Academic Press.

Ward, C.W. 1993. Progress towards a higher taxonomy of viruses. *Rev Virol*, **144**, 419–53.

Wertz, G.W., Perepelitsa, V.P. and Ball, L.A. 1997. Gene rearrangement attenuates expression and lethality of a non-segmented negative strand RNA virus. *Proc Natl Acad Sci USA*, **95**, 3501–6.

Wertz, G.W., Moudy, R. and Ball, L.A. 2002. Adding genes to the RNA genome of vesicular stomatitis virus: positional effects on stability of expression. *J Virol*, **76**, 7642–50.

Wildy, P. 1971. Classification and nomenclature of viruses. First Report of the International Committee on Taxonomy of Viruses. *Monogr Virol*, **5**, 1–65.

Witz, J. 1998. A reappraisal of the contribution of Friedrich Loeffler to the development of the modern concept of virus. *Arch Virol*, **143**, 2261–3.

Zanotto, P.M., Gibbs, M.J., et al. 1996. A reevaluation of the higher taxonomy of viruses based on RNA polymerases. *J Virol*, **70**, 6083–96.

5

The morphology and structure of viruses

ROB W.H. RUIGROK, GUY SCHOEHN, AND JAMES F. CONWAY

INTRODUCTION

Viruses are small quantities of genetic information. This information codes for tools for their multiplication and for a vehicle to go from one site of multiplication to the next. The information can be coded in RNA or DNA. In fact, the information may even be present in the conformation of a particular protein, as in 'prion' proteins, for example, but these are not really viruses. The nature of the viral nucleic acid leads to particular trade-offs that are fundamental to the observed virus morphologies. For the replication of viruses, the genetic information has to be copied by an RNA- or DNA-dependent polymerase. All these polymerases make, on average, one mistake in 10 000 copying steps. This is probably due to the chemical nature of the nucleotide bases, which can exist in two forms, the keto- (lactame-) form and the enol- (lactime-) form (tautomere) (Figure 5.1a). The equilibrium between these two forms is far towards the keto-form, with an equilibrium constant of 10^{-4}, meaning that there is a chance of 10^{-4} that the nucleotide is in the enol-form when the polymerase passes to place the complementary base. Normally, guanines pair with cytidines but not with thymidines (as shown in Figure 5.1b). However, a thymidine in the enol-form can base pair with a keto-guanine and form three hydrogen bonds (Figure 5.1c). The same holds for the other bases: keto-A can pair with enol-C, keto-C with enol-A, and keto-T with enol-G. Therefore, the polymerase will add a wrong base when the template base is in the enol-form. DNA-dependent polymerases have a proofreading activity that corrects these errors in base pairing, leading to error frequencies in DNA organisms of only about 10^{-7} per copied base. This means that DNA virus genomes are rather stable and the genomes of DNA viruses can be large, ranging from about 5 000 (polyomavirus) to 200 000 base pairs (herpes- and poxviruses), the largest genomes belonging to the phycodnaviridae, algal DNA viruses with genomes up to 560 kbp (Yan et al. 2000; Sandaa et al. 2001; van Etten et al. 2002), certain bacteriophages, such as phage G of *Bacillus megaterium*, which packages ~670 kbp (Hutson et al. 1995), and the latest champion, a virus found in ameba with a genome size of about 800 kbp (La Scola et al. 2003). These large viral genomes are bigger than those of the smallest bacteria, such as mycoplasma (580 kbp, Fraser et al. 1995). However, RNA-dependent RNA polymerases usually do not have a proofreading activity (or only a rudimentary form of it). This means that for an RNA virus with a genome of 10 000 nucleotides, on average every offspring virus will have one mutation. Because selection mechanisms cannot function with more than one mutation per offspring virus, this limits the genome size of RNA viruses to about 10–20 000 nucleotides, the only exception being the coronaviruses that have a positive-strand RNA genome of between 27 and 32 kb (Lai and Holmes 2001). Note that the amount of information space that a virus can attribute to coding for its transport vehicle depends on the total amount of information space. Therefore, RNA viruses have capsids with, in general, simpler structures with fewer structural proteins than DNA viruses. Also, because of the genome size, the space inside a DNA virus capsid has to be larger than that for an RNA virus, leading to more elaborate capsids for DNA viruses.

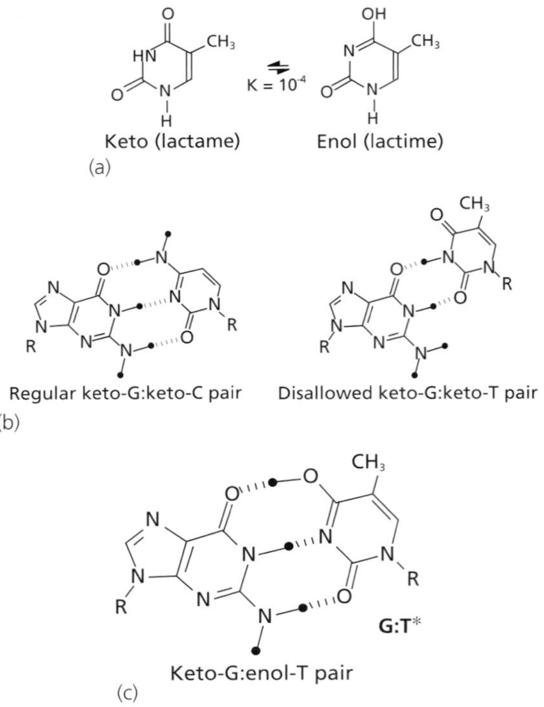

Figure 5.1 (a) *Keto–enol tautomerism of nucleotide bases.* (b) *Allowed and disallowed nucleotide pairs.* (c) *Allowed keto-G:enol-T pair.*

RNA viruses usually only code for the necessary transport and replication proteins, plus often for a protein that counters or avoids the effects of innate immunity. Apart from proteins analogous to those encoded by the RNA viruses, the larger DNA virus genomes also code for a considerable number of ancillary proteins that modify the host metabolism, and also for immunity-modifying factors.

The replication component of RNA viruses may consist of the naked nucleic acid. When positive-strand RNA viruses enter the cell, the vRNA is directly translated into viral proteins. For this effect, the vRNA contains a specific three-dimensional (3D) RNA structure, the internal ribosome entry site (IRES), to which host translation factors bind in order to start viral protein production (Kieft et al. 2001; Sarnow 2003). However, sometimes protein components are needed for the first steps in the replication process. Retroviruses need reverse transcriptase and integrase for insertion of the transcribed DNA into the genome of the host cell, and negative-strand RNA viruses have a viral RNA that does not directly code for proteins but which has to be transcribed into mRNA first. For this function, negative-strand RNA viruses assume a unique structural composite in which the viral RNA is stoichiometrically bound to the nucleoprotein. This helical nucleocapsid, rather than the naked vRNA, is the template for transcription and replication. The viral RNA-dependent RNA polymerase is bound to this helical template,

either directly (influenza virus) or with the help of a phosphoprotein (all nonsegmented negative-strand RNA viruses). This complex structure enters the infected cell and is directly active in transcription. Thus, if a virus needs a virus-specific process at the start of its replication cycle, the proteins needed for this process have to be packed inside the virus particle.

The transport component protects the virus when it is outside a cell. This component contains a receptor-binding protein (or proteins) and sometimes also proteins needed for release from the infected cell. The surface of the virus is also involved in cell entry by membrane fusion (for the membrane or enveloped viruses) or by some other membrane penetration mechanism (for nonenveloped viruses). Because of the limited genome size for encoding protein subunits, viral transport components often exploit symmetry in order to make a 3D structure from many copies of only a few building blocks. There are two major types of symmetry used by viruses: helical symmetry (mainly plant viruses and bacteriophages, bacteriophage tails and the above-mentioned nucleocapsids of negative-strand RNA viruses) and icosahedral symmetry (many small positive-strand RNA viruses, small and large DNA viruses, and bacteriophage heads). The small icosahedral viruses have very simple capsids with only one type of protein, or with three or four closely related proteins. The large icosahedral viruses, such as adenoviruses and herpesviruses, have more complex capsids with several major capsid proteins arranged into topological units, usually pentameric and hexameric, called capsomers, plus a number of small proteins that glue the capsomers together. There are icosahedral viruses with a single protein capsid layer (rhinovirus, hepatitis B virus) and a double protein layer (reoviruses), and there are also icosahedral viruses that have a membrane with proteins both outside and inside the membrane (togaviruses and alphaviruses).

However, many enveloped viruses do not have icosahedral symmetry and formation of the virus particles takes place in a different manner. All negative-strand RNA viruses, the positive-strand coronaviruses and, most likely, the retroviruses (although there is still some debate about this point), are not icosahedral.

An interesting feature of the transport components of certain viruses is that they must be stable enough to form inside the infected cell and to resist attacks in the extra cellular environment, but that they have to fall apart when the virus enters a new cell. This implies that the conditions present during virus formation (encapsidation) must be different from those during decapsidation. Different viruses solve this problem in different ways. Viruses such as HIV undergo cleavage of the GAG polyprotein inside the virion by a virus-encoded protease for maturation. It is the immature, intact GAG polyprotein that is assembled in the infected cell and the mature, cleaved capsid that will fall apart upon cell entry. Influenza viruses code for a membrane channel that allows acidification of the virus interior when it passes through the acidic endosome upon entry. Acidification not only leads to membrane fusion by the hemagglutinin, but it also loosens the interactions between the matrix proteins inside the virus (Hay et al. 1985; Martin and Helenius 1991). Adenoviruses are uncoated in a stepwise fashion: the viral protease is activated by two sequential events, first interaction of the receptor-binding protein with the cellular receptor (an integrin), and then activation of the protease by the reducing environment inside the cytoplasm. This leads to sequential loss of viral proteins and degradation of the core necessary to release the viral DNA for transport through the nuclear pore (Greber et al. 1996).

HELICAL VIRUSES AND HELICAL VIRAL COMPONENTS

One of the symmetries used by viruses in order to build a capsid from repeating units is helical symmetry. The characteristics of a helix are defined mathematically by two parameters: u corresponds to the number of subunits per turn (often not an integral number) and p is the axial rise per unit (Figure 5.2). The pitch (P) of a helix corresponds to the distance along its length that has to be traveled to reach the next subunit, i.e. $P = u \times p$. Helical structures can have a rotation axis coincident with the helix axis, like the tail of bacteriophage T4, which has sixfold symmetry and is made by stacked rings with a rotation angle of 60° between subsequent rings. If a helix is perfect, then a single view of the helix will give all the 3D information of the protein and nucleic acid components that make up the helix, because the same protein can be observed along the helix but in different orientations. Different types of helices can exist in virus particles:

- The nucleic acid can be associated with and protected by many copies of a single protein and form an infectious virus particle. In these helices the protein serves to protect the nucleic acid. Examples are the tobamoviruses (tobacco mosaic virus (TMV); Figure 5.3), tobraviruses (tobacco rattle virus), hordeiviruses (poa

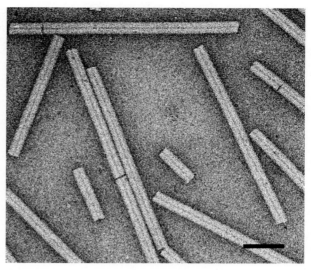

Figure 5.3 *Electron micrograph of tobacco mosaic virus negatively stained with 1% uranyl acetate. The bar corresponds to 100 nm.*

semilatent virus (PSLV) and lychnis ringspot virus (LRSV)), furoviruses (potato mop-top virus (PMTV)) and pecluviruses (peanut clump virus). These viruses are all rod-like positive-strand RNA viruses. Other examples are the badnaviruses, bacilliform double-stranded DNA plant viruses such as sugarcane bacilliform virus (SCBV-IM). Sometimes, proteins with specific functions are added at one or both ends, as is found with single-stranded filamentous DNA bacteriophages such as Pf1 and M13.

- The nucleic acid can be associated with many copies of the same protein and form the matrix for transcription and replication of the nucleic acid, but other proteins and a lipid membrane are needed to complete the virus particle. Good examples of this kind of structure are the nucleocapsids of negative-strand RNA viruses (see under Nonsymmetrical viruses ; Figure 5.9, p. 71). However, under physiological conditions these helical structures are very flexible and do not have defined helical parameters.

- The helix is not associated with the nucleic acid but is part of the virus structure, like the tail of double-stranded bacterial DNA viruses such as bacteriophage T4 that is used for injecting the nucleic acid into the bacterial host cell (Figure 5.4).

In principle a helix can have more than one start (like microtubules), but in the case of a helix associated with nucleic acid the helix has always a single start because as there is only a single nucleic acid molecule.

Methods to study helical virus structures

Electron microscopy (EM) is probably the best method to visualize helical viruses or viral components. TMV

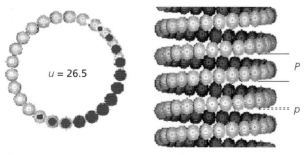

Figure 5.2 *Schematic representation of a helix. P is helical pitch, p corresponds to the axial rise per unit, and u is the number of subunits per helical turn.*

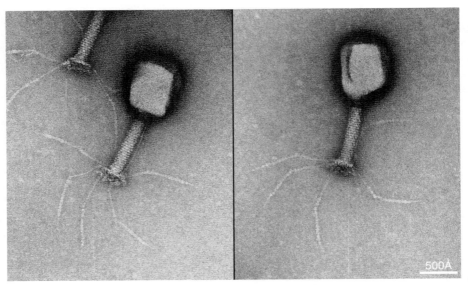

Figure 5.4 *Phage T4 visualized by negative-stain EM. The extended icosahedral head is crumpled by dehydration but the thick contractile tail is well preserved, as are the long tail fibers that extend from the baseplate. Short tail fibers are also visible underneath the baseplate. Figure courtesy of M.E. Cerritelli, N. Cheng, and A.C. Steven, LSBR-NIAMS-NIH.*

was one of the first biological objects to be observed in EM (Horne et al. 1939). For negative-stain EM, virus specimens are first absorbed on to a support film that is transparent to electrons, for example a thin film of evaporated carbon. The embedding of the helix in a layer of stain gives high contrast and makes it possible to visualize the pitch of the helix (Figures 5.3 and 5.4). If the stain stays low on the carbon only one side of the helix is visualized, but the stain may also cover the side of the helix that does not touch the support film. Another method of preparing virus for EM is to evaporate a thin film of metal at an angle over a dried sample on support film. Differences in sample height will lead to differences in metal deposit and, hence, in contrast. Because metal shadowing outlines only one side of the helix, this method gives information on the handedness of the helix (right or left turning). The virus can also be prepared by fast freezing of the virus in a very thin film of buffer – so-called cryo-electron microscopy (cryo-EM), leading to a state of the virus particle that is close to its native form in solution. The picture obtained from cryo-EM is a two-dimensional (2D) projection of the 3D structure of the virus. The disadvantage of this technique is the very low image contrast that makes it necessary to use image analysis in order to enhance the signal-to-noise ratio. In principle, cryo-EM may lead to subnanometer structural information on viruses.

The Fourier transform of the 2D projection of a helix gives a characteristic diffraction pattern in which the information is situated on lines, the layer lines. Analysis of the diffraction pattern leads to total definition of the helical parameters and can be used to recalculate a 3D model of the helical structure. For this approach the cryo-method is the most useful way to prepare the virus

sample for EM. However, this analysis method is difficult and time-consuming. Recently, new algorithms have been developed for the reconstruction of helical filaments using single-particle methods (Egelman 2000; Li et al. 2002). This technique uses iterative real-space reconstruction and is able to overcome most of the problems that can be encountered in helical reconstruction using Fourier analysis, which is more dependent on long-range order.

Another method for the analysis of helical structures is fiber diffraction, for which a sample has to be prepared in which the helices are all aligned in the same direction. Well-aligned fibers can be prepared by drying a gel of purified helical virus under controlled humidity and temperature conditions in a strong magnetic field (Nave et al. 1979, 1981), which is then analyzed by X-ray diffraction. The structure of TMV was solved to a resolution of 3.6 Å with this technique (Namba and Stubbs 1986). TMV contains a single molecule of single-stranded positive-strand RNA plus 2 130 copies of a single coat protein of 17.5 kDa. The pitch of the helix is 23.0 Å, with 16.33 subunits per turn and three nucleotides per protein subunit. The RNA is squeezed in a groove between protein subunits of subsequent helical turns and follows the helical path at a radius of 40 Å.

ICOSAHEDRAL VIRUSES

The high symmetry of the icosahedron offers similar advantages to the helix for capsid architecture, including maximizing packaging volume for the viral genome at a minimal cost in coding space by making use of repeated protein subunits (Crick and Watson 1956). In a simple icosahedron 60 identical subunits are arranged in a closed shell with fivefold axes of symmetry at the 12 vertices, threefold axes on the 20 facets, and twofold axes on the 30 edges (Figure 5.5). Each subunit has equal contacts with its neighbors. However, most icosahedral viruses use elaborate variations on this scheme to construct larger and multifunctional capsids by coding flexibility into the subunits that allow non-identical interactions, as described below, which introduce additional sites of local hexameric symmetry. Consequently, these structures are useful model systems for studying protein folding and assembly, and the flexibility of subunit interfaces.

Viruses from all walks of life have icosahedral capsids, although a spectacular range of variations is observed in their structural details. General principles about assembly, maturation and function of these viruses might best be listed as a menu of strategies from which a combination may be chosen to describe particular cases. For example, the nature of the genome may be RNA or DNA; single- or double-stranded; its recruitment by packaging into a preformed capsid through a specialized

vertex, or capsid assembly around a genomic or pregenomic complex; delivery by capsid entry into the cell or by some membrane-penetrating mechanism from an external membrane-anchored location. Structural variations include possible use of a scaffold for capsid assembly, which may be internal or external; proteolysis of structural proteins during capsid maturation; reorganization of the capsid proteins, which may lead to a change in the capsid diameter; the possible incorporation of a membrane, which may be external to the capsid or internal (or sandwiched between protein shells); host recognition by fibers protruding from the capsid surface or by the capsid surface itself; and so on.

One element remains central to the many aspects of the virus lifecycle, and that is the symmetric capsid. This icosahedral protein complex serves a variety of functions, the most obvious of which is as a protective container for the transport of the viral genome from one cell to another. However, various roles are observed for capsids, including interaction with other virus proteins (connector-tail complex, fibers, tegument, membrane-

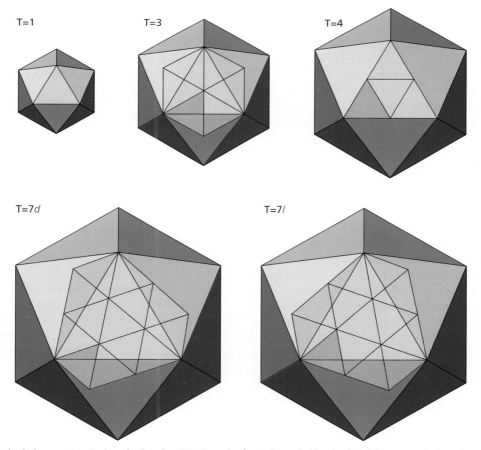

Figure 5.5 *Icosahedral geometry. An icosahedron has 20 triangular facets bounded by the five-fold symmetrical vertices of the icosahedron. By tiling the icosahedral surface with triangles, as shown for different Triangulation numbers 3–7, larger volumes may be enclosed. Additional hexavalent sites are created where triangular vertices meet. Skew symmetries, such as T = 7, may be 'handed' and both laevo (l) and dextro (d) forms are observed in viral capsids (see Figure 5.6, p. 64). The largest T-number observed to date is in the capsid of PBCV-1 (Yan et al. 2000) with T = 169.*

bound glycoproteins), transcriptional compartment, receptor recognition, and genome release through disassembly. The capsid itself may be as simple as a single-species assembly (e.g. hepatitis B virus (HBV)) or include a number of structural components (e.g. herpes simplex virus (HSV)), and generally the complexity is observed to increase with size.

Recent work has revealed some particular elements of capsid structure and function that are common to seemingly quite unrelated viruses. One example is the remarkable similarity in structure between phage PRD1 and the mammalian adenovirus, which extends from capsid architecture to the structures of the major capsid proteins, P3 and hexon, respectively (Benson et al., 1999, 2002). Another example is the similarity between phage T4 and HSV, including the recent discovery of a specialized vertex on the capsid of HSV-1 that is implicated in uptake of the dsDNA genome (Newcomb et al. 2001), analogous to the way in which tailed dsDNA phage capsids package their genome through a unique 'connector' complex prior to attachment of their tail structure. The fold of the capsid protein is also conserved in viruses from a wide variety of sources – for example, the 'jelly roll,' an eight-strand β-barrel, is found in RNA and DNA viruses from bacteria, plants, insects, and animals. In such cases, the study of structure has led not only to an understanding of virus function, but also to the possibility of extensive evolutionary relationships.

An outline of icosahedral architecture is given below, including examples of contrasting systems to highlight connections between structural features and function.

A note on methodology

Electron microscopy has played an important role in visualizing virus structure, starting from the development of the negative-stain technique (e.g. Brenner and Horne 1959), to which the methodology of image reconstruction was subsequently applied (Crowther et al. 1970) for extending structural analyses of icosahedral viruses into three dimensions. Cryo-EM now substitutes for negative staining and avoids dehydration, fixation, and staining artifacts (Adrian et al. 1984). Although EM has been important in studying virus structure, it is equally true that the highly symmetric structure of icosahedral viruses has made them invaluable for the development of 3D structural analysis methods for cryo-EM data. This synergy has led to achievements of subnanometer resolution for several icosahedral capsids (Bottcher et al. 1997; Conway et al. 1997; Mancini et al. 2000; Zhang et al. 2002; Zhou et al. 2000), with the expectation of higher resolution in the future (see Baker et al. 1999b for a recent review of such structural analyses). X-ray crystallography has also been applied to whole capsids (Hogle et al. 1985; Johnson and Chiu

2000), although this kind of analysis remains challenging owing to the large size of the particles leading to large unit cells and, thus, very close packing of diffraction spots. A combination of these two techniques is often employed wherein subunit atomic models from crystallography are placed into a lower-resolution structure of the complex from cryo-EM (Chiu and Rixon 2002; Modis et al. 2002). This hybrid approach, although not atomic in resolution, is nonetheless valuable for situations where crystallization is difficult or impossible. Examples include capsids decorated with antibodies or Fabs (Prasad et al. 1990; Porta et al. 1994; Conway et al. 2003), capsids decorated with receptor fragments (Hewat et al. 2000; Rossmann et al. 1994), and even capsids alone based on subunit models (Speir et al. 1995; Martin et al. 2001; Modis et al. 2002). Another hybrid approach is the use of cryo-EM density maps as phasing models to initiate crystallographic analyses (e.g. Speir et al. 1995; Grimes et al. 1998).

The nonsymmetric components of a virus, such as membranes and nucleic acid, are generally not visualized by these methods and so less is known about the structures they adopt. The problem is one of low signal and high noise; information from many identical copies must be averaged together to yield an interpretable structure by cryo-EM or X-ray crystallography, and this is clearly impossible to do with the nonuniform pieces. Several exceptions have been observed, however, although these are consequences of association with the icosahedral capsid. One is regions of packaged RNA that contact the capsid and which are visualized by crystallography, for example at icosahedral twofold axes of the nodamura viruses, Flock House virus (Fisher and Johnson 1993), and pariacoto virus (Tang et al. 2001), where they appear to influence the interface between capsid proteins and determine in part the T = 3 capsid geometry, and at the transcribing vertices of bluetongue virus cores (Gouet et al. 1999). Another is the highly concentrated dsDNA of bacteriophages, which appears as organized layers spaced ~25 Å apart in cryo-EM images, and as concentric shells of DNA in image reconstructions, which, although somewhat artificial owing to the imposition of symmetry, nonetheless appears to have some bearing on the genome organization within the capsid (Cerritelli et al. 1997; Olson et al. 2001). A similar spacing has been observed for herpes virus DNA (Booy et al. 1991), although the ordering does not appear on the global scale of the phage DNA.

The icosahedral capsid

Icosahedrally symmetric capsids come in various degrees of complexity, from the small and simple, such as capsids of parvoviruses that are built from 60 copies of (essentially) a single protein, to the large and complex, including those of herpesviruses, which comprise 960 copies of the major capsid protein and hundreds of copies of several other structural proteins. Capsids may be multilayered, such as those from rotaviruses and reoviruses, with different copy numbers of the constituent proteins in each layer. How is this variation consistent with icosahedral symmetry, which strictly demands 60 identical asymmetric units? And how might the 960 copies of the major capsid protein of HSV, for example, be subdivided into 60 asymmetric units of 16 copies each and arranged identically to form a closed shell? The prevailing explanation is the concept of 'quasi equivalence' (Caspar and Klug, 1962; Johnson and Speir, 1997), in which identical subunits are placed in slightly different chemical environments according to their position within the asymmetric unit. The different numbers of subunits may be described by a 'triangulation number,' T, which is a count of the number of triangles that may be used to tile an icosahedral facet so that each triangle accounts for the positions of three protein subunits (Figure 5.5). A triangulation number $T = 1$ corresponds to perfect icosahedral symmetry with each subunit in an identical environment. A selection rule determines the allowable triangulation numbers as follows: $T = h^2 + hk + k^2$, where h and k are integers 0, 1, 2, ... The total number of subunits is then 60T. The capsid surface is triangulated by pentavalent positions at the vertices and hexavalent positions elsewhere (except in the case of $T = 1$). Certain T numbers are forbidden, such as $T = 2$, although this number has been used to describe protein shells from dsRNA viruses (yeast L-A virus – Cheng et al. 1994; Caston et al. 1997, and the cores of some multilayer capsids; see below) with 120 copies of a capsid protein subunit arranged as 60 asymmetric dimers. Some extensions to this simple geometric descriptor have been developed to account for more complex structures. One is the pseudo-T number, where the subunits are non-identical, for example in the case of picornaviruses, which have three similar but non-identical capsid subunits arranged in a pseudo-$T = 3$ lattice (Arnold and Rossmann, 1990), and adenovirus, which has pseudo-$T = 25$, where the hexavalent positions are occupied by trimers and the pentamer subunits on the vertices are a different protein. Another is the addition of a second triangulation number, Q, that is used to describe the geometry resulting from one or more additional 'bands' of subunits around the equator in elongated capsids such as that of bacteriophage T4 ($T = 13/Q = 21$) (Aebi et al. 1976).

The concept of quasi equivalence has therefore had to adapt to the various ways in which flexibility between subunits contacts is expressed in virus capsids. In some cases this flexibility involves rather larger departures from symmetry than those originally envisaged. The 'forbidden' $T = 2$ capsid described above is one example. Another is the capsid geometry of SV40, a *Polyomavirus* in which pentameric capsomers occupy both hexavalent and pentavalent sites in a $T = 7$ geometry (Liddington et al. 1991). This architecture, common for all polyoma and papilloma viruses, utilizes just 360 copies of the capsid protein (corresponding in quantity to the forbidden $T = 6$) instead of the expected 420, and involves different conformations for the C-terminal arms that interface with (and invade) neighboring capsomers (Figure 5.6a). A third kind of departure is observed in the hexameric capsomers of some $T = 7$ dsDNA bacteriophages, such as λ, T7, P22, and HK97, which obey 'classic' hexamer and pentamer capsomer structure (Figure 5.6b, c). The hexamers of the early assembly forms of these capsids exhibit a marked departure from local sixfold symmetry, but this is 'cured' upon maturation (Dokland and Murialdo 1993; Conway et al. 1995; Lata et al. 2000). Recently a structure of the procapsid form of an animal virus, HSV-1, has been solved and this shows similar, although less pronounced, changes for the hexameric capsomers during maturation (Heymann et al. 2003; Trus et al. 1996). Yet another example of low quasi equivalence comes from the geminiviruses, plant viruses with double heads of partial $T = 1$ icosahedra fused at a ring of five vertices (Zhang et al. 2001).

The flexibility of capsid proteins at subunit interfaces must also, in some cases, accommodate mismatches in symmetry. A well-known example of this is from tailed bacteriophages, where a 12-subunit connector complex occupies one of the vertices of the capsid, a site of icosahedral fivefold symmetry. The connector is thought to nucleate assembly of the capsid, after which DNA is packaged through it followed by attachment of the tail. The mismatch has been proposed to allow rotation of the 12-fold connector within its fivefold 'bearing' as part of the DNA-packaging (Simpson et al. 2000), in line with rotational functions implicated in other symmetry mismatches (Beuron et al. 1998; Junge et al. 2001; Thomas et al. 1999). However, rotation is not always implicated in symmetry mismatches: for example, it has no obvious role in the mismatch between the penton base of adenovirus and the trimeric fiber that binds to it.

Connectorless capsids may also exhibit large-scale symmetry mismatches, as in the case of some dsRNA viruses which have an inner core that exhibits the forbidden $T = 2$ geometry and is surrounded by an outer layer with $T = 13$ geometry (reovirus – Reinisch et al. 2000; bluetongue virus – Grimes et al., 1998; *Rotavirus* – Lawton et al., 1997; phi6 – Butcher et al. 1997). The subunit interactions between the layers involve non-equivalent contacts that are additional to those within each layer.

Icosahedral capsid protein folds

The most commonly observed fold for capsid proteins is the eight-strand β-barrel mentioned above, first seen in tomato bushy stunt virus (Harrison et al. 1978) and later

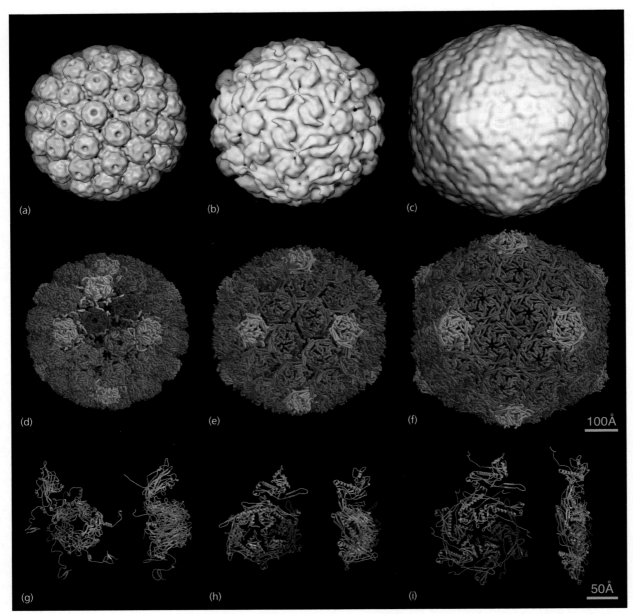

Figure 5.6 *Capsids with T = 7 geometry include polyomaviruses and lambdoid bacteriophages. The atomic model for SV40 (Stehle et al. 1996; PDB Id: 1SVA) is rendered as a surface at 16 Å resolution in panel* **(a)**, *showing the capsomers as protruding knobs in either pentavalent or hexavalent positions and with the right-handed, or T = 7d, configuration. Cryo-EM reconstructions of the procapsid (16 Å – Conway et al. 2001) and mature capsid (24 Å – Conway et al. 1995) of bacteriophage HK97 are shown in panels* **(b)** *and* **(c)**, *respectively. In this case the surface lattice has opposite hand, T = 7l, and the capsomer appearance, although similar to SV40 at the vertices (pentavalent positions), is quite different elsewhere. In particular, the HK97 procapsid shows only local twofold symmetry at the hexavalent sites, whereas the mature capsid shows good six-fold symmetry. The procapsid expands into the mature form during packaging of the dsDNA genome: this remarkable transformation involves a coordinated change in subunit interactions between the 420 copies of the capsid protein. When rendered as tubes, the SV40 capsid* **(d)** *reveals that all capsomers are pentamers, unlike many T = 7 capsids, such as that of HK97, which has a combination of pentamers and hexamers. In* **(d)**, *pentamers at the vertices are colored green, and the rest are red, except for three on a frontmost facet of the icosahedron that are colored blue, purple, and yellow to distinguish them. The HK97 procapsid model* **(e)** *is pseudoatomic, resulting from fitting an atomic model of the mature capsid protein into a 12 Å resolution cryo-EM model of the procapsid (Conway et al. 2001). As for SV40, capsomers at the vertices are green, but the hexameric capsomers are colored as one trimer in red and the other in blue to highlight the local two-fold symmetry. The mature capsid* **(f)** *is from a crystallographic model (Wikoff et al. 2000) and is colored as for the procapsid. Ribbon diagrams of the asymmetric units are shown at the bottom in each case – a top-view at left and a side-view at right – including one subunit from pentavalent capsomers in green and the others in shades to match the views in the middle row. For SV40* **(g)** *the extended carboxy termini are involved in interactions between capsomers. The views of HK97 procapsid* **(h)** *and mature capsid* **(i)** *show the more regular hexon in the mature form, as well as flattening and thinning of the capsomers.*

in picornaviruses and other positive-strand RNA viruses (Rossmann and Johnson 1989) from animals, plants, and insects. It has been seen subsequently in dsDNA viruses, including hexons of adenovirus (Roberts et al. 1986) and phage PRD1 (Benson et al. 1999), and in the enzymatically active cores of dsRNA reoviruses (Grimes et al. 1998; Reinisch et al. 2000), although these also have additional domains that include significant amounts of α-helix. Perhaps surprisingly, the architecturally related yeast L-A virus, which adopts the same arrangement of 60 asymmetric dimers (Cheng et al. 1994; Caston et al. 1997) with similar overall shapes and dimer interface contacts (Naitow et al. 2002), does not, however, share the same fold as the reovirus cores.

Folds with predominantly α-structures are less commonly observed. One example is the capsid of HBV, where the protein dimer interface is a four-helix bundle (Bottcher et al. 1997; Conway et al. 1997; Wynne et al. 1999), including a helix–turn–helix contributed by each of the two subunits (Figure 5.7). A similar motif has also been observed in HIV-1 CA protein dimers (Gamble et al. 1997; Zlotnick et al. 1998), although HIV does not conform to icosahedral symmetry. A recently solved 65 kDa fragment of the 150-kDa major capsid protein of HSV-1 and located in the upper domains of the capsomers is also predominantly α-helical (Bowman et al. 2003). Few structures are available for the capsid proteins of the widespread dsDNA phages, but those for HK97 (Wikoff et al. 2000) (Figure 5.6i) and P22 (Jiang et al. 2003) are similar, although they have no structural homology with any other proteins solved to date.

Capsid assembly

From the descriptions above of icosahedral symmetry and the variety of departures from it, we must suppose that capsid assembly is directed so as to achieve the correct structure in each case (Dokland 2000). Overexpression of capsid proteins sometimes results in multiple and deviant assembly forms, including tubes (e.g. Lepault et al. 2001), and closed shells of various sizes (e.g. Salunke et al. 1989), clearly the result of nonnative conditions and elevated concentration. Assembly of 60-fold subunits to form a specific capsid structure is a complex process involving at least the following steps: onset (e.g. nucleation); accumulation of identical subunits into non-identical positions within a specific architecture; and completion of the capsid by closing the shell. At some stage in this process the non-structural elements, including the genome, must be packaged, and additional maturational events may also occur, including proteolysis of the capsid protein, reorganization of the subunits in the completed capsid, and additional stabilization of the capsid through binding of accessory proteins or some other modification of the subunit interactions. Assembly is generally not well understood, particularly the stages before completion of the capsid.

Innate curvature between subunits offers a framework for constructing a container, although it may be insufficient for specifying a particular geometry or even producing closed surfaces. Smaller icosahedral viruses generally have one capsid protein (or several but with largely similar folds), and these are often capable of self-assembly into virus-like particles in expression systems. Larger capsids, such as that of HSV (Nicholson et al. 1994), assemble with the aid of a scaffold that does not itself obey icosahedral symmetry but which presumably enforces the correct curvature on the assembling subunits and is later removed. Likewise, the outer T = 13 shells of dsRNA viruses are organized by self-assembled T = 2 cores, although these cores are essential to the virus and remain in place. For the *Alphavirus* Sindbis the capsid proteins do not appear to interact strongly with each other, but instead the association of the amino-terminal domain with the genomic ssRNA is the organizing force for assembly (Zhang et al. 2002). In this case, the capsid is surrounded by a membrane penetrated by coiled-coil domains of heterodimeric E1 and E2 glycoproteins that conform to the T = 4 geometry of the underlying capsid. These may also be involved in specifying the correct assembly state of the virus. Similar organization is possible in other alphaviruses, such as Ross River virus and Semliki Forest virus, as well as the more distantly related *Flavivirus*, tick-borne encephalitis virus, which shares structural homology in parts of the glycoprotein.

The necessity for a scaffold appears to be related to capsid diameter, with the limit being approximately 500 Å. Some dsDNA phages of this size, such as λ and P22, require a scaffold, whereas others do not, as is the case for HK97. In the absence of the scaffold protein, phage P22 capsid protein assembles mostly into aberrant particles with T = 4 geometry, as well as some with the normal T = 7 (Thuman-Commike et al. 1998), demonstrating that the flexibility between protein subunit interactions, which serves to allow non-equivalent bonding arrangements in the capsid, must also be controlled to avoid non-productive assembly.

Any internal scaffolding must be expelled to allow space for the genome. In some cases the scaffolding protein is proteolysed, presumably to aid its egress, and often by a virally encoded protease. In the case of HSV, the scaffold and protease genes overlap, ensuring colocalization of protease with the substrate scaffold protein. Phage HK97 apparently has no distinct scaffold protein – one of the largest icosahedral virus to forgo this assembly component – but the capsid protein includes an amino-terminal ~100 residue domain that is proteolysed after assembly and which is proposed to contain the scaffolding function (Conway et al. 1995). In other cases, such as phage P22, the scaffold protein is not proteolysed but none the less exits through holes in the procapsid surface and is recycled to construct new capsids (King and Casjens 1974).

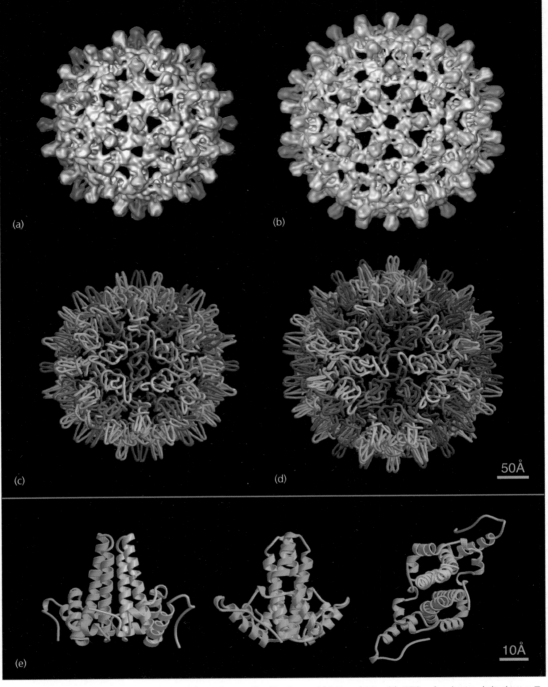

Figure 5.7 *Hepatitis B virus capsids come in two sizes: the smaller T = 3 capsid **(a)** and **(c)** with 180 subunits, and the larger T = 4 capsid **(b)** and **(d)** including 240 subunits. Surface views from cryo-EM reconstructions are shown in the top row at resolutions of 10 and 9 Å for **(a)** and **(b)**, respectively (Conway et al. 1997). The spikes rising from the capsid surface are four-helix bundles, with each of two capsid protein subunits contributing a helix–turn–helix motif to form a tight dimer interface. Unlike the SV40 and HK97 capsids of Figure 5.6, HBV does not have capsomers located on pentavalent and hexavalent sites, but instead the dimers cluster around these positions. The large holes in the capsid are presumably to allow nucleotides to diffuse inwards during reverse transcription of the RNA pregenome, following which the capsid will be enveloped on exiting from the host cell. The middle row shows tube renditions of atomic models of the capsids, based on the crystal structure of the T = 4 capsid (Wynne et al. 1999; PDB Id: 1QGT) but modified to fit the cryo-EM models (Watts et al. 2002). The monomer has three quasiequivalent positions in the T = 3 capsid **(c)**, color-coded as a green–yellow dimer and as a red–red dimer that lies on an icosahedral two-fold symmetry axis. For the T = 4 capsid **(d)** there are four different positions, coded as green–yellow and red–blue dimers. Views of a dimer are shown in **(e)**, where the four-helix bundle is evident. At left and center are two side views, and at right is a top view.*

Smaller capsids assemble around the viral genome or pregenome, whereas larger capsids are assembled first and then the genome is packaged through a specialized vertex, or portal. Packaging into a preformed capsid is driven by an ATP-dependent motor that works against a steadily increasing pressure gradient as the capsid fills. For dsDNA phages such as λ and HK97, the onset of packaging triggers a large-scale irreversible rearrangement of the capsid protein subunits, termed expansion (Figure 5.6b,c). For HK97 this trigger is proposed to be the repulsive force between the incoming DNA and the net negatively charged interior surface of the capsid (Conway et al. 2001). As a consequence of expansion, the HK97 subunits are displaced outwardly by 40 Å and rotate by 40° on average, and the internal volume doubles. Even with this additional volume to fill, the DNA is at high concentrations in these particles, of the order of 500 mg/ml. The capsid, which is round in the precursor form and highly contoured with protruding hexameric and pentameric capsomers, becomes planar and thin walled after expansion. Despite this thinning of the capsid wall, the buried surface area between subunits is estimated to be ~50 percent greater after expansion than before, suggesting that the larger subunit interfaces confer additional stability on the capsid, allowing it to withstand both the internal pressure of the packaged genome and external environmental stress.

Although this expansion transition is common among dsDNA phages, not all capsids that undergo a maturational reshaping necessarily expand. Recent work on HSV capsids indicates a number of conformational rearrangements, which serve to enhance contacts between subunits by closing gaps in the capsid, but with no significant change in its internal volume (Heymann et al. 2003). Another example is Nudaurelia capensis omega virus, a nonenveloped T = 4 RNA virus that infects insects, from which precursor virus-like particles are 16 percent larger than the mature virus, suggesting a maturational shrinkage (Canady et al. 2000). Large-scale structural rearrangements have not been seen in the assembly pathways of other icosahedral RNA viruses, although some plant viruses are observed to have a pH-dependent swollen state that is considered to be a disassembly transition during infection, much as is seen for poliovirus and other picornaviruses as a consequence of receptor binding (Fricks and Hogle 1990; Belnap et al. 2000; Hewat et al. 2002).

Tailed phages often bind one or more accessory proteins to the exterior surface of the capsid after expansion that confer additional stability. Trimers of the viral gpD protein bind to sites of local threefold symmetry on the surface of the T = 7 phage λ capsid, and these are essential for withstanding the internal pressure of packaging the full-length genome (Sternberg and Weisberg 1977). Phage T4 similarly binds the small outer capsid (Soc) protein at most local threefold sites, although it does not form a tight trimeric molecule

(Iwasaki et al. 2000; Olson et al. 2001) as does λ's gpD (Yang et al. 2000). T4 also binds a second accessory protein (highly antigenic outer capsid (Hoc)), which populates local sixfold symmetry positions as a monomer (Iwasaki et al. 2000; Olson et al. 2001) but whose role is unknown. Somewhat akin to both Soc and Hoc is the vp26 protein of herpesvirus, which is dispensable for capsid formation and binds to the tips of hexamers of the major capsid protein vp5, but not to pentamers (Booy et al. 1994). The function of vp26 is unknown. Given its location, it may be expected to interact with a nonsymmetric protein layer called tegument that is between the capsid and the viral envelope (Trus et al. 1999), but this is not supported experimentally (Chen et al. 2001a). Phages HK97 and (probably) HK022 follow a different strategy to that of stabilizing the expanded capsid with accessory proteins. Covalent crosslinks between capsid proteins form autocatalytically as a consequence of expansion (Duda et al. 1995), generating a highly robust shell of interlinked protein rings (Duda 1998; Wikoff et al. 2000). This strategy of rigidifying the capsid is only feasible when the genome is to be released through a prebuilt channel, such as the connector-tail complex, rather than by capsid disassembly.

Different species, similar structures

Several observations of conserved architecture between viruses from quite different sources suggest far-reaching evolutionary relationships. The common features may be at the level of the capsid protein fold, as in the eight-strand β-barrel visualized in bacteriophages, plant, insect, and animal viruses (see Icosahedral capsid protein folds), to the larger-scale morphology of capsid geometry, including the recent intriguing identification of a special DNA packaging vertex on the HSV capsid that is reminiscent of the phage connector (Newcomb et al. 2001). For HSV the parallels with bacteriophages, particularly T4, have been drawn before. Common features include scaffold-assisted assembly, virus-encoded protease to process the immature capsid, maturational reorganization, the binding of accessory proteins, and the passage of the viral genome through a specialized vertex. There are, of course, important differences: the T4 tail, the HSV tegumentation and membrane, different proteins for hexameric and pentameric capsomers in T4, and so on. Possibly the similarities at the gross morphological scale are the results of convergent solutions to similar problems that the viruses face in packaging and delivering their genomes to new host cells. However, in another example, that of adenovirus and phage PRD1, the similarities on the gross scale are matched at the atomic level (Figure 5.8). Both viruses are unusual in the trimeric organization of their major capsid protein at hexavalent positions on a T=25 lattice, and they both employ a different protein for the

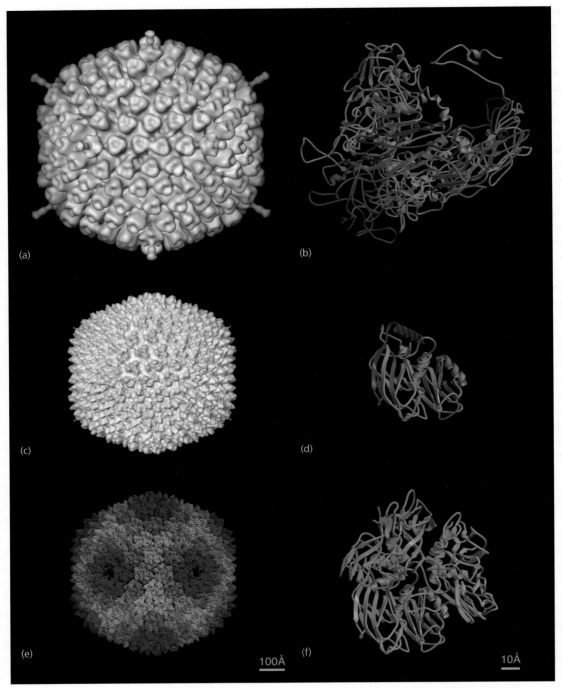

(a)

(b)

(c)

(d)

(e)

(f)

100Å

10Å

Figure 5.8 *Comparison of capsids from the mammalian adenovirus and bacteriophage PRD1. Despite differences in host-cell types, adenovirus and PRD1 share important structural similarities. Surface views of capsids from cryo-EM reconstructions are shown in panel* **(a)***, adenovirus 2 at 25 Å resolution (Stewart et al. 1993; EMDS accession code 1016 – note that full icosahedral symmetry was not evident in the online density map, but has been imposed on the structure viewed here), and panel* **(c)***, PRD1 at 16 Å resolution (San Martin et al. 2002; EMDS accession code 1011). These show the trimeric clustering of subunits on a T = 25 lattice. The adenovirus hexon trimers appear to have considerably more bulk than those of PRD1, which is a smaller capsid that also encloses a membrane. Trimeric spikes are partially visualized in the adenovirus structure, but not in that of PRD1. Atomic models of the major capsid proteins, colored from blue at the amino termini to red at the carboxy termini, are shown in panel* **(b)** *adenovirus hexon (Athappilly et al. 1994; PDB Id: 1DHX), and panel* **(d)** *PRD1 P3 protein (Benson et al. 2002; PDB Id: 1GW7). The adenovirus hexon is considerably larger (967 amino acids) than the PRD1 P3 protein (394 residues), with additional loops that extend upwards, but the core β-barrel is similar. An atomic model of the capsid, built from trimers of P3, is shown in panel* **(e)***, where four adjacent trimers comprising the asymmetric units are colored purple, orange, red, and green. No structures are available yet for the pentameric vertex proteins, which are missing from this image. A single trimer of P3 is rendered as a ribbon diagram in panel* **(f)***.*

pentameric vertices. Also in common is the binding of their receptor recognition molecule, a trimeric fiber, to the respective vertex pentons. The recent crystallographic structure of the PRD1 major capsid protein (Benson et al. 1999) has revealed a fold that is largely identical to that of the equivalent 'hexon' protein of adenovirus, with the exception of the protruding upper domain that is missing in PRD1. This remarkable set of similarities at all levels of structural detail suggests a common ancestry for these two virus proteins, which is further reinforced by a similar protein-primed mechanism of DNA replication initiation (Caldentey et al. 1992). Nonetheless, and not surprisingly, several striking differences are evident between these viruses, in particular the incorporation of a lipid bilayer on the interior of the PRD1 capsid and within which the viral DNA is enclosed. Structural comparisons of other important components, such as the pentameric vertex and trimeric fiber proteins, will be interesting to make when possible. A recent addendum to this fascinating story is the structural analysis of a large algal virus, PBCV1. This virus also incorporates an internal membrane, as does PRD1, but with a diameter of 1900 Å and triangulation number T = 169 its capsid is immensely larger than those of PRD1 and adenovirus (Yan et al. 2000). Nonetheless, the outer surface at 27 Å resolution appears to be populated by trimeric knobs that resemble the adenovirus hexon, and the recently solved structure of its major capsid protein is similar to the PRD1/adenovirus hexon fold (Nandhagopal et al. 2002).

NONSYMMETRICAL VIRUSES

Nonsymmetrical viruses do not have unique structures and cannot be crystallized. As mentioned above, cryo-EM leads to images with rather low signal-to-noise ratios, which can, in principle, be raised by averaging many virus particles if these are identical and can be aligned with each other. This is not possible for viruses that do not have unique structures. For these viruses the negative-staining technique is still often used.

All nonsymmetrical viruses are RNA viruses that have lipid membranes with membrane-embedded glycoprotein spikes. In most cases these spikes are associated with special lipid structures, called rafts (for reviews see Simons and Ehehalt 2002; Schmitt and Lamb 2004; Briggs et al. 2003). Lipid rafts are rich in cholesterol and sphingolipids and are not soluble in Triton X-100 or CHAPS at 4°C (London and Brown 2000), hence their alternative name: detergent-resistant membranes (DRM). The glycoprotein spikes associate with the lipid rafts during maturation in the Golgi apparatus and are transported in the membrane domains to the cell surface. The nonsymmetrical viruses usually also have a small matrix protein (20–30 kDa) that associates with the rafts and the cytoplasmic tails of the membrane-embedded glycoproteins and polymerizes at the interior of the membrane, bringing the rafts together and excluding cellular membrane-embedded proteins. The (encapsidated) genome binds to the layer of matrix protein to form an infectious virus particle. It seems that for the majority of nonsymmetrical viruses, much of the energy for building and maintaining the structure of the virus particle is due to these various and extensive interactions between membranes and proteins.

The glycoproteins are necessary for receptor binding, membrane fusion and, in some cases, for destroying the cell-surface receptors for release of newly formed virus from the infected cell (for those viruses that use sialic acid as receptor, such as influenza and parainfluenza viruses). The proteins that are active in fusion need to undergo a conformational change during which membrane fusion takes place. The trigger for the conformational change can be either low pH, if the virus is internalized through endocytosis (influenza virus and rhabdoviruses), or the trigger can be binding to a virus-specific cell-surface receptor (HIV, paramyxoviruses). The only structures solved for native fusion proteins are those of the hemagglutinins (HA) of influenza A virus and influenza C virus (Wilson et al. 1981; Rosenthal et al. 1998) and that of the fusion protein of Newcastle disease virus (Chen et al. 2001b). There exist now many structures of fusion proteins that correspond to the state of the protein after the conformational change related to membrane fusion. All these structures consist of triple coiled coils with a second layer of helices outside the inner coil (Skehel and Wiley 1998). This probably means that the fusion mechanism for all these viruses is similar, and it may also indicate that the structures before the change have similar features. The only exception may be the fusion-related conformational change of the rhabdovirus glycoproteins. The conformational change of VSV and rabies virus G is reversible, and after the change the fusion peptide is not inserted into the viral membrane, as is the case for influenza virus HA (Gaudin et al. 1995b, 1999).

As mentioned above, there exist neither atomic structures nor 3D EM models for the nonsymmetrical viruses. However, many proteins from these viruses have been crystallized and their structures solved. Table 5.1 gives a list of these structures per virus family. For the retroviruses we have only given the structures of the HIV proteins, although many other protein structures are also known, for example those of SIV proteins.

Negative-strand RNA viruses

The viruses in this group have a genome in the opposite sense to that of mRNA, and for this reason transcription is the first event that takes place after the virus enters the cell. All these viruses have a nucleocapsid in which the viral RNA is tightly and stoichiometrically bound to a nucleoprotein. The interactions between the

Table **5.1** *Structures of proteins of nonsymmetrical viruses*

Protein structure	Nonsymmetrical virus	Reference
Orthomyxoviruses		
Influenza A virus	Native HA (H3)	Wilson et al. 1981
	Uncleaved HA (H3)	Chen et al. 1998
	Native HA (H5, H9)	Ha et al. 2002
	HA after fusion	Bullough et al. 1994
	NA	Varghese et al. 1983
	NS1 (X-ray)	Liu et al. 1997
	NS1 (NMR)	Chien et al. 1997
	M1 pH 5	Sha and Luo 1997
	M1 pH 7	Arzt et al. 2001
Influenza B virus	NA	Burmeister et al. 1992
Influenza C virus	Hemagglutinin-esterase	Rosenthal et al. 1998
Paramyxoviruses		
NDV	HN	Crennell et al. 2000
NDV	Native fusion protein	Chen et al. 2001b
SV5	Fusion protein after fusion	Baker et al. 1999a
hRSV	Fusion protein after fusion	Zhao et al. 2000
Sendai virus	Phosphoprotein polymerization domain	Tarbouriech et al. 2000
Rhabdoviruses		
VSV	Matrix protein	Gaudier et al. 2002
Filoviruses		
Ebola virus	Matrix protein (VP40)	Dessen et al. 2000
	VP40 octamer	Gomis-Rüth et al. 2003
	Glycoprotein (after fusion)	Weissenhorn et al. 1998; Malashkevich et al. 1999
Retroviruses		
HIV	GP120	Kwong et al. 1998
	GP41 after fusion	Weissenhorn et al. 1997; Chan et al. 1997; Tan et al. 1997
	Matrix	Massiah et al. 1994; Matthews et al. 1994; Hill et al. 1996
	Capsid, N-terminal	Gitti et al. 1996; Gamble et al. 1996; Momany et al. 1996
	Capsid, C-terminal	Gamble et al. 1997
	Capsid, intact	Berthet-Colominas et al. 1999
	Nucleocapsid	Morellet et al. 1992; Summers et al. 1992
	Protease	Miller et al. 1989; Navia et al. 1989; Wlodawer et al. 1989
	Reverse transcriptase	Kohlstaedt et al. 1992
	Integrase	Dyda et al. 1994; Eijkelenboom et al. 1995; Lodi et al. 1995; Cai et al. 1997

nucleoprotein molecules determine the helical parameters of the nucleocapsid (Ruigrok and Baudin 1995); see Figure 5.9. They also have matrix proteins with affinities for lipid membranes and for nucleocapsids. All the matrix proteins have a tendency to polymerize, either into well-defined oligomers or into large polymers (Heggeness et al. 1982; Gaudin et al. 1995a, 1997; Ruigrok et al. 2000b; Baudin et al. 2001; Timmins et al. 2003). Polymerization of the matrix proteins probably pulls the glycoproteins in their lipid rafts together to form the virus particle. Interestingly, there are now three structures known of negative-strand RNA virus M proteins, from influenza virus, Ebola virus, and VSV (see Table 5.1), and all are different, suggesting that they are not evolutionarily related. Because the polymerization of the matrix proteins drives the assembly of the negative-strand RNA viruses, the existence of evolutionarily unrelated matrix proteins could imply that the blueprints of viruses from the various families are different.

ORTHOMYXOVIRUSES

We will use the influenza A virus to explain in detail the structure of negative-strand RNA viruses. A schematic

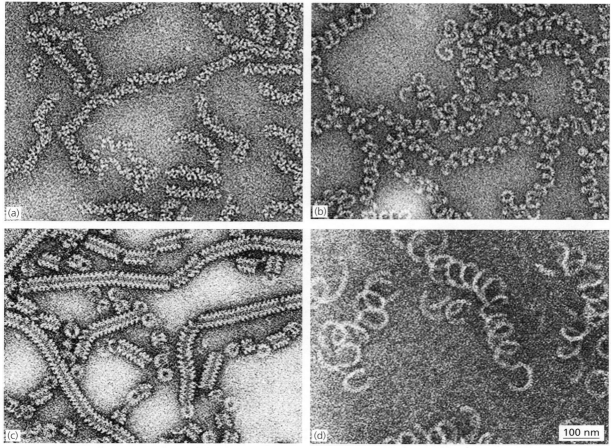

Figure 5.9 *Electron micrographs of negatively stained nucleocapsids of* **(a)** *influenza,* **(b)** *rabies,* **(c)** *measles, and* **(d)** *Marburg viruses. Scale bar = 100 nm.*

drawing of influenza A virus is shown in Figure 5.10 and various electron micrographs in Figure 5.11, p. 73. Influenza virus has a segmented RNA genome consisting of eight segments (seven for influenza C virus), each individually bound to a polymerase complex and each encapsidated by the nucleoprotein (Martín-Benito et al. 2001).

Transport component

Influenza virus has three transmembrane proteins: hemagglutinin (HA), neuraminidase (NA), and the M2 protein. HA is a homotrimer with a stalk part consisting of HA$_2$, which carries the membrane fusion activity, and a more globular head part made up by HA$_1$, which carries the receptor-binding function (Wilson et al. 1981; Skehel and Wiley 2000). NA forms tetramers and consists of a boxlike head that contains the enzymatic receptor-destroying activity, on a long and thin stalk (Varghese et al. 1983; Burmeister et al. 1992). M2 forms a tetrameric membrane channel (Sugrue and Hay 1991; Pinto et al. 1992; Shuck et al. 2000) that is needed for acidification of the interior of the virus as it passes through the endosomal system. Acidification is needed for depolymerization of the matrix protein so that the

individual RNPs can enter the nucleus (Martin and Helenius 1991). Both HA and NA are embedded into lipid rafts, but M2 is not (Scheiffele et al. 1999; Ali et al. 2000; Zhang et al. 2000a, b; Barman et al. 2001).

Replication component

Each RNA segment is individually bound to a heterotrimeric polymerase complex and each is encapsidated by the nucleoprotein (Figure 5.9). The polymerase binds directly to the 3′ and 5′ ends of the RNA, and this complex RNA element forms the promoter for transcription and replication (Hagen et al., 1994; Cianci et al. 1995; Li et al. 2001). Martín-Benito et al. (2001) have made a 3D reconstruction from recombinant and short RNPs that lacked the extensive flexibility and diversity in shape of real viral RNP. The nucleoprotein molecules touch at one extreme side, as was already suggested from negatively stained nucleoprotein polymers (Ruigrok and Baudin 1995). Interestingly, the 3D model also shows extensive contacts between NP molecules and two of the polymerase subunits. Early work suggested that each NP monomer was associated with 20–26 nucleotides (nt) (Compans et al. 1972; Jennings

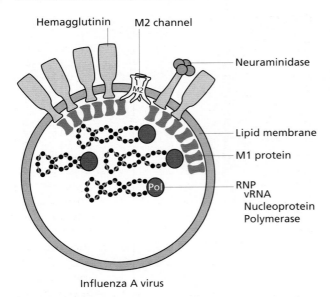

Figure 5.10 *Schematic drawing of an influenza A virus particle.*

et al. 1983). The same group that made the 3D EM reconstruction found that certain lengths of RNA produced recombinant RNP that replicated better than other lengths. These results suggested that the optimal unit of influenza virus RNA that can be encapsidated is not 24 nt per NP monomer, but 48 nt per NP dimer (Ortega et al. 2000). NP binds to the phosphate sugar backbone of the RNA in a sequence-nonspecific manner and, in doing so, prevents RNA secondary structure formation and exposes the nucleotide bases to the outside. In this way, the polymerase can probably read the vRNA without the need for dissociation of NP from the RNA (Baudin et al. 1994; Klumpp et al. 1997).

Connection between replication and transport components

The matrix protein (M1) binds the two components together in the virus particle. M1 consists of two domains, an N-terminal domain that has affinity for membranes and a C-terminal domain that has affinity for the RNP (Baudin et al. 2001). The affinity for membranes appears to be electrostatic and M1 in the virus does not seem to insert into the viral membrane (Ruigrok et al. 2000a). M1 binds to the cytoplasmic tails of the glycoproteins (Jin et al. 1997) and binds also to the M2 membrane channel (Zebedee and Lamb 1989). It is likely that the polymerization of M1 pulls together the fields of lipid rafts with their embedded glycoproteins, and that these fields are subsequently glued together through the M1–M2 interactions. If this model were correct, it would imply that the virus contains more or less rigid and curved protein-membrane sections stuck together at hinge points containing M2 protein. This kind of organization could explain some of the particle shapes of frozen hydrated virus (Figure 5.11a)

and of virus negatively stained with tungstate salts such as sodium silicotungstate (SST) and phosphotungstate (PTA) (Figure 5.11c). A similar model has been proposed for immature HIV particles (Fuller et al. 1997). Such a model also implies that all particles will be slightly different in size and shape. Interestingly, there seem to be about as many copies of M1 protein in a virus particle as there are monomers of the glycoproteins (Ruigrok 1998).

Influenza B and C viruses

The overall shape of influenza B virus seems to be similar to that of the A virus, albeit more spherical than the ellipsoid A virus (Cusack et al. 1985). An interesting detail was observed for the structure of the influenza C virus glycoprotein (Rosenthal et al. 1998). This protein is a trimer of identical subunits. Each subunit consists of two parts (obtained after maturation cleavage by a host protease): a fibrous stalk containing the fusion activity and a more globular head domain carrying the receptor-binding activity, just as in influenza A virus HA (Wilson et al. 1981). However, the influenza C glycoprotein has an extra domain inserted into the receptor-binding domain. This extra domain contains the receptor-destroying activity, and as the influenza C virus does not have a special gene for this function it has not eight but seven gene segments (Compans et al. 1977; Herrler et al. 1981; Desselberger et al. 1980). This single influenza C virus glycoprotein can be organized into a hexagonal surface lattice (Flewett and Apostolov 1967). The influenza C virus glycoprotein is not associated with DRM (Zhang et al. 2000b). Apparently, the structure of the glycoproteins can accommodate additional domains and the different viruses can have their various functions associated with different glycoproteins.

PARAMYXOVIRUSES

The viruses in this large group are all spherical particles that easily deform when negatively stained for EM observation (Figure 5.12, p. 74). The main difference with the influenza viruses is that the genome is not segmented.

Transport component

The paramyxoviruses have trimeric fusion proteins that do not carry the receptor-binding function. This function is found on the H or HN (hemagglutinin–neuraminidase) protein, which has a similar shape to that of influenza virus neuraminidase. Those viruses that use sialic acid as receptor also have a sialidase with receptor-destroying function associated with the HN protein. However, those viruses that bind to other receptors, such as measles virus, do not have a receptor-destroying activity. The glycoproteins of the viruses in this group are also associated with lipid rafts (Manie et al. 2000; Brown et al. 2002; Henderson et al. 2002).

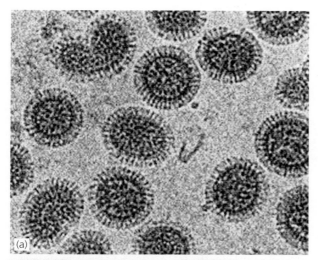

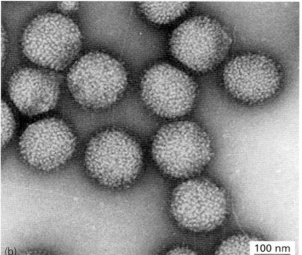

100 nm

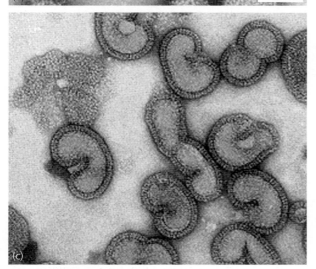

Figure 5.11 *Electron micrographs of influenza B virus (orthomyxoviruses prepared by* **(a)** *fast freezing (cryo-EM),* **(b)** *negative staining with 1% uranyl acetate, and* **(c)** *negative staining with 1% sodium silicotungstate. Scale bar = 100 nm.*

Replication component

The viral RNA is bound to the nucleoprotein with a stoichiometry of six nucleotides per nucleoprotein monomer (Egelman et al. 1989). This N-RNA forms the characteristic herringbone structure that is often used for the identification of paramyxoviruses (Figures 5.9 and 5.12). For some of the viruses in this group this stoichiometry even translates into a 'rule of six': these viruses must have a total number of nucleotides that is a multiple of six (Calain and Roux 1993; Kolakofsky et al. 1998). The proper positioning of the nucleoprotein on to the RNA has an influence on how the polymerase reads the various transcription signals, i.e. on how the polymerase recognizes the nucleotide bases (Iseni et al. 2002). The helical parameters for the nucleocapsids (NC) of the different viruses in this group are not the same: Sendai virus and measles virus have about 13 subunits per helical turn; simian parainfluenza virus 5 (SV-5) NC have 14 subunits; and respiratory syncytial virus (RSV) nucleocapsids contain predominantly ten subunits (Bhella et al. 2002).

The paramyxovirus polymerase is a monomer with polymerase activity that also produces a 5′ cap structure plus the poly-A tail of the viral mRNA. The polymerase is fixed on to the N-RNA template by a tetrameric phosphoprotein (Tarbouriech et al. 2000). The phosphoprotein binds with its C-terminal domain to the C-terminal domain of the nucleoprotein, and the polymerase binds to the oligomerization domain of the phosphoprotein (Curran et al. 1995).

Connection between replication and transport components

As with the influenza viruses, the viral matrix protein makes the connection between the membrane with its embedded spikes and the replication component. Isolated M polymerizes into helical structures depending on the salt concentration (Hewitt and Nermut 1977) and forms orthogonal arrays at the inside of the viral membrane and at the inside of the plasma membrane of infected cells (Büechi and Bächi 1982). The nucleocapsid packs against these arrays to form new virus particles.

RHABDOVIRUSES

This family contains two major groups of bullet-shaped viruses (Figure 5.13), the vesiculoviruses and the lyssaviruses. The viruses in these groups have similar structures, although there are also differences.

Transport component

These viruses have a single, trimeric glycoprotein G that contains the receptor-binding and the fusion activities. The viruses do not have a receptor-destroying activity. Although Brown and Lyles (2003) show interaction of

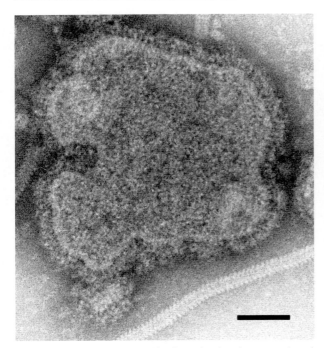

Figure 5.12 *Electron micrograph of measles virus (paramyxoviruses) negatively stained with 1% sodium silicotungstate. Note the helical nucleocapsid in the background. The bar corresponds to 100 nm.*

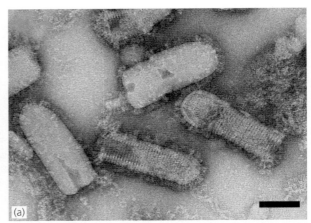

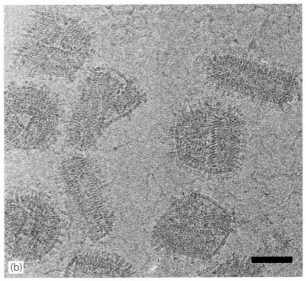

Figure 5.13 *Electron micrographs of VSV (rhabdoviruses) prepared by (a) negative staining with 1% sodium silicotungstate and (b) fast freezing (cryo-EM). Note in (b) that the nucleocapsid is sometimes doubled up to form a more spherical particle. The bar corresponds to 100 nm.*

VSV G with membrane microdomains, there is still debate about whether or not the protein is associated with DRM (discussed in Briggs et al. 2003). It is possible that the membrane domains with which G associates do not have the same structure and composition as detergent-resistant membranes (Owens and Rose 1993; Johnson et al. 1998). For rabies virus, there is also no proof for DRM association from detergent resistance and membrane-floatation experiments (Y. Gaudin, personal communication). The trimeric nature of the rabies virus glycoprotein is clearly visible on EM under slightly acidic conditions (Gaudin et al. 1992). Under these conditions G can also self-associate to form a honeycomb structure, thought to be an intermediate for membrane fusion (Gaudin et al. 1996). Trimerization of the glycoprotein of VSV is also considerably more stable at low pH (Doms et al. 1987).

Replication component

The NC of rabies virus and VSV are loose coils (Figure 5.9) where each N monomer is bound to nine nucleotides (Thomas et al. 1985; Iseni et al. 1998). As for influenza virus and Sendai virus, the nucleoprotein is bound to the sugar phosphate backbone of the RNA and the nucleotide bases are exposed to the outside (Iseni et al. 2000). The polymerase is bound to the N-RNA by the phosphoprotein, which is also an oligomer, but the exact oligomeric state has not yet been clarified (Gigant et al. 2000).

Connection between replication and transport components

The formation of rhabdovirus particles is different from that of the myxoviruses described above. The viral matrix protein associates with the nucleocapsid in the cytoplasm and forms a tightly coiled M–NC complex (Newcomb and Brown 1981; Newcomb et al. 1982; Odenwald et al. 1986). There is a significant increase in the diameter of the helical nucleocapsid upon association with M, owing to slight changes in the angle between N subunits and the tilt angle with respect to the helical axis (Schoehn et al. 2001). The M–NC complex then binds to the cell membrane and, while pushing through it, associates with the glycoprotein spikes (Odenwald et al. 1986). The exact structure of the M–NC complex and the position of the matrix protein is not known. For VSV it has been observed that there is mass inside the nucleocapsid coil, and it has been proposed that at least some of the matrix protein forms a scaffold around which the nucleocapsid is coiled (Brown and Newcomb 1987; Barge et al. 1993). However, this hypothesis on the positioning of the matrix protein is contested by claims that all of M is in contact with the membrane (Chong and Rose 1993). In any case, in contrast to the viruses described above, where the polymerization of the matrix protein leads to membrane curvature and particle shape, for the rhabdoviruses it is the preformed M–NC structure that gives the bullet shape to the rhabdovirus particles.

The VSV particle contains some 1 200 monomers of G, 1 260 monomers of N, and 1 800 monomers of M (Thomas et al. 1985). The rabies virus particle contains much less M – only about 700 copies – whereas it was estimated that there are as many N as G monomers, i.e. some 1 330 copies (Dietzschold et al. 1979; Flamand et al. 1993). Therefore, it would be possible that, in rhabdoviral particles, G associates with N rather than with M. The difference in M protein content between rabies and VSV could mean that there is a difference in structure between the two viruses.

FILOVIRUSES

Filoviruses are long and thin (Figure 5.14), much longer than rhabdoviruses (Feldmann and Klenk 1996; Feldmann and Kiley 1998). There are two groups of filoviruses, Ebola and Marburg. Although many different shapes, such as comma and laureate, have been described, only long and nonbranched particles are seen budding from infected cells (Feldman and Klenk 1996). Because of the high pathogenicity of the virus, only extensively fixed infected cells or purified virus have been used for electron microscopy.

Transport component

The filoviruses have a single glycoprotein with receptor-binding and membrane-fusion activity. This protein is associated with lipid rafts (Bavari et al. 2002).

Replication component

The image of the isolated nucleocapsids in Figure 5.9 was made from nucleoprotein expressed in insect cells. This protein binds to cellular RNA with a stoichiometry of about one N monomer per 12 or 15 nucleotides (Mavrakis et al. 2002). The shape of the N monomers looks somewhat like that of rhabdovirus N, as does the overall appearance of the N RNA. Apart from the nucleoprotein, the polymerase and the phosphoprotein (probably VP35), there is a fourth protein associated with the nucleocapsid of filoviruses, the VP30 protein (Becker et al. 1998; Modrof et al. 2001).

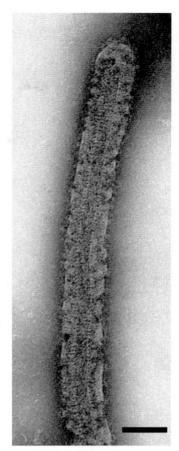

Figure 5.14 *Electron micrograph of an extensively fixed Marburg virus particle (filoviruses) negatively stained with 1% uranyl acetate. The bar corresponds to 100 nm.*

Connection between replication and transport components

The filoviruses have two matrix proteins, VP40 and VP24. VP40 is a two-domain protein (Dessen et al. 2000). The two domains can be dissociated by mutations that destabilize the domain interface, by treatment with low concentrations of urea or by putting the protein in contact with negatively charged lipid membranes (Ruigrok et al. 2000b). When the domains separate, the N-terminal domain associates into ringlike structures and the C-terminal domain binds to membranes (Ruigrok et al. 2000b; Timmins et al. 2003). It is thought that such a conformational change is needed for binding of VP40 to the cell membrane to start particle formation. The diameter of the free Marburg virus nucleocapsid is about 40 nm, whereas the diameter of this structure inside the virus is only 27 nm (Mavrakis et al. 2002). Therefore, whereas the coil diameter of the rhabdovirus nucleocapsid increases as it condenses into the M–NC complex, reducing the length of the structure, for filoviruses the NC diameter decreases, leading to an increase in length. This may be the reason why filoviruses are so long. The *Filovirus* nucleocapsid is also condensed in the cytoplasm, like that of the

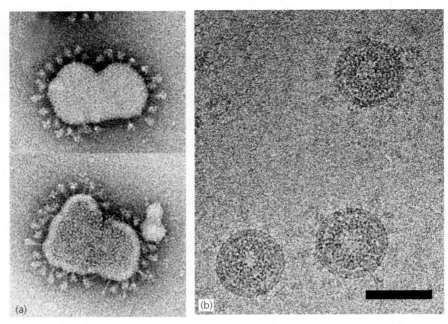

Figure 5.15 *Electron micrographs of Porcine respiratory coronavirus (PRCV) after* **(a)** *negative staining with 1 percent sodium silicotungstate, and* **(b)** *fast freezing (cryo-EM). Note the petalshaped spikes in* **(a)** *and the spherical shape of the particles in* **(b)***. The bar corresponds to 100 nm.*

rhabdoviruses, before it goes into the virus particle (Kolesnikova et al. 2000), and it also seems to be this preformed structure that gives the shape to the virus particle. Between the nucleocapsid and the viral membrane there is an extensive and regular network or scaffold of proteins (Mavrakis et al. 2002; see Figure 5.14). This network is probably made up by the VP40 rings, with or without a contribution of VP24.

CORONAVIRUSES

The coronaviruses, together with the toroviruses and the arteriviruses, form the order of the *Nidovirales*.

Transport component

The name of this group of viruses is derived from its image in negative-stain EM of a spherical particle crowned with petalshaped glycoproteins spikes (S) (Figure 5.15a). S is a trimer (Delmas and Laude 1990). There are two major subgroups of mammalian coronavirus. It seems that S of viruses of subgroup II is cleaved into two parts (like influenza virus HA) and that the trigger for fusion is low pH; and that S of subgroup I viruses is not cleaved and that fusion takes place at neutral pH after interaction with a specific receptor (Hansen et al. 1998; Zelus et al. 2003). However, Gallagher et al. (1991) have isolated different mutants from the same strain of murine hepatitis virus type 4 (group II) with very different pH requirements for fusion, with only a limited number of amino acid substitutions between the mutants. It is possible that the conformational changes

that accompany fusion for the *Coronavirus* S glycoprotein are similar to those of the majority of other viral fusion proteins, because the predicted secondary structure of S also shows two amphiphylic helices per monomer (de Groot et al. 1987; Bosch et al. 2003). The terminal S1 domain is involved in receptor binding (Suzuki and Taguchi 1996), whereas the S2 subunit is involved in membrane fusion (de Groot et al. 1989; Yoo et al. 1991). The *Coronavirus* membrane has at least one other glycoprotein embedded: the small M protein that traverses the membrane three times (Machamer and Rose 1987). For the arteriviruses it has been shown that the membrane can contain several other minor proteins (hemagglutinin esterase (HE), small envelope protein (E), GP(3), and GP(4); Wieringa et al. 2002). It is not known yet whether the coronavirus surface glycoproteins are associated with membrane rafts.

Replication component

Coronaviruses are positive-strand RNA viruses with large genomes of between 27 and 32 kb. This genome size is one of the reasons for the high production of mutant viruses. The viral RNA is capped and polyadenylated (Schochetman et al. 1977; Lomniczi 1977), and upon cell entry the first open reading frame coding for the polymerase is translated. The polymerase then produces subgenomic (sg) copies of the RNA that code for the rest of the viral proteins (Lai and Cavanagh, 1997; van Marle et al. 1999; van Vliet et al. 2002).

Connection between replication and transport components

There is a disagreement in the literature about the function and position of the internal 'nucleocapsid protein' (N). For the arteriviruses it is assumed that N forms a spherical (icosahedral?) shell around the viral RNA. However, no icosahedral reconstructions of these viruses exist, and electron micrographs of thin-sectioned virus particles do not show spherical but rather ellipsoid shapes (Brinton 1999), thereby throwing doubt on the existence of icosahedral symmetry. Older literature on coronaviruses describes N forming helical complexes with vRNA (Macnaughton et al. 1978; Davies et al. 1981) and, because of its positively charged nature, N has been compared with influenza virus nucleoprotein (Laude and Masters 1995). Later work on coronaviruses has suggested that N forms a spherical structure beneath the viral membrane, and that maturation of this structure takes place upon transport of the virus towards the outside of the cell (Risco et al. 1998; Salanueva et al. 1999). The diameter of coronaviruses embedded in vitreous ice is very variable, with no specific size classes (Schoehn, unpublished results), suggesting that the virus does not have icosahedral symmetry.

A number of the characteristics of *Coronavirus* N correspond also to those of the matrix proteins of the negative strand RNA viruses that are also strongly positively charged.

- *Coronavirus* N does not only bind to RNA but also to lipid membranes (Stohlman et al. 1983), a property shared with the positively charged M1 protein of influenza virus that binds to membranes and to naked nucleic acids (Baudin et al. 2001).
- *Coronavirus* N has a tendency to form trimeric complexes (Laude and Masters 1995), a property shared with the MA protein of the retroviruses.
- Detergent-treated influenza virus particles also release helical structures that were initially interpreted to be formed of ribonucleoprotein but which are now thought to consist of oligomeric M1 complexes (Murti et al., 1980, 1992; Ruigrok et al., 1989).
- Experiments with plasmid-expressed proteins suggest that the viral glycoproteins alone can form VLP and leave the cell, but N expressed alone can also form VLP (Vennema et al. 1996), like the matrix proteins of negative-strand RNA viruses and retroviruses.

We only make these comments in order to indicate that, in our opinion, the fine structure of coronaviruses is not yet known in detail.

RETROVIRUSES

As a group, retroviruses are perhaps as variable as the negative-strand RNA viruses. This part of the review will discuss the general principles of retrovirus structures; for more detailed information the reader is referred to Goff (2001) and subsequent chapters in *Fields' Virology*. The structures of virtually all HIV proteins (Table 5.1) and many proteins of other retroviruses have been determined by either crystallography or NMR, but no intact virus or capsid structure has been determined because of a lack of defined symmetry.

Transport component

Retroviruses have a single trimeric glycoprotein (GP160) that, at least for HIV, is associated with lipid rafts (Manes et al. 2000; Ono and Freed 2001) (see Figure 5.16 for a negatively stained SIV particle showing end-on views of the triangular spikes). As for influenza virus HA, GP160 is posttranslationally cleaved into two parts: N-terminal GP120, which is responsible for binding to primary and secondary receptors, and C-terminal GP41, which is membrane anchored and responsible for membrane fusion. GP120 is placed upon GP41, much like the organization of influenza virus HA. GP41 has the same triple coiled coil structure as the fusion proteins of the segmented and nonsegmented negative-strand RNA viruses, implying that the fusion proteins are evolution related and that the fusion processes of all these viruses follow the same mechanism.

Replication component

The replication component of retroviruses consists of the viral RNA bound to the nucleocapsid (NC) protein plus copies of the reverse transcriptase and integrase (see below), necessary for the production of retrotranscribed viral DNA and its integration into the host genome. NC forms a complex with vRNA and facilitates annealing of vRNA with the tRNA primer for reverse transcription (Barat et al. 1993), and prevents the reverse transcriptase stopping at stable stem-loops in the RNA (Wu et al. 1996). In this respect NC has

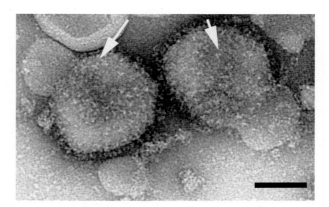

Figure 5.16 *Electron micrograph of simian immunodeficiency virus (SIV, retroviruses) particles negatively stained with 1% uranyl acetate. The arrowheads point out triangular shapes of the trimeric surface glycoprotein. The bar corresponds to 100 nm.*

been named an RNA chaperone (Feng et al. 1999). Although probably structurally different, the function of the retroviral NC protein may be similar to that of the negative strand RNA virus nucleoprotein (see above).

Virus assembly and maturation

The most simple retroviruses code for two polyproteins, Gag and Pol, and a small percentage (about 10 percent) of Gag–Pol proteins when the ribosome reads through the stop codon or when a frame shift occurs at the Gag–Pol boundary, depending on the virus family. More complex viruses have a series of smaller proteins that modulate cellular processes (Goff 2001). The Gag polyprotein consists of the matrix (MA), capsid (CA), and the NC proteins, and Pol consists of the protease (PR), integrase (IN), and the reverse transcriptase (RT). The structure of immature virus was studied from Gag expressed in insect cells or bacteria, which forms virus-like particles (VLP) (Nermut et al. 1994, 2002; Fuller et al. 1997), and from virus with a mutated and inactive protease (Stewart et al. 1990). In immature virus or VLP Gag binds to membranes through the matrix protein (see Figure 5.17) and it forms locally ordered hexagonal lattices (Nermut et al., 1994, 2002; Yeager et al. 1998; Forster et al. 2000; Mayo et al. 2003). However, the spherical structures that are formed are not icosahedral (Fuller et al. 1997; Yeager et al. 1998). Rather, it appears that the Gag polymers bind to membrane patches, leading to shells with local curvature. Somehow, these shells are then joined to form VLP with various diameters (Fuller et al. 1997). The presence of local organization of Gag and curved membrane elements could be similar to what is observed for influenza viruses, where curved M1 membrane shells may be joined by the transmembrane M2 protein (see above). The Gag–Pol proteins are included in the viral bud because the Gag of the Gag–Pol polymerizes with the rest of Gag into the virus. Inside the Gag polymer, nucleic acid (random for

recombinant VLP and viral RNA for intact or PR virus) is bound to the NC part of Gag.

When the virus has budded from the plasma membrane and left the cell, the protease cleaves Gag into MA, CA, and NC, and Pol into PR, IN, and RT. NC remains associated with the viral RNA, MA remains at the membrane and there is no indication that it rearranges at the membrane, but CA forms a new structure inside the virus particle, the capsid (Figures 5.17 and 5.18). The capsid is a closed structure for all the retroviruses, but its form differs by family. As described above for the icosahedral viruses, closed capsids may consist of 12 pentavalent capsomers and a variable number of hexavalent capsomers. The retroviral capsid is also built from CA monomers that are organized into 12 pentavalent and a variable amount of hexavalent units. However, the pentavalent units can be placed at various positions (Ganser et al. 1999; Li et al. 2000). If six pentavalent units are placed close together at one end, six at the opposite end and the rest of the structure consists of hexavalent units, a hollow tube is formed that is indeed sometimes observed in structures formed by purified CA protein in vitro, and which are also observed inside mature HIV (Li et al. 2000; Briggs et al. 2003). Other conical forms are made when the pentavalent units are distributed in an unequal fashion, with five at one end and seven at the other, or other variations (Ganser et al. 1999). All these forms are observed in mature HIV (Briggs et al. 2003). Other retroviruses, such as murine leukemia virus, form rather spherical capsids with a more equal distribution of the pentavalent

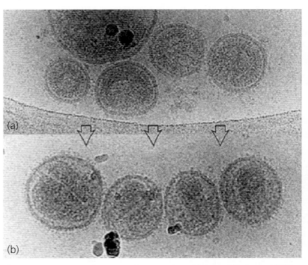

Figure 5.18 *Cryo-electron micrographs of (a) immature and (b) mature Human immunodeficiency virus (HIV, retroviruses) going from immature virus above the arrows to mature virus below. Note the change in shape of the capsid inside the membrane. Photograph courtesy of Stephen Fuller. Reprinted from Fuller, S.D., Wilk, T., et al. Cryo-electron microscopy reveals ordered domains in the immature HIV-1 particle. Current Biology, Vol. 7, pp. 729–38. Copyright (1997), with permission from Elsevier.*

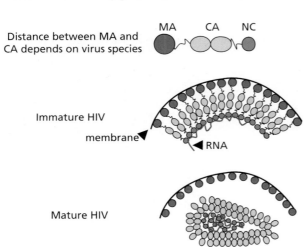

Figure 5.17 *Schematic representation of the changes in HIV capsid structure upon maturation.*

units on a spherical surface, but these capsids are also not all identical and are not icosahedral (Yeager et al. 1998; Kingston et al. 2001). Another observation which goes against the idea that retroviruses have icosahedral structures is that mature and immature viruses do not have diameters with defined values but with rather wide distributions (Fuller et al. 1997; Yeager et al. 1998; Kingston et al. 2001; Briggs et al. 2003). This size variation suggests that smaller viruses can include less nucleic acid than larger viruses, and for HIV it was indeed found that the larger viruses had more than one capsid cone (Briggs et al. 2003).

Some retroviruses do not assemble at the cell membrane but form an immature Gag sphere in the cytoplasm, which subsequently associates with the membrane and the glycoproteins. One could imagine that these viruses are icosahedral, but careful analysis of many different retrovirus families has failed to reveal icosahedral symmetry (S.D. Fuller, personal communication). Another indication that the structures of viruses that assemble at the plasma membrane and those that assemble in the cytoplasm are not essentially different is that a single mutation in MA can change a virus that normally assembles in the cytoplasm into a membrane assembler (Rhee and Hunter 1990).

FINAL COMMENTS

This chapter on virus structures is necessarily incomplete owing to the vastness of the topic. One may look into *Fields' Virology* or similar monumental tomes for additional information. Viruses and virus families may not have been treated here, mainly because none of the authors has worked with them: for example, the nonsymmetrical negative-strand RNA bunya and arenaviruses. However, what has become clear to us during writing this text is that even viruses of the same family can show significant differences in structure, and recent studies also demonstrate that structure may be shared between apparently distant families. We expect that the continuing development of biophysical techniques, especially X-ray crystallography and electron microscopy, will continue to play an important role in defining more details about virus morphology and connecting that information to the dynamics of protein and protein complexes, and their functions. Although we focus on virus structure here, this field also has widespread application to protein structure and function in general, as well as to the burgeoning technologies of nanoparticles and nanomachines.

ACKNOWLEDGMENTS

We thank Stephen Fuller, Hubert Laude, Yves Gaudin, Winfried Weissenhorn, and Alisdair Steven for ideas and discussions. Density maps were made in some cases from atomic coordinates deposited at the Protein Data Bank (PDB – www.pdb.org) and processed by the BSOFT package (Heymann 2001). The adenovirus 2 and PRD1 cryo-EM capsid densities used in Figure 5.8 are from the European Bioinformatics Institute (EBI) Macromolecular Structure Database (EMSD – www.ebi.ac.uk/msd). Surface views were rendered with AMIRA (TGS, San Diego USA). Tube and ribbons views were created with MolScript (Kraulis 1991), BobScript (Esnouf 1997), and Render3D (Merritt and Bacon 1997).

REFERENCES

Adrian, M., Dubochet, J., et al. 1984. Cryo-electron microscopy of viruses. *Nature*, **308**, 32–6.

Aebi, U., Bijlenga, R.K., et al. 1976. Comparison of the structural and chemical composition of giant T-even phage heads. *J Supramol Struct*, **5**, 475–95.

Ali, A., Avalos, R.T., et al. 2000. Influenza virus assembly: effect of influenza virus glycoproteins on the membrane association of M1 protein. *J Virol*, **74**, 8709–19.

Arnold, E. and Rossmann, M.G. 1990. Analysis of the structure of a common cold virus, human rhinovirus 14, refined at a resolution of 3.0 Å. *J Mol Biol*, **211**, 763–801.

Arzt, S., Baudin, F., et al. 2001. Combined results from solution studies on intact influenza virus M1 protein and from a new crystal form of its N-terminal domain show that M1 is an elongated monomer. *Virology*, **279**, 439–46.

Athappilly, F.K., Murali, R., et al. 1994. The refined crystal structure of hexon, the major coat protein of adenovirus type 2, at 2.9 Å resolution. *J Mol Biol*, **242**, 430–55.

Baker, K.A., Dutch, R.E., et al. 1999a. Structural basis for paramyxovirus-mediated membrane fusion. *Mol Cell*, **3**, 309–139.

Baker, T.S., Olson, N.H., et al. 1999b. Adding the third dimension to virus life cycles: three-dimensional reconstruction of icosahedral viruses from cryo-electron micrographs. *Microbiol Mol Biol Rev*, **63**, 862–922.

Barat, C., Schatz, O., et al. 1993. Analysis of the interactions of HIV1 replication primer tRNA (Lys,3) with nucleocapsid protein and reverse transcriptase. *J Mol Biol*, **231**, 185–90.

Barge, A., Gaudin, Y., et al. 1993. Vesicular stomatitis virus M protein may be inside the ribonucleocapsid coil. *J Virol*, **67**, 7246–53.

Barman, S., Ali, A., et al. 2001. Transport of viral proteins to the apical membranes and interaction of matrix protein with glycoproteins in the assembly of influenza viruses. *Virus Res*, **77**, 61–9.

Baudin, F., Bach, C., et al. 1994. Structure of influenza virus RNP. I. Influenza virus nucleoprotein melts secondary structure in panhandle RNA and exposes the bases to the solvent. *EMBO J*, **13**, 3158–65.

Baudin, F., Petit, I., et al. 2001. In vitro dissection of the membrane and RNP binding activities of influenza virus M1 protein. *Virology*, **281**, 102–8.

Bavari, S., Bosio, C.M., et al. 2002. Lipid raft microdomains: a gateway for compartmentalized trafficking of Ebola and Marburg viruses. *J Exp Med*, **195**, 593–602.

Becker, S., Rinne, C., et al. 1998. Interactions of Marburg virus nucleocapsid proteins. *Virology*, **249**, 406–17.

Belnap, D.M., Filman, D.J., et al. 2000. Molecular tectonic model of virus structural transitions: the putative cell entry states of poliovirus. *J Virol*, **74**, 1342–54.

Benson, S.D., Bamford, J.K., et al. 1999. Viral evolution revealed by bacteriophage PRD1 and human adenovirus coat protein structures. *Cell*, **98**, 825–33.

Benson, S.D., Bamford, J.K., et al. 2002. The X-ray crystal structure of P3, the major coat protein of the lipid-containing bacteriophage

PRD1, at 1.65 Å resolution. *Acta Crystallogr D Biol Crystallogr*, **58**, 39–59.

Berthet-Colominas, C., Monaco, S., et al. 1999. Head-to-tail dimers and interdomain flexibility revealed by the crystal structure of HIV-1 capsid protein (p24) complexed with a monoclonal antibody Fab. *EMBO J*, **18**, 1124–36.

Beuron, F., Maurizi, M.R., et al. 1998. At sixes and sevens: characterization of the symmetry mismatch of the ClpAP chaperone-assisted protease. *J Struct Biol*, **123**, 248–59.

Bhella, D., Ralph, A., et al. 2002. Significant differences in nucleocapsid morphology within the Paramyxoviridae. *J Gen Virol*, **83**, 1831–9.

Booy, F.P., Newcomb, W.W., et al. 1991. Liquid-crystalline, phage-like packing of encapsidated DNA in herpes simplex virus. *Cell*, **64**, 1007–15.

Booy, F.P., Trus, B.L., et al. 1994. Finding a needle in a haystack: detection of a small protein (the 12-kDa VP26) in a large complex (the 200-MDa capsid of herpes simplex virus). *Proc Natl Acad Sci USA*, **91**, 5652–6.

Bosch, B.J., van der Zee, R., et al. 2003. The coronavirus spike protein is a class I virus fusion protein: structural and functional characterization of the fusion core complex. *J Virol*, **77**, 8801–11.

Bottcher, B., Wynne, S.A. and Crowther, R.A. 1997. Determination of the fold of the core protein of hepatitis B virus by electron cryomicroscopy. *Nature*, **386**, 88–91.

Bowman, B.R., Baker, M.L., et al. 2003. Structure of the herpesvirus major capsid protein. *EMBO J*, **22**, 757–65.

Brenner, S. and Horne, R.W. 1959. A negative staining method for high resolution electron microscopy of viruses. *Biochim Biophys Acta*, **34**, 103.

Briggs, J.A.G., Wilk, T. and Fuller, S.D. 2003. Do lipid rafts mediate virus assembly and pseudotyping? *J Gen Virol*, **84**, 757–68.

Brinton, M.A. 1999. Arteriviruses. In: Granoff, A. and Webster, R.G. (eds), *Encyclopedia of virology*. San Diego: Academic Press, 89–97.

Brown, E.L. and Lyles, D.S. 2003. Organization of the vesicular stomatitis virus glycoprotein into membrane microdomains occurs independently of intracellular viral components. *J Virol*, **77**, 3985–92.

Brown, J.C. and Newcomb, W.W. 1987. Rhabdoviridae. In: Nermut, M.V. and Steven, A.C. (eds), *Animal virus structure*. Amsterdam: Elsevier, 199–212.

Brown, G., Rixon, H.W. and Sugrue, R.J. 2002. Respiratory syncytial virus assembly occurs in GM1-rich regions of the host-cell membrane and alters the cellular distribution of tyrosine phosphorylated caveolin-1. *J Gen Virol*, **83**, 1841–50.

Büechi, M. and Bächi, T. 1982. Microscopy of internal structures of Sendai virus associated with the cytoplasmic surface of host membranes. *Virology*, **120**, 349–59.

Bullough, P.A., Hughson, F.M., et al. 1994. Structure of influenza haemagglutinin at the pH of membrane fusion. *Nature*, **371**, 37–43.

Burmeister, W.P., Ruigrok, R.W.H. and Cusack, S. 1992. The 2.2 Å resolution crystal structure of influenza B neuraminidase and its complex with sialic acid. *EMBO J*, **11**, 49–56.

Butcher, S.J., Dokland, T., et al. 1997. Intermediates in the assembly pathway of the double-stranded RNA virus phi6. *EMBO J*, **16**, 4477–87.

Cai, M., Zheng, R., et al. 1997. Solution structure of the N-terminal zinc binding domain of HIV-1 integrase. *Nature Struct Biol*, **4**, 567–77.

Calain, P. and Roux, L. 1993. The rule of six, a basic feature for efficient replication of Sendai virus defective interfering RNA. *J Virol*, **67**, 4822–30.

Caldentey, J., Blanco, L., et al. 1992. In vitro replication of bacteriophage PRD1 DNA. Metal activation of protein-primed initiation and DNA elongation. *Nucl Acid Res*, **20**, 3971–6.

Canady, M.A., Tihova, M., et al. 2000. Large conformational changes in the maturation of a simple RNA virus, nudaurelia capensis omega virus (NomegaV). *J Mol Biol*, **299**, 573–84.

Caspar, D.L.D., Klug, A. 1962. Physical principles in the construction of regular viruses. In: *Cold Spring Harbor Symp. Quant. Biol.* 1–24.

Caston, J.R., Trus, B.L., et al. 1997. Structure of L-A virus: a specialized compartment for the transcription and replication of double-stranded RNA. *J Cell Biol*, **138**, 975–85.

Cerritelli, M.E., Cheng, N., et al. 1997. Encapsidated conformation of bacteriophage T7 DNA. *Cell*, **91**, 271–80.

Chan, D.C., Fass, D., et al. 1997. Core structure of gp41 from the HIV envelope glycoprotein. *Cell*, **89**, 263–73.

Chen, D.H., Jakana, J., et al. 2001a. The pattern of tegument-capsid interaction in the herpes simplex virus type 1 virion is not influenced by the small hexon-associated protein VP26. *J Virol*, **75**, 11863–7.

Chen, J., Lee, K.H., et al. 1998. Structure of the hemagglutinin precursor cleavage site, a determinant of influenza pathogenicity and the origin of the labile conformation. *Cell*, **95**, 409–17.

Chen, L., Gorman, J.J., et al. 2001b. The structure of the fusion glycoprotein of Newcastle disease virus suggests a novel paradigm for the molecular mechanism of membrane fusion. *Structure*, **9**, 255–66.

Cheng, R.H., Caston, J.R., et al. 1994. Fungal virus capsids, cytoplasmic compartments for the replication of double-stranded RNA, formed as icosahedral shells of asymmetric Gag dimers. *J Mol Biol*, **244**, 255–8.

Chien, C.Y., Tejero, R., et al. 1997. A novel RNA-binding motif in influenza A virus non-structural protein 1. *Nature Struct Biol*, **4**, 891–5.

Chiu, W. and Rixon, F.J. 2002. High-resolution structural studies of complex icosahedral viruses: a brief overview. *Virus Res*, **82**, 9–17.

Chong, L.D. and Rose, J.K. 1993. Membrane association of functional vesicular stomatitis virus matrix protein in vivo. *J Virol*, **67**, 407–14.

Cianci, C., Tiley, L. and Krystal, M. 1995. Differential activation of the influenza virus polymerase via template RNA binding. *J Virol*, **69**, 3995–9.

Compans, R.W., Content, J. and Duesberg, P. 1972. Structure of the ribonucleoprotein of influenza virus. *Virology*, **10**, 795–800.

Compans, R.W., Bishop, D.H.L. and Meier-Ewert, H. 1977. Structural components of influenza C viruses. *J Virol*, **21**, 658–65.

Conway, J.F., Duda, R.L., et al. 1995. Proteolytic and conformational control of virus capsid maturation: the bacteriophage HK97 system. *J Mol Biol*, **253**, 86–99.

Conway, J.F., Cheng, N., et al. 1997. Visualization of a 4-helix bundle in the hepatitis B virus capsid by cryo-electron microscopy. *Nature*, **386**, 91–4.

Conway, J.F., Wikoff, W.R., et al. 2001. Virus maturation involving large subunit rotations and local refolding. *Science*, **292**, 744–8.

Conway, J.F., Watts, N.R., et al. 2003. Characterization of a conformational epitope on hepatitis B virus core antigen and quasiequivalent variations in antibody binding. *J Virol*, **77**, 6466–73.

Crennell, S., Takimoto, T., et al. 2000. Crystal structure of the multifunctional paramyxovirus hemagglutinin-neuraminidase. *Nature Struct Biol*, **7**, 1068–74.

Crick, F.H.C. and Watson, J.D. 1956. Structure of small viruses. *Nature*, **177**, 473–5.

Crowther, R.A., Amos, L.A., et al. 1970. Three dimensional reconstructions of spherical viruses by Fourier synthesis from electron micrographs. *Nature*, **226**, 421–5.

Curran, J., Boeck, R., et al. 1995. Paramyxovirus phosphoproteins form homotrimers as determined by an epitope dilution assay, via predicted coiled coils. *Virology*, **214**, 139–49.

Cusack, S., Ruigrok, R.W.H., et al. 1985. Structure and composition of influenza virus. A small-angle neutron scattering study. *J Mol Biol*, **186**, 565–82.

Davies, H.A., Dourmashkin, R.R. and Macnaughton, M.R. 1981. Ribonucleoprotein of avian infectious bronchitis virus. *J Gen Virol*, **53**, 67–74.

de Groot, R.J., Luytjes, W., et al. 1987. Evidence for a coiled-coil structure in the spike proteins of coronaviruses. *J Mol Biol*, **196**, 963–6.

de Groot, R.J. and van Leen, R.W. 1989. Stably expressed FIPV peplomer protein induces cell fusion and elicits neutralizing antibodies in mice. *Virology*, **171**, 493–502.

Delmas, B. and Laude, H. 1990. Assembly of coronavirus spike protein into trimers and its role in epitope expression. *J Virol*, **64**, 5367–75.

Desselberger, U., Racianello, V.R., et al. 1980. The 3'- and 5'-terminal sequences of influenza A, B and C viruses are highly conserved and show partial inverted complementarity. *Gene*, **8**, 315–28.

Dessen, A., Volchkov, V., et al. 2000. Crystal structure of the matrix protein VP40 from Ebola virus. *EMBO J*, **19**, 4228–36.

Dietzschold, B., Cox, J.H. and Schneider, L.G. 1979. Rabies virus strains: A comparison study by polypeptide analysis of vaccine strains with different pathogenic patterns. *Virology*, **98**, 63–75.

Dokland, T. 2000. Freedom and restraint: themes in virus capsid assembly. *Structure Fold Des*, **8**, R157–62.

Dokland, T. and Murialdo, H. 1993. Structural transitions during maturation of bacteriophage lambda capsids. *J Mol Biol*, **233**, 682–94.

Doms, R.W., Keller, D.S., et al. 1987. Role for adenosine triphosphate in regulating the assembly and transport of vesicular stomatitis virus G protein trimers. *J Cell Biol*, **105**, 1957–69.

Duda, R.L. 1998. Protein chainmail: catenated protein in viral capsids. *Cell*, **94**, 55–60.

Duda, R.L., Hempel, J., et al. 1995. Structural transitions during bacteriophage HK97 head assembly. *J Mol Biol*, **247**, 618–35.

Dyda, F., Hickman, A.B., et al. 1994. Crystal structure of the catalytic domain of HIV-1 integrase: similarity to other polynucleotidyl transferases. *Science*, **266**, 1981–6.

Egelman, E.H. 2000. A robust algorithm for the reconstruction of helical filaments using single-particle methods. *Ultramicroscopy*, **85**, 225–34.

Egelman, E.H., Wu, S.-S., et al. 1989. The Sendai virus nucleocapsid exists in at least four different helical states. *J Virol*, **63**, 2233–43.

Eijkelenboom, A.P., Lutzke, R.A., et al. 1995. The DNA-binding domain of HIV-1 integrase has an SH3-like fold. *Nature Struct Biol*, **2**, 807–10.

Esnouf, R.M. 1997. An extensively modified version of MolScript that includes greatly enhanced coloring capabilities. *J Mol Graph Model*, **15**, 132–4.

Feldmann, H. and Kiley, M.P. 1998. Classification, structure, and replication of filoviruses. *Curr Topic Microbiol Immunol*, **235**, 1–21.

Feldmann, H. and Klenk, H.-D. 1996. Marburg and Ebola viruses. *Adv Virus Res*, **47**, 1–52.

Feng, Y.X., Campbell, S., et al. 1999. The human immunodeficiency virus type 1 Gag polyprotein has nucleic acid chaperone activity: possible role in dimerization of genomic RNA and placement of tRNA on the primer binding site. *J Virol*, **73**, 4251–6.

Fisher, A.J. and Johnson, J.E. 1993. Ordered duplex RNA controls capsid architecture in an icosahedral animal virus. *Nature*, **361**, 176–9.

Flamand, A., Raux, H., et al. 1993. Mechanisms of rabies virus neutralisation. *Virology*, **194**, 302–13.

Flewett, T.H. and Apostolov, K. 1967. A reticular structure in the wall of influenza C virus. *J Gen Virol*, **1**, 297–304.

Fraser, C.M., Gocayne, J.D., et al. 1995. The minimal gene complement of *Mycoplasma genitalium*. *Science*, **270**, 397–403.

Forster, M.J., Mulloy, B. and Nermut, M.V. 2000. Molecular modelling study of HIV p17gag (MA) protein shell utilising data from electron microscopy and X-ray crystallography. *J Mol Biol*, **298**, 841–57.

Fricks, C.E. and Hogle, J.M. 1990. Cell-induced conformational change in poliovirus: externalization of the amino terminus of VP1 is responsible for liposome binding. *J Virol*, **64**, 1934–45.

Fuller, S.D., Wilk, T., et al. 1997. Cryo-electron microscopy revealsordered domains in the immature HIV-1 particle. *Curr Biol*, **7**, 729–38.

Gallagher, T.M., Escarmis, C. and Buchmeier, M.J. 1991. Alteration of the pH dependence of coronavirus-induced cell fusion: effect of mutations in the spike glycoprotein. *J Virol*, **65**, 1916–28.

Gamble, T.R., Vajdos, F.F., et al. 1996. Crystal structure of human cyclophilin A bound to the amino-terminal domain of HIV-1 capsid. *Cell*, **87**, 1285–94.

Gamble, T.R., Yoo, S., et al. 1997. Structure of the carboxyl-terminal dimerization domain of the HIV-1 capsid protein. *Science*, **278**, 849–53.

Ganser, B.K., Li, S., et al. 1999. Assembly and analysis of conical models for the HIV-1 core. *Science*, **283**, 80–3.

Gaudier, M., Gaudin, Y. and Knossow, M. 2002. Crystal structure of vesicular stomatitis virus matrix protein. *Embo J*, **17**, 2886–92.

Gaudin, Y., Ruigrok, R.W.H., et al. 1992. Rabies glycoprotein is a trimer. *Virology*, **187**, 627–32.

Gaudin, Y., Barge, A., et al. 1995a. Aggregation of VSV M protein is reversible and mediated by nucleation sites: implications for viral assembly. *Virology*, **206**, 28–37.

Gaudin, Y., Ruigrok, R.W.H. and Brunner, J. 1995b. Low-pH induced conformational changes in viral fusion proteins: implications for fusion mechanism. *J Gen Virol*, **76**, 1541–56.

Gaudin, Y., Raux, H., et al. 1996. Identification of amino acids controlling the low-pH-induced conformational change of rabies virus glycoprotein. *J Virol*, **70**, 7371–8.

Gaudin, Y., Sturgis, J., et al. 1997. Conformational flexibility and polymerization of vesicular stomatitis virus matrix protein. *J Mol Biol*, **274**, 5, 816–25.

Gaudin, Y., Tuffereau, C., et al. 1999. Rabies virus-induced membrane fusion. *Mol Membr Biol*, **16**, 21–31.

Gigant, B., Iseni, F., et al. 2000. Neither phosphorylation nor the amino-terminal part of rabies virus phosphoprotein is required for its oligomerization. *J Gen Virol*, **81**, 1757–61.

Gitti, R.K., Lee, B.M., et al. 1996. Structure of the amino-terminal core domain of the HIV-1 capsid protein. *Science*, **273**, 231–5.

Goff, S.P. 2001. Retroviridae: The retroviruses and their replication. In: Knipe, D.M. and Howley, P.M. (eds), *Field's Virology*, 4th edn. Philadelphia: Lippincott, Williams and Wilkins, 1871–939.

Gomis-Rüth, F.X., Dessen, A., et al. 2003. The matrix protein VP40 from Ebola virus octamerizes into pore-like structures with specific RNA binding properties. *Structure (Camb)*, **11**, 423–33.

Gouet, P., Diprose, J.M., et al. 1999. The highly ordered double-stranded RNA genome of bluetongue virus revealed by crystallography. *Cell*, **97**, 481–90.

Greber, U.F., Webster, P., et al. 1996. The role of the adenovirus protease on virus entry into cells. *EMBO J*, **15**, 1766–77.

Grimes, J.M., Burroughs, J.N., et al. 1998. The atomic structure of the bluetongue virus core. *Nature*, **395**, 470–8.

Ha, Y., Stevens, D.J., et al. 2002. H5 avian and H9 swine influenza virus haemagglutinin structures: possible origin of influenza subtypes. *EMBO J*, **21**, 865–75.

Hagen, M., Chung, T.D., et al. 1994. Recombinant influenza virus polymerase: requirement of both 5' and 3' viral ends for endonuclease activity. *J Virol*, **68**, 1509–15.

Hansen, G.H., Delmas, B., et al. 1998. The coronavirus transmissible gastroenteritis virus causes infection after receptor-mediated endocytosis and acid-dependent fusion with an intracellular compartment. *J Virol*, **72**, 527–34.

Harrison, S.C., Olson, A.J., et al. 1978. Tomato bushy stunt virus at 2.9 Å resolution. *Nature*, **276**, 368–73.

Hay, A.J., Wolstenholme, A.J., et al. 1985. The molecular basis of the specific anti-influenza action of amantadine. *EMBO J*, **4**, 3021–4.

Heggeness, M.H., Smith, P.R. and Choppin, P.W. 1982. In vitro assembly of the nonglycosylated membrane protein (M) of Sendai virus. *Proc Natl Acad Sci USA*, **79**, 6232–6.

Henderson, G., Murray, J. and Yeo, R.P. 2002. Sorting of the respiratory syncytial virus matrix protein into detergent-resistant structures is dependent on cell-surface expression of the glycoproteins. *Virology*, **300**, 244–54.

Herrler, G., Nagele, A., et al. 1981. Isolation and structural analysis of influenza C virion glycoproteins. *Virology*, **113**, 439–51.

Hewat, E.A., Neumann, E., et al. 2000. The cellular receptor to human rhinovirus 2 binds around the 5-fold axis and not in the canyon: a structural view. *EMBO J*, **19**, 6317–25.

Hewat, E.A., Neumann, E. and Blaas, D. 2002. The concerted conformational changes during human rhinovirus 2 uncoating. *Mol Cell*, **10**, 317–26.

Hewitt, J.A. and Nermut, M.V. 1977. A morphological study of the M-protein of Sendai virus. *J Gen Virol*, **34**, 127–36.

Heymann, J.B. 2001. Bsoft: Image and molecular processing in electron microscopy. *J Struct Biol*, **133**, 156–69.

Heymann, J.B., Cheng, N., et al. 2003. Dynamics of herpes simplex virus capsid maturation visualized by time-lapse cryo-electron microscopy. *Nature Struct Biol*, **10**, 334–41.

Hill, C.P., Worthylake, D., et al. 1996. Crystal structures of the trimeric human immunodeficiency virus type 1 matrix protein: implications for membrane association and assembly. *Proc Natl Acad Sci USA*, **93**, 3099–104.

Hogle, J.M., Chow, M. and Filman, D.J. 1985. Three-dimensional structure of poliovirus at 2.9 Å resolution. *Science*, **229**, 1358–65.

Horne, R.W., Kausche, G.A., et al. 1939. Electron microscopy of tobacco mosaic virus. Die Sichtbarmachung von pflanzlichem Virus im Übermikroskop. *Naturwissenschaften*, **27**, 292–9.

Hutson, M.S., Holzwarth, G., et al. 1995. Two-dimensional motion of DNA bands during 120° pulsed-field gel electrophoresis. I. Effect of molecular weight. *Biopolymers*, **35**, 297–306.

Iseni, F., Barge, A., et al. 1998. Characterization of rabies virus nucleocapsids and recombinant nucleocapsid-like structures. *J Gen Virol*, **79**, 2909–19.

Iseni, F., Baudin, F., et al. 2000. Structure of the RNA inside the vesicular stomatitis virus nucleocapsid. *RNA*, **6**, 270–81.

Iseni, F., Baudin, F., et al. 2002. Chemical modification of nucleotide bases and mRNA editing depend on hexamer or nucleoprotein phase in Sendai virus nucleocapsids. *RNA*, **8**, 1056–67.

Iwasaki, K., Trus, B.L., et al. 2000. Molecular architecture of bacteriophage T4 capsid: vertex structure and bimodal binding of the stabilizing accessory protein, Soc. *Virology*, **271**, 321–33.

Jennings, P.A., Finch, J.T., et al. 1983. Does the higher order structure of the influenza virus ribonucleoprotein guide sequence rearrangements in influenza virus RNA? *Cell*, **34**, 619–27.

Jiang, W., Li, Z., et al. 2003. Coat protein fold and maturation transition of bacteriophage P22 seen at subnanometer resolutions. *Nature Struct Biol*, **10**, 131–5.

Jin, H., Leser, G.P., et al. 1997. Influenza virus hemagglutinin and neuraminidase cytoplasmic tails control particle shape. *EMBO J*, **16**, 1236–47.

Johnson, J.E. and Chiu, W. 2000. Structures of virus and virus-like particles. *Curr Opin Struct Biol*, **10**, 229–35.

Johnson, J.E. and Speir, J.A. 1997. Quasi-equivalent viruses: a paradigm for protein assemblies. *J Mol Biol*, **269**, 665–75.

Johnson, J.E., Rodgers, W. and Rose, J.K. 1998. A plasma membrane localization signal in the HIV-1 envelope cytoplasmic domain prevents localization at sites of vesicular stomatitis virus budding and incorporation into VSV virions. *Virology*, **251**, 244–52.

Junge, W., Panke, O., et al. 2001. Inter-subunit rotation and elastic power transmission in F0F1-ATPase. *FEBS Lett*, **504**, 152–60.

Kieft, J.S., Zhou, K., et al. 2001. Mechanism of ribosome recruitment by hepatitis C IRES RNA. *RNA*, **7**, 194–206.

King, J. and Casjens, S. 1974. Catalytic head assembling protein in virus morphogenesis. *Nature*, **251**, 112–19.

Kingston, R.L., Olson, N.H. and Vogt, V.M. 2001. The organization of mature Rous sarcoma virus as studied by cryoelectron microscopy. *J Struct Biol*, **136**, 67–80.

Klumpp, K., Ruigrok, R.W.H. and Baudin, F. 1997. Roles of the influenza virus polymerase and nucleoprotein in forming a functional RNP structure. *EMBO J*, **16**, 1248–57.

Kohlstaedt, L.A., Wang, J., et al. 1992. Crystal structure at 3.5 Å resolution of HIV-1 reverse transcriptase complexed with an inhibitor. *Science*, **256**, 1783–90.

Kolakofsky, D., Pelet, T., et al. 1998. Paramyxovirus RNA synthesis and the requirement for hexamer genome length: the rule of six revisited. *J Virol*, **72**, 891–9.

Kolesnikova, L., Mühlberger, E., et al. 2000. Ultrastructural organization of recombinant Marburg virus nucleoprotein: comparison with Marburg virus inclusions. *J Virol*, **74**, 3899–904.

Kraulis, P.J. 1991. MOLSCRIPT: a program to produce both detailed and schematic plots of protein structures. *J Appl Cryst*, **24**, 946–50.

Kwong, P.D., Wyatt, R., et al. 1998. Structure of an HIV gp120 envelope glycoprotein in complex with the CD4 receptor and a neutralizing human antibody. *Nature*, **393**, 648–59.

La Scola, B., Audic, S., et al. 2003. A giant virus in amoebae. *Science*, **299**, 2033.

Lai, M.M.C. and Cavanagh, D. 1997. The molecular biology of coronaviruses. *Adv Virus Res*, **48**, 1–100.

Lai, M.M.C. and Holmes, K.V. 2001. Coronaviridae: The viruses and their replication. In: Knipe, D.M. and Howley, P.M. (eds), *Field's Virology*, 4th edn. Baltimore: Lippincott, Williams and Wilkins, 1163–86.

Lata, R., Conway, J.F., et al. 2000. Maturation dynamics of a viral capsid: visualization of transitional intermediate states. *Cell*, **100**, 253–63.

Laude, H. and Masters, P.S. 1995. The coronavirus nucleocapsid protein. In: Sidell, S.G. (ed.), *The Coronaviridae*. New York: Plenum Press, 141–63.

Lawton, J.A., Zeng, C.Q., et al. 1997. Three-dimensional structural analysis of recombinant rotavirus-like particles with intact and amino-terminal-deleted VP2: implications for the architecture of the VP2 capsid layer. *J Virol*, **71**, 7353–60.

Lepault, J., Petitpas, I., et al. 2001. Structural polymorphism of the major capsid protein of rotavirus. *EMBO J*, **20**, 1498–507.

Li, H., DeRosier, D.J., et al. 2002. Microtubule structure at 8 Å resolution. *Structure (Camb)*, **10**, 1317–28.

Li, M.L., Rao, P. and Krug, R.M. 2001. The active sites of the influenza cap-dependent endonuclease are on different polymerase subunits. *EMBO J*, **20**, 2078–86.

Li, S., Hill, P., et al. 2000. Image reconstruction of helical assemblies of the HIV-1 CA protein. *Nature*, **407**, 409–13.

Liddington, R.C., Yan, Y., et al. 1991. Structure of simian virus 40 at 3.8-Å resolution. *Nature*, **354**, 278–84.

Liu, J., Lynch, P.A., et al. 1997. Crystal structure of the unique RNA-binding domain of the influenza virus NS1 protein. *Nature Struct Biol*, **4**, 896–9.

Lodi, P.J., Ernst, J.A., et al. 1995. Solution structure of the DNA binding domain of HIV-1 integrase. *Biochemistry*, **34**, 9826–33.

Lomniczi, B. 1977. Biological properties of avian coronavirus RNA. *J Gen Virol*, **36**, 531–3.

London, E. and Brown, D.A. 2000. Insolubility of lipids in triton X-100: physical origin and relationship to sphingolipid/cholesterol membrane domains (rafts). *Biochim Biophys Acta*, **1508**, 182–95.

Machamer, C.E. and Rose, J.K. 1987. A specific transmembrane domain of a coronavirus E1 glycoprotein is required for its retention in the Golgi region. *J Cell Biol*, **105**, 1205–14.

Macnaughton, M.R., Davies, H.A. and Nermut, M.V. 1978. Ribonucleoprotein-like structures from coronavirus particles. *J Gen Virol*, **39**, 545–9.

Malashkevich, V.N., Schneider, B.J., et al. 1999. Core structure of the envelope glycoprotein GP2 from Ebola virus at 1.9-Å resolution. *Proc Natl Acad Sci USA*, **96**, 2662–7.

Mancini, E.J., Clarke, M., et al. 2000. Cryo-electron microscopy reveals the functional organization of an enveloped virus, Semliki Forest virus. *Mol Cell*, **5**, 255–66.

Manes, S., del Real, G., et al. 2000. Membrane raft microdomains mediate lateral assemblies required for HIV- infection. *EMBO Rep*, **1**, 190–6.

Manie, S.N., Debreyne, S., et al. 2000. Measles virus structural components are enriched into lipid raft microdomains: a potential cellular location for virus assembly. *J Virol*, **74**, 305–11.

Martin, C.S., Burnett, R.M., et al. 2001. Combined EM/X-ray imaging yields a quasi-atomic model of the adenovirus-related bacteriophage PRD1 and shows key capsid and membrane interactions. *Structure (Camb)*, **9**, 917–30.

Martin, K. and Helenius, A. 1991. Nuclear transport of influenza virus ribonucleoproteins: The viral matrix protein (M1) promotes export and inhibits import. *Cell*, **67**, 117–30.

Martín-Benito, J., Area, E., et al. 2001. Three-dimensional reconstruction of a recombinant influenza virus ribonucleoprotein particle. *EMBO Rep*, **2**, 313–17.

Massiah, M.A., Starich, M.R., et al. 1994. Three-dimensional structure of the human immunodeficiency virus type 1 matrix protein. *J Mol Biol*, **244**, 198–223.

Matthews, S., Barlow, P., et al. 1994. Structural similarity between the p17 matrix protein of HIV-1 and interferon-gamma. *Nature*, **370**, 666–8.

Mavrakis, M., Kolesnikova, L., et al. 2002. Morphology of Marburg virus NP-RNA. *Virology*, **296**, 2, 300–7.

Mayo, K., Huseby, D., et al. 2003. Retrovirus capsid protein assembly arrangements. *J Mol Biol*, **325**, 225–37.

Merritt, E.A. and Bacon, D.J. 1997. Raster3D: photorealistic molecular graphics. *Meth Enzymol*, **277**, 505–24.

Miller, M., Schneider, J., et al. 1989. Structure of complex of synthetic HIV-1 protease with a substrate-based inhibitor at 2.3 Å resolution. *Science*, **246**, 1149–5211.

Modis, Y., Trus, B.L. and Harrison, S.C. 2002. Atomic model of the papillomavirus capsid. *EMBO J*, **21**, 4754–62.

Modrof, J., Möritz, C., et al. 2001. Phosphorylation of Marburg virus VP30 at serines 40 and 42 is critical for its interaction with NP inclusions. *Virology*, **287**, 171–82.

Momany, C., Kovari, L.C., et al. 1996. Crystal structure of dimeric HIV-1 capsid protein. *Nature Struct Biol*, **3**, 763–70.

Morellet, N., Jullian, N., et al. 1992. Determination of the structure of the nucleocapsid protein NCp7 from the human immunodeficiency virus type 1 by 1H NMR. *EMBO J*, **11**, 3059–65.

Murti, K.G., Bean, W.J. Jr. and Webster, R.G. 1980. Helical ribonucleoproteins of influenza virus: an electron microscopic analysis. *Virology*, **104**, 224–9.

Murti, K.G., Brown, P.S., et al. 1992. Composition of the helical internal components of influenza virus as revealed by immunogold labeling/electron microscopy. *Virology*, **186**, 294–9.

Naitow, H., Tang, J., et al. 2002. L-A virus at 3.4 Å resolution reveals particle architecture and mRNA decapping mechanism. *Nature Struct Biol*, **9**, 725–8.

Namba, K. and Stubbs, G. 1986. Structure of tobacco mosaic virus at 3.6 Å resolution: implications for assembly. *Science*, **231**, 1401–6.

Nandhagopal, N., Simpson, A.A., et al. 2002. The structure and evolution of the major capsid protein of a large, lipid-containing DNA virus. *Proc Natl Acad Sci USA*, **99**, 14758–63.

Nave, C., Fowler, A.G., et al. 1979. Macromolecular structural transitions in Pf1 filamentous bacterial virus. *Nature*, **281**, 232–4.

Nave, C., Brown, R.S., et al. 1981. Pf1 filamentous bacterial virus. X-ray fibre diffraction analysis of two heavy-atom derivatives. *J Mol Biol*, **149**, 675–707.

Navia, M.A., Fitzgerald, P.M., et al. 1989. Three-dimensional structure of aspartyl protease from human immunodeficiency virus HIV-1. *Nature*, **337**, 615–20.

Nermut, M.V., Hockley, D.J., et al. 1994. Fullerene-like organization of HIV gag-protein shell in virus-like particles produced by recombinant baculovirus. *Virology*, **198**, 288–96.

Nermut, M.V., Bron, P., et al. 2002. Molecular organization of Mason–Pfizer monkey virus capsids assembled from Gag polyprotein in *Escherichia coli*. *J Virol*, **76**, 4321–30.

Newcomb, W.W. and Brown, J.C. 1981. Role of the vesicular stomatitis virus matrix protein in maintaining the viral nucleocapsid in the condensed form found in native virions. *J Virol*, **39**, 295–9.

Newcomb, W.W., Tobin, G.J., et al. 1982. In vitro reassembly of vesicular stomatitis virus skeletons. *J Virol*, **41**, 1055–62.

Newcomb, W.W., Juhas, R.M., et al. 2001. The UL6 gene product forms the portal for entry of DNA into the herpes simplex virus capsid. *J Virol*, **75**, 10923–32.

Nicholson, P., Addison, C., et al. 1994. Localization of the herpes simplex virus type major capsid protein VP5 to the cell nucleus

requires the abundant scaffolding protein VP22a. *J Gen Virol*, **75**, 1091–9.

Odenwald, W.F., Arnheiter, H., et al. 1986. Stereo images of vesicular stomatitis virus assembly. *J Virol*, **57**, 922–32.

Olson, N.H., Gingery, M., et al. 2001. The structure of isometric capsids of bacteriophage T4. *Virology*, **279**, 385–91.

Ono, A. and Freed, E.O. 2001. Plasma membrane rafts play a critical role in HIV-1 assembly and release. *Proc Natl Acad Sci USA*, **98**, 13925–30.

Ortega, J., Martín-Benito, J., et al. 2000. Ultrastructural and functional analysis of recombinant influenza virus ribonucleoproteins suggests dimerization of nucleoprotein during virus amplification. *J Virol*, **74**, 156–63.

Owens, R.J. and Rose, J.K. 1993. Cytoplasmic domain requirement for incorporation of a foreign envelope protein into vesicular stomatitis virus. *J Virol*, **67**, 360–5.

Pinto, L.H., Holsinger, L.J. and Lamb, R.A. 1992. Influenza virus M2 protein has ion channel activity. *Cell*, **69**, 517–28.

Porta, C., Wang, G., et al. 1994. Direct imaging of interactions between an icosahedral virus and conjugate F(ab) fragments by cryoelectron microscopy and X-ray crystallography. *Virology*, **204**, 777–88.

Prasad, B.V., Burns, J.W., et al. 1990. Localization of VP4 neutralization sites in rotavirus by three-dimensional cryo-electron microscopy. *Nature*, **343**, 476–9.

Reinisch, K.M., Nibert, M.L. and Harrison, S.C. 2000. Structure of the reovirus core at 3.6 Å resolution. *Nature*, **404**, 960–7.

Rhee, S.S. and Hunter, E. 1990. A single amino acid substitution within the matrix protein of a type D retrovirus converts its morphogenesis to that of a type C retrovirus. *Cell*, **63**, 77–86.

Risco, C., Muntion, M., et al. 1998. Two types of virus-related particles are found during transmissible gastroenteritis virus morphogenesis. *J Virol*, **72**, 4022–31.

Roberts, M.M., White, J.L., et al. 1986. Three-dimensional structure of the adenovirus major coat protein hexon. *Science*, **232**, 1148–51.

Rosenthal, P.B., Zhang, X., et al. 1998. Structure of the haemagglutinin-esterase-fusion glycoprotein of influenza C virus. *Nature*, **396**, 92–6.

Rossmann, M.G. and Johnson, J.E. 1989. Icosahedral RNA virus structure. *Annu Rev Biochem*, **58**, 533–73.

Rossmann, M.G., Olson, N.H., et al. 1994. Crystallographic and cryo EM analysis of virion–receptor interactions. *Arch Virol Suppl*, **9**, 531–41.

Ruigrok, R.W.H. 1998. Structure of influenza A, B, and C viruses. In: Nicholson, K.G., Webster, R.G. and Hay, A.J. (eds), *Textbook of influenza*. Oxford: Blackwell Science, 29–42.

Ruigrok, R.W.H. and Baudin, F. 1995. Structure of Influenza virus RNP. II. Purified, RNA-free Influenza ribonucleoprotein forms structures that are indistinguishable from the intact viral ribonucleoprotein particles. *J Gen Virol*, **76**, 1009–14.

Ruigrok, R.W.H., Calder, L.J. and Wharton, S.A. 1989. Electron microscopy of the influenza virus submembranal structure. *Virology*, **173**, 311–16.

Ruigrok, R.W.H., Barge, A., et al. 2000a. Membrane interaction of influenza virus M1 protein. *Virology*, **267**, 289–98.

Ruigrok, R.W., Schoehn, G., et al. 2000b. Structural characterization and membrane binding properties of the matrix protein VP40 of Ebola virus. *J Mol Biol*, **300**, 103–12.

Salanueva, I.J., Carrascosa, J.L. and Risco, C. 1999. Structural maturation of the transmissible gastroenteritis coronavirus. *J Virol*, **73**, 7952–64.

Salunke, D.M., Caspar, D.L. and Garcea, R.L. 1989. Polymorphism in the assembly of polyomavirus capsid protein VP1. *Biophys J*, **56**, 887–900.

San Martin, C., Huiskonen, J.T., et al. 2002. Minor proteins, mobile arms and membrane–capsid interactions in the bacteriophage PRD1 capsid. *Nature Struct Biol*, **9**, 1, 756–63.

Sandaa, R.A., Heldal, M., et al. 2001. Isolation and characterization of two viruses with large genome size infecting *Chrysochromulina ericina* (Prymnesiophyceae) and *Pyramimonas orientalis* (Prasinophyceae). *Virology*, **290**, 272–80.

Sarnow, P. 2003. Viral internal ribosome entry site elements: novel ribosome–RNA complexes and roles in viral pathogenesis. *J Virol*, **77**, 2801–6.

Scheiffele, P., Rietveld, A., et al. 1999. Influenza viruses select ordered lipid domains during budding from the plasma membrane. *J Biol Chem*, **274**, 2038–44.

Schmitt, A.P. and Lamb, R.A. 2004. Escaping from the cell: assembly and budding of negative-strand RNA viruses. *Curr Top Microbiol Immunol*, **283**, 145–96.

Schochetman, G., Stevens, R.H. and Simpson, R.W. 1977. Presence of infectious polyadenylated RNA in coronavirus avian bronchitis virus. *Virology*, **77**, 772–82.

Schoehn, G., Iseni, F., et al. 2001. Structure of recombinant rabies virus N-RNA and identification of the phosphoprotein binding site. *J Virol*, **75**, 490–8.

Sha, B. and Luo, M. 1997. Structure of a bifunctional membrane-RNA binding protein, influenza virus matrix protein M1. *Nature Struct Biol*, **4**, 239–44.

Shuck, K., Lamb, R.A. and Pinto, L.H. 2000. Analysis of the pore structure of the influenza A virus M_2 ion channel by the substituted-cysteine accessibility method. *J Virol*, **74**, 7755–61.

Simons, K. and Ehehalt, R. 2002. Cholesterol, lipid rafts and disease. *J Clin Invest*, **110**, 597–603.

Simpson, A.A., Tao, Y., et al. 2000. Structure of the bacteriophage phi29 DNA packaging motor. *Nature*, **408**, 745–50.

Skehel, J.J. and Wiley, D.C. 1998. Coiled coils in both intracellular vesicle and viral membrane fusion. *Cell*, **95**, 871–4.

Skehel, J.J. and Wiley, D.C. 2000. Receptor binding and membrane fusion in virus entry: the influenza hemagglutinin. *Annu Rev Biochem*, **69**, 531–69.

Speir, J.A., Munshi, S., et al. 1995. Structures of the native and swollen forms of cowpea chlorotic mottle virus determined by X-ray crystallography and cryo-electron microscopy. *Structure*, **3**, 63–78.

Stehle, T., Gamblin, S.J., et al. 1996. The structure of simian virus 40 refined at 3.1 Å resolution. *Structure*, **4**, 165–82.

Sternberg, N. and Weisberg, R. 1977. Packaging of coliphage lambda DNA. II. The role of the gene D protein. *J Mol Biol*, **117**, 733–59.

Stewart, L., Schatz, G. and Vogt, V.M. 1990. Properties of avian retrovirus particles defective in viral protease. *J Virol*, **64**, 5076–92.

Stewart, P.L., Fuller, S.D. and Burnett, R.M. 1993. Difference imaging of adenovirus: bridging the resolution gap between X-ray crystallography and electron microscopy. *EMBO J*, **12**, 2589–99.

Stohlman, S.A., Fleming, J.O., et al. 1983. Synthesis and subcellular localization of the murine coronavirus nucleocapsid protein. *Virology*, **130**, 527–32.

Sugrue, R.J. and Hay, A.J. 1991. Structural characteristics of the M2 protein of influenza A viruses: Evidence that it forms a tetrameric channel. *Virology*, **180**, 617–24.

Summers, M.F., Henderson, L.E., et al. 1992. Nucleocapsid zinc fingers detected in retroviruses: EXAFS studies of intact viruses and the solution-state structure of the nucleocapsid protein from HIV-1. *Protein Sci*, **1**, 563–74.

Suzuki, H. and Taguchi, F. 1996. Analysis of the receptor-binding site of murine coronavirus spike protein. *J Virol*, **70**, 2632–6.

Tan, K., Liu, J., et al. 1997. Atomic structure of a thermostable subdomain of HIV-1 gp41. *Proc Natl Acad Sci USA*, **94**, 12303–8.

Tang, L., Johnson, K.N., et al. 2001. The structure of pariacoto virus reveals a dodecahedral cage of duplex RNA. *Nature Struct Biol*, **8**, 77–83.

Tarbouriech, N., Curran, J., et al. 2000. Tetrameric coiled coil domain of Sendai virus phosphoprotein. *Nature Struct Biol*, **7**, 777–81.

Thomas, D., Newcomb, W.W., et al. 1985. Mass and molecular composition of vesicular stomatitis virus: a scanning transmission electron microscopy analysis. *J Virol*, **54**, 598–607.

Thomas, D.R., Morgan, D.G. and DeRosier, D.J. 1999. Rotational symmetry of the C ring and a mechanism for the flagellar rotary motor. *Proc Natl Acad Sci USA*, **96**, 10134–9.

Thuman-Commike, P.A., Greene, B., et al. 1998. Role of the scaffolding protein in P22 procapsid size determination suggested by $T = 4$ and $T = 7$ procapsid structures. *Biophys J*, **74**, 559–68.

Timmins, J., Schoehn, G., et al. 2003. Oligomerization and polymerization of the filovirus matrix protein VP40. *Virology*, **312**, 359–68.

Trus, B.L., Booy, F.P., et al. 1996. The herpes simplex virus procapsid: structure, conformational changes upon maturation, and roles of the triplex proteins VP19c and VP23 in assembly. *J Mol Biol*, **263**, 447–62.

Trus, B.L., Gibson, W., et al. 1999. Capsid structure of simian cytomegalovirus from cryoelectron microscopy: evidence for tegument attachment sites. *J Virol*, **73**, 2181–92.

Van Etten, J.L., Graves, M.V., et al. 2002. Phycodnaviridae, large DNA algal virus. *Arch Virol*, **147**, 1479–516.

van Marle, G., Dobbe, J.C., et al. 1999. Arterivirus discontinuous mRNA transcription is guided by base pairing between sense and antisense transcription-regulating sequences. *Proc Natl Acad Sci USA*, **96**, 12056–61.

van Vliet, A.L., Smits, S.L., et al. 2002. Discontinuous and non-discontinuous subgenomic RNA transcription in a nidovirus. *EMBO J*, **21**, 6571–80.

Varghese, J.N., Laver, W.G. and Colman, P.M. 1983. Structure of the influenza virus glycoprotein antigen neuraminidase at 2.9 Å resolution. *Nature*, **303**, 35–40.

Vennema, H., Godeke, G.J., et al. 1996. Nucleocapsid-independent assembly of coronavirus-like particles by co-expression of viral envelope protein genes. *EMBO J*, **15**, 2020–8.

Watts, N.R., Conway, J.F., et al. 2002. The morphogenic linker peptide of HBV capsid protein forms a mobile array on the interior surface. *EMBO J*, **21**, 876–84.

Weissenhorn, W., Carfi, A., et al. 1998. Crystal structure of the Ebola virus membrane fusion subunit, Gp2, from the envelope glycoprotein ectodomain. *Mol Cell*, **2**, 605–16.

Weissenhorn, W., Dessen, A., et al. 1997. Atomic structure of an ectodomain from HIV-1 gp41. *Nature*, **387**, 426–30.

Wieringa, R., de Vries, A.A., et al. 2002. Characterization of two new structural glycoproteins, GP_3 and GP_4, of equine arteritis virus. *J Virol*, **76**, 10829–40.

Wikoff, W.R., Liljas, L., et al. 2000. Topologically linked protein rings in the bacteriophage HK97 capsid. *Science*, **289**, 2129–33.

Wilson, I.A., Skehel, J.J. and Wiley, D.C. 1981. Structure of the haemagglutinin membrane glycoprotein of influenza virus at 3 Å resolution. *Nature*, **289**, 366–73.

Wlodawer, A., Miller, M., et al. 1989. Conserved folding in retroviral proteases: crystal structure of a synthetic HIV-1 protease. *Science*, **245**, 616–21.

Wu, W., Henderson, L.E., et al. 1996. Human immunodeficiency virus type 1 nucleocapsid protein reduces reverse transcriptase pausing at a secondary structure near the murine leukemia virus polypurine tract. *J Virol*, **70**, 7132–42.

Wynne, S.A., Crowther, R.A. and Leslie, A.G. 1999. The crystal structure of the human hepatitis B virus capsid. *Mol Cell*, **3**, 771–80.

Yan, X., Olson, N.H., et al. 2000. Structure and assembly of large lipid-containing dsDNA viruses. *Nature Struct Biol*, **7**, 101–3.

Yang, F., Forrer, P., et al. 2000. Novel fold and capsid-binding properties of the λ-phage display platform protein gpD. *Nature Struct Biol*, **7**, 230–7.

Yeager, M., Wilson-Kubalek, E.M., et al. 1998. Supramolecular organization of immature and mature murine leukemia virus revealed by electron cryo-microscopy: Implications for retroviral assembly mechanisms. *Proc Natl Acad Sci USA*, **95**, 7299–304.

Yoo, D.W., Parker, M.D. and Babiuk, L.A. 1991. The S2 subunit of the spike glycoprotein of bovine coronavirus mediates membrane fusion in insect cells. *Virology*, **180**, 395–9.

Zebedee, S.L. and Lamb, R.A. 1989. Growth restriction of influenza A virus by M2 protein antibody is genetically linked to the M1 protein. *Proc Natl Acad Sci USA*, **86**, 1061–5.

Zelus, B.D., Schickli, J.H., et al. 2003. Conformational changes in the spike glycoprotein of murine coronavirus are induced at 37 degrees C either by soluble murine CEACAM1 receptors or by pH 8. *J Virol*, **77**, 830–40.

Zhang, J., Leser, G.P., et al. 2000a. The cytoplasmic tails of the influenza virus spike glycoproteins are required for normal genome packaging. *Virology*, **269**, 325–34.

Zhang, J., Pekosz, A. and Lamb, R.A. 2000b. Influenza virus assembly and lipid raft microdomains: a role for the cytoplasmic tails of the spike glycoproteins. *J Virol*, **74**, 4634–44.

Zhang, W., Mukhopadhyay, S., et al. 2002. Placement of the structural proteins in Sindbis virus. *J Virol*, **76**, 11645–58.

Zhang, W., Olson, N.H., et al. 2001. Structure of the maize streak virus geminate particle. *Virology*, **279**, 471–7.

Zhao, X., Singh, M., et al. 2000. Structural characterization of the human respiratory syncytial virus fusion protein core. *Proc Natl Acad Sci USA*, **97**, 14172–7.

Zhou, Z.H., Dougherty, M., et al. 2000. Seeing the herpesvirus capsid at 8.5 Å. *Science*, **288**, 877–80.

Zlotnick, A., Stahl, S.J., et al. 1998. Shared motifs of the capsid proteins of hepadnaviruses and retroviruses suggest a common evolutionary origin. *FEBS Lett*, **431**, 301–4.

6

Propagation and identification of viruses

DEAN D. ERDMAN

This chapter provides an overview of the main techniques used for propagating and identifying viruses. Detailed descriptions can be found in the appropriate journal citations. In some instances, more general references are made to textbooks of laboratory methods, without necessarily citing specific sections.

SYSTEMS FOR PROPAGATING VIRUSES

Viruses can only replicate in living cells. Therefore, an essential first step in propagating viruses in the laboratory is the provision of a suitable culture system. Cell culture is the most widely used method for propagating viruses, but older techniques, such as tissue or organ culture, may still be used for specialized purposes, as may chick embryo and animal inoculation.

Cell culture

GENERAL

Cell cultures are prepared either as single layers (monolayers) on a glass or plastic surface, or as suspensions, the choice depending on their proposed use. Another choice to be made is the type of cell needed for a particular study. Several international repositories can serve as the starting point for reference cell lines and for microbiological reagents. They include the European Collection of Animal Cell Cultures (www.ecacc.org.uk), the American Type Culture Collection (ATCC)

(www.atcc.org), Statens Seruminstitut (www.ssi.dk/sw162.asp), and Institut Pasteur (www.pasteur.fr/externe). Detailed information on culture media and specialized techniques is also available from these centers, and in other reference works (Lennette et al. 1988, 1995; Schmidt 1989; Freshney 2000; Murray and Baron 1995).

SAFETY

All procedures involving cell lines should be performed in a class II biological safety cabinet under strict aseptic conditions, both to minimize the risk of contaminating cells with bacteria, yeasts, and mycoplasmas and to protect the worker. Cell lines should be considered potentially hazardous. Although continuous (transformed) cell lines are assumed to be free of infectious agents, they may in fact harbor latent viruses that could infect the worker (Barkley 1979). Safety precautions should include the general measures reviewed by Fleming and Richardson (1995), Lennette et al. (1995), Sewell (1995) and in Chapter 66, The laboratory diagnosis of viral infections.

CELL CULTURE MEDIA

Most of the basic culture media used today are chemically defined, but must be supplemented with 1–20 percent serum. This is usually obtained from calf fetuses and must be carefully checked for contamination by viruses, mycoplasma, bacteria, and specific viral antibodies. Serum-free media is also commercially available for specialized applications (e.g. vaccine development). Cells generally grow well at pH 7.0–7.4. Phenol red is often used as an indicator in the medium, changing progressively from purple at pH 7.8 through red at pH 7.4 to yellow at pH 6.5 (Freshney 2000).

Culture media require careful buffering to stabilize the pH under all conditions. In plastic dishes with unsealed lids, in which exposure to oxygen causes the pH to rise, exogenous CO_2 is required by cell lines, particularly at low cell concentrations, to prevent total loss of dissolved CO_2 and bicarbonate from the medium. In tubes or flasks with tight caps, pH can be adjusted by loosening the caps, changing the medium or placing the vessels in a CO_2 incubator with a gas-permeable cap, as dictated by the indicator. The CO_2 level is critical and can be monitored by a gas analyzer. As little as a 1percent increase can result in cell death.

Medium components should be prepared with endotoxin-free water. Water systems are available to produce type I reagent grade water, which minimizes metal and organic ions leaching from storage containers and prevents bacterial and yeast contamination by being used immediately.

Media, media components, and reagents are sterilized by autoclaving if they are heat-stable (e.g. water, salt solutions, amino acid hydrolysates) or by membrane filtration if they are not (e.g. protein or sugar solutions). The type of membrane is important. Cellulose acetate membranes are best for applications involving low protein binding, and cellulose nitrate membranes for general purpose filtration. Cotton pads, membranes of larger pore size, or commercial prefilters should be used for prefiltering, and membranes of 0.22 μm average pore diameter (APD), for sterilization.

TYPES OF CELL CULTURE

Cell cultures may be either primary or continuous. Primary cultures contain mixtures of cells freshly derived from the tissue of origin, which may be obtained either from laboratory animals or from human material procured in the course of surgery. Some specimens (e.g. foreskin) are not derived from pathological tissues. Tissues from young or embryonic animals give better results than those from adults. The tissues are first minced into 3-mm pieces and the cells disaggregated by one or more treatments with a solution of 0.22 percent trypsin and 0.02 percent versene. The cells are then filtered through sterile gauze, washed by centrifugation in cold growth medium (GM), and finally suspended in GM to the desired concentration. The concentration of viable cells is determined by counting a sample diluted in trypan blue, which selectively stains dead or damaged cells. Tubes or flasks are seeded at approximately 3×10^5 viable cells/ml.

Cell lines are also derived from primary cells, but can be repeatedly subcultured. They fall into two categories.

Euploid cells, such as normal human fibroblasts (e.g. MRC-5, WI-38, HFL1), retain their normal karyotype throughout their culture lifespan, rarely give rise to continuous lines and, after approximately 50 generations, stop dividing (Hayflick 1973). They are sometimes called semicontinuous lines. By contrast, aneuploid (or heteroploid) cells, such as those from many human and animal tumors, may give rise to true continuous cell lines (e.g. HEp-2, HeLa, LLC-MK2). Aneuploid cell lines have a chromosome number that is not an exact multiple of the haploid number.

Insect cell lines are continuous cultures derived from, for example, the SF9 ovary (fall armyworm, *Spodoptera frugiperda*) and from mosquitoes (e.g. *Aedes aegypti* and *Ae. albopictus*). The SF9 line, which is grown in special media, is highly susceptible to infection with baculoviruses and can be used for baculovirus expression vectors and other needs. Mosquito lines are used as suspension cultures for the replication of many mosquito-borne viruses. They have special media and subculturing requirements (Lennette et al. 1995).

Suspension cultures can be prepared from many mouse and human leukemias and ascites tumors. They are incubated on shakers or in roller drums or allowed to settle to the bottom of a large culture flask, such as a roller bottle. Alternatively, a spinner apparatus is available that forces normally adherent cells to grow in suspension in a special medium.

Shell vial cultures contain a cell monolayer grown on a coverslip in a 1-dram vial. The vial is then inoculated with the specimen and centrifuged at low speed (700 g for 45 min), which apparently distorts the cell surface and renders it more susceptible to viral attachment. After 1–3 days of incubation, irrespective of any cytopathic effects (CPE), the coverslip is washed briefly, and tested by immunofluorescence assay (IFA), nucleic acid hybridization, or other tests for whichever viruses are suspected. Shell vial cultures have been successfully used as a rapid test for adenovirus (Espy et al. 1987), Cytomegalovirus (CMV) (Gleaves et al. 1989; Buller et al. 1992), varicella-zoster virus (VZV) (Schirm et al. 1989), respiratory syncytial virus (RSV) (Smith et al. 1991), and other respiratory viruses (Matthey et al. 1992; Schirm et al. 1992; Olsen et al. 1993).

Microcultures are cost-efficient systems of growing popularity, having overcome earlier problems with cross-contamination between wells, over-oxygenation, and toxic plastics. Microcultures in 24- to 48- and 96-well plates with sealable lids (or tightly fitting lids for CO_2 incubators) are now commonly used in a variety of viral assays.

In 96-well microtiter plates with flat well bottoms, microcultures are ideal for neutralization tests, tissue culture enzyme immunoassay (EIA), monoclonal antibody testing, and many screening assays (Hierholzer and Bingham 1978; Anderson et al. 1985; Lennette et al. 1995; Murray and Baron 1995). Macrocultures in standard tubes, however, are still used for primary virus isolation because of the ease of setting up stationary or roller cultures in ordinary incubators, of reading the monolayers for CPE and of obtaining sufficient volume of virus culture to use for subpassaging, identification tests, viral genetic analyses, and storage.

Specialized culture systems have been devised to satisfy particular needs. For example, suspension cultures of human peripheral blood lymphocytes are sensitive to the Epstein–Barr herpesvirus, where it is detected by a transformation assay, and, under cocultivation procedures, to the human T-cell leukemia viruses (HTLV) and human immunodeficiency viruses (HIV) (Lennette et al. 1988, 1995; Fields and Knipe 1990; Isenberg 1992). Immortalized human microvascular endothelial cell cultures derived from foreskin are sensitive to a wide variety of viruses under special culture conditions, and have potential use as a model to study the biology of these important cells (Ades et al. 1992). Extracellular matrix systems support the three-dimensional growth of cells as opposed to monolayer cultures. The Matrigel invasion chamber (Collaborative Biomedical Products, Bedford, MA, USA), for instance, can support fastidious cell types and is currently being explored for its use in viral culture and alterations in cell physiology following viral infection (Bissell et al. 1990; Thompson et al. 1991). Finally, large-volume culture systems, such as suspension culture vats, cells on the surfaces of Sephadex beads or other microcarriers, and cells on spirals of Sterilin or other plastic film are used extensively in industry to prepare vaccines, interferons, and monoclonal antibodies (White and Ades 1990).

Mixed cultures of different cell types combined in a single vial have been used successfully to grow a broad range of viruses (Huang and Turchek 2000; Navarro-Marí et al. 1999). A commercial product, Mixed *Fresh-Cells*, available from Diagnostic Hybrids, Inc. (Athens, OH, USA), combines two compatible cell lines optimized for growing particular groups of viruses, e.g. R-Mix for respiratory viruses, E-Mix for enteroviruses and H&V-Mix for herpesviruses. For example, R-Mix consists of a mixed monolayer of mink lung cells (Mv1Lu) and human adenocarcinoma cells (A549) that have been shown in clinical studies to support the detection of influenza A and B viruses, RSV, adenovirus, and parainfluenza viruses 1, 2, and 3 (Barenfanger et al. 2001; St George et al. 2002).

Genetically engineered cell lines offer potential improvements in our ability to grow viruses and to rapidly detect virus infection. Stable transformation of specific virus receptors for HIV-1 (Chesebro and Wehrly 1988) and EBV (Li et al. 1992) into previously nonpermissive cell lines has been shown to permit growth of these viruses. Genetically modified cells that express an easily measured reporter enzyme after infection with a specific virus have also been developed. For example, a transgenic baby hamster kidney cell line (BHKIC-P6LacZ) that contains multiple copies of a virus-inducible HSV promoter sequence linked to the reporter gene *LacZ* developed by Stabell and Olivo (1992) has been used successfully for diagnosis of infections with HSV types 1 and 2 (LaRocco 2000). An FDA-approved diagnostic assay for HSV, based on these cells, is commercially available (ELVIS HSV test; Diagnostic Hybrids, Inc.). For a more comprehensive review of the potential benefits of genetic engineering of cell lines for diagnostic virology, see Olivo (1999).

QUALITY CONTROL

Contamination by bacteria and fungi is an inherent problem of cell culture work. Contamination can be visually detected by appearance of turbidity or color changes due to changes in the pH of the culture medium, or more definitively by microscopic examination of the culture. Detailed protocols for the detection of most bacteria and fungi that would be expected to survive in cell cultures in the presence of the customary antibiotics may be found elsewhere (ATCC 1992). These methods should be incorporated into the quality control program of the media production laboratory to preclude the contamination of cells by detecting organisms in the culture GM.

Contamination by mycoplasmas and viruses is more difficult to detect, because these organisms usually do not cause turbidity or pH changes, may not cause a CPE in the cells, and are able to pass through 0.2 µm filters commonly used for sterile filtration of media and media components. Thus, these agents may be passaged with the cells indefinitely without detection unless specific testing is performed. Primary rhesus monkey kidney (MK), primary African green monkey kidney (AGMK), and primary bovine embryonic kidney cell cultures are particularly notorious for adventitious virus contamination (Hull 1968; Crandell et al. 1978; Schmidt 1989; Eberle and Hilliard 1995). A variety of methods have been described for detection of the mycoplasma species most commonly found in mammalian cell culture, including microbiological culture, DNA staining with fluorescent dyes, mycoplasmal enzymatic assays, IFA, and EIA, hybridization probes, and polymerase chain reaction (PCR) assay. Commercial testing services are widely available for mycoplasmas and viruses and commercial kits, such as the MycoTect test (Invitrogen), MycoSensor PCR Assay (Stratagene), and Mycoplasma Detection Kit (Roche Applied Science) are available that can be incorporated into a quality control program.

Contamination by other cell lines can also occur, the intrusion of HeLa cells into many other lines giving the most problems. Preventative measures that can be taken include working with only one cell line at a time; keeping bottles of medium, trypsin/versene, etc., separate for each cell line; allowing a 'resting' period of approximately 30 min between manipulation of different cell lines in a biological safety cabinet; and decontaminating cabinet surfaces before introducing another cell line to the work area. The species of origin of a cell line can be determined by various immunological, isoenzyme, and cytogenetic tests (ATCC 1992) that are available commercially. Thus, quality control programs for cell culture laboratories must incorporate periodic searches for contaminants of microbiological and cellular origin, because the contaminants may cause irreversible changes in the cell cultures and can completely confound the interpretation of diagnostic tests.

PROPAGATION OF CELLS

Propagating cells by scraping is a physical method of removing adherent cells from the surface of a culture vessel, and is used when enzymatic removal (see below) may be toxic to the cells or may destroy receptors or other important cell surface molecules. The GM is discarded, the cells are physically scraped from the vessel surface with a disposable cell scraper into fresh GM, and the cells are then dispersed by vigorous pipetting to obtain a suspension of single cells. The cells are counted and appropriately diluted for passage to new flasks or other vessels.

Cell counts are used to quantify viable cells for passaging and seeding. They are best performed in the presence of a vital stain, which is excluded by living cell membranes and is incorporated only into dead cells. In the trypan blue vital stain procedure, a sample of the cell suspension is mixed with 0.4 percent dye in physiological saline, placed in the counting chamber of a hemocytometer, and the cells counted at ×100 magnification. The stained (dead) cells and the unstained (living) cells can be counted separately to determine percentage viability if this is desired. Trypan blue and erythrosin B are the dyes most commonly used for dye exclusion tests. Others (e.g. methylene blue, acridine orange, eosin, nigrosin, and safranin) have also been used (Evans et al. 1975). Dyes, such as crystal violet, stain both living and dead cells and are best used to clarify morphology.

Cells can also be propagated by enzyme treatment, a chemical method of detaching adherent cells from the culture vessel with enzymes, such as trypsin, pronase, or collagenase, together with chelating agents, such as versene (tetrasodium ethylenediaminetetraacetic acid (EDTA)). After washing twice with phosphate-buffered saline (PBS), the monolayer is covered with a solution of 0.05 percent trypsin and 0.53 mM versene and placed at room temperature with cell surface down until the cells detach. After vigorously pipetting to break up clumps, the cells are resuspended at the desired concentration in fresh GM.

Cells in suspension cultures are propagated by adding a sample to sufficient GM to give the desired concentration.

For lymphocyte cultures, fresh mononuclear cells can be isolated from whole blood by Ficoll–Hypaque gradient centrifugation and cultured in suspension. Their uses for diagnosis, evaluation of immunity, and detection of disease are numerous, as are the procedures for isolating particular subpopulations of cells from peripheral blood or lymphoid tissues (Markham and Salahuddin 1987; Castro et al. 1988; Coligan and Kruisbeek 1991).

MAINTENANCE OF CULTURES

Once cells have been passaged, routine medium changes are necessary to encourage their viability by feeding them with fresh amino acids, vitamins, glucose, and other metabolic constituents. The initial cell concentration and the metabolic rate of the cells will determine the feeding schedule. Feeding is done with a maintenance medium (MM), which is the regular medium with reduced serum content (1–2 percent serum vs. 10–20 percent used in GM). MM may hold untransformed cell lines at a single cell layer for an extended period, even 2–3 weeks, because it tends not to stimulate mitosis. Diploid cells, with a finite lifespan, can thus be maintained for extended periods without using up the limited number of cell generations available to them.

Cells can also be maintained by subculturing, particularly important for transformed cells, which continue to divide under MM and thus cannot be successfully fed. Transformed (heteroploid) epithelial cells, such as HeLa and HEp-2, metabolize rapidly and should be subcultured twice a week. Alternatively, the seeding concentration of such rapidly proliferating cells may be lowered to reduce subculturing to once a week. Diploid fibroblast cells, such as MRC-5 and WI-38, metabolize slowly and require subculturing only once a week, with a feeding at least once during that week. Suspension cultures must be subcultured, or the volume of medium increased as the cell population reaches approximately 2×10^6 cells/ml, because the viability of suspended cells drops rapidly at higher concentrations.

STORAGE OF CELLS

Cells may be stored by cryopreservation, which provides a ready stock if any is lost through contamination, incubator malfunction, natural senescence, or a genetic drift that may affect their ability to exhibit the expected response in routine assays. Cells are packed by low-speed centrifugation and resuspended in a freeze medium containing serum and dimethylsulfoxide (DMSO) (Schmidt 1989; Mahy and Kangro 1996; Freshney 2000). One-ml volumes are dispensed into cryovials, frozen slowly at approximately 1°C per min, preferably in a controlled-rate freezer, and stored in liquid nitrogen (−165°C).

Cells are recovered from storage by rapidly thawing in a 37°C water bath, diluting the cells with the appropriate medium, and placing them in a cell culture flask. The medium is replaced after 24 h to remove all traces of DMSO. The medium exchange for a suspension culture requires centrifugation and resuspension in fresh medium.

Tissue and organ cultures

Laboratory cultures of pieces of human embryonic lung, kidney, intestine, and other organs have proven essential to the discovery of many viruses, such as the respiratory coronaviruses and rhinoviruses. Organ cultures are explants of whole tissue (approximately 1 mm^3), so many cell types are present in their natural form, and feeding medium must be perfused through the explants to maintain viability. Once inoculated with a clinical specimen, virus may be detected by cessation of ciliary movement (in lung) or by specific tests for the viral products accumulated in the medium (McIntosh et al. 1967; Tyrrell and Blamire 1967; Caul and Egglestone 1977).

Embryonated eggs

The chick embryo is a versatile host system in diagnostic virology, although its use has been diminished by the development of alternate culture and direct detection methods. It is still vital to the isolation of some influenza viruses, and the size and appearance of pocks on the chorioallantoic membrane (CAM) afford a quick diagnostic criterion for poxviruses. The advantages of eggs include ease of handling, production of large amounts of infectious amniotic or allantoic fluids, and lack of antibody production by the host which might hinder virus identification. Disadvantages include the need to obtain sterile eggs of known age (certified germ-free eggs can be virtually unobtainable in some countries) and the need to eliminate all viable bacteria, yeasts, and mycoplasmas from the patient's specimen before inoculation.

Fertile eggs must be incubated at 37°C in 40–70 percent humidity and rotated about every 4 h to keep the embryo floating in the center of the egg. For influenza virus isolation in amniotic or allantoic cavities, 9- to 11-day-old eggs are needed. For poxvirus isolation in the CAM, 12-day-old eggs are best.

Laboratory animals

Many animal systems have been developed to serve as models of human infection and to produce high-titer antisera for diagnostic tests. Others have been developed for propagating viruses that do not grow in cell cultures. Suckling mice (see Gould and Clegg 1985) are required for the recovery of some coxsackie A enteroviruses, and suckling mice, suckling hamsters, rabbits, mosquitoes, or ticks are needed for some arboviruses.

Primates are the most sensitive systems for the hepatitis viruses, with ducks, woodchucks, and mice as alternatives for hepatitis B virus and mice and piglets for hepatitis E virus. In addition, newborn mice or hamsters, young adult guinea-pigs, and primates are required for some of the biosafety level (BSL)-4 agents (e.g. filoviruses, arenaviruses). These highly specialized and dangerous systems are beyond the reach of most laboratories, and the reader should consult other works for details (Lennette et al. 1988, 1995; Isenberg 1992; Murray and Baron 1995).

Animals should be purchased from companies specializing in the breeding of laboratory animals, so that the strain of the species is documented, immunizations for known adventitious organisms are given, and the quality of care (housing, temperature, air filtraton, food, and water) are within the appropriate national guidelines for animal care. The strains of mice and guinea-pigs may be important; often, only a single strain is suitable for a particular virus. Housing of animals in the receiving laboratory is also critical, not only to conform with national regulations on the humane use of animals, but also to minimize the introduction of exogenous microorganisms and cross-contamination.

PREPARATION OF REAGENTS FOR VIRUS IDENTIFICATION

Preparation of viral antigens

Viral antigens may be structural or nonstructural proteins or glycoproteins produced during viral replication, and may be located internally in the virion or be part of the external capsid components. Many are produced in excess during replication and are released into the supernatant fluid as 'soluble' antigens. For some tests, the antigen may simply be the supernatant fluid from the cell culture in which the virus was propagated. For others, intact virus is required at the highest titers achievable, so several freeze–thaw or sonication cycles are applied to the virus culture to disrupt any remaining cells. Again, a particular viral product may need to be enriched in proportion to other products, but not purified in the biochemical sense. For still others, only a specific viral protein can be used in the test, so it must be purified, concentrated, and preserved after removing interfering viral products and medium components. Alternatively, it may be specifically produced by a eukaryotic or prokaryotic gene expression system.

The two most basic concepts are microbiological purity of the starting viral culture and laboratory safety. For purity, starting cultures and final virus products should be proven free of viable bacterial, fungal, and mycoplasmal contamination by appropriate culturing in thioglycolate broth, trypticase soy broth, neopeptone infusion agar streak/pour plates with 5 percent defibrinated sheep blood, Sabouraud glucose agar slants for yeasts, and Hayflick's biphasic medium for mycoplasma. Depending on the test and the day-to-day usage, many antigens can be preserved by adding thiomersal (thimerosal) or sodium azide to the final product to final concentrations of 0.01 and 0.1 percent, respectively. For safety, the routine laboratory precautions discussed in Chapter 66, The laboratory diagnosis of viral infections, must be followed throughout.

For every virus antigen, a parallel 'dummy antigen' should be prepared as a negative control. Dummy antigens are prepared by sham-inoculating cell cultures, eggs, or animals with normal medium and thereafter treating them exactly as for the active preparation.

RELEASING VIRUS FROM CULTURE CELLS

Starting with the highest titers of infectious virus achievable is essential for antigen preparations. Freeze–thaw cycles, sonication and chemical treatments are the most widely used methods for liberating virus from the host cells and for disrupting virions to expose particular antigens (Mahy and Kangro 1996).

For freeze–thawing, cultures with maximal CPE are frozen at $-70°C$ or below, then thawed to a slush, and agitated to dislodge the cells. The procedure is repeated twice and the final material is clarified by low-speed centrifugation.

For sonication, either the cultures may be freeze–thawed but not centrifuged, or the cells may be scraped off the vessel surface with a rubber 'policeman.' The energy level and time are determined in pilot tests; 30–70 watts output for 1–3 min with multiple pulses per minute will generally disrupt the cells without denaturing the antigen. The sonicated material is clarified by low-speed centrifugation.

Chemical treatments may also be used. Alkaline glycine extraction exposes intracellular antigens useful for complement fixation (CF), indirect hemagglutination (IHA), and EIA for many viruses, particularly those that are membrane-associated (Mahy and Kangro 1996). Treating with trypsin or trypsin–versene, followed by sonicating and centrifuging, produces high-titer antigens useful for EIA and hemagglutination (HA) tests for many viruses. Antigens for use in immunofluorescence tests may be prepared from infected cells disaggregated with trypsin and washed.

VIRUS INACTIVATION PROCEDURES

Viruses can be inactivated to permit safe handling. Choice of inactivation strategy is dictated by the lability of the particular virus and the stability of the viral antigens. Three principal methods used for virus inactivation include sonication, β-propiolactone (BPL) treatment, and radiation (Mahy and Kangro 1996).

Sonication can disrupt virus particles and cleave macromolecules if sufficient energy is applied. The

optimum power, number of cycles and length of time must be determined for each virus and test.

BPL treatment is widely used to inactivate viruses because it generally does not interfere with antigen test systems. Cultures are clarified by centrifugation and mixed with BPL in the presence of tris(hydroxymethyl)amino-methane (TRIS) buffer, the final BPL concentration and incubation time having been previously determined in pilot tests. They are then clarified again, adjusted to pH 7.3–7.4 as needed and preserved with thiomersal or sodium azide.

Radiation is a very effective means for inactivating viruses, but must be carried out by people trained and certified for such procedures. The clarified virus/antigen is exposed in an unbreakable container in an ice bath to a ^{60}Co γ source. The dosage required for complete inactivation of the virus (Table 6.1) is estimated from dose–response curves. The product is tested for residual infectivity and for potency (Gamble et al. 1980).

Other virus inactivation methods are useful for specific purposes, but should not be relied upon to insure complete inactivation for some viruses. For immunoperoxidase assays (IPA) and IFA, infected cells may be fixed with acetone for 10 min at $4°C$, which stabilizes viral proteins by partial denaturation and preserves morphological structure and immunological reactivity. Alternatively, viruses can be inactivated with 10 percent formalin at pH 7.0; methanol or ethanol (4 min at $4°C$); acetone/methanol 50:50 (Lennette et al. 1995); 80 percent acetone (Anderson et al. 1985); or photochemically with psoralen and related compounds (Hanson et al. 1978). Copper-catalyzed sodium ascorbate preserves CF and IHA antigens of herpes simplex virus (HSV) (White et al. 1986); certain detergents (e.g. 1 percent Nonidet P-40, 0.1–0.5 percent sodium lauryl sulfate, Tween-20, or Tween-80) can break up virus envelopes without destroying antigenic activity.

ANTIGEN EXTRACTION PROCEDURES

Extraction procedures can free antigens of nonspecific inhibitors, anticomplementary reactions, competing proteins and lipoproteins, and undesired reactions related to the viral host system. For example, HA anti-

Table 6.1 Dosage of ^{60}Co γ-irradiation required for complete inactivation of viruses

Mrad[a]	Viruses inactivated
0.5	Cytomegalovirus
1.5	Influenzavirus
1.6	Herpes simplex virus 1, 2
1.7	Respiratory syncytial virus
2.0	Newcastle disease virus, Rabies virus
2.2	Rotavirus
3.4	Lymphocytic choriomeningitis virus

a) Megarad, or 10^6 rad (rad, radiation absorbed dose).

gens must be free of serum antibodies, host-cell components and microbial contaminants that may agglutinate the erythrocytes used in the assay. Some antigens are enhanced in reactivity by treatment with freeze–thaw cycles, sonication, Tween-80, fluorocarbon, ether, or other organic solvents (Norrby 1962; Chappell et al. 1984). The Tween-80–ether extraction method is found in Mahy and Kangro (1996). The sucrose–acetone–BPL and fluorocarbon methods are briefly described here, by way of example. Alternatively, nonionic detergents, such as Nonidet P-40, high concentrations of salts in the presence of EDTA and β-mercaptoethanol, and other extracting agents can be used to prepare viral antigens (Isenberg 1992; Mahy and Kangro 1996).

The sucrose–acetone–BPL extraction method is useful for the CF and HA antigens of some viruses, including togaviruses (Venezuelan equine encephalomyelitis virus) and flaviviruses (Dengue virus, Japanese B encephalitis virus, Rocio virus, St. Louis encephalitis virus, Yellow fever virus and other formerly group B arboviruses) (Schmidt and Lennette 1971; Chappell et al. 1984). A 40 percent suspension of infected tissue (e.g. mouse brain) is homogenized in borate-saline, pH 9.0 in ice; 1 M TRIS/borate-saline equal to 1/10 the volume of suspension is added, followed by cold BPL drop-wise to a final concentration of 0.1–0.3 percent. After mixing for 1 day in the cold, an equal volume of 17 percent sucrose in distilled water is added, together with 20 volumes of cold acetone chilled to −20°C per volume of homogenate, still in ice and with mixing. After vigorous shaking the tissue is allowed to settle out at −20°C for 30 min, and the supernatant acetone is aspirated. The preparation is again extracted with acetone, keeping the 20:1 ratio. The antigen may be preserved best as a freeze-dried powder, but should be reconstituted in borate-saline and centrifuged at 10 000 g for 1 h before use.

For fluorocarbon extraction, the centrifuged starting material is placed in a stainless steel vessel in an ice bath for high-speed homogenization. Sufficient fluorocarbon (e.g. Genetron; CF_3CCl_3) is added to obtain a 2:1 ratio of antigen to fluorocarbon and the mixture is homogenized at full speed for 4–6 min. The aerosol is allowed to settle in the closed container for 1 h in ice. The suspension is then decanted into bottles or tubes for layer separation at 1000 g for 20 min at 4°C; the supernatant is the treated antigen (Gessler et al. 1956).

Viral antigens can be partially purified by adsorption/elution from erythrocytes or from calcium phosphate gels (Mahy and Kangro 1996). More effective purification is achieved by various types of solid-phase immunological adsorption/elution techniques and by affinity chromatography. Antigens may be immunoaffinity-purified by passing viral cultures (usually after SLS or enzyme treatment to disrupt virions and liberate proteins) through columns containing gel beds coated with specific antibody, or beds of monoclonal antibody-bound protein A–sepharose beads, etc. Other types of affinity chromatography use enzyme- or substrate-bound matrices. The reader is referred to other sources for detailed methods of affinity chromatography (Eisenberg et al. 1982; Wilchek et al. 1984; Chong and Gillam 1985; Harlow and Lane 1988).

SYNTHETIC AND EXPRESSED ANTIGENS

Polypeptides representing discrete viral antigens can be chemically synthesized for use in diagnostic assay and special studies. However, synthetic peptides are typically restricted to single linear epitopes that do not possess the secondary and tertiary structure of more complex antigens. Alternatively, various commercially available recombinant gene expression systems can be used to construct complex viral antigens that may be more suitable for viral diagnostic assays. Prokaryotic expression systems are convenient and inexpensive, but possess different processing pathways which prevent the amino terminal modifications, disulfide bond formation, and glycosylation required for many viral antigens to be active. Eukaryotic expression systems are more complex and expensive, but are closer to the natural mode of replication of the virus. Thus, post-translational modifications necessary for antigenicity are more likely to take place. Many viruses can serve as expression vectors in eukaryotic systems. For example, baculovirus is particularly useful because it can be 'engineered' to incorporate various tag genes which make it possible to purify and identify the virus or its expressed products. Once the gene for the desired antigen has been inserted into the recombinant baculovirus, the virus is grown at 27°C in SF9 or SF21 fall armyworm ovary cells and the desired antigen identified by IFA, EIA, or western blot. The reader is referred to other sources for the details and methods of gene expression systems (Smith and Johnson 1988; Bennink and Yewdell 1990; Vialard et al. 1990; Ausubel and Brent 1991; Jarvis 1991; Taylor et al. 1992; Cox et al. 1993; Alberts et al. 1994).

Preparation of high-titer antisera

High-titer antisera to viruses and viral antigens are readily produced in animals for use in diagnostic assays. Animal-derived antisera were the backbone of early virology, being widely used to distinguish between strains and serotypes and to study the antigenic make up of viruses. Polyclonal antisera of high titer ('hyperimmune sera') is prepared by repeated injection of virus or viral antigen into, for example, rabbits, mice, and guinea-pigs, or larger animals, such as goats and horses. The general procedure is to clarify the preparation by centrifugation, mix it with an equal volume of Freund's incomplete adjuvant or a synthetic muramyl dipeptide adjuvant, inject the mixture into suitable sites between two and four times biweekly, and obtain a blood sample

10–14 days after the final injection. The pre- and post-immunization sera are then tested for the desired antibody. Use of other adjuvants, injection in multiple sites with or without adjuvant, techniques to minimize the development of host-cell antibodies, and preparation of antigen/antibody complexes on solid matrices, such as staphylococcal protein A, are described in other sources (Hierholzer et al. 1991; Lennette et al. 1995; Murray and Baron 1995; Mahy and Kangro 1996).

Preparation of monoclonal antibodies

Monoclonal antibodies have become a vital immunological reagent since their inception in 1975 (Scharff et al. 1981; Peter and Baumgarten 1992; Lennette et al. 1995; Murray and Baron 1995). Many variations in their production have been described, including immunization in vitro and EBV-transformation techniques (Seigneurin et al. 1983; Boss 1986; Foung et al. 1986; Treanor et al. 1988). Suitable methods are described by Goding (1996).

ISOLATION AND IDENTIFICATION OF VIRUSES FROM CLINICAL SPECIMENS

Specimen collection and treatment

To avoid misleading results, it is of the utmost importance that adequate specimens are taken from sites appropriate to the clinical findings and then correctly stored and processed. The type of specimen and the manner of collection depend upon the laboratory methods to be used and on the sites clinically affected (Johnson 1990; Hierholzer 1991, 1993; Lennette et al. 1995). Specimens should ideally be collected within a few days of the onset of symptoms, because most viruses are shed only in the initial stages of illness. Swab specimens are placed in 2 ml of transport medium (e.g. tryptose phosphate broth with 0.5 percent gelatin, veal heart infusion broth or trypticase soy broth), preferably without antibiotics to allow the culture of bacteria and mycoplasmas. Nasopharyngeal aspirates are excellent specimens for respiratory viruses and are collected with a neonatal mucus extractor and mucus trap to which transport medium is added (Waris et al. 1990). According to the circumstances, other specimens may include urine, stool, whole blood, serum, cerebrospinal fluid, biopsy and autopsy specimens, and swabs or scrapings of vesicular lesions. Specimens are placed on wet ice and transported to the laboratory for immediate culturing. If testing is not possible within 5 days of collection, they are frozen on dry ice and stored at −70°C until they can be processed, although this may reduce the amount of viable virus. Before inoculation into the appropriate host system, specimens are treated with antibiotics, mixed vigorously, and clarified by centrifuging at 1000 g for 3 min at 4°C to remove cell debris and bacteria. Many viruses require one or more subpassages for recovery.

Procedures for isolating viruses

CELL CULTURES

Cell cultures should include a continuous human epithelial line (e.g. HEp-2 (Johnston and Siegel 1990); KB, A549 (Woods and Young 1988), HeLa); a human embryonic lung diploid fibroblast cell strain (e.g. HLF, HELF, MRC-5, WI-38); human lung mucoepidermoid cells (NCI-H292) to replace MK cells for most applications (Castells et al. 1990; Hierholzer et al. 1993b); and human rhabdomyosarcoma cells (RD) for the broadest coverage of viruses within practical limitations (Matthey et al. 1992). Treated specimens are adsorbed on to cell monolayers whose GM has been decanted. MM is added and cultures are incubated at 35–36°C up to several weeks, with subpassaging as required. Toxic specimens (urine, stool, tissue homogenates) should be decanted before MM is added.

Some cell types and certain viruses require roller cultures, whereas others do best as stationary cultures during their incubation period. In general, all tube cultures of MK, AGMK, and their derivative cell lines (Vero, BSC-1, LLC-MK2, etc.), all diploid fibroblast cell cultures, and NCI-H292 cells should be rolled in roller drums or agitated on rocker platforms to remove toxic byproducts from the cell surface and to replenish critical nutrients to the cells more quickly. Cultures of human embryonic kidney (HEK), HEp-2, KB, A549, and HeLa do not need to be rolled, except for the isolation of RSV and measles virus.

Small variations in media composition and incubation temperature are also important for the isolation of certain viruses. For instance, viruses may require prior treatment with trypsin (Almeida et al. 1978; Sanchez-Fauquier et al. 1994), or the cells may require trypsin in the MM to render them sensitive to certain viruses (Itoh et al. 1970; Frank et al. 1979; Agbalika et al. 1984; Castells et al. 1990). Cooler incubation temperatures (33–35°C) are best for less invasive viruses, such as coronaviruses, rhinoviruses, and the enteroviruses that cause hemorrhagic conjunctivitis. Finally, whenever MK or AGMK cells are used (e.g. for influenza, measles, or rubella), one should presume that simian adventitious agents are present and may confound the isolation and identification of human viruses (Hull 1968; Eberle and Hilliard 1995).

Viral growth is usually detected as CPE in the infected cell monolayer by scanning at ×40–100 magnification and observing in greater detail at ×200–400 magnification (Figure 6.1). The type of CPE and the time required for it to appear in a particular cell type are suggestive of the type of virus present. Thus, careful

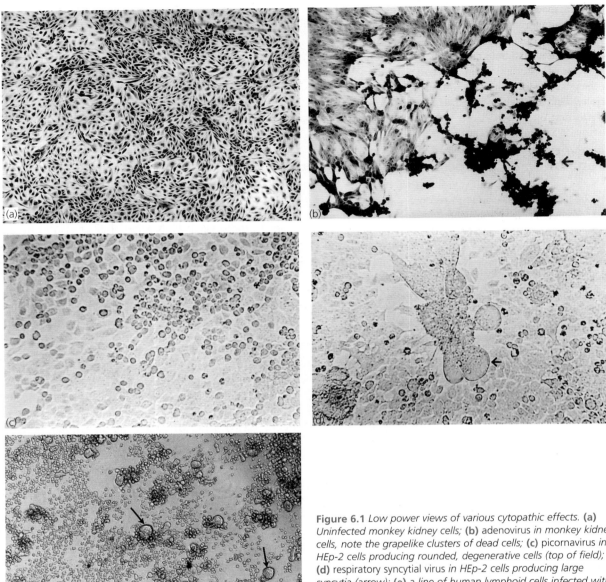

Figure 6.1 *Low power views of various cytopathic effects.* **(a)** *Uninfected monkey kidney cells;* **(b)** *adenovirus in monkey kidney cells, note the grapelike clusters of dead cells;* **(c)** *picornavirus in HEp-2 cells producing rounded, degenerative cells (top of field);* **(d)** *respiratory syncytial virus in HEp-2 cells producing large syncytia (arrow);* **(e)** *a line of human lymphoid cells infected with human immunodeficiency virus (HIV-1). Note syncytia (arrowed). (Part (e) from Collier and Oxford (1993), by permission of Oxford University Press.)*

observation of the monolayers is important for applying the proper identification tests.

EMBRYONATED EGGS

Except for influenza and poxviruses, chick embryos have been largely superseded by cell cultures for virus isolation and identification.

The amniotic route of inoculation is used mainly for primary isolation of influenza viruses, and the allantoic route for serial passages and for obtaining large quantities of virus. Embryos (approximated 10 days old) are inoculated by well-established methods and the fluids are harvested 2–4 days later.

The chorioallantoic membrane (CAM) method is used mainly for poxviruses. The membranes of 12-day-old embryos are inoculated through an opening in the shell about halfway along the long axis of the egg, the CAM having first been pulled away from the shell by applying negative pressure to a second hole drilled over the natural air sac. The CAM is inspected for the appearance of pocks after further incubation for 2–4 days.

For a detailed account of chick embryo methods, see Barrett and Inglis (1985) and Lennette et al. (1995).

LABORATORY ANIMALS

Like chick embryos, animals have largely been superseded by other systems, although they are occasionally used for special purposes, such as the isolation and partial characterization of coxsackieviruses in suckling mice, which can be inoculated both intracerebrally and intraperitoneally (Gould and Clegg 1985).

For use of other animal systems, the reader is referred to chapters dealing with the relevant virus groups in this volume and elsewhere (Lennette et al. 1988, 1995; Murray and Baron 1995).

Recovery and identification of viruses

Table 6.2 summarizes the relative value of a range of methods for isolating and propagating human viruses. Further details may be found in Isenberg (1992), Lennette et al. (1995), and Murray and Baron (1995).

ADENOVIRUSES

Adenoviruses (see Chapter 22, Adenoviruses) are associated with diverse clinical syndromes. They are spread by droplets, fomites, and the fecal–oral route; some serotypes are also spread venereally. Most serotypes replicate readily in HEK, A549, HEp-2, KB, and NCI-H292 cells, with or without rolling, producing grapelike clusters of round, refractile, enlarged cells. Adenoviruses grow in most of the same cells as herpes simplex viruses, but more slowly (3–14 days), depending on serotype, and make more discrete, irregularly shaped cell clusters. Adenoviruses can be adapted to replicate in fibroblast cells, but the CPE develops slowly and infectivity titers are low. Types 40 and 41, associated with infant gastroenteritis, grow best in an Ad5-transformed HEK cell line (Graham-293 cells) or in HEp-2 under a fortified Opti-MEM medium containing 0.4 percent fetal calf serum and 0.1 percent 2-mercaptoethanol. The adenoviruses are among the easier viruses to identify because they are unique in producing in cell culture very large quantities of soluble antigens with many type- and group-specific properties that lend themselves to a wide variety of diagnostic tests. Adenoviruses are distinguished from other viruses by electron microscopy (EM), latex agglutination (LA), IFA, IPA, EIA, time-resolved fluoroimmunoassay (TR-FIA) (Hierholzer et al. 1987; Brown et al. 1990), DNA probes, restriction enzyme analysis (REA) (Adrian et al. 1986), PCR assay (Hierholzer et al. 1993c), and cytological and inclusion-body staining methods. Adenoviruses are serotyped by HI and serum neutralization (SN) tests (Hierholzer 1992).

'ARBOVIRUSES'

The togaviruses (see Chapter 47, Togaviruses), flaviviruses (see Chapter 46, Flaviviruses), arenaviruses (Chapter 49, Arenaviruses), rhabdoviruses, filoviruses (Chapter 50, Filoviruses), and bunyaviruses (Chapter 48, Bunyaviridae) contain most of the agents covered by the term 'arboviruses' and many rare and unusual viruses that cause disease in geographically distinct parts of the world. Arboviruses often have special isolation requirements. Certain arboviruses can be isolated in primary hamster kidney cells, primary chick or duck embryo cells, or derivative cell lines such as AP61 mosquito cells, BHK-21 hamster kidney cells, Vero (African green monkey kidney cells), and LLC-MK2 rhesus monkey kidney cells, after 2–10 days of culture. For example, the Sin Nombre hantavirus is a bunyavirus that can be propagated in the Vero E6 cell line after growth in deer mouse lungs (Elliott et al. 1994). The CPE may not be apparent at first, but becomes generalized in subpassages or forms plaques under agarose. Other arboviruses grow best in mosquito suspension-cell cultures at 20–30°C, in which replication is detected by subpassaging to monolayer cultures, in which CPE may be evident, or by HA/HI, EIA, IFA, CF, SN, or nucleic acid tests for the specific viruses suspected. Still other arboviruses can be recovered only in whole animal systems such as chick embryos, suckling mice or hamsters, or mosquitoes. Fortunately, most diagnostic laboratories will not encounter these viruses, either because of their rarity in most parts of the world or because of their requirement for BSL-3 or -4 containment facilities. The reader is therefore referred to other works that detail the isolation requirements and systems, the specific identification tests and the laboratory precautions for these viruses (Fields and Knipe 1990; Lennette et al. 1988, 1995; Murray and Baron 1995).

CORONAVIRUSES

The human coronaviruses (see Chapter 39, Coronaviruses, toroviruses, and arteriviruses) cause a significant proportion of 'common colds' and are spread by droplet route. Because these viruses are extremely labile and difficult to recover by culture, they are best identified directly in nasal and throat specimens by IFA, EIA, TR-FIA, or reverse transcription (RT)-PCR. The viruses growing in diploid fibroblast cells (229E virus) or in RD cells (OC43 virus) do not cause discernible CPE during their replication phase. Only when viral replication is complete and the virus titer has peaked (at approximately 10^7 tissue culture infective doses (TCID$_{50}$/0.1 ml), after 26–30 h of roller incubation, do changes begin to be evident in the monolayer. For the next several days, CPE develops as a uniform degeneration across the monolayer. The CPE becomes complete concomitant with autolysis of the newly formed virions. By this time, little infectious virus is left in the culture (Hierholzer 1976; Schmidt et al. 1979). The peplomers constitute the primary antigen detected in all tests, including the HI test for strain OC43 (Schmidt et al. 1979; Hierholzer et al. 1994a). Alternatively, the viral RNA can be identified by RT-PCR (Vabret et al. 2001).

The recently identified severe acute respiratory syndrome (SARS) associated coronavirus (SARS-CoV)

Table 6.2 *Isolation and propagation systems for human viruses*

Virus family/group	Cell culture					Organ culture	Embryonated eggs		Laboratory animals		
	Primary	Epithelial	Fibroblast	Vero	Other		Amn/All	CAM	Rodents	Primates	Other
Adenoviridae											
Adenovirus 1–51	+	+	±	+	+	+	–	–	–	–	–
Arenaviridae											
LCM, Lassa virus, others	–	–	±	+	±	–	–	–	+	+	–
Astroviridae											
Astrovirus	±	±	–	–	–	–	–	–	–	–	–
Bunyaviridae											
CE, La Crosse virus	±	–	–	±	+	–	+	+	+	±	+
Hantaviruses	–	–	–	±	–	–	–	–	+	–	–
Other arboviruses	±	–	–	±	+	–	+	+	+	±	+
Caliciviridae											
Norovirus, Sapovirus	–	–	–	–	–	–	–	–	–	±	–
Hepatitis E virus	±	±	–	–	–	–	–	–	+	+	+
Coronaviridae											
Coronaviruses 229E, OC43	±	–	±	–	+	+	–	–	–	–	–
SARS associated coronavirus	+	–	–	+	–	–	–	–	+	+	–
Filoviridae											
Marburg virus, Ebola virus	–	–	±	+	+	–	–	–	+	+	+
Flaviviridae											
Dengue viruses 1–4, JE virus, SLE virus, West Nile virus, Yellow Fever virus, and other arboviruses	+	–	–	+	+	–	+	+	+	±	+
Hepatitis C virus	–	–	–	–	–	–	–	–	–	+	–
Hepadnaviridae											
Hepatitis B virus	±	–	–	–	±	–	–	–	±	+	+
Herpesviridae											
Herpes simplex 1, 2	+	+	+	+	+	+	–	+	+	–	–
Human herpes 6A, 6B, 7, 8	+	–	–	–	–	–	–	–	+	–	–
Varicella-zoster virus (VZV)	+	+	+	±	±	–	–	–	–	–	–
Cytomegalovirus (CMV)	–	–	+	–	+	–	–	–	–	–	–
Epstein–Barr virus (EBV)	–	–	–	–	+	+	–	–	–	–	–
Orthomyxoviridae											
Influenza A, B, C viruses	+	–	–	–	+	+	+	–	±	–	+
Papovaviridae											
Papillomaviruses	–	–	–	–	–	–	–	–	–	–	–
Polyomaviruses BK, JC	+	–	±	±	–	–	–	–	–	–	–

(Continued over)

Table 6.2 Isolation and propagation systems for human viruses (Continued)

Virus family/group	Cell culture					Organ culture	Embryonated eggs		Laboratory animals		
	Primary	Epithelial	Fibroblast	Vero	Other		Amn/All	CAM	Rodents	Primates	Other
Paramyxoviridae											
Parainfluenza viruses 1–3, 4A, 4B	+	+	−	±	+	±	±	−	±	−	+
Mumps virus	+	±	−	+	+	+	+	−	+	±	+
Measles virus	+	−	±	+	+	−	−	−	−	+	−
Respiratory syncytial virus (RSV)	+	+	±	±	+	+	−	−	+	+	+
Human metapneumovirus	+	+	−	+	−	−	−	−	+	+	+
Parvoviridae											
Parvovirus B19	−		−	−	±	±	−	−	−	−	−
Picornaviridae											
Polioviruses 1, 2, 3	+	+	+	+	+	+	−	−	+	+	+
Coxsackie A virus (23 types)	±	−	±	−	+	±	−	−	+	±	+
Coxsackie B virus (6 types)	+	+	+	+	+	+	−	−	+	−	−
Echovirus (31 types)	+	±	±	±	+	+	−	−	−	−	−
Enterovirus 68-71	+	±	±	±	+	−	−	−	−	±	−
Hepatitis A virus	±	−	±	±	±	−	−	−	−	+	−
Rhinoviruses (>100 types)	+	±	+	−	+	+	−	−	−	+	−
Poxviridae											
Vaccinia virus	+	+	+	+	+	−	−	+	+	−	+
Smallpox virus	+	+	+	+	+	−	−	+	−	+	−
Parapoxviruses	+	−	±	−	+	−	−	−	−	−	+
Molluscum contagiosum virus	−	−	−	−	±	−	−	−	−	−	−
Reoviridae											
Reovirus 1, 2, 3	+	±	±	±	+	+	−	−	+	+	+
Colorado tick fever virus	−	−	−	−	±	−	−	−	+	−	−
Rotaviruses	+	−	−	−	+	−	−	−	−	±	±
Retroviridae											
HIV, HTLV	−	−	−	−	+	−	−	−	−	+	−
Rhabdoviridae											
Rabies virus	+	−	−	±	+	−	±	±	+	+	+
VSV, other arboviruses	±	−	−	±	+	−	±	+	+	+	+
Togaviridae											
Sindbis virus, EEE virus, WEE virus, Semliki Forest virus, and other arboviruses	+	−	−	+	+	−	+	+	+	±	+
Rubella virus	+	−	−	+	+	−	−	−	±	±	±

+, Suitable for growth of virus; ±, partially suitable, i.e. some strains do not grow, or titers are low; −, unsuitable; Amn, amniotic cavity; All, allantoic cavity; CAM, chorioallantoic membrane; CE, California encephalitis; EEE, Eastern equine encephalitis; Embry., embryonated; JE, Japanese encephalitis; HIV, human immunodeficiency virus; HTLV, human T-cell leukemia/lymphoma virus; LCM, lymphocytic choriomeningitis; SARS, severe acute respiratory syndrome; SLE, St. Louis encephalitis; VSV, vesiculovirus; WEE, Western equine encephalitis.

is distinct from the other human coronaviruses in that it readily grows in MK, Vero, or Vero E6 cells, but does not grow or grows poorly in most other cell lines (Ksiazek et al. 2003). CPE is focal, with cells giving a rounded, refractile appearance, and is rapidly progressive, leading to detachment of the cell monolayer. Because culture requires BSL-3 procedures and facilities, diagnosis of SARS coronavirus infection is best made by serology (EIA, IFA) or detection of viral RNA by RT-PCR assay.

GASTROENTERITIS VIRUSES

These viruses (see Chapters 41, Human enteric RNA viruses: Astroviruses; and 43, Reoviruses, Orbiviruses, and Coltiviruses) also belong to diverse families and have unique requirements for culture. Rotaviruses will replicate in BSC-1, MA104, and AGMK cells under roller conditions with trypsin treatment. Astroviruses replicate in human CaCo-2 and PLC/PRF/5 cells under a fortified medium with trypsin (Taylor et al. 1997; Brinker et al. 2000). The noroviruses and sapoviruses cannot be isolated in the laboratory (Koopmans and Horzinek 1994; Lennette et al. 1995). The gastroenteritis viruses can be distinguished by EM, EIA, and RT-PCR (Erdman et al. 1989; Coulson et al. 1999; Rabenau et al. 2003).

HEPATITIS VIRUSES

Hepatitis A virus, a picornavirus (see Chapter 53, Hepatitis A and E), replicates in MK cultures in 1–4 weeks, but is noncytolytic. It is detected by EIA or RT-PCR. The hepatitis B virus (see Chapter 55), hepatitis C virus (Chapter 54), hepatitis D virus (Chapter 56), and hepatitis E virus (Chapter 53) do not grow in routine cell cultures and must be diagnosed by antigen (EIA or TR-FIA), or nucleic acid detection assays (Siitari et al. 1983; Balayan 1993; Wilber 1993; Kurstak et al. 1995).

HERPESVIRUSES

The herpesviruses (see Chapters 25–29) are spread by aerosolized droplets, fomites, and direct contact, and cause a wide range of ocular, oropharyngeal, genital, and generalized disease in humans. They have three types of CPE in cell culture. HSV-1 and -2 grow well in many cell types, producing grapelike clusters of round, refractile, enlarged cells often identical to adenovirus CPE in HEK, HEp-2, KB, HeLa, A549, HLF, NCI-H292, primary rabbit kidney, and other cells. At complete CPE, all cells become lysed and detached from the vessel surface. HSV-1 grows fast (1–2 days), makes fewer clusters, and may produce ballooned, multinucleate giant cells with granulated cytoplasm. HSV-2, usually a genital isolate, grows more slowly than type 1. HSV does not require roller cultures, but HEp-2, NCI-H292, and fibroblast cells will probably be on roller or

rocker apparatus for the benefit of other viruses to which these cells are susceptible.

CMV is notably labile. The only herpesvirus that is shed in great amounts in the urine, it replicates slowly (12–30 days) in roller cultures of diploid fibroblast cells. CMV produces giant-cell CPE resembling elongated foci of refractile, swollen cells, somewhat akin to measles CPE.

Varicella-zoster virus (VZV), the cause of chickenpox and herpes zoster (shingles), also grows slowly in fibroblasts on roller culture. It produces a CPE characterized by enlarged, round, glassy cells in small foci in 2–10 days, which is thus distinct from that caused by CMV. VZV can produce large foci of multinucleate giant cells when the individual foci coalesce.

Epstein–Barr virus (EBV) is associated with infectious mononucleosis, Burkitt's lymphoma, and nasopharyngeal carcinoma; human herpesvirus 6 (HHV-6), the cause of roseola infantum (exanthema subitum or 'fourth disease') in children; human herpesvirus 7 (HHV-7), the probable cause of some roseola cases; and human herpesvirus 8 (HHV-8), the cause of AIDS-associated Kaposi's sarcoma (Chang et al. 1994). EBV requires special conditions and cells for successful cultivation in the laboratory. In culture, it infects both B lymphocytes and epithelial cells with the CD21 receptor; HHV-6 grows best in primary CD4$^+$ T lymphocytes rendered more susceptible by the presence of antibody to CD3 (Pellett et al. 1992; Yasukawa et al. 1993; Hall et al. 1994); HHV-7 also replicates in CD4$^+$ T-lymphocytes (Black and Pellett 1993; Lusso et al. 1994; Tanaka et al. 1994). HHV-8 has been difficult to isolate from cell culture, although limited infections of CD19 B lymphocytes, macrophages, and certain endothelial cells has been demonstrated (Blackbourn et al. 2000).

Herpesviruses are readily visualized by EM, the icosahedral nucleocapsid and the baggy envelope being prominent. The viruses are commonly speciated by IFA, EIA, LA, and SN tests and by DNA hybridization and PCR assays (Buller et al. 1992; Drew 1992; Perez et al. 1995).

ORTHOMYXOVIRUSES

Influenza A, B, and C viruses (see Chapter 32, Orthomyxoviruses: influenza) are spread by aerosol droplets and fomites, and are best recovered in roller cultures of primary MK and MDCK cells and in intact chick embryos. Chick embryo cells, MDCK, and other cells require rolling and a fortified medium containing trypsin 2 µg/ml for optimal sensitivity. The CPE may be seen as a combination of syncytia, rounding, and degeneration. The syncytia caused by influenza B virus may be accompanied by vacuolation. Influenza CPE may develop in 4–7 days, but cultures should be blind-passaged and held an additional week. Because the cells rarely become detached and may not have an obvious CPE, virus detection in MK cultures is verified by hemadsorption with chicken or guinea-pig erythrocytes, and in MDCK cells by HA. Some strains of influenza A and B can be isolated only in 9- to 11-day-old chick embryos. The viruses are then typed by HI, IFA, EIA, TR-FIA or RT-PCR assay (Frank et al. 1979; Grandien et al. 1985; Walls et al. 1986; Bucher et al. 1991; Ziegler et al. 1995; Stockton et al. 1998).

Hemadsorption is a fast and convenient method for detecting orthomyxoviruses (influenza A, B, C) and non-RSV paramyxoviruses (parainfluenza 1, 2, 3, 4A, 4B; mumps; measles) in cell cultures. It is even used in the presence of CPE to obtain a quick distinction from other virus groups that may cause similar CPE in the same types of cultures. The supernatant fluid from the cell culture is decanted into a sterile tube at the end of the incubation period (7–10 days), to conserve virus and viral antigens for passaging and testing. The monolayer is washed twice with 2–3 ml of plain Hank's balanced salt solution (HBSS) at room temperature; 1 ml of fresh HBSS is added, followed by 0.2 ml of 0.4 percent mammalian erythrocyte suspension from the appropriate species. The tube is incubated stationary with the fluid covering the monolayer. The test is read three times at 20-min intervals by agitating the tube in a sideways motion and then observing at ×40–100 magnification for erythrocytes firmly attached to the cultured cells (positive) or floating free in the fluid (negative).

PAPOVAVIRUSES

The papovaviruses (see Chapters 23, Papillomavirus; and 24, Polyomaviruses) consist of two genera (*Papillomavirus* and *Polyomavirus*), but only *Polyomavirus* can be isolated in cell culture. The BK polyomavirus can be recovered in NCI-H292 and diploid fibroblast cells, and the JC polyomavirus replicates in primary human fetal glial cells, but both viruses may be missed because their CPE develops slowly and may be ill-defined. It is a granular, degenerative, slowly lytic CPE, similar to that caused by reoviruses. BK virus is identified by hemagglutination inhibition (HI) tests at 4°C with human 'O' erythrocytes and specific antiserum; BK and JC viruses are identified by EIA, SN, hybridization probes or PCR assay. The other genus, papillomaviruses, cannot be propagated in cell culture so are identified in biopsied tissues by antipeptide EIAs and by hybridization probes and PCR (Eklund and Dillner 1995; Ylitalo et al. 1995).

PARAMYXOVIRUSES

The human paramyxoviruses (Chapter 33, General properties of the paramyxoviruses) are parainfluenza types 1, 2, 3, 4A, 4B, mumps, measles (rubeola), RSV and the recently identified human metapneumovirus (hMPV) (van den Hoogen et al. 2001). The parainfluenza and mumps viruses replicate well in roller cultures of NCI-H292 cells under a fortified medium containing trypsin 1.5 µg/ml for optimal sensitivity, and in primary MK cells without trypsin (Meguro et al. 1979; Castells et al.

1990). The CPE induced by these viruses may develop in 4–7 days, and is a combination of syncytia and rounding. The syncytia may be accompanied by a granular degeneration with parainfluenzavirus types 1–4. Mumps virus often gives rise to large syncytia. The cultures must generally be blind-passaged and held an additional week to ensure viral growth. The cells rarely become detached, and may not show obvious CPE at all, so NCI-H292 or MK cultures for these viruses must be hemadsorbed with guinea-pig, human, or monkey erythrocytes at the end of the culture period and then typed by HI, IFA, EIA, TR-FIA or RT-PCR assay (Grandien et al., 1985; Van Tiel et al. 1988; Hierholzer et al. 1989, 1993a; Takimoto et al. 1991; Echevarria et al. 1998).

Measles virus can be grown in a wide range of cell culture systems, but is most successfully isolated in the Epstein–Barr virus-transformed marmoset B lymphoblastoid cell line, B95a (Kobune et al. 1990). CPE is characterized by presence of classical multinucleate giant cells resulting from fusion of adjacent cells. Because the CPE may develop slowly and not be recognized, the monolayers should be screened to ensure detection of the virus. Measles can be identified by HI tests with vervet monkey erythrocytes, IFA, EIA, SN, or RT-PCR assay (Hummel et al. 1992; Nakayama et al. 1995).

RSV produces a distinct syncytial CPE in HEp-2, HeLa, and NCI-H292 cells in 5–12 days in roller cultures. The balled-up syncytia usually become detached from the glass surface and float freely in the medium. Some strains of RSV, particularly of group B, produce more cellular degeneration than syncytia in HEp-2 and NCI-H292 cells. Group A and B strains of RSV are readily identified by IFA, EIA, TR-FIA, or RT-PCR (Freymuth et al. 1991; Waris 1991; Cane et al. 1992; Hierholzer et al. 1994b). Details on paramyxovirus typing are found elsewhere (Popow-Kraupp et al. 1986; Ahluwalia et al. 1987; Akerlind et al. 1988; Anderson et al. 1991).

hMPV produces a delayed cellular degeneration with round and refractile cells and occasional syncytial formation in tertiary MK and LLC-MK2 cells supplemented with 1.5 µg/ml trypsin. The appearance of CPE can take up to 2 to 3 weeks from inoculation of the specimen, or may not be recognized, and therefore cultures should be screened to ensure detection of the virus. HMPV is identified by RT-PCR assay (Boivin et al. 2002; Falsey et al. 2003).

PARVOVIRUSES

The human parvovirus B19 (see Chapter 21, Parvoviruses) causes 'fifth disease' (erythema infectiosum) and is easily spread by aerosolized droplets and fomites in schools, and vertically to the fetus during the first trimester of pregnancy (see Chapter 64, Virus infections in immunocompromised patients). The virus can be grown in specialized erythropoietic stem cell cultures, but not in standard culture systems. Therefore, B19 infection is established by EIA testing of the patient's acute-phase serum for antiviral IgM antibodies or by PCR assay for viral DNA (Heegaard and Brown 2002).

PICORNAVIRUSES

This large family (see Chapter 40, Picornaviruses) includes the enteroviruses (poliovirus 1–3, 23 coxsackie A viruses, six coxsackie B viruses, 31 echoviruses, and five more recent enteroviruses), and the rhinoviruses (approximately 125 serotypes). The enteroviruses are spread by aerosolized droplets, fomites, and the fecal–oral route, whereas the rhinoviruses are spread by aerosols and fomites only (Agbalika et al. 1984; Dick et al. 1987; Mandell et al. 1990). These viruses produce a 'shrunken cell degeneration' CPE in NCI-H292, MK, RD, trypsin-treated MA-104 and diploid fibroblast cells, preferably in roller cultures, although some coxsackie A viruses grow only in the brain of suckling mice. The CPE is often observed as tadpole-shaped, shrunken cells with pyknotic nuclei, beginning in patches at the edges of the monolayer and progressing inward. CPE for polioviruses and some coxsackie B viruses is quite rapid, becoming complete in 1–3 days with all cells detached from the glass. CPE for the remaining enteroviruses and the rhinoviruses generally requires 4–7 days or longer, is often characterized by individual small, rounded, and sometimes refractile cells or by a degenerative appearance across the monolayer, and may never become complete. Subpassaging is helpful. The variable CPE found in enterovirus- or rhinovirus-infected cells is not diagnostically confusing, however, because these viruses do not hemadsorb, rarely hemagglutinate with any species of erythrocytes, and do not interfere with test systems for other viruses. Enteroviruses are distinguished from rhinoviruses by acid- and chloroform-lability tests in which both genera are chloroform-stable, but only enteroviruses are acid-stable, or by group-specific IFA or RT-PCR assay (Hyypia and Stanway 1993; Egger et al. 1995; Halonen et al. 1995; Lipson et al. 2001). The viruses can be serotyped by type-specific SN tests.

POXVIRUSES

Vaccinia and certain other poxviruses (see Chapter 30, Poxviruses) can be isolated in MK, Vero, NCI-H292, and diploid fibroblast cells. Their CPE is characterized as cell fusion with plaques. Plaques ranging from 1 to 6 mm in diameter (depending on the virus) are formed in 2–4 days, during which the infected cells fuse, form cytoplasmic bridging, and then disintegrate. Some poxviruses produce plaques on the CAM of 12-day chick embryos. Identification is accomplished from the type

and size of plaques formed and by EM, HI, EIA, IFA, REA, and PCR.

REOVIRUSES

Reoviruses 1–3 can be isolated from throat and rectal specimens in NCI-H292, MK, and HeLa cells under stationary or roller conditions after 5–14 days of culture, but, unlike other members of the family *Reoviridae* (see Chapter 43, Reoviruses, Orbiviruses and Coltiviruses), have never been clearly associated with human disease. In cell culture they cause a slow lytic degeneration with granulation of the cytoplasm, similar to polyomavirus CPE. MK cultures should be rolled. Reoviruses are easily visualized by EM and serotyped by SN and HI tests with human type 'O' erythrocytes.

RETROVIRUSES

The HIV and HTLV viruses (see Chapter 61, Prions of humans and animals) also require specialized systems for isolation and identification, and will not be recovered by standard culture methods. They are identified by EIA, western blot, or RT-PCR assay (Isenberg 1992; Persing and Smith 1993; Signoret et al. 1993).

RUBELLA

Rubella virus, a togavirus (see Chapter 45, Rubella), was originally detected because of its ability to prevent another virus from infecting the cells in which it was replicating. Current diagnostic testing for rubella may employ specialized cultures in which CPE may become evident. Rubella can, under certain conditions, cause an ill-defined and variable CPE in rabbit cornea, rabbit kidney, and Vero cells. Usually, however, rubella is detected by the interference test, in which replication of another virus (e.g. echovirus 11 or coxsackie virus A9) is inhibited by prior inoculation of the test material. A positive result may be confirmed by HI, EIA, LA, TR-FIA, or RT-PCR assay (Shankaran et al. 1990).

The interpretation of any culture isolation result or of any test used to identify the isolate depends on the methods employed, but viral growth alone should never be considered pathognomonic. The association of an isolate with disease depends on the clinical data obtained with the specimen and on the known epidemiology of the virus. Thus, careful virus isolation and identification test results, coupled with sound epidemiological data are the key to accurate diagnosis of viral infections.

ACKNOWLEDGMENTS

This chapter is adapted and expanded from Hierholzer, J.C. 1998. Propogation and identification of viruses. In: Mahy, B.W.J. and Collier, L. (eds) *Topley & Wilson's Microbiology and Microbial Infections*, 9th edn, Vol. 1. *Virology*. London: Edward Arnold, 57–74.

REFERENCES

Ades, E.W., Hierholzer, J.C., et al. 1992. Viral susceptibility of an immortalized human microvascular endothelial cell line. *J Virol Methods*, **39**, 83–90.

Adrian, T., Wadell, G., et al. 1986. DNA restriction analysis of adenovirus prototypes 1 to 41. *Arch Virol*, **91**, 277–90.

Agbalika, F., Hartemann, P. and Foliguet, J.M. 1984. Trypsin-treated MA-104: a sensitive cell line for isolating enteric viruses from environmental samples. *Appl Environ Microbiol*, **47**, 378–80.

Ahluwalia, G., Embree, J., et al. 1987. Comparison of nasopharyngeal aspirate and nasopharyngeal swab specimens for respiratory syncytial virus diagnosis by cell culture, indirect immunofluorescence assay, and enzyme-linked immunosorbent assay. *J Clin Microbiol*, **25**, 763–7.

Akerlind, B., Norrby, E., et al. 1988. Respiratory syncytial virus: heterogeneity of subgroup B strains. *J Gen Virol*, **69**, 2145–54.

Alberts, B., Bray, D., et al. 1994. *Molecular biology of the cell*, 3rd edn. New York: Garland.

Almeida, J.D., Hall, T., et al. 1978. The effect of trypsin on the growth of rotavirus. *J Gen Virol*, **40**, 213–18.

Anderson, L.J., Hierholzer, J.C., et al. 1985. Microneutralization test for respiratory syncytial virus based on an enzyme immunoassay. *J Clin Microbiol*, **22**, 1050–2.

Anderson, L.J., Hendry, R.M., et al. 1991. Multicenter study of strains of respiratory syncytial virus. *J Infect Dis*, **163**, 687–92.

ATCC. 1992. ATCC quality control methods for cell lines, 2nd edn. Rockville MD: American Type Culture Collection.

Ausubel, F.M. and Brent, R. 1991. *Current protocols in molecular biology*. New York: Green Publishers and Wiley-Interscience.

Balayan, M.S. 1993. Hepatitis E virus infection in Europe: regional situation regarding laboratory diagnosis and epidemiology. *Clin Diagn Virol*, **1**, 1–9.

Barkley, W.E. 1979. Safety considerations in the cell culture laboratory. *Methods Enzymol*, **58**, 36–43.

Barenfanger, J., Drake, C., et al. 2001. R-Mix cells are faster, at least as sensitive and marginally more costly than conventional cell lines for the detection of respiratory viruses. *J Clin Virol*, **22**, 101–10.

Barrett, T. and Inglis, S.C. 1985. Growth, purification and titration of influenza viruses. In: Mahy, B.W.J. (ed.), *Virology: a practical approach*. Oxford: IRL Press, 119–50.

Bennink, J.R. and Yewdell, J.W. 1990. Recombinant vaccinia viruses as vectors for studying T lymphocyte specificity and function. *Curr Top Microbiol Immunol*, **163**, 153–84.

Bissell, D.M., Caron, J.M., et al. 1990. Transcriptional regulation of the albumin gene in cultured rat hepatocytes: role of basement-membrane matrix. *Mol Biol Med*, **7**, 187–97.

Black, J.B. and Pellett, P.E. 1993. Human herpesvirus 7. *Rev Med Virol*, **3**, 217–23.

Blackbourn, D.J., Lennette, E., et al. 2000. The restricted cellular host range of human herpesvirus 8. *AIDS*, **16**, 1123–33.

Boivin, G., Abed, Y., et al. 2002. Virological features and clinical manifestations associated with human metapneumovirus: a new paramyxovirus responsible for acute respiratory-tract infections in all age groups. *J Infect Dis*, **186**, 1330–4.

Boss, B.D. 1986. An improved in vitro immunization procedure for the production of monoclonal antibodies. *Methods Enzymol*, **121**, 27–33.

Brinker, J.P., Blacklow, N.R. and Herrmann, J.E. 2000. Human astrovirus isolation and propagation in multiple cell lines. *Arch Virol*, **145**, 1847–56.

Brown, M., Shami, Y., et al. 1990. Time-resolved fluoroimmunoassay for enteric adenoviruses using the europium chelator 4,7-bis(chlorosulfophenyl)-1,10-phenanthroline-2,9-dicarboxylic acid. *J Clin Microbiol*, **28**, 1398–402.

Bucher, D.J., Mikhail, A., et al. 1991. Rapid detection of type A influenza viruses with monoclonal antibodies to the M protein (M1) by enzyme-linked immunosorbent assay and time-resolved fluoroimmunoassay. *J Clin Microbiol*, **29**, 2484–8.

Buller, R.S., Bailey, T.C., et al. 1992. Use of a modified shell vial technique to quantitate cytomegalovirus viremia in a population of solid-organ transplant recipients. *J Clin Microbiol*, **30**, 2620–4.

Cane, P.A., Matthews, D.A. and Pringle, C.R. 1992. Analysis of relatedness of subgroup A respiratory syncytial viruses isolated worldwide. *Virus Res*, **25**, 15–22.

Castells, E., George, V.G. and Hierholzer, J.C. 1990. NCI-H292 as an alternative cell line for the isolation and propagation of the human paramyxoviruses. *Arch Virol*, **115**, 277–88.

Castro, B.A., Weiss, C.D., et al. 1988. Optimal conditions for recovery of the human immunodeficiency virus from peripheral blood mononuclear cells. *J Clin Microbiol*, **26**, 2371–6.

Caul, E.O. and Egglestone, S.I. 1977. Further studies on human enteric coronaviruses. *Arch Virol*, **54**, 107–17.

Chang, Y., Cesarman, E., et al. 1994. Identification of herpesvirus-like DNA sequences in AIDS-associated Kaposi's sarcoma. *Science*, **266**, 1865.

Chappell, W.A., White, L.A. and Gamble, W.C. 1984. *Production manual for viral, rickettsial, chlamydial, mycoplasmal reagents*, 6th edn. Atlanta, GA: Centers for Disease Control.

Chesebro, B. and Wehrly, K. 1988. Development of a sensitive quantitative focal assay for human immunodeficiency virus infectivity. *J Virol*, **62**, 3779–88.

Chong, P. and Gillam, S. 1985. Purification of biologically active rubella virus antigens by immunoaffinity chromatography. *J Virol Methods*, **10**, 261–8.

Coligan, J.E. and Kruisbeek, A.M. Current protocols in immunology. Vol. 1. New York: Green Publishers and Wiley-Interscience.

Collier, L.H. and Oxford, J.O. 1993. *Human virology*. Oxford: Oxford University Press.

Coulson, B.S., Gentsch, J.R., et al. 1999. Comparison of enzyme immunoassay and reverse transcriptase PCR for identification of serotype G9 rotaviruses. *J Clin Microbiol*, **37**, 3187–93.

Cox, W.I., Tartaglia, J. and Paoletti, E. 1993. Induction of cytotoxic T lymphocytes by recombinant canarypox (ALVAC) and attenuated vaccinia (NYVAC) viruses expressing the HIV-1 envelope glycoprotein. *Virology*, **195**, 845–50.

Crandell, R.A., Hierholzer, J.C., et al. 1978. Contamination of primary embryonic bovine kidney cell cultures with parainfluenza type 2 simian virus 5 and infectious bovine rhinotracheitis virus. *J Clin Microbiol*, **7**, 214–18.

Dick, E.C., Jennings, L.C., et al. 1987. Aerosol transmission of rhinovirus colds. *J Infect Dis*, **156**, 442–8.

Drew, W.L. 1992. Nonpulmonary manifestations of cytomegalovirus infection in immunocompromised patients. *Clin Microbiol Rev*, **5**, 204–10.

Eberle, R. and Hilliard, J. 1995. The simian herpesviruses. *Infect Agents Dis*, **4**, 55–70.

Echevarria, J.E., Erdman, D.D., et al. 1998. Simultaneous detection and identification of human parainfluenza viruses 1, 2, and 3 from clinical samples by multiplex PCR. *J Clin Microbiol*, **36**, 1388–91.

Egger, D., Pasamontes, L., et al. 1995. Reverse transcription multiplex PCR for differentiation between polio- and enteroviruses from clinical and environmental samples. *J Clin Microbiol*, **33**, 1442–7.

Eisenberg, R.J., Ponce de Leon, M., et al. 1982. Purification of glycoprotein gD of herpes simplex virus types 1 and 2 by use of monoclonal antibody. *J Virol*, **41**, 1099–104.

Eklund, C. and Dillner, J. 1995. A two-site enzyme immunoassay for quantitation of human papillomavirus type 16 particles. *J Virol Methods*, **53**, 11–23.

Elliott, L.H., Ksiazek, T.G., et al. 1994. Isolation of the causative agent of hantavirus pulmonary syndrome. *Am J Trop Med Hyg*, **51**, 102–8.

Erdman, D.D., Gary, G.W. and Anderson, L.J. 1989. Development and evaluation of an IgM capture enzyme immunoassay for diagnosis of recent Norwalk virus infection. *J Virol Methods*, **24**, 57–66.

Espy, M.J., Hierholzer, J.C. and Smith, T.F. 1987. The effect of centrifugation on the rapid detection of adenovirus in shell vials. *Am J Clin Pathol*, **88**, 358–60.

Evans, V.J., Perry, V.P. and Vincent, M.M. 1975 *TCA manual*, Vol. 1. Rockville, MD: Tissue Culture Association.

Falsey, A.R., Erdman, D., et al. 2003. Human metapneumovirus infections in young and elderly adults. *J Infect Dis*, **187**, 785–90.

Fields, B.N. and Knipe, D.M. 1990, *Virology*, Vols 1 and 2. 2nd edn. New York: Raven Press.

Fleming, D.O. and Richardson, J.H. 1995. *Laboratory safety: principles and practices*, 2nd edn. Washington DC: American Society for Microbiology Press.

Foung, S.K., Engleman, E.G. and Grumet, F.C. 1986. Generation of human monoclonal antibodies by fusion of EBV-activated B cells to a human–mouse hybridoma. *Methods Enzymol*, **121**, 168–74.

Frank, A.L., Couch, R.B., et al. 1979. Comparison of different tissue cultures for isolation and quantitation of influenza and parainfluenza viruses. *J Clin Microbiol*, **10**, 32–6.

Freshney, R.I. 2000. *Culture of animal cells: a manual of basic technique*, 4th edn. New York: Wiley-Liss.

Freymuth, F., Petitjean, J., et al. 1991. Prevalence of respiratory syncytial virus subgroups A and B in France from 1982 to 1990. *J Clin Microbiol*, **29**, 653–5.

Gamble, W.C., Chappell, W.A. and George, E.H. 1980. Inactivation of rabies diagnostic reagents by gamma radiation. *J Clin Microbiol*, **12**, 676–8.

Gessler, A.E., Bender, C.E. and Parkinson, M.C. 1956. A new and rapid method for isolating viruses by selective fluorocarbon deproteinization. *Trans NY Acad Sci*, **2**, 701–3.

Gleaves, C.A., Hursh, D.A., et al. 1989. Detection of cytomegalovirus from clinical specimens in centrifugation culture by in situ DNA hybridization and monoclonal antibody staining. *J Clin Microbiol*, **27**, 21–3.

Goding, J. 1996. *Monoclonal antibodies: principles and practice*, 3rd edn. London: Academic Press.

Gould, E.A. and Clegg, J.C.S. 1985. Growth, titration and purification of alphaviruses and flaviviruses. In: Mahy, B.W.J. (ed.), *Virology: a practical approach*. Oxford: IRL Press, 44–78.

Grandien, M., Pettersson, C.A., et al. 1985. Rapid viral diagnosis of acute respiratory infections: comparison of enzyme-linked immunosorbent assay and the immunofluorescence technique for detection of viral antigens in nasopharyngeal secretions. *J Clin Microbiol*, **22**, 757–60.

Hall, C.B., Long, C.E., et al. 1994. Human herpesvirus-6 infection in children: a prospective study of complications and reactivation. *N Engl J Med*, **331**, 432–8.

Halonen, P., Rocha, E., et al. 1995. Detection of enteroviruses and rhinoviruses in clinical specimens by PCR and liquid-phase hybridization. *J Clin Microbiol*, **33**, 648–53.

Hanson, C.V., Riggs, J.L. and Lennette, E.H. 1978. Photochemical inactivation of DNA and RNA viruses by psoralen derivatives. *J Gen Virol*, **40**, 345–8.

Harlow, E. and Lane, D. 1988. *Antibodies – a laboratory manual*. Cold Spring Harbor, NY: Cold Spring Harbor Laboratory.

Hayflick, L. 1973. Fetal human diploid cells. In: Kruse, P.F. and Patterson, M.K. (eds), *Tissue culture methods and applications*. New York: Academic Press, 43–5.

Heegaard, E.D. and Brown, K.E. 2002. Human parvovirus B19. *Clin Microbiol Rev*, **15**, 485–505.

Hierholzer, J.C. 1976. Purification and biophysical properties of human coronavirus 229E. *Virology*, **75**, 155–65.

Hierholzer, J.C. 1991. Rapid diagnosis of viral infection. In: Vaheri, A., Tilton, R.C. and Balows, A. (eds), *Rapid methods and automation in microbiology and immunology*. Berlin: Springer-Verlag, 556–573.

Hierholzer, J.C. 1992. Adenoviruses in the immunocompromised host. *Clin Microbiol Rev*, **5**, 262–74.

Hierholzer, J.C. 1993. Viral causes of respiratory infections. *Immunol Allergy Clin N Am*, **13**, 27–42.

Hierholzer, J.C. and Bingham, P.G. 1978. Vero microcultures for adenovirus neutralization tests. *J Clin Microbiol*, **7**, 499–506.

Hierholzer, J.C., Johansson, K.H., et al. 1987. Comparison of monoclonal time-resolved fluoroimmunoassay with monoclonal capture-biotinylated detector enzyme immunoassay for adenovirus antigen detection. *J Clin Microbiol*, **25**, 1662–7.

Hierholzer, J.C., Bingham, P.G., et al. 1989. Comparison of monoclonal antibody time-resolved fluoroimmunoassay with monoclonal antibody capture-biotinylated detector enzyme immunoassay for respiratory syncytial virus and parainfluenza virus antigen detection. *J Clin Microbiol*, **27**, 1243–9.

Hierholzer, J.C., Stone, Y.O. and Broderson, J.R. 1991. Antigenic relationships among the 47 human adenoviruses determined in reference horse antisera. *Arch Virol*, **121**, 179–97.

Hierholzer, J.C., Bingham, P.G., et al. 1993a. Time-resolved fluoroimmunoassays with monoclonal antibodies for rapid identification of parainfluenza type 4 and mumps viruses. *Arch Virol*, **130**, 335–52.

Hierholzer, J.C., Castells, E., et al. 1993b. Sensitivity of NCI-H292 human lung mucoepidermoid cells for respiratory and other human viruses. *J Clin Microbiol*, **31**, 1504–10.

Hierholzer, J.C., Halonen, P.E., et al. 1993c. Detection of adenovirus in clinical specimens by polymerase chain reaction and liquid-phase hybridization quantitated by time-resolved fluorometry. *J Clin Microbiol*, **31**, 1886–91.

Hierholzer, J.C., Halonen, P.E., et al. 1994a. Antigen detection in human respiratory coronavirus infections by monoclonal time-resolved fluoroimmunoassay. *Clin Diagn Virol*, **2**, 165–79.

Hierholzer, J.C., Tannock, G.A., et al. 1994b. Subgrouping of respiratory syncytial virus strains from Australia and Papua New Guinea by biological and antigenic characteristics. *Arch Virol*, **136**, 133–47.

Huang, Y.T. and Turchek, B.M. 2000. Mink lung cells and mixed mink lung and A549 cells for rapid detection of influenza virus and other respiratory viruses. *J Clin Microbiol*, **38**, 422–3.

Hull, R.N. 1968. The simian viruses. *Virol Monogr*, **2**, 1–66.

Hummel, K.B., Erdman, D.D., et al. 1992. Baculovirus expression of the nucleoprotein gene of measles virus and utility of the recombinant protein in diagnostic enzyme immunoassays. *J Clin Microbiol*, **30**, 2874–80.

Hyypia, T. and Stanway, G. 1993. Biology of coxsackie A viruses. *Adv Virus Res*, **42**, 343–73.

Isenberg, H.D. Clinical microbiology procedures handbook. Vol. 2. Washington DC: American Society for Microbiology.

Itoh, H., Morimoto, Y., et al. 1970. Effect of trypsin on viral susceptibility of Vero cell cultures – *Cercopithecus* kidney line. *Jpn J Med Sci Biol*, **23**, 227–35.

Jarvis, D.L. 1991. Baculovirus expression vectors. *Ann NY Acad Sci*, **646**, 240–7.

Johnson, F.B. 1990. Transport of viral specimens. *Clin Microbiol Rev*, **3**, 120–31.

Johnston, S.L. and Siegel, C.S. 1990. Presumptive identification of enteroviruses with RD, HEp-2 and RMK cell lines. *J Clin Microbiol*, **28**, 1049–50.

Kobune, F., Sakata, H. and Suguira, A. 1990. Marmoset lymphoblastoid cells as a sensitive host for isolation of measles virus. *J Virol*, **64**, 700–5.

Koopmans, M. and Horzinek, M.C. 1994. Toroviruses of animals and humans: a review. *Adv Virus Res*, **43**, 233–73.

Ksiazek, T.G., Erdman, D., et al. 2003. A novel coronavirus associated with severe acute respiratory syndrome. *N Engl J Med*, **348**, 1953–66.

Kurstak, E., Kurstak, C., et al. 1995. Current status of the molecular genetics of hepatitis C virus and its utilization in the diagnosis of infection. *Clin Diagn Virol*, **3**, 1–15.

LaRocco, M.T. 2000. Evaluation of an enzyme-linked viral inducible system for the rapid detection of Herpes simplex virus. *Eur J Clin Microbiol*, **19**, 233–5.

Lennette, E.H., Halonen, P. and Murphy, F.A. 1988. *Laboratory diagnosis of infectious diseases: principles and practice. Viral, rickettsial, and chlamydial diseases*, Vol. II. . New York: Springer-Verlag.

Lennette, E.H., Lennette, D.A. and Lennette, E.T. 1995. *Diagnostic procedures for viral, rickettsial and chlamydial infections*, 7th edn. Washington DC: American Public Health Association.

Li, Q.X., Young, L.S., et al. 1992. Epstein–Barr virus infection and replication in a human epithelial cell system. *Nature*, **356**, 347–50.

Lipson, S.M., David, K., et al. 2001. Detection of precytopathic effect of enteroviruses in clinical specimens by centrifugation-enhanced antigen detection. *J Clin Microbiol*, **39**, 2755–9.

Lusso, P., Secchiero, P., et al. 1994. CD4 is a critical component of the receptor for human herpesvirus 7: interference with human immunodeficiency virus. *Proc Natl Acad Sci USA*, **91**, 3872–6.

Mahy, B.W.J. and Kangro, H. (eds) 1996. *Virology methods manual*. London: Academic Press.

Mandell, G.L., Douglas, R.G. and Bennett, J.E. (eds) 1990. *Principles and practice of infectious diseases*. New York: Churchill Livingstone.

Markham, P.D. and Salahuddin, S.Z. 1987. In vitro cultivation of human leukocytes: methods for the expression and isolation of human viruses. *BioTechniques*, **5**, 432–43.

Matthey, S., Nicholson, D., et al. 1992. Rapid detection of respiratory viruses by shell vial culture and direct staining by using pooled and individual monoclonal antibodies. *J Clin Microbiol*, **30**, 540–4.

McIntosh, K., Dees, J.H., et al. 1967. Recovery in tracheal organ cultures of novel viruses from patients with respiratory disease. *Proc Natl Acad Sci USA*, **57**, 933–40.

Meguro, H., Bryant, J.D., et al. 1979. Canine kidney cell line for isolation of respiratory viruses. *J Clin Microbiol*, **9**, 175–9.

Murray, P.R. and Baron, E.J. (eds) 1995. *Manual of clinical microbiology*, 6th edn. Washington DC: American Society for Microbiology Press.

Nakayama, T., Mori, T., et al. 1995. Detection of measles virus genome directly from clinical samples by reverse transcriptase-polymerase chain reaction and genetic variability. *Virus Res*, **35**, 1–16.

Navarro-Marí, J.M., Sanbonmatsu-Gámez, S., et al. 1999. Rapid detection of respiratory viruses by shell vial assay using simultaneous culture of Hep-2, LLC-MK2 and MDCK cells in a single vial. *J Clin Microbiol*, **37**, 2346–7.

Norrby, E. 1962. Hemagglutination by measles virus: a simple procedure for production of high potency antigen for hemagglutination-inhibition (HI) tests. *Proc Soc Exp Biol Med*, **111**, 814–18.

Olivo, P.D. 1999. Application of genetically engineered cell lines to diagnostic virology. In: Lennette, E.H. and Smith, T.F. (eds), *Laboratory diagnosis of viral infections*. New York: Marcel Dekker Inc, 159–75.

Olsen, M.A., Shuck, K.M., et al. 1993. Isolation of seven respiratory viruses in shell vials: a practical and highly sensitive method. *J Clin Microbiol*, **27**, 2107–9.

Pellett, P.E., Black, J.B. and Yamamoto, M. 1992. Human herpesvirus 6: the virus and the search for its role as a human pathogen. *Adv Virus Res*, **41**, 1–52.

Perez, J.L., Niubo, J., et al. 1995. Comparison of three commercially available monoclonal antibodies directed against pp65 antigen for cytomegalovirus antigenemia assay. *Diagn Microbiol Infect Dis*, **21**, 21–5.

Persing, D.H. and Smith, T.F. 1993. *Diagnostic molecular microbiology: principles and applications*. Washington DC: American Society for Microbiology.

Peter, J.H. and Baumgarten, H. 1992. *Monoclonal antibodies*. Berlin: Springer-Verlag.

Popow-Kraupp, T., Kern, G., et al. 1986. Detection of respiratory syncytial virus in nasopharyngeal secretions by enzyme-linked immunosorbent assay, indirect immunofluorescence, and virus isolation: a comparative study. *J Med Virol*, **19**, 123–34.

Rabenau, H.F., Sturmer, M., et al. 2003. Laboratory diagnosis of norovirus: which method is the best? *Intervirology*, **46**, 232–8.

Sanchez-Fauquier, A, Carrascosa, AL, et al. 1994. Characterization of a human astrovirus serotype 2 structural protein (VP26) that contains an epitope involved in virus neutralization. *Virology*, **201**, 312–20.

Scharff, M.D., Roberts, S. and Thammana, P. 1981. Monoclonal antibodies. *J Infect Dis*, **143**, 346–51.

Schirm, J., Meulenberg, J., et al. 1989. Rapid detection of varicella-zoster virus in clinical specimens using monoclonal antibodies on shell vials and smears. *J Med Virol*, **28**, 1–6.

Schirm, J., Luijt, D.S., et al. 1992. Rapid detection of respiratory viruses using mixtures of monoclonal antibodies on shell vial cultures. *J Med Virol*, **38**, 147–51.

Schmidt, N.J. 1989. Cell culture procedures for diagnostic virology. In: Schmidt, N.J. and Emmons, R.W. (eds), *Diagnostic procedures for viral, rickettsial and chlamydial infections*, 6th edn. Washington DC: American Public Health Association, 51–100.

Schmidt, N.J. and Lennette, E.H. 1971. Comparison of various methods for preparation of viral serological antigens from infected cell cultures. *Appl Microbiol*, **21**, 217–26.

Schmidt, O.W., Cooney, M.K. and Kenny, G.E. 1979. Plaque assay and improved yield of human coronaviruses in a human rhabdomyosarcoma cell line. *J Clin Microbiol*, **9**, 722–8.

Seigneurin, J.M., Desgranges, C., et al. 1983. Herpes simplex virus glycoprotein D: human monoclonal antibody produced by bone marrow cell line. *Science*, **221**, 173–5.

Sewell, D.L. 1995. Laboratory-associated infections and biosafety. *Clin Microbiol Rev*, **8**, 389–405.

Shankaran, P., Reichstein, E., et al. 1990. Detection of immunoglobulins G and M to rubella virus by time-resolved immunofluorometry. *J Clin Microbiol*, **28**, 573–9.

Signoret, N., Poignard, P., et al. 1993. Human and simian immunodeficiency viruses: virus–receptor interactions. *Trends Microbiol*, **1**, 328–32.

Siitari, H., Hemmila, I., et al. 1983. Detection of hepatitis-B surface antigen using time-resolved fluoroimmunoassay. *Nature (Lond)*, **301**, 258–60.

Smith, D.B. and Johnson, K.S. 1988. Single-step purification of polypeptides expressed in *Escherichia coli* as fusions with glutathione S-transferase. *Gene*, **67**, 31–40.

Smith, M.C., Creutz, C. and Huang, Y.T. 1991. Detection of respiratory syncytial virus in nasopharyngeal secretions by shell vial technique. *J Clin Microbiol*, **29**, 463–5.

St George, K., Patel, N.M., et al. 2002. Rapid and sensitive detection of respiratory virus infections for directed antiviral treatment using R-Mix cultures. *J Clin Microbiol*, **24**, 107–15.

Stabell, E.C. and Olivo, P.D. 1992. Isolation of a cell line for rapid and sensitive histochemical assay for the detection of herpes simplex virus. *J Virol Methods*, **38**, 195–204.

Stockton, J., Ellis, J.S., et al. 1998. Multiplex PCR for typing and subtyping influenza and respiratory syncytial viruses. *J Clin Microbiol*, **36**, 2990–5.

Takimoto, S., Grandien, M., et al. 1991. Comparison of enzyme-linked immunosorbent assay, indirect immunofluorescence assay, and virus isolation for detection of respiratory viruses in nasopharyngeal secretions. *J Clin Microbiol*, **29**, 470–4.

Tanaka, K., Kondo, T., et al. 1994. Human herpesvirus 7: another causal agent for roseola (exanthem subitum). *J Pediatr*, **125**, 1–5.

Taylor, J., Weinberg, R., et al. 1992. Nonreplicating viral vectors as potential vaccines: recombinant canarypox virus expressing measles virus fusion (F) and hemagglutinin (HA) glycoproteins. *Virology*, **187**, 321–8.

Taylor, M.B., Grabow, W.O. and Cubitt, W.D. 1997. Propagation of human astrovirus in the PLC/PRF/5 hepatoma cell line. *J Virol Methods*, **67**, 13–18.

Thompson, E.W., Nakamura, S., et al. 1991. Supernatants of acquired immunodeficiency syndrome-related Kaposi's sarcoma cells induce endothelial cell chemotaxis and invasiveness. *Cancer Res*, **51**, 2670–6.

Treanor, J.J., Madore, H.P. and Dolin, R. 1988. Development of a monoclonal antibody to the Snow Mountain agent of gastroenteritis. *Proc Natl Acad Sci USA*, **85**, 3616–17.

Tyrrell, D.A. and Blamire, C.J. 1967. Improvements in a method of growing respiratory viruses in organ cultures. *Br J Exp Pathol*, **48**, 217–27.

Van Tiel, F.H., Kraaijeveld, C.A., et al. 1988. Enzyme immunoassay of mumps virus in cell culture with peroxidase-labelled virus-specific monoclonal antibodies and its application for determination of antibodies. *J Virol Methods*, **22**, 99–108.

van den Hoogen, B.G., de Jong, J.C., et al. 2001. A newly discovered human pneumovirus isolated from young children with respiratory tract disease. *Nature Med*, **7**, 719–24.

Vabret, A., Mouthon, F., et al. 2001. Direct diagnosis of human respiratory coronaviruses 229E and OC43 by the polymerase chain reaction. *J Virol Methods*, **97**, 59–66.

Vialard, J., Lalumiere, M., et al. 1990. Synthesis of the membrane fusion and hemagglutinin proteins of measles virus, using a novel baculovirus vector containing the B-galactosidase gene. *J Virol*, **64**, 37–50.

Walls, H.H., Johansson, K.H., et al. 1986. Time-resolved fluoroimmunoassay with monoclonal antibodies for rapid diagnosis of influenza infections. *J Clin Microbiol*, **24**, 907–12.

Waris, M. 1991. Pattern of respiratory syncytial virus epidemics in Finland: two-year cycles with alternating prevalence of groups A and B. *J Infect Dis*, **163**, 464–9.

Waris, M., Ziegler, T., et al. 1990. Rapid detection of respiratory syncytial virus and influenza A virus in cell cultures by immunoperoxidase staining with monoclonal antibodies. *J Clin Microbiol*, **28**, 1159–62.

White, L.A. and Ades, E.W. 1990. Growth of Vero E6 cells on microcarriers in a cell bioreactor. *J Clin Microbiol*, **28**, 283–6.

White, L.A., Freeman, C.Y., et al. 1986. In vitro effect of ascorbic acid on infectivity of herpesviruses and paramyxoviruses. *J Clin Microbiol*, **24**, 527–31.

Wilber, J.C. 1993. Development and use of laboratory tests for hepatitis C infection: a review. *J Clin Immunoassay*, **16**, 204–7.

Wilchek, M., Miron, T. and Kohn, J. 1984. Affinity chromatography. *Methods Enzymol*, **104**, 3–55.

Woods, G.L. and Young, A. 1988. Use of A-549 cells in a clinical virology laboratory. *J Clin Microbiol*, **26**, 1026–8.

Yasukawa, M., Yakushijin, Y., et al. 1993. Specificity analysis of human CD4+ T-cell clones directed against human herpesvirus 6 (HHV-6), HHV-7, and human cytomegalovirus. *J Virol*, **67**, 6259–64.

Ylitalo, N., Bergstrom, T. and Gyllenstein, U. 1995. Detection of genital human papillomavirus by single-tube nested PCR and type-specific oligonucleotide hybridization. *J Clin Microbiol*, **33**, 1822–8.

Ziegler, T., Hall, H., et al. 1995. Type- and subtype-specific detection of influenza viruses in clinical specimens by rapid culture assay. *J Clin Microbiol*, **33**, 318–21.

7

The replication of viruses

DAVID J. ROWLANDS

INTRODUCTION

An essential feature of all viruses is that they are obligate intracellular parasites and are biochemically inert in the extracellular environment. They have no mechanisms for energy generation, protein translation, or a host of other complex biochemical processes that are essential for the maintenance and growth of living cells. Consequently they are totally dependent on the structure and function of cellular machinery to enable the macromolecular synthesis required during the reproductive phase of their life cycles.

Because they co-opt cellular structures and functions to facilitate their own replication, viruses survive successfully with small genome sizes. The number of genes encoded within different viruses ranges from one in the smallest to a few hundred in the largest and most complex. With the largest viruses many of their genes are not required for replication per se, but are involved in the avoidance of host immune defense mechanisms.

From the perspective of their genetic organization, viruses are the most varied organisms in the biosphere. In addition to the wide range in genome size exhibited by different viruses, every conceivable means of nucleic acid genetic storage mechanism seems to have been adopted within the virological spectrum. Viral genomes can be encoded by DNA or RNA, which can be single-stranded or double-stranded, of positive or negative polarity, and comprise single or multiple components. In addition, retroviruses and hepadnaviruses alternate between DNA and RNA as the carrier of their genetic information at different stages in their life cycles.

Despite the wide variation evidenced between viruses, there are a number of features that are common to the replication of all. To be rescued from their inert state in the environment it is essential that viruses can efficiently recognize and bind to appropriate host cells. Having achieved this specific association, the virus must have mechanisms to enable the genome to be introduced to the interior of the cell. This requires breaching cellular membranes and is achieved by markedly different mechanisms in different viruses. Once internalized into the cytoplasm or nucleus, macromolecular synthesis is initiated from the viral template. In most cases the first event is the synthesis of mRNA, although in some RNA viruses the genomic RNA can act directly as mRNA. The mRNA is transcribed by host or viral enzymes, depending on the virus type, and is usually post-transcriptionally modified, again by host or viral enzymes. Viral protein synthesis is entirely dependent on host-cell machinery, although many viruses have mechanisms to subvert the process to their own advantage. The viral protein products are frequently post-translationally modified, again by host or virally encoded enzymes. Virus genome replication frequently occurs in discrete compartments within the cell that are assembled during the infectious process and often involve massive reorganization of the intracellular structure. The assembly of new virus progeny is the penultimate stage of virus replication. It can occur by the spontaneous association of the structural components of the virus in a relatively simple mass action process or, in the case of the larger viruses such as herpesviruses, may involve complex multistep pathways requiring the assembly of templates constructed from proteins that are not incorporated into the mature virus particles. Finally, the progeny virus particles must be released from the infected cell. This can occur by a variety of methods ranging from destructive lysis of the cell to the budding and release of new particles at the cell surface.

As an essential accompaniment to the replication process, many viruses utilize a range of mechanisms to divert or inactivate the innate and adaptive immune responses which would otherwise terminate viral replication either directly, or indirectly through the destruction of the infected cell. In the smaller viruses, these functions are often associated with multifunctional proteins that are also involved in viral replication. With the larger DNA viruses a significant proportion of the genome is devoted to the encoding of a wide range of proteins whose roles are specifically concerned with diverting the immune response mechanisms.

INITIATION OF INFECTION

The roles of virus particles

The essential roles of the virus particle, or virion, are to protect the viral genome from damage in the extracellular and extrahost environments, to efficiently bind to new host cells and to facilitate the delivery of the genome into the new host cell. These requirements place important and sometimes apparently conflicting demands on the structure and function of the virion. To protect the genome the particle must resist, as far as possible, the chemical and physical insults it is likely to encounter in the extrahost environment. It must, therefore, be a stable structure. However, this stability must be reversed during the infection process to allow release of the genome and its delivery into the new cell. In order to accommodate these diverse functions, triggering systems are frequently built into virus particles such that conformational changes occur during the initiation of infection that convert the virion from a protective capsule into an efficient delivery machine. Although these principles apply widely across the virological spectrum, there is great variety in the ways in which they are achieved.

Virus attachment

The first event in the infection process is the attachment of the virus particle to a receptor molecule at the surface of the new host cell. This involves the specific recognition between specialized receptor-binding domains on the virion surface and receptor molecules on the cell. In many cases the specificity of this interaction is a major determinant of cell tropism and can, therefore, be an important factor in defining the pathogenesis of infection. Many cell surface molecules are utilized as receptors for different viruses. In some cases viruses bind to rather nonspecific features of host-cell envelope proteins, for example, sialic acid residues. In other cases the virus/host cell receptor interaction is highly specific and is a major determinant of host and tissue tropism.

For enveloped viruses the first receptor binding protein to be studied in atomic detail was the hemagglutinin (HA) protein of influenza virus (Wiley and Skehel 1987). It is a type 1 envelope protein with a large, highly glycosylated ectodomain exposed at the surface of the virus particle, a single transmembrane domain and a short C terminal domain located on the inside of the viral envelope. The monomeric HA protein trimerizes to form functional spikelike projections from the surface of the virus (Figure 7.1). Each trimer has a stalklike domain adjacent to the membrane and terminates in a globular domain. This globular head contains the receptor binding pockets, three per HA trimer, which engage sialic acid moieties on cell receptor glycoproteins. The specificity for sialic acid is defined by the amino-acid side chains lining the receptor-binding pocket. Although these amino acid residues are necessarily highly conserved across the influenza subtypes, their location within a pocket renders them invisible to antibody recognition. This feature allows the virus to evolve variants able to escape immune responses directed against antigenic sites distributed around the globular domain of HA, while retaining the ability to utilize sialylated host-receptor glycoproteins. A second envelope glycoprotein of influenza virus is the neuraminidase protein. This removes sialic acid residues from host glycoproteins and is important for the release of progeny virus from infected cells which would otherwise be sequestered to membrane surfaces via their HA proteins.

Another virus receptor-binding protein that has received much attention is that of the human immunodeficiency virus (HIV). As for influenza virus, the HIV receptor-binding protein is a type 1 membrane glycoprotein which binds to a 60-kDa envelope glycoprotein, CD4, present at the surfaces of helper T cells and macrophages. The extreme specificity of this recognition process is one of the major factors responsible for the restriction of HIV infection to the higher primates. Although CD4 acts as the primary receptor for HIV, secondary receptors, the chemokine receptors, CXCR4 and CCR5, are engaged post-CD4 binding and are essential for completion of the infection process. Adaptation to either of these coreceptors dictates the cell tropism of different strains of the virus.

Utilization of multiple receptors during the infection process is seen in a wide range of viruses. Several viruses, herpesviruses for example, bind to heparin sulfate found ubiquitously linked to gangliosides at cell surfaces. This nonspecific initial binding probably functions as a means to concentrate virus particles at cell surfaces prior to engagement of more specific receptors

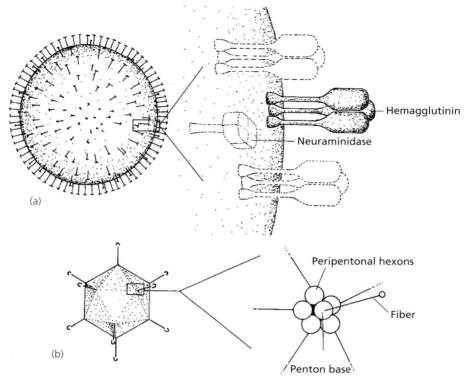

Figure 7.1 *Attachment of viruses to host cells.* **(a)** *Influenza is shown as a typical example of an enveloped virus. The virus membrane is decorated with the trimeric hemagglutinin protein (HA) and the tetrameric neuraminidase protein (N). The cellular receptor binding region of HA is located at the membrane distal 'head' domain of the molecule and associates with sialic acid residues on cell proteins. The N protein is required for release of virus at the end of the replication cycle.* **(b)** *Adenovirus is shown as an example of a naked, nonenveloped virus. The primary receptor binding domain of the virus is located in the knob protein at the ends of the 12 fibers situated at the vertices of the icosohedral capsid. Following initial attachment, conformational changes in the fiber bring the particle closer to the cell surface where a second receptor, an integrin, engages at a site on the penton base. This second receptor interaction is essential for completion of the infection process. The receptor-binding domains of most viruses protrude from the particle surface but in some cases, poliovirus for example, the receptor-binding region of the virus is buried within a groove or 'canyon' in the capsid.*

necessary to complete the infection process. In a further example, the primary receptor binding feature of the nonenveloped adenoviruses is a knob structure located at the tip of long fibrous proteins projecting from the 12 vertices of the icosahedral virus particle (Figure 7.1). After binding of the knob to the primary receptor, the fiber distorts to bring the virus particle closer to the cell surface and allows the engagement of a second receptor as a necessary component of the infection process. The secondary receptors are members of the integrin family, a large family of heterodimeric membrane glycoproteins involved in a range of cellular recognition events. The engagement with integrin molecules initiates viral internalization within endosomes, which is a necessary step in the infection process.

VIRUS ENTRY

All viruses must gain entry to the host-cell cytoplasm and/or nucleus to initiate the infection process. In some cases this occurs directly at the plasma membrane, for others it is subsequent to internalization into endosomes or other invaginated vesicles. However, the crucial step is the transport of the viral genome across a cellular membrane, for even within endosomes the virus is still topologically outside the cytoplasm of the cell. For enveloped viruses the problem of gaining entry is conceptually simple. Fusion of the envelope of the virus with the cell membrane will result in delivery of the viral content directly into the cytoplasm. For non-enveloped viruses, the problem is more complex and different viruses have either evolved mechanisms for the disruption of membranes within vesicles, such as endosomes, to allow the virus particle access to the cytoplasm or they can form pores in cell membranes, which allow the nucleic acid alone to enter the cytoplasm.

Influenza is the classic example of entry of an enveloped virus via endocytosis. The binding of the virus to host-cell receptors initiates the process of endocytosis which draws the attached virus particles into clathrin-coated pits. These pits invaginate into the cell and are pinched off to form endosomal vesicles or endosomes. These migrate within the cytoplasm towards the nucleus, becoming increasingly acidified by the action of proton ATPase during the process. The reduced pH within endosomes triggers conformational changes in HA and facilitate a crucial step in the infection process of enveloped viruses, that of membrane fusion (Weissenhorn et al. 1999). The globular head domains of the HA molecules move away from the central stalk region, which is reorganized into an elongated alpha helical structure terminating in a short hydrophobic region, the fusion peptide. Insertion of this peptide into the endosome membrane and subsequent conformational change brings the viral and cellular membranes into close proximity and initiates the fusion of the two membranes, although the precise details of this process are only now beginning to be understood (Figure 7.2). A key feature of this process is that the fusion peptide is sequestered within the stalk region of the HA trimer and only becomes exposed to facilitate the fusion process following acid-induced reorganization of the structure of the protein within endosomes. Another important feature of the mechanism is that the HA protein is synthesized as a precursor protein, HA0, which must be activated by a maturation cleavage, carried out by a host cell protease, furin, into HA1 and HA2. This cleavage leaves the fusion peptide at the N terminus of HA2 and allows the molecule to undergo acid-induced rearrangement.

The example of influenza illustrates the basic principles that underlie the infection mechanisms of many viruses that gain entry to the cytoplasm via endocytosis (Klasse et al. 1998; Bentz and Mittal 2000). Quasistable components of the virus undergo acid-induced conformational rearrangements to expose specialized features that interact with and modify cellular membranes. Recently the entry mechanisms of the alphaviruses and flaviviruses, two families of enveloped positive-strand viruses, have been elucidated. Although there are important differences from influenza HA in the details of the process, the underlying principles are similar. The surface glycoproteins of these viruses are highly ordered and their interactions define the icosahedral symmetry of the virus particle, in contrast to influenza in which the HA spikes are randomly distributed in the envelope. In addition, the fusion peptide is located internally within an envelope glycoprotein rather than at the N terminus. Marked rearrangements of the envelope proteins result in the insertion of this peptide into the host membrane and draw the host and virus membranes into close apposition to facilitate their fusion, as in the influenza case.

In the examples quoted above, the switch to a fusogenic form of the virus is triggered by acidification in endosomes. Other viruses achieve the same state following receptor or coreceptor engagement. In these cases the acid pH found in endosomes is not necessarily required for virus entry and fusion may occur at the plasma membrane. HIV is a well-studied example of this mechanism in an enveloped virus. As for influenza virus, the receptor binding glycoprotein of HIV is produced as a type 1 envelope protein, gp160, which is subsequently processed into a membrane-associated C-terminal domain, gp41, and a major receptor binding component, gp120. Engagement of the virus with its primary receptor, CD4, occurs via an interaction with gp120. Subsequent engagement of a secondary or coreceptor, which can be CVCR4 or CCR5 depending on the cell tropism of the virus, triggers the conformational changes in gp41 required to convert the protein into a fusogenic state.

Although membrane fusion per se is clearly not an option for nonenveloped viruses, the principle of acid or receptor-induced triggering of conformational changes

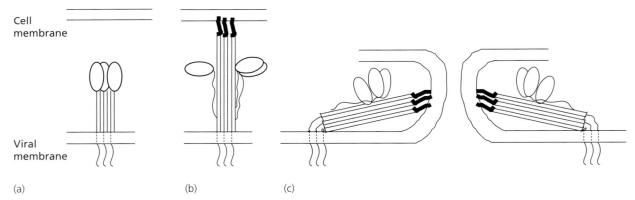

Figure 7.2 *The cell entry process of enveloped viruses. Enveloped viruses gain entry to host cells via fusion of the viral and cellular membranes, thus making the contents of the viral envelope contiguous with the cytoplasm. The diagram illustrates the mechanism for influenza virus, but the principles appear to be the same for most, if not all, enveloped viruses. (a) The virus attaches to the cell by interactions between HA and proteins in the plasma membrane. (b) Conformational changes are induced in the HA molecules and result in the exposure of a hydrophobic 'fusion peptide' sequence, which is projected from the viral membrane and inserts into the cell membrane. In the case of influenza these changes are induced by the reduction in pH in endosomes. Similar conformational changes may be induced by other mechanisms, such as engagement of a second or coreceptor in some viruses. (c) Further conformational changes result in the cellular and viral membranes being brought into close proximity, the reorganized HA being anchored in the cell membrane by the fusion peptide and the viral membrane by the transmembrane domain. This results in membrane fusion, although the details of the final process are not fully understood.*

associated with the infection process still apply. For some viruses, for example the adenoviruses and the reoviruses, the entry process involves the disruption of endosomal membranes so that the virus particles within the vesicles become confluent with the cytoplasm. Although the mechanisms involved in this membrane disruption process are not fully understood, they are clearly preceded by conformational changes in the virus particles.

In many, if not all, picornaviruses only the viral RNA is introduced into the cytoplasm, the proteins of the virion remaining topologically on the outside of the cell. The mechanisms involved are best understood for poliovirus. The receptor for the virus is a type 1 glycoprotein known as CD155 or PVR (poliovirus receptor) and binds within a groove, known as the canyon, which surrounds the fivefold axis of the icosahedral virus capsid. Engagement of the receptor induces major changes in the virus particle, which results in the externalization of the N termini of the VP1 protein and the loss of the small myristoylated internal protein, VP4. The N-terminal amino acid sequence of VP1 has the potential to form an amphipathic helix and this entry intermediate particle associates with membranes via this sequence. Both the externalized N termini of the VP1 proteins and the released VP4 protein are thought to

form channels or pores through which the RNA is transported into the cytoplasm (Hogle 2002). Similar mechanisms probably apply to other picornaviruses but studies with these are less well advanced.

Having breached the membrane and gained entry into the cytoplasm different viruses distribute to different compartments within the cell. Many viruses replicate within the cell nucleus, for example, most DNA viruses and influenza virus. Transport to the nucleus is achieved by association with the microtubule system within the cytoplasm and traveling along this in a retrograde direction to the perinuclear region (Sieczkarski and Whittaker 2002; Greber and Fassati 2003). Either the internal contents of the virus, the genome, and associated proteins, migrate into the nucleus or, as in the case of hepatitis B virus the entire nucleocapsids are transported through nuclear pores.

VIRUS GENE EXPRESSION

As for their strategies of genome organization, viruses have adopted a wide range of mechanisms for gene expression and, of course, the two factors are frequently related. These properties of viruses form the basis of the Baltimore classification of viruses (Baltimore 1971) (Figure 7.3).

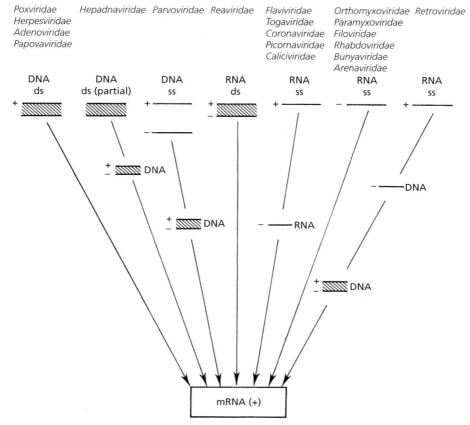

Figure 7.3 *Grouping of viruses by genome composition and pathway of mRNA synthesis.*

Most DNA viruses utilize the basic cellular enzymes for transcription of their mRNAs, although they usually exert strong controls over the specificity of gene expression to their own advantage. A notable exception to this generality is the case of poxviruses, which replicate within the cell cytoplasm and are thus obliged to incorporate virally encoded transcription enzymes in the virus particle.

RNA viruses, on the other hand, invariably encode their own RNA-dependent RNA polymerases (RdRp), which function both as transcriptases to produce mRNAs and as replicases to produce progeny genomes. This is an absolute requirement for RNA viruses as RdRp enzymes are rare in normal cells. For positive-strand RNA viruses, the viral genome functions directly as a mRNA and is translated to produce the virally encoded proteins, including the RdRp. For this reason the naked RNA of positive-strand viruses is itself infectious if appropriately introduced into cells. As a consequence reverse genetics, the in vitro manipulation of cloned cDNAs of viral genomes to introduce specific mutations and their recovery as virus from in vitro transcribed RNA copies, was first developed for positive-strand viruses. This technique has been an immensely useful research tool for dissecting the molecular details of virus replication. Negative-strand viruses, on the other hand, must incorporate the RdRp within the virus particle. This is essential for the transcription of mRNAs required to initiate viral protein synthesis.

DNA viruses

The majority of double-stranded DNA viruses, for example *Papovaviridae*, *Herpesviridae*, and *Adenoviridae*, use the transcription machinery within the host nucleus to synthesize their mRNAs. The initiation of transcription is strictly controlled, often on a temporal basis, in order to co-ordinate the production of viral proteins and to afford maximum advantage to viral biosynthesis. However, some double-stranded DNA viruses, notably the poxviruses, replicate within the cytoplasm. As the host enzymes responsible for transcription and replication are located entirely within the nucleus, these viruses encode all of the enzymes required to carry out these functions. Another important consequence of the cytoplasmic lifestyle is that the enzymes required for mRNA synthesis must be encapsidated along with the viral genome into virus particles in order to initiate the infection process. Consequently, the naked genomes of these viruses are non-infectious when introduced into cells, in contrast to the genomic DNA of nuclear replicating double-stranded DNA viruses.

Single-stranded DNA viruses, such as the *Parvoviridae* must be converted into a double-stranded form before they can act as templates for the synthesis of mRNA. This is accomplished by host polymerase enzymes.

RNA viruses

The genomes of the single-stranded positive-sense RNA viruses, which include the *Picornaviridae*, *Togaviridae*, *Flaviviridae*, *Caliciviridae*, and *Coronaviridae*, are infectious in the absence of any other viral components. The RNA is translated into viral proteins immediately upon delivery into the host cell and the same molecule must function as template for both protein synthesis and, subsequently, for genome replication. The *Picornaviridae* and *Flaviviridae* RNAs are translated into single polyproteins, which are then proteolytically processed into mature protein products, whereas the other viruses produce subgenomic mRNAs. There is a variety of strategies for the production of subgenomic RNAs and their purpose is to control the relative amounts of viral proteins produced; structural proteins generally being required in greater amounts than nonstructural proteins (Figure 7.4).

The single-stranded negative-sense RNA viruses replicate in the cytoplasm. The RNA alone is not infectious as the production of mRNA requires the function of the viral RdRp, an enzyme not found in host cells. The RdRp functions as both transcriptase, to produce viral mRNAs, and as a replicase, to produce progeny genomic RNA later in the growth cycle. It is introduced into the cell along with the genomic RNA as a ribonucleoprotein complex. The mRNAs encoding the different viral proteins are separately transcribed, thus allowing for differential control of the relative amount of each that is produced. In the segmented negative-sense RNA viruses most of the viral genes are encoded on separate RNAs and a successful infection requires the simultaneous delivery of all segments. Each functions as a separate template for transcription and replication. The segmented negative-sense RNA viruses, such as the *Orthomyxoviridae* and the *Bunyaviridae* employ a mechanism known as 'cap snatching' to initiate transcription of their mRNAs. In this process short oligonucleotides are cleaved from the 5′ ends of host mRNAs, including the 5′ terminal CAP structure, and are used to prime transcription of the viral mRNAs. This process occurs in the host-cell nucleus and all of these viruses require a functional host-cell nucleus for their replication.

The double-stranded RNA viruses all have segmented genomes which range in number from two to 11. The double-stranded genomic RNAs are retained within the nucleocapsids at all times during the replication cycle and the particles function as complex transcription machines, ejecting single-stranded RNAs, which can function both as mRNAs and as templates for new viral progeny. Double-stranded RNA is a powerful inducer of innate immune responses, such as the interferon response, and the strategy of these viruses of sequestering the double-stranded genome within particles has

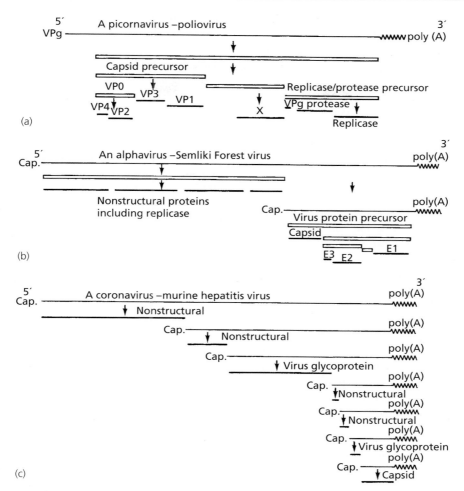

Figure 7.4 *Gene expression strategies of positive-strand RNA viruses.* **(a)** *The picornaviruses, such as poliovirus, translate their genomes as a contiguous polyprotein, which is subsequently proteolytically processed into a series of intermediate and mature proteins. Many of the intermediate products have functional roles different from those of the final cleavage products. The open reading frame for the polyprotein occupies most of the viral sequence and translation is initiated from a highly structured sequence within the 5′ untranslated region of the genome.* **(b)** *The genomic RNA of alphaviruses also functions as a mRNA to produce a polyprotein, but in this case only the nonstructural proteins responsible for virus replication are derived from the virus RNA. During replication, a subgenic mRNA encoding the structural proteins is produced in abundance. The nonstructural protein precursor is processed by viral protease and the structural proteins are processed by cellular enzymes.* **(c)** *The production of subgenomic mRNAs is most evident in the coronaviruses, which synthesize a nested set of subgenomic mRNAs each of which, with minor exceptions, is translated into a single viral protein encoded in the 5′ portion of the sequence.*

obvious relevance for avoidance of these defense mechanisms. The strategy requires that the viral entry mechanism allows for the transport of the entire nucleocapsids into the host-cell cytoplasm and also that there is an accurate packaging mechanism to ensure the incorporation of a full set of genome segments into at least the majority of virus particles.

Reversiviruses

The identification of reverse transcriptase broke the central dogma that stated that information transfer progressed from DNA through RNA to protein and could not travel back up this chain. The reverse transcriptase polymerase is able to copy an RNA template into DNA and its discovery was of great benefit to the expanding field of molecular biology, as well as being of fundamental importance in understanding the life cycle of many significant viruses. Reverse transcriptase is integral to the replication strategies of both the *Retroviridae* and the *Hepadnaviridae*, but it functions at different stages in the life cycles of these two families of viruses. Retrovirus particles contain genomic RNA and are haploid, each particle containing two template molecules. Immediately after infection the encapsidated reverse transcriptase copies the virion RNA into DNA, using a host tRNA as primer. The resulting double-stranded DNA is integrated into the host genomic DNA from where virus-specific mRNAs are transcribed by host transcription mechanisms. In the hepadnaviruses, such as hepatitis B virus, the timing of the reverse transcriptase function is reversed. In these viruses a pregenomic RNA molecule is encapsidated along with the viral polymerase. This then copies the RNA into an incomplete double-stranded circular DNA molecule within the nucleocapsid particle. Upon infection of a new host cell the partial circular DNA is completed and functions as a template for host transcriptase, but without the requirement for integration into the host genome.

mRNA synthesis

The majority of viral mRNAs conform to the paradigm for cellular mRNA structure and function. However, there are some notable exceptions, as will be discussed later. Cellular mRNAs are produced in the nucleus where they undergo a number of processing events before they are exported to the cytoplasm to program protein translation. Viruses that replicate in the nucleus have access to the host-cell mRNA modification machinery, whereas cytoplasmic replicating viruses must encode for the required functions within their genomes. Because of their small size and relative ease of manipulation, viruses have been invaluable agents for the elucidation of many of the molecular mechanisms involved in synthesis, processing, and functioning of mRNAs.

The main steps involved in the synthesis and maturation of host-cell mRNAs can be summarized as follows:

- Initiation of transcription by DNA-dependent RNA polymerase at a defined position on the genomic DNA. The location of the initiation site is defined by promoter binding sequences which are crucial for the control of the nature and amounts of mRNA transcripts produced.
- The cap structure, a modified guanosine residue, is added to the 5′ terminal nucleotide of the nascent transcript.
- The 3′ end of the transcript is extended with a polyadenylate (poly(A)) sequence.
- For most mRNAs, the primary transcript is far longer than the final mature mRNA that is exported to the cytoplasm. A complex series of cleavage and ligation events remove parts of the initial transcript known as introns and splice the remaining exons into the final mRNA.

Capping and polyadenylation

All cellular mRNAs terminate at the 5′ end with a modified nucleotide, 7-methylguanylate (m^7G) which is linked to the 5′ terminal encoded nucleotide of the mRNA by an unusual 5′–5′ linkage. Specialized transferases are responsible for the methylation of the guanyl nucleotide and the addition of the modified nucleotide

to the mRNA. The cap is important for maintaining mRNA stability in the cytoplasm and in the process of initiation of protein synthesis. It is recognized by the cap binding protein, eIF4E, which is one of the components of the eukaryotic translation initiation factor eIF4. The other members of this complex are eIF4A, which may be an RNA helicase and is involved in the migration of the completed complex along the mRNA and eIF4G, which functions as a scaffolding protein to link the cap, via eIF4E, to further initiation factors including the 40S subunit of the ribosome. Once assembled the entire preinitiation complex migrates in a 3′ direction until a translation initiation codon (AUG) in a favorable sequence context is encountered. At this point some initiation factors are released, the 60S ribosomal subunit is engaged to assemble the full 80S ribosome and translation begins.

The 3′ ends of most mRNAs also possess a common feature, the poly(A) tract. This again is nontemplated and is up to 200–250 nucleotides in length. As for the cap, the poly(A) tract is important for mRNA stability within the cell. It is also recognized by the poly(A) tract binding protein (PABP) which, in addition, binds to regions of the initiation factor eIF4G. This interaction effectively results in the circularization of the mRNA and is thought to increase RNA stability and the efficiency at which reinitiation of translation on the mRNA occurs.

Thus, capping and polyadenylation are very important for mRNA function and, with some notable exceptions discussed below, are features of viral, as well as host mRNAs. Viruses that replicate in the nucleus generally make use of the host biochemical machinery present in that compartment of the cell to carry out the capping and polyadenylation modifications of their mRNAs. However, viruses that replicate within the cytoplasm need to supply these functions in addition to the polymerase activity of their transcriptase. The poxviruses are very large DNA viruses that replicate in the cytoplasm and encode all the enzyme functions required for capping and polyadenylation. The best studied member of the family, vaccinia virus provided much of the earliest detailed information on the biochemistry of the capping process. Interestingly, the capping enzyme of vaccinia has multiple roles in the replication of the virus as it also functions as a transcription termination factor of early mRNA synthesis and as an initiation factor in intermediate gene transcription. This illustrates a common theme in virology that virus products often have multiple functions, presumably in the interests of genomic economy. For most of the cytoplasmic replicating RNA viruses, the capping and polyadenylation functions are additional functions associated with the viral RdRp. The importance of this multifunctional polymerase is reflected in the fact that it is often the largest gene encoded by these viruses and accounts for 20 percent of the genome in picornaviruses and 63 percent in rhabdoviruses viruses.

The poly(A) tract found at the $3'$ end of most mRNAs is added by the transcriptase in a stuttering function initiated by specific signal sequences. The most important of these is the conserved consensus sequence AAUAAA situated some 15–30 nucleotides upstream of the polyadenylation site.

Some viruses, such as the *Picornaviridae* and the *Pestivirus* and *Hepacivirus* genera of the *Flaviviridae* have dispensed with the requirement for a cap structure and adopted a different strategy for protein translation as outlined below. In the *Picornaviridae*, the *Flavivirus* genus of the *Flaviviridae* and the *Togaviridae* the poly(A) tract is templated in the genomic RNA while some viruses, the hepaciviruses, pestiviruses, and viruses of the *Reoviridae* family do not have polyadenylated mRNAs.

Control of transcription

The function and nature of every cell is a consequence of it transcription and translation activities, i.e. its gene expression profile. Consequently, the control of transcription and translation are crucial to normal cell function and the same applies, to a greater or lesser extent, to virus gene expression. The three major classes of cellular RNA transcripts, transfer RNAs (tRNA), ribosomal RNAs (rRNA), and messenger RNAs (mRNA) are synthesized by different polymerase enzymes; tRNA by pol I, rRNA by pol III, and mRNA by pol II. It is the profile of mRNA transcripts produced by pol II that defines the gene expression patterns within cells. The rate of transcription of each gene is controlled by specific recognition sequences, termed promoters, which are located at defined distances upstream of the coding sequence for that gene. Promoters are located within 100 base pairs of the start site for transcription of a gene and define the precise position at which transcription of the gene sequence into mRNA is initiated and the frequency of transcription initiation. Within this region two or three short sequences are the most important recognition elements. The most highly conserved of these is the TATA sequence, often referred to as the TATA box. This is located about 30 bases upstream of the initiation site for transcription and artificial movement of this sequence shifts the start site for transcription accordingly. Removal of the TATA box prevents or greatly reduces transcription frequency. Other sequences that are frequently seen in the promoter region are CCAAT and GC boxes. Promoters consist of canonical sequences, like the TATA box, which are involved in DNA-dependent RNA polymerase recognition and specialized sequences that are gene specific and are recognized by highly specific binding proteins, transcription factors, that form complexes with the transcriptase and define the specificity of transcription initiation. Thus the control of gene expression via transcription is dictated by the levels and activities of a range of transcription factors within the cell. The presence and activity of different transcription factors can vary in response to signals received by the cell via a plethora of receptors and transmitted to the transcription machinery in the nucleus by a cascade of biochemical modifications of intermediary signalling molecules. Some of these signalling pathways are initiated by the recognition of viral infection within the cell, e.g. by the presence of double-stranded RNA, and result in the induction of a suite of antiviral response proteins. Many viruses have evolved mechanisms to avoid these responses by either interfering with the cellular signalling pathways or by resisting the inhibitory effects of the induced antiviral response mechanisms.

Another level of transcriptional control is provided by a further series of sequence elements known as enhancers which are present in regions flanking genes. Enhancer sequences are longer than promoters and can be located at considerable distances from the genes whose expression they influence. Moreover they are orientation independent and can be found either upstream or downstream of genes. They are typically 200 nucleotides in length and clearly play important roles in DNA viruses as they are highly conserved and the longest known enhancer sequences have been described in viruses. For example, enhancers in cytomegalovirus range from 400 to 700 nucleotides in length and include the strongest known. They function by altering the structure of DNA to make it more accessible to transcription factors.

DNA viruses that replicate in the nucleus utilize the host pol II-dependent transcriptase activities to express their own genes. DNA viruses that replicate in the cytoplasm, such as the poxviruses, have no access to the host machinery and need to encode their own transcriptase enzymes. In order to initiate the infection process these enzymes must be introduced into the host cell within the virus particle. For this reason the DNA alone of poxviruses is not infectious, in contrast to DNA of herpesviruses and adenoviruses. Sequence analysis of the core polymerase genes of a range of viruses shows considerable conservation between these and host enzymes. In fact, there is significant conservation of certain sequences across the whole biological spectrum from bacteria through to plants and animals. The most striking of these is the triplet GDD which is found in DNA-dependent RNA polymerases, RNA-dependent RNA polymerases, and reverse transcriptases and is involved in the co-ordination of catalytically active magnesium atoms. Other regions of sequence conservation are distributed throughout the polymerase sequences interspersed between more variable regions. Determination of the molecular structures of an ever-increasing range of polymerase enzymes at atomic resolution by X-ray crystallographic techniques is providing insights into their structure/function relationships. From these studies the subdomain components of the enzyme structures are resolved and clarify the patterns of sequence conservation and variation that characterize polymerases from different sources. In addition to the core RNA polymerase enzyme, the functional transcriptase is a complex of a number of proteins with ancillary roles in the transcription process, such as helicase function for unwinding the template during the copying process. The transcriptase complex of vaccinia virus, for example, comprises a total of seven proteins with a combined molecular weight of 500 kDa.

All RNA viruses are transcribed using virus-encoded enzymes. This is because RdRp activities are not available in normal host cells and must be provided by the virus genome. RNA viruses typically have smaller genomes than most DNA viruses and a significant proportion of their genome encodes the RdRp. For example, 19.5 percent of the poliovirus genome, 49.3 percent of the influenza virus genome, 54.5 percent of the Sendai virus genome, and 62.7 percent of the vesicular stomatitis virus (VSV) genome encode this enzyme. RdRps do not have proofreading functions and the replication of RNA viruses is consequently highly error prone. This is likely to be a reason for the small size of RNA virus genomes. Also, for RNA viruses the same polymerase enzyme functions as a transcriptase to produce viral mRNA and as a replicase to produce progeny virus RNA. A wide range of strategies to differentiate the transcriptase and replicase functions exists in RNA viruses, as will be discussed below. RdRp activity was first described and studied in detail for VSV. This is a single-stranded negative-sense RNA virus and encapsidates its polymerase within the virus particle. Removal of the viral envelope with mild detergent releases the ribonucleoprotein core of the virus particle and this is capable of synthesizing viral mRNAs if provided with the four ribonucleotide triphosphate substrates in appropriate buffer conditions. The RdRp component of this functional complex is known as the L protein and has a molecular weight of 241 kDa, comprising 2 109 amino acids. In addition to its function as a polymerase enzyme it also has the enzymatic activities associated with capping and polyadenylation of the mRNA transcripts. In common with the RdRps of other negative-stranded RNA viruses, the VSV L protein can only transcribe mRNAs from a ribonucleoprotein template and is inactive when presented with naked RNA. Thus the transcriptionally active ribonucleoprotein complex comprises the viral RNA genome of 11 000 nucleotides, approximately 1 200 copies of the N or nucleoprotein polypeptide, 500 copies of a phosphoprotein, NS, and 50 copies of the L protein.

Protein encoding and translation strategies

Collectively, viruses have adopted a wide range of strategies for the translation of their genetic information into proteins. The two functional reasons underlying most of the unusual aspects of information transfer in viruses are to maximize the efficiency of information storage in the viral genome and to facilitate control of the expression levels of viral genes. Hepatitis B virus provides a good example of economic storage of protein coding information within a small genome. The circular DNA genome of the virus comprises only 3.2 kbp, but every nucleotide is involved in coding for proteins, most in more than one reading frame.

Eukaryotic mRNAs typically have a 5′ cap structure followed by a short 5′ nontranslated sequence. A complex of translation initiation factors, including the 40S ribosomal subunit, assemble at the cap and migrate along the 5′ nontranslated region until an AUG in a favorable sequence context is encountered, at which point the 60S ribosomal subunit is engaged, the initiation factors are released and translation commences. The optimal initiation sequence for protein synthesis, known as the Kozak sequence (Kozak 1986), is AxxAUGG. In most cases, the translation initiating AUG is the first one encountered by the initiation complex in its migration along the 5′ nontranslated region. Once initiated protein translation proceeds along the mRNA until the ribosome reaches a termination codon near the 3′ end of the message where translation ceases and the ribosome dissociates. Beyond the termination site there is usually a short 3′ nontranslated region terminating in a poly(A) tract. As discussed earlier, there is increasing evidence that the poly(A) tract noncovalently associates with the 5′ end of the mRNA through protein factor interactions and that this pseudocircularization increases the efficiency of mRNA template function.

Although many viral mRNAs conform to this paradigm, there is a fascinating array of exceptions to the norm. These include cap-independent mechanisms for translation initiation, the use of noncanonical initiation codons, proteins encoded in overlapping reading frames, slippage mechanisms to facilitate change of reading frame, RNA editing, and ribosome 'skipping.' In addition, some viruses utilize the normal cellular process of RNA splicing to produce multiple mRNAs from the same genetic sequence, but to an almost profligate degree.

The assembly of a variety of mRNAs derived from a single genomic sequence by splicing mechanisms is restricted to viruses that replicate in the nucleus. In particular, adenoviruses, papovaviruses, and some retroviruses (the lentiviruses, such as HIV) make extensive use of splicing to maximize the information storage and retrieval potential of their genomes (Figure 7.5). Analysis of the mRNA transcript profile of adenoviruses provided the first evidence for RNA splicing which was subsequently shown to be a universal mechanism in eukaryotic gene expression. In the splicing process internal regions within the primary RNA transcript,

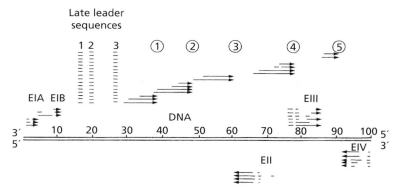

Figure 7.5 *Gene expression strategy of adenoviruses. Adenoviruses demonstrate complex patterns of gene expression. Different mRNAs are produced at early or late stages of infection and the genetic potential of the genome is amplified by the extensive use of RNA splicing. There are five early gene transcription units (the E transcripts) and another five late gene clusters. The 5′ end of each of the late gene mRNAs has a common tripartite leader sequence comprising three spliced sequences.*

known as introns, are removed and the remaining exon sequences are spliced together by an RNA ligation mechanism. If there are a number of splice donor and acceptor sequences within the primary sequence there is the potential to form an array of mature mRNAs that are recombinant assemblages derived from the same primary sequence. An example of this process is the series of T antigens expressed by viruses of the *Polyomaviridae*. For SV40, early in infection two versions of T antigen, large and small T antigens, are produced from differentially spliced mRNAs. Both mRNAs share a common open reading frame at the start of the transcript. At the end of this common sequence, an intron of approximately 350 nucleotides is removed from transcripts destined to be mRNAs for large T antigen and the open reading frame is maintained through the splice site. The mRNA for the small T antigen is produced by the excision of a smaller intron starting from an alternative splice donor sequence, but terminating at the same splice acceptor site as for the large T antigen. In this case the reading frame is not maintained and translation is terminated at the splice acceptor site. Thus the two transcripts encode unrelated amino acid sequences after the common 5′ region. In other members of the *Polyomaviridae*, further alternative T antigen proteins are produced via the use of additional splice donor/acceptor sites. Most of the RNA viruses replicate in the host cytoplasm and hence do not have access to splicing mechanisms. The *Orthomyxoviridae* are an exception to this and, for example, the mRNAs derived from gene segments 7 and 8 of influenza A virus are produced as spliced variants. In each case one protein is translated from the contiguous unspliced transcript and a different protein is encoded in a spliced version of the transcript. In the spliced mRNA, a sequence a little downstream of the translation start site is removed as an intron and the downstream exon is ligated to the 5′ exon in a different reading frame. Thus, the two proteins share a common short N-terminal sequence, but thereafter are completely

different. Additional spliced mRNAs have been demonstrated, but it is unclear whether these are translated into protein products.

Thus, splicing is an important mechanism for deriving the maximum information content from limited genome size. However, this mechanism is not available to cytoplasmic replicating DNA viruses, such as the poxviruses, as no viruses have evolved or acquired the complex enzymatic machinery required to perform the function. In addition, none of the cytoplasmic RNA viruses utilize splicing mechanisms, although these viruses have evolved a number of alternative mechanisms for maximizing genetic storage and control of gene expression and of gaining a competitive advantage over cellular gene expression.

The *Picornaviridae* and the *Pestivirus* and *Hepacivirus* genera of the *Flaviviridae* have evolved a mechanism for the initiation of their protein synthesis that bypasses the normal requirement for recognition of a cap structure by the initiation complex. In these positive-strand RNA viruses the genomic RNA serves as template both for protein translation and for genome replication. They initiate translation via direct association of the initiation complex with a highly conserved RNA sequence located within the 5′ nontranslated region (Figure 7.6). This sequence comprises about 350 nucleotides in the *Flaviviridae* and is nearer 450 nucleotides in the *Picornaviridae*. In both cases the sequences are predicted to possess a high degree of secondary structure and this has been supported by direct biochemical analysis. In addition there is evidence for a considerable amount of conserved tertiary structure. As these RNA structures are able to initiate translation through their ability to associate directly with the initiation complex and so bypass the requirement for a free, capped 5′ end to the mRNA they have been termed internal ribosome entry sites (IRES). The rational for the possession of IRESs may be that they allow for the presence of highly structured sequences at the 5′ end of the RNA that may be

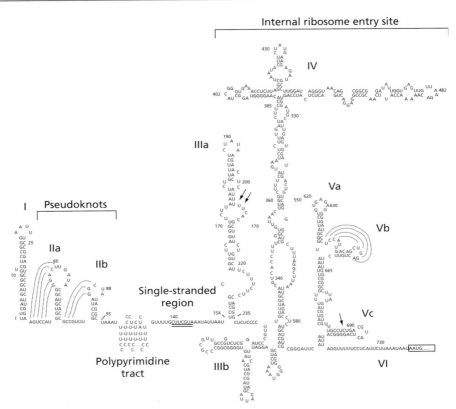

Figure 7.6 *Proposed RNA structure of the 5′ UTR of HAV. Dotted lines represent potential base-pair interactions in putative RNA pseudoknots; the box indicates the 5′ end of the open reading frame. Stem–loops IIIa–VI (nts 155–735) comprise the IRES. Arrows indicate the site of mutations in cell culture-adapted HAV which facilitate translation. Deletion of the underlined sequence (nts 140–144) leads to a temperature-sensitive phenotype. Figure courtesy of Martin and Lemon (2002).*

important for RNA replication. Such sequences would be inhibitory for the normal process of ribosomal scanning through the 5′ nontranslated region to reach the initiating AUG codon. Whether or not this is the primary raison d'être for IRESs, in several picornaviruses they allow the virus to gain a translation advantage over host mRNAs. The enteroviruses, rhinoviruses, and aphthoviruses encode for proteases that specifically cleave the host translation initiation factor eIF4G. This protein forms a bridge linking the cap recognition protein eIF4E to the rest of the translation initiation complex and its hydrolysis by the viral enzymes effectively negates cap-dependent translation in the cell. Thus, the majority of cell protein translation is inhibited leaving the whole translation apparatus available for the virus. Although the cardioviruses do not cleave eIF4G, their IRESs seem to be highly efficient and can outcompete host mRNA translation and also there is recent evidence that one of the viral proteins, 3A, can associate with nascent ribosomes in the nucleus, resulting in modified organelles that preferentially initiate from the virus IRES. IRESs were first described in viruses but there is increasing evidence that some host mRNAs are translated by the same mechanism. In some cases IRESs have been found to be located within viral mRNAs so as to produce a bicistronic message, translation occurring

independently from the 5′ and 3′ portions of the RNA. This has been recognized for some time in certain insect viruses and more recently there is evidence that one of the mRNAs of the herpesvirus, Kaposi's sarcoma virus, is bicistronic, the 3′ open reading frame being translated from an internal IRES.

A number of alternative methods to splicing as a means to maximize information storage have been evolved by viruses that do not have access to splicing machinery. The utilization of alternative translation initiation sites and RNA editing are two methods which are well illustrated by viruses belonging to the *Paramyxoviridae*, for example Sendai virus. Transcripts of the *P* gene of Sendai virus encode three distinct proteins, P, V, and C. The latter is produced as a C terminal nested set of four variant proteins, each initiating at a different in-frame initiation site. The P and C proteins are translated from the primary *P* gene transcript, but initiate at different codons. The frequency at which translation is initiated at different sites is a reflection of their flanking sequence contexts. These include the noncanonical initiation codons ACG and GUG. The *V* gene is produced from a variant transcript in which an extra, nontemplated G residue is added during transcription at a specific RNA editing site. This, of course, alters the reading frame and so the V protein is a hybrid sequence, the N-terminal part shared with P and the C-terminal region derived from an alternative reading frame. A mechanism of RNA editing is also employed during the replication of hepatitis delta virus. The sole open reading frame of this virus encodes the delta antigen which is produced as a long or short form. The long form is translated from transcripts in which an RNA editing event eliminates a stop codon and allows translation to proceed down the mRNA. The long form has a nuclear location signal not present in the short form and so the two proteins are found in different locations in the cell and this differential distribution is important for the regulation of virus replication and encapsidation to a different stages in the life cycle.

The utilization of alternative reading frames within a single sequence by RNA editing, as illustrated above, requires the transcription of subtly modified mRNA transcripts. Another method of utilizing alternative reading frames has been developed in a number of different viruses and relies on manipulation of the translational rather than the transcriptional machinery. This is ribosome slippage in which specific sequence and structural features within the mRNA induce a slowing and stuttering of translation and result in a proportion of ribosomes changing to a different reading frame, thus producing a hybrid protein as in the case of RNA editing. The normal random error rate in translation of eukaryotic mRNA is in the order of 5×10^{-5} per codon, whereas specific frame-shifting in viral mRNAs can exceed 10 percent. Frame-shifting typically occurs at a homopolymeric sequence of the general structure XXXYYYZ followed a short distance downstream in the mRNA by a pseudoknot (Figure 7.7). This is a stem–loop structure in which the stem is formed through the hybridization of complementary sequences in the RNA. The sequences within the loop at the top of the stem–loop also hybridize to sequences adjacent to the stem of the stem–loop. This results in the formation of a pseudo-double-stranded structure which impedes the passage of the translating ribosome and facilitates a single nucleotide slippage at the slippery sequence so that a significant proportion of the ribosomes continue translating the message in the −1 reading frame (Deiman and Pleij 1997; Giedroc et al. 2000). For example, ribosome frame-shifting is utilized by viruses in the *Retroviridae* family to control the levels of reverse trancriptase (*pol*) produced in the infected cell. The *gag* and *pol* proteins are encoded by adjacent regions of the viral RNA, but in different reading frames. A frameshifting event occurs at a frequency of about 10 percent to produce a *gag–pol* fusion protein. The mature *pol* protein is then separated from the *gag–pol* fusion protein by a virus-specific proteolytic event.

Another virus-specific variation on the normal process of protein translation has recently been demonstrated for the picornavirus, foot-and-mouth disease virus. This phenomenon has been termed ribosomal skipping and

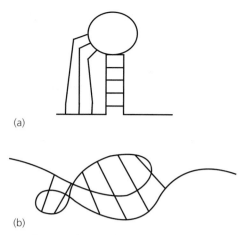

(a)

(b)

Figure 7.7 *Ribosome frameshifting: diagrammatic representation of the structure of a pseudoknot. A pseudoknot is formed when there is complementarity between residues in the loop of a stem–loop structure and residues adjacent to the stem–loop* **(a)**. *The actual folding pattern of such a structure is depicted in* **(b)** *and resembles double-stranded RNA. Translating ribosomes pause when encountering such a structure. This, in conjunction with a nearby 'slippery sequence,' leads to a shift in the translational reading frame by a small proportion of the ribosomes.*

occurs when translation continues along the viral RNA, but fails to create a peptide bond at a specific site (Donnelly et al. 2001). This has the same effect as proteolytic processing of the polyprotein translation product of the virus, as occurs at many positions in the sequence, but in addition it permits a level of translational control not otherwise available to viruses that have a single uninterrupted translation product. The skipping event occurs at a position just after the end of the structural protein coding region and involves a 16 amino acid sequence known as protein 2A and is critically dependent on the 2A sequence. It is postulated that termination of translation at this point through a failure to pass through the skipping position could provide a mechanism for excess production of structural proteins at late stages in the virus replication cycle.

As for host mRNAs, the majority of viral mRNAs are monocistronic and in most cases they are subgenomic. In DNA viruses the mRNAs for individual genes are initiated and terminated at specific sequences within the genome sequence and for nuclear replicating viruses the patterns of gene expression can be further complicated by splicing, as discussed above. For the double-stranded and the negative-sense segmented RNA viruses each genome segment generally encodes a single protein. However, in some segmented RNA viruses some genome segments are ambisense, i.e. the virion-sense and complementary-sense RNAs each encode separate proteins. In the single-stranded negative-sense RNA viruses mRNAs for the different gene products are initiated at specific recognition sites within the viral ribonucleoprotein, but are transcribed in sequence from the 3′ end of the viral RNA. The single-strand positive-sense

Togaviridae produce their structural proteins from a subgenomic message representing the 3' region of the viral genome and in the *Coronaviridae* seven separate subgenomic mRNAs are produced as a 3' nested set (Figure 7.4).

Quantitative and temporal control of viral gene expression

DNA VIRUSES

Most viruses have mechanisms to regulate the production of their proteins during infection, but the patterns of control are far more evident in the DNA viruses than the RNA viruses. Some proteins, such as the structural proteins required for assembly of progeny virions, are required in much larger amounts than the enzymatic proteins involved in the replication process and their production is often modulated accordingly. In addition, many viruses produce different proteins at different stages in the infection process. Typically replication proteins and proteins that modulate the host-cell environment to facilitate virus replication are required early in infection while the synthesis of structural proteins is more important at later stages.

The control of protein synthesis in the adenoviruses is well understood and serves as a good example of the principles that apply to many DNA viruses (Figure 7.5). Transcription is divided into two major phases, early and late. Three of the early genes are transcribed from one of viral DNA strands and two are transcribed from the complementary strand. For all of the adenovirus transcripts multiple alternative initiation, termination, and splicing events result in the production of a variety of proteins from each gene. The first gene expressed when the viral DNA enters the nucleus is E1A. As is often observed with viral proteins the E1A proteins have multiple functions and act as a master gene to both modify the host-cell environment and to orchestrate the transcription of other adenovirus early genes. The E1A proteins have been shown to interact with a large number of host proteins and the functional consequences of all of these interactions are not well understood. However, it is clear that E1A can act as a transactivator to control the transcription of other genes within the early gene cluster via activation of TATA box containing promoters. The activation of these promoters is not through direct interaction with E1A and it does not act as a transcription factor per se. Instead it binds to and modulates the activities of cellular transcription factors and regulatory proteins, such as the TATA box binding protein. It thus facilitates the upregulation of transcription and results in the expression of other early genes. Another important role of E1A is its ability to induce the host cell to progress from a quiescent state into S phase of the cell cycle. This is important for viral replication as the cell environment is far more conducive

to DNA replication when in S phase. It achieves this control through its interaction with the cellular protein, retinoblastoma tumor suppressor protein, pRB. This, in turn, controls the activity of E2F cellular transcription factor and when the inhibitory effects of pRB on this transcription factor are released a number of cellular proteins involved in cell cycle progress are produced. Other members of the early gene families of proteins have important roles in negating the antiviral host responses, both innate and adaptive. For example, E1B binds to p53 and inhibits its proapoptotic activity, E3 blocks immune presentation of viral antigens at the cell surface for recognition by cytotoxic T cells and a series of short RNA transcripts, the VA RNAs, inhibit the protein kinase, PKR. This protein is induced as part of the interferon response and in the presence of double-stranded RNA it phosphorylates the translation initiation factor eIF2α, resulting in the inhibition of protein synthesis. The *E2* genes encode the polymerase and terminal protein responsible for viral DNA replication.

Viral DNA synthesis triggers the switch from early to late transcription although the precise mechanism underlying this change is not fully understood. The major late promoter is minimally active before DNA replication and its activity increases enormously thereafter. It has been shown experimentally that this is a *cis*-active phenomenon and so must reflect a change in the physical nature of the DNA template. This may be due to changes in the profile of associated proteins or, more likely, is due to exposure of the promoter region as a consequence of conformational changes during replication. The five late gene families of proteins are all derived from a single long (29 000 nucleotide) transcript through differential polyadenylation site usage and splicing. All of the late transcripts start with a 200 nucleotide spliced region, the tripartite leader. This sequence confers a translational advantage on the viral transcripts at late times in infection. At these times, the eIF4 transcription factor complex is largely dephosphorylated and this results in an inability to scan through mRNAs from the 5' cap to the translation initiating AUG codon. The tripartite leader allows the ribosome to 'jump' directly from the cap to the initiating AUG without scanning the intervening sequence. An additional translational advantage is gained by the virus late in infection, since at these times newly synthesized host mRNAs are not exported from the nucleus to be translated in the cytoplasm. Viral transcripts are transported to the cytoplasm by a complex of E1B and E4 with cellular factors and this complex may sequester transport factors to the benefit of the viral transcripts and detriment of cellular transcripts.

The general principle of differential expression of viral genes at early and late stages of infection is common to most DNA viruses and many have multifunctional proteins that perform many of the functions outlined above for the E1A protein of adenoviruses. Examples include the T antigens of the papilloma and papovaviruses and ICP4 of herpes simplex virus, which has a negative effect on the expression of other early genes, but is required for the expression of later genes. Splicing is used minimally by the herpesviruses and not at all by the poxviruses, which lack their own splicing mechanisms and replicate in the cytoplasm away from the cellular systems. These viruses possess some of the largest known viral genomes and express their gene products via a complex cascade of transcriptional events. The series of genes expressed during herpesvirus infection are classified as α, β, and γ proteins and there are further subdivisions of β_1 and β_2 classes. The poxviruses encapsidate both the enzymes required for transcription and the transcription factors required to initiate the process for the early genes. Herpes simplex also encapsidates a protein, VP16, that is involved in the initiation of transcription of its early genes. It forms a complex with cellular proteins Oct1 and HCF-1 and together they promote transcription from viral sequences preceded by the motif TAATGARAT, where R is a purine.

RNA VIRUSES

Positive-strand viruses

The genomes of picornaviruses are single, positive-sense RNA strands of between 7.5 and 8.5 kb in length. The 5' end is covalently linked to a small protein, VPg, and the 3' end is polyadenylated. A long 5' nontranslated region precedes a single open reading frame occupying most of the genomic RNA. This is translated into a single polyprotein product which is cleaved by virus-encoded proteases, both co- and post-translation, into a total of about 12 mature products (Figure 7.4). The VPg is not required for mRNA function and is normally cleaved from actively translating genomes by a cellular activity. Although no subgenomic mRNAs are produced and there is no mechanism for temporal control of gene expression differential cleavage at the processing sites of the polyprotein are used to increase the complexity of the gene expression profile (Bedard and Semler 2004). Several 'immature' precursor proteins have functions that are different from those of their component 'mature' cleavage products. The genomic RNAs of the flaviviruses are also translated as a continuous polyprotein and, like the picornaviruses the structural proteins are encoded towards the N terminus, the remainder encoding proteins involved in replication. As with the picornaviruses the polymerase protein is located at the C-terminal end of the polyprotein. The flaviviruses are enveloped and their structural proteins are cleaved from the polyprotein by host signal peptidases in the endoplasmic reticulum. The remaining cleavages are carried out by virus-encoded proteases. Although the translation of most flaviviruses is cap-dependent, viruses in the pestivirus and hepacivirus genera use an IRES to initiate translation.

The gene order of the togaviruses differs from the picornaviruses and flaviviruses in that the nonstructural replication proteins are encoded within the 5' two-thirds of the genomic RNA and the structural proteins are encoded on a separate transcription unit representing the 3' portion of the genome (Figure 7.4). The capped and polyadenylated viral RNA is translated on entry into the host cell to produce the polymerase and associated proteins which copy the input RNA into a complementary negative strand. This is transcribed in its entirety to produce progeny viral RNAs or from an internal promoter to produce a subgenomic mRNA representing the 3' one-third of the genome sequence. This small RNA encodes the structural proteins and is produced in approximately three-fold excess compared with the full length viral RNA. Later in the replication cycle the virion RNA is sequestered by the structural proteins to assemble progeny virions and so the effective concentration of the subgenomic RNA is approximately ten times higher than the viral RNA. As a result, this simple strategy allows for a degree of quantitative and temporal control of the relative synthesis of structural and replication proteins.

The strategy of producing subgenomic mRNAs is carried to its extreme for the positive-stranded viruses in the coronaviruses (Figure 7.4). A total of six to eight mRNAs, depending on the specific virus, are produced in infected cells and represent a 3' nested set, the longest being full-length viral RNA. Most of these RNAs are monocistronic and only produce the protein encoded at the 5' end, the remainder of the RNA remaining translationally silent. Thus, essentially each gene is translated from a separate mRNA. As these are not produced in equivalent amounts this strategy allows for control of the relative amounts of viral proteins produced, although there is no temporal control. Each of the subgenomic RNAs has a common 'leader' sequence at the 5' end and two mechanisms for their synthesis have been proposed. In one model short RNAs representing the leader sequence are transcribed from the 3' end of full-length complementary copies of the virion RNA. These then dissociate from the replication apparatus and prime transcription of the individual subgenomic RNAs from conserved sequences present at each intergenic region. In an alternative model, transcription of negative strands is interrupted at the intergenic sequences and resumes at the 5' leader sequence. Thus a nested set of templates is produced from which the mRNAs are individually transcribed.

Negative-strand viruses

The negative-strand RNA viruses can be broadly divided into those with a continuous genome and those with segmented genomes. Of the single-stranded viruses, VSV is probably the best studied and understood. The obligatory first step in replication is transcription from the virion ribonucleoprotein by the encapsidated L and P proteins, which together constitute the functional transcriptase, to produce a set of mRNAs. Transcription starts at the extreme 3′ end of the RNA to produce a 47 nucleotide leader RNA terminating in a 5′ triphosphate group. After a short pause, transcription is reinitiated to produce the first mRNA. A pause again occurs at the end of the first transcription unit before transcription is again reinitiated at the start of the next gene on the genome. The order of genes on the genome is N, P, M, G, and L and this reflects the order of abundance of each protein that is required for virus replication. Each mRNA is capped by the transcription complex and is polyadenylated from a polyadenylation signal present in each short conserved intergenic sequence. Transcriptase complexes dissociate from the template at a frequency of 20–30 percent at each intergenic junction so that the proportion of each mRNA transcript produced is dependent on its position on the genome. The positional frequency of transcription is maintained if the order of genes on the virion RNA is reversed. This strategy allows for a hierarchy of gene expression but not for temporal control of protein synthesis.

Influenza provides a good example of a segmented negative-strand RNA virus. In common with VSV, the viral polymerase is introduced into the cell as part of the ribonucleoprotein viral core. In contrast, it has no capping activity and the viral mRNA transcripts obtain their 5′ caps from host mRNAs by a process known as cap snatching. The polymerase has a nuclease activity that cleaves host mRNAs at a position about 12 downstream of the cap. These heterogeneous fragments are then used to prime the transcription of the influenza virus mRNAs from the individual viral ribonucleoprotein segments. In addition to acting as templates for mRNA synthesis, the input viral RNA segments act as templates for the synthesis of full-length complementary template RNAs. These are subsequently transcribed into progeny vRNA molecules which can act as fresh templates for further mRNA synthesis. Although the production of template RNAs appears not to be, the synthesis of new vRNAs is regulated. This results in inequality in the abundance of different mRNAs and so control of gene expression on a temporal basis.

Double-stranded viruses

The reoviruses are the best studied of the double-stranded RNA viruses. The virus particles are multi-shelled structures and a core component containing the multisegmented double-stranded RNA genome is introduced intact into the host-cell cytoplasm to initiate infection. At no time during the virus replication cycle is the double-stranded genome exposed to the cytoplasm outside the protein cores. As double-stranded RNA is one of the most potent inducers of host antiviral interferon responses, the sequestering of the genome within

particles is probably an important viral defense mechanism. The icosohedral core particles are, in effect, highly ordered transcription machines which synthesize and export RNA transcripts through pores at the fivefold axes of symmetry. The transcripts are capped by the viral transcription apparatus but, unusually, are not polyadenylated at their 3′ ends. The transcripts are full-length copies of the genome segments and function as mRNAs and as templates for progeny double-stranded genome RNAs, when encapsidated within progeny core particles. The genomes of these viruses comprise ten to 12 segments and their high particle:infectivity ratios suggest that there must be very efficient segment sorting in the assembly of progeny virions, but the mechanism for this is not understood. mRNA transcripts are produced in relative abundance according to their segment lengths, thus giving a measure of control of expression levels. In addition, there appears to be differential efficiency of translation of the different mRNA, as well as a general preference for viral gene translation at later times of infection but, again, the mechanisms for this are unclear.

Protein synthesis, transport, and processing

VIRAL EFFECTS ON HOST PROTEIN SYNTHESIS

Cellular and viral mRNAs, alike, are translated into protein by the ribosome, a machine that is too complex to be encoded by viral genomes. In general, ribosomes are not modified in the infected cell, although recent evidence suggests that one of the nonstructural protein products of viruses of the cardiovirus genus of the *Picornaviridae* may associate with nascent ribosomes to specifically facilitate translation of the viral template. However, many viruses have evolved strategies to usurp cell mRNA translation and to avoid some of the cellular antiviral responses at the level of the initiation of protein synthesis. Disruption of the translation of host mRNAs in a way that permits the continuation of viral protein synthesis allows the virus to maximize its own expression and dominate the host machinery. This is a valuable strategy for viruses that induced acute cytolytic infections to produce a maximum progeny burst size and concomitant death of the cell. Some viruses, such as hepatitis C virus, are able to induce persistent infections without cell death. Clearly, disruption of host-cell protein synthesis would be inappropriate for this viral strategy and such viruses must replicate within a competent, surviving cell.

Different viruses have evolved a variety of mechanisms to inhibit cell protein synthesis while allowing their own gene expression to proceed. As mentioned above, many picornaviruses encode proteases that cleave the important scaffolding protein, eIF4G, which connects the cap-binding protein eIF4E to the remainder of the translation initiation complex. Thus cap-dependent translation is effectively abrogated in the infected cell and the virus overcomes this inhibition by initiating translation via a specialized RNA structure, the IRES. This associates directly with the ribosome and initiation factors without the requirement for cap recognition.

Adenoviruses appear to employ several mechanisms to disrupt cell protein synthesis to their own advantage. Firstly, they can control export of mRNAs from the nucleus. Virus-encoded proteins associate with a cellular RNA transport factor and sequester it in the region of viral replication and transcription. This has the effect of selectively facilitating viral transcript export to the detriment of cellular mRNAs. Secondly, small RNA transcripts known as virus associated (VAI) RNAs are produced in large quantities late in infection and these inhibit the interferon response activated kinase, PKR. Thus the PKR is unable to phosphorylate and inactivate the translation initiation factor eIF2α. As the VAI RNAs are associated with viral transcripts they may selectively protect the virion transcripts from eIF2α phosphorylation. Thirdly, late viral transcripts are able to avoid the inhibition of translation due to phosphorylation of the initiation factor, eIF4F. This is because of a unique property of the so-called tripartite leader sequence common to all late transcripts which allows the translation initiation complex to jump directly from the 5′ cap to the initiating AUG codon without having to scan the intervening sequence. Finally, a late viral protein is able to specifically activate translation of viral transcripts. Rotaviruses produce a protein that interacts with the initiation factor eIF4G to disrupt its interaction with poly(A)-binding protein. This leads to inhibition of translation of polyadenylated cellular transcripts and favoring the nonpolyadenylated viral transcripts.

Infection by a number of viruses leads to reduction in the levels of host mRNAs. In herpesviruses, for example, one of the virus particle-associated proteins that are introduced into the cell during infection seems to be or to activate a nonspecific ribonuclease. This degrades both host and viral mRNAs, but its activity seems to diminish during infection resulting in a selective accumulation of viral transcripts.

PROTEIN TRANSPORT

Viruses make use of the wide range of signalling and transport systems present in host cells to direct their proteins to appropriate compartments. For example, signal sequences are present at the N terminus of proteins destined for secretion into the endoplasmic reticulum, a compartment that is topologically outside the cell. These are relatively short hydrophobic amino acid sequences that associate with the secretory mechanisms and result in the extrusion of the nascent protein through specific pores in the endoplasmic reticulum (ER) membrane. As this occurs concomitantly with

translation ribosomes and polysomes that are synthesizing secreted proteins are intimately associated with the ER membrane. The signal sequence is usually cleaved from the nascent polypeptide by proteases resident in the ER lumen. Proteins destined to become membrane proteins are prevented from being secreted completely by stop transfer sequences and remain anchored to the membrane by hydrophobic stretches of sequence and usually have a C-terminal cytoplasmic domain that may be involved in particle assembly or in signal transduction from interactions involving the extracellular domain. Having been inserted into the ER lumen, the proteins are usually glycosylated and can be transported to various cellular locations as dictated by further recognition signals, often located in the transmembrane domain or cytoplasmic tail. Viruses also use many other intracellular transport systems to distribute their proteins to defined destinations. For example, influenza virus ribonucleoprotein cores interact with cellular proteins to facilitate their transport to and through nuclear pores. Many viral proteins have nuclear location signals and others are able to reversibly shuttle between nucleus and cytoplasm to transport viral components between these compartments. Progeny poxvirus particles are able to stimulate the polymerization of actin and this enables them to be physically pushed through and out of the cell.

PROTEIN PROCESSING
Proteolytic cleavage

Proteolytic cleavages are involved in the replication strategies of many viruses. Practical evidence of their importance is furnished by the success of inhibitors of the virus protease in HIV therapy. Proteolytic cleavages can be broadly divided into two classes, those carried out by host cell proteases and those performed by virus encoded enzymes. The most common examples of the former are the normal modifications of secreted glycoproteins by signal peptidases which remove signal sequences in the ER lumen and signal peptide peptidases which can cleave within the transmembrane portion of the signal sequence. In addition, the surface proteins of many viruses are cleaved by cell surface proteases, such as furins, to prime them for subsequent conformational changes involved in the cell entry process, as discussed earlier. A good example is the HA protein of influenza virus which is synthesized as the precursor protein, HA0. This is activated to a cell fusion competent form by cleavage into HA1 and HA2. Mutations at this cleavage site can influence its susceptibility to cleavage, which in turn can have profound effects on the tissue tropism and pathogenicity of the virus.

Many viruses encode their own proteases which are used in the processing of precursor polyproteins. This is especially important for the single-strand positive-sense RNA viruses, such as the *Flaviviridae* and *Picornaviridae* which translate their entire genome as a single polyprotein (Figure 7.4). This is processed by a cascade of proteolytic cleavages which function in *cis* or in *trans* to produce the final mature proteins. In the *Picornaviridae*, this strategy serves to increase the functional flexibility of a small genome as many of the intermediate proteins produced in the processing cascade have properties and functions that are distinct from those of the final mature products. In addition, the viral proteases are used to cleave specific cellular proteins, such as the translation initiation factor eIF4G, which results in the shut-off of host protein synthesis. In some cases, particularly with the nonenveloped viruses, virus-induced proteolysis also produces maturation cleavages involved in virion assembly. Proteolysis is also important for controlling the complex series of events in the assembly of herpesviruses. Core particles are initially assembled in the nucleus around scaffolding proteins. The scaffolding proteins are then cleaved by a virus protease and removed from the particles prior to packaging of the viral DNA.

Glycosylation

The great majority of secreted eukaryotic proteins, whether they are shed from the cell or remain tethered to cellular membranes by membrane insertion sequences, are post-translationally modified by the addition of carbohydrate residues. Glycosylation probably serves several functions: involvement in the folding process to produce the correct protein conformation, protection of the protein from extracellular enzymes, intercellular recognition, and, in the case of viral glycoproteins, to help mask the protein from immune recognition. Glycosylation of viral membrane proteins is carried by host-cell enzymes in accordance with the same biochemical rules as host proteins. There are two sorts of glycosylation, *N*-linked or *O*-linked of which the former is the dominant form. The recognition signal sequence Asn–X–Ser/Thr is essential for *N*-linked glycosylation, which occurs in the lumen of the ER. The initial step in *N*-linked glycosylation consists of the addition of a multibranched structure consisting of two residues of *N*-acetylglucosamine, nine of mannose, and three of glucose. The glucose residues report on the folding state of the protein, which is released from the chaperone, calnexin, when all have been removed. Further modifications of the carbohydrate chains are carried out in a cell-specific manner in the Golgi apparatus as the protein migrates through the secretory machinery.

Other post-translational modifications

A number of other modifications of viral proteins have been observed. One of the most important is phosphorylation which is used in many host cell and viral examples as a mechanism for inducing reversible conformational changes in proteins, so enabling them to act as molecular switches. Cascades of phosphorylation and dephosphorylation are the most widely used mechanisms for transducing messages from receptor interactions at cell surfaces to effector molecules in the nucleus. Many virus proteins are also modified by phosphorylation which probably alters their interactions with other proteins and/or nucleic acids, but in most cases their function is poorly understood.

A number of viral proteins are known to be modified by fatty acid acylation, the most common being N-terminal myristoylation. The 14 carbon myristic acid is added to the N-terminal amino acid (after removal of the initiation amino acid, *N*-acetyl methionine) of proteins starting with the sequence Gly–X–X–Ser/Thr. It is thought to be important for the interaction of proteins with membranes and may also be involved in 'molecular switching,' in conjunction with phosphorylation. For example, the small internal protein, VP4, of most picornaviruses is myristoylated and there is evidence that the protein interacts with cell membranes to create pores or channels when it is externalized during the infection process. The Nef protein of HIV is also myristoylated and this modification is probably involved in its ability to interact with intracellular membranes to dictate its intracellular localization. It is possible that conformational changes, perhaps induced by phosphorylation, may sequester the N-terminal region, including the myristate moiety, within the structure of the protein and so reversibly alter its distribution within the cell. Other modifications, such as sulfation, poly(ADP) ribosylation, and palmitoylation have been reported but their functions are not well understood. In some cases, proteins involved in viral replication are modified by the addition of nucleosides to enable them to function as primers to initiate nucleic acid synthesis. For example, the small genome linked protein, VPg, of picornaviruses is modified by the addition of one or two uridine residues on the side chain of a highly conserved Tyr residue, after which modification it can function to initiate replication of the viral RNA.

GENOME REPLICATION

DNA viruses

A problem inherent in cellular DNA replication is that of terminal loss. The priming and replication systems in normal cells lead to the loss of small amounts of sequence at each round of replication of the chromosomal DNA. This is overcome by the action of telomerase that adds back sequence to the termini so that there is no loss of important sequence. Viruses do not use this nonspecific addition system and have overcome the problem of terminal loss in several interesting ways. One of the best studied viruses from a replication perspective is SV40 which overcomes the problem by having, in effect, no end. The genome is circular and during replication it produces daughter circles. Most of the enzymes involved in the replication are recruited from the host cell, but the process is initiated and controlled by the multifunctional viral protein, TAg. This binds to the origin of replication sequence as a hexameric complex and opens the complementary DNA strands. It has a helicase function which continues to enlarge the separated domain to allow access by the plethora of proteins involved in normal cell DNA replication. As all DNA is copied in the 3′ to 5′ direction, one strand is replicated discontinuously in a series of small steps (Figure 7.8). These are primed by short RNA sequences synthesized by DNA primase and extended as DNA sequence by Pol α. The RNA primers are excised by RNase H and the single-stranded region thus exposed is filled in by Pol α and joined to the preceding DNA segment by DNA ligase. The opposite strand is extended continuously by Pol δ from a single RNA primers sequence. Thus replication proceeds as two continuously moving forks, one moving in each direction. When they meet, two double-stranded circular DNA molecules have been replicated from one.

Another way of preserving ends is exemplified by the parvoviruses. These single-stranded DNA viruses have inverted repeats at their termini which, therefore, resemble self-priming molecules and are extended to form a hairpin structure. A sequence-specific cleavage occurs near the self complementary loop and the exposed 3′ end is extended to produce a complete double-stranded copy of the genome. Rearrangement of the palendromic end sequences exposes a free 3′ end which is copied back on itself to displace the partner strand as a new single-stranded viral DNA.

Some viruses, such as the adenoviruses, overcome the terminal loss problem by using a protein, to which nucleotides have been covalently attached, as a primer for DNA synthesis. The terminal protein of adenoviruses has a short chain of three nucleotides attached which complement a sequence near the 3′ end of the double-stranded viral DNA. In the presence of the viral polymerase and host factors the end of the DNA is melted and the terminal protein binds via its complementary nucleotides. The complex then jumps back by three nucleotides to bind to a repeat of the recognition sequence located at the extreme 3′ end and then proceeds to copy the entire DNA. Replication proceeds in a single direction, displacing one of the template strands as a single-stranded product (Figure 7.8). This is converted into a double-stranded molecule by the viral polymerase, again using terminal protein as a primer.

The complementary strands of poxvirus DNA are covalently linked so that the molecule is in effect an unbroken hairpin. The herpes virus replication products are continuous concatenated molecules and are cut into genome length units during the encapsidation process.

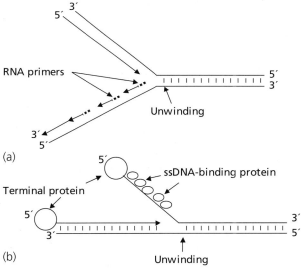

Figure 7.8 Genome replication strategies of DNA viruses. (a) Replication of most double-stranded DNA viral genomes, SV40, for example, proceeds as a replicating fork with each of the parental strands being copied simultaneously. Since DNA polymerase is unidirectional, proceeding from the 3′ end of the template towards the 5′ end, the two parental strands are copied differently, one continuously, the other discontinuously. Discontinuous synthesis is primed by short RNA molecules 9–10 nt long which are subsequently removed when the nascent DNA fragments reach 100–200 nts. The resulting gaps are filled in with deoxyribonucleotides and the discontinuous fragments ligated together. (b) In the adenoviruses, a single nascent strand displaces one of the parental strands during synthesis. DNA synthesis is primed by terminal protein, which is modified by the addition of nucleotides complementary to the 3′ end of the viral sequence. The progeny molecule is encased in single-stranded DNA binding protein and this complex acts as template for synthesis of a complementary strand to recreate the double-stranded genome. Synthesis of the second strand is also primed by terminal protein.

'Reversiviruses'

Retroviruses and hepatitis B viruses alternate between DNA and RNA versions of their genomes at different stages in the replication cycle using reverse transcriptase. In both cases the replication strategies rely on the presence of terminal repeat sequences in the RNA versions of their genomes (Hu and Seeger 1997). Replication starts at a sequence near the 5′ end of the genome RNA. In the case of retroviruses the primer used to initiate replication is a host tRNA, which is extended by the viral reverse trancriptase as a DNA copy. In hepatitis B viruses an N-terminal domain of the polymerase protein acts as a protein primer, recognizing a stem loop structure in the RNA (Figure 7.9). In both cases the nascent DNA molecule is extended to the end of the template RNA at which stage it is transferred to a

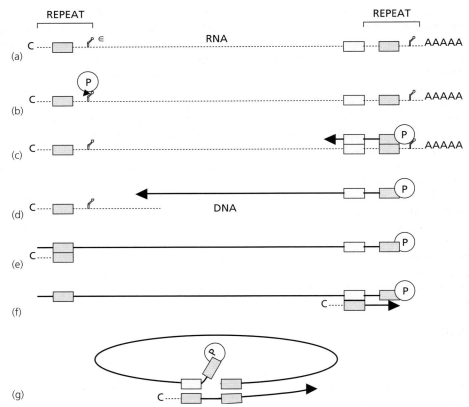

Figure 7.9 *Replication of the hepadnavirus genome. The genomes of hepadnaviruses (e.g. hepatitis B virus (HBV)) and retroviruses alternate between RNA and DNA forms, but at different stages in their life cycles. In both cases, reverse transcriptase copies RNA into a DNA strand and then functions as a DNA-dependent DNA polymerase to synthesize the complementary DNA strand. Repeated sequences at the ends of the molecules are essential for completion of the process. (a) The pregenomic RNA showing terminal repeat sequences (boxed) and the ε structure at which priming of DNA synthesis occurs. (b) The polymerase binds to the ε sequence and primes DNA synthesis via nucleotides linked to its terminal protein domain. (c, d) The replication complex with nascent DNA fragment is transferred to a complementary sequence at the 3′ end of the RNA and DNA synthesis proceeds towards the 5′ end of the template. The RNase H function of the polymerase protein digests the RNA template as synthesis proceeds. (e) A residual RNA fragment remains undigested and this is transferred to a complementary sequence towards the 5′ end of the cDNA to initiate synthesis of the second DNA strand (f). (g) The molecule is then circularized through interactions of the complementary terminal regions and synthesis of the second strand continues. The replication of retroviral genomes is similar in principle, except that a host tRNA is used as the primer for initiation of DNA synthesis.*

repeat sequences at the 3′ end of the RNA from where it is extended to make a complete DNA copy of the genome. In both cases an RNase H activity is associated with the reverse trancriptase and this removes the RNA template. A small residual RNA sequence is used to prime synthesis of the second strand of DNA using the first strand as template. In the retroviruses, the DNA product is integrated into the host genome whereas the hepatitis B virus DNA remains as an episomal circular molecule in the nucleus. In both cases RNA transcripts, both mRNA and viral RNA are produced by host DNA-dependent RNA polymerase.

RNA viruses

HEPATITIS D VIRUS

Hepatitis D virus is unique amongst animal viruses and has a single-stranded circular RNA genome. It encodes

a single viral protein which modifies host-cell polymerase to enable it to make transcripts from the viral genome. The transcript is synthesized as a continuous molecule which is pealed off from the circular template by a 'rolling circle' mechanism. An 83 nucleotide sequence within the viral RNA is highly structured and acts as an RNA enzyme or ribozyme (Shih and Been 2002). This is able to cut the RNA at a specific nucleotide to produce genome length segments of RNA and to ligate the ends to regenerate a circular molecule. The ribozyme functions on both the positive- and negative-sense RNAs.

POSITIVE-STRAND RNA VIRUSES

The genomes of the positive-strand RNA viruses must perform two apparently incompatible functions: to act as mRNA for viral protein translation and as templates for viral replication. As these functions start from opposite ends of the RNA, there is the potential for conformational clashes for molecules performing both functions simultaneously. How this is prevented is only just beginning to be resolved and appears to involve crosstalk between the termini of the RNA by host and protein factors (Gamarnik and Andino 1998). Priming can involve a protein primer, as in the picornaviruses, or the polymerase can initiate synthesis de novo as in the case of hepatitis C virus. Picornavirus RNA replication is primed by the small protein, VPg, which is urydilated by the viral polymerase by a poorly understood mechanism which also involves a conserved stem–loop structure in the RNA, the *cis*-acting replication element (CRE). The primer-independent initiation seen in some viruses appears to require precise structural features of the polymerase to ensure that synthesis starts with the correct nucleotide. Progeny positive-strand RNA is typically produced in large excess ($\times 10$) over negative strand, but the mechanisms governing this imbalance are poorly understood.

NEGATIVE-STRAND RNA VIRUSES

In contrast to positive-strand viruses, the genomic RNA of negative-strand RNA viruses is always found as a ribonucleoprotein complex. This has to function as the template for the transcription of mRNAs and as template for genome replication. The switch from mRNA template to genome template function is determined by the levels of nucleoprotein available in the cell (Portela and Digard 2002). As this increases later in infection so the nascent transcripts are encapsidated and the polymerase functions in an antitermination mode, ignoring the sequence signals important for transcription of individual mRNAs. More recent evidence suggests that for VSV the P and L proteins are important, in addition to the nucleocapsid protein, N, and that different complexes are involved in transcription or replication.

DOUBLE-STRANDED RNA VIRUSES

The replication of the double-stranded RNA viruses occurs entirely within viral core particles. The infecting virus particle is stripped of its outer protein shells to reveal the core particle which contains multiple double-stranded RNA genome segments and the transcription machinery. This transcriptional machine is highly ordered and extrudes nascent positive-strand progeny RNA molecules through pores at the vertices of the icosahedral particle. These act as templates for both translation and for the production of new double-stranded viral genomes. The latter event occurs within newly assembled core particles which can then function to amplify the production of further positive-strand RNAs or to assemble into progeny virus particles. A fascinating and as yet unresolved feature of the double-stranded RNA viruses is that each core particle appears to assemble with a complete set of genome RNA

segments. Part of the supporting evidence for this is that these viruses have very high infectivity to particle ratios, implying that all or most particles must contain a complete set of genome segments. How this selection process is controlled is not known.

RNA synthesis does not require a primer and the crystal structure of the polymerase of the double-stranded RNA phage, $\phi 6$, has demonstrated a novel mechanism for the initiation of replication. The structure of the active site pocket of the enzyme is so constructed that the $3'$ end of the template strand abuts a structural 'wall' which holds it in place to pair with the first substrate molecules. As these are covalently linked the template strand progresses though the active site, effectively pushing the restraining wall from its path. Interestingly, studies of the crystal structure of the polymerase of hepatitis C virus, which also initiates RNA synthesis in a primer-independent fashion, suggest that a similar mechanism operates in that virus (van Dijk et al. 2004).

REFERENCES

Baltimore, D. 1971. Expression of animal virus genomes. *Bacteriol Rev*, **35**, 235–41.

Bedard, K.M. and Semler, B.L. 2004. Regulation of picornaviral gene expression. *Microbe Infect*, **6**, 702–13.

Bentz, J. and Mittal, A. 2000. Deployment of membrane fusion protein domains during fusion. *Cell Biol Int*, **24**, 819–38.

Deiman, B.A.L.M. and Pleij, C.W.A. 1997. Pseudoknots: a vital feature in viral RNA. *Semin Virol*, **8**, 166–75.

Donnelly, M.L.L., Luke, G., et al. 2001. Analysis of the aphthovirus 2A/2B polyprotein 'cleavage' mechanism indicates not a proteolytic reaction, but a novel translational effect, a putative ribosomal 'skip'. *J Gen Virol*, **82**, 1013–25.

Gamarnik, A.V. and Andino, R. 1998. Switch from translation to RNA replication in a positive-stranded RNA virus. *Genes Dev*, **12**, 2293–304.

Giedroc, D.P., Theimer, C.A. and Nixon, P.L. 2000. Structure, stability and function of RNA pseudoknots invoved in stimulating ribosomal frameshifting. *J Mol Biol*, **298**, 167–85.

Greber, U.F. and Fassati, A. 2003. Nuclear import of DNA genomes. *Traffic*, **4**, 136–43.

Hogle, J.M. 2002. Poliovirus cell entry: common structural themes in viral cell entry pathways. *Ann Rev Microbiol*, **56**, 677–702.

Hu, J. and Seeger, C. 1997. RNA signals that control DNA replication in hepadnaviruses. *Semin Virol*, **8**, 205–11.

Klasse, P.J., Bron, R. and Marsh, M. 1998. Mechanisms of enveloped virus entry into animal cells. *Adv Drug Deliv Rev*, **34**, 65–91.

Kozak, M. 1986. Regulation of protein synthesis in virus-infected animal cells. *Adv Virus Res*, **31**, 229–92.

Martin, A. and Lemon, S.M. 2002. The molecular biology of hepatitis A virus. In: Ou, J. (ed.), *Hepatitis viruses*. Norwell: Kluwer Academic Publishers, 23–50.

Portela, A. and Digard, P. 2002. The influenza virus nucleoprotein: a multifunctional RNA-binding protein pivotal to virus replication. *J Gen Virol*, **83**, 723–34.

Shih, I.-H. and Been, M.D. 2002. Catalytic strategies of the hepatitis delta virus ribozymes. *Ann Rev Biochem*, **71**, 887–917.

Sieczkarski, S.B. and Whittaker, G.R. 2002. Dissecting virus entry via endocytosis. *J Gen Virol*, **83**, 1535–45.

van Dijk, A.A., Makeyev, E.V. and Bamford, D.H. 2004. Initiation of viral RNA-dependent RNA polimerization. *J Gen Virol*, **85**, 1065–346.

Weissenhorn, W., Dessen, A., et al. 1999. Structural basis for membrane fusion by enveloped viruses. *Mol Membr Biol*, **16**, 3–9.

Wiley, D.C. and Skehel, J.J. 1987. The structure and function of the hemagglutinin membrane glycoprotein of influenza virus. *Annu Rev Biochem*, **56**, 365–94.

FURTHER READING

Coffin, J.M., Hughes, S.H. and Varmus, H.E. (eds) 1997. *Retroviruses*. Cold Spring Harbor: Cold Spring Harbor Laboratory Press.

Knipe, D.M., Howley, P.M., et al. (eds) 2001. *Field's virology*, 4th edn. New York: Raven Press.

Semler, B.L. and Wimmer, E. (eds) 2002. *Molecular biology of picornaviruses*. Washington: ASM Press.

van Regenmortel, M.H.V. (ed.) 2000. *Virus taxonomy. 7th report of the ICTV*. London: Academic Press.

8

Negative-strand RNA virus replication

RICHARD M. ELLIOTT

As a group, negative-strand RNA viruses include some of the most dreaded human viruses, such as Ebola virus, Lassa fever virus, Crimean-Congo hemorrhagic fever virus and rabies virus, as well as the causes of many common human infections such as influenza, measles, and mumps. Some negative-strand viruses infect domestic animals or plants, causing substantial disease and crop losses, and thus the overall impact of these viruses on human well-being is immense. Negative-strand viruses are united by the coding strategy of their genomes, though they display great variation in both biological and molecular characteristics. In this chapter, an overview of common features in replication is presented; more detailed reviews are provided by the subsequent virus-specific chapters.

CLASSIFICATION OF NEGATIVE-STRAND RNA VIRUSES

By convention, mRNA is termed the plus or positive strand as it contains protein coding information in the directly translatable form. Baltimore (1971) developed a classification scheme for viruses based on the relationship of viral genomic nucleic acid to viral mRNA (Figure 8.1). Hence a strand of genomic nucleic acid that is of equivalent polarity to mRNA is also called positive, and the complement of the positive strand is called negative. Thus viruses could be divided into a series of classes, of which class V comprises the negative-strand

RNA viruses. Although this classification scheme is little used today, the concept of positive- and negative-strand RNA viruses remains. (Note that the terms 'strand' and 'sense,' as in negative strand or negative sense, can be and are used interchangeably).

Viral classification is now under the auspices of the International Committee on Taxonomy of Viruses, which publishes regularly updated reports on classification in both printed (7th Report; Van Regenmortel et al. 2000) and World Wide Web (www.ncbi.nlm.nih.gov/ICTVdb/index.htm) media. There are seven families of negative-strand RNA viruses and three orphan genera that are not yet incorporated into higher taxons (Table 8.1, p. 129). The families can be separated into two groups, those whose genomes comprise a single molecule of RNA (these four families make up the order *Mononegavirales*; see Chapter 119, The Order Mononegavirales) and those that have segmented genomes. Six of the families contain viruses that cause disease in humans, ranging from respiratory tract disease, through encephalitis to hemorrhagic fever. *Bornavirus*, the sole member of the *Bornaviridae* family, has been implicated in neurological disease in horses, and may be linked to psychiatric disease in humans, though this remains controversial (Staeheli et al. 2000). In addition, some viruses in the families *Rhabdoviridae* and *Bunyaviridae* can infect plants. Viruses in the orphan genera *Ophiovirus* and *Tenuivirus* also infect plants and share some similarities with bunyaviruses (van Regenmortel et al.

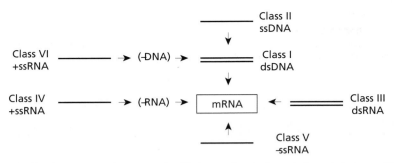

Figure 8.1 *The Baltimore Classification System. Viruses are classified according to the polarity and strategy of their genomes to produce mRNA. By convention, mRNA is designated the positive strand.*

2000). *Hepatitis delta virus* (HDV), the lone virus of the *Deltavirus* genus, is not usually mentioned when discussing negative-strand viruses, but is included in Table 8.1 for completeness. HDV has a 1.7 kb circular, negative-strand RNA genome that is heavily base-paired and more akin to a viroid genome. The genome encodes a single known product, the delta antigen, though this exists in two forms (large and small). HDV is obligatorily dependent on coinfection with *Hepatitis B virus* (HBV) for replication, and uses several HBV proteins to form its viral particle (Lai 1995; Gerin et al. 2002). HDV genome replication is quite distinct from that of the 'classical' negative-strand viruses; it occurs in the nucleus by a rolling-circle mechanism driven by cellular RNA polymerase II. The reader is referred to Chapter 56, Hepatitis delta virus for a detailed description.

OVERVIEW OF NEGATIVE-STRAND VIRUS REPLICATION

The implications for a virus possessing a negative-stranded genome are as follows: the genomic RNA itself cannot be translated into proteins directly, but must serve as the template from which positive-sense mRNA is copied. Since eukaryotic cells do not contain the appropriate enzyme to carry out this process – an RNA-dependent RNA polymerase (RdRp) – the infecting virus must encode and bring into the cell its own RdRp. As a consequence, and in contrast to positive-strand RNA viruses (Chapter 9, Positive-strand RNA virus replication in vertebrate hosts), the isolated genomic RNA of a negative-strand RNA virus is not itself infectious.

All negative-strand RNA viruses share the property that the genomic RNA (and the antigenomic RNA that is synthesized during replication; Figure 8.2, p. 4) is encapsidated by the viral nucleoprotein (N or NP) and is associated with the viral polymerase components to form a ribonucleoprotein complex (RNP) or nucleocapsid. A feature of all negative-strand RNA viruses is that the RNP has helical symmetry. Both genomic and antigenomic RNAs are only found in RNPs and never as naked RNA, implying that encapsidation occurs concurrently during RNA synthesis. Furthermore, only RNP is

the functional template for both transcription and replication.

In simplistic terms, all negative-strand RNA viruses replicate in a similar manner (Figure 8.2). After uncoating of the infecting virion, the genomic RNA (as RNP) is transcribed by the viral RdRp to produce viral mRNAs. These are translated to produce viral proteins, and once sufficient levels of protein have accumulated in the cell, the virus switches to replication mode. The same genomic RNP complex is the template for synthesis of an exact complementary copy of the genomic RNA – the antigenome – that is also encapsidated by the nucleoprotein. (Although this molecule is a positive-sense RNA, encapsidation by N protein prevents access to ribosomes and hence the antigenome cannot function as an mRNA). The antigenomic RNP is then the template for repeated synthesis of new genomic RNA molecules. These can be either packaged into progeny virus particles or act as new templates for further mRNA synthesis, termed secondary transcription. However, there are some key differences in the replication processes between nonsegmented and segmented genomes. In addition, the ambisense coding strategy (Bishop 1986; Nguyen and Haenni 2003) adopted by arenaviruses and some bunyaviruses shows further variation on the theme.

NONSEGMENTED NEGATIVE-STRAND RNA VIRUSES

Although the genomic RNA is packaged into helical RNP and the viruses are enveloped, the four families of nonsegmented negative-strand RNA viruses display a range of morphologies from spherical/pleomorphic (bornaviruses and paramyxoviruses), through bullet-shaped (rhabdoviruses) to filamentous (filoviruses), though variation is seen even within a family. Viruses in all four families share a core complement of genes that are arranged on the genome in a similar order (Strauss et al. 1996). The simplest genome structure is shown by rhabdoviruses (Figure 8.3, p. 130), such as vesicular stomatitis virus (VSV), which has just the core complement: N, P (phosphoprotein, a polymerase subunit), M (matrix), G (surface glycoprotein), and L (RdRp). More

Table 8.1 *Classification of negative-strand RNA viruses*

Family/subfamily/genus	Genome segments/ Size (kb)[a]	Site of replication	Host	Type virus[b] or virus associated with human disease
Order *Mononegavirales*				
Bornaviridae				
Borna disease virus	1/9	Nucleus	Vertebrate	Bornavirus: neuropsychiatric?
Filoviridae				
'Marburg-like viruses'	1/17	Cytoplasm	Vertebrate	Marburg virus: hemorrhagic fever
'Ebola-like viruses'	1/17	Cytoplasm	Vertebrate	Ebola virus: hemorrhagic fever
Paramyxoviridae				
Paramyxovirinae				
Respirovirus	1/15	Cytoplasm	Vertebrate	Human parainfluenza virus type 1: respiratory disease
Morbillivirus	1/16	Cytoplasm	Vertebrate	Measles virus: measles
Rubulavirus	1/15	Cytoplasm	Vertebrate	Mumps virus: mumps
Henipavirus	1/18	Cytoplasm	Vertebrate	Hendra virus: respiratory disease; Nipah virus: encephalitis
Avulavirus	1/15	Cytoplasm	Vertebrate	(Newcastle disease virus)
Pneumovirinae				
Pneumovirus	1/15	Cytoplasm	Vertebrate	Human respiratory syncytial virus: respiratory disease; croup
Metapneumovirus	1/13	Cytoplasm	Vertebrate	Human metapneumovirus: respiratory disease
Rhabdoviridae				
Vesiculovirus	1/11	Cytoplasm	Vertebrate	(Vesicular stomatitis Indiana virus)
Lyssavirus	1/12	Cytoplasm	Vertebrate	Rabies virus: rabies
Ephemerovirus	1/15	Cytoplasm	Vertebrate	(Bovine ephemeral fever virus)
Cytorhabdovirus	1/nc	Cytoplasm	Plant	(Lettuce necrotic yellows virus)
Nucleorhabdovirus	1/14	Cytoplasm	Plant	(Potato yellow dwarf virus)
Novirhabdovirus	1/11	Cytoplasm	Plant	(Infectious hematopoietic necrosis virus)
Bunyaviridae				
Orthobunyavirus	3/12	Cytoplasm	Invertebrate/ vertebrate	La Crosse virus: encephalitis; Oropouche virus: fever
Hantavirus	3/12	Cytoplasm	Vertebrate	Hantaan virus: hemorrhagic fever with renal syndrome; Sin Nombre virus: hantavirus pulmonary syndrome
Nairovirus	3/19	Cytoplasm	Invertebrate/ vertebrate	Crimean-Congo hemorrhagic fever virus: hemorrhagic fever
Phlebovirus	3/12	Cytoplasm	Invertebrate/ vertebrate	Rift Valley fever virus: hemorrhagic fever, retinitis
Tospovirus	3/18	Cytoplasm	Invertebrate/ plant	(Tomato spotted wilt virus)
Arenaviridae				
Arenavirus	2/11	Cytoplasm	Vertebrate	Lassa virus: hemorrhagic fever
Orthomyxoviridae				
Influenzavirus A	8/15	Nucleus	Vertebrate	Influenza A virus: influenza
Influenzavirus B	8/15	Nucleus	Vertebrate	Influenza B virus: influenza
Influenzavirus C	7/12	Nucleus	Vertebrate	Influenza C virus: respiratory disease
Thogotovirus	6/12	Nucleus	Invertebrate/ vertebrate	(Thogoto virus)
Isavirus	8/nc	Nucleus	Fish	(Infectious salmon anemia virus)
Orphan genera				
Ophiovirus	3/12	Cytoplasm	Plant	(Citrus psorosis virus)
Tenuivirus	4/5/18	Cytoplasm	Plant	(Rice stripe virus)
Deltavirus	1 (circular)/1.7	Nucleus	Vertebrate	Hepatitis delta virus: hepatitis

a) Approximate size; nc, not completed.
b) Nonhuman-type viruses are in parenthesis.

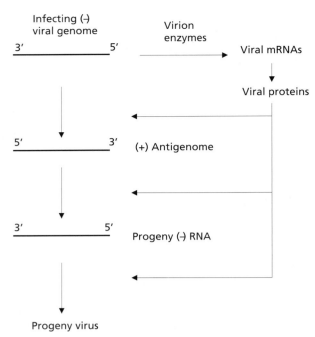

Figure 8.2 *Basic replication of negative-strand RNA viruses. The genome of the infecting virion is transcribed by the viral RdRp to produce viral mRNAs. The viral mRNAs are translated into viral proteins, that in turn are involved in replicating the infecting genome RNA via a complementary positive-strand RNA (the antigenome) and packaging into progeny virions.*

complex genomes such as paramyxoviruses encode other gene products such as additional glycoproteins and also nonstructural proteins. In all cases the genome is bounded by noncoding leader and trailer sequences, and each gene is flanked by transcriptional start and stop sequences. The internal genes are separated by intergenic sequences. Intergenic sequences range from just

2 nt in VSV to more than 60 nt in some paramyxoviruses. The gene stop sequences contain short tracts of U residues that template, via reiterative copying, the addition of a poly(A) tail at the 3′ end of the viral mRNA (Poon et al., 1999; Figure 8.3).

The generally accepted stop–start model of transcription (Banerjee et al. 1977; Emerson 1982), based largely on in vitro studies, is that viral RdRp begins RNA copying at a single promoter site at the 3′ end of the genome (Figure 8.3), and that termination of an upstream gene is required for subsequent transcription of the downstream gene. For VSV, a 47 nt leader RNA is synthesized and then released, and the RdRp initiates synthesis of the first mRNA, for N protein. The RdRp possesses capping activity so that the viral mRNAs have 5′ cap structures (m^7GpppG) similar to host cell mRNAs. After polyadenylation, the mRNA is released and the polymerase reinitiates after the intergenic sequence to synthesize the next mRNA. Transcription of the genome is thus sequential. During transcription, there is attenuation at each initiation step (the RdRp sometimes dissociates from the template and does not reinitiate), such that there is a gradient in the number of copies of each mRNA produced: N mRNA is most abundant and L mRNA the least abundant (Villareal et al. 1976; Iverson and Rose 1981). This is an important regulatory step for the virus in controlling the different amounts of each viral protein needed. For VSV, recombinant viruses have been created by reverse genetics (see later) in which the gene order has been rearranged (Wertz et al. 1998); although viable, such viruses grow less well than wild-type, confirming the importance of mRNA attenuation in viral replication.

Viral proteins are translated from the mRNAs and the amounts of these produced, particularly the N protein,

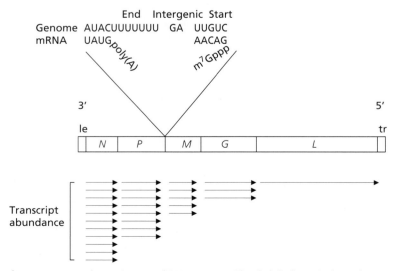

Figure 8.3 *Transcription of a nonsegmented negative strand RNA genome. The rhabdovirus VSV is used as an example. The five viral genes (N, P, M, G, and L) are flanked by leader (le) and trailer (tr) sequences. At each gene junction are found transcription termination and polyadenylation signals (end), an intergenic sequence (just 2 nt in the case of VSV) and a transcription initiation signal (start). There is attenuation of the polymerase at each junction, resulting in a gradient of transcript abundance from the 3′ to 5′ direction.*

are thought to signal the switch from transcription to replication. Sufficient N protein must be available to encapsidate the nascent antigenome RNA. Under these conditions the RdRp does not recognize the mRNA termination or polyadenylation signals but produces a full-length positive-strand RNA molecule that is cotranscriptionally encapsidated by N protein to make a positive-strand RNP. This in turn becomes the template for the synthesis of progeny genomic RNA, which again is cotranscriptionally encapsidated into RNP.

Recent in vivo studies (Whelan and Wertz 2002), however, provide evidence that the VSV polymerase can initiate transcription directly on the *N* gene start, and that prior transcription of leader RNA is not required. Thus the authors hypothesize that the regulation of transcription versus replication is through the polymerase binding to alternative sites on the genome: internally at the *N* gene for transcription and at the extreme 3′ end for replication. While this model has attractions, the factors responsible for which initiation site is used (possibly modification of the template or of the RdRp, or role of host-cell proteins, etc.) remain to be determined.

SEGMENTED GENOME NEGATIVE-STRAND RNA VIRUSES

A significant difference between orthomyxoviruses (e.g. influenza virus) and bunya- and arenaviruses is that the former transcribe and replicate their genomes in the nucleus. This presents an additional dimension to viral replication – transport of viral components in and out of the nucleus. After infection, the influenza virus RNPs must enter the nucleus, newly transcribed mRNAs exit the nucleus to be translated, viral proteins involved in RNP formation must travel back into the nucleus, and progeny negative-strand RNPs must transport out of the nucleus for virus assembly and release through the plasma membrane (Portela and Digard 2002). As orthomyxovirus mRNAs are produced in the nucleus, they can avail themselves of the cellular mRNA splicing machinery; for example, influenza A virus synthesizes differently spliced forms of mRNAs derived from RNA segments 7 and 8. These are translated into different proteins, thus increasing the coding capacity of these genome segments (Lamb and Krug 2001).

mRNA synthesis of all groups of segmented negative-strand RNA viruses is a primer-dependent process (Figure 8.4). The primers are derived from the capped 5′ ends of cellular mRNAs that are cleaved by an endonuclease activity contained within the PB2 protein of influenza virus or the L protein of bunya- and arenaviruses. The capped primers are incorporated into the viral mRNA, such that the viral mRNAs contain short (12–18 nt) nontemplated heterogenous sequences at their 5′ ends (Plotch et al. 1981). Thus these viruses do not need to encode capping functions unlike members of the *Mononegavirales*. This process, termed 'cap-snatching,' occurs in the nucleus for orthomyxoviruses and there-

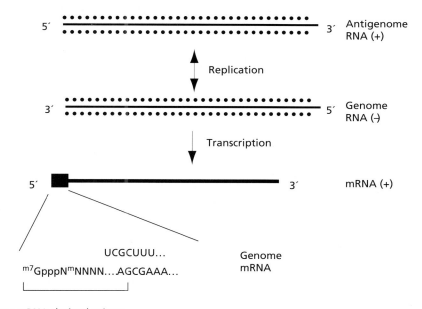

Figure 8.4 *Transcription and replication of a segmented negative-strand RNA virus. The genome and antigenome RNAs are shown encapsidated by nucleocapsid protein. Transcription to produce mRNA is a primer-dependent process where the capped, 5′ ends of host-cell mRNAs are cleaved by a viral endonuclease and the primers incorporated into the viral mRNA. The primers are usually 12–18 nt in length and heterogenous in sequence, though cleavage usually occurs at a base complementary to the 3′ end of the viral genomic RNA. The example shows the 5′ end of an influenza A virus mRNA. Viral mRNAs are truncated relative to the genome RNA, and are not encapsidated by nucleocapsid protein.*

fore needs ongoing host cell transcription; hence ortho-myxovirus replication is inhibited by drugs, such as α-amanitin, which prevent host transcription. By contrast, bunya- and arenaviruses cap-snatch in the cytoplasm from previously synthesized host mRNAs and their replication is not inhibited by α-amanitin. Orthomyxovirus mRNAs are polyadenylated, signaled by a polyU stretch in the genomic RNA. Similar to the RdRp of nonsegmented viruses, the orthomyxovirus polymerase stutters on this sequence to add a poly(A) tail (Poon et al. 1999). By contrast, neither bunya- nor arenavirus mRNAs are polyadenylated (Nguyen and Haenni 2003).

The promoters for mRNA synthesis are located in the terminal untranslated regions of each genome segment. The 3′ and 5′ terminal sequences show a degree of complementarity that permits base-pairing between the ends, creating a panhandle, and accounts for the circular appearance of isolated nucleocapsids (Hsu et al. 1987; Pardigon et al. 1982). The relative strength of each promoter regulates the mRNA transcript abundance from each segment (Barr et al. 2003). Similar to the nonsegmented genome viruses, the concentration of viral N protein is thought to be involved in the switch to replication. RNA replication is a primer-independent event that results in production of full-length positive-strand RNAs (antigenomes) that are assembled into RNPs; these in turn serve as templates for synthesis of progeny genome RNA segments. Like the nonsegmented genome viruses, the newly synthesized genomic RNPs can be packaged into new virions or are involved in secondary transcription. In order to generate an infectious virus particle, one copy of each segment (at least) must be packaged, and there is debate over whether this is a random or specific event. Extraction of viral RNA from purified virions often reveals nonequimolar ratios of RNA, and it could be that virions contain more than just, for example, eight (influenza A virus) or three (bunyavirus) RNA segments. Recent work on influenza A virus has provided evidence for specific packaging signals that span the noncoding/coding region of some segments (Fujii et al. 2003).

AMBISENSE-CONTAINING VIRUSES

A variant of the classic negative-sense coding strategy is displayed by some genome segments of certain bunya-viruses and both segments of arenaviruses (Bishop, 1986; Nguyen and Haenni, 2003; Figure 8.5). Analysis of the genome RNA segments of these viruses reveals two open reading frames (ORF), one negative-sense and one positive-sense. These are separated by an intergenic region that typically shows secondary structure (often a stem-loop). The negative-sense ORF is translated from a subgenomic mRNA transcribed from the infecting genome in the usual manner, with transcription termination occurring at the intergenic structured RNA sequence.

The positive-sense ORF cannot be translated directly from the infecting genome since it is in an RNP form, but from a second subgenomic mRNA that is transcribed from the antigenomic RNA (Figure 8.5). Thus the negative-sense ORF is expressed early, whereas the positive-sense ORF is expressed later in infection, once genome replication has begun, giving the virus a degree of temporal regulation of gene expression. In all other regards, however, ambisense viruses replicate similarly to their strictly negative-sense counterparts.

GENETIC VARIATION, RECOMBINATION, AND REASSORTMENT

A particular feature of all RNA viruses is their genetic variability that is much higher than DNA genome viruses (Holmes 2003). This is because viral RdRp do not contain proofreading activity and thus when incorrect nucleotides are incorporated into the nascent RNA

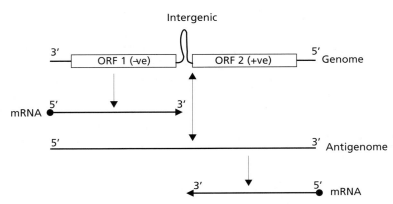

Figure 8.5 *Transcription and replication of an ambisense RNA. The genome RNA contains ORFs in both negative- and positive-sense orientations, separated by an intergenic sequence that usually shows secondary structure. Each ORF is translated from a subgenomic mRNA (transcribed in a primer-dependent manner), with the mRNA for ORF2 being transcribed from the full-length antigenome RNA. This means that the protein encoded by ORF2 is translated relatively late during the replication cycle, after the onset of genome replication itself.*

strand there is no means to correct them. The error frequency of RNA virus polymerases is in the range 10^{-3}–10^{-4}, resulting in rapid evolution of the virus. In fact, the resulting progeny genomes will each probably contain a nucleotide difference from the master or consensus sequence such that, rather than a homogeneous sequence, the virus consists of a population of related sequences known as a quasispecies. A consequence of this rapid evolution is that many progeny genomes will carry lethal mutations. The implications of this are to limit the size of RNA genomes – the bigger the genome the more chance of incorporating a lethal mutation. The positive-strand coronaviruses have the largest known RNA genomes, up to 32 kb (Chapter 39, Coronaviruses, toroviruses, and arteriviruses), and the negative-strand viruses have genomes less than 20 kb. The ability of viruses to evolve and adapt to, for example, host immune pressure is clearly seen with influenza virus where the accumulation of point mutations year on year in the genes encoding the hemagglutinin and neuraminidase surface glycoproteins (antigenic drift) necessitates annual vaccination to maintain protection.

Genetic recombination – the breaking and joining of distinct nucleic acid molecules – has been regarded as a rare occurrence in negative-strand RNA viruses, but evidence is accumulating to suggest that it happens more frequently than previously thought, for instance in hantaviruses, arenaviruses, and paramyxoviruses such as mumps virus and Newcastle disease virus (Chare et al. 2003). However, at present, recombination is not seen as a major evolutionary force in these viruses.

By contrast, genome segment reassortment among the segmented viruses occurs frequently during the course of mixed infection. In this way progeny viruses may contain a genome comprising segments derived from each of the parents, though reasssortment is not entirely random. For as yet unknown reasons, certain genetic constellations are apparently not viable. Reassortment has been studied extensively in influenza viruses, where it is acknowledged as the route by which pandemic influenza virus strains arise – so-called antigenic shift (Reid and Taubenberger 2003). 'New' viruses emerge containing surface antigens not previously experienced by the human population (often the surface genes of an avian influenza virus) and thus the new strains cause havoc among the immunologically naïve population.

MAXIMIZING GENOME CODING POTENTIAL

Although all the viruses discussed in this chapter show the property of a negative-sense coding strategy, the viruses implement this in a number of variations to maximize the protein coding content of their genomes. The genomes encode protein highly efficiently – in general >90 percent of the genome encodes protein. As discussed above, influenza viruses encode different gene products from the same segment by splicing of the transcribed mRNAs. Orthobunyaviruses employ overlapping reading frames to encode two proteins on the S segment, both proteins being translated (unusually for a eukaryotic system) from the same mRNA (Bishop 1996). However, the extreme example of multiple protein expression from a single gene is shown by the paramyxovirus P gene, where up to six distinct proteins may be produced (Curran et al. 1998). Most paramyxoviruses exhibit RNA 'editing' during transcription of their P mRNAs, where nontemplated G residues (usually one, two or four Gs) are inserted, causing a frame-shift in the encoded mRNA. Thus different forms of mRNA are synthesized, encoding different proteins. Coupled with alternate initiation codon usage, including noncanonical AUG codons, a plethora of proteins can be produced from the single P gene. RNA editing also occurs in the glycoprotein mRNA of Ebola virus, producing both full-length and truncated glycoprotein products (Sanchez et al. 1996).

THE MODERN APPROACH TO STUDY RNA VIRUS REPLICATION: REVERSE GENETICS

One of the impediments to detailed analysis of RNA virus replication has been the nature of the genetic material itself; RNA is biochemically more labile than DNA, and techniques to produce specific nucleotide alterations directly in an RNA molecule are not available. In the field of RNA virology, 'reverse genetics' is usually described as the ability to recover (rescue) an infectious virus from cloned complementary DNA. Thus the viral genome can be manipulated at the DNA level using the full gamut of recombinant DNA protocols, and then virus recovered containing defined mutations. The phenotype of the mutant virus can then be related to the genotypic changes (hence **reverse** genetics). Reverse genetics of RNA viruses actually began in 1978 with the recovery of an RNA bacteriophage, Qβ, from cloned cDNA (Taniguchi et al. 1978), and the first animal virus rescued from cDNA was the positive-strand poliovirus in 1981 (Racaniello and Baltimore 1981). However, progress on developing similar methodologies for negative-strand RNA viruses was more difficult, in part because of the requirement to produce a biologically active RNP form isolated components.

A system to manipulate individual genome segments of influenza A virus was reported by Luytjes et al. in 1989, but the first recovery of a negative-strand RNA virus entirely from cDNA was not achieved until 1994: perhaps surprisingly this was rabies virus by Schnell et al. (1994). Since then representatives of paramyxoviruses, filoviruses, bunyaviruses, and orthomyxoviruses have all been rescued entirely from cDNA (Conzelmann 1998; Neumann et al. 2002), and encouraging progress has been made with bornaviruses and arenaviruses (Lee et al. 2000; Perez et al. 2003) to suggest that these will be rescued soon.

These achievements have led to unprecedented progress in understanding detailed aspects of viral replication, structure–function analyses of viral proteins, possibilities for engineering 'designer' vaccines, and in delineating viral–host interactions. These topics are dealt with in detail in the following chapters.

REFERENCES

Baltimore, D. 1971. Expression of animal virus genomes. *Bacteriol Rev*, **35**, 235–41.

Banerjee, A.D., Abraham, G. and Colonno, R. 1977. Vesicular stomatitis virus: mode of transcription. *J Gen Virol*, **34**, 1–8.

Barr, J.N., Elliott, R.M., et al. 2003. Segment-specific terminal sequences of *Bunyamwera bunyavirus* regulate genome replication. *Virology*, **311**, 326–38.

Bishop, D.H.L. 1986. Ambisense RNA genomes of arenaviruses and phleboviruses. *Adv Virus Res*, **31**, 1–51.

Bishop, D.H.L. 1996. Biology and molecular biology of bunyaviruses. In: Elliott, R.M. (ed.), *The Bunyaviridae*. New York: Plenum Press, 19–61.

Chare, E.R., Gould, E.A. and Holmes, E.C. 2003. Phylogenetic analysis reveals a low rate of homologous recombination in negative-sense RNA viruses. *J Gen Virol*, **84**, 2691–703.

Conzelmann, K.K. 1998. Nonsegmented negative-strand RNA viruses: genetics and manipulation of viral genomes. *Annu Rev Genet*, **32**, 123–62.

Curran, J., Latorre, P. and Kolakofsky, D. 1998. Translational gymnastics on the Sendai virus P/C mRNA. *Semin Virol*, **8**, 351–7.

Emerson, S.U. 1982. Reconstitution studies detect a single polymerase entry site on the vesicular stomatitis virus genome. *Cell*, **31**, 635–42.

Fujii, Y., Goto, H., et al. 2003. Selective incorporation of influenza virus RNA segments into virions. *Proc Natl Acad Sci USA*, **100**, 2002–7.

Gerin, J.L., Casey, J.L. and Purcell, R.H. 2002. Hepatitis delta virus. In: Blaine Hollinger, F. (ed.), *Viral hepatitis*. Philadelphia: Lippincott Williams & Wilkins, 169–82.

Holmes, E.C. 2003. Error thresholds and constraints to RNA virus evolution. *Trends Microbiol*, **11**, 543–6.

Hsu, M.T., Parvin, J.D., et al. 1987. Genomic RNAs of influenza viruses are held in a circular conformation in virions and in infected cells by a terminal panhandle. *Proc Nat Acad Sci USA*, **84**, 8140–4.

Iverson, L.E. and Rose, J.K. 1981. Localized attenuation and discontinuous synthesis during vesicular stomatitis virus transcription. *Cell*, **23**, 477–84.

Lai, M.M. 1995. The molecular biology of hepatitis delta virus. *Annu Rev Biochem*, **64**, 259–86.

Lamb, R.A. and Krug, R.M. 2001. *Orthomyxoviridae*: the viruses and their replication. In: Knipe, D.M. and Howley, P.M. (eds), *Fields virology*, 4th edn. Philadelphia, PA: Lippincott Williams and Wilkins, 1487–531.

Lee, K.J., Novella, I.S., et al. 2000. NP and L proteins of lymphocytic choriomeningitis virus (LCMV) are sufficient for efficient transcription and replication of LCMV genomic RNA analogs. *J Virol*, **74**, 3470–7.

Luytjes, W., Krystal, M., et al. 1989. Amplification, expression and packaging of a foreign gene by influenza virus. *Cell*, **59**, 1107–13.

Neumann, G., Whitt, M.A. and Kawaoka, Y. 2002. A decade after the generation of a negative-sense RNA virus from cloned cDNA – what have we learned? *J Gen Virol*, **83**, 2635–62.

Nguyen, M. and Haenni, A.-L. 2003. Expression strategies of ambisense viruses. *Virus Res*, **92**, 141–50.

Pardigon, N., Vialat, P., et al. 1982. Panhandles and hairpin structures at the termini of Germiston virus RNAs (Bunyavirus). *Virology*, **122**, 191–7.

Perez, M., Sanchez, A., et al. 2003. A reverse genetics system for Borna disease virus. *J Gen Virol*, **84**, 3099–104.

Plotch, S.J., Bouloy, M., et al. 1981. A unique cap (^{m7}GpppX^m)-dependent influenza virion endonuclease cleaves capped RNA to generate the primers that initiate viral RNA transcription. *Cell*, **23**, 847–58.

Poon, L.L.M., Pritlove, D.C., et al. 1999. Direct evidence that the poly(A) tail of influenza virus mRNA is synthesized by reiterative copying of a U track in the virion RNA template. *J Virol*, **73**, 3473–6.

Portela, A. and Digard, P. 2002. The influenza virus nucleoprotein: a multifunctional RNA-binding protein pivotal to virus replication. *J Gen Virol*, **83**, 723–34.

Racaniello, V.R. and Baltimore, D. 1981. Cloned poliovirus complementary DNA is infectious in mammalian cells. *Science*, **214**, 916–19.

Reid, A.H. and Taubenberger, J.K. 2003. The origin of the 1918 pandemic influenza virus: a continuing enigma. *J Gen Virol*, **84**, 2285–92.

Sanchez, A., Trappier, S.G., et al. 1996. The virion glycoproteins of Ebola viruses are encoded in two reading frames and are expressed through transcriptional editing. *Proc Natl Acad Sci USA*, **93**, 3602–7.

Schnell, M.J., Mebatsion, T. and Conzelmann, K.-K. 1994. Infectious rabies viruses from cloned cDNA. *EMBO J*, **13**, 4195–203.

Staeheli, P., Sauder, C., et al. 2000. Epidemiology of *Borna disease virus*. *J Gen Virol*, **81**, 2123–35.

Strauss, E.G., Strauss, J.H. and Levine, A.J. 1996. Virus evolution. In: Fields, B.N., Knipe, D.M. and Howley, P.M. (eds), *Fields virology*, 3rd edn. Philadelphia, PA: Raven Press, 153–71.

Taniguchi, T., Palmieri, M. and Weissman, C. 1978. Qβ DNA-containing hybrid plasmids giving rise to Qβ phage formation in the bacterial host. *Nature*, **274**, 223–8.

Van Regenmortel, M.H.V., Fauquet, C.M., et al. 2000. *Virus taxonomy. Seventh Report of the International Committee on Taxonomy of Viruses*. San Diego, CA: Academic Press.

Villareal, L.P., Breindl, M. and Holland, J.J. 1976. Determination of the molar ratios of vesicular stomatitis virus induced RNA species in BHK21 cells. *Biochemistry*, **15**, 1663–7.

Wertz, G.W., Perepelista, V.P. and Ball, L.A. 1998. Gene rearrangement attenuates expression and lethality of a nonsegmented negative strand RNA virus. *Proc Natl Acad Sci USA*, **92**, 8388–92.

Whelan, P.J. and Wertz, G.W. 2002. Transcription and replication initiate on separate sites on the vesicular stomatitis virus genome. *Proc Natl Acad Sci USA*, **99**, 9178–83.

9

Positive-strand RNA virus replication in vertebrate hosts

JO ELLEN BRUNNER AND BERT L. SEMLER

COMMON CHARACTERISTICS ACROSS FAMILIES

Classification and medical significance

This chapter is organized around the features of the intracellular replicative cycle shared by single-stranded, positive-strand RNA viruses that infect vertebrate hosts. Most of the discussion focuses on specific examples of viruses from the families *Picornaviridae*, *Caliciviridae*, *Flaviviridae*, *Togaviridae*, and *Coronaviridae*. Replication of single-stranded, positive-strand RNA plant viruses, a significant proportion of the viruses in this class, will not be covered here. The term positive-strand RNA refers to the taxonomic criterion proposed by Baltimore (Baltimore 1971) to classify viruses, namely, the relationship between the viral genome and the messenger RNA used for translation during the process of viral gene expression. Accordingly, a positive-strand RNA (class IV) virus has a genome that is identical to messenger RNA and competent for translation once released in the cytoplasm of the host cell. This scheme for virus classification does not necessarily take into account the more current genetic information which would form an additional basis for possible reassignments of viruses into superfamilies.

Poliovirus, the prototypic member of *Picornaviridae*, is arguably the most comprehensively studied mammalian single-stranded, positive-strand RNA virus. Much of the information and many of the mechanisms presented here come from the large body of knowledge relating to poliovirus. The majority of the early research concerning the biology and pathogenesis of the virus was motivated by the desire to diminish the human suffering caused by poliomyelitis, and subsequently led to the development of two effective vaccines. As a direct consequence of the widespread application of the Salk and Sabin vaccines during the last five decades, world health officials envision that poliomyelitis may be eradicated worldwide by the end of the year 2005. Ironically, the same scientific research which led to breakthroughs in the understanding of the molecular biology of poliovirus now creates the possibility that this virus could be reconstructed as an agent of bioterrorism in the post-eradication era (Cello et al. 2002).

Human immunodeficiency virus (HIV) is responsible for the current pandemic of acquired immunodeficiency syndrome (AIDS) and the associated climbing levels of worldwide morbidity and mortality. HIV and the other members of the *Retroviridae* are covered in subsequent chapters due to the fact that several aspects of their intracellular replication cycles are unique among single-stranded, positive-strand RNA viruses. Nonetheless, two other viruses of currently increasing medical importance globally, *West Nile virus* (WNV) (*Flaviviridae*) (Briese et al. 1999; Lanciotti et al. 1999; Jordan et al. 2000; Brinton 2002) and severe acute respiratory syndrome virus (SARS-CoV) (representing a new group of *Coronaviridae*) (Marra et al. 2003; Rota et al. 2003) are introduced.

Limited coding capacity of small genomes

The limited coding capacity of the relatively small genomes typical of most single-stranded, positive-strand

RNA viruses (approximately 4–30 kilobases) necessitates gene expression strategies aimed at generating multiple viral proteins or activities from apparent mono- or oligo-cistronic genomic RNAs (Figure 9.1). Viruses in the families *Picornaviridae* and *Flaviviridae* contain a single open reading frame (ORF) within their genomic RNAs which encodes a polyprotein that is processed into functional precursors and mature proteins (Agol et al. 1999; Brinton 2002; Leong et al. 2002). The viral structural proteins are encoded within the 5′ region of the genomic ORF, while the nonstructural proteins are encoded within the 3′ region. Human caliciviruses have small genomes that contain either three [Norwalk-like viruses (NLV)] or two [Sapporo-like viruses (SLV)] ORFs. NLVs express ORF1 as a polyprotein precursor that is cleaved by the viral 3C-like (picornaviruses) proteinase into the nonstructural proteins. ORF2 encodes the single major structural protein, and ORF3 encodes a small basic protein of unknown function (Clarke and Lambden 1997; Robinson et al. 2002). Other families within this class, *Togaviridae* and *Coronaviridae*, with their larger, more complex genomes, follow an expression strategy that involves discontinuous RNA synthesis. For togaviruses, production of subgenomic positive-strand RNA(s) is templated from a full-length negative-strand intermediate RNA (Sawicki and Sawicki 1998a). A polyprotein processed into the nonstructural proteins is encoded by the 5′ end of the genomic RNA. A single subgenomic positive-strand RNA representing the 3′ end of the genome is translated into a polyprotein that is the precursor to the viral structural proteins.

For coronaviruses, the favored model of gene expression involves production of a set of subgenomic negative-strand RNAs, derived from discontinuous transcription of genomic RNA, which will serve as templates for transcription of subgenomic mRNAs (Makino et al. 1988; Sawicki and Sawicki 1998b). As with togaviruses, a polyprotein processed into the nonstructural proteins is encoded by the 5′ two-thirds of the genomic RNA. Coronaviruses generate a nested set of 3′ coterminal subgenomic positive-strand RNAs corresponding to the 3′ end of the genome. Each of these RNAs has at its 5′ end an approximately 70 nt long, capped leader sequence derived from the 5′ end of the genome (Holmes and Enjuanes 2003). The unique portion of the 5′ end of each mRNA is translated to synthesize an individual viral structural or nonstructural protein even though most of these mRNAs contain more than one ORF. Marra et al. identified nine potential ORFs within the SARS-CoV genome that could encode nonstructural proteins unique to this virus (Marra et al. 2003).

Another strategy which in effect amplifies the information encoded by the genome is the production of viral gene products that are multifunctional. The poliovirus precursor polypeptide, 3CD, is involved in protein

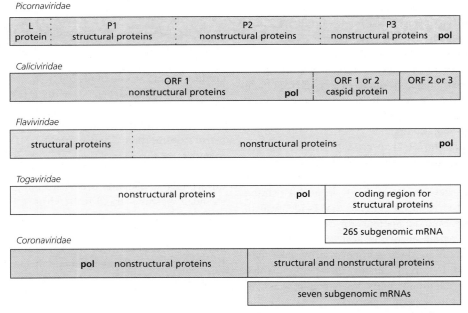

Figure 9.1 *Comparison of genome organization for five positive-strand RNA virus families. Picornaviruses and flaviviruses have a single ORF within their genomic RNAs. The structural proteins are encoded by the 5′ region of the genome and the nonstructural proteins are encoded by the 3′ region. Human caliciviruses have either two or three ORFs. The capsid protein is encoded by the 3′ terminus of ORF1 or ORF2. For togaviruses, a polyprotein processed into the nonstructural proteins is encoded by the 5′ region of the genomic RNA. A single subgenomic positive-strand RNA corresponding to the 3′ region of the genome is translated into a precursor to the viral structural proteins. For coronaviruses, a polyprotein processed into the nonstructural proteins is encoded by the 5′ two-thirds of the genomic RNA. Seven 3′ coterminal subgenomic positive-strand RNAs encode the structural proteins as well as some of the nonstructural proteins.*

processing as well as RNA replication, by way of replication complex formation with host and viral proteins at the 5′ and 3′ ends of the viral genome (Andino et al. 1990, 1993; Herold and Andino 2001). The NS5 protein of the *Flavivirus*, WNV, has methyltransferase and RNA polymerase activities (Brinton 2002). In fact, although the 11 kb genome of WNV is of intermediate length for a positive-strand RNA virus, most of the nonstructural proteins are multifunctional.

Investigators have long recognized that replication of many RNA viruses is cell-type specific, suggesting that there is a dependence on cell-specific factors (Lai 1998). RNA viruses are known to subvert host proteins that are normal components of cellular RNA processing or translation machineries for their own translation, replication, and packaging, another approach by which these viruses overcome the limited coding potential of their genomes (Table 9.1). The most frequently observed cellular proteins thought to be involved in viral RNA synthesis are the heterogeneous nuclear ribonucleoprotein (hnRNP) complex proteins. Several of these RNA-binding proteins, normally involved in assembly of the ribonucleosome and mRNA biogenesis, have been proposed to play a role in the life cycles of different viruses by interacting with viral RNAs in functional complexes (Lai 1998). hnRNP A1 binds to the 3′ untranslated region (UTR) and mediates potential 5′–3′ end crosstalk of the coronavirus mouse hepatitis virus (MHV) RNA.

Within the *Flavivirus* hepatitis C virus (HCV) genome, the 5′ UTR has been shown to interact with several cellular factors: the La autoantigen (Ali and Siddiqui 1997; Spangberg et al. 1999), polypyrimidine tract-binding protein (PTB) (Ali and Siddiqui 1995), hnRNP L (Hahm et al. 1998), eukaryotic initiation factor 3 (eIF3) (Sizova et al. 1998), and poly(rC) binding protein 1 (PCBP1) and poly(rC) binding protein 2 (PCBP2), also known as hnRNP E1 and hnRNP E2, respectively (Spangberg and Schwartz 1999). Human RNA-binding protein (HuR) and hnRNP C have been shown to bind to the 3′ ends of HCV RNAs of both polarities (Spangberg et al. 2000). PTB, also known as hnRNP I, interacts with the pyrimidine-rich region

within the 3′ UTR of the HCV RNA genome (Gontarek et al. 1999). Eukaryotic elongation factor 1 alpha (EF-1α) interacts with the 3′ stem–loop structure of the genomic RNA of WNV (*Flavivirus*) and appears to play a functional role in replication (Blackwell and Brinton 1997).

Picornavirus investigators have determined that the cellular protein PCBP2 interacts with the major stem–loop structure in the internal ribosome entry site (IRES) of the 5′ noncoding region (NCR) of poliovirus positive-strand RNA and is essential for translation initiation (Blyn et al. 1996; Blyn et al. 1997). In addition, the binding of poly(rC) binding protein (PCBP) to the 5′ positive-strand cloverleaf structure in concert with the viral precursor 3CD is required for initiation of negative-strand RNA synthesis (Gamarnik and Andino 1997, 1998; Parsley et al. 1997; Walter et al. 2002).

Conservation of amino acid sequences, functional domains, and common replication strategies

Comparative analysis of amino acid sequences between positive-strand RNA viruses has revealed relationships between disparate groups of plant, animal, and bacterial viruses. Enzymes mediating the expression and replication of virus genomes contain arrays of conserved sequence motifs despite the potential for rapid evolution of RNA genomes (Koonin and Dolja 1993; Steinhauer and Holland 1987) Proteins that include such motifs are the RNA-dependent RNA polymerase (RdRp), a putative RNA helicase, a chymotrypsin-like proteinase and papain-like proteinase, and a methytransferase. Nonetheless, the RdRp is the only universally conserved protein of positive-strand RNA viruses. Evolutionary virologists are developing a concept of the RNA virus genome as a relatively stable foundation of housekeeping genes with a more flexible collection of genes coding for virion components and accessory proteins (Koonin and Dolja 1993). It is thought that all positive-strand RNA viruses and some related double-stranded RNA viruses could have evolved from a common ancestral virus that contained a gene for a RdRp, a chymo-

Table 9.1 *Examples of cellular proteins shown to interact with viral RNAs*

Virus	RNA	Cellular proteins
Poliovirus (*Picornaviridae*)	IRES – 5′ NCR of genome	PCBP2 (hnRNP E2), La, unr, PTB (hnRNP I)
	Cloverleaf – 5′ NCR	PCBP (hnRNP E)
	3′ NCR	Nucleolin
West Nile virus (*Flaviviridae*)	3′ Stem–loop of genome	EF-1α
Hepatitis C virus (*Flaviviridae*)	5′ UTR of genome	La, PTB, hnRNP L, eIF3, PCBP1 (hnRNP E1), PCBP2 (hnRNP E2)
	3′ End of + strand RNA	HuR, hnRNP C
	3′ End of − strand RNA	HuR, hnRNP C
	Pyrimidine-rich region of 3′ UTR of genome	PTB (hnRNP I)
Mouse hepatitis virus (*Coronaviridae*)	3′ UTR of genome	hnRNP A1

trypsin-related proteinase that also functioned as the capsid protein, and perhaps an RNA helicase.

Conservation of functional domains exists within the genomes of positive-strand RNA viruses in the form of *cis*-acting sequence motifs and RNA secondary structures necessary for translation, RNA synthesis, and packaging. The 5′ termini of these viruses typically contain such elements known to participate in binding of viral and host cell factors. Interaction of protein factors and RNA structures is necessary to selectively initiate viral-specific processes such as synthesis of negative-strand intermediate RNA. Binding of protein factors to internal sequence motifs can be a prerequisite to genomic RNA synthesis by implementing the release of single-stranded 3′ termini on negative-strand intermediate RNAs or by participating in a complex that initiates or increases the efficiency of genome replication.

Within the intracellular replicative cycle of most positive-strand RNA viruses, we see asymmetric production of excess genomic positive- over negative-strand RNA. Only a single, nascent negative-strand RNA is copied from a positive-strand RNA template at one time and the full-length duplexed RNA molecule that results from this transcription is referred to as the replicative form (RF). Although genomic positive-strand RNA synthesis may initiate on RF, eventually negative-strand RNA serves as the template for simultaneous synthesis of numerous new genomic RNAs by efficient reinitiation (Figure 9.2). This form of partially duplexed RNA is referred to as the replicative intermediate (RI). The fact that free negative-strand RNA is not recovered from the cytoplasm of the infected cell supports the replication models of RF and RI for picornaviruses, caliciviruses,

flaviviruses, and togaviruses. The transition of the RdRp from competence for negative- to positive-strand RNA synthesis often involves the recruitment of additional host cell factors in temporal conjunction with availability of viral replication proteins.

In addition to demonstrating connection with respect to genomic organization, families within the class of positive-strand RNA viruses show similarity in the morphological types of virus particles assembled (Table 9.2). Viruses with cubic symmetry in the form of naked, icosahedral particles are seen in *Picornaviridae*, *Caliciviridae*, and *Astroviridae* and in the form of enveloped, spherical viruses with icosahedral nucleocapsids in *Togaviridae* and *Flaviviridae*. *Coronaviridae* includes viruses with more complex morphology, that is, spherical viruses with helical nucleocapsids and envelopes with long glycoprotein spikes.

THE INTRACELLULAR REPLICATIVE CYCLE

Initiation of the intracellular replicative cycle

The event that initiates the intracellular replicative cycle is the binding of a viral ligand to a receptor on the surface of a permissive host cell. These receptors, normally bound by cellular ligands, are utilized by virus particles for attachment at the plasma membrane. Host cell receptors thus far identified as the molecules used by positive-strand RNA viruses belong to several groups including the immunoglobulin-related proteins [poliovirus receptor (PVR); intracellular adhesion molecule

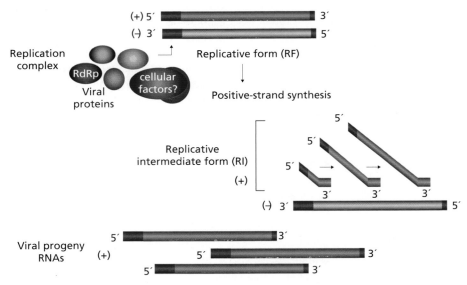

Figure 9.2 *Schematic representation of positive-strand RNA virus genomic RNA synthesis. A replication initiation complex, composed of the RNA-dependent RNA polymerase (RdRp), other viral proteins, and cellular proteins forms on the 3′ end of the negative-strand intermediate RNA or on the duplex RF. Multiples initiations on a single template produce an excess of positive-strand over negative-strand RNAs.*

Table 9.2 *Comparison of positive-strand RNA virus features by family*

Family	Enveloped	Polyprotein	Subgenomic mRNAs
Picornaviridae	No	Yes	No
Caliciviridae	No	Yes	No
Flaviviridae	Yes	Yes	No
Togaviridae	Yes	Yes	Yes
Coronaviridae	Yes	Yes	Yes

(ICAM)-1 – picornaviruses; mouse hepatitis virus receptor (MHVR)/biliary glycoprotein 1 (Bgp1) – coronaviruses], low density lipoprotein-related (LDLR) receptors (LDLR/α2MR/LPR – picornaviruses), integrins (αvβ3 – picornaviruses), receptors involved in complement pathways (CD55 – picornaviruses), as well as miscellaneous other receptors including aminopeptidase-N (coronaviruses), laminin receptor (togaviruses), and glycosaminoglycans (flaviviruses) (Young 2001). Viruses that are transmitted between insect and vertebrate hosts during their natural life cycle, such as some of the flaviviruses, are thought to use highly conserved cell receptor proteins (Brinton 2002). It is thought that alphaviruses and flaviviruses may use various receptor/coreceptor combinations to give the diverse host range (birds, mammals, mosquitos) and tropisms seen in vivo.

Viral ligands differ for each family, primarily based on either the presence or absence of an envelope with embedded glycoproteins. Naked viruses, such as members of the *Picornaviridae*, have a groove, or canyon surrounding each fivefold axis of symmetry in the capsid. These canyons have been shown to be the site of interaction with host cell receptors (Belnap et al., 2000b; He et al. 2000; Xing et al. 2000). Flaviviruses attach to host cells through an interaction between various receptors and the major viral surface protein, the E protein. Within the *Togaviridae*, the alphavirus envelope glycoproteins, E1 and E2, mediate binding of virus particles to host cell receptors. With coronaviruses, although the S protein is likely the main determinant of viral tropism due to specific cell surface glycoprotein binding, members containing the HE glycoprotein may bind to the common surface moiety, 9-O-acetylated neuraminic acid (Schultze and Herrler 1992).

Our understanding of the actual process whereby the virus particle or genomic RNA enters the cell has increased significantly in recent years. Virus particles such as poliovirus are thought to undergo conformational changes in the capsid proteins as the result of receptor binding. These changes expose hydrophobic domains on two of the capsid proteins which subsequently interact with the plasma membrane or endocytotic vesicle membrane, forming a pore through which the genomic RNA may be extruded and relocated into the cytoplasm of the cell (Hogle 2002). The movements of the capsid proteins that occur during this process have been compared with the movements of tectonic plates in the Earth (Belnap et al. 2000a). Human rhinovirus (HRV), a picornavirus, togaviruses (Smit et al. 1999), flaviviruses (Brinton 2002), and coronaviruses (Hansen et al. 1998) are thought to gain entry into the cytoplasm of host cells via the process of receptor-mediated endocytosis. Briefly, receptor-bound particles accumulate in coated pits on the cell surface, which are then endocytosed to form coated vesicles. These vesicles are subsequently uncoated to form acidified endosomes, which creates the environment that triggers low pH-mediated fusion of the viral capsid/envelope with the endosomal vesicle membrane and releases the nucleocapsid into the cytoplasm (DeTulleo and Kirchhausen 1998).

Translation of viral-specific RNAs and processing of polyproteins

Viral gene expression for positive-strand RNA viruses begins with translation of genomic (messenger) RNA in the cytoplasm. The structure of viral messenger RNAs differs somewhat between families with respect to modifications of the termini and presence or absence of an IRES (Table 9.3). Picornavirus genomes are uncapped, have a viral protein VPg(3B), linked to the 5′ end, have either a type I or type II IRES in the 5′ NCR, and are polyadenylated at the 3′ terminus. Caliciviruses also have a VPg, linked to the 5′ end of their 3′ polyadenylated genomes. Togavirus and coronavirus genomes and subgenomic positive-strand RNAs are terminated with a 7-methylguanosine cap at their 5′ end and polyadenylated at the 3′ end. In flaviviruses, two different types of genomic RNAs exist. Viruses in the genus *Flavivirus* are capped with a 7-methylguanosine at the 5′ end but do not contain a 3′ polyadenylate (poly(A)) tract, while hepacivirus and pestivirus genomes are uncapped at the 5′ end, have an IRES in the 5′ NCR, and are not polyadenylated at the 3′ end. *Flaviviridae* is the only family of positive-strand RNA viruses, with members that infect mammalian hosts, that do not have a poly(A) tail at the 3′ end of the genome.

Since most cellular mRNAs are capped at the 5′ end, there are mechanisms which specifically select for translation of viral messages that are capped. In some cases, host-cell factors are involved in the favored recognition of viral mRNAs by the host translational machinery. Each coronavirus subgenomic RNA contains a 5′ leader sequence that enhances translation in lysates from virus-infected cells, suggesting that virus-specific mRNAs may be preferentially translated in the context of decreased host translation, brought about by competition for active ribosomes and degradation of host mRNAs in the infected cell (Tahara et al. 1994).

Although all but the smallest coronavirus mRNAs contain multiple ORFs, only the 5′-most ORF of each

Table 9.3 *Structure of positive-strand viral (genomic) mRNAs*

Family	5′-Linked protein or cap	IRES	3′-Poly(A)
Picornaviridae	VPg	Yes	Yes
Caliciviridae	VPg	?	Yes
Flaviviridae			
Flavi-	7-Methylguanosine cap	No	No
Hepaci-, Pesti-	Uncapped	Yes	No
Togaviridae	7-Methylguanosine cap	No	Yes
Coronaviridae	7-Methylguanosine cap	Yes (some downstream ORFs)	Yes

mRNA is generally translated by a cap-dependent ribosomal scanning mechanism. However, in several coronavirus mRNAs, the second or third ORF is preceded by an IRES and is efficiently translated by allowing ribosomes to bypass the upstream ORF and bind internally to the IRES.

Initiation of translation by cap-independent mechanisms involves some of the cellular proteins that function in cap-dependent translation. In cells infected by some picornaviruses, eIF4G is cleaved by a viral proteinase. The C-terminal fragment created by this cleavage, which contains binding sites for eIF3 and eIF4A, stimulates IRES-mediated translation of poliovirus RNA (Buckley and Ehrenfeld 1987). Several cellular proteins that bind to the picornavirus IRES have been identified. These include PTB (Hellen et al. 1993), PCBP2 (Blyn et al. 1996), the La autoantigen (Meerovitch et al. 1993), and unr (Hunt et al. 1999). It is thought that these cellular proteins may act as RNA chaperones, maintaining the IRES in a structure that allows direct binding to the translation machinery. Several cellular proteins, including PTB (Ali and Siddiqui 1995), the La autoantigen (Ali and Siddiqui 1997), and hnRNP L (Hahm et al. 1998), have been shown to interact with the 5′ NCR of HCV and function in the process of internal initiation of translation.

Polyprotein processing is required for the generation of functional polypeptides utilized by positive-strand RNA viruses. It is also a means by which they amplify the coding capacity of their relatively small genomes. For picornaviruses, almost all of the proteins necessary for a complete intracellular replicative cycle are found within the single long ORF of the genome in the form of intermediates and mature protein products. The full-length polyprotein product encoded by the ORF is never seen since viral-encoded proteinases begin cleavage cotranslationally. The initial processing events of the picornavirus polyprotein differ among the genera with respect to site and proteinase. Primary cleavage of the enterovirus and rhinovirus nascent polyprotein occurs at the P1/P2 junction and is mediated *in cis* by the viral-encoded 2A proteinase (Toyoda et al. 1986). For aphthoviruses, the primary cleavage at the L/P1 junction is thought to occur by enzymatic activity of L *in cis*, while for cardioviruses, the L protein is cleaved from the

P1 region by the 3C proteinase. The 2A proteins of these two genera are not proteinases, but cause their own release at the junction with 2B by an unknown mechanism that appears to be a novel form of peptide bond scission (Palmenberg et al. 1992). In hepatoviruses and parechoviruses, 3C carries out the primary cleavage at the 2A/2B junction (Schultheiss et al. 1994; Stanway and Hyypia 1999). Viral proteinases L, 2A, and 3C (3CD) are active in the nascent picornavirus polypeptide and are involved in their own release by self-cleavage. All subsequent polypeptide cleavages occur *in trans*. For poliovirus, HRV, and coxsackie virus, the precursor, 3CD, is responsible for further processing of P1 following the initial cleavage (Ypma-Wong et al. 1988). The 3D portion of 3CD may be required for recognition of structural motifs in the folded P1 precursor allowing efficient processing by the 3C part of the enzyme (Parsley et al. 1999; Cornell and Semler 2002). The existence of multiple activities in a single proteinase provides another example of maximization of coding capacity of a small RNA genome.

The single large ORF of the flavivirus genome is translated as a polyprotein that is both co- and post-translationally processed by cellular proteases and viral-encoded proteinases. For HCV, the initial processing event of the polyprotein at the NS2/3 junction is mediated by the autoprotease, NS2-3. The NS3 serine protease, with the help of the NS4A cofactor, performs the other cleavages in the nonstructural region of the polyprotein. Cleavages within the structural region of the polyprotein are thought to be effected by the cellular resident endoplasmic reticulum (ER) signal peptidases (Houghton et al. 1994; Reed and Rice 2000).

The togavirus genomic RNA serves as the messenger RNA for translation of the polyprotein that is cleaved by a virally encoded protease (Hardy and Strauss 1989) to form the nonstructural polypeptides. Translation of the polyprotein is initiated at a single AUG near the 5′ end of the genome and proceeds continuously until encountering three termination codons located just downstream of the start of the sequences corresponding to the subgenomic RNA. Several of the alphavirus genomes have an opal stop codon upstream of the nsP4 coding region that is sometimes suppressed to allow read-through and inclusion of nsP4 in the polyprotein.

The final products of translation of the subgenomic mRNA are the capsid protein, released cotranslationally by autoproteolysis, two transmembrane glycoproteins, and a small membrane-embedded protein (Strauss and Strauss 1994) (Figure 9.3).

For MHV, a coronavirus, the structural proteins are each encoded by a separate subgenomic mRNA. However, two polyproteins translated from the replicase gene (gene 1) are processed by the viral-encoded proteinases, papain-like cysteine proteases (PLP1 and PLP2) and chymotrypsin-picornavirus 3C-like protease (3CLp), into at least 15 nonstructural protein products, including the presumed RNA helicase and the RdRp (Denison et al. 1999).

Alteration of the intracellular environment by viral gene products

Positive-strand RNA virus genomes encode nonstructural proteins that induce biochemical and structural changes in the host cell following infection (Figure 9.4). These viral proteins are thus indirectly involved in the process of RNA synthesis since they give rise to modifications in the environment where synthesis occurs. Down-regulation of cellular protein synthesis is one such common consequence of infection by nearly all members of the *Picornaviridae*. Cleavage of eIF4GI, eIF4GII, and poly(A) binding protein (PABP) by picornavirus 2A and/ or 3C proteinases results in cessation of host translation

due to destruction of the eIF4F complex and end-to-end communication in cellular mRNAs (Bushell and Sarnow 2002). For example, the synthesis of poliovirus proteins is not affected since the viral mRNA is translated by internal ribosome binding to the IRES, a mechanism that does not require an intact eIF4F complex. Since optimal function of the poliovirus IRES does require the C-terminal cleavage fragment of eIF4G, the modification of this cellular factor by 2A assists viral replication by inhibiting cellular translation and stimulating IRES-dependent translation. Cleavage of eIF4G in cells infected with foot-and-mouth disease virus (FMDV) is mediated by the viral L protein. Infection of cells with encephalomyocarditis virus and some of the other picornaviruses causes inhibition of cap-dependent translation as well, not by proteolytic cleavage of translation factors but by alteration of the phosphorylation state of two other cellular proteins, 4E-BP1 and 4E-BP2. Dephosphorylation of 4E-BP1, which allows it to bind to eIF4E and thus prevent formation of eIF4F and recognition of capped mRNAs, inhibits translation of cellular messages but does not affect translation of viral mRNA.

Intuitively, in strict consideration of the machinery of RNA synthesis, competition between virus and host may seem minimized by the fact that positive-strand RNA viruses code for their own RdRp. However, down-regulation of cellular transcription mediated by viral gene products would favor the synthesis of viral RNA by increasing the pool of free nucleotides available for the

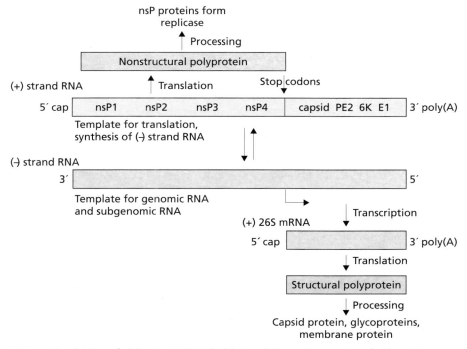

Figure 9.3 *Transcription and replication of alphavirus RNAs including translation and processing of polyprotein precursors. Positive-strand genomic RNA is the template for a full-length negative-strand intermediate RNA. The 5' two-thirds of the genomic RNA encodes a polyprotein processed into the nonstructural proteins. The negative-strand RNA is the template for production of more genomic RNAs as well as the template for production of the 26S subgenomic mRNA that encodes a polyprotein processed into capsid protein, envelope glycoproteins, and membrane protein.*

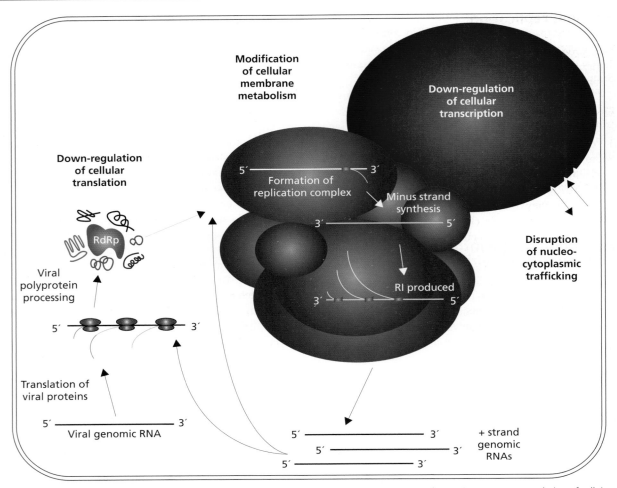

Figure 9.4 *Biochemical and structural changes in the host cell following infection by positive-strand RNA viruses. Down-regulation of cellular protein synthesis favors translation of viral mRNAs. Cellular transcription is often down-regulated, thereby increasing the pool of free nucleotides available for viral RNA synthesis. Excessive proliferation of intracellular membranes provides a matrix for viral RNA synthesis. Disruption of nucleocytoplasmic transport may result in an abundant pool of nuclear proteins in the cytoplasm that may assist with viral protein synthesis, RNA synthesis, assembly, or packaging. Red oval represents the nucleus; blue ovals represent cytoplasmic membranous vesicles.*

viral polymerase. Interestingly, at an intermediate to late time in the course of infection by most picornaviruses, there is a rapid inhibition of host cell RNA synthesis catalyzed by all three classes of DNA-dependent RNA polymerases. Since pol I, pol II, and pol III isolated from such cells are active, the inhibitory mechanism is thought to involve accessory transcription proteins. In fact, cleavage of TATA-binding protein (TBP) and other transcription factors, by poliovirus proteinase 3C and proteinase 2A, has been mechanistically associated with this transcription inhibition (Dasgupta et al. 2002).

During the intracellular replication cycle of positive-strand RNA viruses, modifications of cellular membrane metabolism and function commonly occur. For example, during flavivirus infection, there is extensive reorganization and proliferation of cytoplasmic, perinuclear endoplasmic reticular membranes (Brinton 2002). In picornavirus infection, there is an accumulation of small membranous vesicles thought to be caused by the inhibition of membrane vesicle transport from the endo-

plasmic reticulum to the cell surface. For poliovirus, viral proteins 2B, 3A, 2BC, and 2C are believed to be involved in this process (Cho et al. 1994; Doedens and Kirkegaard 1995). Such modifications of the cytoplasmic environment favor viral replication since the abundant, localized membranes not only provide a subcellular compartment which concentrates cellular and viral proteins but also serve as a matrix upon which viral RNA replication complexes can form.

Even though the positive-strand RNA viruses typically complete their replicative cycle strictly in the cytoplasm, there can be a disruption of nucleocytoplasmic trafficking as the result of viral infection (Gustin and Sarnow 2001, 2002). Alteration in nuclear import, export or both can result in an increase in the levels of nuclear proteins in the cytoplasm available for use in viral translation, replication, and/or packaging. In addition, disruption of signaling to the nucleus can attenuate the antiviral response by preventing transcription of the relevant cellular messages.

Genome replication

The process of RNA-dependent RNA synthesis is foreign to most eukaryotic cells, in which RNA synthesis normally occurs from a DNA template. Eukaryotic DNA-dependent RNA polymerases are formed by multiple subunits. Thus, although the RdRp elongation activity must be encoded by the viral genome, typically there is a dependence on cellular proteins to complete the replicase activity or provide specific selection of the viral template RNA. Cellular factors may serve as part of the RdRp holoenzyme by binding directly to the core enzyme, or they may direct the RdRp to the RNA template by binding directly to the template, or they may carry out both functions by forming a bridge between the RdRp and the RNA template (Lai 1998).

The first structure of an RdRp solved was that of poliovirus 3D^{pol} and it was found to have the same overall configuration as that of the other three types of polymerases, that is, DNA-dependent DNA polymerases, DNA-dependent RNA polymerases, and RNA-dependent DNA polymerases (reverse transcriptases) (Hansen et al. 1997). The native three-dimensional shape of all these polymerases is that of a cupped right hand, with domains corresponding to the thumb, palm, and fingers. The palm domain contains the active site of the enzyme. RdRps may not only be template dependent, but also primer-dependent enzymes as is the case for picornaviruses. The RdRp of poliovirus, 3D^{pol}, copies the viral RNA in the presence of the uridylylated VPg (3B) protein primer.

The first step in RNA synthesis of positive-strand RNA viruses is synthesis of the complementary intermediate negative-strand RNA. With respect to a single strand of viral genomic RNA, it is generally assumed that viral translation is terminated prior to the initiation of negative-strand synthesis, since the ribosomes and RdRp would be unable to travel along the same molecule in opposite directions without colliding. In general, at the beginning of the replication cycle, nascent genomic RNAs may alternate between replication and translation until a sufficient pool of nonstructural proteins has accumulated.

Negative-strand RNA synthesis is presumed to be initiated at the 3′ end of the positive-strand RNA and requires proteins of both viral and cellular origin as well as cis-acting structural and sequence determinants in the genomic RNA. Since some viral RdRp do not bind directly to cis-acting regulatory elements on the viral RNA, initiation of RNA synthesis may depend upon interactions with cellular proteins or viral proteins that bind directly to the viral RNA. It is hypothesized that RNA viruses may assemble RNA transcription or replication complexes which bring noncontiguous regions of viral RNA together, similar to the interaction between enhancer and promoter elements in DNA-dependent RNA synthesis. One end of the viral RNA could function as an enhancer while the other end could serve as a promoter (Lai 1998).

Long-range interactions between the 5′ and 3′ ends of the viral genome mediated through protein–protein contacts have been studied in the context of initiation of negative-strand and/or positive-strand RNA synthesis. For poliovirus, it has been shown that PABP interacts with the cellular protein, PCBP2, and the viral polymerase precursor, 3CD (Herold and Andino 2001). These long-range interactions could bring the two termini of the viral genomic RNA together if PABP were bound to the 3′ poly(A) tail. For HCV, studies indicate that there may be 5′ to 3′ crosstalk between the termini of the RNA of both polarities which may be important for RNA transcription and replication (Huang and Lai 2001).

For single-stranded, positive-strand RNA viruses, RNA synthesis is asymmetric. Genomic RNA synthesis is more efficient than negative-strand synthesis due to multiple initiations on the same negative-strand RNA or RF template. For flaviviruses, the ratio of positive-strand RNA to negative-strand RNA is about 10:1; for poliovirus it is about 40:1.

Initiation of positive-strand synthesis presumably occurs at the 3′ end of the negative-strand RNA. It is not clear if the negative-strand RNA template is single-stranded or in the duplexed RF. Furthermore, it is assumed that the mechanisms for initiation of positive-strand RNA synthesis require cis-acting determinants in the RNA and viral and cellular trans-acting factors and that these mechanisms and factors are, in part, distinct from those used for initiation of negative-strand synthesis. For togaviruses, negative-strand synthesis requires viral protein precursors in replication complexes (Sawicki and Sawicki 1994). When these precursors accumulate and are partially or fully processed, negative-strand synthesis ceases and positive-strand synthesis is initiated. For poliovirus, replication defects due to mutations in specific replication proteins can be rescued in trans, but only when the wild-type viral proteins are supplied in appropriate precursor form (Towner et al. 1999).

Assembly and release of virus particles

Once sufficient viral structural proteins have accumulated, nascent genomic RNAs can function as templates for translation and transcription and as substrates for encapsidation. For Kunjin virus, now considered a subtype of the flavivirus WNV (Scherret et al. 2001), translation is a prerequisite for replication of a nascent RNA, and replication is a prerequisite of encapsidation (Khromykh et al. 2001; Khromykh et al. 1999). The coupling of encapsidation to viral RNA synthesis may account, in part, for the fact that the encapsidation process is highly specific. Selection of a viral RNA for packaging may also depend on the presence of a packaging signal in the RNA. Genomic RNA is selected for encapsidation even in the presence of a molar excess of subgenomic RNA in togaviruses. Sindbis virus contains a structural packaging signal in the 5′ region of the genome, within the coding region for nsP1. For picornaviruses only VPg-linked positive-strand RNA, and not viral mRNA, negative-strand viral RNA, or any cellular RNA, is packaged.

The morphogenetic pathway for formation of mature virions generally involves both assembly intermediates, or substructures, as well as precursor forms of the structural proteins. The first assembly intermediate in the poliovirus pathway, the 5S protomer, consists of one copy each of VP0, VP1, and VP3. Five protomers then assemble to form a pentamer (14S) and pentamers assemble into empty capsids. One assembly model predicts that the viral RNA is threaded into the empty capsid and the final morphogenetic step, cleavage of VP0 to VP2 and VP4, produces the fully mature, infectious virion. In an alternative model, 14S pentamers assemble with virion RNA to form provirions. This pathway suggests that empty capsids, found in infected cells, serve as storage units for 14S pentamers (Nugent and Kirkegaard 1995). For WNV, immature virions, with precursor forms of structural proteins, accumulate in vesicles and are then transported through the host secretory pathway. These precursor interactions may maintain structural proteins in stable conformations until assembly and release of new virions is complete.

Flavivirus virions are transported to the plasma membrane in vesicles and released by exocytosis. For the alphaviruses of *Togaviridae*, nucleocapsids interact with the host cell plasma membrane at sites occupied by viral transmembrane glycoproteins. This leads to binding of additional viral glycoproteins, wrapping of the membrane around the nucleocapsid (budding) and release of the enveloped particle (Garoff et al. 1998).

Coronavirus assembly initiates with binding of the N (nucleocapsid) protein via a specific signal located in the 3′ end of ORF 1b of the genomic RNA. Interaction between the nucleocapsid and the M protein, in the membranes of the ER and Golgi complex, triggers packaging. Virus budding take place in the budding compartment between the ER and Golgi when the E protein interacts with the M protein. Envelope glycoproteins, S and HE, are incorporated into virions through interactions with the M protein. Virions accumulate in secretory vesicles, which eventually fuse with the plasma membrane to release virus (Lai and Holmes 2001).

CONCLUSIONS

RNA viruses are inherently and uniquely interesting due to the fact that, unlike nearly any other biological agent or organism, their genetic blueprint is stored biochemically in the form of RNA instead of DNA. According to the central dogma of molecular biology, the flow of genetic information normally proceeds from DNA to RNA via transcription and from RNA to protein via translation. For positive-strand RNA viruses, this process is more direct since genomic RNA is messenger RNA and can be translated to protein upon release in the cytoplasm of the host cell. These viruses encode their own RdRp for RNA chain elongation activity, although formation of the replicase complex may include other viral as well as cellular factors.

A viral RNA-dependent RNA polymerase is intrinsically more error-prone than a DNA-dependent DNA polymerase and produces a population of viruses, referred to as a quasi species, characterized by members that are not genetically identical (Domingo and Holland 1997). Mutations in the coding region of viral genomic RNA, due to decreased fidelity of the viral polymerase, may be inconsequential, deleterious or even lethal, or may permit survival of the virus. For example, a random single-point nucleotide substitution in viral genomic RNA could result in one of the following five possibilities:

1 no change in amino acid due to redundancy of the genetic code
2 change to a different amino acid similar enough to be inconsequential to overall folding or function of the protein
3 change to a different amino acid dissimilar enough to diminish function due to alteration in protein conformation or catalytic site
4 change to a different amino acid that randomly confers functional benefit in a specific environment, due to improved conformation and/or catalysis, thus allowing survival of the mutant virus
5 change to create an early stop codon or eliminate an existing stop codon
6 no change or conservative change in amino acid with concomitant change in RNA secondary structure that is neutral, harmful or beneficial to function.

Similarly, mutations in the noncoding region of the viral genomic RNA can result in inconsequential, disadvantageous or advantageous functional modifications through alterations in *cis*-acting signals or specific RNA structures required for RNA–RNA or RNA–protein interactions. Thus, paradoxically, long-term survival of an RNA virus with limited coding capacity in a constantly evolving host is accomplished through accidental adaptive modifications that result from slightly unfaithful viral RNA replication by a viral-encoded error-prone polymerase.

REFERENCES

Agol, V.I., Paul, A.V. and Wimmer, E. 1999. Paradoxes of the replication of picornaviral genomes 1. *Virus Res*, **62**, 129–47.

Ali, N. and Siddiqui, A. 1995. Interaction of polypyrimidine tract-binding protein with the 5′ noncoding region of the hepatitis C virus RNA genome and its functional requirement in internal initiation of translation. *J Virol*, **69**, 6367–75.

Ali, N. and Siddiqui, A. 1997. The La antigen binds 5′ noncoding region of the hepatitis C virus RNA in the context of the initiator AUG codon and stimulates internal ribosome entry site-mediated translation 1. *Proc Natl Acad Sci U S A*, **94**, 2249–54.

Andino, R., Rieckhof, G.E. and Baltimore, D. 1990. A functional ribonucleoprotein complex forms around the 5′ end of poliovirus RNA 5. *Cell*, **63**, 369–80.

Andino, R., Rieckhof, G.E., et al. 1993. Poliovirus RNA synthesis utilizes an RNP complex formed around the 5′- end of viral RNA. *EMBO J*, **12**, 3587–98.

Baltimore, D. 1971. Expression of animal virus genomes. *Bacteriol Rev*, **35**, 235–41.

Belnap, D.M., Filman, D.J., et al. 2000a. Molecular tectonic model of virus structural transitions: the putative cell entry states of poliovirus. *J Virol*, **74**, 1342–54.

Belnap, D.M., McDermott, B.M. Jr, et al. 2000b. Three-dimensional structure of poliovirus receptor bound to poliovirus. *Proc Natl Acad Sci U S A*, **97**, 73–8.

Blackwell, J.L. and Brinton, M.A. 1997. Translation elongation factor-1 alpha interacts with the 3′ stem–loop region of West Nile virus genomic RNA. *J Virol*, **71**, 6433–44.

Blyn, L.B., Swiderek, K.M., et al. 1996. Poly(rC) binding protein 2 binds to stem-loop IV of the poliovirus RNA 5′ noncoding region: identification by automated liquid chromatography-tandem mass spectrometry. *Proc Natl Acad Sci U S A*, **93**, 11115–20.

Blyn, L.B., Towner, J.S., et al. 1997. Requirement of poly(rC) binding protein 2 for translation of poliovirus RNA. *J Virol*, **71**, 6243–6.

Briese, T., Jia, X.Y., et al. 1999. Identification of a Kunjin/West Nile-like flavivirus in brains of patients with New York encephalitis. *Lancet*, **354**, 1261–2.

Brinton, M.A. 2002. The molecular biology of West Nile Virus: a new invader of the western hemisphere. *Annu Rev Microbiol*, **56**, 371–402.

Buckley, B. and Ehrenfeld, E. 1987. The cap-binding protein complex in uninfected and poliovirus-infected HeLa cells. *J Biol Chem*, **262**, 13599–606.

Bushell, M. and Sarnow, P. 2002. Hijacking the translation apparatus by RNA viruses. *J Cell Biol*, **158**, 395–9.

Cello, J., Paul, A.V. and Wimmer, E. 2002. Chemical synthesis of poliovirus cDNA: generation of infectious virus in the absence of natural template. *Science*, **297**, 1016–18.

Cho, M.W., Teterina, N., et al. 1994. Membrane rearrangement and vesicle induction by recombinant poliovirus 2C and 2BC in human cells. *Virology*, **202**, 129–45.

Clarke, I.N. and Lambden, P.R. 1997. The molecular biology of caliciviruses. *J Gen Virol*, **78**, 291–301.

Cornell, C.T. and Semler, B.L. 2002. Subdomain specific functions of the RNA polymerase region of poliovirus 3CD polypeptide. *Virology*, **298**, 200–13.

Dasgupta, A., Yalamanchili, P., et al. 2002. Effects of picornavirus proteinases on host cell transcription. In: Semler, B.L. and Wimmer, E. (eds), *Molecular biology of picornaviruses*. Washington, DC: ASM Press, 321–36.

Denison, M.R., Spaan, W.J., et al. 1999. The putative helicase of the coronavirus mouse hepatitis virus is processed from the replicase gene polyprotein and localizes in complexes that are active in viral RNA synthesis. *J Virol*, **73**, 6862–71.

DeTulleo, L. and Kirchhausen, T. 1998. The clathrin endocytic pathway in viral infection. *EMBO J*, **17**, 4585–93.

Doedens, J.R. and Kirkegaard, K. 1995. Inhibition of cellular protein secretion by poliovirus proteins 2B and 3A. *EMBO J*, **14**, 894–907.

Domingo, E. and Holland, J.J. 1997. RNA virus mutations and fitness for survival. *Annu Rev Microbiol*, **51**, 151–78.

Gamarnik, A.V. and Andino, R. 1997. Two functional complexes formed by KH domain containing proteins with the 5′ noncoding region of poliovirus RNA. *RNA*, **3**, 882–92.

Gamarnik, A.V. and Andino, R. 1998. Switch from translation to RNA replication in a positive-stranded RNA virus. *Genes Dev*, **12**, 2293–304.

Garoff, H., Hewson, R. and Opstelten, D.J. 1998. Virus maturation by budding. *Microbiol Mol Biol Rev*, **62**, 1171–90.

Gontarek, R.R., Gutshall, L.L., et al. 1999. hnRNP C and polypyrimidine tract-binding protein specifically interact with the pyrimidine-rich region within the 3′NTR of the HCV RNA genome. *Nucleic Acids Res*, **27**, 1457–63.

Gustin, K.E. and Sarnow, P. 2001. Effects of poliovirus infection on nucleo-cytoplasmic trafficking and nuclear pore complex composition. *EMBO J*, **20**, 240–9.

Gustin, K.E. and Sarnow, P. 2002. Inhibition of nuclear import and alteration of nuclear pore complex composition by rhinovirus. *J Virol*, **76**, 8787–96.

Hahm, B., Kim, Y.K., et al. 1998. Heterogeneous nuclear ribonucleoprotein L interacts with the 3′ border of the internal ribosomal entry site of hepatitis C virus 1. *J Virol*, **72**, 8782–8.

Hansen, G.H., Delmas, B., et al. 1998. The coronavirus transmissible gastroenteritis virus causes infection after receptor-mediated endocytosis and acid-dependent fusion with an intracellular compartment. *J Virol*, **72**, 527–34.

Hansen, J.L., Long, A.M. and Schultz, S.C. 1997. Structure of the RNA-dependent RNA polymerase of poliovirus. *Structure*, **5**, 1109–22.

Hardy, W.R. and Strauss, J.H. 1989. Processing the nonstructural polyproteins of sindbis virus: nonstructural proteinase is in the C-terminal half of nsP2 and functions both *in cis* and *in trans*. *J Virol*, **63**, 4653–64.

He, Y., Bowman, V.D., Mueller, S., et al. 2000. Interaction of the poliovirus receptor with poliovirus. *Proc Natl Acad Sci U S A*, **97**, 79–84.

Hellen, C.U., Witherell, G.W., et al. 1993. A cytoplasmic 57-kDa protein that is required for translation of picornavirus RNA by internal ribosomal entry is identical to the nuclear pyrimidine tract-binding protein. *Proc Natl Acad Sci U S A*, **90**, 7642–6.

Herold, J. and Andino, R. 2001. Poliovirus RNA replication requires genome circularization through a protein–protein bridge 1. *Mol Cell*, **7**, 581–91.

Hogle, J.M. 2002. Poliovirus cell entry: common structural themes in viral cell entry pathways. *Annu Rev Microbiol*, **56**, 677–702.

Holmes, K.V. and Enjuanes, L. 2003. Virology. The SARS coronavirus: a postgenomic era. *Science*, **300**, 1377–8.

Houghton, M., Selby, M. et al. 1994. Hepatitis C virus: structure, protein products and processing of the polyprotein precursor. *Curr Stud Hematol Blood Transfus* (61), 1–11.

Huang, P. and Lai, M.M. 2001. Heterogeneous nuclear ribonucleoprotein a1 binds to the 3′-untranslated region and mediates potential 5′–3′-end cross talks of mouse hepatitis virus RNA. *J Virol*, **75**, 5009–17.

Hunt, S.L., Hsuan, J.J., et al. 1999. Unr, a cellular cytoplasmic RNA-binding protein with five cold-shock domains, is required for internal initiation of translation of human rhinovirus RNA. *Genes Dev*, **13**, 437–48.

Jordan, I., Briese, T. and Lipkin, W.I. 2000. Discovery and molecular characterization of West Nile virus NY 1999. *Viral Immunol*, **13**, 435–46.

Khromykh, A.A., Sedlak, P.L., et al. 1999. Efficient trans-complementation of the flavivirus Kunjin NS5 protein but not of the NS1 protein requires its coexpression with other components of the viral replicase. *J Virol*, **73**, 10272–80.

Khromykh, A.A., Varnavski, A.N., et al. 2001. Coupling between replication and packaging of flavivirus RNA: evidence derived from the use of DNA-based full-length cDNA clones of Kunjin virus. *J Virol*, **75**, 4633–40.

Koonin, E.V. and Dolja, V.V. 1993. Evolution and taxonomy of positive-strand RNA viruses: implications of comparative analysis of amino acid sequences. *Crit Rev Biochem Mol Biol*, **28**, 375–430.

Lai, M.M. 1998. Cellular factors in the transcription and replication of viral RNA genomes: a parallel to DNA-dependent RNA transcription 1. *Virology*, **244**, 1–12.

Lai, M.M. and Holmes, K.V. 2001. *Coronaviridae*: the viruses and their replication. In: Knipe, D.M. and Howley, P.M. (eds), *Fields virology*, vol. 1. Philadelphia, PA: Lippincott, Williams and Wilkins, 1163–78.

Lanciotti, R.S., Roehrig, J.T., et al. 1999. Origin of the West Nile virus responsible for an outbreak of encephalitis in the northeastern United States. *Science*, **286**, 2333–7.

Leong, L.E., Cornell, C.T. and Semler, B.L. 2002. Processing determinants and functions of cleavage products of picornavirus polyproteins. In: Semler, B.L. and Wimmer, E. (eds), *Molecular biology of picornaviruses*. Washington, DC: ASM Press, 187–98.

Makino, S., Soe, L.H., et al. 1988. Discontinuous transcription generates heterogeneity at the leader fusion sites of coronavirus mRNAs. *J Virol*, **62**, 3870–3.

Marra, M.A., Jones, S.J., et al. 2003. The Genome sequence of the SARS-associated coronavirus. *Science*, **300**, 1399–404.

Meerovitch, K., Svitkin, Y.V., et al. 1993. La autoantigen enhances and corrects aberrant translation of poliovirus RNA in reticulocyte lysate. *J Virol*, **67**, 3798–807.

Nugent, C.I. and Kirkegaard, K. 1995. RNA binding properties of poliovirus subviral particles. *J Virol*, **69**, 13–22.

Palmenberg, A.C., Parks, G.D., et al. 1992. Proteolytic processing of the cardioviral P2 region: primary 2A/2B cleavage in clone-derived precursors. *Virology*, **190**, 754–62.

Parsley, T.B., Towner, J.S., et al. 1997. Poly (rC) binding protein 2 forms a ternary complex with the 5′- terminal sequences of poliovirus RNA and the viral 3CD proteinase. *RNA*, **3**, 1124–34.

Parsley, T.B., Cornell, C.T. and Semler, B.L. 1999. Modulation of the RNA binding and protein processing activities of poliovirus polypeptide 3CD by the viral RNA polymerase domain. *J Biol Chem*, **274**, 12867–76.

Reed, K.E. and Rice, C.M. 2000. Overview of hepatitis C virus genome structure, polyprotein processing, and protein properties. *Curr Top Microbiol Immunol*, **242**, 55–84.

Robinson, S., Clarke, I.N., et al. 2002. Epidemiology of human Sapporo-like caliciviruses in the South West of England: molecular characterisation of a genetically distinct isolate. *J Med Virol*, **67**, 282–8.

Rota, P.A., Oberste, M.S., et al. 2003. Characterization of a novel coronavirus associated with severe acute respiratory syndrome. *Science*, **300**, 1394–9.

Sawicki, D.L. and Sawicki, S.G. 1994. Alphavirus positive and negative strand RNA synthesis and the role of polyproteins in formation of viral replication complexes. *Arch Virol Suppl*, **9**, 393–405.

Sawicki, D.L. and Sawicki, S.G. 1998a. Role of the nonstructural polyproteins in alphavirus RNA synthesis. *Adv Exp Med Biol*, **440**, 187–98.

Sawicki, S.G. and Sawicki, D.L. 1998b. A new model for coronavirus transcription. *Adv Exp Med Biol*, **440**, 215–19.

Scherret, J.H., Poidinger, M., et al. 2001. The relationships between West Nile and Kunjin viruses. *Emerg Infect Dis*, **7**, 697–705.

Schultheiss, T., Kusov, Y.Y. and Gauss-Muller, V. 1994. Proteinase 3C of hepatitis A virus (HAV) cleaves the HAV polyprotein P2-P3 at all sites including VP1/2A and 2A/2B. *Virology*, **198**, 275–81.

Schultze, B. and Herrler, G. 1992. Bovine coronavirus uses *N*-acetyl-9-*O*-acetylneuraminic acid as a receptor determinant to initiate the infection of cultured cells. *J Gen Virol*, **73**, 901–6.

Sizova, D.V., Kolupaeva, V.G., et al. 1998. Specific interaction of eukaryotic translation initiation factor 3 with the 5′ nontranslated regions of hepatitis C virus and classical swine fever virus RNAs 1. *J Virol*, **72**, 4775–82.

Smit, J.M., Bittman, R. and Wilschut, J. 1999. Low-pH-dependent fusion of Sindbis virus with receptor-free cholesterol- and sphingolipid-containing liposomes. *J Virol*, **73**, 8476–84.

Spangberg, K. and Schwartz, S. 1999. Poly(C)-binding protein interacts with the hepatitis C virus 5′ untranslated region 1. *J Gen Virol*, **80**, 1371–6.

Spangberg, K., Goobar-Larsson, L., et al. 1999. The La protein from human liver cells interacts specifically with the U- rich region in the hepatitis C virus 3′ untranslated region. *J Hum Virol*, **2**, 296–307.

Spangberg, K., Wiklund, L. and Schwartz, S. 2000. HuR, a protein implicated in oncogene and growth factor mRNA decay, binds to the 3′ ends of hepatitis C virus RNA of both polarities. *Virology*, **274**, 378–90.

Stanway, G. and Hyypia, T. 1999. Parechoviruses. *J Virol*, **73**, 5249–54.

Steinhauer, D.A. and Holland, J.J. 1987. Rapid evolution of RNA viruses. *Annu Rev Microbiol*, **41**, 409–33.

Strauss, J.H. and Strauss, E.G. 1994. The alphaviruses: gene expression, replication, and evolution. *Microbiol Rev*, **58**, 491–562.

Tahara, S.M., Dietlin, T.A., et al. 1994. Coronavirus translational regulation: leader affects mRNA efficiency. *Virology*, **202**, 621–30.

Towner, J.S., Mazanet, M.M. and Semler, B.L. 1999. Rescue of defective poliovirus RNA replication by 3AB-containing precursor polyproteins. *J Virol*, **72**, 7191–200.

Toyoda, H., Nicklin, M.J., et al. 1986. A second virus-encoded proteinase involved in proteolytic processing of poliovirus polyprotein. *Cell*, **45**, 761–70.

Walter, B.L., Parsley, T.B., et al. 2002. Distinct poly(rC) binding protein KH domain determinants for poliovirus translation initiation and viral RNA replication. *J Virol*, **76**, 12008–22.

Xing, L., Tjarnlund, K., et al. 2000. Distinct cellular receptor interactions in poliovirus and rhinoviruses. *EMBO J*, **19**, 1207–16.

Young, A.T. 2001. Virus entry and uncoating. In: Knipe, D.M. and Howley, P.M. (eds), *Fields virology*. Philadelphia, PA: Lippincott Williams and Wilkins, 87–99.

Ypma-Wong, M.F., Dewalt, P.G., et al. 1988. Protein 3CD is the major poliovirus proteinase responsible for cleavage of the P1 capsid precursor. *Virology*, **166**, 265–70.

10

DNA virus replication

SANDRA K. WELLER

INTRODUCTION

The DNA viruses exhibit diverse mechanisms of genome replication that are important to study for many reasons. Viruses provide useful models for the study of eukaryotic DNA replication because of their relative simplicity and ease of study; in fact, much of what we know about eukaryotic DNA replication has come from the study of viral systems. For instance, viruses that rely heavily on host-cell machinery for replication have provided experimental systems that have led to the identification of the components of the cellular replication machinery. Furthermore, viral enzymes involved in replication provide important targets for antiviral therapy, and the study of the mechanisms of viral DNA replication will therefore continue to provide vital information in the development of effective antiviral strategies. DNA viruses exhibit considerable diversity with respect to the molecular mechanisms of DNA replication. This is due to differences not only in genome size and structure but also in the location of viral DNA replication in the cell and the reliance on viral versus host enzymes. In this chapter we will consider DNA viruses of the following families: polyomaviruses, papillomaviruses, parvoviruses, adenoviruses, herpesviruses, and pox viruses (Table 10.1). While the polyoma- and papillomaviruses have circular genomes, the genomes of the other DNA viruses are linear. Among viruses with linear genomes, considerable diversity can be observed with respect to structure: single-stranded for the parvoviruses versus double-stranded for adenoviruses, herpesviruses,

and pox viruses. Diversity in size is also apparent from less than 5 bp in the parvoviruses to approximately 200 kbp for the poxviruses. The diversity in size and structure of viral genomes has important implications in terms of mechanisms of DNA replication. For these reasons, in this chapter, replication strategies of each virus family will be considered separately. First, however, some guiding principles concerning DNA replication in general will be considered.

GENERAL PRINCIPLES OF DNA REPLICATION

DNA synthesis in viral as well as cellular systems involves the incorporation of deoxynucleosides in a template-directed process. Incorporation of deoxynucleosides invariably occurs onto the 3′ OH end of a growing DNA chain, resulting in a 5′ to 3′ polarity of elongation on the growing chain (Kornberg and Baker 1992). Replication generally begins at specific sites on viral genomes known as origins of replication, and many viruses encode specific origin binding proteins responsible for initiation of viral DNA synthesis (Stenlund 2003). DNA replication in DNA viruses is catalyzed by DNA-dependent DNA polymerases which in general require a free 3′ OH end in order to add deoxynucleosides. This is in contrast to DNA-dependent RNA polymerases and RNA-dependent RNA polymerases that are capable of initiating template-directed RNA synthesis de novo and do not require the presence of a free 3′ OH. One implication of this requirement is that viral

Table 10.1 *DNA viruses considered in this chapter*

Virus	Size of viral genome	Structure of viral genome	Location of replication	Replication proteins
Polyomavirus Simian virus 40	~5 000 base pairs	Closed circular double-stranded DNA	Nuclear	Viral and host
Papillomavirus Human and Bovine papillomaviruses	~8 000 base pairs	Closed circular double-stranded DNA	Nuclear	Viral and host
Parvovirus Minute virus of mice, Adeno-Associated Virus	~5 000 bases	Linear single-stranded DNA	Nuclear	Viral and host
Adenovirus Human adenovirus	~36 000 base pairs	Linear double-stranded DNA	Nuclear	Viral and host
Herpesvirus Herpes simplex virus type 1	~150 000 base pairs	Linear double-stranded DNA	Nuclear	Viral primarily (could be some host protein involvement)
Poxvirus Vaccinia virus	~200 000 base pairs	Linear double-stranded DNA	Cytoplasm	Viral

DNA replication is dependent on the presence of a primer; however, it is remarkable how different viruses have evolved novel strategies for priming DNA synthesis. Parvoviruses rely on structural features of the viral genome itself to prime new DNA synthesis whereas adenoviruses utilize a protein priming mechanism. Other DNA viruses utilize a strategy of formation of RNA primers similar to mechanisms used during cellular DNA replication. DNA synthesis for all DNA viruses requires the use of a DNA-dependent DNA polymerase; however, the smaller DNA viruses (polyoma-, papilloma- and parvoviruses) do not have the genetic capacity to encode a large number of viral proteins dedicated to viral replication. These viruses therefore utilize host-cell polymerases, while adenoviruses, herpesviruses, and poxviruses encode their own viral DNA-dependent DNA polymerases as well as additional replication proteins. Poxviruses are unusual in that DNA replication occurs in the cytoplasm and must therefore encode all enzymes and proteins needed for DNA replication.

As mentioned above, DNA replication generally begins at specific sites on viral genomes known as origins of replication with local unwinding or melting of the duplex to provide access to template strands (Stenlund 2003). Origins can increase the efficiency of DNA replication by directly or indirectly recruiting replication machinery leading to the assembly of multiprotein complexes needed for DNA replication. Given the complexity of the environment in which viral genomes replicate and the fact that viral genomes are present as single copy genomes within the host cell, it is important for sufficient concentrations of all of the essential factors to be brought together in one place. It would thus be expected that origin recognition proteins would exhibit highly specific DNA binding. In some systems this specificity is achieved by the initiator protein itself while in others a second viral or cellular protein increases specificity (Table 10.2).

Many viral origins consist of a core origin and auxiliary regions that are important for optimal viral replication. The core origins generally contain binding sites for viral initiator proteins and AT-rich sequences which facilitate melting during initial unwinding reactions. The auxiliary sequences enhance the efficiency of viral DNA replication and interestingly, often contain binding sites for cellular or viral transcription factors. The importance of auxiliary regions was originally discovered in polyoma viruses where the presence of the transcriptional enhancer stimulates DNA replication up to 1 000-fold; however, this has turned out to be a much more general phenomena (Table 10.2). The binding of transcription factors at origins of replication in many cases facilitates the rate limiting steps in the initiation process (Table 10.3). In some cases binding helps to recruit other replication proteins such as polymerases. In other cases, they help to change the activity of initiation proteins. Transcription factors can also cause changes in the global architecture or nucleosome structure of the origin. Thus, specific protein–DNA and protein–protein interactions are very important for initiation and recruitment of replication machinery to occur, and we will see many diverse examples in this chapter.

Table 10.2 *Viral DNA proteins that initiate and participate in DNA replication*

Virus	Origin binding protein(s)	Polymerase(s)	Other replication proteins
Polyomavirus			
Simian virus 40	Large T antigen (helicase activity)	Host cellular DNA polymerases α and δ	Many cellular: RPA, RF-C, RNase H, PCNA, Fen1, DNA ligase I
Papillomavirus			
Human and Bovine Papillomaviruses	E1 protein (helicase activity)	Host cellular DNA polymerases	Many cellular
Parvovirus			
Minute virus of mice	NS1 (helicase activity)	Host cellular DNA polymerases	RPA, PCNA
Adeno-associated virus	Rep 68, Rep 78 (helicase activity)		
Adenovirus			
Human adenovirus	DNA polymerase, preterminal protein complex	Viral	Viral SSB (DBP), Cellular proteins: transcriptional activators (NF1, Oct-1 and topoisomerase)
Herpesvirus			
Herpes simplex virus type 1	UL9, origin-binding protein (helicase activity)	Viral polymerase (UL30) and accessory protein (UL42)	Viral helicase-primase (UL5, UL8, and UL52), viral SSB ICP8
Poxvirus			
Vaccinia virus	?	Viral	Several viral, no cellular

The binding of viral and cellular proteins at an origin of replication is followed by a melting or opening of the duplex. Once a region or regions of the origin are melted or distorted, recruitment of helicases and other replication proteins occurs (Waga and Stillman 1994). The function of the helicase is to unwind the DNA in advance of the replication fork (see Figure 10.1). Helicases translocate along single- or double-stranded DNA in an ATP-dependent fashion. Many DNA and RNA viruses encode helicases (Marintcheva and Weller 2001). The only DNA virus which does not encode its own helicase is adenovirus whose mechanism of replication does not require helicase activity.

In the simplest replication systems, replication proceeds by the formation of two replication forks which synthesize DNA in different directions from the origin (Kornberg and Baker 1992). This requires the use of leading- and lagging-strand DNA replication also known

Table 10.3 *Viral origin recognition proteins*

Virus	Initiator Protein	Binds specifically to ori	Melts ori	Other activities
SV40	Large T antigen	+	+	DNA-stimulated ATPase and helicase activities; recruits RPA, polα-primase, Topo I, and other cellular proteins
Adenovirus	pTP and DNA pol	+ (stimulated by cellular proteins Oct-1 and Nf-1)	+	Priming of DNA synthesis by protein priming
Herpes simplex virus	UL9	+	?	DNA-stimulated ATPase and helicase; binds ICP8 and the UL8 subunit of the viral helicase-primase
Papilloma viruses	E1 and E2	+	+	DNA-stimulated ATPase and helicase (E1); recruits RPA, polα-primase, Topo I, and other cellular proteins
Parvovirus MVM	NS1	+	−	Site-specific endonuclease; DNA-stimulated ATPase and helicase

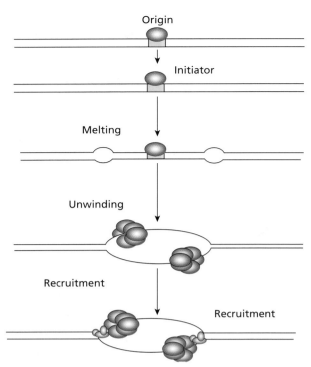

Figure 10.1 *Initiation of DNA replication. DNA replication generally initiates at an origin of replication in four distinct steps. The first step involves specific binding by an origin binding or initiator protein (initiator). In the example shown, specific binding is carried out by a single viral protein, but in some cases additional viral or cellular proteins are required for this initial binding event. In the second step, the initiator protein causes melting or distortion at the origin. The third step, helicase is loaded at the partially unwound origin and in the fourth step additional replication proteins are loaded. In the polyoma- and papillomaviruses, the initiator protein carries out all of these functions, binding, melting, unwinding, and recruitment. SV40 large T antigen and papilloma E1 proteins both form hexameric helicases which also carry out unwinding during the elongation step of DNA replication. (Adapted from Stenlund 2003)*

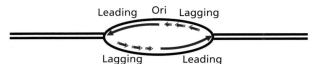

Figure 10.2 *Leading- and lagging-strand DNA synthesis. Since all DNA polymerases synthesize DNA only in a 5' to 3' direction, one strand (the lagging-strand) must elongate in the opposite direction from that of the movement of the fork itself. Lagging-strand DNA synthesis is accomplished by the synthesis of short DNA fragments termed Okazaki fragments. Okazaki fragment synthesis involves first the synthesis of a short RNA primer. In order to produce the final DNA product, an enzyme which removes the RNA primers and a ligase to repair the gaps between adjacent Okasaki fragments are needed. This mode of replication involving leading- and lagging-strand DNA synthesis is utilized by many replication systems including bacterial, eukaryotic, and many viruses. Black lines represent the parental duplex. Solid blue lines represent the nascent DNA strand and the red boxes represent RNA primers.*

to repair the gaps between adjacent Okasaki fragments are needed. This mode of replication involving leading- and lagging-strand DNA synthesis is utilized by many replication systems including bacterial, eukaryotic, and many viruses.

Some eukaryotic viruses have evolved unusual mechanisms for priming DNA synthesis. The parvoviruses have hairpin termini which are self-complementary and the 3' termini can prime DNA synthesis. In adenoviruses, a protein is used to prime DNA synthesis. The first phosphodiester bond is formed between a nucleotide and a serine residue of the virally encode preterminal protein.

Several DNA viruses will be considered in this chapter including *Polyomaviridae, Papillomaviridae, Parvoviridae, Adenoviridae, Herpesviridae,* and *Poxviridae*. All of these virus families utilize the general principles of DNA replication, but each virus illustrates variations which serve to underscore the fascinating diversity among different viruses including genome size, strandedness, the use of novel methods for priming DNA polymerases, and intracellular localization.

POLYOMAVIRUSES

Polyomaviruses infect a wide variety of mammals and include four major species. A polyomavirus originally isolated from mice (murine polyomavirus (MPyV), simian vacuolating virus 40 (SV40) isolated from monkey kidney cells, and two human polyomaviruses, BK polyomavirus (BKPyV) (isolated from an immunosuppressed kidney transplant patient) and JC polyoma virus (JCPyV) from a case of progressive multifocal leukoencephalopathy. Because of the central role the polyomaviruses have played in our understanding of both viral and cellular DNA replications, this genus will be considered first. Because of the small size of

as discontinuous DNA synthesis (Figure 10.2). As mentioned above, all known DNA polymerases must elongate via addition of nucleoside monophosphates to an existing 3' OH group resulting in DNA synthesis which proceeds in a 5' to 3' direction (Kornberg and Baker 1992; Depamphilis 1996). In order for a replication fork to move bidirectionally, both strands must be replicated by a mechanism that involves continuous synthesis on one strand (leading-strand DNA synthesis) and discontinuous synthesis on the other strand (lagging-strand DNA synthesis) (see Kornberg and Baker (1992) for detailed review). Lagging-strand DNA synthesis is accomplished by synthesizing short DNA fragments termed Okazaki fragments. Okazaki fragment synthesis involves first the synthesis of RNA primers; keep in mind that DNA-dependent DNA polymerases are not capable of de novo incorporation of deoxynucleosides into DNA. In order to produce the final DNA product, an enzyme which removes the RNA primers and a ligase

their genomes, their oncogenic properties and the existence of in vitro systems, polyomaviruses have been used extensively as models for eukaryotic DNA replication. Polyomavirus replicates lytically in mouse cells and causes abortive infections of rat and hamster cells in culture. SV40 replicates lytically in monkey and human cells but transforms rodent cells in culture.

General features of SV40 DNA replication

The *Polyomaviridae* have small circular genomes and replicate entirely by theta replication, resulting in interlocked circles that must be separated prior to genome encapsidation (Figure 10.3) (Depamphilis 1996). Polyomaviruses encode only one viral gene product responsible for DNA replication and rely on the host cellular machinery for the rest. SV40 will be discussed here as

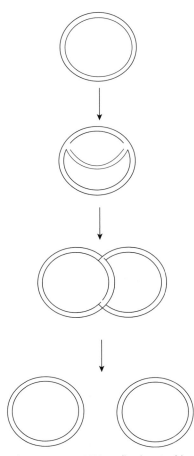

Figure 10.3 *Theta structure DNA replication. In this mode of viral DNA synthesis, double-stranded circular DNA replicates by bidirectional DNA synthesis in opposite directions from the origin of replication. When the forks meet at a point on the genome diametrically opposite to the origin of replication. This results in the formation of a two interlocking daughter molecules. The catenated circles can be resolved into monomer circles by a topoisomerase activity.*

the best studied example of the polyomavirus family. The development of a reconstituted in vitro replication reaction capable of supporting SV40 DNA replication represented an important breakthrough in the study of chromosomal replication and allowed the identification of cellular proteins required for both SV40 and cellular DNA synthesis (Li and Kelly 1984; Waga and Stillman 1994). The detailed study of SV40 DNA replication has revealed many common elements between polyomavirus DNA synthesis and cellular DNA replication including chromatin structure, a common set of proteins comprising the replication machinery and the formation of replication forks which engage in bi-directional replication. In the early 1970s, electron microscopic analysis of replicating viral genomes revealed that SV40 DNA could initiate replication at a single site and that replication proceeded bidirectionally from this site. Replication bubbles could be observed which consisted of two replication forks moving in opposite directions. Bidirectional replication from a single origin was confirmed by elegant biochemical analysis (Hay and Depamphilis 1982). Another interesting feature of polyomavirus DNA replication is that it is tightly regulated; in fact, the study of how initiation and elongation are controlled provides insight into the mechanisms of how eukaryotic DNA replication is regulated.

SV40 GENOME

The SV40 viral genome consists of a single double-stranded circular supercoiled DNA molecule approximately 5 kbp in size (Depamphilis 1996). The genome is complexed with histones both in virions and in infected cells, and the chromatin structure is believed to be similar if not identical to host DNA: four cellular histones H2A, H2B, H3, and H4 are associated with viral DNA. The origin of replication of SV40 is surrounded by noncoding regions which control transcription of early and late genes which are transcribed in opposite directions (Figure 10.4). The early genes of the SV40 encode 'T antigens' – proteins that can be detected by sera from animals bearing SV40-induced tumors. SV40 encodes large and small T antigen while murine polyomavirus encodes small, middle, and large T antigens. These proteins have common N-terminal regions but unique COOH-termini derived from alternative splicing patterns. The only viral protein believed to play a direct role in viral DNA replication is the large T antigen, a multifunctional protein of approximately 90 kDal known to be involved in regulation of transcription, DNA replication, and morphological transformation. The late genes of SV40 encode structural proteins VP1, VP2, and VP3.

At the earliest stages of infection of human or monkey cells, early transcription results in the synthesis of both large and small T antigens. Large T antigen localizes primarily to the nucleus and acts to induce

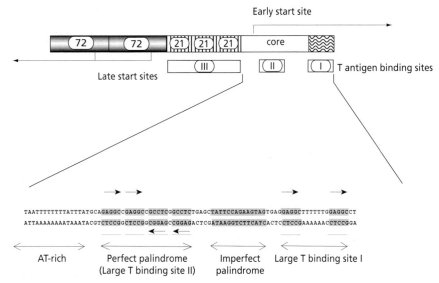

Figure 10.4 *Regulatory regions of SV40. The control region of gene expression in SV40 is shown here. Early and late genes are transcribed in opposite directions. This region contains an origin of DNA replication as well as binding sites for large T antigen. The 72-bp enhancer sequences and the 21-bp repeats are signals which enhance transcription in this region. The minimal origin region is shown below consisting of an AT-rich region, the large T binding site II, an imperfect palindrome and large T binding site I. The pentameric T antigen binding sites are shown in yellow.*

expression of S phase specific cellular genes thereby causing cells to enter S phase. Large T antigen has several functions including down regulation of its own transcription and initiation of viral DNA replication. Once DNA synthesis has initiated, late viral gene expression and assembly of virions proceeds. The binding of large T antigen to the SV40 origin of replication is a critical step and the subject of intensive study.

Origin of replication

As described above, viral origins of replication are discrete DNA segments containing specific sequences to which viral initiator proteins can bind and generally consist of a core region flanked by surrounding auxiliary sequences that can enhance the efficiency of viral DNA replication (Depamphilis 1996; Stenlund 2003). The importance of auxiliary regions was originally discovered in polyomaviruses, but the utilization of auxiliary regions has now turned out to be a general phenomena.

The SV40 origin of replication consists of a core origin region of 64 bp and an extended region containing an enhancer (72 bp) and a series of Sp1 binding sites (21 bp) (Figure 10.4) (Depamphilis 1996). The core region contains a 17-bp AT-rich element, four GAGGC pentanucleotides to which large T antigen binds and the early palindrome (EP). The four pentanucleotides (T antigen binding site II) are arranged as inverted pairs that serve as binding sites for T antigen. The binding of T antigen to site II is believed to bend the DNA. The AT-rich region and the 10-bp early imperfect palindrome are also essential for DNA replication. The AT-rich element is known to undergo

bending independent of protein binding. The AT track can also bind cellular factors such as the transcription factor Oct1. The flanking regions also contain binding sites for cellular transcriptional activators. A second T antigen binding site to the right, site I, is not essential, but can stimulate the efficiency of viral DNA replication in vivo. Other flanking sequences to the left include three copies of the 21-bp repeats containing binding sites for the cellular transcription factor Sp1 and two copies of the 72-bp enhancer. The start sites for the early and late mRNAs are also shown. As will be seen later in this chapter, origins of replication are often situated between promoters, emphasizing a very close relationship between the regulation of transcription and the initiation of viral DNA replications.

Large T antigen

SV40 large T antigen is a 708-aa phosphoprotein that plays multiple functions during the SV40 life cycle. T antigen localizes primarily in the nucleus and in addition to its role in initiation and elongation of viral DNA synthesis it can drive the infected cell into S phase, cause morphological transformation, down-regulate its own transcription, and stimulate late transcription (Fanning and Knippers 1992; Simmons 2000). During DNA replication, T antigen binds the SV40 origin of DNA replication in a sequence-specific manner and its helicase activity unwinds the duplex in an ATP dependent fashion. It is also capable of recruiting cellular replication proteins to the origin through protein–protein interactions. Numerous post-translational modifications have been reported for T antigen including phosphorylation, glycosylation, adenylation, ADP ribosylation, and acylation. It is one of the best studied viral proteins and a large database of mutations that alter various activities of T antigen has been compiled (Fanning and Knippers 1992; Simmons 2000; Ott et al. 2002).

Considerable effort has been given to understanding the structure and function of the 708 residues of SV40 large T. The domain structure of this multifunctional protein is now becoming more clear (Fanning and Knippers 1992; Simmons 2000; Ott et al. 2002; Li et al. 2003a). A minimal sequence-specific DNA binding domain lies in the middle of the protein residues 131–260. The solution structure of the DNA-binding domain has been solved (Li et al. 2003a); interestingly, it is similar to the minimal DNA-binding domain of the papillomavirus replication helicase, E1, described below. Of note is that considerable structural similarity exists despite only an approximately 6 percent identity in the primary amino acid sequence between the two initiator proteins (Li et al. 2003a; reviewed in Stenlund 2003). A zinc-binding domain lies downstream of the DNA-binding domain. The ATPase/helicase domain has been mapped to the C terminus (residues 131–616), and other functional domains which have been mapped include the J domain and binding sites for the cellular cell cycle regulatory proteins Rb and p53.

Mechanism of SV40 DNA synthesis

The binding of an initiator protein to a specific origin of replication is a common theme in the replication of DNA viruses (Depamphilis 1996; Stenlund 2003). A generic reaction of this type is shown in Figure 10.1 in which the initiation process is divided into four separate steps, recognition, melting, unwinding, and recruitment of replication factors.

Initiation At the outset of viral DNA replication, T antigen binds specifically to the SV40 origin of replication as a monomer. In the presence of ATP, individual monomers of T antigen assemble into a single hexamer. In addition to the pentanucleotide binding sites, the EP region is required for hexamer formation. A second hexamer then forms over the origin which causes two types of structural changes: the EP region is melted and the AT track is distorted or twisted (Depamphilis 1996). Following this structural distortion at the origin, T antigen functions as a helicase to unwind the duplex DNA in a reaction which involves ATP hydrolysis. The actual initiation of viral DNA synthesis requires the recruitment of three cellular proteins to the unwound origin: replication protein A (RPA), DNA polymerase α-primase and topoisomerase I (topo I) (Simmons et al. 1996; Gai et al. 2000). T antigen is known to bind RPA and it is believed that DNA unwinding by T antigen produces single-stranded DNA; the interaction between T antigen and RPA results in loading of RPA onto the

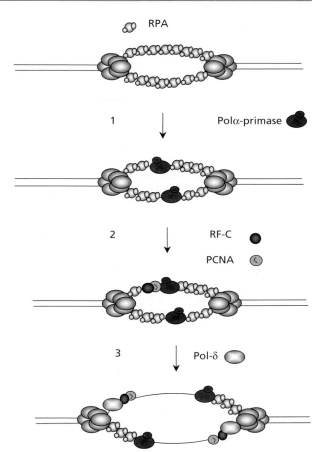

Figure 10.5 *SV40 DNA synthesis. Large T antigen (also depicted in Figure 10.1) recruits cellular proteins to the unwound origin of replication. Once RPA and polymerase α-primase are recruited by T antigen, synthesis of the leading strands is initiated by producing RNA primers which can be extended by pol-α creating an RNA-DNA fragment of approximately 30 nucleotides (Step 1). RF-C binds to the 3' OH of the RNA-DNA fragment in a reaction that requires ATP hydrolysis. RF-C can load PCNA onto the template (Step 2). DNA pol-δ is then recruited and binds to the PCNA–RF-C complex (Step 3). The complex is now able to carry out leading and lagging-strand DNA synthesis.*

single-stranded DNA (Figure 10.5). The DNA polymerase α-primase is responsible for the synthesis of Okazaki fragments. Polymerase α-primase binds specifically to both the RPA and large T antigen assembled at the origin (Ott et al. 2002). Once bound, the primase initiates synthesis of the leading strands by producing RNA primers that can be extended as DNA by polymerase α. Topo I is believed to nick and religate DNA at the origin to relieve torsional strain ahead of the replication fork (Waga and Stillman 1994).

Elongation The 3' OH of the nascent RNA–DNA fragment (about 30 nucleotides) can then be recognized by the replication factor C (RF-C). RF-C promotes the ATP-dependent loading of PCNA onto the template which is followed by the recruitment of DNA polymerase δ. Although pol δ is sufficient for continuous leading strand DNA synthesis in an in vitro reconstitution experiment, in vivo another cellular polymerase, pol ε, appears to be required in addition. Lagging-strand synthesis initiates on the opposite strand again through the action of DNA polymerase α-primase. Thus, leading-strand and lagging-strand replication occurs at each replication fork in the bidirectional origin of replication. The classic problem of how a single replication fork apparatus can synthesize DNA in opposite directions at the same time was solved by the proposal that the template DNA for discontinuous synthesis can be spooled through an immobile replication complex containing all proteins necessary for synthesis of both leading and lagging strands (Wessel et al. 1992; mechanism reviewed in Stenlund 2003). Spooling has been observed by electron microscopic analysis. The DNA fragments produced by lagging-strand synthesis are sealed in a reaction that involves removal of the primers by RNase H (specifically degrades RNA from RNA–DNA hybrids) and the 5'–3' exonuclease *Fen*1. The gaps can then be repaired by DNA polymerase δ and the ends of the DNA fragments joined by DNA ligase I. When replication gets to a point on the circular molecular opposite from the origin of replication, the reaction is terminated in a reaction which involves topoisomerases I and II. These enzymes remove torsional stress which accumulates through the action of the helicase unwinding DNA ahead of the growing fork. Topoisomerase II mediates the separation of the two intertwined (catenated) daughter molecules by the passage of one through the other. Table 10.4 lists the functions of each of these cellular proteins. As mentioned above, it was through the analysis of an in vitro reconstitution experiment with SV40 and large T antigen that the components of the cellular machinery were first identified (Li and Kelly 1984).

When these viruses infect permissive hosts, they initiate a productive cycle of infection; however, there are some cell types that do not support productive infection. Instead, in these cells the viral DNA becomes integrated into that of the host cells, in many cases transforming them. This is known as morphological transformation and occurs through the interaction of viral and cellular proteins (Simmons 2000).

PAPILLOMAVIRUSES

The papillomaviruses are a large family of small double-stranded DNA which are closely related to the polyomaviruses but differ in several important ways (Depamphilis 1996). Papillomaviruses infect mucosal or cutaneous epithelia causing warts and cervical carcinoma. Most of the initial work on DNA replication of these viruses was performed with Bovine papillomavirus

Table 10.4 *Cellular proteins required for SV40 DNA synthesis*

Cellular protein	Molecular mass (kDal)	Function
RPA	70	Binds single-stranded DNA; promotes origin unwinding; stimulates pol-α:primase; cooperates with RF-C and PCNA to stimulate DNA pol-δ
	32	
	12	
DNA pol-α: primase	180	Initiates leading- and lagging-strand synthesis through the synthesis of RNA primers and Okazaki fragments
	70	
	58	
	48	
RF-C	140	Auxiliary factor for DNA pol-δ and -ε; loads PCNA onto DNA; DNA-dependent ATPase
	40	
	38	
	37	
	36.5	
PCNA	36	Processivity factor for DNA pol-δ and -ε
DNA pol-δ	125	Completes leading- and lagging-strand synthesis; processive when bound to PCNA
	48	
DNA pol-ε	255	DNA polymerase which may complete lagging-strand synthesis
	55	
Topoisomerase I	110	Relieves torsional strain in front of replication forks
Fen1	48	5' to 3' exonuclease; removal of RNA primers
RNase H1	89	Endonuclease; cleaves RNA primer
DNA ligase I	125	Ligates Okazaki fragments

(BPV) which has served as a prototype for the papillomaviruses. Recent work with human papillomavirus (HPV) has revealed similarities and differences between BPVs and HPV. Examples from both replication systems will be discussed in this chapter.

General features of papillomavirus DNA replication

Papillomaviruses can be distinguished from polyomaviruses by exhibiting a more complex pattern of replication governed by the differentiation stage of the infected cell. In fact, the life cycle of papillomaviruses is known to be tightly coupled to the cellular differentiation program of the epithelium (Longworth and Laimins 2004). DNA replication actually occurs in three different stages. Three different modes of DNA synthesis during different stages of infection of skin have been reported: amplification, maintenance, and productive replication. The virus first infects proliferating basal epithelial cells, and in these cells the genome enters the nucleus and is amplified as a circular genome to a concentration of approximately 50–100 copies per cell. This replication requires the viral proteins E1 and E2 as well as the cellular replication machinery. This stage is believed to occur by theta mechanism and therefore resembles SV40 DNA replication. These circular DNA episomes are then maintained by a regulated process in which the episomes are replicated once per cell cycle again using an SV40-like mechanism. The final productive stage of DNA replication occurs in the outer layers of the epidermis, in differentiated cells. The shift from maintenance to productive replication is not well understood, but may involve a transition from SV40-like theta replication to a rolling circle mechanism of replication (Flores and Lambert 1997). DNA synthesis during the maintenance and the final productive stage of DNA replication also utilizes E1, E2, and the cellular DNA replication machinery (Broker and Chow 2001; Stenlund 2003). The fact that the productive phase of viral DNA replication occurs in terminally differentiated epithelial cells presents an interesting dilemma in that the cellular replication machinery required for viral replication would not be expected to be present in noncycling terminally differentiated cells (Broker and Chow 2001). Cellular replicative proteins are generally turned off in such cells. During the productive phase of the viral life cycle, papillomaviruses are presumed to be able to induce S-phase-specific viral functions. The viral protein E7 is required for productive infection in these differentiated cells and is believed to function by inducing the synthesis of the cellular replication proteins (Cheng et al. 1995; Broker and Chow 2001). Cellular proteins such as polymerase α and PCNA are likely induced in a manner similar to induction of host DNA synthetic machinery by SV40 T antigen.

The ability to induce the expression of S-phase-specific cellular genes is shared by several DNA viruses. The transcription of such cellular genes is tightly regulated by the Rb-E2f complex (Munger et al. 1989). E2f proteins are transcriptional regulators which bind cellular promoter sequences and stimulate transcription of S-phase-specific cellular genes. The presence of Rb in the E2f complex results in repression of these cellular genes. During the progression into S phase, Rb is phosphorylated resulting in its release from E2f and the induction of cellular genes encoding replication proteins such as histones and polymerases. Several viral proteins including adenoviral E1A, SV40 large T, and the E7 proteins of some human papillomaviruses have been shown to bind to the region of Rb that contacts E2f thereby resulting in activation of the E2f transcription factor. Thus, during productive papillomavirus infection, the E7 protein can stimulate the expression of the cellular DNA synthetic machinery. Following the replication of viral genomes, late viral proteins such as capsid proteins are made and progeny virus are assembled and eventually shed. These stages of replication are believed to be tightly regulated.

PAPILLOMAVIRUS GENOME

The papillomavirus genomes are small double-stranded DNA molecules of approximately 8 kbp (larger than the closely related polymaviruses) (Depamphilis 1996). All ten open reading frames are located on one strand of the viral DNA and all transcription is in a clockwise direction. Open reading frames are designated as either early (E) or late (L) based on their location on the genome. The early region encodes regulatory proteins which are expressed in nonproductively infected cells and also in cells transformed by papillomaviruses. Early genes *E1* and *E2* are required for DNA synthesis (reviewed in Stenlund 2003). At least five other early genes expressed from differentially spliced and partially overlapping mRNAs play various roles in regulation of gene expression and transformation. The late genes *L1* and *L2* encode structural proteins for the viral capsid and are only expressed in productively infected cells.

Origin of replication

The papillomavirus origin of replication lies in a small fragment located between the early open reading frames and a region called the long control region which contains regulatory signals for viral transcription (Stenlund 2003). Thus, as with the polyomaviruses, a relationship between the origin and binding sites for transcription factors exists (Depamphilis 1996). In the case of the papilloma viruses, the definition of the core origin is complicated by the apparent redundancies in this region. In the BPV ori, the core ori is contained in a fragment containing an AT-rich region, a binding site for E1 and

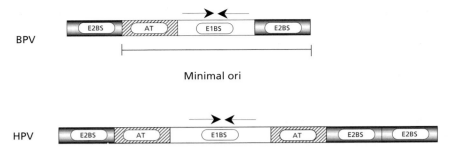

Figure 10.6 *Origin region of papillomavirus. BPV origin contains an AT rich region and a palindromic binding site for the initiator protein E1. However, these two elements are not sufficient for even minimal origin activity which requires at least one binding site for the transcription factor E2. In this case the E2 activator is required for loading of E1 to the origin (see text). In the HPV type origins, two binding sites for the E2 transcription factor are apparently required.*

a binding site for E2 to the right (Figure 10.6) (Chen and Stenlund 2002). However, if the right hand E2 binding site is deleted, replication can occur if the left hand E2 binding site is present. The HPV type origin contains a binding site for the viral replication initiator E1, three copies of a binding site for the viral transcriptional activator E2 and two AT-rich sequences. Thus, as with the polyomavirus origins of replication, both the BPV and HPV origins contain core essential elements flanked by auxiliary sequences which appear to enhance replication activity (Depamphilis 1996).

Replication proteins E1 and E2

E1 is the only viral protein that is directly involved in DNA replication. E2 is a transcription protein which greatly stimulates E1 binding at the origin. E1 proteins from both BPV and HPV share similarities with SV40 large T antigen (Enemark et al. 2000; Hickman et al. 2002). The BPV E1 protein is a 68-kDa nuclear phosphoprotein that binds specifically to the origin of replication. E1 has DNA-dependent ATPase and DNA helicase activities and binds to the origin of replication with weak affinity. E1 also interacts with cellular replication proteins such as the large subunit of DNA polymerase α (reviewed in Broker and Chow 2001). E2 interacts with E1 and facilitates E1 binding to the origin. E2 may also stimulate viral DNA replication by interacting with cellular proteins recruited to the origin such as RPA. E2 also plays a role in genome maintenance.

Mechanism of papillomavirus DNA replication

Initiation   Much of the analysis of papillomavirus initiation has been performed in the BPV system. The availability of an in vitro system in which viral DNA replication occurs in a cell-free extract has been very valuable in our understanding of events which occur during the initiation of DNA replication. It should be kept in mind, however, that such in vitro reactions do not always accurately mimic events which occur in vivo. E1 and E2 proteins interact with one another and form

a complex at the viral origin of replication. E1 is related in sequence and possesses activities analogous to the SV40 large T antigen such as ATPase, helicase, origin binding, and unwinding (Hickman et al. 2002; Stenlund 2003). BPV type 1 E1 binds to an 18-bp inverted-repeat element within the origin DNA with low specificity (Chen and Stenlund 2002). E2 is a dimeric transcription-replication factor that also binds to the origin. E1 and E2 bind cooperatively to the origin of replication to form an active initiation complex. The E2 protein is believed to act as a clamp-loading protein that stabilizes the E1-origin interaction and increases its specificity. A dimer of E1 is first bound together with a dimer of E2 ($E1_2E2_2$) (Chen and Stenlund 2002; Enemark et al. 2000). Binding of a second dimer of E1 occurs by displacing the E2 dimer in an ATP-dependent fashion creating a tetramer of E1. A bend is induced in the DNA by these interactions. Additional monomers of E1 are recruited to the complex eventually forming a hexamer and a double hexamer of E1 at the origin. ATP is required for the formation of the higher order structures. Cell cycle-specific phosphorylation may also be important in this assembly process (Broker and Chow 2001).

The formation of the initiation complex in HPV may differ slightly from BPV in some details; for instance, the HPV-1 E1 appears to be able to bind ori in a stable manner and to initiate replication on its own, at least in vitro. On the other hand, recent evidence suggests that the E1/E2 ratio is important for HPV replication efficiency and that regulation of E1 and E2 protein expression may be important for regulation during various stages of the virus life cycle.

E1 hexamers or double hexamers assemble at the origin, and it is this larger oligomer of E1 that is active in melting or distorting the duplex DNA (Stenlund 2003). This melting step is distinct from the ATP-dependent unwinding which occurs later. Melting is a change in the conformation of the DNA and can be observed by reactivity with single strand-specific agents such as permanganate ions which are able to modify non-base-paired resides. This melting or distortion step is analogous to that described above for melting at the SV40 origin. Once a small region of single-stranded DNA is generated, RPA is recruited and melting occurs. The actual unwinding step involves the double hexamer which is now believed to form a bidirectional helicase. As with SV40, although the two hexamers are believed to unwind DNA in opposite directions, they appear to be held together. A new model for replication is emerging which suggests that instead of the hexameric helicases moving along the viral DNA template during replication in opposite directions, the template is actually drawn through the double hexamer as the DNA is unwound (reviewed in Stenlund 2003). The notion of a helicase which functions by 'pumping' DNA through a double hexamer is not unique to the E1 protein. Similar mechanisms have been proposed for SV40 T antigen and for the *E. coli* replicative helicase DNA B.

Elongation   Little is known about the actual elongation phase of papillomavirus DNA replication. The early stages of DNA replication appear to occur by theta replication, however, it is possible that a switch from theta to rolling circle replication occurs during productive DNA replication (Flores and Lambert 1997). As in SV40 DNA replication, the E1 helicase is presumed to be the replicative helicase (Broker and Chow 2001). E1 also interacts with the polymerase α primase complex. Bidirectional DNA synthesis utilizes the cellular DNA synthetic machinery. In addition to RPA and the polymerase α primase complex, PCNA, RF-C, DNA polymerase δ or ε, and topisomerases I and II are presumably needed for papillomavirus DNA replication (reviewed in Broker and Chow 2001).

PARVOVIRUSES

The *Parvoviridae* are the smallest of the eukaryotic DNA viruses with genomes consisting of linear single stranded DNA molecules of 4 500–5 000 nucleotides. These viruses have been classified as either nondefective or autonomous parvoviruses, genus *Parvovirus*, such as the minute virus of mice (MVM), or defective or dependent parvoviruses, genus *Dependovirus*, such as the adeno-associated viruses (AAV) which rely on co-infection with adenovirus or herpesviruses for productive infection. Members of the autonomous *Parvovirus* genus can replicate productively without the aid of a helper virus. Replication of the autonomous parvoviruses requires that the infected cell enter S phase, since this virus utilizes components of the cell DNA replication machinery for its own replication; however, in contrast to SV40, these viruses cannot induce resting cells to enter S phase. As a result, productive infection is restricted to proliferating cells (Berns 1990; Depamphilis 1996).

General features of parvovirus DNA replication

Parvoviral DNA replication is similar to replication strategies of single-stranded coliphage genomes from bacteria (Berns 1990). The general mechanism has been called a 'rolling hairpin.' The incoming single-stranded DNA molecules form secondary structures at the termini which provide a 3′ OH primer for complementary strand synthesis. A linear duplex intermediate with one covalently closed end is generated. The resolution of this end by a site-specific nick results in the regeneration of the genomic termini. Again, the terminal redundancy can lead to another hairpin which can be elongated to make a double-stranded dimer molecule. Viral DNA replication proceeds through a series of concatemeric duplex intermediates by a strand displacement mode of synthesis involving leading-strand synthesis only. The autonomous and dependent parvoviruses share several features, but differ in some important respects. Both AAV and MVM have palindromic ends, but in MVM, the ends are not identical. Another difference is that in MVM, only the minus or noncoding strand is packaged.

MVM GENOME AND ORIGINS OF REPLICATION

The negative-sense MVM genome is approximately 5 200 bp long and exists primarily as a single-stranded DNA with terminal palindromic units which are predicted to form hairpin and other secondary structures. These terminal palindromic regions act as viral origins of replication during the process of regeneration of terminal sequences from long concatamers (termed junction resolution). They also play a unique role in the rolling hairpin replication mechanism used by this virus (described below) (Berns 1990).

MVM GENE PRODUCTS

The genome encodes two structural proteins VP1 and VP2; a third virion protein VP3 is present in infectious particles and derives from a proteolytic cleavage from VP2. The virus also encodes two nonstructural proteins, NS1 and NS2. NS1 is involved in both viral DNA replication and the transactivation of structural protein expression (Cotmore et al. 1995; Christensen and Tattersall 2002). NS1 is a site-specific nickase, recognizing the origin sequences present in the two viral termini and has been shown to nick and resolve these concatemers into unit length molecules suitable for packaging. The NS1 molecule becomes bound at the 5′ end of the viral DNA after nicking. It also comprises a 3′ to 5′ helicase, similar to the SV40 T antigen and papillomavirus E1 (reviewed in Marintcheva and Weller 2001). Alternate splicing events result in the production of three different versions of NS2 which differ in their C-terminal sequences. NS2 may be involved in DNA replication, although its role is not clear at this time.

Mechanism of replication

Parvoviral DNA replication utilizes a modification of rolling circle replication mechanism dubbed rolling hairpin synthesis (Berns 1990). The genome is replicated through a series of monomeric and concatemeric duplex replicative-form (RF) intermediates. Replication proceeds unidirectionally by leading-strand continuous synthesis of DNA. The incoming viral genome is a linear single-stranded DNA molecule; however, the palindromic origin regions are believed to adopt secondary structures which may be simple hairpins or more complex T- or Y-shaped structures. The ability of the 3′ end to base pair within the terminal palindrome results in the formation of an ideal template-primer structure for the initiation of DNA replication (see Figure 10.7) (Berns 1990). This molecule is converted into a double-stranded intermediate by extension of the 3′ end by the cellular replication machinery resulting in a linear duplex intermediate, the original right-end hairpin is unfolded and copied to form a duplex terminal palindrome. In this model, the unidirectional replication fork shuttles back and forth along the linear genome. This

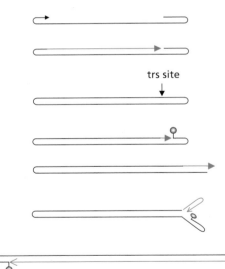

trs site

Figure 10.7 *Model for MVM DNA replication. The 3′ terminus of the virion strand is thought to fold back on itself to provide a primer for initiating synthesis of the complementary strand. When DNA synthesis reaches the right end, it is thought that a ligation event produces a linear duplex molecule with covalently closed termini. The right end can then be nicked by NS1 and the protein becomes covalently associated with the 5′ end, leaving a 3′ OH that copies the right end to a duplex extended form. The right end undergoes a conformational change resulting in the formation of a double hairpinned molecule which can be extended by further DNA synthesis. A dimer molecule is generated in which the monomer viral genomes are inverted with respect to one another. Terminal resolution and strand exchange leads to different orientations of the terminal sequences and eventually one strand is packaged into progeny genomes.*

mechanism involves unfolding and refolding of the two palindromic viral termini in such a way that the advancing replication fork can switch directions backwards and forwards generating a series of dimeric and tetrameric replication intermediates. Duplex copies of the unit-length genome become linked in head-to-head and tail-to-tail configurations.

Initiation   The viral NS1 protein plays a vital role in this mechanism by recognizing origin sequences present in the two viral termini (Cotmore et al. 1995). NS1 recognizes a specific site in the origin region and introduces a nick at an adjacent initiation site. The minimal core origin is approximately 50 bp long and contains three distinct recognition sequences. NS1 binds site specifically to the (ACCA)2 repeat motif in an ATP-dependent manner. Although NS1 can bind by itself, nicking does not occur unless a cellular factor, called parvovirus initiation factor (PIF) is also present. Together, PIF and NS1 form a high-affinity ternary complex capable of nicking and subsequently initiating replication at the origin (Christensen and Tattersall 2002). After nicking, NS1 remains covalently attached to the 5′ end of the nicked DNA thereby freeing the 3′ hydroxyl group to act as a primer for DNA synthesis. The NS1 molecule bound at the 5′ end may also serve as a 3′ to 5′ helicase. Interestingly, it has recently been shown that similar to the SV40 T antigen, NS1 can be regulated by post-translational modification such as phosphorylation. Modification by phosphorylation of NS1 regulates the site-specific binding and DNA unwinding activities of the viral polypeptide (Nuesch et al. 2001). These phosphorylation events also determine the ability of NS1 to nick the left-end MVM origin site-specifically and control strand-displacement synthesis through its progressive helicase function. Multiple cellular kinases are believed to be responsible for these phosphorylation events (Nuesch et al. 2001).

Elongation   DNA replication occurs through a series of monomeric and concatemeric duplex replicative-form intermediates and DNA synthesis by a unidirectional, leading-strand-specific process. The other cellular proteins required for MVM replication are also consistent with a leading-strand synthesis mechanism of DNA replication including RPA and proliferating cellular nuclear antigen (PCNA) (Christensen and Tattersall 2002). Although the cellular polymerase involved in vivo MVM DNA replication has not been identified, a processive leading-strand synthesis reaction has been reconstituted in vitro on a PIF-NS1 initiated origin by the addition of recombinant RF-C, PCNA, RPA and pol δ (Christensen and Tattersall 2002). RF-C is expected to act as a clamp loading protein recognizing the primer-template junction and loading PCNA onto the template to form a sliding clamp which stabilizes DNA polymerase on the template thereby promoting processive chain elongation. Enzymes identified in the SV40 DNA replication system which are involved in the generation or processing of lagging-strand Okazaki fragments (polymerase α-primase, RNase H, ligase I, and MF-I) have not been implicated in parvovirus replication.

ADENO-ASSOCIATED VIRUS (AAV)

In contrast to the MVM autonomous replicating parvovirus, AAV generally requires a co-infecting virus to efficiently replicate. Interestingly however, under conditions of genotoxic stress, AAV is capable of replicating in the absence of helper virus suggesting that whatever functions are provided by the helper viruses can be mimicked in the cell under certain kinds of stress conditions (Yakobson et al. 1989).

AAV genome and origin

Like MVM, AAV is a single-stranded DNA (ssDNA) virus whose genome is approximately 5 kbp and contains inverted terminal repeat (ITR) structures at each end. Trs can self-anneal to form terminal hairpinned structures and serve an important role as primers for DNA synthesis using host-cell synthetic machinery. In addition to containing an origin of replication, TRs also contain the packaging signal and the *cis*-acting elements needed for chromosomal integration (Berns 1990; Im and Muzyczka 1990).

AAV proteins

The 4.7 kbp ssDNA genome of AAV has two open reading frames, rep and cap (Im and Muzyczka 1990). Four viral proteins are encoded by the rep genes, two larger proteins, Rep68 and 78 and two smaller proteins, Rep52 and Rep40. These four gene products are produced by differential use of promoters: Rep68 and 78 are translated from mRNAs initiating at the one viral promoter, and the smaller proteins are translated from mRNAs that originate from another promoter. Differential splicing accounts for the differences between Rep68 and 40 and their longer counterparts, Rep78 and Rep52. Rep 68 and Rep78 are multifunctional proteins involved in DNA replication, transcription, packaging, and proviral integration (Li et al. 2003b). Rep68 and Rep78 exhibit several activities including sequence-specific double-stranded DNA binding, site-specific, single-stranded DNA endonuclease activity and ATP-dependent DNA helicase activities. Interestingly, the smaller Rep proteins 52/40 have been shown to play a role in packaging and this role is inhibited by the larger Reps78/68. In the case of MVM, there are no smaller versions of NS1, and it is not clear how regulation between replication and packaging occurs.

Mechanism of replication
During AAV DNA replication, Rep68 and 78 bind viral Trs and induce a site-specific, single-stranded nick. Rep is thought to form oligomeric structures when bound to DNA containing a specific DNA-binding site (RBE) (Li et al. 2003b). Although a dimer of rep is believed to be required for trs nicking activity, it is thought that larger oligomeric structures then form on DNA, the largest of which appears to contain six Rep molecules (Li et al. 2003b). ATP may stimulate the formation of these higher order structures. A higher order structure containing six Rep molecules is reminiscent of other viral replication proteins which form hexamers upon binding their DNA substrates including SV40 large T antigen and papillomavirus E1 protein (Stenlund 2003; Hickman et al. 2003).

Initiation of replication
Replication of AAV is initiated from the 3′ hairpin primer of the single-stranded input genome. The hairpin exposes a 3′ hydroxyl primer that can be extended by host–cell polymerase to initiate viral DNA synthesis a linear duplex molecule in which one of the ends is covalently joined (Berns 1990). To replicate the covalently closed terminal sequence, the termini are nicked on one of the two strands, and the newly exposed 3′ OH primer that is generated by the nick is used to repair the terminal sequence. This process is similar to the replication of the autonomous DNA viruses and ensures the integrity of the terminal sequences. The helicase activity of Rep68/Rep78 is thought to be involved in unwinding the covalently closed end of the linear viral DNA after it makes the site-specific nick at the trs site. As described above for T antigen, ATP is thought to stimulate multimerization facilitating the formation of double hexamer structures on the origin of DNA synthesis, and these double hexamers are believed to be active for helicase activity. The linear duplex end is then unwound to reform a terminal hairpin, thus providing a 3′-OH primer for strand-displacement synthesis. Elongation from the hairpin primer then generates a single-stranded genome (which is presumably packaged) and a new RF molecule, which again can undergo terminal resolution.

As with MVM, the cellular proteins involved in leading-strand DNA synthesis have also been implicated in the elongation step of AAV DNA replication including RPA, RF-C, PCNA, and a DNA polymerase (Christensen and Tattersall 2002). No requirement for DNA polymerase α-primase has been demonstrated. In an in vitro replication system, purified cellular factors PCNA, RPA, and RF-C and a partially purified fraction containing cellular DNA polymerases are necessary for reconstituting AAV DNA replication. However, investigators were unable to reconstitute activity in assays using combinations of known polymerases, suggesting that an additional cellular factor, which had not been previously identified in the SV40 system, may be necessary for AAV DNA synthesis

Requirement for helper virus In the absence of helper virus, only limited AAV genome replication can occur, and integration of the virus into a specific region of the host chromosome occurs. Interestingly, some transformed cell lines which have been treated with genotoxic agents (heat shock, hydroxyurea, UV light, or carcinogens) can support AAV DNA replication in the absence of helper virus (Yakobson et al. 1989).

Helper activity can be supplied by adenovirus and herpesviruses (including both HSV and HCMV). In the case of Ad, five genetic regions, the E1A, E1B, E4, E2A, and VA regions, are required for complete helper function (Richardson and Westphal 1981). However, none of these genes appears to be directly involved in AAV DNA replication. Genetic analyses have suggested that the role of Ad co-infection is primarily to maximize the synthesis of AAV-encoded gene products and possibly cellular genes that are required for AAV DNA replication. In the case of HSV, the minimal proteins that support AAV are the single-stranded DNA-binding proteins, ICP8 and the three components of the helicase/primase complex (UL5, UL52, and UL8) (Weindler and Heilbronn 1991). Interestingly however, the helicase and primase activities of the HSV proteins are not required for helper activity (Stracker et al. 2004). It has been suggested that the helper activity of the four proteins may be important as a scaffold which can recruit viral and cellular proteins important for AAV replication. Furthermore, it appears that the localization within the nucleus is important for efficiency of AAV replication. Both adenovirus and herpesviruses replicate at discrete sites within the nucleus and are able to subvert host cellular mechanisms to enhance viral replication (discussed below) (Carrington-Lawrence and Weller 2003; Wilkinson and Weller 2003). As discussed above, several viral replication proteins have been shown to interact directly with RPA, including T antigen and E1 of papillomaviruses. AAV rep and MVM NS1 have also been reported to interact with RPA, suggesting that recruitment of RPA and other cellular proteins may be important for parvoviral replication (Christensen and Tattersall 2002; Stenlund 2003; Stracker et al. 2004).

Summary Parvoviruses replication proteins NS1 for MVM and Rep68/78 for AAV act to nick the viral DNA and also as oligomeric helicases. Strand displacement synthesis is then carried out using cellular replication machinery; however, since only leading-strand synthesis occurs, the cellular machinery needed for lagging-strand DNA synthesis does not appear to be involved in parvovirus DNA replication.

ADENOVIRUSES

Adenoviruses cause respiratory infections and conjunctivitis among other ailments and have been isolated from a wide range of mammalian and avian hosts. Human adenoviruses can also cause morphological transformation in rodent cells. Forty-nine human adenovirus serotypes have been identified. All adenoviruses isolated to date contain a linear, double-stranded DNA genome of approximately 35 kbp packaged in a nonenveloped icosahedral capsid (Depamphilis 1996).

General features of adenoviral DNA replication

The linear genome contains two copies of the viral origin within the terminal inverted repeats. Initiation can occur at either end of the viral genome resulting in the formation of a daughter strand and the displacement of one of the parental strands (reviewed in Depamphilis 1996). The displaced parental strand can then serve as a template for the synthesis of a second daughter strand. The DNA replication strategies of this moderately sized DNA virus exhibit several unusual features. For instance, in contrast to the parvo-, polyoma-, and papillomaviruses, adenovirus encodes its own DNA polymerase (pol) and DNA-binding protein (DBP). Another interesting feature is the covalent attachment of a 55 kDa terminal protein (TP) to the 5' end of each strand. The covalent attachment of TP results from that fact that adenovirus utilizes an unusual protein priming mechanism for replication initiation. Three cellular proteins have been shown to stimulate viral DNA synthesis: two transcription factors nuclear factor I (NF1) and Oct-1 and a topoisomerase (NF-II) (de Jong and van der Vliet 1999). Thus this virus is intermediate between the smaller DNA viruses which only encode one viral replication protein, and the larger herpes- and poxviruses which encode not only their own polymerases but most or all (in the case of pox) of the other proteins required for DNA replication. Another interesting feature exhibited by adenovirus will be discussed at the end of this chapter and relates to complex virus–host interactions related to intracellular localization and inactivation of cellular response signals.

As with the SV40 system, the identification of viral and cellular proteins involved in DNA replication was facilitated by the development of a soluble cell-free DNA-replication system. These experiments indicated that adenovirus replication requires three virally encoded proteins: precursor TP (pTP), DNA polymerase (pol) and the DBP. The availability of the reconstituted cell free replication system also allowed the identification of two cellular transcription proteins required for efficient initiation, NF1 and Oct-1 and a third cellular protein, the type I topoisomerase NFII required for efficient elongation in the strand displacement synthesis reaction.

ADENOVIRUS GENOME

The linear double-stranded DNA genome consists of five early transcription units, two delayed early units, and one late unit. Both strands of the viral genome are transcribed although the majority of viral genes are generated from the so-called rightward reading strand. Differential spicing and the use of alternate splicing increase complexity of viral gene expression (Depamphilis 1996).

Origin of replication

The origin of the best studied adenovirus (Ad 2) consists of two distinct regions, a minimal origin region within the first 18 bp and a second region 19–51 which serves to enhance the efficiency of the initiation reaction. The minimal origin (1–18) contains a 10-bp region (bps 9–18) conserved in all adenovirus terminal regions. The minimal origin by itself can only support a limited, basal level of initiation of DNA replication. The auxiliary region contains binding sites for the cellular proteins NF1 and Oct-1. Interestingly, the ori region for another adenovirus, Ad 4, requires only the terminal 18 bp of the viral genome for efficient viral replication. Ad 4 does not seem to require the host factors NF1 and Oct-1 (de Jong and van der Vliet 1999).

Viral proteins involved in DNA synthesis

Adenoviruses encode three viral proteins that are essential for DNA synthesis, the adenovirus polymerase (Ad pol), the pTP and the single-stranded DBP (reviewed in Depamphilis 1996). Sequence analysis reveals that the 140Ad pol is related to the larger family of DNA polymerases. Within this family, the Ad pol is a member of a subfamily of protein-priming DNA polymerases. The polymerase activity of the pol protein is located at the C terminus of the protein (Brenkman et al. 2002). The Ad pol is capable of catalyzing two types of reactions: the covalent addition of dCTP to a hydroxyl residue on a serine in the 80 kDa pTP, and the elongation of a growing DNA chain from the protein primer terminus (de Jong et al. 2003b). It is believed that the switch from a protein- to a DNA-priming polymerization mode may require a conformational change within the polymerase. Biochemical analysis of Ad pol has shown that it replicates DNA in a processive manner and that it has a distributive 3′–5′ exonuclease activity on single-stranded DNA. Both the polymerase and exonuclease activities are decreased when pTP is complexed with Ad pol. This difference in activity depending on association with pTP may explain the switch from protein to DNA-priming mode in that pTP is believed to dissociate from pol before elongation proceeds (de Jong et al. 2003a). Dissociation from pTP is believed to increase processivity of pol. The viral DBP can stimulate the activity of the polymerase and can also increase its processivity.

The 72-kDa single-stranded DBP is essential for DNA replication. This was originally determined by the isolation of temperature sensitive mutations in the DBP gene.

DBP participates in the initiation of DNA synthesis as well as the elongation step. DBP stimulates initiation by enhancing the binding of Pol to the origin of replication (van Breukelen et al. 2003). DBP helps to unwind the double-stranded DNA template and enhances the processivity of Pol by the removal of secondary structures. DBP binds single-stranded DNA in a sequence-independent and cooperative manner. Interestingly, DBP can support the movement of the replication fork over large distances without hydrolysis of ATP. This property of DBP abrogates the need for a helicase during DNA synthesis. In addition to its role in DNA synthesis, DBP plays a role in control of transcription, transformation, and virus assembly. The DNA-binding domain resides in the C terminal 174–529 residues. The N-terminal domain contains the nuclear localization signal.

The 671 amino-acid pTP protein makes many contacts with viral DNA and with other proteins during initiation of viral DNA synthesis. The N terminus interacts with DNA and C-terminal residues interact with Ad DNA pol (de Jong et al. 2003a). pTP also appears to harbor multiple binding sites for Oct 1. The most important single amino acid in pTP is Ser 580, which is covalently coupled to the incoming dCTP (de Jong et al. 2003a). Ad5 pTP contains three protease cleavage sites that are recognized by a virally encoded protease. Cleavage at the TP site most likely occurs after packaging into the viral particle, generating a TP-DNA complex which lacks the N-terminal 349 amino acids of pTP. Another interesting feature of the pTP is its apparent ability to attach to the nuclear matrix. This interaction could provide a scaffold for the recruitment of replication proteins that explains the observation of specific replication foci in the nucleus (see below). Thus the important attributes of pTP include multiple DNA and protein contacts, the presence of Ser 580 which becomes covalently attached to the nascent DNA chain and its ability to undergo cleavage.

Cellular proteins

Oct-1 is a human transcription factor that can stimulate both RNA pol II and pol III transcription from a variety of promoters. It consists of a central bipartite POU DNA binding domain surrounded by activation regions. POU domains can recognize a variety of different promoter DNA sequences. Although adenovirus DNA replication can occur in vitro with only the viral genome and the three virally encoded replication proteins, pTP, pol, and DBP, replication is stimulated up to 200-fold by the addition of the cellular transcription factors Oct-1 and NF1 (de Jong and van der Vliet 1999). The Oct-1 protein interacts with pTP directly and the presence of an Oct-1 binding site in the origin stimulates viral replication in vivo. Oct-1 is believed to enhance the DNA binding of pTP–pol by lowering its dissociation rate leading to a model in which Oct-1 tethers pTP–pol to the replication origin. NF1 is another cellular transcription factor which binds as a dimer to viral and cellular promoters. A type II cellular topoisomerase, nuclear factor II, is also required for adenovirus DNA replication and it thought to relieve overwinding of the template during replication (de Jong and van der Vliet 1999).

Mechanism of viral DNA synthesis

A mechanism for initiation and elongation of viral DNA synthesis has now emerged.

Initiation   The first stage of DNA replication involves the formation of a preinitiation complex comprising NF1, Oct-1, pTP, Pol, and DBP at the origin of replication. The recruitment of viral and cellular proteins to origins of replication is a theme repeated in many other viral and cellular replication systems studied. In the first step of initiation a heterodimer of pTP and pol assembles at the origin of replication in a binding reaction stimulated by the binding of cellular transcription proteins NF1 and Oct-1 to adjacent sites (see Figure 10.8). NF1 and Oct-1 apparently target the pTP-Pol complex to the origin (de Jong and van der Vliet 1999). The DBP can also stimulate the binding of Pol at the origin. The ability of both cellular proteins NF1 and Oct-1 and DBP to stimulate binding of pTP–pol at the origin illustrates the importance of these types of protein–protein interactions in recruitment of the components of a replication machinery to viral origins of replication.

DNA replication is initiated by an unusual protein priming mechanism in which a covalent attachment is formed between the first base and a serine residue in pTP (de Jong et al. 2003b). This reaction is catalyzed by pol, but relies on multiple DNA–protein and protein–protein interactions which act to stabilize the preinitiation complex formed at the adenovirus origin of DNA replication. The pTP and pol must assemble in such a way that the serine-580 in pTP is accessible to the Ad pol catalytic site and the DNA template to react with the first nucleotide to be added, dCTP to give dCMP, in the protein priming reaction (de Jong et al. 2003a). The addition of dCMP is template driven as DNA synthesis is initiated opposite the fourth base of the template strand. In a reaction catalyzed by the Ad polymerase, CMP is covalently bound to the hydroxyl group of a serine residue in the primer pTP. Two more nucleotides are added forming a trinucleotide intermediate (pTP–CAT). Then, in another remarkable reaction, the trinucleotide intermediate jumps back to base pair with template bases 1 to 3 (another CAT triplet). pTP then starts to dissociate from Ad pol (de Jong et al. 2003b).

Elongation and strand displacement synthesis   After dissociation, pol replicates the entire adenovirus genome resulting in strand displacement DNA synthesis of the nontemplate strand. Oct-1 dissoci-

ates as the polymerase elongates past the Oct-1 binding site. Strand displacement elongation synthesis requires DBP and another cellular protein, type I topoisomerase nuclear factor II. At late times after infection, pTP is processed by a virus-encoded protease into the mature TP. The displaced strand is coated by DBP and by virtue of its inverted terminal repeats it can form a panhandle type molecule which contains a stem reminiscent of the duplex of the initial double-stranded DNA template. The duplex can then be recognized by NF1, Oct-1 and the pTP–pol heterodimer and a new cycle of protein primed DNA synthesis can occur (de Jong et al. 2003b).

Summary

In summary, adenovirus DNA replication is of interest because of its intermediate size and coding potential; it encodes many but not all DNA replication proteins. It is thus a relatively simple replication system compared to SV40 and the other smaller DNA viruses which utilizes the very elaborate cellular replication complex. The protein priming mechanism used by adenovirus and the lack of a requirement for a helicase contribute to the simplicity of this system compared to polyoma- and papillomaviruses that utilize cellular polymerases. Other DNA viruses which encode replication machinery such as the herpesviruses and poxviruses are also much more complex. Also of interest are the complex interactions between adenovirus and the host cell.

HERPESVIRUSES

The family *Herpesviridae* encompasses a wide variety of both human and animal pathogens capable of causing medically and economically important diseases in a broad range of hosts. Eight are known to infect humans including herpes simplex virus type 1 (HSV-1) and herpes simplex virus type 2 (HSV-2), Epstein–Barr virus (EBV), cytomegalovirus (HCMV), varicella-zoster virus (VZV), human herpesvirus 6 (HHV-6), human herpesvirus 7 (HHV-7), and Kaposi's sarcoma herpesvirus (KSHV). Herpesviruses, in general, share many aspects of virion structure, genomic organization, and life cycle (described in Chapter 25, Herpesviruses: general properties). For the purposes of this chapter, HSV-1 will be discussed as the primary example of herpesvirus DNA replication; HSV has been studied more extensively than the other herpesviruses, perhaps due to the fact that it is amenable to both genetic and biochemical analysis.

General features of DNA replication

The herpesviruses encode a large number of replication proteins, some of which are functional analogues of cellular replication machinery. Furthermore, the virus appears to have evolved a strategy of DNA replication

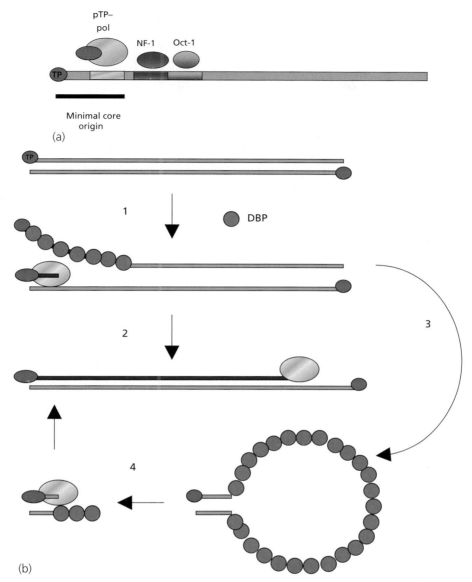

Figure 10.8 *Replication of adenoviral DNA.* **(a)** *The minimal core adenovirus origin of replication consists of the terminal 18 bp of the viral genome which contain the binding site for the pTP–pol heterodimer (9–18 bp). Adjacent to the 9–18 bp region are binding sites for the cellular transcriptional activators NFI (bind residues 25–39) and Oct-1 (binds 39–48), and these proteins facilitate the initiation reaction by binding at the origin and stimulating the association of the pTP–pol heterodimer to the origin. The pTP–pol interaction with the origin is stabilized by interactions with the TP–DNA, between pTP and Oct-1, and Adpol and NF1.* **(b)** *Step 1. The initiation of adenoviral DNA synthesis involves the assembly of a heterodimer consisting of the preterminal protein (pTP) and DNA polymerase (pol) (light green and gold). This heterodimer forms a preinitiation complex with the minimal core origin of replication. DNA replication is initiated by an pol-catalyzed protein priming mechanism in which a covalent bond is formed between the -phosphoryl group of the terminal residue, dCMP, and the hydroxyl group of a serine residue in pTPB. Step 2. The free 3′ OH group of the pTP–dCMP moiety primes elongation in a leading strand type reaction, resulting in the displacement of the non-template strand which becomes coated with DSB, the single-stranded binding protein. The elongation reaction also requires a cellular topoisomerase. Step 3. The displaced strand can form a panhandle reaction due to the complementarity of the inverted repeats at the termini of the adenoviral genome. The short duplex stem can be used to initiate a new round of viral DNA synthesis, steps 3 and 4. At later times in infection pTP (larger green oval) is processed by a virus-encoded protease into the mature TP (smaller green oval) (not shown).*

which utilizes DNA recombination (Wilkinson and Weller 2003). This feature is reminiscent of several of the large DNA bacteriophages including T4 and lambda. The viral genomes are linear molecules which replicate through longer-than-unit-length concatemers. Monomeric genomic units are packaged by cleavage from concatemers in a reaction that occurs in conjunction with the uptake of genomes into preassembled capsids.

HSV GENOME

The genome of HSV is large (152 kbp) and structurally complex, containing two unique regions (U_L and U_S)

that are flanked by the inverted repeat sequences *b* and *c*, respectively. The *a* sequence is present at both termini and an inverted copy is present at the U_L–U_S junction (Figure 10.9a). The HSV genome is capable of genomic inversions in which the U_L and U_S components invert their orientation during replication. HSV-1 is believed to encode over 80 open reading frames. Viral genes are classified as immediate–early, early or late and are transcribed from both strands of the viral genome.

Origins of DNA replication

Three origins of replication have been identified within the HSV genome (Figure 10.9b) (reviewed in Marintcheva and Weller 2001). One origin, OriS, is present in each 'c' component of the short region and thus is present twice in the viral genome and one origin,

OriL, is present in the unique long region between the major DNA binding protein (ICP8) and the DNA polymerase. Both origins contain AT-rich sequences and several recognition sites for UL9, the origin binding protein. OriL contains a near perfect palindrome of 144 bp while OriS contains a shorter palindrome. Both origins are situated between transcriptional initiation sites. OriL, and one copy of OriS, can be deleted without affecting the ability of the virus to multiply, suggesting that viral replication can occur in genomes containing only one copy of the genome.

Viral replication proteins

The HSV-1 genome encodes seven essential replication proteins and several nonessential replication proteins (Table 10.5) (Challberg 1986). These include an origin

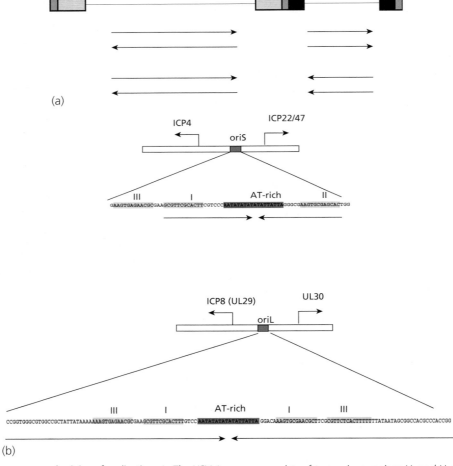

(a)

(b)

Figure 10.9 HSV genome and origins of replication. A. The HSV-1 genome consists of two unique regions U_L and U_S flanked by repeated sequences. U_L is flanked by ab and b'a'; whereas, U_S is flanked by ac and c'a'. During infection, the two unique regions invert relative to each other. The arrows reflect possible orientations of the U_L and U_S segments as a result of genomic inversion. **(b)** HSV-1 Origins of replication. OriS is situated between the immediate early genes ICP4 and ICP22/47. It contains three UL9 binding sites highlighted in yellow (Boxes I, II, and III) and an AT-rich region (highlighted in green). OriS also contains an almost perfect 22-bp palindrome (marked with arrows) OriL is situated between the ICP8 gene (UC29) and the DNA polymerase gene (UL30). It contains four binding sites for the origin recognition protein UL9 highlighted in yellow (Boxes I, II, III, and IV), and AT-rich region (highlighted in green), and a perfect 144-bp palindrome (marked with arrows).

Table 10.5 Herpes simplex virus *replication proteins*

Viral Protein	Function
UL30 (DNA pol)	Synthesis of leading- and lagging-strand DNA; associated 3′ to 5′ proofreading exonuclease; target for several antiviral drugs
UL42	HSV DNA pol processivity factor
UL9	Origin binding; DNA-stimulated ATPase and helicase
UL5, UL8, and UL52	Helicase primase complex; UL8 interacts with ICP8 and HSV pol
ICP8 (UL29)	Viral single-strand DNA-binding protein; binds cooperatively to single-stranded DNA; binds UL42 protein
Thymidine kinase	Phosphorylates thymidine; essential in nondividing cells
Ribonucleotide reductase	Reduces ribose to deoxyribose; essential in nondividing cells
dUTPase	Hydrolyzes dUTP to dUMP; prevents uracil incorporation into DNA
Uracil N glycosylase	Removes uracil from DNA; may be important for DNA repair
Alkaline nuclease (UL12)	Interacts with ICP8 and may promote single-stranded annealing during recombination-dependent DNA replication

binding protein (UL9) and six core replication proteins including a two subunit DNA polymerase (UL30 and UL42), a single-stranded DNA-binding protein (known as ICP8 or UL29) and a three subunit helicase/primase complex (UL5, UL8, and UL52) (Challberg 1986; reviewed in Marintcheva and Weller 2001). Among the eight human herpesviruses and dozens of animal herpesviruses, most encode homologues of the six core replication viral proteins involved in DNA replication, and it is likely that the strategy of replication is also conserved.

UL9

UL9 is a 94-kDa protein possessing the following activities: DNA-dependent nucleoside triphosphatase, DNA helicase on partially double-stranded substrates, ability to form dimers in solution, and cooperative origin-specific DNA binding. The ability of UL9 to bind specifically to origin DNA has been localized to the carboxy-terminal one-third (residues 564–832) of UL9. Protein sequence analysis indicates that the N-terminal domain (residues 1–534) contain seven conserved helicase motifs, characteristic of the SF2 family of helicases. The nuclear localization signal (NLS) of UL9 has been mapped to the C terminal 105 amino acid residues (reviewed in Marintcheva and Weller 2001).

UL30/UL42

UL30 encodes the 140 kDal catalytic subunit of the HSV polymerase, and UL42 encodes the 53 kDal processivity factor. Since no viral DNA synthesis can be detected in the presence of drugs which inhibit the viral polymerase or in cells infected with mutants defective for viral polymerase, it is believed that UL30/UL42 is the sole polymerase needed during viral DNA replication and that it functions as both the leading and lagging strand polymerase. The HSV polymerase has been studied extensively and is the target for antiviral drugs.

UL5/UL8/UL52

The HSV-1 helicase/primase is a three protein heterotrimer consisting of the products of the *UL5*, *UL8*, and *UL52* genes. All three genes are essential in cell culture. The *UL5/UL8/UL52* complex displays DNA-dependent ATPase, primase, and helicase activities (reviewed in Marintcheva and Weller 2001). A subcomplex consisting of UL5/UL52 displays similar activities. The precise function of UL8 within the heterotrimeric complex is not clear. In vitro, the helicase and primase activities do not depend on UL8; however, the ATPase and primase activities of the UL5/UL52 subcomplex can be stimulated in vitro by the addition of UL8. UL8 may also play a role in the proper localization of the UL5/UL8/UL52 complex to the nucleus. Furthermore, since UL8 can interact with other members of the replication machinery including UL9, UL30, and ICP8, it appears that UL8 may act to coordinate complex protein–protein interactions which occur at the replication fork. UL52 contains a motif conserved in many primases which, when altered, abolishes primase but not ATPase and helicase activity. This suggests that the UL52 subunit is likely the primase of the complex; however, recent work indicates that the UL52 subunit may contribute significantly to helicase activity as well (Carrington-Lawrence and Weller 2003). Sequence analysis indicates that UL5 contains seven motifs found in a large superfamily of known and putative helicases, SF1. Thus UL5 is likely to be the helicase of the complex, although it appears that UL52 may also be involved in helicase activity, perhaps by providing at least one DNA binding site.

UL29 or ICP8

ICP8 is the 130 kDa single-stranded binding protein of HSV. ICP8 binds preferentially to ssDNA and exhibits helix-destabilizing activity. ICP8 can also promote strand transfer and is believed to play a role in the high level of recombination exhibited during HSV DNA replication.

Recent work indicates that through its interaction with a viral nuclease (UL12), this two subunit complex may constitute a simple recombinase analogous to the simple red recombinase encoded by bacteriophage lambda (Reuven et al. 2004).

ICP8 is known to interact with other DNA replication proteins such as UL9, UL8, and HSV polymerase, and is believed to be essential for both the initiation and elongation of viral DNA synthesis. ICP8 also plays a role in the localization of viral proteins to replication compartments in infected cell nuclei and in the control of viral gene transcription.

Nonessential viral gene products

In addition to the seven required viral replication proteins, HSV also encodes several nonessential auxiliary proteins such as thymidine kinase, deoxyuridine triphosphatase, ribonucleotide reductase, and uracil N-glycosylase. Some of these proteins participate in nucleotide biosynthesis and others such as dUTPase and uracil-N-glycosylase may be important in preventing misincorporation of uracil residues into the viral genome.

Overall model for HSV DNA replication

Although the exact mechanism of HSV DNA replication is not known, it has long been recognized that the products of DNA replication are larger-than-unit-length concatemers consisting of tandem repeats of the viral genome (reviewed in Marintcheva and Weller 2001). Most of the incoming viral DNA molecules lose their free ends shortly after infection by a process that does not require de novo protein synthesis, and the simplest interpretation of these results is that the viral genome loses its free ends through the formation of a covalently closed circular molecule. It was previously thought that linear virion DNA is rapidly circularized in infected cells and that concatemers were generated by rolling circle replication; however, this model has never been directly confirmed experimentally. Several aspects of this model, including the initial circularization and the rolling circle mechanism, have recently been challenged experimentally, and new models are being considered (Jackson and De Luca 2003). For instance, replicating DNA adopts a complex, possibly branched, structure which could reflect recombination intermediates. It appears that endless viral DNA does not arise as a result of simple end-to-end joining of viral termini by nonhomologous end joining, although it is possible that homologous recombination events may play a role. New models have been proposed suggesting that the viral genome adopts an endless configuration by an intra- or intermolecular homologous recombination events which occur during replication (discussed below) (Wilkinson and Weller 2003).

Initiation   Viral DNA synthesis is believed to initiate at one of the three viral origins of replication. UL9 is essential for HSV DNA replication and has been shown to bind the origins of DNA replication in a cooperative and sequence-specific manner; however, many details of this reaction are still unclear. For instance, although UL9 is believed to be an ATP-dependent DNA helicase, in vitro, it has not been shown to unwind duplex DNA containing an origin of replication. Some distortion at this region can be detected but no actual unwinding (reviewed in Marintcheva and Weller 2001). This is in contrast to SV40 large T antigen that is able to unwind duplex DNA in an ATP-dependent fashion. Recent evidence suggests that UL9 binding at the origin may not be as straightforward as binding to its recognition site within duplex DNA. In in vitro experiments, single-stranded oriS has been reported to fold into a unique conformation, OriS*, which is stably bound by UL9. OriS* contains a stable hairpin formed by complementary base pairing between box I and box III in OriS (Aslani et al. 2001). It has been proposed that that UL9, in conjunction with the single-stranded DNA-binding protein ICP8, can convert OriS to its alternate conformation, OriS*, and form an OBP–OriS* complex. This model has not been tested in vivo however.

Elongation   Once the origin is distorted by UL9 and ICP8, it is believed that the heterotrimeric helicase/primase complex can be recruited (Figure 10.10) (Marintcheva and Weller 2001). Several lines of evidence suggest the ordered assembly of viral replication proteins at the origin. Using immunofluorescence, a subassembly, or scaffold, has been identified consisting of five viral proteins: UL9, ICP8, and the helicase/primase. This scaffold can be detected as ICP8-containing foci in cells infected with wild-type HSV (Burkham et al. 2001). The recruitment of polymerase to this scaffold requires the presence of an active primase subunit (Carrington-Lawrence and Weller 2003). These results suggest that polymerase recruitment to replication foci requires primer synthesis and support the model of an ordered assembly of replication proteins at the replication fork leading to leading and lagging strand DNA synthesis.

Once elongation has begun, leading- and lagging-strand DNA synthesis would be expected to proceed until the replication apparatus either reaches the end of the linear DNA molecule or reaches a nick or gap. Since nicks and gaps have been reported to be present in the viral genome, this may occur soon after elongation has begun. It has recently been proposed that such an event could result in a fundamentally different mode of replication which utilizes a recombination strategy to continue DNA synthesis (Wilkinson and Weller 2003). The ability of replication to begin again after such an event may signal the second stage of replication which would be dependent on cellular or viral recombination

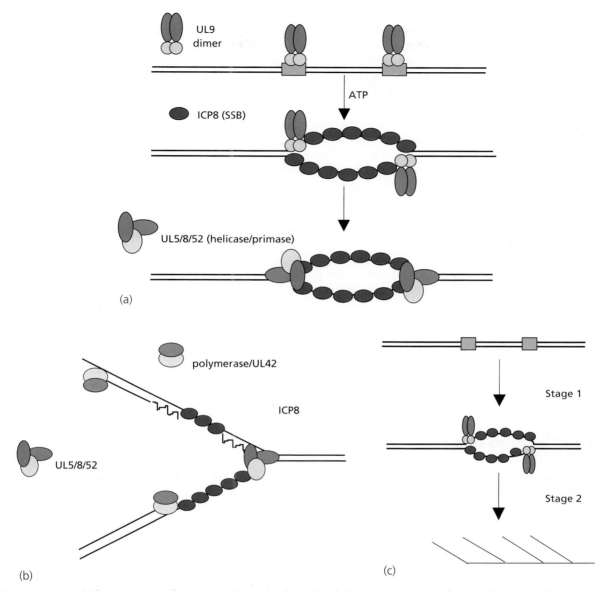

Figure 10.10 *Model for HSV DNA replication.* **(a)** *OriS can be depicted with three recognition sites for UL9, the origin-binding protein (Boxes I, II, and III) and an AT-rich linker positioned between box I and II. According to this model, UL9 dimers bind cooperatively to Boxes I and II and cause either a distortion or an opening of the AT-rich spacer region. In this step UL9 likely acts in conjunction with ICP8. Following the opening, the helicase/primase can be recruited to the complex. UL9, ICP8 and the helicase/primase complex are apparently recruited together during the formation of replication centers [80–82].* **(b)** *An HSV-1 replication fork would be expected to contain the helicase-primase complex (UL5/UL52/UL8) at the fork: UL5 would be expected to unwind duplex DNA ahead of the fork and U52 would be expected to lay down RNA primers which could then be extended by the two subunit DNA polymerase (UL30/UL42). The HSV-1 pol would also be expected to carry out leading-strand synthesis. ICP8 (UL29, SSB) would be expected to bind to ssDNA generated during HSV DNA synthesis. C). In this model, two stages of replication are envisioned, an UL9 dependent step which takes place at origins of replication (Stage 1) and a UL9 independent step which likely involves recombination-dependent replication (Stage 2).*

proteins to 'restart' the replication process. This second stage of replication would not be expected to be dependent on UL9 and, in fact, UL9 is not essential at later times after infection. The later stages of HSV replication are likely to involve recombination although it cannot be ruled out that some rolling circle replication also occurs (Figure 10.10c). The virus encodes a simple recombinase consisting of ICP8 and the viral nuclease UL12 (Reuven et al. 2003). It is possible that viral and cellular recombination proteins are involved during these later stages of viral DNA replication (Wilkinson and Weller 2003). Details of these reactions are the subject of on going studies.

Summary

HSV appears to be unique in the animal DNA viruses in that it exhibits a complex relationship between DNA replication and recombination. In this respect it seems more similar to the large DNA bacteriophages, T4 and λ, which replicate via concatemers of tandemly repeated monomeric units using rolling circle replication as well as multiple pathways to carry out homologous recombination. The seven replication proteins of HSV may work in combination with both viral and cellular recombination proteins during this process, the details of which remain unclear. In summary, it appears that HSV DNA replication occurs in two stages. The first stage involves an origin-UL9 dependent step and in the second stage DNA replication may proceed in an origin-independent manner via a recombination-driven and/or rolling circle mechanism (Wilkinson and Weller 2003).

POXVIRUSES

The poxviruses make up a particularly interesting group of pathogens responsible for devastating human diseases such as smallpox. Poxviruses have been isolated from many animal hosts, and cowpox and vaccinia viruses have been used as vaccines to protect humans from the smallpox virus, variola virus. Poxviruses are unique among the DNA viruses in their ability to replicate entirely within the cytoplasm. They are large complex viruses which exhibit considerable independence from the host cells (Depamphilis 1996).

General features of poxvirus DNA replication

Poxviruses have the largest genomes of any known DNA viruses, and they have been shown to encode all of the proteins needed for DNA replication including DNA polymerase, a processivity factor, two protein kinases, a protein phosphatase, and a DNA ligase (Boyle and Traktman 2004). Although the function of the kinases and phosphatase are not entirely clear, their existence suggests that protein phosphorylation may play an important role in regulating either DNA replication or another step in the virus life cycle. DNA replication occurs in the cytoplasm in specialized foci called viral factories. After fusion of viral and cellular membranes, the inner viral core is localized in the cytoplasm, and early gene expression occurs within these cores. Early mRNAs are extruded from the core where they are translated by host ribosomes. Some of these early proteins encode replication proteins. A secondary uncoating event occurs and viral genomes are released and accessible to replication proteins. Replication occurs in two stages: synthesis of genomes as concatemeric intermediates and resolution of these concaters into mature, monomeric genomes (Depamphilis 1996).

POXVIRUS GENOMES

Poxviruses have linear double-stranded DNA genomes which vary in size from 130 kbp to around 230 kbp. The

vaccinia genome has a very unusual structure: it is composed of a linear duplex of 192 kbp with covalently closed hairpin termini resembling telomeres. The genomes are AT-rich and the inverted terminal hairpin repeats also contain primarily A and T residues (Du and Traktman 1996).

Origins of replication

The termini are believed to contain the origins of replication. In vaccinia, for instance, the telomeric 65 nucleotides can be replicated in infected cells; however, the efficiency of replication increased with the inclusion of additional adjacent sequences. Maximal efficiency was obtained with plasmids containing the 200 terminal bp (Du and Traktman 1996). This region contains the hairpin loop, a region of unique sequences containing a sequence required for genome resolution and a set of 70-bp repeats. The hairpin loop contains 40 base-paired residues and a four-nucleotide loop at the very terminus. In addition, there are some unpaired residues termed extrahelical bases which are asymmetrically located; one strand has ten and the other two. This unusual genomic structure is conserved in all poxviruses. Two isoforms of the genome are found which represent inverted complements of each other and are called flip and flop. The presence of these extrahelical bases and their position within the termini are believed to be important during genome replication.

Viral proteins involved in DNA replication

Several viral proteins have been implicated in viral DNA replication; however, their roles are not well understood (Table 10.6). Genetic analysis has revealed three gene products, E9, D5, and B1 as important since mutants with defects in these genes are defective in DNA synthesis. Another gene, D4, may also be important. Some genes have been identified by sequence analysis. The E9 gene encodes the viral DNA polymerase which is related to alpha family of DNA polymerases. This protein exhibits DNA polymerase as well as 3' to 5' exonuclease activity. A factor which enhances the processivity of the polymerase has been inferred by the observation that infected cell extracts contain a polymerase activity which is highly processive while the purified E9 gene product is distributive. The product of the A20 open reading frame has been reported to be the polymerase processivity factor (Ishii and Moss 2001; Klemperer et al. 2001). Vaccinia also encodes an NTPase (D5 gene) and a protein kinase (B1 gene) whose precise roles in DNA replication are not clear. An early protein H5 appears to be a substrate for the B1 kinase and these two proteins interact with each other, but its role is unclear. Recent evidence suggests that A20 may interact with three other vaccinia proteins, D4, D5, and H5, and that A20 may play an important role in

Table 10.6 *Poxviral proteins that participate in genome replication*

Vaccinia Viral Protein	Function	Expression
DNA polymerase (E9)	Synthesis of viral DNA; associated 3′–5′ exonuclease for proofreading	Early
A20	Processivity factor	Early
D5	NTPase	Early
B1	Serine–threonine kinase	Early
D4	Uracil DNA glycosylase	Early
A50	DNA ligase	Early
Type I topoisomerase (H6)	Unknown but essential	Late (in capsid)
Thymidine kinase ((J2)	Phosphorylates thymidine; essential	Early
Thymidylate kinase (A48)	Phosphorylates TMP	Early
Ribonucleotide Reductase (F4, 14)	Reduces ribose in ribonucleotides to deoxyribose; essential in nondividing cells	Early
dUTPase (F2)	Hydrolyzes dUTP to dUMP	Early
DNase (?)	Has nicking; joining activity	Early

forming or stabilizing the DNA replication complex. Other viral proteins include a DNA ligase which is not essential in tissue culture, and enzymes involved in nucleotide biosynthesis including thymidine kinase, thymidylate kinase, and ribonucleotide reductase. The virus also encodes a Topisomerase I which is found in viral capsids and a dUTPase and a uracil DNA glycosylase which may play roles in DNA replication and/or DNA repair (De Silva and Moss 2003). Details about the precise roles of these proteins are unclear.

Mechanism of DNA replication

Although poxvirus DNA replication is not well understood, models have been suggested based on current evidence. The first step in genome replication is believed to be the introduction of a nick in sequence within the genomic terminus generating a 3′ OH which can be extended by the viral DNA polymerase. Strand displacement synthesis would be expected to extend the template to the terminus. Since the terminus itself is self complementary, a duplex hairpin can form providing a 3′ OH group that can be extended back in the other direction resulting in the formation of a dimeric tail-to-tail concatemer. This process could occur again resulting in the generation of tetrameric or even higher order concatemers. Concatemeric intermediates have been detected experimentally. This model is consistent with leading strand DNA synthesis. As with the herpesviruses, recombination is also a frequent event during poxvirus DNA replication, and it is possible that recombination events such as strand invasion may play a role in viral DNA replication.

It is believed that concatemeric intermediates can be resolved into monomeric units prior to packaging. Plasmids containing the unique resolution sequences can be resolved into linear minichromosomes with authentic hairpin termini after transfection into infected cells. The protein(s) which recognize the resolution sequences has not been identified to date.

Summary

The poxviruses provide a fascinating example of a viral DNA replication system which encodes all of the required proteins. This virus poses unique challenges experimentally which have slowed progress in elucidation of the precise roles of the viral factors.

HOST–VIRUS INTERACTIONS

In recent years it has become clear that viruses rely on the host in previously unknown ways both in terms of localization within the host cell and the utilization of host factors. For instance, viral genomes have been shown to localize to specific sites within the nucleus (Ishov and Maul 1996; Tang et al. 2000). This localization is thought to involve specific interactions with cellular proteins. In addition, several viruses exhibit complex interactions with the cell cycle. Infection with SV40 and papillomaviruses can alter the host-cell cycle by inducing the host-cell DNA synthetic machinery (Munger et al. 1989; Cheng et al. 1995). Since these viruses depend on cellular proteins such as DNA polymerases, RPA, PCNA etc., the induction of the S phase of the cell cycle is essential for genome replication. Other types of interactions involve both the utilization of host cell proteins which benefit their reproductive strategies and in some cases inactivation of cellular response mechanisms which are inhibitory.

Interactions between viral and cellular proteins

Although adeno- and herpesviruses encode their own polymerases and are therefore somewhat more independent of the cell machinery than are the polyoma- and papillomaviruses, these viruses also exhibit very complex interactions with host cell machinery. For instance it has recently been shown that in cells infected with adenovirus, a multiprotein complex consisting of Mre11, Rad50, and NBS1 appears to be inactivated (Stracker et al. 2002). The Mre11 complex is important for double-strand break repair, and infection with adenovirus alters its activity by two mechanisms: spatial reorganization of this complex within the cell and degradation of certain components of this complex. Mutants of adenovirus which fail to inactivate the Mre11 complex have been shown to form concatemers and to replicate inefficiently (Stracker et al. 2002). The evolution of a strategy to promote replication of monomer length molecules by strand displacement as seen in Figure 10.8b belies a complex viral–host interaction in which some cellular pathways remain intact and others are inactivated. Recent work with herpes simplex viruses suggests that this virus inactivates a different cellular pathway, the nonhomologous end joining (NHEJ) pathway (Jackson and DeLuca 2003; Wilkinson and Weller 2003). During the earliest stages of infection, the NHEJ pathway is inactivated by spatial reorganization and by degradation. Another fascinating aspect of virus–host interactions involves the regulation of viral proteins by post-translational modification. We have seen several examples of viral proteins regulated by phosphorylation

using viral and cellular protein kinases (Fanning and Knippers 1992; Nuesch et al. 2001; Ott et al. 2002). Also of interest is the use of molecular chaperones during the viral life cycle. The use of both host-encoded chaperones and virus-specific chaperones has been reported. For instance, it has been shown that in human papillomavirus, E1 protein binding to the origin can be stimulated by the human Hsp70 and Hsp40 chaperone proteins (Lin et al. 2002). Furthermore, SV40 T antigen itself is a functional molecular chaperone J protein. It is expected that chaperones will be implicated in the assembly and function of the replication machinery of many if not all DNA viruses.

Replication within replication compartments or replication centers

Viral DNA replication often takes place within well-defined regions of the cells. In the case of poxviruses, replication occurs within cytoplasmic viral factories. All other DNA viruses replicate in the nucleus, again within well defined regions. In the case of adenovirus and herpesviruses, DNA replication occurs within replication compartments or centers which contain viral genomes and viral and cellular replication proteins. The formation of such compartments may be important for replication efficiency as cellular and viral factors can be concentrated at these sites. Sequestration in such

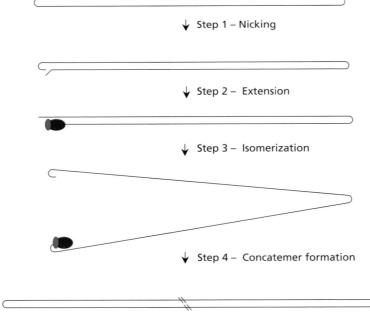

Figure 10.11 *Poxvirus DNA replication. A model for poxviral DNA replication is shown. The parental genome is a linear duplex with covalently closed termini. Step 1. A nick is introduced into the duplex creating a 3' OH group which can be extended by the viral DNA polymerase and processivity factor (shown as ovals). Step 2. Replication proceeds by extension of the primer and copies the left end of the genome. Step 3. Because of the terminal redundancy, the nascent DNA can isomerize to form another hairpin. Step 4. The hairpin structure can be elongated along the length of the genome, around the hairpin and along the complementary strand to form a dimer intermediate.*

compartments may also represent a strategy for limiting access to viral genomes during replication for the purpose of inhibiting apoptosis.

Genomes of several DNA viruses which replicate in the nucleus including SV40, adenoviruses, and herpesviruses (at least HSV and HCMV) appear to localize at sites adjacent to ND10 (Ishov and Maul 1996; Tang et al. 2000; Everett 2001). ND10 are subcellular structures or foci which are defined by those which have been identified including PML containing foci known as ND10 or PML nuclear bodies or PML oncogenic domains (PODs) (Burkham et al. 2001). Viral gene expression is also believed to occur at these sites. ND10 are defined by the accumulation of PM, SP100, SUMO, and other cellular proteins involved in growth control, gene expression, and possibly DNA recombination. ND10 are dynamic structures with many of its constituents able to shuttle between the cytoplasm and the nucleus. The common association of viral DNA genomes with ND10 may indicate that proximity to ND10 or some cellular site associated with ND10 may provide a beneficial environment for viral gene expression and viral DNA replication. Cellular proteins involved in DNA recombination and repair have been shown to localize to ND10 or to ND10-related sites. Ionizing radiation induces the increased expression of PML and the relocalization of ND10 proteins to sites of DNA damage as defined by staining for γH2AX, a marker for dsDNA breaks. The relationship of DNA viruses with the repair/recombination machinery of the cell may be important for viral DNA replication (Wilkinson and Weller 2003). Viral DNA molecules which are located at or near ND10 may have access to cellular recombination and repair proteins. This may confer an advantage for DNA replication.

Viral replication proteins and cellular transformation

Several DNA viruses have been associated with human cancers and morphological transformation. The best studied is SV40 which is known to transform rodent cells in culture. SV40 large T antigen is known to deregulate cellular proliferation pathways and can efficiently immortalize primary rodent cells and transform established rodent cell lines to tumorigenicity (Simmons 2000). The transformation ability of T antigen is caused by its specific interactions with host-cell proteins. The tumor suppressor protein p53 was originally identified by its ability to interact with SV40 large T antigen. T antigen also interacts with another tumor suppressor protein, pRB, and the study of these interactions has greatly improved our understanding of the roles of these cellular proteins in the cell cycle and the role of viral oncogenes transformation. As mentioned above, the N terminus of T antigen has also been shown to contain a

DnaJ domain which is required for efficient viral replication and perhaps for transformation as well. Recently, the N terminus of T antigen has also been shown to interact with the mitotic spindle checkpoint protein Bub1. Perturbations of this spindle checkpoint may result in aneuploidy and genetic instability leading to cell transformation. Thus viral proteins such as large T antigen continue to provide many insights into the host cell and to responses which lead to oncogenesis and cancer (Munger et al. 1989; Cheng et al. 1995; Simmons 2000; Longworth and Laimins 2004).

SUMMARY

The study of viral DNA replication has been important for many reasons. Replication proteins are still the major targets for antiviral therapy, and thus a thorough understanding of viral replication proteins continues to facilitate the development of novel antiviral strategies. In addition, viruses provide useful windows into the cell: most of what is currently known about mammalian DNA replication strategies came about through studies with SV40. The diversity of strategies exhibited by DNA viruses from SV40 and polyomaviruses which rely almost entirely on host-cell machinery to the poxviruses which encode all the proteins required for genome replication have provided a rich field of study. By comparing viral systems, several important principles have emerged and common mechanisms have been identified. Most viral systems require an origin recognition protein, one or more DNA polymerases, proteins that enhance processive DNA synthesis, origin unwinding and helicase functions and a mechanism for priming DNA synthesis. The diversity in priming is perhaps the most interesting: some viruses use RNA primers and discontinuous synthesis of lagging strands reminiscent of cellular DNA replication strategies, whereas others use protein priming or DNA sequence primers. Each mechanism has implications for how ends are replicated and how progeny genomes are produced during encapsidation. Adenovirus genomes replicate and are packaged primarily as monomers, while the herpesviruses replicate as concatemers which must be processed into monomers during encapsidation.

Because viruses need to replicate many copies of their genomes in relatively short periods of time, most DNA viruses have evolved very efficient replication strategies. The evolution of viral replication proteins which can recruit cellular factors results in the concentration of viral and cellular proteins in specialized regions of the cell leading to enhanced replication efficiency. It is anticipated that better understanding of the complex virus–host interactions leading to efficient viral replication will provide additional insights into eukaryotic cell biology as well. Furthermore, the ability of some viruses to transform cells suggests that important lessons of cellular transformation will be learned from the continued study of the replication strategies of DNA viruses.

REFERENCES

Aslani, A., Macao, B., et al. 2001. Complementary intrastrand base pairing during initiation of Herpes simplex virus type 1 DNA replication. *Proc Natl Acad Sci USA*, **98**, 7194–9.

Berns, K.I. 1990. Parvovirus replication. *Microbiol Reviews*, **54**, 316–329.

Boyle, K.A. and Traktman, P. 2004. Members of a novel family of mammalian protein kinases complement the DNA-negative phenotype of a vaccinia virus ts mutant defective in the B1 kinase. *J Virol*, **78**, 1992–2005.

Brenkman, A.B., Breure, E.C. and van der Vliet, P.C. 2002. Molecular architecture of adenovirus DNA polymerase and location of the protein primer. *J Virol*, **76**, 8200–7.

Broker, T.R. and Chow, L.T. 2001. Human papillomaviruses: A window into the mechanism and regulation of eucaryotic cellular DNA replication. *Dev Biol*, **106**, 367–73.

Burkham, J., Coen, D.M., et al. 2001. Interactions of herpes simplex virus type 1 with ND10 and recruitment of PML to replication compartments. *J Virol*, **75**, 2353–67.

Carrington-Lawrence, S.D. and Weller, S.K. 2003. Recruitment of polymerase to herpes simplex virus type 1 replication foci in cells expressing mutant primase (UL52) proteins. *J Virol*, **77**, 4237–47.

Challberg, M.D. 1986. A method for identifying the viral genes required for herpesvirus DNA replication. *Proc Natl Acad Sci USA*, **83**, 9094–8.

Chen, G. and Stenlund, A. 2002. Sequential and ordered assembly of E1 initiator complexes on the papillomavirus origin of DNA replication generates progressive structural changes related to melting. *Mol Cell Biol*, **22**, 7712–20.

Cheng, S., Schmidt, G.D., et al. 1995. Differentiation-dependent up-regulation of the human papillomavirus E7 gene reactivates cellular DNA replication in suprabasal differentiated keratinocytes. *Genes Dev*, **9**, 2335–49.

Christensen, J. and Tattersall, P. 2002. Parvovirus initiator protein NS1 and RPA coordinate replication fork progression in a reconstituted DNA replication system. *J Virol*, **76**, 6518–31.

Cotmore, S.F., Christensen, J., et al. 1995. The NS1 polypeptide of the murine parvovirus minute virus of mice binds to DNA sequences containing the motif [ACCA]2-3. *J Virol*, **69**, 1652–60.

de Jong, R.N. and van der Vliet, P.C. 1999. Mechanism of DNA replication in eukaryotic cells: cellular host factors stimulating adenovirus DNA replication. *Gene*, **236**, 1–12.

de Jong, R.N., Meijer, L.A. and van der Vliet, P.C. 2003a. DNA binding properties of the adenovirus DNA replication priming protein pTP. *Nucleic Acids Res*, **31**, 3274–86.

de Jong, R.N., van der Vliet, P.C. and Brenkman, A.B. 2003b. Adenovirus DNA replication, protein priming, jumping back and the role of the DNA binding protein DBP. *Curr Top Microbiol Immunol*, **272**, 187–211.

Depamphilis, M. 1996. DNA replication. In: Depamphilis, M.L. (ed.), *Eukaryotic cells*. NY: Cold Spring Harbor Laboratory Press.

De Silva, F.S. and Moss, B. 2003. Vaccinia virus uracil DNA glycosylase has an essential role in DNA synthesis that is independent of its glycosylase activity: catalytic site mutations reduce virulence but not virus replication in cultured cells. *J Virol*, **77**, 159–66.

Du, S. and Traktman, P. 1996. Vaccinia virus DNA replication: two hundred base pairs of telomeric sequence confer optimal replication efficiency on minichromosome templates. *Proc Natl Acad Sci USA*, **93**, 9693–8.

Enemark, E.J., Chen, G., et al. 2000. Crystal structure of the DNA binding domain of the replication initiation protein E1 from papillomavirus. *Mol Cell*, **6**, 149–58.

Everett, R.D. 2001. DNA viruses and viral proteins that interact with PML nuclear bodies. *Oncogene*, **20**, 7266–73.

Fanning, E. and Knippers, R. 1992. Structure and function of simian virus 40 large tumor antigen. *Annu Rev Biochem*, **61**, 55–85.

Flores, E.R. and Lambert, P.F. 1997. Evidence for a switch in the mode of human papilloma virus type 16 DNA replication during the viral life cycle. *J Virol*, **71**, 7167–79.

Gai, D., Roy, R., et al. 2000. Topoisomerase I associates specifically with simian virus 40 large-T-antigen double hexamer-origin complexes. *J Virol*, **74**, 5224–32.

Hay, R.T. and DePamphilis, M.L. 1982. Initiation of SV40 DNA replication in vivo: location and structure of 5′ ends of DNA synthesized in the ori region. *Cell*, **28**, 767–79.

Hickman, A.B., Ronning, D.R., Kotin, R.M., and Dyda, F., 2002. Structural unity among viral origin binding protein: crystal structure of the nuclease domain of adeno-associated virus Rep. *Mol Cell*, **101**, 327–37.

Im, D.S. and Muzyczka, N. 1990. The AAV origin binding protein Rep68 is an ATP-dependent site-specific endonuclease with DNA helicase activity. *Cell*, **61**, 447–57.

Ishii, K. and Moss, B. 2001. Role of vaccinia virus A20R protein in DNA replication: construction and characterization of temperature-sensitive mutants. *J Virol*, **75**, 1656–63.

Ishov, A.M. and Maul, G.G. 1996. The periphery of nuclear domain 10 (ND10) as site of DNA virus deposition. *J Cell Biol*, **134**, 815–26.

Jackson, S.A. and DeLuca, N.A. 2003. Relationship of herpes simplex virus genome configuration to productive and persistent infections. *Proc Natl Acad Sci USA*, **100**, 7871–6.

Klemperer, N., McDonald, W., et al. 2001. The A20R protein is a stoichiometric component of the processive form of vaccinia virus DNA polymerase. *J Virol*, **75**, 12298–307.

Kornberg, A. and Baker, T.A. 1992. *DNA replication*. New York: W.H. Freeman and Co.

Li, D., Zhao, R., et al. 2003a. Structure of the replicative helicase of the oncoprotein SV40 large tumour antigen. *Nature*, **423**, 512–18.

Li, J.J. and Kelly, T.J. 1984. Simian virus 40 DNA replication in vitro. *Proc Natl Acad Sci USA*, **81**, 6973–7.

Li, Z., Brister, J.R., et al. 2003b. Characterization of the adenoassociated virus Rep protein complex formed on the viral origin of DNA replication. *Virology*, **313**, 364–76.

Lin, B.Y., Makhov, A.M., et al. 2002. Chaperone proteins abrogate inhibition of the human papillomavirus (HPV) E1 replicative helicase by the HPV E2 protein. *Mol Cell Biol*, **22**, 6592–604.

Longworth, M.S. and Laimins, L.A. 2004. Pathogenesis of human papillomaviruses in differentiating epithelia. *Microbiol Mol Biol Rev*, **68**, 362–72.

Marintcheva, B. and Weller, S.K. 2001. A tale of two HSV-1 helicases: roles of phage and animal virus helicases in DNA replication and recombination. *Prog Nucleic Acid Res Mol Biol*, **70**, 77–118.

Munger, K., Werness, B.A., et al. 1989. Complex formation of human papillomavirus E7 proteins with the retinoblastoma tumor suppressor gene product. *EMBO J*, **8**, 4099–105.

Nuesch, J.P., Christensen, J. and Rommelaere, J. 2001. Initiation of minute virus of mice DNA replication is regulated at the level of origin unwinding by atypical protein kinase C phosphorylation of NS1. *J Virol*, **75**, 5730–9.

Ott, R.D., Wang, Y. and Fanning, E. 2002. Mutational analysis of simian virus 40 T-antigen primosome activities in viral DNA replication. *J Virol*, **76**, 5121–30.

Reuven, N.B., Staire, A.E., et al. 2003. The herpes simplex virus type 1 alkaline nuclease and single-stranded DNA binding protein mediate strand exchange in vitro. *J Virol*, **77**, 7425–33.

Reuven, N.B., Willcox, J.D., et al. 2004. Catalysis of strand exchange by the HSV-1 UL12 and ICP8 proteins: potent ICP8 recombinase activity is revealed upon resection of dsDNA substrate by nuclease. *J Mol Biol*, **342**, 57–71.

Richardson, W.D. and Westphal, H. 1981. A cascade of adenovirus early functions is required for expression of adeno-associated virus. *Cell*, **27**, 133–41.

Simmons, D.T. 2000. SV40 large T antigen functions in DNA replication and transformation. *Adv Virus Res*, **55**, 75–134.

Simmons, D.T., Melendy, T., et al. 1996. Simian virus 40 large T antigen binds to topoisomerase I. *Virology*, **222**, 365–74.

Stenlund, A. 2003. Initiation of DNA replication: lessons from viral initiator proteins. *Nat Rev Mol Cell Biol*, **4**, 777–85.

Stracker, T.H., Carson, C.T. and Weitzman, M.D. 2002. Adenovirus oncoproteins inactivate the Mre11-Rad50-NBS1 DNA repair complex. *Nature*, **418**, 348–52.

Stracker, T.H., Cassell, G.D., et al. 2004. The Rep protein of adeno-associated virus type 2 interacts with single-stranded DNA-binding proteins that enhance viral replication. *J Virol*, **78**, 441–53.

Tang, Q., Bell, P., et al. 2000. Replication but not transcription of simian virus 40 DNA is dependent on nuclear domain 10. *J Virol*, **74**, 9694–700.

van Breukelen, B., Brenkman, A.B., et al. 2003. Adenovirus type 5 DNA binding protein stimulates binding of DNA polymerase to the replication origin. *J Virol*, **77**, 915–22.

Waga, S. and Stillman, B. 1994. Anatomy of a DNA replication fork revealed by reconstitution of SV40 DNA replication in vitro. *Nature*, **369**, 207–12.

Wessel, R., Schweizer, J. and Stahl, H. 1992. Simian virus 40 T-antigen DNA helicase is a hexamer which forms a binary complex during bidirectional unwinding from the viral origin of DNA replication. *J Virol*, **66**, 804–15.

Weindler, F.W. and Heilbronn, R. 1991. A subset of herpes simplex virus replication genes provides helper functions for productive adeno-associated virus replication. *J Virol*, **65**, 2476–83.

Wilkinson, D. and Weller, S. 2003. The role of DNA recombination in herpes simplex virus DNA replication. *IUBMB Life*, **55**, 451–8.

Yakobson, B., Hrynko, T.A., et al. 1989. Replication of adeno-associated virus in cells irradiated with UV light at 254 nm. *J Virol*, **63**, 1023–30.

11

Genetics of vertebrate viruses

CRAIG R. PRINGLE

GENETIC SYSTEMS

The major aim of virus genetics is elucidation of the detailed structure of the genomes of the various types of viruses found in nature and the extent to which the individual components of the virus genome determine the biological and disease-producing potential of viruses. Virus genetics is also concerned with understanding the pattern and origin of the variability of viruses, in terms both of virus evolution and of the temporal changes in antigenicity and pathogenicity of viruses that determine the prevalence and course of virus-associated infectious diseases of humans and animals. Although virus genetics impinges on all aspects of virology, this account will be limited predominantly to a consideration of genome strategy, methods of genetic analysis, and some of the applications of genetic methodology.

Viruses display a diversity of genetic systems unparalleled in any other group of organisms. The viruses considered in this chapter are those that infect humans and higher animals. The genetic systems described here do not include all the known categories, and only occasional reference is made to viruses that infect invertebrates, plants, fungi, protozoa, algae, mycoplasmae, bacteria, and archaea (see Chapter 4, The classification of vertebrate viruses). With the determination of the complete sequences of the genomes of many plant and animal viruses, previously unsuspected phylogenetic relationships are being revealed. For example, cowpea mosaic virus, a plant comovirus with a bipartite positive-sense RNA genome, shows organizational similarity and local sequence homology with the monopartite vertebrate picornaviruses. Tobacco mosaic virus, a monopartite positive-sense RNA virus, and alfalfa mosaic virus and brome mosaic virus, both tripartite genome viruses, show sequence relationships with the animal alphaviruses. On the basis of genome organization and comparison of RNA-dependent RNA polymerase sequences, most plant positive-sense RNA viruses can be classified into two supergroups comprising the picornavirus-like plant viruses (como-, nepo-, and potyviruses), and the *Alphavirus*-like plant viruses (tobamo-, bromo-, carla-, clostero-, cucumo-, furo-, gordei-, ilar-, potex-, tymo-, and tobraviruses) (Koonin and Dolja 1993). The picornavirus-like plant viruses and the animal picornaviruses resemble each other in encoding a number of nonstructural proteins that exhibit similar functions and show some degree of amino acid homology. The *Alphavirus*-like plant viruses are more diverse, but again they encode genes in the same relative order that specify proteins exhibiting significant sequence homology to the three nonstructural proteins of the vertebrate Sindbis virus. There is also an apparent genetic link between the potyviruses of plants and the flaviviruses of animals, in that the putative helicase protein of potyviruses exhibits a closer resemblance to the NS3 protein of flaviviruses, which contains a nucleotide-binding motif, than to the helicases of picornaviruses (Goldbach and de Haan 1993).

Although most viruses are restricted in their host range, several groups of viruses are characteristically less restricted by taxonomic barriers and may multiply in hosts of quite different origin. Some of the arthropod-borne bunyaviruses and rhabdoviruses that infect vertebrates or plants are also able to multiply in their invertebrate vector. Despite the apparent phylogenetic relationships described above, however, no contemporary virus exists that is able to multiply in both vertebrates and plants. Nonetheless, it has been demonstrated experimentally that yeast cells infected artificially can support the replication of vertebrate papillomavirus genomes (Angeletti et al. 2002), and that replication-competent chimeras of plant and animal viruses can be constructed that replicate efficiently in plant protoplasts (Peng et al. 2002).

MOLECULAR PHYLOGENY AND VIRUS EVOLUTION

The existence of plant and animal RNA viruses with similarly ordered genomes encoding proteins with similar amino acid sequences suggests a common ancestry. However, the common ancestors from which these viruses diverged probably appeared subsequent to the separation of the plant and animal kingdoms some 10^9 years ago, and divergent evolution alone cannot account for certain features of these relationships. The coupling of common genes to unique genes in several of these genomes suggests a polyphyletic origin mediated by recombination. Many viral genomes can best be regarded as different assemblages of modules of conserved genes that have arisen by a process of modular evolution. From a phylogenetic analysis of the vertebrate circoviruses and the nanoviruses of plants, both of which have small single-stranded circular DNA genomes, Gibbs and Weiller (1999) concluded that these viruses had not arisen by parallel evolution. Rather, the vertebrate circoviruses had evolved from the plant nanoviruses by a complex recombinational event which involved the incorporation of a gene from an RNA virus, possibly a vertebrate calicivirus, into a plant nanovirus DNA genome. Their hypothesis requires that the circoviruses evolved as a consequence of a host-switch whereby a nanovirus genomic DNA was transferred from a plant to a vertebrate host, perhaps as a consequence of exposure of a vertebrate to infected plant sap or via a vector. The replication-competent DNA persisted, and by a subsequent recombinational event became a virus capable of infecting vertebrate hosts. Because caliciviruses are vertebrate viruses, the hypothesis requires that the host-switch preceded the recombinational event. Unlikely as this scenario may seem, involving the hybridization of a DNA and an RNA virus, there is the precedent of Thogoto virus a negative-sense RNA virus that possess a glycoprotein gene

resembling that of a DNA baculovirus (Morse et al. 1992).

The application of molecular phylogeny analysis to the large and complex DNA-containing herpesviruses has confirmed the ancient origin of these viruses and provided a timescale for their evolution. The branching pattern of the three subfamilies of the mammalian herpesviruses is congruent with that of their corresponding host lineages (McGeoch et al. 1995). Assuming a constant molecular clock, the *Alphaherpesvirinae*, *Betaherpesvirinae* and *Gammaherpesvirinae* subfamilies would have diverged 1.8–2.2×10^8 years ago, at about the time of emergence of mammals from mammal-like reptiles, and the major sublineages within these subfamilies probably arose before the radiation of placental mammals some 6–8×10^7 years ago. Paleontological dating of host lineages has suggested that the contemporary virus lineages within the subfamily *Alphaherpesvirinae* have evolved by a process of co-speciation of viruses with their mammalian hosts (McGeoch and Cook 1994). However, several avian herpesviruses are included in the *Alphaherpesvirinae* and, on the basis of similar assumptions, would have evolved independently with their avian hosts for some 80–120 million years (McGeoch and Davison 1999). Such a timescale, however, would place the origin of the avian viruses in too recent an era, as the ancestors of birds and mammals are considered to have diverged some 310 million years ago. This suggests that the avian herpesviruses may not have evolved with their hosts, but may have resulted from ancient cross-species transmissions of ancestral mammalian alphaherpesviruses to birds (McGeoch et al. 2000). Recently two other major herpesvirus lineages have been identified, one embracing fish and amphibian herpesviruses, and the other represented by unique herpesviruses recovered from bivalve molluscs. If these viruses similarly evolved with their hosts, the fish herpesviruses lineage would have been established some 450 million years ago and the invertebrate herpesvirus lineage perhaps a billion years ago. In contrast to the relationships evident between herpesviruses within the same lineage, there is no obvious relationship between herpesviruses belonging to the three different lineages (avian/mammalian, fish/amphibian, and invertebrate) in terms of amino-acid sequence comparisons, other than those functions that are common to all organisms (e.g. DNA polymerase, helicase, and primase). This extreme divergence perhaps suggests that other mechanisms of herpesvirus evolution remain to be identified. A shared ancestral root for all herpesviruses cannot be assumed, because none of the genes common to these three lineages of herpesviruses are confined to herpesviruses, and could have been acquired independently by gene capture rather than by lineal descent (Davison 2002). On the other hand, a member of the fish/amphibian lineage, Channel catfish virus, possesses a gene distantly related to the ATPase subunit of bacteriophage T4 terminase, a complex of proteins responsible for energy-dependent packaging of nascent genomes into preformed capsid. Although this gene may owe its origin to horizontal exchange, it is possible that herpesviruses share their origins with the ancestors of bacteriophage T4 and other icosahedral double-stranded DNA bacterial viruses (Davison 2002).

The ancestral origins of most other viruses cannot be deduced with any certainty from phylogenetic analysis where there is no linkage to the geological record. Generally there are few virus isolates originating from more than a few decades before the present, and even the direction of evolution cannot be discerned in all cases with any degree of certainty. The antiquity of the retroviruses, however, has been established using polymerase chain reaction methodology to screen for the presence of endogenous retroviruses in a wide range of vertebrate hosts, including amphibian, avian, mammalian, piscine, and reptilian. Phylogenetic analyses have demonstrated that viruses resembling (but not necessarily related to) two (the spumaviruses and the murine leukemialike viruses) of the seven recognized genera of retroviruses are widespread and abundant in vertebrate (but not invertebrate) genomes, whereas viruses resembling the other five genera of retroviruses are restricted to mammals and birds (Herniou et al. 1998). Calculation of the integration dates of some of the numerous families of defective human endogenous retroviruses (HERV) identified recently indicates that most of them are likely to have been part of the human lineage since it diverged from that of the Old World monkeys more than 25 million years ago (Tristem 2000). HERVs probably represent the footprints of ancient germline retroviral infections. Furthermore, HERVs may influence genome regulation through expression of retroviral genes, via genomic rearrangements and the involvement of HERV LTRs in the regulation of gene expression (Sverdlov 2000). Analysis of the human genome has revealed that some 45 percent of it consists of various types of transposable elements, with around 8 percent of human DNA derived from retrovirus-like elements (Paces et al. 2002).

THE STRATEGY OF THE VIRUS GENOME

The 'strategy of the virus genome' is a phrase that has been used to describe collectively the organization and function of the genetic information content of viruses. The mammalian viruses fall into three major categories: the DNA-containing viruses, the RNA and DNA reverse-transcribing viruses, and the RNA-containing viruses (Table 11.1). The DNA viruses range from viruses with small genomes, such as the parvoviruses and the papovaviruses, which depend on host-cell functions for their replication, to large genome viruses such as the nuclear herpesviruses and the cytoplasmic poxviruses,

which have acquired a battery of additional genes that function to mediate replication independently of the host cell and to subvert the immune response of the host. The encoding of genetic information in RNA is unique to viruses (animal, plant, and bacterial), and RNA is the predominant molecular form of the genome in animal and plant viruses. The genomes of more than 90 percent of plant viruses consist of single- or double-stranded RNA. The reverse-transcribing viruses alternate between RNA and DNA forms of the genome; in the retroviruses the genome exists as proviral DNA integrated into the host cell genome and as RNA in the extracellular virion. By contrast, in the DNA-containing hepadnaviruses and the plant caulimoviruses (sometimes referred to as pararetroviruses) the DNA form is present as partially or completely double-stranded DNA in the virion, and the RNA form acts as a replicative intermediate in the infected cell. Exceptionally, recent evidence suggests that the replicative cycle of the foamy viruses (members of the genus *Spumavirus*, one of the seven genera of the family *Retroviridae*) resembles that of pararetroviruses in that the extracellular particles contain full-length double-stranded infectious DNA, as well as RNA (Yu et al. 1999). The spumaviruses differ from hepadnaviruses, however, in that they encode proteases and integrases, and integration is an obligate event in the viral replicative cycle.

The coding potential of viruses

The molecular sizes of the genomes of the vertebrate DNA viruses extend from the 1.7 kb of the circular single-stranded genome of porcine circovirus to the 300 kbp genome of fowlpox virus. (The genomes of the some invertebrate iridoviruses and entomopoxviruses are larger and may extend up to 383 kbp.) In contrast, the RNA viruses are more uniform, varying within a 15-fold range from the 1.7 kb of the single-stranded helper-dependent deltavirus to the 31 kb of certain coronaviruses. This circumstance has been interpreted as a reflection of the low fidelity of viral RNA polymerases, which lack proofreading capability. The consequent high mutability of RNA viruses may impose an upper limit on the size of informational RNA molecules.

Table 11.1 lists the currently recognized vertebrate viruses according to the taxonomy defined in the Seventh Report of the International Committee on Taxonomy of Viruses (ICTV) (Van Regenmortel et al. 2000; see also Chapter 4, The classification of vertebrate viruses). The first column lists viruses by family, and the second column gives an indication of the inherent diversity of the group in terms of the number of distinct genera and their constituent species, as currently listed by the individual specialist study groups of the ICTV. This is of course an imperfect measure of genetic diversity, as the extent of knowledge of any particular

Table 11.1 *The properties of the vertebrate virus genome*

(Order)	Family Subfamily (unassigned genus)	Diversity Genera	Species	Nucleic acid type	Strandedness sense	Configuration	Size	ORF	Particle type	Other features
The DNA viruses										
Parvoviridae		3 (+3 invert)	34 (+5 invert)	DNA	Single (negative or positive)	Linear	4.7–5 kb	2 major	isometric	Nuclear mitosis dependent
Circoviridae		2	4	DNA	Single (negative or ambisense)	Circular	1.8–3.8 kb	3 major (overlaps)	isometric	Nuclear S phase dependent
	(*Anellovirus*)	1	4	DNA	Single (negative)	Circular	2.9–3.8 kb	2 major (overlap)	isometric	High genetic heterogeneity
Papovaviridae		1	12	DNA	Double	Circular	5.2 kb	8 (overlaps)	isometric	Early and late mRNA ex opp. strands
Papillomaviridae		1	7	DNA	Double	Circular	6.8–8.4 kb	9 or 10 (overlaps)	isometric	Early and late mRNA ex same strand
Iridoviridae		1 (+3 invert)	1 (+4 invert)	DNA	Double	Circular (circularly permuted)	150–170 kbp (107 kbp unit)	>40	isometric (enveloped)	Nongenetic Reactivation
Adenoviridae		2	30	DNA	Double	Linear	26–45 kbp	40 (splicing)	Isometric (fibers at vertices)	Covalent-linked protein temporaral gene exp.
Herpesviridae										
	Alphaherpesvirinae	4	23	DNA	Double	Complex linear 4 isomers in HSV	ca. 150 kbp	70–100 splicing rare	isometric	Latency in sensory ganglia
	Betaherpesvirinae	3	7	DNA	Double	Linear	ca. 235 kbp	ca. 200 splicing common	isometric	Latency in lymphoreticular cells
	Gammaherpesvirinae	2	20	DNA	Double	Linear	ca. 170 kbp	ca. 150 splicing common	isometric	Latency in B lymphocytes
	(Ictalurid herpes-like viruses	1	1	DNA	Double	Linear	134 kbp	ca. 80	isometric	Phylogeny uncertain
Asfarviridae		1	1	DNA (inverted term rep.)	Double	Linear, Covalently closed	170–190 kbp	ca. 150	Complex (NC/isometric/env.)	Perinuclear factories nucleus dependent
Poxviridae	*Chordopoxvirinae* (+1 invert subfamily)	8 (3 invert.)	35 (27 invert.)	DNA (cytoplasmic)	Double	Linear, Covalently closed	130–250 kbp	ca. 150–300	complex	Inclusions temporaral expression

(Continued over)

Table 11.1 *The properties of the vertebrate virus genome (Continued)*

Family (Order) / Subfamily (unassigned genus)	Diversity Genera	Species	Nucleic acid type	Strandedness sense	Configuration	Size	ORF	Particle type	Other features
The DNA and RNA reverse-transcribing viruses									
Hepadnaviridae	2	5	DNA (reverse transcription)	Double (incomplete)	Circular (noncovalent link)	3.2 kbp	4 (overlap)	spherical/enveloped	5'-covalent protein
Retroviridae	7	53	RNA* (reverse transcription)	Single (positive sense)	Linear dimer (pseudodiploid)	7–11 kb (monomer)	6–10 (PTC)	spherical/enveloped	tRNA primer high f. recombination
The RNA viruses									
Picornaviridae	6	17	RNA	Single (positive sense)	Linear	7–8 kb	1 (PTC/op)	isometric	5'-covalent VPg IRES and polyC in some
Caliciviridae	4	5	RNA	Single (positive sense)	Linear	7.4–8.3 kb	1, 2 or 3 (PTC/op)	isometric	5'-covalent VPg sgRNA in some
Hepacivirus	1	1	RNA	Single (positive sense)	Linear	7.2	3 (PTC/op)	isometric	Encodes mRNA capping enzyme
Astroviridae	1	7	RNA	Single (positive sense)	Linear	6.8–7.9 kb	3 (PTC/opP)	isometric	sgRNA; polymerase Exp. by ribosomal fr.
Coronaviridae (O. Nidovirales)	2	16	RNA	Single (positive sense)	Linear	28–31 kb	7–10 (nested set)	spherical/enveloped	Amplification of mRNA High fr. recombination
Arteriviridae (O. Nidovirales)	1	4	RNA	Single (positive sense)	Linear	13–16 kb	7–12 (nested set)	spherical/enveloped	as above
Flaviviridae	3	58 (+3?)	RNA	Single (positive sense)	Linear	10–12 kb	1 (PTC)	spherical/enveloped	Most arthropod-borne str. proteins N-terminal
Togaviridae	2	25	RNA	Single (positive sense)	Linear	9–12 kb	1 (and 1 ex sgRNA)	spherical/enveloped	Most arthropod-borne 5'-m7G cap
(Deltavirus)	1	1	RNA	Single (negative sense)	Circular (forms unbranched rod)	1.7 kb	1	spherical	HBV dependent encodes ribozyme
Bornaviridae (O. Mononegavirales)	1	1	RNA	Single (negative sense)	Linear	8.9 kb	6 (spl/opP)	spherical/enveloped	Nuclear Recomb. deficient?
Rhabdoviridae (O. Mononegavirales)	4 (and 2 plant)	23 (and 15 plant)	RNA	Single (negative sense)	Linear	11–15 kb	5–10	rod/bacilliform shaped	Recomb. deficient DI mutants common
Paramyxoviridae (O. Mononegavirales) *Paramyxovirinae*	5	29	RNA	Single (negative sense)	Linear	15–18 kb (n x 6)	9–11 (overlaps)	pleomorphic/env.	Recomb. deficient 'Rule of six' applies
Pneumovirinae	2	5	RNA	Single (negative sense)	Linear	15 n ≠ x 6	8–10	pleomorphic/env.	Recomb. deficient No 'rule of six'

(Continued over)

Table 11.1 *The properties of the vertebrate virus genome (Continued)*

(Order) Family	Subfamily (unassigned genus)	Diversity Genera	Species	Nucleic acid type	Strandedness sense	Configuration	Size	ORF	Particle type	Other features
Filoviridae (O. Mononegavirales)		2	5	RNA	Single (negative sense)	Linear	19 kb	7 (overlaps)	bacilliform/env.	Recomb. deficient GP may be edited
Arenaviridae		1	19	RNA	Single (ambisense)	Linear ×2 (L and S segments)	L – 7.5 kb S – 3.5 kb	4	pleomorphic/env.	Rodent-borne Subunit reassortment
Bunyaviridae		4 (and 1 plant)	87 (and 8 plant)	RNA	Single (negative and ambisense)	Linear ×3, (L, M, and S segments)	L - 6/12 kb M - 3/5 kb S - 1/1.7 kb	6 (overlaps)	spherical/enveloped	Most arboviruses Subunit reassortment
Orthomyxoviridae		5	6	RNA	Single (negative sense)	Linear ×6, 7 or 8 (n = 900– 2350 kb)	10–14.6 kb (total)	10 (spl/op)	spherical/enveloped	Nuclear phase subunit reassortment
Birnaviridae		2 (+1 invert.)	3 (+1 invert.)	RNA	Double	Linear (n = 2715– 3104 kbp)	6 kbp (total)	5 (overlap)	Isometric (single shell)	Subunit reassortment
Reoviridae		5 (+4 pl/inv)	38 (+27 pl/inv)	RNA	Double	Linear 11, or 12 (three size classes)	19–32 kbp (total)	10+ (overlaps)	Isometric (1, 2, or 3 shells)	Subunit reassortment

env, enveloped; exp. expression; invert, invertebrates; opp, opposite; pl/inv, plant and invertebrate; PTC, post-translational cleavage; recomb. recombination; sgRNA, subgenomic RNA; str. structural; term rep, terminal repeat.

taxonomic group is determined to some degree by the extent of its adverse interactions with human and animal populations.

Vertebrate virus genomes, according to virus family, may be linear or circular, single-, or double-stranded, covalently linked to small terminal proteins, or may exist as a unique complement of subunits. The minimum information content of a viral genome can be estimated from the number of nonoverlapping coding triplets if the complete nucleotide sequence is known, or if not, from the ratio of the molecular mass of the genome and the gene products. As a rough estimate the ratio of the molecular mass of genome and gene products is approximately 10:1 for single-stranded genomes and 20:1 for double-stranded genome viruses. Thus, for example, the 4.2×10^6 Mr of the genome of the rhabdovirus vesicular stomatitis Indiana virus (VSIV) is sufficient to code for polypeptides with a total mass of 400 kDa, which approximates closely to the actual 396 kDa of the five gene products of VSV. This is an extreme case, however, because in the genome of this virus the noncoding regions are limited to dinucleotide intergenic junctions, and short leader and trailer regions.

The relationship between linear length and coding capacity is maintained in the larger DNA viruses, but the coding capacity of smaller virus genomes can be considerably expanded by a number of devices operating at the levels of genome organization, mRNA transcription and translation strategies. At the level of genome organization these devices can include overlapping reading frames (almost ubiquitous), and transcription from both DNA strands (*Polyomavirus*); at the level of transcription, mRNA splicing (most nuclear viruses), the generation of mRNA families by alternate splicing (adenoviruses), accessing of multiple open reading frames by RNA editing (paramyxoviruses), use of alternate start sites (adenoviruses and paramyxoviruses) and alternate termination sites (paramyxoviruses and rhabdoviruses), and nontemplated insertion of nucleotides (paramyxoviruses); and at the level of translation, leaky scanning of mRNA (paramyxovvirus *P* gene products), suppression of termination (retrovirus *gag–pol*), ribosomal frameshifting, (several viruses), posttranslational cleavage of polyprotein precursors (picornaviruses, togaviruses, and retroviruses), the presence of internal ribosome entry sites (picornaviruses and flaviviruses), usurpation of host factors (several viruses), and transactivation of host genes (lentiviruses).

Ribosomal frameshifting is observed predominantly in RNA viruses and is often involved in the expression of replicases (Brierle 1995). Slippage of ribosomes into the −1 reading frame (in a 5′ direction) occurs at a specific site comprising two essential elements: a homopolymeric slippage sequence separated by five to eight bases from an RNA pseudoknot structure. Ribosomal frameshifting

may be a strategy to achieve stoichiometry of gene products or to ensure inclusion of replicative enzymes in virions (e.g. by production of *gag–pol* fusions in retroviruses).

The virus classification system known as the Baltimore system (Baltimore 1971) is derived from the obligatory dependence of all viruses on the protein synthesizing machinery of the host cell. Viruses must produce or act as messenger RNA (mRNA) that can be translated by cellular ribosomes. In this classification system the unique relationship of the various forms of the viral genome to mRNA defines virus categories. Class I viruses comprise the double-stranded DNA viruses, class II are the single-stranded DNA viruses, class III are the double-stranded RNA viruses, class IV are the single-stranded positive-sense RNA viruses, and class V are the single-stranded negative-sense RNA viruses. This numbered classification system played a formative role in the development of molecular virology, but is now rarely used. The diverse nature of the viral genome can be rationalized by regarding the genome as an intermediate stage in the cycle of replication of virus nucleic acid that has become sequestered in an extracellular particle. In the Baltimore system a single-stranded RNA molecule is designated as positive sense if it functions as mRNA in protein synthesis, and its complement as the negative-sense strand or anti-message. The retroviruses and some RNA viruses encapsidate the positive-sense RNA strand in the virion, whereas other RNA viruses encapsidate the negative-sense strand or the double-stranded form in the virion. The DNA viruses may be single- or double-stranded, and the positive and negative strands may be encapsidated in separate particles in some of the single-stranded parvoviruses, whereas negative strands are encapsidated exclusively in the recently characterized single-stranded anelloviruses (see Chapter 4, The classification of vertebrate viruses). The only stage in the replication cycle of viral nucleic acids (excluding the replicative intermediates) not represented in known viruses is the RNA:DNA intermediate in the reverse transcription pathway. A small proportion of hepatitis B virus particles, however, do contain DNA/RNA hybrid molecules.

Segmentation of the viral genome

Segmentation of the genome is observed in the arena-, birna-, bunya-, orthomyxo-, and reoviruses. A consequence of segmentation of the genome is the potential for increasing genetic heterogeneity by reassortment of subunits during replication and morphogenesis; the evolution of segmentation in RNA viruses has been equated somewhat fancifully with the evolution of sex, allowing the participation of two, three, or more parents in the production of offspring (Chao 1994). Segmentation and the consequent facility for reassortment may allow the rapid elimination of deleterious mutations and defective genomes. Thus segmentation may be a device evolved to circumvent the assumed limitation on the absolute size of informational RNA molecules imposed by their high mutability. This explanation is difficult to sustain, however, because the total genome sizes of the segmented genome viruses are in the same range as those of nonsegmented genome viruses, and the genome of the largest segmented genome viruses (the 19 kb of the Nairovirus, Crimean–Congo hemorrhagic fever virus) is less than that of the largest nonsegmented genome virus (the 30 kb of murine hepatitis virus, a *Coronavirus*). Segmentation of the genome may more often be a device to facilitate regulation of transcription.

Among mammalian viruses segmentation of the genome is confined to the negative-sense single-stranded RNA viruses and the double-stranded RNA viruses, where the complete complement of genome subunits is contained within a single particle and the infectious unit is a single virion. Segmentation of the genome is common also among the positive-sense single-stranded RNA viruses of plants. These are all multicomponent viruses, however, in which the individual genome subunits are contained in different particles and the infectious unit is a full complement of particles. Genetic reassortment can accompany the maturation of multicomponent viruses and is termed pseudorecombination by plant virologists.

Ambisense encoding of information

Ambisense encoding of genetic information is a phenomenon exhibited by viruses of the family *Arenaviridae*, and by some members of the families *Bunyaviridae* and *Circoviridae*. Ambisense encoding is illustrated diagrammatically in Figure 11.1. In *Punta Toro virus* (family *Bunyaviridae*, genus *Phlebovirus*) the N polypeptide is encoded in a viral complementary

subgenomic RNA corresponding to the 3' half of the S RNA, whereas the NS protein is encoded in a subgenomic viral sense RNA corresponding to the 5' half of the genome; thus the S RNA of punta Toro virus is both positive and negative sense. Ambisense encoding of information is common to members of the genus *Phlebovirus*, but is not observed in the other genera of the *Bunyaviridae*. In the family *Arenaviridae* both segments of the bipartite genome exhibit ambisense encoding of information. The large subunit encodes the *L* gene in the 3' half and the *Z* gene in opposite sense in the 5' half, and the small subunit encodes the *N* gene in the 3' half and the *G* gene in opposite sense in the 5' half. Ambisense encoding may be a device to obtain temporal control of transcription and is not a means of expanding coding capacity.

Reverse transcription, endogenous viruses, and retroid elements

Reverse transcription is not uniquely associated with vertebrate viruses belonging to the families *Retroviridae* and *Hepadnaviridae*. The viruses of plants belonging to the family *Caulimoviridae* also replicate by a reverse transcription route. Comparative analysis of the organization of the RNA associated with vertebrate transposable genetic elements, such as the intracisternal A particles, *VL30* genes and LIMd, and a variety of transposable elements from yeast (Ty), *Drosophila* (copia), *Dictyostelium* (DIRS-1) and maize (B1) revealed structural similarities with the integrated form of the retrovirus genome. Furthermore, the RNA forms of the nucleic acid component of *Drosophila melanogaster copia* transposable element and *Saccharomyces cerevisiae* Ty1 transposable element are present within virus-like particles that have associated reverse transcriptase activity. As a consequence these genetic elements are now ranked as viruses and have been included in the Universal Taxonomy of Viruses as members of a new family – the *Pseudoviridae*

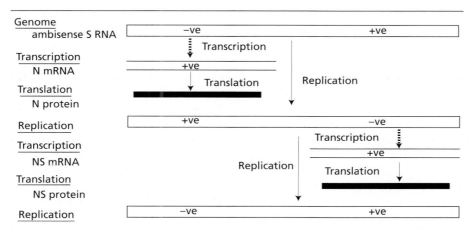

Figure 11.1 *The ambisense encoding of genetic information in the S RNA of Punta Toro virus,* Phlebovirus *(family* Bunyaviridae*). (After Ihara et al. 1984.)*

(Van Regenmortel et al., 2000; see also Chapter 4, The classification of vertebrate viruses).

The common features of the genome maps of these viruses (when linearized in the case of the DNA viruses) are terminal redundancies, which can range from the 17–21 nucleotides of Rous sarcoma virus to the 1123 nucleotides of a human *Spumavirus*, the partial or complete *gag–pol–env* gene order, and the domain structure (protease, reverse transcriptase, integrase) of the polymerase gene. It has been proposed that, during the evolution of these agents, cassettes of genes were added to the basic *gag–pol* core to facilitate adaptation to specific host environments (Hull and Covey 1986). For example, the *env* gene of vertebrate retroviruses is required for protection of the core complex and for cell-to-cell spread, whereas the caulimoviruses have acquired additional genes to facilitate plant-to-plant transmissibility and movement within the plant.

Endogenous retroviruses are defective or nondefective retroviruses transmitted from one generation to the next via the germline, and which probably have evolved in synchrony with their hosts to establish multigenic families. HERVs comprise over 200 distinct groups or subgroups. Although many may have entered the human genome 10–50 million years ago, others appear to have originated from crossinfections at an earlier stage in the evolution of their host. The endogenous feline retrovirus RD114, for example, is thought to have originated as a result of horizontal transfer of an endogenous primate retrovirus, possibly as far back as the Pliocene Age. One view is that HERVs may have played a role in early human evolution by conferring antiviral resistance and altering patterns of gene expression (Sverdlov 2000). Many of the larger mammalian viruses appear to have acquired genes from their host in the course of evolution, but occasionally the reverse can occur. An example is the apparent involvement of a captive retroviral envelope protein, syncytin, in morphogenesis of the human placenta. The syncytin protein is encoded in the *env* gene of a defective endogenous human retrovirus (HERV-W) and its major sites of expression are multinucleate cells in the placenta that originate from fetal trophoblasts. It is presumed that its presence may contribute to normal human placental morphogenesis (Mi et al. 2000).

Infectious nucleic acid

RNA viruses replicate in the cytoplasm, with the exception of the segmented genome orthomyxoviruses and the monopartite negative-sense Bornaviruses (Schneemann et al. 1995), which have nuclear phases. Some others fail to replicate in enucleated cells and are dependent on the presence of a functional nucleus (Pringle 1977). The genome of the positive-sense single-stranded RNA viruses is infectious, because by definition it acts directly on entry as the mRNA for the entire complement of viral proteins, which include the RNA replicase required for replication of the viral genome. The genome of the negative-sense single-stranded RNA viruses, on the other hand, is not infectious because it cannot function as mRNA or be replicated. Mammalian cells do not contain enzymes that can transcribe or replicate RNA templates, and so transcription can be initiated only if the appropriate RNA polymerase is introduced into the cytoplasm of the host cell together with the infecting genome in the form of a nucleocapsid structure.

The DNA of the nuclear DNA viruses is generally infectious, but that of the cytoplasmic poxviruses is not. The poxviruses exhibit the greatest extent of independence of host cell activities of any virus, and the virion contains many enzyme activities, including a viral DNA-dependent RNA polymerase whose presence is essential for infectivity. The discovery of this enzyme by Kates and McAuslan (1967) was crucial to our understanding of the nature of viral genomes and led ultimately to the independent discovery and characterization by Baltimore and Temin and Mitzutani in 1970 of the reverse transcriptase of retroviruses (Baltimore 1971), which is perhaps the greatest single contribution of virology to general biology and which greatly accelerated the exploitation of recombinant DNA technology.

The genomes of retroviruses are also not infectious, probably because preformed virion-associated reverse transcriptase is necessary for initiation of replication. By contrast the proviral DNA form is infectious because it can be transcribed by the host-cell DNA-dependent RNA polymerase to initiate infection. The reverse transcription stage of retrovirus replication takes place in the cytoplasm prior to entry into the nucleus and integration into the host genome.

METHODS OF GENETIC ANALYSIS

Classic genetic analysis of viruses depended on the isolation of spontaneously occurring mutants or the induction of mutations by random mutagenesis followed by nonselective isolation of mutants exhibiting a single conditional lethal phenotype. Further selective screening procedures or systematic characterization of individual mutants were required to identify useful mutations in specific viral genes. Nevertheless, despite the imperfections, many well-defined mutations were identified which played significant roles in the molecular characterization of mammalian viruses, and provisional genetic and physical maps of many viral genomes were obtained by this means (Ramig 1990). The isolation and characterization of revertants is an essential requirement in defining the phenotype of any specific mutant.

Conditional lethal mutants

Conditional lethal phenotypes (temperature sensitivity and host range) have been the favored phenotypes for the isolation of mutations in essential genes. Other phenotypes, such as plaque morphology, drug resistance, enzyme deficiencies, and spontaneous deletions (sometimes presenting as defective interfering particles), have had application in specific circumstances. The conditional lethal mutants employed in animal virology have been temperature-sensitive mutants, cold-sensitive mutants, or temperature-dependent host range mutants. Host range conditional lethal mutants analogous to the suppressible chain-terminating mutants of bacteriophages (amber or nonsense mutations) have played virtually no role in animal virus genetics, although in principle such mutants allow direct identification of the mutated gene product, because a truncated gene product may be present in the nonpermissive host cell and an intact protein in the permissive cell. Host restriction in animal cells is probably due to the absence of a specific receptor, and permissive mammalian cells naturally able to suppress amber mutations by insertion of an amino acid at an amber stop codon have not been identified. Mammalian cells expressing amber-suppressible tRNAs have been engineered, however, and these have been used successfully to isolate mutations of vesicular stomatitis virus following random mutagenesis (White and McGeoch 1987) and by mutagenesis of poliovirus cDNA in vitro (Sedivy et al. 1987).

Spontaneous mutants and random mutagenesis

Spontaneous mutants occur at low frequency, and a variety of mutagens have been employed to increase the frequency of recovery of mutants. Mutagens that have proved effective with human and animal viruses include base analogues (e.g. 5-fluorouracil and 5-azacytidine for RNA viruses and 5-bromodeoxyuridine for DNA viruses), alkylating agents (e.g. ethylmethane sulfonate, diethyl sulfate), intercalating agents (e.g. proflavine and N-nitro-N-nitrosoguanidine), deaminating agents (e.g. nitrous acid), hydroxylamine, ultraviolet light irradiation, and miscellaneous agents (e.g. the antiviral agent ribavirin). The base analogues are incorporated into the viral genome and miscoding during replication produces mutations. The other mutagens induce mutations by direct chemical action on the target nucleic acid. The majority of induced mutations seem to be missense mutations whereby substitution of an amino acid modifies the functional activity of a gene product. Frameshift and nonsense mutations of animal viruses are rare. (Practical protocols for random mutagenesis and isolation of mutants are described by Leppard and Pringle (1996).)

Site-specific and directed mutagenesis

These empirical methods described above have been superseded by the adoption of in vitro methods of site-specific mutagenesis. The methodology for constructing such mutants is similar for all DNA and positive-stranded RNA viruses, although there is an operational distinction between viruses whose genome is small enough to be cloned (as a cDNA in the case of RNA viruses) in its entirety (parvoviruses, polyomaviruses, picornaviruses, retroviruses) and those in which mutagenesis is best carried out with a fragment that, after genetic manipulation, is incorporated into a complete genome, generally by recombination in vivo (adenoviruses, herpesviruses, poxviruses).

A prerequisite for directed mutagenesis is a source of molecularly cloned viral nucleic acid. RNA genomes must be first converted to cDNA by reverse transcription and the larger genomes cleaved with an appropriate restriction endonuclease to generate a library of fragments. Once cloned, directed mutagenesis may make use of existing fortuitous restriction sites or employ synthetic oligonucleotides with specific mismatches flanked by regions of complementarity. Then oligonucleotide-directed mutagenesis can be used to obtain point mutations or precisely located deletions. This can be achieved by cloning wildtype genomic DNA into a single-stranded bacteriophage vector (e.g. M13mp19). The single-stranded phage DNA is isolated and annealed to the mutagenizing oligonucleotide that comprises two noncontiguous complementary sequences flanking the region to be looped out to produce the required deletion, or a mismatched base for the production of point mutations. The annealed oligonucleotide acts as a primer for DNA synthesis in vitro and the resulting double-stranded DNA is circularized with DNA ligase. A mutated genome is recovered by repair synthesis on a single-stranded DNA template or, increasingly, by polymerase chain reaction (PCR). (For a generalized protocol for directed mutagenesis, see Leppard and Pringle (1996).)

PCR-based directed mutagenesis has gained the ascendancy in practice because of its greater flexibility. Synthetic primers are designed to locate on opposite strands on either side of the target site. The region targeted for mutagenesis can be further defined by two opposing internal primers, one of which generates the desired mutation while the other eliminates one of two restriction sites flanking the target site. Two-stage amplification yields DNA that can be cleaved at the sites flanking the target site; only mutated DNA should retain the dispensable restriction site (Figure 11.2). The recovered fragment can then be ligated into an appropriately cleaved plasmid or M13 vector, a process that is facilitated if the restriction sites in the amplified fragment are also unique to the recipient genomic clone. In the case of parvoviruses, polyomaviruses, picornaviruses, and retroviruses, infectious progeny can be generated by direct rescue, i.e. by direct transfection of the reconstructed DNA into susceptible host cells. Transfection of nucleic acid is enhanced variously by

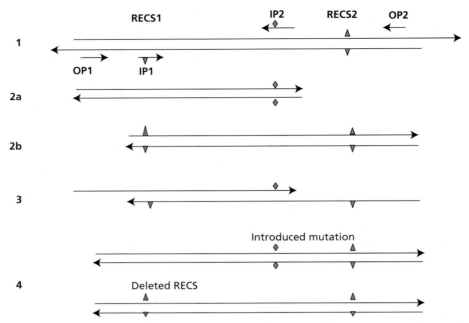

Figure 11.2 *A generalized two-stage protocol for DNA mutagenesis. OP1, OP2, IP1, and IP2 are oligonucleotide outer (OP) and inner (IP) primers with homology to the target DNA at the positions shown; RECS1 and RECS2 are restriction endonuclease cleavage sites. The inner primer IP2 carries the mutation to be introduced into the target region. All DNA strands are shown with the arrowheads directed towards their 3' ends. See the text for further explanation. Where only a single mutation is being introduced, a convenient variation of this protocol is to overlap the internal primers, such that each carries the desired mutation (or its homologue). Cleavage of the second-stage PCR product at sites RECS1 and RECS2 will produce a homogeneous mutated DNA fragment.*

calcium phosphate precipitation, lipofection, electroporation etc. Although picornaviruses can be rescued by transfection of cloned DNA, the process is more efficient if RNA transcribed in vitro is transfected by electroporation. For viruses with larger genomes (adeno-, herpes-, and poxviruses), rescue of the mutated fragment into infectious virus is achieved by cotransfection of the mutated sequence and intact viral genomic DNA into permissive cells. Recombination will occur provided the flanking sequences on either side of the mutated site are sufficient to permit homologous recombination. With the intermediate-sized adenoviruses, viral genomic DNA can be inactivated by cleavage with a single-cutting restriction enzyme such that the genome fragments overlap with the mutant-carrying fragment. In this situation infectious virus can be generated only by a process of homologous recombination, and most of the progeny virus will contain the mutation (Figure 11.3). In the herpesviruses and poxviruses, rescue of directed mutations is mostly confined to genes with phenotypes that are amenable to selection (e.g. enzyme deficiencies, drug resistance, cytopathology) on account of the high background of nonmutated virus in the absence of selection.

Deletion mutants

Operationally, deletion mutants are the simplest to obtain. However, deletion of sequences from a specific

protein-coding gene does not always produce a 'null' phenotype. For example, large stretches of the carboxy terminal region of the attachment (G) protein of respiratory syncytial virus can be deleted without affecting the attachment function or the viability of the virus. Similarly, herpesvirus thymidine kinase retains substantial activity despite loss of the first 45 amino acids. Deletion mutant analysis is particularly useful in defining promoter regions. Specific deletions can be engineered by digesting cloned single-stranded DNA from a single-stranded DNA bacteriophage vector with one or two restriction enzymes and recircularizing to generate two circular molecules, the extent and type of deletion obtained depending on the availability of restriction enzyme sites. Sets of deletion mutations can be obtained by restriction enzyme cleavage of a circular DNA molecule followed by progressive extension of a deletion using an exonuclease and recircularization.

Linker scanning mutagenesis

Linker scanning mutagenesis introduces clustered sets of point mutations at desired locations and allows more refined analysis of *cis*-acting control sequences and characterization of protein-binding sites. This procedure allows rapid screening for mutations and their immediate localization as a result of the appearance of a new restriction site (McKnight and Kingsbury 1982). A limitation of deletion mutant analysis is that if the dele-

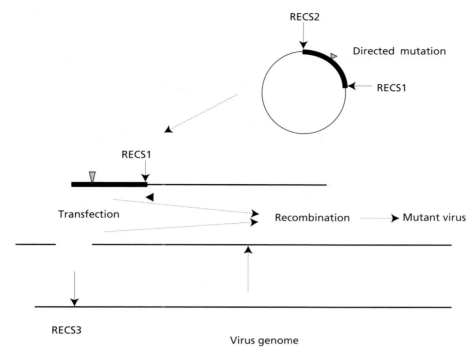

Figure 11.3 *Rescue of a mutated sequence by recombination. A generalized strategy for introduction of mutations into the terminal region of an adenovirus genome. (Similar strategies can be designed to introduce mutations into other regions of the genome.) The cloned adenovirus terminal genome fragment containing the desired mutation is shown as the thick line. Release of the fragment and cleavage of the target virus genome is achieved by digestion with appropriate restriction endonucleases at sites RECS1 and RESC2, and the products are transfected into appropriate susceptible cells (293 cells in the case of adenovirus). Recombination in vivo results in the generation of infectious virus carrying the desired mutation. (See text for further explanation.)*

tion is large it may cause nonspecific effects, for example steric interactions in proteins, or spacing constraints on promoter function.

Linker insertion mutagenesis

Linker insertion mutagenesis does not involve deletion; a linker is inserted at restriction sites within an open reading frame and many sites can be mutagenized by limiting digestion by a frequent cutting restriction enzyme. A linker of 3 bp (or multiples of 3) will maintain the reading frame beyond the insertion, whereas chain termination can be produced in all three reading frames by insertion of other linkers.

COMPLEMENTATION AND OTHER NONGENETIC INTERACTIONS

Interactions between viruses can be classified broadly as either genetic or nongenetic. Nongenetic interactions include complementation, phenotypic mixing, and interference, and will be considered first.

Complementation

Complementation is the ability of the defective gene product of one virus to be substituted by the normal gene product of another, when both viruses are present in the same host cell. Complementation provides a test for nonidentity, whereby mutants of similar phenotype (e.g. temperature sensitivity) can be assigned to different genes without prior knowledge of the existence or function of those genes. Operationally, complementation is measured in terms of a complementation index (CI). The CI can be used to assess the efficiency of complementation, i.e. in the case of temperature-sensitive mutants, the ratio of yield from a mixed infection (A × B) to the sum of the yields of the single infections (A + B) determined at the restrictive temperature. Progeny virus produced as a consequence of complementation between viruses retains the mutant genotype, because the interaction between viruses occurs at the level of gene products only. Consequently, assay of the progeny from a complementation experiment is carried out at the permissive temperature, and a positive CI indicates nonidentity of function. Complementation is normally intergenic in nature, but in the case of multifunctional gene products (e.g. many viral polymerases) intragenic complementation may be observed.

Complementation analysis has had a prominent role in defining gene function in the papovaviruses, adenoviruses, herpesviruses, poxviruses, retroviruses, alphaviruses, flaviviruses, paramyxoviruses, rhabdoviruses, arenaviruses, bunyaviruses, orthomyxoviruses, and reoviruses.

Phenotypic mixing and pseudotype formation

Phenotypic mixing is a form of nongenetic interaction between viruses whereby the structural components (capsid or envelope) may be interchanged partially or completely when two different viruses multiply in the same cell. Phenotypic mixing normally occurs between related viruses, but heterologous phenotypic mixing can occur between unrelated viruses. Viruses that are enveloped on exit from the host cell are prone to phenotypic mixing. The mixing of genomes and structural proteins results in the production of progeny virus particles in which the phenotype does not reflect the genotypic properties of the virus. Phenotypic mixing is thus a transient phenomenon.

Pseudotype formation, the complete investment of the core of one virus by the envelope of another, has provided a convenient means of rapid assay of noncytopathic or fastidious viruses. For example, some of the progeny virus released from cells coinfected with the nonfastidious and rapidly cytopathic rhabdoviruses, vesicular stomatitis virus, or Chandipura virus, and a host-restricted and noncytopathic or slowly cytopathic retrovirus will possess the genome of the lytic virus contained within the envelope of the retrovirus. The pseudotype yield, detected as rapidly plaque-forming virus resistant to neutralization by antiserum to the parental lytic rhabdovirus, provides a means of detection and rapid assay of its nonlytic partner. This technique has been used successfully in studies of host range and for detection and assay of HIV-1, HIV-2, HTLV-I, HTLY-II, mouse mammary tumor virus, bovine leukemia virus, and several avian retroviruses.

Many of the oncogenic avian and mammalian retroviruses exist as replication-defective viruses and are dependent on helper leukemia-associated retroviruses. These oncogenic retroviruses often exist as pseudotypes because their envelope glycoproteins are supplied by the helper virus. Other examples of asymmetric complementation or phenotypic mixing are the commensual association of hepatitis D virus and hepatitis B virus and the adenovirus helper dependence of some parvoviruses.

Interference and defective interfering particles

The ubiquity of nongenetic interactions such as complementation and phenotypic mixing is responsible for the prevalence of defective viruses. Defective viruses accumulate in many laboratory-propagated stocks of viruses and are dependent on the presence of their nondefective progenitor for their survival. It is a characteristic of most

defective viruses that they specifically interfere with the replication of their helper or closely related viruses. Interference occurs at the level of transcription and replication, and is not interferon-mediated. The mechanism of interference varies between viruses belonging to different families and between different defective viruses of the same virus. For example, the majority of the defective interfering (DI) particles of vesicular stomatitis virus, known as panhandle or hairpin DIs, which contain genomes with complementary 5′ ends and incomplete L gene sequences, interfere with the replication of viruses of homologous serotype only, whereas the DI particles that contain internal deletions of the L gene interfere with vesicular stomatitis virus of both homologous and heterologous serotypes. In formal terms, a single mutant or nucleotide substitution can constitute a DI genome, and deletion of sequence is not a necessary characteristic. It has been proposed that the generation of DI virus is a natural phenomenon that moderates the course of viral disease and contributes to the self-limiting nature of most viral diseases (Huang and Baltimore 1970). It has been difficult, however, to obtain evidence of the presence of DI virus in natural infections, although in a few instances the administration of DI particles can alter the outcome of an infection. Mice can be protected from an influenza virus-induced immune-mediated pneumonia by the administration of DI particles. However, the DI particles did not reduce the replication of virus in the lung, but seemed to act by preventing the virus-induced T-cell response that is responsible for consolidation (Morgan and Dimmock 1992).

DI particles have been implicated in the initiation, although not necessarily the maintenance, of persistent infection in vivo and in vitro. For example, a DI particle associated with the tsG31 mutant of vesicular stomatitis virus, possessing a 90 percent deletion of the genome, was a good inducer of persistent infection. Indeed, it has been proposed that persistent infection may be an important force in evolution, maintaining genetic variability in those viruses (such as the negative-sense RNA viruses) unable to acquire variation by genetic recombination. The generation of DI virus is a spontaneous mutational event, which in due course forces a mutational response in the parental virus to counteract the DI-mediated interference, and a cyclical phenomenon of alternating generation of new DI and specific DI interference-resistant viruses ensues. Progressive and extensive mutational change over the whole genome was observed to accompany the propagation of the normally lytic vesicular stomatitis virus as a persistent nonlytic infection in cultured cells, whereas by contrast the virus is genetically stable during cycles of lytic infection. The extensive mutation of the measles virus genome observed in the defective viruses recovered from the brain of patients with subacute sclerosing panencephalitis (SSPE) may be an indication that this phenomenon plays a role in human disease processes.

GENETIC INTERACTIONS

Genetic interactions include recombination, subunit reassortment, and multiplicity reactivation. Their characterization provides information about the evolutionary potential of viruses as well as means of their experimental manipulation.

Recombination in DNA viruses and positive-sense RNA viruses

Recombination occurs as a consequence of the physical interaction of viral genomes in the infected cell. It is a phenomenon common to all DNA-containing viruses, both DNA-containing and RNA-containing retroviruses, and most positive-strand RNA viruses. Recombination between DNA genomes is probably a conventional intramolecular mechanism involving a breakage and reformation of covalent bonds, whereas recombination between RNA genomes is a process mediated by a template switching ('copy-choice') mechanism during minus-strand synthesis. The probability of occurrence of a recombinational event between two genes is proportional to the physical distance separating them on the genome, and genetic maps can be constructed on the basis of recombination frequencies. Temperature-sensitive (ts) mutants have formed the framework for most genetic maps. The recombination frequency (RF) between any pair of temperature-sensitive mutants, A and B, is measured as the frequency (percentage) of wildtype virus generated in multiple infections, such that the RF between any two temperature-sensitive mutants, A and B, is measured as a frequency (percentage), such that $RF = 2 \times 100 \times \text{yield } (A + B)^{RT} - (\text{yield } A^{RT} + \text{yield } B^{RT})/\text{yield } (A + B)^{PT}$, where RT is the restrictive temperature and PT the permissive temperature. The single and mixed infections are carried out at the permissive temperature and yields assayed at the temperatures indicated by the superscript. The factor 2 is included because only the wildtype recombinant is measured by this assay, and it is assumed that the reciprocal recombinant (the double ts mutant) occurs with equal frequency. Using a quantitative PCR assay, Jarvis and Kirkegaard (1992) confirmed that frequencies of the reciprocal recombinants in poliovirus recombination are equivalent, but only when the parental input multiplicities are identical. Linear genetic maps of several DNA viruses (adeno-, herpes-, pox-, and picornaviruses) have been constructed on the basis of two factor crosses to establish relative proximity and three factor crosses to confirm orientation (for a detailed account, see Ramig 1990).

Mutants classified in the same complementation group cluster in the map, and the greatest distance separating mutants in the cluster defines the minimum size of the gene. In the adenoviruses and herpesviruses intertypic crosses, in which the parental ts mutants are derived from viruses of different serotype, have been employed to confirm the linear order of the genetic map and to show that the genetic and physical maps of the genome, constructed on the basis of restriction endonuclease fragment analysis or direct sequencing, are colinear. Recombinants between herpesvirus types 1 and 2 have been isolated from cultured cells, but natural recombinants have not been recovered from patients, suggesting that there are selective constraints preventing such interactions. Paradoxically, although the frequency of recombination is generally lower, natural recombinants occur more frequently in RNA viruses. For example, intertypic recombinants are prominent in the virus recovered from children after vaccination with the trivalent Sabin vaccine, although none of these recombinants has as yet escaped the immune response of the host to become established in nature. Rare heterologous recombinants also occur: for example, the *Alphavirus* known as Western equine encephalitis virus seems to be a recombinant of another *Alphavirus*, Eastern equine encephalitis virus, and a New World relative of Sindbis virus (Hahn and Lustig 1988).

Recombination in RNA viruses is not universal (reviewed by Lai 1992; Wimmer et al. 1993). Low-frequency genetic recombination (up to 0.9 percent) occurs in viruses with positive-strand genomes, and linear genetic maps were derived for both poliovirus and foot-and-mouth disease virus, which were subsequently found to be colinear with physical maps. Homologous recombination does not seem to be site specific, although intertypic recombination in poliovirus and foot-and-mouth disease virus may be influenced by local structural features. The three poliovirus types differ by about 15 percent in their nucleotide sequences, and the frequency of recombination observed between viruses of different subtypes, as expected by a template switching (copy-choice) mode of recombination, is about 100 times less than between viruses belonging to the same serotype.

Large genome sections can be transposed as a result of natural recombination in vivo, and the characterization of the phenotypic properties of recombinants has played a prominent role in the mapping of attenuating mutations in the Sabin poliovirus vaccine strains. Transposition of segments of any size can now be achieved in a more controlled manner by exchange of segments between existing or engineered restriction sites in infectious cDNA clones. This approach also provides a means of direct verification of the association of particular mutations with a specific phenotype. For example, a poliovirus mutant carrying a four-base insertion at position 70 within the 5' untranslated leader region has a small plaque ts phenotype and is deficient in RNA synthesis. Revertants of this mutant retained the four-base insert, and mix-and-match experiments with cDNA located these second site suppressor mutations to a site within the 3C protease gene (Andino et al. 1990). The isolation and characterization of revertants is an essential feature of the characterization of any mutant. The same approach can be used to produce chimeric viruses in order to study the homology and functional compatibility of genetic elements. For example, it has been shown that the 5′ untranslated leader regions of poliovirus and a coxsackie B virus can be interchanged.

The 5′ untranslated region of the genome of picornaviruses contains an internal ribosomal entry site (IRES), and poliovirus can be transformed into a vector by insertion of a foreign gene between tandemly arranged IRES sequences, in which one is derived from a nonhomologous IRES (e.g. from encephalomyocarditis virus (EMCV)) to prevent loss by homologous recombination. A dicistronic virus mimicking the genetic organization of the plant picornavirus cowpea mosaic virus (CPMV) can be created by insertion of the IRES from EMCV between the capsid precursor coding region and the nonstructural protein coding region of the poliovirus genome. Unlike CPMV, however, the two transcriptional units are linked and contained within the same particle.

Exceptionally, high-frequency genetic recombination is observed in mixed infections of coronaviruses, but a linear map of the coronavirus genome has not been produced. This may be a consequence of the complexity of the organization of the *Coronavirus* genome, with its unique 'nested set' configuration of genetic information, whereby subgenomic RNAs with a common 3′ terminus and differential extensions in a 5′ direction are intermediates in mRNA transcription. In addition, the polymerase protein of coronaviruses is encoded in two large open reading frames, from which the gene product is derived by translational frameshifting (ribosomal slippage). The largest *Coronavirus* genome (approximately 31 kb) is much larger than the picornavirus genome (approximately 7.5 kb), but the rate of recombination per nucleotide is similar at approximately 0.1 percent per 100 nucleotides (Lai 1992).

Reverse transcription and recombination

The retrovirus genome is present in the virion in a pseudodiploid form. Two copies of the viral genome are associated head-to-head by hydrogen bonding between short repeats at their 5′ ends. Despite the fact that two genomes are encapsidated in a single virion, only a single provirus is generated under conditions of infection of cells by single virions. The reason for the unique pseudodiploid form of the genome is unknown, except that it does allow for damage repair by recombination during the reverse transcription process. In other viruses

replication is generally accompanied by amplification of the genome, whereas in the replication of retroviruses there is no net gain; the process of reverse transcription results in the conversion of a one pair of single-stranded RNA genomes into one double-stranded DNA provirus (the process has been described as destructive replication). Reverse transcription not only generates a linear DNA copy of the retroviral genome but also produces the long terminal repeats (LTR), which contain the signals necessary for transcription of the integrated DNA, and which together are designated the provirus. At the cell–virus DNA junction there is a 5-bp direct repeat of cellular DNA next to a 3-bp inverted repeat of viral DNA, a structure similar to that present at the termini of several bacterial transposons. A major distinction between the retroviruses and other nuclear DNA viruses is that the former maintain productive infections and do not usually kill the host cell, whereas the latter invariably destroy their host cell and can only become stably integrated in a nonproductive form. (The phenomenon of latency in herpesviruses, however, to some extent blurs this distinction.)

High-frequency recombination is an inherent consequence of retrovirus replication. In crosses of exogenous retroviruses, recombination has been detected both between and within genes and between exogenous and endogenous viruses. The pseudodiploid nature of the genome means that heterozygous genomes can exist and may be intermediates in the generation of stable recombinants. In the replication of retroviruses, the location of the tRNA primer for DNA synthesis near the 5′ ends of the tandemly associated monomers means that the reverse transcriptase must transfer from the 5′ end of one monomer to the 3′ end of the same or the other monomer soon after the initiation of synthesis. Thus every round of synthesis is effectively a recombinational event. Furthermore, the process of reverse transcription itself involves synthesis of negative-strand DNA on the genomic positive-strand RNA template, and simultaneous degradation of the RNA template by the ribonuclease H activity of the enzyme complex, followed by synthesis of a positive DNA strand with internal discontinuities on the negative-strand template. There are abundant opportunities for recombination, either during negative-strand synthesis by a copy choice mechanism, or during positive-strand synthesis by strand displacement and assimilation on to replicating DNA from another genome. Comparison of the inferred amino acid sequences of retroviral proteins suggests that recombination has played an important role in the diversification of the envelope proteins of retroviruses, whereas the polymerase gene seems to have been protected from functionally disruptive recombinational events (McClure et al. 1988).

The extreme variability of the surface proteins of HIV-1 is not mediated by recombination alone. Progressive mutational change plays a role in addition to recombinational events, as does the phenomenon of biased hypermutation (Martinez et al. 1994), see later under Biased hypermutation.

Multiplicity reactivation, marker rescue and cross-reactivation

Multiplicity reactivation occurs when cells are infected with parental viruses which themselves are noninfectious (usually as a result of UV irradiation). At higher multiplicities of infection progeny virus may be released from susceptible cells that contain markers contributed by both parents. Infectivity has been restored by replacement of defective genes by recombination (or reassortment). Multiplicity reactivation is observed only if the inactivating lesions in the two parental viruses are located in different genes. Multiplicity reactivation has been observed between strains of the same virus, and also between viruses of different serotypes. Reactivation between an inactivated parent and an infectious parent is termed crossreactivation, or marker rescue, and is likewise mediated by recombination (or reassortment). Cross-reactivation can be exploited to increase the yield of recombinants (or reassortants) by infecting susceptible cells with a nonplaque-forming virus and a UV-inactivated plaque-forming virus.

Reverse genetics of double-stranded and negative-sense single-stranded RNA viruses

Intermolecular recombination has not been demonstrated unequivocally for any RNA virus with a negative-strand or double-stranded genome, with the exception of the tripartite genome double-stranded RNA phage φ6 (Mindich 1995). It is likely that recombination can occur as a rare event; otherwise it is difficult to account for the origin of some of the DI viruses of vesicular stomatitis virus, influenza A virus, and rotavirus which have truncated and juxtaposed genes, or rare phenomena such as the inversion of genes in the mammalian pneumoviruses, which departs from the otherwise invariant gene order found in other paramyxoviruses.

The double-stranded RNA viruses can exchange genes by reassortment of genome subunits. However, the development of a reverse genetics system to allow controlled mutagenesis of individual genome subunits has proved unexpectedly difficult to achieve. Roner and Joklik (2001) have recently described a reverse genetic system for reovirus type 3, which may be generally applicable to other members of the family *Reoviridae*.

The single-stranded negative-sense RNA viruses as a group do not exhibit genetic recombination, apart from the phenomenon of subunit reassortment in those viruses that have segmented genomes. For long this

prevented the application of molecular genetic analysis to the negative-sense RNA viruses, which include many important animal and human pathogens. However, reverse genetic systems are now available for many members of the nonsegmented genome families *Filoviridae*, *Paramyxoviridae*, and *Rhabdoviridae*, and the segmented genome families *Bunyaviridae* and *Orthomyxoviridae* (reviewed by Neumann et al. 2002). The genomic RNA of negative-strand RNA viruses is not infectious because the negative strand is not translated. However, Luytjes et al. (1989) achieved amplification, transcription, and rescue of synthetic RNA molecules by reconstitution of a biologically active nucleoprotein complex using synthetic RNA and purified core proteins in the presence of helper influenza virus. The packaging of the larger genomic RNAs of the nonsegmented genome viruses (the order *Mononegavirales*) also presented difficulties. The breakthrough came with the construction of a complete infectious cDNA copy of the genome of rabies virus by Schnell et al. (1994), and infectious cDNA clones for many viruses are now available.

Strategies for rescuing negative-sense RNA virus genomes rely on transfection of the cloned copy of the viral genome (usually as the anti-genome) into susceptible host cells, together with a source of T7 RNA polymerase, usually provided by a vaccinia virus recombinant vector, to direct the synthesis from bacteriophage T7 transcription plasmids of RNAs encoding the components of the viral nucleocapsid complex (Figure 11.4). The cloned anti-genomic strand is terminated with a ribozyme sequence. Self-cleavage of the primary transcript then removes the ribozyme sequences, leaving a precise 3′ terminus. The newly transcribed nucleocapsid components first replicate the anti-genomic RNA and then transcribe the newly synthesized negative strand. This results in production of the remaining structural proteins, further replication, and packaging as in a normal infection. Initially it was presumed that expression from an anti-genomic template, rather than genomic RNA, was obligatory to avoid sequestration and functional loss of the L, M, and P mRNAs of rabies virus by annealing to genomic-sense RNA. However, this is not an absolute requirement, and Sendai virus has been rescued from genomic DNA, albeit with reduced efficiency.

Reverse genetic systems for segmented genome viruses were more difficult to exploit because of the difficulty of delivering multiple genomic RNAs. The first successful reverse genetic system was achieved with the tripartite Bunyamwera virus, adapting the methodology developed for nonsegmented genome viruses. Later modified procedures were developed for the reverse genetics of the eight-segmented influenza A virus and influenza B virus, which take account of the nuclear phase in the replication cycle of these viruses. Figure 11.5 illustrates the methodology for the genetic manipulation

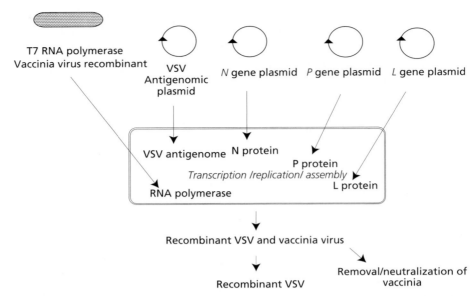

Figure 11.4 *Reverse genetics of nonsegmented negative-sense RNA viruses. The diagram depicts the strategy used to rescue infectious virus from the cDNA clone of a negative-sense RNA virus with a nonsegmented genome: vesicular stomatitis virus (VSV) is used as the example. Plasmids expressing the N, P, and L constituent proteins of transcribing nucleocapsids, and a plasmid containing a full-length cDNA replica of the viral antigenome, all under the control of the T7 RNA polymerase promoter (→), are transfected into susceptible cells. The T7 RNA polymerase is provided by coinfection of the cell substrate with a recombinant vaccinia virus expressing the T7 RNA polymerase. This is sufficient to initiate synthesis of functional nucleocapsids, followed by transcription, replication, assembly, and release of infectious virus.*

and recovery of negative-sense RNA viruses from cDNA clones of segmented genome viruses.

Recombination with host transcripts

Functions essential to replication and maturation can be attributed to no more than half the genes of the herpes simplex virus genome. It is likely that some of the excess coding capacity of the large DNA viruses represents accretion and modification of host genetic material by recombination. It is clear also that the oncogenic retroviruses have acquired their oncogenic potential by incorporation of cellular oncogenes by a recombinational mechanism. It is perhaps surprising, in view of the obligatory proviral phase in the multiplication cycle of these viruses, that these events have been so rare and restricted to experimental propagation of viruses in an inappropriate host.

Although conventional RNA viruses might not be expected to interact with the host-cell genome, there are isolated instances of such interactions for several positive-sense RNA viruses (poliovirus, Sindbis virus, and bovine viral diarrhea virus) and the negative-sense influenza A virus. The latter is the most exceptional because negative-sense RNA viruses do not exhibit intermolecular recombination. None the less, a variant of influenza A virus exists whose *N* gene subunit has an additional sequence exhibiting homology with host ribosomal RNA sequences. Best documented are the several independently derived isolates of the *Pestivirus*, bovine

viral diarrhea virus (BVDV), which have acquired simultaneously a cytopathic (cp) and a virulent phenotype. Molecular analysis of these events suggested that each cp virus evolved from the pre-existing noncytopathic (noncp) virus by a process of RNA recombination. A mechanism based on template switching of the viral polymerase during negative strand synthesis has been proposed to explain this phenomenon. Nonstructural protein NS3 is found exclusively after infection with cp BVDV, whereas uncleaved NS2-3 is characteristic of persistent noncp virus. The mutations that lead to the generation of NS3 from the polyprotein precursor include the precise insertion of cellular sequences, frequently together with large duplications and other genomic rearrangements. Two different kinds of cellular insertion have been identified, either (poly)ubiquitin or part of a cellular polypeptide of unknown function. Cleavage of the polyprotein at the N terminus of NS3 can be mediated by any of the several proteases that cleave ubiquitin in uninfected cells (Meyers and Thiel 1996). The expression of NS3 protein was considered to be strictly correlated with the cp phenotype, but later Qu et al. (2001) isolated a series of non-cp mutants from cp virus that still expressed NS3 protein. Sequence analyses of these noncp revertants uncovered no change in NS3, but all exhibited a single substitution in the NS4B region. Although the mechanism remains to be elucidated, these results illustrate that mutations in NS4B can attenuate BVDV cytopathogenicity despite NS3 production.

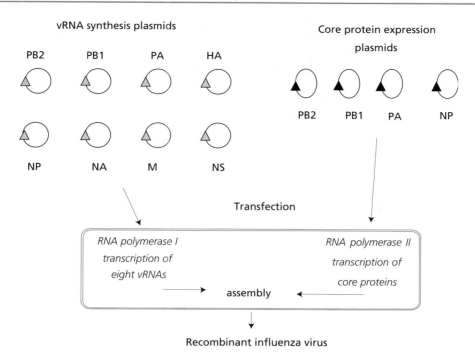

Figure 11.5 *Reverse genetics of segmented genome negative-sense RNA viruses. The diagram depicts the strategy used to rescue infectious virus from cDNA clones of the genome segments of a negative-sense RNA virus; influenza A virus is used as the example. Susceptible cells are transfected with plasmids encoding all eight components of the negative-sense genome under the control of the RNA polymerase I promoter (gray arrow-heads), together with four plasmids expressing the nucleocapsid components (PB1, PB2, PA, and NP) of influenza virus under the control of the RNA polymerase II promoter (black arrow-heads). The viral genomic RNAs are synthesized by cellular RNA polymerase I, and replication and transcription are initiated by synthesis of the viral polymerase (PB1, PB2, and PA) and the nucleoprotein (NP), followed by assembly and release of infectious virus.*

Interactions between cellular RNAs and replicating viral RNA have also been demonstrated in plant viruses, where a replication-competent deletion mutant of CPMV was rescued by recombination in transgenic plants expressing the deleted sequences (Greene and Allison 1994).

Subunit reassortment

All the segmented genome RNA viruses of animals are able to exchange genetic information by a process of subunit reassortment. Reassortment occurs at high frequency between related viruses; for example, all influenza A viruses are able to exchange genome subunits, but influenza A, B, and C viruses do not interact. In the bunyaviruses and the reoviruses restriction on reassortment of genome subunits closely parallels the serological and sequence relationships of the viruses, and does not correlate with the geographic origin of the isolates. In the orthomyxoviruses it is probable that there is random (i.e. unlinked) association of genome subunits and that the low electron microscope particle/plaque-forming unit ratio is a reflection of the imprecision of the maturation process, whereby only some particles receive the essential complement of eight unique subunits.

In the bunyaviruses, with their tripartite genomes, it is possible to undertake complete progeny analysis, because there are only six (2^3–2) nonparental reassortant genotypes, in contrast to the 254 (2^8–2) of influenza A virus, to be assayed. Reassortment appears not to be random and there are preferred associations of subunits even in the case of closely related viruses. The mechanism of restriction appears to operate at the level of gene products, as the terminal sequences of the subunits are identical and do not exhibit the specificity required for nonrandom reassortment. However, in crosses of Bunyamwera virus and Maguari virus, which belong to the Bunyamwera serogroup, once a parental subunit configuration had been broken by reassortment, the restriction on reassortment among progeny virus genomes was relaxed (Pringle 1996).

In the reoviruses, where maturation is efficient and precise, and particle/infectivity ratios are close to unity, reassortment appears to be random. In sharp contrast, if cells were infected (by lipofection) with reovirus infectious cores rather than virions, the progeny was almost exclusively monoreassortant virus (i.e. virus with nine subunits from one parent and one from the other). Lipofection of cells with naked RNA permitted only assortment (i.e. recovery of parental virus), not reassortment (Joklik and Roner 1995). These observations emphasize the complexity of the reassortment process and suggest again that protein–protein interactions, rather than RNA-sequence recognition, determine the specificity of reassortment. A complicating factor in the analysis of reassortment, described in rotavirus progeny analysis but probably true for all segmented genome viruses, is that the phenotype of the reassortants recovered may be modified by the genetic background of the recipient (Chen et al. 1989).

In general, reassortment is restricted to taxonomically related viruses: in the family *Orthomyxoviridae* the boundaries are defined by species, and by serogroups within species in other virus families. Conversely, genetic compatibility, as measured by the ability to reassort genome subunits, may be a useful approach to equating taxons in different virus families. All segmented genome viruses have the potential for rapid adaptation to new hosts, for abrupt generation of viruses with new antigenic characteristics, and for sudden extensions of host range and virulence. Transmission by vectors and multiplication in alternate hosts are also common features of these viruses.

Genetic reassortment plays a major role in the epidemiology of human influenza. Mutation accounts for the progressive genetic and antigenic variation (antigenic drift) of influenza A virus during interpandemic periods, but the appearance of new pandemic strains usually requires the introduction of new genes by reassortment (antigenic shift). Avian viruses seem to provide the reservoir of antigenic variation from which new pandemic strains can be generated. Much evidence suggests that the pig provides the 'mixing vessel' in which avian and human viruses can interact, generating progeny with new antigenic properties and the constellations of genes required to allow transmission to and spread within human hosts. In South China the domestic duck may be the intermediate host carrying viruses from feral ducks to the pig, whereas in North America domesticated turkeys may be a more important intermediate host. Reassortment of influenza A virus seems to have been responsible for the major pandemics afflicting the human population since the beginning of the twentieth century. However, a recent outbreak of a lethal antigenically novel avian-like virus in horses in the Far East, and since 2003 the appearance of various avian influenza A viruses in humans (H5N1 in East Asia, H7N7 in the Netherlands, H7N3 in Canada, and H7N2 in the USA), indicate that avian viruses can spread directly to mammalian species without the need for reassortment or passage through an intermediate host.

Superinfection exclusion and gene capture

The three serotypes of reoviruses exchange genome segments freely during mixed infection both in vitro and in vivo, but little is known about the role of reassortment in the biology of these viruses. In some segmented genome viruses (e.g. some bunyaviruses and orbiviruses), but not in others (e.g. rotaviruses), a phenomenon of superinfection exclusion is observed whereby a superinfecting virus is able to participate in subunit reassortment for only a limited period after primary infection. Superinfection exclusion is also host-dependent. For example, reassortment of the genome subunits of the *Orbivirus*, bluetongue virus, is inhibited if the introduction of the superinfecting virus is delayed by more than 4 h, whereas there is no interference for a period of at least 5 days in asynchronously infected midges.

Natural reassortants of rotaviruses are probably frequent in occurrence, and there is ample evidence for gene capture by the interaction of segmented genome viruses present in alternate hosts. For example, the Au-1 strain of human *Rotavirus* has a VP-4-coding subunit encoding a feline *Rotavirus*-like VP-4, suggesting that genetic interaction between feline and human rotaviruses is not infrequent. Other rotaviruses recovered from humans seem to be reassortants of human, bovine, and a third unidentified parental rotavirus. Likewise, it has been implied that the five serotypes of bluetongue virus present in North America are derived from three distinct gene pools, and that serotype 17 has evolved by a combination of reassortment and genetic drift.

VIRUS VARIABILITY

Like all biological entities that posses the ability to replicate and reproduce themselves, viruses are endowed with an intrinsic variability derived from the error-prone process of nucleic acid replication. This inbuilt variability enables viruses to respond to selective forces and ultimately guarantees their survival.

The quasi-species concept

It is generally accepted that mutation frequencies in most RNA viruses are very high, ranging from 10^{-3} to 10^{-6}, and usually in the range 10^{-4} to 10^{-5}. Consequently, a 10-kb RNA genome will on average carry one or more mutations, and any population of RNA viruses will comprise a heterogeneous swarm of diverse mutants. The term quasi-species was introduced to take account of this phenomenon and the consequent difficulty of defining a viral species (Eigen and Biebricher 1988). A single 'master' sequence may predominate at any one time during replication in a defined environment, but its existence will be transient and dependent on the maintenance of strong external selective forces. The high mutation frequencies of RNA viruses are attributed to the inherent error-proneness of RNA-dependent RNA polymerase and reverse transcriptase, and to the lack of a proofreading function.

Paradoxically, some RNA viruses exhibit great sequence stability during replication in vivo or during propagation in cultured cells. Even the highly variable HIV-1 is more stable during replication in cell culture than the error-proneness of the purified polymerase would predict, indicating the existence of cellular stabilizing factors (Mansky and Temin 1995).

Although the high mutation rates of RNA viruses provide them with great adaptability and may explain why in recent times they have been causes of emerging diseases (e.g. hepatitis C virus, Nipah virus, Hendra virus, severe acute respiratory syndrome (SARS) *Coronavirus*, enterovirus 71, and others) their limited genome size means that they are also subject to major evolutionary constraints. Also gene duplication and lateral gene transfer from their host or other viruses are inherently less likely (Holmes and Rambaut 2004).

Hypermutation

Enhanced frequency mutation mediated by an error-prone polymerase has been described for vesicular stomatis virus (Pringle 1987). Also, hypermutable sites occur in genomes, such as those generating frameshift and other mutations in the attachment (G) protein gene of human respiratory syncytial virus (Cane et al. 1993). Likewise, in DNA viruses mutations in accessory DNA replicating functions have been shown to be responsible for effects on the mutation frequency of herpes simplex virus type 1 (HSV-1) in cultured cells. Mutational loss of HSV-1-encoded dUTPase activity resulted in a fivefold increase in the relative mutant frequency, whereas thymidine kinase-negative mutants reduced the relative mutation rate up to 40-fold (Pyle and Thompson 1994).

Biased hypermutation

Several instances of biased hypermutation have been described. A phenomenon of G→A hypermutation has been observed in retroviruses and hepadnaviruses. Among negative-sense single-stranded RNA viruses, biased A→I hypermutation has been observed to affect mainly the matrix protein gene of measles virus, possibly as a consequence of posttranscriptional enzymatic misreading of A residues (Billeter and Cattaneo 1991); and multiple A→G transitions occur in the attachment protein gene of human respiratory syncytial virus. The latter are characteristic of neutralization escape mutants selected with monoclonal antibodies against the conserved central region of the G protein (Martinez and Melero 2002). A high frequency of frameshift mutations was observed also in the same gene, mediated by the addition or deletion of adenosine residues in some, but not all, runs of such residues. The fidelity of the viral polymerase appeared to be dependent on the template sequence (Cane et al. 1993).

The biased hypermutatiion in which many U residues were substituted by C residues, predominantly in the *M*

(matrix) protein gene of measles virus, was characteristic of isolates of measles virus associated with neurologic conditions such as subacute sclerosing panencephalitis and measles inclusion body encephalitis (MIBE). In the extreme case, 54 percent of U residues were changed to C residues. The phenomenon may be mediated by the presence in the cytoplasm of neural cells of a double-stranded RNA unwindase, an enzyme normally abundant in nuclei. This enzyme (duplex RNA-dependent adenosine deaminase) converts adenosine to inosine ribonucleotide. It is hypothesized that the predominance of U→C misincorporations over A (to I)→G mutations is a consequence of the formation of double-stranded RNA molecules by localized collapse of transcribed mRNA on to the genomic- (negative-) strand template, whereas the collapse of replicating negative-sense RNA on to the positive-sense anti-genome would be less frequent because of the encapsidation of replicating molecules, which is a feature of the synthesis of negative-strand RNA viruses. The phenomenon seems to have clinical significance in that clonal expansion of hypermutated measles viruses was demonstrated throughout the brain of an SSPE patient (Baczko et al. 1993).

Retroviral G→A hypermutation takes place during reverse transcription when the intracellular dTTP concentration greatly exceeds that of dCTP (Vartanian et al. 1997), This results in extensive incorporation of dT opposite rG, leading to G→A substitutions. In vitro the extent of G→A hypermutation can be influenced by manipulation of the dTTP/dCTP ratio. The extreme of such biased hypermutation is observed in the lentiviruses, where misincorporation may reach 60 percent in short stretches. It occurs predominantly during negative-sense DNA strand synthesis, and it has been established that G→A hypermutation can be sustained throughout synthesis of the entire 10-kb negative-sense DNA strand of HIV type 1, resulting in substitution of approximately 31 percent of the G residues (Vartanian et al. 2002).

Gunther et al. (1997) have described two naturally occurring hepatitis B virus genomes from a chronic carrier which exhibited G→A mutations distributed across the whole genome, with a strong dinucleotide preference in the order GpA > GpG > GpC/GpT. The frequency of replacement of guanosine residues by adenosine was 12 and 26 percent. The detection of hypermutation in natural isolates of hepatitis B virus suggested that a minority of hepatocytes might have distorted dNTP pool which, as well as generating hypermutation might be reflected in the fidelity of hepatocyte DNA synthesis and repair.

APPLICATIONS OF GENETIC ANALYSIS IN VIROLOGY

A genetic approach has many actual and potential applications in virology: for example, considered here are the analysis of antigenic properties (epitope mapping), identification of determinants of virulence and drug resistance, interpretation of molecular epidemiology, and the engineering of live virus vaccines.

Epitope analysis

Neutralization escape mutants can be isolated following exposure to, or growth in the presence of, a specific antiserum or an appropriate monoclonal antibody. Specific epitopes can be identified by analysis of the reactivity of neutralization escape mutants with panels of monoclonal antibodies. These epitopes can then be located by nucleotide sequencing of the escape mutants and physical mapping of the mutational changes. Optimally, these changes can then be located on the three-dimensional structure of viral attachment proteins (e.g. the HA protein of influenza A virus; see Chapter 32, Orthomyxoviruses: influenza) or the whole virion (e.g. poliovirus; see Chapter 40, Picornaviruses).

Nonneutralizing monoclonal antibody escape mutants can be obtained by a modification of the selection technique. Infected cell monolayers are reacted with an appropriate murine monoclonal antibody and then treated with an enzyme-linked second antibody (e.g. a horseradish peroxidase rabbit anti-mouse polyclonal serum). Plaques that are unstained represent monoclonal antibody-resistant (MAR) mutants, which can be employed in analysing the antigenic properties of nonstructural and internal components of viruses.

Drug resistance

The isolation of drug resistance mutants can identify the site of action of an antiviral agent and assist in analyzing both the mechanism of action of the drug and the function of the target protein. For example, identification of the function of the M2 protein of influenza virus and confirmation of its presence in the virion were direct results of the isolation of amantidine-resistant mutants of influenza A virus (Hayden and Hay 1992).

The isolation of drug resistance mutants can also provide information of relevance in the treatment of viral disease. For example, molecular analysis of mutants of HIV-1 virus resistant to 3'-azido-3'-deoxythymidine (AZT), nucleoside analogues, and other nonnucleoside reverse transcriptase (RT) inhibitors revealed unpredicted interaction between drugs in patients. In particular, suppression of phenotypic AZT resistance was observed in some viruses with mutations in the RT gene, which conferred resistance to other anti-retroviral drugs. Other combinations of mutations conferred coresistance. A conclusion from such analyses is that certain combinations of antivirals are more likely than others to induce multidrug resistance in the patient, and that it may be possible to design treatment schedules to

reduce this possibility, and even perhaps to reverse the loss of efficacy of AZT (Larder 1994).

Identification of virulence determinants

Analysis of the determinants of the virulence of the three Sabin poliovirus vaccine strains, which were produced by a process of adaptation to growth in nonneural tissue in vitro, provides one of the best examples of the potential of genetic analysis.

Determination of the complete sequence of the type 1 Sabin vaccine strain and its Mahoney virulent progenitor revealed that 56 single-site mutations, resulting in 21 amino acid substitutions, differentiated the two strains. The production of intratypic and intertypic recombinants generated by recombination experiments, the construction of in vitro clones from cDNA, and site-directed mutagenesis led to the conclusion that several mutations, mapped to VP1, VP3 , VP4, 3D^{pol}, and the 3' noncoding region, contributed to the attenuation and temperature-sensitive phenotypes. Although there was a strong correlation between the rct (temperature sensitivity) phenotype and loss of neurovirulence, assay of these recombinants and mutants in transgenic mice expressing the human poliovirus receptor revealed that the determinants of temperature sensitivity and attenuation were separable genetically (Bouchard et al. 1995).

A similar analysis was not possible with the poliovirus type 2, because the progenitor was already avirulent in monkeys. Recognition of virulence determinants in this case relied on comparison of the vaccine virus with a neurovirulent revertant isolated from a vaccine recipient. It was concluded that two major attenuating mutations resided in the 5' NTR (noncoding region) and in VP1.

A similar conclusion was derived from analysis of the type 3 vaccine strain, in which the wildtype (Leon) progenitor and a neurovirulent revertant from a patient were available for comparison. Remarkably, only 10 single-site mutations, resulting in four amino acid substitutions, differentiated the vaccine strain from its virulent progenitor. Two mutations, one located at site 472 in the 5' NTR and the other a ts mutation in the VP3 region, contributed to the attenuation phenotype. Later, a third mutation located in the VP1 region was identified as an additional attenuating factor. The C→U mutation at 472 associated with the attenuated phenotype was observed to revert at high frequency following vaccination. Virus recovered from the gut of a human infant as early as 47 h after vaccination had reverted, and exhibited increased neurovirulence in monkeys. The role of mutation in the 5' NTR region in attenuation was confirmed by mix-and-match type in vitro recombination experiments. Subsequently, mutations at positions 480 and 481 of poliovirus types 1 and 2, respectively, were similarly shown to be involved in the attenuation phenotype

(Figure 11.6). The 5′ NTR mutations locate at different bases in the same inferred secondary structure and may act by destabilizing this stem–loop structure, possibly affecting the translation efficiency of the viruses (Macadam et al. 1994). The other mutations affecting attenuation show no common features, and it is considered that 5′ NTR mutations may be responsible for the greater stability of the three Sabin live attenuated vaccines over their rivals. Similarly, a mutation in the 5′ noncoding region of coxsackie B3 virus has been identified as a determinant of cardiovirulence in mice (Tu et al. 1995).

It is likely for any virus that attenuation may be achieved by more than one route: for example, in the case of human respiratory syncytial virus (HRSV) mutations located in the *L* (polymerase) protein gene, the *F* (fusion) protein gene, or the start region of the *M2* protein gene, all have the potential to attenuate virulence. For this reason the most economical and reliable route to the identification of virulence factors, as exemplified in the case of the Sabin attenuated polioviruses, is to undertake a comparison of the genomic sequences of an existing empirically derived attenuated virus, its progenitor virulent parent, and, optimally, a revertant from the attenuated phenotype to a virulent phenotype. Once identified, critical attenuating mutations can be inserted into the genome of other strains of the same or closely related viruses by site-directed mutagenesis and recombinant virus rescued by recombination or reverse genetics according to the size and nature of the viral genome.

As in the case of the Sabin attenuated polioviruses, often remarkably few mutations distinguish virulent parental virus and attenuated progeny virus. Only 13 amino acid substitutions differentiated a candidate respiratory syncytial virus vaccine, derived semi-empirically by sequential selection of temperature-sensitive mutants under conditions of limiting mutagenesis, from its virulent parent. Comparison of the complete genome sequences of parental virus and first-, second-, and third-stage mutants, combined with testing in adult volunteers, enabled identification of a specific site in the respiratory syncytial virus polymerase protein gene that was a major determinant of attenuation (Tolley et al. 1996).

Attenuation by gene expression control

The location of a major attenuation determinant in the 5′ NTR region of poliovirus indicates that attenuation can be mediated at the level of control of mRNA synthesis, as the internal ribosome entry site of the poliovirus genome is located also in the 5′ region. In the case of nonsegmented negative-sense RNA viruses gene expression is controlled by the linear order of the individual genes and their relative distance from the single 3′-terminal transcriptional promoter. Thus the phenotypes of these viruses can be altered by gene rearrangement (Wertz et al. 1998; Ball et al. 1999) (Figure 11.7).

Flanagan et al. (2001) showed that rearrangement of the genes of vesicular stomatitis virus could eliminate clinical disease in swine, the natural host of the virus, thereby identifying an alternate route to attenuation (Figure 11.7b). Moving the nucleocapsid protein gene away from it normal location adjacent to the single transcriptional promoter site attenuated in stepwise fashion and finally eliminated the potential of the virus to produce disease in an experimental animal (Figure 11.7a). Combining this with relocation of the surface glycoprotein gene closer to the promoter site to increase its level of expression produced a virus that protected vaccinated animals against challenge with virulent virus of the same strain (Flanagan et al. 2000). Remarkably, these rearranged genomes could be propagated indefinitely and retained their altered phenotypes; some internal gene arrangements reduced viability, but others did not (Figure 11.7c). Subsequent work has shown that additional sequences can be inserted and retained in the genome of vesicular stomatitis virus, and that the level of expression of the supernumerary gene is determined by its relative position in the gene order (Wertz et al. 2002).

These results illustrate that negative strand viruses such as vesicular stomatitis virus, which are immune to disruption of gene order by recombination, can serve as stable gene vectors and vaccine delivery agents. The genome of vesicular stomatitis virus will tolerate a 40 percent increase in genome content (Haglund et al. 2002), allowing the insertion of heterologous antigens whose expression can be controlled by their position of insertion, and thereby increasing the scope of this approach to vaccine development. An unresolved question is why the majority of the nonsegmented negative-sense genome viruses (the order *Mononegavirales*) retain a common gene order, rather than any of the several viable permutations of the gene order.

Similar rearrangement of a strictly conserved genome organization without loss of viability has been observed also in the positive-sense RNA coronaviruses (de Haan et al. 2002).

Natural chimeras, transgenes, and genetically engineered vectors

In addition to the natural reassortants and recombinants of influenza viruses, rotaviruses, and picornaviruses encountered in nature, an expanding list of genetically engineered hybrid viruses is being described, e.g. Sindbis/VSV, influenza A/B, and VSV Indiana/VSV New Jersey, among others. The best-documented

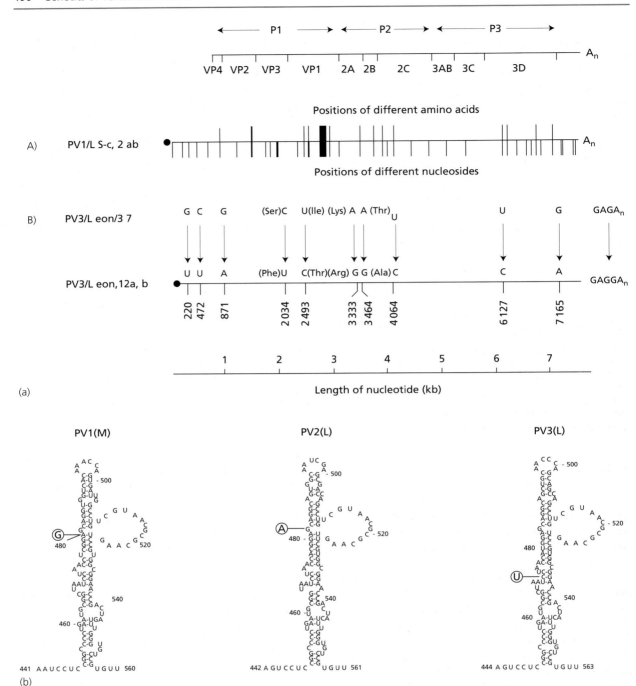

Figure 11.6 (a) *Location of attenuating mutations in the Sabin strains of poliovirus types 1 and 3: (A) the 21 amino acid and 56 nucleotide differences between the virulent parental (P1/Mahoney/41) and vaccine (P1/LSs, Zab) type 1 strains; (B) the four amino acid and ten nucleotide differences between virulent parental (P3/Leon/37) and vaccine (P3/Leon 12a1b) type 3 strains.* **(b)** *Domain V of the 5′ noncoding region of poliovirus types 1, 2, and 3. The attenuating mutations are circled. (Reproduced with permission from Almond 1987).*

chimeras are the adeno–SV40 hybrid viruses, which were inadvertently isolated during the 'adaptation' of adenovirus type 7 to growth in nonpermissive SV40-contaminated African green monkey kidney cells (Grodzicker 1981). Hybrid viruses were obtained in which adenovirus and SV40 virus genetic material was covalently linked. A few adeno–SV40 hybrids were isolated in which an intact adenovirus or SV40 genome was present, whereas others were incomplete and dependent for their existence on an adenovirus helper. Subsequently, helper-dependent and helper-independent adeno2–SV40 hybrids were produced in the same way. The ad2ND1 hybrid contained a nondefective, though incomplete, adenovirus genome covalently linked to

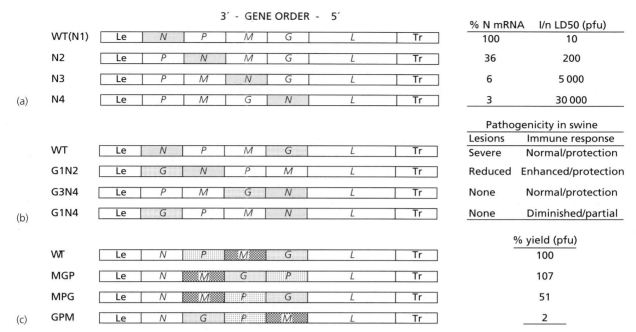

Figure 11.7 *Consequences of rearrangement of the gene order of vesicular stomatitis virus. The order of the components of the genome of vesicular stomatitis virus is indicated diagrammatically: the wildtype (WT) order is noncoding leader (Le), nucleocapsid (N) protein gene, phosphoprotein (P) gene, matrix (M) protein gene, glycoprotein (G) gene, polymerase (L) gene, and noncoding trailer (Tr) region. Panel (a) illustrates that translocation of the nucleoprotein gene down the gene order both attenuates transcription and reduces lethality for mice. Panel (b) indicates that translocation of the glycoprotein gene to a promoter-proximal position can enhance immunogenicity and eliminate clinical disease in the natural host of the virus. Panel (c) indicates that rearrangement of the internal genes can both enhance and reduce viability in cell culture.*

SV40 sequence. The SV40 sequence, which conferred the ability to multiply in monkey cells, varied from 7 to 43 percent, and the dispensable amount of adenovirus genome deleted varied from 4.5 to 7.6 percent. In all the adeno2–SV40 hybrids the insertion point was the same, namely at a site 14 percent from one end of the adenovirus genome.

Continuous passage of papovaviruses at high multiplicity of infection generates particles that have lower buoyant density than competent virions and contain less DNA. The DNA in these particles is circular and may have 10–50 percent of the papovavirus genome deleted. The segment deleted may be substituted by reiterated or nonreiterated host-cell DNA sequences, which may be larger than the segment deleted. These phenomena show that the genome of papovaviruses, and perhaps other DNA viruses, can be modified by the incorporation of host DNA sequences, and on rare occasions can contribute DNA sequences, either by homologous recombination or by illegitimate recombination, to other DNA-containing viruses.

An additional dimension has been added to genetic analysis by the ability to introduce foreign DNA into fertilized murine ova and to raise to maturity transgenic animals that have the foreign DNA integrated chromosomally. Among other things, this technique enables the determinants of tissue specificity to be investigated directly. For example, comparison of the pattern of

tumor development in mice transgenic for genes from SV40, JC, and BK viruses indicated that tissue specificity is determined by early genes.

The construction of recombinant viruses for use as vaccines and gene vectors is probably the most obvious practical outlet for genetic technology. Vaccines of proven worth and safety (e.g. vaccinia virus, fowlpox virus, simian foamy virus, poliovirus, adenovirus, and others) can be employed as vectors for heterologous antigens. This approach to vaccine development (sometimes called vectored antigen delivery) has the advantages of inherent safety, speed, ease of administration and, in contrast to inactivated vaccines, the likelihood of obtaining a balanced cellular and humoral immune response. The potential limitation of pre-existing or induced immunity to the vector has not been a major problem in experimental trials. Control of rabies in wildlife by oral vaccination of red fox populations in Europe using a bait laced with a vaccinia virus/rabies *G protein* gene recombinant virus was the first successful application of this approach (Aubert et al. 1994).

Attenuated vesicular stomatitis viruses have been developed as vectors which can be delivered intranasally and support higher levels of expression than poxvirus vectors. In experimental animals these recombinants have proved effective in inducing humoral and cell-mediated responses to a variety of viral antigens (HIV gag and env; HCV E1 and E2; bovine viral diarrhea E2;

influenza A virus HA; rabbit papilloma virus L1; and respiratory syncytial virus G and F). Vesicular stomatitis vectors with the *G* (attachment) *protein* gene deleted (and expressing the influenza HA protein, or either G or F of respiratory syncytial virus) were protective and nonpathogenic in mice, and had the additional advantage of not inducing neutralizing antibodies to the vector itself (Kahn et al. 2001).

Gene therapy

Viruses have potential as efficient gene delivery vehicles in gene therapy, provided efficient transduction and sustained transgene expression can be achieved without compromising safety. Retroviruses and adenoassociated viruses are favored as gene delivery vehicles because of their low cytopathogenicity and/or tissue specificity. The strategies employed have ranged from complex to simple. The first successful treatment by gene therapy of a disease affecting multiorgan systems in a large mammal employed one of the simplest approaches. Mucopolysaccharidosis VII is a rare inherited disorder in dogs which manifests as ocular defects, cardiac disease, and bone abnormalities leading to loss of mobility by 6 months. This condition is due to a deficiency in the activity of the hepatic enzyme β-glucuronidase. Several 2–3-day-old dogs with this disorder received intravenous injections of Moloney murine leukemia virus carrying a normal canine *β-glucuronidase* gene under the control of a liver-specific promoter (Ponder et al. 2002). Transduced hepatocytes expanded clonally during normal liver growth and secreted normal levels of β-glucuronidase. Dogs treated in this way achieved normal body weight and were fully active at 17 months.

Molecular epidemiology

Recognition of genetic diversity through genome sequencing and phylogenetic analysis plays an increasingly important role in understanding the epidemiology of infectious disease. For example, a high proportion of patients with vaccine-related poliomyelitis exhibit vaccine-derived interserotype recombinant viruses that have also lost their attenuated phenotype (Cherkasova et al. 2002). Study of these isolates revealed a nonrandom distribution of synonymous mutations, conservation of secondary structural features, a relative dearth of mutations affecting the integrity of antigenic determinants, and a frequent occurrence of tripartite intertypic recombinants with either type 1 or type 3 homotypic genomic ends.

Analysis of all available complete genome sequences of dengue viruses revealed that about 10 percent were intrasubtype recombinants (Worobey et al. 1999), thereby discounting the use of partial genome sequences as markers for the whole genome. This phenomenon is a confounding factor in analysis of the circumstances that contribute to the appearance of the lethal hemorrhagic form of dengue fever. In the absence of recombination this complication does not arise. For example, a study of the genetic variability of human RSV, a virus initially assumed to be associated only with seasonal respiratory disease in infancy in temperate climates, established that RSV is a universal respiratory pathogen evolving in a global milieu. Isolates of RSV originating from many parts of the world could be fitted into a genotype classification defined by analysis of viruses recovered from the catchment area of a single hospital in a suburb of Birmingham (Cane and Pringle 1995).

The developing AIDS epidemic is one of the greatest challenges facing mankind. Phylogenetic analysis has established that the origin of the AIDS syndrome was not a unique event, and that the M, N, and O groups of HIV-1 have each arisen as a consequence of independent zoonotic transmission of a simian immunodeficiency virus (SIVcpz) from a subspecies of the common chimpanzee (*Pan troglodytes troglodytes*) to humans. Other explanations for the origin of the M, H, and O groups of HIV-1, such as viral diversification within human populations, are inconsistent with existing phylogenetic data (Gao et al. 1999). The closest relatives of HIV-2 have been found in the sooty mangabey (*Cerocebus atys*), and again phylogenetic evidence suggests independent transmissions to humans. A recent survey has established that a substantial proportion of wild monkeys in West Africa are infected with a diversity of simian immunodeficiency viruses, serologically related to HIV to varying extents, representing a reservoir of potential human pathogens. The emergence of the lentivirus immunodeficiency diseases in humans has been correlated with the increased hunting of primates to provide meat for human consumption (Peeters et al. 2002). On the other hand, a putative evolutionary link has been proposed between HIV-1 and a group of endogenous retroviruses (HERV-K) that are present at about 50 proviral copies per haploid genome and which entered the human genome some 30 million years ago. The connection is based on identification of a functional homolog of the HIV-1 Rev protein encoded in the HERV-K genome, and the presence of a target RNA sequence in the HERV-K LTR region recognized by HIV-1 Rev (Yang et al. 1999), perhaps indicative of previous human encounters with such retroviruses.

Immune evasion

Characterization of the genomes of the large DNA viruses has identified a number of genes that interfere with the immune response of the host. The genome of vaccinia virus comprises about 200 genes, about one-third of which are dispensable for propagation of the virus in cultured cells. These apparently dispensable genes map in the extensive dispensable terminal regions of the vaccinia virus genome, together with host range and virulence markers. Some of these dispensable genes seem to contribute to the survival of the virus in vivo by interfering with specific arms of the immune system, such as complement, interferon, inflammation, cytokines, and cytotoxic T-lymphocyte recognition. The vaccinia virus genome encodes several proteins that have amino acid similarity to components of the complement system, and may prevent complement activation by competitively binding either complement control factors or complement receptors. Analogous genes are present in some herpesviruses.

At least four poxvirus genes interfere with interferon action. However, interference with the interferon response is not restricted to the large genome DNA viruses. Negative-sense RNA viruses also encode proteins that interfere with the interferon response. For example, the *NSs* gene product of bunyamwera virus, identified as a nonessential protein modulating pathogenesis, functions as an interferon induction antagonist to enhance virulence (Weber et al. 2002). Similarly, by construction of deletion mutant and recombinant viruses by reverse genetics it has been established unequivocally that the promoter-proximal *NS1* and *NS2* genes of pneumoviruses, two abundantly transcribed genes of previously unknown function, function as α/β-interferon induction antagonists (Bossert and Konzelmann 2002). Other paramyxoviruses have evolved different mechanisms for counteracting the cellular interferon response. Sendai virus, SV5, and human parainfluenza virus 3 block both type I and type II inferferon responses by targeting the cellular signaling factors (STAT 1 and STAT 2) involved in interferon signaling, an effect which is mediated by one of the alternate products expressed from the virus phosphoprotein gene (Andrejeva et al. 2002).

These are some examples of the continuing value of application of genetic methodology in both fundamental and applied virology.

REFERENCES

Almond, J.W. 1987. The attenuation of poliovirus neurovirulence. *Annu Rev Microbiol*, **41**, 153–80.

Andrejeva, J., Young, D.F., et al. 2002. Degradation of STAT1 and STAT2 by the V proteins of simian virus 40 and human parainfluenza virus type 2, respectively: consequences for virus replication in the presence of alpha/beta and gamma interferon. *J Virol*, **76**, 2159–67.

Angeletti, P.C., Kim, K., et al. 2002. Stable replication of papillomavirus genomes in *Saccharomyces cerevisiae*. *J Virol*, **76**, 3350–8.

Andino, R., Reickhof, G.E., et al. 1990. Substitutions in the protease (3C^{pro}) gene of poliovirus can suppress a mutation in the 5′ noncoding region. *J Virol*, **64**, 607–12.

Aubert, M.F.A., Masson, E., et al. 1994. Oral wildlife rabies vaccination field trials in Europe with recent emphasis on France. *Curr Topic Microbiol Immunol*, **187**, 219–44.

Baczko, K., Lampe, J., et al. 1993. Clonal expansion of hypermutated measles virus in a SSPE brain. *Virology*, **197**, 188–95.

Ball, L.A., Pringle, C.R., et al. 1999. Phenotypic consequences of rearranging the P, M and G genes of vesicular stomatis virus. *J Virol*, **73**, 4705–12.

Baltimore, D. 1971. Expression of animal virus genomes. *Bacteriol Rev*, **35**, 235–41.

Billeter, M.A. and Cattaneo, R. 1991. Molecular biology of defective measles viruses persisting in the human central nervous system. In: Kingsbury, D.W. (ed.), *The paramyxoviruses*. New York: Plenum Press, 323–46.

Bossert, B. and Konzelmann, K.-K. 2002. Respiratory syncytial virus (RSV) nonstructural (NS) proteins as host range determinants: a chimeric bovine RSV with NS genes from human RSV is attenuated in interferon-competent bovine cells. *J Virol*, **76**, 4287–93.

Bouchard, M.J., Lam, D-H.L. and Racaniello, V.R. 1995. Determinants of attenuation and temperature-sensitivity in the type 1 poliovirus Sabin vaccine. *J Virol*, **69**, 4972–8.

Brierle, I. 1995. Ribosomal frameshifting on viral RNAs. *J Gen Virol*, **76**, 1885–92.

Cane, P.A. and Pringle, C.R. 1995. Evolution of subgroup A respiratory syncytial virus: evidence for progressive accumulation of amino acid changes in the attachment protein. *J Virol*, **69**, 2918–25.

Cane, P.A., Matthews, D.A. and Pringle, C.R. 1993. Frequent polymerase errors observed in a restricted area of clones derived from the attachment (G) gene of respiratory syncytial virus. *J Virol*, **67**, 1090–3.

Chao, L. 1994. Evolution of genetic exchange in RNA viruses. In: Morse, S.S. (ed.), *The evolutionary biology of viruses*. New York: Raven Press, 233–50.

Chen, D., Burns, J.W., et al. 1989. Phenotypes of rotavirus reassortants depend upon the recipient genetic background. *Proc Natl Acad Sci USA*, **86**, 3743–7.

Cherkasova, E.A., Korotkova, E.A., et al. 2002. Long-term circulation of vaccine-derived poliovirus that causes paralytic disease. *J Virol*, **76**, 6791–9.

Davison, A.J. 2002. Evolution of the herpesviruses. *Vet Microbiol*, **86**, 69–88.

De Haan, C.A.M., Volders, H., et al. 2002. Coronaviruses maintain viability despite dramatic rearrangements of the strictly conserved genome organisation. *J Virol*, **76**, 12491–502.

Eigen, M. and Biebricher, C.K. 1988. Sequence space and quasispecies distribution. In: Domingo, E., et al. (eds), *RNA genetics*, Vol. 3. . Boca Raton: CRC Press, 211–45.

Flanagan, E.B., Ball, L.A. and Wertz, G.W. 2000. Moving the glycoprotein gene of vesicular stomatitis virus to promoter-proximal positions accelerates and enhances the protective immune response. *J Virol*, **74**, 7895–902.

Flanagan, E.B., Zamparo, J.M., et al. 2001. Rearrangement of the genes of vesicular stomatitis virus eliminates clinical disease in the natural host: new strategy for vaccine development. *J Virol*, **75**, 8107–6114.

Gao, F., Bailes, E., et al. 1999. Origin of HIV-1 in the chimpanzee *Pan troglodytes troglodytes*. *Nature (Lond)*, **397**, 436–41.

Gibbs, M. and Weiller, G.F. 1999. Evidence that a plant virus switched hosts to infect a vertebrate and then recombined with a vertebrate-infecting virus. *Proc Natl Acad Sci USA*, **96**, 8022–7.

Goldbach, R. and de Haan, P.T. 1993. RNA viral supergroups and the evolution of RNA viruses. In: Morse, S.S. (ed.), *The evolutionary biology of viruses*. New York: Raven Press, 105–19.

Greene, A.E. and Allison, R.F. 1994. Recombination between viral RNA and transgenic plant transcripts. *Science*, **263**, 1423–5.

Grodzicker, T. 1981. Adenovirus-SV40 hybrids. In: Tooze, J. (ed.), *DNA tumor viruses*, 2nd edn. Cold Spring Harbor: Cold Spring Harbor Laboratory, 577–614.

Gunther, S., Sommer, G., et al. 1997. Naturally occurring hepatitis B virus genomes bearing the hallmarks of retroviral G→A hypermutation. *Virology*, **235**, 104–8.

Haglund, K., Leiner, I., et al. 2002. High-level primary CD8$^+$ T-cell response to human immunodeficiency virus type 1 gag and env generated by vaccination with recombinant vesicular stomatitis viruses. *J Virol*, **76**, 2730–8.

Hahn, C.S., Lustig, S., et al. 1988. Western equine encephalitis virus is a recombinant virus. *Proc Natl Acad Sci USA*, **85**, 5997–6001.

Hayden, F.G. and Hay, A.J. 1992. Emergence and transmission of influenza A viruses resistant to amantadine and remantadine. *Curr Topic Microbiol Immunol*, **176**, 119–30.

Holmes, E.C. and Rambaut, A. 2004. Virus evolution and the emergence of SARS coronavirus. *Phil. Trans. R Soc. Lond B*, **359**, in press.

Herniou, E., Martin, J., et al. 1998. Retroviral diversity and distribution in vertebrates. *J Virol*, **72**, 5955–66.

Huang, A.S. and Baltimore, D. 1970. Defective virus particles and viral disease processes. *Nature (Lond)*, **226**, 325–7.

Hull, R. and Covey, S.N. 1986. Genome organisation and expression of reverse transcribing elements: variations and a theme. *J Gen Virol*, **67**, 1751–8.

Ihara, T., Akashi, H. and Bishop, D.H.L. 1984. Novel coding strategy (ambisense genomic RNA) revealed by sequence analysis of Punta Toro phlebovirus S-RNA. *Virology*, **136**, 293–306.

Jarvis, T.C. and Kirkegaard, K. 1992. Poliovirus recombination: mechanistic studies in the absence of selection. *EMBO J*, **11**, 3135–45.

Joklik, W.R. and Roner, M.R. 1995. What reassorts when reovirus genome segments reassort? *J Biol Chem*, **270**, 4181–4.

Kahn, J.S., Roberts, A., et al. 2001. Replication-competent or attenuated, nonpropagating vesicular stomatitis viruses expressing respiratory syncytial virus (RSV) antigens protect mice against RSV challenge. *J Virol*, **75**, 11079–87.

Kates, J.R. and McAuslan, B.R. 1967. Poxvirus DNA-dependent RNA polymerase. *Proc Natl Acad Sci USA*, **58**, 134–41.

Koonin, E.V. and Dolja, W. 1993. Evolution and taxonomy of positive-strand RNA viruses: implications of comparative analysis of amino acid sequences. *Crit Rev Biochem Mol Biol*, **28**, 375–430.

Lai, M.M.C. 1992. RNA recombination in animal and plant viruses. *Microbiol Rev*, **56**, 61–79.

Larder, B.A. 1994. Interactions between drug resistance mutations in human immunodeficiency virus type 1 reverse transcriptase. *J Gen Virol*, **75**, 951–7.

Leppard, K.N. and Pringle, C.R. 1996. Virus mutants. In: Mahy, B.W.J. and Kangro, H. (eds), *Virology methods manual*. London: Academic Press, 231–49.

Luytjes, W., Krystal, M., et al. 1989. Amplification, expression and packaging of a foreign gene by influenza virus. *Cell*, **59**, 1107–13.

Macadam, A.T., Stone, D.M., et al. 1994. The 5′ noncoding region and virulence of poliovirus vaccine strains. *Trends Microbiol*, **2**, 449–54.

McClure, M.A., Johnson, M.S., et al. 1988. Sequence comparisons of retroviral proteins: relative rates of change and general phylogeny. *Proc Natl Acad Sci USA*, **85**, 2469–73.

McGeoch, D.J. and Cook, S. 1994. Molecular phylogeny of the *Alphaherpesvirinae* subfamily and a proposed evolutionary timescale. *J Mol Biol*, **238**, 9–22.

McGeoch, D.J., Cook, S., et al. 1995. Molecular phylogeny and evolutionary timescale for the family of mammalian herpesviruses. *J Mol Biol*, **247**, 443–58.

McGeoch, D.J. and Davison, A.J. 1999. The molecular evolutionary history of the herpesviruses. In: Domingo, E., et al. (eds), *Origin and evolution of viruses*. London: Academic Press, 441–65.

McGeoch, D.J., Dolan, A. and Ralph, A.C. 2000. Towards a comprehensive phylogeny for mammalian and avian herpesviruses. *J Virol*, **74**, 10401–6.

McKnight, S.L. and Kingsbury, R. 1982. Transcriptional control signals of a eukaryotic protein-coding gene. *Science*, **21**, 316–24.

Mansky, L.M. and Temin, H.M. 1995. Lower in vivo mutation rate of human immunodeficiency virus type 1 than that predicted from the fidelity of purified reverse transcriptase. *J Virol*, **69**, 5087–94.

Martinez, M.A., Vartanian, J.-P. and Wain-Hobson, S. 1994. Hypermutagenesis of RNA using human immunodeficiency virus type 1 reverse transcriptase and biased dNTP concentrations. *Proc Natl Acad Sci USA*, **91**, 11787–1191.

Martinez, I. and Melero, J.A. 2002. A model for the generation of multiple A to G transitions in the human respiratory syncytial virus genome: predicted RNA secondary structures as substrates for adenosine deaminases that act on RNA. *J Gen Virol*, **83**, 1445–55.

Meyers, G. and Thiel, H-J. 1996. Molecular characterization of pestiviruses. *Adv Virus Res*, **47**, 53–118.

Mi, S., Lee, X.-P., et al. 2000. Syncytin is a captive retroviral envelope protein involved in human placental morphogenesis. *Nature (Lond)*, **403**, 785–9.

Mindich, L. 1995. Heterologous recombination in the segmented dsRNA genome of bacteriophage 6. *Semin Virol*, **6**, 75–83.

Morgan, D.I. and Dimmock, N.J. 1992. Defective interfering virus inhibits immunopathological effects of infectious virus in the mouse. *J Virol*, **66**, 1188–92.

Morse, M.A., Marriott, A.C. and Nuttall, P.A. 1992. The glycoprotein of Thogoto virus (a tick-borne orthomyxo-like virus) is related to the baculovirus glycoprotein gp64. *Virology*, **186**, 640–6.

Neumann, G., Whitt, M.A. and Kawaoka, Y. 2002. A decade after the generation of a negative-sense RNA virus from cloned cDNA – what have we learned? *J Gen Virol*, **83**, 2635–62.

Paces, J., Pavlicek, A. and Paces, V. 2002. HERVd: database of human endogenous retroviruses. *Nucleic Acid Res*, **30**, 205–6.

Peng, C.-W., Peremyslov, V.V., et al. 2002. A replication-competent chimera of plant and animal viruses. *Virology*, **294**, 75–84.

Peeters, M., Courgnaud, V., et al. 2002. Risk to human health from a plethora of simian immunodeficiency viruses in primate bushmeat. *Emerg Infect Dis*, **8**, 1–10.

Ponder, K.P., Melniczek, J.R., et al. 2002. Therapeutic neonatal hepatic gene therapy in mucopolysaccharidosis VII dogs. *Proc Natl Acad Sci USA*, **99**, 13102–7.

Pringle, C.R. 1977. Enucleation as a technique in the study of virus–host interactions. *Curr Topic Microbiol Immunobiol*, **76**, 49–82.

Pringle, C.R. 1987. Rhabdovirus genetics. In: Fraenkel, H. and Wagner, R.R. (eds), *The rhabdoviruses*. New York: Plenum Press, 167–243.

Pringle, C.R. 1996. Bunyavirus genetics. In: Elliott, R.M.E. (ed.), *The bunyaviruses*. New York: Plenum Press, 189–226.

Pyle, R.B. and Thompson, R.L. 1994. Mutations in accessory DNA replicating functions alter the relative mutation frequency of herpes simplex virus type 1 strains in cultured murine cells. *J Virol*, **68**, 4514–24.

Qu, L., McMullan, L.K. and Rice, C.M. 2001. Isolation and characterization of noncytopathic pestivirus mutants reveals a role for nonstructural protein NS4B in viral cytopathogenicity. *J Virol*, **75**, 10651–62.

Ramig, R.F. 1990. Principles of animal virus genetics. In: Fields, B.N., et al. (eds), *Fields' Virology*, 2nd edn. New York: Raven Press, 95–122.

Roner, M.K. and Joklik, W.K. 2001. Reovirus reverse genetics: Incorporation of the CAT gene into the reovirus genome. *Proc Natl Acad Sci USA*, **98**, 8036–41.

Schneemann, A., Schneider, P.A., et al. 1995. The remarkable coding strategy of Borna disease virus: a new member of the nonsegmented negative strand RNA viruses. *Virology*, **210**, 1–8.

Schnell, M.J., Mebatsion, T. and Conzelmann, K.-K. 1994. Infectious rabies virus from cloned cDNA. *EMBO J*, **13**, 4195–203.

Sedivy, J.M., Capone, J.P., et al. 1987. An inducible mammalian amber suppressor: propagation of a poliovirus mutant. *Cell*, **50**, 379–89.

Sverdlov, E.D. 2000. Retroviruses and primate evolution. *Bioessays*, **22**, 161–71.

Tolley, K.P., Marriott, A.C., et al. 1996. Identification of mutations contributing to the reduced virulence of a modified strain of respiratory syncytial virus. *Vaccine*, **14**, 1637–46.

Tristem, M. 2000. Identification and characterization of novel human endogenous retrovirus families by phylogenetic screening of the human genome mapping project database. *J Virol*, **74**, 3715–30.

Tu, Z., Chapman, N.M., et al. 1995. The cardiovirulent phenotype of Coxsackie B3 is determined at a single site in the genomic 5′ nontranslated region. *J Virol*, **69**, 4607–18.

Van Regenmortel, M.H.V., et al. (eds). 2000. *Virus Taxonomy; the 7th Report of the International Committee on Taxonomy of Viruses*. San Diego: Academic Press.

Vartanian, J.P., Plikat, U., et al. 1997. HIV genetic variability is directed and restricted by DNA precursor availability. *J Mol Biol*, **270**, 139–51.

Vartanian, J.P., Henry, M. and Wain-Hobson, S. 2002. Sustained G→A hypermutation during reverse transcription of an entire human immunodeficiency virus type 1 strain Vau group O genome. *J Gen Virol*, **83**, 801–5.

Weber, F., Bridgen, A., et al. 2002. Bunyamwera bunyavirus nonstructural protein NSs counteracts the induction of alpha-beta interferon. *J Virol*, **76**, 7949–55.

Wertz, G.W., Perepelitsa, V.P. and Ball, L.A. 1998. Gene rearrangement attenuates expression and lethality of a nonsegmented negative strand RNA virus. *Proc Natl Acad Sci USA*, **95**, 3501–6.

Wertz, G.W., Moudy, R. and Ball, L.A. 2002. Adding genes to the RNA genome of vesicular stomatitis virus: Positional effects on stability of expression. *J Virol*, **76**, 7642–50.

White, B.T. and McGeoch, D.J. 1987. Isolation and characterisation of conditional lethal nonsense mutants of vesicular stomatitis virus. *J Gen Virol*, **68**, 3033–44.

Wimmer, E., Hellen, C.U. and Cao, X. 1993. Genetics of poliovirus. *Annu Rev Genet*, **27**, 353–436.

Worobey, M., Rambaut, A. and Holmes, E.C. 1999. Widespread intra-serotype recombination in natural populations of dengue virus. *Proc Natl Acad Sci USA*, **96**, 7352–7.

Yang, J., Bogerd, H.P., et al. 1999. An ancient family of human endogenous retroviruses encodes a functional homolog of the HIV-1 rev protein. *Proc Natl Acad Sci USA*, **96**, 13404–8.

Yu, S.F., Sullivan, M.D. and Linial, M.L. 1999. Evidence that the human foamy virus genome is DNA. *J Virol*, **73**, 1565–72.

12

Virus–host cell interactions

L. ANDREW BALL

INTRODUCTION

As obligate intracellular parasites, viruses depend on their host cells at all stages of their infectious cycles. Different viruses impinge on almost every aspect of host-cell metabolism, so virus–host cell interactions are diverse and complex. The details of these interactions have been shaped during the co-evolution of individual viruses and their hosts, and they can be fully understood only within that context. In fact, examination of the defenses mounted by cells and organisms against viral infection, and of the various mechanisms that different viruses have evolved to help them evade these defenses, provides a revealing glimpse into the heart of the host–parasite relationship (Smith 1994).

Experimental studies of virus–cell interactions are usually performed in cell culture, by using purified viruses to infect cultured cells that may be a different type or even a different species from those in which the viruses evolved. Because the consequences of infection can vary greatly from one cell type to another, the link between laboratory studies of virus–cell interactions and the behavior of viruses in their natural state is sometimes tenuous. Nevertheless, experimental studies of virus–host cell interactions have not only enriched our understanding of viral infection but also illuminated many areas of molecular and cellular biology. Among these areas are the mechanisms of receptor function (Nomoto 1992; Haywood 1994; Wimmer 1994) and membrane fusion (White 1992; Bentz 1993; Earp et al. 2005); the pathways and control of macromolecular synthesis,

processing, and transport (Nevins 1989; Ehrenfeld 1993; Gebauer and Hentze 2004); the regulation of cell cycling (Levine 1993; Weinberg 1995); and oncogenic transformation (Teich 1991; Jansen-Durr 1996). This chapter presents a survey of this complex and far-reaching subject, and refers the reader to more detailed coverage of specific topics in other chapters. It also contains an extensive bibliography that includes many review articles to guide those interested in reading further.

Cytopathic effects of viral infection

Infection of susceptible cells with an animal virus usually causes cytological changes that are visible by light microscopy and collectively referred to as the cytopathic effect (CPE) of the virus. The nature of the CPE differs between viruses and from one type of virus–cell interaction to another (described in Types of virus–host cell interactions). In the case of a cytocidal virus infecting a cell monolayer, for example, the CPE frequently includes cell rounding and loss of adherence to the tissue-culture plate, visible consequences of the perturbations of cellular metabolism that presage the death of the cell (Figure 12.1a). In contrast, cells infected with a tumor virus, where the outcome is not cell death but neoplastic transformation, undergo more subtle changes in morphology, although the overall consequences of infection both in cell culture and in animals can be at least as profound (Figure 12.1c).

Viral CPEs are not due simply to the increased load on cellular protein synthesis (which is usually insignificant)

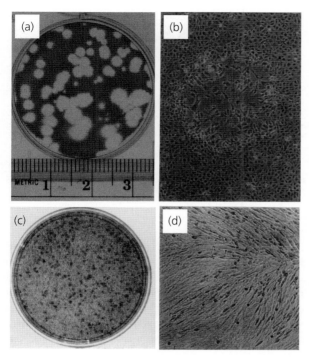

Figure 12.1 (a) *Plaque assay of a lytic virus (vesicular stomatitis virus).* **(b)** *Microphotograph of the typical cytopathic effect (CPE) of a lytic virus (vaccinia virus).* **(c)** *Focus-forming assay of a transforming retrovirus.* **(d)** *Microphotograph of part of a focus of transformed cells. Thanks to Drs. Donald Blair and Karen Joyce Dunn (NIH, NCI) for the photographs shown in (c) and (d).*

nor even to its inhibition, because translation in uninfected cells can be blocked by drugs without inducing a CPE. On the contrary, some aspects of viral CPEs are directly due to the action of specific viral proteins: for example, detachment of adenovirus-infected cells from cell-culture plates results from the penton-base protein of the virion binding to cellular integrins during entry and thereby disrupting their interaction with vitronectin that was responsible for cellular adherence (Wickham et al. 1993). Similarly, some retroviral proteases cause cell rounding by disrupting the cytoskeleton (Luftig and Lupo 1994). However, it also seems that cells can respond to viral infection by launching a specific genetic program that leads to cell death (see Apoptosis), which indicates that some of the consequences of infection are self-inflicted (Razvi and Welsh 1995; Steller 1995; Everett and McFadden 1999). The benefit to the organism of thus limiting the spread of infection outweighs the cost in sacrificed cells (Williams 1994).

QUANTITATIVE ASPECTS OF VIRUS– CELL INTERACTIONS

Multiplicity of infection

Infection is an encounter between two populations: the virus particles and the host cells. The average number of infectious virus particles per cell is called the multiplicity of infection (MOI). When the MOI is very low (10^{-4}, say), only a correspondingly small fraction of the cell population will be infected initially, although the infection can then spread through the cell culture as the virus multiplies. If the spread is contained, by an agarose overlay for example, areas of infected cells (plaques) will develop around each initial infection site, allowing the number of infectious particles (or plaque-forming units (pfu)) in the virus inoculum to be calculated. This is the basis of the plaque assay, an example of which is shown in Figure 12.1a,b. In contrast, when the MOI is high, essentially all the cells will be infected at the outset and the virus will be limited to a single round of synchronous replication. Tumor viruses, which transform cells rather than killing them, produce local foci of transformed cells in culture (Figure 12.1c,d) and can therefore be quantified by an analogous assay that measures the number of infectious particles (or focus-forming units (ffu)) in a tumor virus preparation.

Poisson distribution

The distribution of virus particles among a population of cultured cells is random and can be described mathematically by the Poisson distribution. This formula relates the average MOI (m) to the fraction of cells (P) that actually receive any given number (k) of infectious particles. It shows that an MOI of 1.0 pfu per cell will result in the infection of only 63.2 percent of the population, and that an MOI of $\geqslant 5$ is required to infect at least 99 percent of the cells (Table 12.1).

Ratios of physical particles to plaque-forming units

Not all virus particles in a preparation are capable of forming a plaque; indeed, the particle:pfu ratios for most animal viruses are seldom lower than 10 and sometimes much higher. There are several explanations for this surprising and often overlooked result. First, infection is a multistep process in which the probability of successful completion of each step may be less than 100 percent even for an intrinsically infectious particle. Secondly, the apparent homogeneity of a virus preparation can conceal a substantial level of microheterogeneity: differences in the age of individual particles, their protein composition, and even their genome sequences can influence infectivity. Among the RNA viruses, the high polymerase error rate that results from the absence of proofreading during RNA replication creates a population of genomes whose sequences compose a molecular swarm or quasi-species distribution around a consensus sequence (Smith and Inglis 1987; Holland et al. 1992; Drake 1993; Eigen 1993; Duarte et al. 1994; Domingo and Holland 1997). This concept has profound

Table 12.1 *Poisson distribution: percentage of cells receiving 0, 1, and >1 particles at different MOIs*

Multiplicity of infection (pfu/cell)	Uninfected cells (%)	Singly infected cells (%)	Multiply infected cells (%)
0.0	100.0	0.0	0.0
0.5	60.7	30.3	9.0
1.0	36.8	36.8	26.4
2.0	13.5	27.0	59.5
3.0	5.0	15.0	80.0
5.0	0.67	3.35	96.0
10.0	0.0045	0.045	99.95

$P(k) = (e^{-m}.m^{k}).1/k!$

$P(0) = e^{-m}$

$P(1) = m.e^{-m}$

$P(>1) = 1 - e^{-m}(m+1)$

implications for our understanding of RNA virus evolution (Chapter 2, The origin and evolution of viruses).

Noninfectious virions can nevertheless participate in infection under both natural and experimental conditions. Typically, the number of particles that can undergo receptor binding and other early stages of infection will far exceed the infectious titer, a fact that complicates the study of early events in virus–cell interaction because it is difficult to identify the minority of particles that are on the pathway to productive infection (Wilson 1992). In many cases the genomes of noninfectious particles can engage in complementation and recombination with one another and thus contribute to the outcome of infection. Moreover, some of the most important physiological effects of infection, such as killing of the host cell and the induction of interferon (see Induction and actions of interferons and Chapter 15, The role of cytokines in viral infections), do not depend on the production of viral progeny and can therefore be accomplished by more virus particles than are needed to demonstrate full infectivity (Marcus and Sekellick 1974). The situation is further complicated by the fact that most animal viruses generate defective particles, particularly on repeated passage at high MOI. As their name implies, defective particles are incapable of replication except when supported by coinfection with their parent virus with which they often interfere, thus earning the name defective interfering (DI) particles. Under experimental conditions DI particles can play critical roles in maintaining persistent infections, modulating viral pathogenesis (Chapter 13, Pathogenesis of viral infections), and guiding virus evolution (Chapter 2, The origin and evolution of viruses), and it seems likely that they exert similar effects in nature (Dimmock 1985; Barrett and Dimmock 1986; Whitaker-Dowling and Youngner 1987; Roux et al. 1991; Bangham and Kirkwood 1993).

Single-hit relationships

The fact that preparations of animal viruses have high particle:pfu ratios does not mean that more than one particle per cell is required to initiate a productive infection. The quantitative relationship between virus inoculum and infectivity is generally linear rather than exponential, which shows that infection is a single-hit phenomenon. Combining this observation with a demonstration that the inoculum contains only monomeric virus particles proves that under normal conditions a single virion suffices to infect a cell, although infections that depend on complementation or recombination between viral mutants provide exceptions to this rule. For viruses that have naturally segmented genomes, the quantitative dependence of infectivity on inoculum can supply information on the distribution of genome segments among the individual virus particles.

TYPES OF VIRUS–HOST CELL INTERACTIONS

Viral infections fall into two categories, productive and nonproductive, depending on whether or not viral progeny are produced from the infected cells (Table 12.2). In reality, cellular permissiveness covers a wide spectrum from total nonproductivity, through cases where very low numbers of virions are released, to fully productive situations in which each cell makes hundreds or thousands of infectious particles. Moreover, in the case of latent infections in animals (e.g. by members of the herpesvirus family), infectious virus can re-emerge several years after a nonproductive interaction in one cell type as a fully productive infection in another (Chapters 25, Herpesviruses: general properties and 26, Alphaherpesviruses: herpes simplex and varicella-zoster). As far as the host cell is concerned, its survival is determined not simply by whether the infection is productive, but by the interplay between its genetic program and that of the virus, as described in Cellular responses to viral infection (and see Table 12.2).

Productive infections

The steps in a typical productive viral infection are as follows:

Table 12.2 *Classification of virus–cell interactions*

Consequences for the:				
Virus	Cell	Classification	Specific example	Chapter
Productive	Lethal	Cytolysis	Poliovirus in human cells	40
	Nonlethal	Transformation	Rous sarcoma virus in chicken cells	58
		Persistence	Lymphocytic choriomeningitis virus in mouse cells	49
Nonproductive	Lethal	Apoptosis	Vaccinia virus in Chinese hamster ovary cells	30
	Non lethal	Transformation	Simian virus 40 in mouse cells	24
		Latency	Herpes simplex virus in neural cells	26

1 adsorption of the virus to specific cellular receptors;
2 its penetration across the plasma membrane and into the cell;
3 virus disassembly resulting in partial or complete uncoating of its genome;
4 transcription, translation, and replication of the viral nucleic acid (the order and subcellular location of these steps reflecting the genome strategy of the family to which the virus belongs);
5 assembly of progeny virus particles;
6 their release from the cell.

CYTOCIDAL INFECTIONS

Whether these events kill the host cell depends on the type of virus. For a typical, nonenveloped, cytocidal virus such as poliovirus (Chapter 40, Picornaviruses) which is released when the cell membrane disintegrates, cell death coincides with virus release, although some lytic viruses may be released by an unknown mechanism before the cells burst (Tucker and Compans 1993). In contrast, the release of cytocidal enveloped viruses such as vesicular stomatitis virus (VSV) (see Chapter 51, Rhabdoviruses: rabies), which mature by budding, occurs in a more prolonged manner and precedes the death of the host cell.

PRODUCTIVE TRANSFORMATION

This ability of enveloped viruses to bud from cells without necessarily killing them is exploited by the RNA tumor viruses (Chapter 61, Prions of humans and animals), which establish productive infections in which the host cells undergo neoplastic transformation rather than death (Chapter 17, Viral oncogenicity). By integrating their entire genome into that of the host cell and expressing oncogenes, RNA tumor viruses transform cells to a state of uncontrolled cell division and continuous release of infectious viral progeny.

PERSISTENCE

Persistent infections in cell culture provide situations that are intermediate between these two extremes, and several mechanisms of persistence have been identified (de la Torre and Oldstone 1996). These include carrier cultures, in which for some reason only a specific subpopulation of cells is susceptible to infection; cases in which virus spread is restricted because it can occur only by cell-to-cell contact; and steady states in which infected cells coexist with the virus because they have similar rates of multiplication. In cell culture, temperature-sensitive mutants, DI particles, and interferon have all been implicated in maintaining persistence; the situation in animals is even more complex because it also involves interactions with different cell types, cytokines, and the immune system (Oldstone 1991; Levine et al. 1994; ter Meulen 1994). These aspects are described in detail elsewhere (Chapters 14, The immune response to viral infections and 15, The role of cytokines in viral infections).

Nonproductive infections

Counterintuitively, nonproductive infections are often more challenging than productive ones, both intellectually and medically. In cells that carry receptors for a virus, the initial stages of a nonproductive infection are the same as those listed above for productive situations: receptor binding, penetration, and uncoating. In contrast, cells that lack appropriate receptors are usually not susceptible to infection, although some exceptions to this rule are described in Antibody-mediated enhancement. After these initial stages, however, nonproductive infections can have several different causes, courses, and consequences (see Table 12.2).

APOPTOSIS

In some cases, the early steps of infection trigger the onset of the cell's apoptotic response, resulting in prompt cell death without either virus replication or the production of progeny (Razvi and Welsh 1995; Roulston et al. 1999). Infection of Chinese hamster ovary cells by vaccinia virus provides a good example of this. Several viral genes have been identified whose actions delay the onset of apoptosis (White 1993; Clem and Miller 1994; Ink et al. 1995; Benedict et al. 2002), which suggests that anti-apoptotic mechanisms may be widespread among animal viruses.

NONPRODUCTIVE TRANSFORMATION

Replication of the smaller DNA viruses such as those in the polyoma- and papilloma virus families (Chapter 2,

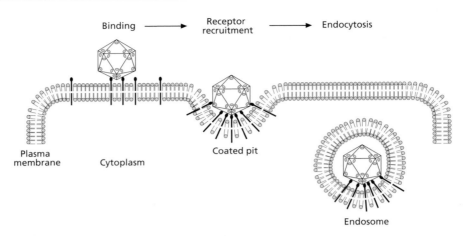

Figure 12.2 *Receptor-mediated endocytic uptake of a virus particle*

The origin and evolution of viruses) depends on viral oncogenes that coax the infected cell into the S phase of the cell cycle and thus establish conditions that are conducive for DNA synthesis. This is particularly critical for papillomaviruses, which replicate only in terminally differentiated, noncycling cells of the epidermis. In this situation, any block in virus replication that allows the cell to survive the infection can lead to integration of the viral oncogenes and consequent neoplastic transformation of the cell (see Table 12.2).

LATENCY

Of all the types of virus–host interactions, those that result in latency are the most perplexing (Garcia-Blanco and Cullen 1991). Members of the alphaherpesvirus family (Chapter 26, Alphaherpesviruses: herpes simplex and varicella-zoster) typically progress from primary productive interactions, often with epithelial cells, to secondary latent infections, usually in neural cells, from which they can re-emerge periodically throughout the life of the infected individual (Wagner 1994). The viral genome remains intact during latency and is maintained as an episome in the nucleus, with at most a small subset of the viral genes being expressed. This situation is best understood for latent infections established by Epstein–Barr virus in B lymphocytes (Masucci and Ernberg 1994; Farrell 1995; Rowe 1999), which can be examined in cell culture. The general mechanisms by which herpesviruses establish, maintain and re-emerge from latency are subjects of intense investigation, but the scarcity of cell culture systems in which these processes can be duplicated renders them difficult to study.

ADSORPTION OF VIRUSES TO HOST CELLS

The first step in virus–cell interaction is a specific noncovalent binding between attachment sites on the surface of the virion and receptors on the plasma membrane of the host cell. Unlike some bacteriophages, all animal viruses carry multiple copies of their attachment proteins or sites, usually arranged in symmetrical or regular arrays on the surface of the virion (Chapter 5, The morphology and structure of viruses). Even the small picornaviruses have 60 receptor-binding sites per virion, and influenza virus has several hundred. What fraction of these sites must be occupied for successful virus binding and uptake is unknown, although it is probably much less than 100 percent and may vary widely among different viruses. Indeed, a current model for the early stages of virus uptake proposes that the initial interaction with one or a few receptor molecules is followed by the recruitment of more receptors that can diffuse laterally in the plasma membrane. This would strengthen the binding, cause invagination of the membrane around the virus particle, and initiate what used to be called 'viropexis,' but is now generally referred to as 'receptor-mediated endocytosis' (Figure 12.2). See Wimmer (1994) for several reviews on all aspects of this subject.

The receptor–virus interaction can fulfil two distinct functions: positioning the virus particle for uptake by the cell and, at least in some cases, promoting virion disassembly. Virus structures have evolved to serve as metastable intermediates between successive cycles of replication, and some receptors not only bind the incoming virus particle but also act as keys to unlock its structure (see Consequences of receptor binding). Of course, the presence of cell surface components that can perform these functions is not due to natural selection of cells for their ability to be infected, but rather to opportunism by viruses whose potential for faster evolution allows them to take advantage of existing host cell molecules with other functions. A remarkable variety of cell surface molecules have been co-opted by different viruses to enable them to bind and enter cells (Table 12.3), and these receptors are described further in the section entitled Cellular receptors for viruses.

Table 12.3 *Some examples of virus receptors*

Virus family	Viruses	Receptors
Coronaviridae	Murine hepatitis virus	Carcinoembryonic antigen family member
	Human coronavirus 229E	Aminopeptidase N
	Human coronavirus OC43	N-acetyl-9-O-acetylneuraminic acid
Herpesviridae	Epstein–Barr virus	B lymphocyte C3d complement receptor (CD21)
	Herpes simplex virus	Heparan sulphate moieties of proteoglycans
Orthomyxoviridae	Influenza A and B viruses	N-acetylneuraminic acid (sialic acid) on glycoproteins and glycolipids
	Influenza C virus	N-acetyl-9-O-acetylneuraminic acid
Paramyxoviridae	Sendai virus	Sialoglycoprotein GP2
	Measles virus	Complement regulator CD46 and SLAM
Picornaviridae	Poliovirus	Poliovirus receptor (immunoglobulin superfamily member)
	Rhinoviruses (major group)	Intercellular adhesion molecule 1 (ICAM-1)
	Rhinoviruses (minor group)	LDL receptor
	Foot-and-mouth disease virus	Integrin (RGD-binding protein)
Reoviridae	Reovirus type 3	β-Adrenergic receptor
Retroviridae	Human immunodeficiency viruses	T-cell surface glycoprotein CD4, galactosyl ceramide, and chemokine co-receptors
	Ectropic murine leukemia virus	Cationic amino acid transporter
	Gibbon ape leukemia virus	Sodium-dependent phosphate symporter
	Feline leukemia virus	Sodium-dependent phosphate symporter
Rhabdoviridae	Vesicular stomatitis virus	Phosphatidylserine and phosphatidylinositol
Togaviridae	Sindbis virus	High-affinity laminin receptor

For references to the original work that described these receptors, see Lentz (1990), Haywood (1994), and Wimmer (1994).

The presence of an appropriate receptor is usually necessary but not always sufficient to allow a particular virus to infect a cell or organism. For example, poliovirus naturally infects only humans and closely related primates because certain cells of these species have a receptor (the poliovirus receptor (PVR)) to which the virus can attach, but the host range of the virus can be extended to mice if they are engineered to express the human gene for PVR (Ren et al. 1990; Nomoto et al. 1994). In contrast, mouse cells expressing CD4, the receptor for human immunodeficiency virus (HIV), can bind the virus but are not infected by it, showing that in some cases there is more to uptake and penetration than simple binding (see Entry accessory factors). Similarly, although receptor distribution is a major determinant of viral tissue tropism, the susceptibility of different tissues in an organism does not simply reflect the tissue distribution of the receptor, because productive infection often requires accessory factors for virus entry (Entry accessory factors), as well as a hospitable intracellular environment for replication. The overall relationship between viral entry mechanisms examined in cell culture and virus spread during a natural infection is a difficult and contentious area of virology.

Viral attachment proteins and sites

In the simplest cases, the task of binding to the host cell has been assigned by evolution to a single species of viral surface protein, such as the hemagglutinin (HA) of influenza virus (Weis et al. 1988) or gp120 of HIV (Weiss 1992), although such attachment proteins usually function as oligomers. In more complex situations such as the picornaviruses, receptor-binding sites on the virion surface are created at the interfaces between two or more viral polypeptides (Colonno 1992; Olson et al. 1993). Larger viruses may show a still higher level of complexity, in which two or more viral surface proteins are involved in a series of progressively tighter interactions with different cell surface components. For example, glycoprotein C of herpes simplex virus (HSV) binds the abundant heparan sulfate moieties of cell surface proteoglycans whereas glycoprotein D binds to mannose-6-phosphate receptors (Spear 1993; Brunetti et al. 1994). Strictly speaking, such downstream components of a multistep entry pathway are best considered 'entry accessory factors' (Entry accessory factors) rather than viral receptors. Nevertheless, the idea of a rapid, relatively low-affinity interaction being followed by a slower, tighter binding, either to a secondary component or to newly recruited primary receptors, is reminiscent of the mechanism by which circulating leukocytes adhere to vascular endothelial cells, by rolling across weak receptors (selectins) before binding irreversibly to integrins (Lawrence and Springer 1991). The speed of the initial binding in three dimensions that is required to capture a passing particle is combined with a slower, two-dimensional search for the interactions that give the overall process its necessary high affinity.

GLYCOPROTEIN SPIKES

Many enveloped viruses display their attachment proteins as surface spikes that project perpendicularly from the viral envelope. These spikes are visible in electron micrographs and consist of oligomers of virus-specified integral membrane glycoproteins. In some, perhaps many, cases, the arrangement of the surface spikes reflects the symmetry of the nucleocapsid underlying the viral envelope (Paredes et al. 1993; Cheng et al. 1995). The three-dimensional structure of one viral attachment glycoprotein, the influenza virus HA, was determined at near-atomic resolution in 1981 and has been influential in shaping ideas of the structure and function of such proteins (Figure 12.3) (Wiley and Skehel 1987). It consists of a bundle of three identical monomers extending 135 Å from the surface of the viral envelope, arranged around a symmetry axis that is parallel to its length. Each monomer contains two disulfide-linked polypeptides, HA1 and HA2, produced by cleavage of the 550 amino acid primary translation product. The globular top of the trimeric bundle has three concave binding sites for sialic acid, the cellular receptor for influenza virus, as well as several antigenic sites that elicit and react with antibodies that neutralize the infectivity of the virus. At its bottom, HA2 anchors the protein by passing through the viral membrane, although the protein whose structure was determined was first made soluble by removal of the transmembrane domain.

A very different picture is presented by glycoprotein E of the flavivirus tick-borne encephalitis virus (TBEV) (Chapter 46, Flaviviruses) (Rey et al. 1995). Like influenza virus HA, this is a type I integral membrane protein that is anchored in the viral envelope by its C terminus. However, rather than forming a protruding spike, the TBEV glycoprotein forms an elongated homodimer that lies flat on the surface of the viral envelope with a symmetry axis that is perpendicular to its length (Figure 12.4). The receptor-binding domain has an immunoglobulin-like folded structure that presents the binding site on the surface of the virion.

CAPSID ATTACHMENT SITES

In nonenveloped viruses, the receptor-binding sites are built into the architecture of the particles and are thus displayed in a symmetry determined by that of the capsid. A technical consequence of this is that individual virus particles with receptors bound at each site can be visualized using cryo-electron microscopy and image reconstruction methods to achieve a resolution of about 25 Å. Figure 12.5a shows a rhinovirus particle decorated with its receptor, intercellular adhesion molecule 1 (ICAM-1) (Olson et al. 1993; Rossmann et al. 1994). Sixty receptor molecules are bound to each virion, arranged in groups of five around each of the 12 axes of five-fold symmetry in the icosahedral particle. The

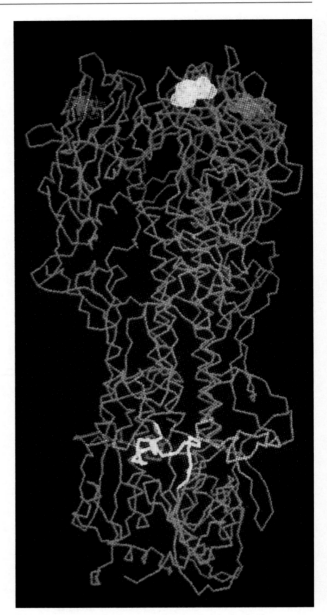

Figure 12.3 *The influenza virus hemagglutinin (HA). The α-carbon backbone of the HA trimer is displayed in blue with the three fusion peptides, located in the stem of the molecule, highlighted in red, yellow, and green. The molecular surfaces of three sialic acid residues are shown (red, yellow, green) in the receptor-binding sites of the globular head domains. The three monomers would be anchored in the viral membrane at the bottom (from White (1992)).*

receptors thus occupy chemically identical binding sites which, in this and some other picornaviruses, lie in a trenchlike depression called the canyon that encircles each fivefold axis. A higher resolution image that shows how a single receptor molecule fits into the canyon has been generated by combining the crystal structure of the rhinovirus particle with the predicted structure of ICAM-1 (Figure 12.5b). It shows that the binding site is created and protected by the juxtaposition of the capsid proteins VP1, VP2, and VP3, parts of which form the

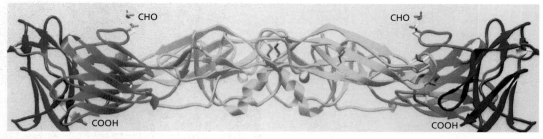

Figure 12.4 *Three-dimensional structure of glycoprotein E of tick-borne encephalitis virus. The dimer is viewed from the side, as it would lie on the surface of the viral membrane (from Rey et al. (1995)).*

walls of the canyon. Ultimately, it may prove possible to co-crystallize a virus–receptor protein complex and directly examine the molecular contacts at atomic resolution.

The specific contacts by which a viral attachment protein binds to its receptor, and hence the amino acid residues involved, are largely fixed by the requirement that they must create a binding surface with steric, electronic, and hydropathic complementarity for the receptor. It is important, therefore, that these residues avoid immune surveillance, because an antibody directed specifically and exclusively against the receptor-binding site would create a barrier to infection that the virus could not circumvent by mutation. This problem has been solved in different ways by different viruses (Chapman and Rossmann 1993). For example, location of the receptor-binding sites in the canyon of rhino- and polioviruses protects them from reach by antibodies which are much bulkier than the receptors (Rossmann 1989). In contrast, the receptor-binding site in foot-and-mouth disease virus is in a surface loop that may avoid antigenic scrutiny by being structurally mobile. Finally, there may be cases where the receptor-binding site mimics the structure of the natural ligand so precisely that the immune system does not recognize it as foreign.

Cellular receptors for viruses

A wide variety of cell surface molecules can be used as receptors by different viruses (Table 12.3). In some cases, a ubiquitous carbohydrate modification is recognized, such as sialic acid or heparan sulfate on a glycoprotein or glycolipid, whereas in other cases it is a specific protein that may be present on the surface of only certain cell types (such as CD4 on T lymphocytes), which thus directs and restricts the tropism of the virus (Lentz 1990; Wimmer 1994). The receptors for poliovirus (PVR), rhinovirus (ICAM-1), and HIV (CD4), among others, belong to the immunoglobulin superfamily of proteins, and contain three to five repeats of the 'immunoglobulin fold,' a structural domain that is characteristic of the immunoglobulins (White and Littman 1989). The three-dimensional structure of two

such domains in a fragment of CD4 that includes the HIV-binding site is illustrated in Figure 12.6 (Harrison et al. 1992; Signoret et al. 1993). Since members of this protein superfamily have been naturally selected for cell surface expression and the ability to bind protein ligands with high specificity, it is easy to understand why they should have been commandeered as viral receptors. Indeed, two very different viruses, HIV and human herpesvirus 7, both use CD4 as their receptor, and the malaria parasite also uses ICAM-1 for cell attachment. The versatility of the immunoglobulin fold as a protein-binding domain is further illustrated by the fact that it sometimes occurs in the other partner in the interaction, the viral attachment protein (Rey et al. 1995).

Just as dissimilar viruses can share the same receptor, so can closely related viruses use different receptors. Human rhinoviruses, of which there are over 100 serotypes, divide into a major group that use ICAM-1 and a minor group that use the low density lipoprotein (LDL) receptor. In this case, the use of different receptors does not seem to influence the outcome of infection, but there are examples where the use of alternative receptors by a single virus can have profound consequences. The ability of HIV to use galactosyl ceramide instead of CD4 to enter cells may be responsible for its infection of the brain and the resulting acquired immunodeficiency syndrome (AIDS)-related dementia (Weiss 1992).

Infection of animals is usually initiated in epithelial cells, which are naturally polarized and express different sets of proteins on their apical and basolateral surfaces (Tucker and Compans 1993; Eaton and Simons 1995). Interaction of viruses with polarized cells whose receptors are distributed asymmetrically can occur only at the cell surface that expresses the receptor, because the intercellular tight junctions prevent access of the virus to the other face of the polarized cell layer. For example, SV40 infection can occur only from the apical surface. Since virus release also often occurs in a polarized manner from epithelial cells, asymmetric receptor distribution can greatly influence the course of infection and the pathway of virus spread in an infected animal (Tucker et al. 1994).

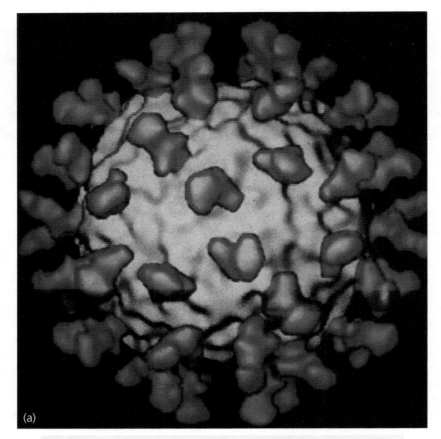

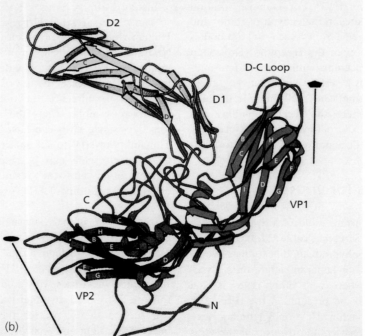

Figure 12.5 *Interaction of rhinovirus with its receptor ICAM-1.* **(a)** *Cryo-EM reconstruction of a virus particle complexed with 60 receptor molecules.* **(b)** *High resolution image of a single receptor-binding site interaction (from Olson et al. (1993)).*

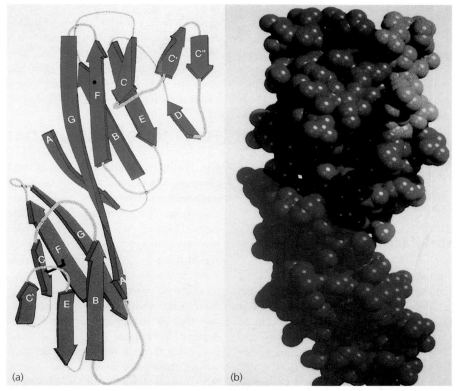

Figure 12.6 *Backbone **(a)** and solid **(b)** representations of the three-dimensional structure of CD4 (D1D2 domains). The D1 domain is in red, the D2 domain is in blue, and the region of D1 implicated in the binding HIV gp120 is yellow (from Wang et al. (1990)).*

Antibody-mediated enhancement

Although the presence of a cognate receptor is usually a prerequisite for infection, some virus–cell interactions can occur through intermediate molecules for which both the virus and the cell have affinity. Paradoxically, virus-specific antibodies can play this role and actually promote virus uptake because some cells express a receptor for the Fc portion of the antibody molecule (Porterfield 1986; Halstead 1994; Tirado and Yoon 2003). In this way, the immune system can collaborate in the spread of infection by circumventing the requirement for a virus-specific receptor (Mason et al. 1994). The pathogenesis of infections by both dengue virus and HIV can be exacerbated by antibody-mediated enhancement of infectivity, but the phenomenon is probably irrelevant for viruses such as polio, in which interaction with the cognate receptor mediates an essential structural change in the virion (Consequences of receptor binding).

Consequences of receptor binding

As mentioned at the start of this section, receptor binding initiates virus entry into the cell and, at least in some cases, destabilizes the structure of the virion so that it begins to disassemble. Before binding to the receptor, poliovirus is stable at pH 2 and can therefore enter the body through the strongly acidic environment of the stomach. However, reaction with PVR causes a major conformational change in the capsid that involves swelling, loss of a small internal protein (VP4), and extrusion of the hydrophobic N terminus of VP1 in preparation for its interaction with membranes (Flore et al. 1990; Racaniello 1992; Gomez Yafal et al. 1993). However, only a few of the poliovirus particles that interact with the receptor are internalized. Substantial numbers of these antigenically altered particles, which can no longer bind the receptor and have therefore lost their infectivity, dissociate from cells during poliovirus infection and may play a role in decoying the immune response. In the case of some rhinoviruses, reaction with the receptor is sufficient to release the viral RNA and produce empty capsids, whereas in other cases this requires exposure to mildly acidic conditions such as those encountered during passage through the endocytic pathway into the cytoplasm (Giranda et al. 1992; Greve and Rossmann 1994) (see Penetration and uncoating). These observations suggest that receptor binding and acid pH may co-operate to initiate picorna-virus disassembly. In the case of HIV, binding to the receptor CD4 causes the release of the viral attachment protein gp120 from the particle, exposing a hydrophobic fusion peptide whose interaction with membranes mediates the next step in viral entry (see Penetration and uncoating).

When the natural function of the receptor is transmembrane signaling, virus binding can trigger a physiological response even without internalization. It is thought that Epstein–Barr virus can activate B lymphocytes by binding to the C3d complement receptor (Hutt-Fletcher 1987). Moreover, this type of effect can be widely disseminated because infected cells often secrete soluble forms of the viral attachment protein. Some of the complex effects of HIV on T-lymphocyte function may be mediated directly by the phosphorylation of CD4 and the consequent transmembrane signaling that is caused by the binding of gp120.

Entry accessory factors

There are many instances in which the ability of a virus to bind to the surface of a cell is sufficient for uptake, but there are others where something else is needed. For example, rodent cells that express human CD4 fail to become infected with HIV unless they also express the human membrane protein fusin, which is required for penetration of the virus–receptor complex into the cell (Feng et al. 1996). In the case of adenovirus, initial receptor binding by the fiber protein must be followed by an interaction between the penton base protein of the virus and cellular integrins in order for internalization to occur (Wickham et al. 1993). The distinction between secondary receptors and entry accessory factors, and the roles that each plays in virus uptake are unclear and will probably remain so until more details of this multistep process are known.

Release from receptors

For viral progeny to spread most effectively, some mechanism is needed to ensure release from receptors expressed by the primary infected cells. In general, a combination of virus-mediated receptor down-regulation and the inhibition of protein synthesis contribute to this requirement, but some viruses that bind to sialic acid also carry specific 'receptor-destroying enzymes' that remove terminal sialic acid residues from oligosaccharides. Along with the HA protein described in the section entitled Viral attachment proteins and sites, particles of influenza A virus and influenza B virus have a second surface glycoprotein (NA) that has neuraminidase (sialidase) activity. Although the presence of this enzyme may allow infecting virions to 'browse' the cell surface during entry, its only essential roles in infection are to prevent infected cells from trapping progeny virus particles and to eliminate the self-aggregation that would otherwise result from HA binding to its own oligosaccharides (Liu et al. 1995). Particles of influenza C virus and some coronaviruses, whose attachment

proteins bind to N-acetyl-9-O-acetylneuraminic acid, carry an esterase that likewise mediates destruction of receptors. In the latter case, and in some paramyxoviruses, the receptor-binding and receptor-destroying activities are both present in the same molecule (HE and HN, respectively), raising interesting questions about their interrelationship and regulation.

PENETRATION AND UNCOATING

Virus particles assemble in cells as very stable structures that are often able to withstand harsh extracellular environments, but when re-exposed to intracellular conditions they spontaneously disassemble. In some cases, binding to the receptor contributes to this dramatic change in virion stability (Consequences of receptor binding), but an important role is played by the paths that viruses follow as they enter cells. Depending on the type of virus, its genome must cross one, two, or three lipid bilayers between binding to the receptor at the plasma membrane and reaching its intracellular destination. During infection, all viral genomes must penetrate the plasma membrane; those of enveloped viruses must also cross the viral membrane, and those that replicate in the nucleus also need to traverse the nuclear membrane. Virion proteins play active roles in these transmembrane passages, and have been sculpted by natural selection to transfer the viral genome to the appropriate cellular compartment. Some stages of virion disassembly and genome uncoating invariably accompany membrane penetration (Hoekstra and Kok 1989; Marsh and Helenius 1989; Carrasco 1994; Greber et al. 1994; Lanzrein et al. 1994; Poranen et al. 2002).

Two pathways of virus entry

Although some viral receptors naturally transport small molecules (see Table 12.3) (Dautry-Varsat and Lodish 1984), it seems that not even the smallest virus is directly carried across the plasma membrane by its receptor. Instead, enveloped viruses transfer their nucleocapsids across membranes by fusing with them, a reaction that achieves simultaneous envelope removal and cell entry. Fusion is mediated by specific virion surface proteins that can fuse lipid bilayers (Viral fusion proteins), and some nonenveloped viruses probably achieve the same result by inserting capsid proteins into a cellular membrane (Uncoating of nonenveloped viruses). For many viruses, both with and without envelopes, activation of the ability to fuse with membranes requires exposure to a mildly acidic environment (pH 5–6); such viruses enter cells by receptor-mediated endocytosis (see Figures 12.2 and 12.7) into endosomes whose contents then become acidified by an ATP-driven proton pump. The result is fusion of the virus with the membrane of the endosome and release of the viral

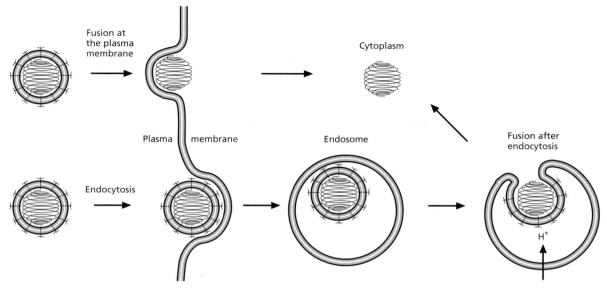

Figure 12.7 *Two pathways of enveloped virus entry: fusion at the plasma membrane or fusion after endocytosis.*

genome into the cytoplasm. Other viruses can fuse without being exposed to low pH, and can therefore enter the cytoplasm directly by fusion with the plasma membrane (Figure 12.7).

Infection by viruses that enter through endosomes can be inhibited by lysosomotropic agents such as ammonium chloride or chloroquine which raise the endosomal pH, whereas viruses that enter at the plasma membrane are insensitive to these reagents. The pathway of entry that leads to a productive infection is thus determined largely by the properties of the viral protein responsible for membrane fusion: whether exposure to low pH is required to activate it. In general, viruses in the herpes-, polyoma-, paramyxo-, retro-, and rotavirus families can enter cells by fusion with the plasma membrane in a pH-independent manner, whereas those in the adeno-, alpha-, bunya-, flavi-, orthomyxo-, picorna-, reo-, and rhabdovirus families need to pass through an acidic endosome. However, there are several individual exceptions to these family rules.

The ability of many viruses to fuse with cellular membranes is responsible for a common cytopathic effect of viral infection: the formation of multinucleated syncytia by cell-to-cell fusion. This is due to the abundant expression of the viral proteins that cause membrane fusion (see Viral fusion proteins) on the surface of infected cells, where they can interact with both infected and uninfected neighbors ('fusion from within'). Cell fusion creates a pathway for the local spread of an infection by which a virus can partly elude the immune system. For respiratory syncytial virus, a member of the paramyxovirus family, the extensive syncytium formation that accompanies infection both in the respiratory tract and in cell culture was used in naming the virus and in diagnosing infections. Another paramyxovirus, Sendai virus, has been widely used by cell biologists as a laboratory reagent to induce the formation of heterokaryons by 'fusion from without.'

Viral fusion proteins

Some viruses (e.g. the paramyxoviruses) have separate envelope glycoproteins for receptor binding and membrane fusion; others (e.g. influenza and the retroviruses) combine the two functions into a single viral protein. Despite their variety of structures, however, the fusion proteins of enveloped viruses have features in common. They all contain two hydrophobic regions: a transmembrane domain by which they are anchored in the viral envelope, and a fusion peptide of 16–26 nonpolar amino acids in the ectodomain of the protein that interacts with the target membrane (Schlesinger and Schlesinger 1987; White 1990, 1992; Doms et al. 1993; Smith and Helenius 2004; Earp et al. 2005). Formation of a bridge between the viral and cellular membranes by means of divalent anchoring is thought to mediate membrane apposition (Figure 12.8), an essential step in fusion (Bentz 1993).

The hydrophobic nature of the fusion peptide must remain masked, both during translation, to allow it to pass through the membrane of the endoplasmic reticulum (ER), and during virus assembly and release, to prevent premature activation of its fusogenic potential. For these reasons, fusion peptide sequences are initially buried, both in the primary sequences and in the oligomeric structure of fusion proteins. A maturational cleavage event, which sometimes occurs after virus release, places the fusion peptide sequence at a newly created N terminus, as in the influenza HA structure where it forms the N terminus of HA2 (see Figure 12.3) or in the HIV gp120/gp41 structure in which it is the N terminus

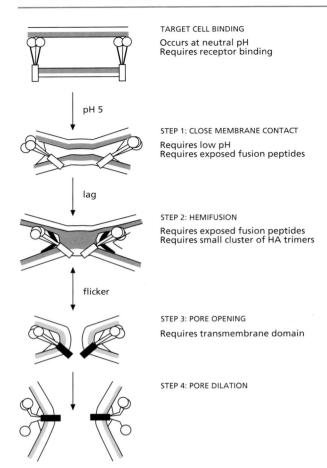

TARGET CELL BINDING

Occurs at neutral pH
Requires receptor binding

pH 5

STEP 1: CLOSE MEMBRANE CONTACT

Requires low pH
Requires exposed fusion peptides

lag

STEP 2: HEMIFUSION

Requires exposed fusion peptides
Requires small cluster of HA trimers

flicker

STEP 3: PORE OPENING

Requires transmembrane domain

STEP 4: PORE DILATION

Figure 12.8 *Steps in HA-mediated membrane fusion (from White (1994)).*

of gp41. However, the two cleavage products remain associated with one another, sometimes by disulfide bonds, in an oligomeric structure that continues to mask the fusion peptide. In the case of influenza HA, rearrangement of the subunits of the trimer is necessary to expose their fusion peptides to the target membrane, and it is likely that a major conformational change of this sort is a common feature of the activation of fusion proteins (see Mechanisms of membrane fusion).

Different viruses prevent premature activation of their fusion proteins in different ways. For Sendai virus, the required cleavage of the fusion protein precursor is mediated by a protease at the membrane of the target cell. For HIV, receptor binding dissociates gp120 and thereby exposes the hydrophobic N terminus of gp41. For Semliki Forest virus, the fusion protein monomer is maintained as an inactive heterodimer with the viral attachment protein until receptor binding and exposure to low pH release it to form the homotrimer that is fusogenic (Kielian 1995). For some paramyxoviruses, fusion requires both the attachment protein HN and the fusion protein F, because binding of HN to its receptor somehow activates the fusion protein, its partner in the viral envelope (Lamb 1993). For influenza A virus,

where exposure to low pH triggers the conformational change that activates HA, the protein is chaperoned during its synthesis and maturation by the viral M2 protein, which acts as a transmembrane proton channel to regulate the pH in the cellular compartments through which the maturing HA must pass (Pinto et al. 1992). Another role for the influenza virus M2 protein as an ion channel is described under Transit to the nucleus.

Mechanisms of membrane fusion

The three-dimensional structure of the neutral form of HA (see Figure 12.3) raised some perplexing questions about how it mediated membrane fusion. Because the receptor-binding site is 135 Å from the transmembrane domain and about 100 Å from the fusion peptide, it was not clear how, after receptor binding, the protein could closely juxtapose the viral envelope in which it was anchored with the target membrane for insertion of the fusion peptide. Some of these problems were solved when it was discovered that a region of HA2 underwent a massive conformational change at the pH of membrane fusion, resulting in a 100 Å relocation of the

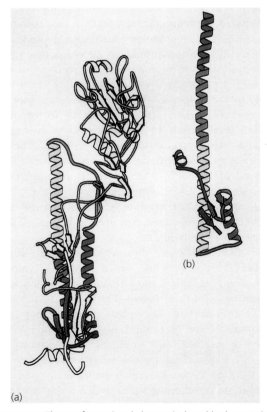

(b)

(a)

Figure 12.9 *The conformational change induced by low pH in influenza virus HA.* **(a)** *The neutral pH form of the HA1,2 monomer is shown in the same orientation as in the HA trimer shown in Figure 12.3.* **(b)** *The low pH form of the HA2 monomer. Corresponding regions are colored identically (from Bullough et al. (1994)).*

fusion peptide to one apex of the molecule (Figure 12.9) (Carr and Kim 1993; Bullough et al. 1994).

In this new location, membrane insertion of the N terminus of HA2 is easy to envisage, although it is not clear whether this and other fusion peptides are inserted into their target membranes vertically, obliquely, or horizontally, as random coils or perhaps as amphipathic α-helices. Unfortunately, the new HA2 structure does not reveal the relative positions of the fusion peptide and the anchor domain, so the way that these regions and the receptor-binding site collaborate to mediate membrane fusion is still unclear (Carr and Kim 1994; Stegman 1994; Hughson 1995; Skehel and Wiley 2000). When last seen in the low pH structure, the C terminus of HA2 was heading in the direction of the fusion peptide (Figure 12.9), raising the possibility that the acid-induced conformational change brings the anchor and fusion peptides (and hence perhaps the viral and cellular membranes) into close proximity with one another. However, there is much yet to be discovered about the mechanism of membrane fusion and several models have been proposed that involve hemifused intermediates (Figure 12.8), inverted micelles, proteinaceous pores, or intermembrane stalks (Stegman 1994). It is interesting that an engineered mutant of HA that is anchored only in the outer membrane leaflet rather than traversing the lipid bilayer mediates only hemifusion, showing that the anchor domain plays different roles in mixing the lipids of the two leaflets (Kemble et al. 1994).

Uncoating of nonenveloped viruses

Nonenveloped viruses are also destabilized during cell entry, by interactions with their receptors (see Consequences of receptor binding), and in some cases by exposure to endosomal pH, reducing conditions or low intracellular calcium ion concentrations. Although entry of nonenveloped viruses into the cytosol cannot be achieved by membrane fusion, it is possible that the hydrophobic N terminus of VP1 of some picornaviruses may play the role of a fusion peptide. It is buried in the capsid structure but becomes exposed when the virus binds to its receptor, and may perhaps be inserted into the cell membrane as a pentamer derived from one of the 12 fivefold axes of the icosahedral virion. The internal protein VP4, which exits the virus particle after receptor binding, is myristylated at its N terminus, and could thereby also interact with membranes. Such a complex might form a hydrophilic transmembrane channel through which the viral RNA could pass into the cytosol (Figure 12.10) (Mosser et al. 1994; Johnson 1996). Despite the external protein symmetry of icosahedral virions and nucleocapsids, it is possible that the asymmetry of the nucleic acid inside confers different properties on some of the capsomers and that these differences are exploited during virion disassembly. Whether the RNA enters the cytosol in a polar manner as depicted in Figure 12.10 remains to be determined. However, the capsid proteins of infecting alphavirus particles are transferred to 28S ribosomal RNA (Singh and Helenius 1992), thus releasing the viral RNA genome for translation. The disassembly of tobacco mosaic virus and cowpea chlorotic mottle virus in plants also occurs cotranslationally, by ribosomes displacing capsid proteins from the viral RNA during the initial round of protein synthesis (Verduin 1992), and a similar possibility exists for extraction of the RNA from positive-strand RNA animal viruses.

For adeno- and reoviruses, whose genomes do not interact directly with ribosomes, partially disassembled subviral particles exit the endosome by lysis or permeabilization of the vesicle membrane. As in the examples described above, it is the acidic environment, sometimes in conjunction with proteolytic cleavage of viral structural proteins, that activates the virus parti-

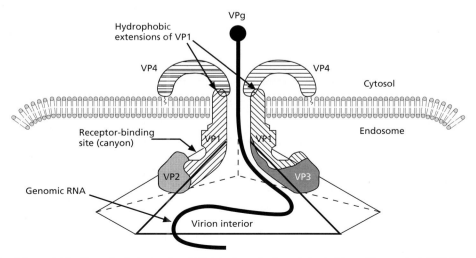

Figure 12.10 *Possible model for the exit of picornavirus RNA into the cytoplasm (adapted from Mosser et al. (1994)).*

Table 12.4 *Initial biosynthetic events in animal virus infections*

Initial biosynthetic event	Virus families	Subcellular location	Origin of enzymes
DNA-dependent DNA synthesis	*Parvo*	Nucleus	Cell
	Hepadna	Nucleus	Virion
RNA-dependent DNA synthesis	*Retro*	Cytoplasm	Virion
DNA-dependent RNA synthesis	*Polyoma*	Nucleus	Cell
	Papilloma	Nucleus	Cell
	Adeno	Nucleus	Cell
	Herpes	Nucleus	Cell
	Baculo	Nucleus	Cell
	Irido	Nucleus	Cell
	Pox	Cytoplasm	Virion
RNA-dependent RNA synthesis	*Orthomyxo*	Nucleus	Virion
	Delta agent	Nucleus	Cell (RNA pol II)
	Paramyxo	Cytoplasm	Virion
	Rhabdo	Cytoplasm	Virion
	Filo	Cytoplasm	Virion
	Bunya	Cytoplasm	Virion
	Reo	Cytoplasm	Virion
	Arena	Cytoplasm	Virion
Protein synthesis	*Picorna*	Cytoplasm	Cell (ribosomes)
	Toga	Cytoplasm	Cell (ribosomes)
	Flavi	Cytoplasm	Cell (ribosomes)
	Corona	Cytoplasm	Cell (ribosomes)
	Calici	Cytoplasm	Cell (ribosomes)
	Noda	Cytoplasm	Cell (ribosomes)

cles to disrupt the endosomal membrane (Dryden et al. 1993).

Transit to the nucleus

Viral genomes that replicate in the nucleus need to travel there from where they entered the cytosol. For a herpesvirus particle infecting a neuron, this may be a journey of several centimeters during which the viral nucleocapsid is transported by axonal flow (Chapter 25, Herpesviruses: general properties). In less extreme cases, transport mechanisms that are thought to involve interactions with the cytoskeleton deliver the viral genome or nucleocapsid to the cytoplasmic face of pores in the nuclear membrane. For adeno- and herpesviruses, whose nucleocapsids are too large to enter the nucleus intact, a final stage of uncoating occurs at the nuclear pores to release the viral DNA into the nucleus. In contrast, most retroviruses require the natural breakdown of the nuclear membrane that occurs during mitosis, and they are therefore restricted to infection of dividing cells.

Influenza virus replicates in the nucleus but assembles its progeny in the cytoplasm and therefore faces unusual problems of compartmentation. The binding of viral nucleocapsids to the matrix protein (M1), which is responsible for their transport out of the nucleus in preparation for virus assembly, must be disrupted at the start of infection in order to permit the incoming viral genome to migrate into the nucleus. This is another function of the viral M2 protein; it creates acid-activated ion channels in the viral envelope which open at the low pH of the endosome to admit ions into the interior of the virion, thereby releasing the viral nucleocapsids from their association with the matrix protein (Hay 1992; Helenius 1992; Marsh 1992). The anti-influenza drug amantadine inhibits this process by blocking the ion channel activity of the M2 protein.

Poxvirus uncoating requires viral gene expression

In the uncoating mechanisms described above, components of the infecting virions played active and essential roles, but the expression of new viral genes was not necessary. Members of the poxvirus family, however, uncoat by a two-stage process in which the second stage depends on viral gene expression (Chapter 31, Poxvirus replication). Vaccinia virus, for example, is taken up by receptor-mediated endocytosis (Hugin and Hauser 1994; Chang et al. 1995). On release of the nucleocapsid core into the cytosol, a viral DNA-dependent RNA polymerase that is part of the core begins to transcribe several viral genes, among them one for a protease that triggers the second stage of uncoating that releases the viral DNA into the cytosol in preparation for genome replication.

EFFECTS ON HOST-CELL METABOLISM

An incoming virus particle faces a formidable challenge in subverting the metabolism of the host cell to its own ends. Depending on the virus, a single copy of its genetic program dominates one that is 10^4–10^6 times larger and already being expressed. To meet this challenge, viruses have evolved a wide variety of ways to manipulate the intracellular environment so that it can better support their replication. These include changes in intermediary metabolism, particularly of deoxyribonucleotides, as well as effects on the synthesis, processing, transport, and turnover of cellular macromolecules. Viruses achieve dominance by combining mechanisms that enhance the expression of viral genes with those that interfere with the host. Many of the latter perturbations have detrimental effects on the infected cell that result in viral pathogenesis and disease (Chapter 13, Pathogenesis of viral infections), but it seems that few if any of them evolved with the primary purpose of causing cellular damage. On the contrary, viruses, like all successful parasites, survive not because they kill the host but because they avoid inducing its premature demise.

The nature of the initial biosynthetic reaction – DNA, RNA, or protein synthesis – and where it occurs in the infected cell depend on the genome strategy of the virus (Table 12.4). Most DNA genomes replicate in the nucleus, whereas most RNA genomes replicate in the cytoplasm, although the pox- and orthomyxoviruses are notable exceptions to this generalization. The retro- and hepadnaviruses are difficult to classify in this regard because their genomes alternate between RNA and DNA during each replication cycle. Whatever the initial biosynthetic reaction, a mechanism that most viruses use to help them attain dominance over the cell is to differentiate their infectious cycles into an early phase, when the viral genomes are present in low copy-number and direct the synthesis of catalytic amounts of viral replication proteins, and a late, postreplicative phase, when the abundant progeny genomes direct the synthesis of stoichiometric amounts of structural proteins.

DNA metabolism

Host-cell DNA replication occurs only during the S phase of the cell cycle, in a tightly regulated manner that is co-ordinated with the cell cycle as a whole. It requires pools of deoxyribonucleotides, replication enzymes, continuous protein synthesis, and access to appropriate anchor points on the nuclear matrix (Challberg and Kelly 1989; Echols 1990; Challberg 1991; Stillman et al. 1992). Viruses perturb this process to different degrees, depending on how much they rely on it for their own

replication. Retroviruses, for example, which integrate DNA copies of their genomes into host chromosomes, ensure their replication by the expression of oncogenes that drive the cell relentlessly through the cell cycle, but do not otherwise affect cellular DNA replication (Chapter 61, Prions of humans and animals). At the other end of the spectrum, the elaborate genomes of herpes- and poxviruses replicate with almost complete autonomy, to the extent that infection by HSV blocks cells from progressing to S phase, and infection by vaccinia virus even causes cellular DNA degradation (Kelly et al. 1988).

DEOXYRIBONUCLEOTIDE BIOSYNTHESIS

Most cells in the body continue to make RNA and protein throughout their lives, but many terminally differentiated cells stop dividing and therefore suppress DNA synthesis. For a virus with a DNA genome to be able to replicate in such cells, it must not only circumvent this suppression or provide the necessary enzymes for DNA replication (or both) but also restore the cellular pools of deoxyribonucleoside triphosphates (dNTPs). Even in dividing cells, the metabolic load imposed by viral DNA synthesis can exceed the capacity of the cell and require continuous replenishment of the dNTP pools. This problem is particularly acute for the poxviruses, which replicate their DNA in the cytoplasm (Chapter 31, Poxvirus replication).

Two distinct mechanisms have evolved to relieve this constraint: DNA viruses with relatively small genomes, such as the polyoma- and adenoviruses, induce cells to enter S phase, when the cellular genes for the necessary enzymes are naturally expressed. This is the basis for the oncogenic potential of viruses in these families (Jansen-Durr 1996), which is described in Chapter 17, Viral oncogenicity. In contrast, larger DNA viruses in the herpes- and poxvirus families have genomes with sufficient capacity to encode viral versions of some of the critical enzymes of nucleotide metabolism. Figure 12.11 shows the major pathways of dNTP biosynthesis in animal cells, with the enzymes encoded by either herpes- or poxviruses (or both) underlined. It is presumed that the genes for these enzymes were acquired from the host during viral evolution and serve to liberate these viruses from dependence on S phase. However, the genes are usually dispensable for virus replication in cultured cells, which are metabolically active and cycling.

Although these virus-specified enzymes catalyze the same reactions as their cellular counterparts, their substrate specificities and regulatory properties are often somewhat different, which makes them feasible targets for the development of antiviral agents (Chapter 70, The emergence and re-emergence of viral diseases). For example, the antiherpetic drugs acyclovir and ganciclovir are analogues of guanosine that can be phosphorylated by the thymidine kinase enzyme of HSV, but not by that

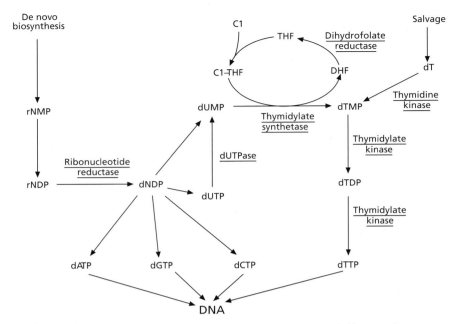

Figure 12.11 *Pathways of deoxyribonucleotide biosynthesis. Underlined enzymes are encoded by some herpes- or poxviruses.*

of the host. Because the 5′-triphosphates of these drugs act as chain terminators during DNA synthesis, they block DNA replication specifically in HSV-infected cells. However, the propensity of viral genomes for mutation and the facile selection of drug-resistant mutants create problems for the long-term use of anti-viral agents that are similar to those encountered with antibiotics. For example, suppression of vaccinia virus replication by hydroxyurea, which inhibits ribonucleo-tide reductase by a radical scavenging mechanism, readily selects for resistant mutants that contain multiple copies of the gene for one of the subunits of the viral enzyme (Slabaugh et al. 1989). Nevertheless, the virus-specific enzymes of nucleotide metabolism that are encoded by the larger DNA viruses provide versatile genetic tools, as well as possible targets for the develop-ment and testing of antiviral agents. The possibility is also being explored of incorporating the HSV thymidine kinase gene into suicide vectors targeted to tumor cells to render them sensitive to acyclovir (Morgan and Anderson 1993).

DNA REPLICATION

As described above, DNA viruses with small genomes stimulate the host cell to provide them with many of the enzymes they need for DNA replication. Polyomaviruses, such as SV40, induce S phase in infected cells by the action of a single viral gene product, large T antigen, which is expressed early in the infectious cycle (Fanning and Knippers 1992). This viral protein binds to the cellular tumor-suppressor protein pRb (Wiman 1993), displacing transcription factors of the E2F family to which it is normally bound (Nevins 1992). These transcription

factors switch on several cellular genes involved in cell cycle control and DNA replication, including the genes for DNA polymerase α, the enzyme that replicates the viral genome. T antigen also binds to another tumor-suppressor protein, p53, and relieves the cell cycle block that is normally imposed by this protein (Ludlow 1993; Ludlow and Skuse 1995). Thus, by expressing a single viral protein, SV40 prepares the cell for DNA replication and gains access to the enzymes necessary to catalyze it. During a productive infection, viral DNA replication will ensue, but the properties of large T antigen are those of an oncogene, and expressed on its own it will transform cells and cause tumors (whence it derives the name of Tumor antigen). In the related papillomaviruses, the inac-tivation of pRb and p53 is delegated to two viral proteins, E7 and E6, respectively (Vousden 1993; Farthing and Vousden 1994).

With DNA genomes three to six times larger than those of the polyomaviruses, adenoviruses (Chapter 22, Adenoviruses) have sufficient genetic capacity to encode three of the proteins necessary for DNA replication: DNA polymerase, a genome-linked terminal protein involved in the initiation of viral DNA synthesis, and a single-stranded DNA binding protein. However, they still need to push the cell into S phase to establish supportive conditions. This push is mediated by two early viral gene products, E1A and E1B, which together perform the functions described above for SV40 T antigen: binding to the tumor-suppressor proteins pRb and p53, respectively (Moran 1993).

In addition to the enzymes of nucleotide metabolism (Figure 12.11), HSV encodes seven proteins that are directly involved in DNA replication (Chapter 26,

Alphaherpesviruses). By providing so much of the replication apparatus itself, HSV gains independence from the cell cycle and attains a degree of autonomy that lets it replicate in highly differentiated cells, such as neurons. Similarly, encoding most or all of their replication machinery enables poxviruses to replicate their DNA in the cytoplasm (Chapter 31, Poxvirus replication).

Two families of animal viruses synthesize DNA by a pathway that has no cellular counterpart, that of reverse transcription of RNA. Retro- and hepadnaviruses both encode an RNA-dependent DNA polymerase (reverse transcriptase) that catalyzes this unique reaction which is central to their mechanisms of genome replication (Chapters 61, Prions of humans and animals; and 56, Hepatitis delta virus). The enzyme is a structural component of virus particles from both families and it catalyzes the initial biosynthetic reactions of their infectious cycles, the synthesis of viral DNA. Retroviruses also encode an integrase enzyme that recombines the proviral DNA into the genome of the host.

Because cellular DNA replication depends on continuous protein synthesis, it is inhibited by many DNA and RNA viruses as a consequence of their effects on translation (see Protein metabolism). The viruses probably benefit from the increased availability of nucleotides. Inhibition also results from the ability of viral DNA molecules to displace cellular DNA from anchor points on the nuclear matrix that are thought to provide the necessary structural framework for DNA replication. It has been suggested that competition for these sites may modulate the interaction between viral and host cell DNA replication (Cook 1991), and, in accordance with this idea, components of the cell's replication machinery are also redistributed within the nucleus following HSV infection (de Bruyn Kops and Knipe 1988).

DNA MAINTENANCE AND TRANSFER

Viral DNAs can be stably maintained in the host cell either by integration into a cellular chromosome, as with the retroviruses, or in the form of extrachromosomal circular episomes, as with papilloma and hepadnavirus DNAs and during latent infections with herpesviruses. In the integrated state, retroviral DNAs use both the origins and the enzymes of the cell for replication, but episomal DNAs contain their own cis-acting replication origins and usually express trans-acting viral proteins to assist in their replication and maintenance. In general, the long-term co-existence of viral and host DNAs in the same cellular compartment creates possibilities for the transfer of genetic information in both directions. Transfers from virus to cell are exemplified by the many instances of cellular transformation mediated by the incorporation of oncogenes from DNA tumor viruses (Teich 1991). Transfers from cell to virus are considered to have been responsible for the acquisition of proto-oncogenes during evolution of the RNA tumor viruses

and for the integration of a cellular retrotransposon into baculovirus DNA (Friesen and Nissen 1990).

DNA MODIFICATION AND DEGRADATION

Unlike bacteria, eukaryotic cells do not generally contain DNA restriction/modification enzyme systems to protect themselves against invading DNA, although a few examples have been found of such enzymes being induced or encoded by viruses of eukaryotes. A family of DNA viruses that infect the green alga Chlorella encode DNA methyltransferases and sequence-specific endonucleases that resemble restriction enzymes of prokaryotes (van Etten et al., 1988, 1991; van Etten and Meints 1999). Cells infected by frog virus 3, an irido-virus, express a cytosine methyltransferase that protects the viral DNA against degradation by a virus-encoded DNase (Murti et al. 1985). Poxviruses, on the other hand, rely on subcellular compartmentation to achieve specific degradation of host DNA. Vaccinia virus particles contain a DNase that enters the host-cell nucleus early in infection and degrades the cellular DNA. The liberated nucleotides are recycled into viral DNA to such an extent that the incorporation of exogenous thymidine via the thymidine kinase pathway is almost completely suppressed during the later stages of viral DNA synthesis. Degradation of cellular DNA also occurs as a result of the induction of apoptosis in response to infection by some viruses (see Apoptosis). During this process, internucleosomal cleavage of chromatin produces a characteristic ladder of DNA fragments that can be resolved by agarose gel electrophoresis. Finally, the genomes of vaccinia virus and HSV encode uracil DNA glycosylases that are thought to be involved in viral DNA base excision repair (Dodson et al. 1994; Millns et al. 1994).

RNA metabolism

Whatever the initial biosynthetic event in infection, sooner or later every virus has to deliver mRNA to the cytoplasm to direct viral protein synthesis. Because the nature of the problem varies with the genetic strategy of the virus, virus families have evolved different mechanisms to ensure efficient transcription of viral genes and to disrupt the expression of host-cell genes (Nevins 1989; Tevethia and Spector 1989).

PREFERENTIAL SYNTHESIS OF VIRAL RNAS

Three general mechanisms have been identified that promote transcription of viral genes at the start of infection:

1 seduction of the cellular RNA polymerase (pol II) by means of a strong promoter/enhancer sequence in the viral DNA (e.g. polyoma- and adenoviruses);
2 import of a new transcription factor that redirects pol II to the viral DNA (e.g. HSV);

3   import of a new RNA polymerase with specificity for the viral genome (e.g. poxviruses and all negative-strand and double-stranded RNA viruses).

These three distinct mechanisms are described below.

Enhancers

Studies of the early SV40 promoter, which directs pol II to transcribe the viral T antigen gene, were the first to discover the *cis*-acting DNA element now known as an enhancer which increases the level of transcription from a minimal promoter on a DNA molecule (Tjian and Maniatis 1994). Enhancers work by recruiting cellular transcription factors which are often differentially expressed in different cell types, so the properties of the viral enhancer can determine which types of cell are able to support replication of the virus (Drapkin et al. 1993). For example, human papillomavirus (Chapter 23, Papillomaviruses) is restricted to replication in keratinocytes partly because the enhancer for its E6 and E7 oncogenes must be recognized by a keratinocyte-specific transcription factor.

Transcription factors

In HSV infection, the viral DNA enters the nucleus together with a virion structural protein called α-*trans*-inducing factor (α-TIF) (or VP16) which is necessary for efficient transcription of the α class of viral genes that are expressed immediately after infection. α-TIF works in conjunction with the cellular transcription factor Oct-1 to recruit pol II to the Oct-1-binding sites (ATGCAAAT) that are present in the promoters for the α-genes (Kristie and Sharp 1993). Among the products of α-gene expression are at least two other transcription factors that change the specificity of the cellular polymerase to prepare it for the next stage of viral gene expression, transcription of the β-genes (Chapters 25, Herpesviruses: general properties; and 26, Alphaherpesviruses). In general, DNA viruses switch transcription from one temporal class of genes to the next by the synthesis of viral factors that act directly or indirectly on the corresponding RNA polymerases. Some of the properties of the SV40 T antigen and the E1A/E1B proteins of adenovirus that provide examples of this were described in the section entitled DNA metabolism. Transcription factors for immediate–early genes (e.g. HSV α-TIF) are synthesized late in the preceding infectious cycle because they themselves are encoded in late viral genes. It is not yet known what prevents them from becoming active until the start of the next infection.

RNA polymerases

Many virus families have genomes that cannot be transcribed by any cellular polymerase and must therefore be presented to the cell in conjunction with a functional virus-specific transcriptase. For example, although poxvirus genomes are composed of double-stranded DNA, infection delivers them to the cytoplasm, which lacks RNA polymerase activity, and anyway their promoter sequences are unrecognizable by the nuclear RNA polymerases (Chapter 31, Poxvirus replication). To ensure transcription of their genes under these conditions, infecting poxvirus particles contain a multisubunit transcription complex that is activated once the viral core reaches the cytoplasm. It is guided specifically to the early viral genes by a viral early transcription factor (VETF) that is bound to early promoters, in conjunction with a polymerase-associated protein (RAP94) that is responsible for recruiting the subunits of the transcription complex during virus assembly in the previous infection (Zhang et al. 1994).

RNA viruses whose genomes consist of either double-stranded RNA or single-stranded negative- or ambisense RNA face the same problem and solve it in the same manner: infection delivers the genome complexed with a virus-encoded RNA-dependent RNA polymerase that transcribes the viral genes (Ishihama and Barbier 1994; O'Reilly and Kao 1998). In many cases, virion-associated enzymes then cap, methylate and polyadenylate the primary transcripts to produce functional mRNAs. The following virus families use this strategy: reo-, orthomyxo-, paramyxo-, rhabdo-, filo-, bunya-, and arenaviruses (see Table 12.4).

PERTURBATIONS OF CELLULAR RNA METABOLISM

Every step of cellular RNA metabolism is disrupted by one virus family or another: transcription, processing, transport from the nucleus to the cytoplasm, translation, and RNA degradation. These effects usually give the viral genes a competitive advantage, although in some cases the advantage may be too slight to be demonstrable during a single infectious cycle. Effects on translation are described in Protein metabolism, the others below.

RNA synthesis

The expression of oncogenes by tumor viruses results in a stimulation of cellular RNA synthesis as a consequence of cell cycling. In contrast, most nononcogenic viruses inhibit cellular transcription, although the mechanisms may be consequences of the inhibition of protein synthesis or the rearrangement of cellular chromatin, or both. The benefit to the virus is presumed to be decreased competition for ribonucleoside triphosphates, and in some cases the increased availability of pol II. Curiously, VSV, a rhabdovirus that replicates entirely in the cytoplasm (Chapter 51, Rhabdoviruses), also inhibits cellular transcription. The 46 nucleotide (nt) VSV leader RNA migrates into the nucleus early in infection, associates with the cellular La protein and can inhibit pol II. However, the idea that leader RNA is responsible for the inhibition of transcription in infected cells has been challenged, and the physiological significance of these effects is unclear.

Influenza virus disrupts cellular RNA synthesis in an unusual manner that is directly related to its own mechanism of transcription (Chapter 32, Orthomyxoviruses: influenza). By endonucleolytic cleavage, the viral RNA polymerase removes 10–13 nt fragments that include the cap from the 5′ ends of newly made cellular transcripts, and uses these fragments to prime the synthesis of viral mRNAs in the nucleus of infected cells (Lamb and Krug, 2001). The effect is to transfer the caps from cellular mRNA precursors to viral messages, thereby labilizing the former and ensuring the translatability of the latter. Bunyaviruses (Chapter 48, *Bunyaviridae*) use a similar cap-snatching mechanism to derive the 5′ ends of their mRNAs, except in this case the cap donors are mature cellular messages that are already in the cytoplasm (Kolakofsky and Hacker 1991).

RNA processing and transport

For viruses that replicate in the nucleus, RNA splicing is usually an important control point in gene expression. In the interests of genetic economy, DNA viruses with small genomes frequently splice their primary transcripts in several different ways, both to derive multiple mRNAs from a single promoter and to access two overlapping reading frames in the same region of the viral genome. Retroviruses use alternative splicing patterns too, but they also need a mechanism to allow the export to the cytoplasm of unspliced RNA to encode some of the viral structural proteins and to be encapsidated into progeny virions. Complex retroviruses, such as HIV, achieve this by the interaction between a viral protein rev, itself the translation product of a spliced message, and a specific RNA sequence in the viral genome (the rev-response element (RRE)). This interaction allows the export of viral RNAs that still contain complete introns and would otherwise be retained in the nucleus (Gait and Karn 1993; Cullen 1994). In simpler retroviruses such as Mason–Pfizer monkey virus, the function of the rev/RRE complex is performed instead by a small *cis*-acting constitutive RNA transport element (CTE) that somehow promotes the export of unspliced viral RNAs to the cytoplasm (Bray et al. 1994; Ernst et al. 1997).

The NS1 protein of influenza virus inhibits splicing of both viral and cellular mRNA precursors by binding to their poly(A) tails and blocking spliceosome function, but in this case the unspliced host cell transcripts are retained in the nucleus, where they provide a source of the capped oligonucleotides that are needed as primers for viral transcription. Phosphorylation of NS1 regulates this inhibition to permit the release of viral mRNAs to

the cytoplasm (Lamb and Krug 2001). Yet another variation is provided by adenovirus, the system in which splicing was originally discovered (Berget et al. 1977; Chow et al. 1977). Splicing is not inhibited in infected cells, and indeed primary adenovirus transcripts are extensively and differentially spliced to access many different open reading frames from a few promoter sites (Chapter 22, Adenoviruses). However, two of the early proteins (E1B and E4) specifically inhibit the export of processed cellular mRNAs from the nucleus and promote that of late viral mRNAs, resulting in the preferential synthesis of viral proteins. It is likely that further studies of the ways that different viruses impinge on the processing and transport of cellular transcripts will deepen our understanding both of virus–cell interactions and of the regulation of mRNA synthesis in uninfected cells (Krug 1993).

RNA degradation

The pathways and control of mRNA degradation in eukaryotic cells are not fully understood (Katze and Agy 1990; Rajagopalan and Malter 1997) but, as with RNA processing and transport, viral genetics provide powerful experimental tools to assist research in this area. Both HSV and vaccinia virus infections increase the rate of host mRNA degradation and thereby inhibit cellular protein synthesis (Rice and Roberts 1983; Strom and Frenkel 1987). The effects are not specific for cellular messages, because viral mRNAs are turned over equally fast, but the greater vigor of viral transcription is better able to compensate for the short mRNA half-lives, which also facilitate the rapid transitions from expression of one temporal class of viral genes to the next. For HSV-1, the ability to induce mRNA labilization has been mapped to the *vhs* gene (for viral host shut-off), which encodes a virus structural protein. The vhs protein in the virion is sufficient to trigger mRNA degradation in some cells, although it is not known whether it works directly as a nuclease or by activating a host cell degradative mechanism. In vaccinia virus, the gene responsible for enhanced mRNA turnover has not been mapped, but mutations that subtly affect the function of the viral RNA polymerase can cause massive nonspecific RNA degradation by producing abundant double-stranded RNA which activates the cellular 2–5A RNase L system for RNA breakdown (Bayliss and Condit 1993) (see Induction and actions of interferons, and Chapter 15, The role of cytokines in viral infections).

Protein metabolism

The synthesis, processing, and transport of viral proteins lie at the heart of the overlap between viral and cellular metabolism, because, whereas most viruses encode specific enzymes or factors that participate in viral transcription and genome replication, they all depend on the host cell for the entire machinery of protein synthesis and transport. One consequence of this is that translation, which is such an effective target for antibacterial agents, is not available as a target for the development of antiviral drugs.

PROTEIN SYNTHESIS

The rate of protein synthesis from a particular mRNA is influenced by many factors (Lodish 1976). In eukaryotic cells, most translational control is exerted at initiation (Merrick 1990; Gale et al. 2000), and a schematic picture of this multistep reaction is shown in Figure 12.12. Because of its complexity, the regulation of this process is not yet fully understood, but the following factors all play a part: the abundance of the mRNA, its 5′ cap structure, the local nucleotide sequence context and secondary structure surrounding its initiation codon, whether it is translated on free or membrane-bound polysomes, and the availability and activity of cellular initiation factors (Hershey 1990, 1993; Kozak 1991a; Wek 1994). Two prominent control points among the latter are eIF4F, the cap-binding complex, and eIF2,

which binds the initiator met-tRNA to the 40S ribosomal subunit. Both of these initiation factors are altered in some virus-infected cells, as described below (Kozak 1986; Schneider and Shenk 1987).

Initiation in uninfected eukaryotic cells usually involves recognition by eIF4F of the 7-methylguanylate cap at the 5′ end of cellular mRNA, followed by association of the mRNA with a complex that contains the 40S ribosomal subunit, met-tRNA$_i$ and eIF2 (Figure 12.12). eIF4F is a cap-dependent RNA helicase that is required for the translation of almost all capped messages. On a very small number of cellular mRNAs and on picornaviral RNAs, initiation occurs at an internal ribosome entry site (IRES), in a manner that is independent of the 5′ cap and eIF4F. In both cases, the 40S subunit then scans in a 3′ direction until it encounters the first AUG codon. If the local sequence context of this AUG is favorable for initiation, the 60S ribosomal subunit joins the complex, eIF2 dissociates and the synthesis of the polypeptide chain begins. Initiation efficiency is influenced most by the identity of the nucleotides in the −3 and +4 positions relative to the AUG, the sequence . . . CRCCAUGG . . . being optimal for initiation, but

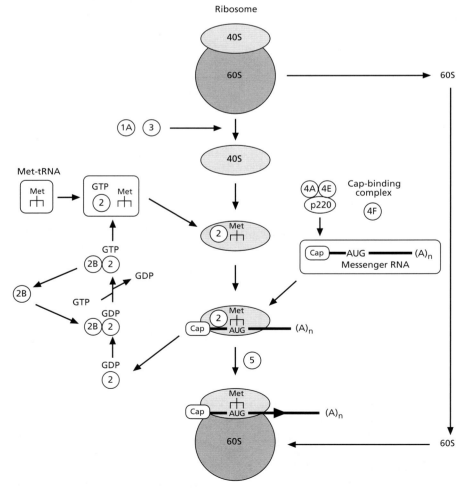

Figure 12.12 *Mechanism of initiation of protein synthesis in animal cells. The numbered circles represent the initiation factors.*

other features of the mRNA 5′ end including its secondary structure can also exert effects (Kozak 1989, 1991a, b, 1992a, b, 1994). Although eukaryotic protein synthesis usually starts at the first AUG codon, if its context is unfavorable for initiation the 40S subunit can continue scanning until it finds the next and starts there instead. In rare instances, alternative initiation codons, including non-AUG codons, are used to derive more than one translation product from a single mRNA, as in the case of the P mRNA of some paramyxoviruses (Curran et al. 1986) (see Chapter 33, General properties of paramyxoviruses). When eIF2 dissociates from the initiation complex it is bound to GDP, but before it can form another met-tRNA-40S subunit complex for another round of initiation, it must exchange this GDP for GTP, a reaction that requires initiation factor eIF2B (Figure 12.12). In several metabolic situations including viral infection, this exchange reaction is a major site at which protein synthesis is regulated, as described below (Hershey 1993).

Host shut-off and the preferential translation of viral mRNAs

The inhibition of host-cell protein synthesis is one of the most obvious metabolic consequences of viral infection, and it has been the focus of much research using several different virus systems (see Ehrenfeld (1993) for reviews). Unfortunately, although it is easy to demonstrate the phenomenon, it has proved difficult to elucidate its mechanisms, because, somewhat surprisingly, viruses shut off host protein synthesis in different ways and even closely related viruses can use completely different mechanisms (Table 12.5). Cytocidal viruses such as polio and vaccinia inhibit host translation profoundly, but retroviruses, which depend on the cell's continued growth and survival, scarcely perturb host protein synthesis at all. Many other viruses lie between these two extremes. Some of the conflicts in the literature on this subject may be because some viruses use more than one mechanism or use different mechanisms when infecting different cell types.

Because viral and host mRNAs compete directly for translation, viruses have evolved mechanisms that favor the synthesis of their own proteins, often at the expense of the cell's. However, the total amount of translation occurring in infected cells is almost always less than that in uninfected cells, because infection generally reduces the overall capacity of the cell for protein synthesis. Rather than simply displacing host mRNAs, viral messages are preferentially translated against the background of a progressive inhibition of total protein synthesis to which they are relatively resistant. For this reason, how viruses inhibit host protein synthesis and the mechanisms they use to achieve preferential translation of their own mRNAs are interdependent.

Several such mechanisms have been identified (Table 12.5). To begin with, the abundance of individual viral mRNAs is usually greater than that of most cellular mRNAs, because of vigorous viral transcription and the high gene copy-number that results from viral genome replication. In the herpes- and poxviruses, this effect is magnified by an increased rate of mRNA breakdown (see RNA metabolism). In addition, many viral mRNAs have a competitive advantage whose structural basis is not fully understood (Garfinkel and Katze 1993; Kozak 1994). Part of the answer lies in the nucleotide sequence context of their initiation codons, but strong contexts, although common, are not ubiquitous in viral mRNAs (Kozak 1986). Their 5′ untranslated regions are usually shorter than those of host mRNAs, and the resulting proximity of the cap to the initiation codon and other undefined structural features of their 5′ ends may also favor translation.

For polio- and rhinoviruses, the mechanism is clear and elegant (Sonenberg 1987; Jackson et al. 1991; Wycoff 1993; Thompson and Sarnow 2000): infection results in the expression of a viral protease (2A), which mediates cleavage of a component (p220 or the γ subunit) of the cellular cap-binding complex, eIF4F (Etchison et al. 1982; Etchison and Fout 1985). The

Table 12.5 *Mechanisms of inhibition of host-cell protein synthesis*

Virus	Mechanism	Reference
Herpes simplex	Degradation of host (and viral) mRNAs	Strom and Frenkel (1987)
Vaccinia	Degradation of host (and viral) mRNAs	Rice and Roberts (1983)
Polio	Inactivation of eIF4F-γ by cleavage	Etchison et al. (1982)
Rhino	Inactivation of eIF4F-γ by cleavage	Etchison and Fout (1985)
Adeno	Inactivation of eIF4F-α by underphosphorylation	Huang and Schneider (1991)
	Inactivation of eIF2B-β by phosphorylation	O'Malley et al. (1989)
Vesicular stomatitis	mRNA abundance	Lodish and Porter (1981)
	Not mRNA abundance	Schnitzlein et al. (1983)
	Affinity for ribosomes	Nuss et al. (1975)
	Interference with eIF2 function	Centrella and Lucas-Lenard (1982)
	Interference with eIF3/4B function	Thomas and Wagner (1983)

result is inactivation of the initiation factor and consequent inhibition of translation of capped mRNAs. Viral RNA is immune to this inhibition because it is translated from an IRES and naturally lacks a 5′ cap (Meerovitch and Sonenberg 1993). In virions, polio- and rhinovirus RNAs carry a covalently attached viral protein (VPg) at their 5′ ends, while the translated form of the viral RNA starts with a 5′-monophosphate, pUp (Chapter 40, Picornaviruses).

It is surprising that cleavage of the cap-binding protein is unique to polio- and rhinoviruses, and does not occur in cells infected with other picornaviruses, despite the fact that all their RNAs contain IRES elements, are translated in a cap-independent manner, and mostly shut-off host protein synthesis (Duncan 1990). Because it is incontrovertible that picornaviruses are all descended from a common ancestor, their use of different shut-off mechanisms suggests either that an ancestral mechanism was replaced in some but not other descendants or that the ancestor did not inhibit host translation and that the present-day mechanisms evolved separately after divergence. Taken with the fact that polio- and herpesvirus mutants that cannot shut off host translation are only partly debilitated for growth (Bernstein et al. 1985; Strom and Frenkel 1987), this evidence suggests that inhibition of host protein synthesis, though beneficial, is not essential for virus replication. Indeed, a general selection method has been developed for the isolation of nonconditional viral mutants that are deficient in host protein shut-off (Francoeur et al. 1987).

The activity of the cap-binding complex is also reduced in adenovirus-infected cells, but in this case it is by reduced phosphorylation of the α subunit (eIF4A, which is the cap-binding protein itself) rather than by cleavage of p220 (Huang and Schneider 1991; Zhang and Schneider 1993). Because adenovirus mRNAs are capped, the rationale for eIF4F inactivation is less obvious than with the picornaviruses. However, it seems that the tripartite leader, a 200-nt RNA segment that is common to the 5′ end of all late adenovirus mRNAs (Chapter 22, Adenoviruses), renders them less dependent for translation on the helicase activity of eIF4F than are cellular messages.

Changes in the level of phosphorylation of another initiation factor, eIF2, are responsible for the regulation of protein synthesis under many different conditions of cellular stress, but in this case it is increased phosphorylation that interferes with initiation. As shown in Figure 12.12, eIF2 needs to exchange its bound GDP for GTP between each round of initiation, and this exchange requires the formation of a complex with eIF2B. Phosphorylation of the α subunit of eIF2 prevents the dissociation of this complex, and, because eIF2B is scarce relative to eIF2, a modest increase in the level of phosphorylation inhibits initiation profoundly. As described in Induction and actions of interferons, this mechanism is part of the cell's response to viral infection

that is enhanced by treatment of cells with interferon. Increases in the phosphorylation of eIF2-α occur in cells infected with adeno- and reoviruses, but it is unclear whether these are part of the virus-mediated inhibition of host mRNA translation or the cell-mediated inhibition of the virus. Nevertheless, this regulatory mechanism is a key point in the balance between viral and cellular protein synthesis, as shown by the fact that vaccinia virus encodes a homologue of eIF2-α, and several other viruses perturb the phosphorylation of eIF2-α in other ways (see Viral mechanisms to evade cellular defenses).

Access to alternative open reading frames

In addition to alternative RNA splicing (see RNA metabolism) and transcriptional editing (Cattaneo 1991; Jacques and Kolakofsky 1991), some viruses use translational frameshifting to express open reading frames that would otherwise be inaccessible in an mRNA. Retroviruses in particular use this mechanism to make proteins that they require only in small amounts, like the gag–pol precursor to the reverse transcriptase in Rous sarcoma virus (Jacks and Varmus 1985). Frameshifting is promoted by specific 'slippery' sequences in the mRNA, which, often in conjunction with adjacent 'hungry' codons and strong RNA secondary structure, persuade ribosomes occasionally to switch reading frames during translation (Brierley 1993). Whether viral infection modulates the intrinsic propensity of the ribosomes for frameshifting is not yet clear. In other retroviruses, synthesis of the gag–pol precursor is achieved by suppression of the termination codon at the end of the gag gene (Chapter 61, Prions of humans and animals).

PROTEIN PROCESSING

During and after their synthesis, viral proteins are processed along many of the same reaction pathways as cellular proteins, and, because they offer such attractive experimental subjects, they have been widely used as model systems for the study of these pathways. There are also several cases in which protein processing reactions are mediated by viral enzymes or modified by viral proteins, and this is a frequent cause of CPEs.

Folding and oligomerization

Viral proteins must adopt the correct tertiary and quaternary structures before they become functional and, in many cases, before they can be transported to their ultimate destinations in the cell. These reactions have been examined in particular detail for viral envelope glycoproteins such as influenza HA, which must undergo glycosylation, folding and trimerization before it can move from the ER, via the compartments of the Golgi apparatus, to the cell surface in preparation for virus assembly (Gething et al. 1986; Doms et al.

1993; Byland and Marsh 2005). Folding is facilitated by interaction with a cellular protein BiP which resides in the lumen of the ER and binds transiently to newly made glycoproteins. BiP belongs to the hsp70 family of cellular proteins that are induced by heat shock and other types of stress, and it functions both to catalyze protein unfolding/refolding and to target misfolded and mutant proteins for degradation (Pelham 1988; Hartl 1996; Paulsson and Wang 2003).

Proteolytic cleavage

Many viral proteins are cleaved during maturation, by either cellular or viral proteases. For example, the activation of viral fusion proteins by cleavage (see Viral fusion proteins) is often catalyzed by members of the furin family of cellular proteases (Klenk and Garten 1994a,b). However, viral proteolysis is used most extensively by the nonsegmented, positive-strand RNA viruses of the picorna-, toga-, and flavivirus families (Chapter 40, Picornaviruses; Chapter 47, Togaviruses; and Chapter 46, Flaviviruses). These viruses synthesize large polyprotein precursors that undergo multiple co- and post-translational cleavages catalyzed by several viral proteases to yield the mature viral proteins (Krausslich and Wimmer 1988; Strauss 1990; Dougherty and Semler 1993; Ryan and Flint 1997; Ryan et al. 1998; ten Dam et al. 1999). They are forced into this strategy of gene expression by a combination of their need to make several different viral proteins from a single mRNA and the reluctance of eukaryotic ribosomes to initiate at more than one site on a message. In contrast, viruses whose transcriptional mechanisms allow them to synthesize individual mRNAs and those with segmented genomes rely less heavily on proteolytic processing.

The assembly of icosahedral and more complex viral structures is also often accompanied by cleavage of structural protein precursors, which imposes a rigid order on the assembly process and can result in large-scale conformational changes in the maturing virion, often coincident with the acquisition of stability and infectivity (Guo 1994). Both in picorna- and in noda-viruses, the final maturational cleavage event occurs inside the assembled virion, and is catalyzed by the interior of the capsid itself. It is interesting that the assembly of helical nucleocapsids generally seems not to involve protein cleavage.

Glycosylation

All enveloped viruses carry surface glycoproteins whose glycosylation is mediated by the normal cellular pathways of carbohydrate attachment and processing. Both *N*- and *O*-linked oligosaccharides are found but viral proteins with the former modification are more common.

Whether glycosylation is required for glycoprotein transport and function varies from one case to another, and probably reflects the different roles that oligosaccharides can play in determining the native structures of individual proteins. In certain cases, however, the influence of glycosylation can be dramatic: the presence or absence of a particular *N*-linked oligosaccharide in influenza HA that partially obstructs the HA1–HA2 cleavage site can have a profound effect on viral virulence because it determines which proteases can cleave the HA precursor, and hence how the virus can spread in the infected animal (Deshpande et al. 1987).

Phosphorylation

Viruses and cells interact with one another by phosphorylation in both directions: the phosphorylation of cellular proteins by viral kinases and the phosphorylation of viral proteins by cellular kinases. Prominent among the former are reactions catalyzed by the tyrosine kinases that are encoded by the oncogenes of Rous sarcoma virus (v-src) and its relatives. In these cases, the major targets of kinase action are cellular proteins involved in cell cycle regulation whose activities are perturbed by phosphorylation. Conversely, cellular kinases can phosphorylate viral proteins and thereby modify their activities. For example, phosphorylation of the P protein of VSV by cellular casein kinase II enables it to form oligomers, which is an essential step in viral transcription (Gao and Lenard 1995).

Other covalent modifications

A wide variety of other covalent modifications of viral proteins have been described in different virus–cell systems, including N-terminal acetylation, acylation (with both palmitate and N-terminal myristate), ADP ribosylation, isoprenylation, methylation, and sulfation. In most cases the cellular enzymes that catalyze these reactions are widely distributed and therefore do not restrict virus replication, but the effects of many of the modifications on the properties of viral proteins have yet to be fully explored.

PROTEIN TRANSPORT

Viral proteins are transported to the appropriate intracellular sites for replication and assembly by interaction with cellular protein trafficking pathways: to the plasma membrane via the ER and Golgi apparatus, to the nucleus, and to other organelles. Despite the disruption of the cytoskeleton and the extensive changes in cell morphology that often accompany infection, these trafficking pathways are generally not disrupted. Many viral proteins contain signals that define their destination in the cell, such as the hydrophobic signal sequences of integral membrane glycoproteins which, by binding to the signal recognition particle, commit the proteins to

ER membrane insertion and transport along the exocytic pathway. Nuclear localization signals, which were first identified in the SV40 T antigen (Kalderon et al. 1984), target the corresponding viral proteins to the nucleus for replication and assembly. Proteins that contain *cis*-acting signals such as these are transported to the appropriate cellular compartment even when they are expressed from a vector in the absence of other viral proteins. In contrast, proteins that lack signals of their own can co-localize by binding with targeted proteins. A striking example of the influence of such signals on virus assembly is provided by the observation that a point mutation in a retroviral matrix protein determines whether the viral nucleocapsids assemble in the cytoplasm or at the plasma membrane (Rhee and Hunter 1990).

PROTEIN DEGRADATION

As described above, viruses in many families encode proteases with new specificities that can cleave cellular as well as viral polypeptides. It is likely that the resulting exposure of new N termini (Varshavsky 1992) to the protein degradation pathways (Hershko and Ciechanover 1992; Rubin and Finley 1995) will enhance the rate of turnover of specific proteins in cells infected with these viruses, although, apart from the cleavage of eIF-4F described above, few specific examples have yet been described.

CELLULAR RESPONSES TO VIRAL INFECTION

Because viruses are a threat to the survival of cells and organisms, it is inevitable that cells and organisms should have evolved defense mechanisms to counteract them. It is similarly inevitable that those viruses with sufficient genetic capacity should have evolved countermeasures to circumvent these defenses. In higher vertebrates, the major defense of organisms against infection is provided by the mucosal, humoral, and cell-mediated arms of the immune system, which are described in Chapter 14, The immune response to viral infections. The major defenses at the cellular level are the interferon (IFN) system (see below and Chapter 15, The role of cytokines in viral infections), RNA interference (Hannon 2002; Ding et al. 2004), and the mechanisms of stress response and apoptosis. The interplay between the processes of virus replication, these cellular responses and the corresponding viral evasion mechanisms determines the outcome of infection at the cellular level.

Induction and actions of interferons

The IFNs are a family of cytokines that elicit profound physiological changes in the cells with which they interact, including the development of resistance to viral infection. In higher vertebrates, the IFN system acts within a few hours of infection, long before the onset of the immune response, to limit the spread of the infection and thus to diminish its severity. Indeed, many of the familiar early symptoms of a viral infection in humans are attributable to IFN action. IFNs are synthesized and secreted by most cell types in response to infection and some other stimuli, and they exert their effects by inducing the expression of several IFN-responsive genes. Understanding the system as a whole, therefore, requires knowledge of the IFN genes, how they are induced, the IFN proteins themselves, and how they interact with their target cells, how these interactions trigger expression of the IFN-inducible genes, and, finally, how the products of these latter genes render the cell resistant to viral infection and mediate their other effects. Although much remains to be learned about this complex and multifunctional regulatory system, intense research in recent years has clarified many important aspects. Here is presented only an overview of the IFN system; for more details the reader should consult Chapter 15, The role of cytokines in viral infections or a review article (Revel and Chebath 1986; Pestka et al. 1987; Samuel 1988, 1991; Staeheli 1990; Sen and Lengyel 1992; Sen and Ransohoff 1993; Johnson et al. 1994; Sen 2001; Malmgaard 2004).

INTERFERONS

Four distinct types of IFNs have been identified and characterized: α, β, γ, and ω. Although their properties overlap to the extent that they are all recognized as IFNs, they are secreted by different cell types in response to different inducers and they exert somewhat different physiological effects on different target cells. In the context of virus–host cell interactions, α, β, and γ IFNs are the most relevant because α and β induce a virus-resistant state in most cell types, whereas IFN-γ primarily modulates aspects of the cell-mediated immune response via its effects on macrophages. Alpha IFNs, which are encoded in a multigene family, are homologous to IFN-β and interact as monomers with the same receptor on the surface of target cells. In contrast, IFN-γ has little homology with the other types and binds as a dimer to two copies of a different cell surface receptor (Walter et al. 1995).

INTERFERON INDUCTION

Alpha and β IFNs are induced and secreted from many different cell types in response to infection by most viruses, as well as some other assaults, and these cytokines act as an early warning system that alerts other cells in the body that infection is imminent. In contrast, IFN-γ is produced only by T lymphocytes and natural killer cells, in response to induction by cognate antigens and other T-cell activators. Induction of IFNs occurs by transcriptional activation of the IFN genes, and,

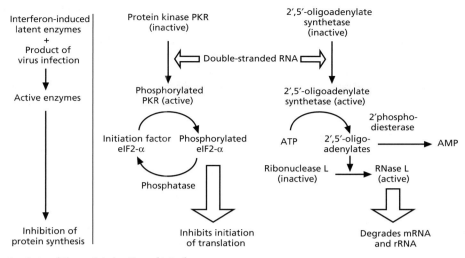

Figure 12.13 *Mechanisms of the antiviral action of interferons.*

although many of the mechanistic details remain obscure, a satisfying picture is emerging for the induction of IFN-β. It has long been known that IFN-β can be induced by treating cells with double-stranded RNA, and indeed the production of double-stranded RNA may be a general mechanism by which viruses induce IFNs. Among the cellular targets for double-stranded RNA is a cytoplasmic protein kinase called PKR, which is also involved in the mechanism of IFN action (see below). On activation by binding to double-stranded RNA, PKR phosphorylates I-κB, the inhibitory subunit of the transcription factor NF-κB (Karin and Hunter 1995). Phosphorylation of I-κB allows NF-κB to enter the nucleus where it recognizes specific DNA binding sites and thereby activates the transcription of several genes, including that for IFN-β (Proud 1995).

INTERFERON ACTION

The binding of IFNs to their corresponding receptors initiates signals that are transmitted to the nucleus of the IFN-treated cell via the JAK/STAT pathway. Signal transduction occurs by the activation of a family of tyrosine kinases (Janus kinases (JAK)) that are associated with the cytoplasmic domains of the transmembrane IFN receptors and activated when the receptors are occupied by binding to IFNs. The activated JAKs phosphorylate a family of transcription factors (signal transducing activators of transcription (STAT)), which then migrate from the cytoplasm to the nucleus. Here they form active complexes that bind to interferon-specific response elements (ISRE) present in the promoter sites upstream of IFN-inducible genes, thereby activating their transcription (Williams 1991; Pellegrini and Schindler 1993). Many other polypeptide ligands that exert a wide variety of physiological effects on cells also transmit their signals to the nucleus via the JAK/STAT pathway. The specificity of the ligand/response relation-

ship seems to be maintained by subtle quantitative, qualitative, and temporal differences in the spectra of JAK activation and STAT phosphorylation that are elicited by the different ligands, although much more work is needed to define fully how the integrity of different signals is maintained (Schindler and Darnell 1995; Aaronson and Horvarth 2002).

Although the IFN system was first discovered by the observation that IFN-treated cells are resistant to viral infection, it has since become clear that this is only one aspect of their altered physiology. IFNs can also have profound antiproliferative and immunomodulatory effects, so the physiology of the IFN response in whole animals is complex. The multiple effects of IFNs are mediated by the IFN-inducible proteins of which scores have been identified, but the roles that many of them play in the altered physiology of the IFN-treated cell are still unknown. Best understood are two inducible enzymes that are responsible, in part, for the resistance of cells to infection by several different viruses. These are the protein kinase (PKR) that is also implicated in the induction of IFN-β (see above), and a family of enzymes called 2′,5′-oligoadenylate (2–5A) synthetases (Figure 12.13).

PKR, a double-stranded RNA-dependent protein kinase

The protein kinase now known as PKR is a 68-kDa polypeptide that is induced by IFN treatment of most types of cultured vertebrate cells (Williams 1999). The enzyme is active only when bound to double-stranded RNA, whereupon it phosphorylates and activates itself, and also phosphorylates the translational initiation factor eIF2-α. This interferes with the initiation of protein synthesis (as described under Protein metabolism and Figure 12.12), which limits viral replication (Hershey 1990, 1993). Untreated cells contain only basal levels of PKR and the enzyme is largely inactive because of the absence of double-stranded RNA. IFN-treated cells contain substantial levels of PKR, but it remains inactive until viral infection produces double-stranded RNA, either as an intermediate of RNA replication or as a byproduct of overlapping transcription. In this way, the effects of IFN are fully manifested only after viral infection, a mechanism that restricts the major physiological consequences to the cells where they will have the greatest effect. Viruses have evolved numerous ways to counteract the effects of IFN in general and PKR in particular (see Viral mechanisms to evade cellular defenses), implying not only that the IFN response significantly restricts virus replication in nature, but also that PKR is a central component in the mechanism of resistance to many viruses.

2–5A synthetases

The 2–5A synthetases that are also induced by IFN treatment catalyze the template-independent oligomerization of ATP to form a series of $2'-5'$-linked oligomers that are referred to collectively as 2–5A (Ball 1982; Player and Torrence 1998; Rebouillat and Hovanessian 1999). Like PKR, the 2–5A synthetases depend on double-stranded RNA for enzyme activity, so full development of this aspect of the IFN response also requires viral infection of IFN-treated cells. The 2–5A oligomers have the general structure $ppp(A^{2'}p^{5'})_nA_{OH}$, and in cells the trimer and tetramer predominate. In general, $2',5'$-phosphodiester bonds are a biochemical rarity, although single such bonds are formed during RNA splicing (Sharp 1994) and also during the priming of cDNA synthesis by bacterial reverse transcriptase (Shimamoto et al. 1995). The only known function of 2–5A oligomers is to activate an endoribonuclease, RNase L, which is present as a constitutive but latent enzyme in most cell types (Bisbal 1997). On activation by 2–5A, RNase L degrades mRNAs and ribosomal RNAs, and thereby inhibits protein synthesis. The degradation of 2–5A itself by a $2'$-phosphodiesterase restores RNase L to its latent state. Thus, in IFN-treated virus-infected cells, PKR and 2–5A synthetase collaborate to restrict virus replication by inhibiting both the initiation and the elongation of polypeptides.

Specificity of IFN action

Although IFN treatment generally induces resistance to a wide range of viruses, the induced gene products play quantitatively different roles in combating infection by different viruses. For example, the 2–5A system seems to be particularly important in the resistance to picornavirus infection, but much less so in the resistance to several other virus families. The murine *Mx* gene is a more extreme example of an IFN-induced resistance mechanism that is effective only against a specific virus family because the Mx protein product makes mice and murine cells resistant to infection by influenza virus, but not by other viruses (Staeheli 1990; Samuel 1991; Haller and Kochs 2002). However, a broader and more complex question is whether IFN action can discriminate generally between viral and cellular events and, if so, how this is achieved. IFN treatment clearly enables organisms and cell cultures to survive viral challenges that would otherwise be lethal, and yet the properties of PKR and 2–5A synthetase provide only a partial explanation for this apparent selectivity. The recognition by these enzymes of double-stranded RNA as a signature of viral infection establishes a mechanism for discriminating between infected and uninfected cells rather than between viral and cellular mRNAs, and in some cases the infected cells are sacrificed to prevent viral replication. In other cases, enzyme activation imposes an indiscriminate but transient suppression of protein synthesis, a situation from which the cell can recover but the virus cannot. Finally, in some situations, the IFN-induced enzymes seem to be preferentially activated in cytoplasmic microenvironments surrounding the viral double-stranded RNA molecules that are responsible for their activation, thus achieving selectivity on the basis of compartmentalization.

It seems likely that combinations of these effects enable PKR and 2–5A synthetase/RNase L, which have no demonstrable specificity for viral mRNAs, nevertheless to discriminate between cellular and viral processes.

VIRAL FACILITATION BY INHIBITION OF THE IFN SYSTEM

Viruses differ in their sensitivity to IFNs, in part because some of them have evolved effective countermeasures against one or more component of the IFN system (see Viral mechanisms to evade cellular defenses). Accordingly, a virus such as vaccinia, which is relatively insensitive, can in some circumstances facilitate the replication of a coinfecting IFN-sensitive virus such as VSV by inhibiting the action of IFN. This contrasts with the more common situation in which coinfecting viruses interfere with one another by a variety of mechanisms that are unrelated to the IFN system (Whitaker-Dowling and Youngner 1987).

Induction and actions of cellular stress proteins

Although viral infection suppresses the synthesis of most cellular proteins by the mechanisms described in the section entitled Protein metabolism, some host cell genes are induced by infection and their proteins are relatively resistant to shut-off. These include the genes that encode the IFNs (see Induction and actions of interferons) and also those for a set of proteins that are generally induced by conditions of metabolic stress, including heat shock (Jindal and Malkovsky 1994; Sarkar and Sen 2004). Some of the cellular stress proteins normally function as molecular chaperones, and certain viruses exploit these properties to assist their own replication and assembly. This is true of some bacteriophages and has also been suggested for several eukaryotic viruses. For example, the cytoplasmic hsp70 protein binds transiently to the poliovirus capsid precursor, perhaps facilitating its folding and assembly. Similarly, BiP protein, which resides in the lumen of the rough endoplasmic reticulum, binds briefly to newly synthesized integral membrane proteins, such as viral glycoproteins, and assists their maturation (Hartl 1996). In addition to these roles, however, the display of virus-induced stress proteins or their peptide fragments on the surface of infected cells may stimulate immune recognition and participate in the activation of the immune response.

Apoptosis

Metazoan organisms have evolved a highly conserved and tightly regulated cellular pathway called 'apoptosis' which, once triggered, leads irreversibly to cell death (Martin et al. 1994; Martin and Green 1995; Steller 1995; Roulston et al. 1999). Apoptosis is the mechanism by which unwanted cells are eliminated during development, but it is also triggered in response to infection by a wide variety of cytocidal viruses (Vaux et al. 1994; Razvi and Welsh 1995; Everett and McFadden 1999). It is characterized by cell rounding, condensation of chromatin, fragmentation of cellular DNA, blebbing of the plasma membrane, and finally break up of the cell contents into membrane-bound apoptotic bodies that are suitable for ingestion by phagocytes. In the context of viral infection, apoptosis serves as an effective defense mechanism for the organism whereby a relatively small number of cells die altruistically to limit virus spread (Williams 1994). This is reminiscent of the self-sacrifice of some IFN-treated infected cells that was described in the section entitled Induction and actions of interferons. The mechanisms by which viruses induce apoptosis have yet to be fully defined, but changes in membrane permeabilities leading to Ca^{2+} influx, the expression of viral proteases with new specificities, and perturbation of the functions of the cellular tumor-suppressor proteins p53 and pRb may all be involved in different situations.

The most persuasive evidence that the effects of apoptosis in virus–host cell interactions are, on balance, detrimental to the virus comes from the observation that several viruses have evolved countermeasures that delay or prevent the onset of apoptosis (Ink et al. 1995; Razvi and Welsh 1995; Gillet and Brun 1996). For example, cowpox virus expresses an inhibitor of an enzyme that is involved in the apoptotic pathway, the interleukin-1β-converting enzyme (ICE) (Kumar 1995), and it thereby blocks both apoptosis and inflammation (Ray et al.

1992). In the absence of an effective apoptotic response, a normally cytocidal virus, such as Sindbis virus, can instead establish a persistent infection (Griffin et al. 1994; Griffin and Hardwick 1997). Conversely, suppression of apoptosis by the adenovirus E1B oncogene is necessary to allow the induction of cell proliferation that is mediated by the E1A oncogene to result in the transformation of adenovirus-infected cells (White 1993).

VIRAL MECHANISMS TO EVADE CELLULAR DEFENSES

During co-evolution with their hosts, different viruses have adopted several different methods of counteracting the various defense mechanisms, an observation that provides compelling evidence for the efficacy of the corresponding host defenses themselves (Smith 1993, 1994; Levy and Garcia-Sastre 2001). As might be expected, inactivation or deletion of the viral genes involved in these evasion mechanisms generally reduces the virulence of the virus. This aspect of the study of virus–host interactions is particularly informative because it provides a window on the relationships as they exist in nature. Moreover, some of the evasion mechanisms have involved the viral acquisition and adaptation of host genes that benefit the virus in much the same way as the acquisition of an oncogene benefits a retrovirus by ensuring cell cycling and concomitant viral replication. These host-derived genes and their products can provide insight into the heart of the virus–host relationship, as well as potential reagents for the experimental and therapeutic manipulation of the host's defense mechanisms (McFadden 1995).

Evasion of immune responses

Many RNA viruses continually evade the immune responses of the host by mutation. The inability of RNA polymerases to correct their mistakes leads to heterogeneous virus populations or quasi species from which antibody-escape mutants are readily selected (Smith and Inglis 1987; Duarte et al. 1994). For viruses that have segmented genomes (e.g. influenza), this effect is reinforced by the potential for reassortment of RNA segments between viruses with different pedigrees (see Chapter 32, Orthomyxoviruses: influenza). With HIV, the continuous generation of antigenic variants within each infected individual eventually overwhelms the ability of the immune system to respond and contributes to the onset of AIDS (see Chapter 61, Prions of animals and humans). In contrast, viruses with double-stranded DNA genomes are usually replicated with much greater fidelity and have therefore resorted to other methods of immune evasion. For example, herpesviruses are hidden from immune surveillance during latent infections (Masucci and Ernberg 1994; Wagner 1994; Lewin 1995), and during lytic growth they specifically inhibit the intracellular transport mechanism by which viral peptide fragments are presented to the cell-mediated immune system (York et al. 1994; Fruh et al. 1995). Adeno-, cytomegalo-, and poxviruses also interfere with peptide presentation, by down-regulating the expression of the major histocompatibility complex class I protein (Smith 1993, 1994). In addition, poxviruses encode a variety of soluble cytokine 'receptors' which are secreted from infected cells to intercept immunostimulatory cytokines (Pickup 1994; Spriggs 1994; Lalani and McFadden 1999) (see also Chapter 15, The role of cytokines in viral infections).

Evasion of complement

The complement system is a major host defense mechanism which, on activation, attacks and permeabilizes the surface membranes of enveloped viruses and infected cells. Complement is activated by two tightly regulated pathways: the classical pathway, which requires an antibody response to the infecting virus, and the alternative pathway, which is antibody-independent. Several members of the pox- and herpesvirus families express cell surface or secreted proteins that interfere either with the complement activation pathways or with the formation of the membrane attack complex itself, which attests to the potential efficacy of complement against these viruses (Isaacs et al. 1992; Smith 1994).

Evasion of interferon

In contrast to the ease with which antibody-resistant mutants can be isolated, IFN-resistant mutants seldom arise even when they are deliberately selected for (Novella et al. 1996), probably because IFNs induce several distinct and overlapping antiviral mechanisms. Nevertheless, viruses vary considerably in their intrinsic sensitivities to IFNs, not only because they differentially activate the IFN-induced enzymes but also because some of them deploy specific IFN evasion mechanisms (McNair and Kerr 1992). For example, among the soluble cytokine receptors secreted from poxvirus-infected cells are proteins that decoy both α and γ IFNs (Smith 1993; Pickup 1994; Spriggs 1994; Alcami and Smith 1996). Intracellularly, reovirus and vaccinia virus express double-stranded RNA-binding proteins that interfere with the activation of PKR, whereas adenovirus and Epstein–Barr virus (EBV) synthesize abundant small RNAs (called virus-associated (VA) RNAs and EBV-encoded early RNAs (EBERs), respectively) that compete with double-stranded RNA for PKR binding, but which fail to activate the kinase (Mathews and Shenk 1991; Mathews 1993). Yet other mechanisms are used by poliovirus, which degrades the activated PKR, and by influenza virus, which activates a latent cellular inhibitor of PKR (Katze 1993, 1995). Its role in uninfected cells has yet to be determined. Finally, vaccinia virus expresses a homologue of eIF2-α, which decoys the kinase and protects the authentic initiation factor against phosphorylation. The variety of mechanisms that have evolved to circumvent the PKR system argues strongly that it can potentially restrict the replication of a wide range of viruses. Viral mechanisms to evade the 2–5A system also exist, but they remain to be fully characterized.

SUMMARY

Their large population sizes and high mutation rates allow viruses to evolve much faster than the host organisms on which they depend for replication. For this reason, they will continue to threaten the health of the rest of the biosphere and to shape the evolution of their hosts. However, as described in this chapter, examination of the intricacies of virus–host interactions provides unique insights into these competitive relationships and illuminates almost every aspect of the biology of the host organisms. The future promises an even richer harvest of experimental and conceptual advances in this area, both enhancing our ability to control and prevent viral diseases and increasing our understanding of the mechanistic and evolutionary relationships between viruses and their hosts.

REFERENCES

Aaronson, D.S. and Horvath, C.M. 2002. A road map for those who don't know JAK-STAT. *Science*, **296**, 1653–5.

Alcami, A. and Smith, G.L. 1996. Receptors for gamma-interferon encoded by poxviruses: implications for the unknown origin of vaccinia virus. *Trends Microbiol*, **4**, 321–6.

Ball, L.A. 1982. 2',5'-oligoadenylate synthetase. In Boyer, P.D. (ed.), *The enzymes*, Vol. XV, Nucleic acids, part B, 3rd edn. New York: Academic Press, 281–313.

Bangham, C.R. and Kirkwood, T.B. 1993. Defective interfering particles and virus evolution. *Trends Microbiol*, **1**, 260–4.

Barrett, A.D. and Dimmock, N.J. 1986. Defective interfering viruses and infections of animals. *Curr Top Microbiol Immunol*, **128**, 55–84.

Bayliss, C.D. and Condit, R.C. 1993. Temperature-sensitive mutants in the vaccinia virus A18R gene increase double-stranded RNA synthesis as a result of aberrant viral transcription. *Virology*, **194**, 254–62.

Benedict, C.A., Norris, P.S. and Ware, C.F. 2002. To kill or be killed: viral evasion of apoptosis. *Nature Immunol*, **3**, 1013–18.

Bentz, J. 1993. *Viral fusion mechanisms*. Boca Raton, FL: CRC Press.

Berget, S.M., Moore, C. and Sharp, P.A. 1977. Spliced segments at the 5' terminus of adenovirus 2 late mRNA. *Proc Natl Acad Sci USA*, **74**, 3171–5.

Bernstein, H.D., Sonenberg, N. and Baltimore, D. 1985. Poliovirus mutant that does not selectively inhibit host protein synthesis. *Mol Cell Biol*, **5**, 2913–23.

Bisbal, C. 1997. RNase L: effector nuclease of an activatable RNA degradation system in mammals. *Prog Mol Subcell Biol*, **18**, 19–34.

Bray, M., Prasad, S., et al. 1994. A small element from the Mason-Pfizer monkey virus genome makes human immunodeficiency virus type 1 expression and replication Rev-independent. *Proc Natl Acad Sci USA*, **91**, 1256–60.

Brierley, I. 1993. Probing the mechanism of ribosomal frameshifting on viral RNAs. *Biochem Soc Trans*, **21**, 822–6.

Brunetti, C.R., Burke, R.L., et al. 1994. Herpes simplex virus glycoprotein D acquires mannose-6-phosphate residues and binds to mannose-6-phosphate receptors. *J Biol Chem*, **269**, 17067–74.

Bullough, P.A., Hughson, F.M., et al. 1994. Structure of influenza haemagglutinin at the pH of membrane fusion. *Nature*, **371**, 37–43.

Byland, R. and Marsh, M. 2005. Trafficking of viral membrane proteins. *Curr Top Microbiol Immunol*, **285**, 219–54.

Carr, C.M. and Kim, P.S. 1993. A spring-loaded mechanism for the conformational change of influenza hemagglutinin. *Cell*, **73**, 823–32.

Carr, C.M. and Kim, P.S. 1994. Flu virus invasion: halfway there. *Science*, **266**, 234–6.

Carrasco, L. 1994. Entry of animal viruses and macromolecules into cells. *FEBS Lett*, **350**, 151–4.

Cattaneo, R. 1991. Different types of messenger RNA editing. *Annu Rev Genet*, **25**, 71–88.

Centrella, M. and Lucas-Lenard, J. 1982. Regulation of protein synthesis in vesicular stomatitis virus-infected mouse L-929 cells by decreased protein synthesis initiation factor 2 activity. *J Virol*, **41**, 781–91.

Challberg, M. 1991. Animal virus DNA replication. *Semin Virol*, **2**, 247–304.

Challberg, M.D. and Kelly, T.J. 1989. Animal virus DNA replication. *Annu Rev Biochem*, **58**, 671–717.

Chang, W., Hsiao, J.-C., et al. 1995. Isolation of a monoclonal antibody which blocks vaccinia virus infection. *J Virol*, **69**, 517–22.

Chapman, M.S. and Rossmann, M.G. 1993. Comparison of surface properties of picornaviruses: strategies for hiding the receptor site from immune surveillance. *Virology*, **195**, 745–56.

Cheng, R.H., Kuhn, R.J., et al. 1995. Nucleocapsid and glycoprotein organization in an enveloped virus. *Cell*, **80**, 621–30.

Chow, L.T., Gelinas, R.E., et al. 1977. An amazing sequence arrangement at the 5′ ends of adenovirus 2 messenger RNA. *Cell*, **12**, 1–8.

Clem, R.J. and Miller, L.K. 1994. Control of programmed cell death by the baculovirus genes p35 and iap. *Mol Cell Biol*, **14**, 5212–22.

Colonno, R.J. 1992. Molecular interactions between human rhinoviruses and their cellular receptors. *Semin Virol*, **3**, 101–8.

Cook, P. 1991. The nucleoskeleton and the topology of replication. *Cell*, **66**, 627–35.

Cullen, B.R. 1994. RNA-sequence-mediated gene regulation in HIV-1. *Infect Agents Dis*, **3**, 68–76.

Curran, J.A., Richardson, C. and Kolakofsky, D. 1986. Ribosomal initiation at alternate AUGs on the Sendai virus P/C mRNA. *J Virol*, **57**, 684–7.

Dautry-Varsat, A. and Lodish, H.F. 1984. How receptors bring proteins and particles into cells. *Sci Am*, **250**, 52–8.

de Bruyn Kops, A. and Knipe, D.M. 1988. Formation of DNA replication structures in herpes virus-infected cells requires a viral DNA-binding protein. *Cell*, **55**, 857–68.

de la Torre, J.C. and Oldstone, M.B. 1996. Anatomy of viral persistence: mechanisms of persistence and associated disease. *Adv Virus Res*, **46**, 311–43.

Deshpande, K.L., Fried, V.A., et al. 1987. Glycosylation affects cleavage of an H5N2 influenza virus hemagglutinin and regulates virulence. *Proc Natl Acad Sci USA*, **84**, 36–40.

Dimmock, N.J. 1985. Defective interfering viruses: modulators of infection. *Microbiol Sci*, **2**, 1–7.

Ding, S.W., Li, H., et al. 2004. RNA silencing: a conserved antiviral immunity of plants and animals. *Virus Res*, **102**, 109–15.

Dodson, M.L., Michaels, M.L. and Lloyd, R.S. 1994. Unified catalytic mechanism for DNA glycosylases. *J Biol Chem*, **269**, 32709–12.

Domingo, E. and Holland, J.J. 1997. RNA virus mutations and fitness for survival. *Annu Rev Microbiol*, **51**, 151–78.

Doms, R.W., Lamb, R.A., et al. 1993. Folding and assembly of viral membrane proteins. *Virology*, **193**, 545–62.

Dougherty, W.G. and Semler, B.L. 1993. Expression of virus-encoded proteinases: functional and structural similarities with cellular enzymes. *Microbiol Rev*, **57**, 781–822.

Drake, J.W. 1993. Rates of spontaneous mutation among RNA viruses. *Proc Natl Acad Sci USA*, **90**, 4171–5.

Drapkin, R., Merino, A. and Reinberg, D. 1993. Regulation of RNA polymerase II transcription. *Curr Opin Cell Biol*, **5**, 469–76.

Dryden, K.A., Wang, G., et al. 1993. Early steps in reovirus infection are associated with dramatic changes in supramolecular structure and protein conformation: analysis of virions and subviral particles by cryo-electron microscopy and image reconstruction. *J Cell Biol*, **122**, 1023–41.

Duarte, E.A., Novella, I.S., et al. 1994. RNA virus quasispecies: significance for viral disease and epidemiology. *Infect Agents Dis*, **3**, 201–14.

Duncan, R.F. 1990. Protein synthesis initiation factor modifications during viral infections: implications for translational control. *Electrophoresis*, **11**, 219–27.

Earp, L.J., Delos, S.E., et al. 2005. The many mechanisms of viral membrane fusion proteins. *Curr Top Microbiol Immunol*, **285**, 25–66.

Eaton, S. and Simons, K. 1995. Apical, basal, and lateral cues for epithelial polarization. *Cell*, **82**, 5–8.

Echols, H. 1990. Nucleoprotein structures initiating DNA replication, transcription, and site-specific recombination. *J Biol Chem*, **265**, 14697–700.

Ehrenfeld, E. 1993. Translational regulation in virus-infected cells. *Semin Virol*, **4**, 199–268.

Eigen, M. 1993. Viral quasispecies. *Sci Am*, **269**, 42–9.

Ernst, R.K., Bray, M., et al. 1997. A structured retroviral RNA element that mediates nucleocytoplasmic export of intron-containing RNA. *Mol Cell Biol*, **17**, 135–44.

Etchison, D. and Fout, S. 1985. Human rhinovirus 14 infection of HeLa cells results in the proteolytic cleavage of the p220 cap-binding complex subunit and inactivates globin translation in vitro. *J Virol*, **54**, 634–8.

Etchison, D., Milburn, S.C., et al. 1982. Inhibition of HeLa cell protein synthesis following poliovirus infection correlates with the proteolysis of a 220,000 dalton polypeptide associated with eukaryotic initiation factor 3 and a cap binding protein complex. *J Biol Chem*, **257**, 14806–10.

Everett, H. and McFadden, G. 1999. Apoptosis: an innate immune response to virus infection. *Trends Microbiol*, **7**, 160–5.

Fanning, E. and Knippers, R. 1992. Structure and function of simian virus 40 large tumor antigen. *Annu Rev Biochem*, **61**, 55–85.

Farrell, P.J. 1995. Epstein–Barr virus immortalizing genes. *Trends Microbiol*, **3**, 105–9.

Farthing, A.J. and Vousden, K.H. 1994. Functions of human papilloma virus E6 and E7 oncoproteins. *Trends Microbiol*, **2**, 170–4.

Feng, Y., Broder, C.C., et al. 1996. HIV-1 entry cofactor: functional cDNA cloning of a seven-transmembrane, G protein-coupled receptor. *Science*, **272**, 872–7.

Flore, O., Fricks, C.E., et al. 1990. Conformational changes in poliovirus assembly and cell entry. *Semin Virol*, **1**, 429–38.

Francoeur, A.M., Poliquin, L. and Stanners, C.P. 1987. The isolation of interferon-inducing mutants of vesicular stomatitis virus with altered viral P function for the inhibition of total protein synthesis. *Virology*, **160**, 236–45.

Friesen, P.D. and Nissen, M.S. 1990. Gene organization and transcription of TED, a lepidopteran retrotransposon integrated within the baculovirus genome. *Mol Cell Biol*, **10**, 3067–77.

Fruh, K., Ahn, K., et al. 1995. A viral inhibitor of peptide transporters for antigen presentation. *Nature*, **375**, 415–18.

Gait, M.J. and Karn, J. 1993. RNA recognition by the human immunodeficiency virus Tat and Rev proteins. *Trends Biochem Sci*, **18**, 255–9.

Gale, M. Jr., Tan, S.L. and Katze, M.G. 2000. Translational control of viral gene expression in eukaryotes. *Microbiol Mol Biol Rev*, **64**, 239–80.

Gao, Y. and Lenard, J. 1995. Multimerization and transcriptional activation of the phosphoprotein (P) of vesicular stomatitis virus by casein kinase-II. *EMBO J*, **14**, 1240–7.

Garcia-Blanco, M.A. and Cullen, B.R. 1991. Molecular basis of latency in pathogenic human viruses. *Science*, **254**, 815–20.

Garfinkel, M.S. and Katze, M.G. 1993. How does influenza virus regulate gene expression at the level of mRNA translation? Let us count the ways. *Gene Expr*, **3**, 109–18.

Gebauer, F. and Hentze, M.W. 2004. Molecular mechanisms of translational control. *Nat Rev Mol Cell Biol*, **5**, 827–35.

Gething, M.J., McCammon, K. and Sambrook, J. 1986. Expression of wild-type and mutant forms of influenza hemagglutinin: the role of folding in intracellular transport. *Cell*, **46**, 939–50.

Gillet, G. and Brun, G. 1996. Viral inhibition of apoptosis. *Trends Microbiol*, **4**, 312–17.

Giranda, V.L., Heinz, B.A., et al. 1992. Acid-induced structural changes in human rhinovirus 14: possible role in uncoating. *Proc Natl Acad Sci USA*, **89**, 10213–17.

Gomez Yafal, A., Kaplan, G., et al. 1993. Characterization of poliovirus conformational alteration mediated by soluble cell receptors. *Virology*, **197**, 501–5.

Greber, U.F., Singh, I. and Helenius, A. 1994. Mechanisms of virus uncoating. *Trends Microbiol*, **2**, 52–6.

Greve, J.M. and Rossmann, M.G. 1994. Interaction of rhinovirus with its receptor ICAM-1. In: Wimmer, E. (ed.), *Cellular receptors for animal viruses*. Cold Spring Harbor, NY: Cold Spring Harbor Laboratory, 195–213.

Griffin, D.E. and Hardwick, J.M. 1997. Regulators of apoptosis on the road to persistent alphavirus infection. *Annu Rev Microbiol*, **51**, 565–92.

Griffin, D.E., Levine, B., et al. 1994. The effects of alphavirus infection on neurons. *Ann Neurol Suppl*, **35**, S23–7.

Guo, P. 1994. Viral assembly. *Semin Virol*, **5**, 1–83.

Haller, O. and Kochs, G. 2002. Interferon-induced Mx proteins: dynamin-like GTPases with antiviral activity. *Traffic*, **3**, 710–17.

Halstead, S.B. 1994. Antibody-dependent enhancement of infection: a mechanism for indirect virus entry into cells. In: Wimmer, E. (ed.), *Cellular receptors for animal viruses*. Cold Spring Harbor, NY: Cold Spring Harbor Laboratory, 493–516.

Hannon, G.J. 2002. RNA interference. *Nature*, **418**, 244–51.

Harrison, S.C., Wang, J., et al. 1992. Structure and interactions of CD4. *Cold Spring Harbor Symp Quant Biol*, **57**, 541–8.

Hartl, F.U. 1996. Molecular chaperones in cellular protein folding. *Nature*, **381**, 571–80.

Hay, A.J. 1992. The action of adamantanamines against influenza A viruses: inhibition of the M2 ion channel protein. *Semin Virol*, **3**, 21–30.

Haywood, A.M. 1994. Virus receptors: binding, adhesion strengthening, and changes in viral structure. *J Virol*, **68**, 1–5.

Helenius, A. 1992. Unpacking the incoming influenza virus. *Cell*, **69**, 577–8.

Hershey, J.W.B. 1990. Overview: phosphorylation and translation control. *Enzyme*, **44**, 17–27.

Hershey, J.W.B. 1993. Introduction to translational initiation factors and their regulation by phosphorylation. *Semin Virol*, **4**, 201–8.

Hershko, A. and Ciechanover, A. 1992. The ubiquitin system for protein degradation. *Annu Rev Biochem*, **61**, 761–807.

Hoekstra, D. and Kok, J.W. 1989. Entry mechanisms of enveloped viruses. Implications for fusion of intracellular membranes. *Biosci Rep*, **9**, 273–305.

Holland, J.J., de la Torre, J.C. and Steinhauer, D.A. 1992. RNA virus populations as quasispecies. *Curr Top Microbiol Immunol*, **176**, 1–20.

Huang, J. and Schneider, R.J. 1991. Adenovirus inhibition of cellular protein synthesis involves inactivation of cap binding protein. *Cell*, **65**, 271–80.

Hughson, F.M. 1995. Structural characterization of viral fusion proteins. *Curr Biol*, **5**, 265–74.

Hugin, A.W. and Hauser, C. 1994. The epidermal growth factor receptor is not a receptor for vaccinia virus. *J Virol*, **68**, 8409–12.

Hutt-Fletcher, L.M. 1987. Synergistic activation of cells by Epstein–Barr virus and B-cell growth factor. *J Virol*, **61**, 774–81.

Ink, B.S., Gilbert, C.S. and Evan, G.I. 1995. Delay of vaccinia virus-Lambinduced apoptosis in non-permissive chinese hamster ovary cells by the cowpox CHOhr and adenovirus E1B 19K genes. *J Virol*, **69**, 661–8.

Isaacs, S.N., Kotwal, G.J. and Moss, B. 1992. Vaccinia virus complement-control protein prevents antibody-dependent complement-enhanced neutralization of infectivity and contributes to virulence. *Proc Natl Acad Sci USA*, **89**, 628–32.

Ishihama, A. and Barbier, P. 1994. Molecular anatomy of viral RNA-directed RNA polymerases. *Arch Virol*, **134**, 235–58.

Jacks, T. and Varmus, H.E. 1985. Expression of the Rous sarcoma virus pol gene by ribosomal frameshifting. *Science*, **230**, 1237–42.

Jackson, R.J., Howell, M.T. and Kaminski, A. 1991. The novel mechanism of initiation of poliovirus RNA translation. *Trends Biochem Sci*, **15**, 477–83.

Jacques, J.P. and Kolakofsky, D. 1991. Pseudo-templated transcription in prokaryotic and eukaryotic organisms. *Genes Dev*, **5**, 707–13.

Jansen-Durr, P. 1996. How viral oncogenes make the cell cycle. *Trends Genet*, **12**, 270–5.

Jindal, S. and Malkovsky, M. 1994. Stress responses to viral infection. *Trends Microbiol*, **2**, 89–91.

Johnson, J.E. 1996. Functional implications of protein–protein interactions in icosahedral viruses. *Proc Natl Acad Sci USA*, **93**, 27–33.

Johnson, H.M., Bazer, F.W., et al. 1994. How interferons fight disease. *Sci Am*, **270**, 68–75.

Kalderon, D., Roberts, B.L., et al. 1984. A short amino acid sequence able to specify nuclear location. *Cell*, **39**, 499–509.

Karin, M. and Hunter, T. 1995. Transcriptional control by protein phosphorylation: signal transmission from the cell surface to the nucleus. *Curr Biol*, **5**, 747–57.

Katze, M.G. 1993. Games viruses play: a strategic initiative against the interferon-induced dsRNA-activated 68,000 Mr protein kinase. *Semin Virol*, **4**, 258–68.

Katze, M.G. 1995. Regulation of the interferon-induced PKR: can viruses cope? *Trends Microbiol*, **3**, 75–8.

Katze, M.G. and Agy, M.B. 1990. Regulation of viral and cellular RNA turnover in cells infected by eukaryotic viruses including HIV. *Enzyme*, **44**, 332–46.

Kelly, T.J., Wold, M.S. and Li, J. 1988. Initiation of viral DNA replication. *Adv Virus Res*, **34**, 1–42.

Kemble, G.W., Danieli, T. and White, J.M. 1994. Lipid-anchored influenza hemagglutinin promotes hemifusion, not complete fusion. *Cell*, **76**, 383–91.

Kielian, M. 1995. Membrane fusion and the alphavirus life cycle. *Adv Virus Res*, **45**, 113–51.

Klenk, H.D. and Garten, W. 1994a. Host cell proteases controlling virus pathogenicity. *Trends Microbiol*, **2**, 39–43.

Klenk, H.D. and Garten, W. 1994b. Activation cleavage of viral spike proteins by host proteases. In: Wimmer, E. (ed.), *Cellular receptors for animal viruses*. Cold Spring Harbor, NY: Cold Spring Harbor Laboratory, 241–80.

Kolakofsky, D. and Hacker, D. 1991. Bunyavirus RNA synthesis: genome transcription and replication. *Curr Top Microbiol Immunol*, **169**, 143–59.

Kozak, M. 1986. Regulation of protein synthesis in virus-infected animal cells. *Adv Virus Res*, **31**, 229–92.

Kozak, M. 1989. The scanning model for translation: an update. *J Cell Biol*, **108**, 229–41.

Kozak, M. 1991a. An analysis of vertebrate mRNA sequences: intimations of translational control. *J Cell Biol*, **115**, 887–903.

Kozak, M. 1991b. Structural features in eukaryotic mRNAs that modulate the initiation of translation. *J Biol Chem*, **266**, 19867–70.

Kozak, M. 1992a. Regulation of translation in eukaryotic systems. *Annu Rev Cell Biol*, **8**, 197–225.

Kozak, M. 1992b. A consideration of alternative models for the initiation of translation in eukaryotes. *Crit Rev Biochem Mol Biol*, **27**, 385–402.

Kozak, M. 1994. Determinants of translational fidelity and efficiency in vertebrate mRNAs. *Biochimie*, **74**, 815–21.

Krausslich, H.-G. and Wimmer, E. 1988. Viral proteinases. *Annu Rev Biochem*, **57**, 701–54.

Kristie, T.M. and Sharp, P.A. 1993. Purification of the cellular C1 factor required for the stable recognition of the oct-1 homeodomain by the herpes simplex virus α trans-inducing factor (VP16). *J Biol Chem*, **268**, 6526–34.

Krug, R.M. 1993. The regulation of export of mRNA from nucleus to cytoplasm. *Curr Opin Cell Biol*, **5**, 944–9.

Kumar, S. 1995. ICE-like proteases in apoptosis. *Trends Biochem Sci*, **20**, 198–202.

Lalani, A.S. and McFadden, G. 1999. Evasion and exploitation of chemokines by viruses. *Cytokine Growth Factor Rev*, **10**, 219–33.

Lamb, R.A. 1993. Paramyxovirus fusion: a hypothesis for changes. *Virology*, **197**, 1–11.

Lamb, R.A. and Krug, R.M. 2001. *Orthomyxoviridae*: the viruses and their replication. In: Fields, B.N., Knipe, D.M., et al. (eds), *Fields' virology*, 4th ed. New York: Raven Press, 1487–531.

Lanzrein, M., Schlegel, A. and Kempf, C. 1994. Entry and uncoating of enveloped viruses. *Biochem J*, **302**, 313–20.

Lawrence, M.B. and Springer, T.A. 1991. Leukocytes roll on a selectin at physiologic flow rates: distinction from and prerequisite for adhesion through integrins. *Cell*, **65**, 859–73.

Lentz, T.L. 1990. The recognition event between virus and host cell receptor: a target for antiviral agents. *J Gen Virol*, **71**, 751–66.

Levine, A.J. 1993. The tumor suppressor genes. *Annu Rev Biochem*, **62**, 623–51.

Levine, B., Hardwick, J.M. and Griffin, D.E. 1994. Persistence of alphaviruses in vertebrate hosts. *Trends Microbiol*, **2**, 25–8.

Levy, D.E. and Garcia-Sastre, A. 2001. The virus battles: IFN induction of the antiviral state and mechanisms of viral evasion. *Cytokine Growth Factor Rev*, **12**, 143–56.

Lewin, D.I. 1995. Herpes, EBV survive by antigenic stealth. *J NIH Res*, **7**, 49–53.

Liu, C., Eichelberger, M.C., et al. 1995. Influenza type A virus neuraminidase does not play a role in viral entry, replication, assembly, or budding. *J Virol*, **69**, 1099–106.

Lodish, H.F. 1976. Translational control of protein synthesis. *Annu Rev Biochem*, **45**, 39–72.

Lodish, H.F. and Porter, M. 1981. Vesicular stomatitis virus mRNA and inhibition of translation of cellular mRNA. Is there a P function in vesicular stomatitis virus? *J Virol*, **38**, 504–17.

Ludlow, J.W. 1993. Interactions between SV40 large-tumor antigen and the growth suppressor proteins pRB and p53. *FASEB J*, **7**, 866–71.

Ludlow, J.W. and Skuse, G.R. 1995. Viral oncoprotein binding to pRB, p107, p130, and p300. *Virus Res*, **35**, 113–21.

Luftig, R.B. and Lupo, L.D. 1994. Viral interactions with the host–cell cytoskeleton: the role of retroviral proteases. *Trends Microbiol*, **2**, 178–82.

Malmgaard, L. 2004. Induction and regulation of IFNs during viral infections. *J Interferon Cytokine Res*, **24**, 439–54.

Marcus, P.I. and Sekellick, M.J. 1974. Cell killing by viruses. I. Comparison of cell-killing, plaque-forming, and defective-interfering particles of vesicular stomatitis virus. *Virology*, **57**, 321–38.

Marsh, M. 1992. Keeping the viral coat on. *Curr Biol*, **2**, 379–81.

Marsh, M. and Helenius, A. 1989. Virus entry into animal cells. *Adv Virus Res*, **36**, 107–51.

Martin, S.J. and Green, D.R. 1995. Protease activation during apoptosis: death by a thousand cuts? *Cell*, **82**, 349–52.

Martin, S.J., Green, D.R. and Cotter, T.G. 1994. Dicing with death: dissecting the components of the apoptosis machinery. *Trends Biochem Sci*, **19**, 26–30.

Mason, P.W., Rieder, E. and Baxt, B. 1994. RGD sequence of foot-and-mouth disease virus is essential for infecting cells via the natural receptor but can be bypassed by an antibody-dependent enhancement pathway. *Proc Natl Acad Sci USA*, **91**, 1932–6.

Masucci, M.G. and Ernberg, I. 1994. Epstein–Barr virus: adaptation to a life within the immune system. *Trends Microbiol*, **2**, 125–30.

Mathews, M.B. 1993. Viral evasion of the cellular defense mechanisms: regulation of the protein kinase DAI by RNA effectors. *Semin Virol*, **4**, 247–57.

Mathews, M.B. and Shenk, T. 1991. Adenovirus virus-associated RNA and translational control. *J Virol*, **65**, 5657–62.

McFadden, G. 1995. *Viroceptors, virokines and related immune modulators encoded by DNA viruses*. New York: Demos Publications.

McNair, A.N. and Kerr, I.M. 1992. Viral inhibition of the interferon system. *Pharmacol Ther*, **56**, 79–95.

Meerovitch, K. and Sonenberg, N. 1993. Internal initiation of picornavirus RNA translation. *Semin Virol*, **4**, 217–28.

Merrick, W.C. 1990. Mechanism of translation initiation in eukaryotes. *Enzyme*, **44**, 7–16.

Millns, A.K., Carpenter, M.S. and DeLange, A.M. 1994. The vaccinia virus-encoded uracil DNA glycosylase has an essential role in viral DNA replication. *Virology*, **198**, 504–13.

Moran, E. 1993. Interaction of adenoviral proteins with pRB and p53. *FASEB J*, **7**, 880–5.

Morgan, R.A. and Anderson, W.F. 1993. Human gene therapy. *Annu Rev Biochem*, **62**, 191–217.

Mosser, A.G., Sgro, J.Y. and Rueckert, R.R. 1994. Distribution of drug resistance mutations in type 3 poliovirus identifies three regions involved in uncoating functions. *J Virol*, **68**, 8193–201.

Murti, K.G., Goorha, R. and Granoff, A. 1985. An unusual replication strategy of an animal iridovirus. *Adv Virus Res*, **30**, 1–19.

Nevins, J.R. 1989. Mechanisms of viral-mediated trans-activation of transcription. *Adv Virus Res*, **37**, 35–83.

Nevins, J.R. 1992. E2F: a link between the Rb tumor suppressor protein and viral oncoproteins. *Science*, **258**, 424–9.

Nomoto, A. 1992. Cellular receptors for virus infection. *Semin Virol*, **3**, 77–133.

Nomoto, A., Koike, S. and Aoki, J. 1994. Tissue tropism and species specificity of poliovirus infection. *Trends Microbiol*, **2**, 47–51.

Novella, I.S., Cilnis, M., et al. 1996. Large population transmissions of vesicular stomatitis virus in interferon-treated cells select variants of only limited resistance. *J Virol*, **70**, 6414–17.

Nuss, D.L., Oppermann, H. and Koch, G. 1975. Selective blockage of initiation of host protein synthesis in RNA virus-infected cells. *Proc Natl Acad Sci USA*, **72**, 1258–62.

Oldstone, M.B. 1991. Molecular anatomy of viral persistence. *J Virol*, **65**, 6381–6.

Olson, N.H., Kolatkar, P.R., et al. 1993. Structure of a human rhinovirus complexed with its receptor molecule. *Proc Natl Acad Sci USA*, **90**, 507–11.

O'Malley, R.P., Duncan, R.F., et al. 1989. Modification of protein synthesis initiation factors and the shut-off of host protein synthesis in adenovirus-infected cells. *Virology*, **168**, 112–18.

O'Reilly, E.K. and Kao, C.C. 1998. Analysis of RNA-dependent RNA polymerase structure and function as guided by known polymerase structures and computer predictions of secondary structure. *Virology*, **252**, 287–303.

Paredes, A.M., Brown, D.T., et al. 1993. Three-dimensional structure of a membrane-containing virus. *Proc Natl Acad Sci USA*, **90**, 9095–9.

Paulsson, K. and Wang, P. 2003. Chaperones and folding of MHC class I molecules in the endoplasmic reticulum. *Biochim Biophys Acta*, **1641**, 1–12.

Pelham, H. 1988. Heat shock proteins: coming in from the cold. *Nature*, **332**, 776–7.

Pellegrini, S. and Schindler, C. 1993. Early events in signalling by interferons. *Trends Biochem Sci*, **18**, 338–42.

Pestka, S., Langer, J.A., et al. 1987. Interferons and their actions. *Annu Rev Biochem*, **56**, 727–77.

Pickup, D.J. 1994. Poxviral modifiers of cytokine response to infection. *Infect Agents Dis*, **3**, 116–27.

Pinto, L.H., Holsinger, L.J. and Lamb, R.A. 1992. Influenza virus M2 protein has ion channel activity. *Cell*, **69**, 511–28.

Player, M.R. and Torrence, P.F. 1998. The 2–5A system: modulation of viral and cellular processes through acceleration of RNA degradation. *Pharmacol Ther*, **78**, 55–113.

Poranen, M.M., Daugelavicius, R. and Bamford, D.H. 2002. Common principles in viral entry. *Annu Rev Microbiol*, **56**, 521–38.

Porterfield, J.S. 1986. Antibody-dependent enhancement of viral infectivity. *Adv Virus Res*, **31**, 335–55.

Proud, C.G. 1995. PKR: a new name and new roles. *Trends Biochem Sci*, **20**, 241–6.

Racaniello, V.R. 1992. Interaction of poliovirus with its cell receptor. *Semin Virol*, **3**, 473–82.

Rajagopalan, L.E. and Malter, J.S. 1997. Regulation of eukaryotic messenger RNA turnover. *Prog Nucleic Acid Res Mol Biol*, **56**, 257–86.

Ray, C.A., Black, R.A., et al. 1992. Viral inhibition of inflammation: cowpox virus encodes an inhibitor of the interleukin-1β converting enzyme. *Cell*, **69**, 597–604.

Razvi, E.S. and Welsh, R.M. 1995. Apoptosis in viral infections. *Adv Virus Res*, **45**, 1–60.

Rebouillat, D. and Hovanessian, A.G. 1999. The human 2′,5′-oligoadenylate synthetase family: interferon-induced proteins with unique enzymatic properties. *J Interferon Cytokine Res*, **19**, 295–308.

Ren, R., Costantini, F., et al. 1990. Transgenic mice expressing a human poliovirus receptor: a new model for poliomyelitis. *Cell*, **63**, 353–62.

Revel, M. and Chebath, J. 1986. Interferon-activated genes. *Trends Biochem Sci*, **11**, 166–70.

Rey, F.A., Heinz, F.X., et al. 1995. The envelope glycoprotein from tick-borne encephalitis virus at 2Å resolution. *Nature*, **375**, 291–8.

Rhee, S.S. and Hunter, E. 1990. A single amino acid substitution within the matrix protein of a type D retrovirus converts its morphogenesis to that of a type C retrovirus. *Cell*, **63**, 77–86.

Rice, A.P. and Roberts, B.E. 1983. Vaccinia virus induces cellular mRNA degradation. *J Virol*, **47**, 529–39.

Rossmann, M.G. 1989. The canyon hypothesis. Hiding the host cell receptor attachment site on a viral surface from immune surveillance. *J Biol Chem*, **264**, 14587–90.

Rossmann, M.G., Olson, N.H., et al. 1994. Crystallographic and cryo EM analysis of virion–receptor interactions. *Arch Virol Suppl*, **9**, 531–41.

Roulston, A., Marcellus, R.C. and Branton, P.E. 1999. Viruses and apoptosis. *Annu Rev Microbiol*, **53**, 577–628.

Roux, L., Simon, A.E. and Holland, J.J. 1991. Effects of defective interfering viruses on virus replication and pathogenesis in vitro and in vivo. *Adv Virus Res*, **40**, 181–211.

Rowe, D.T. 1999. Epstein–Barr virus immortalization and latency. *Front Biosci*, **4**, D346–71.

Rubin, D.M. and Finley, D. 1995. The proteasome: a protein-degrading organelle? *Curr Biol*, **5**, 854–8.

Ryan, M.D. and Flint, M. 1997. Virus-encoded proteinases of the picornavirus super-group. *J Gen Virol*, **78**, 699–723.

Ryan, M.D., Monaghan, S. and Flint, M. 1998. Virus-encoded proteinases of the *Flaviviridae*. *J Gen Virol*, **79**, 947–59.

Samuel, C.E. 1988. Mechanisms of the antiviral action of interferons. *Prog Nucl Acid Res Mol Biol*, **35**, 27–72.

Samuel, C.E. 1991. Antiviral actions of interferon: interferon-regulated cellular proteins and their surprisingly selective antiviral activities. *Virology*, **183**, 1–11.

Sarkar, S.N. and Sen, G.C. 2004. Novel functions of proteins encoded by viral stress-inducible genes. *Pharmacol Ther*, **103**, 245–59.

Schindler, C. and Darnell, J.E. Jr. 1995. Transcriptional responses to polypeptide ligands: the JAK-STAT pathway. *Annu Rev Biochem*, **64**, 621–51.

Schlesinger, M.J. and Schlesinger, S. 1987. Domains of virus glycoproteins. *Adv Virus Res*, **33**, 1–44.

Schneider, R.J. and Shenk, T. 1987. Impact of virus infection on host cell protein synthesis. *Annu Rev Biochem*, **56**, 317–32.

Schnitzlein, W.M., O'Banion, M.K., et al. 1983. Effect of intracellular vesicular stomatitis virus mRNA concentration on the inhibition of host cell protein synthesis. *J Virol*, **45**, 206–14.

Sen, G.C. 2001. Viruses and interferons. *Annu Rev Microbiol*, **55**, 255–81.

Sen, G.C. and Lengyel, P. 1992. The interferon system. A bird's eye view of its biochemistry. *J Biol Chem*, **267**, 5017–20.

Sen, G.C. and Ransohoff, R.M. 1993. Interferon-induced antiviral actions and their regulation. *Adv Virus Res*, **42**, 57–102.

Sharp, P.A. 1994. Split genes and RNA splicing. *Cell*, **77**, 805–15.

Shimamoto, T., Inouye, M. and Inouye, S. 1995. The formation of the 2′,5′-phosphodiester linkage in the cDNA priming reaction by bacterial reverse transcriptase in a cell-free system. *J Biol Chem*, **270**, 581–8.

Signoret, N., Poignard, P., et al. 1993. Human and simian immunodeficiency viruses: virus–receptor interactions. *Trends Microbiol*, **1**, 328–33.

Singh, I. and Helenius, A. 1992. Nucleocapsid uncoating during entry of enveloped animal RNA viruses into cells. *Semin Virol*, **3**, 511–18.

Skehel, J.J. and Wiley, D.C. 2000. Receptor binding and membrane fusion in virus entry: the influenza hemagglutinin. *Annu Rev Biochem*, **69**, 531–69.

Slabaugh, M.B., Roseman, N.A. and Mathews, C.K. 1989. Amplification of the ribonucleotide reductase small subunit gene: analysis of novel joints and the mechanism of gene duplication in vaccinia virus. *Nucleic Acids Res*, **12**, 7073–88.

Smith, A.E. and Helenius, A. 2004. How viruses enter animal cells. *Science*, **304**, 237–42.

Smith, D.B. and Inglis, S.C. 1987. The mutation rate and variability of eukaryotic viruses: an analytical review. *J Gen Virol*, **68**, 2729–40.

Smith, G.L. 1993. Vaccinia virus glycoproteins and immune evasion. *J Gen Virol*, **74**, 1725–40.

Smith, G.L. 1994. Virus strategies for evasion of the host response to infection. *Trends Microbiol*, **2**, 81–8.

Sonenberg, N. 1987. Regulation of translation by poliovirus. *Adv Virus Res*, **33**, 175–204.

Spear, P.G. 1993. Entry of alphaherpesviruses into cells. *Semin Virol*, **3**, 167–80.

Spriggs, M. 1994. Poxvirus-encoded soluble cytokine receptors. *Virus Res*, **33**, 1–10.

Staeheli, P. 1990. Interferon-induced proteins and the antiviral state. *Adv Virus Res*, **38**, 147–200.

Stegman, T. 1994. Anchors aweigh. *Curr Biol*, **4**, 551–4.

Steller, H. 1995. Mechanisms and genes of cellular suicide. *Science*, **267**, 1445–9.

Stillman, B., Bell, S.P., et al. 1992. DNA replication and the cell cycle. *CIBA Found Symp*, **170**, 147–56.

Strauss, J.H. 1990. Viral proteinases. *Semin Virol*, **1**, 307–84.

Strom, T. and Frenkel, N. 1987. Effects of herpes simplex virus on mRNA stability. *J Virol*, **61**, 2198–207.

Teich, N. 1991. Viral oncogenes, parts I and II. *Semin Virol*, **2**, 305–409.

ten Dam, E., Flint, M. and Ryan, M.D. 1999. Virus-encoded proteinases of the *Togaviridae*. *J Gen Virol*, **80**, 1879–88.

ter Meulen, V. 1994. Pathogenesis of persistent virus infections. *Semin Virol*, **5**, 259–324.

Tevethia, M.J. and Spector, D.J. 1989. Heterologous transactivation among viruses. *Prog Med Virol*, **36**, 120–90.

Thomas, J.R. and Wagner, R.R. 1983. Inhibition of translation in lysates of mouse L-cells infected with vesicular stomatitis virus: presence of a defective ribosome-associated factor. *Biochemistry*, **22**, 1540–6.

Thompson, S.R. and Sarnow, P. 2000. Regulation of host cell translation by viruses and effects on cell function. *Curr Opin Microbiol*, **3**, 366–70.

Tirado, S.M. and Yoon, K.J. 2003. Antibody-dependent enhancement of virus infection and disease. *Viral Immunol*, **16**, 69–86.

Tjian, R. and Maniatis, T. 1994. Transcriptional activation: a complex puzzle with few easy pieces. *Cell*, **77**, 5–8.

Tucker, S.P. and Compans, R.W. 1993. Virus infection of polarized epithelial cells. *Adv Virus Res*, **42**, 187–247.

Tucker, S.P., Wimmer, E. and Compans, R.W. 1994. Expression of viral receptors and the vectorial release of viruses in polarized epithelial cells. In: Wimmer, E. (ed.), *Cellular receptors for animal viruses*. Cold Spring Harbor, NY: Cold Spring Harbor Laboratory, 323–40.

van Etten, J.L. and Meints, R.H. 1999. Giant viruses infecting algae. *Annu Rev Microbiol*, **53**, 447–94.

van Etten, J.L., Xia, Y.N., et al. 1988. Chlorella viruses code for restriction and modification enzymes. *Gene*, **74**, 113–15.

van Etten, J.L., Lane, L.C. and Meints, R.H. 1991. Viruses and viruslike particles of eukaryotic algae. *Microbiol Rev*, **55**, 586–620.

Varshavsky, A. 1992. The N-end rule. *Cell*, **69**, 725–35.

Vaux, D.L., Haecker, G. and Strasser, A. 1994. An evolutionary perspective on apoptosis. *Cell*, **76**, 777–9.

Verduin, B.J.M. 1992. Early interactions between viruses and plants. *Semin Virol*, **3**, 423–32.

Vousden, K. 1993. Interactions of human papillomavirus transforming proteins with the products of tumor suppressor genes. *FASEB J*, **7**, 872–9.

Wagner, E.K. 1994. Herpesvirus latency. *Semin Virol*, **5**, 189–258.

Walter, M.R., Windsor, W.T., et al. 1995. Crystal structure of a complex between interferon-γ and its soluble high-affinity receptor. *Nature*, **376**, 230–5.

Wang, J., Yan, Y., et al. 1990. Atomic structure of a fragment of human CD4 containing two immunoglobulin domains. *Nature*, **348**, 411–18.

Weinberg, R.A. 1995. The retinoblastoma protein and cell cycle control. *Cell*, **81**, 323–30.

Weis, W., Brown, J.H., et al. 1988. Structure of the influenza virus haemagglutinin complexed with its receptor, sialic acid. *Nature*, **333**, 426–31.

Weiss, R.A. 1992. Human immunodeficiency virus receptors. *Semin Virol*, **3**, 79–84.

Wek, R.C. 1994. eIF-2 kinases: regulators of general and gene-specific translation initiation. *Trends Biochem Sci*, **19**, 491–6.

Whitaker-Dowling, P. and Youngner, J.S. 1987. Viral interference-dominance of mutant viruses over wild-type virus in mixed infections. *Microbiol Rev*, **51**, 179–91.

White, E. 1993. Regulation of apoptosis by the transforming genes of the DNA tumor virus adenovirus. *Proc Soc Exp Biol Med*, **204**, 30–9.

White, J.M. 1990. Viral and cellular membrane fusion proteins. *Annu Rev Physiol*, **52**, 675–97.

White, J.M. 1992. Membrane fusion. *Science*, **258**, 917–24.

White, J.M. 1994. Fusion of influenza virus in endosomes: role of the hemagglutinin. In: Wimmer, E. (ed.), *Cellular receptors for animal viruses*. Cold Spring Harbor, NY: Cold Spring Harbor Laboratory, 281–301.

White, J.M. and Littman, D.R. 1989. Viral receptors of the immunoglobulin superfamily. *Cell*, **56**, 725–8.

Wickham, T.J., Mathias, P., et al. 1993. Integrins $\alpha_v\beta_3$ and $\alpha_v\beta_5$ promote adenovirus internalization but not virus attachment. *Cell*, **73**, 309–19.

Wiley, D.C. and Skehel, J.J. 1987. The structure and function of the hemagglutinin membrane glycoprotein of influenza virus. *Annu Rev Biochem*, **56**, 365–94.

Williams, B.R. 1991. Transcriptional regulation of interferon-stimulated genes. *Eur J Biochem*, **200**, 1–11.

Williams, G.T. 1994. Programmed cell death: a fundamental protective response to pathogens. *Trends Microbiol*, **2**, 463–4.

Williams, B.R. 1999. PKR; a sentinel kinase for cellular stress. *Oncogene*, **18**, 6112–20.

Wilson, T.M.A. 1992. Early events in RNA virus infection. *Semin Virol*, **3**, 419–527.

Wiman, K.G. 1993. The retinoblastoma gene: role in cell cycle control and cell differentiation. *FASEB J*, **7**, 841–5.

Wimmer, E. 1994. *Cellular receptors for animal viruses*. Cold Spring Harbor, NY: Cold Spring Harbor Laboratory.

Wycoff, E.E. 1993. Inhibition of host cell protein synthesis in poliovirus-infected cells. *Semin Virol*, **4**, 209–16.

York, I.A., Roop, C., et al. 1994. A cytosolic herpes simplex virus protein inhibits antigen presentation to CD8[+] T lymphocytes. *Cell*, **77**, 525–35.

Zhang, Y. and Schneider, R.J. 1993. Adenovirus inhibition of cellular protein synthesis and the specific translation of late viral mRNAs. *Semin Virol*, **4**, 229–36.

Zhang, Y., Ahn, B.Y. and Moss, B. 1994. Targeting of a multicomponent transcription apparatus into assembling vaccinia virus particles requires rap94, an RNA polymerase-associated protein. *J Virol*, **68**, 1360–70.

13

Pathogenesis of viral infections

NEAL NATHANSON AND KENNETH L. TYLER

INTRODUCTION

Viral pathogenesis deals with the interaction between a virus and its host. Included within the scope of pathogenesis are the stepwise progression of infection from virus entry through dissemination to shedding, the defensive responses of the host, and the mechanisms of virus clearance or persistence. Pathogenesis also encompasses the disease processes that result from infection, variations in viral pathogenicity, and the genetic basis of host resistance to infection or disease. A subject this broad cannot be treated in a single chapter, and this presentation focuses on the dissemination of viruses and their pathogenicity, while other aspects of pathogenesis will be dealt with in Chapters 7, 12, 14, 15, 16, and 17. Several detailed reviews of viral pathogenesis have recently been published (Tyler and Nathanson 2001; Nathanson et al. 2002).

SEQUENTIAL STEPS IN VIRAL INFECTION

One of the cardinal differences between viral infection of a simple cell culture and infection of an animal host is the structural complexity of the multicellular organism. The virus must overcome a number of barriers to accomplish the stepwise infection of the host, beginning with entry, followed by dissemination, localization in a few target tissues, shedding, and transmission to other hosts (Figures 13.1 and 13.2).

Entry

SKIN AND MUCOUS MEMBRANES

Some viruses (such as papillomaviruses, poxviruses, and herpes simplex viruses) will replicate in cells of the skin or mucous membranes. It is likely that infections with these viruses are initiated at breaks in the epithelium, just as the skin must be scratched to facilitate a take by vaccinia virus. Mucous membranes represent a minimal physical barrier to infection, but are bathed in mucus that contains immunoglobulin and provides protection by virtue of its viscous nature. Following infection of the skin, viruses may spread further by passage of intact virions or virus-infected macrophages and dendritic cells to the regional lymph nodes.

The epidermis consists of several layers of cells including, from the deepest to the most superficial: the basal germinal layer of dividing cells (malpighian stratum), the granular layer of dying cells (stratum granulosum), and the superficial layer of keratin (stratum corneum). Most viruses that replicate in the skin grow in the germinal cells, and some viruses, such as papillomaviruses, have a selective tropism for these cells (Lowy and Howley 2001). Poxviruses and herpes simplex viruses will also replicate in fibroblasts and macrophages in the dermis (Blank et al. 1951; Roberts 1962b). Some adenoviruses, coxsackievirus A24, and enterovirus type 70 are regularly associated with conjunctivitis, and the conjunctiva may represent a primary portal of entry in such instances. Table 13.1 lists representative viruses that invade via the skin and mucous membranes.

UROGENITAL TRACT

A considerable number of viruses cause sexually transmitted disease, which is usually acquired by exposure to virus-containing secretions. Infection is initiated either

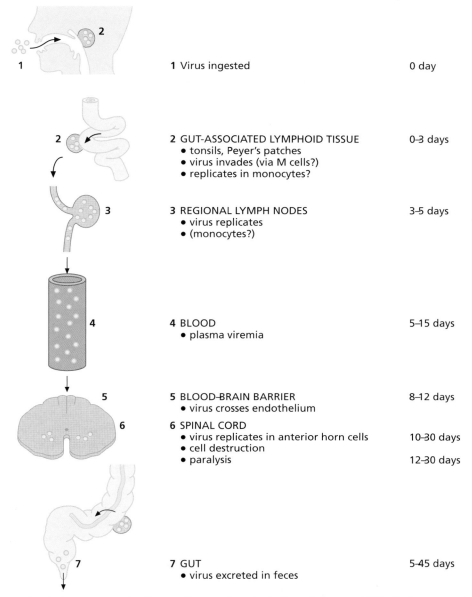

1 Virus ingested	0 day
2 GUT-ASSOCIATED LYMPHOID TISSUE	0–3 days
• tonsils, Peyer's patches	
• virus invades (via M cells?)	
• replicates in monocytes?	
3 REGIONAL LYMPH NODES	3–5 days
• virus replicates	
• (monocytes?)	
4 BLOOD	5–15 days
• plasma viremia	
5 BLOOD–BRAIN BARRIER	8–12 days
• virus crosses endothelium	
6 SPINAL CORD	
• virus replicates in anterior horn cells	10–30 days
• cell destruction	
• paralysis	12–30 days
7 GUT	5–45 days
• virus excreted in feces	

Figure 13.1 *Spread of* poliovirus, *an example of a virus that can disseminate through the blood (after Nathanson et al. 2002)*

by penetration through breaks in the skin or by direct invasion of the superficial epithelium of the mucous membranes (Pomerantz et al. 1988; Tan et al. 1993).

Some sexually transmitted viruses, such as hepatitis B virus (HBV) and human immunodeficiency virus (HIV), are associated with persistent viremia. Thus, contaminated blood, semen, or secretions may introduce HBV directly into the circulation via breaks in skin and membranes. HIV may be trapped on the surface of dendritic cells (Langerhans cells) in the epidermis and then transported to draining lymph nodes where it infects $CD4^+$ T lymphocytes. Also, HIV may infect T lymphocytes in the submucosal tissues, which are the first infected cells detected in experimental vaginal infection of macaques with simian immunodeficiency virus (SIV).

TRANSCUTANEOUS AND INTRAVENOUS INJECTION

Although the skin is a formidable barrier, mechanical injection that breaches the barrier is a natural route of entry for many viruses.

Arboviruses

Many animal viruses are maintained in nature by a cycle that involves a vector and a vertebrate host (Monath 1988), including over 500 individual viruses mainly in the families *Bunyaviridae*, *Flaviviridae*, *Reoviridae*, *Rhabdoviridae*, and *Togaviridae*. When the infected vector takes a blood-meal, virus contained in the salivary gland is injected. Although most viruses that are transmitted by an insect vector replicate in the vector, there are a few instances in

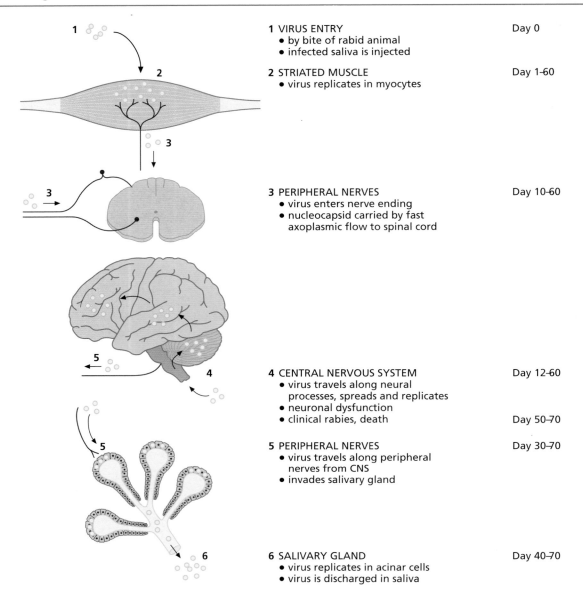

1 VIRUS ENTRY   Day 0
  • by bite of rabid animal
  • infected saliva is injected

2 STRIATED MUSCLE   Day 1–60
  • virus replicates in myocytes

3 PERIPHERAL NERVES   Day 10–60
  • virus enters nerve ending
  • nucleocapsid carried by fast
    axoplasmic flow to spinal cord

4 CENTRAL NERVOUS SYSTEM   Day 12–60
  • virus travels along neural
    processes, spreads and replicates
  • neuronal dysfunction
  • clinical rabies, death   Day 50–70

5 PERIPHERAL NERVES   Day 30–70
  • virus travels along peripheral
    nerves from CNS
  • invades salivary gland

6 SALIVARY GLAND   Day 40–70
  • virus replicates in acinar cells
  • virus is discharged in saliva

Figure 13.2 *Spread of rabies virus, an example of a virus that spreads through the neural route only (after Nathanson et al. 2002).*

Table 13.1 *Representative viruses that invade via skin and mucous membranes (modified after Nathanson et al. 2002).*

Site of entry	Route	Virus family	Representative example
Skin	Minor breaks	*Papillomaviridae*	Papillomaviruses
		Herpesviridae	Herpes simplex virus 1
		Poxviridae	Ectromelia virus
Conjunctiva	Contact	*Picornaviridae*	Enterovirus 70
		Adenoviridae	Adenoviruses
Oropharynx	Contact	*Herpesviridae*	Epstein–Barr virus
Genital tract	Contact	*Retroviridae*	HIV
		Papillomaviridae	Papillomaviruses
		Herpesviridae	Herpes simplex virus 2
Rectum	Contact	*Retroviridae*	HIV

which the vector acts only as a flying pin and apparently carries the virus mechanically from one vertebrate host to another. Examples are myxoma virus of rabbits and rabbit papillomatosis virus (Fenner 1983; Dalmat 1958).

Intramuscular injection: rabies

Rabies is the only virus that is maintained in many of its natural cycles by the bite of a sick animal (Baer 1991). Following transcutaneous and intramuscular injection, the virus may either enter the distal processes of peripheral nerves directly or replicate in striated muscle. It can then cross the neuromuscular junction and spread along peripheral nerves to the central nervous system.

Injection or transfusion

Virus may be transmitted accidentally by repeated use of contaminated needles, injection of a virus-contaminated therapeutic, transfusion with virus-contaminated blood or blood products, or tattooing. The agents most frequently involved are those that produce persistent viremias, such as hepatitis B, C, D viruses, cytomegalovirus, and human immunodeficiency virus. Contaminated needles play a major role in transmission, either by parenteral injection of drugs by abusers in developed countries, or by reuse of needles in developing countries. Following parenteral injection, virus appears to be widely disseminated, replicating in those cells for which it has a tropism.

OROPHARYNX AND GASTROINTESTINAL TRACT

The oropharynx and gastrointestinal tract are important portals of entry for many viruses, and enteric viruses may invade the host at a variety of sites from the oral cavity to the colon (Table 13.2). Some viruses produce localized infections that remain confined to the gastrointestinal tract, whereas others disseminate to produce systemic infection. Most enteric viruses, such as rotaviruses, infect the epithelium of the small or large intestine (Saif 1990; Little and Shadduck 1982) (Figure 13.3), but some enteroviruses, such as poliovirus, replicate in the lymphoid tissue of the gut and nasopharynx.

There are numerous barriers to infection via the enteric route. First, much of the ingested inoculum will remain trapped in the luminal contents and never reach the wall of the gut. Secondly, the lumen constitutes a hostile environment because of the acidity of the stomach, the alkalinity of the small intestine, the digestive enzymes found in saliva and pancreatic secretions, and the lipolytic action of bile. Thirdly, the mucus that lines the intestinal epithelium presents a physical barrier protecting the intestinal surface. Fourthly, phagocytic scavenger cells and secreted antibodies in the lumen can reduce the titer of infectious virus.

Acid labile viruses, such as rhinoviruses, cannot infect by the intestinal route. Viruses that are successful in using the enteric portal tend to be resistant to acid pH, proteolytic attack, and bile, and some may actually exploit the hostile environment to enhance their infectivity (Clark et al. 1981; Estes et al. 1981). hepatitis A and B viruses illustrate this point – both viruses are excreted in the bile into the intestinal tract, but hepatitis A virus survives and is excreted in an infectious form in the feces while hepatitis B virus is inactivated. As a consequence, only hepatitis A is transmitted as an enterovirus.

Lower gastrointestinal tract

The importance of anal intercourse as a risk factor for hepatitis B and HIV infection has led to the recognition that some viruses can gain entry through the lower gastrointestinal tract. HIV has been detected in bowel epithelium (Levy 1998), but the exact mechanism of HIV infection through the anocolonic portal remains to be determined.

RESPIRATORY TRACT

Respiratory infection may be initiated either by virus contained in aerosols that are inhaled by the recipient

Table 13.2 *Representative enteric viruses that do and do not cause gastroenteritis (modified after Nathanson et al. 2002).*

Disease	Replicate in the pharynx and/or gastroenteric tract	Virus family	Representative example
Gastroenteritis	Yes	*Astroviridae*	Astroviruses
	Yes	*Caliciviridae*	Norwalk virus
	Yes	*Coronaviridae*	Transmissible gastroenteritis virus of swine
	Yes	*Rotaviridae*	Rotaviruses
	Yes	*Parvoviridae*	Canine parvoviruses
	Yes	*Adenoviridae*	Adenoviruses 40,41
No enteric illness (± systemic illness)	Yes	*Picornaviridae*	Poliovirus
	Yes	*Picornaviridae*	Coxsackieviruses
	Yes	*Picornaviridae*	Enteroviruses
	No	*Picornaviridae*	Hepatitis A virus
	Yes	*Adenoviridae*	Adenoviruses

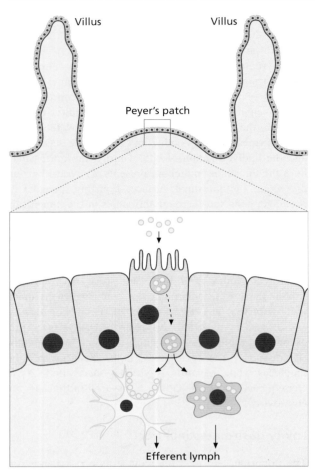

Figure 13.3 *Virus invasion of the intestine, showing the pathway taken by reovirus in the mouse. The virus binds to M cells, is carried by transcytosis to the basolateral surface, where it infects dendritic cells and macrophages in the lamina propria. This well-studied experimental model probably resembles many natural infections (after Wolf et al. 1981).*

host, or by virus that is contained in nasopharyngeal fluids and is transmitted by hand-to-hand contact. Important groups of viruses transmitted by the respiratory route include rhinoviruses, myxoviruses, adenoviruses, herpesviruses, and poxviruses (Table 13.3).

Aerosolized droplets are deposited at different levels in the respiratory tract depending upon their size: those over 10 μm diameter are deposited in the nose, those 5–10 μm in the airways, and those <5 μm in the alveoli (Lippmann et al. 1980). Once deposited, the virus must bypass several effective barriers to initiate infection. These barriers include phagocytic cells in the respiratory lumen, a covering layer of mucus, and ciliated epithelial cells that clear the respiratory tree of foreign particles. The temperature of the respiratory tract varies from 33°C in the nasal passages to 37°C (core body temperature) in the alveoli. Viruses (such as rhinoviruses) that can replicate well at 33°C, but not at 37°C, are limited to the upper respiratory tract and, conversely, viruses that replicate well at 37°C, but not at 33°C (such as

influenza virus), mainly infect the lower respiratory tract. Most respiratory viruses initiate infection by replicating in epithelial cells lining the alveoli or the respiratory tree, but some viruses will also replicate in phagocytic cells located either in the respiratory lumen or in subepithelial spaces (Douglas et al. 1966; Roberts 1962a).

Spread

Once infection is established at the site of entry, most viruses will spread locally by cell-to-cell transmission of infection. Some viruses remain localized near their site of entry while others spread widely. One determinant of dissemination is the pattern of viral release from polarized epithelial cells. Viruses that are released only at the apical surface of infected cells tend to remain localized, while those that are released at the basal surface tend to disseminate (Tucker and Compans 1992; Jourdan et al. 1997). Usually, the first step in dissemination of the infection is the transport of virus via the efferent lymphatic drainage from the initial site of infection to the regional lymph nodes, either as free virions or in virus-infected phagocytic cells.

VIREMIA

The single most important route of dissemination is the circulation, which can potentially carry viruses to any site in the body. There are several sources of viremia. Virus may enter with the efferent lymphatic flow, or may be shed from infected endothelial cells or circulating mononuclear leukocytes (Charles et al. 1998; Fish et al. 1998). Viruses can circulate either free in the plasma phase of the blood (plasma viremia) or associated with formed elements (cell-associated viremia), and these two types of viremia have quite different characteristics and implications.

Passive viremia is used to describe the entry of a virus inoculum directly into the circulation following injection, without any preceding replication (Figure 13.4). Passive viremia typically occurs about 3–6 h after injection and disappears within 12–24 h. It has been estimated that about 0.1 percent of the virus in a subcutaneous inoculum enters the bloodstream (Griot et al. 1993b; Pekosz et al. 1995).

Active viremia is used to designate viremia caused by the active replication of virus in the host. In some instances, active viremia may occur in two phases, a primary viremia in which virus spreads from a focal site of entry and a secondary viremia generated after infection has occurred and virus has initially replicated in peripheral tissues, such as endothelium, tissue macrophages, liver, muscle, or other sites (Oaks et al. 1998). An example of an active viremia is shown in Figure 13.5, in which the virus appears in the plasma a few days after infection and lasts for about 1 week.

Table 13.3 *Representative viruses that invade via the nasopharynx or respiratory tract, according to localization of disease (modified after Nathanson et al. 2002).*

Localization of disease	Virus family	Representative example
Upper respiratory	*Picornaviridae*	Rhinoviruses
	Adenoviridae	Adenoviruses
Lower respiratory	*Coronaviridae*	Bovine coronaviruses
	Orthomyxoviridae	Influenza viruses
	Paramyxoviridae	Respiratory syncytial virus
	Bunyaviridae	Sin Nombre virus
No respiratory illness	*Togaviridae*	Rubella virus
(± systemic illness)	*Paramyxoviridae*	Mumps virus
	Bunyaviridae	Hantaan virus
	Arenaviridae	Lassa fever virus
	Reoviridae	Reovirus
	Papovaviridae	Murine polyomavirus
	Herpesviridae	Varicella-zoster virus
	Poxviridae	Variola virus

The initial lag period is the interval required for tissue replication and shedding into the circulation. Termination of viremia is often quite abrupt and coincides with the appearance of neutralizing antibody in the serum. When an infected animal is treated with an immunosuppressive regime, the viremia may not be cleared quickly, but persist for longer periods (Nathanson and Cole 1971).

Plasma viremia reflects a dynamic process in which virus continually enters the circulation and is removed. The rate of turnover of virus within the plasma compartment is best expressed as transit time, the average duration of a virion in the blood compartment. Typically, transit times range from 1–60 min and tend to decrease as the size of the virions increases (Mims 1964). Circulating viruses are removed by the phagocytic cells of the reticuloendothelial system, principally in the liver (Kupffer cells), and to a lesser extent in the lung, spleen, and lymph nodes. The fate of viruses that are ingested by Kupffer cells is quite variable and may be an important determinant of pathogenesis. Ingested virions may be degraded, may transit macrophages to underlying parenchyma without replicating, or may replicate in macrophages with or without spread of infection to underlying parenchymal cells. Once the host has developed circulating antibody, plasma virus is very rapidly neutralized in the circulation (Figure 13.5), and virus–antibody complexes bind to Fc receptors, facilitating removal by sessile macrophages lining the circulation. Under these circumstances, transit time is reduced by several fold (Igarishi et al. 1999; Zhang et al. 1999; Mittler et al. 1999).

Although plasma viremias are usually shortlived, there are notable exceptions. Some viruses are bound by antibody, but the immune complex retains infectivity. In these instances, such as Aleutian disease virus (a parvovirus) and lactic dehydrogenase virus (a togavirus), plasma infectivity may resist neutralization with exogenous antibody but may be reduced by the addition of anti-Ig antibodies (Notkins et al. 1966; Porter and Larsen 1967). Other exceptions are instances where the infected host is tolerant of the viral antigens and fails to develop a sufficient level of antibody to clear viremia. Examples are hepatitis B virus and lymphocytic choriomeningitis virus (Figure 13.6).

A number of viruses replicate in cells that are found in the circulation, particularly monocytes, B or T lymphocytes, or (rarely) erythrocytes (Table 13.4). Under these circumstances, the viremia is cell-associated, although some virus may also be found free in the plasma compartment. Cell-associated viremias may be of short duration, as in the case of ectromelia and other poxviruses. However, in many instances of cell-associated viremia, virus titers are low, virus may be difficult to isolate from the blood, and viremia persists

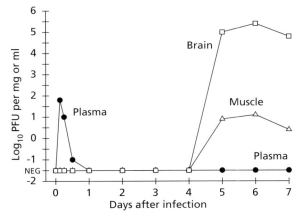

Figure 13.4 *Passive viremia, after injection of La Crosse virus in weanling mice. Viremia appears as a sharp peak limited to the first 12 h and stands out in profile since there is no active viremia in mice of this age. Even this transient viremia was sufficient to deliver enough virus to the target organ to initiate a lethal encephalitis (data from Pekosz et al. 1995).*

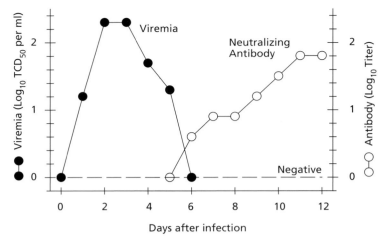

Figure 13.5 *Active plasma viremia after intramuscular injection of poliovirus in monkeys. Viremia lasts for about 1 week, and the clearance of viremia coincides with the appearance of neutralizing antibody in the serum (data from Nathanson and Bodian 1961).*

for the life of the host rather than terminating when neutralizing antibody appears (Figure 13.7).

Human immunodeficiency virus provides an important instance of cell-associated viremia (Hsia and Spector 1991; Bagasra et al. 1993; Levy 1998). HIV infects both CD4[+] T lymphocytes and monocytes in the blood, but most infected cells are CD4[+] T lymphocytes. The frequency of infected peripheral blood CD4[+] T lymphocytes varies from 0.2 to 10 percent in asymptomatic persons to between 2 and 60 percent in symptomatic patients, and 50–90 percent of infected T lymphocytes contain the genome in a latent state. In typical asymptomatic individuals, there are about 5 000 infected cells per ml blood. In addition to infected cells, free infectious HIV is also present in the plasma, the amount varying with the stage of disease. In typical asympto-

matic individuals, it has been estimated that there are about 100 tissue culture infectious doses (TCD) per ml plasma, considerably fewer than the number of infected cells.

Antibody-dependent enhancement of infection is a special aspect of cell-associated viremia, which has been described mainly for dengue and other flaviviruses (Halstead and O'Rourke 1977; Gollins and Porterfield 1984). Dengue virus replicates primarily in monocytes, but it does not enter these cells readily. However, in the presence of low concentrations of antibody, infection is markedly enhanced, presumably because the virus–antibody complex is bound to Fc receptors on monocytes, enhancing viral entry.

Tissue invasion from the blood

There are several ways in which a virus might cross the vascular wall (Johnson and Mims 1968; Johnson 1998), but the precise mechanism for penetrating the blood–tissue barrier is unknown in most instances.

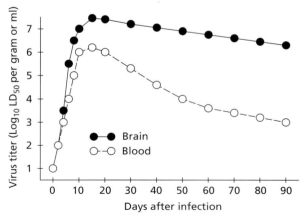

Figure 13.6 *Persistent plasma viremia associated with immunological hyporesponsiveness to the viral antigens. Adult mice were infected with lymphocytic choriomeningitis virus (LCMV) intracerebrally and were immunosuppressed with aminopterin on days 4 and 6 after infection. Mice infected in the same way but not treated with aminopterin died of acute choriomeningitis about 8 days after infection (data from Hotchin 1962).*

- In many tissues, the capillary endothelial cells are not joined by tight junctions, and viruses can pass between them. One example is the fenestrated capillaries of the choroid plexus of the central nervous system. Penetration at this site provides access to the epithelial cells of the choroid plexus and can be followed by entry into the cerebrospinal fluid and spread to the ependymal cells lining the ventricles (Herndon et al. 1974).

- Virus may be transported through endothelial cells by a process of endocytosis, translocation of virus-containing vesicles, and subsequent release by exocytosis at the basal surface of the endothelial cell (Johnson and Mims 1968; Pathek and Webb 1974).

- Some viruses are capable of replicating within endothelial cells and are released from these cells into the surrounding tissues. Examples include selected picorna-

Table 13.4 *Viruses that replicate in circulating blood cells, a representative list*

Cell type	Virus family	Representative virus	Duration viremia	References
Monocytes	*Flaviviridae*	Dengue	acute	Halstead and O'Rourke (1977)
	Togaviridae	Rubella	acute	Chantler and Tingle (1982)
	Paramyxoviridae	Measles	acute	Esolen et al. (1993)
	Arenaviridae	LCMV	persistent	Matloubian et al. (1993)
	Retroviridae	HIV	persistent	Collman et al. (1989)
		Ovine visna maedi	persistent	Gendelman et al. (1985)
		EIAV	persistent	Oaks et al. (1998)
	Herpesviridae	Cytomegalo	persistent	Taylor-Weideman et al. (1991)
	Poxviridae	Mousepox	acute	Fenner (1949)
		Rabbit myxoma	acute	Fenner (1983)
B lymphocytes	*Retroviridae*	Murine leukemia	persistent	Kozak and Ruscetti (1992)
	Herpesviridae	Epstein–Barr	persistent	Ho (1981)
T lymphocytes	*Retroviridae*	HIV	persistent	Bagasra et al. (1993)
		HTLV-I	persistent	Depper et al. (1984)
	Herpesviridae	Human herpes 6, 7	acute	Takahashi et al. (1989)
Erythroblasts	*Reoviridae*	Colorado tick fever	acute	Oshiro et al. (1978)

EIAV, equine infectious anemia virus; HIV, human immunodeficiency virus; HTLV, human T-cell leukemia virus; LCMV, lymphocytic choriomeningitis virus.

viruses, retroviruses, alphaviruses, and parvoviruses (Johnson 1965; Baringer and Nathanson 1972; Friedman et al. 1981; Pitts et al. 1987).

● Viruses that cause a cell-associated viremia may invade by an alternate mechanism, namely, as passengers in infected lymphocytes or monocytes, a mechanism that has been suggested for tissue invasion of HIV and other lentiviruses (Haase 1986).

Infected mononuclear cells can cross the blood–tissue barrier as part of their normal trafficking pattern, or may be actively recruited into sites of inflammation.

NEURAL SPREAD

Some viruses can disseminate by spreading through the axons of peripheral nerves (Table 13.5). Although less

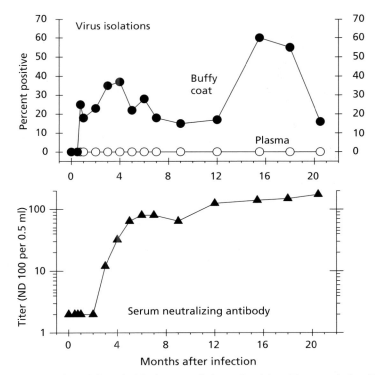

Figure 13.7 *Cell-associated viremia in sheep infected with visna maedi virus, a Lentivirus. Virus was isolated by cocultivation of buffy coat cells with indicator cells and was never isolated from the plasma. The frequency of virus isolations was unrelated to the appearance or titer of neutralizing antibody (data from Petursson et al. 1976).*

Table 13.5 *Viruses that spread by the neural route, a representative list*

Virus family	Representative virus	Notes	References
Picornaviridae	Poliovirus	Neuroadapted clones only; natural isolates are viremogenic	Nathanson and Bodian (1961); Bodian (1955)
Flaviviridae	Yellow fever	Neuroadapted clones only; natural isolates are viremogenic	Strode (1951)
Alphaviridae	VEE	Hematogenous invasion of peripheral nerves	Charles et al. (1995)
	Semliki Forest	Age-specific olfactory invasion	Oliver and Fazakerley (1998)
Coronaviridae	Mouse hepatitis	Neural spread after intranasal infection	Perlman et al. (1989); Barnett and Perlman (1993)
Rhabdoviridae	Rabies	Exclusively neural	Baer (1991)
Reoviridae	Reo	Type 3 uses neural route	Tyler et al. (1986)
		Type 1 spreads by the hematogenous route	Morrison et al. (1991)
Herpesviridae	Herpes simplex 1, 2	Exclusively neural in adults; pantropic in newborns	Cook and Stevens (1973)
	Pseudorabies	Used for neural pathways	Enquist (1994)

Venezuelan equine encephalitis virus (VEE).

important than viremia, neural spread plays an essential role for certain viruses (such as rabies viruses and several herpesviruses), while other viruses (such as poliovirus and reovirus) can utilize both mechanisms of spread (Johnson 1998). Different strains of the same virus may differ markedly in their ability to use the neural route (Nathanson and Bodian 1961; Tyler et al. 1986; Ren et al. 1990; Barnett and Perlman 1993), as shown in Table 13.6. Also, different viral variants may utilize different neuronal pathways (Card et al. 1998).

It seems certain that viruses enter neurons by mechanisms similar to those involving entry into other cell types. The uncoated nucleocapsid is then carried passively along axons or dendrites, probably by fast axoplasmic flow (Maratou et al. 1998; Ohka et al. 1998). After the transport process, the virus may replicate in the perikaryon, but this is a much slower process and is not required for neural spread. There are several lines of evidence for this reconstruction of neural spread:

- Neural transection will block neural spread (Table 13.6) and the rate of movement (>5 cm per day) is similar to the rate of axoplasmic transport (>10 cm per day) (Kristensson et al. 1971; Tyler et al. 1986; Tsiang 1993).
- Drugs, such as colchicine, which block fast axoplasmic transport by disrupting microtubules, also block the transport of viral genomes (Tsiang 1979).
- Temperature-sensitive strains of herpesvirus (which cannot replicate at body temperature) are able to move from a peripheral site of inoculation to a sensory ganglion, such as the trigeminal ganglion, and may be recovered by culturing the explanted ganglion at temperatures that are permissive for temperature-sensitive clones (Sederati et al. 1993).
- Several days after initiation of neural spread, the nucleocapsids of viruses, such as rabies virus, herpes simplex virus, and pseudorabies virus (an alphaherpes virus), may be seen within axons (Rabin et al. 1968).

Localization or tropism

One of the salient features that distinguishes viruses is their tropism within the animal host (see Figures 13.1 and 13.2). The names of individual viral diseases often reflects the organs or tissues that are involved. Thus, smallpox, poliomyelitis, and hepatitis each have their characteristic features. Localization of infection, or viral tropism, is regulated both by viral dissemination and cellular susceptibility. Disease localization may not correspond to the distribution of infection since it reflects both the spread of the virus and the host response to infection.

VIRAL DISSEMINATION

The localization of a virus is determined at several phases of infection, including penetration at the portal of entry, systemic spread by viremia or the neural route, and the invasion of local organs or tissues.

Table 13.6 *Different mode of dissemination of a neurotropic and a pantropic strain of the same virus*

	Neuroadapted MV strain		Pantropic Mahoney strain	
	Control	Block	Control	Block
Paralysis	25/26	0/11	19/19	18/20
Site of initial paralysis				
Injected leg	24	–	3	5
Other	1	–	16	13
Incubation to paralysis	5 days	–	7 days	7.5 days

Comparison of a neuroadapted and a natural pantropic isolate of poliovirus following intramuscular injection in cynomolgus macaques. The neuroadapted virus spreads only by the neural route, causes initial paralysis in the injected limb and fails to paralyse after a nerve block, while the pantropic strain spreads by viremia, does not cause localised initial paralysis, and is not impeded by nerve block. (Data from Nathanson and Bodian 1961).

Portal of entry

The physical characteristics of a virus that influence its ability to survive in the external environment play a role in circumscribing the portal of entry. Thus, many picornaviruses are enteroviruses that are capable of surviving in the hostile environment of the enteric tract, but some picornaviruses, such as the rhinoviruses, are acid labile, cannot survive gastric acidity, and are confined to the respiratory tract. The biological characteristics of the virus also plays a role in its initial localization. Again, the rhinoviruses replicate well at 33°C, the temperature of the nasopharynx, while influenza virus has a replication optimum of 37°C that permits it to infect the lower respiratory tract. These limiting factors are particularly important for the localization of viruses that fail to spread systemically.

Viremia and neural spread

Viremia plays a key role in systemic spread of most viruses (Figures 13.1 and 13.2), and the viremogenicity of the specific viral strain determines its likelihood of reaching target organs. Conversely, the inability to initiate viremia explains the local nature of the infections caused by many respiratory and enteric viruses. The importance of viremia in determining localization is illustrated in Table 13.7, which indicates that in adult mice La Crosse virus (a bunyavirus) has the capability of initiating a lethal encephalitis after intracerebral injection of a minimal dose (approximately 1 plaque forming unit (pfu)), but fails to cause illness after subcutaneous injection of $>10^7$ pfu because no viremia is produced. Likewise, poliovirus, in spite of its high potential to induce paralysis, is estimated to cause only one paralytic case per 150 human infections, presumably because it rarely generates sufficient viremia to reach the spinal cord (Figure 13.8).

For viruses that spread primarily by the neural route, the ability to disseminate is also an important determinant of localization (Gromeier and Wimmer 1998). For instance, herpes simplex virus is capable of initiating a very severe encephalitis in humans if the virus reaches the central nervous system. However, most infections are either silent, or limited to mucocutaneous lesions, and encephalitis occurs at a rate of less than one case per 1 000 primary infections, indicating that the virus rarely reaches its potential target in sufficient dose to localize in the brain.

CELLULAR RECEPTORS

Most viruses are quite selective in the cell types that are infected in vivo and this selectivity plays a significant role in localization. One major determinant of cellular susceptibility is the presence of viral receptors, namely, molecules on the cellular surface that act as receptors for the specific virus, usually by binding a protein on the virion surface (the viral attachment protein). From studies of many viral receptors (Figure 13.9), several generalizations can be made (Wimmer 1994a; Dimitrov 2000):

- Although receptors have been identified for only a small proportion of viruses, it is generally thought that specific receptors are necessary for efficient infection by most viruses. Presumably viruses have evolved to utilize, as receptors, cellular surface molecules that subserve other functions required for normal cellular activity.
- A variety of molecules, including glycoproteins, glycolipids, and glycosaminoglycans, can serve as viral receptors. The domain of the receptor that binds the virus may be either a polypeptide sequence or a carbohydrate moiety, often located at the external tip of the receptor molecule.
- Different viruses employ different cellular receptors, although a few receptors are used by more than one virus.
- Many viruses are capable of utilizing more than a single cellular molecule as a receptor.
- Different isolates of the same virus may prefer different receptors, and a specific virus isolate may alter its receptor preference by selection of a mutant viral attachment protein during serial passage in animals or cell cultures (Borza and Hutt-Fletcher 2002).
- In some instances, viral entry requires two or more different coreceptors on the cell surface. Usually, both coreceptors are necessary and neither alone is sufficient.

Table 13.7 *The relative virulence of viruses depends on variables such as the route of entry and age of the host.*

Virus clone	PFU per LD_{50}			
	IC infection suckling mice[a]	SC infection suckling mice	IC infection adult mice	SC infection adult mice
Wild-type La Crosse original	~1	~1	~1	$>10^7$
Attenuated B.5 clone	~1	$>10^5$	$>10^6$	$>10^7$

Illustrated by two variants of La Crosse virus, a bunyavirus, when injected by different routes in suckling and adult mice. One clone, La Crosse/original, is a wild-type isolate and the other clone, B.5, is a laboratory-derived attenuated strain. Note that the two viruses exhibit striking differences in virulence upon intracerebral injection of adult mice or subcutaneous injection of suckling mice, but that both appear similar in their high virulence for suckling mice inoculated intracerebrally and similar in their low virulence for adult mice inoculated subcutaneously. Virulence is expressed as the ratio of pfu per LD_{50}; the lower the number the more virulent the virus. IC, intracerebral; SC, subcutaneous (data from Endres et al. 1990).

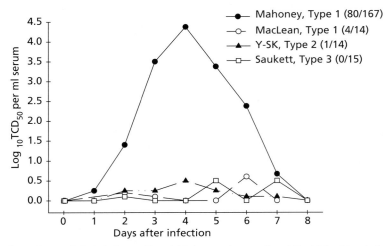

Figure 13.8 *Viremia as a determinant of viral virulence. Type 1 Mahoney virus produced the highest level of viremia and the highest frequency of paralysis (48%) while the other three (low viremia) strains produced an aggregate paralytic rate of 12% (the frequency of paralysis is shown in parentheses) (data from Bodian 1954).*

- Entry of a virus into a potential host cell is a multi-step process in which binding to the receptor is only the initiating event.
- Not all cells that express the viral receptor are capable of supporting the complete cycle of viral replication.

These generalizations are illustrated by human immunodeficiency virus (HIV) (Levy 1998; Weiss

1994). The CD4 molecule is a type I glycoprotein, which is expressed by certain subsets of T lympho-cytes and monocytes/macrophages, and subserves signaling between lymphoid and monocytic cells. CD4 has four immunoglobulin-like domains in its extra-cellular amino terminus, and the outermost of these domains contains a region that binds a specific site on gp120, the surface glycoprotein of HIV. The primary cellular targets of HIV are CD4[+] T lymphocytes and

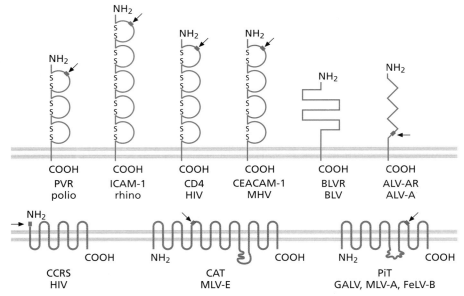

Figure 13.9 *Molecular backbone cartoons of some glycoprotein viral receptors. Receptors diverge widely in their structure and in their physiological function. The amino and carboxy termini are shown, together with important disulfide bonds and the probable domains that bind virus. ALV-AR, avian leukosis virus A receptor; BLVR, bovine leukemia virus receptor; CAT, cationic amino acid transporter; CCR5, chemokine receptor 5; CEACAM, carcinoembryonic antigen-related cell adhesion molecule; ICAM, intercellular adhesion molecule; PiT, inorganic phosphate transporter; PVR, poliovirus receptor; Viruses: polio, poliovirus; rhino, rhinovirus, major group; HIV, human immunodeficiency virus; MHV, mouse hepatitis virus (a coronavirus); BLV, bovine leukemia virus; ALV-A, avian leukosis virus A; MLV-E, murine leukemia virus E; GALV, gibbon ape leukemia virus; MLV-A: murine leukemia virus A; FeLV-B; feline leukemia virus B (after Wimmer 1994b; Weiss and Tailor 1995; Holmes, 1997).*

monocytes/macrophages and the distribution of CD4 explains this cellular localization.

However, the expression of CD4 on the surface of a cell is not sufficient to assure viral entry. HIV utilizes a coreceptor, several members of the family of chemokine receptors, most frequently CCR5 or CXCR4 (Berger et al. 1999). HIV-1 strains can utilize either CCR5 or CXCR4 or, in some instances, both coreceptors. CCR5 is expressed on macrophages, while CXCR4 is expressed on T-lymphocyte cell lines, explaining why some HIV-1 strains will infect macrophages but not T-cell lines, while the reverse is true for other HIV-1 strains (Figure 13.10). Furthermore, there are important biological distinctions between HIV-1 isolates that use R5 or X4 coreceptors. Under natural conditions, infections are mainly initiated by R5 viruses, while X4 viruses are more frequent in patients with advanced AIDS. In experimental infections of monkeys, R5 viruses preferentially infect lymph nodes while X4 viruses replicate preferentially in gut-associated lymphoid tissue (Harouse et al. 1999).

Poliovirus offers another example of localization determined by receptors (Wimmer et al. 1994; Freistadt 1994; Evans and Almond 1999). It was long known that poliovirus would only replicate in primate tissues, and it had been deduced that this was because a putative poliovirus receptor (PVR) was expressed only by primate cells, since nonprimate mammalian cells would support poliovirus replication if transfected with viral RNA, thereby bypassing the requirement for a viral receptor. Using this conceptual framework, the PVR

was cloned and sequenced, and when transfected into rodent cells it rendered them permissive for the virus (Mendelsohn et al. 1989). Furthermore, when transgenic mice were created that expressed the PVR, the animals developed typical clinical and pathological poliomyelitis after intracerebral injection of human poliovirus (Ren et al. 1990).

However, the relationship of the PVR to viral localization appears to be more complex, since the PVR alone may not confer cellular susceptibility. Thus, the PVR is expressed quite ubiquitously in human tissues, but most of these tissues are not infected by the virus. Also, PVR transgenic mice cannot be readily infected by the oral route (the natural route of infection in primates) and pantropic strains of poliovirus that are viremogenic in primates fail to cause viremia in these mice (Ren and Racaniello 1992).

OTHER MECHANISMS OF CELLULAR LOCALIZATION

Cellular susceptibility may be determined at post-entry steps in the replication cycle. Some viruses are quite fastidious and can replicate only in selected cell types, thus accounting for their selective tropism. For example, some of the murine leukemia viruses appear to require enhancers or promoters that are supplied only in certain cell types (Evans and Morrey 1987). In these instances, genetic studies have mapped the viral determinants of replication to the unique 3′ (U3) noncoding region of the viral genome (Hopkins et al. 1989).

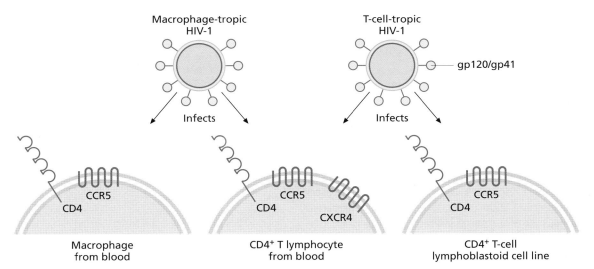

Figure 13.10 *HIV-1 is an example of a virus that requires a primary receptor and a coreceptor to infect target cells efficiently. The primary receptor is the CD4 molecule, a protein expressed on the surface of certain subsets of lymphocytes (so called CD4+ cells). The gp120 spike glycoproteins of all HIV strains can bind to human CD4. In addition, virus entry requires a coreceptor, which is either CCR5 or CXCR4. These proteins are members of a large family of molecules that serve as chemokine receptors on the surface of lymphoid cells or macrophages. Some HIV-1 isolates are macrophage-tropic because their gp120 spikes use CCR5, a chemokine receptor that is expressed on the surface of macrophages, while other isolates are T-cell-tropic because they utilize the CXCR4 molecule, another chemokine receptor expressed on the surface of T-cell lines. Both kinds of viruses can replicate on peripheral blood mononuclear cells (PBMC), lymphocytes freshly cultured from peripheral blood, since these cells express both coreceptors. By the same token, some HIV-1 isolates (not shown) are dual-tropic since they can utilize both coreceptors. (Recent studies have shown that macrophages express low levels of CXCR4 at concentrations insufficient for entry of T-cell-tropic HIV-1.)*

A number of enveloped viruses encode glycoproteins that require cleavage to activate either their viral attachment function or their fusion function. Absent proteolytic cleavage virions are not infectious. An example is Newcastle disease virus, a paramyxovirus of birds. Virulent isolates of Newcastle disease virus encode a fusion protein that is readily cleaved by furin, a proteolytic enzyme present in the Golgi apparatus, so that the protein is activated during maturation prior to reaching the cell surface, and before budding of nascent virions. This makes it possible for virulent strains of the virus to infect many avian cell types, thereby increasing its tissue host range, and causing systemic infections that are often lethal. In contrast, avirulent strains of Newcastle disease virus encode a variant fusion protein that is not cleaved during maturation in the Golgi, so that nascent virus requires activation by an extracellular protease. The required protease is found only in the respiratory or enteric tracts, thereby limiting tropism to surface cells and conferring an attenuated phenotype on the virus (Nagai 1995).

LOCALIZATION OF VIRAL PATHOLOGY

Pathological lesions were traditionally used to trace the spread of viral infections. However, the pathological process initiated by viral infections does not always co-localize at the sites of viral replication. Some viruses kill all cells in which they replicate and, in such instances, viral disease tends to mirror the localization of viral replication. In contrast, certain viruses will destroy some, but not all, of the cells in which they replicate. For instance, viruses that are cytocidal because they trigger a cascade of events leading to cellular apoptosis may replicate in a noncytodical fashion in cells in which apoptosis is blocked by the protective effect of the bcl-2 proto-oncogene (Griffin et al. 1994).

A number of viruses initiate immune-mediated cellular pathology in which CD8[+] T lymphocytes attack cells that present viral peptides associated with MHC class I proteins. If the virus infects both cells that do and do not express MHC class I molecules, then the MHC negative cells are not attacked. This phenomenon is thought to explain the sparing of neurons after infection by certain viruses, since neurons do not express class I molecules (Rall et al. 1995). Immune-mediated lesions may be even more indirect, such as those that are caused by antigen–antibody complexes. In this instance, the lesions are seen in locations such as the glomerulus of the kidney, which cannot handle the large accumulations of macromolecular complexes, while the virus has replicated at sites distant from the kidney (Oldstone 1975). Dengue hemorrhagic fever is thought to be initiated by the antiviral immune response that leads to a consumptive coagulopathy (Rothman and Ennis 1999).

For oncogenic viruses, the tumors may represent a distant echo of virus localization (Figure 13.11).

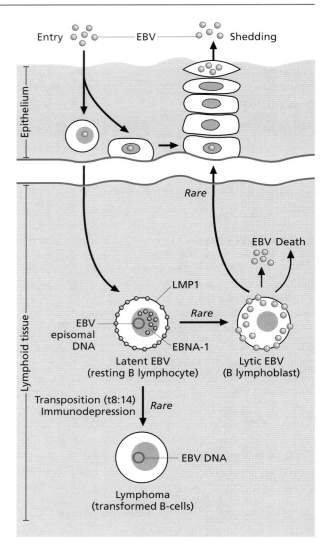

Figure 13.11 *The localization of pathological lesions may only be a remote echo of the distribution of the causal virus, as exemplified by this diagrammatic summary of possible pathogenesis of EBV and Burkitt's lymphoma. The virus initially infects epithelial cells and B lymphocytes. In epithelial cells, EBV causes both latent and lytic infection, the latter resulting in virus shedding into the oral cavity. EBV persists in resting B cells as a latent infection which is rarely activated to produce new virus. During latent persistence in lymphocytes, several EBV genes are expressed, particularly EBNA-1 (EB nuclear antigen) and LMP1 (latent membrane protein) which immortalizes B cell clones. In a few infected people, persistently infected B cells undergo further transformation into tumor cells, producing a variety of lymphomas, such as Burkitt's lymphoma, which is frequently associated with a chromosomal transposition (t8:14) that up-regulates the c-myc oncogene (after Nathanson et al. 2002).*

Epstein–Barr virus (EBV) infects epithelial cells and B cells (Burkitt 1958; Epstein et al. 1964; Hutt-Fletcher 1999; Cohen 2000). EBV causes both a latent and a lytic infection in epithelial cells from which it is shed into the oral cavity. Latently infected B cells are immortalized, and – rarely – these B cells undergo further transformation into lymphomas by virtue of additional genetic events such as chromosomal transposition (t8:14). Lymphoma cells often carry EBV DNA as nuclear episomes.

Shedding

Acute viral infections are characterized by brief periods of intensive virus shedding into respiratory aerosols, feces, urine, or other bodily secretions or fluids. Persistent viruses are often shed at relatively low titers, but this may be adequate for transmission over the prolonged duration of infection.

GASTROINTESTINAL AND RESPIRATORY TRACT

The course of shedding of enteric viruses can be readily followed. For instance, poliovirus is shed in the pharynx for 2–4 weeks and in the feces for 1–2 months after infection, although viremia only lasts about 1 week (Figure 13.5). Respiratory viruses may be transmitted by aerosols generated by coughing or sneezing or by virus-containing nasopharyngeal fluids that are transmitted by hand-to-hand contact. Most acute respiratory viruses are excreted over a relatively short period and infected persons are potential transmitters for only about 1 week (Figure 13.12). Transmission may begin a few days before onset of symptoms (Douglas et al. 1966).

SKIN, MUCOUS MEMBRANES, ORAL AND GENITAL FLUIDS, SEMEN, AND MILK

Although many viruses replicate in the skin, relatively few are spread from skin lesions. Exceptions are herpes simplex (labial transmission), varicella-zoster (rarely

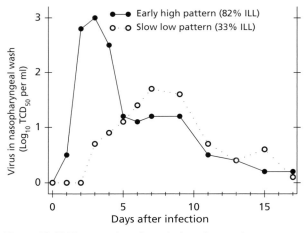

Figure 13.12 *The excretion of a typical respiratory virus, rhinovirus type 15, following inoculation of human volunteers by the transnasal route. The subjects demonstrated either an early onset high concentration pattern associated with a high frequency of respiratory symptoms, or a late onset low concentration pattern associated with a low frequency of symptoms (data from Douglas et al. 1966).*

spread from zoster to cause chickenpox), papillomaviruses, and Ebola virus, a filovirus which causes hemorrhagic fever (Peters 1997). Those viruses, such as herpes simplex type 2 and papillomaviruses, which cause sexually transmitted disease, are often shed from lesions of the genital mucous membranes. In addition, some viruses, such as rabies virus and mumps virus, replicate in the salivary glands and are discharged into the saliva to enter the oral cavity.

Several viruses are shed in the semen, including hepatitis B and human immunodeficiency virus (Alter et al. 1977; Levy 1998). A number of viruses are excreted in colostrum and milk, including cytomegalovirus, mumps, rubella, and ovine visna maedi virus (de Boer and Houwers 1979) and HIV.

BLOOD AND URINE

Blood is also an important source of transmitted virus, particularly for those viruses that produce persistent plasma or cell-associated viremias. Hepatitis B, C, D viruses, human immunodeficiency virus, HTLV-1, HTLV-2, and cytomegalovirus are among the important human pathogens shed in this manner. Arboviruses usually cause short-term acute viremias, and are transmissible only if an appropriate vector ingests a blood meal during this brief interval. In view of the limited amount of blood taken, the viremia must reach considerable levels if it is to be transmitted.

A number of viruses have been isolated from the urine, but viruria is probably not important for transmission of most viruses. A special exception are certain zoonotic viruses, such as the arenaviruses and the hantaviruses, which cause lifelong virurias in their natural rodent hosts, leading to human infection through exposure to aerosolized dried urine (Gonzalez-Scarano and Nathanson 1990). Cytomegalovirus spreads readily among young children in enviroments contaminated by urine (such as creches and play centers).

SURVIVAL IN THE ENVIRONMENT

The probability that a virus will be transmitted depends both upon the intensity and duration of shedding, and upon its ability to survive in the environment. Viruses differ in their ability to survive in aerosols and, somewhat surprisingly, under conditions of low humidity, enveloped viruses appear to be better able to retain viability than do nonenveloped viruses (deJong and Winkler 1968). To be excreted in an infectious form, enteric viruses must survive the harsh environment of the lower gastrointestinal tract.

Transmission

Once shed, there are several means by which a virus is transmitted from host to host in a propagated chain of infection. Probably the most important mechanism is contamination of the hands of the infected transmitter from feces, oral fluids, or respiratory secretions expelled during coughing or sneezing. The virus is then passed by hand-to-hand contact leading to oral, gastro-intestinal, or respiratory infection. A second common route is inhalation of aerosolized virus. A third significant mechanism involves direct person to person contact (oral–oral, genital–genital, oral–genital, or skin–skin). Finally, indirect person-to-person transmission can occur via blood or contaminated needles. Common source transmissions are less frequent but can produce dramatic outbreaks, via contaminated water, food products, or biologicals, such as blood products and vaccines.

The success of a virus, as a life form, can be defined as its ability to be perpetuated over the millenia. In turn, perpetuation of a virus depends in part upon its efficient transmission, particularly for viruses that cause only acute infections. The relative transmissibility of a virus in different populations is reflected in the age-specific profile of immune individuals, as illustrated in Figure 13.13 for hepatitis A virus. For viruses that can persist in individual hosts, perpetuation is determined by transmission over the lifetime of the host, and in some instances, by the ability to be vertically passed to offspring of the host, either by transplacental or peri-natal routes, or as germline genes. If transmissibility is reduced sufficiently, then a given virus will disappear from a defined population. This can happen in nature, when a virus spreads so widely in a specific population that it eliminates most susceptibles and burns out. Transmissibility can also be reduced by immunization which, under certain circumstances, can be used to eradicate a virus from its host population. Smallpox is the seminal example of planned eradication (Fenner et al. 1988), and the elimination of wild poliovirus

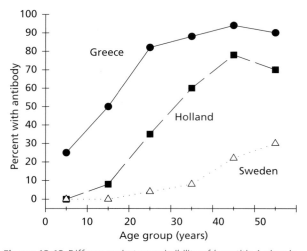

Figure 13.13 *Differences in transmissibility of hepatitis A virus in three European countries, as reflected in the different age-specific profiles of antibody prevalence (data from Frosner et al. 1979).*

from the western hemisphere is another important illustration.

VIRULENCE OF VIRUSES

Virulence refers to the ability of a virus to cause illness or death in an infected host, relative to other isolates or variants of the same agent. From the beginning of experimental virology, it has been recognized that different strains of a given virus may vary in their ability to cause disease. The study of virulence variants can provide important insights into pathogenesis, and varia-tion in viral phenotype must be given consideration in design and interpretation of in vivo studies of the dis-semination, localization, and pathological consequences of viral infection. Study of virulence also has practical implications because it carries the potential for develop-ment of attenuated live virus variants that can be used as vaccines, a principle that was initially recognized by Jenner in 1798 when he introduced vaccinia virus for the prevention of smallpox (Fenner et al. 1988).

There are two distinct approaches to the study of viru-lence. If virulence is regarded as a property of the virus, it is possible to map the genetic determinants that underlie the virulence phenotype. The other approach to virulence is through a study of pathogenesis, which describes the differences in infections with viral variants of different virulence. Pathogenic measures of virulence may be quantitative, involving the rate of viral replica-tion or number of cells infected. Alternatively, differ-ences in virulence may be qualitative, since variants of a single virus may differ markedly in their cellular tropism, their mode of dissemination in the infected host, or the disease phenotype that they produce.

Measures of viral virulence

RELATIVE NATURE OF VIRAL VIRULENCE

Virulence is not an absolute property of a virus strain but depends upon the dose of virus, the route of infec-tion, and the age, gender, and genetic susceptibility of the host. Two viruses that differ in virulence in one experimental paradigm may exhibit similar degrees of virulence in another paradigm. This point is illustrated in Table 13.7, which compares a virulent wild-type clone with a laboratory-derived attenuated clone of California serogroup bunyaviruses. When the two viruses are injected intracerebrally in adult mice, the differences in their virulence are striking. One plaque forming unit (pfu) of the wild-type virus will initiate a fatal encepha-litis, whereas 10^6 pfu of attenuated clone B.5 fails to cause any illness. On the other hand, both viruses are highly virulent when injected intracerebrally in suckling mice (approximately 1 plaque-forming unit (pfu) of either virus is lethal) and cannot be distinguished.

CLINICAL, PATHOLOGICAL, AND FUNCTIONAL INDICATORS OF DISEASE

The conventional measure of viral virulence is the production of disease in the host, using as an endpoint either death or some specific constellation of signs and symptoms caused by the infection. This is illustrated in Table 13.8, which compares the paralytic rate following primary infection with wild-type virus versus the rate following oral poliovirus vaccine. An alternative measure of virulence is an assessment of virus-induced pathological lesions. Also, laboratory tests, that reflect virus-induced pathophysiological changes, can be used as surrogate markers of virulence. For instance, the severity of hepatitis can be assessed by the serum titer of alanine aminotransferase that signals release of hepatocellular proteins, and the severity of human immunodeficiency virus infection by the reduction in the the blood concentration of CD4$^+$ T lymphocytes.

For a precise estimation of virulence, it is important to adjust for virus dose, which can conveniently be done by titrating different virus strains in a permissive cell culture system, as well as in animals. The ratio of plaque forming units per 50 percent lethal dose (pfu per LD$_{50}$) can then be compared for different virus variants (Figure 13.14).

Experimental manipulation of virulence

A prerequisite to the study of virulence is the availability of viral variants differing in their virulence phenotype. In some instances natural isolates may differ in virulence, for instance, serotype 1 and serotype 3 reoviruses, which vary remarkably in their biological properties even though reassortants between them are readily constructed. In many instances, laboratory manipulation must be used to obtain virulence variants.

PASSAGE IN ANIMAL HOSTS

In general, passage by a defined route in a particular species enhances the virulence of the virus when assessed under the conditions of passage, but often reduces the virulence in other animals or by alternate routes of infection. Human polioviruses on occasion have been adapted to mice; repeated mouse passage of monkey neurovirulent isolates produces variants that often have high intracerebral and intraspinal virulence

for mice, but may exhibit relatively low intracerebral virulence for monkeys (Racaniello 1988).

PASSAGE IN CELL CULTURE

Passage in cell culture frequently leads to the selection of attenuated virus strains. A prominent example was Theiler's successful search for an attenuated variant of yellow fever virus, culminating in the selection of the 17D strain (Theiler and Smith 1937). Experience with cell passage has led to several common observations: (1) apparently identical passage protocols can yield stocks with different degrees of attenuation so that there is an element of unpredictability in this approach to attenuation; (2) viral stocks often represent a swarm of genetically diverse variants that differ in their degree of attenuation; and (3) attenuated variants may be temperature sensitive even when they were not selected for this phenotype.

MUTAGENESIS AND TEMPERATURE-SENSITIVE MUTANTS

A standard strategy for the production of attenuated variants is the treatment of a virus with a mutagen. One convenient way to select mutants is to look for viral variants that are temperature sensitive (ts), and that will replicate well at the permissive temperature of 33–37°C, but not at an elevated nonpermissive temperature, such as 40°C, where the nonmutagenized parent virus will still replicate well. Many ts mutants have reduced virulence in animals. Reduced virulence is not necessarily a direct consequence of temperature sensitivity, since the body temperature of the host is frequently within the range of permissive temperatures. It is more likely that such ts mutants are also host range restricted in certain cell types even at the permissive temperature, thus explaining their in vivo attenuation. Although random mutagenesis is a convenient way to produce attenuated viruses, it has the drawback that there may be mutations in several viral genes that are silent in cell culture, but influence the in vivo phenotype, complicating conclusions about the mechanism of attenuation.

Many viruses can be cold adapted by passage at a reduced temperature (traditionally 25°C) and such variants are often attenuated in animals (Maassab and DeBorde 1985). Cold-adapted variants of influenza virus replicate as well at 37°C and much better at 25°C than wild-type virus, but are usually temperature sensitive at

Table **13.8** *Virulence expressed as the comparative ability of different strains of a virus to produce clinical illness*

Virus	Paralytic case rate per 1 000 000 primary infections (range)	Relative rates	Study period
Wild-type (mainly type 1)	7 000 (2 000–20 000)	~10 000	1931–1954
OPV (mainly type 3)	0.62	1	1961–1978

The paralytic rate following infection with wild-type polioviruses is compared to the rate following infection with attenuated oral polioviruses (OPV).
Data from Schonberger et al. 1976; Nathanson and Martin 1979; Nathanson 1984; Nkowane et al. 1987.

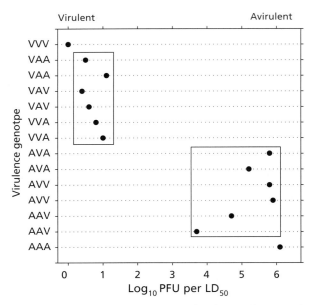

Figure 13.14 *Quantitative comparison of virulence using a panel of California serogroup viruses. Virulence is expressed as the ratio of plaque forming units per 50% lethal dose (pfu per LD$_{50}$) plotted on a log scale. Reassortants were made between a virulent (genotype VVV for the large, intermediate, and small gene segments, respectively) and an avirulent clone (genotype AAA). Reassortants bearing a large gene segment derived from the virulent parent had a virulent phenotype and those bearing a large segment derived from the avirulent parent had an avirulent phenotype (data from Griot et al. 1994).*

40°C, and have markedly reduced pneumopathogenicity when tested intranasally in ferrets. Cold-adapted influenza viruses have mutations in many or all of their eight gene segments, but reassortant viruses bearing only a few segments from cold-adapted variants exhibit the cold-adapted attenuated phenotype.

DESIGNED MUTATIONS

With the development of methods for introducing mutations into DNA, it has become possible to design mutants of many DNA and RNA viruses. Several different kinds of mutations can be introduced, including point mutations that result in substitution of a single or several individual amino acids, construction of genetic chimeras between two viral variants by exchange of genetic sequences, or inactivation of an open reading frame either by introduction of a stop codon, insertion of a selectable marker cassette, or deletion of part of the open reading frame. In some instances, noncoding domains of the viral genome carry major determinants of virulence, which can be mapped by similar methods (Almond 1991; Minor 1993; Racaniello et al. 1993).

An example of the use of these methods is provided by human and simian immunodeficiency viruses (HIV and SIV), where genetic modifications have been utilized to address various aspects of virulence (Levy 1998). For instance, chimeric viruses have been used to

map macrophage tropism to the *env* gene and point mutations have been used to map tropism within the fine structure of the V3 loop of the gp120 envelope protein. Introduced stop codons and deletions have been used to explore the role of the *nef* gene of SIV, with the finding that *nef* deletions do not affect the ability of the virus to replicate in cell culture, but markedly reduce the ability of a virulent clone, mac 239, to induce AIDS in rhesus monkeys (see below).

SELECTION OF ATTENUATED VARIANTS

In selecting variants of reduced virulence, several points should be kept in mind. First, as noted above, most virus pools consist of a mixture of variants, which may differ markedly in their biological phenotype. Thus, it is necessary to plaque purify and characterize a number of stocks prior to selecting virus variants for study. Secondly, the mutations of greatest interest are those that specifically impair virulence in vivo without affecting the ability of a virus to replicate in a defined reference cell culture system. Such mutants can be considered to be 'host range' variants in contrast to 'global' mutants that impair replication in all cell hosts.

With the development of panels of monoclonal antibodies for most viruses, it has become possible to select variants that escape neutralization. Such variants often represent point mutations and occur naturally at a frequency of about 10^{-5} depending on the virus (Steinhauer and Holland 1987). When a panel of such monoclonal antibody-resistant (MAR) variants are tested in vivo, it is often observed that a few of the escape mutants are attenuated. Variants selected in this manner generally have mutations in the viral attachment protein since this is the typical target of neutralizing monoclonal antibodies.

Pathogenic mechanisms of virulence

There are many sequential steps in a viral infection and a difference in the comparative replication of two virus variants at any one of these steps could explain their relative degrees of virulence. In practice, attenuated variants will usually replicate or spread less briskly in one or several tissues associated with the pathogenic process. Also, variant viruses may differ qualitatively in their cell and tissue tropism or in their mode of dissemination.

VIREMIA

A reduction in viremia can be an important mechanism for the reduction in virulence. An example is shown in Figure 13.8 that compares poliovirus strains of different virulence. The Mahoney strain of type 1 poliovirus caused a much higher viremia and paralytic rate than did several other strains that were less viremogenic.

NEURAL SPREAD

Rabies viruses are obligatory neurotropes and disseminate only by neural spread. The attenuation of rabies virus has been investigated using MAR mutants. Some of the MAR variants in one epitope group were markedly attenuated, and one attenuating mutation was mapped to a single amino acid residue (at position 333) in the rabies glycoprotein (Tuffereau et al. 1989). After intramuscular injection, an attenuated mutant spreads to the brain at a rate similar to virulent parent CVS virus, but within the central nervous system the attenuated clone spreads to relatively few neurons, while the virulent virus spreads rapidly to many contiguous neurons (Jackson 1991). The difference between virulent and attenuated MAR viruses lay in their differential efficiency of entry into neuronal cells, probably associated with differences in the binding of their glycoproteins to cellular receptors (Dietzschold et al. 1983).

TROPISM AND HOST RANGE

Different variants of a single virus can exhibit differences in their tropism for organs, tissues, and cell types, which confers a multidimensional character upon virulence. Thus, a variant virus may be reduced in its ability to cause one type of pathology but enhanced in its ability to cause another. Human immunodeficiency virus (HIV) presents an example of tropism differences (Table 13.9). Most strains of HIV can be classified into two categories, according to their ability to replicate in T-cell lines (T-tropic) or in primary macrophages (M-tropic) (Levy 1998). Tropism has been mapped to the V3 domain on the envelope glycoprotein (gp120) and is associated with coreceptor preference. HIV utilizes members of the chemokine receptor family as a coreceptor. M-tropic viruses preferentially utilize CCR5 while T-tropic viruses preferentially utilize CXCR4 as a coreceptor. Most viruses isolated shortly after infection are M-tropic, while most viruses isolated from patients with severe AIDS are T-tropic. It is inferred that M-tropic viruses are preferentially transmitted for reasons yet to be elucidated, while T-tropic viruses replicate preferentially in T lymphocytes, particularly in patients lacking immune defenses.

VIRULENCE FOR TARGET ORGANS

Different variants of a specific virus may show different degrees of virulence for a key target organ. The three attenuated strains of poliovirus used in the oral poliovirus vaccine provide an example (Table 13.10). The type 3 strain has the greatest virulence since it causes more cases of paralytic poliomyelitis in vaccine recipients than does either the type 1 or type 2 strains. The type 2 strain is clearly the most viremogenic in children. However, after intracerebral injection of monkeys, the type 3 strain produces very severe spinal cord lesions at a higher frequency than do the type 1 or type 2 strains. In this instance, virulence for the target organ (the spinal cord), rather than viremogenicity, appears to be the most important determinant of virulence after virus feeding.

TUMORIGENESIS

When applied to tumor viruses, virulence can be expressed in several different ways. The most common differences among the oncogenic viruses involve either the latent period from infection to development of a neoplasm, or the cell type that is transformed. In general, the transforming retroviruses can be divided into two major classes, according to whether they cause tumors with a long latency or are acutely transforming. The long latency viruses are often replication competent and do not carry a transduced oncogene. They act as insertional mutagens when their proviruses are integrated into the host DNA. On rare occasion, insertion occurs at a site where the promoter, enhancer, or terminator sequences in the viral genome can influence the transcriptional rate of a proto-oncogene. Up-regulation of such a proto-oncogene then leads to transformation of the infected cell, which can result in neoplasia usually after a long latency.

Murine leukemia viruses (MuLV) are replication-competent long latency oncogenic retroviruses. Different MuLV isolates induce different kinds of neoplasms, involving T lymphocytes, B lymphocytes, erythroid, or myeloid precursor cells. Genetic studies, including the production of viral chimeras, has mapped the genetic determinants to the viral U3 region, a

Table 13.9 *Isolates of a single virus may vary in their host range*

| Viral biotype | HIV-1 isolate | Growth in each cell type | | |
		Peripheral blood T lymphocytes	Monocyte-derived macrophages	T cell line Sup-T1
T-tropic	IIIB	++++	+	++++
	DV	++++	++	++++
M-tropic	SF162	++++	+++	−
	89.6	++++	+++	−

HIV (human immunodeficiency virus) strains can be classified into two major biotypes, M-tropic (replicating in macrophages) and T-tropic (replicating in T-lymphocyte cell lines) as shown for several different virus strains.
Data from Collman et al. 1989; Collman and Nathanson 1992.f

Table 13.10 *Virulence for the target organ appears to be the major determinant of the relative in vivo virulence of the three oral polio-virus vaccine strains.*

	Type 1	Type 2	Type 3
In vivo virulence (poliomyelitis in OPV recipients)	22	13	62
Viremogenicity (frequency of viremia)	0/16	17/19	0/16
Neurovirulence (percent severe lesions)	0.05%		1.15%

Top line. The type 3 vaccine strain causes paralytic poliomyelitis at a rate that is about threefold higher than the type 1 and fivefold higher than the type 2 strain. Cases of paralytic poliomyelitis in recipients of oral poliovirus vaccine (OPV), United States, 1961–1984. Data from Schonberger et al. 1976; Nkowane et al. 1987.
Middle line. The type 2 strain generates viremia more effectively than either of the other strains indicating that it has a much higher potential for invading the spinal cord. Frequency of viremia in infants fed oral poliovirus vaccine. Data from Horstmann et al. 1964.
Bottom line. On direct intraspinal injection of monkeys, the type 3 strain causes severe spinal cord lesions at a rate that is much higher than the rate associated with the type 1 strain. Data from Nathanson and Horn 1992.

noncoding part of the viral genome that is just upstream from the transcriptional start site and has a domain that contains a number of transcriptional enhancer sites (Hopkins et al. 1989). Tropism is thought to correlate with relative ability to replicate in different target cells, and this has been borne out, at least in part, by in vivo studies of the relative replication rates of different MuLVs in different tissues (Evans and Morrey 1987).

Genetic determinants of virulence

Viral virulence is encoded in the viral genome and expressed through structural proteins, nonstructural proteins, or noncoding sequences. A large body of information about virus variants has established several important points:

- The use of mutants has made it possible to identify the role of individual genes and proteins as determinants of the biological behavior of many viral variants.
- There is no 'master' gene or protein that determines virulence, and attenuation may be associated with changes in any of the structural or nonstructural proteins, or in the noncoding regions of the genome.
- The virulence phenotype can be altered by very small changes in the genome, if they occur at 'critical sites.' At such sites, a single point mutation leading to the substitution of a specific amino acid or base is often sufficient to alter virulence. For most viruses with small genomes (<20 kb) only a few discrete 'critical sites' have been discovered, usually fewer than 10 per genome.
- It is possible to create variants with attenuating mutations at several critical sites and these may be more attenuated than single point mutants. Also, reversion to virulence is less frequent in variants with several discrete attenuating mutations.
- Attenuating mutations are often host range mutations that affect replication in some cells, but not in others. This is partly a reflection of the fact that most well characterized mutants have been deliberately selected

because they replicate well in a standard cell culture system.
- Although many attenuating mutations have been sequenced, relatively few have been characterized at a biochemical or structural level as to their mechanism of action.

These generalizations may be illustrated with examples from a few selected virus groups.

POLIOVIRUSES

Polioviruses are single-stranded RNA viruses of positive polarity, with a genome that contains a relatively long 5' and a shorter 3' nontranslated region (NTR) flanking a single open reading frame of about 7 kb that encodes a single polyprotein that is cleaved into four structural proteins (VP1-VP4) and several nonstructural proteins.

Virulence studies have focused on the three attenuated strains of types 1, 2, and 3 poliovirus that constitute the oral poliovirus vaccine (OPV) originally developed by Sabin (1985). The three vaccine strains are about 10 000-fold less virulent than wild-type poliovirus (Table 13.8), and they can be compared to the wild-type viruses from which they were derived. However, the genomes of wild-type parental viruses and their vaccine progeny differ at a considerable number of sites (reflecting their complex passage history) and many of these differences are not relevant to the attenuated phenotype. Virulent revertants of the vaccine strains occur on passage in humans or in cell culture and are better suited to genetic analysis, since there are relatively few sequence differences between them and the vaccine strains. Using reverse genetics (Racaniello and Baltimore 1981), infectious DNA clones of poliovirus genomes can be used to construct chimeric viruses and these clones can then be transfected into permissive cells to reconstitute mutated infectious virus.

The 5' nontranslated region (NTR)

The attenuation of the vaccine strains of poliovirus is due to critical sites, both in the 5' NTR upstream from the long open reading frame and in selected structural and nonstructural proteins (Racaniello 1988; Minor 1992, 1993; Racaniello et al. 1993). Each of the three strains of OPV carry point mutations in the 5′ NTR, at positions 480, 481, or 472, in types 1, 2, and 3, respectively. Attenuating mutations at these sites are associated with reduced neurovirulence in monkeys, and reduced ability to replicate in the central nervous system of transgenic mice bearing the poliovirus receptor. Attenuated variants are temperature-sensitive host range mutants that replicate well in primate fibroblast cell lines, such as HeLa cells, but have reduced ability to replicate in neuroblastoma cells (La Monica and Racaniello 1989). The bases at attenuating sites in the 5′ NTR are thought to be involved in an RNA stem loop based on computer models of their predicted secondary structure. It is believed that the stem structure at positions 470–540 is involved in the binding of ribosomal complexes at the initiation of translation. Presumably, initiation factors must differ, either quantitatively or qualitatively, in different cell types to explain the cellular host range restriction of the vaccine strains.

Structural or nonstructural proteins

Each of the OPV strains carries at least one mutation that is associated with an alteration in a viral structural or nonstructural protein and confers temperature sensitivity and reduced neurovirulence, and these mutations involve different proteins for the three OPV strains. For type 1 OPV, mutations associated with increased virulence are found in the virus capsid proteins, and in the nonstructural 3D polymerase (Bouchard et al. 1995; Georgescu et al. 1995). For type 2 OPV, it appears that neurovirulence in the mouse is associated with virus capsid protein VP1 (Ren et al. 1991; Macadam et al. 1993). For type 3 OPV, sites in virus capsid proteins VP3 and VP1 confer temperature sensitivity and neuroattenuation (Tatem et al. 1992). It is not clear how mutations in the structural proteins produce attenuation, but it has been suggested that these are involved in structural transitions that occur either during virion assembly or virion uncoating.

BUNYAVIRUSES

Bunyaviruses are negative-strand (or ambisense) RNA viruses with a trisegmented genome. The large (L) RNA segment encodes the viral polymerase; the middle (M) RNA segment encodes two glycoproteins (G1 and G2) and a nonstructural protein, Ns_m; the small (S) segment encodes the nucleoprotein (N) and a nonstructural protein, Ns_s. Most studies of virulence have utilized members of the California serogroup that will reassort readily with each other. Beginning with two parent viruses, panels of reassortants containing all possible combinations of gene segments can be constructed. In addition, monoclonal antibody-resistant (MAR) mutants

have been used to identify variants in the major G1 glycoprotein that are associated with differences in virulence. Attenuation can involve either the ability of the virus to replicate in the central nervous system (neurovirulence) or its ability to cause viremia and reach the central nervous system (neuroinvasiveness).

The middle RNA segment and glycoprotein G1

A detailed comparison has been made of two California serogroup viruses, wild-type La Crosse virus and a laboratory passaged strain of Tahyna virus which exhibited reduced neuroinvasiveness, but high neurovirulence (Griot et al. 1993a). The reduction in neuroinvasiveness of the attenuated virus is associated with low viremogenicity that, in turn, is associated with a reduced ability to replicate in striated muscle, the major extraneural site of replication of this group of viruses. Attenuation maps to the M RNA segment encoding the viral glycoproteins suggesting that there is an alteration in the entry phase of infection of myocytes (but not of neurons). These viruses plaqued equally well on BHK-21 cells. However, on a murine myocyte cell line (C2C12), viral variants bearing the M RNA segment of the attenuated parent failed to plaque while variants bearing the M RNA segment of the virulent parent plaqued well (Griot et al. 1994).

MAR mutants of La Crosse virus are readily obtained, using antibodies directed against the major (G1) glycoprotein, and a mutant at one epitope site (but not at other sites) exhibited reduced neuroinvasiveness with wild-type neurovirulence (Gonzalez-Scarano et al. 1985). Furthermore, the attenuated clone showed strikingly reduced fusion efficiency at acid pH compared to parental wildtype La Crosse virus. These observations suggested that attenuation might be associated with an alteration in glycoprotein G1 that reduced efficiency in the infection of myocytes.

The large RNA segment and the viral polymerase

An attenuated California serogroup virus clone, B.5, obtained by passage in BHK-21 cells, showed a striking reduction in its ability to replicate in the central nervous system of adult mice. Using reassortant analysis (Figure 13.14) clone B.5 was shown to bear an attenuated L RNA segment (Endres et al. 1990). This clone is a temperature-sensitive host range mutant that replicates poorly in C1300 NA neuroblastoma and other murine cell lines, although it grows well in BHK-21 cells. Presumably, clone B.5 has a mutant polymerase that restricts viral replication in neurons and certain other cell types.

REOVIRUSES

Reoviruses are double-stranded ten-segmented RNA viruses. The gene segments and the proteins that they encode have been characterized in detail. The large number of segments have made reoviruses an attractive model system for study of the genetic determinants of viral phenotypes (Virgin et al. 1997). These studies have been facilitated by major differences in the biological phenotypes of naturally occurring reovirus serotypes, particularly serotypes 1 and 3. Table 13.11 illustrates the use of reassortants to map virulence phenotypes to reovirus gene segments.

Biological functions have been ascribed to many of the reovirus genes and proteins. Most of the virulence determinants represent qualitative differences between type 1 Lang and type 3 Dearing (T1L and T3D) in tissue and organ tropism rather than quantitative differences in disease severity.

- The S1 segment encodes the σ1 protein, which is the viral attachment protein that binds to receptors on permissive cells, and is a major target for neutralizing and hemagglination inhibiting (HI) antibodies. T1L and T3D viruses differ markedly in the disease that they cause in suckling mice. T1L disseminates through the blood and causes an ependymitis in the brain, while T3D disseminates through the neural route and causes a neuronotropic encephalitis in the brain. The S1 segment is the major determinant of dissemination and brain cell tropism (Table 13.11). In addition, the S1 segment is a determinant of replication in cardiac myocytes and myocarditis, of replication levels in the intestine, and of differences in reovirus strains to induce apoptosis and perturb the cell cycle.
- The M1 segment encoding the μ2 protein influences replication in cardiac myocytes and myocarditis.

- The M2 segment encoding the μ1 protein affects the protease sensitivity of the virion, and quantitative neurovirulence.
- The L1 segment encoding λ3 protein influences replication in cardiac myocytes and myocarditis.
- The L2 segment encoding λ2 protein acts as a guanylyl transferase in cell culture and influences replication levels in the intestine, titers of shed virus, and horizontal transmission between mice.

Viral virulence genes of cellular origin

Since 1985 a new class of virus-encoded proteins has been recognized that contribute to the virulence of viruses by mimicking normal cellular proteins (McFadden 1995). This group of 'cell-derived' genes has been identified primarily within the genomes of large DNA viruses that probably have a greater capacity to maintain accessory genes than do viruses with small genomes. Because these genes are homologues of cellular genes, it is hypothesized that they were acquired by recombination and modification. Thus, from an evolutionary viewpoint, they resemble viral oncogenes.

Cell-derived viral genes encode proteins that enhance virulence by many different mechanisms. 'Virokines' are secreted from virus-infected cells and mimic cytokines, thereby perturbing normal host responses. 'Viroceptors' resemble cellular receptors for cytokines (including antibodies or complement components) that are thereby diverted from their normal cellular targets. Some virus-encoded proteins interfere with antigen presentation and

Table 13.11 *Mapping virulence to a specific viral gene segment*

Pattern of spread	Outer capsid gene segments			Core gene segments					Nonstructural gene segments		Clone
	M2	S1	S4	L2	L1	L3	M1	S2	M3	S3	
Viremia	L	L	L	L	L	L	L	L	L	L	T1L
	D	L	L	L	L	L	L	L	D	D	R
	L	L	L	D	D	D	D	D	L	D	R
	L	L	D	L	L	L	L	L	L	L	R
	D	L	D	D	D	D	D	D	D	D	R
	D	L	L	D	D	D	L	D	D	D	R
	D	L	D	D	D	D	D	D	L	D	R
Neural	D	D	D	D	D	D	D	D	D	D	T3D
	D	D	D	D	D	D	D	D	D	L	R
	L	D	L	L	D	L	L	L	L	L	R
	L	D	L	L	L	L	L	L	L	L	R
	L	D	L	D	L	L	L	L	L	L	R

The *S1* gene segment of reovirus determines whether the virus spreads by viremia or by the neural route, since it was the only gene segment that cosegregated with the mode of spread. Two viruses, type 1 Lang (T1L) and type 3 Dearing (T3D) were used to derive reassortant clones (R) that were genotyped (L or D indicates origin of each gene segment) and were tested for their mode of spread. Adapted from Tyler et al. 1986.

immune induction (Smith et al. 1997; Lafon 2002; Jackson and Ramsay 2001), while others prevent apoptosis or interrupt intracellular signalling initiated by cytokines or interferons. A brief review of selected cell-derived genes that have been described for pox and herpes viruses will serve as examples of this group of viral genes and illustrate how they contribute to viral virulence.

POXVIRUSES

Tumor induction

Several poxviruses cause either benign or malignant tumors. However, it appears that the mechanism of oncogenesis is different from that associated with classic DNA or RNA tumor viruses, since there is no evidence that viral sequences are incorporated into the genome of transformed cells. Virus strains may gain or lose tumorigenicity quite independent of their ability to replicate, and continued productive replication of the virus appears to be required for tumor growth. It was postulated in the 1960s that these viruses might produce a growth factor that accounted for their induction of tumors (Kato et al. 1963). A large body of research has now documented that several poxviruses encode a protein that can be classified as a member of the epidermal growth factor (EGF)-like family of growth factors (McFadden et al. 1995). Shope fibroma virus and malignant rabbit fibroma virus both encode a very similar protein (Shope fibroma growth factor (SFGF)), while myxoma virus encodes a related myxoma growth factor (MGF). These proteins contain the shared functional domains (six characteristically spaced cysteines) shared by members of the EGF family. Furthermore, when these genes are deleted from the virus genomes, the MGF-negative or SFGF-negative viruses replicated normally in cell culture, but showed much reduced ability to induce tumors in rabbits (Opgenorth et al. 1992).

Receptors for tumor necrosis factor

Tumor necrosis factor (TNF) is a potent pro-inflammatory cytokine that is produced by activated macrophages and T cells. TNF acts by binding to a class of cellular receptors that are type 1 integral membrane proteins characterized by multiple cysteine-rich exodomains. Through their receptors on myeloid and lymphoid cells, the TNFs exert complex pleiotropic effects on immune networks and host responses to infection. A number of poxviruses encode a protein designated T2 that is a soluble form of the cellular p75 TNF receptor (Smith and Goodwin 1995). It is presumed that this protein binds free TNF, thereby modulating TNF-mediated cellular responses to infection. It is postulated that T2 could enhance replication of poxviruses in vivo by down-modulating the antiviral defenses of the infected host, although T2 might simultaneously favor the host by reducing the severity of virus-induced inflammatory lesions.

Vaccinia virus complement control protein (VCP)

The complement system is a complex group of proteins that act in a cascade that forms one of the initial host defenses against microbial pathogens. The system is a potent one that, uncontrolled, has the potential to cause severe damage, and is therefore tightly regulated by several different mechanisms, including C4-BP, a plasma protein that binds C4b2a, one of the complexes formed in the course of complement activation. Vaccinia virus encodes a protein, vaccinia virus complement control protein or VCP, that is homologous to C4-BP (Isaacs and Moss 1995). VCP binds human C4b and a VCP−mutant of vaccinia virus fails to inhibit complement-mediated lysis of sensitized sheep erythrocytes, while wild-type vaccinia virus has an inhibitory effect (Kotwal et al. 1990). When wild-type and VCP− vaccinia viruses were compared in vivo, the VCP− mutant was less virulent upon intracerebral injection of mice and, as shown in Figure 13.15, produced smaller skin lesions after intradermal inoculation in rabbits (Isaacs et al. 1992).

HERPES SIMPLEX VIRUSES

Herpes simplex virus (HSV) complement receptors

The importance of the complement cascade and its regulation already have been mentioned. C3b, one of the intermediates in the cascade, plays a key role in initiating the formation of the membrane attack complex (the last part of the complement cascade) so that its regulation is important. A number of cell types,

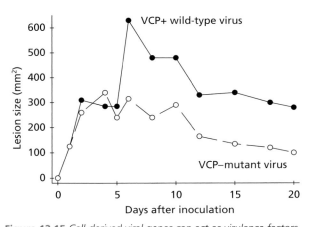

Figure 13.15 *Cell-derived viral genes can act as virulence factors. The skin lesions (median of three rabbits) produced by a wild-type vaccinia virus expressing the vaccinia complement control gene (VCP+) are more extensive than the lesions caused by the same virus from which the gene had been deleted (VCP−) (data from Isaacs et al. 1992).*

including monocytes/macrophages, neutrophils, and some T cells, express receptors for C3b, that down-modulate the complement cascade by reducing the levels of C3b and enhancing its inactivation by cleavage to iC3b. Glycoprotein C (gC) of HSV-1 binds C3b and iC3b, thereby providing protection against complement-mediated neutralization of HSV, and against complement-mediated lysis of HSV-infected cells (Harris et al. 1990; York and Johnson 1995). Although it has not yet been demonstrated that gC− mutants are less virulent in vivo, the conservation of gC in natural isolates of HSV suggests that this protein (and its complement-binding activity) play a role in HSV survival in nature.

HSV Fc receptors

HSV-infected cells express receptors (FcR) for the Fc domain of the immunoglobulin (IgG) molecule (Baucke and Spear 1979). A considerable body of work (York and Johnson 1995) has identified glycoproteins gE and gI of HSV as the molecules that bind IgG. It has been suggested that the presence of Fc receptors on the HS virion or on the surface of virus-infected cells would lead to bipolar bridging of the IgG molecule that might reduce secondary effects of antibody binding, such as the ability to initiate the complement cascade. Comparison of an FcR-deficient mutant, expressing an altered gE protein, with wild-type HSV, has shown that FcR-deficient virus is more susceptible to complement-mediated neutralization and lysis of virus-infected cells, as shown in Figure 13.16 (Frank and Friedman 1989; Dubin et al. 1991). Furthermore, gE− HSV exhibits reduced virulence in mice (Rajcani et al. 1990).

PERSISTENT INFECTIONS

A number of viruses are capable of producing infections that persist for the lifetime of the host (Ahmed and Chen 1999). In order to persist, a virus must achieve a delicate balance such that it maintains its genome without killing the host. In addition, the virus must evade immune surveillance mechanisms that are sufficiently potent to be able to clear many acute viral infections (Ploegh 1998).

Immune clearance of acute virus infections

If the duration of an acute infection is defined as the time between acquisition of infection to total clearance, then length ranges from about 1 week (for rhinoviruses) to about 6 months (for hepatitis B virus). Before considering immune evasion, it is useful to recapitulate briefly the mechanisms by which the immune response eliminates an acute infection. Effector T lymphocytes with specificity for the antigenic determinants of an infecting virus can destroy virus-infected cells, produce antiviral

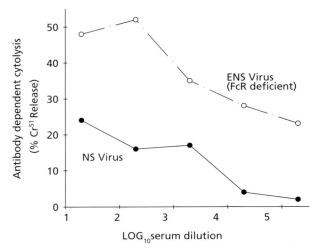

Figure 13.16 *Cell-derived viral genes can act as virulence factors. Glycoprotein gE of herpes simplex virus, which functions as an Fc receptor (FcR), influences the susceptibility of HSV-infected cells to antibody-dependent cell-mediated cytotoxity (ADCC). Target cells infected with the NS (FcR+) strain of HSV show lower percent lysis than cells infected with an FcR-deficient mutant of NS virus (strain ENS), indicating that the viral-encoded FcR can reduce the susceptibility of HSV-infected cells to ADCC (data from Dubin et al. 1991).*

cytokines, such as interferon, and recruit phagocytic cells to the sites of infection. B lymphocytes differentiate into plasma cells that secrete antiviral antibodies which can neutralize virions, initiate complement-mediated virolysis, and opsonize virus so that it is efficiently phagocytosed (Figure 13.5) (Binder and Griffin 2001). To persist, a virus must evade these mechanisms (Igarishi et al. 1999).

Mechanisms of persistence

Many different genera of both RNA and DNA viruses include members that can cause persistent infections. Furthermore, the same viruses may cause either acute self-limited or persistent infections, depending upon the circumstances of infection. Lytic viruses that kill the cells in which they replicate tend to use different strategies than nonlytic viruses that can be shed from cells over long periods of time without cell death. The strategies of persistence can be classified into three major categories, which are outlined in Figure 13.17. For each viral strategy, there is a corresponding strategy for evasion of the immune response.

- *High titer replication* requires that virus either be noncytocidal or that there is rapid replacement by cellular proliferation of target cells. Immune surveillance is unable to eliminate the virus, due to tolerance, immune complex formation, viral mutation, or another mechanism.
- *Latency* requires that the viral genome can persist in a nonreplicating mode, either integrated into the

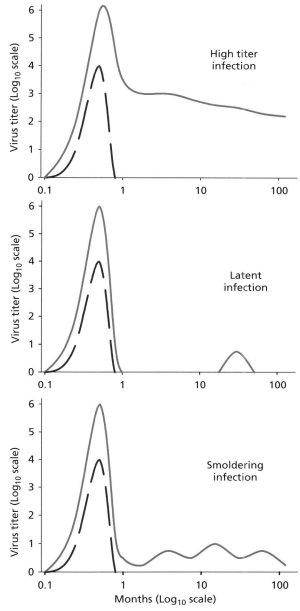

Figure 13.17 *Patterns of virus persistence. For reference, an acute infection is shown by dashed line in all panels.* High titer infection: *An acute phase is often apparent, following which the titer drops but persists at a high level for a long time.* Latent infection: *An acute infection is followed by disappearance of replicating virus which persists only as a latent genome. Periodic recrudescence occurs, during which replication of the virus may be accompanied by signs of disease, followed by another period of latency. Intervals between recrudescences may last from weeks to many years, and some infected individuals may never experience a recrudescence.* Smoldering infection: *An acute infection of varying severity is followed by marked reduction in overt virus replication, but infectious virus may be frequently recovered indicating that true latency has not occurred (after Nathanson et al. 2002).*

genome of the host cell or as an episome. Immune surveillance may be competent to eliminate the virus which can be activated but can only replicate for brief

intervals. Alternately, recurrence may be associated with intermittent reduction of immune defenses.

- *Smoldering infections* involve continuous productive infection and cell-to-cell transmission at a low level. Usually, potentially effective immune surveillance is circumvented by mechanisms such as antigenic variation, infectious immune complexes, or intercellular bridges.

HIGH-TITER PERSISTENT INFECTIONS

Nonlytic viruses

Many viruses can replicate productively without causing cell death, and a number of them can cause persistent infections. In such instances, the initial dynamics resemble those of an acute infection, following which the virus titer decreases somewhat, but then reaches a setpoint that may be maintained indefinitely or gradually decline. Examples of this pattern are hepatitis B virus HBV and lymphocytic choriomeningitis virus (LCMV) of mice (Buchmeier and Zajac 1999).

High-titer persistence is often characterized by tolerance, an apparent absence of virus-specific immunity. The mechanisms by which the tolerance can be induced include deletion of forbidden clones of naive T lymphocytes in the thymus and exhaustion of peripheral virus-specific T lymphocytes in the presence of excess antigen. Tolerance may be limited to specific components of the effector limb of the immune response. For instance, hepatitis B virus persistence is characterized by absence of antiviral antibody against HbsAg while anti-HBcAg may be induced. LCMV persistence is characterized by absence of cellular immune responses while virus-specific antibody is produced. The presence of persistent high titers of virions and viral antigens may overwhelm either antibody or CD8[+] lymphocytes, so that assays must be interpreted with caution. Thus, in persistently infected mice, anti-LCMV antibodies circulate as immune complexes and not as free antibody, which originally led to the mistaken view that antibody was not induced in persistently infected mice.

Evidence for the role of immune tolerance in maintaining viral persistence is provided by the experimental termination of persistence by intravenous injection of virus-specific CD8[+] cells. Figure 13.18, summarizing an experiment with LCMV, exemplifies this phenomenon. Similar results have been obtained with HBV, where CTLs specific for HBs epitopes cleared virus from hepatocytes.

Lytic viruses

It is unusual for high titer persistence to be produced by a cytolytic virus, but the primate lentiviruses represent an important exception. Figure 13.19 shows the persistent viremia produced by simian immunodeficiency virus (SIV). The main target cells for these lentiviruses are

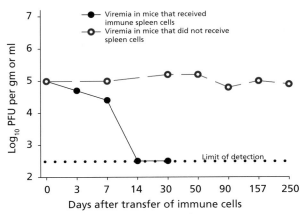

Figure 13.18 *Immune T lymphocytes can clear a persistent virus infection, implying that (in some instances) persistence involves escape from the cellular arm of the immune response. In this example, LCMV causes persistent lifelong infection of mice. When such mice are treated by adoptive immunization of CTLs from an immune donor ($10^{7.3}$ spleen cells from adult mice immunized by infection 60 days prior to transfer), the virus is cleared. The specificity of the process is shown by the requirement for syngeneic donor lymphocytes and by the ability of clones of $CD8^+$ T lymphocytes specific for an individual viral epitope to clear infection. The rate of clearance differs for different organs and tissues, implying some differences in the action of effector cells and in the mechanisms of immune evasion (after Ahmed et al. 1987).*

$CD4^+$ lymphocytes which undergo lytic infection. It has been calculated that the continuous destruction of $CD4^+$ cells results in a reduction of the average half-life of these cells from 75 to 25 days. However, the bone marrow is able to respond to the abnormal rate of destruction by increasing the production of naive $CD4^+$

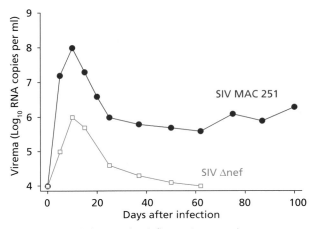

Figure 13.19 *Viral genes that influence immune clearance can alter in vivo infection. SIV mac 251 wildtype is compared with a mutant engineered to delete the nef gene, a regulatory gene that reduces expression of MHC class I molecules on the plasma membrane, permitting escape of virus-infected cells from immune attack. The figure shows the typical course of viremia in individual animals infected with wild-type and Δnef viruses (after Connor et al., 1998).*

cells, at a rate sufficient to maintain a reasonable concentration of circulating $CD4^+$ cells. The compensatory replenishment of target cells permits this generally lytic virus to persist at a high titer for an extended period of time, although eventually the bone marrow is unable to compensate and CD4 levels drop, leading to functional immunodeficiency.

In contrast to most high-titer persistent infections, lentiviruses induce immune responses rather than tolerance. The immune response to lentiviruses is quite effective, as judged by its ability to rapidly contain the acute phase of infection, resulting in a reduction from peak viremia at about 6 weeks to a setpoint at about 3–6 months which may be as much as 1 000-fold lower than the peak viremia. Once this setpoint is reached, a dynamic equilibrium is established between virus production and clearance. The half-life of individual SIV virions is <30 min in the absence of immunity and about 10 min in infected animals with an established immune response. It has been calculated that to maintain virus titers of 10^2 to 10^4 infectious virions per ml plasma requires the production of 10^{10} to 10^{12} new infectious virions daily. In this instance, high titer persistence is maintained by an extraordinary rate of virus production that exceeds the rate at which a potent immune response can clear the virus.

LATENCY

Latent infections are produced by a considerable number of herpesviruses, including herpes simplex viruses (HSV), varicella-zoster virus (VZV), Epstein–Barr virus (EBV), and cytomegalovirus (CMV) of humans. There is a characteristic sequence of events following primary infection. Initially the virus replicates in permissive cells at the portal of entry. The virus is lytic and destroys permissive target cells. Once immune induction has occurred, the virus is cleared and appears to be eliminated.

However, the viral genome persists in a latent form. Latency occurs in one or more cell types – such as neurons – that are distinct from the permissive cell types that support productive lytic infection. Neurons appear to be restrictive or permissive, depending upon their physiological state (Stevens 1994). Under conditions of restriction, the virus undergoes the early steps of entry and uncoating, but further steps in replication are blocked. In the absence of active replication, the viral genome is maintained in one of several forms, depending upon the specific virus and host cell. In some instances, the double-stranded DNA genome integrates into the host genome, while in other examples the genome persists as a non-integrated episome, in the nucleus or cytoplasm.

If latency occurs in cell types such as neurons that do not divide, then there is no need to replicate the latent genome. If the latent genome is maintained in dividing cells, then the genome must be replicated or it will be diluted to extinction. If the genome is integrated into the host genome then it will be automatically replicated during the cell cycle. Episomal DNA can also be replicated by the enzymes involved in copying cellular genomes. However, there are no parallel mechanisms for RNA, so RNA viruses cannot assume a latent state unless they undergo reverse transcription to DNA intermediates. Latent viral genomes can be detected by in situ polymerase chain reaction (PCR) methods that – at their most sensitive – can detect as little as one genome per infected cell.

Latency maintains the viral genome for the lifetime of the infected host. Activation of latent infections occur at irregular intervals, and may never occur in some infected individuals. Activation of latent genomes can be initiated by a number of stimuli, characteristic for each virus. For instance, herpes simplex virus (HSV) can be activated by fever, sunburn, and trigeminal nerve injury. Most of these stimuli appear to act upon the primary sensory neurons in which latent HSV genomes are maintained. However, on occasion, waning of the immune response can serve as a trigger for activation of some herpesviruses.

Following reactivation of HSV, the viral genome may be transported by axoplasmic spread in both centripetal and centrifugal directions. Centrifugal spread, toward the periphery, conducts the virus to the skin where it may replicate and spread, causing herpes labialis (fever blister or cold sore). After spreading for a few days, host defenses prevent further spread, and the skin lesion heals. Centripetal spread from the trigeminal ganglion conducts the HSV genome to the central nervous system, where, in some instances, it can spread to cause an encephalitis that may be devastating.

Typically, viruses that cause latent infections induce a brisk and potent immune response that clears the initial infection. However, latently infected cells do not express viral proteins, permitting escape from immune surveillance. Furthermore, when the latent infection is activated, immune surveillance limits its spread. Latent viruses cannot be spread from host to host, but virus produced during activation may be spread to another host. For instance, activation of latent varicella zoster virus (VZV) produces characteristic skin lesions in older adults. Seronegative children exposed to virus aerosolized from these lesions can develop chicken pox, the primary form of VZV infection.

SMOLDERING INFECTIONS

Smoldering infections fall between the extremes of high titer persistence and latency. Infectious virus is produced, but at minimal levels that may require special methods for detection and isolation. Virus continues to spread from infected to uninfected cells, but often at an indolent tempo. If the virus is pathogenic, it may produce a gradually progressive chronic disease

(McCune 2001). There is a detectable immune response to the virus and, in some instances, the response may be hypernormal, due to the continuous presence of viral antigens. The ability of a virus to spread in the presence of a potentially effective immune response is a paradoxical phenomenon, and involves a variety of strategies several of which may operate in any given example (Billeter et al. 1994; Cattaneo et al. 1987). Some of the more important strategies are described below.

Immunologically privileged sites

There are a few organs and tissues that favor virus persistence, particularly the brain and kidney. The brain has classically been considered an immunologically privileged site because immunological effector mechanisms may spare cells bearing foreign antigens if these cells are located in the brain (in contrast to foreign cells in other sites). There are at least two factors that account for virus persistence in the brain. First, the blood–brain barrier limits the trafficking of lymphocytes through the brain and, secondly, neurons express little if any MHC class I molecules rendering them relatively poor targets for virus-specific cytolytic T lymphocytes (CTL).

The kidney is the other tissue that frequently harbors persistent viruses, such as JC and BK polyomaviruses, and cytomegalovirus. Also, LCMV is cleared more slowly from the kidney than from other tissues, even the brain. However, there is no clear explanation why virus in the kidney should be able to evade immunological surveillance, although it has been speculated that lymphocytes may not readily cross the subendothelial basement membrane to access infected glomerular epithelial cells.

Intercellular bridges

In some instances, the process of entry of viruses into cells can be shortcircuited, so that a transient intercellular bridge is formed. Intercellular bridges permit the viral genome to pass from cell to cell without having to survive in the extracellular environment (Figure 13.20), thus providing a means of avoiding neutralizing antibody. This phenomenon is probably operative in a progressive fatal disease called subacute sclerosing panencephalitis (SSPE). In SSPE a defective variant of measles or rubella virus spreads gradually from neuron to neuron in spite of extraordinarily high titers of neutralizing antibody in the extracellular fluid of the brain parenchyma (Cattaneo et al. 1987; Billeter et al. 1994).

Suppression of MHC class I expression

A number of viruses, including adenoviruses and lentiviruses, encode specific proteins that are capable of down-regulating the expression of MHC class I mole-

Spread by extracellular virions

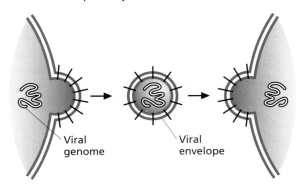

Viral
genome

Viral
envelope

Spread by intercellular bridge

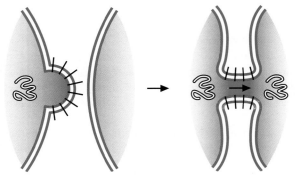

Figure 13.20 *Cell-to-cell transmission of a virus by intercellular bridges, a hypothetical reconstruction. Top, normal cell-to-cell spread of an enveloped virus as free extracellular virions. Bottom, cell-to-cell spread of the viral genome through a transient intercellular bridge. This phenomenon has been invoked to explain the spread of measles and rubella viruses during persistent infection of the brain.*

cules (Brodsky et al. 1999). Virus-infected target cells are rendered relatively less sensitive to virus-specific CTL attack, permitting them to continue to produce virions for an extended period of time.

Infectious immune complexes

In some instances where a virus persists in the presence of an active immune response, infectivity in the blood circulates in the form of immune complexes that are composed of infectious virions coated by virus-specific antibodies. Immune complexes can be demonstrated by the addition of anti-IgG antisera that will neutralize the infectivity. The molecular mechanism by which an antibody-coated virion can retain its infectivity has never been well elucidated. One possibility is that the complex is bound to Fc receptors on macrophages and internalized in vacuoles in which the complex dissociates, followed by infection of the macrophage. Consistent with this hypothesis, several of the persistent viruses (lymphocytic choriomeningitis virus, lactic dehy-

drogenase virus, and Aleutian disease virus) for which infectious complexes have been demonstrated, target macrophages as a major host cell.

Antigenic variation

During the course of persistent infection, there may be a selection for viral variants that are able to escape neutralization (Lutley et al. 1983). This phenomenon has been observed with several persistent lentiviruses such visna/maedi virus of sheep and equine infectious anemia virus. Equine infectious anemia virus (EIAV) is a lentivirus that produces a lifelong persistent infection of horses – the virus may be isolated from the blood even though the animals develop neutralizing antibody. Newly infected horses undergo discrete episodes of acute anemia, associated with bursts of viral replication. In each instance, the virus isolated during the episode of illness resists neutralization by serum obtained at the time of virus isolation (Table 13.12). However, the same serum can neutralize virus isolated at earlier times in infection. In other words, there is sequential replacement of virus with newly emerging variants that can escape neutralization. Ponies that survive repeated episodes of illness finally develop such a broad neutralization response that they can suppress all potential variants, thereby modulating, but not clearing, the smoldering infection. A similar evolution of virus during persistent infection has recently been shown to be a common phenomenon in persistent HIV-1 infections (Richman et al. 2003).

Escape mutants can also be selected by the cellular immune response (Aebischer and Mokophidis 1991; Allen et al. 2000; Ciurea et al. 2001). Most evidence for this phenomenon has been derived from experimental models (Schmitz et al. 1999; Evans et al. 1999; Allen et al. 2000), but it is possible that similar mechanisms play a role in naturally occurring persistent infections. Figure 13.21 shows an example where a macaque successfully immunized was able to contain a virulent challenge virus until a breakthrough occurred (Barouche et al. 2002). Analysis of viral isolates demonstrated that the breakthrough was associated with the emergence of a point mutation in the immunodominant epitope that was responsible for cellular immune control of infection.

Persistent viral infections often cause chronic diseases (McCune 2001). Some representative examples are set forth in Table 13.13.

HOST DETERMINANTS OF SUSCEPTIBILITY AND RESISTANCE

The outcome of the virus–host interaction is determined in part by host variables that can be conveniently considered under two categories, physiological factors and genetic determinants.

Table 13.12 *A smoldering infection associated with antigenic variation of the persistent virus*

Virus isolate (day of infection)	Fever spike (day of infection)	Neutralization index (log$_{10}$) of serum collected on the indicated day after infection					
		0 days	20 days	44 days	62 days	83 days	155 days
0 days		0	0	0.7	2.5	3.2	3.2
20 days	21	0	0	1.0	1.5	1.5	2.5
44 days	44	0	0	0	3.5	5.4	>5.4
62 days	62	0	0	0	0	2.0	2.0
83 days	83	0	0	0	0	0	3.5
155 days	155	0	0	0	0	0	0

Equine infectious anemia virus (EIAV) infection is associated with periodic febrile episodes. One infected horse experienced several fever spikes each lasting about 5 days, during which virus was isolated from the blood and was subsequently tested for neutralizability. Each virus isolate was neutralized by sera collected after the time of the isolate, but not by sera collected at or prior to the time of isolation. Likewise, each serum neutralized all the virus isolates made prior to the date of the serum, but none of the isolates made thereafter. This is evidence of continual antigenic drift of the virus, which probably explains the burst of replication associated with each fever spike, as well as the persistence of the virus in the face of an active neutralization response. After Kono et al. 1973.

Physiological factors

The host response to a viral infection may be influenced by a variety of physiological variables such as age, sex, stress, and pregnancy, all of which have been shown to influence the outcome of infection with some viruses (Brinton 1996). Age is perhaps the most consistently important variable in this category.

In general, very young animals are more susceptible than adult hosts to acute viral infections, and are more likely to undergo severe or fatal illness (Jubelt et al. 1980; Ogata et al. 1991; Tucker et al. 1993). However, it is important to recognize that in most mammalian species, young animals born of immune mothers receive maternal antibody either in utero by the transplacental route and/or postnatally, in colostrum and milk, or both. Furthermore, newborns have a special transport system that permits them to absorb intact immunoglobulin from the gut lumen into the circulation. The innate high susceptibility of infants born of non-immune mothers is revealed only in those rare instances where a virus has disappeared from an isolated community so that all age groups lack immune protection. A classical example is measles, which can be a devastating disease with a mortality of up to 25 percent in non-immune infants (Panum 1940; Morely 1969), but which is relatively benign in most societies where almost all women of childbearing age have acquired active immunity from natural infection or from measles vaccine. The mechanisms of enhanced susceptibility of newborn animals have been obscure, but recently it has been shown that an alphavirus induces apoptosis in neurons of newborn mice, but does not kill neurons from older mice in which enhanced expression of the cellular oncogene, bcl-2, blocks apoptosis (Levine et al. 1993).

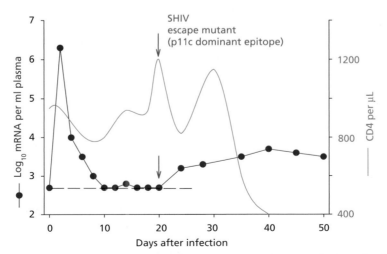

Figure 13.21 *Selection of viral variants that can escape the cellular immue response is one mechanism of viral persistence. In this example a monkey was immunized with a potent vaccine against SHIV (chimeric SIV–HIV virus) and then infected with a virulent SHIV strain. The monkey contained the infection quite effectively until the SHIV broke through due to emergence of a SHIV variant with a point mutation in an immunodominant epitope (data from Barouche et al. 2002).*

Table 13.13 *Diseases associated with persistent viral infections, selected examples*

Virus family/genus	Virus	Host	Disease
Oncogenic viruses			
Retroviridae	MuLV	Mice	Hematopoietic, lymphoreticular neoplasms
Hepadnaviridae	HBV	Humans	Hepatocellular carcinoma
Papillomaviridae	HPV	Humans	Cervical carcinoma
Herpesviridae	EBV	Humans	Burkitt's lymphoma
High titer persistence			
Arenaviridae	LCMV	Mice	Glomerulonephritis, vasculitis
Parvoviridae	Aleutian disease	Mink	Glomerulonephritis, vasculitis
Latent infections			
Herpesviridae	HSV	Humans	Cold sores, encephalitis
	CMV	Humans	Pneumonitis, retinitis, encephalitis
	EBV	Humans	Mononucleosis
	VZV	Humans	Herpes zoster
Smoldering infections			
Morbillivirus	Measles virus	Humans	Subacute sclerosing panencephalitis
	CDV	Dogs	Encephalitis, demyelination
Retrovirus	HTLV I	Humans	Tropical spastic paraparesis
Polyomavirus	JC	Humans	Progressive multifocal leukoencephalopathy
Lentivirus	VMV	Sheep	Interstitial pneumonitis, demyelination
	EIAV	Horses	Episodic hemolytic anemia
	HIV	Humans	AIDS

JC, the initials of the patient from whom virus was isolated; EIAV, equine infectious anemia virus; CDV, canine distemper virus; CMV, cytomegalovirus; EBV, Epstein–Barr virus; HBV, hepatitis B virus; HIV, human immunodeficiency virus; HTLV-1, human T cell leukemia virus; LCMV, lymphocytic choriomeningitis virus; MuLV, murine leukemia virus; VMV, visna maedi virus; VZV, varicella zoster virus.

Less commonly, advanced age can also be associated with increased susceptibility to viral infection. St. Louis encephalitis is an example of this phenomenon (Table 13.14). In one epidemic, the ratio of encephalitis cases to infections was about 0.2 per 1 000 for children aged 0–9 years and about 3.0 per 1 000 for adults aged 60 and over. Another example is varicella zoster virus, which usually produces primary infections in childhood followed by latent infections of the spinal ganglia. Reactivations of latent infections, in the form of herpes zoster, rarely occur before age 50 (except in individuals with other debilitating illnesses), but are much more common over 60 years of age.

Host genes

Studies with inbred animals have documented that the outcome of infections often varies in different strains of mice (Brinton 1996), and genetic analyses have been conducted to determine the form of inheritance of susceptibility, and also to map the chromosomal location of the responsible genetic loci (Lodmell 1983; Oktsuka and Taguchi 1997). Several generalizations may be made, based on numerous studies of a wide variety of viruses:

- Most genetic loci control susceptibility to a specific family of viruses and not to all viruses.
- Susceptibility can often be mapped to a single autosomal locus, but multiple loci have been identified in some instances.
- When a single genetic locus has been identified, susceptibility may be either dominant or recessive.
- Where loci have been mapped, they are usually distant from the major histocompatibility locus, and in most such instances, the mechanism of susceptibility is not immunological.
- The exact mechanism of susceptibility has not been well defined in most instances, although there are some examples that map to the MHC, implying an

Table 13.14 *Age is one of the physiological variables that can determine host susceptibility*

Age group	Encephalitis rate per 100 000	Case-fatality rate per 100	Percent with SLE antibody
0–9	8	0	41%
10–19	13	0	29%
20–29	15	0	38%
30–39	14	0	36%
40–49	17	0	26%
50–59	28	13%	38%
60+	78	27%	25%

Age distribution of St. Louis encephalitis showing that attack rates increased strikingly in the older age groups, although the frequency of infection was similar for all ages.
Data from Luby et al., 1967; Henderson et al., 1970.

immunological explanation (Miyazawa et al. 1992; Poskophidis et al. 1994).

An example of genetically determined host susceptibility is shown in Table 13.15, in which there is a single autosomal genetic locus and resistance is dominant (Haller et al. 1980). In this instance, the genetic determinant, called the *Mx* locus, has been shown to influence the response to influenza viruses and is related to differential ability to mount an interferon response (Pavlovic et al. 1992; Staeheli et al. 1993). Thus, treatment with anti-interferon antibody abrogates resistance, and renders all strains of mice equally susceptible.

It is difficult to investigate genetic determinants of host susceptibility in an outbred population. Classical studies of myxoma virus in outbred rabbit populations (Fenner 1983) have clearly demonstrated genetic determinants that became manifest under the selective pressure of a virulent virus. Likewise, individual monkeys exhibit marked differences in susceptibility to Simian immunodeficiency virus (SIV) that correlates with ex vivo infectibility of their T lymphocytes (Goldstein et al. 2000). If it is assumed that there are human homologues for most mouse genes, then it may be inferred that the outcome of viral infections in humans is also influenced by genetic determinants. Consistent with this presumption are observations that human responses to standardized virus inocula may be somewhat variable (Table 13.10 and Figure 13.12).

Recent studies of HIV-1 have provided substantial evidence of a number of human genetic determinants of susceptibility to infection or to the rate of progression to overt AIDS (Liu et al. 1996; Kaslow et al. 1996; Migueles et al. 2000; Moore et al. 2002). The most striking of these is a polymorphism in the gene that encodes the chemokine receptor, CCR5, which is the major coreceptor for HIV-1. Some people have a deletion in the gene ($\Delta 32$ deletion) such that no CCR5

Table 13.16 *Differences in host susceptibility have been defined for a few viruses of humans*

HIV-1 antibody	Parameter	Total	CCR5 +/+	CCR5 +/−	CCR5 −/−
Positive	Number	1343	1148	195	0
	Percent	100%	85%	15%	0%
Negative	Number	612	508	87	17
	Percent	100%	83%	14%	3%

In this example, the chemokine receptor CCR5 acts as a coreceptor for most wildtype HIV isolates. A naturally occurring mutation ($\Delta 32$) in the CCR5 gene abrogates the expression of CCR5 and homozygous carriers of the mutation are resistant to HIV-1. Subjects at high risk of HIV exposure were divided into those who were HIV-infected and those who were not, and tested for their CCR5 status (CCR5 +/+, +/−, or −/−). There was a striking absence of CCR5$^{-/-}$ persons in the HIV-infected group and an excess of CCR5$^{-/-}$ persons (above the 1% expectancy) in the HIV-uninfected group.
After Dean et al. 1996.

protein is expressed, and these individuals are at very low risk of HIV infection (Table 13.16). People who are heterozygous for the $\Delta 32$ deletion can be infected but, on average, have prolonged incubation periods to the onset of AIDS by comparison with CCR5$^+$ homozygous individuals.

ACKNOWLEDGMENTS

Many of the updates from the previous edition of this chapter were drawn from several chapters and illustrations in Nathanson et al. (2002).

REFERENCES

Aebischer, T. and Mokophidis, D. 1991. In vitro selection of lymphocytic choriomeningitis virus escape mutants by cytotoxic T lymphocytes. *Proc Natl Acad Sci USA*, **88**, 11047–51.

Ahmed, R., Jamieson, B. and Porter, D.D. 1987. Immune therapy of a persistent and disseminated viral infection. *J Virol*, **61**, 3920–9.

Ahmed, R. and Chen, I.S.Y. (eds) 1999. *Persistent viral infections*. New York: John Wiley and Sons.

Allen, T.M., O'Connor, D.H., et al. 2000. Tat-specific cytotoxic T lymphocytes select for SIV escape variants during resolution of primary viraemia. *Nature*, **407**, 386–90.

Almond, J.W. 1991. Poliovirus neurovirulence. *Semin Neurosci*, **3**, 101–8.

Alter, H.J., Purcell, R.H. and Gerin, J.L. 1977. Transmission of hepatitis B surface antigen positive saliva and semen. *Infect Immun*, **16**, 928–33.

Baer, G.M. (ed.) 1991. *The natural history of rabies*. Boca Raton: CRC Press.

Bagasra, O., Seshamma, T., et al. 1993. High percentages of CD4-positive lymphocytes harbor the HIV-1 provirus in the blood of certain infected individuals. *AIDS*, **7**, 1419–25.

Baringer, J.R. and Nathanson, N. 1972. Parvovirus hemorrhagic encephalopathy of rats: electron microscopic observations of the vascular lesions. *Lab Invest*, **27**, 514–22.

Barnett, E.M. and Perlman, S. 1993. The olfactory nerve and not the trigeminal nerve is the major site of CNS entry for mouse hepatitis virus, strain JHM. *Virology*, **194**, 185–91.

Barouche, D.H., Kunstman, J., et al. 2002. Eventual AIDS vaccine failure in a rhesus monkey by viral escape from cytotoxic T lymphocyte. *Nature*, **415**, 335–9.

Table 13.15 *Genetic determinants of host susceptibility can be delineated in inbred strains of mice*

Mouse strain	Genotype	Mortality dead/total	Log$_{10}$ virus titer in blood
Not treated			
A/J	r/r	4/4	6.0
A2G	R/R	0/4	3.7
F1 (A/J × A2G)	R/r	0/4	3.5
Treated with anti-interferon antiserum			
A/J	r/r	4/4	6.0
A2G	R/R	4/4	6.3
F1 (A/J × A2G)	R/r	4/4	6.5

A/J mice are susceptible and A2G mice are resistant to a hepatotropic strain of influenza virus, and the F1 hybrid is also resistant, indicating that a single dominant autosomal gene determines resistance. In addition, treatment with anti-interferon antiserum abrogates resistance, suggesting that the effect is mediated through the action of interferon.
Data from Haller et al. (1980).
R, resistant; r, susceptible.

Baucke, R.B. and Spear, P.G. 1979. Membrane proteins specified by herpes simplex virus. V. Identification of an Fc-binding glycoprotein. *J Virol*, **32**, 779–89.

Berger, E.A., Murphy, P.M. and Farber, J.M. 1999. Chemokine receptors as HIV-1 coreceptors: roles in viral entry, tropism, and disease. *Annu Rev Immunol*, **17**, 657–700.

Billeter, M.A., Cattaneo, R., et al. 1994. Generation and properties of measles virus mutations typically associated with subacute sclerosing panencephalitis. *Ann NY Acad Sci*, **724**, 367–77.

Binder, G.K. and Griffin, D.E. 2001. Interferon-γ-mediated site-specific clearance of alphavirus from CNS neurons. *Science*, **293**, 303–6.

Blank, H., Burgoon, C.F., et al. 1951. Cytologic smears in diagnosis of herpes simplex, herpes zoster, and varicella. *J Am Med Assoc*, **146**, 1410–12.

Bodian, D. 1954. Viremia in experimental poliomyelitis. I. General aspects of infection after intravascular inoculation with strains of high and low invasiveness. *Am J Hyg*, **60**, 339–57.

Bodian, D. 1955. Emerging concepts of poliomyelitis infection. *Science*, **122**, 105–8.

Borza, C.M. and Hutt-Fletcher, L.M. 2002. Alternate replication in B cells and epithelial cells switches tropism of Epstein–Barr virus. *Nature Med*, **8**, 594–9.

Bouchard, M.J., Lam, D.-H. and Racaniello, V.R. 1995. Determinants of attenuation and temperature sensitivity in the Type 1 poliovirus Sabin vaccine. *J Virol*, **69**, 4972–8.

Brinton, M.A. 1996. Host factors controlling susceptibility to viral diseases. In: Nathanson, N. (ed.), *Viral pathogenesis*. Philadelphia: Lippincott-Raven Publishers, 303–28.

Brodsky, F.M., Lem, L., et al. 1999. Human pathogen subversion of antigen presentation. *Immunol Rev*, **168**, 199–215.

Buchmeier, M.J. and Zajac, A.J. 1999. Lymphocytic choriomeningitis virus. In: Ahmed, R. and Chen, I.S.Y. (eds), *Persistent virus infections*. New York: John Wiley and Sons, 575–605.

Burkitt, D. 1958. A sarcoma involving the jaws in African children. *Br J Surg*, **45**, 218–23.

Card, J.P., Levitt, P. and Enquist, L.W. 1998. Different patterns of neuronal infection after intracerebral injection of two strains of pseudorabies virus. *J Virol*, **72**, 4434–41.

Cattaneo, R., Rebman, G., et al. 1987. Altered ratios of measles virus transcripts in diseased human brains. *Virology*, **160**, 523–6.

Chantler, J.K. and Tingle, A.J. 1982. Isolation of rubella virus from human lymphocytes after acute natural infection. *J Infect Dis*, **145**, 673–7.

Charles, P.C., Walters, E., et al. 1995. Mechanism of neuroinvasion of Venezuelan equine encephalitis virus in the mouse. *Virology*, **208**, 662–71.

Charles, P.C., Guida, J.D., et al. 1998. Mouse adenovirus type-1 replication is restricted to vascular endothelium in the CNS of susceptible strains of mice. *Virology*, **245**, 216–28.

Ciurea, A., Nunziker, H., et al. 2001. CD4+ T-cell epitope escape mutant virus selected in vitro. *Nature Med*, **7**, 795–800.

Clark, S.M., Roth, J.R. and Clark, M.L. 1981. Tryptic enhancement of rotavirus infectivity: mechanism of enhancement. *J Virol*, **39**, 816–22.

Cohen, J.I. 2000. Epstein–Barr virus infection. *New Engl J Med*, **343**, 481–92.

Collman, R., Hassan, N.F., et al. 1989. Infection of monocyte-derived macrophages with human immunodeficiency virus type 1 (HIV-1). Monocyte- and lymphocyte-tropic strains of HIV-1 show distinctive patterns of replication in a panel of cell types. *J Exp Med*, **170**, 1149–63.

Collman, R. and Nathanson, N. 1992. Human immunodeficiency virus type-1 infection of macrophages. *Semin Virol*, **3**, 185–202.

Connor, R.I., Montefiori, D.C., et al. 1998. Temporal analyses of virus replication, immune responses, and efficacy in rhesus macaques immunized with a live attenuated simian immunodeficiency virus vaccine. *J Virol*, **72**, 7501–9.

Cook, M.L. and Stevens, J.G. 1973. Pathogenesis of herpetic neuritis and ganglionitis in mice: evidence of intra-axonal transport of infection. *Infect Immun*, **7**, 272–88.

Dalmat, H. 1958. Arthropod transmission of rabbit papillomatosis. *J Exp Med*, **108**, 9–20.

Dean, M., Carrington, M., et al. 1996. Genetic restriction of HIV-1 infection and progression to AIDS by a deletion allele of the CKR5 structural gene. *Science*, **273**, 1856–62.

de Boer, G.F. and Houwers, D.J. 1979. Epizootiology of maedi/visna in sheep. In: Tyrrell, D.A.J. (ed.), *Aspects of slow and persistent virus infections*. The Hague: Martinus Nijhoff, 198–220.

DeJong, J.G. and Winkler, K.C. 1968. The inactivation of poliovirus in aerosols. *J Hyg*, **66**, 557–65.

Depper, J.M., Leonard, W.J., et al. 1984. Augmented T cell growth factor receptor expression in HTLV-1-infected human leukemic T cells. *J Immunol*, **133**, 1691–5.

Dietzschold, B., Wunner, W.H., et al. 1983. Characterization of an antigenic determinant of the glycoprotein that correlates with pathogenicity of rabies virus. *Proc Natl Acad Sci USA*, **80**, 70–4.

Dimitrov, D.S. 2000. Cell biology of virus entry. *Cell*, **101**, 697–702.

Douglas, R.G. Jr., Cate, T.R., et al. 1966. Quantitative rhinovirus shedding patterns in volunteers. *Am Rev Respir Dis*, **94**, 159–67.

Dubin, G., Socolof, E. and Frank, I. 1991. Herpes simplex virus type 1 Fc receptor protects infected cells from antibody-dependent cellular cytotoxicity. *J Virol*, **65**, 7046–50.

Endres, M.J., Valsamakis, A., et al. 1990. Neuroattenuated bunyavirus variant: derivation, characterization, and revertant clones. *J Virol*, **64**, 1927–33.

Enquist, L.W. 1994. Infection of the mammalian nervous system by pseudorabies virus (PRV). *Semin Virol*, **5**, 221–31.

Epstein, M.A., Achong, B.G. and Barr, Y.M. 1964. Virus particles in cultured lymphoblasts from a Burkitt's lymphoma. *Lancet*, **1**, 252–3.

Esolen, L.M., Ward, B.J., et al. 1993. Infection of monocytes during measles. *J Infect Dis*, **168**, 47–52.

Estes, M.K., Graham, D.Y. and Mason, B.B. 1981. Proteolytic enhancement of rotavirus infectivity: molecular mechanisms. *J Virol*, **39**, 879–88.

Evans, L. and Morrey, J. 1987. Tissue-specific replication of Friend and Moloney mouse leukemia viruses in infected mice. *J Virol*, **61**, 1350–7.

Evans, D.J. and Almond, J.W. 1999. Cell receptors for picornaviruses as determinants of cell tropism and pathogenesis. *Trends Microbiol*, **6**, 198–202.

Evans, D.T., O'Connor, D.H., et al. 1999. Virus specific cytotoxic T lymphocyte responses select for amino acid variation in simian immunodeficiency virus Env and Nef. *Nature Med*, **5**, 1270–6.

Fenner, F. 1949. Mousepox (infectious ectromelia of mice): a review. *J Immunol*, **63**, 341–73.

Fenner, F. 1983. Biological control as exemplified by smallpox eradication and myxomatosis. *Proc Roy Soc*, **218**, 259–85.

Fenner, F., Henderson, D.A., et al. 1988. *Smallpox and its eradication*. Geneva: World Health Organization.

Fish, K.N., Soderberg-Naucler, C., et al. 1998. Human cytomegalovirus persistently infects aortic endothelial cells. *J Virol*, **72**, 5661–8.

Frank, I. and Friedman, H. 1989. A novel function of the herpes simplex virus type 1 Fc receptor: participation of bipolar bridging of antiviral immunoglobulin. *J Virol*, **63**, 4479–88.

Freistadt, M. 1994. Distribution of the poliovirus receptor in human tissue. In: Wimmer, E. (ed.), *Cellular receptors for animal viruses*. Cold Spring Harbor: Cold Spring Harbor Laboratory Press, 445–62.

Friedman, H., Macarek, E. and MacGregor, R.A. 1981. Virus infection of endothelial cells. *J Infect Dis*, **143**, 266–73.

Frosner, G.G., Papaevangelou, G., et al. 1979. Antibody against hepatitis A in seven European countries. I. Comparison of prevalence data in different age groups. *Am J Epidemiol*, **110**, 63–9.

Gendelman, H.E., Narayan, O., et al. 1985. Slow, persistent replication of lentiviruses: role of tissue macrophages and macrophage precursors in bone marrow. *Proc Natl Acad Sci USA*, **82**, 7082–90.

Georgescu, M.-M., Tardy-Panit, M., et al. 1995. Mapping of mutations contributing to the temperature sensitivity of the Sabin 1 vaccine strain of poliovirus. *J Virol*, **69**, 5278–86.

Goldstein, S., Brown, C.R., et al. 2000. Intrinsic susceptibility of rhesus macaque peripheral CD4+ T cells to simian immunodeficiency virus in vitro is predictive of in vivo viral replication. *J Virol*, **74**, 9388–95.

Gollins, S.W. and Porterfield, J.S. 1984. Flavivirus infection enhancement in macrophages: radioactive and biological studies on the effect of antibody on viral fate. *J Gen Virol*, **65**, 1261–72.

Gonzalez-Scarano, F., Janssen, R., et al. 1985. An avirulent G1 glycoprotein variant of La Crosse bunyavirus with defective fusion function. *J Virol*, **54**, 757–63.

Gonzalez-Scarano, F. and Nathanson, N. 1990. Bunyaviruses. In: Fields, B.N. and Knipe, D.M. (eds), *Virology*. New York: Raven Press, 1195–228.

Griffin, D.E., Levine, B., et al. 1994. Age-dependent fatal encephalitis: alphavirus infection of neurons. *Arch Virol*, **9S**, 31–9.

Griot, C., Gonzalez-Scarano, F. and Nathanson, N. 1993a. Molecular determinants of the virulence and infectivity of California serogroup bunyaviruses. *Ann Rev Microbiol*, **47**, 117–38.

Griot, C., Pekosz, A., et al. 1993b. Polygenic control of neuroinvasiveness in California serogroup viruses. *J Virol*, **67**, 3861–7.

Griot, C., Pekosz, A., et al. 1994. Replication in cultured C2C12 muscle cells correlates with the neuroinvasiveness of California serogroup bunyaviruses. *Virology*, **201**, 399–403.

Gromeier, M. and Wimmer, E. 1998. Mechanism of injury-provoked poliomyelitis. *J Virol*, **72**, 5056–60.

Haase, A.T. 1986. Pathogenesis of lentivirus infections. *Nature*, **322**, 130–6.

Haller, O., Arnheiter, H., et al. 1980. Host gene influences sensitivity to interferon action selectively for influenza virus. *Nature*, **283**, 660–2.

Halstead, S.B. and O'Rourke, E.J. 1977. Dengue viruses and mononuclear phagocytes. I. Infection enhancement by non-neutralizing antibody. *J Exp Med*, **146**, 201–17.

Harouse, J.M., Gettle, A., et al. 1999. Distinct pathogenic sequelae in rhesus macaques infected with CCR5- or CXCR4-tropic strains of SHIV. *Science*, **284**, 816–20.

Harris, S.L., Frank, I. and Lee, A. 1990. Glycoprotein C of herpes simplex virus type 1 prevents complement-mediated cell lysis and virus neutralization. *J Infect Dis*, **162**, 331–7.

Henderson, B.E., Pigford, C.A., et al. 1970. Serologic survey for St. Louis encephalitis and other group B arbovirus antibodies in residents of Houston, Texas. *Am J Epidemiol*, **91**, 87–98.

Herndon, R.M., Johnson, R.T. and Davis, L.E. 1974. Ependymitis in mumps virus meningitis: electron microscipic studies of the cerebrospinal fluid. *Arch Neurol*, **30**, 475–9.

Ho, M. 1981. The lymphocyte in infections with Epstein–Barr virus and cytomegalovirus. *J Infect Dis*, **143**, 857–62.

Holmes, K.V. 1997. Localization of virus infections. In: Nathanson, N., et al. (eds), *Viral pathogenesis*. Philadelphia: Lippincott-Raven Publishers.

Hopkins, N., Golemis, E. and Speck, N. 1989. Role of enhancer regions in leukemia induction by nondefective murine C type retroviruses. In: Notkins, A.L. and Oldstone, M.B.A. (eds), *Concepts in viral pathogenesis*. New York: Springer Verlag, 41–9.

Horstmann, D.M., Opton, E.M., et al. 1964. Viremia in infants vaccinated with oral poliovirus vaccine (Sabin). *Am J Hyg*, **79**, 47–63.

Hotchin, J. 1962. The biology of lymphocytic choriomeningitis infection: virus-induced immune disease. *Cold Spring Harbor Symp Quant Biol*, **27**, 479–500.

Hsia, K. and Spector, S.A. 1991. Human immunodeficiency virus DNA is present in a high percentage of CD4+ lymphocytes of seropositive individuals. *J Infect Dis*, **164**, 470–5.

Hutt-Fletcher, L. 1999. Epstein–Barr virus. In: Ahmed, R. and Chen, I.S.Y. (eds), *Persistent viral infections*. New York: John Wiley and Sons, 243–68.

Igarishi, T., Endo, Y., et al. 1999. Emergence of a highly pathogenic simian/human imunodeficiency virus in a rhesus macaque treated with anti-CD8 mAb during a primary infection with a nonpathogenic virus. *Proc Natl Acad Sci USA*, **96**, 14049–54.

Isaacs, S.N., Kotwal, G.J. and Moss, B. 1992. Vaccinia virus complement-control protein prevents antibody-dependent complement-enhanced neutralization of infectivity and contributes to virulence. *Proc Natl Acad Sci USA*, **89**, 628–32.

Isaacs, S.N. and Moss, B. 1995. Inhibition of complement activation by vaccinia virus. In: McFadden, G. (ed.), *Viroceptors, virokines, and related immune modulators encoded by DNA viruses*. Austin: RG Landes Co, 55–66.

Jackson, A. 1991. Biological basis of rabies virus neurovirulence in mice: comparative pathogenesis study using the immunoperoxidase technique. *J Virol*, **65**, 537–40.

Johnson, R.T. 1965. Virus invasion of the central nervous system. A study of Sindbis virus infection in the mouse using fluorescent antibody. *Am J Pathol*, **46**, 929–43.

Johnson, R.T. 1998. *Viral infections of the nervous system*. Philadelphia: Lippincott-Raven Press.

Johnson, R.T. and Mims, C.A. 1968. Pathogenesis of virus infections of the nervous system. *New Engl J Med*, **278**, 23–92.

Jackson, R.J. and Ramsay, A.J. 2001. Expression of mouse interleukin-4 by a recombinant ectromelia virus suppresses cytolytic lymphocyte responses and overcomes genetic resistance of mousepox. *J Virol*, **75**, 1205–10.

Jourdan, N., Maurice, M., et al. 1997. Rotavirus is released from the apical surface of cultured human intestinal cells through nonconventional vesicular transport that bypasses the Golgi apparatus. *J Virol*, **71**, 8267–78.

Jubelt, B., Narayan, O. and Johnson, R.T. 1980. Pathogenesis of human poliovirus infection in mice. II. Age-dependency of paralysis. *J Neuropathol Exp Neurol*, **39**, 149–59.

Kaslow, R.A., Carrington, M., et al. 1996. Influence of combinations of human major histocompatibility complex genes on the course of HIV-1 infection. *Nature Med*, **2**, 405–11.

Kato, S., Miyamoto, H. and Takahashi, M. 1963. Shope fibroma and rabbit myxoma viruses. II. Pathogenesis of fibromas in domestic rabbits. *Biken J*, **6**, 135–43.

Kono, Y., Kobayashi, K. and Fukunaga, Y. 1973. Antigenic drift of equine infectious anemia virus in chronically infected horses. *Arch Virusforsch*, **41**, 1–10.

Kotwal, G.J., Isaacs, S.N., et al. 1990. Inhibition of the complement cascade by the major secretory protein of vaccinia virus. *Science*, **250**, 827–30.

Kozak, C.A. and Ruscetti, S. 1992. Retroviruses in rodents. In: Levy, J.A. (ed.), *The Retroviridae*. New York: Plenum Press, 405–81.

Kristensson, K., Lycke, E. and Sjostand, J. 1971. Spread of herpes simplex virus in peripheral nerves. *Acta Neuropathol*, **17**, 44–53.

Lafon, M. 2002. Immunology. In: Jackson, A.C. and Wunner, W.H. (eds), *Rabies*. New York: Academic Press, 351–69.

La Monica, N. and Racaniello, V.R. 1989. Differences in replication of attenuated and neurovirulent polioviruses in human neuroblastoma cell line SH-SY5Y. *J Virol*, **63**, 2357–60.

Levine, B., Huang, Q., et al. 1993. Conversion of lytic to persistent alphavirus infection by the bcl-2 cellular oncogene. *Nature*, **361**, 739–42.

Levy, J.A. 1998. *HIV and the pathogenesis of AIDS*. Washington: ASM Press.

Lippmann, M., Yeates, D.B. and Albert, R.E. 1980. Deposition, retention, and clearance of inhaled particles. *Br J Ind Med*, **37**, 337–62.

Little, L.M. and Shadduck, J.A. 1982. Pathogenesis of rotavirus infection in mice. *Infect Immun*, **38**, 755–63.

Liu, R., Paxton, W.A., et al. 1996. Homozygous defect in HIV-1 coreceptor accounts for resistance of some multiply-exposed individuals to HIV-1 infection. *Cell*, **86**, 367–77.

Lodmell, D. 1983. Genetic control of resistance to street rabies virus in mice. *J Exp Med*, **157**, 451–60.

Lowy, D.R. and Howley, P.M. 2001. Papillomaviruses. In: Knipe, D.M. and Howley, P.M. (eds), *Virology*. Philadelphia: Lippincott Williams & Wilkins, 2231–64.

Luby, J.P., Miller, G., et al. 1967. The epidemiology of St. Louis encephalitis in Houston, Texas. *Am J Epidemiol*, **86**, 584–97.

Lutley, R., Petursson, G., et al. 1983. Antigenic drift in visna: virus variation during long-term infection of Icelandic sheep. *J Gen Virol*, **64**, 1433–40.

Maassab, H.F. and DeBorde, D.C. 1985. Development and characterization of cold-adapted viruses for use as live virus vaccines. *Vaccine*, **3**, 355–69.

Macadam, A.J., Pollard, S.R., et al. 1993. Genetic basis of the attenuation of the Sabin type 2 vaccine strain of poliovirus in primates. *Virology*, **192**, 18–26.

Maratou, E., Theophilidis, G. and Arsenakis, M. 1998. Axonal transport of herpes simplex virus-1 in an in vitro model based on the isolated nerve of the frog *Rana ridibunda*. *J Neurosci Meth*, **79**, 75–8.

Matloubian, N., Kolhekar, S.R., et al. 1993. Molecular determinants of macrophage-tropism and viral persistent: importance of single amino acid changes in the polymerase and glycoprotein of lymphocytic choriomeningitis virus. *J Virol*, **67**, 7340–9.

McCune, J.M. 2001. The dynamics of CD4 T-cell depletion in HIV disease. *Nature*, **410**, 980–7.

McFadden, G. (ed.) 1995. *Viroceptors*. Austin: R.G. Landes Co.

McFadden, G., Graham, K. and Opgenorth, A. 1995. Poxvirus growth factors. In: McFadden, G. (ed.), *Viroceptors, virokines, and related immune modulators encoded by DNA viruses*. Austin: R.G. Landes Co, 1–16.

Mendelsohn, C.L., Wimmer, E. and Racaniello, V.R. 1989. Cellular receptor for poliovirus: molecular cloning, nucleotide sequence, and expression of a new member of the immunoglobulin superfamily. *Cell*, **56**, 855–69.

Migueles, S.A., Sabbaghain, M.S., et al. 2000. HLA B*5701 is highly associated with restriction of virus replication in a subgroup of HIV-infected long term nonprogressors. *Proc Natl Acad Sci USA*, **97**, 2709–14.

Mims, C.A. 1964. Aspects of the pathogenesis of virus diseases. *Bacteriol Rev*, **28**, 30–71.

Minor, P.D. 1992. The molecular biology of poliovaccines. *J Gen Virol*, **73**, 3065–77.

Minor, P.D. 1993. Attenuation and reversion of the Sabin strains of poliovirus. *Dev Biol Stand*, **78**, 17–26.

Mittler, J.E., Markowitz, M., et al. 1999. Improved estimates for HIV-1 clearance rate and intracellular delay. *AIDS*, **13**, 1415–17.

Miyazawa, M., Nishio, J., et al. 1992. Influence of MHC genes on spontaneous recovery from Friend retrovirus-induced leukemia. *J Immunol*, **148**, 644–7.

Monath, T.R. (ed.) 1988. *The arboviruses: epidemiology and ecology*. Boca Raton: CRC Press.

Moore, C.B., John, M., et al. 2002. Evidence of HIV-1 adaptation to HLA-restricted immune responses at a population level. *Science*, **296**, 1439–43.

Morely, D. 1969. The severe measles of West Africa. *Proc Roy Soc Med*, **57**, 846–9.

Morrison, L.A., Sidman, R.L. and Fields, B.N. 1991. Direct spread of reovirus from intestinal lumen to the central nervous system through the autonomic vagal nerve fibers. *Proc Natl Acad Sci USA*, **88**, 2852–6.

Nagai, Y. 1995. Virus activation by host proteinases: a pivotal role in the spread of infection, tissue tropism, and pathogenicity. *Microbiol Immunol*, **39**, 1–9.

Nathanson, N. 1984. Eradication of poliomyelitis in the United States. *Rev Infect Dis*, **4**, 940–5.

Nathanson, N. and Bodian, D. 1961. Experimental poliomyelitis following intramuscular virus injection. I. The effect of neural block on a neurotropic and a pantropic strain. *Bull Johns Hopkins Hosp*, **108**, 308–19.

Nathanson, N. and Cole, G.A. 1971. Immunosuppression: a means to assess the role of the immune response in acute virus infection. *Fed Proc*, **30**, 1822–30.

Nathanson, N. and Horn, S.D. 1992. Neurovirulence tests of type 3 oral poliovirus vaccine manufactured by Lederle Laboratories, 1964–1988. *Vaccine*, **10**, 469–75.

Nathanson, N. and Martin, J.R. 1979. The epidemiology of poliomyelitis: enigmas surrounding its appearance, epidemicity, and disappearance. *Am J Epidemiol*, **110**, 672–92.

Nathanson, N., Ahmed, R., et al. 2002. *Viral pathogenesis and immunity*. Philadelphia: Lippincott Williams & Wilkins.

Nkowane, B.M., Wassilak, S.G.F., et al. 1987. Vaccine-associated paralytic poliomyelitis, United States: 1973 through 1984. *J Am Med Assoc*, **257**, 1335–40.

Notkins, A.L., Mahar, S., et al. 1966. Infectious virus–antibody complexes in the blood of chronically infected mice. *J Exp Med*, **124**, 81–97.

Oaks, J.L., McGuire, T.C., et al. 1998. Equine infectious anemia virus is found in tissue macrophages during subclinical infection. *J Virol*, **72**, 7263–9.

Ogata, A., Nagashima, K., et al. 1991. Japanese encephalitis virus neurotropism is dependent on the degree of neuronal immaturity. *J Virol*, **65**, 880–6.

Ohka, S., Yang, W.X., et al. 1998. Retrograde transport of intact poliovirus though the axon via the fast axonal transport system. *Virology*, **250**, 67–75.

Oktsuka, N. and Taguchi, F. 1997. Mouse susceptibility to mouse hepatitis virus infection is linked to viral receptor genotype. *J Virol*, **71**, 8860–3.

Oldstone, M.B.A. 1975. Virus neutralization and virus-induced immune complex disease. *Prog Med Virol*, **19**, 84–119.

Oliver, K.R. and Fazakerley, J.K. 1998. Transneuronal spread of Semliki Forest virus in the developing mouse olfactory system is determined by neuronal maturity. *Neuroscience*, **82**, 867–77.

Opgenorth, A., Strayer, D. and Upton, C. 1992. Deletion of the growth factor gene related to EGF and TGFα reduces virulence of malignant rabbit fibroma virus. *Virology*, **186**, 175–91.

Oshiro, L.S., Dondero, D.V., et al. 1978. The development of Colorado tick fever virus within cells of the haemopoietic system. *J Gen Virol*, **39**, 73–9.

Panum, P.L. 1940. *Observations made during the epidemic of measles on the Faroe Islands in the year 1846*. New York: American Public Health Association.

Pathek, S. and Webb, H.E. 1974. Possible mechanisms for the transport of Semliki Forest virus into and within mouse brain: an electron microscopic study. *J Neurol Sci*, **23**, 175–84.

Pavlovic, J., Haller, O. and Staeheli, P. 1992. Human and mouse Mx proteins inhibit different steps of the influenza virus multiplication cycle. *J Virol*, **66**, 2564–9.

Pekosz, A., Griot, C., et al. 1995. Protection from La Crosse virus encephalitis with recombinant glycoproteins: role of neutralizing anti-G1 antibodies. *J Virol*, **69**, 3475–81.

Perlman, S., Jacobsen, G. and Afifi, A. 1989. Spread of a neurotropic murine coronavirus into the CNS via the trigeminal and olfactory nerves. *Virology*, **170**, 556–60.

Peters, C.J. 1997. Viral hemorrhagic fevers. In: Nathanson, N. (ed.), *Viral pathogenesis*. Philadelphia: Lippincott-Raven Publishers, 779–800.

Petursson, G., Nathanson, N., et al. 1976. Pathogenesis of visna. I. Sequential virologic, serologic, and pathologic studies. *Lab Invest*, **35**, 402–12.

Pitts, O., Powers, M. and Billelo, J. 1987. Ultrastructural changes associated with retroviral replication in central nervous system capillary endothelial cells. *Lab Invest*, **56**, 401–9.

Ploegh, H.L. 1998. Viral strategies of immune invasion. *Science*, **280**, 248–53.

Pomerantz, R.J., de la Monte, S.M., et al. 1988. Human immunodeficiency virus (HIV) infection of the uterine cervix. *Ann Intern Med*, **108**, 321–7.

Porter, D.D. and Larsen, A.E. 1967. Aleutian disease of mink: infectious virus–antibody complexes in the serum. *Proc Soc Exp Biol Med*, **126**, 680–2.

Poskophidis, D., Lechner, F., et al. 1994. MHC class I and non-MHC-linked capacity for generating an antiviral CTL response determines susceptibility to CTL exhaustion and establishment of virus persistence in mice. *J Immunol*, **152**, 4976–83.

Rabin, E., Jenson, A. and Melnick, J. 1968. Herpes simplex virus in mice: electron microscopy of neural spead. *Science*, **162**, 126–9.

Racaniello, V.R. 1988. Poliovirus neurovirulence. *Adv Vir Res*, **34**, 217–46.

Racaniello, V.R. and Baltimore, D. 1981. Cloned poliovirus complementary DNA is infectious in mammalian cells. *Science*, **214**, 914–19.

Racaniello, V.R., Ren, R. and Bouchard, M.J. 1993. Poliovirus attenuation and pathogenesis in a transgenic mouse model for poliomyelitis. *Dev Biol Stand*, **78**, 109–16.

Rajcani, J., Herget, U. and Kaerner, H.C. 1990. Spread of herpes simplex virus (HSV) strains SC16, ANG, ANGpath and its GlyC minus and GlyE minus mutants in DBA-2 mice. *Acta Virol*, **34**, 305–20.

Rall, G.F., Mucke, L. and Oldstone, M.B.A. 1995. Consequences of cytotoxic T lymphocytes interaction with major histocompatibility complex class I-expressing neurons in vivo. *J Exp Med*, **182**, 1201–12.

Ren, R., Constantini, F.J., et al. 1990. Transgenic mice expressing a human poliovirus receptor: a new model for poliomyelitis. *Cell*, **63**, 353–62.

Ren, R., Moss, E.G. and Racaniello, V.R. 1991. Identification of two determinants that attenuate vaccine-related type 2 poliovirus. *J Virol*, **65**, 1377–82.

Ren, R. and Racaniello, V.R. 1992. Poliovirus spreads from muscle to the central nervous system by neural pathways. *J Infect Dis*, **166**, 747–52.

Richman, D.D., Wrin, T., et al. 2003. Rapid evolution of the neutralizing antibody response to HIV type 1 infection. *Proc Natl Acad Sci USA*, **100**, 4144–9.

Roberts, J.A. 1962a. Histopathogenesis of mousepox. I. Respiratory infection. *Br J Exp Pathol*, **43**, 451–61.

Roberts, J.A. 1962b. The histopathogenesis of mousepox. II. Cutaneous infection. *Br J Exp Pathol*, **43**, 462–70.

Rothman, A.L. and Ennis, F.A. 1999. Immunopathogenesis of dengue hemorrhagic fever. *Virology*, **267**, 1–6.

Sabin, A.B. 1985. Oral poliovirus vaccine: history of its development and use and current challenge to eliminate poliomyelitis from the world. *J Infect Dis*, **151**, 420–36.

Saif, L.J. 1990. Comparative aspects of enteric virus infection. In: Saif, L.J. and Theil, K.W. (eds), *Viral diarrheas of man and animals*. Boca Raton: CRC Press, 9–31.

Schmitz, J.E., Kuroda, M.J., et al. 1999. Control of viremia in simian immunodeficiency virus infection by CD8+ lymphocytes. *Science*, **283**, 857–60.

Schonberger, L.B., McGowan, J.E. Jr. and Gregg, M.B. 1976. Vaccine-associated poliomyelitis in the United States, 1961–1972. *Am J Epidemiol*, **104**, 202–11.

Sederati, F., Margolis, T.P. and Stevens, J.G. 1993. Latent infection can be established with drastically restricted transcription and replication of the HSV-1 genome. *Virology*, **192**, 687–91.

Smith, C.A. and Goodwin, R.G. 1995. Tumor necrosis factor receptors in the poxvirus family: biological and genetic implications. In: McFadden, G. (ed.), *Viroceptors, virokines and related immune modulators encoded by DNA viruses*. Austin: RG Landes Co, 29–40.

Smith, G., Symons, J.A., et al. 1997. Vaccinia virus immune evasion. *Immunol Rev*, **159**, 137–54.

Staeheli, P., Pitossi, F. and Pavlovic, J. 1993. Mx proteins: GTPases with antiviral activity. *Trend Cell Biol*, **3**, 268–72.

Steinhauer, D.A. and Holland, J.J. 1987. Rapid evolution of RNA viruses. *Ann Rev Microbiol*, **41**, 409–33.

Stevens, J.G. 1994. Overview of herpesvirus latency. *Semin Virol*, **5**, 191–6.

Strode, G.K. (ed.) 1951. *Yellow fever*. New York: McGraw-Hill.

Takahashi, K., Sonoda, S. and Higashi, K. 1989. Predominant CD4 T-lymphocyte tropism of human herpes 6-related virus. *J Virol*, **63**, 3161–3.

Tan, X., Pearce-Pratt, R. and Phillips, D.M. 1993. Productive infection of a cervical epithelial cell line with human immunodeficiency virus: implications for sexual transmission. *J Virol*, **67**, 6447–52.

Tatem, J.M., Weeks-Levy, C., et al. 1992. A mutation present in the amino terminus of Sabin 3 poliovirus VP1 protein is attenuating. *J Virol*, **66**, 3194–7.

Taylor-Wiedeman, J., Sissons, J.G.P., et al. 1991. Monocytes are a major site of persistence of human cytomegalovirus in peripheral blood mononuclear cells. *J Gen Virol*, **72**, 2059–64.

Theiler, M. and Smith, H.H. 1937. Effect of prolonged cultivation in vitro upon pathogenicity of yellow fever virus. *J Exp Med*, **65**, 767–86.

Tsiang, H. 1979. Evidence for an intraaxonal transport of fixed and street rabies virus. *J Neuropathol Exp Neurol*, **38**, 286–95.

Tsiang, H. 1993. Pathophysiology of rabies virus infection of the nervous system. *Adv Vir Res*, **42**, 375–412.

Tucker, S.P. and Compans, R.W. 1992. Virus infection of polarized epithelial cells. *Adv Vir Res*, **42**, 187–247.

Tucker, P.C., Strauss, E.G., et al. 1993. Viral determinants of age-dependent virulence of Sindbis virus for mice. *J Virol*, **67**, 4605–10.

Tuffereau, C., Leblois, H., et al. 1989. Arginine or lysine in position 333 of ERA and CVS glycoprotein is necessary for rabies virulence in adult mice. *Virology*, **172**, 206–12.

Tyler, K.L. and Nathanson, N. 2001. Pathogenesis of viral infections. In: Knipe, D.E. and Howley, P.M. (eds), *Fields' Virology*. Philadelphia: Lippincott Williams & Wilkins, 199–243.

Tyler, K., McPhee, D. and Fields, B.N. 1986. Distinct pathways of viral spread in the host determined by reovirus S1 gene segment. *Science*, **233**, 770–4.

Virgin IV, H.W., Tyler, K.L. and Dermody, T.S. 1997. Reovirus. In: Nathanson, N. (ed.), *Viral pathogenesis*. Philadelphia: Lippincott-Raven Publishers, 669–702.

Weiss, R.A. 1994. Human receptors for retroviruses. In: Wimmer, E. (ed.), *Cellular receptors for animal viruses*. Cold Spring Harbor: Cold Spring Harbor Laboratory Press, 15–32.

Weiss, R.A. and Tailor, C.S. 1995. Retrovirus receptors. *Cell*, **82**, 531–3.

Wimmer, E. 1994a. Introduction. In: Wimmer, E. (ed.), *Cellular receptors for animal viruses*. Cold Spring Harbor: Cold Spring Harbor Laboratory Press, 1–15.

Wimmer, E. (ed.) 1994b. *Cellular receptors for animal viruses*. Cold Spring Harbor: Cold Spring Harbor Laboratory Press.

Wimmer, E., Harber, J.J., et al. 1994. Poliovirus receptors. In: Wimmer, E. (ed.), *Cellular receptors for animal viruses*. Cold Spring Harbor: Cold Spring Harbor Laboratory Press, 101–28.

Wolf, J.L., Rubin, D., et al. 1981. Intestinal M cells: a pathway for entry of reovirus into the host. *Science*, **212**, 471–2.

York, I.A. and Johnson, D.C. 1995. Inhibition of humoral and cellular immune recognition by herpes simplex viruses. In: McFadden, G. (ed.), *Viroceptors, virokines, and related immune modulators encoded by DNA viruses*. Austin: RG Landes Co, 89–110.

Zhang, L., Dailey, P.J., et al. 1999. Rapid clearance of simian immunodeficiency virus particles from plasma of rhesus macaques. *J Virol*, **73**, 855–60.

14

The immune response to viral infections

ANTHONY A. NASH AND BERNADETTE M. DUTIA

Viruses and the immune system are continually involved in a sophisticated game of hide and seek. Whereas many virus infections are readily controlled by the immune response, some have evolved strategies to evade detection and persist in their host. This balance in the host–pathogen relationship is maintained by the immune system; a breakdown in immune surveillance can lead to recurrent infections and clinical disease.

The immune system employs a variety of strategies to combat virus infection. These can be divided into innate or 'nonspecific' defenses, which include interferon (IFN), natural killer (NK) cells, and macrophages, and adaptive or specific immunity that involves T cells and antibodies. The evolution of T-cell and antibody receptor diversity has probably been critical for the survival of higher vertebrates; it has enabled the host to match evolutionary mutations in structure used by viruses to evade host defenses (Janeway 1992; Zinkernagel 1995; Litman et al. 1999; Janeway and Medzhitov 2002).

Immunological defenses are marshaled at strategic areas in the body where entry of virus is favored. For example, IgA at mucosal surfaces functions by blocking virus adsorption and penetration, macrophages are located throughout the body in various tissues and IFN is produced by most cells in response to viral infection. Once the outer defenses are breached, viruses and viral antigens become channeled into the lymphoid system where they encounter T and B cells. A critical event in this process is the uptake and presentation of antigens by specialized antigen-presenting cells, which include dendritic cells (DC), macrophages, and B lymphocytes. From such encounters, antiviral T cells are generated that target and rapidly destroy infected cells, and antiviral antibodies are produced that protect the host from viremia and reinfection. How the immune response recognizes and kills virus-infected cells, how virus is neutralized by antibody and complement, and how these responses can have pathological outcomes will be discussed. These events will be contrasted with the evasion strategies employed by viruses.

INNATE IMMUNE DEFENSES

The innate defenses restrict early infection and limit spread to other tissues. Because this first line defense is mobilized within minutes or a few hours, it may hold the balance in the host response to virus infection. A key early surveillance mechanism against virus infection is mediated by Toll-like receptors (TLR) found on macrophages, DCs, and polymorphonuclear cells. TLR are a family of receptors with an extracellular domain containing leucine-rich repeats and an intracellular domain homologous to the cytoplasmic tail of the interleukin (IL)-1 receptor (Takeda et al. 2003). Signaling through TLR's leads to activation of NF-κB resulting in the production of pro-inflammatory cytokines. Of the current 11 TLR's, TLR-3 and TLR-7 are of interest here as they recognize dsRNA (TLR-3) and ssRNA (TLR-7) (Diebold et al. 2004). Restricting the early

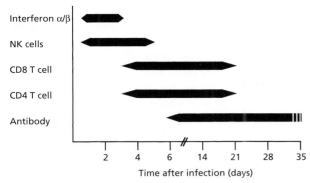

Figure 14.1 *Time scale of the innate and adaptive immune response.*

infection is the province of IFNs α and β, NK cells, and macrophages. The inflammatory response that follows this early encounter with viruses signals its location to the specific immune system, which becomes effective after a few days to a week. Only then will T cells home to the site of infection and antibody be active in limiting virus spread. A time scale for the evolution of the immune response is shown in Figure 14.1.

Antiviral properties of IFN

IFN is a first line of defense against viruses. There are two major families of IFN. Type I IFN, which includes IFN-α (leucocyte-type) encoded by 13 genes and IFN-β (fibroblast-type) encoded by a single gene on human chromosome 9 (mouse chromosome 4). Other type I IFN genes include human IFN-ω, IFN-τ/ε (trophoblast), and the recently described IFN-κ (LaFleur et al. 2001), and IFN-λ (IL-28/IL-29 family) (Kotenko et al. 2003). IFN-α/β is induced within hours of infection and initiates the antiviral state in neighboring cells via the IFN-α/β receptor. This results in the activation of a number of genes associated with the antiviral response as well as anti-proliferative and immunomodulatory activities. In contrast, type II IFN or IFN-γ is produced following antigenic or mitogenic activation of T cells and NK cells. IFN-γ binds to the type II IFN receptor and mediates a similar cascade of gene activation to type I IFN (for reviews see Vilcek and Sen 1996 and Goodbourn et al. 2000) (see also Chapter 15, The role of cytokines in viral infections).

The antiviral response mediated by IFN involves three well described mechanisms, although several others probably exist. Of these protein kinase R (PKR) and 2′–5′ oligo adenylate synthetase are the best characterized. dsRNA-dependent PKR is activated by viral dsRNA and acquires a central role in initiating a number of interactions. PKR phosphorylates the α-subunit of eIF2 preventing the recycling of initiation factors resulting in a block in translation of viral RNA (Clemens and Elia 1997). PKR also mediates apoptosis via Bcl-2 and caspase-dependent mechanisms, thereby thwarting virus infection (Lee et al. 1997). In addition,

PKR plays a role in signal transduction via NF-κB, important for activation of the *IFN-β* gene (Williams 1999). Although a key protein in a number of cellular events, PKR is not essential for IFN-mediated antiviral responses, as mice lacking PKR are still able to resist viral infection (Abraham et al. 1999).

2′–5′ oligoadenylate synthetase catalyses the synthesis of short oligomers (2′–5′ A oligomers) from ATP that act as potent activators of the latent endonuclease RNase L. This endonuclease mediates cleavage of ssRNA thereby inhibiting protein synthesis (Silverman 1999). This IFN mechanism is known to be effective against vaccinia virus and reovirus.

Mx proteins are found in all vertebrate species. They are readily induced by type I IFN and function by inhibiting transcription of a range of RNA viruses including orthomyxoviruses and paramyxoviruses.

Other IFN-dependent mechanisms clearly exist, since mice deficient in PKR, RNase L, and Mx (triple gene knock-out) still retain antiviral activity (Zhou et al. 1999). Other likely mechanisms include dsRNA-dependent adenosine deaminase (ADAR) and caspases 1, 3, and 8.

IFNs play a major role in the immunomodulation of innate and adaptive immune responses. IFN-α/β is an important activator of major histocompatibility complex (MHC) class I and NK cell activity. IFN-γ is a powerful inducer of MHC class I and class II expression, as well as the machinery involved in antigen presentation, for example, proteosomes and TAP-1 and TAP-2 peptide transporters. This augments the activity of cytotoxic T cells (CTL) making them more efficient killers of virus infected cells (see section entitled T lymphocytes and immunity to viruses). Other roles for IFN-γ include directing CD4$^+$ T cells towards a Th1 phenotype, and activating the antiviral state of macrophages.

The importance of type I IFNs in antiviral immunity stems from three experimental approaches: (1) the local administration of IFN to sites such as the nasal passage which protects against rhinovirus infection (Merigan et al. 1973); (2) the administration of anti-IFN antibodies to neutralize IFN-α/β in mice which leads to an increased susceptibility to infection with vesicular stomatitis virus (VSV) and herpes simplex virus (HSV) (Gresser et al. 1976); and (3) the use of IFN receptor gene knock-out mice. The last demonstrates, quite dramatically, the importance of IFN in arresting viral replication in vivo. A variety of RNA viruses (lymphocytic choriomeningitis virus (LCMV), VSV, Theiler's murine encephalomyelitis virus), and DNA viruses (vaccinia, herpesviruses) show increased replication and pathogenic effects in IFN-α/β receptor knock-out mice (van den Broek et al. 1995).

NK cells in antiviral immunity

NK cells are large granular lymphocytes distinct from T- and B-cell lineages. Human NK cells are characterized by the presence of CD16 and CD56 markers. Mouse NK cells have NK1 or NK2 and asialo-GM1 markers that are used to study their function in vivo. A population of NK1.1, CD8$^+$ cells has been described, which have important regulatory functions in the immune response (Vicari and Zlotnik 1996). NK cells produce a number of cytokines involved in antiviral immunity (see Chapter 15, The role of cytokines in viral infections), including IFN-γ, tumor necrosis factor α (TNF-α), tumor growth factor β1 (TGF-β1), granulocyte–macrophage colony-stimulating factor (GM-CSF), and IL-1β (Trinchieri 1989; Perussia 1991).

NK cells display a number of receptors involved in the activation and inhibition of NK cell function. Activation receptors include NKp30, NKp44, and NKp46 on human NK cells and Ly49D and Ly49H on mouse NK cells. These receptors are involved in recognition of virus infected cells with NKp46 recognizing influenza hemagglutinin and Ly49H recognizing m157 of murine cytomegalovirus (Mandelboim et al. 2001; Arase et al. 2002). Other activation receptors include LFA-1 and CD2 members. In addition, NK cells have receptors for a number of cytokines known to be important in activation and proliferation, for example, type I IFN, IL-2, IL-12, IL-15, and IL-18.

In order to protect normal cells from overt NK cell activation and damage, NK cells also carry a variety of inhibitory receptors. This includes the killer cell immunoglobulin-like receptors (KIR), immunoglobulin-like inhibitory receptors (ILT), and lectin-like heterodimers CD94–NKG2A. These receptors bind most MHC class I molecules and deliver inhibitory signals to the cells via immunoreceptor tyrosine-based inhibitory motifs (ITIM). This ability to regulate NK-cell activation has been exploited by some viruses by mimicking inhibitory receptors thereby confusing NK cells at sites of infection (see section Interference with MHC function and NK cell recognition, below).

NK cells can also recognize IgG antibody-coated cell surfaces via FcγRIII (CD16) and kill target cells. This process, known as antibody-dependent cell cytotoxicity (ADCC), is a highly efficient mechanism for activating NK cells and precipitating rapid destruction of virus-infected cells. Cell killing is mediated by a perforin-dependent mechanism (Kagi and Lederman 1994).

NK cells seem to be rapidly mobilized following virus infection. They are detected at sites of infection within 2 days of virus entry, and their appearance is related to a rise in type I IFN levels in the blood. Initial encounter of NK cells with virus-infected cells results in a 'bystander' proliferation mediated by cytokines such as IL-15 and type I IFN. The latter is known to induce blastogenesis in NK cells, probably via up-regulation of IL-15 (Nguyen et al. 2002). After the initial phase of nonspecific activation, there appears to be a more selective amplification of NK cells. In murine cytomegalovirus infection there is a preferential selection for Ly49H-expressing NK cells that appear around day 4–6

following recognition of m157 encoded by the virus (Dokun et al. 2001; Arase et al. 2002). This specific expansion of NK cells is only seen during murine cytomegalovirus (MCMV) infection in resistant mouse strains. Conversely, m157 also interacts with Ly49I, an inhibitory molecule on NK cells. This interaction predominates in MCMV-susceptible mouse strains which lack Ly49H. Around day 6 of MCMV infection there follows a contraction of NK-cell expansion at a time when there is a rise in the adaptive immune response.

Mice vary in susceptibility to MCMV. Resistance to infection is controlled by both *H-2* and non-*H-2* genes. The latter was identified as a single autosomal dominant gene called *Cmv-1* (Scalzo et al. 1992). This gene is located on chromosome 6 and is linked to the NK cell complex, which includes *NK1.1* and *Ly49* genes. Depletion of NK cells in mice bearing the *Cmv-1* gene increases viral replication, proving the link between this gene and NK cell activity (Scalzo et al. 1990). The *Cmv-1* gene has now been identified as Ly49H which targets the m157 protein on MCMV infected cells.

An interesting series of experiments involves the role of NK cells in immunity to vaccinia. Athymic nude mice are highly susceptible to vaccinia but are resistant to vaccinia virus expressing the *IL-2* gene. The mechanism of resistance in this instance involves activation of NK cells by IL-2 to produce IFN-γ, which mediates protection, probably via macrophage activation (Karupiah et al. 1990).

In humans, NK cells are considered to play an important role in immunity to herpesvirus infections. A single NK cell-deficient patient has been reported with severe herpesvirus infections, including cytomegalovirus (CMV) and varicella-zoster virus (VZV) (Biron et al. 1989, 1999).

The key role of macrophages and DCs in immunity to viruses

Macrophages are strategically located throughout the body as a first line of defense against infectious agents. Their importance in virus infections is often underestimated; nevertheless, they have potent antiviral activity and serve to limit virus spread. Macrophage antiviral activity can be broadly divided into intracellular and extracellular defense mechanisms. Macrophages are major producers of IFN-α found in the blood stream following infection. Other antiviral molecules produced by macrophages include:

- TNF-α, which functions either by inducing genes coding for 2'–5'A synthetase and Mx, or by selectively killing virus-infected cells, via apoptosis (Wong and Goeddel 1986).
- Arginase, which depletes local arginine concentrations and effectively aborts HSV infection (Bonina et al. 1984; Mistry et al. 2001).

- Nitric oxide synthase, which is induced following IFN-γ activation of macrophages and leads to the generation of nitric oxide which inhibits the replication of vaccinia virus and HSV (Karupiah et al. 1993).

For many viruses, the hostile environment of a phagolysosome leads to a loss of infectivity. Here, both oxygen-dependent and oxygen-independent mechanisms are likely to contribute to the inactivation of certain viruses. Viruses can be targeted for intracellular destruction by phagocytosis of infected cells or by opsonization of virus–antibody complexes via the Fc receptor; the latter is an efficient way of removing virus from the blood stream. Macrophages can also kill virus-infected cells either by direct contact or, more efficiently, by ADCC through recognition of IgG antibody. In herpesvirus infections, neutrophils have also been implicated in the destruction of infected cells via ADCC.

Despite the hostile nature of macrophages, some viruses selectively exploit these cells for growth and survival; they include lactate dehydrogenase virus, maedi-visna virus, human immunodeficiency virus (HIV), and CMV.

DCs play a major role in the induction of the adaptive immune response (see section entitled T lymphocytes and immunity to viruses). However, it is now apparent that multiple subsets of DCs exist, some of which may have specialized functions in the control of virus infection (Shortman and Liu 2002). An example is the plasmacytoid-derived DC-2 which is a major producer of type I IFN (Siegal et al. 1999). They have been found during influenza virus, HSV, and CMV infections where they appear at sites of infection and in lymphoid tissue associated with infection. During influenza virus infection, DC-2 cells make large amounts of IFN-α which results from endosomal recognition of viral RNA by TLR-7 and activation through MyD88 (Diebold et al. 2004). One role for DC-2 cells is to orchestrate the innate immune response through production of IFN-α. This almost certainly involves activation of NK cells and NKT cells. NK cell–DC interactions are known to be important in the response to MCMV infection (Andrews et al. 2003). This interaction is independent of DC-2 cells and favors a subset of DCs in the mouse that are CD8$^+$.

Collectins and the complement system

Collectins are soluble proteins found in serum, lung, and nasal secretions that can act as a first line of defense against infectious agents (Epstein et al. 1996). They include mannose-binding lectin (MBL) (also known as mannose-binding protein), conglutinin, and lung surfactant proteins A and D (SP-A, SP-D). The basic structural unit is composed of a collagen stalk and a globular head with a lectin-binding domain. Each unit exists as a trimer or multimeric complex. These structural features are similar to the first complement protein C1q. The collectins constitute a primitive antibody-like defense able to target diverse carbohydrate structures on pathogens and yet distinguish self from nonself structures. MBL interacts with HIV, influenza virus, and hepatitis B virus (HBV), and is capable of activating the classical complement pathway to neutralize the virus (Malhotra and Sim 1995; Reading et al. 1997; Hakozaki et al. 2002).

Complement proteins can also directly target viruses or virus-infected cells. Human serum is particularly efficient in the neutralization of certain retroviruses (e.g. murine leukemia virus (MLV)). Human C1q binds the p15E protein of MLV, resulting in activation of the complement system and neutralization of the virus by a process termed virolysis, i.e. damage to the virion envelope (Bartholomew et al. 1978). Classical complement pathway is also activated by CMV-infected cells (Spiller and Morgan 1998) and by cell-free humanT-lymphotropic virus type 1 (HTLV-1) (Ikeda et al. 1998). Sindbis virus is also able to activate the classical complement pathway, but can also directly activate the alternative pathway, i.e. via C3. Other important roles for complement involve interaction with antibody: these events are discussed in the section entitled The role of antibodies in immunity to viruses. C3a and C5a are both inflammatory mediators and as such can serve as signals for alerting inflammatory cells to sites of infection. This is probably one of the reasons why some viruses e.g. herpesviruses and poxviruses carry genes able to subvert C3 activation (see section entitled Viral strategies for evading the immune response). A summary of the complement activation pathways and their functions is shown in Figure 14.2.

The significance of the complement system in antiviral immunity has been difficult to evaluate. In humans and animals, natural deficiencies of complement components do not predispose the host to severe virus infection (Lachmann and Rosen 1979). Experimental approaches have involved the administration of cobra venom factor to exhaust endogenous C3 and hence incapacitate the complement system and the use of complement deficient, i.e. gene knock-out mice. Although most virus infections studied were not affected by depletion of C3, with Sindbis virus an increased viremia was observed in the depleted mice (Hirsch et al. 1980).

Summary of innate immunity

Innate immunity performs an essential role in the early stages of virus infection. Components of the system act rapidly and initiate the cascade of events that focus the specific immune response on the infected area. Factors released in the processes described above lead to an upregulation of adhesion and MHC molecules on local blood vessels, which enable lymphocytes to extravasate and enter the parenchyma. Chemoattractants produced

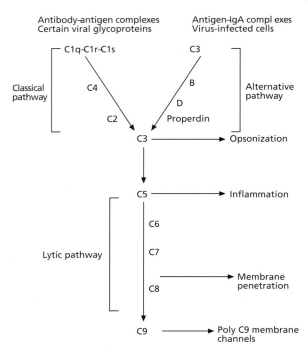

Figure 14.2 *Activation of the complement cascade by virus infection.*

by mast cells, macrophages, NK cells, and complement components recruit lymphocytes, which can then interact with antigen-presenting cells both at the site of infection and in the local lymph nodes.

T LYMPHOCYTES AND IMMUNITY TO VIRUSES

T lymphocytes are central for inducing immunological responses and, in many instances, for the recognition and destruction of virus-infected cells. A deficiency or complete absence of T cells in a host often predisposes to severe or fatal disease. This is particularly so in patients who are severely immunocompromised during organ transplantation. These individuals are at particular risk from reactivating herpesviruses, such as CMV and Epstein–Barr virus (EBV). The complex interrelationship between HIV and humans is another example of an apparent selective immunodeficiency of CD4$^+$ T cells leading inexorably to opportunistic infection in which CMV becomes a life-threatening infection.

Our understanding of the importance of T cells in viral infections stems from studies in animal models. In mice, selective immunodeficiency states can be 'manufactured' using gene knock-out technology (Doherty 1993a). These enable specific questions to be addressed on the function of different T-cell populations and their products (for example, cytokines and receptors). A similar approach involves the use of monoclonal antibodies to interfere selectively with the function of lymphocytes and other cells and cytokines. The advantage of these techniques is

that cell activity can be interrupted before or during an infection, thus permitting examination of the induction and effector capacity of the immune response. The inbred nature of laboratory mice also enables specific T-cell populations and clones to be adoptively transferred to syngeneic recipients and their function monitored. This approach has implications for immunotherapy in humans, in whom protection of high risk transplant patients from CMV disease can be achieved by the transfer of selective anti-CMV T-cell clones derived from the patient prior to immunosuppression (Riddell and Greenberg 1994).

These powerful techniques emphasize the importance of α/β T-cell receptor populations, in particular the role of CD8$^+$ T cells in immunity and immunopathology of virus infections. The significance of γ/δ T cells in anti-viral immunity is still unclear although they are found at sites of virus infection, suggesting a role in defense (Born et al. 1991). They have a more restricted receptor repertoire than α/β T cells and are thought to recognize different restriction elements, including CD1 molecules (Sciammas et al. 1994). In this section we focus on the activities of α/β T cells.

Central role for CD4$^+$ T cells in the induction of the immune response to viruses

As with any antigenic challenge, the initial events in the induction of immunity involve the uptake of virus or viral proteins by DCs and processing to peptides for presentation by MHC class II molecules (Watts and Powis 1999). Briefly, antigen is internalized in endosomes and subjected to proteolytic degradation. These endosomal compartments then fuse with vesicles carrying MHC class II molecules to the cell membrane. MHC class II arises in the endoplasmic reticulum (ER) complexed with the invariant chain. The invariant chain serves two important functions: (1) to target MHC class II to the trans-Golgi and (2) to block the MHC class II cleft from binding peptides prematurely in the ER. On fusing with endosomes, a combination of the acidic pH and MHC class II M molecules (a nonclassic MHC class II molecule) dissociates the invariant chain and allows peptides of around 15 amino acids in length to associate with MHC molecules (Busch and Mellins 1996). Recognition of this structure on the antigen-presenting cell is by the T-cell receptor (TCR) and CD4 molecule on T cells. Additional secondary interactions between cell surface receptors, for example B7 and CD28, LFA-1 and ICAM 1/2, LFA-3, and CD2, lead to signal transduction and the production of IL-2 and IL-2 receptors, resulting in clonal expansion of the interacting CD4$^+$ T cell (Dustin and Springer 1991; Montoya et al. 2002). These events initiate the T helper cell response, which catalyses the induction of CD8$^+$ CTLs, activates NK cells and macrophages, and is critical for induction of the

T-dependent antibody response. Many of these amplifying events involve cytokines and the interaction with key cell surface molecules CD40 and CD40L (T-cell ligand) and B7.1 and CD28. B lymphocytes are the other major antigen-presenting cells in the immune system and are particularly effective at presenting to memory T cells. Figure 14.3 outlines the various helper interactions mediated by CD4 T cells.

Recognition of virus-infected cells by CD8$^+$ T lymphocytes

CD8$^+$ T cells recognize a complex of MHC class I with a foreign (virus) peptide on infected cells. The process by which viral antigens are processed and presented is referred to as the endogenous antigen-presenting pathway (Lehner and Cresswell 1996). Briefly, newly synthesized viral proteins are degraded in part by a complex of proteolytic enzymes called the proteosome. Small peptides generated by this process are actively transported via peptide transporters (TAP1 and 2) to the ER where they associate with the MHC class I heavy chain. Peptides may be trimmed by enzymes in order to fit snugly into the MHC cleft which accommodates peptides of around nine amino acids. The light chain (β2-microglobulin) associates with the heavy chain and the trimolecular complex is transported to the cell surface. The evolutionary advantage of this process is that peptides derived from intracellular pathogens can be processed at an early stage in the infection, well before replication or assembly of new virions has occurred. If they can be recognized by the immune system the infectious agent can be rapidly eliminated.

The fact that viral immediate early and early antigens can be recognized by T cells supports this view.

Selection for the relevant peptides can occur at three stages in this processing pathway: (1) the proteosome, i.e. where peptide cleavage occurs according to the enzymatic specificity within the proteosome; (2) the peptide transporters that show a preference for selecting certain C-terminal amino acids; and (3) the MHC molecule for which many allelic forms exist, all differing at the peptide-binding groove/cleft.

Because MHC class I molecules occur on virtually all nucleated cells, viruses will have difficulty avoiding the attentions of cytotoxic CD8 T cells. They have, however, evolved some intriguing strategies to disrupt antigen presentation, discussed below (see section entitled Viral strategies for evading the immune response). One strategy adopted by HIV involves antigenic variation and T-cell receptor antagonism. Mutation in antigenic peptides is a feature of HIV infection. Changes can occur that affect (1) peptide binding to MHC class I molecules, (2) peptide recognition by the TCR, and (3) peptide processing by proteosomes. In (3), alterations to amino acids flanking either side of an antigenic peptide could alter peptide processing. Altered peptides affecting TCR recognition can antagonize the T-cell response to the unmutated antigenic peptides (Klenerman et al. 1996).

T cells in antiviral immunity

The importance of particular T-cell subsets in immunity to viruses depends on several, often interrelated, factors, including the nature of the infecting virus, dose of infecting agent, route of infection, and age of the host.

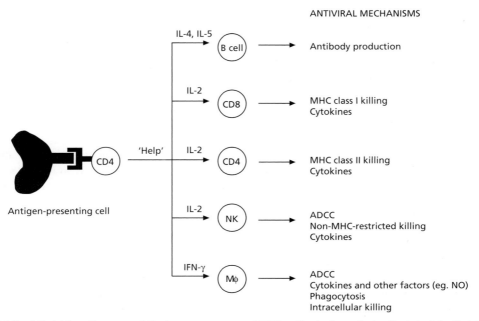

Figure 14.3 *CD4 T cell 'help' for other arms of the immune response. ADCC, antibody-dependent cell cytotoxicity; IL, interleukin; MHC, major histocompatibility complex; Mφ, macrophage.*

Since 1976, a vast amount of information has been generated on the role of T cells in a number of virus infections, including the well-studied examples of influenza virus, LCMV, vaccinia virus, HSV, and HBV. A more detailed analysis of the immune response to selected virus families is provided in the section entitled Examples of immune responses to specific viruses. These studies indicate a direct role for CD4 and CD8 T cells in recovery from infection, which is emphasized in studies on mice deficient in MHC class I and II genes.

Targeted disruption of β2-microglobulin resulted in low levels of MHC class I expression. These mice have normal CD4 T cells but are severely lacking in CD8 T cells. Such deficient mice infected with LCMV had an impaired ability to clear the infection, stressing the importance of CD8 T cells in this process. In contrast, when these mice were infected with influenza, Sendai or vaccinia viruses they cleared the infection normally. This was surprising, because previous experiments on the adoptive transfer of CD4 or CD8 T cells from infected mice had indicated that CD8 T cells were central to recovery and that CD4 T cells contributed to pathology of the lung infection (Leung and Ada 1982). Not all antiviral CD4 T-cell responses are pathological in outcome, many play an important role in recovery from infection through interaction with B cells and in activating cell-mediated immune responses. In cutaneous HSV infection of mice, a clear role for CD4 T cells exists in clearing virus from the epidermis. The mechanism of protection involves IFN-γ and macrophage recruitment and activation, and resembles a delayed hypersensitivity response (Nash and Cambouropoulos 1993). Similarly, control of vaccinia virus infection of ovaries and VSV infection of the central nervous system (CNS) is mediated by an infiltrating CD4 Th1 response, but not by a CD4 Th2 response (Maloy et al. 2000).

Mice deficient in MHC class II molecules had a deficient CD4 response but normal numbers of CD8 T cells. Infection of these animals with influenza virus resulted in the generation of a virus-specific CD8 T-cell response and recovery from infection (Bodmer et al. 1993). This and previous observations on HSV infection in CD4 T-cell-deficient mice (Nash et al. 1987) indicate that virus-specific CD8 T cells can be induced in a 'helperless' environment. It is interesting that, in mice with a CD4 disrupted gene, there is a failure to maintain a LCMV-specific CD8 T-cell response, leading to persistence of the virus (Battegay et al. 1994). These data argue in favor of a role for CD4 T cells in the maintenance of a continuing CD8 T-cell response and of T-cell memory. In fact, the number of memory T cells arising from an infection is related to the extent of the CD8 T-cell expansion during the primary response (Marshall et al. 2001). The maintenance of T-cell memory is related to the presence of cytokines such as IL-7 and IL-15 (Becker et al. 2002; Tan et al. 2002) and not the continued presence of antigen (Murali-Krishna et al. 1999).

How do CD4 and CD8 T cells mediate antiviral immunity in vivo? Following recognition of the relevant restriction element (MHC class I or II molecules) and T-cell activation, the effector activity of T cells involves cytolysis of the infected cell or control of infection by cytokines, or both. Cytolysis can occur via perforin and the fragmentins, e.g. granzymes, Fas–Fas ligand interaction and tumor necrosis factor (TNF) (Doherty 1993b). The key cells in cytolysis are the CD8 T cells; 'killer' CD4 T cells have been described in measles and HSV infections but are clearly limited to target cells expressing MHC class II molecules (Yasukawa and Zarling 1984). The major cytokines in antiviral immunity include IL-2, IFN-γ, and TNF.

The importance of cytolytic mechanisms in vivo has been demonstrated by targeted gene disruption. Mice deficient in perforin expression are susceptible to LCMV infection. Susceptibility is correlated with a considerably reduced ability of CD8 T cells to lyse infected target cells in vivo. However, some lytic activity is still detected which is attributed to Fas-mediated cell death (Kagi and Lederman 1994). In murine gamma-herpesvirus infection, perforin does not seem to be essential for antiviral immunity mediated by CD8 T cells (Usherwood et al. 1997).

In many virus infections the destruction of certain tissue cells by cytolytic mechanisms may be an unacceptable price for the host to pay. Consequently, nondestructive mechanisms that eliminate the virus but spare the cell are biologically advantageous. Cytokines clearly fulfill this role and are now viewed in a much more positive light as effector molecules in viral infections (Ramshaw et al. 1992; Ramsey et al. 1993) (see also Chapter 15, The role of cytokines in viral infections). Perhaps the best characterized is IFN-γ. A striking illustration of cytokine-mediated antiviral immunity is seen in HBV transgenic mice where clearance of virus is mediated in the absence of cell death, thereby 'curing' the infected cell (Guidotti et al. 1999) (see also section entitled Immune response to hepatitis B, below).

THE ROLE OF ANTIBODIES IN IMMUNITY TO VIRUSES

In general, antibodies appear 5–7 days after virus infection. The first antibody class to appear is IgM, which is usually of low affinity. Such antibodies are effective in controlling the spread of virus in the blood stream. As the antibody response evolves and affinity maturation proceeds (a process involving B cell proliferation leading to somatic mutation of immunoglobulin V regions and immunoglobulin class switching) IgG becomes the dominant class in serum and is characterized by increased affinity for viral antigens (Wabl and Steinberg 1996). Such antibodies are the major defense against reinfection by virus, which becomes neutralized by a variety of mechanisms (see section entitled Destruction of infected cells, below). The main antibody defense at mucosal surfaces involves IgA, which occurs as a dimeric immunoglobulin with a secretory piece which protects them against the hostile environment of the gut and other mucosal sites. As discussed in the section entitled Destruction of infected cells below, antibodies form an important link with the innate immune response where they focus and activate the complement system and interact with a variety of phagocytic cells and lymphocytes via receptors for the Fc region of IgG (FcγR) and complement (CR). This combined response leads to neutralization of virus or lysis of virus-infected cells or phagocytosis.

Mechanisms of antibody-mediated neutralization of virus

The process whereby antibody neutralizes a virus is extremely varied and depends on the nature of the viral epitope, the class of antibody, and the nature of the infected cell (for review, see Dimmock 1995 and Klasse and Sattentau 2002). This process falls into two parts: neutralization at the cell surface and neutralization within the cell. A summary of the various antiviral mechanisms involving antibody is shown in Figure 14.4.

An obvious mechanism involves the blockade of virus ligand–cell receptor interaction. However, this event is quite rare, because a build-up of antibody on the virion surface is necessary in order to occupy all the available attachment sites, thus making the process inefficient from the viewpoint of the host defenses. Steric hindrance of receptor–anti-receptor interaction occurs with antibody neutralization of rhinoviruses. Here the antibodies attach to the rim of a 'canyon' or pit on the virion which is the site for binding to ICAM-1 on the cell membrane (Rossman 1989). In the early stages of the immune

response, when antibodies have a low affinity for viral antigens, activation of the complement system can augment neutralization. This is illustrated with mono-clonal antibodies that neutralize only in the presence of complement. The rapid build-up of complement on the virion membrane can lead to steric hindrance of virus–cell interaction or lysis of the virion envelope.

Another form of antibody-mediated neutralization involves inhibition of penetration of the virion. This might involve interfering with the fusion of the virion envelope with the cell membrane, as seen with HIV (Dimmock 1995). This process is probably the main mechanism of neutralization of paramyxoviruses and herpesviruses.

Even when a virus has entered the cell it is still subject to neutralization by antibody. For example, fusion with the endosome is a key mechanism used by influenza virus to enter the cytoplasm. To achieve this, hemagglutinin undergoes a major conformational rear-rangement to engage and fuse with the endosomal membrane. Antibodies have been implicated in inhi-biting this process (Wharton et al. 1995). Certain none-nveloped viruses enter the cell by adsorptive endocy-tosis, and changes in local pH lead to acidification and eventual uncoating. Poliovirus undergoes a series of changes resulting in a reduced sedimentation coefficient from 160S to 140S to 80S. Several neutralizing anti-bodies have been defined that inhibit this progression, blocking uncoating (Vrijsen et al. 1993). A similar process occurs with adenovirus, in which the anti-hexon antibody inhibits the pH-dependent changes required for fusion with the endosome and infectivity (Wohlfart 1988). In rare instances, antibody can neutralize infec-tivity after uncoating has taken place. With influenza virus, transcription is blocked by a failure of the ribonu-cleoprotein to function (Armstrong and Dimmock 1992).

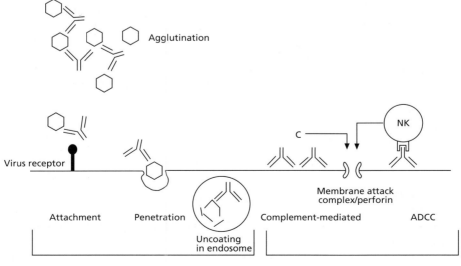

Figure 14.4 *Antiviral effector mechanisms mediated by antibodies. ADCC, antibody-dependent cell cytotoxicity; C, complement; NK, natural killer.*

Other direct effects of antibody

In neurons infected with Sindbis virus, replication is inhibited following antibody binding to viral glycoproteins on the cell membrane. This occurs with neutralizing and nonneutralizing monoclonal antibodies and is independent of complement and ADCC. The mechanism is unclear but may involve up-regulation of some cytoplasmic defense system (Levine et al. 1991; Levine and Griffin 1992).

Neutralization by IgA is a highly effective method of inhibiting virus invasion at mucosal surfaces. This can take place at two levels: extracellular and intracellular neutralization of virus. The latter is thought to occur in polarized cells in which IgA passes through via the poly-Ig receptor from the luminal to the apical surface. It is speculated that, during this process, vesicles containing IgA interact with those containing virus, leading to neutralization (Mazanec et al. 1992, 1993).

Antibodies can inhibit the release of some viruses from the infected cell. Examples include the herpesviruses in which antibodies to glycoprotein H of HSV-1 can block virus egress. Antibodies are also effective in blocking virus-induced cell fusion, thereby inhibiting syncytial (giant cell) formation.

Destruction of infected cells

Antibody can contribute to the destruction of virus-infected cells in two ways: complement-dependent lysis and ADCC.

Usually, a high density of membrane-bound antibody (calculated to be of the order of 5×10^6 IgG molecules/cell) is required for complement-mediated lysis of measles virus-infected cells. Clearly, such mechanisms are likely to be effective late in the infectious cycle. It is interesting that in most cases of antibody-targeted complement-mediated lysis it is the alternative complement pathway that becomes activated and not the classical pathway as one might have predicted (Sissons 1984).

ADCC is a highly efficient process, requiring only small quantities of bound IgG (10^3 molecules/cell). With HSV-1-infected cells ADCC is effective early on, before new progeny virus is assembled and released (Kohl 1991). The types of cell involved in this process have been discussed in the sections entitled Antiviral properties of IFN and NK cells in antiviral immunity, above.

Significance of antiviral antibody mechanisms in vivo

It is likely that all the antibody mechanisms discussed above contribute to immunity in the host. Studies with monoclonal antibodies have allowed dissection of the role of specific mechanisms. Antibodies that neutralize viruses in vitro are also effective at inhibiting their replication in vivo. This is illustrated by the inactivation of respiratory syncytial virus (RSV) by Fab fragments directed against the F protein of the virus (Crowe et al. 1994). This observation has formed the basis for the therapeutic use of 'humanized' anti-F protein antibodies in the treatment of RSV infections.

Nonneutralizing monoclonals against some viruses (e.g. HSV-1) can also protect against infection when passively administered to mice. The antibodies function in the absence of an active complement system (i.e. in C5-deficient mice), indicating a likely role for ADCC (Kohl 1991).

Passive delivery of antibody is an important natural process in the protection of the newborn. Transplacental transport of IgG antibodies offers an important initial defense against microbial invasion, allowing the infant's immune system time to develop. Likewise, antibodies delivered via colostrum are a major defense against rotavirus infections.

Despite the obvious advantages of antiviral antibodies in preventing infection, individuals with natural deficiencies in antibody are generally not prone to severe virus infections. Exceptions include echovirus infections, in which individuals with X-linked agammaglobulinemia (XLA) are prone to chronic infections of the CNS and muscles that can prove fatal (McKinney et al. 1987).

Summary of T- and B-cell immunity

T and B lymphocytes form an integrated system that tailors the immune response specifically to the relevant virus infection. In addition to specificity, the system retains a memory of the viruses to which it has been exposed, so that the host can be protected better on subsequent encounter. Central to the specific response is the CD4 T cell, which produces growth factors that induce the proliferation and differentiation of both T and B lymphocytes to magnify an immune response. In addition, 'help' from CD4 T cells enables B cells to produce higher affinity antibodies as the response progresses, which are more potent in binding to virus proteins. Such antiviral antibodies can neutralize free virions, and are therefore effective in infections in which there is a cell-free viremia. CTLs then complement antibody by destroying cells that have already been infected. In influenza virus infection, CTLs are necessary to resolve an initial infection; however, antiviral antibody prevents virus spreading in the body and provides subsequent protection from reinfection with the same virus strain.

IMMUNOPATHOLOGY IN VIRUS INFECTION

In any virus infection there is a likelihood of pathological damage to tissues by the immune system. The mechanisms associated with damage are varied and depend on the nature of the virus, its tissue tropism, and the antigenic load associated with the infection. Examples of virus-induced immunopathology are listed in Table 14.1.

Antibody-mediated pathology

Antibody-mediated damage can be divided into immune complex diseases and enhancement of virus infectivity. Antibody-dependent enhancement (ADE) of virus infection is a process whereby virus-specific antibodies enhance the entry of virus into macrophages via interaction with Fc and/or complement receptors (Porterfield 1986; Tirado and Yoon 2003). The phenomenon is observed with many diverse virus infections, for example, flaviviruses to poxviruses, with the common theme that they target macrophages as a site of infection, that they preferentially induce a weak neutralizing antibody response in the infected host, and that they are associated with persistent, viremic infections. ADE has been implicated in a number of human and animal viral diseases. The most compelling examples include dengue virus, Aleutian mink disease virus (AMDV), and feline infectious peritonitis virus (FIPV) (Weiss and Scott 1981; Halstead 1982). In dengue virus infection, children aged <1 year are particularly susceptible, probably because of waning protective maternal antibody leading to infectious immune complexes resulting in exacerbation of infection. This enhancement of infectivity can lead to dengue hemorrhagic fever or dengue shock syndrome (Halstead 1988), the latter resulting in exces-

sive procoagulant release by monocytes. ADE can also be seen in individuals subsequently infected with another dengue virus subtype to which there are cross-reactive antibodies. One of the major problems associated with the development of vaccines to a number of viruses, for example FIPV, lentiviruses, dengue virus, AMDV, is the potential for ADE in natural virus challenges. In several situations the induction of antibodies following vaccination resulted in exacerbations of disease following subsequent virus challenge, for example FIPV (Vennema et al. 1990).

In immune complex disease there is usually a large excess of virus antigen which circulates as complexes with antibody and becomes deposited in tissues such as the kidney or blood vessels, leading to complement activation and inflammation. In persistent LCMV infection, only a weak neutralizing antibody response is generated and immune complexes become lodged in the kidney, resulting in glomerulonephritis (Oldstone et al. 1975). Chronic HBV carriers are also prone to glomerulonephritis and polyarteritis nodosa, an inflammatory disease of blood vessels initiated by deposition of virus–antibody complexes (Lai et al. 1991).

T-cell-mediated immune pathology

Damage mediated by T cells can occur via cytolysis of infected cells or by cytokine liberation. The widely used example of T-cell-mediated pathology in virus infection involves LCMV. In adult mice, infection of the CNS

Table 14.1 *Examples of antibody and T-cell-mediated immune pathology in virus infections*

Virus	Host	Comments
T-cell-mediated effects		
LCMV	Mouse	CD8 T-cell damage during virus infection of CNS
Hepatitis B	Humans	CD8 T-cell destruction of chronically virus-infected hepatocytes
HSV	Mouse	CD4 T-cell-mediated stromal keratitis
EBV	Humans	Infectious mononucleosis
Alcelaphine herpesvirus 1	Cattle	Malignant catarrhal fever
Theiler's murine encephalomyelitis	Mouse	CD4 T-cell-mediated demyelination
Measles	Humans	Rash dependent on T-cell immunity
Immune complex disease		
Aleutian mink disease	Mink	High risk of immune complex disease in kidney and blood vessels
LCMV	Mouse	Nonneutralizing antibody in a persisting virus infection leads to glomerulonephritis
Hepatitis B	Humans	Rash, glomerulonephritis, polyarteritis nodosa
Feline infectious peritonitis	Cat	Disseminated intravascular coagulation triggered by immune complexes
Other antibody effects		
Dengue	Humans	Antibody-dependent enhancement of infection link to dengue hemorrhagic fever
Rabies	Humans/animals	Antibody enhancement linked to early death syndrome

EBV, Epstein–Barr virus; HSV, herpes simplex virus; LCMV, lymphocytic choriomeningitis virus.

results in severe pathological changes mediated by CD8 T cells. Treatment of mice with anti-CD8 antibodies protects against disease. The damage is not related to massive cell destruction, but is attributed to cerebral edema arising from damage to the blood–brain barrier (Buchmeier et al. 1980). CD8 CTLs are thought to underlie the damage to hepatocytes seen in chronic HBV carriers.

Delayed type hypersensitivity mediated by CD4 T cells (Th1 cells) has been associated with several types of virus-triggered immunopathology; for example, lung damage in experimental influenza virus infection (Leung and Ada 1982) and deep stromal disease of the eye in HSV-1 infection (Doymaz and Rouse 1992). CD4 T cells have also been implicated in RSV vaccination pathology. Vaccination of mice with the G protein of RSV induces a CD4 Th2 cell response, which, on challenge with RSV, initiates eosinophilic infiltration in the lung (Alwan et al. 1994). This type of pathology was identified in patients who received an ineffective formalin-inactivated RSV vaccine and subsequently became infected with RSV.

In EBV-induced infectious mononucleosis there is amplification of lymphocytes and an outpouring of cytokines (see section entitled Immune response to herpesviruses, below). An exaggerated form of infectious mononucleosis is malignant catarrhal fever seen in cattle infected with alcelaphine herpesvirus-1. This fatal disease is associated with intense proliferation of T cells resulting from a dysregulation of the cytokine response (Reid et al. 1984).

Immune-mediated pathology is a feature of infection of the CNS by a number of different viruses. Theiler's murine encephalomyelitis virus, a picornavirus, establishes a chronic infection in glial cells and induces a chronic delayed-type hypersensitivity response. Activated macrophages recruited to the CNS are believed to secrete factors such as TNF-α that kill local glial cells and result in areas of demyelination around infected cells (Chamorro et al. 1986; Clatch et al. 1986). Similarly, Semliki Forest virus (an alphavirus) causes demyelinating immunopathology, but in this case the culprit is believed to be virus-specific CD8 T cells that kill infected oligodendrocytes (Subak-Sharpe et al. 1993). Sheep infected with the maedi-visna retrovirus often develop a chronic inflammatory condition that can result in accumulation of mononuclear cells and accompanying pathological changes in various organs, including the CNS, respiratory tract, bones, and joints (Sigurdsson et al. 1962; Oliver et al. 1981).

Summary of immunopathology

The immune system is often likened to a double-edged sword, capable of efficient protection from infectious agents but sometimes causing damage to healthy tissue

in the process. When the intricate series of checks and balances that regulate immune control of the host–virus relationship is upset (for example by excessive secretion of a viral protein in a persistent infection), an inappropriate response can often be deleterious. In some virus infections (for example hepatitis B, see below, section entitled Immune response to hepatitis B) the disease has a large immunopathological component, and therapy for such diseases is the focus of much research.

EXAMPLES OF IMMUNE RESPONSES TO SPECIFIC VIRUSES

General mechanisms of immunity to viruses have been outlined above; however, it is useful to consider certain case histories to illustrate how different components of the immune response are integrated. Picornaviruses are chosen as examples of acute virus infection in which antibody plays an important role. The three other virus families cause persistent and chronic infection in which the immune system has failed to clear the virus and the infection continues in the face of a continuing immune response. The outcome of HBV infection can be virus clearance or, in up to 10 percent of cases, a chronic infection with continuing virus production over long periods of time. Here, the continuing immune response causes immunopathological damage manifested as liver disease. Retroviruses and herpesviruses establish persistent infections where the virus cannot be eliminated from the host by the immune system. In the case of herpesviruses, the virus is generally in a latent form with restricted expression of viral genes presenting fewer targets to the immune system. An intact CTL response is crucial in controlling occasional reactivation and productive virus infection but does not clear latent virus. Retroviruses also establish latent infections where they do not need to transcribe viral genes but generally this is accompanied by chronic virus production. Both herpesviruses and retroviruses illustrate an equilibrium between virus replication and antiviral immunity where the virus persists but damage to the host is limited by the immune system. This equilibrium is a compromise which enables both virus and host to survive, but if breached by a breakdown in the immune system, for example in an immunosuppressed host, it can lead to serious disease. These four examples broadly cover the spectrum of viral disease ranging from acute self-limiting viral disease to life-long, chronic conditions.

Immune response to retroviruses

Retroviruses (Chapter 58, Retroviruses and associated diseases in humans) have several unique characteristics that make recognition by host defenses particularly difficult. Their life cycle involves reverse transcription of viral RNA into DNA, which is then integrated into the host genome. Once integrated, the virus may remain transcriptionally inactive and become methylated along with the surrounding cellular DNA. This ability to exist in the host genome without expressing viral protein makes the retrovirus invisible to the immune system. Indeed, it is estimated that 5–10 percent of the mammalian genome consists of elements introduced by reverse transcription, 10 percent of which are retrovirus-like. Most of these endogenous retroviruses cause no harm to their host, but coexist and are propagated along with host DNA and inherited by any offspring.

Vertical transmission via the germ cells is a mode of spread unique to retroviruses, and enables the virus to influence the host's immune system in early development. Retrovirus proteins expressed early in development are recognized as 'self' by the developing immune system and the responding T cells are purged from the immune repertoire. The adult animal does not therefore possess lymphocytes capable of recognizing and eliminating infected cells expressing this antigen. Ronchese and colleagues (1984) showed that mice carrying endogenous Moloney murine leukemia virus (MoMLV) did not develop antibody or cytotoxic T lymphocyte responses to the antigenically cross-reactive murine sarcoma virus. Mice infected with MoMLV had a lower than normal complement of CTL precursor cells, suggesting that clonal deletion of virus-specific cells had taken place.

In a different murine retrovirus system, mouse mammary tumor virus (MMTV) uses superantigens which bind to specific TCRs to delete reactive T cells in infected mice. This virus is transmitted from infected mothers to offspring via milk and, in susceptible mouse strains, virus integration leads to the formation of mammary tumors. The virus targets B lymphocytes and DCs where reverse transcription, integration, and gene expression lead to expression of viral superantigen (SAg) which primes an SAg specific T-cell response. The virus uses the immune system to enhance its infection in two ways – it binds directly to TLR-4 on B cells and DC resulting in the cellular activation necessary for efficient infection of B cells (Rassa et al. 2002) and in up-regulation of its receptor on DC (Burzyn et al. 2004); expression of SAg on infected B cells leads to T-cell-driven proliferation of infected cells. Continued expression of the SAg eventually leads to deletion of reactive T cells. Later in infection, the virus targets epithelial cells of the exocrine secretory organs from where it can be transmitted to offspring. Antibody is important in determining the outcome of infection. Passive immunization of susceptible mice with neutralizing antibody can prevent infection (Mpandi et al. 2003). A strong neutralizing antibody response leads to decreased mammary gland infection, development of tumors, and infection of progeny. There is a correlation between a strong antibody response and resistance to MMTV infection. Antibody plays an important role in maintaining a balance so

that infection of exocrine glands, which is necessary for transmission of the virus, occurs but levels of infection are sufficiently controlled to prevent rapid tumor development (Finke et al. 2003).

Much effort has been expended in recent years on the investigation of immune responses to human retroviruses, research that has been driven partly by the HIV epidemic. HIV, a retrovirus of the genus *Lentivirus*, is therefore the most intensively studied retrovirus, although care must be taken when extrapolating from HIV to other retrovirus infections.

There is a growing body of evidence that the interaction of HIV with the immune system represents a unique situation. Acute HIV infection causes cytolytic infection of CD4 T cells, particularly those at mucosal sites, a common point of entry for the virus. The predominant CD4 T cell at those sites is the memory CD4 T cell expressing CCR5, the coreceptor for HIV in most natural infection. This results in a severe depletion of these cells which continues throughout the course of the infection. The tropism of HIV for CD4 T cells also presents particular problems for the immune system. HIV-specific CD4 T cells are particularly good targets for virus infection as activated rapidly expanding T cells are highly susceptible to HIV infection. This activation of the CD4 T-cell response presents the virus with more targets to infect and maintain the chronic infection. (Douek et al. 2003).

HIV-specific CD8 T-cell responses are present throughout the course of infection before the onset of acquired immunodeficiency syndrome (AIDS) but are unable to clear HIV infection in the majority of cases. The major problem for CD8 CTL control of HIV infection lies in the high levels of mutation rate associated with high levels of HIV replication, which results in escape epitope mutation such that at any time the CTL pool may be directed against, and indeed continuously stimulated by, epitopes which represent a very minor portion of the current HIV population. HIV infection leads to down-modulation of MHC class I on infected cells contributing to the failure of CD8 T cells to recognize and kill infected cells. Depletion of the CD4 T-cell numbers leads to loss of available CD4 T-cell help for CTL responses. Another reason for the failure of CD8 T cells to control infection may be inactivation; there is evidence that during chronic HIV infection where there is chronic stimulation of CD8 T cells, the cells loose responsiveness to antigen, for example, they often have TCRs of low functional avidity and inappropriate signaling, even those against well-conserved epitopes on one of the outer loops of gp120. This is also seen with other virus infections such as CMV and EBV. Regulatory CD4 T cells can cause functional impairment of virus specific CD8 CTLs in Friend murine leukemia virus (FrMLV) infection (Dittmer et al. 2004), and it is possible that a similar mechanism may occur in HIV infection.

HTLV-1 also targets CD4 T cells, although in this case CD8 T cells are also infected, albeit at a lower level. However, HTLV-1 is not associated with severe immunodeficiency but with adult T cell leukemia/lymphoma and a number of chronic inflammatory diseases. HTLV-1 varies little in sequence and does not present the immune system with the escape mutation scenario found in HIV infection, rendering CTL control of infection much more efficient.

An important role for antibody can be demonstrated in equine infectious anemia virus (EIAV). Episodes of disease coincide with viremia, which is brought under control by the antibody response. Disease then remits until a new virus variant emerges that cannot be neutralized by the previous antibodies; there follows another disease episode. With time, the episodes of disease become less severe, until the horse enters an asymptomatic carrier state. In this phase the disease is under effective immune control, as demonstrated by the fact that immunosuppression induces relapse.

Evasion of the antibody response is an interesting feature of HIV infection. The receptor-binding protein of HIV, gp120, is a prime target for an antibody response; however, the high degree of glycosylation and the tight conformation of this protein restrict the access of antibodies to the highly conserved receptor binding domains within the protein. In addition, the high degree of variability in the exposed faces of gp120 and the conformation-dependence of most anti-gp120 antibodies render most of the antibodies raised to be ineffective against the vast majority of the circulating virus population. One of the exposed loops, thought to contain an important neutralizing determinant, is exceptionally variable, enabling rapid escape from any effective neutralizing antibody response. Soluble gp120 is secreted in large amounts during infection, and it has been suggested that this may act as a decoy to raise an antibody response, but the conformation of gp120 on the virion is different, so the antibodies are not neutralizing. This may explain why there is a large amount of virus-specific antibody in infected individuals but the vast majority is not neutralizing.

In conclusion, while antibodies can contribute to limiting the disease process in retrovirus infection, they are generally ineffective at clearing the infection. The CTL response seems to be more important than the antibody response in protection against most retroviruses

Immune response to picornaviruses

Picornaviruses are small nonenveloped RNA viruses with a relatively simple structure consisting of an icosahedral capsid comprising four proteins and a single strand of positive-sense RNA. Members of this family are very diverse and can cause a wide range of diseases, which are usually acute infections in which the virus replicates in the host over a short time period and generally does not persist. There are some exceptions: for example, Theiler's murine encephalomyelitis virus can remain in the CNS for the lifetime of the host (Lipton et al. 1984). Others do not generally persist but can do so on rare occasions: for example, some cattle infected with foot-and-mouth disease virus go on to become chronic virus secretors.

Most picornavirus infections occur at mucosal surfaces, so the first line of defense for the host lies in the acidic mucus, which contains a number of proteases. Sensitized B cells may secrete antibody of the IgA isotype, which is transported through mucosal cells and secreted from the luminal surface. Challenge with a virus of a strain previously encountered by the immune system will result in neutralization of the virus by secreted antibody before it is able to gain access to the epithelial surface. Stimulation of IgA is the rationale behind the oral polio vaccine: it is more effective than the inactivated virus given systemically because it stimulated gut immunity directly, leading to an effective mucosal antibody response.

The replication of rhinoviruses is confined to the epithelial surface of the upper respiratory tract, and occurs so quickly that by the time the immune system has raised a response, the infection has already resolved. The object of the immune system here is to prevent reinfection. Rhinoviruses exist in hundreds of different serotypes, so there is little chance of preventing reinfection with viruses other than the initial strain. This explains the high incidence of, and poor protection against, the common cold.

In the course of systemic picornavirus infection, the virus penetrates the mucosal surface and can invade the blood stream. The viremia is not cell-associated, making the virions particularly susceptible to neutralization by serum antibody. Poliovirus infection illustrates this very well. After initial replication in the small intestine and mucosal-associated lymphoid tissue (tonsils, Peyer's patches, and lymph nodes of the neck) poliovirus can be detected in the blood. The relatively rare neurological disease (poliomyelitis) occurs following virus invasion of the CNS via the blood or through retrograde transport inside neurons. The experimental administration of neutralizing antibodies can prevent the paralytic disease in both monkeys and humans.

Both B and T cells are involved in the generation of an effective antibody response, because in the absence of T cell help only low affinity antibodies can be made, and there is no immunological memory. In recent years, the contribution made by T lymphocytes in immunity to picornavirus infections has been studied extensively. CD4 T cells involved in providing immunological 'help' for the antibody response are often cross-reactive between virus serotypes, and sometimes between different members of the picornavirus family.

The importance of T cell help can be illustrated by experiments performed in the mouse poliovirus model. Poliovirus does not normally infect mice, but using transgenic mice expressing the human poliovirus receptor they become susceptible to infection of the CNS. T cell clones have been raised against poliovirus proteins, and the transfer of these cell lines with immune B cells was able to protect the mice from lethal infection (Mahon et al. 1995). Transfer of immune B cells alone had no effect emphasizing the importance of T cells in protection. The T-cell lines secreted interferon-γ and this seemed to stimulate the preferential secretion of the IgG2a isotype antibody.

There have been several reports of CTLs in picornavirus infections (reviewed by Usherwood and Nash 1995). These are usually of the CD8 phenotype, although specific CD4 CTLs are also known to exist. Their role in the protection against picornavirus infection is unclear at present, although CD8 T cells are known to contribute to viral clearance in Theiler's virus in both susceptible and resistant mouse strains (Pullen et al. 1993; Begolka et al. 2001).

Immune responses to coxsackie B virus have been implicated in virus associated myocarditis and diabetes. Molecular mimicry (where an antiviral response cross-reacts with host antigens) is thought to be involved in the etiology of these diseases. Antisera generated against synthetic peptide sequences derived from coxsackie B3 protein and the cellular adenine nucleotide translocator cross reacted with both proteins, and antibodies which reacted with the peptides were present in patients with inflammatory cardiomyopathy. Removal of immunoglobulin from patients has been demonstrated to improve the clinical situation and, in a severe combined immunodeficiency (SCID) mouse model, human PBL have been shown to transfer disease symptoms (Schwimmbeck et al. 2004). Other evidence implicates both CD4 and CD8 T cells in coxsackie virus induced myocarditis (Henke et al. 1995). However, there is also evidence that direct viral damage is involved in disease, and limiting viral replication can limit disease (Horwitz et al. 2000). Similarly, autoreactive T cells clearly are associated with coxsackie B virus induced diabetes but there is evidence that T cells do not initiate the disease process. Phagocytosis of infected pancreatic β cells by macrophages has been observed prior to T-cell infiltration. Subsequent antigen presentation by these cells may drive an autoimmune response (Horwitz et al. 2004).

Because of their small genome (7–8.5 kb) it has been possible to map mutations that affect antibody binding sites and T-cell recognition elements for a number of picornaviruses (Usherwood and Nash 1995). In several members of the family, antibody binding sites are present on all three external capsid proteins (for example poliovirus, human rhinovirus), whereas in others, only two proteins are thought to be involved (for example, hepatitis A virus). There does not seem to be a close association between the position of T and B cell epitopes on a given virus protein.

Immune response to hepatitis B

Over 300 million people worldwide are chronically infected with HBV. HBV infection of adults is often asymptomatic, and in most cases the infection is completely cleared. However, in 5–10 percent of adults, the virus establishes a persistent infection. Neonatal infection also occurs, resulting in a degree of immunological tolerance to the virus; over 90 percent of such children become chronically infected. The persistent infection is associated with liver disease and cirrhosis in 25 percent of carriers and can progress to hepatocellular carcinoma. Reports indicate that the lifetime risk to males infected with HBV at birth of developing hepatocellular carcinoma approaches 40 percent (Beasley et al. 1981). The different outcomes of HBV infection illustrate the varied effects of alterations in the equilibrium between virus replication and the antiviral immune response.

Activation of innate nonspecific mechanisms represents a key step in the control of the initial burst of HBV replication. These mechanisms are highly efficient causing an 80 percent drop in the quantity of HBV DNA prior to the onset of the antigen-specific adaptive immune system. NK and NK-T cells are the major component of this response (Kakimi et al. 2000), but the interferon system and liver Kupffer cells play a role. During acute, self-limiting viral hepatitis, antibodies can be detected that are specific for the viral envelope (HBsAg), core antigens (HBcAg and HBeAg), and the viral polymerase (Chisari and Ferrari 1995). Antibodies to HBsAg in serum are neutralizing and are thought to play an important role in viral clearance by binding to cell free virus and preventing spread to other susceptible cells. Induction of anti-HBsAg alone during prophylactic vaccination is often sufficient to completely prevent infection.

Strong CD4 T-cell responses to HBeAg and HBcAg are seen in the peripheral blood of almost all patients with acute hepatitis. Historically, HBeAg is seen as a marker of acute infection but sensitive assays indicate replicating virus remains after removal of HBeAg. The CD4 response to the envelope is much less vigorous, the reason for which is not understood. The CD4 response in self-limiting acute hepatitis is predominantly Th1 while T-cell clones from chronically infected patients produce mainly Th2 responses (Bertoletti et al. 1997; Penna et al. 1997).

CD8 CTLs are known to be crucial in the control of the infection and strong responses to HBsAg, HBcAg and polymerase are found in patients who control HBV. Multiple epitopes are recognized. Activated HBV-specific CTL can persist long after recovery from active HBV infection, suggesting that low levels of persistent infection maintain and are controlled by the CTL response. CD8 CTL responses in chronically infected patients are difficult to detect by classical cytotoxicity assays in both peripheral blood and the liver. Clearance in these patients via spontaneous or interferon induced remission is associated with a boost in this response. Use of MHC class I tetramer technology, which allows direct detection of virus-specific CTLs, has shown that CTLs specific for residues 18–27 of HBcAg comprise up to 1.3 percent of circulating CTLs in acutely infected patients. This is accompanied by a CTL response directed against a number of other viral epitopes. In contrast, in chronically infected HBeAg positive patients, these are barely detectable (Jung and Pape 2002). Tetramer staining shows that, in patients with a high rate of HBV replication and liver inflammation, the numbers of intrahepatic HBcAg-specific CTLs are similar to those in patients without disease, but they are accompanied by large numbers of nonspecific CD8 cells meaning that specific CTLs are present at low frequencies. Thus comparable numbers of intrahepatic virus specific CTLs could be associated with either protection or pathology raising the possibility that there is a functional defect in CTLs in chronic HBV infection (Maini et al. 1999).

HBV does not infect mice or rats but lines of transgenic mice which express HBV and can mimic chronic liver infection have been invaluable in understanding the role of the immune response in control of infection. Transfer of virus specific CTLs into these mice showed that, in addition to killing infected cells, these CTLs eliminate virus from many other infected cells noncytolytically by release of IFN-γ and TNF-α (Guidotti and Chisari 2001). Studies in chimpanzees have confirmed the importance of IFN-γ and TNF-α in removing HBV replicative intermediates from the cytoplasm and closed circular form from the nucleus of HBV infected cells (Guidotti et al. 1999). The transgenic mouse model has been used to show the importance of type I interferons in control of infection and to dissect the pathways involved in clearance. Studies show that neutrophils induce matrix metalloproteinase (MMP) which leads to recruitment of antigen nonspecific mononuclear cells. Elimination of MMPs does not affect viral clearance but prevents damage to the liver by nonspecific mechanisms (Sitia et al. 2004).

Current evidence suggests that both T cell and antibody responses to HBV are necessary to clear HBV and that CTLs act not only by lysing infected cells, but also by releasing cytokines such as IFN-γ and TNF-α that reduce the intracellular virus load without killing the infected cell. The reasons why some HBV infections of adults become chronic, while the majority are limited and cleared by the immune system, are not understood. Model systems provide support for the possibility that outcome is determined by the size of the inoculum and replication rate of the infecting virus. If this is high, then even with a fully activated immune response, viral persistence may be favored (Jung and Pape 2002). It is likely that persistence is determined by multiple mechanisms. The immune system also seems to contribute to the chronic liver pathology by causing destruction of hepatocytes, resulting in a high rate of mitosis and therefore an increased risk of damaging mutations.

Immune response to herpesviruses

There are three subfamilies in the *Herpesviridae*, each with different biological and genetic characteristics (see Chapters 25, Herpesviruses:general properties; 26, Alphaherpesviruses; 27, Betaherpesviruses; 28, Human herpesvirus 8; and 29, Gammaherpesviruses). A central feature of the biology of these viruses is their ability to establish latent infections in either the nervous or immune system. Herpesviruses commonly have numerous immune evasion strategies which allow them sufficient time to progress from the site of primary infection and establish and maintain latency.

HSV is the prototype of the alphaherpesviruses. The natural history of HSV involves infection at mucosal surfaces followed by transmission to the peripheral nervous system where the virus remains latent in neurons. Periodic reactivation occurs with reinfection of epithelial cells which may present as recrudescent disease. HSV lesions are often more severe in immunocompromised individuals, emphasizing the importance of the immune system in controlling disease.

Components of the innate immune system including NK cells, type I interferon, and complement, play a role in the control of HSV infection in vivo but are not sufficient to prevent symptomatic infection. Antibody has been shown to interfere with virus entry to, and movement from, the nervous system (Simmons and Nash 1985), and the existence of immune evasion mechanisms directed against antibody function emphasizes the importance of antibody in neutralization of infectious virus and in antibody mediated cytoxicity. However, T lymphocytes provide the major control mechanism for both primary and recurrent infection.

DCs play a central role in stimulating the T-cell response to HSV. They are readily infected with the virus which inhibits their function as antigen presenting cells (APC) and their migration from the skin. However, infected DCs are potent producers of IFN-α which may act as a danger signal to stimulate uptake and presentation by surrounding DCs (Pollara et al. 2004). These uninfected DCs from the lesion site cross-present viral antigens and stimulate both CD4 and CD8 T cells.

A clear role for CD4 T cells is identified by their clearance of virus from the mouse epidermis. CD4 T cells are potent producers of IFN-γ which stimulates macrophage function. IFN-γ may also be important in counteracting the action of viral immune evasion molecules. HSV-specific CD4 CTL clones are present in skin lesions and are capable of killing infected cells in vitro. The human CD4 T-cell response is broadly directed including targets from all stages of the virus life cycle (Koelle and Corey 2003).

CD8 T cells also participate in resolution of peripheral lesions (van Lint et al. 2004), but in the nervous system they assume a more important role and regulate virus replication in neurons without destroying these cells (Simmons and Tscharke 1992). Evidence suggests that within the human trigeminal ganglia, HSV infection is associated with a chronic immune reaction which influences reactivation (Theil et al. 2003). The CD8 T-cell response appears to be narrower than the CD4 response but as with CD4 T cells, the glycoproteins gB and gD are major targets (Koelle and Corey 2003).

The betaherpesviruses are typified by human and murine cytomegaloviruses, but also include human herpesviruses 6 and 7. The initial infection by CMV is via epithelial surfaces and involves a persistent or latent phase in cells of the myeloid lineage. MCMV can also establish latent infection in other cell types, probably endothelial cell or histiocytes. (Reddehase et al. 2002). cytomegaloviruses in general cause asymptomatic infection in immunocompetent hosts but are important pathogens in immunocompromised individuals.

There is a clear role for NK cells in early protection against lethal MCMV infection. An NK cell receptor which confers resistance to MCMV infection by binding directly to a viral protein expressed on the surface of MCMV infected cells and selectively killing the infected cells has been identified (Arase et al. 2002; Smith et al. 2002). The NK-cell response is limited to the first 3 days of infection and thereafter the CD8 T-cell response dominates recovery from primary infection. In MCMV, the CD8 T-cell response is against an immediate–early (IE) antigen IE1. A single antigenic peptide is recognized in the context of H-2L^d (MHC class I restriction molecule) of BALB/c mice. Immunization with this peptide is sufficient to confer protection against MCMV infection. Likewise, adoptive transfer of T-cell clones specific for the antigenic peptide also eliminates productive infection in most tissues (Koszinowski et al. 1990). In mice lacking CD8 T cells, CD4 T cells can take over this function. In this case, CD4 T cells derived from CD8-deficient animals can confer protection, unlike those from immunocompetent mice. Thus, the immune system appears to be able to compensate, to some extent, for lack of specific function under certain circumstances, however, this compensation does not appear to be complete. For example, mice depleted of CD4 T cells cannot eliminate virus from the salivary gland. Thus, both CD8 and CD4 cells are essential for an efficient immune response to MCMV (Krmpotic et al. 2003). CTL responses to human cytomegalovirus (HCMV) are also directed against one major target, the tegument protein pp65, although the major IE protein may be important in some individuals. CD8 T-cell responses are critical in control of HCMV infection but, like MCMV, CD4 T cells also play a role (Gamadia et al. 2003). Studies in B cell knock-out mice show that antibody is important in protecting from reactivation while CD8, CD4, and NK cells are important in both primary and recurrent infections.

The principal feature of the gammaherpesviruses is a tropism for either B or T lymphocytes. The best studied member is EBV, which targets and establishes latent infection in B cells. This virus also has the ability to transform B cells in vitro and is associated with lymphoproliferative disease. The main immunological surveillance is by CD8 T cells, which target predominantly B cells expressing the latent viral antigens EBNA-3 and LMP (Rickinson and Kieff 2001). Immunosuppression as seen in transplantation affects this balance by reducing the number of EBV-specific CD8 T cells, which results in the appearance of B cell lymphomas.

Murine gammaherpesvirus 68 (MHV-68) infection of laboratory mice has provided an opportunity for studying the immune response to a gammaherpesvirus in its natural host. This virus establishes a latent infection in B cells, DCs, macrophages, and lung epithelial cells and, like EBV, is associated with lymphoproliferative disease and an infectious mononucleosis-like syndrome (Nash et al. 2001). The availability of gene knock-out mice with targeted deletions in genes affecting immune function has made it possible to study the role of individual aspects of the immune response to MHV-68 infection. Studies in mice which lack a type I interferon response have shown that type I interferons are critical in the early control of infection (Dutia et al. 1999). MHV-68, like Kaposi's sarcoma herpesvirus and herpesvirus saimiri encodes a regulator of complement activation which has been shown to play a role in control of persistent replication and virulence in mice lacking IFN-γ responses (Kapadia et al. 2002).

During the primary infection, the virus replicates in alveolar epithelial cells. CD8 T cells clear the productive infection in the lung. A critical event is splenomegaly. This is dependent on CD4 T cells and is accompanied by a transient high load of latently infected cells. Although CD4 T cells are not essential for clearance of the initial lung infection, they are crucial for long term control of infection. Mice lacking CD4 T cells initially clear the infection, but within 3–4 months there is a recurrence of infectious virus in the lung and mice develop severe lung pathology (Cardin et al. 1996). The critical role of CD4 T cells seems to come not from providing help for antibody production or to CD8 T cells. Infection of mice lacking B cells shows that antibody is not essential for control of acute or latent infection although levels of latency are very low in these mice (Usherwood et al. 1996). Depletion of CD8 T cells and IFN-γ in B-cell-deficient mice has identified a critical role for IFN-γ produced by CD4 T cells in control of latent infection (Christensen et al. 1999). Mice lacking CD4 T cells have normal numbers of

CD8 T cells (Stevenson et al. 1998). The exact role of IFN-γ remains to be determined as mice lacking an IFN-γ response, while exhibiting pathological changes (Dutia et al. 1997), do not succumb to infection.

VIRAL STRATEGIES FOR EVADING THE IMMUNE RESPONSE

In order to survive in the host for a prolonged period a virus must either hide from or evade the antiviral immune response. As mentioned above in the section entitled Immune response to retroviruses, viruses such as MMTV that contain a superantigen, can induce a state of tolerance against themselves. A similar situation has been reported with lymphocytic choriomeningitis virus infection, in which an overwhelming infection is thought to 'exhaust' the immune response; the virus then infects the thymus so that newly emerging T lymphocytes are tolerant to virus antigens (Moskophidis et al. 1993). Some sites in the body are regarded as immunologically privileged, meaning that the ability of the immune system to respond to foreign proteins present in them is impaired. Some viruses have exploited such shelters, and preferentially infect sites such as the CNS (Fazakerley and Buchmeier 1993).

As with any rapidly replicating organism, viruses can evolve quickly in response to a changing environment. In the case of eukaryotic viruses, the immune system is a potent selective pressure, so, in order to survive, many viruses have acquired ways either of evading recognition or of obstructing the effector arms of the immune response. Most RNA viruses have high mutation rates due to errors produced by virus polymerases that lack proof-reading functions. A mutation rate of 10^{-4}–10^{-5} per base per replication cycle is typical (Holland et al. 1992). Any mutant virus that is recognized less efficiently by the immune system will dominate the virus population in the face of a stringent immune response. For example, the retrovirus HIV has a highly variable surface protein, gp120, which is the target for antiviral antibodies. Many serotypes of influenza virus exist, which have been selected by their ability to evade neutralizing antibody responses. Periodically, an antigenic shift occurs, when reassortment between two distinct influenza virus isolates result in antigenically distinct progeny that may give rise to pandemics as the virus replicates in a nonimmune population (Webster et al. 1992).

DNA viruses have less plastic genomes, often of sufficient size to accommodate genes acquired from host cells that may allow them to subvert immune attack strategies. There are also examples of convergent evolution whereby viral genes have apparently evolved to mimic cellular genes involved in immune regulation. As should be clear from the preceding sections of this chapter, many facets of the immune system are involved in the antiviral response, and the following section details how each part of the immune network may be subverted by viruses.

The literature underpinning this field has risen dramatically over the past few years. Consequently, we refer the reader to several excellent reviews that go into far greater detail on the viral genes and their mechanisms of action (Tortorella et al. 2000; Alcami and Koszinowski 2000; Alcami 2003; Benedict et al. 2002; Yewdell and Hill 2002; Goodbourn et al. 2000; Orange et al. 2002; Favoreel et al. 2003)

Inhibitors of inflammation

Inflammation is the first response to virus-induced tissue damage, which releases many cytokines necessary to attract immune cells. Vaccinia virus encodes a steroid-synthesizing enzyme, 3β-hydroxysteroid dehydrogenase, which is transcribed early in infection. It is not known which steroids are synthesized by this enzyme; several glucocorticoids are, however, anti-inflammatory and it is known that this gene contributes to viral virulence. Several poxviruses possess serine protease inhibitors (serpins), which are thought to interfere with the pathways leading to the production of lipoxygenase metabolites and IL-1β production, both of which are important pro-inflammatory factors. African swine fever virus (ASFV) directly inhibits the activation of pro-inflammatory cytokines in pig macrophages through the expression of an IκB homologue (A238L). This protein interferes with cytokine transcription by inhibiting the function of NFκB (see Alcami and Koszinowski 2000 and Tortorella et al. 2000)

Inhibition of interferon

Type I interferon released from infected cells can both induce enzymes that destroy intracellular viral nucleic acid and prevent translation of viral mRNA. Proteins made by reovirus and vaccinia virus can complex with double-stranded RNA (dsRNA) and inhibit dsRNA-dependent protein kinase (PKR) activation. Small RNAs made by adenovirus, HIV-1, and EBV are able to bind to PKR and inhibit its activation. Another protein produced by vaccinia virus acts as an alternative substrate for PKR, preventing it from phosphorylating eIF-2a. The normal cellular control mechanisms for PKR regulation are subverted by influenza virus, resulting in the repression of PKR by another cellular factor, p58. By contrast, poliovirus induces the phosphorylation and degradation of PKR. Another strategy used by viruses to disrupt interferon response involves inhibiting the activation of the JAK/STAT signaling pathway. SV5 specifically targets STAT1 for proteasome-mediated degradation. Other viruses target STAT2 (human parainfluenza virus) or JAK1(murine polyomavirus). Poxviruses have yet another mechanism for inhibiting interferon responses involving the expression

Viral interference with apoptosis

For some DNA viruses, survival in the cell is of paramount importance. To this end they have exploited strategies for disrupting apoptotic mechanisms by the use of decoy proteins with anti-apoptotic activity. Bcl-2 homologues are a feature of many herpesviruses and function as a powerful inhibitor of apoptosis. In the process of apoptosis caspase activation is a critical event. The cytokine response modifier A (CrmA) of cowpox virus is a potent inhibitor of caspase 1 and caspase 8 activity, following a variety of death inducing stimuli. Adenovirus also encodes an inhibitor of caspase 8.

Both NK cells and cytotoxic T cells kill target cells through TNF's and FasL interaction with TNF receptor (TNFR) family molecules. Poxviruses counter this by production of secreted viral TNFR which neutralizes cytotoxic cytokines. The gammaherpesviruses, Kaposi's sarcoma associated herpesvirus (KSHV) and herpesvirus saimiri (HSV) encode molecules called vFLIPS that interfere with the Fas-associated death domains (FADD)–caspase interaction blocking induction of apoptosis (see Benedict et al. 2002).

Humoral factors: complement and antibody

As mentioned in the section entitled Collectins and the complement system, above, the complement cascade is activated by a C3-convertase that can be induced by either cross-linked antibody or the surface of particular pathogens, the end result being the deposition of a membrane attack complex that causes lysis of cells or virus. Proteins encoded by some poxviruses and herpesviruses contain short consensus repeats (SCR), which are present in many complement control proteins, for example CD46 and CD55. Viral homologues of CD46, CD55, CR1, and CB4P are known to bind to C3b and C4b, inhibiting the C4b2a C3 convertase. Purified EBV virions have also been reported to accelerate the decay of C3 convertase. The *ORF4* gene of MHV-68 is present as a membrane-bound and secreted protein and functions as a regulator of complement activation. Virus lacking ORF4 is attenuated in infected mice, suggesting this viral gene product functions in vivo as a virulence determinant. Similarly, HVS possesses a protein with four SCRs that is both secreted by, and present on, infected cells and virions. HVS also has a homologue of CD59, a cellular factor that accelerates the decay of the membrane attack complex. Some viruses, HCMV and HIV, actually hijack host CD59 and incorporate this into the viral envelope. A protein present on the infected cell and on the virion of HSV-1, glycoprotein C, can bind C3b and C3bi, inhibiting initiation of the complement cascade.

Two herpesviruses, HCMV and HSV-1, are known to code for Fc receptor homologues. It is thought that these bind antibody molecules in such a way that their Fc portion cannot activate the classical complement pathway or be available for engagement by Fc receptors on phagocytes. The presence of bound immunoglobulin on the cell surface may also hinder the attachment of antibodies specific for virus antigens (see Favoreel et al. 2003; Alcami and Koszinowski 2000).

Interference with MHC function and NK cell recognition

As described in the section entitled Recognition of virus-infected cells by CD8[+] T lymphocytes, above, cytotoxic lymphocytes recognizing MHC class I in association with a viral peptide represent an important defense mechanism against viruses. Not surprisingly some viruses have developed ways of manipulating the CTL response, by interfering with normal antigen presentation mechanisms through MHC class I. This can be achieved at various levels in the infected cell including resistance to the catalytic processes of the proteosome, for example EBNA-1 of EBV, blockade of peptide transport by TAP proteins, for example HSV, and inhibition of maturation, assembly and migration of MHC class I molecules, for example human and mouse CMV.

The down-regulation of MHC class I expression by viruses might well disrupt CD8 T-cell recognition. However, NK cells take advantage of reduced MHC class I expression and become activated, killing virus infected cells (see section entitled NK cells in antiviral immunity). In order to thwart the attentions of NK cells, CMV encodes a MHC class I homologue (UL18 HCMV and m144 MCMV) that becomes expressed on the surface of infected cells and serves to engage Ly49 inhibitory molecules or killer inhibitory receptors (KIR) resulting in the inactivation of NK-cell killing. Another strategy used by HCMV involves the induced expression of HLA-E by a peptide generated by the viral protein UL40. HLA-E serves to protect infected cells from NK-cell attack.

Some of the DNA viruses have developed strategies to disrupt MHC class II expression. For example, adenoviruses and some herpesviruses block MHC class II transcription. HCMV US2 protein interferes post-translationally with MHC class II by translocating DRα and the DMα chain to the cytosol for proteosome-mediated degradation. HIV Nef protein interacts with the endocytic mechanisms and initiates the rapid internalization of CD4 and MHC class I molecules from the cell surface. This process brings Nef into contact with the proton pump in MHC class II containing vesicles leading to acidification and interference with peptide presentation. A similar mechanism exists for the E5 protein of papillomavirus (see Yewdell and Hill 2002; Tortorella et al. 2000; Orange et al. 2002).

Subversion of cytokine and chemokine function

The cytokine system represents the communication network coordinating the character and magnitude of the immune response. Viruses target cytokines at two levels. One involves production of viral cytokines homologues that mimic normal cytokine activity. The second involves viral cytokine receptors and binding proteins. KSHV encodes a vIL-6 and EBV produces a vIL-10, both cytokine homologues have the potential to act as growth factors for B cells with implications for the biology of these B cell tropic viruses. Poxviruses encode vTGF-β (fowlpox virus) and vSEMA, a semaphorin homologue (vaccinia virus). However, the function of these cytokine homologues has still to be determined. Both poxviruses and herpesviruses encode vTNF receptors that are secreted from infected cells and act to neutralize soluble TNF. Poxviruses also encode a variety of secreted binding proteins, for example vIL-18BP which can inhibit IL-18 induced IFN-γ and NK cell responses.

A second major immunological network involves chemokines and the role played in trafficking leukocytes to sites of inflammation and in regulating movement in and out of lymphoid compartments. The herpesviruses and poxviruses have an elaborate armory for disrupting or utilizing the chemokine network. One viral strategy involves production of viral chemokine homologues. KSHV encodes vMIP homologues that act as chemokine antagonists that attract Th2 cells and also have angiogenic activity. These activities aid the virus by disrupting the induction of protective Th1 responses and also recruiting cells to sites of infection for the purpose of virus infection.

Many gammaherpesviruses and some poxviruses encode viral chemokine receptors (vCKR). Over expression of these receptors can lead to cell transformation. A more relevant biological role for these receptors could be in transient cell proliferation and cell migration.

A third group of proteins with direct chemokine inhibitory activity are the chemokine-binding proteins. These proteins have no homology to chemokine receptors yet have evolved a high affinity for chemokines. Some binding proteins have a restricted affinity for CC chemokines, whereas the M3 protein of MHV-68 targets C, CC, CXC, CX3C chemokines. M3 functions in vivo by inhibiting lymphocyte migration to sites of infection and also plays a role in the establishment of latency, presumably by interfering with T-cell recognition of latently infected cells (for a review of this section see Alcami 2003)

CONCLUDING REMARKS

Viruses of humans and animals and their immune systems have evolved together over millions of years, each shaping the other. As protective mechanisms become more efficient and sophisticated, so do the strategies used by viruses to favor their survival. Because of their short replication time and their ability to mutate and evolve rapidly, viruses have been able to exploit niches inaccessible to immune cells. Some viruses have appropriated cellular genes coding for proteins that have a role in immune regulation, whereas others synthesize their own mimics to fool the hapless lymphocyte.

In most cases, however, the immune system can limit the damage caused during virus infections. From the perspective of the virus it is a distinct advantage if the host remains healthy, as this will assist its dissemination. Thus, acute infections (for example, rhinoviruses) may replicate quickly, causing a mild, self-limiting disease that can spread to a new host before the immune system eliminates it. The strategy adopted by viruses causing chronic infections is different: the virus can be disseminated over a much longer period of time but it must evade the immune response. Some herpesviruses (for example, HHV-6) seem to have mastered the art of persisting in a large proportion of the population for long periods without causing disease except in special circumstances. Infections such as these can be considered to have reached an amicable compromise with the host's immune system, causing little disease yet enabling the virus to spread. Viruses causing more severe disease may be those that have recently spread to their host species and have not yet evolved a mutually acceptable relationship.

REFERENCES

Abraham, N., Stojdl, D.F., et al. 1999. Characterisation of transgenic mice with targeted disruption of the catalytic domain of the double-stranded RNA-dependent protein kinase PKR. *J Biol Chem*, **274**, 5053–62.

Alcami, A. 2003. Viral mimicry of cytokines, chemokines and their receptors. *Nature Rev Immunol*, **3**, 36–50.

Alcami, A. and Koszinowski, U.H. 2000. Viral mechanisms of immune evasion. *Immunol Today*, **21**, 447–55.

Alwan, W.H., Kozlowska, W.J. and Openshaw, P.J. 1994. Distinct types of lung disease caused by functional subsets of antiviral T cells. *J Exp Med*, **179**, 81–9.

Andrews, D.M., Scalzo, A.A., et al. 2003. Functional interactions between dendritic cells and NK cells during virus infection. *Nat Immunol*, **4**, 175–81.

Arase, H., Mocarski, E.S., et al. 2002. Direct recognition of cytomegalovirus by activating and inhibitory NK cell receptors. *Science*, **296**, 1323–6.

Armstrong, S.J. and Dimmock, N.J. 1992. Neutralization of influenza virus by low concentrations of HA-specific polymeric IgA inhibits viral fusion activity but activation of the ribonucleoprotein is also inhibited. *J Virol*, **66**, 3823–32.

Bartholomew, R.M., Esser, A.F. and Muller-Eberhard, H.J. 1978. Lysis of oncornaviruses by human serum isolation of the viral complement (CI) and identification as p15E. *J Exp Med*, **147**, 844–53.

Battegay, M., Moskophidis, D., et al. 1994. Enhanced establishment of a virus carrier state in adult CD4+ T cell-deficient mice. *J Virol*, **68**, 4700–4.

Beasley, R.P., Lin, C.-C., et al. 1981. Hepatocellular carcinoma and hepatitis B virus: a prospective study of 22,707 men in Taiwan. *Lancet*, **2**, 1129–33.

Becker, T.C., Wherry, E.J., et al. 2002. Interleukin 15 is required for proliferation renewal of virus-specific memory CD8 T cells. *J Exp Med*, **195**, 1541–8.

Begolka, W.S., Haynes, L.M., et al. 2001. CD8-deficient SJL mice display enhanced susceptibility to Theiler's virus infection and increased demyelinating pathology. *J Neurovirol*, **7**, 409–20.

Benedict, C.A., Norris, P.S. and Ware, C.F. 2002. To kill or be killed: viral evasion of apoptosis. *Nature Immunol*, **3**, 1013–18.

Bertoletti, A., D'Elios, M.M., et al. 1997. Different cytokine profiles of intrahepatic T cells in chronic hepatitis B and hepatitis C virus infections. *Gastroenterology*, **112**, 193–9.

Biron, C.A., Byron, K.S. and Sullivan, J.A. 1989. Severe herpesvirus infections in an adolescent without natural killer cells. *N Engl J Med*, **320**, 1731–5.

Biron, C.A., Nguyen, K.B., et al. 1999. Natural killer cells in antiviral defense: Function and regulation by innate cytokines. *Annu Rev Immunol*, **17**, 189–220.

Bodmer, H., Obert, G., et al. 1993. Environmental modulation of the autonomy of cytotoxic T lymphocytes. *Eur J Immunol*, **23**, 1649–54.

Bonina, L., Nash, A.A., et al. 1984. T-cell macrophage interaction in arginase mediated resistance to herpes simplex virus. *Virus Res*, **1**, 501–5.

Born, W.K., Harshen, K., et al. 1991. The role of g/d T lymphocytes in infection. *Curr Opin Immunol*, **3**, 455–9.

Buchmeier, M.J., Welsh, R.M., et al. 1980. The virology and immunology of lymphocytic choriomeningitis virus infection. *Adv Immunol*, **30**, 275–331.

Burzyn, D., Rassa, J.C., et al. 2004. Toll-like receptor 4-dependent activation of dendritic cells by a retrovirus. *J Virol*, **78**, 576–84.

Busch, R. and Mellins, E.D. 1996. Developing and shedding inhibitions: how MHC class II molecules block maturity. *Curr Opin Immunol*, **8**, 51–8.

Cardin, R.D., Brooks, J.W., et al. 1996. Progressive loss of CD8+ T cell-mediated control of a gamma-herpesvirus in the absence of CD4+ T cells. *J Exp Med*, **184**, 863–71.

Chamorro, M., Aubert, C. and Brahic, M. 1986. Demyelinating lesions due to Theiler's virus are associated with ongoing central nervous system infection. *J Virol*, **57**, 992–7.

Chisari, F.V. and Ferrari, C. 1995. Hepatitis B virus immunopathogenesis. *Annu Rev Immunol*, **13**, 29–60.

Christensen, J.P., Cardin, R.D., et al. 1999. CD4⁺ T cell-mediated control of a gamma-herpesvirus in B cell-deficient mice is mediated by IFN-gamma. *Proc Natl Acad Sci USA*, **96**, 5135–40.

Clatch, R.J., Lipton, H.L. and Miller, S.D. 1986. Characterisation of Theiler's murine encephalomyelitis virus (TMEV)-specific delayed-type hypersensitivity responses in TMEV-induced demyelinating disease: correlation with clinical signs. *J Immunol*, **136**, 920–7.

Clemens, M.J. and Elia, A. 1997. The double-stranded RNA-dependent protein kinase PKR: structure and function. *J Interferon Chemokine Res*, **17**, 503–24.

Crowe, J.E., Murphy, B.R., et al. 1994. Recombinant human respiratory syncytial virus (RSV) monoclonal antibody Fab is effective therapeutically when introduced directly into the lungs of RSV-infected mice. *Proc Natl Acad Sci USA*, **91**, 1386–90.

Diebold, S.S., Kaisho, T., et al. 2004. Innate antiviral responses by means of TLR-7 mediated recognition of single-stranded RNA. *Science*, **303**, 1529–31.

Dimmock, N.J. 1995. Update on the neutralisation of animal viruses. *Rev Med Virol*, **5**, 165–79.

Dittmer, U., He, H., et al. 2004. Functional impairment of CD8⁺ T cells by regulatory T cells during persistent retroviral infection. *Immunity*, **20**, 293–303.

Doherty, P.C. 1993a. Virus infections in mice with targeted gene disruption. *Curr Opin Immunol*, **5**, 479–83.

Doherty, P.C. 1993b. Cell-mediated cytotoxicity. *Cell*, **75**, 607–12.

Dokun, A.O., Groh, V., et al. 2001. Specific and non-specific NK cell activation during virus infection. *Nat Immunol*, **2**, 951–6.

Douek, D.C., Picker, L.J. and Koup, R.A. 2003. T cell dynamics in HIV-1 infection. *Annu Rev Immunol*, **21**, 265–304.

Doymaz, M.Z. and Rouse, B.T. 1992. Immunopathology of herpes simplex virus infections. *Curr Top Microbiol Immunol*, **179**, 121–36.

Dustin, M.L. and Springer, T.A. 1991. Role of adhesion receptors in transient interactions and cell locomotion. *Annu Rev Immunol*, **9**, 27–66.

Dutia, B.M., Clarke, C.J., et al. 1997. Pathological changes in the spleens of gamma interferon receptor-deficient mice infected with murine gammaherpesvirus: a role for CD8 T cells. *J Virol*, **71**, 4278–83.

Dutia, B.M., Allen, D.J., et al. 1999. Type I interferons and IRF-1 play a critical role in the control of a gammaherpesvirus infection. *Virology*, **261**, 173–9.

Epstein, J., Eichbaum, Q., et al. 1996. The collectins in innate immunity. *Curr Opin Immunol*, **8**, 29–35.

Favoreel, H.W., van de Weille, G.R., et al. 2003. Virus complement evasion strategies. *J Gen Virol*, **84**, 1–15.

Fazakerley, J.K. and Buchmeier, M.J. 1993. Pathogenesis of virus-induced demyelination. *Adv Virus Res*, **42**, 249–324.

Finke, D., Luther, S.A. and Acha-Orbea, H. 2003. The role of neutralizing antibodies for mouse mammary tumor virus transmission and mammary cancer development. *Proc Natl Acad Sci USA*, **100**, 199–204.

Gamadia, L.E., Remmerswaal, E.B., et al. 2003. Primary immune responses to human CMV: a critical role for IFN-gamma-producing CD4+ T cells in protection against CMV disease. *Blood*, **101**, 2686–92.

Goodbourn, S., Didcock, L. and Randall, R.E. 2000. Interferons: cell signaling, immune modulation, antiviral responses and virus counter measures. *J Gen Virol*, **81**, 2341–64.

Gresser, I., Tovey, M.G., et al. 1976. Role of interferon in the pathogenesis of virus diseases as demonstrated by the use of anti-interferon serum. II. Studies with herpes simplex, Moloney sarcoma, vesicular stomatitis, Newcastle disease and influenza viruses. *J Exp Med*, **144**, 1316–24.

Guidotti, L.G. and Chisari, F.V. 2001. Noncytolytic control of viral infections by the innate and adaptive immune response. *Annu Rev Immunol*, **19**, 65–91.

Guidotti, L.G., Rochford, R., et al. 1999. Viral clearance without destruction of infected cells during acute HBV infection. *Science*, **284**, 825–9.

Hakozaki, Y., Yoshiba, M., et al. 2002. Mannose-binding lectin and the prognosis of fulminant hepatic failure caused by HBV infection. *Liver*, **22**, 29–34.

Halstead, S.B. 1982. Immune enhancement of virus infection. *Prog Allergy*, **31**, 301–64.

Halstead, S.B. 1988. Pathogenesis of dengue: challenges to molecular biology. *Science*, **239**, 476–81.

Henke, A., Huber, S., et al. 1995. The role of CD8+ T lymphocytes in coxsackievirus B3-induced myocarditis. *J Virol*, **69**, 6720–8.

Hirsch, G.L., Winkelstein, J.A. and Griffin, D.E. 1980. The role of complement in viral infections. *J Immunol*, **124**, 2507–10.

Holland, J.J., de la Torre, J.C. and Steinhauer, D.A. 1992. RNA virus populations as quasispecies. *Curr Top Microbiol Immunol*, **176**, 1–20.

Horwitz, M.S., La Cava, A., et al. 2000. Pancreatic expression of interferon-gamma protects mice from lethal coxsackievirus B3 infection and subsequent myocarditis. *Nat Med*, **6**, 693–7.

Horwitz, M.S., Ilic, A., et al. 2004. Coxsackieviral-mediated diabetes: induction requires antigen-presenting cells and is accompanied by phagocytosis of beta cells. *Clin Immunol*, **110**, 134–44.

Ikeda, F., Haragucji, Y., et al. 1998. Human complement component c1q inhibits the infectivity of cell-free HTLV-1. *J Immunol*, **161**, 5712–19.

Janeway, C.A. 1992. The immune system evolved to discriminate self from non-infectious self. *Immunol Today*, **13**, 11–16.

Janeway, C.A. and Medzhitov, R. 2002. Innate immune recognition. *Annu Rev Immunol*, **20**, 197–216.

Jung, M.C. and Pape, G.R. 2002. Immunology of hepatitis B infection. *Lancet Infect Dis*, **2**, 43–50.

Kagi, D. and Lederman, B. 1994. Cytoxicity mediated by T cells and natural killer cells is greatly impaired in perforin-deficient mice. *Nature (London)*, **369**, 31–7.

Kakimi, K., Guidotti, L.G., et al. 2000. Natural killer T cell activation inhibits hepatitis B virus replication in vivo. *J Exp Med*, **192**, 921–30.

Kapadia, S.B., Levine, B., et al. 2002. Critical role of complement and viral evasion of complement in acute, persistent, and latent gamma-herpesvirus infection. *Immunity*, **17**, 143–55.

Karupiah, G., Blanden, R.V. and Ramshaw, I.A. 1990. Interferon-γ is involved in the recovery of athymic nude mice from recombinant vaccinia virus/IL-2 infection. *J Exp Med*, **172**, 1495–502.

Karupiah, G., Xie, Q.-W., et al. 1993. Inhibition of viral replication by interferon γ-induced nitric oxide synthase. *Science*, **261**, 1445–8.

Klasse, P.J. and Sattentau, Q.J. 2002. Occupancy and mechanism in antibody-mediated neutralization of animal viruses. *J Gen Virol*, **83**, 2091–108.

Klenerman, P., Phillips, R. and McMichael, A. 1996. Cytotoxic T cell antagonism in HIV-1. *Semin Virol*, **7**, 31–40.

Koelle, D.M. and Corey, L. 2003. Recent progress in herpes simplex virus immunobiology and vaccine research. *Clin Microbiol Rev*, **16**, 96–113.

Kohl, S. 1991. Role of antibody-dependent cellular cytotoxicity in defense against herpes simplex virus infections. *Rev Infect Dis*, **13**, 108–14.

Koszinowski, U.H., del Val, M. and Reddehasse, M.J. 1990. Cellular and molecular basis of the protective immune response to cytomegalovirus infection. *Curr Top Microbiol Immunol*, **154**, 189–220.

Kotenko, S.V., Gallagher, G., et al. 2003. IFN-lambdas mediate antiviral protection through a distinct class II cytokine receptor complex. *Nat Immunol*, **4**, 69–77.

Krmpotic, A., Bubic, I., et al. 2003. Pathogenesis of murine cytomegalovirus infection. *Microbes Infect*, **5**, 1263–77.

Lachmann, P.J. and Rosen, F.S. 1979. Genetic defects of complement in viral infection. *Semin Immunopathol*, **1**, 339–53.

LaFleur, D.W., Nardelli, B., et al. 2001. Interferon-kappa, a novel type I interferon expressed in human keratinocytes. *J Biol Chem*, **276**, 39765–71.

Lai, K.N., Li, P.K.Y., et al. 1991. Membranous nephropathy related to hepatitis B in adults. *N Engl J Med*, **324**, 1457–63.

Lee, S.B., Rodriguez, D., et al. 1997. The apoptosis pathway triggered by the interferon-induced protein kinase PKR requires the basic domain, initiates upstream of Bcl-2, and involves ICE-like proteases. *Virology*, **231**, 81–8.

Lehner, P.J. and Cresswell, P. 1996. Processing and delivery of peptides presented by MHC class I molecules. *Curr Opin Immunol*, **8**, 59–67.

Leung, K.N. and Ada, G.L. 1982. Different functions of subsets of effector T cells in murine influenza virus infection. *Cell Immunol*, **67**, 312–24.

Levine, B. and Griffin, D.E. 1992. Persistence in mouse brains after recovery from acute alphavirus encephalitis. *J Virol*, **66**, 6429–35.

Levine, B., Hardwick, J.M., et al. 1991. Antibody-mediated clearance of alpha virus infection from neurons. *Science*, **254**, 856–60.

Lipton, H., Kratchovil, J., et al. 1984. Theiler's virus antigen detected in mouse spinal cord $2^1/_2$ years after infection. *Neurology*, **34**, 1117–19.

Litman, G.W., Anderson, M.K. and Rast, J.P. 1999. Evolution of antigen-binding receptors. *Annu Rev Immunol*, **17**, 109–47.

Mahon, B.P., Katrak, K., et al. 1995. Poliovirus-specific CD4 Th1 clones with both cytotoxic and helper activity mediate protective humoral immunity against a lethal poliovirus infection in transgenic mice expressing the human poliovirus receptor. *J Exp Med*, **181**, 1285–92.

Maini, M.K., Boni, C., et al. 1999. Direct ex vivo analysis of hepatitis B virus-specific CD8+ T cells associated with the control of infection. *Gastroenterology*, **117**, 1386–96.

Malhotra, R. and Sim, R.B. 1995. Collectins and viral infection. *Trends Microbiol*, **3**, 240–4.

Maloy, K.L., Burkhart, C., et al. 2000. CD4+T cell subsets during virus infection: protective capacity depends on effector cytokine secretion and on migratory capability. *J Exp Med*, **191**, 2159–70.

Mandelboim, O., Lieberman, N., et al. 2001. Recognition of haemagglutinins on virus-infected cells by NKp46 activates lysis by human NK cells. *Nature*, **409**, 1055–60.

Marshall, D.R., Turner, S.J., et al. 2001. Measuring the diaspora for virus-specific CD8+ T cells. *Proc Natl Acad Sci USA*, **98**, 6313–18.

Mazanec, M., Kaetzel, C.S., et al. 1992. Intracellular neutralization of virus by immunoglobulin A antibodies. *Proc Natl Acad Sci USA*, **89**, 6901–5.

Mazanec, M.B., Nedrud, J.G., et al. 1993. A three-tiered view of the role of IgA in mucosal defense. *Immunol Today*, **14**, 430–5.

McKinney, R.E. Jr, Katz, S.L. and Wilfert, C.M. 1987. Chronic enteroviral meningoencephalitis in agammaglobulinaemic patients. *Rev Infect Dis*, **9**, 334–56.

Merigan, T.C., Reed, S.E., et al. 1973. Inhibition of respiratory virus infection by locally applied interferon. *Lancet*, **1**, 563.

Mistry, S.K., Zheng, M., et al. 2001. Induction of arginase I and II in cornea during herpes simplex virus infection. *Virus Res*, **73**, 177–82.

Montoya, M.C., Sancho, D., et al. 2002. Cell adhesion and polarity during immune interactions. *Immunol Rev*, **186**, 68–82.

Moskophidis, D., Laine, E. and Zinkernagel, R.M. 1993. Peripheral clonal deletion of antiviral memory CD8+ T cells. *Eur J Immunol*, **23**, 3306–11.

Mpandi, M., Otten, L.A., et al. 2003. Passive immunization with neutralizing antibodies interrupts the mouse mammary tumor virus life cycle. *J Virol*, **77**, 9369–77.

Murali-Krishna, K., Lau, L.L., et al. 1999. Persistence of memory CD8 T cells in MHC class I-deficient mice. *Science*, **286**, 1377–81.

Nash, A.A. and Cambouropoulos, P. 1993. The immune response to herpes simplex virus. *Semin Virol*, **4**, 181–6.

Nash, A.A., Jayasuriya, A., et al. 1987. Different roles for L3T4+ and Lyt2+ T cell subsets in the control of an acute herpes simplex virus infection of the skin and nervous system. *J Gen Virol*, **68**, 825–33.

Nash, A.A., Dutia, B.M., et al. 2001. Natural history of murine gamma-herpesvirus infection. *Philos Trans R Soc Lond B Biol Sci*, **356**, 569–79.

Nguyen, K.B., Salazar-Mather, T.P., et al. 2002. Coordinated and distinct roles for IFN-alpha beta, IL-12 and IL-15 regulation of NK cell responses to viral infection. *J Immunol*, **165**, 4279–87.

Oldstone, M.B., Welsh, R.M. and Joseph, B.S. 1975. Pathogenic mechanisms of tissue injury in persistent viral infections. *Ann NY Acad Sci*, **256**, 65–72.

Oliver, R.E., Gorham, J.R., et al. 1981. Ovine progressive pneumonia: pathologic and virologic studies on the naturally occurring disease. *Am J Vet Res*, **42**, 1554–9.

Orange, J.S., Fassett, M.S., et al. 2002. Viral evasion of natural killer cells. *Nature Immunol*, **3**, 1006–12.

Penna, A., Del-Prete, G., et al. 1997. Predominant T-helper 1 cytokine profile of hepatitis B virus nucleocapsid-specific T cells in acute self-limited hepatitis B. *Hepatology*, **25**, 1022–7.

Perussia, B. 1991. Lymphokine activated killer cells, natural killer cells and cytokines. *Curr Opin Immunol*, **3**, 49–55.

Pollara, G., Jones, M., et al. 2004. Herpes simplex virus type-1-induced activation of myeloid dendritic cells: the roles of virus cell interaction and paracrine type I IFN secretion. *J Immunol*, **173**, 4108–19.

Porterfield, J.S. 1986. Antibody dependent enhancement of viral infectivity. *Adv Virus Res*, **31**, 335–55.

Pullen, L.C., Miller, S.D., et al. 1993. Class-I deficient resistant mice intracerebrally inoculated with Theiler's virus show an increased T cell response to virus antigens and susceptibilty to demyelination. *Eur J Immunol*, **23**, 2287–93.

Ramsey, A.J., Ruby, J. and Ramshaw, I.A. 1993. A case for cytokines as effector molecules in the resolution of virus infection. *Immunol Today*, **14**, 155–7.

Ramshaw, I.A., Ruby, J., et al. 1992. Expression of cytokines by recombinant vaccinia viruses: a model for cytokines in virus infections in vivo. *Immunol Rev*, **127**, 157–82.

Rassa, J.C., Meyers, J.L., et al. 2002. Murine retroviruses activate B cells via interaction with toll-like receptor 4. *Proc Natl Acad Sci USA*, **99**, 2281–6.

Reading, P.C., Morey, L.S., et al. 1997. Collectin-mediated antiviral host defense of the lung:evidence from influenza virus infections in mice. *J Virol*, **71**, 253–8.

Reddehase, M.J., Podlech, J. and Grzimek, N.K. 2002. Mouse models of cytomegalovirus latency: overview. *J Clin Virol*, **25**, Suppl 2, S23–36.

Reid, H.W., Buxton, D., et al. 1984. Malignant catarrhal fever. *Vet Rec*, **114**, 581–4.

Rickinson, A.B. and Kieff, E. 2001. Epstein-Barr virus. In: Knipe, D.M., Howley, P.M., et al. (eds), *Fields' Virology*, 4th edn. Philadelphia: Lippincott, Williams and Wilkins, 2575–627.

Riddell, S.R. and Greenberg, P.D. 1994. Therapeutic reconstitution of human viral immunity by adoptive transfer of cytotoxic T lymphocyte clones. *Curr Top Microbiol Immunol*, **189**, 9–34.

Ronchese, F., D'Andrea, E., et al. 1984. Tolerance to viral antigens in Mov-13 mice carrying endogenized Moloney-murine leukaemia virus. *Cellular Immunol*, **83**, 379.

Rossman, M.G. 1989. The canyon hypothesis. Hiding the host cell receptor attachment site on a viral surface from immune surveillance. *J Biol Chem*, **264**, 14587–90.

Scalzo, A.A., Fitzgerald, N.A., et al. 1990. Cmv-1, a genetic locus that controls murine cytomegalovirus replication in the spleen. *J Exp Med*, **171**, 1469–83.

Scalzo, A., Fitzgerald, N.A., et al. 1992. The effect of the Cmv-1 resistance gene, which is linked to the natural killer cell gene complex, is mediated by natural killer cells. *J Immunol*, **149**, 581–9.

Schwimmbeck, P.L., Bigalke, B., et al. 2004. The humoral immune response in viral heart disease: characterization and pathophysiological significance of antibodies. *Med Microbiol Immunol (Berl)*, **193**, 115–19.

Sciammas, R., Johnson, R.M., et al. 1994. Unique antigen recognition by a herpesvirus-specific TCR-gamma delta cell. *J Immunol*, **152**, 5392–7.

Shortman, K. and Liu, Y.J. 2002. Mouse and human dendritic cell subtypes. *Nat Rev Immunol*, **2**, 151–61.

Siegal, F.P., Kadowaki, N., et al. 1999. The nature of the principal type I interferon-producing cells in human blood. *Science*, **284**, 1835–7.

Sigurdsson, B., Palsson, P.A. and van Bogaert, L. 1962. Pathology of visna transmissible demyelinating disease in sheep in Iceland. *Acta Neuropathol*, **1**, 343–62.

Silverman, R.H. 1999. 2-5A-dependent RNase L: a regulated endoribonuclease in the interferon system. In: D'Alessio, G. and Riordan, J.F. (eds), *Ribonucleases: structure and function*. New York: Academic Press, 515–51.

Simmons, A. and Nash, A.A. 1985. Role of antibody in primary and recurrent herpes simplex infection. *J Virol*, **53**, 944–8.

Simmons, A. and Tscharke, D.C. 1992. Anti-CD8 impairs clearance of HSV from the nervous system: implications for the rate of virally infected neurons. *J Exp Med*, **175**, 1337–44.

Sissons, J.G.P. 1984. Antibody and complement lysis of virus infected cells. In: Oldstone, M.B.A. and Notkins, A.L. (eds), *Concepts in viral pathogenesis*, vol. 39. New York: Springer-Verlag.

Sitia, G., Isogawa, M., et al. 2004. MMPs are required for recruitment of antigen-nonspecific mononuclear cells into the liver by CTLs. *J Clin Invest*, **113**, 1158–67.

Smith, H.R., Heusel, J.W., et al. 2002. Recognition of a virus-encoded ligand by a natural killer cell activation receptor. *Proc Natl Acad Sci USA*, **99**, 8826–31.

Spiller, O.B. and Morgan, B.P. 1998. Antibody-independent activation of the classical complement pathway by cytomegalovirus-infected fibroblasts. *J Infect Dis*, **178**, 1532–8.

Stevenson, P.G., Belz, G.T., et al. 1998. Virus-specific CD8(+) T cell numbers are maintained during gamma-herpesvirus reactivation in CD4-deficient mice. *Proc Natl Acad Sci USA*, **95**, 15565–70.

Subak-Sharpe, I., Dyson, H. and Fazakerley, J.K. 1993. In vivo depletion of CD8 T cells prevents lesions of demyelination in Semliki Forest virus infection. *J Virol*, **67**, 7629–33.

Takeda, K., Kaisho, T. and Akira, S. 2003. Toll-like receptors. *Annu Rev Immunol*, **21**, 335–76.

Tan, J.T., Ernst, B., et al. 2002. Interleukin (IL) -15 and IL-7 jointly regulate homeostatic proliferation of memory phenotype CD8+ cells but are not required for memory phenotype CD4+ cells. *J Exp Med*, **196**, 1523–32.

Theil, D., Derfuss, T., et al. 2003. Latent herpesvirus infection in human trigeminal ganglia causes chronic immune response. *Am J Pathol*, **163**, 2179–84.

Tirado, S.M.C. and Yoon, K.-J. 2003. Antibody-dependent enhancement of virus infection and disease. *Viral Immunol*, **16**, 69–86.

Tortorella, D., Gewurz, B.E., et al. 2000. Viral subversion of the immune system. *Annu Rev Immunol*, **18**, 861–926.

Trinchieri, G. 1989. Biology of natural killer cells. *Adv Immunol*, **47**, 187–376.

Usherwood, E.J. and Nash, A.A. 1995. Lymphocyte recognition of picornaviruses. *J Gen Virol*, **76**, 499–508.

Usherwood, E.J., Stewart, J.P., et al. 1996. Absence of splenic latency in murine gammaherpesvirus 68-infected B cell deficient mice. *J Gen Virol*, **77**, 2819–25.

Usherwood, E.J., Brooks, J.W., et al. 1997. Immunological control of murine gammaherpesvirus infection is independent of perforin. *J Gen Virol*, **78**, 2025–30.

van den Broek, M.F., Muller, U., et al. 1995. Immune defense in mice lacking type I and/or type II interferon receptors. *Immunol Rev*, **148**, 8–18.

van Lint, A., Ayers, M., et al. 2004. Herpes simplex virus-specific CD8+ T cells can clear established lytic infections from skin and nerves and can partially limit the early spread of virus after cutaneous inoculation. *J Immunol*, **172**, 392–7.

Vennema, H., de Groot, R.J., et al. 1990. Early death after feline infectious peritonitis virus challenge due to recombinant vaccinia virus immunization. *J Virol*, **64**, 1407–9.

Vicari, A.P. and Zlotnik, A. 1996. Mouse NK11 T cells: a new family of T cells. *Immunol Today*, **17**, 71–5.

Vilcek, J. and Sen, G.C. 1996. Interferons and other cytokines. In: Fields, B.N., Knipe, D.M., et al. (eds), *Fields' virology*, 3rd edn. New York: Raven-Lippincott, 375–400.

Vrijsen, R., Mosser, A. and Boeye, A. 1993. Postadsorption neutralization of poliovirus. *J Virol*, **67**, 3126–33.

Wabl, M. and Steinberg, C. 1996. Affinity maturation and class switching. *Curr Opin Immunol*, **8**, 89–92.

Watts, C. and Powis, S. 1999. Pathways of antigen processing and presentation. *Rev Immunogenetics*, **1**, 60–74.

Webster, R.G., Bean, W.J., et al. 1992. Evolution and ecology of influenza A viruses. *Microbiol Rev*, **56**, 152–79.

Weiss, R.C. and Scott, F.W. 1981. Antibody-mediated enhancement of disease in feline infectious peritonitis: comparisons with dengue hemorrhagic fever. *Comp Immunol Microbiol Infect Dis*, **4**, 175–89.

Wharton, S., Calder, L., et al. 1995. Electron microscopy of antibody complexes of influenza virus haemagglutinin in the fused pH conformation. *EMBO J*, **14**, 240–6.

Williams, B.R. 1999. PKR; a sentinel kinase for cellular stress. *Oncogene*, **18**, 6112–20.

Wohlfart, C. 1988. Neutralization of adenoviruses: kinetics, stoichiometry and mechanisms. *J Virol*, **62**, 2321–8.

Wong, G.H. and Goeddel, D.V. 1986. Tumour necrosis factors alpha and beta inhibit virus replication and synergize with interferons. *Nature (London)*, **323**, 819–22.

Yasukawa, M. and Zarling, J.M. 1984. Human cytotoxic T cell clones directed against herpes simplex virus-infected cells. Lysis restricted by HLA class II MB and DR antigens. *J Immunol*, **133**, 422–7.

Yewdell, J.W. and Hill, A.B. 2002. Viral interference with antigen presentation. *Nature Immunol*, **3**, 1019–25.

Zinkernagel, R.M. 1995. Immunology taught by viruses. *Science*, **271**, 173–8.

Zhou, A., Papanjape, J.M., et al. 1999. Interferon action in triply deficient mice reveals the existence of alternative antiviral pathways. *Virology*, **258**, 435–40.

15

The role of cytokines in viral infections

PAULA M. PITHA AND MYRIAM S. KÜNZI

INTRODUCTION

The pathological manifestation of viral disease is the result of complex interactions between the direct cytopathic effect of viral infection and the local and systemic immune responses to infection. Cytokine production is responsible for common manifestations of viral diseases such as fevers, chills, and myalgia, and the cytokine response has been associated with complications secondary to some viral infections, such as immunosuppression and dementia. It is also now clear that cytokines produced either directly in infected cells or indirectly by lymphocytes and macrophages activated by the immune response to viral proteins play an important role both in the outcome of the viral infection and in its virulence. These proteins can inhibit viral replication either directly by inducing the antiviral state in the host cells or indirectly by increasing the activation of macrophage and NK cell responses, expression of major histocompatibility antigens, initiating inflammatory responses, and stimulating the development of cytotoxic T cells, as well as the differentiation of B cells into antibody-producing plasma cells.

Recently, a new dimension of complexity has been added to the virus-mediated immune response by the finding that certain viruses have evolved mechanisms that allow them to overcome some of the components of the host-induced cytokine response by producing proteins that mimic cytokines or their receptors. Other viruses have developed defense mechanisms that enable

them to interfere with the transcriptional activation of cytokine genes or with their mechanisms of action. Thus, many of the viral genes that are not required directly for viral replication may be essential for pathogenicity of the virus in vivo. These aspects of viral escape from immune surveillance are discussed elsewhere in this volume (Chapter 14, The immune response to viral infections).

Local immune responses seem to be especially important in the development of cell-mediated immunity and antibody production. During the early stages of viral infection, innate cytokines such as interferon (IFN)-α and -β play a critical, but not overlapping role, in the stimulation of NK cell functions. The cytokine expression profile defined as Th1, associated with the production of IFN-γ, interleukin (IL)-2, and IL-12, leads predominantly to cell-mediated immunity. The Th2 profile of cytokine expression, in which IL-4, IL-5, IL-6, and IL-10 are produced, results in the production of virus-specific antibodies. Depending on the type of infection, the T-helper (Th)1 or Th2 response can be local or systemic, as has been suggested for human immunodeficiency virus type 1 (HIV-1) infection. This chapter deals with the role of cytokines in the early inflammatory responses and the outcome of viral infection. Particular emphasis is given to the viral infections of the central nervous system (CNS), HIV-1, herpesvirus and hepatitis virus infections, where there is clear evidence of a close relationship between cytokine production, viral replication, and pathogenicity. The use of recombinant viruses to examine the effect of a selected cytokine is also discussed. Finally the current knowledge of the immune response triggered by the ligation of Toll receptors is summarized, since there is accumulating evidence that these are recognized not only by bacterial envelopes and double-stranded RNA and DNA, but also by viral proteins.

CYTOKINES INDUCED DURING VIRAL INFECTIONS

Interferons

IFNs have a broad antiviral action against many viruses and play a critical role in innate immunity. They are the earliest defense mounted by the host during viral infection, until immune mechanisms can be fully engaged. An important element of the extensive cytokine network, IFNs also play a crucial role in the modulation of the immune system (de Maeyer and de Maeyer-Guignard 1991). Functionally, IFNs can be divided into two groups: type I IFNs, IFN-α, IFN-β, IFN-ω and IFNκ and type II IFN, IFN-γ (Table 15.1). Recently, a new group of antiviral proteins that are induced as response to viral infection and share the antiviral properties with type I IFNs, IFNλ (Kotenko et al. 2003; Sheppard et al. 2003) has been identified.

Normally silent, IFN A and B genes are rapidly induced in response to viral infection, while a distinct feature of IFNκ is its constitutive expression. A deficiency in the IFN system can lead to fulminate viral disease (Levin and Hahn 1985). Human type I IFN

genes lack introns and map to the short arm of chromosome 9. There are more than 20 IFN-α genes and pseudogenes, five IFN-ω genes, but only one IFN-β and IFNκ gene (Diaz 1995). The single IFN-γ gene contains three introns and maps to the long arm of chromosome 12. Whereas IFN-α is a family of nonglycosylated monomeric proteins (Allan and Fantes 1980), IFN-β, IFN-ω and IFN-γ are N-glycosylated. Functionally, IFN-β is a dimer, whereas IFN-γ is a tetramer. Synthesis of IFN-α takes place mainly in cells of lymphoid origin, while IFN-β is synthesized in fibroblasts, epithelial cells, and macrophages. IFN-ω is induced in leukocytes and trophoblasts and IFNκ is expressed in keratinocytes and dendritic cells. Production of IFN-γ is a specialized function of T lymphocytes, although NK cells and macrophages can produce IFN-γ as well. Competitive binding studies (Merlin et al. 1985) indicate that a common receptor for IFN-α, -β and -ω, as well as the receptor for IFN-γ, are encoded by genes mapping to chromosome 21.

IFNs exert their multiple effects through binding to cell-specific receptors and receptor-mediated transduction pathways results in the induction of IFN-stimulated genes (ISG) (Darnell et al. 1994). The type I IFNs, IFN α, β, ω and κ bind to a common receptor consisting of two subunits that both map to human chromosome 21. Type II IFN, IFN-γ binds to a distinct set of receptors that also consists of two subunits. The recently identified IFN λ binds to a heterodimeric receptor that consists of IL-10Rβ and orphan class II receptor chain, IL-28Rα (Sheppard et al. 2003; Kotenko et al. 2003). The gene arrays analysis has shown that the type I IFN binding to its receptor results in a major transcriptional

Table 15.1 *Human interferons*

Name	Genes	Proteins	Producer cells	Effect
IFN-α	>20 No introns Chromosome 9	Nonglycosylated 166 aa Monomer	Lymphoid cells Macrophages	Antiviral state ISG induction MHC I induction
IFN-β	1 No introns Chromosome 9	N-glycosylated 166 aa Dimer	Fibroblasts Epithelial cells Macrophages	Antiviral state ISG induction MHC I induction
IFN-ω	5 No introns Chromosome 9	N-glycosylated 172 aa . . .	Leucocytes Trophoblasts	Similar to IFN-α
IFN-γ	1 3 introns Chromosome 12	N-glycosylated 146 aa Tetramer	T cells Macrophages NK cells	2′,5′-OAS induction IL-1 enhancement MHC I induction, MHC II induction
IFNκ	No introns Chromosome 9	180 aa	Keratinocytes, DC	Antiviral Cytokine induction
IFN λ	3 6 introns Chromosome 19	Glycosylated	Most tissues	Antiviral activity 2′,5′-OAS, Mx induction MHC I induction

aa, amino acid; DC, dendritic cells; IFN, interferon; ISG, interferon-stimulated gene; MHC, major histocompatibility complex; 2′,5′-OAS, 2′,5′-oligoadenylate synthetase.

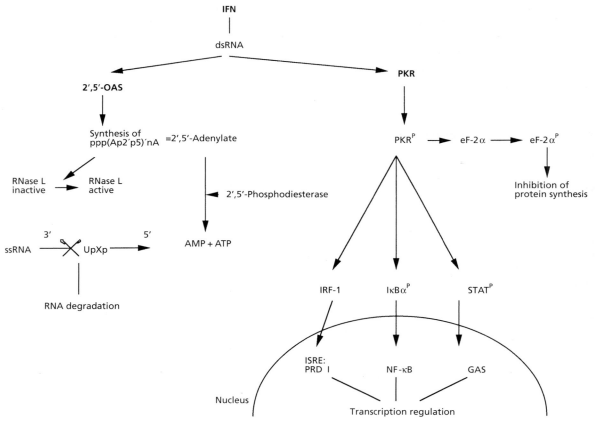

Figure 15.1 *Double-stranded (ds) RNA-dependent interferon-stimulated antiviral activities. GAS, γ-interferon-activated sequence; IκBα, inhibitor protein binding NF-κB transcription factors; IRF-1, interferon responsive factor 1; ISRE/PRD 1, interferon-sensitive response element/positive regulatory domain 1; P, phosphorylated; STAT, signal transduction activator transducer; UpXp, (by convention) a short RNA sequence in which the phosphorylated base uridine is followed by any other phosphorylated base (A, C, or G).*

activation and expression of more than 100 cellular genes, including genes encoding proteins with antiviral properties, growth-regulating proteins, and components of ubiquitin pathway (Samuel 1991; Malakhova et al. 2003).

The IFN-induced signaling pathway involves activation of several Janns-activated kinase (JAK) kinases that are associated with IFN receptors and by the consequent tyrosine phosphorylation cascade they activate the pre-existing transcriptional factors called signal transducers and activators of transcription (STAT). Phosphorylated STAT proteins, bind to importin and accumulate in the nucleus assembled in multimeric complexes where they interact with interferon-responsive elements present in the 5′ flanking region of interferon-stimulated genes (ISGs) (Levy 1995). Although both IFN-α and -β bind to the same receptors induction of distinct gene(s) by IFN-β was reported suggesting a possible existence of yet unidentified cofactor. Type I and type II IFNs are essential for antiviral defense and they are not functionally redundant (Muller et al. 1994). Both types of IFNs modulate the expression of major histocompatibility complex (MHC) antigens. It is via that mechanism that IFN-α/β increases the susceptibility of fibroblasts

infected with vaccinia virus or lymphocytic choriomeningitis virus (LCMV) to cytotoxic T lymphocyte (CTL) lysis (Bukowski and Welsh 1985). Type I and type II IFNs modulate MHC II antigen expression, IFN-γ and tumor necrosis factor (TNF)-α are the most powerful inducers of MHC II antigens. IFN-γ enhances expression of MHC II antigens on accessory cells, stimulates the interaction of these cells with T cells and promotes CTL development. Murine IFN-α and IFN-β can block IFN-γ-mediated class II antigen up-regulation (de Maeyer and de Maeyer-Guignard 1991).

IFNs act via a paracrine loop. Virus-induced IFNs are secreted by the cell and activate neighboring cells into an antiviral state characterized by the expression of a number of ISGs. Several of the proteins encoded by ISGs have direct antiviral activities (Samuel 1991). The antiviral activities of 2′,5′-oligoadenylate synthetase (2′,5′-OAS), PKR protein kinase, and Mx proteins have been well characterized (Figure 15.1). The 2′,5′-OAS pathway comprises three enzymes. 2′,5′-OAS, upon activation by double-stranded RNA, polymerizes ATP into pppA(2′p5′A)n, (2′,5′A) (Kerr and Brown 1978). 2′,5′A in turn activates a cellular endonuclease, 2′,5′-OAS-dependent RNaseL (Williams and Silverman 1985;

Zhou et al. 1993). RNaseL is present in the cells in an inactive form. When activated by 2',5'A, it degrades both cellular and viral RNAs at UU or AU nucleotides. 2',5'-Phosphodiesterase (Lengyel 1982) catalyzes the degradation of 2',5'A. Expression of 2',5'-OAS (40 kDa) in cells leads to the establishment of an antiviral state which results in the selective inhibition of the replication of picornaviruses, such as mengovirus and encephalomyocarditis virus (Chebath et al. 1987). The antiviral effect of the 2',5'-OAS system is specific for picornaviruses and no inhibition of VSV or HSV-1 has been observed.

Activation of the IFN-induced kinase, PKR, depends on the presence of dsRNA. The phosphorylation of the α subunit of protein synthesis initiation factor eF-2 (Samuel 1979; Berry et al. 1985) by PKR has been implicated in the inhibition of viral protein synthesis (Pathak et al. 1988). The crucial role of PKR in the antiviral effect of IFN is further indicated by the observation that a number of viruses have developed mechanisms to negate the function of PKR. Among these adenovirus encodes small RNAs, VA-RNA, which are synthesized in the late stages of the replication cycle and interfere with the activation of PKR and phosphorylation of eF-2a (Davies et al. 1989). Vaccinia virus encodes a specific PKR inhibitory factor (SKIF) (Akkaraju et al. 1989).The reovirus encoded protein G3 binds dsRNA and inhibits the activation of PKR by competing for dsRNA (Imani and Jacobs 1988). Poliovirus, on the other hand, inactivates PKR by inducing the autophosphorylation of PKR and its subsequent degradation. In addition to its antiviral effect PKR is also implicated in the control of cell proliferation (Samuel 1991).

The Mx proteins are GTPases and the molecular mechanism and the antiviral activity of Mx proteins depends on specific MX protein, its cellular localization of the type of viral infection. The antiviral activity of MX is dependent on its oligomerization, GTP binding, and hydrolysis. Athough originally identified as inhibitor of influenza virus infection (Haller et al. 1979; Samuel 1991). It has recently been shown that the Mx protein inhibits also additional RNA viruses, including measles and hantavirus replication (Frese et al. 1995).

The IFN induced RNA-specific adenosine deaminase-ADAR1 catalysis A-I editing and recent studies described an extensive A-I (G) hypermutation editing for several viral RNA.

ISG 20 was recently identified as single-stranded RNA endonuclease and its role in the antiviral effect of IFN against VSV and EMC was implicated (Espert et al. 2003).

These and possibly other IFN-regulated proteins confer on IFN its broad antiviral spectrum. In addition to the above-described IFN-mediated viral inhibition, IFN has been shown to block other steps of the viral life cycle. IFN-α inhibits cytomegalovirus (CMV) at the level of transcription of viral immediate–early (IE) genes, in particular that of the major genes *IE1*, *IE2*, and *IE3* (Martinotti and Gribaudo 1992). Whereas both IFN-α and IFN-γ inhibit adenovirus early gene expression, only IFN-γ inhibits late transcription (Mistchenko et al. 1989). IFN-α inhibits HIV-1 at many steps of its life cycle, but predominantly at the level of reverse transcription in acutely infected T cells and monocytes (Shirazi and Pitha 1992, 1993) and at the level of virus assembly in chronically infected cells (Pitha 1991). Inhibition of virus assembly and maturation is the major mechanism by which IFN blocks the replication of murine retroviruses (Pitha 1980). Stimulation of HLA class 1 expression on measles virus infection is mediated by IFN-β.

The availability of purified and recombinant IFN preparations has made possible the clinical use of IFN-α for the treatment of papillomavirus infections of the larynx, the anogenital regions, and the skin (Fingerote et al. 1995). IFN-α has also become the treatment of choice for chronic hepatitis B and hepatitis C virus infections. Hepatitis virus replication is inhibited by IFN-induced 2',5'-OAS in mouse peritoneal macrophages. The antiviral effect of 2',5'-OAS is not sufficient, however, to prevent the hepatocellular injury associated with hepatitis virus infection (Fingerote et al. 1995). Intranasal use of IFN-α for rhinovirus infections causes substantial damage to the nasal mucosa (Finter et al. 1991; Gutterman 1994). The major role of IFN-γ in antiviral defense is to modulate the immune response to viral infection. IFN-γ has, however, a direct antiviral effect, possibly through the induction of 2',5'-OAS (de Maeyer and de Maeyer-Guignard 1991). In mice, IFN-γ controls T cell-mediated viral clearance in acute cutaneous and ocular infection with herpes simplex (HSV-1) and in poxvirus infection. In macrophages, IFN-γ inhibits HSV-1 and vaccinia virus replication by inducing the production of nitric oxide in the infected cells (Karupiah et al. 1993). The growth of hepatitis virus is restricted in mice by IFN-γ-activated macrophages (Vassao et al. 1994). IFN-γ is also necessary for a normal antigen-specific immunoglobulin G2a response, as demonstrated in mice lacking the IFN-γ receptor (Huang et al. 1993). Intraperitoneal infection with mouse cytomegalovirus or herpes simplex virus (HSV) results in inflammatory infiltrates, consisting mainly of macrophages with increased expression of IFN-γ and TNF-α. CMV titers are increased in IFN-γ-depleted mice and in mice with severe combined immunodeficiency (SCID) (Heise and Virgin 1995). The antiviral effect of IFN-γ has also been demonstrated by the observation that the replication of recombinant vaccinia virus expressing IFN-γ is markedly inhibited, compared to that of wild-type virus (Ramshaw et al. 1992). The virulence of poxvirus infection is increased in mice lacking IFN-γ, and one of the myxoma virus genes implicated in the growth of the virus in vivo encodes the IFN-γ receptor (Upton et al. 1987).

Viruses have, however, evolved mechanisms to evade the antiviral effects of IFN. Many viruses have developed mechanisms by which they negate the function of RNA-activated protein kinase (PKR) (Reich et al. 1988). By contrast, flaviviruses (e.g. West Nile virus and Kunjin virus) induce expression of intercellular adhesion molecule-1 (ICAM-1) by two distinct mechanisms. First, induction is mediated by type I IFNs and occurs only in quiescent fibroblasts in G0 phase; the second induction is cytokine-independent and occurs within hours of viral challenge. The induction of cell–cell contact via ICAM-1 expression early in infection may significantly enhance the ability of the virus to spread before the immune response is triggered (Shen et al. 1995).

Cross-talk between IFNs and other cytokines is an essential component of the immune response

The experimental evidence suggests that both the innate and the acquired immune response involves cytokine-mediated amplification and cross-talk network. Thus the antiviral response seems to undergo the amplification step in which the IFN-β induced during the initial response to infection stimulates the expression of transcription factors that are required for the induction of expression of the IFN-α family of proteins resulting in much robust antiviral response.

In addition to the antiviral function, the IFN-α/β-mediated signaling pathway affects also the immune responses through the modulation of expression of several cytokines. Thus, while IFN-γ promotes expression of IL-12, IFN-α/β down-regulates IL-12 expression in monocytes and dendritic cells. IFN-α/β mediates induction of IL-15 that promotes survival of activated NK cells and their accumulation (Biron 2001). In human cells but not in mice, IFN-α/β activates IFN-γ and Th1 development of CD4$^+$ cells. Altogether these results indicate that IFN-α/β stimulates the signaling pathway for the innate regulation of adaptive immunity.

Tumor necrosis factor

TNF-α (cachectin) and -β (lymphotoxin) are two related peptides encoded by linked genes mapping within the MHC (Spies et al. 1986). Although TNF-α is secreted mainly by macrophages/monocytes and TNF-β by T cells, they compete for a common receptor. TNF-α, like IFN, can establish an antiviral state, and TNF-α-mediated induction of 2',5'-OAS has been demonstrated in a number of cell lines (Mestan et al. 1988). IFN-γ and IFN-β synergize with TNF-α to increase levels of 2',5'-OAS and viral inhibition (Mestan et al. 1988). Studies in vivo, with mice as a model for encephalomyocarditis virus (EMCV) infection, have shown that TNF-α alone is not sufficient to inhibit viral replication, but requires

combined treatment with IFN-γ (Czarniecki 1993). The same requirement has been observed with murine CMV (Anderson et al. 1993). The direct antiviral effect of TNF-α has been well documented with recombinant vaccinia virus expressing TNF-α (Ramshaw et al. 1992). In contrast, the replication of retroviruses, such as simian immunodeficiency virus (SIV) and HIV, is activated by TNF-α (Lairmore et al. 1991). Although IL-6 mRNA levels are increased in response to TNF-α, IL-6 alone does not seem to contribute to the TNF-α-induced antiviral state (Jacobsen et al. 1989).

Both RNA and DNA viruses can induce TNF-α expression in peripheral blood mononuclear cells (PBMC) and macrophages. Influenza virus increases TNF-α mRNA levels in monocytes (Nain et al. 1990), respiratory syncytial virus (RSV) stimulates TNF-α secretion in macrophages (Franke-Ullman et al. 1995) and human herpesvirus-6 (HHV-6) triggers TNF-α secretion in PBMCs (Flamand et al., 1991). TNF-α secretion by PBMCs from patients with chronic hepatitis B virus infection correlates with the level of virus replication. TNF-α inhibits replication of vesicular stomatitis virus (VSV) in WISH cells and replication of EMCV in HeLa cells. Another mechanism by which TNF-α limits viral spread is by enhancing viral cytotoxicity. TNF-α induces cytolysis of HSV-1 and HSV-2-infected rat embryo cells (Koff and Fann 1986). Cytolysis is also observed with either TNF-α or TNF-β in VSV or adenovirus-2-infected A549 cells. In vivo, however, adenovirus *E1A* gene encodes a 14.7 kDa protein which suppresses TNF-α-mediated cytolysis and thereby allows escape from the antiviral effects of TNF-α (Laster et al. 1994). Furthermore, co-expression of the adenovirus 14.7 kDa protein in a recombinant vaccinia virus expressing TNF-α inhibits the TNF-α-mediated attenuation of vaccinia virus virulence (Tufariello et al. 1994). Also, one of the genes in the terminal repeat of myxoma virus involved in modulating the replication of the virus in vivo encodes a soluble TNF-α receptor. Because induction of TNF-α is an essential part of the cellular defense against myxoma virus infection, the virus is able to neutralize the effect of TNF-α. Induction of TNF-α, as well as IFN-γ and IL-1 during dengue virus infection in macrophages may result in permeability of vascular endothelial cells and plasma leakage, which are characteristic of the hemorrhagic fever secondary to dengue virus infection. Not all viruses, however, can induce TNF-α. HSV-1, for instance, is a strong inducer, whereas Epstein–Barr virus (EBV) down-regulates the levels of TNF-α mRNA and protein in PBMCs (Gosselin et al. 1992).

Interleukin-1

The interleukin-1 (IL-1) family is composed of two cytokines, IL-1α and IL-1β, and one inhibitor, IL-1 receptor antagonist (IL-1ra). Although IL genes are highly conserved across species, they share little homology with one another and their regulation is different. Both IL-1α and IL-1β are synthesized as membrane-bound precursors of 270 aa, cleaved by proteases to yield circulating soluble proteins. IL-1 is produced mainly by macrophages, but T and B cells, dendritic cells, fibroblasts, epithelial cells, and astrocytes can synthesize IL-1 as well. IL-1 has no direct antiviral activity but, together with IL-2, induces IFN-γ synthesis and thus contributes indirectly to the antiviral immune response. IFN-α has been reported to down-regulate IL-1β in bone marrow stromal cells, while stimulating expression of the IL-1 receptor, thereby contributing to the myelosuppression associated with viral infections (Arman et al. 1994). Not all viral infections result in the induction of IL-1. Whereas influenza virus induces substantial IL-1 activity in macrophages, RSV induces IL-1 inhibitor activity (Roberts et al. 1986). In situ hybridization studies have shown that HIV-1, herpesviruses, EBV and CMV, adenovirus, and chronic hepatitis B virus (HBV) infection induce *IL-1β* and *IL-6* genes, not, however, in the infected cells themselves but in macrophages and epithelial cells adjacent to the infected cells (Devergne et al. 1991). IL-1, together with TNF-α and IL-6, is a key cytokine expressed during inflammation. In mice, cerebral expression of IL-1α and -1β and TNF-α correlates with the onset of neurodegenerative processes secondary to scrapie infection (Campbell et al. 1994). Although both adult T cell leukemia (ATL) and human T-cell lymphotrophic virus type 1 (HTLV-1)-associated myelopathy/tropical spastic paraparesis (HAM/TSP) are associated with HTLV-1 infection, the difference in virus-induced cytokine expression may underlie the differences in pathogenesis between the two diseases: IFN-γ, TNF-α, and IL-1β expression is induced in HAM/TSP, whereas elevated levels of transforming growth factor β (TGF-β) are secreted by leukemic cells in ATL (Tendler et al. 1991).

Interleukin-6

IL-6 is produced by T and B cells, macrophages, fibroblasts, and endothelial cells. During viral infection, *IL-6* seems to play an essential role in antibody production, since it induces B cells to differentiate into antibody-producing cells. Mice with targeted disruption of the *IL-6* gene have a reduced number of IgA-producing cells. Expression of IL-6 enhances systemic and mucosal antibody responses in mice infected with a recombinant fowlpox virus expressing influenza virus hemagglutinin and IL-6 (Ramsay et al. 1994). In contrast, IFN-γ expression in those animals inhibits antibody responses, but not cell-mediated immunity (Leong et al. 1994). Both RNA and DNA viruses induce IL-6 expression. Thus, HTLV-I transactivator protein, Tax, induces IL-6 expression through the direct activation of the IL-6 NF-κB site (Mori et al. 1994). Chronic virus-producing, but not chronic latent, hepatitis B infection increases serum

IL-6 activity, and IL-6 levels are further enhanced during acute exacerbation of the disease (Kakumu et al. 1991). Dengue virus, which is transmitted through mosquito bites, induces a rapid expression of IL-6 in fibroblasts, as well as granulocyte/macrophage colony stimulation factor (GM-CSF) and IFN-β. IFN protects uninfected cells from infection and limits virus spread (Kurane et al. 1992). Elevated serum levels of IL-6, IL-1 and TNF-α are also found in patients with dengue hemorrhagic fever (Hober et al. 1993). HIV-1 transactivating protein tat can induce IL-6 production in uninfected PBMCs in vitro and IL-6-dependent IgG and IgA synthesis (Rautonen et al. 1994). In the presence of IL-4, HIV-1 infection induces an autocrine IL-6 loop in B cells. Acquired immune deficiency syndrome (AIDS)-associated Kaposi's sarcoma positive PEL cells express the IL-6 receptor and use IL-6 as an autocrine growth factor (Masood et al. 1994). Macaque monkeys infected with a lethal variant of SIV (SIVsmm/PBj-14) show a marked increase in both IL-6 mRNA in inflamed tissues and IL-6 protein in serum (Birx et al. 1993).

Virally induced IL-6 participates in inflammatory reactions together with IL-1 and TNF-α. Live or inactivated RSV induces increased levels of IL-6, as well as TNF-α mRNA in alveolar macrophages. The combination of these two cytokines (IL-6 and TNF-α) does not seem, however, to have a direct antiviral effect but modulates the inflammatory response to RSV infection (Becker et al. 1991). In a similar manner, live or UV-irradiated coxsackie virus B3 (CVB3) stimulates the release of IL-6, IL-1, and TNF-α in infected human monocytes, and supernatants from CVB3-infected monocytes are cytotoxic to heart cells, suggesting that these cytokines induced by viral infection may contribute to the pathology of CVB3-induced myocarditis. In patients with cerebrospinal inflammation, however, it is acute bacterial meningitis and not viral meningitis (such as is caused by mumps virus) that is associated with increased IL-6 activity (Torre et al. 1992).

Interleukin-7, 8, and 10

IL-7 is a 177 aa protein secreted by thymic stroma cells and acts as a T-cell growth and differentiation factor and a macrophage activation factor. IL-7 also augments an *env*-specific CTL response in HIV-1 infected individuals in a dose- and time-dependent manner and promotes the maturation of precursor CTLs independently of IL-2. IL-8 is a member of a large family of factors secreted by macrophages and endothelial cells which act as mediators in inflammation. Constitutive expression of IL-8 and IL-6 by tracheobronchial and nasal epithelial cells is significantly increased upon viral infection (Adler et al. 1994). RSV, in particular, induces the release of IL-8 and IL-6 in the human epithelial cell line A549 in a time- and viral load-dependent manner. In addition, proinflammatory cytokines, such as TNF-α and IL-1

Table 15.2 *Virus-induced modulation of cytokine effects*

Virus	Viral gene	Cellular homologue	Effect
Poxviruses	MGF	EGF/TGF-α	Cell growth
	T2	TNF receptor	TNF inhibition
	T7	IFN-γ receptor	IFN-γ inhibition
	Unmapped	IL-1 receptor	IL-1 inhibition
EBV	BCRFI = vIL-10	IL-10	Escape from immune surveillance
Adenovirus	E1A = 14 ± 7 kDa protein	. . .	Suppresses TNF lysis
	E1B = 19 kDa protein		Counteracts TNF effects
	VA RNA		Inhibits IFN-α/β

synergistically enhance IL-8 secretion in RSV-infected A549 cells (Arnold et al. 1994). IL-10, appropriately termed cytokine synthesis inhibitory factor, inhibits the production of IFN-γ, and secretion of IL-1, IL-6, and TNF-α by macrophages. An open reading frame from EBV, *BCRFI*, shows extensive homology with IL-10, and it has been suggested that viral IL-10 expression enables infected cells to escape from immune surveillance (Moore et al. 1990) (Table 15.2).

Interleukin-4 and 12

IL-4 is a 20 kDa glycoprotein, B cell growth and differentiation factor which is secreted by Th2 cells and plays an essential role in the initiation of humoral immunity. IL-12, also known as NK cell stimulatory factor (Kobayashi et al. 1989), is a heterodimer which stimulates IFN-γ production. It has become clear now that IL-12 and IL-4 play pivotal roles in the differentiation of naive T cells into Th1 and Th2 subsets. Although viruses tend to trigger cell-mediated immunity, not all do so. CNS infection with live measles virus induces IL-4 expression and Th2 cell activation (Ward and Griffith 1993). Sindbis virus, which causes acute encephalomyelitis in mice, also triggers a Th2 response in the brain, characterized by increased expression of IL-4, IL-16, IL-10, and TGF-β in the brain (Wesselingh et al. 1994). IL-4 and IL-12 also seem to have an enhancing effect on HIV-1 replication, as is described in detail later under Role of cytokines in specific viral infections. The role of IL-4 and IL-12 in the Th1 and Th2 immune responses is explored more fully later in this chapter (see Th1–Th2 shift, below).

MODULATION OF THE IMMUNE RESPONSE

Th1–Th2 shift

As mentioned earlier, T lymphocytes are required for cell-mediated immune responses and antibody production by B cells. This dual role is controlled by two distinct Th cell subsets. Th1 cells produce IL-2 and IFN-γ and direct cell-mediated immunity, whereas Th2 cells produce IL-4, IL-6, and IL-10 and promote antibody production for humoral immunity. IL-12, secreted by macrophages and B cells, stimulates the production of IFN-γ in T cells and NK cells. IL-12 has been shown to act directly on CD4[+] naive T cells derived from T receptor transgenic mice to induce IFN-γ production and T-cell differentiation towards Th1 development (Seder et al. 1993). In contrast, IL-4 has been shown, in the same system, to drive Th2 cell development and Th2-specific cytokine expression. Moreover, Th2-specific cytokines, IL-4 and IL-10, inhibit IL-12 production in human macrophages and, thereby, the Th1 response. As both IL-12 and IL-10 are produced by macrophages, these can either promote or inhibit Th1 cell development, depending on the relative production of either cytokine by these cells. IFN-α stimulates production of Th1 cells and IFN-γ blocks Th2 development (Sher et al. 1992). Th1 and Th2 responses play important roles in viral clearance. In mice, Th1 clones are protective against lethal challenges with influenza virus, whereas Th2 clones are not protective and delay viral clearance (Graham et al. 1994). A switch from Th1 to Th2 responses has been suggested as playing a role in HIV infection and progression to AIDS. According to this model, HIV-specific T cell responses of the Th1 type would keep the infection under control. An increased viremia would result in a Th2 response, antibody production, and progression to AIDS. In this model, any stimulus or pathogen that could promote a switch from Th1 to Th2 would act as a cofactor in the progression to AIDS. If this model holds true, treatment with exogenous IL-12 might support and maintain Th1 cell function and thus delay the progression of the disease. This question is being explored in a number of clinical trials.

ROLE OF CYTOKINES IN SPECIFIC VIRAL INFECTIONS

HIV replication and pathogenicity

Human immunodeficiency virus (HIV-1) (Chapter 60) is recognized as the etiological agent of the slowly progressing immune deficiency in humans that culminates in the development of AIDS (Barré-Sinoussi et al. 1983). The rate of progression of this lentiviral infection and the onset of the disease seem to depend on viral determinants (multiplicity of infection, virus strain, or isolate), the interaction of HIV-1 with the host immune system and a number of cofactors, such as secondary viral and bacterial infections, cytokines, or stress factors. The primary targets of HIV-1 infection are CD4$^+$ cells, especially T cells and the cells of the myeloid lineage, monocytes and macrophages.

Initial infection with HIV-1 is followed within 3–5 weeks by an acute phase characterized by influenza-like symptoms, lymphadenopathy, plasma viremia, and a significant decrease in circulating CD4$^+$ cells. During the acute phase, HIV-1 disseminates to other tissues, particularly to the lymph nodes. The generation of an immune response at those sites results in the suppression of HIV-1 levels in the blood and restoration of the CD4$^+$ cells. Infection then enters a state of clinical latency, when little virus can be detected in plasma. However, viral replication takes place in lymph nodes, where it continues to infect the CD4$^+$ cells (Pantaleo et al. 1993). Recent studies from several laboratories have shown that, during these seemingly asymptomatic stages, virus-infected T cells are rapidly cleared from the circulation by the vigorous immune response (Coffin 1995; Ho et al. 1995). The high replication rate of HIV-1 results in the death of lymphocytes that are continuously being replenished by the immune system. This leads to the gradual decrease in CD4$^+$ T cells and the deterioration of the immune response. In the final stages of infection, HIV-1 reappears in the blood as a consequence of a breakdown of lymph node ultrastructure; the paucity of CD4$^+$ cells and the lack of appropriate immune response facilitate numerous opportunistic infections and the development of neoplasia.

Effect of HIV infection on cytokine gene expression

The production of cytokines by macrophages and T cells is part of the inflammatory response to viral infection, which is essential for lymphocyte activation, generation of cytotoxic cellular responses, and antibody production.

Increased levels of TNF-α, IL-1, IL-6, transforming growth factor β (TGF-β), and IFN-α and IFN-β have been found in the sera of AIDS patients (Birx et al. 1990; Breen et al. 1990). However, in vitro, the spontaneous and lipopolysaccharide (LPS)-stimulated production of TNF-α, IL-1, and IL-6 does not seem to be significantly different in peripheral blood lymphocytes (PBL) isolated from AIDS and uninfected donors (D'Addario et al. 1990; Molina et al. 1990; Yamato et al. 1990). In another set of reports, an increase in TNF-α production in PBLs has been observed with the progression of

HIV-1 infection (Rossol et al. 1992). An increase in the relative levels of TNF-α, IL-1, and IL-6 mRNAs has also been observed in LPS-stimulated alveolar macrophages isolated from individuals with AIDS, compared with the levels of mRNAs present in macrophages isolated during the early stages of HIV infection. Polyclonal activation of B cells (Reickmann et al. 1991) and increased levels of IL-6 may be associated with the higher frequency of B cell malignancies seen in AIDS patients.

Increased levels of IFN-α and IFN-γ (acid-labile IFN-α) were found both in pre-AIDS and in AIDS patients, but the frequencies and levels were higher in AIDS patients (Künzi and Pitha 1995). Elevated levels of IFN-α serum have been associated with a poor prognosis (Voth et al. 1990). It is not clear, however, what type of cell is responsible for IFN-α production in people infected with HIV-1 because, in vitro, HIV-1 infection of PBL does not result in the induction of IFN gene expression. PBMC isolated from individuals infected with HIV-1 or from AIDS patients has impaired IFN production upon stimulation with double-stranded RNA, NDV or HSV-1 (Fitzgerald-Bocarsky et al. 1989). This impairment in IFN production seems to occur at the transcriptional level (Gendelman et al. 1990).

In contrast, HIV-1 infection in vitro seems to induce cytokine expression. Thus, stimulation of HIV-1-infected monocytes with bacterial antigens from *Pneumocystis carinii* or *Mycobacterium avium* results in enhanced expression of TNF-α, IL-1, IL-6 and IL-8 mRNAs, compared to those present in stimulated but uninfected controls (Newman et al. 1993; Kandil et al. 1994). Both enhanced and unaltered cytokine expression have, however, been reported in HIV-1-infected monocytes stimulated with LPS, and no difference in cytokine production between HIV-1-infected and uninfected monocytes has been observed after stimulation with endotoxin or double-stranded RNA (Gendelman et al. 1990; Molina et al. 1990). A large variability in reported results suggests that inducible expression of cytokine genes may depend both on genetic determinants and on the nature of the inducer.

The molecular mechanism by which HIV-1 infection alters spontaneous and inducible cytokine gene expression is not clear. However, as most of the cytokines (whose expression is up-regulated by HIV-1 infection) contain an NF-κB enhancer in their promoter and NF-κB-specific binding is essential for transcription activation, it is likely that the binding of the HIV-1 or gp120 to the CD4 receptor induces change in the signaling pathways, such as those leading to the activation of NF-κB heterodimers, that alter both the constitutive and the inducible expression of the cytokine genes.

Effect of cytokines on HIV-1 replication

Transcription of HIV-1 is controlled by cellular and viral transactivators that bind to regulatory sequences present both in the long terminal repeat (LTR) of HIV-1 provirus and in the untranslated leader sequence of viral RNAs. Activation of viral transcription occurs upon binding of virally encoded tat protein to the tat-binding region present in all viral mRNAs (Rosen et al. 1985; Cullen and Greene 1989). In contrast, DNA elements present in the HIV-1 LTR, such as NF-κB enhancer (Nabel and Baltimore 1987), play a major role in the activation of the promoter by cellular and extracellular factors. Additional regulation of the inducible response is mediated through specific interaction between nuclear transactivators and the AP-1, NFAT, LBP-1, HLP-1, and TCF-1 DNA-binding sequences (Jones et al. 1988).

Many inflammatory cytokines stimulate HIV-1 transcription from the LTR and affect HIV-1 replication (Butera 1993; Poli and Fauci 1993). This observation is of biological importance, because cytokines are released during the immune response to HIV-1 infection and increased cytokine expression can be detected in lymph nodes in the vicinity of the focus of infection (Emille et al. 1991). The local environment in the infected lymph nodes allows for extensive interactions between activated B cells and T cells, resulting in the production of a variety of cytokines secreted in both an autocrine and a paracrine fashion. The profile of cytokines induced at the site of infection can then not only determine the nature of the immune response (cellular immunity mediated by CTL response versus antibody response) but also directly affects HIV-1 replication and thus positively or negatively enhances the progression of disease.

Cytokine-mediated up-regulation of HIV-1 replication

Of the stimulatory cytokines, TNF-α probably has the most significant effect on HIV-1 replication and a direct role in the pathogenicity of HIV-1 infection has been attributed to it. In vitro, TNF-α can up-regulate the transcriptional activity of HIV-1 LTR and the effect is mediated by the induction of NF-κB binding in the nucleus (Duh et al. 1989; Osborn et al. 1989). It has been shown that the TNF-α-mediated signal transduction pathway begins with the binding of TNF-α to one of the membrane receptors TNF-Rβ (55 kDa) and proceeds through sphingomyelinase and ceramide (Schutze et al. 1992). The TNF-α-mediated activation is not limited to the HIV-1 LTR. TNF-α can also effectively induce the expression of poorly expressed (latent) HIV-1 provirus in both T cells and monocytes. An interesting feature of TNF-α activation from the point of view of HIV-1 replication is that it is independent of transactivation mediated by the virus-encoded transactuator, tat. TNF-α can effectively rescue transcription and viral replication of a mutant HIV-1 provirus in which the tat region is deleted and therefore transcriptionally inactive (Popik and Pitha 1993). These results point to the existence of an alter-

native pathway in HIV-1 transcription regulation that is independent of tat. Because elevated levels of TNF-α can be detected in the serum in the later stages of HIV-1 infection, it is assumed that TNF-α is one of the factors that contribute to the progression of the disease and to some of the clinical signs, such as AIDS-associated weight loss (Serwadda et al. 1985). The ability of TNF-α to activate HIV-1 replication in a tat-independent manner has important implications for the antiviral strategies aimed at eliminating tat transactivation. Effective inhibition of HIV-1 replication requires both tat and NF-κB inhibition, and, in the presence of TNF-α, the drug RO5 that blocks tat transactivation is not effective (Popik and Pitha 1994). Thus, the presence of TNF-α in the serum and the ability of TNF-α to transactivate HIV-1 replication in a tat-independent fashion may be one of the reasons why the drug RO5 was ineffective in clinical trials.

Several other cytokines up-regulate HIV-1 transcription and HIV-1 provirus in vitro. In vitro, IL-1 stimulates transcription of a latent HIV-1 provirus in both T cells and monocyte lines (Poli et al. 1994). The induction was associated with the stimulation of NF-κB activities. IL-3 and the proteins of the colony stimulating factor (CSF) family, GM-CSF and M-CSF, up-regulate HIV-1 replication in primary macrophages and in monocyte and myeloid cell lines (Gendelman et al. 1990). It is interesting that CSF-mediated stimulation does not seem to be mediated entirely through NF-κB binding, as the region upstream of the NF-κB enhancer is also required for activation (Zack et al. 1990). IL-6 is another cytokine that has been implicated in the upregulation of HIV-1 replication (Poli et al. 1994). In contrast to the other cytokines, IL-6-mediated enhancement does not seem to take place at the transcriptional level, but occurs at the post-transcriptional level. The exact mechanism of this enhancement is not known. Of importance from a biological point of view is the synergy between IL-6 and TNF-α or IL-1 which leads to a significant enhancement of HIV-1 replication (Poli et al. 1990, 1994).

Cytokine-mediated down-regulation of HIV-1 infection

Recent data indicate that progression to AIDS is accompanied by a shift from a Th1 cytokine response and production of IL-2 and IFN-γ to a Th2 cytokine response, with production of IL-4, IL-6, and IL-10. In vivo, production of IFN-γ during the Th1 response may play a role in the down-regulation of HIV-1 infection. Although in vitro HIV-1 infection in macrophages does not induce IFN-α or IFN-β production, IFN-α can be detected in serum during the later stages of HIV-1 infection. The biological role in vivo of this IFN is not known, but IFN-α, IFN-β, and IFN-γ can effectively inhibit HIV-1 replication in vitro.

In vitro, IFNs inhibit HIV-1 replication both in primary cells and in established T cells and monocytic cell lines (Yamamoto et al. 1986; Kornbluth et al. 1989; Poli et al. 1989; Gendelman et al. 1990). In a single cycle infection in T cells (Shirazi and Pitha 1992) or in IFN-producing cells (Bednarik et al. 1989), IFN inhibits early steps in HIV-1 replication and HIV-1 transcripts cannot be detected in these cells (Shirazi and Pitha 1993). Furthermore, in primary macrophages, Type 1 IFNs decrease the levels of integrated provirus (Kornbluth et al. 1990). Hence, in multiple infection cycles or in chronic infection, IFN inhibited HIV-1 replication at the post-translational level and decreased the levels of virus released into the culture medium, but did not substantially affect the synthesis of viral RNA and proteins in infected cells. The mechanism by which IFN inhibits HIV-1 replication at the preintegrational step is not clear. Inhibition of the early replication steps has been observed in cells constitutively producing low levels of IFN-β, and it has been suggested that inhibition occurs at the level of viral uptake.

IFN also inhibits the activation of HIV-1 provirus by external stimuli in vitro. Poli et al. (1989) have shown that TNF-α-mediated stimulation of HIV-1 provirus is inhibited by IFN-α, and it has been suggested that the IFN-mediated block is at the level of virus maturation and assembly. Activation of a *tat*-defective provirus by 12-*O*-tetradecanylphorbol 13-acetate (TPA) or by HSV-1 is also inhibited in the presence of IFN. However, the inability of these inducers to activate HIV-1 provirus in the presence of IFN occurs at the transcriptional level, and is associated with the alteration of NF-κB-specific binding (Popik and Pitha 1991, 1992).

Several studies have shown that, although HIV-1 infection does not induce IFN type I synthesis in vitro, it can modulate the levels of at least two dsRNA-dependent enzymes, 2',5'-OAS and RNaseL, and induce expression of Mx protein. It has also been shown that the activation of PKR by tat-binding region (Edery et al. 1989) inhibits the translation of HIV-1 mRNAs and that inhibition of protein synthesis correlates with phosphorylation of eF-2. Yet none of these IFN-induced proteins seems to play a significant role in the IFN-mediated inhibition of HIV-1 replication. Neither small nor large 2',5'-OAS can be detected in HIV-1-infected cells (Popik and Pitha, unpublished). Productive HIV-1 infection leads to a decrease, not an increase, in cellular PKR activity. It has been suggested that the binding of the cellular protein tat region binding protein (TRBP) to the tat-binding region interferes with recognition of the dsRNA structure and prevents induction of PKR (Park et al. 1994) in HIV-1-infected cells. Together, these results indicate that IFN can inhibit many steps of the HIV-1 replication cycle with differing efficiency and they suggest that, in vivo, IFN may have a broad spectrum of action (Figure 15.2).

Cytokines with both stimulatory and inhibitory effects on HIV-1 replication

The wide range of biological properties of certain cytokines is often manifested by their bifunctional effects. This is also true of their effects on HIV-1 replication. TGF-β pretreatment can stimulate HIV-1 replication in primary T cells and in myeloid and monocytic cell lines (Lazdins et al. 1991; Poli et al. 1991). However, when TGF-β is applied to infected cultures, it inhibits PMA, TNF, and IL-6-mediated stimulation of HIV-1 replication (Poli et al. 1991). IL-4 is another cytokine with a bifunctional effect on HIV-1 replication: it can either induce or inhibit HIV-1 replication in myeloid cells. In undifferentiated monocytes, IL-4 stimulates HIV-1 replication, as well as the proliferation of the cells (Kazazi et al. 1992; Foli et al. 1995) whereas, in differentiated macrophages, IL-4 suppresses HIV-1 replication (Novak et al. 1990). In T cells, however, IL-4 does not affect HIV transcription. This indicates that differences in host cells and types of infection, as well as the timing of exposure to cytokines, may determine the outcome of the cytokine effects.

Herpesvirus infections

Herpesviruses selectively regulate proinflammatory cytokine synthesis. Human herpesvirus-6 infection induces high levels of IL-1β and TNF-β in wildtype cultures, but inhibits the induction of IL-6. In the same cells, EBV inhibits TNF-α secretion (Gosselin et al. 1992). The pattern of cytokine expression during herpes simplex virus-induced keratitis (HSK) has been well studied in the mouse and human cornea. HSV-1 infection in murine keratinocytes induces transient expression of TNF-α, IL-6, and IL-1, a cytokine profile that is characteristic of a transient inflammatory response (Sprecher and Becker 1992). Exogenous IL-10, a cytokine with inflammatory suppressive activity, also significantly decreases IL-6 levels in HSV-1-infected murine cornea and sharply reduces the incidence of blindness secondary to the HSV-1-induced inflammatory response, even though IL-1α levels are not decreased (Tumpey et al. 1994). At low concentrations, IFN-γ and TNF-α induce a synergistic antiviral effect against HSV-1 in human corneal cells (Chen et al. 1994). Cells isolated from eyes in the active phase of HSK have been found to be of the CD4$^+$ Th1 subset, secreting IL-2, IFN-γ, and TNF-α, but not IL-4 or IL-10 (Niemialtowski and Rouse 1992). Treatment with monoclonal antibodies specific for IFN-γ or IL-2 reduces the severity of HSV-1-induced corneal inflammation in mice, and inhibition of IFN-γ production by UV-irradiation enhances IL-4 production, as well as zosteriform skin lesions (Hendricks et al. 1992; Yasumoto et al. 1994). These findings indicate that Th1 and Th2 responses define the pathogenicity of HSV-1 in

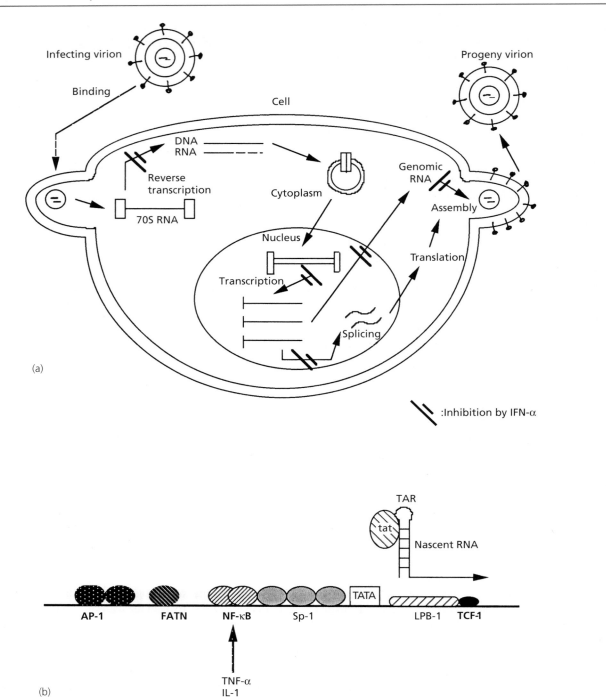

Figure 15.2 (a) *IFN-α inhibition of the HIV-1 life cycle.* **(b)** *Cytokine activation of HIV long terminal repeats.*

the cornea and the skin. HSV-1 and -2 activate macrophages and induce IFN-α/β production, which synergizes with TNF-α in an autocrine manner to protect macrophages from herpetic infection (Ellerman-Eriksen et al. 1994).

EBV infection is associated with acute, self-limiting, infectious mononucleosis, chronic infectious mononucleosis, and lymphoproliferative disease (LPD). In all acute forms of EBV infection, IFN-γ, TNF-α, IL-2, and IL-6 are elevated (Linde et al. 1992). EBV-associated LPDs are a common complication of primary immunodeficiency and are associated with elevated serum levels of IL-4 and, to a lesser extent, IL-5, IL-10, and IFN-γ (Mathur et al. 1994). Cyclosporin A, used in immunosuppressive therapy, increases EBV-associated lymphoproliferative disorders by inducing

IL-6 expression in T cells and by increasing the number of EBV-immortalized B cells expressing viral lytic antigens. Exposure to EBV stimulates IL-6 expression in B cells and in monocytes (Tanner and Menezes 1994).

EBV-infected B cells express IL-10 and B-cell regulatory factor (BCRF) 1, the viral homologue of IL-10, and expression of both viral and cellular cytokines is maintained during transformation. Inhibition of viral IL-10 (vIL-10) expression with antisense oligonucleotides at the time of viral challenge prevents EBV B-cell transformation. Conversely, transformation is rescued by exogenous cellular IL-10. These observations indicate that EBV-encoded *IL-10* is a latency gene involved in B cell transformation (Miyazaki et al. 1993). EBV has been implicated in the etiology of Sjögren's syndrome, a disease characterized by lymphocytic infiltration, squamous cell metaplasia and a decrease in goblet cell numbers in the conjunctival epithelium of the eye. Although the marker for latent EBV infection, EBNA-1 or EBV IL-10 is not expressed at a higher frequency than in the normal eye, HLA-DR, ICAM-1, and IL-6 expression is significantly increased in Sjögren's syndrome (Jones et al. 1994).

Infections with hepatitis viruses

Hepatitis virus clearance and persistence hinge upon the intricate, and as yet not fully understood, modulation of virus-induced cytokines. Monocytic production of IL-6, the mediator of acute-phase protein synthesis in hepatocytes, is decreased in chronic HBV infection, whereas it is normal in chronic hepatitis C virus (HCV) and in acute hepatitis A virus (HAV), HBV and HCV infections. Exacerbation of chronic HBV induces expression of IL-6 and TNF-α which correlates with an increase in HBV DNA levels in serum (Kakumu et al. 1991; Sheran et al. 1991). Moreover, IL-6 contains recognition sites for the segment of the HBV envelope protein through which the virus binds to cell surfaces (Neurath et al. 1992).

HBV is not cytopathic, but it evokes a strong lymphomononuclear inflammatory response in the liver during acute and chronic infections. Transgenic mice whose hepatocytes do not secrete HBV, but retain the antigen in the endoplasmic reticulum, are highly susceptible to liver damage induced by bacterial lipopolysaccharide, a potent inducer of inflammatory cytokines. The effect seems to be mediated by both IFN-γ and TNF-α. Hepatocellular injury and induction of inflammatory cytokines coincide with a reduction in HBV steady-state mRNA content (Gilles et al. 1992). TNF-α induces two other proinflammatory cytokines, IL-8 and IL-6, in patients with chronic HBV. Inflammatory cytokines appear to down-regulate HBV expression by both TNF-α-dependent and TNF-α-independent pathways. Administration of exogenous recombinant TNF-α, IL-2,

IFN-α, and IFN-β has been shown to reduce steady-state levels of HBV RNA in transgenic mice. TNF-α antibodies block the effect of TNF-α and IL-2, but not that of IFNs. Administration of exogenous IFN-γ, IL-1, IL-3, IL-6, or TNF-α has no effect on the HBV RNA levels (Guidotti et al. 1994). De-regulation of the inflammatory cascade can have disastrous effects, as illustrated by fulminant hepatic failure, characterized by a striking elevation of IL-6, TNF-α, IL-1Rα, and IL-1β levels (Sekiyama et al. 1994). IFN-γ and HBV X protein increase the rate of transcription of intercellular adhesion molecule 1 (ICAM-1), a molecule critically important to adhesion-dependent leukocyte functions, such as antigen presentation and target cell lysis (Hu et al. 1992). IFN-γ initially also activates HBV-specific class I restricted CTL, suppressing expression of the HBV gene.

Chronic hepatitis B, C, or D may lead to cirrhosis, hepatocellular failure or hepatocellular carcinoma. IFN-α has recently become the treatment of choice for chronic hepatitis, because HBV and HCV infections respond well to treatment with it. Sustained loss of HBV DNA and HBV nucleocapsid and surface antigens leads to the restoration of normal liver function. However, the relatively high prevalence of resistance of HBV to IFN is of concern. It was shown that the terminal domain of HBV polymerase is responsible for the resistance of the virus to IFN-α and IFN-γ. Individuals infected with several HCV quasi species seem to be less responsive to IFN therapy than are those with a single major species (Gutterman 1994; Dusheiko 1995).

CYTOKINE RESPONSES TO VIRAL INFECTIONS OF THE CENTRAL NERVOUS SYSTEM

There is increasing evidence that local cytokine production induced as a response to viral infection of cells of the CNS or infiltrating lymphoid cells plays a crucial role in the pathogenicity and outcome of viral infection in this location (Benveniste 1992).

Local synthesis of TNF-α within the CNS seems to be especially damaging. TNF-α damages glial cells and has a direct toxic effect on neurons. In vitro, TNF-α induces demyelination of oligodendrocytes, whereas the closely related TNF-β kills oligodendrocytes by inducing apoptosis. Production of both TNF-α and TNF-β in the CNS results in the death of myelin-producing oligodendrocytes. TNF-α can also act indirectly by stimulating microglia and astrocytes to produce nitric oxide and the neurotoxic metabolites of arachidonic acid (Benveniste 1995). TNF-α also stimulates synthesis of other cytokines such as GM-CSF, G-CSF, and M-CSF, which enhance inflammatory responses as well as the synthesis of IL-6 (Doherty et al. 1989; Moskophidis et al. 1991; Campbell et al. 1994). IL-6 enhances inflammation in the CNS, as well as stimulating the proliferation of B cells and their differentiation into antibody-producing cells.

The local immune responses in the CNS and the outcome of the infection are affected by the cytokines induced in situ, whether directly in infected cells (Sebire et al. 1993; Wesselingh et al. 1994), as a response to viral infection (e.g. IFNs, TNF-α or IL-6 in astrocytes or microglia) or by infiltrating T cells and macrophages during local inflammation (Shankar et al. 1992; Gillespie et al. 1993).

It is interesting that the profile of cytokines synthesized in the CNS seems to be determined by the type of infecting virus rather than by the type of host cells. Thus, infection of neurons with LCMV leads to synthesis of TNF-α, IL-1, IL-6, and IFN-γ, generating a strong CTL response (Campbell et al. 1994). The strong Th1 cytokine response and induction of cytotoxic T cells leads ultimately to death, whereas viral replication alone is regulated by the presence of IFNs. The association of LCMV pathogenicity with the immune response provided the first clear evidence that viral pathogenicity may be mediated by the immune response of the host (Rowe 1954). In contrast, the infection of neurons with the Sindbis virus (an alphavirus closely related to Western equine encephalitis virus), which causes acute encephalomyelitis in mice, results in generation of the Th2 cytokine response (Wesselingh et al. 1994). Increases in mRNAs and IL-1, IL-4, IL-6, IL-10, and TNF-α proteins have been observed during the early stages of acute infection in mice, followed by the appearance of antiviral antibodies and clearance of virus from the CNS (Tyor et al. 1989; Levine et al. 1991). Although it has been suggested that the CNS may provide an environment that favors B-cell antibody response, it is difficult at present to generalize this finding. Thus, recovery from acute HSV infection depends on a T-cell response, whereby the MHC class I-restricted CD8[+] cytotoxic T lymphocytes control HSV infection in the brain (Schmidt and Rouse 1992; Nash and Cambouropoulos 1993). Secretion of IFN-γ from activated T cells is critical for clearing of herpes virus infection (Raniero et al. 1990; Lucin et al. 1992). Recently, it has been shown that the T cell inflammatory response and production of IFN-γ persist in trigeminal ganglia long after HSV-1 has established the latent phase of infection (Cantin et al. 1995). This observation may indicate that the prolonged production of IFN-γ and possibly also of other cytokines (e.g. TNF-α) (Schmidt and Rouse 1992) may block or suppress HSV-1 replication after reactivation from latency (Cunningham and Merigan 1983; Torseth and Merigan 1986).

De-regulated local production of cytokines in the brain has also been observed in patients with AIDS dementia complex (ADC), which afflicts 30–50 percent of all people infected with HIV-1 (Johnson et al. 1988). In the CNS, HIV-1 can be found primarily in infiltrating

monocytes and macrophages, as well as in resident microglia (Koenig et al. 1986; Wiley et al. 1986), but there is evidence for major damage to neurons (Ketzler et al. 1990). There is no explanation at present for the cause of this extensive neurological impairment. It has been suggested that cytokines produced in macrophages and glial cells in response to HIV-1 infection (Gelbard et al. 1994) may either directly damage the neurons or alter the function of astrocytes and, consequently, neuronal function (Benveniste 1992, 1995).

Analysis of the cerebrospinal fluid from ADC patients has shown elevated levels of IL-1, TNF-α, IL-6, and neopterin, an indicator of the presence of IFN-γ (Grimaldi et al. 1991). With the exception of IFN-γ, all these substances are the products of activated macrophages and microglia. IFN-γ is most likely to be produced by infiltrating CD8[+] cells (Tyor et al. 1992). The expression of cytokine mRNA in the brain has been analyzed (Wesselingh et al. 1993). The results reveal a strong association between increased levels of TNF-α mRNA and ADC. As discussed above, TNF-α induces many abnormalities in the CNS and so its over-production may be one of the causes of the neuron dysfunction in ADC. It is interesting that an increased number of TNF-α-producing cells was also observed in patients with other neurological disease, such as multiple sclerosis (Benveniste 1995). These data suggest that TNF-α may play a major role in inflammatory disorders of the CNS.

DIRECTED CYTOKINE EXPRESSION WITH RECOMBINANT VIRUSES

The role of individual cytokines in response to viral infection has been studied by using recombinant cytokines administered systematically. This approach does not mimic well conditions in vivo, in which cytokines are acting locally and presumably in much higher concentrations (Biron et al. 1990). Results from experiments with transgenic animals expressing IL-2 (Ishida et al. 1989), IL-4 (Tepper et al. 1990), IL-5 (Tominaga et al. 1991), or GM-CSF (Lang et al. 1987) have often been difficult to interpret, because of the widely spread expression. More clear-cut results have been obtained with experiments in which animals with a homozygous deletion of a given cytokine or its receptor are used (e.g. IFN-γR nu/nu mice (Huang et al. 1993), IL-6 nu/nu mice) or when production of cytokines is suppressed by monoclonal antibodies (Leist et al. 1989).

Recently, a new technique has been used, whereby a cytokine gene inserted in a nonessential part of a recombinant virus is able to target cytokine production directly to the focus of infection. This makes it possible to determine the effect of local cytokine production on viral replication and the immunological consequences of cytokine overproduction. The most common type of virus for cytokine delivery has been vaccinia virus (Ramshaw et al. 1992), although HSV-1 (Mester et al. 1995) and mouse cytomegalovirus (Burnes, personal communication, 1995) have also been used.

Vaccinia virus is a complex DNA virus that replicates in the cytoplasm. Foreign DNA can easily be inserted into the virus under the control of a viral promoter (Davidson and Moss 1989), and foreign proteins are processed and transported with fidelity (Moss and Flexner 1987). Furthermore, a large region of this virus DNA genome is not essential for replication. Insertion of the *IL-2* gene into vaccinia virus enhances neither T cell-mediated immunity nor the immune response, but it decreases the virulence of the virus and enables immune-suppressed mice to resolve infection (Ramshaw et al. 1992). Enhancement of NK cell cytotoxic activity is an important factor in the clearance of infection in nude mice, and it has been found that IFN-γ plays an essential role in IL-2-mediated recovery. Since no host response was demonstrated that explained the rapid clearance of IFN-γ-expressing virus, these authors concluded that the observed inhibition in viral replication is caused by the direct antiviral effect of IFN. Similarly, the recombinant virus expressing TNF-α was rapidly cleared without any detectable involvement of the host immune system. Furthermore, local production of TNF-α was not toxic and no pathogenicity induced by TNF-α could be detected. Thus, TNF-α, like IFN-γ, seems to inhibit viral replication by the direct antiviral effect (Sambhi et al. 1991). These results indicate that overproduction of Th1 cytokines inhibits viral replication. Inhibition of viral replication is localized and limited to the recombinant virus and does not affect the coinoculated control virus (Ramshaw et al. 1992).

To determine the effect of Th2 cytokines on the course of viral infection, recombinant viruses expressing Th2 cytokines have been constructed. In normal mice, recombinant virus encoding IL-4 replicates more efficiently than control virus, whereas expression of IL-5 or IL-6 has no apparent antiviral effect. However, vectors encoding IL-5 and IL-6 significantly increase terminal differentiation of IgA-committed B cells and mucosal IgA antibody response in vivo (Ramsay and Kohonen-Corish 1993; Ramsay et al. 1994). Expression of IL-6 augments both the primary systemic antibody and the mucosal antibody responses. In contrast, expression of IFN-γ significantly inhibits antibody responses without affecting the general cell-mediated immune response (Leong et al. 1994). Furthermore, the vectors expressing IL-6 are able to reconstitute the IgA and IgG responses in IL-6-deficient mice (Ramsay et al. 1994). These results indicate that IL-6 plays a critical role in the induction of mucosal immunity.

Herpes simplex virus type 1 (HSV-1) has also been used for targeted delivery of cytokine genes. Weir and Elkins (1993) inserted a human IFN A gene into a replication-incompetent herpesvirus and showed that IFN expressed in infected monocytes is able to inhibit HIV-1

replication. Murine IFN A has been inserted in both replication-competent and incompetent HSV-1. HSV-1-derived IFN A gene expression did not inhibit HSV-1 replication in vitro. However, preinfection of the cells with the nonreplicating HSV–IFN vector provided complete protection against a subsequent viral challenge (Mester et al. 1995). Replication-defective vectors derived from HSV-1 have also been used for delivering genes to neurons (Fink et al. 1992), suggesting their usefulness for analyzing cytokine effects within the nervous system. In summary, these approaches suggest a novel and highly effective approach to the study of local cytokine effects in viral infections and to the effectiveness of virus-derived vectors in vaccine development and cytokine gene therapy.

CONCLUSION

It is evident that viral infection induces a complex host response mediated by the induction of genes encoding various cytokines and lymphokines, as well as stress proteins. This response can be induced directly in the infected cells or indirectly in cells of lymphoid origin tethered to the focus of infection during the immune response. The primary function of these cytokines is either to inhibit viral replication or to activate the cells mediating the cellular and humoral immune responses. However, inflammatory cytokines, produced during the immune response, are not always beneficial to the host and can contribute to the pathogenicity and side-effects of viral infections. The detrimental effect of cytokines can be most clearly demonstrated in conditions in which infection is localized to a specific organ or system such as the CNS. Then, production of even relatively low levels of cytokines, such as TNF-α, can have profoundly toxic effects and result in the death of neurons or the dysfunction of oligodendrocytes.

Several viruses have developed ways to eliminate or overcome the effect of cytokines. This again demonstrates the great plasticity of some viral genomes and their ability to adapt. Thus, HIV-1 has modified its regulatory region to resemble the promoter of some of the inflammatory cytokines, and can therefore use several of the inflammatory cytokines to stimulate its own replication. Other viruses, such as the poxviruses, carry several genes that encode soluble cytokine receptors. Others, such as adenovirus, have developed a specific mechanism that can allow them to inhibit the effects of cytokines. Some of the HIV-1-encoded accessory proteins may carry similar functions. Expression of viral genes that inhibit cytokine induction and function seems to be essential for the replication of many of these viruses in vivo, because the replication and pathogenicity of mutants with 'mimicry' functions deleted are usually considerably diminished. One of the main objects of future research should, therefore, be to characterize these cytokine-inhibiting viral functions. This would help not only to understand the role that a given cytokine plays in a particular viral infection but also to generate attenuated, nonpathogenic viruses that could be used for vaccine development. However, the real challenge will be to use the mechanisms that viruses have developed to avoid the immune response as selective tools to eliminate viral infections.

REFERENCES

Adler, K.B., Fischer, B.M., et al. 1994. Interactions between respiratory epithelial cell and cytokines: relationship to lung inflammation. *Ann NY Acad Sci*, **725**, 128–45.

Akkaraju, G.R., Whitaker-Dowling, P., et al. 1989. Vaccinia specific kinase inhibitory factor prevents translational inhibition by double-stranded RNA in rabbit reticulocyte lysate. *J Biol Chem*, **264**, 10321–5.

Allan, G. and Fantes, K. 1980. A family of structural genes for human lymphoblastoid (leukocyte-type) interferon. *Nature (Lond)*, **287**, 408–11.

Anderson, K.P., Lie, Y.S., et al. 1993. Effects of tumor necrosis factor-alpha treatment on mortality in murine cytomegalovirus-infected mice. *Antiviral Res*, **21**, 343–55.

Arman, M.J., Keller, U., et al. 1994. Regulation of cytokine expression by interferon-alpha in human bone marrow structural cells: inhibition of hematopoietic growth factors and induction of interleukin-1 receptor antagonist. *Blood*, **84**, 4142–50.

Arnold, R., Humbert, B., et al. 1994. Interleukin-8, interleukin-6 and soluble tumor necrosis factor receptor type I release from a human pulmonary epithelial cell line (A549) exposed to respiratory syncytial virus. *Immunology*, **82**, 126–33.

Barré-Sinoussi, F., Chermann, J.-C., et al. 1983. Isolation of a T-lymphotropic retrovirus from a patient at risk for acquired immune deficiency syndrome (AIDS). *Science*, **220**, 868–71.

Becker, S., Quay, J. and Soukup, S. 1991. Cytokine (tumor necrosis factor, IL-6 and IL-8) production by respiratory syncytial virus-infected human alveolar macrophages. *J Immunol*, **147**, 4307–12.

Bednarik, D.P., Mosca, J.D., et al. 1989. Inhibition of human immunodeficiency virus (HIV) replication by HIV-*trans*-activated α2-interferon. *Proc Natl Acad Sci USA*, **86**, 4958–62.

Benveniste, E.N. 1992. Inflammatory cytokines within the central nervous system: sources, function and mechanism of action. *Am J Physiol*, **263**, C1–C16.

Benveniste, E.N. 1995. Role of cytokines in multiple sclerosis, autoimmune encephalitis and other neurological disorders. In: Aagarwal, B.B. and Puri, P.K. (eds), *Human cytokines: their role in research and therapy*. Cambridge, MA: Blackwell Science, 195–216.

Berry, M.J., Knutson, G.S., et al. 1985. Purification and substrate specificities of the double-stranded RNA-dependent protein kinase from untreated and interferon-treated mouse fibroblasts. *J Biochem*, **260**, 11240–7.

Biron, C.A., Young, H.A. and Kasaian, M.T. 1990. Interleukin 2-induced proliferation of murine natural killer cells in vivo. *J Exp Med*, **171**, 173–88.

Birx, D.L., Redfield, R.R., et al. 1990. Induction of interleukin-6 during human immunodeficiency virus infection. *Blood*, **76**, 2303–10.

Birx, D.L., Lewis, M.G., et al. 1993. Association of IL-6 in the pathogenesis of acutely fatal SIVsmm-PBj-14 in pigtailed macaques. *AIDS Res Hum Retrovir*, **9**, 1123–9.

Breen, E., Rezal, A., et al. 1990. Infection with HIV is associated with elevated IL-6 levels and production. *J Immunol*, **144**, 480–4.

Bukowski, J.F. and Welsh, R.M. 1985. Interferon enhances the susceptibility of virus-infected fibroblasts to cytotoxic T cells. *J Exp Med*, **161**, 257–62.

Butera, S. 1993. Cytokine involvement in viral permissiveness and the progression of HIV disease. *J Cell Biochem*, **53**, 336–42.

Campbell, I.L., Hobbs, M.V., et al. 1994. Cerebral expression of multiple cytokine genes in mice with lymphocytic choriomeningitis. *J Immunol*, **152**, 716–23.

Cantin, E.M., Hinton, D.R., et al. 1995. Gamma interferon expression during acute and latent nervous system infection by herpes simplex virus type 1. *J Virol*, **69**, 4898–905.

Chebath, J., Benech, P., et al. 1987. Constitutive expression of (2′–5′) oligo A synthetase confers resistance to picornavirus infection. *Nature (Lond)*, **330**, 587–8.

Chen, S.H., Oakes, J.E. and Lausch, R.N. 1994. Synergistic anti-herpes effect of TNF-alpha and IFN-gamma in human corneal epithelial cells compared with that in corneal fibroblasts. *Antiviral Res*, **25**, 201–13.

Coffin, J.M. 1995. HIV population dynamics in vivo: implications for genetic variation, pathogenesis, and therapy. *Science*, **267**, 483–9.

Cullen, B.R. and Greene, W.C. 1989. Regulatory pathways governing HIV-1 replication. *Cell*, **58**, 423–6.

Cunningham, A.L. and Merigan, T.C. 1983. γ-Interferon production appears to predict time of recurrence of herpes labialis. *J Immunol*, **130**, 2397–400.

Czarniecki, C.W. 1993. The role of tumor necrosis factor in viral disease. *Antiviral Res*, **22**, 223–58.

D'Addario, M., Roulston, A., et al. 1990. Coordinate enhancement of cytokine gene expression in human immunodeficiency virus type 1-infected promonocytic cells. *J Virol*, **64**, 6080–9.

Darnell, J.E., Kerr, I.M. and Stark, G.R. 1994. Jak-STAT pathways and transcriptional activation in response to IFNs and other extracellular signaling proteins. *Science*, **264**, 1415–20.

Davidson, A.J. and Moss, B. 1989. Structure of vaccinia virus early promoters. *J Mol Biol*, **210**, 771–84.

Davies, M.V., Furtado, M., et al. 1989. Complementation of adenovirus virus-associated RNA I gene deletion by expression of a mutant eukaryotic translation initiation factor. *Proc Natl Acad Sci USA*, **86**, 9163–7.

de Maeyer, E. and de Maeyer-Guignard, J. 1991. Interferons. In: Thomson, A.W. (ed.), *The Cytokine Handbook*. London: Harcourt Brace Jovanovich, 215–39.

Devergne, O., Peuchmaur, M., et al. 1991. In vivo expression of IL-1 beta and IL-6 genes during viral infection in humans. *Eur Cytokine Netw*, **2**, 183–94.

Diaz, M.O. 1995. The human type 1 interferon gene cluster. *Semin Virol*, **6**, 143–9.

Doherty, P.C., Allan, J.E. and Clark, I.A. 1989. Tumor necrosis factor inhibits the development of viral meningitis or induces rapid death depending on the severity of inflammation at time of administration. *J Immunol*, **142**, 3576–80.

Duh, E.J., Maury, W.J., et al. 1989. Tumor necrosis factor α activates human immunodeficiency virus-1 through induction of a nuclear factor binding to the NF-κB sites in the long terminal repeat. *Proc Natl Acad Sci USA*, **86**, 5974–8.

Dusheiko, G.M. 1995. Treatment and prevention of chronic viral hepatitis. *Pharmacol Ther*, **65**, 47–73.

Edery, I., Petryshyn, R. and Sonenberg, N. 1989. Activation of double-stranded RNA-dependent kinase (dsI) by the TAR region of HIV-1 mRNA: a novel translational control mechanism. *Cell*, **56**, 303–12.

Ellerman-Eriksen, S., Christensen, M.M. and Mogensen, S.C. 1994. Effect of mercuric chloride on macrophage-mediated resistance mechanisms against infection with herpes simplex virus type 2. *Toxicology*, **93**, 269–87.

Emille, D., Peuchmaur, M., et al. 1991. Production of interleukins in human immunodeficiency virus 1-replicating lymph nodes. *J Clin Invest*, **86**, 148–59.

Fingerote, R.J., Cruz, B.M., et al. 1995. A 2′,5′-oligoadenylate analogue inhibits murine hepatitis virus strain 3 (MHV-3) replication in vitro but does not reduce MHV-3-related mortality or induction of procoagulant activity in susceptible mice. *J Gen Virol*, **76**, 373–80.

Fink, D.J., Sternberg, L.R., et al. 1992. In vivo expression of β-galactosidase in hippocampal neurons by HSV-mediated gene transfer. *Hum Gene Ther*, **3**, 11–19.

Finter, N.B., Chapman, S., et al. 1991. The use of interferon-alpha in virus infections. *Drugs*, **42**, 749–65.

Fitzgerald-Bocarsky, P., Feldman, M., et al. 1989. Deficient interferon-gamma production and natural NK activity in AIDS patients with HIV-2 infection. *J Infect Dis*, **160**, 1084–5.

Flamand, L., Gosselin, J., et al. 1991. Human herpesvirus 6 induces interleukin-1b and tumor necrosis factor alpha, but not interleukin-6 in peripheral blood mononuclear cell cultures. *J Virol*, **65**, 5105–10.

Foli, A., Saville, M.W., et al. 1995. Effects of the Th1 and Th2 stimulatory cytokines interleukin-12 and interleukin-4 on human immunodeficiency virus replication. *Blood*, **86**, 2114–23.

Franke-Ullman, G., Pfortner, C., et al. 1995. Alteration of pulmonary macrophage function by respiratory syncytial virus infection in vitro. *J Immunol*, **154**, 268–80.

Frese, M., Kochs, G., et al. 1995. MxA protein mediates resistance to hantavirus. *J Interferon Cytok Res*, **15**, Suppl. 1, S231.

Gelbard, H.A., Nottet, H.S.L.M., et al. 1994. Platelet-activating factor: a candidate human immunodeficiency virus type 1-induced neurotoxin. *J Virol*, **68**, 4628–35.

Gendelman, H.E., Baca, L.M., et al. 1990. Regulation of HIV replication in infected monocytes by IFN-α: mechanisms for viral restriction. *J Immunol*, **145**, 2669–76.

Gilles, P.N., Guerrette, D.L., et al. 1992. HBsAg retention sensitizes the hepatocyte to injury by physiological concentrations of interferon-gamma. *Hepatology*, **16**, 655–63.

Gillespie, J.S., Cavanagh, M.A., et al. 1993. Increased transcription of interleukin-6 in the brains of mice with chronic enterovirus infection. *J Gen Virol*, **74**, 741–3.

Gosselin, S., Flamand, L., et al. 1992. Infection of peripheral blood mononuclear cells by herpes simplex and Epstein–Barr viruses: differential induction of interleukin-6 and tumor necrosis factor-α. *J Clin Invest*, **89**, 1849–56.

Graham, M.B., Braciale, V.L. and Braciale, T.J. 1994. Influenza virus-specific CD4+ T helper type 2 T lymphocytes do not promote recovery from experimental virus infection. *J Exp Med*, **180**, 1273–82.

Grimaldi, L.M.E., Martion, G.V., et al. 1991. Elevated alpha-tumor necrosis factor levels in spinal fluid from HIV-1-infected patients with central nervous system involvement. *Ann Neurol*, **29**, 21–5.

Guidotti, L.G., Guilhot, S. and Chisari, F.V. 1994. Interleukin-2 and alpha/beta interferon down-regulate hepatitis B virus gene expression in vivo by tumor necrosis factor-dependent and -independent pathways. *J Virol*, **68**, 1265–70.

Gutterman, J.U. 1994. Cytokine therapeutics: lessons from interferon α. *Proc Natl Acad Sci USA*, **91**, 1198–205.

Haller, O., Arnheiter, H., et al. 1979. Genetically determined, interferon-dependent resistance to influenza virus in mice. *J Exp Med*, **149**, 601–12.

Heise, M.T. and Virgin, H.W. 1995. The T-cell-independent role of gamma interferon and tumor necrosis factor alpha in macrophage activation during murine cytomegalovirus and herpes simplex virus infection. *J Virol*, **69**, 904–9.

Hendricks, R.L., Tumpey, T.M. and Finnegan, A. 1992. IFN-gamma and IL-2 are protective in the skin but pathologic in the corneas of HSV-1 infected mice. *J Immunol*, **149**, 3023–8.

Ho, D.D., Neumann, A.U., et al. 1995. Rapid turnover of plasma virions and CD4 lymphocytes in HIV-1 infection. *Nature (Lond)*, **373**, 123–6.

Hober, D., Poli, L., et al. 1993. Serum levels of tumor necrosis factor-alpha (TNF-alpha), interleukin-6 (IL-6) and IL-1 beta in dengue infected patients. *Am J Trop Med Hyg*, **48**, 324–31.

Hu, K.Q., Yu, C.H. and Vierling, J.M. 1992. Up-regulation of intercellular adhesion molecule 1 transcription by hepatitis B virus X protein. *Proc Natl Acad Sci USA*, **89**, 11441–5.

Huang, S., Hendriks, W., et al. 1993. Immune response in mice that lack the interferon-γ receptor. *Science*, **259**, 1742–5.

Imani, F. and Jacobs, B.L. 1988. Inhibitory activity for the interferon-induced protein kinase is associated with the reovirus serotype 1 sigma 3 protein. *Proc Natl Acad Sci USA*, **80**, 7887–91.

Ishida, I., Nishi, M., et al. 1989. Effects of deregulated expression of human interleukin-2 in transgenic mice. *Int Immunol*, **1**, 113–19.

Jacobsen, M., Mestan, J., et al. 1989. Beta-interferon subtype induction by tumor necrosis factor. *Mol Cell Biol*, **9**, 3037–42.

Johnson, R.T., McArthur, J.C. and Narayan, O. 1988. The neurobiology of human immunodeficiency virus infections. *FASEB J*, **2**, 2970–81.

Jones, D.T., Monroy, D., et al. 1994. Sjögren's syndrome: cytokine and Epstein–Barr viral gene expression within the conjunctival epithelium. *Invest Ophthalmol Vis Sci*, **35**, 3493–504.

Jones, K.A., Luciw, P.A. and Duchange, N. 1988. Structural arrangements of transcription control domains within the 5′-untranslated leader regions of the HIV-1 and HIV-1 promoters. *Genes Dev*, **2**, 1101–14.

Kakumu, S., Shinagawa, T., et al. 1991. Serum interleukin-6 levels in patients with chronic hepatitis B. *Am J Gastroenterol*, **86**, 1804–8.

Kandil, O., Fishman, J.A., et al. 1994. Human immunodeficiency virus type 1 infection of human macrophages modulates the cytokine response to *Pneumocystis carinii*. *Infect Immun*, **62**, 644–50.

Karupiah, G., Fredrickson, T.N., et al. 1993. Importance of interferons in recovery from mousepox. *J Virol*, **67**, 4214–26.

Kazazi, F., Mathijs, J.M., et al. 1992. Recombinant interleukin 4 stimulates human immunodeficiency virus production by infected monocytes and macrophages. *J Gen Virol*, **73**, 941–9.

Kerr, I.M. and Brown, R.E. 1978. pppA2′p5′A: an inhibitor of protein synthesis synthesized with an enzyme fraction from interferon treated cells. *Proc Natl Acad Sci USA*, **75**, 256–60.

Ketzler, S., Weis, S., et al. 1990. Loss of neurons in the frontal cortex in AIDS brains. *Acta Neuropathol*, **80**, 92–4.

Kobayashi, M., Fitz, I., et al. 1989. Identification and purification of natural killer cell stimulatory factor (NKSF), a cytokine with multiple biological effects on human lymphocytes. *J Exp Med*, **170**, 827–45.

Koenig, S., Gendelman, H.E., et al. 1986. Detection of AIDS virus in macrophages in brain tissue from AIDS patients with encephalopathy. *Science*, **233**, 1089–93.

Koff, W.C. and Fann, A.V. 1986. Human tumor necrosis factor-α kills herpes virus infected but not normal cells. *Lymphokine Res*, **5**, 215–21.

Kornbluth, R.S., Oh, P.S., et al. 1989. Interferons and bacterial liposaccharides protect macrophages from productive infection by human immunodeficiency virus in vitro. *AIDS*, **3**, 301–13.

Kornbluth, R.S., Oh, P.S., et al. 1990. The role of interferons in the control of HIV replication in macrophages. *Clin Immunol Immunopathol*, **54**, 200–19.

Kotenko, S.V., Gallagher, G., et al. 2003. IFN lambdas mediate antiviral protection through a distinct class II cytokine receptor complex. *Nat Immunol*, **4**, 1, 69–77.

Künzi, M.S. and Pitha, P.M. 1995. Identification of human immunodeficiency virus primary isolates resistant to interferon-α and correlation of prevalence to disease progression. *J Infect Dis*, **171**, 822–8.

Kurane, I., Janus, J. and Ennis, F.A. 1992. Dengue virus infection of human skin fibroblasts in vitro production of IFN-beta, IL-6 and GMCSF. *Arch Virol*, **124**, 21–30.

Lairmore, M.D., Post, A.A., et al. 1991. Cytokine enhancement of simian immunodeficiency virus (SIV/mac) from a chronically infected T-cell line (HuT-78). *Arch Virol*, **121**, 43–53.

Lang, R.A., Metcalf, D., et al. 1987. Transgenic mice expressing a haemopoietic growth factor gene (GM-CSF) develop accumulations of macrophages, blindness and a fatal syndrome of tissue damage. *Cell*, **51**, 675–86.

Laster, S.M., Wold, W.S.M. and Gooding, L.R. 1994. Adenovirus proteins that regulate susceptibility to TNF also regulate the activity of PLA$_2$. *Semin Virol*, **5**, 431–42.

Lazdins, J.K., Klimkait, T., et al. 1991. In vitro effect of transforming growth factor-β on progression of HIV-1 infection in primary mononuclear phagocytes. *J Immunol*, **147**, 1201–7.

Leist, T.P., Eppler, M. and Zinkernagel, R.M. 1989. Enhanced virus replication and inhibition of lymphocytic choriomeningitis virus disease in anti-γ interferon-treated mice. *J Virol*, **63**, 2813–19.

Lengyel, P. 1982. Biochemistry of interferons and their actions. *Annu Rev Biochem*, **51**, 251–82.

Leong, K.H., Ramsay, A.J., et al. 1994. Selective induction of immune responses by cytokines coexpressed in recombinant fowlpox virus. *J Virol*, **68**, 8125–30.

Levin, S. and Hahn, T. 1985. Interferon deficiency syndrome. *Clin Exp Immunol*, **60**, 267–73.

Levine, B., Hardwick, J.M., et al. 1991. Antibody-mediated clearance of alphavirus infection from neurons. *Science*, **254**, 856–60.

Levy, D.E. 1995. Interferon induction of gene expression through the JAK-Stat pathway. *Semin Virol*, **6**, 81–9.

Linde, A., Andersson, B., et al. 1992. Serum levels of lymphokines and soluble cellular receptors in primary Epstein–Barr virus infection and in patients with chronic fatigue syndrome. *J Infect Dis*, **165**, 994–1000.

Lucin, P., Pavic, I., et al. 1992. Gamma interferon-dependent clearance of cytomegalovirus infection in salivary glands. *J Virol*, **66**, 1977–84.

Malakhova, O.A., Yan, M., et al. 2003. Protein ISGylation modulates the JAK-STAT signaling pathway. *Genes Dev*, **17**, 455–60.

Martinotti, M.G. and Gribaudo, G. 1992. Effects of interferon alpha on murine cytomegalovirus replication. *Microbiologia*, **15**, 183–6.

Masood, R., Lunardi-Iskandar, Y., et al. 1994. Inhibition of AIDS-associated Kaposi's sarcoma cell growth by DAB389-interleukin-6. *AIDS Res Hum Retrovir*, **10**, 969–75.

Mathur, A., Kamat, D.M., et al. 1994. Immunoregulatory abnormalities in patients with Epstein–Barr virus-associated B cell lymphoproliferative disorders. *Transplantation*, **57**, 1042–5.

Merlin, G., Falcoff, E. and Aguet, M. 1985. ^{125}I-labelled human interferons alpha, beta and gamma: comparative receptor-binding data. *J Gen Virol*, **66**, 1149–52.

Mestan, J., Brockhaus, M., et al. 1988. Antiviral activity of tumor necrosis factor. Synergism with interferons and induction of $(2',5')A_n$-synthetase. *J Gen Virol*, **69**, 3113–20.

Mester, J.C., Pitha, P.M. and Glorioso, J.C. 1995. Antiviral activity of herpes simplex virus vectors expressing murine α1-interferon. *Gene Therapy*, **2**, 187–96.

Mistchenko, A.S., Diez, R.A. and Falcoff, E. 1989. Inhibitory effect of interferon-gamma on adenovirus replication and late transcription. *Biochem Pharmacol*, **38**, 1971–8.

Miyazaki, I., Cheung, R.K. and Dosh, H.M. 1993. Viral interleukin-10 is critical for the induction of B cell growth transformation by Epstein–Barr virus. *J Exp Med*, **178**, 439–47.

Molina, J.M., Scadden, D.T., et al. 1990. Human immunodeficiency virus does not induce interleukin-1, interleukin-6, or tumor necrosis factor in mononuclear cells. *J Virol*, **64**, 2901–6.

Moore, K.W., Vieira, P., et al. 1990. Homology of cytokine synthesis inhibitory factor (IL-10) to the Epstein–Barr virus gene BCRFI. *Science*, **248**, 1230–4.

Mori, N., Shirakawa, F., et al. 1994. Transcriptional regulation of the human interleukin-6 gene promoter in human T-cell leukemia virus type 1-infected T-cell lines: evidence for the involvement of NF-κB. *Blood*, **84**, 2904–11.

Moskophidis, D., Frei, K., et al. 1991. Production of random classes of immunoglobulins in brain tissue during persistent viral infection paralleled by secretion of interleukin-6 (IL-6) but not IL-4, IL-5, and gamma interferon. *J Virol*, **65**, 1365–9.

Moss, B. and Flexner, C. 1987. Vaccinia virus expression vectors. *Annu Rev Immunol*, **5**, 305–24.

Muller, U., Steinhoff, U., et al. 1994. Functional role of type I and type II interferons in antiviral defense. *Science*, **264**, 1918–21.

Nabel, G. and Baltimore, D. 1987. An inducible transcription factor activates expression of human immunodeficiency virus in T-cells. *Nature (Lond)*, **326**, 711–13.

Nain, M., Hinder, F., et al. 1990. Tumor necrosis factor-α production in influenza A virus-infected macrophages and potentiating effect of lipopolysaccharide. *J Immunol*, **147**, 1921–8.

Nash, A.A. and Cambouropoulos, P. 1993. The immune response to herpes simplex virus. *Semin Virol*, **4**, 181–6.

Neurath, A.R., Strick, N. and Sproul, P. 1992. Search for hepatitis B virus cell receptors reveals binding sites for interleukin-6 on the virus envelope. *J Exp Med*, **175**, 461–9.

Newman, G.W., Kelley, T.G., et al. 1993. Concurrent infection of human macrophages with HIV-1 and *Mycobacterium avium* results in decreased cell viability, increased *M. avium* multiplication and altered cytokine production. *J Immunol*, **151**, 2261–72.

Niemialtowski, M.G. and Rouse, B.T. 1992. Predominance of Th1 cells in ocular tissues during herpetic stromal keratitis. *J Immunol*, **149**, 3035–9.

Novak, R.M., Holzer, T.J., et al. 1990. The effect of interleukin 4 (BSF-1) on infection of peripheral blood monocyte-derived macrophages with HIV-1. *AIDS Res Hum Retrovir*, **6**, 973–6.

Osborn, L., Kunkel, S. and Nabel, G.J. 1989. Tumor necrosis factor α and interleukin 1 stimulate the human immunodeficiency virus enhancer by activation of the nuclear factor κB. *Proc Natl Acad Sci USA*, **86**, 2336–40.

Pantaleo, G., Grailosi, C. and Fauci, A.S. 1993. The role of lymphoid organs in the pathogenesis of HIV infection. *Semin Immunol*, **5**, 157–63.

Park, H., Davis, M.V., et al. 1994. TAR RNA-binding protein is an inhibitor of the interferon-induced protein kinase, PKR. *Proc Natl Acad Sci USA*, **91**, 4713–17.

Pathak, V.K., Schindler, D. and Hershey, J.W.B. 1988. Generation of a mutant form of protein synthesis initiation factor eIF-2 lacking the site of phosphorylation of eIF-2 kinase. *Mol Cell Biol*, **8**, 993–5.

Pitha, P.M. 1980. The effect of interferon in mouse cells infected with MuLV. *Ann NY Acad Sci*, **350**, 301–13.

Pitha, P.M. 1991. Multiple effects of interferon on HIV-1 replication. *J Interfer Res*, **11**, 313–18.

Poli, G. and Fauci, A.S. 1993. Cytokine modulation of HIV expression. *Semin Immunol*, **5**, 165–73.

Poli, G., Orenstein, J.M., et al. 1989. Interferon-α but not AZT suppresses HIV expression in chronically infected cell lines. *Science*, **244**, 575–7.

Poli, G., Bressler, P., et al. 1990. Interleukin 6 induces human immunodeficiency virus expression in infected monocytic cells alone and in synergy with tumor necrosis factor α by transcriptional and post-transcriptional mechanisms. *J Exp Med*, **172**, 151–8.

Poli, G., Kinter, A.L., et al. 1991. Transforming growth factor β suppresses human immunodeficiency virus expression and replication in infected cells of the monocyte/macrophage lineage. *J Exp Med*, **173**, 589–97.

Poli, G., Kinter, A.L. and Fauci, A.S. 1994. Interleukin 1 induces expression of the human immunodeficiency virus alone and in synergy with interleukin 6 in chronically infected U1 cells; inhibition of inductive effects by the interleukin 1 receptor antagonist. *Proc Natl Acad Sci USA*, **91**, 108–12.

Popik, W. and Pitha, P.M. 1991. Inhibition by interferon of herpes simplex virus type 1-activated transcription of tat-defective provirus. *Proc Natl Acad Sci USA*, **88**, 9573–7.

Popik, W. and Pitha, P.M. 1992. Transcriptional activation of the Tat-defective human immunodeficiency virus type-1 provirus: effect of interferon. *Virology*, **189**, 435–47.

Popik, W. and Pitha, P.M. 1993. Role of tumor necrosis factor alpha in activation and replication of the tat-defective human immunodeficiency virus type 1. *J Virol*, **67**, 1094–9.

Popik, W. and Pitha, P.M. 1994. The presence of Tat protein or tumor necrosis factor alpha is critical for herpes simplex virus type 1-induced expression of human immunodeficiency virus type 1. *J Virol*, **68**, 1324–33.

Ramshaw, I., Ruby, J., et al. 1992. Expression of cytokines by recombinant vaccinia viruses: a model for studying cytokines in virus infection in vivo. *Immunol Rev*, **127**, 157–82.

Ramsay, A.J. and Kohonen-Corish, M. 1993. Interleukin-5 expressed by a recombinant virus vector enhances specific soluble IgA response in vivo. *Eur J Immunol*, **23**, 3141–5.

Ramsay, A.J., Husband, A.J., et al. 1994. The role of interleukin-6 in mucosal IgA antibody responses in vivo. *Science*, **264**, 561–3.

Raniero, D.E., Stasio, P. and Taylor, M.W. 1990. Specific effect of interferon on the herpes simplex virus type 1 transactivation event. *J Virol*, **64**, 2588–93.

Rautonen, J., Rautonen, R., et al. 1994. HIV type 1 Tat protein induces immunoglobulin and interleukin 6 synthesis by uninfected peripheral blood mononuclear cells. *AIDS Res Hum Retrovir*, **10**, 781–5.

Reich, N.C., Pine, R., et al. 1988. Transcription of interferon-stimulated genes is induced by adenovirus particles, but suppressed by E1A gene products. *J Virol*, **62**, 114–19.

Reickmann, P., Poli, G., et al. 1991. Activated B lymphocytes from human immunodeficiency virus-infected individuals induce virus expression in infected T cells and a promonocytic cell line, U1. *J Exp Med*, **173**, 1–5.

Roberts, N.F. Jr., Prill, A.M. and Mann, T.N. 1986. Interleukin and interleukin 1 inhibitor production by human macrophages exposed to influenza virus or respiratory syncytial virus: respiratory syncytial virus is a potent inducer of inhibitor activity. *J Exp Med*, **163**, 511–19.

Rosen, C.A., Sodroski, J.G. and Haseltine, W.A. 1985. The location of *cis*-acting regulatory sequences in the human T cell lymphotropic virus type III (HTLV-III/LAV) long terminal repeat. *Cell*, **41**, 813–23.

Rossol, S., Glanni, G., et al. 1992. Cytokine-mediated regulation of monocyte/macrophage cytotoxity in human immunodeficiency virus-1 infection. *Med Microbiol Immunol*, **181**, 267–81.

Rowe, W.P. 1954. Studies on pathogenesis and immunity in lymphocytic choriomeningitis infection of the mouse. *Naval Med Res Inst Rep*, 005-048.14.01.

Sambhi, S.K., Kohonen-Corish, M. and Ramshaw, I.A. 1991. Local production of tumour necrosis factor encoded by recombinant vaccinia virus is effective in controlling viral replication in vivo. *Proc Natl Acad Sci USA*, **88**, 4025–9.

Samuel, C.E. 1979. Mechanism of interferon action. Phosphorylation of protein synthesis initiation factor eIF-2 in interferon-treated human cells by a ribosome-associated kinase possessing site specificity similar to hemin-required rabbit reticulocyte kinase. *Proc Natl Acad Sci USA*, **76**, 600–4.

Samuel, C.E. 1991. Antiviral actions of interferon. Interferon-regulated cellular proteins and their surprising selective antiviral activities. *Virology*, **183**, 1–11.

Schmidt, D.S. and Rouse, B.T. 1992. The role of T cell immunity in control of herpes simplex virus. *Curr Top Microbiol Immunol*, **179**, 57–74.

Schutze, S., Potthoff, K., et al. 1992. TNF activates NF-κB by phosphatidylcholine-specific phospholipase C-induced 'acidic' sphingomyelin breakdown. *Cell*, **71**, 765–76.

Sebire, G., Emilie, D., et al. 1993. In vitro production of IL-6, IL-1-beta, and tumor necrosis factor-alpha by human embryonic microglial and neural cells. *J Immunol*, **150**, 1517–23.

Seder, R.A., Gazzinell, R., et al. 1993. Interleukin 12 acts directly on CD4+ T cells to enhance priming for interferon-γ production and diminishes interleukin 4 inhibition of such priming. *Proc Natl Acad Sci USA*, **90**, 10188–92.

Sekiyama, K.D., Yoshiba, M. and Thomson, A.W. 1994. Circulating proinflammatory cytokines (IL-1 beta, TNF-alpha and IL-6) and IL-1 receptor antagonist (IL-1Ra) in fulminant hepatic failure and acute hepatitis. *Clin Exp Immunol*, **98**, 71–7.

Serwadda, D., Sewankambo, N.K., et al. 1985. Slim disease: a new disease in Uganda and its association with HTLV-III infection. *Lancet*, **2**, 849–52.

Shankar, V., Kao, M., et al. 1992. Kinetics of virus spread and changes in levels of several cytokine mRNAs in the brain after intranasal infection of rats with Borna disease virus. *J Virol*, **66**, 992–8.

Shen, J., Devery, J.M. and King, N.J. 1995. Early induction of interferon-independent virus-specific ICAM-1 (CD45) expression by flavivirus in quiescent but not proliferating fibroblasts: implications for virus–host interactions. *Virology*, **208**, 437–49.

Sheppard, P., Kindsvogel, W., et al. 2003. IL-28, IL-29 and their class II cytokine receptor IL-28R. *Nat Immunol*, **4**, 1, 63–8.

Sher, A., Gazzinelli, R.T., et al. 1992. Role of T-cell derived cytokines in the downregulation of immune responses in parasitic and retroviral infection. *Immunol Rev*, **127**, 183–204.

Sheran, N., Lau, S., et al. 1991. Increased production of tumor necrosis factor alpha in chronic hepatitis B virus infection. *J Hepatol*, **2**, 241–5.

Shirazi, Y. and Pitha, P.M. 1992. Alpha interferon inhibits early stages of the human immunodeficiency virus type 1 replication cycle. *J Virol*, **66**, 1321–8.

Shirazi, Y. and Pitha, P.M. 1993. Interferon α-mediated inhibition of human immunodeficiency virus type 1 provirus synthesis in T-cells. *Virology*, **193**, 303–12.

Spies, T., Morton, C.C., et al. 1986. Genes for the tumor necrosis factors α and β are linked to the major histocompatibility complex. *Proc Natl Acad Sci USA*, **83**, 8699–702.

Sprecher, E. and Becker, Y. 1992. Detection of IL-1 beta, TNF-alpha and IL-6 gene transcription by the polymerase chain reaction in keratinocytes, Langerhans cells and peritoneal exudate cells during infection with herpes simplex virus-1. *Arch Virol*, **126**, 253–69.

Tanner, J.E. and Menezes, J. 1994. Interleukin-6 and Epstein–Barr virus induction by cyclosporin A: potential role in lymphoproliferative disease. *Blood*, **84**, 3956–64.

Tendler, C.J., Greenberg, S.J., et al. 1991. Cytokine induction in HTLV-1 associated myelopathy and adult T cell leukemia: alternate molecular mechanisms underlying retroviral pathogenesis. *J Cell Biochem*, **46**, 302–11.

Tepper, R.I., Levinson, D.A., et al. 1990. IL-4 induces allergic-like inflammatory disease and alters T cell development in transgenic mice. *Cell*, **62**, 457–67.

Tominaga, A., Takaki, S., et al. 1991. Transgenic mice expressing a B cell growth and differentiation factor gene (interleukin-5) develop eosinophilia and autoantibody production. *J Exp Med*, **173**, 429–36.

Torre, D., Zeroli, C., et al. 1992. Cerebrospinal fluid levels of IL-6 in patients with acute infections of the central nervous system. *Scand J Infect Dis*, **24**, 787–91.

Torseth, J.W. and Merigan, C.T. 1986. Tumor necrosis factor α and β inhibit virus replication and synergize with interferons. *Nature (Lond)*, **323**, 819–22.

Tufariello, J., Cho, S. and Horwitz, M.S. 1994. The adenovirus E3 14.7 kilodalton protein which inhibits cytolysis by tumor necrosis factor increases the virulence of vaccinia virus in a murine pneumonia model. *J Virol*, **68**, 453–62.

Tumpey, T.M., Elner, V.M., et al. 1994. Interleukin-10 treatment can suppress stromal keratitis induced by herpes simplex virus type 1. *J Immunol*, **153**, 2258–65.

Tyor, W.R., Moench, T.R. and Griffin, D.E. 1989. Characterization of the local and systemic B cell response of normal and athymic nude mice with Sindbis virus encephalitis. *J Neuroimmunol*, **24**, 207–15.

Tyor, W.R., Glass, J.D., et al. 1992. Cytokine expression in the brain during AIDS. *Ann Neurol*, **31**, 349–60.

Upton, C., DeLange, E.M. and MacFadden, G. 1987. Tumorigenic poxviruses genomic organization and DNA sequence of the telomeric region of Shope fibroma virus genome. *Virology*, **160**, 20–30.

Vassao, R.C., Mello, I.G. and Pereira, C.A. 1994. Role of macrophages, interferon-gamma and procoagulant activity in the resistance of genetic heterogeneous mouse populations to mouse hepatitis virus infection. *Arch Virol*, **137**, 277–88.

Voth, R., Rossol, S., et al. 1990. Differential gene expression of IFNα and tumor necrosis factor-α in peripheral blood mononuclear cells from patients with AIDS related complex and AIDS. *J Immunol*, **144**, 970–5.

Ward, B.J. and Griffin, D.E. 1993. Changes in cytokine production after measles virus vaccination: predominant production of IL-4 suggests induction of a Th2 response. *Clin Immunol Immunopathol*, **67**, 171–7.

Weir, J.P. and Elkins, K.L. 1993. Replication-incompetent herpesvirus vector delivery of an interferon α gene inhibits human immunodeficiency virus replication in human monocytes. *Proc Natl Acad Sci USA*, **90**, 9140–4.

Wesselingh, S.L., Power, C., et al. 1993. Intracerebral cytokine messenger RNA expression in acquired immunodeficiency syndrome dementia. *Ann Neurol*, **33**, 576–82.

Wesselingh, S.L., Levine, B., et al. 1994. Intracerebral cytokine mRNA expression during fatal and nonfatal alphavirus encephalitis suggests a predominant type 2 T cell response. *J Immunol*, **152**, 1289–97.

Wiley, C.A., Schrier, R.D., et al. 1986. Cellular localization of human immunodeficiency virus infection within the brains of acquired immune deficiency syndrome patients. *Proc Natl Acad Sci USA*, **83**, 7089–93.

Williams, B.R.G. and Silverman, R.H. 1985. *The 2-5A system*. New York: Alan R Liss.

Yamamoto, J.K., Barre-Sinoussi, F., et al. 1986. Human alpha- and beta-interferon but not gamma suppress the in vitro replication of LAV, HTLV-III and ARV-2. *J Interfer Res*, **6**, 143–52.

Yamato, K., El-Hajjaoul, Z., et al. 1990. Modulation of interleukin 1β RNA in monocytoid cells infected with human immunodeficiency virus 1. *J Clin Invest*, **86**, 1109–16.

Yasumoto, S., Mori, Y., et al. 1994. Ultraviolet-B irradiation alters cytokine production by immune lymphocytes in herpes simplex virus-infected mice. *J Dermatol Sci*, **8**, 218–23.

Zack, J.A., Arrigo, S.J. and Chen, I.S.Y. 1990. Control of expression and cell tropism of human immunodeficiency virus type 1. *Adv Virus Res*, **38**, 125–46.

Zhou, A., Hassel, B.A. and Silverman, R.H. 1993. Expression cloning of 2–5A-dependent RNase: a uniquely regulated mediator of interferon action. *Cell*, **72**, 753–65.

16

Viral evasion of the host immune response

ANTONIO ALCAMI

INTRODUCTION: AN INTIMATE RELATIONSHIP BETWEEN VIRUSES AND THEIR HOSTS

Viruses depend on the cell for replication and production of new virus particles, and thus viruses have established a complex interaction with the cellular machinery for nucleic acid replication and protein synthesis, and have 'learned' how to take advantage of cellular compartments to generate virus particles. The viral replication cycle and morphogenesis of virus particles can be observed in vitro in cell culture. However, in real life, viruses replicate in an animal host that is well prepared with a variety of defense mechanisms to prevent viral infection. In turn, viruses have evolved many different strategies to counteract host defenses.

The immune evasion strategies used by different virus families are related to the 'lifestyle' of the virus, which depends on the nature and replication of their genetic material, cell tropism, mechanism of transmission, and ability to persist in the infected host. Some viruses such as human immunodeficiency virus (HIV) infect immune cells and may cause immunosuppression. RNA viruses take advantage of the high mutation rate of the RNA polymerases to generate variants that escape recognition by the host immune system. Herpesviruses establish latency, a viral stage that maintains the viral genome

with minimal expression of viral proteins, avoiding recognition by the host immune system and allowing viral persistence for the life of the host. In this case, intermittent phases of reactivation generate newly synthesized virus particles to ensure transmission to other individuals and virus persistence in the host population. Recent investigations during the last few years have shown that viruses not only hide to avoid immune recognition but they take a very active role to interfere with specific molecular mechanisms of immunity. Large DNA viruses, such as poxviruses and herpesviruses, may accommodate between 100 and 200 genes in their genomes and have the capacity to code for a large number of proteins that interfere with the immune antiviral response.

Viral strategies of immune evasion block the development of innate (nonspecific) or adaptive (antigen-specific) immune responses. The innate response constitutes the first line of immune defense since it does not require previous encounters with the viral agent, and is rapidly activated during the first hours after infection. Innate responses include interferons (IFN), the complement system or natural killer (NK) cells. The adaptive immune response consists of antibodies and cytotoxic T cells (CTL) which are directed against specific antigens encoded by the viral invaders. This response requires days or even weeks to develop and induces immunological memory, so that the host will respond more rapidly and efficiently to viruses that have been experienced previously. The inflammatory response illustrates how innate responses may favor specific immune responses. As a result of viral infection and tissue damage, the inflammatory response is triggered which is characterized by an increased permeability of blood vessels and the production of soluble mediators such as cytokines and chemokines which induce the migration of immune cells into areas of infection. The end result is a massive infiltration of cells and soluble factors that protect the host from viral infection and trigger antigen-specific cellular and humoral responses that will offer further protection mechanisms.

The activation of the immune response requires the cooperation of T helper (Th) lymphocytes which differentiate into Th1 and Th2 cells that produce specific sets of cytokines. Th1 cells produce cytokines such as interleukin (IL)-2 and interferon (IFN)-γ that promote cellular pro-inflammatory responses associated with the maturation of macrophages and CTLs. Other cytokines such as IL-12 play an important role by inducing Th1 and NK cells to produce IFN-γ. By contrast, Th2 cells promote the humoral response inducing the differentiation of B cells to produce antibodies. In addition, Th2 cells produce IL-4 and IL-10 which may reduce cellular inflammatory responses. Whereas cellular immune responses are thought to play a critical role in viral elimination once viral infection has been established, the antibody response plays an important role in preventing the early stages of infection.

We have just started to understand the complex interaction of viruses with their hosts and how viruses achieve an equilibrium leading to the survival of both virus and host. Viruses are fully dependent on the host for their replication and production of progeny virus, and thus they should avoid high virulence that may lead to extermination of the host. Much of the pathology associated with viral diseases may be the result of an unbalanced virus–host interaction, and in some cases it represents uncontrolled attempts of the immune system to destroy the virus that lead to damage of the host. It has become clear that a more profound knowledge of the interaction of viruses with their host will help us to understand the molecular mechanisms of viral pathogenesis.

The study of the interaction of viruses with the host immune system is a research area that has expanded enormously in recent years and it is not possible to cover all aspects in depth in a chapter. Here I provide a general view of the different strategies used by viruses to evade the host immune response. Basic concepts of viral immune evasion are discussed and illustrated with representative examples. More information can be found in review articles (Alcami and Koszinowski 2000; Johnson and Hill 1998; Katze et al. 2002; Seet et al. 2003; Tortorella et al. 2000).

INHIBITION OF HUMORAL IMMUNITY

Genetic variability

The production of antibodies specific to viral antigens that neutralize virus particles is an important mechanism to prevent viral infection. One of the first mechanisms of immune evasion identified in viruses was the accumulation of mutations that translate into antigenic variability, a mechanism that has special relevance in viruses with RNA genomes (Flint et al. 2000). In contrast to DNA polymerases, RNA polymerases have low fidelity and introduce a high rate of mutations as the genetic material is copied. As a consequence, viral RNA genomes consist of a collection of RNA species (quasi species) carrying point mutations. These mutations translate into viral epitopes that are recognized with lower affinity by antibodies that neutralize the infectivity of the viral particles. An example of this strategy is found in rhinoviruses, which exist in the human population in the form of 160 serotypes. Neutralizing antibodies raised after the infection with one particular serotype do not protect from infection by other viral serotypes. Genetic variability may also generate variant peptide sequences that have lost the ability to bind to major histocompatibility complex (MHC) molecules, thus evading recognition by the cellular immune system as well.

Influenza virus is one of the best examples to illustrate genetic variability as a mechanism to escape immune recognition (Flint et al. 2000). The genome of influenza virus consists of eight RNA fragments encoding different proteins, including the virion surface proteins known as hemaglutinin (HA) and neuraminidase (NA). Coinfection of the same host with influenza viruses bearing different subtypes of HA and NA may generate virus particles containing new combinations of genomic fragments. This results in a sudden change of antigenic properties, known as antigenic shift, that facilitates the immediate evasion of neutralizing humoral responses in the majority of the population. This phenomenon may lead to pandemics such as that of 1918 in which more than 20 million people died. At the same time, influenza virus accumulates point mutations continuously due to the low fidelity of its RNA polymerase, a phenomenon known as antigenic drift. These limited changes are responsible for the flu epidemics of each season.

Fc receptors

Some viruses encode receptors for the Fc domain of immunoglobulin G (IgG) to evade the action of antibodies (Johnson and Hill 1998) (Figure 16.1). The glycoproteins gE and gI from herpes simplex virus (HSV) form a heterodimeric complex that functions as an Fc receptor. It has been proposed that gE–gI interacts with antibodies

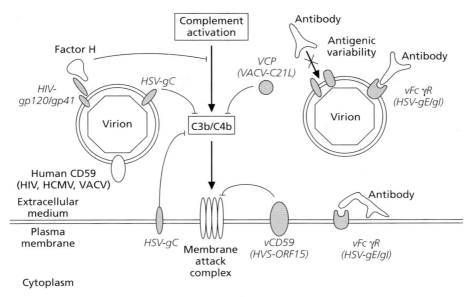

Figure 16.1 *Viral mechanisms to evade the complement and antibody responses*

that recognize specific HSV antigens and inhibit complement-mediated antibody neutralization and antibody-dependent cellular cytotoxicity by cells carrying Fc receptors (Frank and Friedman 1989; Lehner et al. 1975). The spike protein of the coronaviruses mouse hepatitis virus, bovine coronavirus, and transmissible gastroenteritis virus display Fc receptor activity (Oleszak et al. 1993).

Complement system

The complement system constitutes one of the major defense systems against pathogens. Viral antigens or antigen–antibody complexes may activate the complement cascade, a complex family of proteins that are sequentially activated and culminates with the formation of a membrane attack complex leading to the destruction of infected cells or the envelope of virus particles in those viruses with an outer lipid membrane.

Herpesviruses and poxviruses encode proteins with amino acid sequence motifs found in complement regulatory proteins and bind critical factors in the complement activation pathways, such as C3b and C4b, and inhibit their activity (Favoreel et al. 2003; Johnson and Hill 1998; Kotwal et al. 1990) (Figure 16.1). The HSV membrane glycoprotein gC binds the complement factor C3 and protects cellfree virus from complement-mediated neutralization and inhibits the lysis of HSV-infected cells by antibody and complement (Lubinski et al. 1999). The poxviruses variola virus, vaccinia virus (VACV), and cowpox virus (CPXV) encode a secreted protein, known as viral complement control protein (VCP), that blocks the classical and alternative pathways of complement activation (Kotwal et al. 1990; Rosengard et al. 2002). Inactivation of the *VCP* gene in VACV causes virus attenuation in animal models, demonstrating an important role of this protein in preventing host

defense mechanisms and a role for complement in antiviral immunity (Isaacs et al. 1992). Interestingly, inactivation of the CPXV VCP, known as inflammation modulatory protein (IMP), caused a substantial increase in the inflammatory response in infected mice compared to wild type CPXV infections (Miller et al. 1997). This illustrated that inhibition of the inflammatory response by viral proteins may reduce tissue damage and reduce the pathology associated with viral infection.

The complement system has the potential to cause extensive damage in the host cells and is therefore strictly controlled by both soluble and membrane proteins that block its activity. A strategy used by HIV is to recruit the soluble factor H that inhibits complement activation by interacting with the gp120–gp41 complex (Stoiber et al. 1996). Herpesvirus saimiri (HVS), a virus that infects monkeys, encodes a homologue of the inhibitor of the membrane attack complex CD59 that protects the infected cells from complement-mediated lysis (Rother et al. 1994). An alternative strategy is adopted by human retroviruses, VACV and human cytomegalovirus (HCMV). Instead of encoding homologues of host proteins, these viruses incorporate into the virion envelope host complement regulatory proteins, such as CD56 and CD59, that confer complement resistance to the virus particle (Saifuddin et al. 1995; Spear et al. 1995; Vanderplasschen et al. 1998).

EFFECTS ON SOLUBLE MEDIATORS OF THE IMMUNE SYSTEM

Modulation of IFN functions

IFNs were discovered because of their ability to protect cells from viral infection. IFNs can be classified as type I (α and β) and type II (γ), and represent one of the first antiviral defense mechanisms to be activated after infection. The finding in recent years of anti-IFN strategies encoded by most viruses highlights the key role of IFNs against viral infection (Figure 16.2). IFNs are produced and secreted in response to viral infection and bind specific receptors which trigger intracellular pathways that activate antiviral mechanisms (Goodbourn et al. 2000; Katze et al. 2002). Two major pathways that induce an antiviral state in cells are up-regulated by IFN: the double-stranded RNA (dsRNA)-dependent protein kinase (PKR) and the 2′-5′ oligoadenylate system (2′-5′ OAS) that activates RNase L. In addition, IFNs have immunomodulatory activity that can influence the type of immune response mounted in response to infection.

Viruses block the activity of IFN at three different levels: (i) blockade of IFN binding to specific receptors;

(ii) inhibition of signal transduction pathways induced by IFN; and (iii) inhibition of antiviral effector functions induced by IFN (Figure 16.2).

SECRETED VIRAL IFN RECEPTORS (IFNRS) AND IFN BINDING PROTEINS (IFNBPS)

Poxviruses encode proteins that are secreted from infected cells and bind with high affinity type I or type II IFN and prevent their interaction with IFNRs (Alcami 2003; McFadden and Murphy 2000) (Figure 16.2). This mechanism inhibits the initiation of IFN-mediated biological effects that lead to the establishment of an antiviral state in the cell or the activation of immune functions. Soluble receptors or binding proteins for other cytokines have been identified, mainly in the poxvirus family. Of particular relevance for IFN activity is the poxvirus IL-18 binding protein (vIL-18BP) which blocks the activity

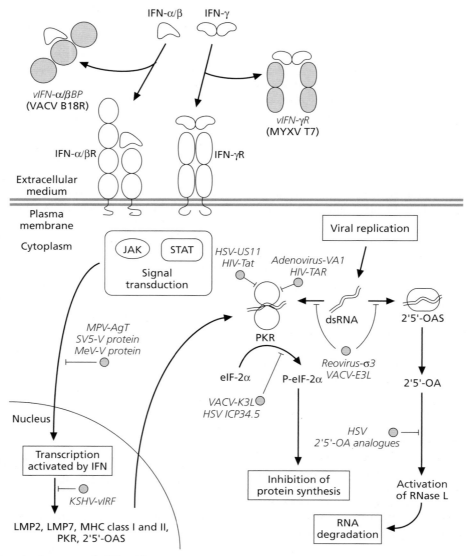

Figure 16.2 *Viral mechanisms to evade IFN activity*

of IL-18, a cytokine required together with IL-12 for the induction of IFN-γ (see below).

The viral IFN-γR (vIFN-γR) was first identified in myxoma virus (MYXV) and later in other members of the poxvirus family including VACV and CPXV (Alcami and Smith 1995; Mossman et al. 1995; Upton et al. 1992). The vIFN-γR has sequence similarity to the IFN binding domain of the cellular IFN-γR. The role of vIFN-γR during viral infection has been demonstrated by the attenuated phenotype a MYXV mutant lacking this IFN inhibitor (Mossman et al. 1996). A recent report describes a secreted IFN-γBP encoded by fowlpox virus that has no sequence similarity to known cellular IFN-γRs (Puehler et al. 2003). Because the IFN-γR of birds has not yet been characterized at the molecular level, this interesting finding raises the possibility that this virus may have hijacked an avian IFN-γR of different structure to the mammalian counterparts.

VACV and various poxviruses encode a secreted IFN-α/β receptor or binding protein (vIFN-α/βBP) that has very limited sequence similarity to the cellular counterparts (Colamonici et al. 1995; Symons et al. 1995). The vIFN-α/βBP has the unique property of binding to the cell surface after secretion (Alcami et al. 2000). The expression of viral decoy IFN-α/βRs at the cell surface of infected tissues will prevent the activation of IFN-mediated pathways more efficiently. A VACV mutant lacking the *vIFN-α/βBP* gene is attenuated in mice and its ability to grow in tissues and spread to other organs is impaired (Symons et al. 1995).

INTERFERENCE WITH SIGNAL TRANSDUCTION INDUCED BY IFNS

The interaction of IFNs with specific receptors at the cell surface triggers a complex cascade of intracellular pathways through janus kinase (JAK) and signal transducers and activators of transcription (STAT) pathways (Goodbourn et al. 2000; Katze et al. 2002) (Figure 16.2). These signaling events result in the up-regulation of cellular proteins that limit viral replication in several ways. Some of the genes upregulated by IFN are the low-molecular-weight protein (LMP) 2 and LMP7 subunits of the proteasome, involved in the generation of viral peptides for MHC class I molecules, the molecules that present viral peptides to T cells. Other genes upregulated by IFNs are protein kinase dsRNA (PKR) and 2′5′-OAS which confer an antiviral state in cells.

Some viral proteins interfere with the IFN signaling cascade (Goodbourn et al. 2000; Katze et al. 2002). For example, the T antigen of murine polyomavirus (MPV) binds to and inactivates JAK1 (Weihua et al. 1998), whereas the protein V from simian virus 5 (SV-5) interacts with STAT1 and induces its degradation by the proteasome (Didcock et al. 1999). Other paramyxovirus V proteins target different components of the IFN signaling pathway. Type II human parainfluenza virus V protein targets STAT2, mumps virus V protein targets

both STAT1 and STAT3, and measles virus (MeV) V protein causes a defect in STAT nuclear accumulation and STAT-inducible transcription (Nishio et al. 2002; Palosaari et al. 2003; Parisien et al. 2001; Ulane et al. 2003). Kaposi's sarcoma-associated herpesvirus (KSHV) uses a different mechanism by encoding a homologue of the IFN regulatory factor (IRF) that represses the IFN-mediated transcriptional activation of host genes (Zimring et al. 1998).

VIRAL MODULATION OF IFN EFFECTOR FUNCTIONS

One of the best-characterized antiviral effects of IFN is the induction of the PKR and 2′5′-OAS pathways that lead to the blockade of viral gene expression in the cell (Gale and Katze 1998; Goodbourn et al. 2000; Katze et al. 2002) (Figure 16.2). The replication and transcription of viral genomes leads to the formation of dsRNA that activates PKR, which phosphorylates the translation initiation factor 2α (eIF-2α) causing its inactivation and the subsequent arrest of protein synthesis in infected cells. Viral mechanisms that prevent the activation of PKR include: (i) proteins encoded by reovirus (σ3) and VACV (E3L) that bind dsRNA; (ii) RNAs encoded by adenovirus (VAI) and HIV (TAR) that bind PKR but do not activate the enzyme; and (iii) proteins encoded by HSV (US11) and HIV (Tat) that bind directly to PKR and inactivate the enzyme. An alternative strategy to block the PKR pathway is to prevent the phosphorylation of eIF-2α. VACV and other poxviruses encode an eIF-2α homologue, the K3L protein in VACV, that acts as a substrate of PKR and prevents phosphorylation of eIF-2α. An alternative strategy is illustrated by the HSV IC34.5 protein which activates protein phosphatase 1α that removes the phosphate groups from eIF-2α.

The formation of dsRNA during viral replication also activates the enzyme 2′5′-OAS, producing 2′5′-OA which in turn activates RNase L and the degradation of RNA within the infected cell, causing the blockade of viral replication. HSV produces analogues of 2′5′-OA which bind RNaseL and inhibit this pathway (Goodbourn et al. 2000). The proteins σ3 from reovirus and E3L from VACV bind dsRNA and thus inhibit the activation of 2′5′-OAS as well as PKR (see above).

Modulation of cytokine networks

Cytokines are a family of molecules that initiate and orchestrate the immune response, and include growth factors, IFNs, tumor necrosis factor (TNF), ILs, and chemokines. Cytokines are normally secreted from cells, although some are expressed at the cell surface, and activate specific responses in cells expressing the appropriate receptors. Immune cells use this complex network of ligands and receptors to orchestrate the immune response. In this way, the production of a particular cytokine after viral infection will determine the type of immune and inflammatory response that takes place. In addition, some cytokines such as IFN and TNF may act directly on infected cells and restrict virus replication.

The importance of cytokines in antiviral defense is highlighted by the number of mechanisms that viruses encode to block their activity (Alcami and Koszinowski 2000; Tortorella et al. 2000). The purpose of many of the viral anticytokine strategies is to down-regulate the immune responses to infection. However, it is important to consider that some viruses replicate in immune cells and these may be taking advantage of the effects that cytokines have on cell physiology to enhance the ability of cells to support viral replication, thus promoting viral replication rather than evading the immune system. Viruses may block the synthesis and maturation of cytokines or may modulate cytokine signaling in the target cells. Large DNA viruses such as poxviruses and herpesviruses have captured in their genomes genes encoding host cytokines and cytokine receptors (Alcami 2003; McFadden and Murphy 2000; Seet et al. 2003) (Figures 16.3 and 16.4).

VIRAL MODULATION OF CYTOKINE EXPRESSION AND ACTIVATION

Mechanisms that modulate the synthesis of cytokines have been described (Figure 16.3). African swine fever virus (ASFV) replicates in macrophages, one of the major cytokine producers in the immune system, and offers a good example to illustrate the control of cytokine production by viruses. ASFV encodes an IκB homologue that interacts with the transcription factors nuclear factor κB (NF-κB) and nuclear factor activated T cell (NFAT) and prevents the transcription of cytokine genes (Miskin et al. 1998). During virus entry into cells, the interaction of MeV with its cellular receptor CD46, a complement regulatory protein that protects cells from lysis by complement, blocks the production of IL-12, a potent inducer of IFN-γ and cellular responses. The CPXV protein cytokine response modifier A (CrmA) was found to inhibit the IL-1β converting enzyme (ICE) or caspase 1, which proteolytically cleaves the precursor form of proinflammatory cytokine IL-1β (pro-IL-1β) to generate mature, active IL-1β (Ray et al. 1992). CPXV CrmA may also prevent the maturation of IL-18, which is also proteolytically cleaved by ICE, and is an inhibitor of apoptosis (see below).

VIRAL MODULATION OF CYTOKINE SIGNAL TRANSDUCTION

There are several examples of viruses that inhibit cytokine-induced intracellular pathways, such as some of the anti-IFN mechanisms discussed above. The interaction of TNF and Fas ligand (FasL) with their receptors induce signaling that lead to an apoptotic response that some viruses are able to block (see below). Adenoviruses interfere with signaling induced by TNF at different levels (Mahr and Gooding 1999). The poxvirus VACV encodes two intracellular proteins (A52R and A46R) that block signaling mediated by Toll-like and IL-1 receptors by mimicking intracellular regulatory domains of these receptors (Bowie et al. 2000; Harte et al. 2003). The Toll-like receptor pathway is important in NF-κB activation and amplification of inflammatory signals.

Lastly, some viruses may subvert cytokine-mediated signaling for their own benefit. The latent membrane

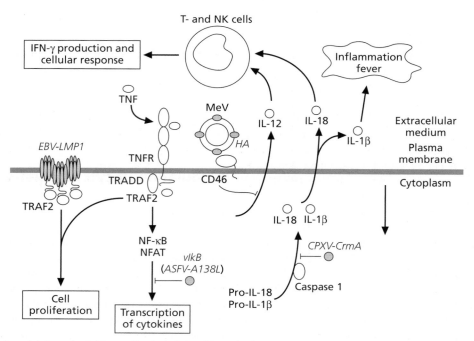

Figure 16.3 *Viral modulation of cytokine synthesis and signal transduction*

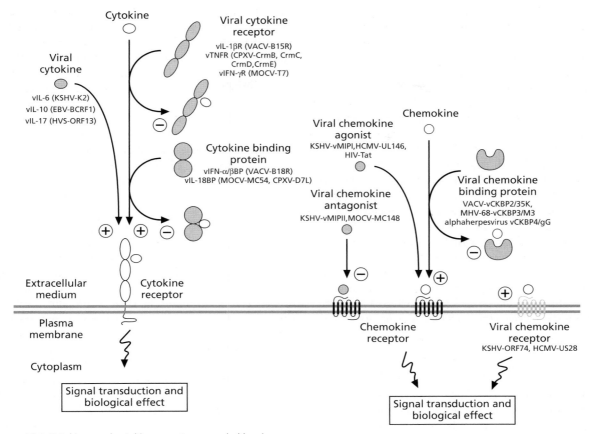

Figure 16.4 *Cytokines and cytokine receptors encoded by viruses*

protein 1 (LMP1) of Epstein–Barr virus (EBV), a virus that establishes latency in B cells, best illustrates this (Figure 16.3). LMP1 is a membrane protein that lacks sequence similarity to members of the TNF receptor (TNFR) superfamily but has a short cytoplasmic sequence that binds TNFR activating factors (TRAF), components of the TNFR and CD40 transduction machinery. During the immune response, binding of trimeric TNF to its receptor induces receptors multimerization and recruitment of TRAFs followed by the initiation of a signaling cascade leading to either B cell proliferation or the induction of apoptosis. In EBV-infected cells, the recruitment of TRAFs by LMP1 induces biological responses such as cell proliferation that may enhance virus replication (Farrell 1998). In this way, EBV takes advantage of a B-cell activation pathway to ensure survival of the infected cell that carries the latent viral genome.

Molecular mimicry: viral cytokines and cytokine receptors

The sequence of the genome of large DNA viruses (poxviruses and herpesviruses) showed that some viral proteins have sequence similarity to ligands and receptors of the cytokine family (Alcami 2003; McFadden and

Murphy 2000; Seet et al. 2003) (Figure 16.4). The sequence similarity suggests that, during evolution, viruses may have 'stolen' host genes that play critical roles in the immune system and incorporated them into their genomes. Viruses may have later modified the function of these host proteins for their own benefit since very often the biological properties of the viral proteins differ from their cellular counterparts.

VIRAL CYTOKINES

Viral cytokines act normally as agonists, driving the immune response in a direction that will be more beneficial for the virus (Figure 16.4). The VACV epidermal growth factor homologue (VGF) was the first viral cytokine identified. VGF activates cell growth and promotes viral replication, but an immune-related function has not been ascribed to it (McFadden et al. 1994). The EBV-encoded IL-10 homologue (vIL-10) was the first viral cytokine identified with immunomodulatory activity (Hsu et al. 1990). Genes encoding related vIL-10s have also been identified in other viruses. It has been shown that the EBV vIL-10 suppresses cellular immunity by inhibiting the production of IFN-γ, but has lost the immunostimulatory properties of the host counterpart. Other viral cytokines are the IL-6 homologue (vIL-6) encoded by KSHV (Moore et al. 1996) and the IL-17 homologue (vIL-17) encoded by HVS (Yao et al. 1995). In addition to their immunomodulatory activity, vIL-6 and vIL-17 may also promote the proliferation of B and T cells, respectively. These are the major host cell types for these viruses and their increased presence in infected tissues may favor viral replication.

The identification of semaphorin homologues (vSEMAs) in poxvirus and herpesvirus genomes was somehow surprising because semaphorins were described as chemoattractants and chemorepellents involved in axonal guidance during nervous system development, and only CD100 had been identified as a semaphorin involved in the immune system (Spriggs 1999). Investigations on the vSEMA encoded by VACV and ectromelia virus (ECTV) led to the identification of a specific receptor in macrophages that triggers expression of cytokines. The pro-inflammatory activity of vSEMA has been observed in mice infected with a VACV expressing an active protein (Gardner et al. 2001). However, the precise role of vSEMA in immune modulation during viral infection remains to be determined.

SECRETED VIRAL CYTOKINE RECEPTORS

Viral genes encoding soluble cytokine receptors have been identified mainly in the poxvirus family and a few examples have been recently described in the herpesvirus family (Figure 16.4). Viral cytokine receptors lack the transmembrane and cytoplasmic domains of the host counterparts, are secreted in large quantities from infected cells and have the ability to bind with high affinity the cognate cytokine and to block its activity. The poxvirus soluble cytokine receptors were initially identified because of their sequence similarity to the extracellular binding domain of their host counterparts. A second class of cytokine receptors, known as binding proteins, have very limited sequence similarity to the host cytokine receptors and were identified in cytokine binding or activity assays.

The soluble TNFR (vTNFR) M-T2 encoded by MYXV was the first viral cytokine receptor identified (Smith et al. 1991). Four different genes encoding vTNFRs were subsequently identified in other poxviruses such as CPXV, VACV, and ECTV, and were designated CrmB, CrmC, CrmD, and CrmE (Hu et al. 1994; Loparev et al. 1998; Saraiva and Alcami 2001; Smith et al. 1996). These vTNFRs have different molecular size, are produced at different times of infection, and in some cases show distinct binding properties. The reasons for the existence in poxvirus genomes of such a variety of vTNFRs apparently targeting the same ligand are unknown. Further complexity has been added by the recent description of a secreted protein encoded by Tanapox virus that binds TNF but has no sequence similarity to TNFRs (Brunetti et al. 2003). It appears that different poxviruses encode related, but distinct, proteins

to block TNF activity extracellularly. Clinical isolates of HCMV, but not laboratory strains, encode a membrane TNFR homologue (UL144) related to herpesvirus entry mediator (HVEM) that is retained intracellularly (Benedict et al. 1999). No ligand has been identified for this protein and its function remains to be determined. Maybe this membrane TNFR subverts TNF-mediated pathways in the infected cell.

Another member of the TNFR superfamily has been recently identified in CPXV and ECTV: a secreted and shorter version of CD30 (vCD30) (Panus et al. 2002; Saraiva et al. 2002). Viral cytokine receptors function as decoy receptors and, accordingly, vCD30 blocks the interaction of CD30 to CD30 ligand (CD30L). However, in this case, the ligand is only expressed at the cell surface and vCD30 induces reverse signaling in CD30L-expressing cells. The function of vCD30 in the context of infection has not been elucidated, but vCD30 has been shown to down-regulate type 1 cytokine-mediated inflammatory responses in mice, a property that may help the virus to evade an efficient antiviral response (Saraiva et al. 2002).

The viral IL-1β receptor (vIL-1βR) is related to the human type II IL-1R and acts as a decoy receptor (Alcami and Smith 1992; Spriggs et al. 1992). In contrast to the membrane IL-1Rs encoded by the host, the vIL-1βR binds exclusively IL-1β and not IL-1α or IL-1 receptor antagonist. Deletion of this gene in VACV causes attenuation when the virus is administered intracranially (Spriggs et al. 1992) but leads to enhanced virulence associated with fever and accelerated death in mice infected through the respiratory route, a natural route of poxvirus transmission (Alcami and Smith 1992; Alcami and Smith 1996). The enhanced virulence observed after deletion of the vIL-1βR from VACV illustrates that the role of some viral immunomodulatory proteins may be to reduce pathology induced by excess production of cytokines, in this case IL-1β, during infection rather than to cause immunosuppression.

VIRAL CYTOKINE-BINDING PROTEINS

IL-18 is a pro-inflammatory cytokine that is required, together with IL-12, for induction of IFN-γ and the generation of an efficient cellular response against viral infection. The viral IL-18 binding protein (vIL-18BP) encoded by several poxviruses is homologue of the human IL-18BP but has no sequence similarity to membrane IL-18 receptors (Figure 16.4). The vIL-18BP is an effective scavenger of IL-18 and down-regulates IFN-γ production and NK responses in ECTV-infected mice (Born et al. 2000; Smith et al. 2000). Interestingly, the vIL-18BP is also expressed by molluscum contagiosum virus (MOCV), a poxvirus that causes benign skin tumors and persists in the skin for months without inducing an inflammatory response (Smith et al. 2000; Xiang and Moss 1999). The vIL-18BP is the only cytokine receptor encoded by MOCV and may be responsible in part for the lack of inflammation in MOCV lesions.

The EBV-encoded colony stimulating factor 1 binding protein (vCSF-1BP) has limited sequence similarity to the cellular counterpart and is the only secreted cytokine binding protein identified in herpesvirus (Strockbine et al. 1998). It has been proposed that vCSF-1BP may modulate the response of macrophages during EBV infection. An interesting example of a viral secreted cytokine binding protein that binds ligands that interact with different host receptors is the orf virus-encoded protein that binds granulocyte–macrophage colony stimulating factor (GM-CSF) and IL-2. The role of this protein during infection of Orf virus, which causes skin lesions in sheep, goat, and man, has not been defined (Deane et al. 2000).

Modulation of chemokine networks

Chemokines are a family of small molecular size cytokines that induce cell migration and other biological effects, such as cell differentiation and angiogenesis, and control the trafficking of cells of the immune system throughout the body (Baggiolini 1998). There are more than 40 chemokines identified that can be structurally classified as CC, CXC, C or CX3C, according to the number of amino acids found between the first cysteine residues. Chemokines mediate their biological effects by binding and signaling through G-protein coupled receptors, proteins that have seven transmembrane domains. More than 20 chemokine receptors have been identified. Chemokines also interact with glycosaminoglycans (GAG) to enable their presentation at the surface of the endothelium and the establishment of chemokine gradients in tissues. There is recent evidence that chemokine–GAG interactions are required for the activity of chemokines in vivo (Proudfoot et al. 2003). The immune system makes the decision of which type of immune cell will migrate in response to infection or inflammation depending on the chemokine that is produced and the cell type that expresses the appropriate receptor. Thus the chemokine system plays a critical role in determining the type of immune response initiated after infection.

Viruses, mainly herpesviruses and poxviruses, utilize three mechanisms to modulate chemokine activity: expression of chemokine homologues, of chemokine receptor homologues, and of secreted chemokine binding proteins (Alcami 2003; Lalani et al. 2000; McFadden and Murphy 2000; Murphy 2001) (Figure 16.4). The function of these viral proteins during the infectious cycle is diverse and is discussed below (Figure 16.4).

VIRAL CHEMOKINE HOMOLOGUES

Some viruses encode chemokine homologues that are secreted from infected cells and function as agonists or antagonists (Figure 16.4). The chemokine homologues vMIP-II from KSHV and MC148 from MOCV bind to chemokine receptors but do not transduce signals (Boshoff et al. 1997; Damon et al. 1998; Kledal et al. 1997; Krathwohl et al. 1997). These antagonists block the binding of endogenous chemokines to their specific receptor and inhibit the migration of immune cells into infected tissues. By contrast, some viral chemokines have agonistic activity and induce cell migration into areas of infection, and thus their function may be unrelated to immune evasion. Viruses encoding chemokine agonists take advantage of the chemokine system to recruit to areas of infection immune cells that represent good targets for viral replication in order to enhance viral dissemination. HCMV UL146, known as vCXC-1, induces neutrophil chemotaxis by binding to CXCR2 and may account for the association of neutrophils with HCMV infections (Penfold et al. 1999). Human herpesvirus 6 (HHV-6) U83 induces monocyte migration that may favor the establishment of viral latency and persistence in the infected host (Zou et al. 1999). Another example of chemokine mimetics is the protein Tat from HIV that shows limited sequence similarity to chemokines. HIV Tat is a chemoattractant for monocytes and may enhance replication and spread of HIV in infected individuals (Albini et al. 1998). Direct evidence for a role of viral chemokine agonists in vivo comes from studies with murine cytomegalovirus (MCMV) mutants lacking the chemokine genes M131/129. The MCMV chemokine is encoded by the m131 orf and is expressed as a protein fused to the m129 orf. The isolated synthetic m131 product attracts activated macrophages by engaging a receptor related to human CCR3 (Saederup et al. 1999). A mutant MCMV lacking the function shows reduced spread to salivary glands, indicating that monocyte attraction serves for virus trafficking.

The role of the viral chemokines encoded by KSHV in viral dissemination has not been fully defined but they may play a role in pathogenesis due to their angiogenic properties that may cause the enhanced vascularization observed in Kaposi's sarcoma lesions (Boshoff et al. 1997). In addition, the KSHV chemokines are chemoattractants for Th2 polarized T cells and may influence the type of immune response initiated after viral infection (Dairaghi et al. 1999; Endres et al. 1999; Sozzani et al. 1998; Stine et al. 2000).

An interesting addition to chemokine mimicry by viruses is the glycoprotein G (gG) of respiratory syncytial virus which has partial sequence similarity to fractalkine and chemokine-like activity (Tripp et al. 2001). This property of gG may be used to facilitate virus entry into cells and to modulate the host immune response.

VIRAL CHEMOKINE RECEPTOR HOMOLOGUES

There are many examples of chemokine receptor homologues in members of the herpesvirus family and some in the poxvirus family (Figure 16.4). These proteins are expressed at the surface of infected cells and their ability to neutralize large amounts of chemokine may be limited. Some viral chemokine receptors have been found to bind chemokines and to transduce signals, and they may function to modulate the physiological state of the cell by activating chemokine-mediated signaling pathways. The ORF74 protein from KSHV is constitutively active and binding of chemokines can modulate the activation status of the receptor (Arvanitakis et al. 1997; Rosenkilde et al. 1999). Expression of this receptor in cell culture induces cell proliferation and may favor the persistence of KSHV. Transgenic mice expressing ORF74 develop Kaposi's sarcoma-like lesions (Arvanitakis et al. 1997; Yang et al. 2000). The possibility that expression of KSHV ORF74 may contribute to neoplasia through a paracrine effect has been proposed but may be difficult to demonstrate in KSHV-infected individuals. ORF74 is one of the best examples to illustrate the direct effect that viral immunomodulatory proteins may have on the pathology caused by viral infection. Four chemokine receptor homologues are encoded by HCMV: UL78, UL33, US27 and US28. MCMV encodes the viral chemokine receptors M33 and M78, which are homologous to their counterparts in HCMV. HCMV US28 can modify the chemokine environment of infected cells by sequestering and internalizing chemokines and depleting them from the medium (Bodaghi et al. 1998). Similarly, HHV-6 UL51 reduces extracellular accumulation of chemokines by sequestration, but also by a novel mechanism of down-regulation of CCL5 (RANTES) transcription (Milne et al. 2000). The potential contribution of viral chemokine receptors to pathology is also illustrated by the fact that HCMV US28 expression on the cell surface mediates cell adhesion, vascular smooth muscle cell migration, and it is thought to be related to vascular disease (Streblow et al. 1999). Evidence for a role for viral chemokine receptors in virus replication in vivo was demonstrated first for MCMV M33 (Davis-Poynter et al. 1997).

VIRAL CHEMOKINE BINDING PROTEINS (VCKBP)

The third class of viral chemokine inhibitors are the vCKBPs from poxviruses and herpesviruses that sequester chemokines in solution without apparent sequence similarity to host chemokine receptors (Seet and McFadden 2002; Smith et al. 2003) (Figure 16.4).

The MYXV M-T7 protein (vCKBP-1) is a soluble vIFN-γR with sequence similarity to human IFN receptors that was later found to interact also with chemokines. MYXV M-T7 binds a broad spectrum of chemokines and it has been proposed that it prevents the interaction of chemokines with GAGs and their correct presentation to leukocytes (Lalani et al. 1997). vCKBP-2

was identified in the medium from cultures infected with MYXV, VACV, or CPXV (Alcami et al. 1998; Graham et al. 1997; Smith et al. 1997). In this case, the protein binds CC chemokines with high affinity and neutralizes their effect by preventing the binding of chemokines to specific receptors in leukocytes. The protein M3 (vCKBP-3) encoded by murine gammaherpesvirus 68 (MHV-68) was found to bind a broad range of chemokines, including C, CC, CXC, and CX3C chemokines, and to block their interaction with cellular receptors (Parry et al. 2000; van Berkel et al. 2000). More recently, another family of vCKBPs has been identified in alphaherpesviruses (Bryant et al. 2003). gG is a membrane protein, present in the virions of some alphaherpesviruses, that is proteolytically cleaved and released to the extracellular space. Broad spectrum chemokine binding activity has been found in gG encoded by some alphaherpesviruses. This vCKBP blocks the interaction of chemokines to both specific chemokine receptors and GAGs.

The vCKBPs have amino acid sequences unrelated to chemokine receptors or other vCKBPs. Interestingly, the existing experimental data indicates that vCKBPs mimic the interaction of chemokines to their membrane receptors, in spite of the lack of amino acid sequence similarity (Alexander et al. 2002; Beck et al. 2001; Seet et al. 2001; Webb et al. 2003). The crystal structure of the poxvirus 35 kDa and MHV-68 M3 vCKBPs have been reported (Alexander et al. 2002; Carfi et al. 1999).

The generation of relevant virus mutants lacking specific vCKBPs and the infection of rabbits or mice suggest that these proteins may block chemokine-mediated leukocyte infiltration into infected areas in vivo (Graham et al. 1997; Lalani et al. 1999; Mossman et al. 1996; Reading et al. 2003; van Berkel et al. 2002). Interestingly, expression of the vCKBP-2 from VACV attenuates the virus in a murine intranasal model, probably due to a reduced inflammatory reaction to infection (Reading et al. 2003). In addition, MHV-68 M3 has been proposed to be required by the virus to establish virus latency and to enable persistence of the virus in the host (Bridgeman et al. 2001).

EVASION OF ANTIGEN PRESENTATION AND THE CELLULAR RESPONSE

The variability of viral antigens, discussed above in the context of the humoral response, is also relevant in the evasion of CTL recognition. Peptides derived from mutated viral proteins may lose their ability to bind to MHC molecules and be presented to the immune system. However, those viruses such as herpesviruses that establish infections for the life of the host but have a very low mutation rate must identify alternative mechanisms to persist in the presence of a vigorous immune response (Figure 16.5).

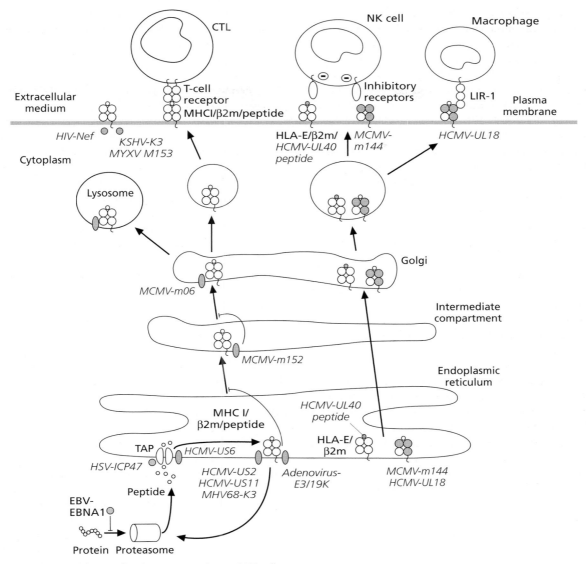

Figure 16.5 *Viral inhibition of antigen presentation and NK cell response*

Blockade of antigen presentation mediated by MHC class I molecules

MHC class I molecules display peptides at the cell surface derived from proteins expressed in the cell for recognition by the immune system (Figure 16.5). Viral proteins synthesized in the infected cell are degraded in the cytosol mostly by the proteasome, the major intracellular proteolytic complex, and the peptides generated are translocated to the lumen of the endoplasmic reticulum (ER) by transporters associated with antigen processing (TAP). The peptides associate with MHC class I molecules and β2-microglobulin to form a complex that is transported to the cell surface through the Golgi apparatus. The presentation of peptides derived from viral proteins activate specific CTLs that may destroy the infected cell. Herpesviruses are particularly well prepared with mechanisms that inhibit almost

every step of the antigen presentation pathway (Figure 16.5) (Fruh et al. 1999; Johnson and Hill 1998; Yewdell and Hill 2002).

The nuclear antigen EBNA1 encoded by EBV has a long segment of repeated glycine and alanine residues that prevents protein degradation by the proteasome (Levitskaya et al. 1995). The HSV protein ICP47 and the HCMV US6 bind to TAP and inhibit peptide translocation from the cytosol to the ER lumen (Ahn et al. 1997; Hengel et al. 1997; Lehner et al. 1997; York et al. 1994). While ICP47 is a cytosolic protein, US6 is a transmembrane glycoprotein that binds TAP on the lumenal side of the ER. In the ER, MHC class I molecules associate with TAP as part of a peptide loading complex that includes tapasin. The adenovirus E3/19K protein binds TAP and interferes with the ability of tapasin to bring class I molecules and TAP together (Bennett et al. 1999).

The degradation of newly synthesized MHC class I molecules is an alternative mechanism. The HCMV US2 and US11 proteins are membrane glycoproteins that interact with lumenal domain of MHC class I molecules and cause them to be transported back to the cytosol, where MHC class I molecules are ubiquitinylated and destroyed by the proteasome (Wiertz et al. 1996a; Wiertz et al. 1996b). The molecular mechanism behind this immune evasion strategy has attracted much interest because it sheds light on an important transport system from the ER to the cytosol. The K3 protein of MHV-68 is a ubiquitin ligase that ubiquitylates the cytoplasmic tail of ER-resident class I molecules and targets them for destruction in the cytosol (Boname and Stevenson 2001). The related K3 and K5 proteins encoded by KSHV also targets class I, but in this case the viral proteins target cell surface class I molecules for degradation (see below).

Several viruses block trafficking of class I molecules to the cell surface. The adenovirus E3/19K protein and the m152 protein from MCMV block the transport of peptides complexed to MHC class I molecules and β2-microglobulin (β2m) at different levels (Jefferies and Burgert 1990; Ziegler et al. 1997). The m06 protein from MCMV binds MHC class I molecules and directs them to the lysosome for degradation, due to the presence of a di-leucine motif in its cytoplasmic tail (Reusch et al. 1999). HIV Nef removes MHC class I molecules from the cell surface and directs them to the trans-Golgi network, due to the interaction of Nef with the PACS-1 protein which sorts molecules to the trans-Golgi network (Piguet et al. 2000). The KSHV K3 and K5 proteins ubiquitylate MHC class I and this signals class I internalization from the plasma membrane for endosomal degradation (Hewitt et al. 2002). A related protein encoded by MYXV, named M153, has been shown to target class I molecules both at the cell surface and in the post-Golgi compartment for retention and degradation in the lysosome. MYXV M153 has also been implicated in the depletion from the cell surface of CD4, the coreceptor in MHC class II-restricted antigen-induced T-cell activation, and Fas, which triggers apoptosis after interaction with FasL (Guerin et al. 2002; Mansouri et al. 2003).

The significance of the viral interference with CTL function is not clear in the context of the infected host since most of these mechanisms have been identified in cell cultures in vitro. A modest role for MCMV m152 in CTL escape in vivo has been reported, but no major effect on the virus replication was observed (Krmpotic et al. 2002). In the case of MHV-68, a mutant virus lacking K3 grows normally in the initial lung infection but does not establish latency in the spleen, which is controlled by CTLs (Stevenson et al. 2002). The in vivo advantage of CTL escape mutants in simian immunodeficiency virus (SIV) and HIV expressing mutant CTL epitopes has been established (Allen et al. 2000;

Goulder et al. 2001). Also, there is evidence that the ability of SIV Nef to down-regulate class I molecules is important in vivo (Munch et al. 2001).

Blockade of antigen presentation by class II MHC molecules

In contrast to MHC class I molecules, which present peptides derived from newly synthesized proteins, MHC class II molecules present peptides derived from exogenous antigens that are internalized and degraded in the lysosome. Only a few viral proteins have been found to block this pathway of antigen presentation. The US2 protein from HCMV induces the degradation of MHC class II molecules in the proteasome and HIV Nef interferes with the transport of MHC class II molecules to compartments where they associate with peptides before they reach the cell surface (Tomazin et al. 1999). HCMV US3 has also been shown to cause intracellular MHC class I retention (Hegde et al. 2002).

Evasion of the lysis of virus-infected cells by NK cells

NK cells constitute one of the first lines of defense against viruses. These cells posses specific activating receptors that recognize carbohydrate at the cell surface and induce their cytolytic activity. The NK cells also express other receptors, known as inhibitory receptors, that recognize MHC class I molecules and transduce a signal that blocks their cytotoxic machinery. In this way, NK cells recognize healthy cells expressing normal levels of MHC class I molecules and destroy cells that do not express class I molecules. The down-regulation of MHC class I molecules by some viruses prevents the specific recognition of the infected cell by CTLs, but may have dramatic consequences by increasing the susceptibility of virus-infected cells to NK cell lysis (Orange et al. 2002).

To solve this problem, some viruses encode homologues of MHC class I molecules (Figure 16.5). The MCMV protein m144 forms a complex with β2-microglobulin and is expressed at the cell surface where it interacts with NK cells and induces inhibitory signals that prevent the lysis of the infected cell (Farrell et al. 1997). A virus lacking m144 is attenuated in mice but is similar to wild-type virus in mice depleted of NK cells, suggesting that m144 controls NK activity in vivo. The role of the HCMV protein UL18, a class I homologue, in evasion of NK cell lysis is controversial (Reyburn et al. 1997). The demonstration that HCMV UL18 interacts with a receptor in macrophages suggested that these class I homologues may also modulate the activation of other immune cells that play a critical role against viral infections (Cosman et al. 1997). MOCV, unlike other poxviruses, establishes persistent infections in the skin and encodes an MHC class I homologue of unknown function (Senkevich and Moss 1998).

HLA-E is an MHC class I molecule that presents peptides derived from signal sequences from other MHC class I molecules, interacts with an inhibitory receptor in NK cells, NKG2A, and prevents lysis mediated by NK cells (Figure 16.5). In this way, HLA-E 'informs' the NK cells on global levels of MHC class I expression in the cell. To compensate for the low levels of MHC class I molecules in the infected cell, HCMV encodes a signal peptide, present in the UL40 protein, that specifically binds HLA-E. In this way, normal levels of HLA-E-peptide complexes at the cell surface are present in the infected cell and protect it from NK cell attack (Tomasec et al. 2000).

The MCMV protein m152 interferes with class I antigen presentation (see above). In addition, it was found that m152 also reduces the cell surface levels of the class I-like molecules RAE and H60, which serve as ligands for the NK cell activating receptor NKG2D (Krmpotic et al. 2002). An MCMV mutant lacking m152 was more susceptible to NK cell lysis.

A soluble form of HCMV UL16 binds to a family of human glycosylphosphatidylinositol-linked receptors and MHC class I-related proteins know as UL16 binding proteins (ULBP). The NK cell activating receptor NKG2D binds ULBPs, and this interaction is blocked in the presence of soluble UL16 (Cosman et al. 2001). These data suggest a mechanism by which UL16 may inhibit NK cell function.

Viral inhibition of dendritic cell (DC) functions

Antigen presenting cells (APC), usually DCs, capture antigen at the site of infection and migrate to the lymph nodes where they interact and activate naïve T cells. The T cells acquire a mature phenotype and can migrate to infected tissues where they can activate effector functions with antiviral properties, such as cytolytic activity or the release of antiviral cytokines. The inhibition of DC function by viruses is predicted to have a major impact in antiviral immunity.

By infecting DCs viruses may interfere with class I MHC processing and presentation would inhibit the role of DCs in immunity. A number of reports have shown that some viruses interfere with the maturation of DCs, which is necessary for DCs to present antigens to T cells and to activate them. DCs infected by MeV inhibit rather than promote the proliferation of T cells and express the apoptosis inducing ligand TRAIL (Grosjean et al. 1997; Vidalain et al. 2000). The interference of MeV with DC function is thought to be largely responsible for the generalized immunosuppression associated with MeV infection. Inhibition of DC maturation has been reported for HSV, MCMV, and HCMV (Andrews et al. 2001; Moutaftsi et al. 2002; Salio et al. 1999).

APOPTOSIS

Apoptosis or programmed cell death can be activated in several ways, including by TNF superfamily members, irradiation, inhibitors of cell cycle or infectious agents such as viruses. The sequential activation of a family of proteases known as caspases plays a central role in the control of the apoptotic response (Figure 16.6). Apoptosis can be considered an innate mechanism of defense against viral infection that limits virus replication. In addition, CTLs and NK cells destroy virus-infected cells by inducing apoptosis as a result of the production of cytokines such as TNF, the activation of Fas at the cell surface by FasL or the secretion of perforin that enables other secreted proteins (granzymes) to enter the cell. Although the apoptotic response limits virus replication when activated at early times of infection, the induction of apoptosis may also favor the release of virus particles and viral dissemination within the host under some circumstances. Many cellular proteins involved in the control of apoptosis are targets of viral anti-apoptotic mechanisms (Figure 16.6) (Benedict et al. 2002; Everett and McFadden 1999).

Blockade of signaling through TNFR and Fas

The soluble vTNFRs encoded by poxviruses, discussed above, prevent the binding of TNF to its receptor and the induction of TNF-mediated apoptosis (Alcami 2003; McFadden and Murphy 2000; Seet et al. 2003) (Figure 16.6). The interaction of TNFRs and Fas with their respective ligands induces the binding of cytoplasmic factors that interact through death domains (DD) and death effector domains (DED) present in adaptor proteins, such as TRADD (TNF-receptor-activated death domain) and FADD (Fas-associated death domain), and in some caspases. These factors initiate a cascade of interactions that culminate with the activation of caspases and the induction of apoptosis. MOCV and KSHV encode vFLIPs (FLICE or caspase 8-inhibitory proteins) that have death domains and prevent signal transduction through receptors for TNF and FasL (Bertin et al. 1997; Thome and Tschopp 2001). The HCMV *UL36* gene product vICA associates with caspase 8 and blocks its activation, but its sequence is unrelated to FLIPs (Skaletskaya et al. 2001). Adenoviruses produce a number of proteins encoded by the E3 region that inhibit TNF- and Fas-mediated apoptosis (Wold et al. 1999). The adenovirus receptor internalization and degradation (RID) complex, formed by the E3/10.4K and E3/14.5K proteins, induces internalization and subsequence degradation in lysosomes of TNFR and Fas. As a result of this, the infected cell becomes resistant to TNFR- and Fas-mediated apoptosis (Burgert et al. 2002; McNees and Gooding 2002).

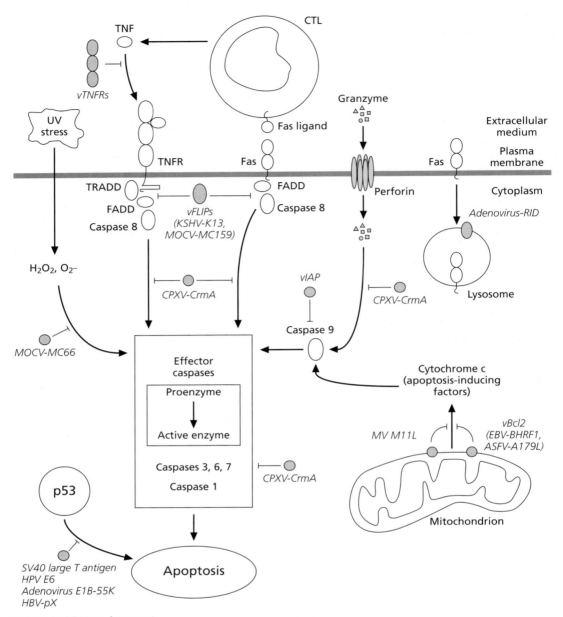

Figure 16.6 *Viral inhibition of apoptosis*

Inhibition of caspases

Caspases are proteolytic enzymes that are critical for the induction of apoptosis, and many viral proteins have been described to inhibit their activity (Figure 16.6). The CrmA protein encoded by CPXV, VACV and other poxviruses blocks caspase 1 and caspase 8, which play critical roles in major pro-apoptotic pathways, and prevents apoptosis initiated by several stimuli including TNF, FasL, and granzyme B (Miura et al. 1995; Talley et al. 1995; Tewari et al. 1995). In addition, CrmA inhibits the proteolytic maturation of IL-1β and, presumably, IL-18, cytokines that are cleaved by caspase 1 (Ray et al. 1992). The enzymatic activity of caspases is regulated by a family of inhibitor of apoptosis proteins (IAP)

that were originally identified in baculoviruses, a family of insect viruses (Clem and Miller 1994). IAP homologues are not frequently found in mammalian viruses, with the exception of ASFV (Neilan et al. 1993). The adenovirus E3-14.7K protein inhibits caspase 8 through interactions with a small GTPase and dynein (Lukashok et al. 2000).

Inhibition of mitochondrial pathways of caspase activation

Apoptosis can also be controlled at the level of mitochondria, as a result of loss of extracellular viral signals or by signals affecting the cell cycle (Rathmell and Thompson 2002). The release of cytochrome c, which resides in the space between the inner and outer membranes of the mitochondria, oligomerizes APAF1 and recruits pro-caspase 9 forming a protein complex known as the apoptosome and activates caspase 9 leading to apoptosis. Bcl2 is a cellular protein that resides in the outer mitochondrial membrane and inhibits the release of cytochrome c from the mitochondria. A number of viruses encode Bcl-2 homologues to prevent the induction of apoptosis, including adenovirus, ASFV, and the gammaherpesviruses EBV, KSHV and MHV-68 (Afonso et al. 1996; Cheng et al. 1997; Gangappa et al. 2002; Henderson et al. 1993; Sarid et al. 1997) (Figure 16.6). The HCMV protein UL37 shares no sequence similarity to Bcl-2 but resides in the mitochondria and is functionally similar to Bcl-2 (Goldmacher et al. 1999). Recently, the MYXV protein M11L has been shown to closely associate with a component of the mitochondrial permeability transition pore and to prevent apoptosis (Everett et al. 2002). A related protection of mitochondrial membrane potential has also been observed with VACV, but the viral protein responsible for it has not been identified (Wasilenko et al. 2001).

Other anti-apoptotic mechanisms

The tumor suppressor p53 limits cell proliferation by inducing apoptosis or cell cycle arrest. p53 stimulates transcription of genes involved in apoptotic pathways, and viruses can disrupt apoptosis by inactivating p53 (Figure 16.6). The simian virus 40 (SV40) large T antigen sequesters p53 in an inactive complex (Lane and Crawford 1979; Linzer and Levine 1979). The human papillomavirus (HPV) E6 protein and adenovirus E1B-55K protein promote ubiquitylation and degradation of p53 by different mechanisms (Scheffner et al. 1990; Steegenga et al. 1998; Werness et al. 1990). The hepatitis B virus (HBV) pX protein binds p53 and inhibits p53-mediated apoptosis (Wang et al. 1995). An alternative mechanism is represented by the glutathione superoxide MC66 encoded by MOCV which protects infected cells from peroxide radicals and ultraviolet radiation, and perhaps from peroxide radicals induced by TNF, macrophages, and neutrophils (Shisler et al. 1998).

CONCLUSIONS AND FUTURE PERSPECTIVES

In the past, viral immunology studies have characterized the host mechanisms to prevent and eliminate viral infections. The ability of many viruses to evade the host immune response by antigenic variation was shown many years ago. However, it is in the last ten years that we have become more aware of the many viral proteins that have evolved to block host specific mechanisms of antiviral immunity. There are numerous viral proteins without an ascribed function and it is likely that many of

these proteins encode new viral immune evasion strategies, which may only be evident in the infected host. The fact that we have not identified these viral functions may reflect our limited knowledge of the molecular mechanisms of immunity.

The reasons why a virus blocks a particular immune mechanism is not clear, and may depend on the replication and transmission mechanisms adopted by the virus. Many questions need to be resolved in the future. We need to determine which viral genes are required for the initial steps of the infection or for efficient transmission to another host in the presence of an active immune system. The apparent complexity and redundancy of these viral proteins may only be understood in the context of viral infection in the host. The lack of good animal models of infection for many viruses is limiting our understanding of the function of viral immune evasion strategies in vivo.

A better knowledge of the interaction of viruses with the host defense mechanisms will help us to understand the mechanisms of viral pathogenesis. Very often, the pathology observed in viral infections is not due to viral replication but a consequence of the immune and inflammatory responses to infection that may cause damage in the host. Moreover, some viral proteins may directly cause the pathological effects during infection. Some human inflammatory and autoimmune diseases are the result of an uncontrolled production of immune mediators such as TNF and IL-1 that constantly activate the immune response. We are finding examples of viral proteins that may enhance these immunopathological responses in the infected host.

The deletion of viral immune evasion proteins from the viral genome causes viral attenuation in most cases due to increased host defenses. However, enhanced viral virulence has been observed in VACV and CPXV when some of these viral functions have been deleted from the genome. These include the soluble vIL-1βR, IMP, and the 35 kDa vCKBP (Alcami and Smith 1992; Miller et al. 1997; Reading et al. 2003). These surprising observations suggest that the function of some of the viral immune evasion proteins is not to promote viral replication but to 'protect' the host from the detrimental effects of an over-reactive immune system, mediated in these examples by IL-1β, complement or chemokines, respectively. An enhanced host survival will be beneficial since the virus fully depends on the host for its replication. The complex interaction of each virus with the immune system is unique, and a better understanding of this interaction will lead to new strategies to control viral replication and the design of more efficient viral vaccines.

The fact that viruses have co-existed with their hosts during evolution and are able to survive in the presence of potent host defense mechanisms suggests that viruses know the mechanisms of immunity better than us. Viruses point at those molecules that play a critical role in defense against pathogens, one of the primary aims of the immune system, and thus viruses offer us a unique opportunity to identify basic mechanisms of immunity. Moreover, viruses may help us to understand the function of some of the large number of human genes recently identified in the human genome. The study of viral mechanisms of immune evasion is fascinating and will increase our understanding of the complex interaction of viruses with the host immune system.

ACKNOWLEDGMENTS

Research in the author's laboratory is funded by grants from the Wellcome Trust and the European Union.

REFERENCES

Afonso, C.L., Neilan, J.G., et al. 1996. An African swine fever virus Bcl-2 homolog, 5-HL, suppresses apoptotic cell death. *J Virol*, **70**, 4858–63.

Ahn, K., Gruhler, A., et al. 1997. The ER-luminal domain of the HCMV glycoprotein US6 inhibits peptide translocation by TAP. *Immunity*, **6**, 613–21.

Albini, A., Ferrini, S., et al. 1998. HIV-1 Tat protein mimicry of chemokines. *Proc Natl Acad Sci USA*, **95**, 13153–8.

Alcami, A. 2003. Viral mimicry of cytokines, chemokines and their receptors. *Nature Rev Immunol*, **3**, 36–50.

Alcami, A. and Koszinowski, U.H. 2000. Viral mechanisms of immune evasion. *Immunol Today*, **21**, 447–55.

Alcami, A. and Smith, G.L. 1992. A soluble receptor for interleukin-1 beta encoded by vaccinia virus: a novel mechanism of virus modulation of the host response to infection. *Cell*, **71**, 153–67.

Alcami, A. and Smith, G.L. 1995. Vaccinia, cowpox, and camelpox viruses encode soluble gamma interferon receptors with novel broad species specificity. *J Virol*, **69**, 4633–9.

Alcami, A. and Smith, G.L. 1996. A mechanism for the inhibition of fever by a virus. *Proc Natl Acad Sci USA*, **93**, 11029–34.

Alcami, A., Symons, J.A., et al. 1998. Blockade of chemokine activity by a soluble chemokine binding protein from vaccinia virus. *J Immunol*, **160**, 624–33.

Alcami, A., Symons, J.A. and Smith, G.L. 2000. The vaccinia virus soluble alpha/beta interferon (IFN) receptor binds to the cell surface and protects cells from the antiviral effects of IFN. *J Virol*, **74**, 11230–9.

Alexander, J.M., Nelson, C.A., et al. 2002. Structural basis of chemokine sequestration by a herpesvirus decoy receptor. *Cell*, **111**, 343–56.

Allen, T.M., O'Connor, D.H., et al. 2000. Tat-specific cytotoxic T lymphocytes select for SIV escape variants during resolution of primary viraemia. *Nature*, **407**, 386–90.

Andrews, D.M., Andoniou, C.E., et al. 2001. Infection of dendritic cells by murine cytomegalovirus induces functional paralysis. *Nat Immunol*, **2**, 1077–84.

Arvanitakis, L., Geras-Raaka, E., et al. 1997. Human herpesvirus KSHV encodes a constitutively active G-protein-coupled receptor linked to cell proliferation. *Nature*, **385**, 347–50.

Baggiolini, M. 1998. Chemokines and leukocyte traffic. *Nature*, **392**, 565–8.

Beck, C.G., Studer, C., et al. 2001. The viral CC chemokine-binding protein vCCI inhibits monocyte chemoattractant protein-1 activity by masking its CCR2B-binding site. *J Biol Chem*, **276**, 43270–6.

Benedict, C.A., Butrovich, K.D., et al. 1999. Cutting edge: a novel viral TNF receptor superfamily member in virulent strains of human cytomegalovirus. *J Immunol*, **162**, 6967–70.

Benedict, C.A., Norris, P.S. and Ware, C.F. 2002. To kill or be killed: viral evasion of apoptosis. *Nat Immunol*, **3**, 1013–18.

Bennett, E.M., Bennink, J.R., et al. 1999. Cutting edge: adenovirus E19 has two mechanisms for affecting class I MHC expression. *J Immunol*, **162**, 5049–52.

Bertin, J., Armstrong, R.C., et al. 1997. Death effector domain-containing herpesvirus and poxvirus proteins inhibit both Fas- and TNFR1-induced apoptosis. *Proc Natl Acad Sci USA*, **94**, 1172–6.

Bodaghi, B., Jones, T.R., et al. 1998. Chemokine sequestration by viral chemoreceptors as a novel viral escape strategy: withdrawal of chemokines from the environment of cytomegalovirus-infected cells. *J Exp Med*, **188**, 855–66.

Boname, J.M. and Stevenson, P.G. 2001. MHC class I ubiquitination by a viral PHD/LAP finger protein. *Immunity*, **15**, 627–36.

Born, T.L., Morrison, L.A., et al. 2000. A poxvirus protein that binds to and inactivates IL-18, and inhibits NK cell response. *J Immunol*, **164**, 3246–54.

Boshoff, C., Endo, Y., et al. 1997. Angiogenic and HIV-inhibitory functions of KSHV-encoded chemokines. *Science*, **278**, 290–4.

Bowie, A., Kiss-Toth, E., et al. 2000. A46R and A52R from vaccinia virus are antagonists of host IL-1 and toll-like receptor signaling. *Proc Natl Acad Sci USA*, **97**, 10162–7.

Bridgeman, A., Stevenson, P.G., et al. 2001. A secreted chemokine binding protein encoded by murine gammaherpesvirus-68 is necessary for the establishment of a normal latent load. *J Exp Med*, **194**, 301–12.

Brunetti, C.R., Paulose-Murphy, M., et al. 2003. A secreted high-affinity inhibitor of human TNF from Tanapox virus. *Proc Natl Acad Sci USA*, **100**, 4831–6.

Bryant, N.A., Davis-Poynter, N., et al. 2003. Glycoprotein G isoforms from some alphaherpesviruses function as broad-spectrum chemokine binding proteins. *EMBO J*, **22**, 833–46.

Burgert, H.G., Ruzsics, Z., et al. 2002. Subversion of host defense mechanisms by adenoviruses. *Curr Top Microbiol Immunol*, **269**, 273–318.

Carfi, A., Smith, C.A., et al. 1999. Structure of a soluble secreted chemokine inhibitor vCCI (p35) from cowpox virus. *Proc Natl Acad Sci USA*, **96**, 12379–83.

Cheng, E.H., Nicholas, J., et al. 1997. A Bcl-2 homolog encoded by Kaposi sarcoma-associated virus, human herpesvirus 8, inhibits apoptosis but does not heterodimerize with Bax or Bak. *Proc Natl Acad Sci USA*, **94**, 690–4.

Clem, R.J. and Miller, L.K. 1994. Control of programmed cell death by the baculovirus genes p35 and iap. *Mol Cell Biol*, **14**, 5212–22.

Colamonici, O.R., Domanski, P., et al. 1995. Vaccinia virus B18R gene encodes a type I interferon-binding protein that blocks interferon alpha transmembrane signaling. *J Biol Chem*, **270**, 15974–8.

Cosman, D., Fanger, N., et al. 1997. A novel immunoglobulin superfamily receptor for cellular and viral MHC class I molecules. *Immunity*, **7**, 273–82.

Cosman, D., Mullberg, J., et al. 2001. ULBPs, novel MHC class I-related molecules, bind to CMV glycoprotein UL16 and stimulate NK cytotoxicity through the NKG2D receptor. *Immunity*, **14**, 123–33.

Dairaghi, D.J., Fan, R.A., et al. 1999. HHV8-encoded vMIP-I selectively engages chemokine receptor CCR8. Agonist and antagonist profiles of viral chemokines. *J Biol Chem*, **274**, 21569–74.

Damon, I., Murphy, P.M. and Moss, B. 1998. Broad spectrum chemokine antagonistic activity of a human poxvirus chemokine homolog. *Proc Natl Acad Sci USA*, **95**, 6403–7.

Davis-Poynter, N.J., Lynch, D.M., et al. 1997. Identification and characterization of a G protein-coupled receptor homolog encoded by murine cytomegalovirus. *J. Virol.*, **71**, 1521–9.

Deane, D., McInnes, C.J., et al. 2000. Orf virus encodes a novel secreted protein inhibitor of granulocyte-macrophage colony-stimulating factor and interleukin-2. *J Virol*, **74**, 1313–20.

Didcock, L., Young, D.F., et al. 1999. The V protein of simian virus 5 inhibits interferon signalling by targeting STAT1 for proteasome-mediated degradation. *J Virol*, **73**, 9928–33.

Endres, M.J., Garlisi, C.G., et al. 1999. The Kaposi's sarcoma-related herpesvirus (KSHV)-encoded chemokine vMIP-I is a specific agonist for the CC chemokine receptor (CCR) 8. *J Exp Med*, **189**, 1993–8.

Everett, H. and McFadden, G. 1999. Apoptosis: an innate immune response to virus infection. *Trends Microbiol*, **7**, 160–5.

Everett, H., Barry, M., et al. 2002. The myxoma poxvirus protein, M11L, prevents apoptosis by direct interaction with the mitochondrial permeability transition pore. *J Exp Med*, **196**, 1127–39.

Farrell, H.E., Vally, H., et al. 1997. Inhibition of natural killer cells by a cytomegalovirus MHC class I homologue in vivo. *Nature*, **386**, 510–14.

Farrell, P.J. 1998. Signal transduction from the Epstein-Barr virus LMP-1 transforming protein. *Trends Microbiol*, **6**, 175–7, discussion 177–8.

Favoreel, H.W., Van de Walle, G.R., et al. 2003. Virus complement evasion strategies. *J Gen Virol*, **84**, 1–15.

Flint, S.J., Enquist, L.W., et al. 2000. *Principles of virology*. Washington, DC: ASM Press.

Frank, I. and Friedman, H.M. 1989. A novel function of the herpes simplex virus type 1 Fc receptor: participation in bipolar bridging of antiviral immunoglobulin G. *J Virol*, **63**, 4479–88.

Fruh, K., Gruhler, A., et al. 1999. A comparison of viral immune escape strategies targeting the MHC class I assembly pathway. *Immunol Rev*, **168**, 157–66.

Gale, M. Jr. and Katze, M.G. 1998. Molecular mechanisms of interferon resistance mediated by viral-directed inhibition of PKR, the interferon-induced protein kinase. *Pharmacol Ther*, **78**, 29–46.

Gangappa, S., van Dyk, L.F., et al. 2002. Identification of the in vivo role of a viral bcl-2. *J Exp Med*, **195**, 931–40.

Gardner, J.D., Tscharke, D.C., et al. 2001. Vaccinia virus semaphorin A39R is a 50-55 kDa secreted glycoprotein that affects the outcome of infection in a murine intradermal model. *J Gen Virol*, **82**, 2083–93.

Goldmacher, V.S., Bartle, L.M., et al. 1999. A cytomegalovirus-encoded mitochondria-localized inhibitor of apoptosis structurally unrelated to Bcl-2. *Proc Natl Acad Sci USA*, **96**, 12536–41.

Goodbourn, S., Didcock, L. and Randall, R.E. 2000. Interferons: cell signalling, immune modulation, antiviral responses and virus countermeasures. *J Gen Virol*, **81**, 2341–64.

Goulder, P.J., Brander, C., et al. 2001. Evolution and transmission of stable CTL escape mutations in HIV infection. *Nature*, **412**, 334–8.

Graham, K.A., Lalani, A.S., et al. 1997. The T1/35kDa family of poxvirus-secreted proteins bind chemokines and modulate leukocyte influx into virus-infected tissues. *Virology*, **229**, 12–24.

Grosjean, I., Caux, C., et al. 1997. Measles virus infects human dendritic cells and blocks their allostimulatory properties for CD4+ T cells. *J Exp Med*, **186**, 801–12.

Guerin, J.L., Gelfi, J., et al. 2002. Myxoma virus leukemia-associated protein is responsible for major histocompatibility complex class I and Fas-CD95 down-regulation and defines scrapins, a new group of surface cellular receptor abductor proteins. *J Virol*, **76**, 2912–23.

Harte, M.T., Haga, I.R., et al. 2003. The poxvirus protein A52R targets Toll-like receptor signaling complexes to suppress host defense. *J Exp Med*, **197**, 343–51.

Hegde, N.R., Tomazin, R.A., et al. 2002. Inhibition of HLA-DR assembly, transport, and loading by human cytomegalovirus glycoprotein US3: a novel mechanism for evading major histocompatibility complex class II antigen presentation. *J Virol*, **76**, 10929–41.

Henderson, S., Huen, D., et al. 1993. Epstein-Barr virus-coded BHRF1 protein, a viral homologue of Bcl-2, protects human B cells from programmed cell death. *Proc Natl Acad Sci USA*, **90**, 8479–83.

Hengel, H., Koopmann, J.O., et al. 1997. A viral ER-resident glycoprotein inactivates the MHC-encoded peptide transporter. *Immunity*, **6**, 623–32.

Hewitt, E.W., Duncan, L., et al. 2002. Ubiquitylation of MHC class I by the K3 viral protein signals internalization and TSG101-dependent degradation. *EMBO J*, **21**, 2418–29.

Hsu, D.H., de Waal Malefyt, R., et al. 1990. Expression of interleukin-10 activity by Epstein-Barr virus protein BCRF1. *Science*, **250**, 830–2.

Hu, F., Smith, C.A. and Pickup, D.J. 1994. Cowpox virus contains two copies of an early gene encoding a soluble secreted form of the type II TNF receptor. *Virology*, **204**, 343–56.

Isaacs, S.N., Kotwal, G.J. and Moss, B. 1992. Vaccinia virus complement-control protein prevents antibody-dependent complement-enhanced neutralization of infectivity and contributes to virulence. *Proc Natl Acad Sci USA*, **89**, 628–32.

Jefferies, W.A. and Burgert, H.G. 1990. E3/19K from adenovirus 2 is an immunosubversive protein that binds to a structural motif regulating the intracellular transport of major histocompatibility complex class I proteins. *J Exp Med*, **172**, 1653–64.

Johnson, D.C. and Hill, A.B. 1998. Herpesvirus evasion of the immune system. *Curr Top Microbiol Immunol*, **232**, 149–77.

Katze, M.G., He, Y. and Gale, M. Jr. 2002. Viruses and interferon: a fight for supremacy. *Nat Rev Immunol*, **2**, 675–87.

Kledal, T.N., Rosenkilde, M.M., et al. 1997. A broad-spectrum chemokine antagonist encoded by Kaposi's sarcoma-associated herpesvirus. *Science*, **277**, 1656–9.

Kotwal, G.J., Isaacs, S.N., et al. 1990. Inhibition of the complement cascade by the major secretory protein of vaccinia virus. *Science*, **250**, 827–30.

Krathwohl, M.D., Hromas, R., et al. 1997. Functional characterization of the C—C chemokine-like molecules encoded by molluscum contagiosum virus types 1 and 2. *Proc Natl Acad Sci USA*, **94**, 9875–80.

Krmpotic, A., Busch, D.H., et al. 2002. MCMV glycoprotein gp40 confers virus resistance to CD8+ T cells and NK cells in vivo. *Nat Immunol*, **3**, 529–35.

Lalani, A.S., Graham, K., et al. 1997. The purified myxoma virus gamma interferon receptor homolog M-T7 interacts with the heparin-binding domains of chemokines. *J Virol*, **71**, 4356–63.

Lalani, A.S., Masters, J., et al. 1999. Role of the myxoma virus soluble CC-chemokine inhibitor glycoprotein, M-T1, during myxoma virus pathogenesis. *Virology*, **256**, 233–45.

Lalani, A.S., Barrett, J.W. and McFadden, G. 2000. Modulating chemokines: more lessons from viruses. *Immunol Today*, **21**, 100–6.

Lane, D.P. and Crawford, L.V. 1979. T antigen is bound to a host protein in SV40-transformed cells. *Nature*, **278**, 261–3.

Lehner, P.J., Karttunen, J.T., et al. 1997. The human cytomegalovirus US6 glycoprotein inhibits transporter associated with antigen processing-dependent peptide translocation. *Proc Natl Acad Sci USA*, **94**, 6904–9.

Lehner, T., Wilton, J.M. and Shillitoe, E.J. 1975. Immunological basis for latency, recurrences and putative oncogenicity of herpes simplex virus. *Lancet*, **2**, 60–2.

Levitskaya, J., Coram, M., et al. 1995. Inhibition of antigen processing by the internal repeat region of the Epstein–Barr virus nuclear antigen-1. *Nature*, **375**, 685–8.

Linzer, D.I. and Levine, A.J. 1979. Characterization of a 54K dalton cellular SV40 tumor antigen present in SV40-transformed cells and uninfected embryonal carcinoma cells. *Cell*, **17**, 43–52.

Loparev, V.N., Parsons, J.M., et al. 1998. A third distinct tumor necrosis factor receptor of orthopoxviruses. *Proc Natl Acad Sci USA*, **95**, 3786–91.

Lubinski, J., Wang, L., et al. 1999. In vivo role of complement-interacting domains of herpes simplex virus type 1 glycoprotein gC. *J Exp Med*, **190**, 1637–46.

Lukashok, S.A., Tarassishin, L., et al. 2000. An adenovirus inhibitor of tumor necrosis factor alpha-induced apoptosis complexes with dynein and a small GTPase. *J Virol*, **74**, 4705–9.

Mahr, J.A. and Gooding, L.R. 1999. Immune evasion by adenoviruses. *Immunol Rev*, **168**, 121–30.

Mansouri, M., Bartee, E., et al. 2003. The PHD/LAP-domain protein M153R of myxomavirus is a ubiquitin ligase that induces the rapid internalization and lysosomal destruction of CD4. *J Virol*, **77**, 1427–40.

McFadden, G. and Murphy, P.M. 2000. Host-related immunomodulators encoded by poxviruses and herpesviruses. *Curr Opin Microbiol*, **3**, 371–8.

McFadden, G., Graham, K. and Opgenorth, A. 1994. Poxvirus growth factors. In: McFadden, G. (ed.), *Viroceptors, virokines and related immune modulators encoded by DNA viruses*. Georgetown, Texas: R. G. Landes Company, 1–15.

McNees, A.L. and Gooding, L.R. 2002. Adenoviral inhibitors of apoptotic cell death. *Virus Res*, **88**, 87–101.

Miller, C.G., Shchelkunov, S.N. and Kotwal, G.J. 1997. The cowpox virus-encoded homolog of the vaccinia virus complement control protein is an inflammation modulatory protein. *Virology*, **229**, 126–33.

Milne, R.S., Mattick, C., et al. 2000. RANTES binding and down-regulation by a novel human herpesvirus-6 beta chemokine receptor. *J Immunol*, **164**, 2396–404.

Miskin, J.E., Abrams, C.C., et al. 1998. A viral mechanism for inhibition of the cellular phosphatase calcineurin. *Science*, **281**, 562–5.

Miura, M., Friedlander, R.M. and Yuan, J. 1995. Tumor necrosis factor-induced apoptosis is mediated by a CrmA-sensitive cell death pathway. *Proc Natl Acad Sci USA*, **92**, 8318–22.

Moore, P.S., Boshoff, C., et al. 1996. Molecular mimicry of human cytokine and cytokine response pathway genes by KSHV. *Science*, **274**, 1739–44.

Mossman, K., Upton, C., Buller, R.M.L. and McFadden, G. 1995. Species specificity of ectromelia virus and vaccinia virus interferon-γ binding proteins. *Virology*, **208**, 762–9.

Mossman, K., Nation, P., et al. 1996. Myxoma virus M-T7, a secreted homolog of the interferon-gamma receptor, is a critical virulence factor for the development of myxomatosis in European rabbits. *Virology*, **215**, 17–30.

Moutaftsi, M., Mehl, A.M., et al. 2002. Human cytomegalovirus inhibits maturation and impairs function of monocyte-derived dendritic cells. *Blood*, **99**, 2913–21.

Munch, J., Stolte, N., et al. 2001. Efficient class I major histocompatibility complex down-regulation by simian immunodeficiency virus Nef is associated with a strong selective advantage in infected rhesus macaques. *J Virol*, **75**, 10532–6.

Murphy, P.M. 2001. Viral exploitation and subversion of the immune system through chemokine mimicry. *Nat Immunol*, **2**, 116–22.

Neilan, J.G., Lu, Z., et al. 1993. An African swine fever virus gene with similarity to the proto-oncogene bcl-2 and the Epstein-Barr virus gene BHRF1. *J Virol*, **67**, 4391–4.

Nishio, M., Garcin, D., et al. 2002. The carboxyl segment of the mumps virus V protein associates with Stat proteins in vitro via a tryptophan-rich motif. *Virology*, **300**, 92–9.

Oleszak, E.L., Perlman, S., et al. 1993. Molecular mimicry between S peplomer proteins of coronaviruses (MHV, BCV, TGEV and IBV) and Fc receptor. *Adv Exp Med Biol*, **342**, 183–8.

Orange, J.S., Fassett, M.S., et al. 2002. Viral evasion of natural killer cells. *Nat Immunol*, **3**, 1006–12.

Palosaari, H., Parisien, J.P., et al. 2003. STAT protein interference and suppression of cytokine signal transduction by measles virus V protein. *J Virol*, **77**, 7635–44.

Panus, J.F., Smith, C.A., et al. 2002. Cowpox virus encodes a fifth member of the tumor necrosis factor receptor family: A soluble, secreted CD30 homologue. *Proc Natl Acad Sci USA*, **99**, 8348–53.

Parisien, J.P., Lau, J.F., et al. 2001. The V protein of human parainfluenza virus 2 antagonizes type I interferon responses by destabilizing signal transducer and activator of transcription 2. *Virology*, **283**, 230–9.

Parry, C.M., Simas, J.P., et al. 2000. A broad spectrum secreted chemokine binding protein encoded by a herpesvirus. *J Exp Med*, **191**, 573–8.

Penfold, M.E., Dairaghi, D.J., et al. 1999. Cytomegalovirus encodes a potent alpha chemokine. *Proc Natl Acad Sci USA*, **96**, 9839–44.

Piguet, V., Wan, L., et al. 2000. HIV-1 Nef protein binds to the cellular protein PACS-1 to downregulate class I major histocompatibility complexes. *Nat Cell Biol*, **2**, 163–7.

Proudfoot, A.E., Handel, T.M., et al. 2003. Glycosaminoglycan binding and oligomerization are essential for the in vivo activity of certain chemokines. *Proc Natl Acad Sci USA*, **100**, 1885–90.

Puehler, F., Schwarz, H., et al. 2003. An interferon-gamma-binding protein of novel structure encoded by the fowlpox virus. *J Biol Chem*, **278**, 6905–11.

Rathmell, J.C. and Thompson, C.B. 2002. Pathways of apoptosis in lymphocyte development, homeostasis, and disease. *Cell*, **109**, S97–107.

Ray, C.A., Black, R.A., et al. 1992. Viral inhibition of inflammation: cowpox virus encodes an inhibitor of the interleukin-1 beta converting enzyme. *Cell*, **69**, 597–604.

Reading, P.C., Symons, J.A. and Smith, G.L. 2003. A soluble chemokine-binding protein from vaccinia virus reduces virus virulence and the inflammatory response to infection. *J Immunol*, **170**, 1435–42.

Reusch, U., Muranyi, W., et al. 1999. A cytomegalovirus glycoprotein re-routes MHC class I complexes to lysosomes for degradation. *EMBO J*, **18**, 1081–91.

Reyburn, H.T., Mandelboim, O., et al. 1997. The class I MHC homologue of human cytomegalovirus inhibits attack by natural killer cells. *Nature*, **386**, 514–17.

Rosengard, A.M., Liu, Y., et al. 2002. Variola virus immune evasion design: expression of a highly efficient inhibitor of human complement. *Proc Natl Acad Sci USA*, **99**, 8808–13.

Rosenkilde, M.M., Kledal, T.N., et al. 1999. Agonists and inverse agonists for the herpesvirus 8-encoded constitutively active seven-transmembrane oncogene product, ORF-74. *J Biol Chem*, **274**, 956–61.

Rother, R.P., Rollins, S.A., et al. 1994. Inhibition of complement-mediated cytolysis by the terminal complement inhibitor of herpesvirus saimiri. *J Virol*, **68**, 730–7.

Saederup, N., Lin, Y.C., et al. 1999. Cytomegalovirus-encoded beta chemokine promotes monocyte-associated viremia in the host. *Proc Natl Acad Sci USA*, **96**, 10881–6.

Saifuddin, M., Parker, C.J., et al. 1995. Role of virion-associated glycosylphosphatidylinositol-linked proteins CD55 and CD59 in complement resistance of cell line-derived and primary isolates of HIV-1. *J Exp Med*, **182**, 501–9.

Salio, M., Cella, M., et al. 1999. Inhibition of dendritic cell maturation by herpes simplex virus. *Eur J Immunol*, **29**, 3245–53.

Saraiva, M. and Alcami, A. 2001. CrmE, a novel soluble tumor necrosis factor receptor encoded by poxviruses. *J Virol*, **75**, 226–33.

Saraiva, M., Smith, P., et al. 2002. Inhibition of type 1 cytokine-mediated inflammation by a soluble CD30 homologue encoded by ectromelia (mousepox) virus. *J Exp Med*, **196**, 829–39.

Sarid, R., Sato, T., et al. 1997. Kaposi's sarcoma-associated herpesvirus encodes a functional bcl-2 homologue. *Nat Med*, **3**, 293–8.

Scheffner, M., Werness, B.A., et al. 1990. The E6 oncoprotein encoded by human papillomavirus types 16 and 18 promotes the degradation of p53. *Cell*, **63**, 1129–36.

Seet, B.T. and McFadden, G. 2002. Viral chemokine-binding proteins. *J Leukoc Biol*, **72**, 24–34.

Seet, B.T., Singh, R., et al. 2001. Molecular determinants for CC-chemokine recognition by a poxvirus CC- chemokine inhibitor. *Proc Natl Acad Sci USA*, **98**, 9008–13.

Seet, B.T., Johnston, J.B., et al. 2003. Poxviruses and immune evasion. *Annu Rev Immunol*, **21**, 377–423.

Senkevich, T.G. and Moss, B. 1998. Domain structure, intracellular trafficking, and beta2-microglobulin binding of a major histocompatibility complex class I homolog encoded by molluscum contagiosum virus. *Virology*, **250**, 397–407.

Shisler, J.L., Senkevich, T.G., et al. 1998. Ultraviolet-induced cell death blocked by a selenoprotein from a human dermatotropic poxvirus. *Science*, **279**, 102–5.

Skaletskaya, A., Bartle, L.M., et al. 2001. A cytomegalovirus-encoded inhibitor of apoptosis that suppresses caspase-8 activation. *Proc Natl Acad Sci USA*, **98**, 7829–34.

Smith, C.A., Davis, T., et al. 1991. T2 open reading frame from Shope fibroma virus encodes a soluble form of the TNF receptor. *Biochem Biophys Res Commun*, **176**, 335–42.

Smith, C.A., Hu, F.Q., et al. 1996. Cowpox virus genome encodes a second soluble homologue of cellular TNF receptors, distinct from CrmB, that binds TNF but not LT alpha. *Virology*, **223**, 132–47.

Smith, C.A., Smith, T.D., et al. 1997. Poxvirus genomes encode a secreted, soluble protein that preferentially inhibits beta chemokine activity yet lacks sequence homology to known chemokine receptors. *Virology*, **236**, 316–27.

Smith, V.P., Bryant, N.A. and Alcami, A. 2000. Ectromelia, vaccinia and cowpox viruses encode secreted interleukin-18-binding proteins. *J Gen Virol*, **81**, 1223–30.

Smith, V.P., Bryant, N.A. and Alcami, A. 2003. Soluble chemokine binding proteins encoded by viruses. In: Mahalinham, S. (ed.), *Chemokines in viral infections*. Georgetown, TX: Eureka.

Sozzani, S., Luini, W., et al. 1998. The viral chemokine macrophage inflammatory protein-II is a selective Th2 chemoattractant. *Blood*, **92**, 4036–9.

Spear, G.T., Lurain, N.S., et al. 1995. Host cell-derived complement control proteins CD55 and CD59 are incorporated into the virions of two unrelated enveloped viruses. Human T cell leukemia/lymphoma virus type I (HTLV-I) and human cytomegalovirus (HCMV). *J Immunol*, **155**, 4376–81.

Spriggs, M.K. 1999. Shared resources between the neural and immune systems: semaphorins join the ranks. *Curr Opin Immunol*, **11**, 387–91.

Spriggs, M.K., Hruby, D.E., et al. 1992. Vaccinia and cowpox viruses encode a novel secreted interleukin-1-binding protein. *Cell*, **71**, 145–52.

Steegenga, W.T., Riteco, N., et al. 1998. The large E1B protein together with the E4orf6 protein target p53 for active degradation in adenovirus infected cells. *Oncogene*, **16**, 349–57.

Stevenson, P.G., May, J.S., et al. 2002. K3-mediated evasion of CD8⁺ T cells aids amplification of a latent gamma-herpesvirus. *Nat Immunol*, **3**, 733–40.

Stine, J.T., Wood, C., et al. 2000. KSHV-encoded CC chemokine vMIP-III is a CCR4 agonist, stimulates angiogenesis, and selectively chemoattracts TH2 cells. *Blood*, **95**, 1151–7.

Stoiber, H., Pinter, C., et al. 1996. Efficient destruction of human immunodeficiency virus in human serum by inhibiting the protective action of complement factor H and decay accelerating factor (DAF, CD55). *J Exp Med*, **183**, 307–10.

Streblow, D.N., Soderberg-Naucler, C., et al. 1999. The human cytomegalovirus chemokine receptor US28 mediates vascular smooth muscle cell migration. *Cell*, **99**, 511–20.

Strockbine, L.D., Cohen, J.I., et al. 1998. The Epstein-Barr virus BARF1 gene encodes a novel, soluble colony-stimulating factor-1 receptor. *J Virol*, **72**, 4015–21.

Symons, J.A., Alcami, A. and Smith, G.L. 1995. Vaccinia virus encodes a soluble type I interferon receptor of novel structure and broad species specificity. *Cell*, **81**, 551–60.

Talley, A.K., Dewhurst, S., et al. 1995. Tumor necrosis factor alpha-induced apoptosis in human neuronal cells: protection by the antioxidant N-acetylcysteine and the genes bcl-2 and crmA. *Mol Cell Biol*, **15**, 2359–66.

Tewari, M., Telford, W.G., et al. 1995. CrmA, a poxvirus-encoded serpin, inhibits cytotoxic T-lymphocyte-mediated apoptosis. *J Biol Chem*, **270**, 22705–8.

Thome, M. and Tschopp, J. 2001. Regulation of lymphocyte proliferation and death by FLIP. *Nat Rev Immunol*, **1**, 50–8.

Tomasec, P., Braud, V.M., et al. 2000. Surface expression of HLA-E, an inhibitor of natural killer cells, enhanced by human cytomegalovirus gpUL40. *Science*, **287**, 1031.

Tomazin, R., Boname, J., et al. 1999. Cytomegalovirus US2 destroys two components of the MHC class II pathway, preventing recognition by CD4+ T cells. *Nat Med*, **5**, 1039–43.

Tortorella, D., Gewurz, B.E., et al. 2000. Viral subversion of the immune system. *Annu Rev Immunol*, **18**, 861–926.

Tripp, R.A., Jones, L.P., et al. 2001. CX3C chemokine mimicry by respiratory syncytial virus G glycoprotein. *Nat Immunol*, **2**, 732–8.

Ulane, C.M., Rodriguez, J.J., et al. 2003. STAT3 ubiquitylation and degradation by mumps virus suppress cytokine and oncogene signaling. *J Virol*, **77**, 6385–93.

Upton, C., Mossman, K. and McFadden, G. 1992. Encoding of a homolog of IFN-γ receptor by myxoma virus. *Science*, **258**, 1369–72.

van Berkel, V., Barrett, J., et al. 2000. Identification of a gammaherpesvirus selective chemokine binding protein that inhibits chemokine action. *J Virol*, **74**, 6741–7.

van Berkel, V., Levine, B., et al. 2002. Critical role for a high-affinity chemokine-binding protein in gamma-herpesvirus-induced lethal meningitis. *J Clin Invest*, **109**, 905–14.

Vanderplasschen, A., Mathew, E., et al. 1998. Extracellular enveloped vaccinia virus is resistant to complement because of incorporation of host complement control proteins into its envelope. *Proc Natl Acad Sci USA*, **95**, 7544–9.

Vidalain, P.O., Azocar, O., et al. 2000. Measles virus induces functional TRAIL production by human dendritic cells. *J Virol*, **74**, 556–9.

Wang, X.W., Gibson, M.K., et al. 1995. Abrogation of p53-induced apoptosis by the hepatitis B virus X gene. *Cancer Res*, **55**, 6012–16.

Wasilenko, S.T., Meyers, A.F., et al. 2001. Vaccinia virus infection disarms the mitochondrion-mediated pathway of the apoptotic cascade by modulating the permeability transition pore. *J Virol*, **75**, 11437–48.

Webb, L.M., Clark-Lewis, I. and Alcami, A. 2003. The gammaherpesvirus chemokine binding protein binds to the N terminus of CXCL8. *J Virol*, **77**, 8588–92.

Weihua, X., Ramanujam, S., et al. 1998. The polyoma virus T antigen interferes with interferon-inducible gene expression. *Proc Natl Acad Sci USA*, **95**, 1085–90.

Werness, B.A., Levine, A.J. and Howley, P.M. 1990. Association of human papillomavirus types 16 and 18 E6 proteins with p53. *Science*, **248**, 76–9.

Wiertz, E.J., Jones, T.R., et al. 1996a. The human cytomegalovirus US11 gene product dislocates MHC class I heavy chains from the endoplasmic reticulum to the cytosol. *Cell*, **84**, 769–79.

Wiertz, E.J., Tortorella, D., et al. 1996b. Sec61-mediated transfer of a membrane protein from the endoplasmic reticulum to the proteasome for destruction. *Nature*, **384**, 432–8.

Wold, W.S., Doronin, K., et al. 1999. Immune responses to adenoviruses: viral evasion mechanisms and their implications for the clinic. *Curr Opin Immunol*, **11**, 380–6.

Xiang, Y. and Moss, B. 1999. IL-18 binding and inhibition of interferon gamma induction by human poxvirus-encoded proteins. *Proc Natl Acad Sci USA*, **96**, 11537–42.

Yang, T.Y., Chen, S.C., et al. 2000. Transgenic expression of the chemokine receptor encoded by human herpesvirus 8 induces an angioproliferative disease resembling Kaposi's sarcoma. *J Exp Med*, **191**, 445–54.

Yao, Z., Fanslow, W.C., et al. 1995. Herpesvirus saimiri encodes a new cytokine, IL-17, which binds to a novel cytokine receptor. *Immunity*, **3**, 811–21.

Yewdell, J.W. and Hill, A.B. 2002. Viral interference with antigen presentation. *Nat Immunol*, **3**, 1019–25.

York, I.A., Roop, C., et al. 1994. A cytosolic herpes simplex virus protein inhibits antigen presentation to CD8+ T lymphocytes. *Cell*, **77**, 525–35.

Ziegler, H., Thale, R., et al. 1997. A mouse cytomegalovirus glycoprotein retains MHC class I complexes in the ERGIC/cis-Golgi compartments. *Immunity*, **6**, 57–66.

Zimring, J.C., Goodbourn, S. and Offermann, M.K. 1998. Human herpesvirus 8 encodes an interferon regulatory factor (IRF) homolog that represses IRF-1-mediated transcription. *J Virol*, **72**, 701–7.

Zou, P., Isegawa, Y., et al. 1999. Human herpesvirus 6 open reading frame U83 encodes a functional chemokine. *J Virol*, **73**, 5926–33.

17

Viral oncogenicity

JAMES C. NEIL AND JOHN A. WYKE

INTRODUCTION

A brief history of tumor virology

The incidence of tumors in animals and humans often shows geographical variation. This clustering sometimes reflects genetic differences in the populations at risk but more often results from environmental factors that vary between populations. Features of the environment that enhance the risk of tumor development (i.e. carcinogens) comprise physical factors (such as ultraviolet and other irradiation that impinges on and penetrates the body), chemical factors (ingested or contaminating the body surface), and infectious agents. Of the last, the most important are viruses. Viruses that produce tumors in animals have been known since the early 1900s, but it is only in recent decades that they have excited great interest. The reasons for this are twofold.

First, as diverse viruses were increasingly implicated as causes of cancer in animals of all vertebrate classes, it was hoped that they might also be important in the etiology of human neoplasia. This concept was attractive, not least because it suggested that, if the causative organisms could be identified and characterized, the incidence of cancer might be reduced by the prophylactic measures so successful against other infectious agents. The development of a tumor is usually a rare outcome of virus infection but it has nevertheless been estimated that up to 20 percent of human tumors have a viral risk factor (zur Hausen 1991) (Figure 17.1). Only one family of RNA-containing viruses, the retroviruses, has well-established oncogenic members (Table 17.1),

but representatives of all the major subdivisions of DNA-containing viruses (except the parvoviruses) in vertebrates have been implicated in neoplasia. Examples are given in Tables 17.2 and 17.3, p. 332, but, because all these agents receive attention elsewhere in this volume, this chapter will concentrate on general principles rather than specific details.

The second reason for an interest in viruses was their promise as tools for studying the basic mechanisms underlying neoplastic change. This idea rested on several earlier developments in laboratory research. Inbreeding of laboratory animals produced some strains with high incidence of various virus-associated neoplasms. In addition, inbred strains permitted transplantation studies, which demonstrated that a single donor cell could produce a tumor in the recipient animal. This finding focused attention on changes that occurred at a subcellular level and provided the rationale for studying oncogenesis in vitro rather than in the whole animal. This switch in emphasis was facilitated by the development of tissue culture techniques and, at the same time, it was found that tissue culture was an ideal way to measure the cytopathic effects of viruses, so that animal virologists could adopt the quantitative approach developed in studies on bacteriophages.

A correlation soon emerged between the ability of viruses readily to cause solid mesenchymal tumors in animals and their induction of morphological transformation of cultured cells (Figure 17.2, p. 333). This finding had important implications, not widely appreciated at the time. Following Theodor Boveri's proposals in 1914, the notion that tumors were clones of cells whose altered

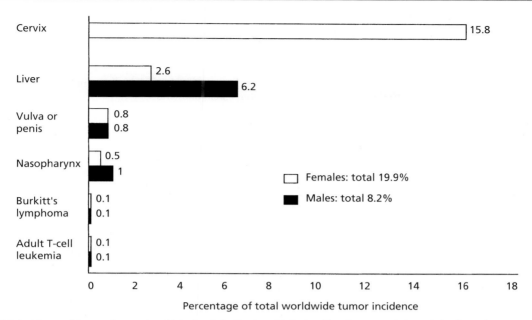

Figure 17.1 *Incidence of human tumors in which virus infection is a risk factor. The viruses most strongly implicated are papillomaviruses – tumors of cervix and external genitalia (Chapter 23, Papillomaviruses); HBV – primary liver tumors (Chapter 56, Hepatitis delta virus); EBV – Burkitt's lymphoma and nasopharyngeal carcinoma (Chapter 29, Gamma herpesviruses: Epstein–Barr virus); and human T-cell leukemia viruses – adult T-cell leukaemia (Chapter 58, Retroviruses and associated diseases in humans). (Modified, with permission, from zur Hausen 1986.) Note that these estimates do not include recent changes in cancer incidence due to HIV infection (Chapters 58, Retroviruses and associated diseases in humans and 60, Human immunodeficiency virus).*

properties result from accumulated mutations was accepted by many scientists (Baltzer 1964). However, before molecular genetic technology was developed, they could not conceive ways of identifying, among the thousands of genes in every somatic cell, the putative subsets that were mutated. Tumor viruses seemed to offer a way round this impasse. Some of them possessed only a few genes among which, it was argued, were those that

Table 17.1 *Some RNA viruses implicated in cancers of animals and humans*

Virus classification	Virus	Associated tumors	Other risk factors
Retroviridae			
Alpharetroviruses	ALVs; Rous sarcoma virus	Various sarcomas, some carcinomas, lymphomas, and leukemias	Genetic susceptibility affecting virus penetration replication and spread
Betaretroviruses	MMTV	Mammary adenocarcinomas, T-cell lymphoma	Pregnancy (altered hormone levels)
	JSRV	Pulmonary adenoma	. . .
	Mason–Pfizer monkey virus	Fibrosarcomas	. . .
Gammaretroviruses	MLV, murine sarcoma virus	Lymphomas, leukemias, and sarcomas	Genetic susceptibility to viral infection and spread
	Reticuloendotheliosis virus (avian)	Lymphomas and leukemias	. . .
	FeLV, feline sarcoma virus	Lymphosarcomas (mainly T cell), myeloid leukemias, fibrosarcomas	Age at exposure, immunosuppression
Deltaretroviruses	HTLV-I, HTLV-II	Adult T-cell leukemia	. . .
	BLV	Lymphosarcoma (B cell)	. . .
Lentiviruses	HIV	B lymphomas, Kaposi's sarcoma	EBV, KSHV
	Simian immunodeficiency virus	B lymphomas	Simian herpesvirus
	Feline immunodeficiency virus	B lymphomas	FeLV
Flaviviridae	HCV	Hepatocellular carcinoma	. . .

ALV, avian leukosis virus; BLV, bovine leukemia virus; BPV, bovine papillomavirus; EBV, Epstein–Barr virus; FeLV, feline leukemia virus; HBV, hepatitis B virus; HIV, human immunodeficiency virus; HPV, human papilloma virus; HTLV, human T-cell leukemia virus; HVS, herpesvirus saimiri; JSRV, jaagsiekte sheep retrovirus; MLV, murine leukemia virus; MMTV, mouse mammary tumor virus; SIV, simian immunodeficiency virus; WHV, woodchuck hepatitis virus.

Table 17.2 *Some oncogenic small DNA viruses of animals and humans*

Virus family	Virus	Host of origin	Associated tumors	Other risk factors
Hepadnaviridae	Hepatitis B group	Humans, apes, rodents, ducks	Primary hepatocellular carcinoma	In humans: alcohol, smoking, fungal toxins, other viruses
Papovaviridae	Polyoma	Mouse	Various carcinomas and sarcomas	. . .
	SV40	Monkey	Sarcomas, mesothelioma (in rodents, man?)	. . .
	BK and JC	Human	None in humans; neural tumors in rodents and monkeys	. . .
	Papilloma	Human	Genital, laryngeal and skin warts; may progress to:	. . .
			Cervical carcinoma	Smoking, herpes simplex viruses, immunosuppression
			Laryngeal carcinoma	X-irradiation, smoking
			Skin carcinoma	Sunlight, genetic disorders
		Cattle	Genital, alimentary, skin warts; may progress to:	. . .
			Alimentary carcinoma	Carcinogens and immunosuppressants in bracken fern
			Skin carcinoma	Sunlight, genetic predisposition (lack of pigmentation)
		Other mammals	Papillomas; may progress to carcinomas	Experimentally, carcinogens such as methylcholanthrene

transformed cells in vitro and induced tumors in vivo. Identification of these viral cancer genes (oncogenes) should help define the molecular basis of cancer, because they might have functional analogues among the cellular genes required for neoplasia. Although naive in hindsight, this concept proved correct for the retroviruses used widely by laboratory workers. Indeed, for the retroviruses, its significance exceeded expectations, for in many cases the viral oncogenes were descended from cellular cognates, the proto-oncogenes. These, in turn, have been convincingly implicated in the genesis of a range of animal and human tumors of both viral and nonviral etiology. The

Table 17.3 *Some oncogenic large DNA viruses of animals and humans*

Virus family	Virus	Host of origin	Associated tumors	Other risk factors
Adenoviridae	Types 2, 5, 12	Human	None in humans; sarcomas in hamsters	. . .
Herpesviridae	Frog herpesvirus	Leopard frog	Adenocarcinomas	Ambient temperature
	Marek's disease	Fowl	Neurolymphomatosis (T cell)	Genetic predisposition, MHC and non-MHC loci
	Herpesvirus ateles and saimiri	Monkeys	Lymphoma, leukemia	. . .
	EBV	Human	Burkitt's lymphoma, Hodgkin's disease, immunoblastic lymphoma	Malaria, HIV, immunodeficiency
			Nasopharyngeal carcinoma	Salted fish in infancy, HLA type
	Herpes simplex (types 1 and 2)	Human	Cervical neoplasia	Papillomaviruses, smoking, immunodeficiency
	Cytomegalovirus	Human	Cervical neoplasia	Immunodeficiency, HLA type
	Kaposi's sarcoma herpesvirus (KSHV/HHV8)	Human	Kaposi's sarcoma, primary effusion lymphoma/ Castleman's disease	HIV
Poxviridae	Shope fibroma	Rabbit	Fibroma	. . .
	Yaba monkey tumor virus	Monkey	Nodular fibromatous hyperplasia	Not relevant; progressive tumors never develop
	Molluscum contagiosum	Human	Nodular epidermal hyperplasia	. . .

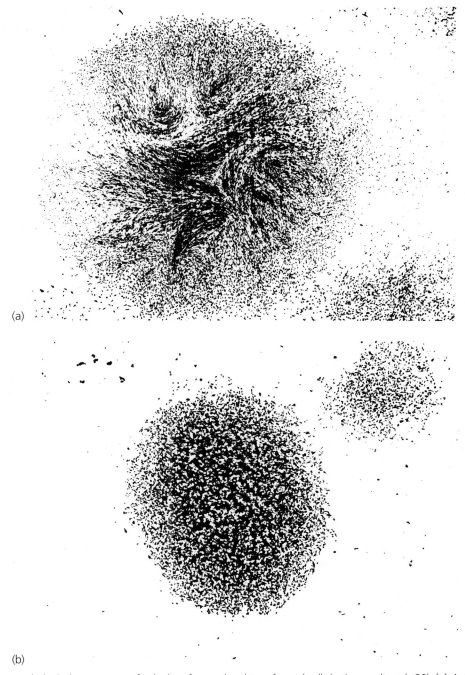

(a)

(b)

Figure 17.2 *The morphological appearance of colonies of normal and transformed cells in tissue culture (×20).* **(a)** *A colony of BHK-21/C13, a cell line derived from Syrian hamster kidney. Note that the colony is flat and the cells are lined in parallel array.* **(b)** *The same cell line after transformation by* Polyomavirus. *The cells are piled on one another and lack orientation.*

DNA tumor viruses have also provided vital insights into the cancer process because their oncogenes encode proteins that interfere with cellular checkpoint controls of proliferation and survival which have in a similar fashion proved to be of general relevance in human cancer.

These concepts gave rise to a large amount of work, reviewed elsewhere (Bishop 1991; Vogelstein and Kinzler 1992). This chapter summarizes in turn the two broad divisions of tumor virology:

1 studies on the molecular mechanisms of virus-induced neoplasia
2 attempts to implicate viruses in the aetiology of cancer.

These divisions, however, share concepts and techniques, and are increasingly considered together (Minson et al. 1994). Such a unitary approach is particularly important when attempting to combat virus-associated cancer, as outlined in the third part of this chapter.

Paradoxically, the tumor viruses themselves are now being developed as part of our anticancer armory.

Cancer – a disorder of cellular controls

The development of a fertilized egg into a multicellular organism and the subsequent maintenance of its form and function require complex controls over cell proliferation and cell death, and the expression of differentiated cell functions. These attributes of cells result from an interplay between stimuli from outside the cell and its current program of activity. Many of these stimuli are mediated by chemical signals classified according to their origin; endocrine signals originate from distant cells, paracrine signals from cells in the neighborhood of the recipient, and autocrine signals from the recipient cell itself. Whatever their origin and consequence, these signals have an effect only if the recipient cell has appropriate cell surface or internal receptors for the signal, an appropriate machinery of second messengers to process it and the metabolic capacity to respond.

Perturbations in these controls can lead to local increases in tissue mass. These may be the response of a normal cell to abnormal stimuli, leading to cell hypertrophy or, if the cells can multiply, to hyperplasia. On the other hand, the cells themselves may be altered, so their growth and behavior are no longer controlled in the same way as their normal counterparts and they become neoplastic. We might expect neoplasia to result from a change in any of the components of the system by which the cell responds to external signals, and there is now considerable evidence that in neoplastic cells mutations exist that change the function of various components in the signaling pathway controlling cell proliferation. As we shall see, viral oncogenes frequently act to stimulate growth in this way.

However, the oncogenes represent only one facet of the genetic basis of cancer. The requirement for recessive mutations in cancer was long suspected, both from the occurrence of inherited cancer syndromes (Knudson 1993) and from classic in vitro cell fusion studies where the transformed phenotype was often found to be extinguished in hybrid cells (Harris 1985). It was suspected that the genes underlying these phenomena might play a role in commitment to terminal differentiation, with loss of function leading to a block at an immature, highly proliferative stage. Although there is evidence to support this hypothesis for a number of genes, the most widely implicated tumor suppressor genes appear to play quite different roles in controlling cell cycle progression ('gatekeepers') or in maintaining the integrity of the genome ('caretakers') (Shields and Harris 2000). Given the fundamental nature of these roles, the discovery that the archetypal tumor suppressor, p53, is dispensable for normal development was a surprise to the field. Mice lacking functional p53 are ostensibly normal, but are prone to develop tumors, particularly lymphomas (Donehower et al. 1992). In its normal physiological role, p53 orchestrates cellular responses to genotoxic damage; induction of p53 leads to cell cycle arrest and allows repair synthesis to occur. Whilst this phenomenon is a partial explanation for the protective role of p53, there is another important facet to the story. Cells in which p53 is induced may also undergo programmed cell death or apoptosis as a consequence (Yonish-Rouach et al. 1991). This cell suicide mechanism, which plays vital roles in normal development and morphogenesis, also serves as a brake to cancer development. For cancer to develop, it seems that cells must acquire mutations which block cell death as well as those which drive cellular proliferation (Liebermann et al. 1995).

In practice, the simple binary classification of cancer genes as oncogenes or tumor suppressors is no longer tenable as some genes display facets of both, with gain or loss of function of a single gene contributing to tumor development in different cellular contexts (Lee and Farnham 2000; Wotton et al. 2002). The p53 protein itself is functionally complex, as some mutant forms act as dominant negative inhibitors of the wild-type counterpart, hence acquiring oncogene-like properties (Vogelstein and Kinzler 1992). Also, certain oncogenes (e.g. c-*myc*) actually induce growth stasis or apoptosis instead of proliferation when overexpressed in a cellular environment unfavorable for growth (Evan et al. 1992). Such mechanisms serve to protect multicellular organisms from cancers and explain the need for multiple genetic events to transform normal cells to full malignancy.

THE PATHOGENESIS OF TUMOR VIRUSES

Reasoning from first principles, we can envisage many ways by which features of virus infection might favor the development of tumors. The interactions between viruses and their hosts are such that it is clear that most of these mechanisms exist in one or another naturally occurring cancer. Indeed, the genesis of a given neoplasm may be influenced by more than one mechanism, because they are not mutually exclusive.

Direct oncogenic mechanisms

A first major category of pathogenic mechanism is direct or intrinsic, in which the tumor cells, or at least their ancestral lineage, are infected by the causative virus. Although this mechanism was presumed to be involved in studies of tumor viruses in vitro, only one aspect of it was useful to the experimenter – that in which all or part of the virus genome persisted in the tumor lineage. Genome persistence provides a marker that pinpoints crucial events in tumorigenesis, either because a specific portion of the virus is always present or because the genome is inserted in a specific region of the host chromosome DNA.

The consistent presence of a viral gene, either free in the cell or integrated randomly in host DNA, suggests that it directly contributes to the neoplastic phenotype. These viral oncogene functions can supersede those of the cell and invariably mediate either oncogenicity by the virus or its presumed counterpart in vitro, cell transformation (see Figure 17.2).

THE RETROVIRAL ONCOGENES

The oncogenes of most retroviruses play no part in virus replication. Indeed, many replace portions of viral replicative genes in the virus genome. These oncogenes (v-onc) are related to sequences in normal host cells from which they are believed to evolve after capture (transduction) of the cellular gene, known as a proto-oncogene (c-onc), during some ancestral infection (Table 17.4). Such transduction is observed in certain naturally occurring tumors; however, because it is sporadic, and because oncogene transduction appears to confer no advantage on the virus for transmission (Onions et al. 1987), it appears to represent an evolutionary dead-end. However, for the 'simple' retroviruses such as the alpha and gammaretroviruses, de novo oncogene transduction can in some circumstances be observed in a high proportion of tumors (Neil et al. 1984; Miles and Robinson 1985; Tsatsanis et al. 1994). Transduction has major implications for understanding the mechanism of neoplasia because, if cell proto-oncogenes can mediate neoplasia when incorporated within a virus genome, they might also be able to do so in other circumstances. A considerable body of evidence now suggests that this is the case, some of the earliest data coming from work on the mode of tumor virus pathogenesis described next.

Since the first glimpses of oncogenes in rapidly transforming retroviruses, it has been apparent that their products can be demonstrated in many different cellular

Table 17.4 *Examples of genes transduced by retroviruses in cancer*

Viral oncogene	Location, structural features of gene product	Normal function of host-cell gene[a]	Transducing virus[b]	Associated tumors
v-*sis*	Secreted growth factor	B chain PDGF	GaLV/FeLV	Sarcoma
v-*erb*-B		EGF receptor	ALV	Erythroblastosis
v-*kit*		SCF receptor	FeLV	Fibrosarcoma
v-*fms*		CSF-1 receptor	FeLV	Fibrosarcoma
v-*ros*			ALV	Fibrosarcoma
v-*Notch1*	Transmembrane receptors		FeLV	T-cell lymphoma
v-*mpl*		Thrombopoietin receptor	MLV	Myeloproliferative disease
v-*sea*			ALV	Erythroblastosis
v-*tcr*		T-cell receptor β-chain	FeLV	T-cell lymphoma
v-*abl*			MLV/FeLV	B-cell leukemia, fibrosarcoma
v-*fes*/v-*fps*			FeLV/ALV	Fibrosarcoma
v-*fgr*	Plasma membrane tyrosine kinases		FeLV	Fibrosarcoma
v-*ryk*			ALV	. . .
v-*src*			ALV	Fibrosarcoma
v-*yes*			ALV	Fibrosarcoma
v-Ha-*ras*	Plasma membrane G proteins		MLV	Sarcoma
v-Ki-*ras*			MLV	Sarcoma
v-*mos*	Cytoplasmic serine/ threonine kinase		MLV	Sarcoma
v-*raf*/v-*mil*			MLV/ALV	Sarcoma, carcinoma
v-*crk*	Cytoplasmic adapter		ALV	Sarcoma
v-*erb*-A	Cytoplasm/nucleus	Thyroid hormone receptor	ALV	Erythroblastosis
v-*maf*			ALV	Fibrosarcoma
v-*myb*			ALV	Myeloblastosis
v-*myc*			ALV, FeLV	Myelocytomatosis, lymphoma
v-*qin*	Nuclear transcription factors		ALV	Fibrosarcoma
v-*rel*		NFκB transcription factor	REV	Reticuloendotheliosis
v-*fos*		AP-1 transcription factor	MLV	Sarcoma
v-*jun*		AP-1 transcription factor	ALV	Sarcoma

a) CSF-1, colony stimulating factor type 1; EGF, epidermal growth factor; PDGF, platelet-derived growth factor; SCF, stem cell factor.
b) ALV, avian leukosis virus; FeLV, feline leukemia virus; GaLV, gibbon ape leukemia virus; MLV, murine leukemia virus; REV, reticuloendotheliosis virus.

sites; their functions, where elucidated, identify these as components of pathways of growth control signaling and response. The captured versions of these cellular genes are released from normal transcriptional and translation controls when expressed as part of the viral genome. Furthermore, if the viral version of the gene is truncated or mutated, functional controls may be lost. Thus, retroviral oncogenes are in some cases altered forms of growth factors (e.g. v-*sis*), transmembrane growth factor receptors (some of which are protein tyrosine kinases such as v-*erb*-B) or 'G proteins' that couple ligand–receptor interactions to intracellular signaling events (e.g. the *ras* gene family). Others are second messengers, such as the intracellular protein tyrosine kinases and serine–threonine kinases. The oncogenes whose products are located in the nucleus can affect DNA synthesis or, more probably, gene expression; examples are v-*jun* and v-*fos*, which encode nuclear proteins that assemble as heterodimers to form a well characterized transcription factor complex (AP-1). It is easy to appreciate that mutations altering the expression of one of these genes, or their products, might short-circuit normal cell controls and lead to unregulated growth and behavior. However, it remains a major challenge to understand the detailed mechanism of many of these perturbations. For a comprehensive listing of the known oncogenes and their properties, the reader is referred elsewhere (Hesketh 1997).

The leukemogenic deltaretroviruses bovine leukemia virus (BLV), human T-cell leukemia viruses (HTLV) (HTLV-I, HTLV-II), and simian T-cell leukemia virus (STLV-I) form a discrete subgroup where a normal constituent of the viral genome is implicated in transformation. They contain a region, called p*X*, which encodes Tax and Rex, along with a series of minor gene products. The Tax protein is the most clearly implicated in the process of in vitro transformation by these viruses. It acts on the long terminal repeat (LTR) of the integrated provirus, usually to increase viral transcription, through interaction with cellular transcription factors (Figure 17.3); as a result of this activity, it can also modulate the transcription of cellular genes (see Chapter 58, Retroviruses and associated diseases in humans). However, it should be noted that tumors are rare and late consequence of HTLV infection, and that most tumors have downregulated the expression of Tax and other viral proteins (Matsuoka 2003). In this context, the deltaretroviruses must be considered as initiating factors, with largely unknown mutations to cellular genes playing a rate-limiting role in the leukemogenic process.

A further example of a retroviral product that plays a direct role in oncogenesis is provided by the Friend spleen focus-forming virus (SFFV), an unusual defective isolate encoding a truncated envelope protein that binds to and activates the erythropoietin receptor in the absence of its natural ligand (Ruscetti 1999). Another is the recently characterized jaagsiekte sheep retrovirus (JSRV), a betaretrovirus which has been shown to be the causal agent of the sporadic epithelial tumor, ovine pulmonary adenomatosis. Transformation of fibroblast cells in vitro is mediated by the viral envelope gene, although it as yet unclear whether this activity is sufficient to explain the malignant potential of JSRV (Chow et al. 2003).

THE ONCOGENES OF DNA TUMOR VIRUSES

The observation that SV40 T antigen binds tightly to a cellular protein, p53 (Lane and Crawford 1979; Linzer and Levine 1979) was the first step towards the elucidation of a transformation mechanism common to many of the DNA tumor viruses. Binding results in the inactivation or degradation of the cellular target protein. Furthermore, T antigen also binds and inactivates a second tumor suppressor, pRb. The p53 and Rb pathways are common targets for many of the DNA virus oncoproteins, although the mechanisms by which their functions are subverted are varied and may be direct or indirect (see Table 17.5, p. 338).

The transforming genes of SV40 and the other small DNA viruses of the papovavirus group bear no close relationship to cellular gene products, but interact with key factors controlling host cell replication to create a permissive environment for the virus to replicate its own genome. If the viral replication cycle fails to proceed past the expression of these early gene products, the result is a persistently infected, transformed cell. In this abortive mode of replication, the host cell is induced to multiply abnormally and will present few viral antigens to the host immune system, with obvious advantages to the virus in establishing latent or persistent infection. There are other mechanisms by which DNA tumor virus oncogenes can interfere with cell growth regulation, as shown by polyomavirus middle T antigen which interacts in subtle ways to activate nonreceptor tyrosine kinases at the plasma membrane (Kiefer et al. 1994). Moreover, polyomavirus small t antigen interferes with p53 indirectly by uncoupling responses to its upstream activator, Arf (Lomax and Fried 2001). Also, cell lifespan, and hence susceptibility to transformation, can be increased by activation of telomerase as reported for human papillomavirus (HPV) E6 (Klingelhutz et al. 1996). For hepatitis B virus (HBV), analysis of viral oncogenic functions has been hampered by the lack of tractable in vitro systems. However, both p*X* and the large envelope protein preS can transactivate cellular genes (Rossner 1992), while the pX protein has been reported to bind and inactivate p53 (Truant et al. 1995).

While transformation by the papovaviruses is a consequence of abortive infection, the oncogenic herpesviruses have evolved latent infection as an essential feature of the normal life cycle. In the minimal state, the virus expresses only those functions necessary to maintain and ensure replication of its episomal DNA genome

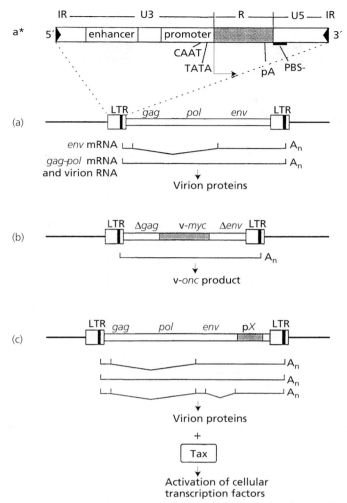

Figure 17.3 *Chapter 58, Retroviruses and associated diseases in humans, considers retroviruses at length. This figure and Figure 17.4 give only enough detail to appreciate their pathogenesis.* **(a*)** *Detail of a typical retroviral LTR. Each LTR resembles an insertion sequence, having an inverted repeat (IR) at its extremities. A direct repeat (R) derives from either end of the virion RNA, with a cap site at its 5' end (large arrow) and a polyadenylation signal (pA) close to its 3' end. The 3' boundary is marked by a primer binding site (PBS) to which is bound the tRNA primer for reverse transcription of virion RNA. The remainder of the LTR comprises U3 and U5 regions, derived respectively from the 3' and 5' ends of viral RNA. U3 contains a promoter region, with characteristic 'CAAT' and 'TATA' boxes that regulate proviral transcription. Upstream (5') to the promoter is an enhancer with a nonpolar stimulatory effect on gene expression.* **(a)** *A retroviral provirus (boxes) integrated in cell DNA (thick line). LTRs flank and control the expression of coding regions that comprise, in replication-competent retroviruses, at least three genes,* gag, pol, *and* env, *expressed through unspliced or spliced polyadenylated mRNAs.* **(b)** *A retroviral provirus bearing a viral oncogene (v-onc), in this case the v-myc in the avian myelocytomatosis virus 29. In transducing v-myc the virus has lost the pol gene and portions of* gag *and* env, *so it can be propagated only if these missing functions are provided in trans in the same cell by a 'helper' virus of the sort shown in* **(a)**. **(c)** *A simplified diagram of the human T-cell leukemia virus. The oncogene region of this virus (pX) encodes Tax, Rex, and a series of other minor products (p30, p12), which have no known cellular counterparts. Tax interacts with cellular transcription factors to transactivate a range of cellular genes, including IL-2 and its receptor.*

in the host cell. For the best characterized oncogenic herpesvirus, Epstein–Barr virus (EBV), a subset of six viral gene products has been implicated in the efficient immortalization of B cells, including a series of nuclear proteins (EBNAs) and two membrane proteins (LMP1 and 2), and the same gene products are expressed in EBV-positive immunoblastic lymphomas which arise in immunosuppressed transplant recipients and patients with the acquired immunodeficiency syndrome (AIDS). A key effector of transformation is LMP1 that appears

to mimic the action of a constitutively active tumor necrosis factor (TNF) family receptor (Eliopoulos and Young 2001). A more limited subset of EBV proteins (EBNA1, LMP1 and -2) is expressed in nasopharyngeal carcinoma cells, while Burkitt's lymphoma cells express only EBNA1 (Rickinson 1994).

The human adenoviruses are oncogenic only in rodents, but have served as important models of cell transformation. Again, their major effectors (E1A, E1B, E4Orf6) appear to operate by similar principles, by

Table 17.5 *Selected DNA tumor virus oncogenes and mechanisms of action*

Virus	Effector	Target/mechanism
SV40	Large T antigen	Binds, inactivates p53, Rb
Polyoma	Middle T antigen	Binds activates src family kinases
	Small T antigen	Inhibits Arf/p53 activation
HPV	E6	p53 binding, degradation
	E7	Rb binding
BPV	E6	p53 binding
HBV	pX	Binds inactivates p53
Adenovirus	E1A	Rb
	E1B	Bak, Bax binding; inhibition of apoptosis
	E4Orf6	p53 binding
EBV	LMP1	Activation of NFκB, JNK pathways
	LMP2	Recruit src, syk tyrosine kinases
	EBNA5/LP	cdk6/D2 activation (inactivates Rb)
KSHV	LANA	p53, Rb binding
	v-cyclin	Phosphorylation/ inactivation of Rb

BPV, bovine papillomavirus; HBV, hepatitis B virus; HPV, human papillomavirus; SV40, simian virus 40.

binding to and inactivating p53 (Shen and White 2001; Tauber and Dobner 2001) and Rb (Gallimore and Turnell 2001) or inhibiting their downstream effectors (Shen and White 2001).

The large DNA tumor viruses encode many products that affect growth and survival of the infected cell, and others that allow infected cells to evade the host immune response. These include homologues of cellular genes encoding cytokines as well as regulators of apoptosis and cell-cycle progression. Many of these products have the theoretical potential to contribute to neoplastic transformation, but the term 'oncogene' is usually reserved for those products that have been implicated directly in the initiation or maintenance of oncogenic transformation. Despite their potency in various in vitro transformation assays, most DNA tumor viruses are weakly oncogenic, particularly in their natural hosts. This may be explained in part by the efficiency of the host immune response in controlling virus replication and destroying potential tumor cells that express virus-coded cell surface antigens or T-cell epitopes. However, immunosuppression reveals the malignant potential of these infections. EBV-induced malignancies are a significant complication in patients undergoing organ transplant or in the context of human immunodeficiency virus (HIV)-induced immunosuppression (Holmes and Sokol 2002). In a similar fashion, the indirect effects of HIV potentiate the carcinogenic effects of HPV infection (Hawes et al. 2003) and have increased the prevalence

of Kaposi's sarcoma to the point where it is now one of the most common virus-associated malignancies (Boshoff and Weiss 2001).

A summary of the targets and mechanisms of action of DNA tumor virus oncoproteins is given in Table 17.5. Note, however, that these are in general a small subset of the binding interactions and effects of these multifunctional viral proteins.

INSERTIONAL MUTAGENESIS

Many retroviruses lack an oncogene but induce clonal tumors in which their genome is integrated as a DNA provirus in a specific region of the host chromosome (Figure 17.4). This insertion is mutagenic, so it changes the sequence of DNA in that region, and can have either of two results: activation of a gene or its ablation. In most cases proviral insertion activates a nearby gene, either by qualitative alteration or by augmentation of its expression (Peters 1990; Kung et al. 1991). In some cases the activated gene proves to be the cellular counterpart of a known retrovirus oncogene. Thus, B-cell lymphomas induced by avian leukosis virus (ALV) and T-cell lymphosarcoma induced by feline leukemia virus (FeLV) often contain a c-*myc* gene activated by insertional mutagenesis. In ALV-induced erythroleukemia, on the other hand, it is the c-*erb*-B proto-oncogene that is activated. These findings support a role for proto-oncogenes in neoplasia, and in the latter case also appear to represent an intermediate stage in the process of oncogene transduction (Nilsen et al. 1985).

By extrapolation from the observed activation of known proto-oncogenes by proviral insertion, it can be argued that, when an inserted virus consistently integrates into a limited region of the host genome in a series of tumors, the affected region harbors a putative oncogene. In this way a large number of loci have been identified, of which the activation is characteristic of certain virus-induced tumors; the available evidence as to the nature of these loci strongly supports the concept that their activation is relevant to neoplasia.

Although the first example of insertional mutagenesis came from avian lymphomas (Neel et al. 1981), much recent work to identify new oncogenes has been in the laboratory mouse. Moreover, the use of this facet of retroviral oncogenesis as a gene discovery tool by 'tagging' of target genes has enjoyed a renaissance since the completion of the draft human and mouse genome sequences (Neil and Cameron 2002). The target gene at a common insertion site can in some cases be difficult to determine, not least because retroviral *cis*-activation of target genes can in some cases operate over a great distance (up to 300 kb) (Lazo et al. 1990; Hanlon et al. 2003).

The strategy of retroviral tagging is complemented by the parallel development of techniques for the manipulation of the mouse genome. Thus, the introduction of

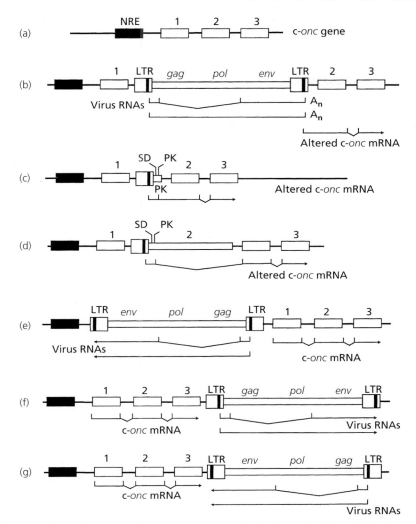

Figure 17.4 *Modes of insertional mutagenesis. The examples given show insertional mutagenesis by a retroviral provirus, but WHV (Buendia 1994) and others may have comparable effects.* **(a)** *Diagram of a proto-oncogene (c-onc) comprising three exons (open boxes), the first of which is largely noncoding, and an upstream negative regulatory element (NRE) (closed box), which helps to ensure that the gene is often poorly transcribed.* **(b)** *Insertion of a provirus between exons 1 and 2 of the c-onc gene. Expression of c-onc is elevated by 'promoter insertion,' regulatory elements in the 3' LTR driving transcription of a viral c-onc hybrid message.* **(c)** *Insertion of a truncated provirus, with c-onc transcription initiating in the 5' LTR. In this instance the transcript is not spliced at the donor site (SD) for generating subgenomic viral mRNA, so it includes the sequence (PK) 3' to SD that permits packaging of the RNA into virions. This altered c-onc mRNA may thus be incorporated in an infectious virion, and infection leading to reverse transcription and genetic recombination with another viral RNA could generate a virus containing a transduced onc gene.* **(d)** *Another example of promoter insertion by a truncated provirus. In this case the packaging signal is spliced out of the mRNA so, like subgenomic viral mRNA, it is unlikely to be incorporated into virions.* **(e)** *Proviral insertion 5' to c-onc, but in the opposite transcriptional orientiation, precluding enhancement of onc expression by the viral promoter. The virus thus acts either through the effect of its enhancer alone or by distancing c-onc from the 'upstream' NRE.* **(f and g)** *Proviral insertion 3' to c-onc in either transcriptional orientation. In these instances it appears that the virus can augment proto-oncogene expression only by virtue of its enhancer.*

mutant proto-oncogenes into the mouse germline has confirmed their oncogenic potential, whilst their inactivation by homologous recombination has provided valuable insights into their normal functions (Meuwissen et al. 2001). Insertional mutagenesis is also a prominent oncogenic mechanism for at least one representative of the hepadnaviruses; woodchuck hepatitis virus (WHV) often activates the c-*myc* or N-*myc* genes in the genesis of liver tumors that arise without the extensive cirrhosis that precedes HBV-associated cancers (Buendia 1994).

By contrast, there is only fragmentary evidence for insertional mutagenesis in HBV-associated tumors. The reasons for the marked difference in mode of action between two similar viral agents are unknown.

So far we have focused on the capacity of integrated viruses to activate genes. The converse of this process, gene disruption by retroviral insertion, underlies some developmental mutations in laboratory mice (Lock et al. 1991). In such cases it is possible to reveal the disruptive effects of a single insertion by back-crossing to generate a homozygous mutation. In somatic cells, gene ablation is an improbable outcome because it requires inactivating insertions at both alleles. Nevertheless, there are instances in which retroviral insertions have been shown to ablate gene function in tumor cells. Examples include the inactivation of p53 by insertion of Friend murine leukemia virus (MLV) in erythroleukemia (Ben-David et al. 1988) and the targeting of the neurofibromin gene (*NF1*) by BXH-2 virus in myeloid leukemia (Largaespada et al. 1995).

At first sight, mutagenic ablation might be thought to be more likely because it is less specific than activation, and so insertion anywhere within the coding region would destroy the integrity of the gene. However, mutational activation seems to operate by such a variety of mechanisms that it, too, can result from insertion at many locations near the activated gene (Figure 17.4). In the classic example of avian B-cell lymphomas, c-*myc* transcription is driven by the viral promoter in an LTR situated 5′ to the gene (Figure 17.4b). However, the subsequent discovery of enhancers in retroviral LTRs, their nonpolar action over long distances, and their effects predominantly on the nearest promoters now indicate that, in different circumstances, a viral LTR can augment activity of a gene either 5′ or 3′ to itself in either orientation (Figure 17.4e–g). Moreover, it is theoretically possible that an inserted provirus may activate a gene by simply separating it from *cis*-acting cellular repressors.

Although the focus of most current research is on the γ-retroviruses that infect the laboratory mouse, the mechanism of insertional mutagenesis is relevant in tumors induced by other members of the γ-retrovirus and β-retrovirus families. While FeLV appears to target a similar set of genes to MLV (Tsatsanis et al. 1994), a very different pattern emerges for mouse mammary tumor virus (MMTV), which frequently targets genes of the *Wnt* and *Fgf* families (Kapoun and Shackleford 1997). The relevance of insertional mutagenesis to human cancer has also come into focus recently with the observation of leukemia in gene therapy subjects which appear to have been induced by integration at the *LMO2* oncogene. This observation has led to a renewed interest in the specificity and consequences of retroviral integration in the host genome (Baum et al. 2003).

OTHER EVIDENCE IMPLICATING PROTO-ONCOGENES IN NEOPLASIA

A detailed consideration of the molecular and cell biology of neoplasia is outside the scope of this chapter, but the following brief survey is intended to provide some understanding of the basis of viral oncogenicity.

Two major lines of investigation have further incriminated proto-oncogenes in cancer.

1 DNA from certain tumor cells, but not DNA from their normal counterparts, can induce morphological transformation of, or confer tumorigenicity upon, appropriate recipient cells in culture. The genes responsible are often mutant members of the *ras* oncogene family, first encountered as the v-*onc* genes of certain murine sarcoma viruses. However, as with insertional mutagenesis by viruses, DNA 'transfection' has revealed further novel putative oncogenes whose properties, where known, are compatible with a role in neoplasia (Bishop 1987).

2 Many cancers display characteristic karyological abnormalities, typically deletions, translocations or amplification of identifiable regions of chromosomes. In some cases the genes affected by translocation and amplification are the cellular relatives of known v-*onc* genes; again a number of novel loci are deemed guilty by association (Rabbitts 1994).

In short, proto-oncogenes have been incriminated in neoplasia by a variety of phenomena, and some genes have been implicated in several ways. The mutations suffered by proto-oncogenes in tumor cells – be they single base changes, transduction or gross disruption by viruses or massive, microscopically visible aberrations in karyotype – have one (or both) of two effects: they change either the expression of the gene or the nature of its product.

'HIT AND RUN' MECHANISMS

The pattern of virus persistence in a tumor may be complex but is amenable to study. The same cannot be said for those instances in which a virus is implicated in tumor formation in vivo or cell transformation in vitro but in which it is impossible to demonstrate either persistence of a specific portion of the viral genome or integration in a limited region of host DNA. The virus in such cases is presumed to act transiently. It may operate by one of the mechanisms detailed above but the genes involved are required only in the early stages of tumor evolution and unknown selective pressures against the virus eliminate it during tumor progression.

The absence of bovine papillomavirus type 4 from the alimentary carcinomas that it causes may reflect such a mechanism, because at least some papillomaviruses are known to carry transforming genes. On the other hand, this virus, as proposed for herpes simplex viruses and cytomegalovirus in cervical cancer, may act as a mutagen, through an ephemeral association of its genome with cell DNA or, possibly, through the action of viral enzymes (Minson 1984; Macnab 1987). The mechanisms in either case are hard to study and investigators have invoked this 'hit and run' explanation only after eliminating other possibilities (McDougall 2001).

Indirect mechanisms

The second major category of pathogenic mechanism is also frustrating for the student of in vitro systems but is clinically significant, whether operating alone or in concert with mechanisms outlined above. In these indirect, or extrinsic, mechanisms neither the cells of the tumor nor their ancestral lineage need ever have been infected by the causative virus; instead, tumors arise in response to virus infection of other cells, the nature of the response taking several forms.

Cell death or impaired function as a direct or indirect effect of virus infection can have different consequences depending on the type of cell affected. If the immune system is compromised the outgrowth of cells might be permitted from many tissues that had acquired neoplastic potential by various means; in practice, however, immunosuppression leads to increases in the incidences of a relatively small spectrum of tumors, a significant proportion of which are associated with viral risk factors (Figure 17.1). Cell death, or untoward cell proliferation, among hemopoietic tissues can also upset delicate homoeostatic cellular interrelations, and compensatory proliferation in other lineages may favor independent neoplastic alterations in these reactive cells.

A number of tumor viruses cause immune impairment (Table 17.6), probably by a variety of mechanisms. Immunosuppression by some viruses may be due to cytotoxicity, reflecting, in the case of avian reticuloendotheliosis viruses, the burden of intracellular unintegrated viral DNA. The immunosuppressive effect of HIV could also result simply from cytopathic effects on $CD4^+$ T cells, but the extent of infection does not seem sufficient to account for the degree of immune impairment. Various theories of HIV immunosuppression have been elaborated, including virus-induced autoimmune attack, T-cell apoptosis following nonspecific immunosuppression, cytokine dysregulation, and cell destruction due to chronic antiviral immune responses (Zinkernagel and Hengartner 1994). Two points should be noted at this juncture:

1 with the possible exception of HIV and its relatives, the tumor viruses that are immunosuppressive also seem to have efficient and direct means of inducing neoplasia
2 immunosuppression is the only indirect mode of viral carcinogenesis that does not necessarily involve cell proliferation as an early stage.

Death or damage to nonhemopoietic cells may likewise favor neoplastic change, but in uninfected cells of the same lineage that are dividing in an attempt at tissue regeneration. This is one way in which chronic hepatitis B or hepatitis C infections may increase the risk of primary liver cancer (Slagle et al. 1994).

Virus infection may also stimulate cells to produce growth factors of various types. In some cases, the viruses themselves carry growth factor-like genes, such as the EBV *BCRF1* gene which has homology with IL-10 (Morein and Merza 1991). When the producing cell itself possesses receptors for these factors, their effects can be autocrine with the virus acting directly, as

described above. An example of such a process is the stimulation of IL-2 and its receptor by HTLV-I in infected T cells (Ruben et al. 1988).

A further example of viral interplay with host immunoregulatory systems is provided by the MMTVs, which encode superantigens. Endogenous MMTVs in the mouse genome express these polymorphic proteins that stimulate developing T cells via the Vβ of the αβTCR, leading to clonal deletion of reactive cells and a consequent bias in the Vβ repertoire of mature T cells. This phenomenon may be regarded as an aberrant outcome of viral sequestration in the mouse germline. However, it seems that the expression of these ligands on B cells is an important early event in establishment of infection by MMTV, because this may stimulate mature T cells to release growth factors that drive proliferation of the infected cell. Along the way, the virus usurps the host immune response to favor its own dissemination (Acha-Orbea and MacDonald 1995).

The potential stimulatory effects of viral antigens may also be due to their mimicry of ligands for receptors on a range of cell types. If these receptors modulate normal cell growth and behavior, chronic unscheduled binding of ligand analogues may lead to hyperplasia and then neoplasia. Such effects probably are widespread, and the oncogene of the spleen focus-forming component of Friend murine leukemia retrovirus is perhaps the best characterized example. This oncogene has no cell counterpart, being derived entirely from virus envelope gene sequences, but it appears to interact with the erythropoietin receptor, replacing the requirement for exogenous growth factors (Ruscetti 1999).

IMPLICATION OF VIRUSES IN THE ETIOLOGY OF CANCER

The pathogenic strategies just discussed are clearly crucial to the concepts of the genesis of virus-associated tumors but are only part of this complex process. Experimental, clinical, and epidemiologic observations all suggest that malignancy results from a step-by-step accumulation of stable cellular alterations whose occurrence reflects, and is greatly accelerated by, exposure to multiple risk factors. The age of the animal and the duration, intensity, and frequency of exposure to risk factors are important elements in tumor evolution, and these variables tend to obscure any causal relationship between virus infection and the eventual development of malignancy. We must take account of these other components if we are to understand the etiologic significance of viruses.

The influence of risk factors on viral carcinogenesis can be considered by dividing them into three major, but overlapping, categories:

1 factors associated with the virus infection and its effect on host cells

Table 17.6 *Viral functions implicated in cancer*

| | Virus group (and representatives) | | | | | | | | |
| | Retroviruses | | | | | Hepadna | Papova SV40; | Papilloma | Herpes |
Function	α: ALV	γ:MLV; FeLV	β:MMTV; JSRV	δ:HTLV; BLV	Lenti:HIV; SIV	HBV; WHV	polyoma	HPV; BPV	EBV; KSHV; HVS
Viral gene product stimulates proliferation	–	+/–	+	+	+/–	+	+	+	+
Insertional mutagenesis	+	+	+ (MMTV)	–	+/–	+ (WHV)	–	+/–	–
Generalized immunosuppression	+	+	–	–	+	–	–	–	–

ALV, avian leukosis virus; BLV, bovine leukemia virus; BPV, bovine papillomavirus; EBV, Epstein–Barr virus; FeLV, feline leukemia virus; HBV, hepatitis B virus; HIV, human immunodeficiency virus; HPV, human papilloma virus; HTLV, human T-cell leukemia virus; HVS, herpesvirus saimiri; JSRV, jaagsiekte sheep retrovirus; MLV, murine leukemia virus; MMTV, mouse mammary tumor virus; SIV, simian immunodeficiency virus; WHV, woodchuck hepatitis virus.

2 factors that determine the evolution and properties of neoplastic cells

3 factors that affect the host response to both virus and tumor.

We can consider in turn the interplay of these factors during three arbitrary stages of tumor development:

1 the successful infection of the organism by a virus and, when the virus acts by a direct means, its infection of the tumor cell lineage

2 the conversion within the tumor cell lineage of a normal cell to neoplastic growth and behavior

3 the survival and growth of its descendants to form a detectable tumor.

An assessment of the relative importance of the different risk factors at each stage of tumor development

is shown in the histogram in Figure 17.5. In this diagram the three stages of development are shown on the abscissa, which is thus a time scale axis; it is, however, impossible to draw this to scale. Stage 2 is probably the longest period; important stage 2 events probably often precede those in stage 1.

Virus infection/transmission

An animal becomes infected with an oncogenic virus by one of three routes (Weiss 1984). The first is genetic transmission, by which most individuals, of many species, have acquired endogenous retroviruses during evolution. These viruses seem to be nonessential but innocuous passengers in the genomes of their hosts and they are often xenotropic (i.e. capable of replication

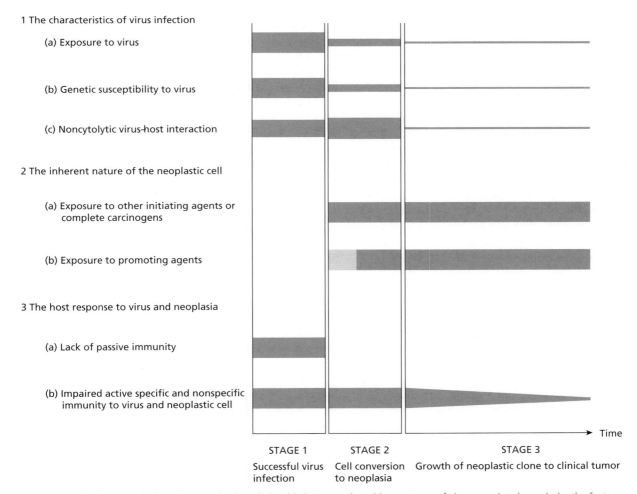

RISK FACTORS AFFECTING

1 The characteristics of virus infection

    (a) Exposure to virus

    (b) Genetic susceptibility to virus

    (c) Noncytolytic virus–host interaction

2 The inherent nature of the neoplastic cell

    (a) Exposure to other initiating agents or complete carcinogens

    (b) Exposure to promoting agents

3 The host response to virus and neoplasia

    (a) Lack of passive immunity

    (b) Impaired active specific and nonspecific immunity to virus and neoplastic cell

Time

STAGE 1   STAGE 2   STAGE 3
Successful virus   Cell conversion   Growth of neoplastic clone to clinical tumor
infection   to neoplasia

Figure 17.5 *Risk factors in viral carcinogenesis: the relationship between the arbitrary stages of virus-associated neoplasia, the features of the neoplastic process, and the risk factors that influence each feature. The stages of neoplasia are shown on the abscissa. The breaks in the time axis indicate that these stages vary in length and they are not shown to scale (in general, stage 1 is likely to be relatively short and stage 2 is usually the longest period). The risk factors affecting any of the three features characterizing virus-associated neoplasia are shown on the ordinate and they may operate at different, and often more than one, stages of the disease process. The thickness of the bars indicates the relative importance of each risk factor at each stage of neoplasia, broken lines indicating periods at which the risk factors are of no or uncertain significance. (Modified, with permission, from Wyke and Weiss 1984.)*

only in other species). A clear exception to this harmlessness is that certain strains of mice harbor endogenous viruses that are ecotropic (i.e. they can infect mouse cells). Moreover, these viruses evolve by recombination with other defective endogenous proviruses, generating variants with enhanced leukemogenicity (Stoye et al. 1991). Comparable variants of altered, if not augmented, pathogenicity can also arise by recombination of FeLV with endogenous cat retroviruses (Neil et al. 1991). In both mice and cats the recombinant viruses reveal altered viral envelope glycoproteins, some of which have an increased propensity to bind to and stimulate proliferation of immune-responsive and other cells.

The second route, congenital transmission of exogenous viruses across the placenta or oviduct, is important in the case of leukemogenic avian, feline, and bovine retroviruses. However, for these and many others the third route, horizontal transmission peri- and postnatally is also significant. Whereas the papovaviruses are hardy, the enveloped herpesviruses and retroviruses are far more labile; their horizontal spread is therefore more efficient when animals are grouped together and make close contact with carriers. Moreover, such conditions increase the risk of repeated exposure to high doses of virus early in life, a pattern which, in turn, appears to encourage the eventual appearance of neoplasia.

With regard to the routes of transmission, the pattern of virus spread is also greatly influenced by its site of replication in the animal. Thus, for FeLV and EBV, free virus is shed in the buccal cavity and transmitted in saliva. Marek's disease virus of fowls, on the other hand, replicates in feather follicle epithelium and is spread in dander, whereas BLV and HTLV remain cell-associated and require the transmission of whole cells. In the case of the last two viruses, iatrogenic transfer and 'flying pin' arthropod vectors might be expected to be significant routes of infection, and epidemiologic data support this notion.

Genetic susceptibility to viruses

All viruses require the means to enter a cell, express their genomes, and assemble progeny for spread to other cells. Interspecies variation in the susceptibility of cells to viruses – often associated with severe constraints on the virus life cycle – are taken for granted but there can also be pronounced variation within a species. In cases of virus-associated neoplasia, such variation is indicated by clustering of tumor incidence. Clusters are often due to variation in the other risk factors discussed here, but difference in virus susceptibility is a likely cause when clustering is demonstrably familial. In domestic animals, where breeding is often controlled and one male can sire many dispersed offspring, it is easier to discern familial clusters. The clusters of, for example, bovine leukosis, reflect genetic factors that are not well defined, but in

other instances the basis for the underlying enhanced susceptibility is better understood. The species in which this has been studied most comprehensively is, of course, the laboratory mouse (Rosenberg and Jolicoeur 1997).

The need for entry of virus into cells provides a crucial barrier to infection; in many cases, efficient penetration is highly specific, not only for the whole animal but also for particular types of cell within the host. Retroviruses enter cells whose surfaces bear receptors to which the viral envelope glycoprotein can bind. In chickens, receptors are found on a wide range of cell types but their specificity (and hence host susceptibility to virus) reveals genetically determined polymorphisms between individual birds (Payne 1992). Other receptors are of limited distribution within the host: human CD4 lymphocyte antigen is an important component of the HIV-1 receptor, this stringency explaining in part the tropism of HIV-1 for a particular T-cell subset (Dalgleish et al. 1984). These receptors do not of course exist merely to facilitate virus penetration and, indeed, not all binding sites serve this role. They clearly have structural or other functional purposes on the cell surface. For the mammalian type C retroviruses, related families of transmembrane transporter proteins for basic amino acids and phosphate have been identified as mediators of viral entry (Cunningham and Kim 1994). However, the relevance of these to oncogenesis seems to be slight, as there is little evidence of effects on cell growth and viability emanating from virus binding to these receptors.

EBV gains entry to B cells via binding to the complement receptor molecule CR2 (Nemerow et al. 1987). Other oncogenic DNA virus receptors have yet to be definitively identified. Once inside cells, viruses may do some damage, which will, however, be greatly limited by any further restrictions on their replication and spread. For instance, retroviruses are subject to both physiological and genetic constraints after penetration. For the type C retroviruses, stable integration of a complete DNA transcript of the virion RNA genome can occur only in cells that synthesize DNA; on the other hand, the early gene functions of polyomaviruses can themselves stimulate DNA synthesis. The host range restrictions of ectropic MLV mediated by the mouse Fv-1 locus also operate during this early part of the infectious cycle. Recently, the retroviral LTR (see Figure 17.4) has attracted considerable attention and there is a wealth of evidence to suggest that its potency varies with cell type. Cellular factors interact *in trans* with the LTR enhancer to modulate the level of transcripts mediated by this element in a given cell and hence the extent of viral replication, the oncogenic potential of the virus, and its cell tropism (Tsichlis and Lazo 1991). Thus, the pathogenesis of, for example, retrovirus-induced mouse leukemia is a very complex process in which both the virus and the tumor cell evolve. When virus infection of an appropriate host results in proviral insertion at a specific site, the expression is stimulated by one or more of a range of cell genes. The amplitude of this expression may depend on the potency of the viral LTR in that cell (Morrison et al. 1995).

Noncytolytic virus–host interactions

Some tumor-associated viruses, such as HBV and many retroviruses, can be released by cells without compromising viability, but for many others cytolysis is necessary for escape of virus. Cytolysis is, of course, incompatible with direct mechanisms of virus oncogenesis, so neoplasia is likely to be a rare and aberrant consequence of infection by these viruses. In such cases, either the host restricts the later stages of virus replication or the virus is defective in directing these events, but, in both instances, viral functions needed to induce neoplasia are retained.

Two other properties of tumor viruses are worth mentioning here: virus integration and latent virus infection. The viruses of all families that include directly oncogenic members can exist as DNA within the cell, inserted in the host chromosome. This may be a rare outcome of infection or, as with retroviruses, an essential part of the virus life cycle. Virus integration is obligatory for oncogenesis by insertional mutagenesis, but there seems to be no reason why it should be required for other forms of oncogenesis. Indeed, as virus genomes are absent from some tumors for which viruses are considered risk factors, integration is presumably not essential – at least in the later stages of tumor evolution. Poxviruses, although not true tumor viruses, need special consideration because they can induce proliferating lesions, probably through the action of viral genes that encode molecules resembling cell growth factors (Opgenorth et al. 1992) but the lesions produced do not progress to full-blown cancer. Nevertheless, infection can be fatal due to concomitant inflammatory disease. It is possible that poxviruses fail to induce tumors because they replicate in the cytoplasm, never integrate, and so do not achieve a sufficiently stable association with the host cell. A number of RNA viruses also achieve persistent infections, yet they rarely, if ever, integrate and only one representative (hepatitis C virus (HCV)) has so far been incriminated in neoplasia. Integration is clearly important in achieving a stable infection but may have additional undefined significance.

Latency is a characteristic of two families of oncogenic viruses: the retroviruses and the herpesviruses. Prolonged latent infection is a common sequel of primary FeLV infection in cats. It is associated with a humoral and cellular immune response and can be abolished by treatment with immunosuppressive agents (Rojko et al. 1982). Without such insults, however, this form of latent infection tends to resolve in recovery with subsequent immunity (Pacitti and Jarrett 1985). Latent infection with BLV has also been described but in this case a non-immunoglobulin plasma protein seems to be involved in virus suppression (Gupta and Ferrer 1982). Like those of many endogenous retroviruses, latent exogenous genomes may be in the configuration of inactive chromatin, which is highly methylated. This has practical significance because tumor cells do not usually express their resident viral genomes unless the animals are immunosuppressed or the cells are cultured, with or without agents intended to activate silent genomes. At the mechanistic level, the role of latency in neoplasia is not obvious, but, like integration, it may serve primarily to ensure persistence of the viral genome, thus facilitating its interactions with the other risk factors germane to neoplasia.

EBV latency is a paradigm for this mode of infection by the γ-herpesviruses and appears to be critical to virus persistence and central to its involvement in tumors (Rickinson and Kieff 1996). Human peripheral blood cells can be transformed and immortalized by EBV infection in vitro. These latently infected cells express a subset of the EBV genome comprising six nuclear proteins (EBNA1, EBNA2, EBNA-LP, EBNA3A, EBNA3B, and EBNA3C), as well as two oncogenic membrane proteins (LMP1, 2) and small EBV RNAs (EBER). EBV-positive tumor cells display a restricted subset of these genes. The minimal expression pattern is exemplified by Burkitt's lymphoma, where viral expression is restricted to a EBNA-1 and EBERs. A more complex pattern is observed in nasopharyngeal carcinoma, which includes the oncogenic latent membrane proteins (LMP-1,2) as well as EBERs and EBNA-1. A variation on this theme is seen in EBV-associated lymphoproliferative diseases of transplant recipients and AIDS patients, which express EBNA-2 in addition to the list for nasopharyngeal carcinoma. These distinctive patterns reflect the critical role of the immune system in containing EBV infection and the consequences of its compromise in neoplastic disease and immunosuppressed states. They probably also reflect differences in the relationship of EBV to tumor initiation and maintenance in these diverse neoplastic diseases.

A similar pattern is emerging for Kaposi's sarcoma-associated herpesvirus (KSHV), where HIV appears to be the primary cofactor, revealing its latent oncogenic properties and enabling a wider range of viral products to be expressed in the tumor cell (Schulz and Neil 2002).

Viruses and the multistep development of neoplasia

Many of the viruses that transform cells in vitro carry oncogenes of which the activity is under the control of powerful viral regulatory elements (see Figure 17.4). Oncogenes – perhaps aided by a spreading virus infection – are very potent carcinogens that rapidly induce tumors in host animals. In some circumstances, however, oncogene-mediated viral carcinogenesis is far less efficient and the appearance of a neoplastic cell phenotype requires other genetic or epigenetic events such as the loss of tumor suppressor genes or the acquisition of additional, activated oncogenes. There is abundant evidence for this. Some tumor viruses carry more than one oncogene, each of which contributes to their tumor-inducing capacity. In the example of the retrovirus avian erythroblastosis virus, *erb*-B encodes a transmembrane protein [epidermal growth factor (EGF) receptor] and *erb*-A a nuclear protein (thyroid hormone receptor) (see Table 17.4). Other examples are the presence of the c-*myc* nuclear oncogene and the protein kinase oncogene *mil/raf* in avian carcinoma virus Mill Hill virus 2 (ACMHV-2), and the presence of two nuclear oncogenes, *myb* and *ets* in avian myeloblastosis virus (AMV).

Further evidence of the cooperative action of multiple genes in lymphoma development comes from the γ-retroviruses, in which multiple different insertional mutagenic events can be observed in a single tumor (Tsichlis et al. 1985; Tsatsanis et al. 1994). Furthermore, mice carrying an activated oncogene in the germline may show greatly accelerated tumor onset when infected with the virus, and activation of cooperating genes by insertional mutagenesis occurs at high frequency. Further evidence of the cooperative action of these genes is provided by the strongly synergistic effect on tumor development of crossing mice carrying different activated oncogenes (e.g. c-*myc* and *pim*-1) (Jonkers and Berns 1996). Similarly, MMTV appears to be capable of mediating multiple mutational hits by insertion at synergistic oncogenes of the *Wnt* and *Fgf* families (MacArthur et al. 1995). The relatively unrestricted replication of these agents in the persistently infected host may account for their unusual propensity for insertional mutagenesis.

In naturally occurring cancer, the requirement for multiple cellular changes is mirrored in the time- and risk-factor-dependent pattern of tumor development. Many clinically important tumor viruses, particularly those of humans, need the operation of additional chemical, physical, or infectious risk factors to initiate or promote neoplasia (see Tables 17.1, 17.2 and 17.3). Because these viruses are incomplete carcinogens, it is not certain whether they act as initiators or promoters of oncogenesis.

Viruses have often been considered initiators, for a number of reasons. Initiation in experimental systems is a dose-dependent, irreversible event with many hallmarks of mutation (Montesano and Slaga 1983), and direct models of virus oncogenesis either induce or introduce mutant genes. Moreover, virus infection is often observed early in life in the susceptible individual, perhaps before exposure to other likely risk factors. However, aside from instances of possible transient effects, virus-induced cancer is often associated with persistent infections, virus integration, and possibly latency. Infection early in life may simply be a prerequisite for achieving persistence, a prolonged exposure to virus that can be significant in two ways. First, it may increase the chance of crucial, if rare, virus–cell interactions. Second, and this seems particularly relevant to viruses that act indirectly, it may enhance the possibility that other environmental risk factors that may be encountered can be influenced by a chronic viral tumor-promoting activity. Some instances, however, are not clearcut. Consider, for example, tumor induction by EBV and HTLV-I: both seem to stimulate a proliferation of lymphoid cells that is strictly neoplastic (in that it is driven from within the cell and results from a 'mutation') but which resembles hyperplasia in being polyclonal. These viruses seem to behave as tumor promoters, and subsequent clonal events such as c-*myc* translocation in EBV-associated Burkitt's lymphoma are more likely to be the result of initiation. It seems that the concepts of initiation and promotion that have been so fruitful in studying experimental carcinogenesis are not so readily applicable to viral cancer. The consequences of virus infection are, however, clearly capable of contributing to several stages of neoplasia.

The host response

The ability of the infected animal to limit both virus infection and the multiplication of neoplastic cells is of great importance in virus-associated neoplasia, particularly the leukemias in which the tumors themselves are prone to perturb both specific and nonspecific immune regulation. Establishment of virus persistence increases the chance of viral pathogenic mechanisms coming into play; persistence can often be achieved by exposing a young animal, with waning maternal immunity, to large and possibly repeated doses of virus, resulting in impaired ability to limit the extent of the infection. Episodes of immune impairment later in life, due to nutritional or hormonal factors, disease or other physiological stresses, can reinforce this effect or even favor infection of a previously virus-free animal. When the viral risk factor is itself an immunosuppressant (see Figure 17.5) the problem is exacerbated, and, once a tumor burden develops, it may reinforce the predisposing impairment.

An intimate association with compromised immunity is often seen in the natural history of virus carcinogenesis. Examples from avian, feline, and human hemopoietic neoplasms, in which the virus infection contributes wholly or partially to the immunosuppression, have been given above. In other instances, another risk factor is responsible. Thus, an immunosuppressant in bracken fern seems to be important in the etiology of papillomavirus-associated alimentary carcinomas in cattle (Jarrett 1985; Beniston et al. 2001). In humans, iatrogenic immunosuppression is associated with an increased incidence of certain tumors, many of which had prior association with a virus risk factor. Indeed, so striking is this that Kinlen has suggested that all human tumors of which the incidence increases in immunosuppressed patients may have a viral component in their cause (Kinlen 1992). In short, the host response seems to be more important in controlling virus infection than other aspects of cell neoplasia.

The search for new viruses

There are three important motifs in naturally occurring viral cancers in animals and humans:

1 virus
2 immune impairment
3 co-carcinogen.

The first two components appear to be particularly important in most animal tumors, whereas the third is of greater importance in humans. These must all be considered in assessing the roles of other potential tumor viruses.

The most profitable tumors for study are those showing clustering that can be familial, geographical, or social/occupational, implying important genetic or environmental risk factors, both of which can point to viruses. Another important clue is any evidence of increased tumor prevalence in immunosuppressed individuals.

Both intact animals and tumors must be examined for characteristics of virus infection. Virus isolation from tumor material may require culture of tumor cells to demonstrate any latent virus, perhaps with addition of hormones, or of chemicals such as bromo- or iododeoxyuridine to activate endogenous viruses, or $5'$-azacytidine which inhibits cytosine methylation. Virus can sometimes also be detected by electron microscopy or immunological techniques. It is important to try to discover an appropriate cell type for virus propagation in vitro because the tumor itself is often an unsuitable host. The complexity of the mammalian genome was a barrier to solving this problem by subtractive hybridization methods, but polymerase chain reaction (PCR)-based techniques can now identify small amounts of foreign DNA in tumor cells (representational difference analysis). This strategy led to the discovery of a new human herpesvirus (KSHV) in Kaposi's sarcoma cases (Chang et al. 1994).

Isolation of a candidate virus provides the opportunity for a more detailed study of its association with the tumor. If, however, isolation fails, much can be learned by comparison with known tumor viruses together with the screening of tumor cells for molecular evidence of viral infection and examination of intact animals for epidemiological clues. If infection with a virus is common in a population, features of the infection peculiar to the tumor-bearing hosts should be sought. Is the infection unusually persistent? Is the serological response abnormal? Is the virus in the tumor defective? Are unusual viral antigens expressed? Even when a virus cannot be identified, a specific tumor antigen may be an important clue to a viral etiology.

Epidemiological evidence is crucial in humans, in whom it is impossible to test a causal role for the agent by virus inoculation. Case–control studies can associate the virus with the tumor, and laboratory investigations will establish the features of high- and low-risk groups. Retrospective and, ideally, prospective studies of high-risk groups can establish a temporal relationship between virus infection, other risk factors, and tumor development. This knowledge can then serve as a basis for the management of the tumor.

PRINCIPLES OF THE MANAGEMENT OF VIRUS-ASSOCIATED CANCER

Although little is known of many aspects of the pathogenesis of virus-associated tumors, the knowledge that a virus is implicated can be used to try to manage the disease at any of three arbitrary stages of virus neoplasia described earlier (Figure 17.5). Two points should be remembered. First, a wider range of prophylactic measures can be applied in veterinary medicine (where the health of the herd can override the survival of the individual) than in human practice. Second, for all tumors in which a virus is implicated, the detection of virus infection at any stage of the disease might be of diagnostic or prognostic use. This is clearly the case in the few diseases in which infection often leads to tumor formation. However, even when neoplasia is rare, detailed knowledge of the role played by the virus might identify features of the infection that are characteristic of hosts at high risk.

Prevention of virus infection

Before infection, steps can be taken to:

- decrease the concentration of virus in the hosts' environment
- increase the natural (genetic) resistance of host populations
- increase the resistance of the hosts by active or passive immunization.

THE SOURCE OF VIRUS

This is determined by the density of symptomatic or asymptomatic carriers in the population, the ability of the virus to survive outside its host, and whether other animals act as natural reservoirs for the virus. Many tumor viruses are species-specific and in practice only the first two factors are amenable to prophylactic measures.

The identification of carriers often requires specialized techniques to detect virus infection. It is thus costly and further action is effective only when the carrier can be killed, cured, or isolated from the susceptible population.

For these reasons, identification of human carriers poses ethical problems but can be important for several groups of patients. The first are those whose habits place them at particular risk, for example intravenous drug abusers in the case of HIV and HBV infections and the sexually promiscuous in the case of papillomavirus and herpesvirus infections. The second are those who have acquired iatrogenic infections, such as HIV and HBV from contaminated blood products. The third are mothers infected with HTLV, where breast milk can be a very important but avoidable means of transmission.

Identification of carriers can be useful in the control of avian, feline, and bovine lymphoid leukemias. A small proportion of cats infected with FeLV do not develop immunity and remain viremic. Such animals can either be removed from colonies or identified before introduction into virus-free groups. Eradication of enzootic bovine leukosis is greatly assisted by tests for virus carriers, whose lineage can be maintained free of virus by the transfer of well-washed embryos (with the zona pellucida intact) to virus-negative recipients.

Improved hygiene to reduce the source of the virus is probably of little significance within susceptible host populations but, in combination with appropriate husbandry, can reduce the dissemination of disease between local concentrations of animals such as the spread of ALV from one poultry farm to another. Many tumor viruses are highly susceptible to chemical disinfectants, drying, and other inactivating agents, but horizontal and congenital spread depend on such intimate contact between hosts that disinfection is impracticable. Papillomas and enzootic bovine leukosis are exceptions to this because the causal viruses can be spread on the instruments of stockmen and veterinarians. Another possible measure, applicable to BLV and HTLV-I, is the control of insects that may spread infection. The social and hygiene practices in many Western countries delay some EBV infections until puberty or later, but these increase the incidence of infectious mononucleosis. A delay in the age of acquisition of EBV infection in Africa and Asia might reduce the incidence of Burkitt's lymphoma or nasopharyngeal carcinoma, but this has not yet been demonstrated. However, one virus-associated human neoplasm for which a change in habits should reduce incidence is carcinoma of the uterine cervix. As with other venereally transmitted infections, the spread of papillomavirus and herpes simplex virus (HSV) type 2 has been favored by promiscuity and changes in contraceptive practices.

THE GENETIC SUSCEPTIBILITY OF HOST ANIMALS

The selective breeding of genetically resistant stock is possible only in animals, and particularly in those that have a short generation time. It has been successful in reducing the incidence of avian lymphoid leukosis; the causal virus exists in the field as two major subtypes, characterized by the presence of particular glycoproteins on the viral envelope. These glycoproteins interact with specific cell surface receptors to allow the viruses to penetrate the host cells. Strains of domestic chicken have been bred that lack the surface receptors for the field strains of ALF and these birds are resistant to infection (Crittenden and Motta 1969). Some strains partly resistant to lymphoid leukosis apparently permit infection but not tumor development. A similar genetic resistance is seen in the production of Marek's disease lymphomas.

IMMUNITY TO VIRUS INFECTION

Although a number of commercial vaccines exist for oncogenic viruses of animals, proposals to produce vaccines against human oncogenic viruses are controversial, for several reasons.

- In many instances the role of the virus in the tumor is uncertain; indeed, proof of a causal role may rely on the prophylactic effect of vaccination. This leads to the dilemma of whether to embark on such measures before they can be shown to be necessary.
- Tumor production may be a rare outcome of infection by a widespread and not very pathogenic virus.
- The presence of many latently infected carriers and the frequent acquisition of infection early in life (e.g. with human herpesviruses) will limit vaccine efficacy.
- Because tumors can result from an aberrant virus–cell interaction, a traditional type of vaccine, based on inactivated or attenuated virus, may itself pose a risk of oncogenicity. This last objection might be overcome by the use of purified immunogens either produced by genetically manipulated portions of viral genomes or synthesized in the laboratory.

However, the first two considerations suggest that the returns (in terms of improved health of the human population) may justify the outlay only if three conditions are fulfilled:

1 the virus causes significant disease in addition to its oncogenic potential (as is the case with HIV and HBV)
2 the populations concerned are clearly defined, small and at high risk
3 the virus is the only clearly defined risk factor in the genesis of a common tumor (as with EBV-associated nasopharyngeal carcinoma).

The first successful commercial vaccines against a neoplasm were produced for Marek's disease and have proved of great value to the poultry industry. Avirulent strains of the virus, either natural or artificially attenuated, have been used as vaccine, as has a related herpesvirus of turkeys; continual modification of the vaccine, however, has been necessary to try to keep up with the emergence of highly virulent strains (Schat

1987). The vaccine virus strains establish a latent infection and induce tumor-associated surface antigens in lymphoid cells, sometimes with minor cytopathic effects and neuritis. There is, however, no immunosuppression and vaccinated birds resist challenge with oncogenic virus (Calnek et al. 1979), apparently by an immunity directed against both viral and tumor antigens.

Approaches to vaccination against human herpesviruses have been more conservative, most efforts being directed to the testing of recombinant subunit vaccines in animal models. Using recombinant subunit vaccines based on viral surface glycoproteins, protection against infectious virus challenge has been achieved against EBV in a cottontop tamarin model, and against HSV in mice (reviewed in Morein and Merza 1991). While it would be desirable to eradicate both these viruses from the human population, the case for large-scale vaccination is not clearcut.

Recombinant subunit vaccines based on HBV surface antigen have been available since 1982 and have proved effective in reducing the incidence of infection in selected at-risk groups. However, these measures have had little impact on the overall incidence of infection in the population, leading to calls for mass vaccination programs to be extended (Rizzetto and Zanetti 2002).

Vaccines made from ground-up wart tissue have long been used for prophylaxis and therapy of papillomas in animals. This empirical approach illustrates the potential for vaccination against papillomavirus infection, but is clearly incompatible with modern quality-control standards for human medicine. More recently, recombinant gene products of bovine papillomavirus, both early and late genes, have been efficacious in preventing warts and in accelerating rejection (Campo 1995). Translation of these results to human vaccination is complicated by the multiplicity of HPV types and our limited knowledge of the natural history of HPV infections (Galloway 1994).

A number of commercial vaccines have been developed for feline leukemia, including inactivated virus, infected cell extracts, and recombinant subunit *env* vaccines (Jarrett 1994), and attempts to produce a BLV vaccine are also under way.

Although prophylactic vaccination is also considered highly desirable as a means of containing the HIV epidemic, trials of candidate subunit vaccines to date have failed to demonstrate efficacy. Experiments with animal lentivirus models such as simian and feline immunodeficiency viruses have shown only weak protection or short-term suppression of virus replication with conventional subunit or inactivated virus vaccines, and the problem of vaccine escape due to strain variation is significant (Mwau and McMichael 2003).

ANTIVIRAL THERAPY

Another approach to the control of oncogenic viruses (one popular with the pharmaceutical industry) is to try to limit the infection – usually after it is clinically evident – with antiviral chemotherapy. This, too, poses problems inherent in the close symbiosis between viruses and their host cells, because drugs must be devised that are selectively toxic for the virus. One approach is to direct research to the development of inhibitors of processes essential to the virus but dispensable by the cell, such as reverse transcriptase. Within these constraints, some widely used and moderately effective drugs have been developed against, for instance, herpesviruses and retroviruses. These drugs may assist in the control of virus replication but in their current modes of use have shown no beneficial effect on tumor development or on established cancers. For example, the most widely used antiretroviral agent, azidothymidine, was first tested as a potential anticancer agent but its long-term use in AIDS patients does not appear to reduce, and might conceivably increase, the incidence of non-Hodgkin's lymphoma (Pluda et al. 1990).

The use of interferons to control virus-associated cancers was considered an exciting prospect in the last decade but clinical trials have, in general, been disappointing. Striking exceptions have been the effects of interferon-α in virus-associated laryngeal and genital papillomas and in hairy cell leukemias. However, effects other than antiviral activity may be involved in the former examples (Gangemi et al. 1994) while in the latter case the ability of interferon to induce cell differentiation seems to be the most likely mechanism (Vedantham et al. 1992).

Prevention of cell conversion to neoplasia

The problems of tackling viral infection suggest that other potentially avoidable risk factors (see Tables 17.1, 17.2, and 17.3), which tend to operate in association, might provide easier targets for preventive measures. Such hopes, however, seem largely misplaced. In humans these risk factors include habits (notably smoking), dietary factors (which may be even harder to eliminate than smoking unless, like aflatoxin contamination, their deleterious effects are obvious), and other diseases. The most striking example of the last is malaria, a risk factor in Burkitt's lymphoma in certain tropical areas but also a major disease problem in its own right in many parts of the world. Indeed, the reduction or elimination of some of these risk factors would have benefits far beyond the postulated decrease in cancer incidence. This is so self-evident that there must be doubt as to whether the incentive of cancer prevention per se will succeed where other imperatives have failed.

Therapy of virus-associated cancers

Once a virus-infected cell has become neoplastic, the prevention of further tumor growth depends on therapy rather than prophylaxis. But with virus-associated tumors, the detection of infection at any stage of the disease might itself influence prognosis. In cases in which neoplasia is a rare outcome of virus infection, knowledge of the role played by the virus might identify features characteristic of hosts at high risk. Such knowledge has been used, for instance, in attempts at early diagnosis of nasopharyngeal carcinoma by screening populations at risk in China for EBV-specific salivary IgA (Zeng et al. 1982).

When viral etiology is established, immunotherapy might be considered as a means of achieving regression. Indeed, early experimentation demonstrated that most virally induced tumors were quite readily rejected, unlike those without obvious viral etiology (Klein and Klein 1977). However, these experiments involved the inoculation of immunocompetent animals with tumors expressing readily detectable viral antigens. By contrast, the human malignancies most tightly linked to virus infection are seen in the context of obviously impaired immunity (e.g. AIDS or transplant patients) or express very little if any viral antigens [e.g. HTLV-I-associated adult T-cell leukemia (ATL), Burkitt's lymphoma]. Moreover, the latter tumors may have arisen in individuals with specific deficits in their immunological repertoire, as suggested by associations with specific types of major histocompatibility complex. In these contexts, immunotherapy seems much less promising and it may be necessary instead to consider the means of repairing the defective response. One way to achieve this may be to create tumor cell vaccines by transfection with co-receptor or cytokine genes. Ironically, the retroviruses have recently found a role as vectors to mediate this type of gene therapy for cancer (Vieweg and Gilboa 1995).

Papillomavirus-associated neoplasms have long been treated with extracts of tumors. For example, treatment of bovine ocular squamous cell carcinoma (a common neoplasm in light-skinned cattle in areas of high sunlight) with an allogeneic tumor extract resulted in remissions (Hoffmann et al. 1981). However, it is not clear whether viral antigens were targets in the regression of this malignancy. As discussed earlier, the possibility that vaccines against HPV-16 and 18 might be able to cause regression of cervical carcinoma is now under experimental trial (Frazer 2002).

Finally, if viral genes can be shown to play a role in the maintenance of the tumor state, then direct inhibition of their expression or even their downstream effectors may be a route to therapy. For example, antisense inhibition of NF-κB was found to limit the growth of HTLV Tax-transformed cells in a mouse tumor model, while antisense to Tax itself was ineffective (Kitajima et al. 1992).

CONCLUSIONS

In recent years, research on tumor viruses has identified some of the genetic lesions that underlie neoplasia and

has led to some remarkable advances in basic cancer research. These studies are now influencing areas of cell biology and biochemistry that seem far removed from their virological origins. At the same time, however, tumor viruses have become more important to the virologist. We now appreciate that viruses are often one of a complex of risk factors that predisposes to a significant proportion of human disease. Although the part they play often results from an insidious and intractable pathogenic process, they are, in theory, avoidable risk factors. As such, they may provide the key to the management of many cancers.

REFERENCES

Acha-Orbea, H. and MacDonald, H.R. 1995. Superantigens of mouse mammary tumour virus. *Ann Rev Immunol*, **13**, 459–86.

Baltzer, F. 1964. Theodor Boveri. *Science*, **144**, 809–15.

Baum, C., Dullmann, J., et al. 2003. Side effects of retroviral gene transfer into hematopoietic stem cells. *Blood*, **101**, 2099–114.

Ben-David, Y., Prideaux, V.R., et al. 1988. Inactivation of the p53 oncogene by internal deletion or retroviral integration in erythroleukemia cell lines induced by Friend murine leukemia virus. *Oncogene*, **3**, 179–85.

Beniston, R.G., Morgan, I.M., et al. 2001. Quercetin, E7 and p53 in papillomavirus oncogenic cell transformation. *Carcinogenesis*, **22**, 1069–76.

Bishop, J.M. 1987. The molecular genetics of cancer. *Science*, **235**, 305–11.

Bishop, J.M. 1991. Molecular themes in oncogenesis. *Cell*, **64**, 235–48.

Boshoff, C. and Weiss, R.A. 2001. Epidemiology and pathogenesis of Kaposi's sarcoma-associated herpesvirus. *Philos Trans R Soc Lond B Biol Sci*, **356**, 517–34.

Buendia, M.A. 1994. Hepatitis B viruses and liver cancer: the woodchuck model. In: Minson, A., Neil, J. and McCrae, M. (eds), *Viruses and cancer*. Cambridge, UK: Cambridge University Press, 174–87.

Calnek, B.W., Carlisle, J.C., et al. 1979. Comparative pathogenesis studies with oncogenic and nononcogenic Marek's disease viruses and turkey herpesvirus. *Am J Vet Res*, **40**, 541–8.

Campo, M.S. 1995. Infection by BPV and prospects for vaccination. *Trends Microbiol Sci*, **3**, 92–7.

Chang, Y., Cesarman, E., et al. 1994. Identification of herpesvirus-like DNA sequences in AIDS-associated Kaposi's sarcoma. *Science*, **266**, 1865–9.

Chow, Y.H., Alberti, A., et al. 2003. Transformation of rodent fibroblasts by the jaagsiekte sheep retrovirus envelope is receptor independent and does not require the surface domain. *J Virol*, **77**, 6341–50.

Crittenden, L.B. and Motta, J.V. 1969. A survey of genetic resistance to leukosis-sarcoma viruses in commercial stocks of chickens. *Poultry Sci*, **48**, 1751–7.

Cunningham, J.M. and Kim, J.W. 1994. Cellular receptors for type C retroviruses. In: Wimmer, E. (ed.), *Cellular receptors for animal viruses*. Cold Spring Harbor, New York: Cold Spring Harbor Press, 49–59.

Dalgleish, A.G., Beverley, P.C., et al. 1984. The CD4 (T4) antigen is an essential component of the receptor for the AIDS retrovirus. *Nature*, **312**, 763–7.

Donehower, L.A., Harvey, M., et al. 1992. Mice deficient for p53 are developmentally normal but susceptible to spontaneous tumours. *Nature*, **356**, 215–21.

Eliopoulos, A.G. and Young, L.S. 2001. LMP1 structure and signal transduction. *Semin Cancer Biol*, **11**, 435–44.

Evan, G.I., Wyllie, A.H., et al. 1992. Induction of apoptosis in fibroblasts by c-*myc* protein. *Cell*, **69**, 119–28.

Frazer, I. 2002. Vaccines for papillomavirus infection. *Virus Res*, **89**, 271–4.

Gallimore, P.H. and Turnell, A.S. 2001. Adenovirus E1A: remodelling the host cell, a life or death experience. *Oncogene*, **20**, 7824–35.

Galloway, D.A. 1994. Human papillomaviruses: a warty problem. *Infect Agents Dis*, **3**, 187–93.

Gangemi, J.D., Piris, L., et al. 1994. HPV replication in experimental models: effects of interferon. *Antiviral Res*, **24**, 175–90.

Gupta, P. and Ferrer, J.F. 1982. Expression of bovine leukemia virus genome is blocked by a nonimmunoglobulin protein in plasma from infected cattle. *Science*, **215**, 405–7.

Hanlon, L., Barr, N.I., et al. 2003. Long-range effects of retroviral activation on c-myb over-expression may be obscured by silencing during tumor growth in vitro. *J Virol*, **77**, 1059–68.

Harris, H. 1985. Suppression of malignancy in hybrid cells: the mechanism. *J Cell Sci*, **79**, 83–94.

Hawes, S.E., Critchlow, C.W., et al. 2003. Increased risk of high-grade cervical squamous intraepithelial lesions and invasive cervical cancer among African women with human immunodeficiency virus type 1 and 2 infections. *J Infect Dis*, **188**, 555–63.

Hesketh, R. 1997. *The oncogene and tumour suppressor gene facts book*. London: Academic Press.

Hoffmann, D., Jennings, P.A. and Spradbrow, P.B. 1981. Autografting and allografting of bovine ocular squamous carcinoma. *Res Vet Sci*, **31**, 48–53.

Holmes, R.D. and Sokol, R.J. 2002. Epstein–Barr virus and post-transplant lymphoproliferative disease. *Pediatr Transplant*, **6**, 456–64.

Jarrett, W.F.H. 1985. The natural history of bovine papillomavirus infection. *Adv Viral Oncol*, **5**, 83–102.

Jarrett, O. 1994. Transmission and control of feline leukaemia virus. In: Minson, A., Neil, J. and McCrae, M. (eds), *Viruses and cancer*. Cambridge, UK: Cambridge University Press, 235–46.

Jonkers, J. and Berns, A. 1996. Retroviral insertional mutagenesis as a strategy to identify cancer genes. *Biochim Biophys Acta*, **1287**, 29–57.

Kapoun, A.M. and Shackleford, G.M. 1997. Preferential activation of Fgf8 by proviral insertion in mammary tumors of Wnt1 transgenic mice. *Oncogene*, **14**, 2985–9.

Kiefer, F., Courtneidge, S.A. and Wagner, E.F. 1994. Oncogenic properties of the middle T antigens of polyomaviruses. *Adv Cancer Res*, **64**, 125–57.

Kinlen, L.J. 1992. Immunosuppressive therapy and acquired immunological disorders. *Cancer Res*, **52**, 5474–6.

Kitajima, I., Shinohara, T., et al. 1992. Abalation of transplanted HTLV-I Tax-transformed tumors in mice by antisense inhibition of NF-kappa-B. *Science*, **258**, 1792–5.

Klein, G. and Klein, E. 1977. Rejectability of virus-induced tumors and nonrejectability of spontaneous tumors: a lesson in contrasts. *Transplant Proc*, **9**, 1095–104.

Klingelhutz, A.J., Foster, S.A. and McDougall, J.K. 1996. Telomerase activation by the E6 gene product of human papillomavirus type 16. *Nature*, **380**, 79–82.

Knudson, A.G. Jr. 1993. The genetic predisposition to cancer. *Birth Defects*, **25**, 15–27.

Kung, H.-J., Boerkel, C. and Carter, T.H. 1991. Retroviral mutagenesis of cellular oncogenes: a review with insights into the mechanisms of insertional activation. *Curr Top Microbiol Immunol*, **171**, 1–25.

Lane, D.P. and Crawford, L.V. 1979. T antigen is bound to a host protein in SV40-transformed cells. *Nature*, **278**, 261–3.

Largaespada, D.A., Shaughnessy, J.D. Jr, et al. 1995. Retroviral integration at the Evi-2 locus in BXH-2 myeloid leukemia cell lines disrupts Nf1 expression without changes in steady-state Ras-GTP levels. *J Virol*, **69**, 5095–102.

Lazo, P.A., Lee, J.S. and Tsichlis, P.N. 1990. Long-distance activation of the *myc* protooncogene by provirus insertion in Mlvi-1 or Mlvi-4 in rat T-cell lymphomas. *Proc Natl Acad Sci U S A*, **87**, 170–3.

Lee, T.A. and Farnham, P.J. 2000. Exogenous E2F expression is growth inhibitory before, during, and after cellular transformation. *Oncogene*, **19**, 2257–68.

Liebermann, D.A., Hoffman, B. and Steinman, R.A. 1995. Molecular controls of growth arrest and apoptosis: p53-dependent and independent pathways. *Oncogene*, **11**, 199–210.

Linzer, D.I.H. and Levine, A.J. 1979. Characterization of a 54K Dalton cellular SV40 tumour antigen in SV40-transformed cells and uninfected embryonal carcinoma cells. *Cell*, **17**, 43–52.

Lock, L.F., Jenkins, N.A. and Copeland, N.G. 1991. Mutagenesis of the mouse germline using retroviral insertion. *Curr Top Microbiol Immunol*, **171**, 27–41.

Lomax, M. and Fried, M. 2001. Polyoma virus disrupts ARF signaling to p53. *Oncogene*, **20**, 4951–60.

MacArthur, C.A., Shankar, D.B. and Shackleford, G.M. 1995. Fgf-8, activated by proviral insertion, cooperates with the Wnt-1 transgene in murine mammary tumorigenesis. *J Virol*, **69**, 2501–7.

Macnab, J.C.M. 1987. Herpes simplex virus and human cytomegalovirus: their role in morphological transformation and genital cancers. *J Gen Virol*, **68**, 2525–50.

Matsuoka, M. 2003. Human T-cell leukemia virus type I and adult T-cell leukemia. *Oncogene*, **22**, 5131–40.

McDougall, J.K. 2001. 'Hit and run' transformation leading to carcinogenesis. *Dev Biol*, **106**, 77–82.

Meuwissen, R., Jonkers, J. and Berns, A. 2001. Mouse models for sporadic cancer. *Exp Cell Res*, **264**, 100–10.

Miles, B.D. and Robinson, H.L. 1985. High-frequency transduction of c-*erbB* in avian leukosis virus-induced erythroblastosis. *J Virol*, **54**, 295–303.

Minson, A., Neil, J. and McCrae, M. (eds) 1994. *Viruses and cancer*. Cambridge: Cambridge University Press.

Minson, A.C. 1984. Cell transformation and oncogenesis by herpes simplex virus and human cytomegalovirus. *Cancer Sur*, **3**, 91–111.

Montesano, R. and Slaga, T.J. 1983. Initiation and promotion in carcinogenesis: an appraisal. *Cancer Sur*, **2**, 613–21.

Morein, B. and Merza, M. 1991. Vaccination against herpesviruses, fiction or reality? *Scand J Infect Dis*, **23**, 110–18.

Morrison, H.L., Soni, B. and Lenz, J. 1995. Long terminal repeat enhancer core sequences in proviruses adjacent to c-*myc* in T-cell lymphomas induced by a murine retrovirus. *J Virol*, **69**, 446–55.

Mwau, M. and McMichael, A.J. 2003. A review of vaccines for HIV prevention. *J Gene Med*, **5**, 3–10.

Neel, B., Hayward, W.S., et al. 1981. Avian leukosis virus-induced tumors have common proviral integration sites and synthesize discreet new RNAs: oncogenesis by promoter insertion. *Cell*, **23**, 323–34.

Neil, J.C. and Cameron, E.R. 2002. Retroviral insertion sites and cancer: fountain of all knowledge? *Cancer Cell*, **2**, 253–5.

Neil, J.C., Hughes, D., et al. 1984. Transduction and rearrangement of the *myc* gene by feline leukaemia virus in naturally occurring T-cell leukaemias. *Nature*, **308**, 814–20.

Neil, J.C., Fulton, R., et al. 1991. Feline leukaemia virus: generation of pathogenic and oncogenic variants. *Curr Top Microbiol Immunol*, **171**, 67–93.

Nemerow, G.R., Mold, C., et al. 1987. Identification of gp350 as the viral glycoprotein mediating attachment of Epstein–Barr virus (EBV) to the EBV/C3d receptor of B cells: sequence homology of gp350 and C3 complement fragment C3d. *J Virol*, **61**, 1416–20.

Nilsen, T., Maroney, P.A., et al. 1985. c-*erbB* activation in ALV-induced erythroblastosis: novel RNA processing and promoter insertion results in expression of an amino-truncated EGF receptor. *Cell*, **41**, 719–26.

Onions, D., Lees, G., et al. 1987. Recombinant feline viruses containing the *myc* gene rapidly produce clonal tumours expressing T-cell antigen receptor gene transcripts. *Int J Cancer*, **40**, 40–5.

Opgenorth, A., Strayer, D., et al. 1992. Deletion of the growth factor gene related to EGF and TGF alpha reduces virulence of malignant rabbit fibroma virus. *Virology*, **186**, 175–91.

Pacitti, A.M. and Jarrett, O. 1985. Duration of the latent state in feline leukaemia virus infections. *Vet Rec*, **117**, 472–4.

Payne, L.N. 1992. Biology of avian retroviruses. In: Levy, J.A. (ed.), *The Retroviridae*. New York: Plenum Press, 299–404.

Peters, G. 1990. Oncogenes at viral integration sites. *Cell Growth Diff*, **1**, 503–10.

Pluda, J.M., Yarchoan, R., et al. 1990. Development of non-Hodgkins's lymphoma in a cohort of patients with severe human immunodeficiency virus infection on long-term antiretroviral therapy. *Ann Intern Med*, **113**, 276–82.

Rabbitts, T.H. 1994. Chromosomal translocations in human cancer. *Nature*, **372**, 143–9.

Rickinson, A.B. 1994. EBV infection and EBV-associated tumours. In: Minson, A., Neil, J. and McCrae, M. (eds), *Viruses and cancer*. Cambridge: Cambridge University Press, 81–100.

Rickinson, A.B. and Kieff, E. 1996. Epstein–Barr virus. In: Fields, B.N., Knipe, D.M. and Howley, P.M. (eds), *Fields virology*. Philadelphia, PA: Lippincott-Raven, 2397–446.

Rizzetto, M. and Zanetti, A.R. 2002. Progress in the prevention and control of viral hepatitis type B: closing remarks. *J Med Virol*, **67**, 463–6.

Rojko, J.L., Hoover, E.A., et al. 1982. Reactivation of latent feline leukemia virus infection. *Nature (Lond)*, **298**, 385–8.

Rosenberg, N. and Jolicoeur, P. 1997. Retroviral pathogenesis. In: Coffin, J.M., Hughes, S.H. and Varmus, H.E. (eds), *Retroviruses*. Cold Spring Harbor, New York: Cold Spring Harbor Laboratory Press, 475–586.

Rossner, M.T. 1992. Review: hepatitis B virus X-gene product: a promiscuous transcriptional activator. *J Med Virol*, **36**, 101–17.

Ruben, S., Poteat, H., et al. 1988. Cellular transcription factors and regulation of IL-2 receptor gene expression by HTLV-I Tax gene product. *Science*, **241**, 89–92.

Ruscetti, S.K. 1999. Deregulation of erythropoiesis by the Friend spleen focus-forming virus. *Int J Biochem Cell Biol*, **31**, 1089–109.

Schat, K.A. 1987. Marek's disease: a model for protection against herpesvirus-induced tumours. *Cancer Sur*, **6**, 1–37.

Schulz, T.F. and Neil, J.C. 2002. Viruses and leukemia. In: Henderson, E.S., Lister, T.A. and Greaves, M.F. (eds), *Leukemia*. Philadelphia, PA: W.B. Saunders, 200–25.

Shen, Y. and White, E. 2001. p53-dependent apoptosis pathways. *Adv Cancer Res*, **82**, 55–84.

Shields, P.G. and Harris, C.C. 2000. Cancer risk and low-penetrance susceptibility genes in gene-environment interactions. *J Clin Oncol*, **18**, 2309–15.

Slagle, B.L., Becker, S.A. and Butel, J.S. 1994. Hepatitis viruses and liver cancer. In: Minson, A., Neil, J. and McCrae, M. (eds), *Viruses and cancer*. Cambridge, UK: Cambridge University Press, 149–71.

Stoye, J.P., Moroni, C. and Coffin, J.M. 1991. Virological events leading to spontaneous AKR thymomas. *J Virol*, **65**, 1273–85.

Tauber, B. and Dobner, T. 2001. Adenovirus early E4 genes in viral oncogenesis. *Oncogene*, **20**, 7847–54.

Truant, R., Antunovic, J., et al. 1995. Direct interaction of the hepatitis B virus HBx protein with p53 leads to inhibition by HBx of p53 response element-directed transactivation. *J Virol*, **69**, 1851–9.

Tsatsanis, C., Fulton, R., et al. 1994. Genetic determinants of feline leukemia virus-induced lymphoid tumors: patterns of proviral insertion and gene rearrangement. *J Virol*, **68**, 8294–303.

Tsichlis, P.N. and Lazo, P.A. 1991. Virus–host interactions and the pathogenesis of murine and human oncogenic retroviruses. *Curr Top Microbiol Immunol*, **171**, 95–172.

Tsichlis, P.N., Gunter-Strauss, P. and Lohse, M.A. 1985. Concerted DNA rearrangements in Moloney leukemia virus-induced thymomas: a potential synergistic relationship in oncogenesis. *J Virol*, **56**, 258–67.

Vedantham, S., Gamliel, H. and Golomb, H.M. 1992. Mechanism of interferon action in hairy cell leukemia: a model of effective cancer biotherapy. *Cancer Res*, **52**, 1056–66.

Vieweg, J. and Gilboa, E. 1995. Considerations for the use of cytokine-secreting tumor cell preparations for cancer treatment. *Cancer Invest*, **13**, 193–201.

Vogelstein, B. and Kinzler, K.W. 1992. p53 function and dysfunction. *Cell*, **70**, 523–6.

Weiss, R.A. 1984. Experimental biology and assay of RNA tumor viruses. In: Weiss, R., Teich, N., et al. (eds), *RNA tumor viruses*. Cold Spring Harbor Laboratory, New York: Cold Spring Harbor Laboratory Press, 209–60.

Wotton, S., Stewart, M., et al. 2002. Proviral insertion indicates a dominant oncogenic role for Runx1/AML1 in T-cell lymphoma. *Cancer Res*, **62**, 7181–5.

Yonish-Rouach, E., Resnitsky, D., et al. 1991. Wild type p53 induces apoptosis of myeloid leukaemic cells that is inhibited by IL-6. *Nature*, **352**, 345–7.

Zeng, Y., Zhang, L.G. and Li, H.Y. 1982. Serological mass survey for early detection of nasopharyngeal carcinoma in Wuzhou City, China. *Int J Cancer*, **29**, 139–41.

Zinkernagel, R.M. and Hengartner, H. 1994. T-cell-mediated immunopathology versus direct cytolysis by virus: implications for HIV and AIDS. *Immunol Today*, **15**, 262–7.

zur Hausen, H. 1986. Intracellular surveillance of persistent viral infections: human genital cancer results from deficient cellular control of papilloma viral gene expression. *Lancet*, **2**, 489–91.

zur Hausen, H. 1991. Viruses in human cancers. *Science*, **254**, 1167–73.

18

The epidemiology of viral infections

ARNOLD S. MONTO

INTRODUCTION

Epidemiology describes the occurrence of illness in populations and, by means of specific study designs, facilitates analysis of the risk factors that determine its distribution. Such investigations are often observational and do not involve experimentation or intervention but, rather, they gather and interpret events as they occur in nature. In the process, the occurrence of diseases is quantified according to their characteristics. Hypotheses concerning etiology and other variables are generated and are tested using statistical techniques. Epidemiology also provides experimental approaches for evaluating the efficacy of interventions such as vaccines to prevent or drugs to treat disease. Infectious diseases were the primary concern of epidemiologists for many years, and concepts were developed to evaluate the infectious process in populations. Now, most epidemiologists work on noncommunicable diseases, and methods originally developed to study acute infections are being used to evaluate etiology and risk factors for conditions such as coronary heart disease and cancer.

Whilst similar methods are now employed to study both communicable and noncommunicable diseases, the unique nature of replicating agents makes certain techniques more relevant to infectious illnesses, especially in examining questions of etiology. Debate has raged about the appropriateness of separating causes of diseases into 'necessary' and 'contributing' (Susser 1973). For example, it is impossible to produce a case of polio without the poliovirus, although contributing factors may be involved in determining the consequences of the infection, i.e. whether disease develops and how severe it is. Epidemiological approaches may also be required to evaluate some of the basic characteristics of infectious agents in humans, such as the infectious dose, which is important in terms of both the amount of pathogen required to initiate infection and the ease and likelihood of transmission. When animal models are available, many of these variables can be estimated. Results may or may not be applicable to humans, so epidemiological studies are needed for confirmation. They are essential when no animal model is available.

When dealing with viral infections (as opposed to those caused by other infectious agents), epidemiological principles are modified only because of characteristics of the pathogens. Most reflect differences in the ability of the agents to persist in the environment (typically more limited with viruses) and the comparative lack of the intermediate hosts that exist with animal parasites. Features such as the possibility of persistent infection and induction of chronic disease and malignancies are not unique to viruses, but are certainly more characteristic of infection with some of them than with other types of agents. In this chapter, the examination of the epidemiology of viral infections emphasizes the elements that are unique to viruses, but the discussion is not limited to them. More general issues are also covered and viral infections serve as illustrations of the principles and methods discussed.

CLASSIFYING MECHANISMS OF VIRAL TRANSMISSION

Direct transmission

In the cycle of infection, the period during transmission of the agent from one host to the next is when the virus is exposed to the environment and therefore most vulnerable. Systems have been developed to divide the transmission mechanisms of infectious agents into different categories and subcategories. There are classification systems based on portals of entry and exit of the agent to and from the host (Fox et al. 1970). That shown in Table 18.1 is based on duration and route in transit from one host to the next, but some categories are limited to specific portals such as the skin or the respiratory tract (American Public Health Association 1985). The major division is between direct transmission, which is essentially immediate, and indirect transmission, which is delayed. Direct contact generally implies no exposure of the agent to the environment. This type of transmission occurs during sexual intercourse, as with human immunodeficiency virus (HIV) or hepatitis B, or during direct skin contact, as with herpes gladiatorum, a herpes simplex infection of wrestlers transmitted as they rub their skin against that of an opponent (Belongia et al. 1991). In most cases, virus-containing fluids are involved and the viruses are often cell associated. Direct contact includes, by extension, vertical transmission which may take place transplacentally, during the birth process or in breast milk. All these extended mechanisms are documented for HIV, which can be transmitted directly but is not well transmitted when the agent

comes in contact with the environment (Friedland and Klein 1987).

Droplets of various sizes are expelled as part of respiratory discharges; the larger droplets, greater than 5 μm in diameter, settle out rapidly and do not spread further than about 1 m, rendering this form of transmission essentially immediate. Thus, even though the previously and the newly infected hosts are not in contact with each other, this is also considered to be a form of direct transmission, because of the limited transit time of this class of infected droplets which do not stay in the air for long periods. Agents potentially destroyed by longer exposure to the environment can still be transmitted by this mechanism. Rhinoviruses are spread by large droplets. As a result, rhinovirus disease transmission, which generally peaks in the autumn when schools reopen, is in fact a summation of mini-outbreaks produced by concurrent dissemination of many different serotypes (Monto et al. 1987). Some large droplets evaporate to become aerosols that may stay suspended and remain infectious for long periods. Influenza is spread by both large droplet and aerosol; a single viral subtype is generally responsible for outbreaks (Couch et al. 1966), in contrast to the relatively limited nature of transmission via large droplets alone. The childhood exanthemata, measles, mumps, and chickenpox, are transmitted mainly by large droplets, which explains why outbreaks may take months to run their course in a partially immune population.

Indirect transmission

Indirect transmission covers many diverse mechanisms that have in common only the fact that there can be a delay, often prolonged, in the infectious agent reaching a new host. Indirect transmission is divided into three categories (Table 18.1). Vehicles are varied nonliving entities, ranging from inanimate objects to water and biological products such as milk, urine, or human tissue on or in which the infectious agent remains in transit to a new host. Personal inanimate objects, such as combs, blankets, and writing materials serving as vehicles for transmission of infective agents, are termed fomites. Many important viruses can be transmitted by fomites, including the agents of measles, chickenpox, and smallpox, but the period in transit cannot be long. Again, the issue is one of survival during exposure to environmental extremes. Because infections known to be transmitted from person to person can also be spread via freshly contaminated fomites, the definition of a contagious disease was extended to include this route, which is sometimes termed 'indirect contact.' Thus, a contagious disease is one transmitted by direct or indirect contact. In reality, contagious agents are transmitted mainly directly, especially by large droplets. Only infrequently are fomites involved,

Table 18.1 Principal mechanisms of transmission

Principal mechanisms
Direct (essentially immediate)
Contact (touching, kissing, sexual intercourse, etc.)
Large droplet – limited distance
Indirect
Vehicle-borne
Indirect contact – fomites
Other inanimate objects and biological substances (water, milk, urine, stool, etc.)
Vectorborne
Mechanical – without multiplication
Biological – with multiplication
Dusts and airborne droplet nuclei (aerosols)

because this route is a relatively inefficient means of transmission.

Whereas some viruses transmitted by vehicle are spread in water, urine, and milk, this kind of transmission is more common with bacteria that can survive in the environment for prolonged periods. The spread of picornaviruses (Chapter 40, Picornaviruses), other enteric viruses (Chapters 41, Human enteric RNA viruses: astroviruses, and 42, Human enteric RNA viruses: noroviruses and sapoviruses) and hepatitis A and E viruses (Chapter 53, Hepatitis A and E) has been related to exposure to infected water. These viruses, known to be associated with fecal contamination, may be spread not only by drinking water itself but also by ingesting shellfish which filter and concentrate the virus (Hedstrom and Lycke 1964; Portnoy et al. 1975). Transmission from infected urine occurs with a number of the viruses whose primary hosts are sylvatic, such as the arenavirus Machupo (Chapter 49, Arenaviruses). Likewise, hantaviruses such as the agents of Korean hemorrhagic fever and the hantavirus pulmonary syndrome (Chapter 48, *Bunyaviridae*), recently described in southwestern USA may be transmitted from infected urine or feces (Johnson et al. 1966; Childs et al. 1994). For these, and for other agents similarly transmitted, rodents are the reservoir of infection. They often live close to or in human dwellings and infect humans via their excreta.

Vector transmission is divided into mechanical and biological categories. Mechanical transmission implies that the vector, typically an arthropod, is involved only in providing transport for the agent, i.e. moving it from one site to another without multiplication taking place. This occurs with certain enteric bacteria, in which the pathogen may adhere to the surface of the vector. It rarely takes place with viruses because the agents would be inactivated by the environmental exposure. No multiplication of the agent occurs, so it is not an efficient form of transmission. In contrast, biological transmission is highly efficient. Most of the large group of viruses transmitted by this mechanism were formerly termed the arthropod-borne or arboviruses (Chapters 46, Flaviviruses; and 47, Togaviruses). They are now divided into different families, such as the flaviviruses and the togaviruses (Westaway et al. 1985a, b). By definition, arboviruses are transmitted by mosquitoes, ticks, or other arthropods, and, in the process, the quantity of virus increases, thus enhancing the probability of infection. Multiplication takes place in the body of the arthropod, and, for example, is released from the salivary glands during a mosquito bite. There has been speculation that nonarboviruses, such as hepatitis B, might be mosquito transmitted, because epidemiological data suggested that distribution was related to mosquito density (Papaevangelou and Kourea-Kremastinou 1974). However, multiplication has never been demonstrated, so the likelihood of a bite producing transmission is low

even if infected blood has been taken up (Berquist et al. 1976).

Infected dusts are rarely involved in transmitting viral infections by the airborne route, because desiccation usually inactivates them if they stay exposed to the environment for prolonged periods. Certain respiratory viral infections such as influenza and coxsackie virus A21 are commonly transmitted by small droplets or droplet nuclei (Couch et al. 1966). The droplet nuclei are formed from large droplets as they evaporate while suspended in the air around a spicule of dust. In most cases it has not been possible to demonstrate by air sampling the presence of virus in aerosols, but this mechanism is assumed to operate because of the ability of a virus to infect large numbers. These are the true viral aerosols: the small droplets are able to stay in the air and remain suspended long enough to infect occupants of an entire naval vessel or aircraft with influenza, or to transmit smallpox from one infected person to another through the air-conditioning system of a hospital (Wehrle et al. 1970; Moser et al. 1979). The small droplets also have the ability to reach into the lower respiratory tract, which influences the character of illness that results.

The issue of whether aerosol spread occurs affects control strategies. Natural smallpox was eradicated by ring vaccination, that is, vaccinating those exposed to a case. However, aerosol transmission may rarely occur naturally and could take place in a terrorist incident. The difference in results of mathematical models about how many individuals should be vaccinated in anticipation of an incident is in large part a result of different opinions about how many susceptibles a case can infect (Fauci 2002).

QUANTIFICATION OF CHARACTERISTICS OF VIRAL INFECTION

Infectious dose and secondary attack rate

Epidemiology provides definitions that help to quantify the occurrence of infection and disease in a population. Experimental infection of laboratory animals is always accompanied by quantification; similarly, for work in human infection and disease, quantification is needed. However, because the situation is typically observational and not experimental, different terms and definitions are used. For example, to calculate the infectious dose required to initiate infection in animals, a 50 percent infectious dose (ID_{50}) is determined by inoculation of serial dilutions. Except for certain self-limited infections such as those caused by the rhinoviruses, such experimental studies cannot be carried out in humans (Tyrrell et al. 1960). Even when experimental infection of humans is ethically possible, there are always questions concerning their comparability with those that occur naturally. Such questions apply to experimental studies of influenza, where large droplet inoculation in the nose does not mimic the aerosol spread of natural infection in which the lower respiratory tract is exposed.

The epidemiological measure historically used to approximate indirectly the infectivity of an agent in humans is the so-called secondary attack rate (SAR). It is more than a measure of infectivity: it describes numerically the communicability of a contagious disease, which is in part related to the ID_{50} of the virus but is also affected by loss of viability during transmission and the susceptibility of the recipient. An index or primary case is identified in a family or other similar semi-closed group. Cases that subsequently occur in the group during the incubation period (the time between inoculation and development of illness) are regarded as secondary; those that occur before are considered co-primary, i.e. a separate introduction into the group. The denominator for the calculation is based on the total number in the group less the index or co-primary cases. Other variations are possible, especially when using laboratory data to identify those truly at risk of infection or illness – i.e. those without prior evidence of infection such as antibody and therefore susceptible to infection. The classic calculation of the SAR is most appropriate for diseases with relatively long incubation periods, such as rubella and mumps. A problem arises with diseases of shorter incubation period (approximately 2–4 days), such as influenza and the common cold, in which it is difficult to distinguish between co-primary and secondary cases because they are only days apart or may overlap. It is possible mathematically to model transmission: if infection rates are known for sufficient numbers of families to be representative of the community, statistical methods can be used to adjust the observed, or so-called apparent, SAR by the probability of acquiring from the community a new infection that had seemed to be a secondary case (Longini et al. 1982). Among infections of high SAR are measles and chickenpox. Rubella is less contagious, thus leaving residual susceptibles among young women entering childbearing age (Sever et al. 1964).

Pathogenicity and virulence

'Pathogenicity' sometimes compares the capacity of different organisms to cause disease, whereas 'virulence' compares the severity of disease caused by different strains of the same organism (see Chapter 13, Pathogenesis of viral infections). Here, these terms are specified somewhat differently. In the epidemiological sense, 'pathogenicity' is the proportion of total infections that produce overt disease, which varies from virus to virus and may be affected by host factors (e.g. prior infection with the agent). 'Virulence' here indicates the capacity

of a pathogen to produce severe disease. The likelihood of a fatal outcome is calculated as the case-fatality rate or ratio. It is not a true rate, which should cover a specific period, but is in fact a proportion, the denominator being represented by all recognized cases and the numerator by all deaths included in the denominator. Case fatality is high in many hantavirus and filovirus infections; it still is 100 percent in clinical cases of rabies, with rare and often questionable exceptions (Hattwick et al. 1972; Peters et al. 1994). There have been attempts to quantify virulence other than as case fatality, which has the disadvantage of not being a fixed quantity but one that can be reduced in most situations by appropriate treatment. Also, many diseases with the capacity to produce severe illness infrequently cause death; thus the measure is not a good indication of virulence. A persistent problem in quantifying severity is defining exactly what is meant by this term. In contrast, death as an endpoint is unambiguous. Polio is an illustration of the relative independence of pathogenicity and virulence; the disease is potentially very severe or virulent if it occurs, but only 0.1–1 percent of infections are symptomatic. Therefore the virus would be considered of relatively low pathogenicity but of relatively high virulence (Melnick and Ledinko 1951).

OBSERVATIONAL EPIDEMIOLOGY

Viral infections in person, place, and time

Many epidemiological studies of infections involve description of the occurrence of disease and identification of factors that appear to be related to their distribution. Description is the first phase of an epidemiological investigation. It accepts that there is in fact an infection problem and permits development of hypotheses concerning etiology, risk factors, and other variables determining distribution. These relationships may be investigated further in analytical studies. Occurrence of the infectious disease can be described on the basis of a number of criteria. For some conditions, a case definition may be used: a list of signs and symptoms that are required before a case is recognized. Laboratory confirmation may or may not be included in this definition. Sometimes the aim is to identify inapparent infections as well as cases of disease. Here the criteria may be based on laboratory data only, such as virus identification or significant change in antibody titer.

PERSONAL FACTORS

Descriptions of infections or diseases are made in terms of their occurrence in person, place, and time. Whilst temporal, geographical, and personal factors are interrelated, it is useful to examine each separately as a systematic way of describing the occurrence of an infectious disease. Age is the most important personal determinant of disease because of development and ageing of the immune system, accumulation of exposures over time, and behavioral changes that affect the likelihood of exposure to infectious agents. It is impossible to generalize how age affects pathogenicity or virulence. Hepatitis A and polio are typically mild in young children and become increasingly virulent as children become young adults. Polio emerged as a recognized problem in northern and western Europe only at the end of the nineteenth century. It was called infantile paralysis because it infected mainly the very young, but as time passed it also caused disease in older children. In developing countries the process is being repeated; polio infections often occur in the first 6 months of life, modified by the universal presence of maternal antibody, but the disease is now also present in older children (Nathanson and Martin 1979). Hepatitis A has had a similar progression as the age at the time of infection has changed. In contrast, respiratory viruses such as respiratory syncytial virus (RSV) and parainfluenza produce the most severe disease in young children. In the USA, the median age of infants hospitalized because of RSV is 3 months (Parrott et al. 1973).

The proportion of those infected who develop overt disease also falls with increasing age, in part as the result of repeated exposure to those agents that have the capacity to reinfect with regularity (Monto and Lim 1971). Previous exposures result in a spectrum of outcomes ranging from asymptomatic infection to disease of diminished severity. Other personal factors affecting outcomes of infection are listed in Table 18.2.

Position in the family affects the occurrence of infections best transmitted in that setting (e.g. the respiratory viruses and enteric agents such as the rotaviruses). An only child in a family will experience lower rates of respiratory infection until other siblings are born (Monto and Ross 1977). Other exposures, such as in day care, may increase the probability of the youngest child acquiring an agent which can then be introduced into and spread within the family (Bartlett et al.

Table 18.2 *Examples of personal factors important in viral illness*

Personal factors
Age and gender
Position in family – birth order
Income
Education
Crowding
Socioeconomic status
Occupation – exposures
Genetic and related factors
Immunity
Nutrition

1985). There is evidence that this pattern of occurrence is common with hepatitis A; in fact, community-wide outbreaks of hepatitis A have frequently been traced to day care transmission (Matson et al. 1989). Occupational exposure plays a role in the acquisition of, for example, sylvatic or jungle yellow fever by people working in the forest. The risk from rabies among veterinarians is another type of occupational exposure, but such infections do not result in further dissemination.

FACTORS RELATED TO PLACE

Place of occurrence of viral infection may be related to purely local biological or physical factors. Regional characteristics such as climate and resident flora and fauna determine whether transmission can take place. Most arboviruses are found in specific locations, determined by the distribution of the appropriate vectors or animal hosts. Sometimes the range of a particular agent is quite limited, minor ecological variation producing a niche where transmission can take place. Similarly, agents that are transmitted mainly among animals are limited to the range of that particular animal. Humans are often infected only incidentally, having been in the area where transmission is occurring to the animal hosts or vectors. Infections of animals in which humans are not involved in the major cycle of transmission but are occasionally infected are termed zoonoses.

Other physical or biological environmental factors determine whether common source outbreaks, such as those produced by hepatitis A or E from contaminated water, can occur at a particular location. Generally, special situations in the area, such as sewage outflows or substandard wells are responsible. The presence of an individual in certain locations such as a hospital could result in transmission of hepatitis B in those parts of the world where nosocomial transmission still occurs. In certain areas of Africa where the Ebola virus is present, being in a hospital adds greatly to risk (Baron et al. 1981). Events seemingly associated with place are often equally related to person or to time. Clusters of illnesses are sometimes detected, indicating that transmission of infection is taking place in a particular location. For a cluster to be recognized the transmission must occur over a limited period of time. Such a cluster may involve everyone in that location or may be limited to certain individuals. Reports of clusters are an important alert that unusual transmission is taking place. The first cases of acquired immune deficiency syndrome (AIDS) were detected as simultaneous clusters, in several cities, of a disease producing Kaposi's sarcoma or opportunistic infections in young homosexual men (Gottlieb et al. 1981; Friedman-Kien et al. 1982). The existence of these clusters focused attention on an infectious etiology of the disease, which at the time was thought by some to have other causes such as exposure to environmental toxins or to drugs. HIV transmission was later found to be the explanation.

TEMPORAL FACTORS: CLASSIFICATION OF OUTBREAKS

Time of occurrence may be the most systematically evaluated of the three factors. Much of the terminology used in epidemiology has a temporal component. The terms epidemic, endemic, and sporadic do not have any statistical definitions but simply mean, respectively, occurrence of an infection at a higher than expected frequency, at the expected frequency, or only rarely and in seemingly unconnected fashion. Another term frequently used, also without statistical definition, is pandemic, meaning an epidemic appearing in many geographic locations at about the same time. The term has been used for influenza outbreaks occurring on a global scale following appearance of variants with a new hemagglutinin or a new hemagglutinin and new neuraminidase. It is now appropriately applied to HIV/AIDS which has involved all continents in its inexorable spread (World Health Organization/Global Program on AIDS 1994). The years this has taken contrasts with the months needed for an influenza pandemic to involve the whole world. This contrasting pattern is related to differences in transmission characteristics between HIV, spread by direct contact, and influenza, transmitted by droplet and airborne routes.

The characteristics of outbreaks are described according to the occurrence of cases over time. These characteristics are generally studied by creating an epidemic curve, with cases on the ordinate and time (in days or hours, depending on the speed of development) on the abscissa. Figure 18.1 shows the pattern of a point source outbreak of Norovovirus infection in which all individuals were exposed at the same time and either became infected and ill with diarrheal disease or remained well (Warner et al. 1991). The group exposed was large (3 000 people) and the attack rate, at 48 percent, was high. The times of onset were divided into 4-h intervals. The suspect meal in question was consumed at noon on

Monday; illnesses reported earlier are viewed as baseline cases of diarrhea unrelated to the exposure. Such cases are typical in investigations of a common illness such as gastroenteritis, which can be produced by many agents. The time from the exposure to the peak of the outbreak is the mean incubation period of the pathogen, in this case 40 h. The peak occurred during the 4-h period beginning at 5 a.m., Wednesday.

If the source remains infectious for a time, the outbreak may continue. The new cases are still being infected from the source and the outbreak may now be better termed common rather than point source. A contaminated well is an example of a common source. With viruses such as hepatitis A or Norwalk-like agents, cases may arise in lower numbers even when the source is no longer infectious. Such continued occurrence is possible only for viruses that can also spread from person to person, a different type of transmission. Pure point source outbreaks assume exposure from one site or at one point in time, the time from exposure to peak being the median incubation period. In contrast, in propagated source outbreaks the infectious agents spread exclusively from person to person. Spread may be by different transmission mechanisms, often large droplet. Even with influenza, which may be transmitted by the more efficient airborne route, one person can infect only two or three individuals, and the outbreak takes 6–10 weeks (or more) to move through a community. It should be remembered that the incubation period of the infection is only 2–4 days, so many generations of spread occur until the outbreak has run its course (Monto and Kioumehr 1975).

Many infectious diseases such as hepatitis A and rubella do not occur at uniform levels in populations but undergo predictable changes in frequency. Certain terms are used to describe these changes. Seasonal variation describes the phenomenon, well recognized with the respiratory viruses, of much higher frequency in colder than in warmer months. Other seasonal variations are less obvious, with rubella generally increasing (before vaccine control) in the spring and hepatitis A in the fall. In temperate zones, transmission of rotavirus takes place almost exclusively during cold weather. Figure 18.2 shows 5 years of data from the study of young children hospitalized for diarrhea in Washington DC (Brandt et al. 1983). Hospitalizations over all are most common in colder months. Cyclical variation refers to changes of frequency over periods of years, with gradual increases in intensity of transmission. Hepatitis A, for example, has a cycle of 5–7 years. This means that, when intensity of transmission is increasing, illness in the autumn is more frequent than in the previous autumn. The term 'cycle' also implies that there is not only a waxing but also a waning period. In contrast, the term 'secular' is used to indicate long-term trends, which can be unidirectional in nature. The time periods involved must be long, generally more than 10 years.

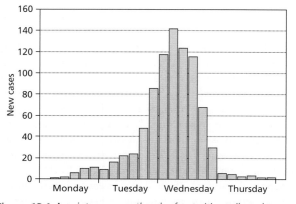

Figure 18.1 *A point source outbreak of enteritis attributed to Norvovirus after a meal eaten at noon, Monday. Onset of illness (moving means) shown in intervals of 4 h (from Warner et al. 1991).*

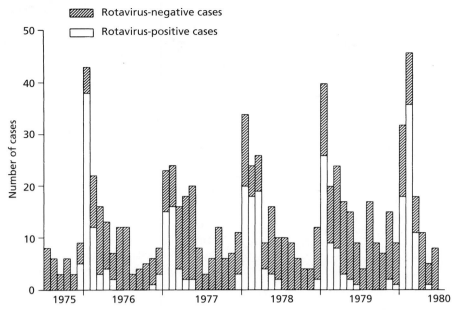

Figure 18.2 *Distribution by month over a 5-year period of children hospitalized for gastroenteritis and the proportions rotavirus-positive. Children's Hospital National Medical Center, Washington DC (from Brandt et al. 1983).*

Incidence and prevalence

INCIDENCE

Two critical terms used in epidemiology that have temporal definitions are incidence and prevalence. 'Incidence' is the number of new cases of a disease arising during a fixed period in a population of given size; for example, 1 000 or 10 000 individuals. Incidence is sometimes further specified as either a cumulative incidence which expresses incidence as a risk or probability, or as an incidence density which does so as a rate.

These terms, whilst often used interchangeably, provide two types of information (Kleinbaum et al. 1982). Risk is the probability of a disease-free person developing the disease of interest over a defined time and not dying from any other disease during that period. As a probability, risk can have values between zero and one. Risk is measured as cumulative incidence, the proportion of the study population becoming ill in a given period: for example, 'the risk of becoming ill with influenza-like illness in the study population was 12.8/ 1 000 persons per year.' The need to specify a period can be appreciated by looking at the extreme case of mortality from all causes. If a cohort of 1 000 subjects is followed for 120 years, the risk of dying during this period will be 1 000/1 000 per 120 years. However, during any 1 year of this period, the risk of dying will be much smaller. Thus, when applied to a vectorborne infection, risk of acquiring dengue over a 4-month mosquito season in an endemic area might be 10/100, but only 1.2/100 for a given week. The term attack rate is a cumulative incidence measure used to describe the number in a defined population who become infected or ill during the period of transmission of an agent; for example, the number of children infected with measles in the course of a school outbreak, using the number of susceptible children as the denominator of the proportion. This is more properly termed a risk, and is an example of cumulative incidence. The secondary attack rate, described above, is also an example of such a risk.

In contrast to risk, the incidence rate, sometimes called incidence density, describes the occurrence of new cases in the population per unit of time. Incidence density is most useful for testing epidemiological hypotheses when a long time is needed to follow a cohort to estimate risk, as in most chronic conditions and in some population-based studies of infection. The rate over a period of time is typically estimated using person-time as the denominator of the rate calculation. Person-time is the amount of time each study subject contributes to a study before becoming ill or leaving the study for some reason. Sometimes new individuals may be added to the study population. Figure 18.3 illustrates the calculation of person-time. Among ten people who were followed over differing periods of time, two cases of disease developed. In the incidence density calculation, eight subjects completed the study, each contributing 12 person-months or a total of 96 person-months. Subjects 3 and 7 contributed 6 and 10 person-months, respectively, before becoming ill. The number of new cases (two) divided by the total number of person-months (112) yields a rate of 2/112 or 1.78/100 person-months. Dividing person-months by 12 would give person-years. Thus, the above translates to a rate of 1.78/8.33 person-months or 21/100 person-years. The same data could be used for an incidence density calculation for ten subjects at risk. The data would give a rate

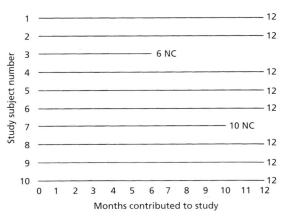

Figure 18.3 *Hypothetical 1-year study of ten individuals. Two new cases (NC) of disease developed during this period, giving a risk calculation of 2/10 per year and a rate calculation of 2.1/10 person-years.*

of two new cases per ten persons at risk, or 20/100 per year. The differences between the risk and rate calculations, while small, would have been greater with more cases developing or if the study had been carried out for a longer period.

PREVALENCE

The other important term, prevalence, is used less often when dealing with acute illnesses. Most often, the concept is defined as point prevalence, the point here being an arbitrary point in time. In prevalence, it is not new but existing cases that are identified, thus the ideal would be to enumerate them as a simultaneous count. Again the denominator is the population at risk from which the cases are drawn. Enumeration of all cases of AIDS existing in the population of interest at one time, whatever their date of onset, would provide a prevalence rate (Elandt-Johnson 1975).

Prevalence is often used in viral epidemiology when doing serological surveys based on collecting one specimen per person. Serum banks have been established to reflect past experience with infectious diseases in a population. Ideally, the specimens should be representative of the population from which they have been drawn. Antibody present at a specific titer in a population sample collected to represent all age groups will indicate the pattern of past infection. For certain agents, such as arboviruses present intermittently in a geographical area, and for other more common agents such as measles in isolated populations, age-specific prevalence will indicate when infection was last present in that population, the years of birth of the youngest cohort with antibody indicating the last period of spread of the agent (Black 1989). Documenting the occurrence of influenza A subtypes over the last century is another example of use of antibody prevalence. Antibody present in sera, collected before the appearance of a new subtype of type A, has been taken as evidence for

the spread of that subtype many years before (Masurel and Marine 1973). When seroepidemiology is carried out with paired sera, change in antibody titer can be sought between two specimens collected from the same individual. The results are the equivalent to incidence, not prevalence, because they indicate that a new infection has occurred in the interval. This is also the case when examining IgM antibody in a single specimen for agents such as hepatitis A, known to produce that antibody for only a short time and thus indicating recent infection.

Monitoring and surveillance

The descriptive variables time, place, and person are employed in monitoring and surveillance of viral disease. For infections that occur regularly the intention is to detect unusual increases. The expected frequency of these conditions, identified either by laboratory tests or on the basis of standard case definitions of illness, can be calculated. An example of the latter involves the use in the USA of reported deaths from pneumonia and influenza (P&I) from 121 cities. The reports are based on a list of specific causes of death, not on the laboratory detection of influenza infection, and are calculated weekly as a proportion of total deaths. Results of the method are shown in Figure 18.4, with distribution of isolates by type in each of the influenza seasons. The P&I mortality curve has three components: the expected value, the threshold value (1.65 S.D. above the expected) and the actual values observed in the various cities. The expected values are a mathematical expression of past observed values derived from observations of periods without influenza transmission (Serfling 1963). They are higher in winter months than in summer, because of other noninfluenza causes of pneumonia deaths that increase at the same time, such as those caused by primary bacterial infections. As can be seen in Figure 18.4, in some years the observed mortality considerably exceeds the threshold level for several weeks. Typically, these are years in which there is considerable transmission of type A(H3N2) virus (Eickhoff et al. 1961). In some years (not shown in the figure), excess mortality has also occurred with type B transmission, but this is observed less frequently (Nolan et al. 1980). When examining the data in Figure 18.4, it is important to realize that the mortality data are the result of clinical diagnoses at the time of death, i.e. without laboratory evidence that the death was related to influenza. Thus the data for laboratory surveillance on which the annual distribution of isolates is based can be viewed as an independent determination. Only influenza produces this characteristic increase in mortality. The phenomenon is remarkable because the data are collected nationally in a country as large as the USA, in which outbreaks do not necessarily occur synchronously in different regions (Glezen et al. 1982). Similar systems

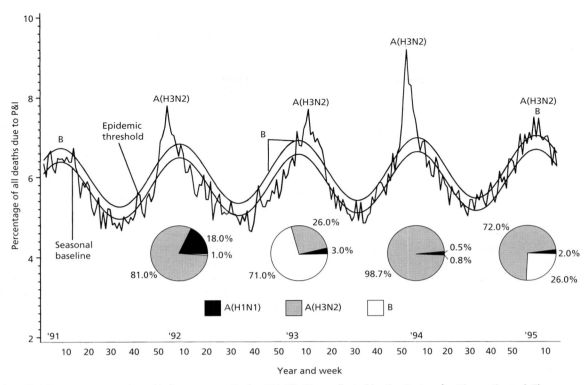

Figure 18.4 *Data on pneumonia and influenza mortality for 121 US cities, collected by the Centers for Disease Control. The curve indicates the observed mortality data, superimposed on the seasonal baseline and epidemic threshold. Also shown are the distributions of influenza isolates from specimens collected independently during the four seasons.*

are in use in other parts of the world, the data on virus circulation being based on collection of specimens in standard surveillance systems based in physicians' practices (Johnson et al. 1991).

Other diseases only rarely increase in frequency sufficiently to become noticeable in data collected nationally. Most infections are likely to be more localized, and the detection of outbreaks is based on the recognition of the unusual occurrence of cases in time, place or person. Outbreaks are variously defined according to expected occurrence; for some entities a single case may be so unusual as to produce an outbreak investigation. Rabies cases in areas of developed countries where this disease is unusual will be investigated on the basis of a single event. The virus causing hantavirus pulmonary syndrome was recognized and identified as a newly emerging pathogen in southeastern USA on the basis of deaths and severe illnesses clustered in time, place, and, in part, person (Centers for Disease Control 1994). The regional nature of the outbreak contributed to its recognition; had the same number of cases occurred in a wider area, they would have gone unnoticed. As with other similar situations, prospective surveillance initiated after identification of the 'new' virus suggested that it had occurred at low frequency in the past, and that recognition was due to an unusual natural event that produced a cluster of cases; in the case of the hantavirus pulmonary syndrome, the increase in food available for

the rodent hosts resulted in their proliferation and an increased likelihood of interfacing with humans. The spread of West Nile virus through much of the United States is an example of a contrary situation. It represented a new introduction into a continent where it had not existed before and was originally recognized because of the clustering of cases. However, the extensive subsequent spread is a result in part because of lack of immunity in the population (Petersen et al. 2002).

Primary analytical methods

CASE–CONTROL STUDIES

The descriptive phases of epidemiological investigations generate hypotheses about factors influencing the occurrence of a disease. Analytical studies then follow, and may involve formal outbreak investigations or more elaborate longitudinal studies. The investigations have in common the use of specific study designs. These designs are divided into case–control and cohort studies. In the first, cases of the disease or outcome being studied are identified and controls without the particular outcome are selected by matching or similar methods to be comparable to the cases in age and other characteristics. Past exposures or risk factors are then examined to determine if they are associated with the disease (Schlesselman 1982). In contrast, in the cohort design individuals are selected according to characteristics other than presence of the disease or infection of interest. They are followed over time and cases of the disease outcome are observed (Breslow and Day 1987).

Case–control studies can be relatively straightforward in their design and produce results quickly because all the exposures and outcomes have already occurred. The investigation of an outbreak of an infectious disease is generally case–control in nature, one group having the disease and the comparison group not having it. For example, an outbreak of vomiting and diarrhea occurred in a group outing on an American lake where food was served in common and where many had gone swimming (Koopman et al. 1982). Individuals who developed disease according to a case definition were compared with those who did not. The food intake and other exposures of the cases and the controls were then compared. There was no significant difference between cases and controls in terms of foods consumed or other relevant characteristics. However, swimming in the lake, especially with the head submerged, was the risk factor that was more common in those who developed diarrhea compared to those who did not, and the differences were statistically significant. Furthermore, some samples, when available, showed rises in titer for the Norvovirus, suggesting that it was the agent responsible. In this sort of outbreak investigation, the group studied is small. However, it is very important that the cases and controls have similar possibilities of exposure; in this case, people not at the lake would be ineligible.

Larger and more elaborate case–control studies were used to confirm the role of rubella as a cause of congenital anomalies. The original description of clusters of congenital anomalies involving the eyes, and then the heart, ears, and other organs occurring in children whose mothers had experienced rubella in pregnancy allowed development of an etiological hypothesis (Gregg 1941; Swan et al. 1946). The clusters seemed to be related to the epidemic behavior of rubella, since frequency of the abnormality increased cyclically when rubella was widespread (Sever et al. 1965). Many of the initial studies were simply a series of cases. For the analytical studies, cases were children with certain types of abnormalities

identified at birth or shortly thereafter and controls were children without abnormalities born in the same locations. Pregnancy histories of mothers of both case and control children were obtained; because rubella and other conditions of interest do not generally result either in a doctor being consulted or in hospitalization, data are generally obtained by interviewing the mothers. This has a disadvantage of introducing potential recall bias: mothers know whether their children had birth defects or were normal and, if the former, are more likely to remember every event that might possibly have been related to the defect (Klemetti and Saxen 1967). Methods can sometimes be developed to try to validate these reported events. If possible, medical or other records collected before the birth are used. By their very nature, case–control studies are nearly always retrospective: cases and controls are identified on the basis of the outcome, and the prior factors determining the development or nondevelopment of the disease are compared. Table 18.3 lists some of the advantages and disadvantages of the basic study designs. Accurate recall of previous events is an inherent problem with case–control studies because of knowledge of the outcome. The design has other attractive features: it is highly cost efficient, especially for outcomes that are relatively rare. Cases can be gathered easily and, because they have already occurred, the study can be carried out quite quickly. Another inherent problem of the design, however, is the selection of controls. Controls should be similar to the cases in all characteristics except the disease in question. This is often difficult to achieve and questions are always raised about this point. Typically there are two choices of populations from which to draw controls: hospital databases or the community. Each has its own advantages and disadvantages. In the study of infectious diseases, controls must have similar probabilities of exposure to the infections as the cases. In terms of, for example, rubella, cases and controls must have the same opportunity to be exposed and to experience rubella, which varies by both time and place in intensity of transmission. The case–control studies concluded that there was a high level of association between rubella in the first trimester of pregnancy and

Table 18.3 *Advantages and disadvantages of study designs*

Advantages	Disadvantages
Case–control	
Efficiency – results rapidly available	Selection of comparable controls
Superior for rare outcome	Recall problems
Relatively inexpensive	Validity of recorded data
Cohort studies	
Reduction in potential bias	Duration – may be long
Greater ability to generalize results	Greater expense
No necessity to select healthy comparable controls	Uncertainty of adequate numbers and loss to follow-up
	Rare diseases require large numbers

fetal malformations. That association was very strong and suggested that the risk of fetal malformation was greater than 50 percent in some studies, in one case 80 percent (Pitt 1957; Ingalls et al. 1960) (see also Chapter 45, Rubella).

COHORT STUDIES

Cohort studies are generally undertaken after case–control studies indicate the likelihood of an association between a particular exposure and disease outcome. With rubella, these studies began relatively early, because of recognition of biases associated with obtaining histories on the cases. Such investigations are typically prospective in nature, and allow collection of data as new events occur, thus minimizing the possibility of recall bias. However, they must generally be larger with sufficient participants to allow for reasonable numbers of dropouts, and must last long enough to achieve the necessary numbers of events. As a precondition, the outcome of interest must be so frequent that the group followed does not need to be too large or followed for too long. For all these reasons, cohort studies are carried out less frequently than case–control studies because they are more expensive and problematic in terms of producing the required number of observations. However, when feasible, they are powerful evidence for confirming results of case–control studies, as many sources of bias can be avoided and there is not the problem of selecting comparable controls.

In this design the cohort is the population unit selected for study. The only requirement is that the selection cannot be on the basis of disease outcome or anything that might be closely related to the disease. Typically the unit may be individuals in an occupational group, such as nurses or physicians or people living in a certain area. In the case of rubella, two kinds of cohort studies have been carried out (Manson et al. 1960; Sever et al. 1969). In the most powerful design, all children born during specific periods in particular hospitals were studied. Because all children born at the appropriate time were eligible, there was no need to identify controls, and all adverse outcomes of pregnancy could be followed in the cohort. Some mothers would have been exposed to rubella and might therefore give birth to children born with malformations. Most would not.

Another cohort design attempts to minimize the number of nonexposed women who would have to be included. This method identifies an exposure cohort (mother exposed to rubella) and a comparison cohort of mothers not exposed. Note that the selection here is based not on the outcome, congenital abnormalities, as would be the situation in a case–control study, but on exposures, so this remains a cohort study. There is no issue of recall bias because the comparison group is selected on documented lack of exposure. However, it has the potential problem of not being as representative as if all individuals, rather than a selected subgroup, were followed up. Estimates of the risk of maternal rubella in the first trimester in producing malformations was as low as 7–17 percent in some cohort studies, although others felt that, depending on length of follow-up and definitions used it might actually be higher (Jackson and Fisch 1958; Lundstrom 1962). This reduction in risk estimation had public health implications before the vaccine era, because pregnancies were often terminated after maternal rubella. From an epidemiological standpoint, cohort studies are better than case–control studies in providing data and results that can be generalized to the population of interest so that appropriate decisions can be made.

OTHER USES OF ANALYTICAL STUDIES

Although vaccines are usually evaluated by randomized controlled trials, an experimental study design involving an intervention, observational designs can also be employed successfully to evaluate the effectiveness of vaccines. The term 'efficacy' is generally employed for results of randomized trials; 'effectiveness' is used to indicate the results of observations when the intervention is in general use, especially when the outcome is not a laboratory-confirmed infection but a clinical diagnosis. The latter sort of study is the only type possible when, as is the case in North America for influenza vaccine for the elderly, ethical considerations preclude use of a placebo and questions still exist as to the value of the preparation. The observational design does not require that vaccine be denied to part of the group, as would be the case if a placebo were employed. The purpose of using inactivated influenza vaccine in older people is to prevent serious complications of the disease, especially those requiring hospitalization. However, unless a large population can be followed, these hospitalizations do not occur sufficiently often to allow the use of the cohort design. For this reason, two multi-year case–control studies were carried out, one in the USA and the other in Canada (Foster et al. 1992; Fedson et al. 1993; Ohmit and Monto 1995). The exact designs varied, but in both cases the influenza season was identified and possible influenza complications were defined from hospital records. Recognizing the need for generalization of results, both studies were designed to select their controls not from hospitals but from comparable community residents. In both, the vaccine was found to be significantly effective in preventing hospitalization, and, in the Canadian study, in preventing deaths in the influenza seasons coded as being related to respiratory diseases. Another study used a cohort design to confirm these findings (Nichol et al. 1994). As expected, many people needed to be followed up. The effectiveness of the vaccine was comparable with that in the previous case–control investigations. That several differently designed nonexperimental studies came to similar conclusions is convincing evidence that the results in a single investigation were not simply a chance occurrence.

Observational studies to confirm etiology

Koch's postulates in their various forms were the first systematic approach for determining that a pathogen caused a disease (Rivers 1937). They were formulated after early observations that simply isolating an agent from an individual with a particular disease did not necessarily mean that the agent caused that disease. The postulates were based on experiments, provided that disease could be reproduced in laboratory animals. They did not allow for asymptomatic infection because they stated that the agent should always produce disease. They also assumed that the potential pathogen had a unique role in producing a disease: only one hepatitis virus could produce hepatitis. We now know that clinical syndromes can frequently be caused by a variety of agents and that clinical manifestations of infection vary greatly in terms of age and other factors, so it might not seem that the same pathogen was involved. In addition, many viruses may not infect experimental animals at all or, if they do, will not produce diseases comparable to those in humans. For this reason, Koch's postulates have been complemented (or modified) by epidemiological studies, usually observational, to confirm etiology. Typically, case–control designs are used, because they are easy to carry out and require smaller numbers of observations. Studies of this sort are particularly necessary when dealing with agents that produce chronic infections.

Another problem occurs when a potential pathogen is shed for prolonged periods from people who have had an illness in the past, or after an asymptomatic infection. Agents may be isolated from individuals who develop another illness, and thought, incorrectly, to cause the current instead of the preceding illness. This misconception can occur with the herpesviruses. At the very least, an agent must be identified significantly more frequently in cases with the disease than in comparable controls. This analytical design assumes that asymptomatic or chronic infection will occur and that some controls will be virus positive, but not as frequently as cases. Etiological association of infectious mononucleosis with Epstein–Barr virus (EBV) was difficult to accomplish, because of continuing shedding of the virus (Hallee et al. 1974). Even more difficult has been the demonstration of the association of hepatitis B virus with primary hepatocellular carcinoma, because of the long period between infection and development of the disease (Beasley 1982).

When observational approaches, rather than experimentation, are used to demonstrate etiology, additional standards are generally applied to assist in deciding that there is a statistically significant etiological relationship

between a disease and an agent or other potential precipitation factor. These standards were developed to evaluate the relationship between environmental exposure and chronic diseases, specifically cigarette smoking and lung cancer. They apply equally to viral infection (Hill 1965). There must always be a proper temporal relationship: the putative etiological factor is present before the disease occurs. This point is not particularly difficult to understand; in fact, there is often a tendency to assume an etiological role on the basis of a simple temporal relationship. It is further required that the etiological agent must have a scientifically logical role in the disease it is thought to cause. In other words, hepatitis B virus has a logical role in producing chronic liver disease, whereas it would be difficult to hypothesize such a role for the influenza virus. Strength of the association is also critical; i.e. if the associations are strongly statistically significant, an etiological role is more likely. Most critical, as illustrated by the examples given above, is reproducibility of results. Consistent results from different study designs are strong evidence of an etiological association.

The road to demonstrating etiology involves an initial hypothesis and a series of studies. Such a road can be followed in the demonstration in North America of the role of aspirin in the production of Reye's syndrome. The syndrome is a combination of encephalopathy and acute liver abnormalities involving mitochondrial damage. It was recognized for many years to be an unusual complication of various infections, mainly influenza and chickenpox, occurring a few days after the acute illness. Why it happened in a small proportion of infected children was unknown. Descriptive studies suggested that aspirin ingestion might be involved, but this notion was rejected by many investigators because of lack of a clear dose–response relationship (Starko et al. 1982). However, the characteristics of aspirin intoxication provided a credible scientific basis for the relationship. A series of independent case–control studies demonstrated such a statistically strong and consistent role for aspirin that the last study was suspended in the pilot phase and an educational program was begun (Halpin et al. 1982; Waldman et al. 1982; Hurwitz et al. 1985). Cohort studies were not carried out because Reye's syndrome was too rare to allow use of that design and the associations in the case–control studies were so strong.

EXPERIMENTAL EPIDEMIOLOGY

Simulations

Although most contributions of epidemiology to our understanding of viral infections are observational, experimental approaches are often useful in understanding relationships not defined by other methods. Two will be considered: one involving actual interventions and the other involving simulations. The latter method has mainly been applied to modeling transmission and epidemics mathematically and identifying the effects of various interventions that might be used to prevent or interrupt the outbreaks of infection. Mathematical models have evolved from rather simple approaches ranging from the use of balls to simulate individuals (Monte Carlo models) to elaborate computer structures designed to resemble a community with families and schools that mix with each other. The two basic types are deterministic models, which use differential equations, and stochastic models, which use random number generation to approximate the manner in which events take place naturally (Abbey 1952; Bailey 1957). The latter type of simulation is now easier with use of powerful computers so that many replications can be carried out. One of the first infections to be studied with these methods was influenza. Simulations were performed to determine the effects of, for example, vaccinating school age children with influenza vaccine (Elveback et al. 1976; Longini et al. 1977). As demonstrated in one experiment, vaccination of school age children increased immunity, sometimes termed herd immunity, in the segment of the population most responsible for introducing the virus into families and spreading it in the community (Monto et al. 1970). The result was not only protection of the vaccinated children but also interruption of transmission, which indirectly protected the rest of the community. Simulation modeling has also been applied to HIV transmission and AIDS forecasting, and has been particularly valuable, given the long-term nature of the infection and the difficulty in predicting spread (Hethcote et al. 1991). Most recently, it has been especially useful in assessing the effects that vaccination could have on the future occurrence of the disease.

Controlled trials

The most accepted intervention study in infectious disease epidemiology is the randomized controlled trial. Traditionally, the intervention has been vaccination, although more recently antivirals have frequently been studied. Methods for randomized clinical trials have been the subject of a number of reviews and comments, and the many issues and approaches will not be discussed here (Spilker 1991). The endpoint for acute illnesses is generally prevention of the disease. The efficacy of hepatitis B vaccine was evaluated by antibody production and prevention of acute disease in populations of homosexual males (Szmuness et al. 1975). The design was a randomized, controlled trial. The group chosen for study was at high risk of infection and the study could be concluded in a short period of time. Potentially eligible participants were screened and only those without antibody were included. The frequencies of infection and disease at various periods after vaccina-

tion were compared in those who received the active preparation and those who received placebo. The results demonstrated the value of this vaccine in primary prevention. In addition to protecting against acute infection in adults living in developed countries, the vaccine is now used in developing countries, not only to prevent the acute illness but mainly to prevent primary hepatocellular carcinoma. If this tumor decreases in frequency as a result of vaccination, it will be ultimate proof of etiology. Similarly, with Reye's syndrome, education about the role of aspirin in the disease resulted in decreased use. Reye's syndrome has nearly disappeared in areas where it was previously common, adding further evidence for an etiological connection (Remington et al. 1986). Certain potential etiological relationships have bedeviled investigators for many years. It was thought that certain viral infections trigger attacks of asthma in sensitive children. The data are better for children than for adults, and, in both, rhinoviruses seem to be the virus most frequently involved (Mcintosh et al. 1973; Minor et al. 1974). Development of PCR techniques which can identify rhinoviruses which cannot be cultivated has helped to document this relationship (Johnston et al. 1995a). A similar situation applies to triggering exacerbations of chronic respiratory disease in the elderly although the relationship here is more tenuous. If use of an antiviral to prevent or treat rhinoviral infection also reduces episodes of the chronic condition, it would be the final demonstration of an etiological relationship.

EPIDEMIOLOGICAL CHARACTERISTICS OF RESPIRATORY VIRUSES

Causes of common respiratory illnesses

Many viruses are responsible for the bulk of respiratory infections. Although the agents are very different from a virological standpoint, they do share epidemiological characteristics. Being surface infections, they do not produce long-lasting immunity. Instead they have the capacity to reinfect, even without antigenic change (Glezen et al. 1986). Other than influenza (Chapter 32, Orthomyxoviruses: influenza), which can produce severe disease in older children and adults, some viruses such as parainfluenza and RSV (see Chapter 36, Respiroviruses: parainfluenza virus), may cause severe disease in infants and young children on initial infection and mild or inapparent infection indistinguishable from the common cold in older people. Thus, older siblings who introduce a particular infection to the family may contract a mild illness, while the younger child may experience bronchiolitis or pneumonia. RSV is the principal cause of severe lower respiratory illness in young children. The mean age for hospitalization, which occurs in a small proportion of infected children, is 3 months

(Parrott et al. 1973). This early age of onset prompted the hypothesis, later proven to be incorrect, that maternal antibody, which is always present to this ubiquitous virus, is responsible for the pathogenesis of the disease. It has now been shown that children born with the highest titers of maternal antibody are those least likely to develop severe disease (Glezen et al. 1981). As a result, maternal immunization is being examined as a way of modifying the initial infantile infection and the use of immune globulin is being examined for prophylaxis and treatment. Parainfluenza virus types 1 and 2 are the major agents of laryngotracheobronchitis (croup). The peak age for these initial, recognizable infections is later than that for RSV, and the protective effect of maternal antibody was never in doubt (Monto 1973).

Rhinoviruses (Chapter 40, Picornaviruses) and coronaviruses (Chapter 39, Coronaviruses, toroviruses, and arteriviruses), in contrast to RSV and parainfluenzaviruses, produce only coldlike symptoms regardless of whether they infect children or adults. Rhinoviruses, as the principal agents of the common cold, infect individuals many times throughout life. Even in the first years of age, when attention is usually directed to the other agents that may produce lower respiratory infection, the rhinoviruses are more commonly isolated (Monto et al. 1986). Data on the annual incidence of respiratory infections due to all causes were collected from residents of the small community of Tecumseh, Michigan (Monto and Sullivan 1993). These data are shown as curves in Figure 18.5, with results arranged by gender. As can be seen, there is a suggestion of sparing of infants aged <1 year, because of the presence of maternal antibody. Thereafter the frequencies fall off with increasing age, rising again in young adulthood when individuals start their families and are exposed to young children. The higher frequency of illnesses in

females as compared to males is well recognized. In women who work outside the home, the frequency of illness in those aged 20–34 years is higher than in those who do not. Thus continual exposure to children must be a major factor. The age-specific frequency of rhinoviruses roughly parallels these curves. This similarity is a result of the major role of rhinoviruses in the etiology of the common cold and other frequent respiratory illnesses (Monto et al. 1987). Coronaviruses are responsible for illnesses similar to those caused by rhinoviruses. Because they are difficult to isolate and occur much less frequently than the rhinoviruses, much less information is available on their occurrence in populations. Newer tests involving antigen detection may increase our knowledge of their behavior and distribution (MacNaughton 1982).

Respiratory virus infections differ in their seasonality (Monto and Sullivan 1993). Although, overall, viral respiratory infections increase in frequency in cold weather in many geographic areas, isolation of rhinoviruses peaks in the period after schools reopen: children come into contact with each other for long periods and can spread these viruses that require relatively close contact for transmission. Rhinoviruses account for most of the respiratory illnesses in the community at that time. In other geographic areas, although the autumn peak is prominent, another peak of infection in the spring is also recognized (Hendley et al. 1969). Other respiratory viruses have different periods of spread in different regions. In many areas, RSV transmission peaks in winter or early spring and parainfluenza virus in spring and late autumn, the exact occurrence varying by place and by year. Outside the temperate zones, periods of activity are different and must be defined locally. Because person-to-person transmission is always involved, the agents take weeks to move through even a small community.

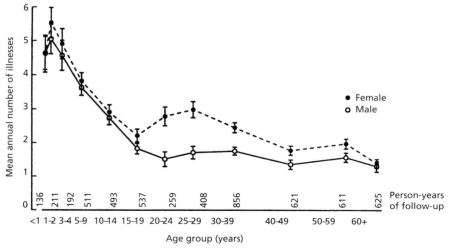

Figure 18.5 *Mean number of respiratory illnesses per person-year (95 percent confidence intervals) in males and females living in Tecumseh, Michigan (from Monto and Sullivan 1993).*

INFLUENZA

Influenza (Chapter 32, Orthomyxoviruses: influenza) is potentially serious in all individuals who develop disease. Infection rates are highest in children and adults who are sufficiently ill to seek medical advice (Monto et al. 1985). However, the elderly and those with chronic illnesses experience the most severe disease, often with complications such as pneumonia (Chin et al. 1960). Reasons for the susceptibility of older individuals are varied, and probably related to depressed cell-mediated immunity (Phair et al. 1978). Because of the danger of illness in older people and those with chronic conditions, vaccination programs in many countries are not intended to prevent infection in the young. Rather, older people are vaccinated as a means of preventing hospitalization or death. As a result, disease in the young, who sustain the major burden of a complicated infection, is not affected, and outbreaks continue. An exception is Japan, where a former policy was designed to limit spread by vaccinating school-age children (Dowdle et al. 1980).

Influenza, like other respiratory agents, is seasonal, no obvious transmission taking place in warmer months of the year in the temperate zones, although asymptomatic infections have been detected serologically, particularly with type A viruses. Outbreaks of influenza in cold seasons can be recognized by various indicators, including increased visits to physicians or school absenteeism. These indicators can be found during major outbreaks of all types and subtypes of influenza; they are a reflection of the high infection frequency in the general population. Transmission of influenza types A(H3N2) and B can also be detected by the ability of these viruses to be fatal in older people and those with high risk conditions. Such deaths, as complications of the primary viral infection, generally occur 2 weeks after the initial episode, so excess mortality is a delayed indication of transmission.

Although seasonal outbreaks of influenza may be caused by one viral type or subtype, mixed or sequential outbreaks of different types may also occur. The viruses appear at various other times in tropical climates, either throughout the year or during the rainy season, and such regions are likely to be the source of new strains. Pandemics of type A influenza take place at irregular intervals following sudden changes in the viral hemagglutinin or the neuraminidase, or both ('antigenic shift'). For a time, it was thought that new viruses with pandemic potential emerged at regular intervals, approximately every 10 years. In retrospect, these conclusions were based on confusion concerning whether a shift in surface antigens had occurred during the period 1918–1956, and observations during only a limited period thereafter. It had always been assumed that, when a type A strain with new surface antigen or antigens emerged, it would totally replace the previous A subtype. In 1977, the A(H1N1) subtype reappeared 20 years after it had been completely replaced in 1957 by type A(H2N2). The type A(H3N2) viruses have been circulating since 1968 and, instead of replacing these viruses, both subtypes have co-circulated since that time. Type A(H1N1) has largely been restricted to the younger segment of the population and type A(H3N2) has occurred in all age groups (Masurel 1976; Kendal et al. 1977).

When pandemics of influenza have followed a shift in type A antigens, the same age-specific morbidity and mortality patterns have been observed as in the annual epidemics of influenza but at much higher frequency. However, in 1918, the pandemic viruses thought, on the basis of serological epidemiology, to be related to swine influenza, produced unusually high mortality in young adults, a group usually experiencing significant morbidity, but little mortality. At least 20 million people died worldwide during this pandemic, which is still a unique and unexplained event, possibly related to unusual bacterial superinfections (Shope 1936). Even with the identification of the hemagglutinin of the 1918 virus, reasons for its higher pathogenesis have not emerged (Taubenberger et al. 1997). Recent pandemic strains of influenza first caused outbreaks of disease in humans in southern China. There, the combination of high population density and animals, especially domestic ducks and pigs, living in close contact with humans, often in the same dwellings, might have been responsible (Kawaoka et al. 1993). Many domestic animals have their own type A influenza viruses, but such infections are not true zoonoses because these viruses are not pathogenic for humans. A recent exception was the spread in Hong Kong of A(H5N1) virus from chickens to humans (Subbarao et al. 1998; Claas et al. 1998).

New pandemic viruses seem to result from reassortment made possible by the segmented genome of the influenza virus. The gene segments coding for the surface antigens of the animal strains replace the comparable segments of the strains pathogenic for humans. The result is a new virus with internal components from the old pathogenic virus but with new hemagglutinin and sometimes a new neuraminidase from the animal strain. Type B influenza viruses do not infect animals, and pandemics of type B do not occur, strengthening the hypothesis of the animal origin of pandemic type A variants. Thus, the only changes seen with type B viruses are gradual year-to-year variations, referred to as 'antigenic drift.' The same drift also occurs with type A strains over the years, in addition to the episodic shift associated with pandemics. This regular drift makes it necessary to incorporate fresh strains in the vaccine, because efficacy drops if there is not a good match between circulating variants and in the vaccine strains. Updating is usually done annually with type A(H3N2) and not as often with type A(H1N1) and type B viruses, reflecting more rapid changes in type A(H3N2).

VIRUSES INFECTING THE GASTROINTESTINAL TRACT

Agents of diarrheal disease

Diarrheal disease in industrialized countries is of varied etiology. Unlike respiratory illnesses, in which viruses are the principal pathogens, enteric illnesses are sometimes of bacterial or parasitic origin, especially when they occur as outbreaks. Much of the disease that occurs more regularly in families is of viral origin and its frequency increases in the cold season, reflecting greater opportunities for transmission (Monto and Koopman 1980). Rotaviruses are the main cause of dehydrating diarrheal disease in young children throughout the world (see Chapter 44, Rotaviruses). Although infants and young children in developing countries may die of these infections if they are not rehydrated with salt-containing solutions (orally or sometimes intravenously), the disease is rarely so severe in the developed world, mainly because of such factors as better nutrition (Black et al. 1981). These are surface infections that recur throughout life. Whilst initial infections in infants may be severe, re-infections usually produce mild illness or asymptomatic infection. As with the respiratory viruses, this has implications for spread within families.

Paradoxically, the pattern of occurrence of rotavirus infection is more like that of the respiratory viruses than of other enteric agents, although transmission clearly takes place by the fecal–oral route; whereas large amounts of virus are shed in the stools, none has been detected in the upper respiratory tract. As with respiratory viruses it is possible to examine the role of the family and the community in determining the occurrence of infection. All rotavirus types are seasonal in the temperate zones, most illness occurring in the colder months (Brandt et al. 1982; Vesikari et al. 1992). Rotavirus vaccines, prepared from live-attenuated strains, have been and continue to be developed for use in infants (see Chapter 44, Rotaviruses). Because of the need for multiple types, there has been at least a potential problem with interference, a phenomenon common to live attenuated vaccines, with difficulty in producing immunity simultaneously to several types. The purpose of vaccination is not necessarily to prevent infection or illness completely, but to render it more like re-infection, thus preventing severe dehydration.

Rotaviruses are responsible for only some of the enteric illnesses experienced in the community during the cold season. Identifying the etiological agents of other common illnesses has been complicated by the difficulty or impossibility of growing many of them in cell culture. Norvovirus, now recognized to be a calicivirus, is one of a group of viruses causing water-related outbreaks (see Chapter 42, Human enteric RNA viruses: norvoviruses and sapoviruses). A variety of exposures are involved, including drinking and swimming in water containing the virus, especially when the head is submerged; contaminated seafood has also been implicated (Gunn et al. 1980; Kaplan et al. 1982). Person-to-person transmission also occurs, increasing the potential for spread in families and the community.

Immune electron microscopy was the basic method for identifying rise in antibody titer and reagents had to be prepared by inoculating human volunteers (Herrmann et al. 1985).

The recent cloning of the Norwalk agent will allow better understanding of its epidemiology as reagents become available for testing sera. Similarly the enteric adenoviruses, types 40 and 41, originally detected only by electron microscopy can now be identified by enzyme immunoassay (EIA) (Johansson et al. 1985). The association of these viruses with enteric disease in infants is an example of use of the case–control design. The respiratory adenoviruses, which could at that time be easily cultivated in cell culture, were isolated in equal numbers from the stools of cases (children hospitalized with diarrhea) and controls (children hospitalized with other conditions). However, adenoviruses that could not be cultivated in routine cell cultures were significantly more commonly detected in children with disease than in controls (Brandt et al. 1985). It has been suggested that an autumnal increase in enteric illness is related to these adenoviruses, but such seasonality could not be demonstrated in hospital-based studies.

Polio and enteric hepatitis viruses

The enteroviruses are generally transmitted by the fecal–oral route. Some exceptions exist, however, such as coxsackie virus A21, an unusual cause of respiratory infection that can spread by aerosol. The dynamics and characteristics of this infection were well studied in the military, in whom it had presented an occasional problem. Polio is the best known of the enteroviruses, producing a potentially serious disease in a small proportion of those infected. Global elimination of polio is underway, by use of the live-attenuated vaccine administered universally and repeatedly to young children. The method is based on the known transmission pattern of the vaccine virus, which resembles that of the wild virus in being shed in large quantities and for long periods in the stool of inoculated children (Hull et al. 1994). The shed virus can be transmitted to contacts, especially other children, and to adults in the family. By inoculating children regularly (annually or more frequently) as part of a mass vaccination program, it is possible to spread the vaccine viruses in the environment so that children who are missed by the vaccine program are indirectly exposed to them. This approach, which combines herd immunity, or increasing the level of antibody in a population so that susceptibles are rare and transmission is interrupted, together with the special characteristics of transmissibility of the live polio vaccine, has resulted in the elimination of transmission of wild polio virus in the Americas. The procedure is now being applied in other parts of the developing world (Centers for Disease Control 1995).

Hepatitis A is classified as an enterovirus; it shares epidemiological characteristics with other enteroviruses but is unusual in having a relatively long incubation period (median 28 days) (Lemon 1985). Spread in the developed countries typically occurs from person to person in the family or in settings such as day care centers for children, especially when they are not toilet trained. Much of the infection in North America has been traced to these day care outbreaks, from which spread continues in families and older individuals (Hadler and McFarland 1986). In developing countries and in special situations in the industrialized world, spread can often occur through contaminated water or by consuming uncooked shellfish from contaminated waters. Other food transmission is possible whenever there is fecal contamination. In the developing world, infection occurs at an early age and is often asymptomatic. In the industrialized countries, infection is delayed and often will not occur at all, rendering much of the population susceptible if exposed. Travelers to developing countries generally do not have protective antibodies from past exposure, and are thus at increased risk. One solution, before vaccine became available, was use of immune globulin, which gives temporary protection. There are now vaccines that can protect individuals from developed countries who will be exposed in the developing world. Such infection has been a major risk, especially for people exposed for long periods in areas with poor standards of hygiene (Wagner et al. 1993). Hepatitis E has epidemiological characteristics similar to those of hepatitis A, and increasing availability of reagents will allow better understanding of its behavior in populations. Some outbreaks of disease thought to be due to hepatitis A are now recognized to have been, in all probability, caused by hepatitis E (Wong et al. 1980).

VIRAL INFECTIONS WITH BLOODBORNE TRANSMISSION

Hepatitis B and related viruses

Hepatitis B was, before the discovery of HIV, the most extensively studied bloodborne pathogen. During the course of many viral infections, there is often a phase of viremia; however, bloodborne transmission is unlikely when viremia lasts for only a period of hours. The probability of such transmission is increased when viremia persists for days or, as is the case with some infected with hepatitis B, for years. The likelihood that infection will persist decreases with increasing age at time of exposure. Thus, perinatal infection is most likely to result in chronic viremia. The transmission of hepatitis B by blood or blood products was documented well before the virus or its antigens were identified (Sawyer et al. 1944). During the Second World War, yellow fever vaccine used by the US military was stabilized by the addition of human albumin. Those who received the vaccine developed hepatitis and, by epidemiological evidence, it became clear that it was contaminated by what is now known to be hepatitis B virus. On initial study, the cases of hepatitis that were detected did not seem to bear any temporal relationship to an exposure to persons with infection or to a common event. Then it was realized that vaccination might be the common source. Because vaccinations had been administered over a long period, cases were occurring in an apparently unrelated fashion. Plotting of duration since vaccination resulted in a typical epidemic curve, with cases distributed around the long median incubation period of approximately 120 days from exposure.

Hepatitis B is transmissible not only through blood and blood products but also through sexual contact. Simply living in a family with an infected person slightly increases the probability of transmission. It is not clear exactly how this occurs. The virus is present in various body fluids, in addition to blood and semen (Irwin et al. 1975). Transmission requires only very small amounts of blood, so leakage through minor abrasions and tears may be responsible. Hepatitis B was known to be more common in certain professional groups such as dentists, almost certainly because of exposure to small amounts of infected blood commonly lost in dental procedures rather than through virus present in saliva (Mosley et al. 1975). It was especially common among homosexual men, especially those with multiple partners. In fact, the trial of hepatitis B vaccine was conducted in uninfected sexually active homosexual men, because exposure was predictable (Szmuness et al. 1980). The transmission was clearly sexual, but how much of it involved transfer of small quantities of highly infectious blood and how much other infected bodily fluids was difficult to quantify. Various specific sexual practices such as anal intercourse were identified as risk factors even before the study of HIV transmission (Szmuness et al. 1975).

A particular problem with hepatitis B, especially in eastern Asia (including China) and in sub-Saharan Africa, is that transmission is mainly vertical and children become infected at birth from transplacental and direct exposure to maternal blood (Stevens et al. 1975). When infection occurs at this age, it is likely to persist, and thus may be carried to the next generation. Hepatitis C shares many features with hepatitis B, including its transmission by blood and blood products. Risk groups differ somewhat with, for example, less sexual transmission (Alter et al. 1989).

Human immunodeficiency virus

When human immunodeficiency virus (HIV) was first described, its epidemiology was found to be remarkably similar to that of hepatitis B (see Chapter 55, Hepatitis B). Differences are related to the natural history of the disease and to the far lower transmissibility of HIV under most conditions. A persistently high level of viremia allows hepatitis B virus transmission to occur with relative ease for long periods. In contrast, transmission of HIV is most likely early in the infectious process when there is viremia of high titer, or later in the development of AIDS itself when the level of viremia increases again. The early period is probably the most important for transmission, because at that time individuals may not know they are infected and remain sexually active (Jacquez et al. 1994). Because of its importance, the epidemiology of HIV has been studied intensively over the period since the virus was identified and many characteristics of its distribution are now well established. Much attention has been given to the role that various behaviours play in transmission, since, in the developed countries, antibody tests have ensured that blood and blood products are safe and transmission by that route of infection no longer occurs. Among homosexual men, receptive anal intercourse is the prime risk factor, but other sexual practices are possibly to blame, if not nearly as risky. Heterosexual intercourse can also transmit the virus efficiently, but male-to-female transmission is accomplished more easily than the reverse (Padian et al. 1991). As with hepatitis B, injecting drug use appears to be an independent risk factor for transmission. Transmission also occurs through breast milk and artificial insemination. In one controversial case, the argument for transmission of virus to the patients of an HIV-infected dentist was strengthened by the similarity of the viral nucleic acids in the various cases, a technique sometimes referred to as molecular epidemiology (Crandall 1995).

In the developed countries, the disease has predominantly been one of males, both homosexual and bisexual men and injecting drug users. Heterosexual transmission has often involved sexual partners of these individuals. In the USA, African-Americans and other minority groups are increasingly involved. In developing countries, the male to female ratio often is 1:1, and the prevalence of infection in the general population, especially in certain countries of Africa, is high. The infection has entered south and southeast Asia, where transmission has been rapid. Mathematical epidemiology has been used to study the relative probability of different transmission mechanisms when several may be involved, and to predict the course of the pandemic. Simulations have been particularly valuable in trying to understand how altering transmission by vaccination or behavior modification will affect the course of the epidemic in different regions.

ZOONOSES AND VECTORBORNE INFECTION

Zoonoses not involving arthropods

Many, but not all, of the vectorborne viral infections are also zoonoses and are discussed together. The zoonoses are human infections in which the principal reservoirs of the viral agent are wild and domestic mammals, birds, and possibly other species such as reptiles. Cycles of infection can be maintained in these reservoirs without the involvement of humans, in whom infection occurs incidentally. Zoonoses not involving arthropod-vector transmission are listed in Table 18.4, with animal reservoir and route transmission. Rabies (see Chapter 51, Rhabdoviruses: rabies) is an example of a zoonosis not involving vectors. In most of the world, rabies is widely distributed in a variety of mammals, the predominant species varying from region to region. In North America, foxes, skunks, and raccoons are mainly involved (Anderson et al. 1984). Of these, only raccoons frequently invade human habitations but in most cases transmission remains within the particular species. Transmission sometimes involves domestic animals such as dogs or cats, who, because of their activities outside the home, will occasionally come in contact with the wildlife hosts. Insectivorous bats also maintain rabies in their own colonies but, because they often live in human dwellings, direct transmission to humans occasionally occurs. Vaccination of domestic pets is used to create a barrier between wildlife rabies and humans; it is highly effective, with the possible exception of preventing direct bat transmission. There have been several years in the USA without a single case of human rabies, even though extensive transmission in animals still occurs. In other parts of the developed world, the species involved in maintaining wildlife rabies differ. In Europe, foxes are often involved, and attempts are now being made to control transmission in these hosts by drops of baited food containing vaccine (Brochier et al. 1991). This is possible only when the geographic areas are relatively limited. In remote areas, many more species are involved and control is impractical.

Some parts of the world, typically islands such as Great Britain and Hawaii, are rabiesfree; because potential hosts are present in the wild, exclusion of animals who might be responsible for importation is a critical part of control activity. In many developing countries, rabies of domestic animals is common, especially of dogs which are barely domesticated and often form feral packs. Transmission from dog to dog does occur, as well as from dog to humans. This is in contrast to the typical situation in the developed world, where the dog, as well as humans who become infected, are 'dead-end hosts'; that is, they are generally not responsible for any further transmission. The few human cases that occur in indus-

Table 18.4 *Zoonotic viral infections without arthropod transmission*

	Virus and disease	**Animal reservoir**	**Mode of transfer**
Rhabdoviruses	Rabies virus	Foxes, skunks, bats, raccoons, mongooses, dogs, cats, etc.	Bite. Possibly saliva through abraded skin or airborne
Arenaviruses	Lymphocytic choriomeningitis virus	*Mus musculus*	Contact with urine, feces or other infected fluids. Rarely person-to-person or nosocomial spread. Possible airborne distribution
	Junin–Argentine hemorrhagic fever	*Calomys musculinus*	
	Machupo–Bolivian hemorrhagic fever	*Calomys callosus*	
	Guanarito virus disease–Venezuelan hemorrhagic fever	*Sigmodon hispidus*	
	Lassa fever	*Mastomys natalensis*	
Bunyaviruses/ hantaviruses	Hantaan virus		Contact with urine, feces, and saliva. May be aerosolized or enter through abraded skin
	Korean hemorrhagic fever virus	Field mice	
	Seoul virus	Urban rats	
	Sin Nombre virus		
	Hantavirus pulmonary syndrome	Deer mice and other rodents	
Puumulavirus	Nephropathia epidemica virus	Voles	
Filoviruses	Marburg virus	Reservoir not clear	Contact with infected monkeys
	Ebola virus	Reservoir not clear	Blood and other personal contact after infection in humans
Poxviruses	Cowpox virus, Monkeypox virus	Cows, monkeys, sheep	Animal skin lesion to abraded human skin
	Contagious pustular dermatitis (orf)		
Herpesvirus	Herpesvirus B	Rhesus monkeys	Saliva by bite or contact
Orthomyxovirus	Swine influenza virus	Pigs	Close contact
Picornavirus	Encephalomyocarditis	Rodents and monkeys	Possible contamination by urine and feces

trialized countries are often imports from developing countries, where exposure of travelers to infected domestic animals is more likely. Molecular techniques, based on differences in viral nucleic acid structure in rabies viruses transmitted in different parts of the world, are often used to determine the source of exposure (Smith et al. 1992). The few cases and intensive study of those that do occur have allowed recognition of unusual sources of infection, such as a transplanted cornea obtained from a cadaver whose death was caused by undetected rabies (Houff et al. 1979).

Zoonoses not involving arthropods are typical of infections produced by arenaviruses and hantaviruses. With both, rodents and other wildlife hosts are responsible for transmission and maintenance of infection. Sometimes the rodents become diseased, but in most cases the infections are inapparent. Humans become involved incidentally and have no further role in maintenance of the chain of transmission. Viruses such as the arenaviruses (Machupo, the cause of Bolivian hemorrhagic fever, and Junin, the cause of Argentine hemorrhagic fever), as well as the hantaviruses (producing Korean hemorrhagic fever and the hantavirus pulmonary syndrome in North America) are limited geographically by the area ranged by the rodents primarily infected. Human-to-human transmission is rare; most human infection appears to result from exposure to rodent urine heavily contaminated with virus, and possibly other animal products such as feces or saliva (Peters et al. 1974; Mercado 1975). The rodents often live in or near dwellings, and humans may be exposed via aerosol or through abraded skin. Increases in frequency of the disease, which, for example, led to the recognition of the hantavirus pulmonary syndrome in southwestern USA, are related to changes in the environment affecting numbers and activities of the rodent host (Hjelle et al. 1994). It is suggested that an overproduction of pine nuts, the rodents' principal food, led to the emergence of the disease in the Four Corners area of the USA.

Yellow fever and dengue

The term 'arbovirus' was used for many years to describe a large group of enveloped, lipid-containing viruses that had in common transmission by arthropods (Theiler 1957). This diverse group of viruses has many epidemiological features in common (see Chapters 46, Flaviviruses; 47, Togaviruses; and 48, Bunyaviridae). The principal vector is the mosquito, although there are important infections involving ticks and other arthropods. Many are also zoonoses, in which the infection is maintained in wild or domestic animals (the reservoirs), humans being involved only occasionally as dead-end hosts. Because of the nature of the vectors and the reservoirs, particular arboviruses are often geographically limited in distribution. Certain mosquitoes cannot exist outside the tropical or subtropical areas, so climate becomes a major determinant, as does other vector behavior, including preferences in multiplication sites, sources of blood meals, and flight distances. The introduction of West Nile virus from the Middle East and subsequent spread throughout much of North America shows that geographic limitations are not absolute (Petersen et al. 2002).

A list of some important arthropod-borne viral infections, according to the geographical area of their occurrence is given in Table 18.5. Two important infections, both transmitted preferentially by the mosquito *Aedes aegypti*, which can be spread from human to human by the vector, are yellow fever and dengue. Thus, unlike many other arboviruses, dengue and (in this context) yellow fever are not zoonoses. The mosquito is closely associated with human dwellings in urban areas of the tropics and subtropics, but does not persist in areas with cold winter seasons. Urban outbreaks are typical, because infected humans are ready sources for the transmission of viruses to others. In certain regions, outbreaks of the infections are a regular seasonal occurrence. Control of yellow fever was accomplished in many cities of the Americas before availability of insecticides by eradicating the vector from urban areas. Early control of yellow fever transmission made possible the construction of the Panama Canal. With no urban yellow fever, sylvatic or jungle yellow fever was detected in areas without the usual vectors. The same virus caused the disease, which was found to have a zoonotic host, i.e. subhuman primates. It could be transmitted to humans, especially to people working or living in the forests, by hemagogus mosquitoes. *Aedes aegypti* has recently returned to many cities from which it had been eliminated, and, with it, urban outbreaks of yellow fever.

Several vaccines have been developed to control outbreaks of yellow fever and for primary prevention in endemic areas. The most successful, the 17-D vaccine, is a live-attenuated preparation that confers long-term protection.

Dengue is currently the most important arthropod-borne virus because of its widespread distribution in large parts of the tropics and subtropics and the potential there for extensive outbreaks of life-threatening disease. Urbanization in these regions has led to an

Table **18.5** *Arthropod-borne viruses of global importance and their vectors*

	Diseases	Family/genus	Vector
Tropics and subtropics	Yellow fever	*Flaviviridae/Flavivirus*	*Aedes* and hemagogus mosquitoes
	Dengue	*Flaviviridae/Flavivirus*	*Aedes aegypti* and *A. albopictus*
	Sandfly fever	*Bunyaviridae/Phlebovirus*	Phlebotomine sandflies
American	Eastern, Western, Venezuelan equine encephalitis	*Togaviridae/Alphaviruses*	*Aedes* and *Culex* mosquitoes
	St. Louis encephalitis	*Flaviviridae/Flavivirus*	*Culex* mosquitoes
	California encephalitis	*Bunyaviridae/Bunyavirus*	*Aedes* mosquitoes
	California tick fever	*Reoviridae/Orbivirus*	*Dermacentor* ticks
Eurasian	Tick-borne encephalitis (Russian spring–summer/central European)	*Flaviviridae/Flavivirus*	Ixodid ticks
	Crimean hemorrhagic fever (Crimean–Congo)	*Bunyaviridae/Nairovirus*	*Hyalomma* ticks
	Omsk haemorrhagic fever	*Flaviviridae/Flavivirus*	*Dermacentor* ticks
	Japanese B encephalitis	*Flaviviridae/Flavivirus*	*Culex* mosquitoes
African	Rift Valley fever	*Bunyaviridae/Phlebovirus*	*Culex* and *Aedes* mosquito
	Chikungunya fever	*Togaviridae/Alphavirus*	*Aedes aegypti* and others
	West Nile fever	*Flaviviridae/Flavivirus*	*Culex* mosquitoes
Australasian	Murray Valley encephalitis	*Flaviviridae/Flavivirus*	*Culex* mosquitoes
	Ross River fever	*Togaviridae/Alphavirus*	*Aedes* and *Culex* mosquitoes

increase in the probability of dengue infection because the virus is transmitted by the vector mosquito from one human host to another without the involvement of a zoonotic reservoir. The high concentration of susceptibles in the sprawling cities results in large-scale outbreaks. The vector *A. aegypti* is well adapted to multiplying in the small pools of water that are frequently found in these areas, especially in seasons with heavy rainfall. In its acute form, dengue is debilitating with high fever and deep pain; and infection can result in dengue hemorrhagic fever/dengue shock syndrome (DHF/DDS). These are life-threatening conditions, which affect mainly children. There are four types of dengue virus, and infection with one type produces only partial immunity to another type. The principal hypothesis to explain the pathogenesis of dengue hemorrhagic fever is based on epidemiological observations (Halstead 1970). The disease is widespread when a second outbreak of infection, typically caused by type 2, follows shortly after another outbreak caused by a different type. Reinfection appears to be the common factor; this occurs mainly in children, and maternal antibody may play a role in infants. A number of immunological characteristics of the disease support this hypothesis, although there is some evidence that the syndrome can be produced on initial infection in individuals without maternal antibody (Barnes and Rosen 1974). In recent years, dengue has been spreading, especially in the Americas. This is of particular concern in the USA because *A. aegypti* is present in the southern states.

Other arboviruses

For arboviruses that are principally zoonoses, disease in humans is generally sporadic or occasional. In North America, eastern equine encephalitis (EEE) is an example of an agent that occurs sporadically, during the summer. Many of the infections are inapparent. Symptomatic infection occurs only occasionally, but may manifest as severe encephalitis with residual mental retardation. The reservoir is wild and domestic birds; maintenance of infection does not require either humans or horses, both of which are dead-end hosts. With arboviruses in the temperate zones there is always the question of persistence through the winter (overwintering) during the period when there is no vector activity. Migrating birds infected by the virus winter in areas where mosquitoes are present and are responsible for the continued transmission of the agent. They return, some being infected, in the spring (Lord and Calisher 1970). With other arboviruses there is some evidence that animals in hibernation may serve to overwinter the virus (Reeves 1974).

In the Eurasian land mass, tick-borne encephalitis (TBE), also called Russian spring–summer encephalitis, is an important, though uncommon, sporadic disease associated with forested areas. The reservoir is small mammals and, to a lesser extent, birds; humans moving into sites where transmission is occurring become infected incidentally. Transovarian transmission can take place in ticks in which the virus is passed to the next generation, further maintaining the infection. In contrast, the most important arbovirus of eastern and southeast Asia, Japanese encephalitis, may be responsible for large numbers of cases of relatively severe encephalitis in humans. This disease is mosquito transmitted and occurs in rice-growing regions which generally have a high mosquito density. The principal reservoir is pigs, also common in the region. Because vector control in these areas has been difficult, emphasis has been placed on vaccination.

VIRUSES AND CHRONIC DISEASES

Persistent infection is well documented for many DNA viruses and some RNA viruses. The herpesvirus group is well known for producing persistent infections, for example recurrent cold sores or genital ulcers caused by herpes simplex virus and herpes zoster due to varicella-zoster virus. The retroviruses, including HIV, are also characterized by long-term chronic infection. It is difficult to establish the role of various viruses to late, seemingly unrelated, events such as the development of cirrhosis and primary hepatocellular carcinoma (PHC) or carcinoma of the cervix. Relating these conditions to viral infections requires the application of epidemiological study designs. For hepatitis B and the production of primary hepatocellular carcinoma, the studies were mainly conducted in Taiwan, where there is a combination of high prevalence of chronic infection and a health care system that allowed a longitudinal study of health care workers. A problem in any of these evaluations is the long time between the infection, which may have been acquired perinatally, and development of the tumor, which can occur many decades later. Demonstration of viral antigen in the tumor is of help, but is not conclusive proof of etiology where the population has a history of widespread infection with the agent. The major epidemiological evidence for etiology has come from a series of case–control and cohort studies that noted a strong association between the persistent infection and primary hepatocellular carcinoma even after controlling for potential confounding variables (Beasley 1988). Similar work is now underway to investigate the link between hepatitis C and PHC.

Epidemiological approaches have also provided evidence of involvement of certain types of papilloma virus in carcinoma of the cervix (Chapter 23, Papillomaviruses). Descriptive epidemiological studies have long suggested that an infectious entity, probably sexually transmitted, was involved in etiology. Attention was first focused on behavioral differences and on herpes simplex virus. Case–control studies revealed that herpes antibody titers were higher in people with tumors than in those without (Rawls et al. 1970). It was possible to identify viral components in excised tumor, and other factors seemed to confirm the relationship. However, the link was not well sustained in studies controlling for confounding factors, such as sexual activity. When it became easier to work with papillomaviruses, epidemiological studies confirmed the specificity of the association with certain types. Moreover, it was possible to replicate the relationship in different studies in different parts of the world and to demonstrate the strength of the association with the specific papilloma types in question (Reeves et al. 1987). Vaccine control now appears possible (Koutsky et al. 2002).

Research into the long-term consequences of viral infection is very important, because it brings together acute and chronic outcomes affecting the health of populations. Examples include the relationship of EBV to the later development of nasopharyngeal carcinoma and Burkitt's lymphoma. Work in this area is diverse, and ranges from efforts to relate acute respiratory infection to later chronic bronchitis and emphysema to studies attempting to relate infectious agents to the pathogenesis of atherosclerosis. All these investigations must use appropriate epidemiological methods, especially as these techniques are a recognized component of other investigations of risk factors for chronic disease.

REFERENCES

Abbey, H. 1952. An examination of the Reed Frost theory of epidemics. *Hum Biol*, **24**, 201–33.

Alter, H.J., Purcell, R.H., et al. 1989. Detection of antibody to hepatitis C virus in prospectively followed transfusion recipients with acute and chronic non-A, non-B hepatitis. *N Engl J Med*, **321**, 1494–500.

American Public Health Association. 1985. *Control of communicable diseases of man*, 14th edn. In Beneson, A.S. (ed.). Washington DC: APHA, 457–9.

Anderson, L.J., Nicholson, K.G., et al. 1984. Human rabies in the United States, 1960 to 1979: epidemiology, diagnosis, and prevention. *Ann Intern Med*, **100**, 728–35.

Bailey, N.T.J. 1957. *The mathematical theory of epidemics*. London: Griffin.

Barnes, W.J.S. and Rosen, L. 1974. Fatal hemorrhagic disease and shock associated with primary dengue infection on a Pacific island. *Am J Trop Med Hyg*, **23**, 495–506.

Baron, R.C., McCormick, J.B. and Zubeir, O.A. 1981. Ebola virus disease in southern Sudan: hospital dissemination and intrafamilial spread. *Bull WHO*, **61**, 997–1003.

Bartlett, A.V., Moore, M., et al. 1985. Diarrheal illness among infants and toddlers in day care centers. II. Comparison with day care homes and households. *J Pediatr*, **107**, 503–9.

Beasley, R.P. 1982. Hepatitis B virus as the etiologic agent in hepatocellular carcinoma – epidemiologic considerations. *Hepatology*, **2**, 215–65.

Beasley, R.P. 1988. Hepatitis B virus. The major etiology of hepatocellular carcinoma cancer. *Cancer*, **61**, 1942–56.

Belongia, E.A., Goodman, J.L., et al. 1991. An outbreak of herpes gladiatorum at a high school wrestling competition. *N Engl J Med*, **325**, 906–10.

Berquist, K.R., Maynard, J.E., et al. 1976. Experimental studies on the transmission of hepatitis B by mosquitoes. *Am J Trop Med Hyg*, **25**, 730–2.

Black, F.L. 1989. Epidemiology and control. In: Evans, A.S. (ed.), *Measles in viral infections of humans*. New York and London: Plenum Medical, 457.

Black, R.E., Merson, M.H., et al. 1981. Incidence and severity of rotavirus and *Escherichia coli* diarrhea in rural Bangladesh. Implications for vaccine development. *Lancet*, **1**, 141–3.

Brandt, C.D., Kim, H.W., et al. 1982. Rotavirus gastroenteritis and weather. *J Clin Microbiol*, **16**, 478–82.

Brandt, C.D., Kim, H.W., et al. 1983. Pediatric viral gastroenteritis during eight years of study. *J Clin Microbiol*, **18**, 71–8.

Brandt, C.D., Kim, H.W., et al. 1985. Adenoviruses and pediatric gastroenteritis. *J Infect Dis*, **151**, 437–43.

Breslow, N.E. and Day, N.E. 1987. *The design and analysis of cohort studies. Statistical methods in cancer research*, Vol. II. Lyon: International Agency for Research on Cancer.

Brochier, B., Kieny, M.P., et al. 1991. Large-scale eradication of rabies using recombinant vaccinia-rabies vaccine. *Nature (London)*, **354**, 520–2.

Centers for Disease Control. 1994. Hantavirus pulmonary syndrome – United States, 1993. *Morbid Mortal Weekly Rep*, **43**, 45–8.

Centers for Disease Control. 1995. Progress toward poliomyelitis eradication – South East Asia region, 1988–1994. *Morbid Mortal Weekly Rep*, **44**, 791–801.

Childs, J.E., Ksiazek, T.G., et al. 1994. Serologic and genetic identification of *Peromyscus maniculatus* as the primary rodent reservoir for a new hantavirus in the southwestern United States. *J Infect Dis*, **169**, 1271–80.

Chin, T.D.Y., Foley, J.F., et al. 1960. Morbidity and mortality characteristics of Asian strain influenza. *Public Health Rep*, **75**, 149–58.

Claas, E.C.J., Osterhaus, A.D.M.E., et al. 1998. Human influenza A (H5N1) virus related to a highly pathogenic avian influenza virus. *Lancet*, **351**, 472–7.

Couch, R.B., Cate, T.R., et al. 1966. Effect of route of inoculation on experimental respiratory viral disease in volunteers and evidence for airborne transmission. *Bacteriol Rev*, **30**, 517–31.

Crandall, K.A. 1995. Intraspecific phylogenetics: support for dental transmission of human immunodeficiency virus. *J Virol*, **69**, 2351–6.

Dowdle, W.R., Millar, J.O., et al. 1980. Influenza immunization policies and practices in Japan. *J Infect Dis*, **141**, 258–64.

Eickhoff, T.C., Sherman, I.L. and Serfling, R.E. 1961. Observations on excess mortality associated with epidemic influenza. *JAMA*, **176**, 104–10.

Elandt-Johnson, R.C. 1975. Definition of rates: some remarks on their use and misuse. *Am J Epidemiol*, **102**, 261–71.

Elveback, L.R., Fox, J.P., et al. 1976. An influenza simulation model for immunization studies. *Am J Epidemiol*, **103**, 152–65.

Fauci, A.S. 2002. Smallpox vaccination policy – the need for dialogue. *New Engl J Med*, **346**, 1319–20.

Fedson, D.S., Wajda, A., et al. 1993. Clinical effectiveness of influenza vaccine in Manitoba. *JAMA*, **270**, 1956–61.

Foster, D.A., Talsma, A., et al. 1992. Influenza vaccine effectiveness in preventing hospitalization for pneumonia in the elderly. *Am J Epidemiol*, **136**, 296–307.

Fox, J.P., Hall, C.E. and Elveback, L.R. 1970. *Epidemiology, man and disease*. London: Macmillan.

Friedland, G.H. and Klein, R.S. 1987. Transmission of the human immunodeficiency virus. *N Engl J Med*, **317**, 1125–35.

Friedman-Kien, A.E., Laubenstein, L.J., et al. 1982. Disseminated Kaposi's sarcoma in homosexual men. *Ann Intern Med*, **96**, 693–700.

Glezen, W.P., Paredes, A., et al. 1981. Risk of respiratory syncytial virus infection for infants from low-income families in relationship to age, sex, ethnic group, and maternal antibody level. *J Pediatr*, **98**, 708–15.

Glezen, W.P., Payne, A.A., et al. 1982. Mortality and influenza. *J Infect Dis*, **146**, 313–21.

Glezen, W.P., Taber, L.H., et al. 1986. Risk of primary infection and reinfection with respiratory syncytial virus. *Am J Dis Child*, **140**, 543–6.

Gottlieb, M.S., Schroff, R., et al. 1981. *Pneumocystis carinii* pneumonia and mucosal candidiasis in previously healthy homosexual men: evidence of a new acquired cellular immunodeficiency. *N Engl J Med*, **305**, 1425–31.

Gregg, N.M. 1941. Congenital cataract following German measles in the mother. *Trans Ophthal Soc Aust*, **3**, 35–46.

Gunn, R.A., Terranova, W.A., et al. 1980. Norwalk virus gastroenteritis aboard a cruise ship: an outbreak on five consecutive cruises. *Am J Epidemiol*, **112**, 820–7.

Hadler, S.C. and McFarland, L. 1986. Hepatitis in day care centers. Epidemiology and prevention. *Rev Infect Dis*, **154**, 231–7.

Hallee, T.J., Evans, A.S., et al. 1974. Infectious mononucleosis at the US military academy: a prospective study of a single class over four years. *Yale J Biol Med*, **47**, 182–95.

Halpin, T.J., Holtzhauer, F.J., et al. 1982. Reye's syndrome and medication use. *JAMA*, **248**, 687–91.

Halstead, S.B. 1970. Observations relating to pathogenesis of dengue hemorrhagic fever. VI. Hypotheses and discussion. *Yale J Biol Med*, **42**, 350–62.

Hattwick, M.A.W., Weis, T.T., et al. 1972. Recovery from rabies: a case report. *Ann Intern Med*, **76**, 931–42.

Hedstrom, C. and Lycke, E. 1964. An experimental study on oysters as virus carriers. *Am J Hyg*, **79**, 134–42.

Hendley, J.O., Gwaltney, J.M. and Jordan, W.S. 1969. Rhinovirus infections in an industrial population. IV. Infections within families of employees during two fall peaks of respiratory illness. *Am J Epidemiol*, **89**, 184–96.

Herrmann, J.E., Nowak, N.A., et al. 1985. Detection of Norwalk virus in stools by enzyme immunoassay. *J Med Virol*, **17**, 127–33.

Hethcote, H.W., Van Ark, J.W. and Longini, I. 1991. A simulation model for AIDS in San Francisco. I. Model formulation and parameter estimation. *Math Biosci*, **106**, 203–22.

Hill, A.B. 1965. The environment and disease: association or causation? *Proc R Soc Med*, **58**, 295.

Hjelle, B., Jenison, S., et al. 1994. A novel hantavirus associated with an outbreak of fatal respiratory disease in the southwestern United States: evolutionary relationships to known hantaviruses. *J Virol*, **68**, 592–6.

Houff, S.A., Burton, R.C., et al. 1979. Human-to-human transmission of rabies virus by corneal transplant. *N Engl J Med*, **30**, 603–4.

Hull, H.F., Ward, N.A., et al. 1994. Paralytic poliomyelitis: seasoned strategies, disappearing disease. *Lancet*, **343**, 1331–7.

Hurwitz, E.S., Barrett, M.J., et al. 1985. Public health service study on Reye's syndrome and medications. *N Engl J Med*, **313**, 849–57.

Ingalls, T.H. and Babbott, F.L. 1960. Rubella: its epidemiology and teratology. *Am J Med Sci*, **239**, 363–83.

Irwin, G.R., Allen, A.M., et al. 1975. Hepatitis B antigen in saliva, urine, and stool. *Infect Immun*, **11**, 142–5.

Jackson, A.D.M. and Fisch, L. 1958. Deafness following maternal rubella: results of a prospective investigation. *Lancet*, **2**, 1241–4.

Jacquez, J., Koopman, J.S., et al. 1994. Role of the primary infection in epidemic HIV of gay cohorts. *J Acquired Immune Defic Syndr*, **7**, 1169–84.

Johansson, M.E., Uhnoo, I., et al. 1985. Enzyme-linked immunosorbent assay for detection of enteric adenovirus 41. *J Med Virol*, **17**, 19–27.

Johnson, K.M., Kuns, M.L., et al. 1966. Isolation of Machupo virus from wild rodent *Calomys callosus*. *Am J Trop Med Hyg*, **15**, 103–6.

Johnson, N., Mant, D., et al. 1991. Use of computerised general practice data for population surveillance: comparative study of influenza data. *Br Med J*, **302**, 763–5.

Johnston, S.L., Pattemore, P.K., et al. 1995. Community study of role of viral infections in exacerbations of asthma in 9–11 year old children. *Br Med J*, **310**, 1225–9.

Kaplan, J.E., Gary, G.W., et al. 1982. Epidemiology of Norwalk gastroenteritis and the role of Norwalk virus in outbreaks of acute nonbacterial gastroenteritis. *Ann Intern Med*, **96**, 756–61.

Kawaoka, Y., Bean, W.J., et al. 1993. The roles of birds and pigs in the generation of pandemic strains of human influenza. In: Hannoun, C., Kendal, A.P., et al. (eds), *Options for the control of influenza II*. Amsterdam: Elsevier Science, 187–91.

Kendal, A.P., Joseph, J.M., et al. 1977. Laboratory-based surveillance of influenza virus in the United States of 1977–1978. I. Periods of prevalence of H1N1 and H3N2 influenza A strains; their relative rates of isolation. *Am J Epidemiol*, **110**, 449–61.

Kleinbaum, D.G., Kupper, L.L. and Morgenstein, L.L. 1982. *Epidemiologic research: principles and quantitative methods*. Belmont, CA: Lifetime Learning Publications.

Klemetti, A. and Saxen, L. 1967. Prospective versus retrospective approach in the search for environmental causes for malformations. *Am J Public Health*, **57**, 2071–5.

Koopman, J.S., Eckert, E.A., et al. 1982. Norwalk virus enteric illness acquired by swimming exposure. *Am J Epidemiol*, **115**, 173–7.

Koutsky, L.A., Ault, K.A., et al. 2002. A controlled trial of human papillomavirus type 16 vaccine. *New Engl J Med*, **347**, 1645–51.

Lemon, S.M. 1985. Type A viral hepatitis: new developments in an old disease. *N Engl J Med*, **313**, 1059–67.

Longini, I.M., Ackerman, E. and Elveback, L.R. 1977. An optimization model for influenza A epidemics. *Math Biosci*, **38**, 141–57.

Longini, I.M., Koopman, J.S., et al. 1982. Estimating household and community transmission parameters for influenza. *Am J Epidemiol*, **115**, 736–51.

Lord, R.D. and Calisher, C.H. 1970. Further evidence of southward transport of arboviruses by migratory birds. *Am J Epidemiol*, **92**, 73–8.

Lundstrom, R. 1962. Rubella during pregnancy. A follow-up study of children born after an epidemic of rubella in Sweden, 1951, with additional investigations on prophylaxis and treatment of maternal rubella. *Acta Paediat*, **133**, 1–110.

McIntosh, K., Ellis, E.F., et al. 1973. The association of viral and bacterial respiratory infections with exacerbations of wheezing in young asthmatic children. *J Pediatr*, **82**, 578–90.

MacNaughton, M.R. 1982. Occurrence and frequency of coronavirus infections in humans as determined by enzyme-linked immunosorbent assay. *Infect Immun*, **38**, 419–23.

Manson, M.M., Logan, W.P.D. and Loy, R.M. 1960. *Rubella and other virus infections during pregnancy. Reports on public health and medical subjects, No. 101*. London: Ministry of Health/Her Majesty's Stationery Office.

Masurel, N. 1976. Swine influenza virus and the recycling of influenza A viruses in man. *Lancet*, **2**, 244–7.

Masurel, N. and Marine, W.M. 1973. Recycling of Asian and Hong Kong influenza A virus hemagglutinins in man. *Am J Epidemiol*, **97**, 44–9.

Matson, D.O., Estes, M.K., et al. 1989. Human calicivirus-associated diarrhea in children attending day care centers. *J Infect Dis*, **159**, 71–8.

Melnick, J.L. and Ledinko, N. 1951. Social serology: antibody levels in a normal young population during an epidemic of poliomyelitis. *Am J Hyg*, **54**, 354–82.

Mercado, R. 1975. Rodent control programmes in areas affected by Bolivian hemorrhagic fever. *Bull WHO*, **52**, 691–6.

Minor, T.E., Dick, E.C., et al. 1974. Viruses as precipitants of asthmatic attacks in children. *JAMA*, **227**, 292–8.

Monto, A.S. 1973. The Tecumseh study of respiratory illness. V. Patterns of infection with the parainfluenzaviruses. *Am J Epidemiol*, **97**, 338–48.

Monto, A.S. and Kioumehr, F. 1975. The Tecumseh study of respiratory illness. IX. Occurrence of influenza in the community, 1966–1971. *Am J Epidemiol*, **102**, 553–63.

Monto, A.S. and Koopman, J.S. 1980. The Tecumseh Study. XI. Occurrence of acute enteric illness in the community. *Am J Epidemiol*, **112**, 323–33.

Monto, A.S. and Lim, S.K. 1971. The Tecumseh study of respiratory illness. III. Incidence and periodicity of respiratory syncytial virus and *Mycoplasma pneumoniae* infections. *Am J Epidemiol*, **94**, 290–301.

Monto, A.S. and Ross, H. 1977. Acute respiratory illness in the community: effect of family composition, smoking, and chronic symptoms. *Br J Prev Soc Med*, **31**, 101–8.

Monto, A.S. and Sullivan, K.M. 1993. Acute respiratory illness in the community: frequency of illness and the agents involved. *Epidemiol Infect*, **110**, 145–60.

Monto, A.S., Davenport, F.M., et al. 1970. Modification of an outbreak of influenza in Tecumseh, Michigan, by vaccination of schoolchildren. *J Infect Dis*, **122**, 16–25.

Monto, A.S., Koopman, J.S. and Longini, I.M. 1985. The Tecumseh study of illness. XIII. Influenza infection and disease, 1976–1981. *Am J Epidemiol*, **121**, 811–22.

Monto, A.S., Koopman, J.S. and Bryan, E.R. 1986. The Tecumseh study of illness. XIV. Occurrence of respiratory viruses, 1976–1981. *Am J Epidemiol*, **124**, 359–67.

Monto, A.S., Bryan, E.R. and Ohmit, S. 1987. Rhinovirus infections in Tecumseh, Michigan: frequency of illness and numbers of serotypes. *J Infect Dis*, **156**, 43–9.

Moser, M.R., Bender, T.R., et al. 1979. An outbreak of influenza aboard a commercial airliner. *Am J Epidemiol*, **110**, 1–7.

Mosley, J.W., Edwards, V.M., et al. 1975. Hepatitis B virus infection in dentists. *N Engl J Med*, **293**, 729–34.

Nathanson, N. and Martin, J.R. 1979. The epidemiology of poliomyelitis: enigmas surrounding its appearance, epidemicity, and disappearance. *Am J Epidemiol*, **110**, 672–92.

Nichol, K.L., Margolis, K.L., et al. 1994. The efficacy and cost effectiveness of vaccination against influenza among elderly persons living in the community. *New Engl J Med*, **331**, 778–84.

Nolan, T.F., Goodman, R.A., et al. 1980. Morbidity and mortality associated with influenza B in the United States 1978–1980. A report from the Centers for Disease Control. *J Infect Dis*, **142**, 360–2.

Ohmit, S.E. and Monto, A.S. 1995. Influenza vaccine effectiveness in preventing hospitalization among the elderly during influenza type A and B seasons. *Int J Epidemiol*, **24**, 1240–8.

Padian, N.S., Shiboski, S.C. and Jewell, N.P. 1991. Female-to-male transmission of human immunodeficiency virus. *JAMA*, **266**, 1664–7.

Papaevangelou, G. and Kourea-Kremastinou, T. 1974. Role of mosquitoes in transmission of hepatitis B virus infection. *J Infect Dis*, **130**, 78–80.

Parrott, R.H., Kim, H.W., et al. 1973. Epidemiology of respiratory syncytial virus infection in Washington, DC. *Am J Epidemiol*, **98**, 289–300.

Peters, C.J., Kuehne, R.W., et al. 1974. Hemorrhagic fever in Cochabamba, Bolivia, 1971. *Am J Epidemiol*, **99**, 425–33.

Peters, C.J., Sanchez, A., et al. 1994. Filoviruses as emerging pathogens. *Semin Virol*, **5**, 147–54.

Petersen, L.R., Roehrig, J.T. and Hughes, J.M. 2002. Outlook: West Nile Virus encephalitis. *New Engl J Med*, **347**, 1225–6.

Phair, J., Kauffman, C.A., et al. 1978. Failure to respond to influenza vaccine in the aged: correlation with B-cell number and function. *J Lab Clin Med*, **92**, 822–8.

Pitt, D.B. 1957. Congenital malformations and maternal rubella. *Med J Aust*, **1**, 233–9.

Portnoy, B.L., Mackowiak, P.A., et al. 1975. Oyster-associated hepatitis: failure of shellfish certification program to prevent outbreaks. *JAMA*, **233**, 1065–8.

Rawls, W.E., Iwamoto, K., et al. 1970. Herpesvirus type 2 antibodies and carcinoma of the cervix. *Lancet*, **2**, 1142–3.

Reeves, W.C. 1974. Overwintering of arboviruses. *Prog Med Virol*, **17**, 193–220.

Reeves, W.C., Caussy, D., et al. 1987. Case–control study of human papillomaviruses and cervical cancer in Latin America. *Int J Cancer*, **40**, 450–4.

Remington, P.L., Rowley, D., et al. 1986. Decreasing trends in Reye's syndrome and aspirin use in Michigan 1979–1984. *Pediatrics*, **77**, 93–8.

Rivers, T. 1937. Viruses and Koch's postulates. *J Bacteriol*, **33**, 1–12.

Sawyer, W.A., Meyer, K.F., et al. 1944. Jaundice in army personnel in the western region of the United States and its relation to vaccination against yellow fever. *Am J Hyg*, **39**, 337–430; **40**, 35–107.

Schlesselman, J.J. 1982. *Case–control studies: design, conduct, analysis*. New York: Oxford University Press.

Serfling, R.E. 1963. Methods for current statistical analysis of excess pneumonia-influenza deaths. *Pub Health Rep*, **78**, 494–506.

Sever, J.L., Hardy, J.B., et al. 1969. Rubella in the collaborative perinatal research study. II. Clinical and laboratory findings in children through 3 years of age. *Am J Dis Child*, **118**, 123–32.

Sever, J.L., Nelson, K.B. and Gilkeson, M.R. 1965. Rubella epidemic, 1964: effect on 6000 pregnancies. I. Preliminary clinical and laboratory findings through the neonatal period: a report from the collaborative study on cerebral palsy. *Am J Dis Child*, **110**, 395–407.

Sever, J.L., Schiff, G.M. and Huebner, R.J. 1964. Frequency of rubella antibody among pregnant women and other human and animal populations. *Obstet Gynecol*, **23**, 153–9.

Shope, R.E. 1936. The incidence of neutralizing antibodies for swine influenza virus on the sera of human beings of different ages. *J Exp Med*, **63**, 669–84.

Smith, J.S., Orciari, L.A., et al. 1992. Epidemiologic and historical relationships among 87 rabies virus isolates as determined by limited sequence analysis. *J Infect Dis*, **166**, 296–307.

Spilker, B. 1991. *Guide to clinical trials*. New York: Raven Press.

Starko, K.M., Ray, C.G., et al. 1982. Reye's syndrome and salicylate use. *Pediatrics*, **66**, 859–64.

Stevens, C.E., Beasley, R.P., et al. 1975. Vertical transmission of hepatitis B antigen in Taiwan. *N Engl J Med*, **292**, 771–4.

Subbarao, K., Klimov, A., et al. 1998. Characterization of an avian influenza A (H5N1) virus isolated from a child with a fatal respiratory illness. *Science*, **279**, 393–6.

Susser, M. 1973. *Causal thinking in the health sciences*. New York: Oxford University Press.

Swan, G., Tostevin, A.L. and Black, G.H.B. 1946. Final observations on congenital defects in infants following infectious diseases during pregnancy with special reference to rubella. *Med J Aust*, **2**, 889–908.

Szmuness, W., Much, M.I., et al. 1975. On the role of sexual behavior in the spread of hepatitis B infection. *Ann Intern Med*, **83**, 489–95.

Szmuness, W., Stevens, C.E., et al. 1980. Hepatitis B vaccine: demonstration of efficacy in a controlled clinical trial in a high-risk population in the United States. *N Engl J Med*, **303**, 833–41.

Taubenberger, J.K., Reid, A.H., et al. 1997. Initial genetic characterization of the 1918 'Spanish' influenza virus. *Science*, **275**, 1793–6.

Theiler, M. 1957. Action of sodium deoxycholate on arthropodborne viruses. *Proc Soc Exp Biol Med*, **96**, 380–2.

Tyrrell, D.A., Bynoe, M.L., et al. 1960. Some virus isolations from common colds. I. Experiments employing human volunteers. *Lancet*, **1**, 235–7.

Vesikari, T., Ruuska, T., et al. 1992. Protective efficacy against serotype 1 rotavirus diarrhea by live oral rhesus-human reassortant rotavirus vaccines with human rotavirus VP7 serotype 1 or 2 specificity. *Pediatr Infect Dis J*, **11**, 535–42.

Wagner, G., Lavanchy, D., et al. 1993. Simultaneous active and passive immunization against hepatitis A studied in a population of travellers. *Vaccine*, **11**, 1027–32.

Waldman, R.J., Hall, W.N., et al. 1982. Aspirin as a risk factor in Reye's syndrome. *JAMA*, **247**, 3089–94.

Warner, R.D., Carr, R.W., et al. 1991. A large nontypical outbreak of Norwalk virus: gastroenteritis associated with exposing celery to nonpotable water and with *Citrobacter freundii. Arch Intern Med*, **151**, 2419–24.

Wehrle, P.F., Posch, J., et al. 1970. An airborne outbreak of smallpox in a German hospital and its significance with respect to other recent outbreaks in Europe. *Bull WHO*, **43**, 669–79.

Westaway, E.G., Brinton, M.A., et al. 1985a. Flaviviridae. *Intervirology*, **24**, 183–92.

Westaway, E.G., Brinton, M.A., et al. 1985b. Togaviridae. *Intervirology*, **24**, 125–39.

Wong, D.C., Purcell, R.H., et al. 1980. Epidemic and enteric hepatitis in India: evidence for a non-A, non-B hepatitis virus etiology. *Lancet*, **2**, 876–8.

World Health Organization/Global Programme on AIDS. 1994. *The current global situation of the HIV/AIDS Pandemic*. Geneva: WHO.

19

The order *Mononegavirales*

ANDREW J. EASTON AND CRAIG R. PRINGLE

INTRODUCTION – THE UNIVERSAL SYSTEM OF VIRUS TAXONOMY

The *Universal System of Virus Taxonomy* has been developed to its present state by the International Committee on Taxonomy of Viruses (ICTV) through a series of seven reports (see Chapter 4, The classification of vertebrate viruses), the most recent of which was published in 2000 (van Regenmortel et al. 2000) and an eighth report is reaching completion. The system of taxonomy adopted by the ICTV is sufficiently flexible to withstand the stress of the continual discovery of new viruses from an ever-increasing diversity of host organisms. A hierarchy of five taxa, ranked as orders, families, subfamilies, genera, and species, has been developed. Taxonomic categories below the species level, such as subspecies, strains, variants, genotypes, etc., are not included in this taxonomy and are defined according to the practical needs in each particular field. The concept and definition of the category of virus species is central to the structure of the taxonomy, and the nature of the virus species is discussed separately in Chapter 4, The classification of vertebrate viruses.

The highest taxon, the order, comprises a group of families that have certain features in common. In the 7th Report of the ICTV only three orders are recognized. The taxon below the order is the family and 68 families are recognized at present. As yet only nine of these 68 families have been grouped into each of the three orders. However, it is anticipated that the number of orders will increase in parallel with refinement of the methods of characterization of viruses. Orders are designated by names with the suffix *-virales*, families by the ending *-viridae*, and sub-families by the ending *-virinae*. The first order described in virus taxonomy was the order *Mononegavirales*, which contains the families of nonsegmented single-stranded negative-sense RNA viruses (Pringle 1991, 1997; Pringle and Easton 1997). The other orders currently recognized are the order *Caudovirales*, comprising the three families of tailed phages – *Myoviridae*, *Siphoviridae*, and *Podoviridae* (Maniloff and Ackermann 1998) and the order *Nidovirales* comprising the positive-sense RNA viruses with nested-set genomes – the families *Coronaviridae* and *Arteriviridae* (see Chapter 20, The order *Nidovirales*).

The orders *Mononegavirales* and *Nidovirales* were established to embrace families of viruses exhibiting similar features of genomic organization and replicative strategies. In the case of the order *Caudovirales*, different criteria were required since any preexisting phylogenetic relationships were obscured by a combination of great geological age, large population sizes, and extensive horizontal gene transfer. Nonetheless, relationships are still evident in respect of common aspects of morphology, replication, and assembly, which can be utilized to provide an operationally useful classification. This emphasizes a fundamental aspect of the *Universal System of Virus Taxonomy*; namely, it is hierarchical and consistent with phylogenetic relationships but not dependent on them. To some extent this is exemplified also in the case of the order *Mononegavirales*, which was established initially to accommodate three families (*Filoviridae, Paramyxoviridae, Rhabdoviridae*) with clear phylogenetic links, and subsequently expanded to include a fourth family (*Bornaviridae*) on the basis of similar genomic organization rather than close phylogenetic relationship. The following list presents the current taxonomy of the order *Mononegavirales*. The convention is now that all taxonomic names, including those of virus species, should be rendered in italics with an initial capital letter when used in a taxonomic context. The names can be used without italics in other contexts.

> *Bornaviridae*
>> *Bornavirus*
>>> *Borna disease virus*
>
> *Filoviridae*
>> *Marburgvirus*
>>> *Lake Victoria marburgvirus*
>> *Ebolavirus*
>>> *Zaire ebolavirus*
>
> *Paramyxoviridae*
>> *Paramyxovirinae*
>>> *Avulavirus*
>>>> *Newcastle disease virus*
>>> *Henipavirus*
>>>> *Hendra virus*
>>> *Morbillivirus*
>>>> *Measles virus*
>>> *Respirovirus*
>>>> *Sendai virus 1*
>>> *Rubulavirus*
>>>> *Mumps virus*
>> *Pneumovirinae*
>>> *Pneumovirus*
>>>> *Human respiratory syncytial virus*
>>> *Metapneumovirus*
>>>> *Turkey rhinotracheitis virus*
>
> *Rhabdoviridae*
>> *Cytorhabdovirus*
>>> *Lettuce necrotic yellows virus*
>> *Ephemerovirus*
>>> *Bovine ephemeral fever virus*
>> *Lyssavirus*
>>> *Rabies virus*
>> *Novirhabdovirus*
>>> *Infectious hematopoietic necrosis virus*
>> *Nucleorhabdovirus*
>>> *Potato yellow dwarf virus*
>> *Vesiculovirus*
>>> *Vesicular stomatitis Indiana virus*

THE ORDER *MONONEGAVIRALES*

Background

The order *Mononegavirales* was established to accommodate all known viruses with nonsegmented negative-sense single-stranded RNA genomes as indicated by the derivation of the name (mono – single, nega – negative-sense, -virales – viruses). Initially that comprised viruses classified in the families *Filoviridae, Paramyxoviridae,* and *Rhabdoviridae*. The features that distinguished these three families were predominantly morphological and biological. Later, molecular characterization of *Borna disease virus* (the type species and sole representative of the family *Bornaviridae*) revealed that this virus possessed a nonsegmented, negative-sense single-stranded RNA virus genome (De la Torre 1994; Schneemann et al. 1995). It differs substantially from the other three families in several respects, the most fundamental being the intranuclear site of transcription and replication. Entry by receptor-mediated endocytosis is followed by transport of viral ribonucleoprotein to the nucleus where transcription and replication occur. The features common to the four families are listed in Table 19.1, and the characteristics which distinguish each family are listed in Table 19.2. (Detailed descriptions and references can be found in Chapters 33–38 and 50–52.)

Table 19.1 *Common properties of the members of the order* Mononegavirales

Common properties
Negative-sense nonsegmented single-stranded RNA in the virion
Conservation of gene order
Virion-associated RNA polymerase mediates transcription and replication
Genome transcribed into 6–10 discrete mRNAs from a single 5′-terminal promoter, with the exception of *Borna disease virus* where two primary transcripts are post-transcriptionally processed by the host-cell mRNA splicing machinery
Replication occurs by synthesis of a complete positive-sense RNA antigenome
Nucleoprotein is the functional template for the synthesis of replicative and mRNA
Independently assembled nucleocapsids are enveloped at the cell surface at sites containing virus proteins, except in the case of *Borna disease virus*
All cytoplasmic, except viruses in the genera *Bornavirus* and *Nucleorhabdovirus*
Gene boundaries marked by an end/intergenic/start configuration in all except *Borna disease virus*
None exhibit genetic recombination
Occur in invertebrates, plants and vertebrates

Table 19.2 *Characteristic features of the four families of the order* Mononegavirales

Family *Bornaviridae*

Spherical particles of 90 nm diameter, with 50–60 nm diameter electron dense core, and outer membrane with 7 nm-long spike projections

Nuclear

Spherical 50–60 nm diameter nucleoprotein core

Genome size: 8.9 kb

Six major open reading frames encoding presumptive 3′-NP (p40)-P (p24)/NS? (p10)-M (p16)-G (p56)-L (p180). Complex pattern of mRNA transcription involving 3 initiation sites and 4 termination sites, mRNA splicing at two introns

Wide host range, horses and sheep regarded as main natural hosts. Associated with neurological disease and behavioural abnormalities

Family *Filoviridae*

Filamentous forms with branching, sometimes U-shaped, 6-shaped or ring-shaped. A unique diameter of 80 nm and varying lengths extending up to 14 000 nm, with spike projections of 10 nm approximately. Infectious particle length is 790 nm for Lake Victoria marburgvirus and 970 nm for Zaire ebolavirus

All cytoplasmic

Helical nucleocapsid, 50 nm diameter, with an axial space of 20 nm diameter and a helical periodicity of 5 nm approximately

Genome size: 18.9–19.1 kb

Seven proteins are encoded in the genome in the order 3′-NP (nucleoprotein)-VP35 (phosphoprotein)-VP40 (matrix protein)-GP (glycoprotein)-VP30(?)-VP24(?)-L (polymerase)-5′. Most genes are separated by nonconserved intergenic sequences, but some genes overlap in a highly conserved pentamer junction region

Biology enigmatic: only two antigenically unrelated viruses known; transmitted by the bloodborne route; restricted to primates; reservoir species unknown

Family *Paramyxoviridae*

Pleomorphic, some roughly spherical, 150 nm in diameter, filamentous forms common in some. All cytoplasmic

Helical nucleocapsid; 13–18 nm diameter, 5.5–7 nm pitch

Genome size: all in the range15.4–15.9 kb, with the exception of the 18 kb of the recently discovered *Hendra virus* and *Nipah virus*

The family comprises two phylogenetically distinct subfamilies; the genome size of viruses in the sub-family Paramyxovirinae conforms to 'the rule of six' (i.e. the nucleotide number is divisible by six), whereas this rule does not apply in the subfamily Pneumovirinae

Seven to nine proteins are encoded in the Paramyxovirinae (of which two to four are derived from overlapping reading frames in the *P* gene), and 9 to 11 in the Pneumovirinae, The virion proteins common to all genera are three nucleocapsid–associated proteins (N or NP, P and L), three membrane-associated proteins (M, G or H or HN, and F). Variable proteins include several non-structural proteins (C, NS1, NS2), a cysteine-rich zinc-binding protein (V), a small integral membrane protein (SH), and a transcription processivity protein (M2). Genes non-overlapping except in the case at the M2/L junction in some pneumoviruses

Found only in vertebrates; no arthropod vectors known. Horizontal transmission, mainly by the airborne route. Predominantly associated with respiratory infections

Family *Rhabdoviridae*

Bullet-shaped or bacilliform; 100–430 nm in length and 45–100 nm in diameter. Surface spikes 5–10 nm in length × 3 nm in diameter

Helical nucleocapsid, 50 nm diameter, unwinding to helical structure of 20 × 700 nm (VSV)

Cytoplasmic with the exception of plant viruses of the genus Nucleorhabdovirus, which multiply in the nucleus and form nuclear inclusions

Genome size: 11–15 kb

Generally have five structural proteins (3′-N-P-M-G-L-5′) plus an additional presumptive non-structural protein in some. Exceptionally, members of the genus Ephemerovirus have up to ten genes encoding glycoproteins of uncertain function

Wide host range, different species infect plants, invertebrates and vertebrates. Some multiply in invertebrates and plants, some in invertebrates and vertebrates, but none in plants and vertebrates. May be vertically transmitted in arthropods (Sigman virus), otherwise transmitted horizontally

General properties

Conventional transmission electron microscopic analysis shows that the virions are large enveloped structures with a prominent fringe of peplomers, 5–10 nm long and spaced 7–10 nm apart, in all except the *Bornaviridae*. The morphologies are variable, but in general distinguish the families. Virion Mr is $300–1\,000 \times 10^6$. S_{20w} is 550–1 045 (plant rhabdoviruses have larger S_{20w} values). Virion buoyant density in CsCl is 1.18–1.22 g/cm³. Virus infectivity is rapidly inactivated by heat treatment at 56°C, or following UV- or X-irradiation, or exposure to lipid solvents.

Virions contain one molecule of linear, non-infectious, negative-sense, single-stranded RNA, 8.9–19 kb in size, (M_r of $3–5 \times 10^6$), which comprises about 0.5–2.0 percent of the particle weight. The viral RNA lacks a capped 5′ terminus, or a covalently associated protein. The 3′ terminus of viral RNA lacks a poly(A) tract. The immediate 5′ and 3′ terminal regions exhibit inverse complementarity, and there are conserved motifs in the terminal regions of all four families. Full-length positive-sense (anti-genomic) RNAs are found in infected cells. The genome comprises a linear sequence of genes, with limited overlaps in some viruses, and with short terminal noncoding regions. There are conserved motifs in the transcription start and end signals in all families and the intergenic regions, which lie between the transcribed genes, range from two to several hundred nucleotides. Exceptionally, genetic information may be encoded in additional reading frames in the *P* genes of respiroviruses and morbilliviruses. Splicing of some mRNA and overlapping start/stop signals are characteristic of bornaviruses.

There are a limited number of proteins in relation to the large particle size. The 5–7 structural proteins comprise envelope glycoprotein(s), a matrix protein, a major RNA-binding protein, other nucleocapsid-associated protein(s), and a large molecular weight polymerase protein, plus in some viruses, several additional nonstructural proteins, which may be phosphorylated. The glycoproteins may have a covalently associated fatty acid proximal to the lipid envelope. The matrix protein is nonglycosylated in all except the bornaviruses in which it is *N*-glycosylated and expressed on the surface of virions and may function as an attachment protein. Enzymatic activities associated with the virions may include RNA polymerase, polyadenylate transferase, mRNA transferase, and neuraminidase.

Virions are composed of about 15–25 percent lipids, their composition reflecting that of the region of the host cell membrane where virions bud. Generally, phospholipids represent about 55–60 percent, and sterols and glycolipids about 35–40 percent of the total lipids. Virions are composed of about 3 percent carbohydrates by weight, which are present as *N*- and *O*-linked glycan chains on surface proteins and on glycolipids. When made in mammalian cells the oligosaccharide chains are generally of the complex type, in insect cells they are of noncomplex types.

In the *Filoviridae*, *Paramyxoviridae*, and *Rhabdoviridae*, discrete mRNAs are transcribed by sequential interrupted synthesis. Transcription is polar with stepwise attenuation. Generally genes do not overlap, the exceptions being the *M2* and *L* genes of respiratory syncytial virus (family *Paramyxoviridae*, subfamily *Pneumovirinae*, genus *Pneumovirus*), the *VP30* and *VP24*

genes of *Lake Victoria marburgvirus* (family *Filoviridae* genus *Marburgvirus*) and the *VP35/VP40*, *GP/VP30*, and *VP24/L* genes of *Zaire ebolavirus* (family *Filoviridae*, genus *Ebolavirus*). The site of multiplication is the cytoplasm, with the exception of plant viruses classified in the genus *Nucleorhabdovirus*. The *P* genes of respiroviruses and morbilliviruses are exceptional in that additional open reading frames may be utilized via alternative non-AUG start codons, and mRNA editing occurs by insertion of nontemplated nucleotides to change the reading frame for the expression of *P* gene products. In the filovirus *Zaire ebolavirus*, a nontemplated insertion event during transcription of the glycoprotein gene generates the membrane-inserted glycoprotein seen in virions, whereas the faithfully transcribed mRNA encodes a secreted form of the glycoprotein lacking the membrane anchor. This does not appear to occur in the other filovirus, *Lake Victoria marburgvirus*. In the *Bornaviridae*, the site of multiplication is the nucleus and transcription is complex with splicing of mRNA and overlapping transcriptional stop/start signals.

Replication occurs by synthesis of a complete positive sense anti-genomic RNA. Genomic and anti-genomic RNAs are present only as nucleocapsids. The mRNAs of bornaviruses are capped, but synthesis is not inhibited by α-amanitin suggesting that a cap-snatching mechanism is not involved. In the filoviruses, paramyxoviruses and rhabdoviruses, maturation of the independently assembled helical nucleocapsid occurs by budding through host membranes with investment by a host-derived lipid envelope containing transmembrane proteins. The process of assembly and maturation of bornaviruses is not understood at present.

Membrane glycoproteins are involved in antibody-mediated neutralisation. Virus serotypes are defined by the surface antigens. Filoviruses are an exception in that they are poorly neutralized in vitro. In bornaviruses antibodies to both the glycosylated matrix protein and the gp94 envelope protein neutralize infectivity.

The host ranges vary from restricted to unrestricted. Filoviruses have only been isolated from primates. Paramyxoviruses occur only in vertebrates and no vectors are known. Rhabdoviruses infect invertebrates, vertebrates, and plants. Some rhabdoviruses multiply in both invertebrates and vertebrates, some in invertebrates and plants, but none in all three. In human hosts the pathogenic potential tends to be characteristic of the family: i.e. hemorrhagic fever (*Filoviridae*); respiratory and neurological diseases (*Paramyxoviridae*); mild febrile to fatal neurological diseases (*Rhabdoviridae*). Bornaviruses have been isolated from horses, cattle, sheep, rabbits, rats, cats, ostriches, and man. The pathology associated with virus infection is variable. Infection of animals is associated with conditions ranging from behavioral disturbances to severe nonpurulent encephalomyelitis, and there is some evidence of association of bornavirus infection with neuropsychiatric illness in man. Cytopathology varies from none (bornaviruses and filoviruses) to rapidly lytic (rhabdoviruses and paramyxoviruses); syncytium formation is common in paramyxoviruses.

BRIEF DESCRIPTIONS OF THE FOUR FAMILIES COMPRISING THE ORDER *MONONEGAVIRALES*

The family *Bornaviridae*

The family *Bornaviridae* is represented by *Borna disease virus*, a species of some antiquity. Borna disease takes its name from the town of Borna in Saxony, Germany, where extensive outbreaks of fatal neurological disease in horses, and occasionally sheep, have occurred at least since 1895. The viral etiology of the disease was established in 1925, but it was not recognized to be a negative-sense RNA virus until 1995. As yet, no other virus with comparable molecular characteristics has been isolated. Borna disease was considered to be sporadically endemic only in Central Europe, but it may have spread worldwide in recent times. In horses, the outcome of infection is often death, and surviving animals may exhibit permanent sensory or motor deficiencies. No data are available that might identify reservoir hosts facilitating the spread of the virus, and there is no evidence for vectorborne transmission. The question of the involvement of Borna disease virus in human neuropsychiatric illness remains unresolved, but experimental infection of a primate (the tree shrew *Tupaia*) appeared to induce aberrant social behaviour and altered response to environmental stimuli (see also: Chapter 52, Borna disease virus).

The family *Filoviridae*

The family *Filoviridae* comprises two genera, *Ebolavirus* and *Marburgvirus*. *Marburgvirus* is represented by a single species, now designated *Lake Victoria marburgvirus*, whereas *Ebolavirus* is represented by four distinct species *Cote d'Ivoire ebolavirus*, *Reston ebolavirus*, *Sudan ebolavirus*, and *Zaire ebolavirus*. All these viruses, except for *Reston ebolavirus*, which does not appear to be pathogenic for humans, have been associated with outbreaks of acute and often fatal hemorrhagic fever in Central Africa. The virions exhibit similar filamentous pleomorphic morphology and virus infectivity is poorly neutralized in vitro. There is virtually no cross-reactivity between the two genera. The amino acid homology of the surface glycoproteins of ebolaviruses and marburgviruses is approximately 30 per cent, compared with 55–66 percent between ebolavirus species. The natural reservoirs of filoviruses are unknown, but no vector appears to be involved in transmission (see also: Chapter 50, Filoviruses).

The family *Paramyxoviridae* – subfamily *Paramyxovirinae*

The family *Paramyxoviridae* is divided into two subfamilies; the *Paramyxovirinae* containing the five genera *Avulavirus, Henipavirus, Morbillivirus, Respirovirus*, and *Rubulavirus*; and the *Pneumovirinae* containing the two genera *Pneumovirus* and *Metapneumovirus*. The features exhibited by all members of the *Paramyxovirinae* are the following: identical genome organisation consisting of six (seven in some rubulaviruses) transcriptional elements; nucleocapsid diameter of 18 nm, 5.5 nm pitch; genome length a multiple of six nucleotides; a 3' leader of approximately 55 nucleotides with the first three nucleotides (ACC) absolutely conserved; conserved transcription start and stop signals; RNA editing site in the *P/V* gene; fusion and attachment functions segregated to separate glycoproteins (F and HN or H) that exhibit sequence relatedness across the subfamily.

The avian pathogen *Newcastle disease virus* was long regarded as representative of all paramyxoviruses, but as molecular characterization of other paramyxoviruses progressed it became apparent that *Newcastle disease virus* possessed unique properties. Consequently, it has been reassigned as the sole member of the new genus *Avulavirus* and it is anticipated that other avian paramyxoviruses may be reassigned to this genus when more molecular information is available. The genus *Respirovirus* comprises *Sendai virus, Human parainfluenza viruses 1* and *3, Bovine parainfluenza virus 3*, and *Simian virus 10*. The genus *Morbillivirus* comprises *Measles virus, Canine distemper virus, Rinderpest virus*, and *Peste-des-petits-ruminants virus*. In addition, *Cetacean morbillivirus* and *Phocine distemper virus*, two viruses from marine mammals, have been added to the *Morbillivirus* genus recently. The genus *Rubulavirus* comprises *Mumps virus, Human parainfluenza viruses 2* and *4, Porcine rubulavirus, Simian virus 5, Simian virus 41*, and three viruses isolated from bats – *Mapuera virus*, Menangle virus, and Tioman virus. The avian paramyxoviruses are currently grouped with the rubulaviruses but this is expected to alter with the advent of molecular characterization of these viruses. Recently two other viruses isolated from bats in South-east Asia and Australia – Hendra virus and Nipah virus – proved to be related to each other but quite distinct from the bat rubulaviruses and indeed other paramyxoviruses. As a consequence these viruses have been assigned to a new genus *Henipavirus*. These viruses are distinguished by their larger genome size (18 kb compared with the uniform 15–16 kb of all other paramyxoviruses). The size of the *Henipavirus* gene products is similar to those of other viruses in the subfamily, with the exception of the P protein which is approximately 100 amino acids longer than the longest P protein previously characterized. The size, sequence, and domain structure of the Hendra virus L protein are very similar to those of other viruses in the subfamily. Extensive phylogenetic analyses of both full-length L protein and the more conserved domain III sequences confirmed that Hendra virus is a member of the subfamily *Paramyxovirinae* and is more closely related to morbilliviruses and respiroviruses (see below and Figure 19.1a). However, the L proteins of the two henipaviruses and Tupaia paramyxovirus (an as yet unclassified paramyxovirus isolated from the tree shrew

Tupaia belangeri in Thailand) differ from the L proteins of other negative-sense RNA viruses in one important respect. The four-amino acid sequence GDNQ, that is absolutely conserved among all known *L* genes of negative-sense RNA viruses is replaced by GDNE (Figure 19.1b). This sequence resides in the highly conserved and functionally important C motif of domain III of all negative-sense RNA virus polymerases.

The subfamily *Paramyxovirinae* is an ever-expanding taxonomic group; Salem virus, isolated in North America from a horse, and Tupaia paramyxovirus are in the process of characterization and their place in the

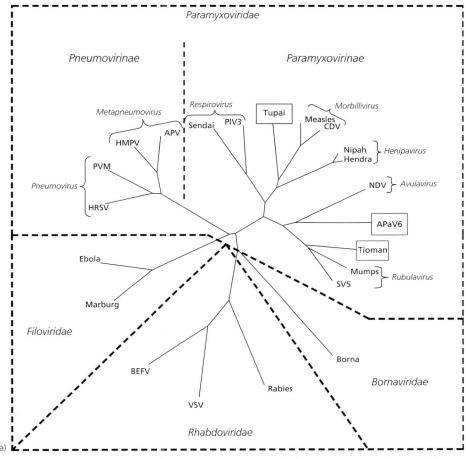

Figure 19.1 (a) *Unrooted phylogenetic tree of members of the order* Mononegavirales. *The tree was constructed using the CLUSTALX programme with the sequences of the conserved domain III region of the* L *polymerase proteins (Poch et al. 1989, 1990). The ICTV classification designations of the viruses are indicated. For the* Paramyxoviridae, *the two subfamilies and five genera are also indicated. The unclassified Tupaia paramyxovirus (Tupai), avian parainfluenzavirus type 6 (ApaV6) and Tioman virus (Tioman) are indicated.*
(b) *Alignment of the domain III region sequences of members of the order* Mononegavirales. *The four conserved polymerase motifs (A–D) are indicated. The conserved GDNQ motif is highlighted. The viruses are:* Sendai virus (Sendai; Middleton et al. 1990), *human parainfluenza virus type 3 (HPIV-3; Galinski et al. 1988), Tupai paramyxovirus (Tupai; Accession number NP_054697), Measles virus (measles; Bankamp et al. 1999), Canine distemper virus (CDV; Sidhu et al. 1993), Nipah virus (Nipah; Chan et al. 2001), Hendra virus (Hendra; Wang et al. 2000), Newcastle disease virus (NDV; Yusoff et al. 1987), avian paramyxovirus 6 (ApaV6; Accession number NP_150063), Tioman virus (Tioman; Chua et al. 2002), Mumps virus (Mumps; Okazaki et al. 1992), Simian virus 5 (SV5; Higuchi et al. 1992), Human respiratory syncytial virus (HRSV; Tolley et al. 1996), pneumonia virus of mice (PVM; L. Thorpe and A. Easton, unpublished), Human metapneumovirus (HMPV; Accession number AF371337), avian pneumovirus (APV; Randhawa et al. 1996), Marburg virus (Marburg; Muhlberger et al. 1992), Ebola virus, strain Zaire (Ebola; Volchkov et al. 2000), Rabies virus (Rabies; Conzelmann et al. 1990), Vesicular stomatitis Indiana virus (VSV; Schubert et al. 1984), Bovine ephemeral fever virus (BEFV; Walker et al. 1994), Borna disease virus (Borna; Briese et al. 1994). (Adapted from Pringle, C.R. 2004.* Mononegavirales. *In Fauquet, C.M. et al. (eds)* Virus Taxonomy, VIII Report of the ICTV. *London: Elsevier/Academic Press, pp. 609–14.) (Continued over).*

Figure 19.1 Alignment of the domain III region sequences of members of the order Mononegavirales *(Continued). For full caption see previous page.*

(b)

A

```
Sendai : FLTTDLKKYCLNWRFESTALFGQRCNEIFGFKTFNWMHPVLERCTIVGDPYCPVADRMHR-QLQDHADSGIFIHNPRGGIEGYCQKLWTLISMSAIHLAAVRVGVRVSA
PIV3   : FLTTDLKKYCLNWRYESTALFGETCNOIFGLNKLFNWLHPRLEGSTLYVDYPCPPSDKEHY-SLEDHDSGFYVHNPRGGIEGFCQKLWTLISISAIHLAAVRIGVRTA
Tupai  : FLTTDLQKFCLNWRYETSAIYAQRLDEIYGLPNFFEWLHKRLERSTLYVCDPSCPPKLAKHV-DLDTMPNEHIFIKNMGGIEGYSQKLWTIATIPYLYLSAYEVGVRTA
Measles: FITTDLKKYCLNWRYETISLFAQRLNEIYGLPSFFQWLHKRLETSVLYVSDPHCPPPDLDAHV-PLCKVPNDQIFIKYPMGGIEGYCQKLWTISTIPYLYLAAYESGVRIAS
CDV    : FITTDLKKYCLNWRYETISIFAQRLNEIYGLPSFFQWLHRRLEQSILYVSDPHCPPPDLDRHV-DLNTAPNSQIFIKYPMGGVEGYCQKLWTISTIPYLYLAAHESGVRIAS
Nipah  : FLTTDLKKFCLNWRYESMAIFAERLDEIYGLPGFFNWMHKRLERSVIVVADPNCPPNIDKHM-ELEKTPEDDIFIHYPKGGIEGYSQKTWTIATIPFFLSAYETNTRIAA
Hendra : FLTTDLKKFCLNWRYESMAIFAERLDEIYGLPGFFNWMHKRLEKSVIVVADPNCPPDIGKHI-NLDDTPEDDIFIHSPKGGIEGYSQKTWTIATIPFFLSAYETNTRIAA
NDV    : FITTDLQKYCLNWRYQTIKLFAHAINQLMGLPHFFEWIHLRLMDTTMFVGDPFNPPSDPTDC-DLSRVPNDIYVSARGGIEGLCQKLWTMISIAAIQLAAARSHCRVAC
ApaV6  : FLTTDLQKYCLNWRYTVVKPFAQRLNQLFGIPHGFEWIHLRLMNTTMFVGDPHNVPQFSSTH-DLESQENDGIFIVSPRGGIEGLCQKMWTMISIAAIHiAATESGCRVAS
Tioman : FLTTDLSKYCLNWRYQSIILFAKSMNQLYGYNHLFEWIHLRLMRSTLYVGDPFNPPRNLTSA-DLDLVENGDIFIVSPRGGIEGLCQKLWTMISIAVIVLSATEAGTRVMS
Mumps  : FLTTDLKKYCLNWRYQVIIPFARTLNSMYGIPHLFEWIHLRLMRSTLYVGDPFNPPSDPTQL-DLDTALNDDIFIVSPRGGIEGLCQKAWTMISIAVIILSATESGTRVMS
SV5    : FLTTDLKKYCLQWRYQTIIFAQSLNRMYGYNHLFEWIHLRLMRSTLYVGDPFNPPSDPTGL-DLDKVINGDIFIVSPRGGIEGLCQKLWTMISIAVIILSATESGTRVMS
RSV    : SIITDLSKFNQAFRYETSCICSDVLDELHGTQSLFSWLHLTIPHVTIICTYRHAPYIRDHIVDLNVDEQSGLYRYMGGIEGWCQKLWTTEAISLLDLSLKGKFSITA
PVM    : SLITDLSKFNQAFRYESSCCVSDLLDELHGTQSLFSWLHLTVPLTTMTYRHAPPDTGNNY-NVDDIAEQSGLYRYHMGGIEGWCQKLWTTEAIALLDLDVSVKTRCQMTS
HMPV   : SIVTDLSKFNQAFRYETTAICADVADELHGTQSLFCWLHLIVPMTTMICAYRHAPPETKGEY-DIDKIEEQSGLYRYHMGGIEGWCQKLWTMEAISLLDVVSVRNRVQLTS
APV    : SIVTDLSKFNQAFRYETTSVCADVADELHGTQSLFCWLHLTVSSTTMICTYRHAPPDTGGIY-DIDQIPEQSGLYRFHMGGIEGWCQKMWTMEAISLLDVVSVRNRVQLTS
Marburg: SFVTDLEKYNLAFRYEFTRHFIDYCNRCYGVKNLFDWMHFLIPLCYMHVSDFYSPPHCVTED-NRNNPPDCANAYHYHLGGIEGLQQKLWTCISCAQITLVELKTKLKIKS
Ebola  : SFVTDLEKYNLAFRYEFTAPFIEYCNRCYGVKNVFNWMHYTIPQCYMHVSDYYNPPHNLTLE-NRDNPPEGPSSYRGHMGGIEGLQQKLWTSISCAQISLVEIKTGFKLRS
Rabies : AFHLDYEKWNNHQRLESTEDVFSVLDQVFGLKRVFSRTHEFFQKAWIYSDRSDLIGLREDQIYCLDASNGPTCWNGQDGGLEGLRQKGWSLVSLLMIDRESQIRNTRTKI
VSV    : ANHIDYEKWNNHQRKLSNGPVFRVMGQFLGYPSLIERTHEFFEKSLIYNGRPDLMRVHNN--LINSTSQRVCWQGQEGGLEGLRQKGWSIINYLMIERSRVRNTRVKI
BEFV   : ANNIDYEKWNNYQRIESNGPVFTVMGRFLGLPNLFTRTHEFFQKSLIYNQRPDLMMVRGRE--CLNRLGVKVCWEGQKQGGLEGLRQKGWSILNYLMIERSVRNTRVKI
Borna  : VINLDYSSWCNGFRPELQAPICRQLDQMFNCGYFFRTGCTLPCFTTFIIQDRFNPPYSLSGE---PVEDGVTCAVGTKTMGEGMRQKLWTILTSCWEIIALREINVTFNI
```

B

```
Sendai : ----ITKYFGALRHVMFDVGHELKLNETIISSKMFVYSKRIIYDGKILPQCLKALTKCVFWSETLVDENRSACSNISTSIA
PIV3   : ----VVRFFDSLREVMDDLGHELKLNETIISSKMFIYSKRIIYDGKILPQALKALSRCVFWSETVIDETRSASSNLATSFA
Tupai  : VVQGDNEVGAITKRVKSSLPYSVKKRMSTQM---ALEFFDRLRWNFSMVGHNLKASETIISSHFFVYSKRIIYDGVCMTQGLKAVARCVFWSETIVDETRSACSNISTSLA
Measles: LVQGDNQTIAVTKRVPSTWPYNLKKREAARV---TRDYFVILRQRLHDIGHHLKANETIVSSHFFVYSKRIIYDGVCMTQGLKAVARCVFWSETIVDETRAACSNISTSLA
CDV    : LVQGDNQTIAVTKRVPSTWSYALKKSEASRV---TTEYFIALRQRLHDVGHHLKANETIISSHFFVYSKGIIYDGMLISQSLKSIARCVFWSETIVDETRAACSNIATTMA
Nipah  : IVQGDNESIAITQKVHPNLPYKVKKEICAKQ---AQLYFERLRMNLRALGHNLKATETIISTHLFIYSKKIHYDGAVLSQALKSMSRCCFWSETLVDETRSACSNISTTIA
Hendra : IVQGDNESIAITQKVHPNLPYKVKKEICARQ---AQLYFDRLRMNLRALGHNIKATETIISTHLFVYSKKIHYDGAVLSQALKSMSRCCFWSETLVDETRSACSNISTTIA
NDV    : MVQGDNQVIAVTREVRSDDSPEMVLTQLHQA---SDNFFKELIHVNHLIGHNLKDRETIRSDTFFIYSKRIFKDGAILSQVLKNSSKLVMVSGDLSENTVMSCANIASTVA
ApaV6  : MVQGENQAIAITTEIEEGEDASVASIRLKEI---SERFFRVFREINRGIGHNLKVQETIHSESFFVYSKRIFFEGKILSQLLKNASRLLVSETVGENCVGNCSNISSTVA
Tioman : LVQGDNQAMAITTMVPRGLPHHEKKRIAYEN---SQTFIRRLRENNLGMGHHLKEQETIVSSEFLIYSKRIINGRILNQSLKNVSKLCLIADILGESTQTSCSNLATTVM
Mumps  : MVQGDNQAIAITTRVVRSLSHSEKKEQAYKA---SKLFFERLRANNHGIGHHLKEQETILSSDFFIYSKRVFYQGRILTQALKNVSKMCLTADILGDCSQASCSNLATTVM
SV5    : MVQGDNQAIAVTTRVPRSLPTLEKKTIAFRS---CNLFFERLKCNNFGLGHHLKEQETIISSHFFVYSKRIFYQGRILTQALKNASKLLCITADVLGECTQSSCSNLATTVM
RSV    : LINGDNQSIDISKPVRLMEGQTHAQADYLL---AINSLKLLYKEYAGIGHKLKGTETYISRDMQFMSKTIQHNGVYYPASIKKVLRVGPWINTILDDFKVSLESIGSLTQ
PVM    : LINGDNQSIDISKPTRL-GTRTQSEADYDL---AINSLRLISAAYKGIGHKLKEGETYISRDLQFISKVIQSEGVMHPTPIKKILRVGPWINTILDDIKTSESIGSLTQ
HMPV   : LLNGDNQSIDVSKPVKLSEGLDEVKADYSL---AVKMLKEIRDAYRNIGHKLKEGETYISRDLQFMSKTIQSEGVMYPAAIKKVLRVGPWINTILDDIKTSAEIGSLCQ
APV    : LLNGDNQSIDVSKPVRLTGAQTEIQADYSL---AIKMLTAVRDAYYNIGHKLKEGETYVSRDIQFMSKTIQSEGWMYPAAIKKVLRVGPWINTILDDIKTSMEAIGSLCQ
Marburg: SVMGDNQCITTLSLFPIDAPNDYQENEAELN---AARVAVELAITTGYSGIFLKPEETFVHSGFIYFGKKQYLNGVQLPQSLKTMARCGPLSDSIFDDLQGSLASIGTSFE
Ebola  : AVMGDNQCITVLSVFPLETDADEQEQSAEDN---AARVAASLAKVTSACGIFLKPDETFVHSGFIYFGKKQYLNGVQLPQSLKTAARMAPLSDAIFDDLQGTLASIGTAFE
Rabies : LAQGDNQVLCPTYMLSPGLSQEGLLYELERISRNALSIYRAVEEGASKLGLIIKKEETMCSYDFLIYGKTPLFRGNILVPESKRWARVSCVSNDQIVNLANIMSTVSTNAL
VSV    : LAQGDNQVICTQYKTKSSRNVELQGALNQMVSNNEKIMTAIKIGTGKLGLLINDDETMQSADYLNYGKIPIFRGVIRGLETKRWSRVTCVTNDQIPTCANIMSSVSTNAL
BEFV   : LAQGDNQTISMCYKTESWQNEEELDNHIKNMVSNNNQIMQAIINGTEKIGLRINLDETMTSADYINYGKVPIIEGTIKGLPTKRWSRVNFTSNDQLPSTSTVINSSSTNAL
Borna  : LGQGDNQTIIIHKSASQNNQLL----------AERALGALYKHARLAGHNLKVEECWVSDCLYEYGKLFFRGVPVPGCKLQLSRVTDSTGELFPNLYSKLACLTSSCL
```

C

D

existing taxonomy is still uncertain. Paramyxoviruses have been isolated frequently from reptiles, including snakes, lizards, and turtles. Preliminary molecular characterization of 18 reptilian viruses, isolated from 18 species of snakes belonging to three different families, suggests that these viruses should be classified in a new genus within the subfamily *Paramyxovirinae* (Franke et al. 2001) (see also: Chapters 33 and 36–38).

The family *Paramyxoviridae* – subfamily *Pneumovirinae*

Members of this subfamily are distinguished by the possession of 8 or 10 transcriptional elements, smaller open reading frames, an additional unglycosylated nucleocapsid-associated M2 (sometimes designated 22k) protein, an extensively *O*-linked G (attachment) protein, an unedited *P* gene and in some members, two 3′-terminal nonstructural protein genes (*NS1* and *NS2*). The open reading frames encode proteins with little amino acid sequence homology with those of any of the *Paramyxovirinae* except in the *F* and *L* genes. The nucleocapsid diameter is 13–14 nm and the pitch is 7 nm. The G protein is structurally unrelated to the HN or H proteins of the *Paramyxovirinae* and exhibits a high level of strain variability with as little as 53 percent identity between strains.

The subfamily *Pneumovirinae* comprises two genera: *Pneumovirus* and *Metapneumovirus*. The genus *Pneumovirus* includes three virus species: *Human respiratory syncytial virus*, *Bovine respiratory syncytial virus*, and *Pneumonia virus of mice*. The bovine and human respiratory syncytial viruses share considerable sequence and antigenic relatedness, with the F and HN proteins exhibiting 81 percent identity. They differ predominantly in their hosts. Murine pneumonia virus (sometimes still given as Pneumonia virus of mice) differs from the other two species to a greater extent, with amino acid sequence relationships varying from almost nil in the case of the NS1 and NS2 proteins to 60 percent identity in the case of the nucleoprotein (NP). Pneumonia virus of mice lacks the *M2/L* gene overlap present in the genome of human respiratory syncytial virus and the pneumonia virus of mice *P* gene encodes several additional proteins by using alternative AUG translation initiation codons. Gene transfer experiments have established that the functions of the proteins encoded by the 3′-terminal *NS1* and *NS2* genes, which have no homologues in other paramyxoviruses, are involved in suppression of the antiviral interferon response of infected cells.

The second genus *Metapneumovirus* was originally assigned to accommodate the avian virus *Turkey rhinotracheitis virus* (also known as avian pneumovirus), and has recently been extended by the inclusion of a human virus (designated provisionally as human metapneumo-virus), which closely resembles its avian counterpart in molecular properties, but exists in the same biological niche as human respiratory syncytial virus. The metapneumoviruses lack the 3′-terminal *NS1* and *NS2* genes characteristic of other pneumoviruses and exhibit a displacement of the *SH-G* and *F-M2* gene pairs in the gene order. This is rather remarkable since the same relative gene order is conserved throughout the order *Mononegavirales*, except for the two virus species making up the genus *Metapneumovirus* and some genetically engineered recombinant rhabdoviruses (see below). All of the pneumoviruses lack a neuraminidase and all, except pneumonia virus of mice, a hemagglutinating activity. In contrast to the *Paramyxovirinae*, in none of the known pneumoviruses is the genome size a multiple of six nucleotides (see also: Chapter 37, Pneumovirus and metapneumovirus).

The family *Rhabdoviridae*

The rhabdoviruses infecting vertebrates are bullet-shaped or cone-shaped, whereas the rhabdoviruses infecting plants appear bacilliform when fixed prior to negative staining or bullet-shaped or pleomorphic if unfixed. The virions are 100–430 nm long and 45–100 nm in diameter. The nucleocapsid of rhabdoviruses contains RNA polymerase activity and is infectious, whereas the naked negative-sense RNA genome is not. Some putative plant viruses, identified solely by electron microscopy appear to lack envelopes. The family consists of six genera: *Vesiculovirus*, *Lyssavirus*, *Ephemerovirus*, *Novirhabdovirus*, *Cytorhabdovirus*, and *Nucleorhabdovirus*. The genomic RNA has a 5′-terminal phosphate and is not polyadenylated. The ends of the genome have inverted complementary sequences, a feature consistent with the mechanism of replication of rhabdoviruses. Defective RNAs are easily detected because the size of the encapsidated RNA determines the linear dimension of the virus particle. Defective RNAs are dependent on infectious virus but they also interfere specifically with replication, and are responsible for reduction of virus yields by autointerference in virus passaged at high multiplicity.

Currently, nine species and at least 19 tentative species have been assigned to the genus *Vesiculovirus*. These viruses originate from mammals, fish and insects. *Vesicular stomatitis Indiana virus* is the type species of the genus and represents the basic organisational pattern for the entire order *Mononegavirales*. The 11.2 kb genome encodes a 3′-leader sequence of 47 nucleotides that precedes the N, P, M, G, and L open reading frames, which are separated by minimal intergenic dinucleotides, and terminates in a 54 nucleotide trailer region. There is a common 3′-AUACUUUUUU sequence preceding each intergenic region and a UUGUCNNU sequence at the beginning of each gene.

The leader region is transcribed and a Le RNA may be present in the nuclei of infected cells. The viruses in this genus show varying degrees of amino acid identity in N protein comparisons. *Vesicular stomatitis Indiana virus* has been employed widely as a model system in virus research since all the gene products are structural proteins and can be isolated from purified virions. The genus *Lyssavirus* contains *Rabies virus* and another six rabies-related viruses, four of which originate from bats. Until recently the island continent of Australia was considered to be rabies-free prior to the isolation of *Australian bat lyssavirus* from both pteropid and insectivorous bats. Phylogenetic analysis of the genomes of these viruses suggest that they may have been endemic in Australia prior to European colonization. The 11.9 kb rabies virus genome comprises a 60 nucleotide leader region followed by the five basic rhabdovirus genes, separated by di- or pentanucleotides and followed by a 70 nucleotide trailer. (Exceptionally, the Pasteur strain includes a 423 nucleotide pseudogene region between the *G* and *L* genes which is transcribed within the G mRNA). The rabies viruses are neurotropic and all the viruses in the genus show some antigenic cross-reactivity. The viruses classified in the genus *Ephemerovirus* depart significantly from the standard rhabdovirus pattern. There are three species in the genus: *Bovine ephemeral fever virus*, *Adelaide river virus*, and *Berrimah virus*. The 14.9-kb genome of *Bovine ephemeral fever virus* encodes ten genes in the order 3′-N–P–M–G–Gns–α1–α2–β–γ–L-5′, with intergenic regions of between 26 and 53 nucleotides. Adelaide river virus has intergenic regions of 1 to 4 nucleotides, lacks the γ gene and has a β–L overlap. The functions of the products of the *α1*, *α2*, *β*, and *γ* genes have not been identified. Gns is a nonvirion glycoprotein and may be analogous to the soluble G proteins of some paramyxoviruses and ebolaviruses, but it does not induce neutralizing antibodies and is not protective, causes economically important enzootic disease of cattle and is transmitted by, and replicates in, hematophagous arthropods. The genus *Novirhabdovirus* comprises three virus species infecting aquatic hosts: *Infectious hematopoietic necrosis virus*, *Hirame rhabdovirus*, and *Viral hemorrhagic septicemia virus*. These viruses encode the standard rhabdovirus complement of five structural protein genes, plus a sixth nonvirion (NV) protein gene of unknown function located between the *G* and *L* genes. There is a 60 nucleotide leader sequence, a 100 nucleotide trailer, and single nucleotide intergenic regions. The N protein sequence identity between these species is about 34 percent and there is no cross-neutralisation. The genus *Cytorhabdovirus* comprises eight species of plant rhabdoviruses, which multiply in the cytoplasm in association with thread-like structures (viroplasms). They are transmitted by arthropod vectors (predominantly leafhoppers and aphids), and most appear to be able to multiply in the arthropod vector as well as the host plant. The gene

order of the type species, *Lettuce necrotic yellows virus*, is 3′-N–P(4a)–4b–M–G–L–5′ with an 84 nucleotide leader and a 187 nucleotide trailer. The *4b* gene is thought to encode a nonstructural protein. The genus *Nucleorhabdovirus* comprises seven species of plant viruses, which multiply in the nucleus of plant cells forming large granular inclusions. Virus morphogenesis occurs at the inner nuclear envelope and enveloped particles accumulate in the perinuclear space. The genome order is similar to that of the cytorhabdoviruses, except that the nonstructural protein gene is designated *SC4*, and there is an additional gene between the *G* and *L* genes in *Rice yellow stunt virus* which encodes a virion-associated protein. There is a 114 nucleotide leader and a 160 nucleotide trailer. Like the cytorhabdoviruses, the nucleorhabdoviruses are predominantly transmitted by leafhoppers and aphids.

In addition to the rhabdoviruses assigned to genera, there at least six serogroups of rhabdoviruses whose taxonomic affiliations are indeterminate at present. There are also more than 37 ungrouped animal viruses that have been propagated and characterized to varying extents, and another 58 plant viruses of uncertain status because their identification is based often on morphological evidence only. Some of the ungrouped animal viruses, such as the arthropod-borne Obodhiang virus and Kotonkan virus previously included in the genus *Lyssavirus*, have been excluded from earlier classifications as knowledge of their uniqueness accrues. Perhaps the most significant of the ungrouped animal rhabdoviruses is Sigma virus, which is transmitted vertically through the germ cells of *Drosophila* spp. conferring CO_2 sensitivity on the infected insect. Both host and viral genes contribute to maintenance of the virus in the host. The Sigma virus genome has an *M–G* gene overlap, variable intergenic regions, and encodes a sixth gene of unknown function, but with motifs related to reverse transcriptase motifs, located between the *P* and *M* genes (see also Chapter 51, Rhabdoviruses: rabies).

Table 19.3 provides a diagrammatic representation of the 3′ to 5′ characteristic arrangement of the transcriptional elements of the genomes of viruses classified in the four families comprising the order *Mononegavirales*.

THE CONSERVATION OF GENE ORDER

The conservation of a preferred gene order is one of the striking and unifying features of the order *Mononegavirales* (Table 19.3). The order of their genes is the major determinant of the relative levels of gene expression, since genes that are close to the 3′ promoter site are transcribed at higher levels than those that occupy more distal positions. Genetic manipulation of an infectious cDNA clone of vesicular stomatitis Indiana virus resulted in production of viable viruses with rearrangements of gene order, which left the viral nucleotide sequence otherwise unaltered (Ball et al. 1999). The

Table 19.3 A diagrammatic representation of the 3' to 5' arrangement of the transcriptional units in the genomes of viruses classified in the four families (Bornaviridae, Filoviridae, Paramyxoviridae, and Rhabdoviridae) comprising the order Mononegavirales. Genes encoding polypeptides of presumed homologous function are aligned vertically

Family	Genus	Virus	3'	Gene order	5'
Subfamily					
Bornaviridae	*Bornavirus*	BDV	le	N (P) (M) (G)	L tr
Filoviridae	*Ebolavirus*	ZEBOV	le	N P (M1) GP/SP (?) (M2)	L tr
	Marburgvirus	MARV	le	N P (M1) G (?) (M2)	L tr
Rhabdoviridae	*Vesiculovirus*	VSV	le	N P M G	L tr
	Lyssavirus	RV	le	N P M G Ps	L tr
	Cytorhabdovirus	LNYV	le	N P 4b M G	L tr
	Nucleorhabdovirus	SYNV	le	N P Sc4 M G	L tr
	Novirhabdovirus	IHNV	le	N P M G NV	L tr
	Ephemerovirus	BEFV	le	N P M G Gns (α1,α2,β,χ,0)	L tr
	''	ARV	le	N P M G Gns (α1,α2,0)	L tr
	Unassigned	SiV	le	N P (RT) M G	L tr
Paramyxoviridae					
Paramyxovirinae	*Avulavirus*	NDV	le	N P/V M F H	L tr
	Henipavirus	HeV	le	N P/C/V M F H	L tr
	Morbillivirus	MV	le	N P/C/V M F H	L tr
	Respirovirus	SeV	le	N P/C/V M F H/N	L tr
	Rubulavirus	MuV	le	N P/V M F H/N	L tr
Pneumovirinae	*Metapneumovirus*	TRTV	le	N P M1 F M2 SH G	L tr
	Pneumovirus	RSV	le	N P NS1 NS2 M1 SH G F M2	L tr
	''	PVM	le	N P/(C) NS1 NS2 M1 SH G F M2	L tr

Abbreviations: viruses; BDV: Borna disease virus; VSV: vesicular stomatitis virus; SYNV: Sonchus yellow net virus; SlV: Sigma virus; RV: rabies virus; IHNV: infectious hematopoietic virus; BEFV: bovine ephemeral fever virus; ARV: Adelaide river virus; ZEOV: Zaire ebola virus; MARV: Marburg virus; MV: measles virus; MuV: mumps virus; SeV: Sendai virus; TRTV: turkey rhinotracheitis virus; RSV: respiratory syncytial virus; PVM: pneumonia virus of mice; LNYV: lettuce necrotic yellows virus; transcriptional units; le: noncoding leader region; NS: nonstructural protein gene; N: nucleoprotein gene; P: phosphoprotein gene; V and C: dispensible nonstructural protein genes; sc4, 4b and (RT): genes of unknown function; M and M1: nonglycosylated matrix protein gene; (M): glycosylated matrix protein gene; F: fusion protein gene; SH: small hydrophobic protein gene; G (or H or HN): glycosylated (or hemagglutinin or hemagglutinin/neuraminidase) attachment protein gene; M2: nonglycosylated (BDV excepted) envelope protein gene; NV: nonvirion protein gene; Ps: pseudogene; Gns: presumptive duplicated G sequence; α1, α2, β, χ: glycoprotein gene products of unknown function; L: large (polymerase) protein gene; tr: noncoding trailer region. (Modified from Pringle and Easton (1997).)

three central genes in the gene order, which encode *P*, *M*, and *G*, were rearranged in all six possible configurations. All six rearrangements were propagated stably as infectious virus and each rearrangement had changed the expression levels of the encoded proteins in accordance with their relative proximity to the 3′ promoter. Similarly, translocation of the *N* gene away from its promoter proximal location to successive positions down the gene order reduced N mRNA and protein expression in a step-wise manner (Wertz et al. 1999). Remarkably, some of the viruses with rearranged genomes replicated as well as or slightly better than the unrearranged wild type virus. Despite the highly conserved gene order of the *Mononegavirales*, gene rearrangement is neither lethal nor necessarily detrimental.

Furthermore, moving the attachment protein gene (*G*) from fourth to first position in the gene order of vesicular stomatitis virus increased expression of the G protein and enhanced the kinetics and level of antibody response in mice infected with this gene order variant (Flanagan et al. 2000). Similar experiments have shown that vesicular stomatitis Indiana virus can tolerate the insertion of duplicated or heterologous genes into the gene order (Wertz et al. 2002), thereby opening up new routes to vaccine development. In general, the nonstandard gene rearrangements and the inserted genes were stably maintained in the modified genomes on repeated passage. The absence of a mechanism for homologous recombination in negative-sense RNA viruses may be responsible for the maintenance of a preferred gene order in evolution, but the reason for choice of the particular gene order adopted by the *Mononegavirales* is an enigma.

PHYLOGENY OF THE ORDER *MONONEGAVIRALES*

The determination of the nucleotide sequences of specific genes, and in many cases the complete genomes, of many members of the order *Mononegavirales* has allowed an analysis of the molecular phylogeny of this group of viruses (Figure 19.1a). While in principle a phylogenetic analysis can be performed with any of the genes shared by all members of the *Mononegavirales*, it is most appropriate to use sequences of internal proteins as these are least affected by the selective pressure of antibody surveillance in the host. Of the internal protein genes, the most conserved is that encoding the RNA polymerase, the L protein. A comparison of the polymerase protein genes of a number of nonsegmented viruses identified four conserved domains (Poch et al. 1989, 1990; Le Mercier et al. 1997). Domain III contains four conserved motifs, including the GDNQ motif associated with polymerase activity (Figure 19.1b). A phylogenetic tree constructed using the sequences of the RNA polymerase conserved domain III of a representative selection of viruses is shown in Figure 19.1a. This analysis shows clearly the phylogenetic divisions of the different virus groups represented in the ICTV classification system. The families *Paramyxoviridae*, *Bornaviridae*, *Rhabdoviridae*, and *Filoviridae* segregate into different lineages, presumably linked by a common ancestor. Within the family *Paramyxoviridae*, the two subfamilies *Paramyxovirinae* and *Pneumovirinae* can be seen to segregate and within each the genera are clearly distinct, though related. Molecular phylogeny has confirmed the relationship of the viruses assigned to the order *Mononegavirales* on the basis of a number of physical and biochemical parameters and now allows a rapid classification of newly isolated viruses. This approach has recently led to the identification of new genera, the genus *Avulavirus* and the genus *Henipavirus*. Figure 19.1 also shows the phylogenetic relationship of three currently unassigned viruses to the other members of the *Paramyxovirinae*. *Avian paramyxovirus 6* appears to be related most closely to *Newcastle disease virus* (also known as *avian paramyxovirus 1*), whereas Tioman virus and Tupaia paramyxovirus are closest to the rubulaviruses and morbilliviruses, respectively.

REFERENCES

Ball, L.A., Pringle, C.R., et al. 1999. Phenotypic consequences of rearranging the *P*, *M* and *G* genes of vesicular stomatitis virus. *J Virol*, **73**, 4705–12.

Bankamp, B., Bellini, W.J. and Rota, P.A. 1999. Comparison of L proteins of vaccine and wild-type measles viruses. *J Gen Virol*, **80**, 1617–25.

Briese, T., Schneemann, A., et al. 1994. Genomic organization of Borna disease virus. *Proc Natl Acad Sci USA*, **91**, 4362–6.

Chan, Y.P., Chua, K.B., et al. 2001. Complete nucleotide sequences of Nipah virus isolates from Malaysia. *J Gen Virol*, **82**, 2151–5.

Chua, K.B., Wang, L.F., et al. 2002. Full length genome sequence of Tioman virus, a novel paramyxovirus in the genus Rubulavirus isolated from fruit bats in Malaysia. *Arch Virol*, **147**, 1323–48.

Conzelmann, K.K., Cox, J.H., et al. 1990. Molecular cloning and complete nucleotide sequence of the attenuated rabies virus SAD B19. *Virology*, **175**, 485–99.

de la Torre, J.C. 1994. Molecular biology of Borna disease virus: Prototype of a new group of animal viruses. *J Virol*, **68**, 7669–75.

Flanagan, E.B., Ball, L.A. and Wertz, G.W. 2000. Moving the glycoprotein gene of vesicular stomatitis virus to promoter-proximal positions accelerates and enhances the protective immune response. *J Virol*, **74**, 7895–902.

Franke, J., Essbauer, S., et al. 2001. Identification and molecular characterization of 18 paramyxoviruses isolated from snakes. *Virus Res*, **80**, 67–74.

Galinski, M.S., Mink, M.A. and Pons, M.W. 1988. Molecular cloning and sequence analysis of the human parainfluenza 3 virus gene encoding the L protein. *Virology*, **165**, 499–510.

Higuchi, Y., Miyahara, Y., et al. 1992. Sequence analysis of the large (L) protein of simian virus 5. *J Gen Virol*, **73**, 1005–10.

Le Mercier, P., Jakob, Y. and Tordo, N. 1997. The complete Mokola virus genome sequence: structure of the RNA-dependent RNA polymerase. *J Gen Virol*, **78**, 1571–6.

Maniloff, J. and Ackermann, H.-W. 1998. Taxonomy of bacterial viruses: establishment of tailed virus genera and the order *Caudovirales*. *Arch Virol*, **143**, 2051–63.

Middleton, Y., Tashiro, M., et al. 1990. Nucleotide sequence analyses of the genes encoding the HN, M, NP, P and L proteins of two host range mutants of Sendai virus. *Virology*, **176**, 656–7.

Muhlberger, E., Sanchez, A., et al. 1992. The nucleotide sequence of the L gene of Marburg virus, a filovirus: homologies with paramyxoviruses and rhabdoviruses. *Virology*, **187**, 534–47.

Okazaki, K., Tanabayashi, K. and Takeuchi, K. 1992. Molecular cloning and sequence analysis of the mumps virus gene encoding the L protein and the trailer sequence. *Virology*, **188**, 926–30.

Poch, O., Sauvaget, I., et al. 1989. Identification of conserved motifs among the RNA-dependent polymerase encoding elements. *EMBO J 8*, **4**, 3867–74.

Poch, O., Blumberg, B.M., et al. 1990. Sequence comparison of 5 polymerases (L-proteins) of unsegmented negative-strand RNA viruses – theoretical assignment of functional domains. *J Gen Virol*, **71**, 1153–62.

Pringle, C.R. 1991. The order *Mononegavirales. Arch Virol*, **117**, 137–40.

Pringle, C.R. 1997. The order *Mononegavirales* – current status. *Arch Virol*, **142**, 2321–6.

Pringle, C.R. and Easton, A.J. 1997. Monopartite negative strand RNA genomes. *Semin Virol*, **8**, 49–57.

Randhawa, J.S., Wilson, S.D., et al. 1996. Nucleotide sequence of the gene encoding the viral polymerase of avian pneumovirus. *J Gen Virol*, **77**, 3047–51.

Schneemann, E., Schneider, P.A., et al. 1995. The remarkable coding strategy of Borna disease virus: a new member of the nonsegmented negative strand RNA viruses. *Virology*, **210**, 1–9.

Schubert, M., Harmison, G.G. and Meier, E. 1984. Primary structure of the vesicular stomatitis virus polymerase (L) gene: evidence for a high frequency of mutations. *J Virol*, **51**, 505–14.

Sidhu, M.S., Husar, W., et al. 1993. Canine distemper terminal and intergenic non-protein coding nucleotide sequences: completion of the entire CDV genome sequence. *Virology*, **193**, 66–72.

Tolley, K.P., Marriott, A.C., et al. 1996. Identification of mutations contributing to the reduced virulence of a modified strain of respiratory syncytial virus. *Vaccine*, **14**, 1637–46.

Van Regenmortel, M.H.V., Fauquet, C.M. and Bishop, D.H.L. (eds) 2000. *Virus Taxonomy; the 7th Report of the International Committee on Taxonomy of Viruses*. San Diego: Academic Press.

Volchkov, V.E., Chepurnov, A.A., et al. 2000. Molecular characterization of guinea pig-adapted variants of Ebola virus. *Virology*, **277**, 147–55.

Walker, P.J., Wang, Y., et al. 1994. Structural and antigenic analysis of the nucleoprotein of bovine ephemeral fever rhabdovirus. *J Gen Virol*, **75**, 1889–99.

Wang, L.F., Yu, M., et al. 2000. The exceptionally large genome of Hendra virus: support for creation of a new genus within the family *Paramyxoviridae*. *J Virol*, **74**, 9972–9.

Wertz, G.W., Perepelitsa, V.P. and Ball, L.A. 1999. Gene rearrangement attenuates expression and lethality of a nonsegmented negative strand RNA virus. *Proc Natl Acad Sci USA*, **95**, 3501–6.

Wertz, G.W., Moudy, R. and Ball, L.A. 2002. Adding genes to the RNA genome of vesicular stomatitis virus: positional effects on stability of expression. *J Virol*, **76**, 7642–50.

Yusoff, K., Millar, N.S., et al. 1987. Nucleotide sequence analysis of the L gene of Newcastle disease virus: homologies with Sendai and vesicular stomatitis viruses. *Nucleic Acids Res*, **15**, 3961–76.

20

The order *Nidovirales*

ERIC J. SNIJDER, STUART G. SIDDELL, AND ALEXANDER E. GORBALENYA

INTRODUCTION

Nidovirus infections in both animals and man result in a variety of diseases that may range from relatively benign to fatal. The order *Nidovirales* (Figure 20.1) is comprised of the genus *Coronavirus*, which together with the genus *Torovirus* forms the *Coronaviridae* family, and the families *Arteriviridae* and *Roniviridae*. The biological and pathogenic properties of individual coronaviruses, toroviruses, and arteriviruses are summarized in Chapter 39. In this chapter, we present a comparative overview of nidoviruses that has three major goals. First, this broader approach presents our knowledge of human coronaviruses in an evolutionary perspective, thus preparing the ground for further expansion of a cluster of viruses that contains pathogens responsible for emerging infections. Second, it highlights the parallels and homologies amongst nidoviruses and, as such, forms a common framework for studies on animal models and human nidovirus infections. Third, it provides an overview of both unique and conserved nidovirus properties, thus highlighting potential targets for the development of reagents to detect and combat nidovirus infections.

Over the past 20 years, molecular biology and genetics have contributed enormously to the characterization of viruses and, at the same time, changed the face of virus taxonomy. It has become increasingly evident that the comparative analysis of virus genomes provides a better foundation for comprehensive virus taxonomy than more traditional parameters, such as virion morphology or host range. This realization has resulted in the reclassification of specific viruses (or groups of viruses) and also in the introduction of higher order taxa to recognize evolutionary ties that surpass the level of the virus family.

Besides the order *Nidovirales*, only two other virus orders have been recognized thus far. The order *Caudovirales* unites several families of tailed DNA viruses of bacteria (bacteriophages) and the order *Mononegavirales* (Chapter 19) is comprised of three virus families with a negative-strand RNA genome that consists of one single-stranded RNA segment. The order *Nidovirales* was established by the International Committee on the Taxonomy of Viruses (ICTV) in 1996 (Cavanagh 1997). At that time, it united the newly established family *Arteriviridae* with the pre-existing family *Coronaviridae* (containing the genera *Coronavirus* and *Torovirus*). As will be explained below, the inclusion of these groups of positive-strand RNA viruses in the order *Nidovirales* recognized striking similarities at the level of genome organization and expression, and the intriguing phylogenetic clustering of their giant replicase polyproteins, the precursors to the key enzymes that drive virus replication (Gorbalenya et al. 1989; den Boon et al. 1991). More recently, and on the same grounds, the order *Nidovirales* was expanded to include the family *Roniviridae* (Walker et al. 2004; Spaan et al. 2005), which currently comprises a single genus, *Okavirus*. Whereas other known nidoviruses infect

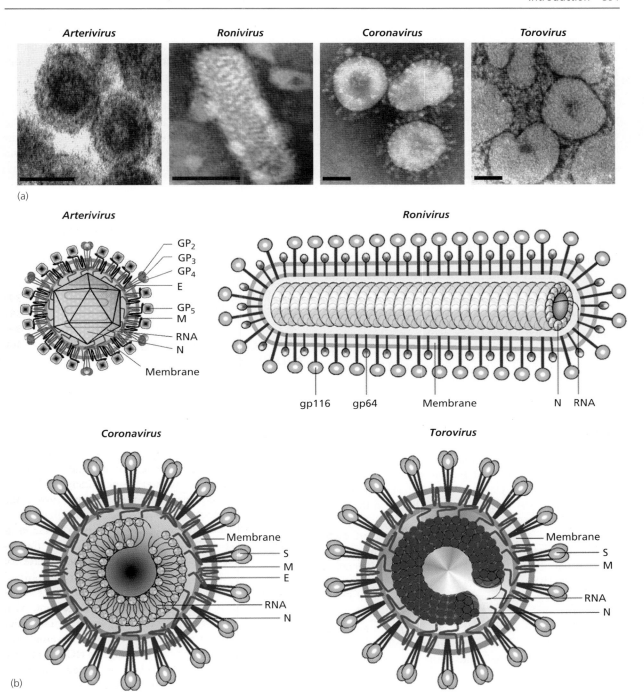

Figure 20.1 *Electron micrographs* **(a)** *and schematic representations* **(b)** *of nidovirus structure.* **(a)** *Characteristic images of negatively stained arterivirus, ronivirus, coronavirus, and torovirus particles, as captured with a transmission electron microscope. The diverse size and different structural features of representatives of the four main nidovirus branches are evident. Images were reproduced (with permission) from Snijder and Meulenberg (1998), arterivirus; Spann et al. (1995), ronivirus; Dr. Fred Murphy, Centers for Disease Control and Prevention (CDC), Atlanta, USA, coronavirus; and Weiss et al. (1983), torovirus. Bar is 50 nm.* **(b)** *Schematic representation of arterivirus, ronivirus, coronavirus, and torovirus virion structure. The different symmetries of the nucleocapsid structures and virions are indicated (see Chapter 39 for more details). Viral membrane proteins present in the virion envelope are depicted. Note that some viruses have been found to contain additional envelope proteins, e.g. the hemagglutinin esterase (HE) protein identified in certain coronaviruses and toroviruses. The stoichiometry of the virion components is shown (more or less) arbitrarily. N, nucleocapsid protein; M, membrane protein; S, spike protein; E, envelope protein; GP or gp, glycoprotein.*

vertebrate hosts (mostly mammals and some avian hosts), roniviruses infect invertebrates, specifically prawns. Nevertheless, their molecular biological features and elements of their genetic plan clearly link them to arteriviruses and coronaviruses (Cowley et al. 2000). The expansion of the *Nidovirales* with new viruses, and the extensive characterization of a few nidoviruses over recent years, have resulted in a refinement and partial revision of the framework of specific and conserved features that defines this virus order.

MAJOR NIDOVIRUS BRANCHES AND THEIR PROTOTYPE VIRUSES

For obvious reasons, the best-studied nidoviruses are the viruses that either cause significant disease in humans or livestock and/or are most easily studied in cell culture or small animal model systems. In the family *Coronaviridae* (Lai and Cavanagh 1997; Lai and Holmes 2001), the prototype of the genus *Coronavirus* is the avian *Infectious bronchitis virus* (IBV), although *Murine hepatitis virus* (MHV), has probably been more extensively studied. Modest attention has also been paid to the two human common cold viruses, HCoV-229E and HCoV-OC43. The recent emergence of a third human coronavirus, which was identified as the cause of severe acute respiratory syndrome (SARS), has boosted research on human coronaviruses in general (Drosten et al. 2003; Ksiazek et al. 2003; Peiris et al. 2003a). Currently, many aspects of SARS-coronavirus (SARS-CoV) and the disease that it causes are being characterized at an unprecedented rate (Stadler et al. 2003; Peiris et al. 2003b; Berger et al. 2004; Ziebuhr 2004a). The identification of a fourth human coronavirus (NL63 and HKU1) (van der Hoek et al. 2004; Fouchier et al. 2004; Woo et al. 2005), which are relatively closely related to previously identified group 1 and group 2 coronaviruses, respectively, was recently reported, and the detection of additional human coronaviruses can be expected now that the significance of this group of viruses has been recognized in the wake of the SARS outbreak.

Animal coronaviruses that have been studied quite extensively because of the respiratory and/or enteric disease that they cause in livestock or companion animals are IBV, *Bovine coronavirus* (BCoV), porcine *Transmissible gastroenteritis virus* (TGEV), and *Feline coronavirus* (FCoV or FIPV). In the genus *Torovirus* (Snijder and Horzinek 1993), the *Equine torovirus* (EToV) (or Berne virus) is the sole representative, thus far, that can be amplified and studied in cultured cells. Bovine, porcine, and possibly human toroviruses have been identified but have not yet been propagated in cell culture. The name coronavirus is derived from the solar corona-like (Latin *corona*: crown) appearance of virus particles in negatively stained electron micrographs, whereas the name torovirus is derived from the curved tubular (Latin *torus*: lowest convex molding in the base of a column) morphology of the torovirus nucleocapsid structure (Figure 20.1a).

The outcome of arterivirus infection can range from an asymptomatic, persistent carrier-state to lethal hemorrhagic fever. The arterivirus family (Plagemann 1996; Snijder and Meulenberg 1998; Snijder and Meulenberg 2001) currently consists of a single *Arterivirus* genus with four virus species, of which the prototype

Equine arteritis virus (EAV) is the best-studied representative in terms of molecular biology. Arteritis (inflammation of an artery), one of the disease symptoms caused by EAV, gave the arterivirus family its name. EAV and the *Porcine reproductive and respiratory syndrome virus* (PRRSV), of which different genotypes emerged in Europe and North America during the late 1980s, are the two arteriviruses that cause significant disease in livestock. Arteriviruses spread primarily via the respiratory route, but sexual transmission by persistently infected animals is an important secondary cause of infection in the case of EAV and PRRSV.

In the family *Roniviridae* (for *ro*d-shaped *ni*dovirus), the prototype of the genus *Okavirus* is the Gill-associated virus (GAV) (Spann et al. 1995; Cowley et al. 2000) of which the black tiger prawn (*Penaeus monodon*) appears to be the natural host. GAV can cause devastating infections in cultured prawns, where it targets the lymphoid organ (or 'oka') in particular.

KEY COMMON FEATURES OF NIDOVIRUSES

Nidoviruses are enveloped, positive-strand RNA viruses that share a similar genome organization and similar replication strategy (Figure 20.2) that is driven by the gene encoding the large nonstructural or 'replicase' proteins. Phylogenetic analysis of key domains in the nidovirus replicase gene revealed that these elements are much more closely related to each other than to the corresponding sequences in the genomes of other positive-strand RNA viruses (see below and Figure 20.3 for details). Thus, the nidovirus replicase represents a separate lineage in RNA virus evolution (den Boon et al. 1991; Gorbalenya and Koonin 1993; Gorbalenya et al. 1989).

Nidoviruses have diverged profoundly since they originated from their common root. They differ significantly in terms of the size of their genome, virion morphology, host range, and various biological properties. However, a number of features, although not diagnostic of this virus order alone, are thought to be common to nidoviruses. Still, it should be noted that, in particular for toroviruses and roniviruses, many of these properties have not been studied in great detail and the list below may be subject to future updates.

- Nidoviruses have positive-strand RNA genomes consisting of one single-stranded, linear RNA molecule that contains a 5′ cap structure and a 3′ poly(A) tail.
- The general nidovirus genome organization (with some exceptions) is: 5′ untranslated region – replicase – envelope proteins – nucleocapsid protein – 3′ untranslated region (however, note that the ronivirus N protein gene is located upstream of the envelope protein gene (Cowley et al. 2004)).

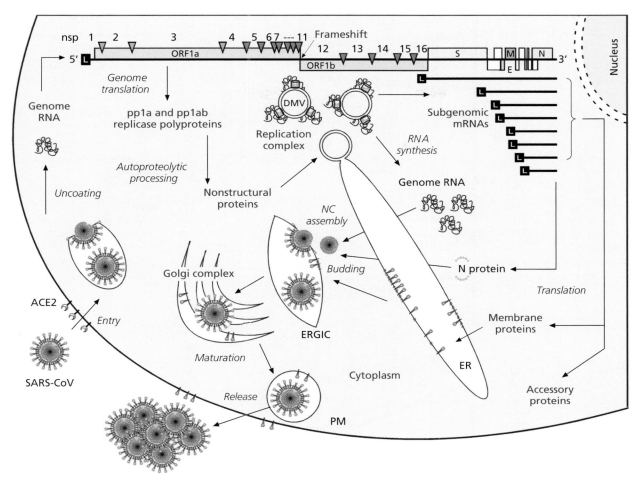

Figure 20.2 *Overview of the nidovirus life cycle, using SARS-CoV as an example. Depicted is the cytoplasmic replication cycle of a typical coronavirus (see text and Chapter 39 for more details). Infection starts with binding of the virus to a specific receptor on the host cell's plasma membrane (PM) (in this case angiotensin-converting enzyme 2 (ACE2)), entry by fusion of viral envelope and cellular membrane, and release of the viral plus-strand RNA genome into the cytoplasm. Subsequently, the genome is translated by host ribosomes to produce the polyprotein precursors (pp1a and pp1ab) to the nonstructural proteins (nsp) that drive viral RNA synthesis. Following limited autoproteolysis of these 'replicase' polyproteins, a complex for viral RNA synthesis is assembled on cytoplasmic double-membrane structures (double-membrane vesicles (DMVs)). This complex produces minus-strand RNAs (not shown) that serves as template for genome replication and the synthesis of a nested set of subgenomic mRNAs. The latter, which contain a common leader sequence (L) identical to the 5' end of the genome, are translated to express the genes that are encoded in the 3'-proximal third of the genome. Translation of the smallest subgenomic mRNA yields the viral nucleocapsid protein (N) that assembles into new nucleocapsid (NC) structures together with newly generated genome RNA. Other subgenomic mRNAs encodes viral envelope proteins that are (largely cotranslationally) inserted into membranes of the host cell's exocytic pathway and migrate towards the site of virus assembly (the ER–Golgi intermediate compartment (ERGIC) in the case of coronaviruses). Following budding of the NC through membranes that contain viral envelope proteins, the new virion ends up in the lumen and, while undergoing additional maturation steps in, for example, the Golgi complex, leaves the cell via the exocytic pathway.*

- The nidovirus replicase gene comprises two large and overlapping open reading frames (ORF) that encode the replicase polyproteins pp1a and pp1ab. Expression of the downstream ORF1b is mediated by programmed −1 ribosomal frameshifting (FS).

- An RNA structure (slippery sequence plus RNA pseudoknot) mediates programmed ribosomal frameshifting in the ORF1a/1b overlap region (Brierley et al. 1989).

- In the infected cell, nidovirus gene expression is mediated by a set of at least three 3' co-terminal subgenomic mRNAs that are thought to be produced from a set of complementary templates of the same sizes. Generally, only the ORFs contained within the 5' unique regions of each mRNA, i.e. the regions not found in the next smallest mRNA are expressed.

- Viral RNA synthesis occurs on intracellular, virus-induced (double) membrane structures.

- Nidovirus particles contain a lipid envelope.

- The envelope of nidovirus particles contains an integral, triple-spanning membrane (m) protein.

- Nidovirus particles are assembled intracellularly, by budding into the lumen of membrane-bound organelles.

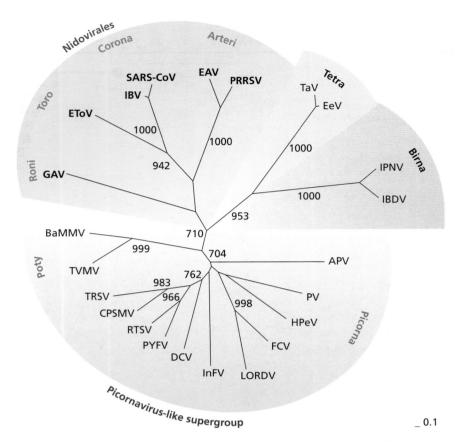

Figure 20.3 *Unrooted phylogenetic tree of RNA-dependent RNA polymerase (RdRp) domains of* Nidovirales *and other (super)groups of positive-strand and double-stranded RNA viruses. The most conserved part of RdRps from representative viruses in the* Picornaviridae, Dicistroviridae, Sequiviridae, Comoviridae, Caliciviridae, Potyviridae, Coronaviridae, Roniviridae, Arteriviridae, Birnaviridae, Tetraviridae, *and unclassified insect viruses was aligned. An unrooted neighbor-joining tree was inferred by the ClustalX1.81 program. For details of the analysis, see Gorbalenya et al. (2002). All bifurcations with support in >700 out of 1 000 bootstraps are indicated. Different groups of viruses are highlighted with different colors. The tree was modified from Gorbalenya et al. (2002) and Spaan et al. (2005). Virus families/groups and abbreviations of viruses included in the analysis:* Coronaviridae: *avian infectious bronchitis virus (IBV), severe acute respiratory syndrome virus (SARS-CoV) and equine torovirus (EToV);* Arteriviridae, *equine arteritis virus (EAV) and porcine reproductive and respiratory syndrome virus strain VR-2332 (PRRSV);* Roniviridae: *gill-associated virus (GAV);* Picornaviridae, *human poliovirus type 3 Leon strain (PV) and parechovirus 1 (HPeV); iflavirus, infectious flacherie virus (InFV); unclassified insect viruses, Acyrthosiphon pisum virus (APV);* Dicistroviridae, *Drosophila C virus (DCV);* Sequiviridae, *rice tungro spherical virus (RTSV), and Parsnip yellow fleck virus (PYFV);* Comoviridae, *cowpea severe mosaic virus (CPSMV) and tobacco ringspot virus (TRSV);* Caliciviridae, *feline calicivirus F9 (FCV), and Lordsdale virus (LORDV);* Potyviridae, *tobacco vein mottling virus (TVMV) and barley mild mosaic virus (BaMMV);* Tetraviridae, *Thosea asigna virus (TaV) and Euprosterna elaeasa virus (EeV);* Birnaviridae, *infectious pancreatic necrosis virus (IPNV) and infectious bursal disease virus (IBDV).*

Nidoviruses also share a number of unique features that could be considered as genetic markers of this order. All of them are associated with the replicase gene, which contains a conserved series of key functional domains (a constellation abbreviated as M–3CLpro-M–FS–RdRp–ZF–HEL–NendoU; see below) including:

- A cluster of domains, encoded by ORF1a, consisting of a main proteinase (3C-like proteinase; 3CLpro), which has a chymotrypsin-like fold and substrate specificity resembling that of picornavirus 3C proteinases, and flanking transmembrane (M) domains (M-3CLpro-M);

- An ORF1b-encoded protein that combines an N-terminal (putative) multinuclear zinc-finger (ZF) domain with a C-terminal NTP-binding/5′-to-3′-helicase domain (HEL);
- An ORF1b-encoded uridylate-specific endoribonuclease (NendoU).

The exact role of these unique genetic markers in the nidovirus life cycle remains largely unknown. The presence of a common 'leader' sequence at the 5′ end of all viral mRNA species (Spaan et al. 1983; Baric et al. 1983; Lai et al. 1984; de Vries et al. 1990) was initially considered a major hallmark of nidoviruses, but recently proved to be a property that is not universally conserved amongst members of this virus order (Cowley et al. 2002; van Vliet et al. 2002).

MAIN DIFFERENCES BETWEEN MAJOR NIDOVIRUS BRANCHES

Despite the common features of their genome and molecular biology (see also below), evolutionary distances within the order *Nidovirales* are vast and there are major differences between the virus families and genera that are united in this taxon. A striking difference that separates the arteriviruses from other nidoviruses is the smaller size of their genome (12.7 to 15.7 kb versus more than 27 kb for the other nidoviruses). Accordingly, the arterivirus replicase polyproteins are less than half the size of their coronavirus, torovirus, and ronivirus counterparts. Despite this difference, coronaviruses and arteriviruses share a common property that is not conserved in toroviruses and roniviruses, as they have a common leader sequence at the 5′ end of all viral mRNAs, genomic and subgenomic.

Most of all, however, the features that distinguish the various nidovirus branches from each other are found at the level of virion structure and the properties of structural proteins (see Figure 20.1 and Chapter 39 for details). Arterivirus are spherical with a diameter of about 60 nm and lack prominent surface projections. Coronavirus particles have a diameter of 120–140 nm (including the extended peplomers). Toroviruses have a virion size similar to coronaviruses, while the bacilliform ronivirus particles are 150–200 nm long, have a diameter of 20–30 nm, and are also studded with prominent peplomers projecting approximately 11 nm from the surface. The nucleocapsid structure is helical–spherical for coronaviruses, helical–tubular for toroviruses and roniviruses, and isometric for arteriviruses. The nucleocapsid proteins of the four virus groups do not appear to share any common ancestry and their sizes range from 50 to 60 kDa for coronaviruses to only 12–14 kDa for arteriviruses. Also, the number of viral envelope proteins is quite variable, ranging from a single, post-translationally cleaved spike glycoprotein in roniviruses to a combination of six integral envelope proteins in arteriviruses. Whereas coronaviruses, toroviruses, and roniviruses carry a prominent spike structure (an oligomer of the S protein) on their surface, such structures have not been observed for arteriviruses. However, a common feature of all nidoviruses is the presence of an integral, triple-spanning membrane (M) protein in the viral envelope, which plays a crucial role during virus assembly.

A final difference that should be highlighted is the presence of genes encoding so-called 'accessory proteins' in coronavirus genomes. In the case of arteriviruses, toroviruses, and probably also roniviruses, all genes downstream of the replicase gene encode structural proteins. However, in coronaviruses several nonstructural proteins are encoded in this part of the genome.

These genes differ (in terms of position and protein encoded) between the different subgroups that are recognized among coronaviruses (for example, see the small undesignated genes dispersed among the *S*, *E*, *M*, and *N* protein genes in the 3′ proximal region of the SARS-CoV genome in Figure 20.2). A common feature, however, is that these genes appear to be dispensable for replication in cell culture. This suggests that the products of these genes exert their function at the level of the interaction with the host and may be important for the virus in, for example, countering antiviral responses triggered by the infection.

GENERAL SCHEME OF THE NIDOVIRUS LIFE CYCLE

Our knowledge of the nidovirus life cycle is largely based on cell culture-based studies with a limited number of viruses from the arterivirus and coronavirus families. Consequently, the description that follows (and the example of the SARS-CoV life cycle presented in Figure 20.2) should not be considered as definitive for all nidoviruses.

Nidoviruses attach to their host cell by binding to a receptor on the cell surface. These host molecules are mostly proteins, but in some cases carbohydrates may be involved. A number of cellular receptors have been identified and studied in detail for coronaviruses (Yeager et al. 1992; Williams et al. 1991; Li et al. 2003) and for the arterivirus PRRSV (Vanderheijden et al. 2003). Fusion of the nidoviral and cellular membrane is mediated by one of the major surface glycoproteins. Since the spike (S) protein of several coronaviruses displays fusion activity at neutral pH, fusion of the viral envelope and the plasma membrane is considered to be one route of entry for this virus group. However, endocytosis of coronaviruses has been described, which is the same infection route used by arteriviruses. Fusion of the viral envelope and a cellular membrane (either plasma membrane or endosome) results in the release of the viral nucleocapsid into the cytoplasm of the host cell (see Chapter 39 for details). Uncoating of the viral genome, which must precede genome translation, has not been studied in any detail.

The nidovirus genome is translated by host ribosomes that bind to the cap structure at the 5′ end of the genomic RNA and subsequently scan the template to find the translation initiation codon of replicase ORF1a. Following ORF1a translation, 60–80 percent of the ribosomes terminate at the ORF1a stop codon. However, the remaining ribosomes shift into the −1 reading frame just upstream of the ORF1a stop codon, at a specific heptanucleotide sequence (the slippery sequence), and continue translation in replicase ORF1b (Brierley et al. 1989; Snijder et al. 1990a; den Boon et al. 1991; Cowley et al. 2000). Consequently, genome translation leads to the synthesis of two replicase polyproteins, pp1a and pp1ab, with pp1ab being a carboxyl-extended version of pp1a. The −1 frameshift is stimulated by an RNA pseudoknot structure (i.e. two stem–loop structures that interact by base-pairing between sequences in the loops of the two hairpins) that probably induces a ribosomal pause over the slippery sequence. Due to the ribosomal frameshift mechanism, the ratio between translation of ORF1a and ORF1b is constant, which is thought to be an important part of the regulation of nidovirus replicase expression.

Nascent replicase polyproteins have never been detected in nidovirus-infected cells due to the speed of autoproteolytic processing, which seems to be initiated before the completion of ORF1a translation. The processing of the N-terminal 20–25 percent of the pp1ab polyprotein, is controlled by one or more so-called accessory proteinases that initiate autoproteolysis, while the main proteinase (3CLpro) is responsible for the processing of the downstream and most conserved part of the polyproteins (reviewed by Ziebuhr et al. (2000)). The accessory proteinase domains are located in the ORF1a-encoded region of the replicase and belong to the papainlike superfamily of cysteine proteinases (Gorbalenya et al. 1991). They are either autoproteinases that liberate the replicase subunit of which they are part (arteriviruses), or they can cleave up to three sites in the N-terminal half of pp1a (coronaviruses). The C-terminal half of pp1a and the ORF1b-encoded part of pp1ab are cleaved at eight to 11 sites by the viral main proteinase, which belongs to the chymotrypsin-like superfamily of proteinases (Gorbalenya et al. 1989; Snijder et al. 1996; Ziebuhr et al. 2003; Anand et al. 2002; Barrette-Ng et al. 2002). Replicase proteolysis is a crucial and probably highly regulated process, which should produce the right cleavage products in the right amounts at the right moment. The number of mature replicase products (nonstructural proteins or nsps) ranges from 12 or 13 in arteriviruses to 16 in most coronaviruses. By analogy with other RNA viruses, it may be expected that certain processing intermediates also have specific functions in the nidovirus life cycle.

Either during or shortly after translation, and possibly regulated by proteolytic cleavages, most of the nidovirus replicase proteins associate with intracellular membranes to form a membrane-bound complex for RNA synthesis ('replication complex'), a common feature of animal positive-strand RNA viruses. A number of ORF1a-encoded subunits contain hydrophobic domains and become transmembrane proteins, although they cannot be classified as 'conventional' membrane proteins (e.g. a signal sequence is lacking) and their mode of membrane insertion is unclear. For arteriviruses, it has been shown that the expression of two of these proteins (nsp2 and nsp3) suffices to induce the formation of specific double membrane vesicles, which seem to be derived from the endoplasmic reticulum and carry the viral replication complex (Pedersen et al. 1999; Snijder et al. 2001). Similar structures have been identified in cells infected with coronaviruses (Gosert et al. 2002), although other studies implicated late endosomes (van der Meer et al. 1999) or autophagosomes (Prentice et al. 2004) in the formation of the coronavirus replication complex. Other replicase subunits lack hydrophobic sequences, but immunofluorescence and electron microscopy has revealed that most of them co-localize with the ORF1a-encoded transmembrane subunits. Thus, the latter are likely to form a membrane-bound scaffold for the replication complex.

The first step in viral RNA synthesis is the recognition of RNA signals that promote the association of the 3′ end of the viral genome with a complex of viral enzymes that includes the RNA-dependent RNA polymerase encoded in the 5′-proximal part of replicase ORF1b. This 'RdRp complex' initiates the synthesis of full-length minus-strand RNA (or antigenome), which in turn will be the template for the synthesis of novel genome RNA. For the latter process, recognition signals present in the 3′ end of the antigenome must be used (see Chapter 39 for details). The amplification of the viral RNA is asymmetric and results in the production of much more plus- than minus-strand RNA. In coronavirus-infected cells, the structures engaged in viral RNA synthesis have been characterized. Approximately 70 percent of the RNA structures that accumulate in infected cells are multi-stranded intermediates (replicative intermediates) and 30 percent are double-stranded structures (replicative forms). These estimates describe, essentially, the structures involved in plus-strand synthesis. The structures engaged in minus-strand synthesis have not yet been characterized, although it is known that minus-strand templates are unstable and turnover during viral replication (Sawicki et al. 2001).

The newly synthesized genome RNA may be utilized in translation, replication, subgenomic mRNA synthesis, and/or encapsidation. First, genome RNA is used for translation of replicase ORFs 1a and 1b, thus yielding the polyprotein precursors of the main components of the viral replicase/transcriptase complex. Second, genome RNA serves as template for antigenome synthesis in the asymmetric cycle of genome replication described above. Third, genome RNA is assumed to be the template to produce subgenome-length minus strands that are used as templates for subgenomic mRNA synthesis. A nested set of subgenomic mRNAs is produced to express the viral structural proteins (and sometimes also accessory proteins) from genes located in the 3′-proximal third of the genome (the region downstream of ORF1b), which remains inaccessible for ribosomes translating the genome RNA. The synthesis of nidovirus subgenomic mRNAs was studied extensively and this will be discussed in a separate paragraph below. Finally, the de novo synthesized genomes can be used for encapsidation into progeny virions at the end of the infection cycle.

Following the accumulation of the structural proteins, the components for new virus particles have to assemble in the infected cell. New genomes first associate with the cytoplasmic nucleocapsid protein to form nucleocapsid structures. The viral envelope proteins are inserted into intracellular membranes, mostly by conventional cotranslational translocation. Subsequently, the envelope proteins are targeted to the site of virus assembly (usually membranes between the endoplasmic reticulum and Golgi complex; see Chapter 39 for details). Here, they meet up with the nucleocapsid structure and trigger a budding process that results in the envelopment of the nucleocapsid by host membrane impregnated with viral envelope proteins. As a result of budding, the newly formed virus particle is located in the lumen of the membrane compartment, after which it can leave the cell by following the exocytic pathway towards the plasma membrane. During this process, additional maturation of viral proteins and/or carbohydrates attached to these proteins occurs, in particular during transit through the Golgi complex.

THE NIDOVIRUS REPLICASE/ TRANSCRIPTASE

The synthesis of nidovirus-specific RNAs is mediated by a molecular machinery known as replicase/transcriptase (for simplicity often referred to as 'replicase'), which has not been characterized in detail for any nidovirus. Much of what is currently known about this macromolecular complex derives from comparative sequence analysis (reviewed in (Gorbalenya 2001); see below) that implicated ORF1a and 1b in encoding the key elements of the nidovirus replicase/transcriptase. This prediction has only recently been verified experimentally using genetic methods for the arterivirus EAV and the coronaviruses HCoV-229E and MHV (van Dinten et al., 1997, 1999; Tijms et al. 2001; Thiel et al. 2001; Seybert et al. 2005; Ivanov et al. 2004; Siddell et al. 2001).

The nidovirus replicase gene forms the backbone of the unique genetic plan that unites the different nidovirus subgroups (den Boon et al. 1991; Gorbalenya and Koonin 1993; Gorbalenya et al. 1989). From the end of the 1980s and through the 1990s, sequence analysis of different coronavirus, arterivirus, and torovirus genomes revealed a genetic plan consisting of nontranslated regions at the 5′ and 3′ ends of the genome that flank six to 11 ORFs, some of which are partly overlapping. The 5′-proximal two-thirds of the nidovirus genome is dominated by the replicase ORFs that encode the large pp1a and pp1ab polyproteins. These polyproteins are organized around a conserved framework of a dozen replicative domains and are autocatalytically processed to numerous products at conserved interdomain junctions (Ziebuhr et al. 2000). The other ORFs, whose number varies in different viruses, are located further downstream and a nested set of subgenomic mRNAs is generated to allow their expression.

The first nidovirus genome to be fully sequenced was that of the coronavirus IBV (Boursnell et al. 1987). Pairwise and profile comparisons of the IBV pp1a/pp1ab with replicative proteins of positive-strand RNA viruses and selected cellular proteins (Gorbalenya et al. 1988, 1989) tentatively identified a total of eight domains and 13 sites of proteolytic autoprocessing in pp1a/pp1ab. This analysis proved to be quite accurate and was largely confirmed by subsequent experimental studies. In the ORF1a-encoded sequence, a 3CLpro was recognized that is flanked by two highly hydrophobic, presumably transmembrane domains. Downstream of the ORF1a/1b ribosomal frameshift site, sequences encoding a putative RdRp and a putative superfamily 1 helicase (HEL1), the latter linked to an upstream-positioned Cys/His-rich domain predicted to form a multi-nuclear Zn-finger (ZF), were correctly identified.

Three domains identified in IBV, namely 3CLpro, RdRp, and HEL1, were (distant) variants of domains that are ubiquitous in the replicative polyproteins of positive-strand RNA viruses. Like their counterparts in other viruses, the IBV RdRp and HEL1 domains were postulated to play a central role in RNA synthesis. These domains, along with 3CLpro, were found to possess unique structural properties (Gorbalenya et al. 1988, 1989). RdRp has a replacement of Gly by Ser in the GDD signature that is otherwise absolutely conserved in positive-strand RNA viruses. The substitution of this Gly residue was later found to be a common feature of all nidoviruses. HEL1 is uniquely associated with ZF in the same protein and evidence for an important role of the ZF domain in HEL1 activity and other functions has emerged (van Dinten et al. 2000; Seybert et al. 2005). Nidovirus 3CLpro has several unique features (Barrette-Ng et al. 2002; Anand et al. 2002) and the two flanking hydrophobic domains have not been observed elsewhere. Furthermore, these and other (nidovirus-specific) conserved domains are positioned in a very specific and unique order within the replicase. Taken together, these observations confirmed that coronaviruses were the prototype of a separate supergroup (an informal rank above the family level) of positive-strand RNA viruses.

Since most unique features of the proposed IBV replicase organization were derived from the analysis of weak sequence similarities, independent validation of these findings was important and became possible upon publication of the sequence of MHV (Bredenbeek et al. 1990; Gorbalenya et al. 1991; Lee et al. 1991; Bonilla et al. 1994). These analyses confirmed and extended the predictions made for IBV and also revealed that the most N-terminal ~2 000 amino acids of the replicase are poorly conserved between coronaviruses. Among the few conserved features identified in this region were the so-called X domain and two papainlike proteinase (PLpro) domains (Gorbalenya et al. 1991) that are part of the same protein (nsp3) (see Figure 20.2). The X domain was shown to be a homologue of a functionally uncharacterized domain previously identified in the vicinity of the HEL1 domain in replicative polyproteins of the *Togaviridae* (Dominguez et al. 1990). It was subsequently shown to be a unique property of PLpros to contain a homologue of the Zn-ribbon domain that is commonly associated with a cellular transcription elongation factor (Herold et al. 1999). The presence of this Zn-ribbon, which is essential for the proteolytic activity of PLpro, implies a role in RNA synthesis for the nsp3 protein that contains this domain.

Further insight into the organization and evolution of coronavirus replicative polyproteins was gained by a study of the equine torovirus EToV (Berne virus) (Snijder et al. 1990a), which was found to have a coronaviruslike genome organization, including the characteristic RdRp–ZF–HEL1 domains encoded by ORF1b and a frameshifting signal at the ORF1a/1b junction. These results unequivocally established the relationship between toroviruses and coronaviruses, even though these viruses have different virion morphologies. The comparison also led to new assignments. In the C-terminal part of the ORF1b-encoded protein, a unique conserved domain of unknown function was delineated (Snijder et al. 1990a). Secondly, a surprising similarity was found between the C-terminal region of EToV pp1a and an accessory protein encoded by ORF2 in group 2 coronaviruses such as MHV (Snijder et al. 1991). This observation indicated that some replicative proteins are optional (since they are not conserved in all corona- and toroviruses) and that they can be subject to reshuffling, possibly through RNA recombination.

In 1991, the publication of the first complete arterivirus sequence, that of EAV, revealed several remarkable features of this virus group (den Boon et al. 1991). At that time, this virus, together with alphaviruses and rubiviruses, was considered to be part of the *Togaviridae* family. Although EAV has distinct virion morphology and a genome size approximately half that of an average coronavirus genome, it proved to share numerous features with coronaviruses. In particular, the ORF1b-encoded polyprotein, expressed through ribosomal frameshifting, contained distant homologues of the four previously identified conserved domains in corona- and toroviruses. Likewise, the pp1a polyprotein contained a characteristic domain set consisting of PLpro domains, as well as a 3CLpro domain embedded between two hydrophobic domains (den Boon et al. 1991).

However, at the same time, arteriviruses were also found to possess specific features. All conserved arterivirus domains were found to be smaller than their coronavirus counterparts, and the sequence similarities between ORF1a-encoded sequences of corona- and arteriviruses were so weak that a relationship could not be rigorously established (Ziebuhr et al. 2000). Unlike their coronavirus counterparts and the related picornavirus enzymes, the arterivirus 3CLpro was shown to employ Ser as the catalytic nucleophile (Snijder et al. 1996; Barrette-Ng et al. 2002). Importantly, though, the replicase domains of arteriviruses, like those of the corona- and toroviruses, were found to have no strong sequence similarities to other virus groups. All these observations were most compatible with a pronounced divergent evolution of arteriviruses and coronaviruses from a common ancestor (den Boon et al. 1991). Accordingly, these families were united in a coronavirus-like supergroup (Gorbalenya and Koonin 1993; Snijder and Horzinek 1993), which was subsequently recognized as the order *Nidovirales* (Cavanagh 1997).

The most recent, and most unexpected, extension of the nidovirus order was triggered by the sequence analysis of RNA viruses infecting prawns in Australia and Southeast Asia, GAV and Yellow head virus (YFV). The phylogenetic relationship between GAV and nidoviruses became evident from comparative sequence analyses of the replicase polyproteins, which again revealed striking similarities in organization and mode of expression (Cowley et al. 2000). Comparative sequence analysis identified ORF1b-encoded putative helicase and RdRp domains, ordered as in other nidoviruses and carrying specific sequence signatures, such as the GDD to SDD replacement in the RdRp. Collectively, the data argued that the replicases of GAV (infecting invertebrates) and other nidoviruses (infecting vertebrates) have a common ancestor. On the other hand, the presence of a number of regions with low sequence similarity in the ORF1b-encoded sequence and, in particular, the extremely poor pp1a conservation also suggested that GAV has diverged significantly from the vertebrate nidoviruses. Indeed, the only region in pp1a with significant sequence similarity proved to be a 3CLpro domain, again flanked by hydrophobic (probably membrane-spanning) domains (Ziebuhr et al. 2003).

Finally, the impulse given to the analysis of the nidovirus replicase by the SARS outbreak of 2003 should be mentioned. The relatively distant position of the SARS-coronavirus (SARS-CoV) among previously identified coronaviruses, and the impact of the disease that it causes, resulted in renewed in-depth analyses of all genes and proteins of coronaviruses (Rota et al. 2003; Marra et al. 2003; Thiel et al. 2003; Snijder et al. 2003; Stadler et al. 2003; Yan et al. 2003; Ziebuhr 2004b). At the level of the replicase, distant relationships between cellular enzymes involved in RNA metabolism and five nidovirus domains were tentatively identified (Snijder et al. 2003; von Grotthuss et al., 2003; Yan et al. 2003) and partially verified by subsequent experimental analysis (Ivanov et al. 2004; Bhardwaj et al. 2004). Thus, it was proposed that adenosine diphosphate-ribose1″-phosphatase (ADRP) activity is associated with the coronavirus X-domain (Gorbalenya et al. 1991) and cyclic phosphodiesterase (CPD) activity with the domain found at the C-terminal region of pp1a in EToV and in the ORF2 protein of group 2 coronaviruses (Snijder et al.

1991). New functional assignments were also made for an array of domains conserved in the carboxyl-terminal region of pp1ab (now named nsp14, 15, and 16 in coronaviruses) that is comprised of a 3'-to-5' exonuclease (ExoN), a uridylate-specific endoribonuclease (NendoU), and an *S*-adenosylmethionine-dependent ribose 2'-*O*-methyltransferase (2'-*O*-MT). These three domains are conserved in coronaviruses, toroviruses, and roniviruses, but only the NendoU domain is present in arteriviruses. It was proposed that these five nidovirus enzymes might cooperate in a manner described for their cellular homologues. In this cooperation NendoU, ExoN, and 2'-*O*-MT might provide specificity and the CPD and ADRP may modulate the pace of the reaction(s) in a single or several pathways. The expected functional hierarchy of the five nidovirus enzymes may be reflected in their level of evolutionary conservation, with the most conserved NendoU playing a key role in the initiation of a cascade of reactions (Snijder et al. 2003).

In summary, the comparison of nidovirus replicases leads to the conclusion that the basis of nidovirus common ancestry lies in the enzymatic functions that drive virus replication. Comparative analysis of pp1a and pp1ab (particularly between coronaviruses and arteriviruses) reveals a remarkable colinearity in organization, which contrasts with the overall low sequence similarity and size difference. As our understanding of the genetic blueprints for the different nidovirus branches continues to be refined, novel details of the nidovirus-specific replication machinery are coming to light. Despite many overall similarities, the enormous evolutionary distance between the different groups united in the order *Nidovirales* guarantees that many minor and possibly also major differences will emerge during the coming years. Advanced bioinformatics, structural studies, biochemistry, virus genetics, and molecular virology each play a specific and valuable role during the functional dissection of this unique positive-strand RNA virus replicase.

SUBGENOMIC RNA SYNTHESIS

The synthesis of one or multiple subgenomic mRNAs is a mechanism that many positive-strand RNA viruses have evolved to selectively express structural and accessory proteins from ORFs other than those encoding the major replicase subunits (reviewed in Miller and Koev (2000)). In nidoviruses, these ORFs are located downstream of the replicase ORFs 1a and 1b. Accordingly, nidovirus RNA synthesis also entails, in addition to the replication of the full-length genome, the production of a set of subgenomic mRNAs. The nidovirus genome and subgenomic mRNAs form a 3' co-terminal nested set of three to 10 mRNAs, depending on the particular virus species. The 5'-proximal part of each subgenomic mRNA encompasses a specific ORF (or sometimes several ORFs) from the 3'-proximal genome region,

which thus becomes accessible for translation by host ribosomes.

For a long time, it was thought that the hallmark of nidoviruses (mostly coronaviruses at that time) was the fact that the viral subgenomic mRNAs are composed of regions that are noncontiguous in the viral genome (Spaan et al. 1983; Baric et al. 1983; Lai et al. 1984). All subgenomic mRNAs of coronaviruses, and later also arteriviruses (de Vries et al. 1990), were found to carry a common 5' leader sequence, which is a copy of the 5'-terminal sequences of the genomic RNA. Thus, these subgenomic mRNAs (and the genome) share both 5'- and 3'-terminal sequences. In some respects, their mosaic nature resembles that of eukaryotic mRNAs generated by splicing.

More recently, however, it has become clear that the generation of subgenomic mRNAs containing noncontiguous sequences is not universal amongst the nidoviruses. First, evidence was obtained that makes it unlikely that ronivirus subgenomic mRNAs contain a common leader sequence (Cowley et al. 2002). Shortly afterwards, it was found that only one of the subgenomic mRNAs (RNA 2) of the torovirus EToV shares a short 5'-proximal leader sequence with the genome, whereas the smaller subgenomic mRNAs (like those of roniviruses) do not contain such a common leader sequence (van Vliet et al. 2002). Thus, there are differences in the mechanisms used to generate nidovirus subgenomic mRNAs and more studies are needed to identify the unique aspects of roniviruses and toroviruses RNA synthesis. However, the differences described above, rather than being viewed as fundamental, may transpire to be 'variations on a theme.' Thus, we will describe the discontinuous mode of subgenomic RNA synthesis used by coronaviruses and arteriviruses, which has been studied in much more detail, as a basis for identifying mechanistic principles that, eventually, may be related back to the unique nidovirus replicase functions that have been identified recently.

Despite the similarities between the structure of spliced eukaryotic mRNAs and the subgenomic mRNAs of coronaviruses and arteriviruses, the underlying mechanisms that generate these RNAs probably differ dramatically. The coronavirus/arterivirus subgenomic RNAs are generated in the cytoplasm of the infected cell via a unique mechanism that does not involve the post-transcriptional processing of a larger precursor to convert it into a smaller mature product (Jacobs et al. 1981; den Boon et al. 1995b; Yokomori et al. 1992), as is the case with host mRNAs generated by splicing (a nuclear process). Rather, nidovirus subgenomic RNAs derive from a process of discontinuous RNA synthesis that appears to be a variant of the similarity-assisted RNA recombination that can operate during genome replication (for a review, see Nagy and Simon (1997)).

Over the years, different models have been proposed to explain the discontinuous step in arterivirus and coronavirus subgenomic RNA synthesis (reviewed in van der Most and Spaan (1995), Brian and Spaan (1997), Lai and Cavanagh (1997), Snijder and Meulenberg (1998, 2001), Lai and Holmes (2001)). In the two most prominent models (commonly referred to as 'leader-primed transcription' and 'discontinuous minus strand synthesis', see Figure 20.4), it is proposed that short conserved transcription-regulating sequences (TRS) play a key role in connecting the common leader sequence to each of the subgenomic RNA 'bodies' (the variable part of the mRNA that is identical to a part of the 3'-proximal region of the genome). These TRS elements are present at the 3' end of the leader (leader TRS) and at the 5' end of each of the regions in the genome that corresponds to a subgenomic RNA body (body TRSs).

In the subgenomic RNA, a copy of the TRS connects the leader and body regions that are noncontiguous in the genome. Base-pairing between the leader TRS (+TRS) (in the genome) and the complement of the body TRSs (−TRS) (in the nascent minus strand) was shown to be essential for subgenomic mRNA synthesis (van Marle et al. 1999; Pasternak et al. 2001, 2003; Zuniga et al. 2004; Curtis et al. 2004).

According to the 'leader-primed transcription' model, subgenomic RNA synthesis would be primed by free leader molecules whose +TRS would base-pair with one of the body TRS complements in the anti-genome. Subsequently, using the anti-genome template, the leader primer would be extended with the body part to complete the subgenomic mRNA (Spaan et al. 1983;

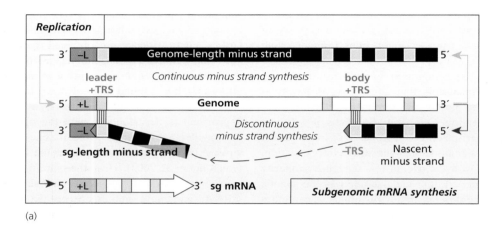

(a)

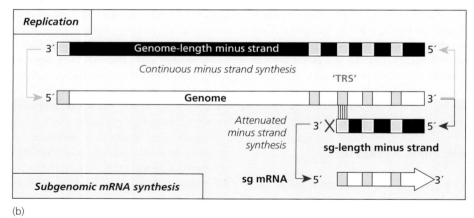

(b)

Figure 20.4 *Models for subgenomic mRNA synthesis from minus-strand subgenome-length templates in different nidoviruses.* **(a)** *Model for coronaviruses and arteriviruses, which have a common 5' leader sequence on all viral mRNAs. Discontinuous extension of minus-strand RNA synthesis (Sawicki and Sawicki 1995) has been proposed as the mechanism to produce subgenome-length minus-strand templates for subgenomic mRNA synthesis. Obviously, minus-strand RNA synthesis can also be continuous (top), yielding the genome-length minus-strand required for replication. During discontinuous minus-strand synthesis (bottom), the replicase/transcriptase is proposed to be attenuated at one of the body TRSs in the 3'-proximal part of the genome. Subsequently, the nascent minus strand, with the complement of the body TRS at its 3' end, is redirected to the 5'-proximal part of the template, where its 3' end can base-pair with the complementary leader TRS. Next, the subgenome-length minus-strand is completed by extension with the antileader sequence and used as template for mRNA synthesis.* **(b)** *Ronivirus subgenomic mRNAs and all but the largest subgenomic mRNAs of toroviruses do not contain a common 5' leader sequence (Cowley et al. 2002; van Vliet et al. 2002), although conserved ('body TRS-like') sequences are found upstream of each of the genes in the 3' proximal part of their genome. It is thought that these viruses may employ a variant of the mechanism explained in* **(a)**, *in which attenuation of minus-strand RNA synthesis does occur, but the discontinuous step required for antileader addition does not take place. Rather, the attenuated minus-strand RNA can serve directly as template for subgenomic mRNA production.*

Baric et al. 1983; Lai et al. 1984). This model was partly based on the fact that complements of subgenomic RNAs (subgenome-length minus strands) were initially not detected in cells infected with MHV (Lai et al. 1982). However, after the subsequent discovery of such molecules in coronavirus- and arterivirus-infected cells (Sethna et al. 1989; Sawicki and Sawicki 1990; den Boon et al. 1996), an alternative model for subgenomic mRNA synthesis was proposed (Figure 20.4a) (Sawicki and Sawicki 1995). According to this model, the discontinuous step in subgenomic RNA synthesis does not occur during plus, but during minus-strand RNA synthesis. The body TRSs in the plus-strand template would attenuate minus-strand synthesis, after which the nascent minus strand, having a TRS complement at its $3'$ end, would be transferred to base-pair with the leader TRS, which may be presented as part of a stem–loop structure (Chang et al. 1996; van Marle et al. 1999; van den Born et al. 2004). The subgenome-length minus strands would then be completed by extension with the complement of the leader sequence and subsequently be used as templates for the synthesis of subgenomic mRNAs. In recent years, this model, which was originally proposed by Sawicki and Sawicki, has gained considerable experimental support from both biochemical and genetic studies (Baric and Yount 2000; Sawicki et al. 2001; Pasternak et al. 2001).

The mechanism of discontinuous subgenomic RNA synthesis, as proposed for coronaviruses and arteriviruses, is a unique strategy for the generation of viral subgenomic transcripts. It contrasts with a mechanism used by many other RNA viruses that have been found to produce subgenomic mRNAs by internal initiation of transcription from 'promoters' in the antigenome (Miller et al. 1985). However, the mechanism used by coronaviruses and arteriviruses may share similarities with that of other positive-strand RNA viruses that employ premature termination (attenuation) of minus-strand RNA synthesis (reviewed in White (2002)). Also in the latter case, subgenome-length minus strands are produced that serve as the templates for subgenomic mRNA synthesis, but their synthesis does not involve the discontinuous extension of the nascent minus-strand RNA.

One of the most interesting questions that remains to be resolved is whether attenuation of minus-strand RNA synthesis is used by roniviruses and toroviruses (van Vliet et al. 2002). This property might explain the conservation in torovirus (Snijder et al. 1990b; van Vliet et al. 2002) and ronivirus (Cowley et al. 2002) genomes of sequences that appear to be the equivalent of the body TRSs of coronaviruses and arteriviruses. Whereas in coronaviruses and arteriviruses the attenuation step would be followed, according to the model of Sawicki and Sawicki, by extension of the nascent minus strand with the antileader sequence, the attenuated minus-strand products of roniviruses and toroviruses may be directly used as templates for subgenomic mRNA synthesis (Figure 20.4b). Thus, attenuation of minus-strand RNA synthesis may be the common feature that unites the mechanisms used to produce subgenomic mRNAs in different nidoviruses, while the process of discontinuous RNA synthesis may be restricted to coronaviruses and arteriviruses. This conclusion provokes, of course, the question of the functions of the coronavirus and arterivirus common leader sequence at the level of, for example, regulation of RNA synthesis and mRNA translation and, obviously, of alternative mechanisms used by nidoviruses that generate mRNAs that lack a common leader sequence.

NIDOVIRUS EVOLUTION

Comparative genomics and the phylogenetic analysis of nidovirus replicative domains clearly established nidoviruses as a distinct evolutionary lineage among positive-strand RNA viruses. The main nidovirus branches have diverged profoundly from each other in the course of evolution. This is evident from the enormous diversity among nidovirus enzymes, which exceeds that of their cellular homologues. For instance, nidovirus main proteinases have evolved several variants of the most conserved part of the enzyme (Gorbalenya et al. 1989; den Boon et al. 1991; Anand et al. 2002; Barrette-Ng et al. 2002; Ziebuhr et al. 2003). In nidovirus proteinases, the otherwise uniform catalytic site may include either a serine or a cysteine nucleophile and other structural variations not encountered in the cellular homologues that were identified in the three main kingdoms of life. Low replicase fidelity and, in particular, a high frequency of RNA recombination have been implicated in the generation of the nidovirus diversity. To achieve this diversity in the restricted and relatively slowly evolving environment of the infected host cell, these mechanisms must have been at work over a considerable period of time, possibly many millions of years (Koonin and Gorbalenya 1989). Given the considerable diversity of the conserved replicase among nidoviruses, it may not be surprising to see that three families of nidoviruses employ seemingly unrelated sets of structural protein genes that evolve faster than the replicases of the same origin. It has been hypothesized that a major split in nidovirus evolution, giving rise to viruses with remarkably different genome sizes, may have been coupled with the acquisition of different nucleocapsid protein genes by corona- and arteriviruses (Godeny et al. 1993).

How did the nidovirus genetic plan come to life? How have nidoviruses evolved replicative polyproteins of such outstanding complexity? There are two basic ways to increase complexity – either by acquiring domains from an outside source or by duplication of a pre-existing domain of the parental genome. These processes depend on intergenomic and intragenomic recombination, respectively. For example, most nidoviruses encode two or more papainlike proteinase (PLpro) domains that form family-specific branches that are well separated from their relatives of other origin (Ziebuhr et al. 2000). This implies that an amplification of PLpro domains has contributed to the enlargement of the nidovirus genome (den Boon et al. 1995a; Ziebuhr et al. 2001). However, it remains an open question how many of such events occurred and when they took place – in the ancestral nidovirus lineage or later, in individual nidovirus branches.

The nidovirus-replicative domains show remote sequence similarity with replicative proteins of other (super)groups of positive-strand RNA viruses. In particular, the coronavirus ADRP and nidovirus HEL1 domains cluster with homologues encoded by viruses from the *Alphavirus*-like supergroup (Gorbalenya et al. 1988; Gorbalenya et al. 1991). In contrast, the coronavirus RdRp and main proteinase (3Clpro) domains have specific affinity with homologous enzymes in plant potyviruses (Gorbalenya et al. 1989, 2002) and the coronavirus PLpros may be grouped with the leader proteinase (Lpro) of animal aphthoviruses (Gorbalenya et al. 1991). Both poty- and aphthoviruses belong to the picornavirus-like supergroup. Sequence affinity with the potyvirus 3CLpro was also documented for the ronivirus main proteinase (Cowley et al. 2000; Ziebuhr et al. 2003). Furthermore, and in apparent contradiction to the relationships cited above, the main proteinase of arteriviruses clusters with homologues encoded by plant sobemo- and luteoviruses (Snijder et al. 1996; Ziebuhr et al. 2000). Moreover, all these proteins also have complex, albeit very distant, relationships to a variety of cellular homologues (prototypes).

These mosaic relationships between different groups of positive-strand RNA viruses suggests that their replicative domains are derived from several common gene pools and that their genomes have been built by reshuffling these domains. This hypothesis implies that the nidovirus replicative polyproteins may, in fact, be of chimeric origin. On the other hand, no evidence has been obtained so far that any of the nidovirus-replicative domains is evolutionarily interleaved with related domains of other origin. Thus, it remains possible that all or some of these similarities to members of other virus supergroups have been preserved in the course of a continuous process of profound evolution of positive-strand RNA viruses, including nidoviruses, from a common root (Gorbalenya and Koonin 1993). More analyses and new sequences are needed for a more detailed reconstruction of the evolution of nidovirus genomes in general and the nidovirus replicase gene in particular.

From a practical perspective, the vast genetic diversity of nidoviruses presents the basis for designing molecular probes of different selectivity and constitutes a formidable challenge in the development and application of therapeutics. The first genome-based and immunochemical probes for the detection of multiple and individual nidoviruses have been developed by targeting their most and least conserved components, respectively. The list of functions that are unique and well conserved in the order *Nidovirales* or its separate branches is constantly growing and provides targets for specific drugs. To be effective, these drugs must be able to cope with viruses that have shown an amazing structural plasticity during their evolution.

REFERENCES

Anand, K., Palm, G.J., et al. 2002. Structure of coronavirus main proteinase reveals combination of a chymotrypsin fold with an extra alpha-helical domain. *EMBO J*, **21**, 3213–24.

Baric, R.S. and Yount, B. 2000. Subgenomic negative-strand RNA function during mouse hepatitis virus infection. *J Virol*, **74**, 4039–46.

Baric, R.S., Stohlman, S.A. and Lai, M.M.C. 1983. Characterization of replicative intermediate RNA of mouse hepatitis virus: presence of leader RNA sequences on nascent chains. *J Virol*, **48**, 633–40.

Barrette-Ng, I.H. 2002. Structure of arterivirus nsp4 – the smallest chymotrypsin-like proteinase with an alpha/beta C-terminal extension and alternate conformations of the oxyanion hole. *J Biol Chem*, **277**, 39960–6.

Berger, A., Drosten, C., et al. 2004. Severe acute respiratory syndrome (SARS) – paradigm of an emerging viral infection. *J Clin Virol*, **29**, 13–22.

Bhardwaj, K., Guarino, L. and Kao, C.C. 2004. The severe acute respiratory syndrome coronavirus Nsp15 protein is an endoribonuclease that prefers manganese as a cofactor. *J Virol*, **78**, 12218–24.

Bonilla, P.J., Gorbalenya, A.E. and Weiss, S.R. 1994. Mouse hepatitis virus strain A59 RNA polymerase gene ORF 1a: heterogeneity among MHV strains. *Virology*, **198**, 736–40.

Boursnell, M.E., Brown, T.D.K., et al. 1987. Completion of the sequence of the genome of the coronavirus avian infectious bronchitis virus. *J Gen Virol*, **68**, 57–77.

Bredenbeek, P.J., Pachuk, C.J., et al. 1990. The primary structure and expression of the second open reading frame of the polymerase gene of the coronavirus mhv-a59; a highly conserved polymerase is expressed by an efficient ribosomal frameshifting mechanism. *Nucl Acid Res*, **18**, 1825–32.

Brian, D.A. and Spaan, W.J.M. 1997. Recombination and coronavirus defective interfering RNAs. *Semin Virol*, **8**, 101–11.

Brierley, I., Digard, P. and Inglis, S.C. 1989. Characterization of an efficient coronavirus ribosomal frameshifting signal – requirement for an RNA pseudoknot. *Cell*, **57**, 537–47.

Cavanagh, D. 1997. *Nidovirales*: a new order comprising *Coronaviridae* and *Arteriviridae*. *Arch Virol*, **142**, 629–33.

Chang, R.Y., Krishnan, R. and Brian, D.A. 1996. The UCUAAAC promoter motif is not required for high-frequency leader recombination in bovine coronavirus defective interfering RNA. *J Virol*, **70**, 2720–9.

Cowley, J.A., Dimmock, C.M., et al. 2000. Gill-associated virus of *Penaeus monodon* prawns: an invertebrate virus with ORF1a and ORF1b genes related to arteri- and coronaviruses. *J Gen Virol*, **81**, 1473–84.

Cowley, J.A., Dimmock, C.M. and Walker, P.J. 2002. Gill-associated nidovirus of *Penaeus monodon* prawns transcribes 3'-coterminal subgenomic mRNAs that do not possess 5'-leader sequences. *J Gen Virol*, **83**, 927–35.

Cowley, J.A., Cadogan, L.C., et al. 2004. The gene encoding the nucleocapsid protein of Gill-associated nidovirus of *Penaeus monodon* prawns is located upstream of the glycoprotein gene. *J Virol*, **78**, 8935–41.

Curtis, K.M., Yount, B., et al. 2004. Reverse genetic analysis of the transcription regulatory sequence of the coronavirus transmissible gastroenteritis virus. *J Virol*, **78**, 6061–6.

den Boon, J.A., Snijder, E.J., et al. 1991. Equine arteritis virus is not a togavirus but belongs to the coronaviruslike superfamily. *J Virol*, **65**, 2910–20.

den Boon, J.A., Faaberg, K.S., et al. 1995a. Processing and evolution of the N-terminal region of the arterivirus replicase ORF1a protein: identification of two papainlike cysteine proteases. *J Virol*, **69**, 4500–5.

den Boon, J.A., Spaan, W.J.M. and Snijder, E.J. 1995b. Equine arteritis virus subgenomic RNA transcription: UV inactivation and translation inhibition studies. *Virology*, **213**, 364–72.

den Boon, J.A., Kleijnen, M.F., et al. 1996. Equine arteritis virus subgenomic mRNA synthesis: analysis of leader-body junctions and replicative-form RNAs. *J Virol*, **70**, 4291–8.

de Vries, A.A.F., Chirnside, E.D., et al. 1990. All subgenomic mRNAs of equine arteritis virus contain a common leader sequence. *Nucl Acid Res*, **18**, 3241–7.

Dominguez, G., Wang, C.Y. and Frey, T.K. 1990. Sequence of the genome RNA of Rubella virus – evidence for genetic rearrangement during togavirus evolution. *Virology*, **177**, 225–38.

Drosten, C., Gunther, S., et al. 2003. Identification of a novel coronavirus in patients with severe acute respiratory syndrome. *N Engl J Med*, **348**, 1967–76.

Fouchier, R.A.M., Hartwig, N.G., et al. 2004. A previously undescribed coronavirus associated with respiratory disease in humans. *Proc Natl Acad Sci USA*, **101**, 6212–16.

Godeny, E.K., Chen, L., et al. 1993. Complete genomic sequence and phylogenetic analysis of the lactate dehydrogenase-elevating virus (LDV). *Virology*, **194**, 585–96.

Gorbalenya, A.E. 2001. Big nidovirus genome: when count and order of domains matter. *Adv Exp Biol Med*, **494**, 1–17.

Gorbalenya, A.E. and Koonin, E.V. 1993. Comparative analysis of the amino acid sequences of the key enzymes of the replication and expression of positive-strand RNA viruses. Validity of the approach and functional and evolutionary implications. *Sov Sci Rev Sect D*, **11**, 1–84.

Gorbalenya, A.E., Koonin, E.V., et al. 1988. A novel superfamily of nucleoside triphosphate-binding motif containing proteins which are probably involved in duplex unwinding in DNA and RNA replication and recombination. *FEBS Lett*, **235**, 16–24.

Gorbalenya, A.E., Koonin, E.V., et al. 1989. Coronavirus genome: prediction of putative functional domains in the non-structural polyprotein by comparative amino acid sequence analysis. *Nucl Acid Res*, **17**, 4847–61.

Gorbalenya, A.E., Koonin, E.V. and Lai, M.M.C. 1991. Putative papain-related thiol proteases of positive-strand RNA viruses. Identification of rubi- and aphthovirus proteases and delineation of a novel conserved domain associated with proteases of rubi-, alpha- and coronaviruses. *FEBS Lett*, **288**, 201–5.

Gorbalenya, A.E., Pringle, F.M., et al. 2002. The palm subdomain-based active site is internally permuted in viral RNA-dependent RNA polymerases of an ancient lineage. *J Mol Biol*, **324**, 47–62.

Gosert, R., Kanjanahaluethai, A., et al. 2002. RNA replication of mouse hepatitis virus takes place at double-membrane vesicles. *J Virol*, **76**, 3697–708.

Herold, J., Siddell, S.G. and Gorbalenya, A.E. 1999. A human RNA viral cysteine proteinase that depends upon a unique Zn^{2+}-binding finger connecting the two domains of a papain-like fold. *J Biol Chem*, **274**, 14918–25.

Ivanov, K.A., Hertzig, T., et al. 2004. Major genetic marker of nidoviruses encodes a replicative endoribonuclease. *Proc Natl Acad Sci USA*, **101**, 12694–9.

Jacobs, L., Spaan, W.J.M., et al. 1981. Synthesis of subgenomic mRNAs of mouse hepatitis virus is initiated independently: evidence from UV transcription mapping. *J Virol*, **39**, 401–6.

Koonin, E.V. and Gorbalenya, A.E. 1989. Evolution of RNA genomes: does the high mutation rate necessitate high rate of evolution of viral proteins? *J Mol Evol*, **28**, 524–7.

Ksiazek, T.G., Erdman, D., et al. 2003. A novel coronavirus associated with severe acute respiratory syndrome. *N Engl J Med*, **348**, 1953–66.

Lai, M.M.C. and Cavanagh, D. 1997. The molecular biology of coronaviruses. *Adv Virus Res*, **48**, 1–100.

Lai, M.M.C. and Holmes, K.V. 2001. *Coronaviridae*. In: Knipe, D.M. and Howley, P.M. (eds), *Fields' virology*, Vol. 1. Philadelphia, PA: Lippincott, Williams & Wilkins, 1163–85.

Lai, M.M.C., Patton, C.D. and Stohlman, S.A. 1982. Replication of mouse hepatitis virus: negative-stranded RNA and replicative form RNA are of genome length. *J Virol*, **44**, 487–92.

Lai, M.M.C., Baric, R.S., et al. 1984. Characterization of leader RNA sequences on the virion and mRNAs of mouse hepatitis virus, a cytoplasmic RNA virus. *Proc Natl Acad Sci USA*, **81**, 3626–30.

Lee, H.J., Shieh, C.K., et al. 1991. The complete sequence (22 kilobases) of murine coronavirus gene 1 encoding the putative proteases and RNA polymerase. *Virology*, **180**, 567–82.

Li, W.H., Moore, M.J., et al. 2003. Angiotensin-converting enzyme 2 is a functional receptor for the SARS coronavirus. *Nature*, **426**, 450–4.

Marra, M.A., Jones, S.J.M., et al. 2003. The genome sequence of the SARS-associated coronavirus. *Science*, **300**, 1399–404.

Miller, W.A. and Koev, G. 2000. Synthesis of subgenomic RNAs by positive-strand RNA viruses. *Virology*, **273**, 1–8.

Miller, W.A., Dreher, T.W. and Hall, T.C. 1985. Synthesis of brome mosaic virus subgenomic RNA in vitro by internal initiation on (−)-sense genomic RNA. *Nature*, **313**, 68–70.

Nagy, P.D. and Simon, A.E. 1997. New insights into the mechanisms of RNA recombination. *Virology*, **235**, 1–9.

Pasternak, A.O., van den Born, E., et al. 2001. Sequence requirements for RNA strand transfer during nidovirus discontinuous subgenomic RNA synthesis. *EMBO J*, **20**, 7220–8.

Pasternak, A.O., van den Born, E., et al. 2003. The stability of the duplex between sense and antisense transcription-regulating sequences is a crucial factor in arterivirus subgenomic mRNA synthesis. *J Virol*, **77**, 1175–83.

Pedersen, K.W., van der Meer, Y., et al. 1999. Open reading frame 1a-encoded subunits of the arterivirus replicase induce endoplasmic reticulum-derived double-membrane vesicles which carry the viral replication complex. *J Virol*, **73**, 2016–26.

Peiris, J.S.M., Lai, S.T., et al. 2003a. Coronavirus as a possible cause of severe acute respiratory syndrome. *Lancet*, **361**, 1319–25.

Peiris, J.S.M., Yuen, K.Y., et al. 2003b. Current concepts: the severe acute respiratory syndrome. *N Engl J Med*, **349**, 2431–41.

Plagemann, P.G.W. 1996. Lactate dehydrogenase-elevating virus and related viruses. In: Fields, B.N., Knipe, D.M. and Howley, P.M. (eds), *Fields' virology*. Philadelphia, PA: Lippincott-Raven Publishers, 1105–20.

Prentice, E., Jerome, W.G., et al. 2004. Coronavirus replication complex formation utilizes components of cellular autophagy. *J Biol Chem*, **279**, 10136–41.

Rota, P.A., Oberste, M.S., et al. 2003. Characterization of a novel coronavirus associated with severe acute respiratory syndrome. *Science*, **300**, 1394–9.

Sawicki, S.G. and Sawicki, D.L. 1990. Coronavirus transcription: subgenomic mouse hepatitis virus replicative intermediates function in RNA synthesis. *J Virol*, **64**, 1050–6.

Sawicki, S.G. and Sawicki, D.L. 1995. Coronaviruses use discontinuous extension for synthesis of subgenome-length negative strands. *Adv Exp Biol Med*, **380**, 499–506.

Sawicki, D., Wang, T. and Sawicki, S. 2001. The RNA structures engaged in replication and transcription of the A59 strain of mouse hepatitis virus. *J Gen Virol*, **82**, 385–96.

Sethna, P.B., Hung, S.L. and Brian, D.A. 1989. Coronavirus subgenomic minus-strand RNAs and the potential for mRNA replicons. *Proc Natl Acad Sci USA*, **86**, 5626–30.

Seybert, A., Posthuma, C.C., et al. 2005. A complex zinc finger controls the activities of nidovirus helicases. *J Virol*, **79**, 696–704.

Siddell, S.G., Sawicki, D.L., et al. 2001. Identification of the mutations responsible for the phenotype of three MHV RNA-negative ts mutants. *Adv Exp Biol Med*, **494**, 453–8.

Snijder, E.J. and Horzinek, M.C. 1993. Toroviruses: replication, evolution and comparison with other members of the coronavirus-like superfamily. *J Gen Virol*, **74**, 2305–16.

Snijder, E.J. and Meulenberg, J.J.M. 1998. The molecular biology of arteriviruses. *J Gen Virol*, **79**, 961–79.

Snijder, E.J. and Meulenberg, J.J.M. 2001. Arteriviruses. In: Knipe, D.M. and Howley, P.M. (eds), *Fields' virology*. Philadelphia, PA: Lippincott, Williams & Wilkins, 1205–20.

Snijder, E.J., den Boon, J.A., et al. 1990a. The carboxyl-terminal part of the putative Berne virus polymerase is expressed by ribosomal frameshifting and contains sequence motifs which indicate that toro- and coronaviruses are evolutionarily related. *Nucl Acid Res*, **18**, 4535–42.

Snijder, E.J., Horzinek, M.C. and Spaan, W.J.M. 1990b. A 3′-coterminal nested set of independently transcribed mRNAs is generated during Berne virus replication. *J Virol*, **64**, 331–8.

Snijder, E.J., den Boon, J.A., et al. 1991. Comparison of the genome organization of toro- and coronaviruses: evidence for two nonhomologous RNA recombination events during Berne virus evolution. *Virology*, **180**, 448–52.

Snijder, E.J., Wassenaar, A.L.M., et al. 1996. The arterivirus nsp4 protease is the prototype of a novel group of chymotrypsin-like enzymes, the 3C-like serine proteases. *J Biol Chem*, **271**, 4864–71.

Snijder, E.J., van Tol, H., et al. 2001. Non-structural proteins 2 and 3 interact to modify host cell membranes during the formation of the arterivirus replication complex. *J Gen Virol*, **82**, 985–94.

Snijder, E.J., Bredenbeek, P.J., et al. 2003. Unique and conserved features of genome and proteome of SARS-coronavirus, an early split-off from the coronavirus group 2 lineage. *J Mol Biol*, **331**, 991–1004.

Spaan, W.J.M., Delius, H., et al. 1983. Coronavirus mRNA synthesis involves fusion of non-contiguous sequences. *EMBO J*, **2**, 1839–44.

Spann, K.M., Vickers, J.E. and Lester, R.J.G. 1995. Lymphoid organ virus of *Penaeus monodon* from Australia. *Dis Aqua Organ*, **23**, 127–34.

Spaan, W.J.M., Cavanagh, D., et al. 2005. *Nidovirales*. In: Fauquet, C.M., Mayo, M.A., et al. (eds), *Virus taxonomy, VIIIth report of the ICTV*. London: Elsevier/Academic Press, 935–43.

Stadler, K., Masignani, V., et al. 2003. SARS – beginning to understand a new virus. *Nat Rev Microbiol*, **1**, 209–18.

Thiel, V., Herold, J., et al. 2001. Viral replicase gene products suffice for coronavirus discontinuous transcription. *J Virol*, **75**, 6676–81.

Thiel, V., Ivanov, K.A., et al. 2003. Mechanisms and enzymes involved in SARS coronavirus genome expression. *J Gen Virol*, **84**, 2305–15.

Tijms, M.A., van Dinten, L.C., et al. 2001. A zinc finger-containing papain-like protease couples subgenomic mRNA synthesis to genome translation in a positive-stranded RNA virus. *Proc Natl Acad Sci USA*, **98**, 1889–94.

van den Born, E., Gultyaev, A.P. and Snijder, E.J. 2004. Secondary structure and function of the 5′-proximal region of the equine arteritis virus RNA genome. *RNA*, **10**, 424–37.

van der Hoek, L., Pyrc, K., et al. 2004. Identification of a new human coronavirus. *Nature Med*, **10**, 368–73.

van der Meer, Y., Snijder, E.J., et al. 1999. Localization of mouse hepatitis virus nonstructural proteins and RNA synthesis indicates a role for late endosomes in viral replication. *J Virol*, **73**, 7641–57.

van der Most, R.G. and Spaan, W.J.M. 1995. Coronavirus replication, transcription, and RNA recombination. In: Siddell, S.G. (ed.), *The Coronaviridae*. New York, NY: Plenum Press, 11–31.

van Dinten, L.C., den Boon, J.A., et al. 1997. An infectious arterivirus cDNA clone: identification of a replicase point mutation which abolishes discontinuous mRNA transcription. *Proc Natl Acad Sci USA*, **94**, 991–6.

van Dinten, L.C., Rensen, S., et al. 1999. Proteolytic processing of the open reading frame 1b-encoded part of arterivirus replicase is mediated by nsp4 serine protease and is essential for virus replication. *J Virol*, **73**, 2027–37.

van Dinten, L.C., van Tol, H., et al. 2000. The predicted metal-binding region of the arterivirus helicase protein is involved in subgenomic mRNA synthesis, genome replication, and virion biogenesis. *J Virol*, **74**, 5213–23.

van Marle, G., Dobbe, J.C., et al. 1999. Arterivirus discontinuous mRNA transcription is guided by base-pairing between sense and antisense transcription-regulating sequences. *Proc Natl Acad Sci USA*, **96**, 12056–61.

van Vliet, A.L., Smits, S.L., et al. 2002. Discontinuous and non-discontinuous subgenomic RNA transcription in a nidovirus. *EMBO J*, **21**, 6571–80.

Vanderheijden, N., Delputte, P.L., et al. 2003. Involvement of sialoadhesin in entry of porcine reproductive and respiratory syndrome virus into porcine alveolar macrophages. *J Virol*, **77**, 8207–15.

von Grotthuss, M., Wyrwicz, L.S. and Rychlewski, L. 2003. mRNA cap-1 methyltransferase in the SARS genome. *Cell*, **113**, 701–2.

Walker, P.J., Bonami, J.R., et al. 2004. *Roniviridae*. In: Fauquet, C.M. and Mayo, M.A. (eds), *Virus taxonomy, VIIIth report of the ICTV*. London: Elsevier/Academic Press, 973–7.

Weiss, M., Steck, F. and Horzinek, M.C. 1983. Purification and partial characterization of a new enveloped RNA virus (Berne virus). *J Gen Virol*, **64**, 1849–58.

White, K.A. 2002. The premature termination model: a possible third mechanism for subgenomic mRNA transcription in (+)-strand RNA viruses. *Virology*, **304**, 147–54.

Williams, R.K., Jiang, G.S. and Holmes, K.V. 1991. Receptor for mouse hepatitis-virus is a member of the carcinoembryonic antigen family of glycoproteins. *Proc Natl Acad Sci USA*, **88**, 5533–6.

Woo, P.C., Lau, S.K., et al. 2005. Characterization and complete genome sequence of a novel coronavirus, coronavirus HKU1, from patients with pneumonia. *J Virol*, **79**, 884–95.

Yan, L., Velikanov, M., et al. 2003. Assessment of putative protein targets derived from the SARS genome. *FEBS Lett*, **554**, 257–63.

Yeager, C.L., Ashmun, R.A., et al. 1992. Human aminopeptidase-N is a receptor for human coronavirus-229e. *Nature*, **357**, 420–2.

Yokomori, K., Banner, L.R. and Lai, M.M.C. 1992. Coronavirus mRNA transcription: UV light transcriptional mapping studies suggest an early requirement for a genomic-length template. *J Virol*, **66**, 4671–8.

Ziebuhr, J. 2004a. Molecular biology of severe acute respiratory syndrome coronavirus. *Curr Opin Microbiol*, **7**, 412–19.

Ziebuhr, J. 2004b. The coronavirus replicase. *Curr Topic Microbiol Immunol*, **287**, 57–94.

Ziebuhr, J., Snijder, E.J. and Gorbalenya, A.E. 2000. Virus-encoded proteinases and proteolytic processing in the *Nidovirales*. *J Gen Virol*, **81**, 853–79.

Ziebuhr, J., Thiel, V. and Gorbalenya, A.E. 2001. The autocatalytic release of a putative RNA virus transcription factor from its polyprotein precursor involves two paralogous papain-like proteases that cleave the same peptide bond. *J Biol Chem*, **276**, 33220–32.

Ziebuhr, J., Bayer, S., et al. 2003. The 3C-like proteinase of an invertebrate nidovirus links coronavirus and potyvirus homologs. *J Virol*, **77**, 1415–26.

Zuniga, S., Sola, I., et al. 2004. Sequence motifs involved in the regulation of discontinuous coronavirus subgenomic RNA synthesis. *J Virol*, **78**, 980–94.

PART II

SPECIFIC VIRUSES AND VIRAL INFECTION

21

Parvoviruses

PETER TATTERSALL AND SUSAN F. COTMORE

CHARACTERISTICS OF THE VIRUSES

INTRODUCTION

As their name implies, parvoviruses, from the Latin *parvus* meaning small, are amongst the smallest of the known animal viruses, having nonenveloped icosahedral protein virions approximately 250 Å in diameter. These particles, which comprise only DNA and protein, are quite dense and extremely rugged. They can survive many inactivation procedures, including most used to protect the blood supply, and remain fully viable at ambient temperatures for months or years. Some members of the family are major pathogens of insects and domestic animals, but only one, human parvovirus B19, has so far been identified as a human pathogen, and is the causative agent of fifth disease (erythema infectiosum). Many parvoviruses are essentially apathogenic, and over the past few years this characteristic has helped them gain recognition as effective vectors for the safe delivery of vaccines or therapeutic genes.

In the known biosphere, only parvoviruses have DNA genomes that are both single-stranded and linear. Parvoviruses package a single genomic molecule between 4 and 6 kb in length, which terminates in short palindromic sequences that can fold back on themselves to create duplex hairpin telomeres. These terminal hairpins are essential for the virus's unusual replication strategy,

and hence serve as an invariant hallmark of the family. DNA replication proceeds through a series of duplex intermediates in the host cell, via a characteristic unidirectional strand-displacement mechanism called 'rolling-hairpin' synthesis, organized by the major viral nonstructural protein. Transmitted as single-stranded progeny, parvoviruses do not arrive in their host cell with a complementary copy of their genome sequence against which environmental damage can be corrected. This may well contribute to the observation that their genetic mutation rates are higher than those seen in double-stranded DNA viruses, and approach those more commonly associated with some RNA viruses. However, their tendency to drift genetically is held severely in check by the compact nature of the genome, and the structural constraints on its few gene products, which ensure that only a limited spectrum of mutations are compatible with progeny viability.

Parvovirus particles exhibit $T = 1$ icosahedral symmetry, but are generally constructed from 2–4 capsid protein size classes, usually called VP1 to VP4. Of these, VP1 is the longest, at 80–96 kDa, while the remainder comprise a nested set of polypeptides derived from its carboxy terminus (VP2 64–85 kDa, VP3 60–75 kDa, and VP4 49–52 kDa), with VP2 or VP3 being the principal capsid component. Particles are built up from 60 equivalent copies of this large carboxy-terminal core sequence, and the amino-terminal extensions carried by some of the polypeptides are alternately concealed or exposed at the particle surface during different stages of the infectious cycle, displaying stage-specific trafficking signals or effector domains. Notably, VP1-specific sequences from most genera contain the enzymatic core of a phospholipase A2 (PLA2) molecule, which is essential for infectious entry and appears to be a unique feature of this family (Zadori et al. 2001). Virions lack essential lipids, and none of the viral proteins are known to be glycosylated, but they are modulated post-translationally by important phosphorylation events. Parvovirus virions are exceptionally stable, and quite simple antigenically. In nature only a single serotype of any particular species is generally found circulating in its host population, and this has led to the use of individual serotype, defined by neutralization of infectivity in cell culture, hemagglutination-inhibition, or specific enzyme-linked immunosorbent assay (ELISA), as the major criterion for taxonomic species demarcation (Tattersall et al. 2005). Just two antigenic sites, defined by mutations that confer resistance to neutralization by monoclonal antibodies, have been identified for canine parvovirus (CPV). Despite their differences in capsid serology, the nonstructural proteins of most species in a genus do show antigenic cross-reactivity, so that genera-specific infections can often be diagnosed serologically.

While adeno-associated viruses (AAV), from the genus *Dependovirus*, generally require coinfection with a helper adenovirus or herpesvirus in order to complete their replication cycle, the great majority of family members are capable of helper-independent, so-called 'autonomous,' replication. Viral genomes typically contain just two gene cassettes, of which one encodes the nonstructural proteins (called Rep in the AAVs and NS in other species), which are essential for viral gene expression and DNA replication, while the other encodes the overlapping set of capsid polypeptides. The limited coding potential of these genomes therefore renders them highly dependent on the synthetic machinery provided by the host cell for their own, preferential, replication. In contrast to most other DNA viruses, parvoviruses do not encode proteins that can coerce resting cells to enter cell division. Nevertheless, they do require host cells to enter S phase in order to provide the extensive deoxynucleotide triphosphate pools and active cellular DNA synthetic apparatus required for their replication, and that are not present in interphase cells. As a consequence, autonomously replicating parvoviruses cannot grow in resting cell populations, and amplify best in populations of rapidly dividing cells, both in vitro and in vivo. This lack of any encoded positive growth regulators means that parvoviruses are universally nontumorigenic, and indeed, for reasons that are not yet clear, they are often specifically oncosuppressive, exhibiting an enhanced ability to replicate in transformed cells.

AAVs overcome their limited gene repertoire by resorting to a pattern of latent infection in which they generally integrate into the host-cell genome, only switching to a productive life cycle when their host cell becomes infected with a 'helper' virus. In this situation, the helper inadvertently activates resident AAV genes, while also reprogramming the host's cell cycle for its own use, sending the cell into S phase. Resulting helper virus replication is paralleled, or even overtaken, by that of the resident AAV, culminating in cell death and the release of infectious progeny of both viruses. In recent years, this capacity of AAV to integrate, or otherwise persist in host cells, has been exploited for the safe and efficient delivery of a wide range of therapeutic genes, so that AAVs are now among the most promising vector systems available for long-term gene substitution or correction strategies. In most of these vectors all of the viral genes are deleted to accommodate the therapeutic transgene, so that these constructs cannot give rise to infectious progeny.

Characteristics of the viral life cycle inevitably dictate the types of disease parvoviruses are able to induce. On one hand, AAVs have been selected for their ability to remain essentially invisible over prolonged periods of time, and to specifically exploit coinfection with potentially tumorigenic helper viruses, while the helper-independent viruses require cells of specific differentiated phenotypes which must also be undergoing cell division, and hence DNA replication, of their own volition. These viruses are therefore parasites of specific, rapidly dividing cell populations, and generally only give rise to overt disease in situations where large numbers of their target cells continue to replicate in the adult, or where the timing of organ development in the fetus means that transiently replicating cell populations, once damaged, can no longer be effectively regenerated, resulting in fetal or neonatal death, or teratogenesis. In healthy adults, the immune response mounted against otherwise innocuous viruses can also sometimes exacerbate the pathogenesis of infection, as manifest, for instance, by the rashes and polyarthropathy which often follow infection of otherwise healthy people by human parvovirus B19.

HISTORY AND TAXONOMIC RELATIONSHIPS WITHIN THE FAMILY *PARVOVIRIDAE*

In 1970 the taxonomic family, *Parvoviridae*, was established to encompass all small nonenveloped viruses with approximately 5 kb linear, self-priming, single-stranded DNA genomes. Although genome sequences were not then available to confirm their phylogenetic relationships, the DNA sequence data amassed since that time confirm that all viruses in the family share a common evolutionary history. As delineated in Table 21.1, the family *Parvoviridae* is currently divided into two subfamilies on the basis of host range: the *Parvovirinae*,

Table 21.1 *Taxonomic structure of the family* Parvoviridae

Subfamily *Parvovirinae*	Subfamily *Densovirinae*
Genus	Genus
Parvovirus	*Densovirus*
Erythrovirus	*Iteravirus*
Dependovirus	*Brevidensovirus*
Amdovirus	*Pefudensovirus*
Bocavirus	

which infect vertebrate hosts, and the *Densovirinae*, infecting insects and other arthropods (Tattersall et al. 2005). This chapter will focus exclusively on members of the *Parvovirinae* subfamily. These are currently divided into five genera, as detailed in the phylogenetic tree in Figure 21.1, but we will mostly consider the properties of species belonging to the three major genera, namely the dependoviruses, predominantly the helper-dependent AAVs, and the autonomously replicating parvoviruses and erythroviruses. The latter include the human pathogen, parvovirus B19, and are named for the striking tropism of this agent for cells of the erythroid lineage.

The genus *Parvovirus*

In 1959, a small stable virus, subsequently named *Kilham rat virus* (KRV), was isolated from lysates of an experimental rat tumor (Kilham and Olivier 1959). In the following decade a number of other physically similar agents were identified as contaminants of laboratory tumors that were being serially transplanted in normal or immunosuppressed rodents, and as contaminants of cell cultures or other virus stocks in routine laboratory use (Tattersall and Cotmore 1986). Although lacking known host species, some of these isolates were injected into rodents where they caused a broad spectrum of pathology, which varied with the virus serotype and age of the host, from apparently asymptomatic viremia to teratogenesis and fetal or neonatal death (Toolan 1961). Concurrently, an infectious agent responsible for epidemics of enteritis, panleukopenia, and congenital cerebellar ataxia in domestic cats was identified, called *Feline panleukopenia virus* (FPV), and it soon became apparent that this shared the same characteristic size and genome structure as the so-called 'rodent' parvoviruses isolated in the laboratory (Kilham et al. 1967; Gorham et al. 1966). Transplacental transmission has been described for several viruses in the genus, and under experimental conditions their host range can often be extended to include a large number of vertebrate species. Since the capsids of most species hemagglutinate red blood cells of one or other mammalian species, this provides a facile assay for virion detection and quantitation. These viruses, listed in Table 21.2, are now all classified in the genus *Parvovirus*, with the

murine virus, *Minute virus of mice* (MVM) (occasionally referred to as *Mice minute virus* (MMV)), as the type species.

Much of our knowledge of the whole parvovirus family, and the nature of parvoviral infections, has been derived from the study of these autonomously replicating viruses, which generally grow efficiently in cell culture and are readily susceptible to experimental manipulation. Mature virions of most species in the genus contain DNA strands that are predominantly negative-sense with respect to transcription, while one virus, LuIII, packages approximately equimolar positive and negative-sense strands. This unusual variability is less significant than at first suspected, since it is caused by differential rates of initiation from the two viral replication origins, rather than by any strand-specific packaging signal or mechanism. The linear single-stranded DNA genome, 5.0–5.3 kb in length, has hairpin structures at both the 5′ and 3′ ends. However, the 3′-terminal, or left-end, hairpin is 121 nucleotides (nt) in length, while the 5′, or right-end, structure is 248 nts long, and the left- and right-end hairpins are quite different from one another, both in sequence and predicted secondary structure. The intervening single-stranded region of the genome contains two mRNA transcription units, with promoters at map units 4 and 38 (where map units represent 1 percent segments of the genome, starting from the left-hand end) and a single functional polyadenylation site, located close to the right-hand end.

The genus *Dependovirus*

The mid-1960s also saw the discovery of a group of physically similar, but defective viruses, which were dubbed 'adeno-associated viruses' because they were common contaminants of laboratory adenovirus stocks. Populations of mature dependovirus virions contain equivalent numbers of positive and negative-sense single DNA strands, each approximately 4.7 kb in length, packaged into separate virions. The genome has three mRNA promoters, at map units 5, 19, 40, and inverted terminal repeats (ITR) of 145 nts, of which the first 125 nts form an imperfect palindrome that folds to create the hairpin-like telomeres. To date, no AAVs have been associated with disease, although they appear to be ubiquitously infectious in humans and primates, and are commonly isolated from adenovirus-infected tissues. At the time of writing, nine distinct full-length AAV genomes have been sequenced (Table 21.1), but this number is likely to expand rapidly as more potential host species are examined. The best characterized *Dependovirus* is the type species, AAV2, but AAV1, AAV2, AAV3, and AAV4 are extensively homologous at the DNA level. While AAV serotypes 2 and 3 have frequently been isolated from humans, serotypes 1 and 4 are simian isolates, and AAV6 appears to be a recombinant between AAV1 and

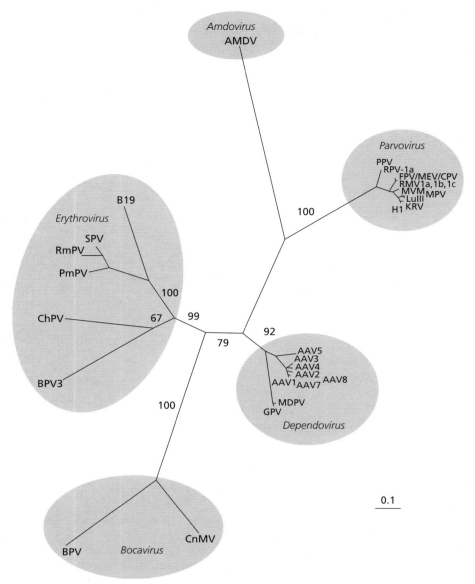

Figure 21.1 *Phylogenetic relationship between the nonstructural genes of members of the subfamily* Parvovirinae. *The tree was constructed with programs included in the Phylip package (courtesy of Z. Zadori and P. Tijssen).*

AAV2, and is now regarded as a strain of AAV1, since it is specifically neutralized by AAV1-specific antiserum. AAV5 is somewhat less related and has only been isolated once, from humans, where it appears to circulate in conjunction with a herpesvirus helper. Two further closely-related but distinct serotypes, AAV7 and AAV8, were recently isolated from monkeys, and more disparate avian (AAAV) and snake (SAAV) isolates have also recently been cloned and sequenced. For these viruses, efficient replication is dependent upon helper adenoviruses or herpes viruses, both in vitro, and by serological correlation, in vivo. However, in vitro, under certain conditions such as exposure to genotoxic agents or the synchronization of cell replication with hydroxyurea, AAV growth can be detected in the absence of helper viruses.

Originally, as the name *Dependovirus* implies, the genus comprised only helper-dependent viruses, but phylogenetic analysis, as illustrated in Figure 21.1, now places the autonomously replicating *Duck parvovirus* and *Goose parvovirus* (GPV) firmly within this genus. The *Duck parvovirus* species currently comprises two closely related strains, Muscovy duck parvovirus (MDPV) and Barbarie duck parvovirus (BDPV). These avian parvovirus species also have much larger ITRs, of between 444 and 457 nts, than those of the AAVs. They also differ from the AAVs in exhibiting marked pathogenicity in their natural hosts. The epidemics they cause in commercial flocks of domestic fowl led to their initial identification, in Hungary, where the diseases they elicit have significant agricultural impact.

Table 21.2 *Members of the subfamily* Parvovirinae

Species	Acronym
Genus *Parvovirus*	
Minute virus of mice	(MVM)
Feline panleukopenia virus strains:	
Feline parvovirus	(FPV)
Canine parvovirus	(CPV)
Mink enteritis virus	(MEV)
Raccoon parvovirus	(RPV)
Hamster parvovirus	(HaPV)
H-1 parvovirus	(H-1PV)
Kilham rat virus strains:	
Kilham Rat virus	(KRV)
H-3 virus	(H-3V)
LuIII virus	(LuIIIV)
Mouse parvovirus 1	(MPV-1)
Porcine parvovirus	(PPV)
Rat minute virus 1	(RMV-1)
Rat parvovirus 1	(RPV-1)
Genus *Dependovirus*	
Adeno-associated virus 1 strains:	
Adeno-associated virus 1	(AAV-1)
Adeno-associated virus 6	(AAV-6)
Adeno-associated virus 2	(AAV-2)
Adeno-associated virus 3	(AAV-3)
Adeno-associated virus 4	(AAV-4)
Adeno-associated virus 5	(AAV-5)
Adeno-associated virus 7	(AAV-7)
Adeno-associated virus 8	(AAV-8)
Avian adeno-associated virus	(AAAV)
Serpentine adeno-associated virus	(SAAV)
Bovine parvovirus 2	(BPV-2)
Duck parvovirus strains:	
Barbarie duck parvovirus	(BDPV)
Muscovy duck parvovirus	(MDPV)
Goose parvovirus	(GPV)
Genus *Erythrovirus*	
Human parvovirus B19 strains:	(B19V)
B19-Au, B19-Wi, B19-A6, B19-LaLi, and B19-V9	
Simian parvovirus	(SPV)
Pig-tailed macaque parvovirus	(PmPV)
Rhesus macaque parvovirus	(RmPV)
Bovine parvovirus type 3	(BPV-3)
Chipmunk parvovirus	(ChpPV)
Genus *Amdovirus*	
Aleutian mink disease virus strains:	(AMDV)
ADV-G (Gorham)	(ADV-G)
ADV-Utah	(ADV-U)
ADV-Pullman	(ADV-P)
Genus *Bocavirus*	
Bovine parvovirus 1	(BPV)
Canine minute virus	(CnMV)

The genus *Erythrovirus*

Human parvovirus B19, the only known human pathogenic member of the *Parvoviridae*, was discovered serendipitously in 1975 as an antigen present in a serum sample bearing the laboratory code 'B19,' from an apparently healthy donor whose blood was being screened for hepatitis reactivity (Cossart et al. 1975). Electron microscopy revealed that the antigen was associated with a virus particle of approximately 23 nm diameter, and the isolate was initially described as 'parvovirus-like' merely because of its size and appearance. Although around 60 percent of normal adults were subsequently found to have antibody to B19 virus (Cohen et al. 1983), suggesting common childhood exposure, the infection was initially thought to be asymptomatic. However, 5 years later the same antigen was identified in the blood of two soldiers suffering from mild fever, and in the next year a survey of sera archived at King's College Hospital, London, suggested an etiologic role for the virus in a type of transient aplastic crisis experienced by children with sickle cell anemia (Pattison et al. 1981). B19 virus has since been shown to be responsible for transient aplastic crisis in patients with a variety of hemolytic anemias. In 1983, the virus was linked sero-epidemiologically to erythema infectiosum (EI), a widespread childhood rashlike disease also referred to as fifth disease (Anderson et al. 1983), and in the next year it was shown that intrauterine transmission of B19 from an infected mother could sometimes lead to hydrops fetalis, particularly in the second trimester of pregnancy. By 1984, the B19 genome had been characterized, cloned, and sequenced (Summers et al. 1983; Cotmore and Tattersall 1984; Shade et al. 1986), allowing it to be placed firmly in the subfamily *Parvovirinae*. However, these analyses revealed that B19 was phylogenetically distant from viruses in the two existing genera (Dependovirus and Parvovirus), so that soon afterward the new genus Erythrovirus was created, with B19 virus as its type species. Populations of mature B19 virions contain equal numbers of positive and negative sense DNA strands of around 5.5 kb, with inverted terminal repeats of 383 nts in which the first 365 nts are palindromic and fold into complex hairpin telomeres. To date this virus cannot be efficiently propagated in any established cell line, so that virus stocks have predominantly been isolated from viremic human sera. Productive infection does occur in some primary erythroid progenitor cells present in primary human bone marrow explants stimulated with erythropoietin (EPO), which has allowed some aspects of the molecular biology of the virus to be studied, and recently an infectious clone of the viral genome was created in a bacterial plasmid (Zhi et al. 2004). This gives rise to limited progeny virus after transfection into the EPO-stimulated erythroid cells, allowing hope for future rapid advances in the genetic dissection of viral gene products and synthetic processes.

Additional erythroviruses have also been identified in other primate species (listed in Table 21.2), and these viruses appear to share the exquisite tissue specificity of B19 for erythroid progenitor cells and accordingly give rise to similar disease spectra (O'Sullivan et al. 1994; Green et al. 2000). Subsequently, a more distantly related virus was isolated from Manchurian chipmunks (Yoo et al. 1999), and while this could potentially provide a useful, nonprimate, model system for studying erythrovirus infection, currently little is known about this virus. Recent advances in viral diagnostics using polymerase chain reaction (PCR) technology have also allowed the identification of related viral sequences in sera from healthy bovines, suggesting that these animals likely harbor another apathogenic or weakly pathogenic erythrovirus species (Allander et al. 2001).

The *Amdovirus* and *Bocavirus* genera

Recently the taxonomy of the *Parvoviridae* has been rationalized to more closely reflect their phylogeny by clustering viruses according to the similarity of the gene sequences of their encoded proteins. As shown in Figure 21.1, this has led to the reapportioning of some disparate autonomously replicating viruses from the genus *Parvovirus* into two new genera: the *Amdoviruses*, containing a single outlying species, *Aleutian mink disease virus* (AMDV); and the *Bocaviruses*, which currently has two members, *Bovine parvovirus* (BPV) and *Canine minute virus* (CnMV). Despite their phylogenetic isolation, most features of these viruses are shared with members of the genus *Parvovirus*. Mature AMDV virions contain a negative-strand DNA of 4 748 nts, with different palindromic sequences at each terminus. Permissive replication is observed in cell culture for only one isolate, ADV-G, which replicates in Crandell feline kidney cells, although restricted replication is also observed in cells bearing Fc receptors, such as macrophages, where the virus's ability to infect may be antibody-dependent (Dworak et al. 1997). There are several highly pathogenic strains of AMDV, and evidence of infection with this virus has been detected in most mustelids, skunks, and raccoons, being of particular economic impact for the mink industry. Virion structure differs slightly from members of the genus *Parvovirus*. Apart from its divergent DNA sequence, the major distinguishing features of AMDV are its VP1 N-terminus, which is much shorter than those of other *Parvovirinae*, and does not contain the phospholipase 2A enzymatic core, and the fact that in vivo its capsid proteins are highly susceptible to proteolysis, so that intact particles contain few full-length polypeptides (Aasted et al. 1984).

The *NS1* and *VP1* genes of the *Bocaviruses*, BPV and CnMV are 34 to 41 percent similar to one another, but their genomes are very distinct from all other viruses in the *Parvovirinae* subfamily. Somewhat larger than other parvoviral genomes, at 5.5 kb, the genomes of *Bocaviruses*, like those of members of the *Parvovirus* and *Amdovirus* genera, have unique termini. BPV is also notable because it packages 90 percent negative-sense and 10 percent positive-sense DNA and because it encodes a 22.5-kDa nuclear phosphoprotein, NP-1, that is distinct from any other parvovirus-encoded polypeptide.

STRUCTURE AND ORGANIZATION OF PARVOVIRUS COMPONENTS

Structure and assembly of the capsid

Parvoviruses elaborate empty capsids and full virions that are nonenveloped, 18–26 nm in diameter, and exhibit T = 1 icosahedral symmetry. The largest capsid polypeptide is routinely designated VP1, the next VP2, and so on, and they constitute a nested set of polypeptides that share a common carboxy-terminal sequence. Sixty copies of this core sequence are assembled to form the particle, with the majority being derived from either VP2 or VP3 polypeptides, but with the VP1 molecules contributing between nine and 12 copies, which are essential for infectivity. The virion has an M_r of about 5.5–6.2×10^6, with an S_{20w} of 110–122S, and a buoyant density of 1.39–1.43 g/cm^3 in CsCl. The infectious particle comprises between 70 and 80 percent protein, with the remainder being DNA, and mature virions are stable in the presence of lipid solvents, upon exposure to pH 3–9 and, for most species, incubation at 56°C for at least 60 min. The three-dimensional structures of several parvoviruses, namely CPV, FPV, MVM, porcine parvovirus (PPV), AAV2 and galleria mellonella densovirus (*Gm*DNV), have been determined to near atomic resolution by X-ray crystallography. The common core structural feature is an eight-stranded antiparallel β-barrel, a structure shared with many viral structural polypeptides, in which the β-strands are connected by elaborate and highly variable loops that make up most of the viral surface (Chapman and Rossmann 1993). The amino-terminal peptide domains of the larger proteins are submolar, so that their disposition cannot be deduced from X-ray data. Viral genomes are thought to be packaged vectorially in a 3' to 5' direction into pre-assembled 'empty' particles, whose X-ray structure appears almost identical to that of the infectious virion. Viral preparations frequently contain large numbers of these empty capsids, which have a density of 1.32 g/cm^3 in CsCl and a sedimentation coefficient of 70S, as well as the 'full,' DNA-containing virions, subgenomic defective DNAs ($p = 1.33$–1.39 g/cm^3), and particle-assembly intermediates of various densities.

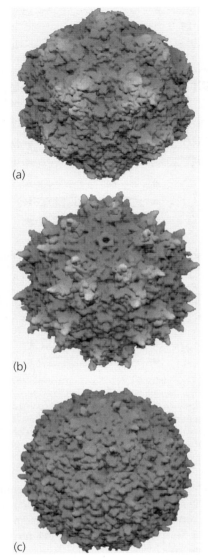

(a)

(b)

(c)

Figure 21.2 *Space-filling models of the capsid structures of* (a) *canine parvovirus (CPV),* (b) *adeno-associated virus 2 (AAV-2), and* (c) *Galleria mellonella* densovirus *(GmDNV). Each model is drawn to the same scale and is shaded according to distance from the viral center. In each case, the view is down a two-fold axis at the center of the virus, with three-fold axes left and right of center, and five-fold axes above and below (courtesy of M. Chapman).*

The parvoviral capsid shell displays icosahedral symmetry, but its surface topology can vary substantially between genera, as illustrated in Figure 21.2 for members of the *Parvovirus*, *Dependovirus*, and *Densovirus* genera. In general, there is an elevated 'spike' surrounding each of the twenty three-fold symmetry axes in the particle, deep depressions at the two-fold axes. A hollow cylindrical structure surrounds each of the 12 icosahedral five-fold axes, which contains a central pore that connects the inside of the virion with the particle exterior. In B19 virus and AMDV, for which there is cryo-electron microscopic imaging and/or low

resolution X-ray data, these pores appear occluded, and in full virions of MVM or CPV, from the genus *Parvovirus*, each pore contains a single copy of the glycine-rich, amino-terminus-proximal sequence from a VP2 molecule, positioned so that the amino-terminal 25 amino acids are externalized (Tsao et al. 1991; Agbandje-McKenna et al. 1998). On the outer virion surface these cylindrical structures are themselves encircled by deep canyonlike depressions of unknown function. Neutralizing antibody-binding sites generally map to the three-fold spike, or to its shoulders, and sequences that determine viral host range and oligosaccharide recognition and, in some viruses, receptor binding, lie in the two-fold depression and up the adjacent edge of the three-fold spike. In virions some of the single-stranded DNA also displays icosahedral symmetry, so that about a third of the genome can be visualized, by crystallography, within the particle shell. This DNA is oriented with its bases pointing outwards, forming a number of hydrogen bonds with amino acids of the inner surface of the capsid shell (Xie and Chapman 1996; Agbandje-McKenna et al. 1998).

A single molecule of the viral replication initiator protein (called Rep 68/78 in AAV, but NS1 in most other members of the family) is located on the outside of newly released virions, covalently attached to the extreme 5′ terminus of the genome by a short single-stranded DNA 'tether' sequence which projects through the capsid shell at an unknown location (Cotmore and Tattersall 1989).

Structure of the parvoviral genome

Infectious particles contain a single copy of the linear, nonpermuted, monopartite DNA genome, in which a relatively long single-stranded coding region (approximately 5 kb) is bracketed by short (121–418 nts) palindromic terminal sequences, capable of folding into hairpin duplexes. These duplex viral telomeres, which can be structurally quite complex, are critical for both DNA replication and encapsidation. While they are the essential hallmarks of the parvoviral genome, they vary markedly in size and structure between genera and even between species within the same genus.

With the exception of members of the *Densovirus* and *Pefudensovirus* genera of insect parvoviruses, the viral genome is monosense, that is, it codes for protein only on one strand. On this strand, designated the positive strand, the genes are organized into two separate expression cassettes. By convention, transcription is represented as proceeding left to right on the DNA, placing the 5′ end of the positive strand and the 3′ end of the negative at the left side of the genetic map, as illustrated in Figures 21.3–21.5. The open reading frames (ORF) within the left cassette give rise to a small number of nonstructural proteins which are involved in gene

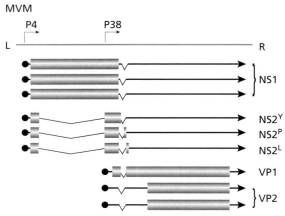

Figure 21.3 *Gene organization and transcription scheme for members of the* Parvovirus *genus, as shown for* Minute virus of mice *(MVM). Encoded polypeptides are shown as horizontal cylinders. The left ends of the mRNAs (thick lines) are the sites of the mRNA caps (filled circles), the right ends are the polyadenylation sites (arrowheads); introns are indicated by thin carets. Rightward arrows marked with a P indicate the start sites for transcripts driven by promoters whose location is shown in map units from the left-hand end.*

regulation and DNA replication, while those encompassed by the right cassette program synthesis of the overlapping set of capsid proteins.

PARVOVIRUS GENOMES

For MVM, the type species of the *Parvovirus* genus, alternate splicing events orchestrate viral gene expression, as shown in Figure 21.3 (Morgan and Ward 1986; Pintel et al. 1983). Transcripts encoding the NS proteins are all made from the promoter at 4 map units. Singly-spliced transcripts encode only the multifunctional replication initiator protein, NS1, while further P4-derived transcripts are spliced into an alternate reading frame by removal of the major intron, and encode small nonstructural polypeptides, in order of abundance, NS2P, NS2Y, and NS2L, the extreme carboxy termini of which are different due to the use of alternative 5′ and 3′ splice sites bordering the small intron (Cotmore and Tattersall 1990; Morgan and Ward 1986). One function of NS1 is to up-regulate the P4 promoter itself, and this positive feedback loop appears to be a part of the 'hard-wiring' of infection that insures rapid viral takeover of the cell. A second promoter at 38 map units is *trans*-activated by NS1, as infection progresses (Clemens and Pintel 1988), and drives synthesis of the structural gene transcripts. All P38 transcripts contain a 280 nt 5′ untranslated region located upstream of the minor splice region, and the use of the same alternative 5′ splice sites that are present in the P4 transcripts, regulates synthesis of the capsid proteins. A transcript that employs the downstream 5′ and 3′ splice sites encodes the minor VP1 polypeptide, translation of which initiates at a methionine codon between the two alternate 5′ splice sites. In

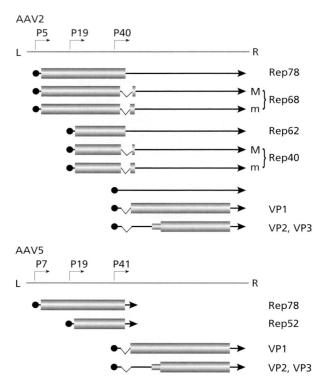

Figure 21.4 *Gene organization and transcription scheme for members of the* Dependovirus *genus, as shown for adeno-associated virus 2 (AAV-2) (top) and adeno-associated virus 5 (AAV5) (bottom), annotated as described for Figure 21.3. The narrower cylinder represents the N-terminal region of VP2, translation of which is initiated at a weak, in-frame, ACG start codon.*

the more abundant transcripts, which employ the upstream 5′ splice site, this initiation codon is spliced out, and translation of the major coat protein VP2 initiates from a start codon nearly 400 nts further downstream of the splice.

Although parvoviruses may encode several smaller accessory nonstructural proteins, such as the NS2 species

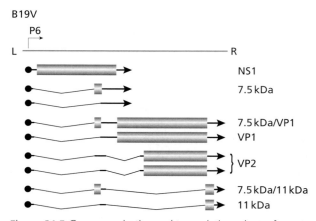

Figure 21.5 *Gene organization and transcription scheme for members of the* Erythrovirus *genus, as shown for human parvovirus B19 (B19V), annotated as described for Figures 21.3 and 21.4.*

depicted in the MVM map, only the replication initiator protein, NS1, is absolutely required for replication in all cell types (Bodendorf et al. 1999; Cater and Pintel 1992; Naeger et al. 1990). NS1, or Rep68/78 as it is known in AAV, is an ATP-dependent, site-specific DNA-binding protein with helicase activity, which initiates replication at specific viral origin sequences by introducing a site-specific single-strand nick, thus providing a base-paired 3′ nucleotide to serve as a primer for successive rounds of strand displacement DNA synthesis (Cotmore and Tattersall 1996). The *trans*-esterification reaction that creates this nick leaves NS1/Rep covalently attached to the 5′ nucleotide at the nick site, where it may serve as the 3′ to 5′ replicative helicase. All replicons that use this type of replication mechanism encode their own initiator proteins, and two protein motifs in NS1, representing a putative metal ion coordination site and the active site tyrosine of the nickase, can be traced from the *Parvoviridae* to their prokaryotic 'cousins,' the *Microviridae* (Koonin and Ilyina 1993). MVM NS1 is an 83-kDa nuclear phosphoprotein which self-associates in the presence of ATP to form an oligomeric complex that is capable of binding to a consensus DNA motif found both in the viral origins and at many other locations throughout the genome (Cotmore et al. 1995; Christensen et al. 1995). However, it is only able to nick the DNA in the context of the viral origins, where it encounters the appropriate consensus nick sequence and specific host-derived accessory proteins (Christensen et al. 1997; Cotmore et al. 2000).

Parvoviral replication initiators have evolved into highly pleiotropic proteins, playing multiple roles in the viral life cycle. In addition to their site-specific nicking function, they act as potent transactivators of viral gene transcription, binding to their recognition sequences in viral promoters and activating transcription through acidic carboxy-terminal domains (Legendre and Rommelaere 1994). In MVM, NS1-binding sites are reiterated so frequently that any sequence of 100 base pairs or more contains a site, and some carry multiple tandem and inverted reiterations (Cotmore et al. 1995). This suggests that NS1 likely plays a significant role in viral chromatin structure and progeny strand packaging.

DEPENDOVIRUS GENOMES

Dependoviruses generally have three transcriptional promoters. These are located at 5, 19, and 40 map units along the genome of the type species, AAV2, and transcribe viral mRNAs, as shown in Figure 21.4, in a temporally regulated fashion throughout infection (Mouw and Pintel 2000; Marcus et al. 1981). P5 transcripts are the first to be expressed, followed by those from P19 and P40, whose protein products are required later in the viral life cycle. P5 transcripts encode the replication initiator proteins Rep78 and Rep68, which appear to serve almost identical functions although they

differ slightly in sequence due to splicing of the centrally positioned intron. Spliced messages link the body of *Rep* to a small carboxy terminal segment downstream of the major 3′ splice site, to make the smaller Rep68 protein. In unspliced messages, the sequence encoding the Rep protein body continues on through most of the intron, producing the larger Rep78 protein. Likewise, P19 transcripts encode two Rep forms, Rep52 and Rep48, which differ similarly at their carboxy termini. P40 transcripts are also spliced to alternative 3′ splice sites, and since the downstream acceptor is more efficient than the upstream one, major and minor spliced species are again generated. As an interesting counterpoint to the situation described above for the parvoviruses, in AAV2 the minor VP1 polypeptide initiates from a start codon located between the two 3′ splice sites, rather than between the two 5′ sites, as in MVM. The other AAV2 capsid proteins are then translated from the major, differentially spliced, transcript that lacks the initiation codon used for VP1. The major, and smallest, capsid protein, VP3, initiates from the first AUG codon in this transcript, while the less abundant VP2 species initiates from an upstream in-frame ACG codon. As a result, capsid proteins, VP1, 2, and 3, accumulate in an approximately 1:1:10 ratio, each having identical carboxy-terminal sequences but with VP1 being 137 residues longer than VP2, which is in turn 65 residues longer than VP3. While all AAV2 transcripts coterminate at the right end of the genome, AAV5 has recently been shown to exhibit an additional level of transcriptional control, as shown in the lower panel of Figure 21.4. Here most of the transcripts encoding nonstructural genes, driven in this case by promoters at 7 and 19 map units, terminate at a central polyadenylation site, located just downstream of the P41 promoter. Cleavage and polyadenylation at this internal site precludes alternative splicing in the Rep transcripts, so that only a single form of the P5 and p19 products are generated (Qiu et al. 2004).

ERYTHROVIRUS GENOMES

The human erythrovirus B19 employs a genetic strategy distinct from those of the other genera, as shown in Figure 21.5, in that it contains only one promoter, at 6 map units (Ozawa et al. 1987). An unspliced transcript terminating at a central polyadenylation site encodes NS1, while a set of full length transcripts that are spliced in the NS region, encode VP1 and VP2. Two small ORFs can also be accessed by alternatively spliced mRNAs, giving rise to 7.5- and 11-kDa nonstructural proteins. The 11-kDa protein contains three proline-rich regions that conform to consensus SH3 (Src homology 3) ligand sequences (Fan et al. 2001); however, functions for these two protein species remain to be defined. B19 uses two alternative polyadenylation sites, situated similarly to those present in AAV5, as discussed above.

Alternative use of poly(A) sites appears to be controlled by the host cell in a way that suggests that it may act as a major factor in viral tropism (Liu et al. 1992). In a productive infection of erythroid precursors, transcripts terminating at both sites are observed, and give rise to the full array of viral gene products. However, in transfected, nonpermissive cells the central polyadenylation site predominates, and viral gene expression may be largely confined to the synthesis of NS1. This situation is predicted to lead to cytopathogenesis due to the toxic nature of NS1 (Moffatt et al. 1998; Ozawa et al. 1988; Poole et al. 2004), without the production of progeny virus, and may explain in vivo observations of tissue destruction in the absence of B19 growth.

MECHANISMS OF INFECTION

Early events

Steps involved in delivering the viral genome to the host nucleus are illustrated in Figure 21.6, specifically for members of the genus *Parvovirus* such as MVM. In general, viruses need to achieve a sequence of interactions with the host cell to bring about infection, starting with adsorption to one or more cell surface receptors, internalization (generally in some sort of vesicle), transfer across the cell's delimiting lipid bilayer into the cytoplasm, uncoating leading to exposure of the viral genome, and delivery to the appropriate cellular replication compartment. This pathway is so complex

and multifaceted that, while entry is not the only determinant of tropism, it often plays a major role in cell specificity.

Rather than using a single molecule as a cell surface receptor, many viruses employ two more-or-less separate classes of molecules: an 'attachment' receptor, or co-receptor, which effectively accumulates virus in the vicinity of the cell surface; and an infectious-entry receptor that mediates entry into the cytoplasm. While some parvoviruses are known to employ this strategy, the extent to which they rely on multiple surface interactions appears to vary from species to species, and within a species from host cell to host cell, so that few general rules are apparent. MVM binds to sialoglycoproteins present at about 5×10^5 copies per cell on murine fibroblasts, and both binding and infection are neuraminidase-sensitive, indicating a critical role for specific oligosaccharide side chains in these steps. However, at present it is not clear if these comprise one specific cell surface molecule that mediates MVM entry, in addition to others that merely effect attachment, or if all 5×10^5 receptors are equipotent. In contrast, FPV and CPV virions can bind to neuraminidase-sensitive N-glycolyl neuramininic acid side chains on some host-cell types, which presumably only function as attachment receptors, since infectious entry is insensitive to neuraminidase and is now known to be mediated by binding to host species-specific protein domains on cell surface transferrin receptor (TfR) molecules (Parker and Parrish 2000). AAVs also use a variety of surface receptors, many of which are widely distributed, but nevertheless fine

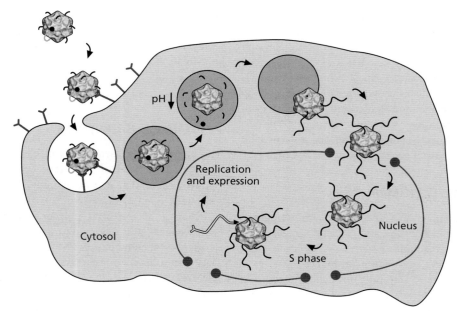

Figure 21.6 *Entry pathway for a generic parvovirus, as described in the text predominantly for MVM. Short black lines extruding from the virion represent VP2 N-termini, and the single line with a terminal ball represents the tether sequence and its covalently attached NS1 molecule. Longer, gray lines represent the VP1-specific N-terminal extruded upon entry into the cytosol, and the thin double line attached to nuclear virions represents the emerging genome in the process of being converted into double-stranded DNA. See text for additional details.*

details of these interactions have a major impact on effective cell tropism. AAV2 and AAV3 bind the ubiquitous glycosaminoglycan, heparan sulfate, albeit with slightly different specificities (Summerford and Samulski 1998). This may not be all that is required to mediate entry, since AAV2 has also been shown to interact specifically with either α_v, β_5 integrin or basic fibroblast growth factor receptor 1 in ways that ultimately enhance viral gene transduction and hence may function by promoting entry (Summerford et al. 1999; Qing et al. 1999). AAV4 and AAV5 do not bind heparan sulfate, but instead use cell surface carbohydrates carrying the α 2–3 form of neuraminic acid for cell attachment, AAV4 preferentially binding O-linked carbohydrates while AAV5 prefers N-linked forms (Kaludov et al. 2001). AAV5 then appears to recruit platelet derived growth factor (PDGF) receptors as its primary receptor (Di Pasquale et al. 2003). This is an unexpected finding, since AAVs generally maintain a low profile in their host, and might be expected to enter cells by stealth, whereas PDGF receptors normally respond to ligand-induced cross-linking by autophosphorylating their cytoplasmic tyrosine kinase domains, leading directly to activation of many growth factor response pathways in the host cell. It will be interesting to see whether AAV5 binding does indeed induce receptor-mediated activation, and if so, whether such changes are important in infectious entry by this virus. Finally, the human parvovirus B19 binds to cells of the erythroid lineage via the erythrocyte glycolipid globoside P antigen (Brown et al. 1993). However, a number of cell types that express globoside are not susceptible to infection, suggesting that there could be additional infectious entry receptor(s) for B19 virus.

Following receptor binding, all parvoviruses are rapidly internalized from the cell surface by receptor-mediated endocytosis, predominantly via clathrin-coated pits, and enter an endosome compartment that is sensitive to lysosomotropic agents such as bafilomycin, indicating that low endosomal pH is somehow essential for infection. While members of the genus *Parvovirus* remain sensitive to bafilomycin for up to 6 h after internalization, AAV2 appears to transit into a pH-independent compartment much faster, suggesting that aspects of their penetration mechanisms may be different. Exposure to low pH might be required during entry because it induces essential conformational changes in the virion, because it insures normal endosomal trafficking, or because the viruses specifically need to transit a hydrolase-rich late endosomal/lysosomal compartment to ensure successful entry. Which of these possibilities pertains is currently unclear and is likely to vary between viral species. Indeed, for MVM all three of these processes may be important. Thus, as illustrated in Figure 21.6, phosphoserinerich amino-terminal peptides from MVM VP2 molecules are displayed at the surface of mature virions, and in some cell types these peptides are known to

mediate nuclear export (Maroto et al. 2004), so that removal of all such signals during entry may be essential for the success of subsequent nuclear translocation. This suggests that infectious entry may occur via a late endosomal or lysosomal route, since these are rich in proteases and nucleases, and such exposure would also explain why genomes lose their covalently-linked 5′ NS1 molecules, and the nucleotide 'tether' sequence, prior to arrival in the nucleus (Cotmore and Tattersall 1989).

MVM particles also appear to be stabilized by an acid environment. Amino-terminal sequences of VP1 are known to be essential for entry, but this region is highly protease-sensitive and is sequestered within the virion prior to its entry into the cell. However, the VP1-specific region can become accessible at the particle surface following conformational transitions, inducible in vitro by heating, which are potentiated by the removal of VP2 amino termini, but stabilized by exposure to pH 6.5 or below. Such transitions externalize the VP1 N-terminus and the viral DNA, while leaving the DNA still firmly attached to the otherwise intact particle via its left-end hairpin (Cotmore et al. 1999). Enhanced virion stability during exposure to low pH could thus serve to protect essential hydrolase-sensitive viral structures within an obligate late endosomal/lysosomal entry compartment.

Vesicle trafficking is a complex process that leads to particle delivery to many different cell locations, and trafficking studies typically compound this problem by the use of high multiplicities of input virus needed for signal detection. For example, AAV5 has been reported to enter early endosomelike structures and the cisternae of the trans-Golgi network, but also to accumulate in lysosomes, particularly when applied at high multiplicities (Bantel-Schaal et al. 2002). The high particle-to-infectivity ratios of many viruses also add to this problem, since most of the internalized viruses may enter dead-end circuits that never provide access to the nucleus. This conundrum is well illustrated by recent studies with CPV, which is internalized via an interaction with surface TfRs and presumably remains physically associated with its receptor for at least 4 h, since infectious entry can be blocked throughout that period by intracytoplasmic injection of antibodies directed against the cytoplasmic tails of the receptor (Parker and Parrish 2000). The normal cellular uptake and complex recycling patterns of TfRs have been well studied, and are known to depend upon the presence of a YTRF (Tyr–Thr–Arg–Phe) motif in its cytoplasmic tail. However, when these sequences were deleted or mutated, or polar residues introduced into the TfR transmembrane domain, which vastly increased receptor degradation, virus infection remained efficient (Hueffer et al. 2004). This suggests that infectious entry may involve a minority of TfRs that take, or are directed by the virus to take, an atypical pathway.

Exactly where, or how, these viruses penetrate the endosomal bilayer remains open to conjecture, but CPV infectivity can be blocked by the intracytoplasmic injection of various antibodies directed against structural determinants in the capsid, indicating that there must be an essential, capsid-associated, cytoplasmic phase (Vihinen-Ranta et al. 2000). VP1 amino-termini carry a PLA2 active site, which is highly conserved among the *Parvoviridae* and appears to be essential for infectivity at some stage following endosomal accumulation, although its role and site-of-action remain to be completely elucidated (Zadori et al. 2001). However, anti-VP1 specific antibodies injected into the cytoplasm have been shown to block CPV infectivity, suggesting that structural transitions leading to exposure of this peptide must accompany entry into the cytoplasmic compartment in vivo, perhaps during transit through the bilayer, as suggested in Figure 21.6.

The VP1-specific N-terminal region also contains karyopherin-alpha binding sequences, which probably serve to traffic particles to the nuclear pore (Lombardo et al. 2002). Parvoviral particles are very stable and are small enough to be transported through the nuclear pore, so that during infectious entry, viral DNA may remain encapsidated until it is inside the nucleus. Docking of intact particles at the nuclear pore, and/or their translocation into the nucleus has yet to be demonstrated for members of the *Parvovirinae* during natural infection. However, this is likely since recombinant AAV particles have been repeatedly observed in the nucleus, and CPV virions microinjected into the cytoplasm accumulated in the nucleus over a period of 2 h or more where they could be detected with antibodies specific for intact particles (Vihinen-Ranta et al. 2000). Surprisingly, the protracted accumulation of intact recombinant AAV2 virions in the nuclei of liver cells has recently been associated with poor expression of virally-coded transgenes, whereas exactly similar genomes pseudotyped into AAV6 or AAV8 coats were uncoated more rapidly and transcribed more efficiently. This has led to the hypothesis that, for optimal expression, AAV virions must be trafficked to a specific site in the nucleus, where uncoating is efficiently induced by interaction with unidentified nuclear factors, and that AAV2 particles fail to achieve this intranuclear translocation (Thomas et al. 2004).

Parvoviruses are unable to induce resting cells to enter S phase, and it is not until infected cells enter S phase of their own volition that viral transcription normally initiates. Since the viral promoters are packaged as single-stranded DNA, acquisition of a complementary strand necessarily precedes viral gene expression, and its synthesis likely represents the first S phase dependent step in the viral life cycle. Initial transcription of MVM also depends upon the availability of the host transcription factor E2F to activate its P4 promoter, so that viral transcription is optimized for expression during S phase (Deleu et al. 1999). As early MVM gene products accumulate, host-cell DNA synthesis is terminated and progression through the cell cycle is suspended, but the molecular mechanisms underlying these interactions have yet to be elucidated. In contrast to the helper independent parvoviruses, productive AAV infection relies upon the ability of its helper virus to drive resting cells into S phase, and even in the absence of cellular replication some viral transcription may occur at high input multiplicities, from duplex episomes generated by the annealing of opposite sense input strands (Nakai et al. 2000), as will be discussed later.

DNA replication

Parvoviral DNA is replicated through a series of duplex, concatemeric intermediates by a strand displacement mechanism called rolling hairpin replication (RHR), depicted in Figure 21.7 (Cotmore and Tattersall 1996; Tattersall and Ward 1976). The replication fork is aphidicolin-sensitive, requires PCNA, is unidirectional and results in the synthesis of a single, continuous DNA strand, indicating that synthesis is probably mediated predominantly by DNA polymerase δ and its accessory proteins (Ni et al. 1998; Christensen and Tattersall 2002). Short imperfect palindromic sequences at each end of the genome repeatedly fold and unfold during this process, first creating duplex hairpin telomeres in which the 3′ nt of each strand is paired to an internal base to create a DNA primer, and then unfolding to allow the hairpin to be copied. Together with a few flanking nucleotides, these palindromes contain all of the *cis*-acting information needed for both viral replication and packaging. During RHR they effectively serve as 'toggle-switches,' reversing the direction of synthesis at each end of the linear genome, thus adapting the more ancient rolling-circle replication strategy (Ilyina and Koonin 1992) for the amplification of a linear chromosome.

Since MVM packages negative-sense strands predominantly, and hence the 3′ end of the DNA is always at left end of the incoming genome, it is easier to describe the rolling hairpin process for this virus, but exactly parallel steps ensue for incoming positive strands of all genera, except that replication would initiate at the right-end of such genomes. Thus, for MVM in step (i) of Figure 21.7, the base-paired 3′ nucleotide of the left-end hairpin is used by a host polymerase to prime conversion of virion DNA to the first duplex intermediate. This generates a monomer length duplex molecule in which the two strands are covalently continuous at the viral left-end telomere. Synthesis of this intermediate precedes viral gene expression. The cellular replication fork assembled on such viral templates appears to be unable to displace and copy the right-end hairpin sequence, so the 3′ end of the new DNA strand is ligated to the 5′ end of the hairpin by a host ligase, creating a covalently continuous duplex molecule (Cotmore and Tattersall 1996) (step ii). Replication

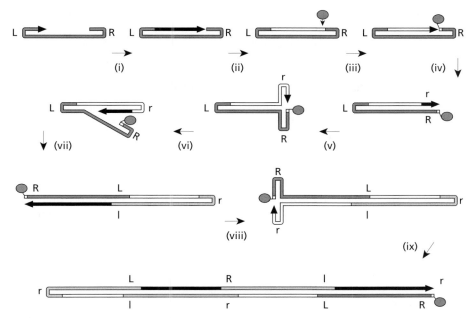

Figure 21.7 *Parvoviral 'rolling hairpin' DNA replication scheme. The viral genome is represented by continuous line, shaded dark gray for the original genome, light gray for progeny genomes, and black for newly synthesized DNA, the 3' end of which is indicated by the arrowhead. The gray sphere represents an NS1 molecule. The letters L and R represent left-end and right-end palindromic sequences, respectively. Upper and lower case represent 'flip' and 'flop' versions of these sequences, respectively, which are inverted complements of one another. See text for further explanation.*

beyond this point requires expression of the viral initiator protein, NS1 in MVM or Rep68/78 in AAV, which nicks the ligated strand, as illustrated in Figure 21.7, step (iii), in a reaction that is assisted by a host DNA-bending protein from the HMG1 family. This requirement for HMG1 appears to vary somewhat between genera, being essential for the MVM right-end telomere, but merely enhancing initiation at the AAV2 hairpins (Costello et al. 1997; Cotmore and Tattersall 1998). Nicking is achieved by a transesterification reaction, which liberates a base-paired 3' nt that supports the assembly of a new replication fork, while leaving NS1 covalently attached to the 5' end of the DNA at the nick, where it is believed to function as the 3' to 5' replicative helicase of the subsequent replication fork (Christensen and Tattersall 2002; Smith and Kotin 1998; Wu et al. 1999; Zhou et al. 1999). NS1 also recruits the cellular RPA (replication protein A) complex, which binds and stabilizes single-stranded DNA, while AAV appears to favor adenovirus single-stranded binding protein, although in either case the availability of such factors appears rate-limiting for the progress of this strand displacement mechanism (Ward et al. 1998; Christensen and Tattersall 2002).

A complex sequence of melting and reannealing reactions then ensues, step (iv–v) Figure 21.7, in which the replication fork, assisted by the initiator protein, first unfolds and copies the hairpin, in a process called 'hairpin transfer,' thus replacing the original sequence of the terminus with its inverted complement (step iv).

Since the terminal sequences are imperfect palindromes, and this inversion occurs with every round of replication, progeny genomes comprise equal numbers of each terminal orientation, dubbed 'flip' and 'flop.' In MVM the entire sequence of reactions from the introduction of the NS1-mediated nick to the generation of a duplex extended-form telomere is referred to as 'hairpin resolution,' while in AAV the equivalent sequence of events is called 'terminal resolution' (Snyder et al. 1990; Cotmore and Tattersall 1996). A general rule seems to be that viruses with identical termini, like the AAVs and B19, replicate both termini by hairpin resolution, and thus have flip and flop forms of each telomere, while viruses with disparate termini, like MVM, replicate the right-end by hairpin resolution and the left by an asymmetric mechanism, called junction resolution, which conserves a single sequence orientation and uses different structural arrangements and cofactors to activate the NS1 nickase, as discussed below.

The extended-form duplex termini generated in step (iv), Figure 21.7, are then melted out and the strands reformed into hairpinned 'rabbit ear' structures, in a process facilitated by the direct binding of NS1 to symmetrical copies of its duplex recognition sequence surrounding the axis of the extended palindrome (Willwand et al. 2002; Ward and Berns 1995) (step v). This allows the 3' nucleotide of the newly synthesized DNA strand to pair with an internal base, thus priming synthesis of additional linear sequences (step vi). The result of rolling hairpin synthesis is the accumulation of palindromic duplex dimeric (step vii) and tetrameric (step ix) concatemers, in which alternating unit length genomes are fused in left-end–left-end and right-end–right-end orientations. Although such concatemers are generated during AAV replication, they tend to be heterogeneous because both ends of the genome can be excised by equivalent reactions, whereas in MMV, left-end–left-end dimer duplexes accumulate, awaiting resolution by the more complex, and apparently slower, junction resolution process.

During junction resolution, left-end sequences are replicated and separated asymmetrically, so that new termini are created in a single sequence orientation, designated 'flip.' This effectively allows the two arms of the hairpin to be dedicated to different roles in the viral life cycle, the outboard arm supporting resolution, while the inboard arm potentially provides upstream elements for the nearby transcriptional P4 promoter. The 121 base left-end telomere of MVM has an important unpaired 'bubble' element in the hairpin stem, where a trinucleotide on the inboard arm opposes a mismatched dinucleotide. During rolling hairpin synthesis this hairpin is unfolded and copied to form the left-end–left-end junction, which links monomer genomes in the dimer intermediate (Figure 21.7, step vii), and within which these asymmetric bubble nucleotides segregate to opposite sides of the junction. It is this duplex junction structure, rather than a single hairpinned terminus, which contains the replication origin required for copying and separating MVM left-end sequences. The junction contains one candidate nick site for NS1 on each arm of the palindrome, located on opposite strands, but only the origin on the arm carrying the 'bubble' dinucleotide has the precise spatial organization required for nicking to occur. This is because, at the left-end origin, activation requires a cellular protein, called parvoviral initiation factor (PIF), to bind the viral DNA in exact juxtaposition to NS1 (Christensen et al. 1999). This interaction occurs only across the dinucleotide, and not the trinucleotide, bubble spacer element. PIF effectively stabilizes the binding of NS1 to its recognition element in the active origin, allowing it to use its 3′ to 5′ helicase activity to melt the duplex DNA at the adjacent nick site (Christensen et al. 2001). This is an essential prerequisite for nicking because, like other rolling-circle initiator proteins, NS1 is only able to nick its cognate site if this is presented as single-stranded DNA. The formation of individual nicking complexes and the biochemistry of these reactions have studied extensively, but are largely outside the scope of this article, and the interested reader is referred to the more detailed discussions in the references cited above.

Following introduction of a single nick in the active arm of the junction, the 3′ to 5′ helicase activity of NS1 destabilizes the palindrome, frequently promoting its rearrangement into a cruciform intermediate that is essential for junction resolution. Replication forks that assemble after the junction reconfigures into this cruciform synthesize DNA in the flip orientation, creating a heterocruciform structure, which then undergoes a form of hairpin transfer. Ultimate resolution of the resulting, partially single-stranded, product requires the introduction of an NS1-mediated nick in the 'inactive' arm of the junction introduced as this is transiently presented in single-stranded form to the nickase (Cotmore and Tattersall 2003). Operationally, whether or not this final single-strand nick occurs is thought to depend upon the efficiency of hairpin resolution at the right end of the genome, since forks returning from the right end could recreate the partially resolved duplex junction before the single strand nick occurs. Thus the speed of initiation at the right-end of the genome influences the products generated at the left-end of the genome, a theme which becomes important when considering which strands are ultimately packaged, as discussed below. Although junction resolution appears complex, it uses a series of reactions that are characteristic of parvoviral replicons and their replicator proteins, and may represent a way of resolving junctions so that each arm could be dedicated to a different activity. That this might indeed be the case is suggested by studies with MVM genomes that have been mutated to present an active origin on both arms of the left telomere. Such mutations are invariably lethal, but allow the selection of viable variants in which the origin associated with the inboard arm has been inactivated by a variety of secondary mutations, suggesting that restricting cleavage at the inboard site is essential (Burnett and Tattersall 2003).

Capsid assembly and packaging

Late in infection, viral capsid gene expression predominates because NS1/Rep is able to strongly *trans*-activate the P38 promoter (Rhode 1985; Labow et al. 1986). As illustrated for MVM in Figure 21.8, VP1 and VP2 are synthesized in approximately the ratio required for capsid assembly. Partially assembled capsid subunits, probably in the form of trimers, exhibit a structure-dependent nuclear localization signal on a VP-common β-strand that will eventually form part of the internal surface of the capsid. This directs translocation of the intermediates into the nucleus, where they are assembled into empty capsids, which are believed to be the precursors of full virions. For AAV2 assembly appears to occur within the nucleoli, which also become highly disorganized in many other parvovirus infections (Singer and Rhode 1978; Wistuba et al. 1997). In MVM infection of murine cells some aspect of the continued synthesis and assembly of the capsid precursors requires the small nonstructural polypeptide NS2 (Cotmore et al.

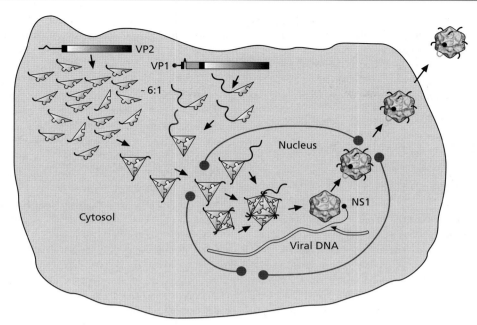

Figure 21.8 *Assembly and packaging pathway for a generic parvovirus, as described in the text predominantly for MVM. Lines and blocks at top left indicate the P38-driven transcripts and their encoded protein sequences. The core VP sequence that is the building block for the particle is shown as a gray gradient-filled box in the coding diagram, and a triangular icon as its translated form. Shading of VP components and identity of other symbols are described in the legend to Figure 21.6. See text for additional details.*

1997). Significantly, when empty capsids are assembled, the VP1 and VP2 N-termini are internalized, so that both the VP1-specific and VP-common nuclear localization signals are hidden within the particle, while the VP2 N-termini, which contain a nuclear export signal discussed later, are also effectively concealed from the export machinery. Thus empty capsids appear to be entirely neutral with regard to intercompartmental trafficking.

As assembled capsids accumulate, progeny single-stranded DNA synthesis begins to predominate over duplex DNA amplification. How this switch is controlled is unknown, but progeny synthesis is entirely dependent upon the availability of preformed capsids, and most of the single-stranded monomeric DNA in the cell appears to be encapsidated. Exactly how DNA strands are selected for packaging remains uncertain, but the minimal requirement appears to be the presence of an active nick site (Nony et al. 2003; Musatov et al. 2002; Huser et al. 2003). Since the viral initiator proteins, NS1 and Rep68/78, become covalently attached to the DNA at such sites, and because these proteins bind efficiently to intact capsids (Dubielzig et al. 1999), they may well mediate the initial interactions. Selection of positive or negative sense DNA is not directed by strand-specific packaging signals, but rather reflects the relative efficiencies of the viral replication origins associated with the two genomic termini (Chen et al. 1989; Cotmore and Tattersall 2005). However, since packaging requires ongoing viral DNA synthesis, it is not simply a process of melting out and sequestering preformed DNA strands

(Myers and Carter 1980; Zhou and Muzyczka 1998). Strands are packaged vectorially, in a 3′ to 5′ direction, driven in AAV2 by the helicase activity of the small Rep proteins, Rep40 and Rep52 (King et al. 2001). As DNA is translocated into the MVM particle, approximately 25 amino acids of a VP2 N-terminus becomes externalized through the pore in each of the 12 cylindrical turrets protruding from the capsid surface at the fivefold symmetry axes (Agbandje-McKenna et al. 1998; Xie et al. 2002; Cotmore et al. 1999). This region of the VP2 polypeptide carries a series of phosphorylated serine residues and can be shown to function as a nuclear export signal, causing full virions to be translocated into the cytoplasm, and hence out of the cell via an as yet unknown route, prior to lysis (Maroto et al. 2000; Maroto et al. 2004). Thus, the act of packaging converts a trafficking-neutral capsid to a nuclear export competent virion.

NS2 is involved in this early exit pathway, even in cells where it is not required for capsid assembly, and part of this function appears to be mediated via a binding motif for the nuclear export protein, Crm1, located in its central exon (Ohshima et al. 1999; Miller and Pintel 2002; Bodendorf et al. 1999). During normal infection, NS2 is predominantly cytoplasmic, but mutations in the Crm1 binding site reveal it to be a constitutively nuclear protein, which is normally transported out of the nucleus via a Crm1-dependent pathway. Early virion release is impaired in such mutants, but it is not yet clear whether Crm1-complexed NS2 simply acts by inducing essential changes in the cellular environment, or whether it acts through a direct interaction with the particle. Ultimately infections are generally lytic, and cells remain actively synthesizing viral DNA until necrotic or apoptotic lysis occurs at about 16–20 h after entry into S phase (Ran et al. 1999; Rayet et al. 1998), which results in significant release of residual progeny virions.

HOST RANGE

Tissue and host species specificity

Lytic growth is modulated by developmentally regulated factors operating in the host at the cellular level. Significant differences in target tissue specificity clearly exist between different parvovirus species. These can often be explained by the use of a different cell surface receptor repertoire by each virus serotype, as discussed elsewhere in this chapter, although postentry blocks to viral growth have also been identified in some virus–host combinations. However, differences in pathogenic potential exist not only between virus serotypes, but between virus strains of the same serotype, as seen within the MVM, PPV, FPV, and AMDV species. The prototype strain of MVM, MVMp, productively infects murine fibroblasts, but cannot establish infection efficiently in T lymphocytes. The isolation of a second strain of minute virus of mice, MVMi, as an immunosuppressive agent from a murine lymphoma (Bonnard et al. 1976), indicated that a mutable genetic component of the virus played a role in determining the type of differentiated cell the virus can lytically infect. For MVM, this discrimination is mediated by a region of the viral capsid called the allotropic determinant, which acts in *cis* with the genome it encapsidates (Gardiner and Tattersall 1988a,b). The determinant involves a small group of amino acids that map near the surface of the virion, grouped along the edge of the spike at the threefold symmetry axis and down into the depression at the two-fold axis (Agbandje-McKenna et al. 1998). Here a coordinated change in just two amino acid residues in the capsid of the lymphotropic murine virus MVMi allows it to extend, or even switch, its host range, gaining the ability to replicate productively in murine fibroblasts (Ball-Goodrich and Tattersall 1992).

Genetically and pathogenically distinct strains of PPV also exhibit allotropic specificity determined in a similar way, which controls their ability to replicate in particular porcine cell lines in vitro (Bergeron et al. 1996), and AMDV replication has been similarly linked to a cluster of capsid residues (Fox et al. 1999). Studies on MVM, PPV, and AMDV strains have shown that infection of the 'wrong' host cell is profoundly restricted at an, as yet, unidentified step, which occurs after virus internalization from the cell surface, but before the onset of transcription and DNA amplification. Significantly, while

each MVM strain is reciprocally restricted in each other's host cell, both strains replicate efficiently in somatic cell hybrids between the two host-cell types, implying that restricted infections fail to establish because of the absence of a differentiated host factor in the restrictive host that is usually exploited by the restricted strain in its permissive cell type. However, the molecular identities of the host factors that mediate these strain-specific tropisms remain elusive, and may well vary between virus–host combinations.

While control of species host range among viruses from the FPV/CPV group is determined by a similar cluster of surface amino acid changes in the capsid (Chang et al. 1992; Parrish 1991; Truyen and Parrish 1992), these changes are now known to act via species-specific interactions with the viral cell surface receptor, recently shown to be the TfR (transferrin receptor). Thus, while all of the viruses can bind to feline and human TfR, and use these receptors to enter and infect cells, canine cell infection is a specific property of CPV and depends on the ability of this virus to bind the canine TfR (Govindasamy et al. 2003; Parker et al. 2001; Hueffer et al. 2003). The specific contact established between CPV or FPV capsids and the TfR also appears to be important, since modifications introduced into either the virus or receptor can allow cell surface binding to occur without leading to infection (Hueffer et al. 2004). For these viruses, the critical step likely involves receptor-mediated internalization of the virus in a way which selectively leads to its successful translocation across the endosomal bilayer, but how or where this operates remains uncertain.

The situation for MVM appears to be substantially different. Both fibrotropic and lymphotropic strains of MVM bind to sialoglycoproteins present at about 5×10^5 copies per cell on murine fibroblasts, and compete for binding to these receptors (Spalholz and Tattersall 1983). While all of these receptors could be equipotent, it is still possible that different minor classes of specific cell surface molecules mediate cytoplasmic delivery of MVMi and MVMp, while the more abundant species merely effect surface attachment. Thus a cytoplasmic delivery mechanism, like that conjectured for CPV, remains a possibility for MVM whereby both virus strains are internalized into endosomes on a variety of receptors, but can only penetrate the bilayer successfully from a particular receptor species. Precedent for this type of restriction has been documented for the 'small plaque' mutants of polyomavirus (Bauer et al. 1999), which vary from wildtype in binding avidly to entry-incompetent receptors. However, restriction to the extent seen for MVM, which would require most of the virus to be bound on incompetent receptors, has yet to be described. Alternatively, capsid-mediated MVM host range restriction could operate at a later stage in the life cycle, and involve a selective interaction between the virion and cell type-specific host molecules that mediate nuclear entry, viral uncoating, or the assembly of the initial viral transcription templates. In this respect, it is interesting to note that recent studies suggest that the uncoating of recombinant AAV particles shows virus species-specificity in rat liver cells, with AAV6 and AAV8 virions being uncoated much more efficiently than their AAV2 counterparts, possibly because the latter are not delivered to nuclear loci containing host factors that mediate this transition (Thomas et al. 2004).

Tissue specificity can also be mediated in MVM after the onset of infection, by sequences that map to a region in the nonstructural gene containing the splice control regions for the major intron (Rubio et al. 2001; Gardiner and Tattersall 1988b; Colomar et al. 1998). Splicing efficiency at this intron, which can be modulated by single nucleotide mutations in the putative splice branch point region, determines the relative levels of NS1 and NS2 transcripts generated during infection, with growth in fibroblasts apparently requiring the more efficient NS2 splice configuration, while the opposite is true for growth in lymphocytes. However, the level at which this tropism operates remains to be determined. The absolute ability to express NS2 has also been identified as a host range determinant, since MVMp NS2-null mutants, which cannot express any of this protein, are completely defective for growth in murine fibroblasts, although they are able to replicate in a number of cell types, notably transformed human fibroblasts (Naeger et al. 1990). At present it is not clear whether this phenomenon represents a true host species restriction or if transformation of a normally nonpermissive host cell can sometimes complement for the lack of NS2, thus rendering the cell permissive for NS2-null virus replication.

Oncotropism

The affinity of parvoviruses for dividing cells is also reflected in their ability to interfere with, and suppress, another type of rapid cellular proliferation in their hosts, namely, neoplastic disease. Infection with autonomous parvoviruses has been shown to suppress tumor formation by a large number of viruses and carcinogens. For example, KRV suppresses leukemia induction in rats by Moloney murine leukemia virus (MoMLV) (Bergs 1969), and H1 infection of hamsters suppresses tumor formation by either adenovirus or dimethylbenzanthracene (Toolan and Ledinko 1968; Toolan et al. 1982). Similarly, AAV2 has been shown to inhibit the oncogenicity of tumor viruses and transformed cells (de la Maza and Carter 1981; Katz and Carter 1986), although in this case the effects may predominantly reflect the complex interactions between AAVs and their helper viruses.

Despite their apparent lack of natural infectivity for humans, rodent parvoviruses can grow in many human cell lines in vitro, and this is especially true if the cells are transformed by agents such as gamma-rays, nitro-

quinolines, or SV40 (Cornelis et al. 1988). Extensive studies over the past two decades, focusing on MVM and H1, have defined in vitro analogues of this oncotropism, and have established that it is a cell-intrinsic, rather than an immune-mediated phenomenon. Sensitization to parvovirus-mediated cell killing has been demonstrated following transformation of rodent and human fibroblasts, human keratinocytes and human mammary epithelium. Transforming agents used have varied from activated oncogenes such as h-*ras* and v-*src*, to c-*myc* and papovaviral T antigens (Rommelaere and Cornelis 1991). The biochemical basis for such sensitization is complex, and can take several forms. In some cells it manifests as a dramatic, transformation-associated increase in viral DNA amplification, while in others it can present as transcriptional up-regulation of the P4 promoter, combined with a significant lowering of the threshold concentration of viral NS proteins above which cell survival is drastically impaired (Caillet-Fauquet et al. 1990). In *ras*-transformed cells, a significant proportion of this P4 promoter up-regulation is known to be controlled by two separate transcription factor-binding sites upstream of its TATA box, one specific for members of the CREB/ATF family, while the other binds factors belonging to the Ets family (Perros et al. 1995; Perros et al. 1999; Fuks et al. 1996). Transformation-induced modulation of normal cell cycle control thus appears to promote viral replication, and pathogenicity, by impinging upon several different processes in the viral life cycle. Since it clearly does not relate entirely to their requirement for rapidly dividing cells, it is not clear why the parvoviruses should exhibit these oncotropic properties, particularly those controlled by the P4 promoter. It may be that this property has been fortuitously selected for by its natural growth in developing, particularly neonatal, hosts, where aspects of the intracellular milieu of its target cell populations may be mimicked by some of the events that contribute to transformation in the adult cell types. In support of this possibility, is the recent observation that *LacZ* expression is controlled in a cell-type-specific and differentiation-dependent pattern during embryogenesis in mice transgenic for an MVM P4-driven β-galactosidase reporter gene, indicating that P4 is markedly responsive to developmental signals (Davis et al. 2003).

Persistence: latency and cryptic infection

The first direct evidence for parvoviral latency came from the observation that adenovirus infection of some primary human embryonic kidney cultures would yield infectious AAV particles that were not detectable in the original adenovirus stock. Subsequently, it was shown that propagation of human Detroit 6 cells, infected with AAV in the absence of adenovirus, led to the gradual disappearance of demonstrable AAV, which could then be recovered by subsequent adenovirus infection. This led to the hypothesis that AAV could persist in cells in a latent, inheritable form (Berns et al. 1975). The advent of Southern blotting allowed the identification of AAV genomes in such cells, integrated into chromosomal DNA as tandem repeats (Cheung et al. 1980). Subsequent studies have shown that the integration of AAV genes is dependent upon the presence of the *Rep* genes. While the *Rep* gene products up-regulate their own synthesis during coinfection of AAV2 with a helper adenovirus, when AAV2 infects on its own this feed-back effect of Rep is reversed and Rep production is shut down. However, between 1 000 and 4 000 Rep molecules are produced per cell, and this is enough to catalyze the integration of the viral genome into a specific site at chromosome 19q13.3-qter in the human genome (Kotin et al. 1990). Specific integration at this chromosomal locus requires the interaction of Rep with a target DNA sequence that has key features in common with the origin of AAV DNA replication embedded in each viral terminal repeat (Kotin et al. 1992). When the chromosome 19 sequence, known as AAVS1, is placed in a plasmid, it can serve as a substrate for Rep-dependent DNA replication in an in vitro system (Urcelay et al. 1995), and when present as a 'knock-in' transgene in the mouse X-chromosome, it will direct site-specific integration of AAV2 in murine cells (Young et al. 2000). Cloned into an Epstein–Barr virus (EBV) episome and transfected into human cells, the AAVS1 sequence supports site-specific AAV2 integration in vivo, which provides a system where integration can be genetically manipulated (Giraud et al. 1994). Studies using this system have confirmed that AAVS1 must be able to function as an AAV replication origin in order to serve as an integration target site (Linden et al. 1996). In addition, it appears to be important that chromatin associated with the AAVS1 locus is in an open configuration, as shown by the presence of a nearby active gene, encoding slow skeletal troponin T (Dutheil et al. 2000), a DNase I hypersensitive site (Lamartina et al. 2000), and an upstream insulator element that blocks the spread of heterochromatin over the locus (Ogata et al. 2003). In the absence of the Rep 68/78 protein, AAV2 still integrates into the host genome, but at multiple, and apparently random, sites, although there still seems to be a bias towards actively transcribed genes (Nakai et al. 2003). It seems likely that these integration events involve pre-existing double-strand breaks in the host chromosome (Song et al. 2001).

Early studies showed that the autonomously replicating parvoviruses do not integrate into host DNA during a normal infection cycle (Richards and Armentrout 1979). While no stable cell lines carrying integrated genomes resulting from helper-independent parvoviral infections have been reported, MVM has been shown to integrate site-specifically into an episomal EBV-based shuttle vector in a permissive cell, provided the left-end viral replication origin, containing a nick site for NS1, is present (Corsini et al. 1997). Interestingly, no integration was detected into episomes harboring a functional right-end origin. Isolation of such integrants was achieved by recovering the targeted shuttle vector by transfection of DNA derived from the dying cell culture into a bacterial host. This suggests that the reason stable integrants cannot normally be obtained from parvovirus-infected cell cultures is that such interactions, if or when they occur, do not confer protection against subsequent lytic infection, and thus the integrants cannot survive as clonal lines. Significantly, it has also been shown recently that MVM genomes that lack active *NS1* genes also integrate efficiently in a nonsite-specific fashion, at an efficiency that is comparable to that of Rep-negative AAV (Hendrie et al. 2003). Thus, random integration is possibly a feature common to all parvoviral genomes in situations where they are unable to express their NS genes and kill their host cell.

Although the helper-independent parvoviruses are inherently lytic, they are also exquisitely dependent on the host cell-cycle program, because while they are unable to force cells to proliferate, they require their host to enter S phase to support replication and transcription. This leads to another potential form of persistence, in noncycling cells, which has been dubbed cryptic infection, to distinguish it from the latent infections described previously for AAV. In cryptic infection, the viral life cycle does not proceed further than nuclear sequestration of the incoming virion, and is thus completely silent with respect to viral gene expression. Thus, in resting peripheral blood lymphocyte cultures, infectious virus has been observed to remain sequestered and initiate replication only after the addition of phytomitogens (Paul et al. 1979). This type of interaction is inherently unstable, and cannot persist by vertical transmission, in vitro or in vivo, because when a cryptically infected host cell enters S phase, in response to an exogenous signal, its resident virus will initiate replication, express its genes, and the cell would subsequently die (Tattersall and Gardiner 1990).

The application of highly sensitive PCR techniques to patient-derived material has recently led to the realization that B19 genomes are retained at low levels in a variety of tissues in infected individuals over the course of many years (Soderlund-Venermo et al. 2002). Possibly such viruses emerge at intervals, and boost host immunity, explaining why anti-B19 antibody titers are routinely maintained for life. At present, it has not been established whether the B19 genomes found in each of these situations persist as cryptic or latent state, as intact virions, integrated proviruses or episomal complexes.

PATHOGENESIS OF PARVOVIRAL INFECTION

INFECTIONS WITH MEMBERS OF THE *PARVOVIRUS*, *AMDOVIRUS*, AND *BOCAVIRUS* GENERA

Epidemiology

Parvoviruses are generally widely disseminated in their natural hosts. In part this is due to their high level viremias and efficient transmission via bodily secretions and excretions, and in part to the fact that infectious particles are exceptionally rugged, so that they survive outside their host for extended periods. Thus when CPV, a new virus in the feline panleukopenia serotype, emerged as a pathogen of dogs in 1978, it spread through most of the world within a few months, probably because it remained fully viable in fecal material transported on the shoes of airline passengers. Exactly how long shed virions retain viability in nature is undocumented, but they are resistant to most normal ambient temperature ranges, for instance, the half-life for MVM infectivity is in excess of 9 months at refrigerator temperatures. Statistics for virus distribution in wild animal populations are not readily available, but many, such as MPV and H1, are known to be widespread. Infection is generally acute and self-limiting, with transient viremias that last for 7–10 days while the host seroconverts, but some viruses, such as KRV, persist despite high neutralizing antibody titers, so that infected individuals may routinely shed virus for many months (Robey et al. 1968). With the advent of sensitive PCR technology it has become apparent that even following acute, apparently self-limiting infections in immune-competent hosts, low levels of viral DNA are routinely retained in some tissues for many years, although whether this DNA is episomal, cryptic, or integrated is uncertain.

Wild populations of the natural host generally have a high incidence of neutralizing antibody, so that most mothers transmit immunity to their offspring. Thus, infection of neonatal or nursing animals as maternal antibody wanes leads to an active, long-lasting immune response, rather than overt disease. As a consequence, clinically manifest infection is a rare event under endemic conditions, and is generally observed only in immunocompromised individuals. However, in veterinary medicine, vaccination of the entire population is a routine procedure because in domestic animal populations, epizootic and even panzootic, crises may develop if a virus is introduced into an immunologically naive host population.

Pathogenesis

Since their discovery at the end of the 1950s, viruses from the genus *Parvovirus* have been recognized as potential pathogens, although many of them have coevolved with their host to such an extent that infection generally remains subclinical. The spectrum of parvovirus disease thus ranges from acute lethal infections, through slowly progressing, sometimes chronic, illness, to transient subclinical malaise. Somewhat surprisingly, there are no known members of the genus *Parvovirus* that productively infect humans, although several can enter and initiate infection in normal human tissues in culture, or replicate productively in transformed human cell lines.

The types of pathology associated with viral infection can be readily understood by considering a few basic biological principles that control the viral life cycle. Firstly, parvoviruses all exhibit tissue specificity, which limits their lytic potential to cells of particular differentiated types, although this specificity may vary widely between virus species. As discussed previously, tissue specificity is frequently mediated by the presence or absence of appropriate cell surface receptors and coreceptors. However, it also commonly occurs at later stages in the infectious cycle, since the limited genetic complexity of these viruses means that they are peculiarly dependent upon exploiting the synthetic pathways of their chosen host. Disease potential is also controlled by their lack of growth control genes, so that, unlike most DNA viruses, they have no mechanism for forcing noncycling host cells to enter S phase, even though they depend absolutely upon cell functions expressed transiently during this phase of the cell cycle. Thus productive viral replication, and even viral gene expression, is restricted to proliferating cell populations. As lytic parasites of dividing cell populations, their ability to cross the placenta means that they can be potent teratogenic agents, causing fetal and neonatal abnormalities by destroying specific cell populations that are rapidly proliferating during the course of normal development. Indeed, the first autonomous parvoviruses were discovered because of their teratogenic potential in laboratory rodents. These same tissues are often quiescent, and therefore resistant, in the adult.

The age of the infected host thus profoundly influences susceptibility, since it determines the availability of mitotically active cells of the correct differentiated type. Age also influences the viruses' pathologies by determining the degree to which tissue regeneration can take place, so that viruses that replicate in tissues or organs capable of efficient regeneration, such as the liver in a young animal, lead to acute but self-limiting disease with no permanent damage, while the destruction of tissues with limited regenerative potential, such as the developing cerebellum, leaves permanent defects (reviewed in more detail in Siegl 1984, 1988).

INFECTION OF FETAL AND NEONATAL HOSTS

Fetuses and neonates are particularly susceptible to disease. If infection occurs early in pregnancy, the effects on the fetus tend to be generalized, and often fatal, thus viruses infecting pigs, cows, rodents, and mink are commonly associated with fetal wastage. By the late pregnancy, and in neonatal animals, infection tends to be less devastating, coinciding with the increasing ability of the developing host to mount an effective immune response. As the patterns of cell division and differentiation change during development, infection also becomes more organ-specific and leads to distinct syndromes. Thus, infection with FPV or some of the rodent parvoviruses late in gestation specifically induces cerebellar ataxia by lytically targeting, or inducing apoptosis in, cells in the outer germinal layer of the differentiating cerebellum. Newborn mink infected with AMDV develop a severe, potentially fatal, respiratory distress syndrome, resulting from destruction of the type 2 alveolar pneumocytes that are proliferating during this period, while puppies infected with CPV in a time window between 8 days before and 5 days after birth show evidence of viral replication in the developing myofibers, leading to a fatal interstitial myocarditis (reviewed in Bloom and Young 2001). Most dramatically, lytic replication of some rodent parvoviruses in osteogenic tissues that are active during the perinatal period can lead to severe craniofacial and dental deformities, the so-called osteolytic syndrome, which results in offspring with small flat faces, microcephalic heads, protruding eyes and tongue, missing or abnormal teeth, and fragile bones (Siegl 1984, 1988).

INFECTIONS OF MATURE HOSTS

In older animals, more tissues are mitotically quiescent, so that acute disease is generally limited. However, some adult tissues, such as gut epithelium and the lymphopoietic system do retain large numbers of cycling cells. The small subset of autonomous parvoviruses that are capable of effectively targeting these cells, most notably viruses from the FPV/MEV/CPV complex, typically cause fatal disease in adult animals involving extensive destruction of gut epithelium and reticuloendothelial cells, while less extreme forms of leukopenia are also associated with PPV, BPV, and some rodent virus infections. Hepatitis is another common outcome of parvoviral disease in the post neonate, associated with protracted mitotic activity in the maturing liver, or damage-induced cell proliferation in adult tissue. While overt liver disease is a major symptom of GPV infections of goslings, hepatic damage associated with most viruses is rarely lasting because hepatocytes regenerate efficiently following immune clearance of the infecting virus. Patterns of acute disease in the adult thus directly reflect the replicating target tissues available at that time, and are often different from the patterns established by the same virus in the fetus or neonate (Siegl 1984, 1988).

A second, chronic, type of disease may also result from viral infection in the mature animal, associated with the immune response of the host. Thus, AMDV gives rise to a persistent infection in adult mink involving the antigen-presenting cells of the immune system, which ultimately results in immune-complex mediated glomerular nephritis. As a result, while vaccination is generally protective against most acute parvoviral disease, it can be contraindicated for viruses such as AMDV where it actually serves to intensify the pathology (Bloom and Young 2001).

INFECTIONS OF IMMUNOCOMPROMISED HOSTS

Infection of normal and mutant mice with MVM has shown that otherwise lethal pathogenic interactions between the virus and its host are effectively controlled by the host's immune system. Thus, MVMi is essentially apathogenic in adult animals (Segovia et al. 1995), but susceptible newborn mice, with immature immune systems, develop lethal myeloid depression. In vitro, the virus readily kills committed granulocyte–macrophage and erythroid progenitors, as well as pluripotent hematopoietic progenitors, derived from the bone marrow of normal mice (Segovia et al. 1991). Moreover, infection of adult SCID mice, homozygous for the severe combined immunodeficiency mutation, results in a profound leukopenia by the end of the first month and death within 4 months (Segovia et al. 1999). In these animals, the virus causes a novel dysregulation of hemopoiesis, in which primitive hemopoietic progenitors are targeted. This results in severe leukopenia, although circulating platelet and erythrocyte numbers remain stable. In the bone marrow of infected mice, granulocyte–macrophage lineage cells are seen to be markedly depleted, but erythroid progenitors undergo a twofold absolute increase (Segovia et al. 1999), indicating that compensatory mechanisms are mounted specifically by the erythroid lineage in order to maintain effective erythropoiesis. Thus, in immunocompromised adult hosts, complex pathological responses to MVMi infection can emerge that are not apparent in normal mice, a situation that parallels human erythrovirus infections of similarly immunocompromised individuals, as discussed later.

Use as vectors for gene therapy and vaccine delivery

Autonomous parvovirus vectors intended for eventual therapeutic use in humans have been modeled to date on three rodent parvoviruses, MVM, H1, and LuIII, and fall into two main classes. In the first type, the entire coding region of the virus is replaced with transgene encoding sequence, a strategy also employed in the majority of AAV vectors currently in use, discussed below. In the autonomous viruses, these complete coding replacement vectors, mostly based on an infectious clone of LuIII, have been constructed using either the endogenous viral P4 promoter, or a heterologous mammalian promoter, to drive transgene expression (Maxwell et al. 2002). In the latter case, the only viral components remaining in the vector sequence are the terminal regions, which are used to replicate and package the construct driven by nonstructural and capsid proteins provided in *trans* from a helper plasmid. These vectors have been tested for their efficiency at transducing reporter genes, such as luciferase, into a variety of target cell types. Since helper plasmids can be organized to express VP1 and VP2 species from different parental viruses to construct a single packaged vector, these vectors have been used to map viral tropic determinants to individual structural protein species (Maxwell and Maxwell 2004; Maxwell et al. 1995).

The second type of vector retains the nonstructural gene of the virus and has the transgene substituted for sequences normally encoding the capsid proteins. These capsid replacement vectors, although crippled for the production of progeny, retain the replicative and cytotoxic functions of NS1, and therefore are designed to target cells for transgene expression concomitant with cell destruction. This arrangement also allows for high level transgene expression, both by virtue of being driven off the strongly transactivated P38 promoter and because vector genomes can replicate upon uncoating in the target cell, thus extensively amplifying the P38 transcription templates. In addition to transducing reporter transgenes, vectors of this type have been constructed to express suicide genes, as well as various cytokines, such as IL2, IL4, IP-10, or MCP-3 and other immunomodulatory molecules (Cornelis et al. 2004; Russell et al. 1992; Wetzel et al. 2001; Giese et al. 2002). The rationale behind such vectors is to exploit the natural oncotropism of the parental virus to specifically target transgene expression to tumor cells, with the anticipated result of selectively killing tumor cells or augmenting host antitumor immune responses (Haag et al. 2000; Giese et al. 2002; Cornelis et al. 2004).

The unique life cycle of the autonomous parvoviruses has also been exploited to construct vaccine vectors capable of eliciting lifelong immunity in mice following a single inoculation. By transducing antigen genes into resting lymphocytes, these vectors appear to establish cryptic infection, during which sporadic vector activation primes and continually boosts both humoral and cell-mediated Th1-like immune responses (Palmer et al. 2004).

A consistent problem faced in the successful production of parvoviral vectors has been the generation of contaminating replication competent virus following cotransfection of vector and helper plasmids. This presumably occurs as a result of recombination between NS and capsid gene sequences present in the separate vector and helper plasmids, and considerable effort has been expended to abrogate this phenomenon. Success in this has been achieved by reducing the overlap between the two viral components, and where this is impractical, by altering the DNA sequence underlying the coding sequence through the overlap, by introducing deleterious mutation into one copy of the homologous region, or combinations of these approaches (Dupont et al. 2001; Brandenburger and Velu 2004; Palmer and Tattersall 2000; Brown et al. 2002), such that vector stocks can now be generated with extremely low or undetectable contamination with replication competent virus.

INFECTIONS WITH THE *DEPENDOVIRUS* GENUS

Epidemiology

AAVs were first identified in the mid-1960s as 20-nm particles often found contaminating human and monkey adenovirus preparations. Currently, there are seven recognized human/simian serotypes, of which AAV2, AAV3, and AAV5 were isolated directly from human tissue. More specifically, serotypes 2 and 3 are frequently isolated from multiple tissues in conjunction with adenoviruses, whereas AAV5, the most distantly related member of the group by DNA and protein sequence criteria, has been isolated once, from a condylomatous genital wart, where its natural helper was likely a herpes virus (Georg-Fries et al. 1984). Antibodies against all three are found in about 50 percent of adults, with peak titers occurring between the ages of 10 and 20 (Blacklow et al. 1968a; Georg-Fries et al. 1984). In contrast, AAV4 is probably derived from a simian reservoir, since antibodies to it are very common in nonhuman primates, but are detected at much lower frequencies in humans, with a peak incidence of about 10 percent between the ages of 2 and 5 (Blacklow et al. 1968b). Antibodies reactive to AAV1 are found in a high proportion of both human and simian populations, so that its reservoir is questionable. AAV6 appears to be a hybrid recombinant between AAV1 and AAV2, which can be neutralized with anti-AAV1 sera (Rutledge et al. 1998). The remaining serotypes, AAV7 and AAV8, were isolated from Rhesus monkey tissues. Neutralizing antibodies directed against them are rare in the human population and, when present, are of low titer (Gao et al. 2002).

A surprisingly diverse series of unique AAV proviruses have also been rescued from the tissues of various nonhuman primates with, for example, a single lymph node from one rhesus monkey yielding several quite distinct viruses. This heterogeneity appears to result from AAV sequence evolution within an individual animal due, in part, to extensive homologous recombination between a limited set of coinfecting parental viruses, leading to the formation of swarms of quasispecies (Gao et al. 2003). Interstrain and interserotype genome recombination of this type has also been observed for members of other parvoviral genera

(Lopez-Bueno et al. 2003; Gottschalck et al. 1991), and is likely a common source of diversity in situations where multiple related viruses are able to infect the same host tissue.

AAV-like sequences have also been found throughout the *Mammalia*, commonly being detected in conjunction with species-specific adenoviruses. Recently, avian and snake viruses, AAAV and SAAV, have been cloned and sequenced (Bossis and Chiorini 2003; Farkas et al. 2004). Since they are not associated with pathology, such contaminants are rarely noticed, but are likely ubiquitous throughout the higher vertebrates.

Pathogenesis

AAV infection appears to occur predominantly via respiratory, fecal–oral, and conjunctival routes (Schmidt et al. 1975; Blacklow et al. 1967), although sexual transmission has also been suggested (Han et al. 1996; Georg-Fries et al. 1984). Despite the demonstrable presence of low levels of AAV DNA in many tissues, and their high seroprevalence, no study has convincingly linked AAV to any human disease. Studies designed to investigate the teratogenic potential and tissue distribution of AAVs following transplacental infection in mice and rhesus monkeys similarly failed to suggest pathologic sequelae, and recent interest in these viruses as vectors for gene therapy, discussed below, means that there have now been a large number of detailed animal studies of vector AAVs (predominantly AAV2) in mice, rats, rabbits, and dogs, without identifying reasons for clinical concern. In addition, AAV infection has been shown to inhibit transformation of cells by adenoviruses both in vitro and in animal models in vivo, leading to the suggestion that these ubiquitous viruses might even carry out a form of cancer surveillance in the human population. Results of some serological studies appear compatible with this possibility (Sprecher-Goldberger et al. 1970, 1971; Mayor et al. 1976; Georg-Fries et al. 1984; Han et al. 1996), but the idea still remains controversial.

Use as recombinant vectors for gene therapy

AAV vectors are currently being evaluated in clinical trials for the gene therapy of cystic fibrosis, hemophilia B, and muscular dystrophy (Wagner et al. 2002; Kay et al. 2000; Greelish et al. 1999; Aitken et al. 2001), while many, more preliminary, studies are currently probing their potential use to alleviate a broad range of genetic disorders. The simplicity of the AAVs, their apparent lack of pathogenicity or immune stimulation, and their broad tissue specificities, coupled with their ability to integrate into the host genome and thus achieve stable vertical transmission in dividing cells,

render them exceptionally attractive for this purpose. Moreover, they can theoretically be made to integrate preferentially into a single locus in the human genome, on chromosome 19 (19q13-qter), thus limiting the danger of insertional mutagenesis associated with other viral vectors (such as retroviruses) that integrate randomly into host DNA. However, integration into this specific locus requires low level expression of the *Rep* gene, and most AAV vectors explored to date have this sequence deleted in order to avoid its potential cyto-toxicity and to increase the genetic capacity of the vector. Thus they resemble the complete coding replacement vectors discussed above for the autonomous parvoviruses. In the absence of *Rep*, vector genomes still integrate with high efficiency into host DNA, but at apparently random sites, that may be the result of insertion into pre-existing double-stranded breaks (Zentilin et al. 2001; Miller et al. 2003).

Since integration generally appears to require on-going DNA synthesis, it may well be restricted to target cells that are able to enter S phase. This is an important consideration for many gene therapy applications where gene delivery to nondividing cells is required. Surprisingly, however, studies with AAV vectors have shown that relatively stable transgene expression can also be achieved without cell division or integration. Instead, incoming positive- and negative-sense viral genomes appear to become uncoated and rearranged in nondividing cells, where they can be shown to reside as transcriptionally active, monomeric, or concatemeric duplex episomes. It is likely that incoming parental plus and minus strands, derived from separate virions, can anneal during or after uncoating to create these duplexes (Nakai et al. 2000), although various repair strategies can also be invoked, rendering cell division unnecessary for vector persistence and expression. Linear forms of these duplex episomes are commonly observed, particularly in cells with defective repair pathways (Song et al. 2001), but the hyper-recombinogenic nature of the AAV ITR generally results in concatemerization and ultimately circularization of the duplexes, in the absence of either *Rep* or cellular S-phase-dependent DNA replication (Yang et al. 1999).

Recognizing the potential cell cycle independence and transcriptional potency of duplex genomes has also led to the development of 'self-complementary' (scAAV) vectors (McCarty et al. 2001). These have one mutated ITR, which cannot be nicked, flanked by an inverted pair of genomes that are approximately half as long as the wild-type virus and end in a competent ITR, so that progeny are excised and packaged as self-complementary sequences separated by a single, uncleavable, hairpin. As predicted, when used to transduce various nondividing mouse tissues, such as liver, muscle, or brain, these vectors routinely gave more rapid gene expression and higher transduction efficiencies than their single-stranded counterparts. This may, in part, also reflect enhanced genome survival, since naked single-stranded DNA is likely susceptible to rapid degradation in the host nucleus, making immediate conversion into duplex forms a priority for effective transgene delivery. However, viral capsids exhibit a strict DNA packaging limit, which means that sequences of more than about 5 kb cannot be encapsidated. Since scAAV vectors must carry two copies of the transgene, they have even more limited payloads, of around 2 150 basepairs of nonviral sequence, and hence can only transduce small proteins, ribozymes or anti-sense RNAs.

The transgene size limitation, which might be thought to severely restrict the usefulness of all AAV vectors can, in fact, be overcome by packaging single or multiple exons of large genes, bracketed by intronic sequences, into separate recombinant AAVs. Upon coinfection of the same nucleus, the recombinant genomes can circularize and recombine, creating concatemeric episomes in which the various gene sequences are transcribed in order, and the resulting mRNAs spliced, to yield the desired transgene product (Sun et al. 2000; Yan et al. 2000).

One further potential limitation to the use of AAV vectors is tissue specificity or, more accurately, the levels of therapeutic transgene expression that can be achieved in specific target tissues, since low level expression in most cells is possible with the original AAV2-based constructs. As discussed previously, AAV2 exhibits broad tissue specificity, using a variety of cell surface molecules including heparin sulfate proteoglycan, human fibroblast growth factor receptor and α_v,β_5 integrin as receptors or coreceptors, but it has subsequently become apparent that capsids from other AAV serotypes might prove more efficient for gene delivery to certain tissues. For example, AAV5 particles, which enter by binding to sialic acid residues and polypeptides from the PDGF family, appear to be more efficient at binding and delivering transgenes to cells of the airway epithelia, offering prospects for improved transgene delivery to the lungs (Walters et al. 2001; Rooney et al. 2002), while AAV6 and AAV8 are more efficient than AAV2 in transducing the liver (Grimm and Kay 2003; Gao et al. 2002). In the latter case, the improvement is apparently due to intranuclear uncoating efficiencies, which mean that AAV2 genomes are released slowly and are likely degraded prior to duplex episome formation (Thomas et al. 2004). Efforts to fine-tune the AAV particle to maximize gene delivery to particular cell types has thus led to an explosion of interest in the alternate capsid hypervariable regions available in nature, discussed above, and in the mapping and experimental manipulation of receptor-binding sites on the capsid surface, generating capsids that are targeted to alternate cell surface molecules. Use of such custom-designed AAVs may also ultimately overcome the problem of widespread immunity to the traditional serotypes in the human community, opening the possibility of delivering these rugged, resistant particles by in vivo, systemic routes, rather than the more technically demanding localized or ex vivo applications in current use.

Research on the use of AAV vectors to redress specific clinical conditions is expanding rapidly, although a description of these applications is beyond the scope of this chapter and has been extensively reviewed elsewhere (Carter et al. 2004). Suffice it to mention here that recombinant AAV vectors have been demonstrated to be efficacious in the treatment of many animal disease models, including those for cystic fibrosis, hemophilia, muscular dystrophy, rheumatoid arthritis, and lysosomal storage diseases, as well as several ophthalmic diseases and diseases of the central nervous system. Thus the AAVs appear to offer promise as remarkably versatile and unusually safe gene vectors, while the intense research interest in their biology that this has generated continues to reveal fascinating and unexpected details of their life cycle. With such interest and analysis, it seems likely that a whole family of vectors, fine-tuned to particular tissues and diseases, could rapidly become available.

INFECTIONS WITH THE *ERYTHROVIRUS* GENUS

Epidemiology of B19 virus

The human erythrovirus B19 is distributed globally, and infection is common, so that in Europe, the United States, and Asia around 60 percent of adults have anti-B19 IgG antibodies. It is mostly endemic, potentially emerging at any time during the year, although, in temperate climates, extended outbreaks commonly occur in late winter to early summer. These are particularly apparent in children of elementary school age, but infection continues at a lower rate throughout life. Once infected, immunity generally persists for life, and is a reliable marker of past exposure. In a typical study in England and Wales, anti-B19 IgG was found in 5–15 percent of children between the ages of 1 and 5 years, 50–60 percent of people 16–40 years old, and in excess of 85 percent of people over 70 (Cohen and Buckley 1988).

B19 virus is transmitted primarily via respiratory droplets, and virus can be detected in throat swabs during the week following infection, although exactly where the virus is replicating locally during this time is not known. Transient high titer viremias ensue during which virus can be present at concentrations of up to 10^{12} particles/ml of blood, depending upon the genetic make-up of the patient, as discussed later. However, the incidence of virus in donated blood is generally very low, with only around one in 20 000 to one in 40 000 units containing significant titers of virus, even in an epidemic season (Cohen et al. 1990), so that infection via transfusion of individual blood units is rare. In contrast, blood products prepared from pools of donated blood can present a problem because B19 is small enough to escape removal by filtration, and is resistant to the heat and solvent treatments traditionally used to inactivate potential microbiological contaminants in such products. As a result, virus from a few viremic blood units appear to have been widely disseminated in blood products such as Factor VIII (Mortimer et al. 1983b), efficiently transmitting B19 virus infection. Thus, the incidence of B19 virus infection among hemophiliacs has historically been high (up to 90 percent), and the probability of infection correlates with the amount of clotting factor received (Azzi et al. 1999; Rollag et al. 1991). Since 2002, producers of plasma derivatives have quantitated and controlled B19 DNA in their source materials, to minimize the risk of transmission.

Diagnosis of B19 infection

Since the virus cannot be propagated effectively in tissue culture, diagnosis of acute infection relies on serologic tests and on the direct demonstration of viral DNA by hybridization or PCR (Zerbini et al. 2002). Antiviral antibodies can be measured with commercial enzyme-linked IgG or IgM capture assays, which usually employ recombinant particles as a target. The presence of IgM antibodies is indicative of recent infection, since these reliably appear within a few days of the onset of infection and persist for 2 or 3 months. Retrospective information on B19 virus infection is obtained by serological survey, with IgG and IgA antibodies typically persisting for life, possibly in response to the reactivation of latent virus. Diagnosis of persistent infection relies on DNA tests, because antibody production may be low or absent in these cases. DNA hybridization using an essentially full-length probe is sensitive enough to detect serum B19 virus levels during acute transient aplastic crisis or in chronically immunosuppressed patients, but the levels of viremia that occur during infection of normal individuals may be missed, as the technique has a baseline detection limit of around 10^6 genomes per ml. The advent of PCR-mediated gene-amplification greatly increased the sensitivity of B19 DNA detection, although this technique readily generates false-positives due to contamination. PCR results can sometimes be difficult to interpret, because low levels of virus routinely persist for months after infection in serum, bone marrow, skin, or synovial tissue from otherwise normal individuals, so that low level detection does not necessarily indicate acute infection. Moreover, the oligonucleotide primers selected may not detect extreme sequence variants of B19, such as the V9/A6 variants discussed later, whereas DNA hybridization does.

Clinical manifestations of B19 virus infection

Many cases of B19 virus infection are asymptomatic. Its most common clinical presentation in hematologically normal children is erythema infectiosum, a mild febrile illness that often presents as a 'slapped cheeks' rash or as a 'lacy' reticulate rash covering the trunk and arms. This common childhood infection was originally called fifth disease, being the fifth in a classic list of childhood rubelliform illnesses, and was well known to pediatricians for the 80 years prior to the recognition of parvovirus B19 as its sole etiologic agent (Anderson et al. 1983, 1984). The rash may be evanescent, and recurrences can be provoked by exposure to sunlight, emotion, heat, or exercise, but it frequently escapes detection in people with dark skin. About 10 percent of EI cases in children have been associated with arthropathy, although retrospective sero-epidemiological studies suggest that an equal number of arthropathies may occur in infected children not presenting with classic EI rash symptoms. Joint pains can persist for months, to a year or more, and are sometimes diagnosed as juvenile rheumatoid arthritis. In adults the classic rash symptoms are somewhat rare, although more prevalent in women than men, and arthralgia and inflammatory arthritis are much more frequent consequences of B19 infection, occurring in about 50 percent of patients. Specifically, nearly two-thirds of female and one-third of male adults experiencing a primary B19 virus infection also experience moderately severe symmetrical polyarthritis involving peripheral finger, wrist, ankle, or knee joints. This effectively means that around 15 percent of new cases of arthritis are the result of B19 virus infections. While arthropathies can sometimes be prolonged and severe enough to fulfill the diagnostic criteria for rheumatoid arthritis, B19 virus infection does not lead to articular erosion, and the arthropathy typically resolves within a few months even in more severe cases.

A characteristic biphasic clinical course of viremia followed by immune complex disease, has been described in both natural and experimental B19 virus infections of normal, otherwise healthy, individuals. In a study of human adult volunteers, viremia was detected 1 week after experimental intranasal infection of seronegative individuals, and was accompanied by a mild, flu-like illness with fever, malaise, myalgia, and itching (Anderson et al. 1985). During the viremic phase, virus is excreted from the respiratory tract, which likely represents the natural mode of transmission. Viremia is coincident with a transient, but absolute, reticulocytopenia and accompanying lymphopenia, neutropenia, and thrombocytopenia. Since the erythrocyte half-life in normal, healthy individuals is several times longer than this period of profound virus-induced bone marrow failure, frank anemia does not develop, and while the hematological consequences of B19 virus infection are diagnostic, they are not clinically significant. Toward the middle of the second week following infection, virus-specific IgM levels rise, coincident with a fall in detectable circulating virus and the restoration of normal hematological parameters. A brief overshoot of reticulocyte numbers often prefaces this return to normality. IgM, which normally persists for 2–3 months, is followed by IgG, appearing at around 2 weeks after infection and persisting thereafter. The appearance of IgG ushers in the second phase of symptoms beginning 17–18 days after infection, which appear to be the result of immune complex formation. These include both the lacy rashes typical of EI and arthralgia, which normally last for 3–4 days, but can be protracted. Although the major protective immune response to B19 virus is humoral, some studies of cellular immune responses have been reported. These demonstrate that infected individuals mount a robust Th1-like CD4$^+$ T-cell response to viral components, and generate CD8$^+$ cytotoxic T cells that can kill cells pulsed with peptides derived from the B19 NS1 protein sequence (Klenerman et al. 2002).

Ongoing or recent B19 virus infection has also been linked to some forms of idiopathic thrombocytopenic purpura, myocarditis, acute fulminant liver failure accompanied by aplastic crisis, neuropathy, complex regional pain syndrome, neuralgic amyotrophy, and virus-associated hemophagocytic syndrome, although a causal etiology for B19 in these syndromes has not been firmly established. Viral entry and early gene expression can occur in some tissues, such as hepatocytes, that are not susceptible to productive infection. In such cases NS1-mediated apoptosis can sometimes be demonstrated in vitro, and provides a credible biological basis for the clinical observations (Poole et al. 2004). These possible disease associations are discussed in more detail elsewhere (Young and Brown 2004), although the full spectrum of virus-induced disease has still to be unraveled.

The major risk for serious pathologic outcome in normal individuals arises from exposure to B19 virus during pregnancy. A clear connection has been established between B19 virus infection, especially during the second trimester, and the development of non-immune hydrops fetalis, a potentially lethal condition for the fetus that occurs in approximately one of 3 000 pregnancies, and of which 10–20 percent are now believed to be due to B19 virus infection. About 50 percent of pregnant women lack circulating anti-B19 IgG, and thus are potentially susceptible to primary infection, and prospective studies suggest that the risk of transplacental transmission for infected women is about 30 percent, with a 5–9 percent risk of fetal loss. Thus most B19 virus infections during pregnancy do not lead to fetal loss. However, the virus replicates productively in dividing cells of the erythroid lineage, so that transplacental infection of the fetus during the second trimester, in particular, leads to destruction of the rapidly proliferating erythroblasts that

are present in erythroid sinuses in the liver at this stage of fetal development. In hydrops cases, fetal infection results in severe anemia, high-output cardiac failure, fluid accumulation and death, although intrauterine transfusion of packed red cells can substantially lower the mortality rate. Fetal B19 virus infection may also cause fetal or congenital anemia, abortion, or stillbirth, although the risk of these occurring as a consequence of a primary B19 virus infection is apparently quite low. Surprisingly, this clear association between fetal pathology and B19 virus has not led, to date, to demand for a protective vaccine. Non-infectious empty recombinant B19 particles have been found to be immunogenic in normal volunteers, and might prevent fetal hydrops if 'at risk,' seronegative women were immunized early in pregnancy. Vaccine-mediated expression of the highly-immunogenic VP1-specific polypeptide, which carries phospholipase A2 activity on the outside of recombinant particles, might possibly be of concern, although such sequences could presumably be mutated or eliminated from a vaccine construct with relative ease.

Since B19 pathogenesis results predominantly from the destruction of rapidly proliferating eythroid precursors, in individuals with genetic defects that result in a shortened erythrocyte half-life and an expanded erythroblast population, anemia develops rapidly, reaches exceptionally high levels, and can require intervention. Thus transient aplastic crisis has been observed as an inevitable consequence of B19 virus infection in patients with single gene defects such as sickle cell anemia, α- or β-thalassemia, hereditary spherocytosis, stomatocytosis, or elliptocytosis, deficiencies in glucose-6-phosphate dehydrogenase, pyruvate kinase, or pyrimidine-5-nucleotidase, as well as in other hematopoietically compromised conditions, such as cold and heat antibody-mediated or chronic autoimmune hemolytic anemia, paroxysmal nocturnal hemoglobinuria, or malarial infection (Heegaard and Brown 2002). The aplastic crisis can be resolved by medical intervention, such as red cell transfusion. Otherwise it will run its course until the humoral immune response clears the virus and erythropoiesis is restored. This type of crisis only occurs once in the life of a patient and, although self-limiting, can cause severe, life-threatening anemia that can precipitate congestive heart failure, cerebrovascular events, and acute splenic sequestration (Smith-Whitley et al. 2004).

Finally, failure to produce neutralizing antibodies to B19 virus can occur in a variety of immunodeficiency states with congenital, iatrogenic, or infectious causes. Typical EI rashes do not develop in such patients, but there are high titers of circulating virus, and its persistence can lead to pure red cell aplasia, with depletion of serum reticulocytes and erythroid precursors from the bone marrow. Pure red cell aplasia of this type has been seen in Nezelof syndrome, an inherited combined immunodeficiency disorder, in patients being treated with cytotoxic chemotherapy or immunosuppressive drugs, often after organ transplantation, and in patients infected with human immunodeficiency virus (Heegaard and Brown 2002). Immunosuppression can sometimes reactivate latent virus infections, although which tissues serve as the virus reservoir is not currently known. Persistent infection usually responds well to parenteral administration of commercial immune globulin, which invariably contains anti-B19 antibodies because of their prevalence in the donor population, but such intervention commonly leads to the rashes and arthropathy seen in acute infection. More detailed accounts of the clinical outcomes of B19 virus infection are to be found in recent reviews (Heegaard and Brown 2002; Young and Brown 2004).

Genomic polymorphism in B19

The DNA sequence of B19 was first determined from a bacterially cloned copy of a viral genome, B19-Au, isolated in Georgia, USA, from the serum of a child with homozygous sickle cell disease undergoing transient aplastic crisis (Shade et al. 1986), and this has become the reference sequence. Since that time a large number of isolates have been sequenced, or partially sequenced throughout the world, and, until 1999, all genomes appeared highly conserved. In general, they showed less than 2 percent nucleotide divergence, spread throughout the entire virus although certain regions, such as the *NS* gene, were particularly conserved. Minor antigenic and genetic differences between isolates were sometimes observed, manifest as differences in monoclonal antibody specificity, restriction fragment polymorphism, or single-stranded conformational polymorphism, but these did not appear to correlate with differences in the tissue specificity of the virus or its disease spectra. However, B19 diagnosis commonly relies on the identification of viral DNA by PCR, and this test inevitably favors the detection of conserved genomes.

Accordingly, in 1999, the blood of a French child suffering from transient aplastic anemia was found to contain a new type of virus, called V9, which eluded detection by the then-current PCR technique (Nguyen et al. 1999). At the nucleotide level, the isolate was more than 11 percent divergent from published B19 sequences (Heegaard et al. 2001), although certain regions were relatively conserved and allowed the design of new PCR assays using primers that would detect both V9 and B19 DNA. An extensive prospective study conducted in France between 1999 and 2001 subsequently revealed that V9-related viruses circulate beside B19 viruses at a significant frequency (11.4 percent) in the French population. Such genomes were surprisingly absent from large groups of North American and Danish samples analyzed at that time, suggesting that such variants might be epidemiologically linked to a particular geographic area, in this case France. An extraordinary aspect of V9 is that, despite its DNA sequence divergence, it is 96–97 percent

homologous to B19-Au at the protein level. Thus, the great majority of its nucleotide changes are silent mutations that do not affect the amino acid sequence of the viral proteins, which therefore react with most anti-B19 antibodies (Heegaard et al. 2001). Another new variant, designated A6, has since been isolated in America, which is 88 percent similar to B19 virus and 92 percent similar to V9 at the nucleotide level (Nguyen et al. 2002), and an essentially similar mutant was detected in Finland, where it was called K71 or Lali (Hokynar et al. 2002). At present there is no established explanation for the emergence of these hypermutated variants, however, relationships between specific genotypic variants and specific disease states have been looked for, but not found.

In vitro cellular correlates of B19 pathology

Parvovirus B19 binds to the blood group P antigen, a neutral glycolipid called globoside that is expressed predominantly on human erythrocytes and erythroid progenitors. This functions as a productive cell surface receptor for B19, consistent with its observed tropism (Brown et al. 1993). In the human population, about one in 200 000 individuals genetically lack P antigen, and show no serologic evidence of past B19 virus infection. Bone marrow cultures derived from these individuals fail to support the growth of B19 virus in vitro, even at a high multiplicity of infection (Brown et al. 1994), indicating that the presence of P antigen is necessary for infection. However, it may not be sufficient. Thus, while P antigen is present on a number of cells such as fetal myocytes, megakaryocytes, endothelial cells, as well as the hepatocytes discussed previously, these cell types do not appear to be permissive for B19 replication, suggesting that additional factors may be required for complete replication. Some studies indicate that entry coreceptors, such as β-integrins, may be required, but intracellular permissivity factors are also indicated, since in culture many nonpermissive cells appear to support early, but not late, transcription (Liu et al. 1992). This abrogates capsid protein synthesis, but still allows expression of the potentially cytotoxic NS1 molecule of the virus (Moffatt et al. 1998; Ozawa et al. 1988), which in vitro can be shown to induce caspase-mediated cell death (Poole et al. 2004).

Development of a cell culture system that supports productive B19 replication has been extremely difficult, and at present, there is no animal model for the virus. In primary human bone marrow cultures, B19 virus inhibits colony formation by late erythroid progenitors and the more primitive burst-forming erythroid progenitors, while leaving differentiation of myeloid precursors unperturbed (Mortimer et al. 1983a). It appears from both in vivo and in vitro studies, that the pluripotent erythrogenic stem cell is resistant to virus infection, while in the presence of erythropoietin, B19 virus will grow in later progenitors derived from human bone marrow, fetal liver, and peripheral or umbilical blood. Infection of such erythroid precursors in vitro with B19 leads to a cytopathic effect characterized by the presence of giant pronormoblasts, which appear to be equivalent to the 'lantern cells' that can be observed in vivo in the bone marrow of patients undergoing B19-associated transient aplastic crisis. These cells exhibit large eosinophilic nuclear inclusion bodies and cytoplasmic vacuolization, and electron microscopy reveals nuclei with marginated chromatin that contains virus particles. While such explanted cells cannot be maintained in long-term culture, B19 virus has also been shown to propagate in a small number of permanent cell lines of megakaryoblastoid and erythroleukemic origin, although net synthesis of virus has not been achieved in these systems (Heegaard and Brown 2002).

An infectious plasmid clone of B19 has recently been constructed, and shown to give rise to detectable levels of infectious progeny when transfected into the erythropoietin-responsive cell line UT7/Epo-S1 in vitro (Zhi et al. 2004). It seems likely that mutational analysis of this clone should allow rapid progress in understanding the molecular biology of this ubiquitous human fellow traveler, which will hopefully also inform our understanding of B19 pathology. At the core of this pathology is the destruction of rapidly proliferating erythroid precursors, which derives from the narrow tissue tropism of the virus and its absolute dependence on the presence of rapidly dividing cell populations. Thus, despite the organizational differences between individual genera in the *Parvovirinae*, the pathogenic potential of B19 follows the same underlying biological principles that determine disease throughout the autonomously replicating viruses from this family.

ACKNOWLEDGMENTS

The authors thank Zoltan Zadori and Peter Tijssen for the phylogenetic analysis presented in Figure 21.1, and Michael Chapman for the parvovirus images shown in 21.2. The authors were supported by NIH grants CA29303 and AI26109 from NCI and NIAID, respectively.

REFERENCES

Aasted, B., Race, R.E. and Bloom, M.E. 1984. Aleutian disease virus, a parvovirus, is proteolytically degraded during in vivo infection in mink. *J Virol*, **51**, 7–13.

Agbandje-McKenna, M., Llamas-Saiz, A.L., et al. 1998. Functional implications of the structure of the murine parvovirus, minute virus of mice. *Structure*, **6**, 1369–81.

Aitken, M.L., Moss, R.B., et al. 2001. A phase I study of aerosolized administration of tgAAVCF to cystic fibrosis subjects with mild lung disease. *Hum Gene Ther*, **12**, 1907–16.

Allander, T., Emerson, S.U., et al. 2001. A virus discovery method incorporating DNase treatment and its application to the identification of two bovine parvovirus species. *Proc Natl Acad Sci USA*, **98**, 11609–14.

Anderson, M.J., Jones, S.E., et al. 1983. Human parvovirus, the cause of erythema infectiosum (fifth disease)? *Lancet*, **1**, 1378.

Anderson, M.J., Lewis, E., et al. 1984. An outbreak of erythema infectiosum associated with human parvovirus infection. *J Hyg (Lond)*, **93**, 85–93.

Anderson, M.J., Higgins, P.G., et al. 1985. Experimental parvoviral infection in humans. *J Infect Dis*, **152**, 257–65.

Azzi, A., Morfini, M. and Mannucci, P.M. 1999. The transfusion-associated transmission of parvovirus B19. *Transfus Med Rev*, **13**, 194–204.

Ball-Goodrich, L.J. and Tattersall, P. 1992. Two amino acid substitutions within the capsid are coordinately required for acquisition of fibrotropism by the lymphotropic strain of minute virus of mice. *J Virol*, **66**, 3415–23.

Bantel-Schaal, U., Hub, B. and Kartenbeck, J. 2002. Endocytosis of adeno-associated virus type 5 leads to accumulation of virus particles in the Golgi compartment. *J Virol*, **76**, 2340–9.

Bauer, P.H., Cui, C., et al. 1999. Discrimination between sialic acid-containing receptors and pseudoreceptors regulates polyomavirus spread in the mouse. *J Virol*, **73**, 5826–32.

Bergeron, J., Hebert, B. and Tijssen, P. 1996. Genome organization of the Kresse strain of porcine parvovirus: identification of the allotropic determinant and comparison with those of NADL-2 and field isolates. *J Virol*, **70**, 2508–15.

Bergs, V.V. 1969. Rat virus-mediated suppression of leukemia induction by Moloney virus in rats. *Cancer Res*, **29**, 1669–72.

Berns, K.I., Pinkerton, T.C., et al. 1975. Detection of adeno-associated virus (AAV)-specific nucleotide sequences in DNA isolated from latently infected Detroit 6 cells. *Virology*, **68**, 556–60.

Blacklow, N.R., Hoggan, M.D. and Rowe, W.P. 1967. Isolation of adenovirus-associated viruses from man. *Proc Natl Acad Sci USA*, **58**, 1410–15.

Blacklow, N.R., Hoggan, M.D., et al. 1968a. Epidemiology of adenovirus-associated virus infection in a nursery population. *Am J Epidemiol*, **88**, 368–78.

Blacklow, N.R., Hoggan, M.D. and Rowe, W.P. 1968b. Serologic evidence for human infection with adenovirus-associated viruses. *J Natl Cancer Inst*, **40**, 319–27.

Bloom, M.E. and Young, N. 2001. Parvoviruses. In: Knipe, D.M. and Howley, P.M. (eds), *Fields' Virology: Fourth Edition (Eds*, 4th edn. Philadelphia: Lippincott, Williams & Wilkins, 2361–79, Chapter 70.

Bodendorf, U., Cziepluch, C., et al. 1999. Nuclear export factor CRM1 interacts with nonstructural proteins NS2 from parvovirus minute virus of mice. *J Virol*, **73**, 7769–79.

Bonnard, G.D., Manders, E.K., et al. 1976. Immunosuppressive activity of a subline of the mouse EL-4 lymphoma. Evidence for minute virus of mice causing the inhibition. *J Exp Med*, **143**, 187–205.

Bossis, I. and Chiorini, J.A. 2003. Cloning of an avian adeno-associated virus (AAAV) and generation of recombinant AAAV particles. *J Virol*, **77**, 6799–810.

Brandenburger, A. and Velu, T. 2004. Autonomous parvovirus vectors: preventing the generation of wild-type or replication-competent virus. *J Gene Med*, **6**, S203–11.

Brown, C.S., DiSumma, F.M., et al. 2002. Production of recombinant H1 parvovirus stocks devoid of replication-competent viruses. *Hum Gene Ther*, **13**, 2135–45.

Brown, K.E., Anderson, S.M. and Young, N.S. 1993. Erythrocyte P antigen: cellular receptor for B19 parvovirus. *Science*, **262**, 114–17.

Brown, K.E., Hibbs, J.R., et al. 1994. Resistance to parvovirus B19 infection due to lack of virus receptor (erythrocyte P antigen). *N Engl J Med*, **330**, 1192–6.

Burnett, E. and Tattersall, P. 2003. Reverse genetic system for the analysis of parvovirus telomeres reveals interactions between transcription factor binding sites in the hairpin stem. *J Virol*, **77**, 8650–60.

Caillet-Fauquet, P., Perros, M., et al. 1990. Programmed killing of human cells by means of an inducible clone of parvoviral genes encoding non-structural proteins. *EMBO J*, **9**, 2989–95.

Carter, B.J., Burstein, H. and Peluso, R.W. 2004. Adeno-associated virus and AAV vectors for gene delivery. In: Templeton, N.S. (ed.), *Gene and cell therapy: therapeutic mechanisms and strategies*, 2nd edn. New York: Marcel Dekker, Chapter 5.

Cater, J.E. and Pintel, D.J. 1992. The small non-structural protein NS2 of the autonomous parvovirus minute virus of mice is required for virus growth in murine cells. *J Gen Virol*, **73**, 1839–43.

Chang, S.F., Sgro, J.Y. and Parrish, C.R. 1992. Multiple amino acids in the capsid structure of canine parvovirus coordinately determine the canine host range and specific antigenic and hemagglutination properties. *J Virol*, **66**, 6858–67.

Chapman, M.S. and Rossmann, M.G. 1993. Structure, sequence, and function correlations among parvoviruses. *Virology*, **194**, 491–508.

Chen, K.C., Tyson, J.J., et al. 1989. A kinetic hairpin transfer model for parvoviral DNA replication. *J Mol Biol*, **208**, 283–96.

Cheung, A.K., Hoggan, M.D., et al. 1980. Integration of the adeno-associated virus genome into cellular DNA in latently infected human Detroit 6 cells. *J Virol*, **33**, 739–48.

Christensen, J. and Tattersall, P. 2002. Parvovirus initiator protein NS1 and RPA coordinate replication fork progression in a reconstituted DNA replication system. *J Virol*, **76**, 6518–31.

Christensen, J., Cotmore, S.F. and Tattersall, P. 1995. Minute virus of mice transcriptional activator protein NS1 binds directly to the transactivation region of the viral P38 promoter in a strictly ATP-dependent manner. *J Virol*, **69**, 5422–30.

Christensen, J., Cotmore, S.F. and Tattersall, P. 1997. A novel cellular site-specific DNA-binding protein cooperates with the viral NS1 polypeptide to initiate parvovirus DNA replication. *J Virol*, **71**, 1405–16.

Christensen, J., Cotmore, S.F. and Tattersall, P. 1999. Two new members of the emerging KDWK family of combinatorial transcription modulators bind as a heterodimer to flexibly spaced PuCGPy half-sites. *Mol Cell Biol*, **19**, 7741–50.

Christensen, J., Cotmore, S.F. and Tattersall, P. 2001. Minute virus of mice initiator protein NS1 and a host KDWK family transcription factor must form a precise ternary complex with origin DNA for nicking to occur. *J Virol*, **75**, 7009–17.

Clemens, K.E. and Pintel, D.J. 1988. The two transcription units of the autonomous parvovirus minute virus of mice are transcribed in a temporal order. *J Virol*, **62**, 1448–51.

Cohen, B.J. and Buckley, M.M. 1988. The prevalence of antibody to human parvovirus B19 in England and Wales. *J Med Microbiol*, **25**, 151–3.

Cohen, B.J., Mortimer, P.P. and Pereira, M.S. 1983. Diagnostic assays with monoclonal antibodies for the human serum parvovirus-like virus (SPLV). *J Hyg (Lond)*, **91**, 113–30.

Cohen, B.J., Field, A.M., et al. 1990. Blood donor screening for parvovirus B19. *J Virol Meth*, **30**, 233–8.

Colomar, M.C., Hirt, B. and Beard, P. 1998. Two segments in the genome of the immunosuppressive minute virus of mice determine the host-cell specificity, control viral DNA replication and affect viral RNA metabolism. *J Gen Virol*, **79**, 581–6.

Cornelis, J.J., Becquart, P., et al. 1988. Transformation of human fibroblasts by ionizing radiation, a chemical carcinogen, or simian virus 40 correlates with an increase in susceptibility to the autonomous parvoviruses H-1 virus and minute virus of mice. *J Virol*, **62**, 1679–86.

Cornelis, J.J., Salome, N., et al. 2004. Vectors based on autonomous parvoviruses: novel tools to treat cancer? *J Gene Med*, **6**, S193–202.

Corsini, J., Tal, J. and Winocour, E. 1997. Directed integration of minute virus of mice DNA into episomes. *J Virol*, **71**, 9008–15.

Cossart, Y.E., Field, A.M., et al. 1975. Parvovirus-like particles in human sera. *Lancet*, **1**, 72–3.

Costello, E., Saudan, P., et al. 1997. High mobility group chromosomal protein 1 binds to the adeno-associated virus replication protein (Rep) and promotes Rep-mediated site-specific cleavage of DNA, ATPase activity and transcriptional repression. *EMBO J*, **16**, 5943–54.

Cotmore, S.F. and Tattersall, P. 1984. Characterization and molecular cloning of a human parvovirus genome. *Science*, **226**, 1161–5.

Cotmore, S.F. and Tattersall, P. 1989. A genome-linked copy of the NS-1 polypeptide is located on the outside of infectious parvovirus particles. *J Virol*, **63**, 3902–11.

Cotmore, S.F. and Tattersall, P. 1990. Alternate splicing in a parvoviral nonstructural gene links a common amino-terminal sequence to downstream domains which confer radically different localization and turnover characteristics. *Virology*, **177**, 477–87.

Cotmore, S.F. and Tattersall, P. 1996. Parvovirus DNA replication. In: DePamphilis, M. (ed.), *DNA replication in eukaryotic cells*. Cold Spring Harbor, New York: Cold Spring Harbor Laboratory Press, 799–813, Chapter 28.

Cotmore, S.F. and Tattersall, P. 1998. High-mobility group 1/2 proteins are essential for initiating rolling-circle-type DNA replication at a parvovirus hairpin origin. *J Virol*, **72**, 8477–84.

Cotmore, S.F. and Tattersall, P. 2003. Resolution of parvovirus dimer junctions proceeds through a novel heterocruciform intermediate. *J Virol*, **77**, 6245–54.

Cotmore, S.F. and Tattersall, P. 2005. Genome packaging sense is controlled by the efficiency of the nick site in the right-end replication origin of parvoviruses MVM and LuIII. *J Virol*, **79**, 2287–300.

Cotmore, S.F., Christensen, J., et al. 1995. The NS1 polypeptide of the murine parvovirus minute virus of mice binds to DNA sequences containing the motif [ACCA]2-3. *J Virol*, **69**, 1652–60.

Cotmore, S.F., D'Abramo, A.M. Jr., et al. 1997. The NS2 polypeptide of parvovirus MVM is required for capsid assembly in murine cells. *Virology*, **231**, 267–80.

Cotmore, S.F., D'Abramo, A.M. Jr., et al. 1999. Controlled conformational transitions in the MVM virion expose the VP1 N-terminus and viral genome without particle disassembly. *Virology*, **254**, 169–81.

Cotmore, S.F., Christensen, J. and Tattersall, P. 2000. Two widely spaced initiator binding sites create an HMG1-dependent parvovirus rolling-hairpin replication origin. *J Virol*, **74**, 1332–41.

Davis, C., Segev-Amzaleg, N., et al. 2003. The P4 promoter of the parvovirus minute virus of mice is developmentally regulated in transgenic P4-LacZ mice. *Virology*, **306**, 268–79.

de la Maza, L.M. and Carter, B.J. 1981. Inhibition of adenovirus oncogenicity in hamsters by adeno-associated virus DNA. *J Natl Cancer Inst*, **67**, 1323–6.

Deleu, L., Pujol, A., et al. 1999. Activation of promoter P4 of the autonomous parvovirus minute virus of mice at early S phase is required for productive infection. *J Virol*, **73**, 3877–85.

Di Pasquale, G., Davidson, B.L., et al. 2003. Identification of PDGFR as a receptor for AAV-5 transduction. *Nat Med*, **9**, 1306–12.

Dubielzig, R., King, J.A., et al. 1999. Adeno-associated virus type 2 protein interactions: formation of pre-encapsidation complexes. *J Virol*, **73**, 8989–98.

Dupont, F., Karim, A., et al. 2001. A novel MVMp-based vector system specifically designed to reduce the risk of replication-competent virus generation by homologous recombination. *Gene Ther*, **8**, 921–9.

Dutheil, N., Shi, F., et al. 2000. Adeno-associated virus site-specifically integrates into a muscle-specific DNA region. *Proc Natl Acad Sci USA*, **97**, 4862–6.

Dworak, L.J., Wolfinbarger, J.B. and Bloom, M.E. 1997. Aleutian mink disease parvovirus infection of K562 cells is antibody-dependent and is mediated via an Fc(gamma)RII receptor. *Arch Virol*, **142**, 363–73.

Fan, M.M., Tamburic, L., et al. 2001. The small 11-kDa protein from B19 parvovirus binds growth factor receptor-binding protein 2 in vitro in a Src homology 3 domain/ligand-dependent manner. *Virology*, **291**, 285–91.

Farkas, S.L., Zadori, Z., et al. 2004. A parvovirus isolated from royal python (*Python regius*) is a member of the genus *Dependovirus*. *J Gen Virol*, **85**, 555–61.

Fox, J.M., McCrackin Stevenson, M.A. and Bloom, M.E. 1999. Replication of Aleutian mink disease parvovirus in vivo is influenced by residues in the VP2 protein. *J Virol*, **73**, 8713–19.

Fuks, F., Deleu, L., et al. 1996. Ras oncogene-dependent activation of the P4 promoter of minute virus of mice through a proximal P4 element interacting with the Ets family of transcription factors. *J Virol*, **70**, 1331–9.

Gao, G.P., Alvira, M.R., et al. 2002. Novel adeno-associated viruses from rhesus monkeys as vectors for human gene therapy. *Proc Natl Acad Sci USA*, **99**, 11854–9.

Gao, G., Alvira, M.R., et al. 2003. Adeno-associated viruses undergo substantial evolution in primates during natural infections. *Proc Natl Acad Sci USA*, **100**, 6081–6.

Gardiner, E.M. and Tattersall, P. 1988a. Evidence that developmentally regulated control of gene expression by a parvoviral allotropic determinant is particle mediated. *J Virol*, **62**, 1713–22.

Gardiner, E.M. and Tattersall, P. 1988b. Mapping of the fibrotropic and lymphotropic host range determinants of the parvovirus minute virus of mice. *J Virol*, **62**, 2605–13.

Georg-Fries, B., Biederlack, S., et al. 1984. Analysis of proteins, helper dependence, and seroepidemiology of a new human parvovirus. *Virology*, **134**, 64–71.

Giese, N.A., Raykov, Z., et al. 2002. Suppression of metastatic hemangiosarcoma by a parvovirus MVMp vector transducing the IP-10 chemokine into immunocompetent mice. *Cancer Gene Ther*, **9**, 432–42.

Giraud, C., Winocour, E. and Berns, K.I. 1994. Site-specific integration by adeno-associated virus is directed by a cellular DNA sequence. *Proc Natl Acad Sci USA*, **91**, 10039–43.

Gorham, J.R., Hartsough, G.R., et al. 1966. Studies on cell culture adapted feline panleukopenia virus. Virus neutralization and antigenic extinction. *Vet Med Small Anim Clin*, **61**, 35–40.

Gottschalck, E., Alexandersen, S., et al. 1991. Nucleotide sequence analysis of Aleutian mink disease parvovirus shows that multiple virus types are present in infected mink. *J Virol*, **65**, 4378–86.

Govindasamy, L., Hueffer, K., et al. 2003. Structures of host range-controlling regions of the capsids of canine and feline parvoviruses and mutants. *J Virol*, **77**, 12211–21.

Greelish, J.P., Su, L.T., et al. 1999. Stable restoration of the sarcoglycan complex in dystrophic muscle perfused with histamine and a recombinant adeno-associated viral vector. *Nat Med*, **5**, 439–43.

Green, S.W., Malkovska, I., et al. 2000. Rhesus and pig-tailed macaque parvoviruses: identification of two new members of the erythrovirus genus in monkeys. *Virology*, **269**, 105–12.

Grimm, D. and Kay, M.A. 2003. From virus evolution to vector revolution: use of naturally occurring serotypes of adeno-associated virus (AAV) as novel vectors for human gene therapy. *Curr Gene Ther*, **3**, 281–304.

Haag, A., Menten, P., et al. 2000. Highly efficient transduction and expression of cytokine genes in human tumor cells by means of autonomous parvovirus vectors; generation of antitumor responses in recipient mice. *Hum Gene Ther*, **11**, 597–609.

Han, L., Parmley, T.H., et al. 1996. High prevalence of adeno-associated virus (AAV) type 2 rep DNA in cervical materials: AAV may be sexually transmitted. *Virus Genes*, **12**, 47–52.

Heegaard, E.D. and Brown, K.E. 2002. Human parvovirus B19. *Clin Microbiol Rev*, **15**, 485–505.

Heegaard, E.D., Panum Jensen, I. and Christensen, J. 2001. Novel PCR assay for differential detection and screening of erythrovirus B19 and erythrovirus V9. *J Med Virol*, **65**, 362–7.

Hendrie, P.C., Hirata, R.K. and Russell, D.W. 2003. Chromosomal integration and homologous gene targeting by replication-incompetent vectors based on the autonomous parvovirus minute virus of mice. *J Virol*, **77**, 13136–45.

Hokynar, K., Soderlund-Venermo, M., et al. 2002. A new parvovirus genotype persistent in human skin. *Virology*, **302**, 224–8.

Hueffer, K., Govindasamy, L., et al. 2003. Combinations of two capsid regions controlling canine host range determine canine transferrin receptor binding by canine and feline parvoviruses. *J Virol*, **77**, 10099–105.

Hueffer, K., Palermo, L.M. and Parrish, C.R. 2004. Parvovirus infection of cells by using variants of the feline transferrin receptor altering clathrin-mediated endocytosis, membrane domain localization, and capsid-binding domains. *J Virol*, **78**, 5601–11.

Huser, D., Weger, S. and Heilbronn, R. 2003. Packaging of human chromosome 19-specific adeno-associated virus (AAV) integration sites in AAV virions during AAV wild-type and recombinant AAV vector production. *J Virol*, **77**, 4881–7.

Ilyina, T.V. and Koonin, E.V. 1992. Conserved sequence motifs in the initiator proteins for rolling circle DNA replication encoded by diverse replicons from eubacteria, eucaryotes and archaebacteria. *Nucleic Acids Res*, **20**, 3279–85.

Kaludov, N., Brown, K.E., et al. 2001. Adeno-associated virus serotype 4 (AAV4) and AAV5 both require sialic acid binding for hemagglutination and efficient transduction but differ in sialic acid linkage specificity. *J Virol*, **75**, 6884–93.

Katz, E. and Carter, B.J. 1986. Effect of adeno-associated virus on transformation of NIH 3T3 cells by ras gene and on tumorigenicity of an NIH 3T3 transformed cell line. *Cancer Res*, **46**, 3023–6.

Kay, M.A., Manno, C.S., et al. 2000. Evidence for gene transfer and expression of factor IX in haemophilia B patients treated with an AAV vector. *Nat Genet*, **24**, 257–61.

Kilham, L. and Olivier, L.J. 1959. A latent virus of rats isolated in tissue culture. *Virology*, **7**, 428–37.

Kilham, L., Margolis, G. and Colby, E.D. 1967. Congenital infections of cats and ferrets by feline panleukopenia virus manifested by cerebellar hypoplasia. *Lab Invest*, **17**, 465–80.

King, J.A., Dubielzig, R., et al. 2001. DNA helicase-mediated packaging of adeno-associated virus type 2 genomes into preformed capsids. *EMBO J*, **20**, 3282–91.

Klenerman, P., Tolfvenstam, T., et al. 2002. T lymphocyte responses against human parvovirus B19: small virus, big response. *Pathol Biol (Paris)*, **50**, 317–25.

Koonin, E.V. and Ilyina, T.V. 1993. Computer-assisted dissection of rolling circle DNA replication. *Biosystems*, **30**, 241–68.

Kotin, R.M., Siniscalco, M., et al. 1990. Site-specific integration by adeno-associated virus. *Proc Natl Acad Sci USA*, **87**, 2211–15.

Kotin, R.M., Linden, R.M. and Berns, K.I. 1992. Characterization of a preferred site on human chromosome 19q for integration of adeno-associated virus DNA by non-homologous recombination. *EMBO J*, **11**, 5071–8.

Labow, M.A., Hermonat, P.L. and Berns, K.I. 1986. Positive and negative autoregulation of the adeno-associated virus type 2 genome. *J Virol*, **60**, 251–8.

Lamartina, S., Sporeno, E., et al. 2000. Characteristics of the adeno-associated virus preintegration site in human chromosome 19: open chromatin conformation and transcription-competent environment. *J Virol*, **74**, 7671–7.

Legendre, D. and Rommelaere, J. 1994. Targeting of promoters for *trans* activation by a carboxy-terminal domain of the NS-1 protein of the parvovirus minute virus of mice. *J Virol*, **68**, 7974–85.

Linden, R.M., Ward, P., et al. 1996. Site-specific integration by adeno-associated virus. *Proc Natl Acad Sci USA*, **93**, 11288–94.

Liu, J.M., Green, S.W., et al. 1992. A block in full-length transcript maturation in cells nonpermissive for B19 parvovirus. *J Virol*, **66**, 4686–92.

Lombardo, E., Ramirez, J.C., et al. 2002. Complementary roles of multiple nuclear targeting signals in the capsid proteins of the parvovirus minute virus of mice during assembly and onset of infection. *J Virol*, **76**, 7049–59.

Lopez-Bueno, A., Mateu, M.G. and Almendral, J.M. 2003. High mutant frequency in populations of a DNA virus allows evasion from antibody therapy in an immunodeficient host. *J Virol*, **77**, 2701–8.

Marcus, C.J., Laughlin, C.A. and Carter, B.J. 1981. Adeno-associated virus RNA transcription in vivo. *Eur J Biochem*, **121**, 147–54.

Maroto, B., Ramirez, J.C. and Almendral, J.M. 2000. Phosphorylation status of the parvovirus minute virus of mice particle: mapping and biological relevance of the major phosphorylation sites. *J Virol*, **74**, 10892–902.

Maroto, B., Valle, N., et al. 2004. Nuclear export of the non-enveloped parvovirus virion is directed by an unordered protein signal exposed on the capsid surface. *J Virol*, **78**, 10685–94.

Maxwell, I.H. and Maxwell, F. 2004. Parvovirus LuIII transducing vectors packaged by LuIII versus FPV capsid proteins: the VP1 N-terminal region is not a major determinant of human cell permissiveness. *J Gen Virol*, **85**, 1251–7.

Maxwell, I.H., Spitzer, A.L., et al. 1995. The capsid determinant of fibrotropism for the MVMp strain of minute virus of mice functions via VP2 and not VP1. *J Virol*, **69**, 5829–32.

Maxwell, I.H., Terrell, K.L. and Maxwell, F. 2002. Autonomous parvovirus vectors. *Methods*, **28**, 168–81.

Mayor, H.D., Drake, S., et al. 1976. Antibodies to adeno-associated satellite virus and herpes simplex in sera from cancer patients and normal adults. *Am J Obstet Gynecol*, **126**, 100–4.

McCarty, D.M., Monahan, P.E. and Samulski, R.J. 2001. Self-complementary recombinant adeno-associated virus (scAAV) vectors promote efficient transduction independently of DNA synthesis. *Gene Ther*, **8**, 1248–54.

Miller, C.L. and Pintel, D.J. 2002. Interaction between parvovirus NS2 protein and nuclear export factor Crm1 is important for viral egress from the nucleus of murine cells. *J Virol*, **76**, 3257–66.

Miller, D.G., Petek, L.M. and Russell, D.W. 2003. Human gene targeting by adeno-associated virus vectors is enhanced by DNA double-strand breaks. *Mol Cell Biol*, **23**, 3550–7.

Moffatt, S., Yaegashi, N., et al. 1998. Human parvovirus B19 nonstructural (NS1) protein induces apoptosis in erythroid lineage cells. *J Virol*, **72**, 3018–28.

Morgan, W.R. and Ward, D.C. 1986. Three splicing patterns are used to excise the small intron common to all minute virus of mice RNAs. *J Virol*, **60**, 1170–4.

Mortimer, P.P., Humphries, R.K., et al. 1983a. A human parvovirus-like virus inhibits haematopoietic colony formation in vitro. *Nature*, **302**, 426–9.

Mortimer, P.P., Luban, N.L., et al. 1983b. Transmission of serum parvovirus-like virus by clotting-factor concentrates. *Lancet*, **2**, 482–4.

Mouw, M.B. and Pintel, D.J. 2000. Adeno-associated virus RNAs appear in a temporal order and their splicing is stimulated during coinfection with adenovirus. *J Virol*, **74**, 9878–88.

Musatov, S., Roberts, J., et al. 2002. A *cis*-acting element that directs circular adeno-associated virus replication and packaging. *J Virol*, **76**, 12792–802.

Myers, M.W. and Carter, B.J. 1980. Assembly of adeno-associated virus. *Virology*, **102**, 71–82.

Naeger, L.K., Cater, J. and Pintel, D.J. 1990. The small nonstructural protein (NS2) of the parvovirus minute virus of mice is required for efficient DNA replication and infectious virus production in a cell-type-specific manner. *J Virol*, **64**, 6166–75.

Nakai, H., Storm, T.A. and Kay, M.A. 2000. Recruitment of single-stranded recombinant adeno-associated virus vector genomes and intermolecular recombination are responsible for stable transduction of liver in vivo. *J Virol*, **74**, 9451–63.

Nakai, H., Montini, E., et al. 2003. AAV serotype 2 vectors preferentially integrate into active genes in mice. *Nat Genet*, **34**, 297–302.

Nguyen, Q.T., Sifer, C., et al. 1999. Novel human erythrovirus associated with transient aplastic anemia. *J Clin Microbiol*, **37**, 2483–7.

Nguyen, Q.T., Wong, S., et al. 2002. Identification and characterization of a second novel human erythrovirus variant, A6. *Virology*, **301**, 374–80.

Ni, T.H., McDonald, W.F., et al. 1998. Cellular proteins required for adeno-associated virus DNA replication in the absence of adenovirus coinfection. *J Virol*, **72**, 2777–87.

Nony, P., Chadeuf, G., et al. 2003. Evidence for packaging of rep-cap sequences into adeno-associated virus (AAV) type 2 capsids in the absence of inverted terminal repeats: a model for generation of rep-positive AAV particles. *J Virol*, **77**, 776–81.

O'Sullivan, M.G., Anderson, D.C., et al. 1994. Identification of a novel simian parvovirus in cynomolgus monkeys with severe anemia. A paradigm of human B19 parvovirus infection. *J Clin Invest*, **93**, 1571–6.

Ogata, T., Kozuka, T. and Kanda, T. 2003. Identification of an insulator in AAVS1, a preferred region for integration of adeno-associated virus DNA. *J Virol*, **77**, 9000–7.

Ohshima, T., Nakajima, T., et al. 1999. CRM1 mediates nuclear export of nonstructural protein 2 from parvovirus minute virus of mice. *Biochem Biophys Res Commun*, **264**, 144–50.

Ozawa, K., Ayub, J., et al. 1987. Novel transcription map for the B19 (human) pathogenic parvovirus. *J Virol*, **61**, 2395–406.

Ozawa, K., Ayub, J., et al. 1988. The gene encoding the nonstructural protein of B19 (human) parvovirus may be lethal in transfected cells. *J Virol*, **62**, 2884–9.

Palmer, G.A. and Tattersall, P. 2000. Autonomous parvoviruses as gene transfer vehicles. *Contrib Microbiol*, **4**, 178–202.

Palmer, G.A., Brogdon, J.L., et al. 2004. A nonproliferating parvovirus vaccine vector elicits sustained, protective humoral immunity following a single intravenous or intranasal inoculation. *J Virol*, **78**, 1101–8.

Parker, J.S. and Parrish, C.R. 2000. Cellular uptake and infection by canine parvovirus involves rapid dynamin-regulated clathrin-mediated endocytosis, followed by slower intracellular trafficking. *J Virol*, **74**, 1919–30.

Parker, J.S., Murphy, W.J., et al. 2001. Canine and feline parvoviruses can use human or feline transferrin receptors to bind, enter, and infect cells. *J Virol*, **75**, 3896–902.

Parrish, C.R. 1991. Mapping specific functions in the capsid structure of canine parvovirus and feline panleukopenia virus using infectious plasmid clones. *Virology*, **183**, 195–205.

Pattison, J.R., Jones, S.E., et al. 1981. Parvovirus infections and hypoplastic crisis in sickle-cell anaemia. *Lancet*, **1**, 664–5.

Paul, P.S., Mengeling, W.L. and Brown, T.T. Jr. 1979. Replication of porcine parvovirus in peripheral blood lymphocytes, monocytes, and peritoneal macrophages. *Infect Immun*, **25**, 1003–7.

Perros, M., Deleu, L., et al. 1995. Upstream CREs participate in the basal activity of minute virus of mice promoter P4 and in its stimulation in ras-transformed cells. *J Virol*, **69**, 5506–15.

Perros, M., Fuks, F., et al. 1999. Atypical nucleoprotein complexes mediate CRE-dependent regulation of the early promoter of minute virus of mice. *J Gen Virol*, **80**, 3267–72.

Pintel, D., Dadachanji, D., et al. 1983. The genome of minute virus of mice, an autonomous parvovirus, encodes two overlapping transcription units. *Nucleic Acids Res*, **11**, 1019–38.

Poole, B.D., Karetnyi, Y.V. and Naides, S.J. 2004. Parvovirus B19-induced apoptosis of hepatocytes. *J Virol*, **78**, 7775–83.

Qing, K., Mah, C., et al. 1999. Human fibroblast growth factor receptor 1 is a co-receptor for infection by adeno-associated virus 2. *Nat Med*, **5**, 71–7.

Qiu, J., Nayak, R. and Pintel, D.J. 2004. Alternative polyadenylation of adeno-associated virus type 5 RNA within an internal intron is governed by both a downstream element within the intron 3′ splice acceptor and an element upstream of the P41 initiation site. *J Virol*, **78**, 83–93.

Ran, Z., Rayet, B., et al. 1999. Parvovirus H-1-induced cell death: influence of intracellular NAD consumption on the regulation of necrosis and apoptosis. *Virus Res*, **65**, 161–74.

Rayet, B., Lopez-Guerrero, J.A., et al. 1998. Induction of programmed cell death by parvovirus H-1 in U937 cells: connection with the tumor necrosis factor alpha signalling pathway. *J Virol*, **72**, 8893–903.

Rhode 3rd, S.L. 1985. *trans*-Activation of parvovirus P38 promoter by the 76K noncapsid protein. *J Virol*, **55**, 886–9.

Richards, R.G. and Armentrout, R.W. 1979. Early events in parvovirus replication: lack of integration by minute virus of mice into host cell DNA. *J Virol*, **30**, 397–9.

Robey, R.E., Woodman, D.R. and Hetrick, F.M. 1968. Studies on the natural infection of rats with the Kilham rat virus. *Am J Epidemiol*, **88**, 139–43.

Rollag, H., Patou, G., et al. 1991. Prevalence of antibodies against parvovirus B19 in Norwegians with congenital coagulation factor defects treated with plasma products from small donor pools. *Scand J Infect Dis*, **23**, 675–9.

Rommelaere, J. and Cornelis, J.J. 1991. Antineoplastic activity of parvoviruses. *J Virol Meth*, **33**, 233–51.

Rooney, C.P., Denning, G.M., et al. 2002. Bronchoalveolar fluid is not a major hindrance to virus-mediated gene therapy in cystic fibrosis. *J Virol*, **76**, 10437–43.

Rubio, M.P., Guerra, S. and Almendral, J.M. 2001. Genome replication and postencapsidation functions mapping to the nonstructural gene restrict the host range of a murine parvovirus in human cells. *J Virol*, **75**, 11573–82.

Russell, S.J., Brandenburger, A., et al. 1992. Transformation-dependent expression of interleukin genes delivered by a recombinant parvovirus. *J Virol*, **66**, 2821–8.

Rutledge, E.A., Halbert, C.L. and Russell, D.W. 1998. Infectious clones and vectors derived from adeno-associated virus (AAV) serotypes other than AAV type 2. *J Virol*, **72**, 309–19.

Schmidt, O.W., Cooney, M.K. and Foy, H.M. 1975. Adeno-associated virus in adenovirus type 3 conjunctivitis. *Infect Immun*, **11**, 1362–70.

Segovia, J.C., Real, A., et al. 1991. In vitro myelosuppressive effects of the parvovirus minute virus of mice (MVMi) on hematopoietic stem and committed progenitor cells. *Blood*, **77**, 980–8.

Segovia, J.C., Bueren, J.A. and Almendral, J.M. 1995. Myeloid depression follows infection of susceptible newborn mice with the parvovirus minute virus of mice (strain i). *J Virol*, **69**, 3229–32.

Segovia, J.C., Gallego, J.M., et al. 1999. Severe leukopenia and dysregulated erythropoiesis in SCID mice persistently infected with the parvovirus minute virus of mice. *J Virol*, **73**, 1774–84.

Shade, R.O., Blundell, M.C., et al. 1986. Nucleotide sequence and genome organization of human parvovirus B19 isolated from the serum of a child during aplastic crisis. *J Virol*, **58**, 921–36.

Siegl, G. 1984. Biology and pathogenicity of autonomous parvoviruses. In: Berns, K.I. (ed.), *The parvoviruses*. New York: Plenum, 297–362, Chapter 8.

Siegl, G. 1988. Patterns of parvoviral disease in animals. In: Pattison, J.R. (ed.), *Parvoviruses and human disease*. Boca Raton: CRC Press, 43–68, Chapter 3.

Singer, I.I. and Rhode 3rd, S.L. 1978. Ultrastructural studies of H-1 parvovirus replication. VI. simultaneous autoradiographic and immunochemical intranuclear localization of viral DNA synthesis and protein accumulation. *J Virol*, **25**, 349–60.

Smith, R.H. and Kotin, R.M. 1998. The Rep52 gene product of adeno-associated virus is a DNA helicase with 3′-to-5′ polarity. *J Virol*, **72**, 4874–81.

Smith-Whitley, K., Zhao, H., et al. 2004. Epidemiology of human parvovirus B19 in children with sickle cell disease. *Blood*, **103**, 422–7.

Snyder, R.O., Samulski, R.J. and Muzyczka, N. 1990. In vitro resolution of covalently joined AAV chromosome ends. *Cell*, **60**, 105–13.

Soderlund-Venermo, M., Hokynar, K., et al. 2002. Persistence of human parvovirus B19 in human tissues. *Pathol Biol (Paris)*, **50**, 307–16.

Song, S., Laipis, P.J., et al. 2001. Effect of DNA-dependent protein kinase on the molecular fate of the rAAV2 genome in skeletal muscle. *Proc Natl Acad Sci USA*, **98**, 4084–8.

Spalholz, B.A. and Tattersall, P. 1983. Interaction of minute virus of mice with differentiated cells: strain-dependent target cell specificity is mediated by intracellular factors. *J Virol*, **46**, 937–43.

Sprecher-Goldberger, S., Dekegel, D., et al. 1970. Incidence of antibodies to adenovirus-associated viruses in patients with tumours or other diseases. *Arch Ges Virusforsch*, **30**, 16–21.

Sprecher-Goldberger, S., Thiry, L., et al. 1971. Complement-fixation antibodies to adenovirus-associated viruses, cytomegaloviruses and herpes simplex viruses in patients with tumors and in control individuals. *Am J Epidemiol*, **94**, 351–8.

Summerford, C. and Samulski, R.J. 1998. Membrane-associated heparan sulfate proteoglycan is a receptor for adeno-associated virus type 2 virions. *J Virol*, **72**, 1438–45.

Summerford, C., Bartlett, J.S. and Samulski, R.J. 1999. AlphaVbeta5 integrin: a co-receptor for adeno-associated virus type 2 infection. *Nat Med*, **5**, 78–82.

Summers, J., Jones, S.E. and Anderson, M.J. 1983. Characterization of the genome of the agent of erythrocyte aplasia permits its classification as a human parvovirus. *J Gen Virol*, **64**, 2527–32.

Sun, L., Li, J. and Xiao, X. 2000. Overcoming adeno-associated virus vector size limitation through viral DNA heterodimerization. *Nat Med*, **6**, 599–602.

Tattersall, P. and Cotmore, S.F. 1986. The rodent parvoviruses. In: Bhatt, P.N., Jacoby, R.O., et al. (eds), *Viral and mycoplasma infections of laboratory rodents: effect on biomedical research*. New York: Academic Press, 305–48.

Tattersall, P. and Gardiner, E.M. 1990. Autonomous parvovirus host–cell interactions. In: Tijssen, P. (ed.), *The Parvoviruses*, Vol. 1. Boca Raton: CRC Press, 111–22, Chapter 7.

Tattersall, P. and Ward, D.C. 1976. Rolling hairpin model for replication of parvovirus and linear chromosomal DNA. *Nature*, **263**, 106–9.

Tattersall, P. and Bergoin, M. 2005. The Parvoviridae. In: Fauquet, C.M., Mayo, M.A., et al. (eds), *Virus taxonomy, VIIIth Report of the ICTV*. London: Elsevier/Academic Press.

Thomas, C.E., Storm, T.A., et al. 2004. Rapid uncoating of vector genomes is the key to efficient liver transduction with pseudotyped adeno-associated virus vectors. *J Virol*, **78**, 3110–22.

Toolan, H.W. 1961. A virus associated with transplantable human tumors. *Bull NY Acad Med*, **37**, 305–10.

Toolan, H.W. and Ledinko, N. 1968. Inhibition by H-1 virus of the incidence of tumors produced by adenovirus 12 in hamsters. *Virology*, **35**, 475–8.

Toolan, H.W., Rhode 3rd, S.L. and Gierthy, J.F. 1982. Inhibition of 7,12-dimethylbenz(a)anthracene-induced tumors in Syrian hamsters by prior infection with H-1 parvovirus. *Cancer Res*, **42**, 2552–5.

Truyen, U. and Parrish, C.R. 1992. Canine and feline host ranges of canine parvovirus and feline panleukopenia virus: distinct host cell tropisms of each virus in vitro and in vivo. *J Virol*, **66**, 5399–408.

Tsao, J., Chapman, M.S., et al. 1991. The three-dimensional structure of canine parvovirus and its functional implications. *Science*, **251**, 1456–64.

Urcelay, E., Ward, P., et al. 1995. Asymmetric replication in vitro from a human sequence element is dependent on adeno-associated virus Rep protein. *J Virol*, **69**, 2038–46.

Vihinen-Ranta, M., Yuan, W. and Parrish, C.R. 2000. Cytoplasmic trafficking of the canine parvovirus capsid and its role in infection and nuclear transport. *J Virol*, **74**, 4853–9.

Wagner, J.A., Nepomuceno, I.B., et al. 2002. A phase II, double-blind, randomized, placebo-controlled clinical trial of tgAAVCF using maxillary sinus delivery in patients with cystic fibrosis with antrostomies. *Hum Gene Ther*, **13**, 1349–59.

Walters, R.W., Yi, S.M., et al. 2001. Binding of adeno-associated virus type 5 to 2,3-linked sialic acid is required for gene transfer. *J Biol Chem*, **276**, 20610–16.

Ward, P. and Berns, K.I. 1995. Minimum origin requirements for linear duplex AAV DNA replication in vitro. *Virology*, **209**, 692–5.

Ward, P., Dean, F.B., et al. 1998. Role of the adenovirus DNA-binding protein in in vitro adeno-associated virus DNA replication. *J Virol*, **72**, 420–7.

Wetzel, K., Menten, P., et al. 2001. Transduction of human MCP-3 by a parvoviral vector induces leukocyte infiltration and reduces growth of human cervical carcinoma cell xenografts. *J Gene Med*, **3**, 326–37.

Willwand, K., Moroianu, A., et al. 2002. Specific interaction of the nonstructural protein NS1 of minute virus of mice (MVM) with [ACCA](2) motifs in the centre of the right-end MVM DNA palindrome induces hairpin-primed viral DNA replication. *J Gen Virol*, **83**, 1659–64.

Wistuba, A., Kern, A., et al. 1997. Subcellular compartmentalization of adeno-associated virus type 2 assembly. *J Virol*, **71**, 1341–52.

Wu, J., Davis, M.D. and Owens, R.A. 1999. Factors affecting the terminal resolution site endonuclease, helicase and ATPase activities of adeno-associated virus type 2 Rep proteins. *J Virol*, **73**, 8235–44.

Xie, Q. and Chapman, M.S. 1996. Canine parvovirus capsid structure, analyzed at 2.9 A resolution. *J Mol Biol*, **264**, 497–520.

Xie, Q., Bu, W., et al. 2002. The atomic structure of adeno-associated virus (AAV-2), a vector for human gene therapy. *Proc Natl Acad Sci USA*, **99**, 10405–10.

Yan, Z., Zhang, Y., et al. 2000. *Trans*-splicing vectors expand the utility of adeno-associated virus for gene therapy. *Proc Natl Acad Sci USA*, **97**, 6716–21.

Yang, J., Zhou, W., et al. 1999. Concatamerization of adeno-associated virus circular genomes occurs through intermolecular recombination. *J Virol*, **73**, 9468–77.

Yoo, B.C., Lee, D.H., et al. 1999. A novel parvovirus isolated from Manchurian chipmunks. *Virology*, **253**, 250–8.

Young, N.S. and Brown, K.E. 2004. Parvovirus B19. *N Engl J Med*, **350**, 586–97.

Young, S.M. Jr., McCarty, D.M., et al. 2000. Roles of adeno-associated virus Rep protein and human chromosome 19 in site-specific recombination. *J Virol*, **74**, 3953–66.

Zadori, Z., Szelei, J., et al. 2001. A viral phospholipase A2 is required for parvovirus infectivity. *Dev Cell*, **1**, 291–302.

Zentilin, L., Marcello, A. and Giacca, M. 2001. Involvement of cellular double-stranded DNA break binding proteins in processing of the recombinant adeno-associated virus genome. *J Virol*, **75**, 12279–87.

Zerbini, M., Gallinella, G., et al. 2002. Diagnostic procedures in B19 infection. *Pathol Biol (Paris)*, **50**, 332–8.

Zhi, N., Zadori, Z., et al. 2004. Construction and sequencing of an infectious clone of the human parvovirus B19. *Virology*, **318**, 142–52.

Zhou, X. and Muzyczka, N. 1998. In vitro packaging of adeno-associated virus DNA. *J Virol*, **72**, 3241–7.

Zhou, X., Zolotukhin, I., et al. 1999. Biochemical characterization of adeno-associated virus rep68 DNA helicase and ATPase activities. *J Virol*, **73**, 1580–90.

Adenoviruses

WILLIE RUSSELL

The term adenoviruses was coined in 1956 (Enders et al. 1956) to describe infectious agents that had been isolated from human adenoids (Rowe et al. 1953) and were similar to those associated with outbreaks of respiratory disease in military recruits (Hilleman and Werner 1954). The virus family was initially characterized in terms of crossreactivity in serological tests and it soon became apparent that adenoviruses sharing this common antigen were to be found in a wide variety of species. Fundamental studies on adenoviruses and their interactions with their host cells were greatly stimulated by the discovery by Trentin and his colleagues (Trentin et al. 1962) that some human adenovirus serotypes could induce tumors in hamsters. However, later studies could not demonstrate any association with human tumors. This finding, coupled with the observations that adenoviruses did not appear to be associated with any serious morbidity and that they could readily be grown in a wide variety of cell lines, led to their being used extensively as model laboratory systems to study the molecular basis of virus infection (for a review, see Russell 2000).

PROPERTIES OF THE VIRUSES

Classification

Adenoviruses have been characterized primarily on the basis of a common genus-specific antigen and a very characteristic morphology. Serotypes are classified by their ability to induce specific neutralizing antibodies. A serotype can therefore be defined as one that either exhibits no cross-reaction in neutralization with other animal typing antisera or shows a homologous:heterologous neutralization ratio of >16 (in both directions). For ratios of 8 or 16, a serotype assignment is made on the basis of other serological, biophysical, or biochemical differences.

Four families are now recognized using phylogenetic calculations based on distance matrix or parsimony analysis coupled with protein or DNA alignment on any suitable gene. These are the *Mastadenoviridae* isolated from mammals (bovine, canine, caprine, equine, human, murine, ovine, porcine, simian); the *Aviadenoviridae* isolated from birds (duck, fowl, goose, pheasant, turkey); the *Atadenoviridae* isolated from some bovines, birds, and snakes, and the *Siadenoviridae* isolated from frogs, fish, and turkeys, giving a total of at least 170 different viruses. However, the most intensively studied adenoviruses are the 51 serotypes isolated from humans (Russell and Benko 1998; Benko et al. 2000).

Morphology and structure

The virions are non-enveloped, 80–110 nm in diameter and their capsids have icosahedral symmetry (Figures 22.1 and 22.2). They have 240 nonvertex capsomeres (hexons) 8–10 nm in diameter and 12 vertex capsomeres (pentons). The pentons consist of penton bases and attached knobbed fibers, each in close association with a ring of five hexons; these are termed the peripentonal hexons. Each of the penton bases has one (or occasionally two) fibers that protrude 9–30 mm from the capsid. Several other structural polypeptides (IIIa, VI, VIII, IX) are associated with the capsid and serve to cement the hexons and to link the capsid to the core (Stewart et al. 1993). The latter consists of a double-stranded DNA genome with a covalently linked terminal

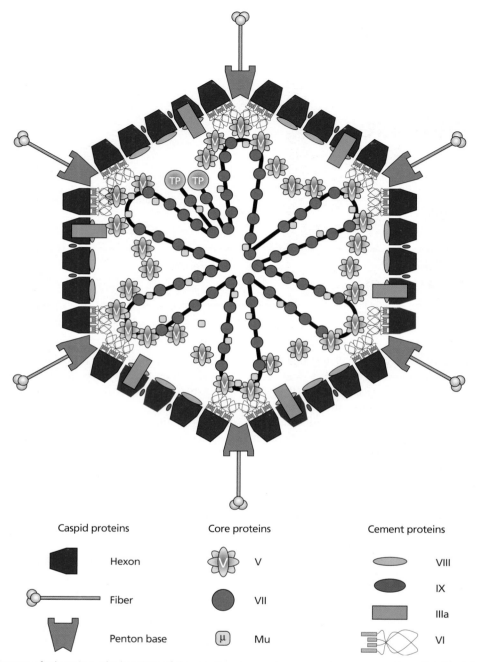

Figure 22.1 *Structure of adenovirus. The locations of the capsid and cement components are reasonably well defined. By contrast, the dispositions of the core components are largely conjectural. (Redrawn from Figure 1 of Russell (2000), with permission of the Society for General Microbiology)*

protein (TP) in tight association with three other polypeptides, V, VII, and mu (Figure 22.1). The structure of this nucleoprotein core has not been established and the core polypeptides are shown in hypothetical locations in Figure 22.1. The major capsid protein, the hexon, has been crystallized and its three-dimensional structure shown to be based on a composite of three identical and interlocking polypeptide chains that form a triangular tower superimposed on a pseudohexagonal base (Stewart and Burnett 1995). The fiber knob has also been crystallized and a structure obtained (van

Raaij 1999). The virus is stable between pH 6.0 and 9.5, is resistant to chloroform, ether, and fluorocarbons, and on heating to 56°C disintegrates, releasing core structures (Russell et al. 1967).

On examination by electron microscopy, some preparations of adenoviruses are seen to be contaminated by small round adeno-associated viruses (Figure 22.2). These ssDNA parvoviruses belong to the family *Dependoviridae* (see Chapter 21, Parvoviruses) and require adenoviruses (or herpesviruses) for their replication.

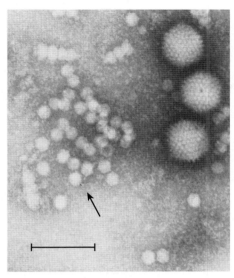

Figure 22.2 *Three adenovirus virions with dependoviruses (arrowed), negatively stained with phosphotungstic acid. Scale bar, 100 nm.*

Genome structure and function

The adenovirus virion contains a single linear dsDNA genome of approximately 20–25 kb. A virus-coded terminal protein is covalently linked to the 5′ end of each DNA strand. The genome of the prototype human adenovirus type 2 has 35 937 bp and contains inverted terminal repeats (ITR) of 103 bp. A large number of other adenoviruses have been completely sequenced and all contain ITRs, but of variable length. Viruses replicate in the nuclei of a wide variety of cells of the species that they normally infect, giving a characteristic pattern of nuclear staining. Some adenoviruses can infect cells of other species; such infections are often abortive and, under suitable conditions, may give rise to morphological transformation and thereby provide model systems for oncogenesis (see below).

Entry of virus is by attachment of the fiber via its knob (Figure 22.1) to cell receptors, the major one being termed coxsackie adenovirus receptor (CAR) (Bergelson et al. 1997). Some human serotypes can also utilize sialoglycoproteins as receptors (Arnberg et al. 2002). It is interesting that human adenovirus 41 has two fibers and only one recognizes the CAR. Since this virus readily infects cells of the gastrointestinal tract and produces diarrhea, it seems likely that one of the fibers may adsorb to enterocytes. Internalization of the virus particles with the penton bases interacting with cellular integrins via clathrin-coated vesicles is followed by transfer into endosomes. Thereafter, the virus capsid is partially disrupted by a virus-coded protease (Greber et al. 1996) and then transported to the nuclear pores where the virus DNA, probably in close association with the core components, is delivered into the nucleus and becomes attached to the nuclear matrix via the viral

terminal protein (Fredman and Engler 1993). A series of nuclear and nucleolar perturbations then follow in which transcription and virus DNA replication are prominent (see Russell and Matthews 2003)

The adenovirus genome becomes available for transcription using cellular transcription factors that are abundant in the nuclear matrix. This process is well regulated and involves the synthesis of four major classes of 'early' transcripts (E1–E4), minor 'intermediate' transcripts, and late transcripts (L1–L5). The last are initiated at the 'major late promoter' and, allied to a tripartite leader formed by a series of splicing events, drive the synthesis of most of the structural proteins; the 'early' transcripts are also subject to complex splicing mechanisms. The overall nature of transcriptional regulation has not been completely elucidated but it has been suggested that as well as splicing control, the topology of the virus genome can be affected by the core proteins limiting template availability for transcription. After synthesis of the early transcripts and synthesis of 'early' proteins [e.g. virus DNA-binding protein (DBP)], further alterations in template topology and availability could permit virus DNA replication, thereby creating new progeny templates for late transcription (see Figure 22.3). However, all these transcriptional events are subject to other regulatory controls of a quite complex nature (see Russell 2000).

Virus DNA replication

Adenovirus DNA synthesis is initiated at either end of the linear double-stranded DNA and three 'early' viral proteins are required together with at least three cellular proteins. The initial event involves the interaction of one of the early proteins, the precursor of the terminal protein (pTP), with specific terminal DNA sequences followed by association with another early protein (polymerase) and then the formation of an ester bond between the phosphate of dCMP (C being the first nucleotide in the DNA sequence) and a serine residue in pTP. This can then function as a primer to extend a progeny DNA strand using one strand of the virus DNA as template; this process utilizes the viral polymerase and the cooperation of three other proteins, two of them cellular. The latter (NF1 and NF3) are also transcription factors and bind to specific sequences in the viral DNA, presumably facilitating the formation of the initiation complex. The other early virus protein, the DBP, also plays a role in virus DNA initiation as well as facilitating strand separation during elongation and binding to the progeny DNA strands. A third cellular protein (NF2) seems to be required for complete elongation of the progeny strand and appears to be equivalent to cellular topoisomerase I. Synthesis of the second strands takes place after that of the first strands and the formation of

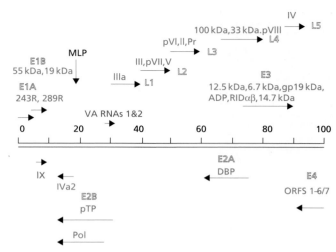

Figure 22.3 *Transcription of the adenovirus genome. The early (E) transcripts are outlined in green. The components of each cassette are named in a conventional manner, e.g. some are merely numbered as open reading frames (orfs) and others defined by their molecular weights or by the number of amino acids. The late (L) transcripts are outlined in blue. MLP refers to the major late promoter. The transcripts IX, IVa2 and the VA RNAs are transcribed late but independently of the MLP. The VA RNAs are not translated and play a significant role in combating cellular defense mechanisms. Arrows indicate the direction of transcription. (From Figure 2 of Russell (2000), with permission from the Society for General Microbiology.)*

a 'panhandle' structure formed by the interacting ITRs, thus allowing replication by a similar mechanism – for a recent review see Liu et al. (2003).

Polypeptides and maturation of the virion

Translation of the adenovirus transcripts begins quite early in infection and continues uninterrupted in concert with virus assembly for up to about 40 hours when both cellular and virus protein synthesis are shut off. In tissue culture systems this process is very inefficient and normally a vast excess of virus capsid proteins are made.

A number of adenovirus genomes have been completely sequenced and the dispositions of the polypeptide genes have been mapped. While there are some differences in the number and position of the polypeptides on the genome across the adenovirus family, on the whole there is good conservation of genome structure. It is also apparent that, by virtue of its splicing mechanisms, the genome makes efficient use of template information and synthesizes about 40 different polypeptides, 13 of these being incorporated into the mature virus particle (see Figure 22.1). Three of the nonstructural proteins synthesized early in infection are involved in virus DNA replication and are derived from the E2 transcription region. The remainder of these 'early' nonstructural proteins seem to function as modulators of the host cell, so that virus transcription and replication are favored, and to counteract the host immune response. It should be noted that not all the 'late' genes are structural: a major product of ca. 100 kDa seems to function as a chaperone for other structural proteins but is not itself encapsidated.

Two other gene products, polypeptides IX and IVa2, are regulated independently of the others and, whereas IX is clearly a structural component, the evidence that IVa2 is structural is not very strong.

The maturation of adenovirus is intimately linked to the functioning of the adenovirus gene-coded 23 kDa protease (Webster et al. 1989). This enzyme is synthesized late in infection and performs cleavages, leading to maturation, on six virus structural proteins: IIIa, pVI, pVII, pVIII, pTP, and protein p-mu. The enzyme is a cysteine protease of an unusual subset and recognizes consensus sequences (M,L,I)XGX↓G or (M,L,I)XGG↓X (Webster et al. 1989). It also has the remarkable characteristic of requiring for activation a disulfide-bonded dimer of an 11-residue peptide derived from the C terminus of polypeptide pVI (Webster et al. 1993). Investigations have also shown that, in an in vitro assay, pVI will bind to the principal capsid component, the hexon, but binding is very significantly enhanced whenever pVI is cleaved by the protease (Matthews and Russell 1995). This suggests that a primary maturation event is the interaction of adenovirus protease with pVI in a 'young' virion, i.e. that formed by the introduction of virus DNA and associated proteins into the precapsid. The protease is then activated, allowing cleavage of pVI to VI accompanied by tight binding to hexons, probably also with conformational changes leading to the proteolytic cascade that marks virion maturation. The encapsidation process is also governed by the presence in the virus DNA of a packaging sequence at the conventional left end and seems to involve the binding of the virus-coded IVa2 protein (Zhang et al. 2001).

These events take place in the cell nucleus and many thousands of virions can be assembled, often in paracrystalline arrays. In some cells the assembly process seems to be inefficient, so that many structural proteins (mostly capsomers) are made in excess and these can also form paracrystalline structures. Release of the virus results from permeabilization of nuclear membranes largely mediated by one of the nonstructural virus proteins (Tollefson et al. 1996). Abortive infections by adenovirus can occur whereby some of the early genes are expressed and, given the appropriate circumstances, can lead to morphological transformation and tumor formation in some animal model systems. There are also indications that adenoviruses can persist in vivo, engendering life-long immunity – see Lukashok and Horwitz (1998).

Antigens

As noted above, adenoviruses can be characterized on the basis of their crossreacting (or 'group') antigens and further subdivided into serotypes based on neutralization. Most adenoviruses can hemagglutinate rat or monkey cells and this characteristic has been used to subgroup the human adenoviruses and to confirm serospecificity (Table 22.1). These subgroups also correlate to some extent with clinical patterns (see Table 22.2) and with the ability to induce tumors in hamsters. The utility of these serological assays has undoubtedly been enhanced by the relatively large amount of antigens (mostly associated with the capsomers) released during infection.

The serotype-specific antigens are located on the surface of the virions and are responsible for the formation of the neutralizing antibodies. Both hexons and fibers can induce neutralizing antibodies, whereas pentons and fibers appear to function in hemagglutination. The hexon serotype-specific antigens can be assigned to the tower regions of the structure whereas the genus-specific antigens seem to reside on the basal surfaces of the hexons at the region where they interact with each other and with polypeptide VI.

A range of hexon and fiber monoclonal antibodies has been prepared and has been instrumental in defining type and group specificities as well as antigenic relationships both within and between subgroups (Watson et al. 1988).

Classification of adenoviruses by serological procedures was later supplemented by restriction enzyme analysis of virus DNA extracted from infected cells. By using a defined and limited range of restriction enzymes, patterns characteristic of adenovirus serotypes can be obtained; furthermore, this approach allows further analysis of serotypes into defined 'genotypes' – see Kajon et al. (1996). However, with the increasing availability of sequence data it has become possible to apply phylogenetic analyses to adenovirus classification and this has now become the method of choice and can even be applied in the absence of isolation of the infectious virus (e.g. Benko et al. 2002).

CLINICAL AND PATHOLOGICAL ASPECTS

Adenoviruses are widespread in many species and can be isolated from both sick and healthy individuals. Antibodies can be detected in almost all humans, reflecting infection early in childhood and possibly lifelong persistence in adenoid and lung tissues. Mortality and morbidity associated with infection are relatively low and undoubtedly ensure that the virus retains its biological niche. Nevertheless, pneumonia and gastrointestinal disease can be serious especially when immunological status is impaired – as is the case for patients with the acquired immunodeficiency syndrome (AIDS) and those undergoing transplantation procedures.

Clinical manifestations

Adenovirus infections are mostly asymptomatic but may be associated with diseases of the respiratory, ocular,

Table 22.1 *Subgrouping of human adenoviruses: hemagglutination and oncogenicity*

Subgroup[a]	Serotypes	Species giving hemagglutination titers	Oncogenicity in hamsters
A	12, 18, 31	Rat (incomplete)	High
B	3, 7, 11, 14, 16, 21, 34, 35	Monkey	Weak
C	1, 2, 5, 6	Rat (incomplete)	No
D	8, 9, 37	Rat, mouse, human, guinea pig, dog	No
	10, 19, 26, 27, 36, 38, 39	Rat, mouse, human	
	13, 43	Rat, mouse, human, monkey	
	15, 22, 23, 30, 44–47	Rat, mouse, monkey	
	17, 24, 32, 33, 42	Rat, mouse	
	20, 25, 28, 29	Rat, monkey	
E	4	Rat (incomplete)	No
F	40, 41	Rat (atypical)	No

a) The subgrouping is based on a variety of criteria: differential hemagglutination, fiber length, oncogenic potential in rodents, percentage DNA homology, G+C content of viral DNAs, and the ability to recombine with other members of the subgroup (see Horwitz 1990 for a more detailed explanation). Table derived from information presented by Hierholzer (1992) and Horwitz (1990).

Table 22.2 *Subgrouping of human adenoviruses: association with disease*

Syndrome	A	B	C	D	E	F
Upper respiratory illness	. . .	All	. . .	. . .	. . .	. . .
Lower respiratory illness	. . .	3, 7, 21	. . .	. . .	4	. . .
Pertussis syndrome	. . .	. . .	5	. . .	. . .	. . .
Acute respiratory disease	. . .	7, 21	. . .	. . .	4	. . .
Pharyngoconjunctival fever	. . .	3, 7	. . .	. . .	4	. . .
Epidemic keratoconjunctivitis	. . .	. . .	. . .	8, 19, 37	. . .	. . .
Acute hemorrhagic conjunctivitis	. . .	11	. . .	. . .	. . .	. . .
Acute hemorrhagic cystitis	. . .	7, 11, 21, 35	. . .	. . .	. . .	. . .
Immunocompromised host disease	31	All	All	29, 30, 37, 43, 45	. . .	. . .
Infant gastroenteritis[a]	31	. . .	2	. . .	. . .	40, 41
Central nervous system disease	. . .	3, 7	. . .	. . .	. . .	. . .
Sexually transmitted disease[b]	. . .	. . .	2	19, 37	. . .	. . .

a) Gastroenteritis is due predominantly to types 40 and 41 and to a lesser extent to types 2 and 31.
b) Penile and labial ulcers and urethritis. Table derived mainly from information presented by Hierholzer (1992) and Horwitz (1990).

and gastrointestinal systems (Table 22.2). Volunteers have been infected by rubbing virus into their conjunctivae or by administration of aerosols but, in general, it has been difficult to demonstrate unequivocally that the viruses cause disease, because they can be found in apparently normal tonsils and adenoids. Infections with human adenovirus serotypes 1, 2, 3, 5, and 6 usually take place in early childhood, giving mild respiratory infections. It has been suggested that these infections may well induce sufficient immunological defenses to modulate the progress of subsequent infections by related serotypes. The importance of adenoviruses in pediatric respiratory tract infection is not as great as that of respiratory syncytial and parainfluenza viruses, and it has been estimated that only about 5–10 percent of pediatric respiratory infection can be attributed to them. Nevertheless, acute respiratory infections occur in children and in immunocompromised children disseminated disease (with some mortality) has been reported, particularly in association with types 3 and 7 and even with type 5 (Munoz et al. 1998). Adenoviruses have also been reported to account for 10 percent of pneumonia in children and are a particular threat in developing countries where there is malnutrition and exposure to measles (for a review see Wadell 2000). Respiratory infections may also be important in military recruits, of whom 30–80 percent may become infected, usually with types 4, 7, 14, or 21; up to 20 percent may require hospitalization. This morbidity had such an effect on training schedules that the US government invested heavily in the development of appropriate vaccines. Explosive outbreaks have also been reported in boarding schools and other institutions where young people live in close association.

Pharyngoconjunctival fever is another well-defined clinical syndrome that is characterized by conjunctivitis, fever, pharyngitis, and enlargement of the adenoids. This is usually associated with types 3, 4, and 7 and can be disseminated via poorly chlorinated swimming pools.

Epidemic keratoconjunctivitis ('shipyard eye') was first associated with adenovirus type 8, but other serotypes (e.g. 19 and 37) have also been incriminated in this syndrome. Adenovirus type 11 has been associated with hemorrhagic cystitis in school-age boys and cases have been reported after renal and bone marrow transplantation. Adenoviruses are often a serious problem in patients undergoing immunosuppressive treatment and in AIDS patients. Indeed, a range of new serotypes was first isolated from patients with AIDS (e.g. the latest serotypes 50 and 51 – see Schnurr and Dondero 1993; De Jong et al. 1999), suggesting that persistent long-term infection by adenoviruses kept under control by immune surveillance may be the usual situation.

The role of adenoviruses in gastrointestinal disease is, however, much more important; infection of the colon and the gut can cause severe diarrhea and acute gastroenteritis, especially in developing countries. Serotypes 40 and 41 seem to be mainly responsible for these outbreaks and the viruses can be detected in large numbers in the feces of infected children. Up to 15 percent of children hospitalized with acute gastroenteritis can be attributed to these enteric adenoviruses, second only to rotaviruses as the cause of infantile viral diarrhea. It is interesting that fecal shedding of adenoviruses appears to be a characteristic of all serotypes, but types 40 and 41 are particularly associated with enteric disease. The tropisms of these serotypes differ from those of others in that they fail to infect standard tissue cell lines such as HeLa and HEp-2 and require primary human kidney cells or the adenovirus-transformed human cell line 293 (Graham et al. 1977).

Adenovirus infections are common in many animal species. As in humans, they appear to be mostly asymptomatic and there is therefore a paucity of information on the mode and mechanics of virus transmission. There is some evidence that sometimes a virus that is asymptomatic in its natural host can produce disease in other species. Thus epidemics of reduced laying and production of soft shell or shell-less eggs in some chicken flocks have been attributed to a duck adenovirus (EDS'76). As in humans, most of the animal adenoviruses can be isolated from the tissues of healthy animals and there is very little evidence that they cause disease in wild populations. Nevertheless, two serotypes of canine adenovirus (CAdV) do seem to cause different patterns of disease: CAdV-1 is responsible for infectious canine hepatitis and, along with CAdV-2, is among the viruses causing the 'kennel cough' syndrome. Epizootic infections with CAdV-1 in foxes, bears, wolves, coyotes, and skunks have also been reported. CAdV-2, on the other hand, seems to be confined to infections of the canine respiratory tract (reviewed by Russell and Benko 1998).

Epidemiology

Adenovirus infections are widespread and appear to be transmitted primarily by the fecal–oral rather than the respiratory route. The latter may, however, be more important for the lower numbered human serotypes. Seasonal variation of adenovirus epidemics is well recognized. Most outbreaks of pharyngoconjunctival fever in school-age children occur in summer; by contrast, epidemics in military recruits appear almost exclusively in the winter.

Infections with adenoviruses occur early in life: by 5 years of age almost all children have been infected by at least one, generally a low-numbered serotype. The epidemiology of individual serotypes has been elucidated in more detail by using restriction enzyme analysis to distinguish between isolates of type-specific viruses. In this way, the provenance of particular genotypes within these serotypes (e.g. Ad8, Ad19, Ad37) can be traced in the population. Such studies suggest that some genotypes may be associated with increased morbidities. They also indicate that multiple persistent infections probably provide opportunities for recombinational events (for a review see Wadell 2000).

Pathogenesis and pathology

In susceptible cells, adenoviruses cause early rounding and aggregation, followed by the appearance of characteristic basophilic nuclear inclusions. In organ cultures of human embryonic nasal mucosa and trachea, they infect and destroy the ciliated epithelium and it is likely that the same process occurs in vivo. Although organs outside the respiratory tract may be affected (eg liver and kidney) during severe adenovirus infection, replication rarely occurs unless the patient is immunologically compromised.

Considerable progress has been made in our understanding of adenovirus pathogenesis by studies in cotton rats (*Sigmodon hispidus*). These animals are susceptible to intranasal infection with human adenovirus type 5 (and other members of subgroup C), developing pulmonary histopathology very similar to that in human cases. The virus replicates in the bronchiolar epithelial cells, but in situ hybridization also shows early gene expression in macrophages/monocytes and in both alveoli and hilar lymph nodes. It is interesting that only early gene expression is needed to produce the pathology, of which there is an 'early' and a 'late' phase (for a review see Ginsberg 1999).

It is now well established that at the molecular level host pathology is largely governed by the success or otherwise of the ability of the invading virus to evade the host protective responses. In general, host cells have a range of strategies to combat infection: these can be considered as innate and adaptive. In the first category can be included the natural antimicrobial peptides (defensins) released by epithelial cells. Some tissues on receiving the appropriate signal (e.g. when a virus particle interacts with the plasma membrane) are able to release multiple chemokines which in turn recruit neutrophils and invoke an inflammatory response. One key factor in regulating the innate response is the activation of the cellular transcription factor NFκB (Dixit and Mak 2002).

Interferons are an important component of the innate response but adenoviruses are generally refractive to interferons mainly because their early gene products can down-regulate components of the cellular pathways that are activated by interferons. Another mechanism that can be utilized by cells under attack is to commit suicide by switching on their apoptosis circuits. A key regulator of these events is the tumor suppressor p53 which controls both cell cycle arrest and apoptosis (Ljungman 2000). Once again, early virus gene products can interfere with these pathways in a variety of ways (for a review see Russell 2000).

Immune response

The response to adenovirus infection by the immune system is efficient and well orchestrated and undoubtedly accounts for the generally low levels of morbidity. Cell-mediated responses are mounted but the virus can counteract most of these by means of products expressed from the early genes. For example, one of these is an abundant transmembrane protein which binds class I major histocompatibility complex (MHC) antigens and retains the complex in the endoplasmic reticulum. Since surface expression of class I antigens complexed with viral peptides is required for recognition and lysis by virus-specific cytotoxic T cells (CTL), this strategy effectively thwarts the host CTL response. Although CTLs are one means by which the host eliminates virus-infected cells, there are others, involving secretion of cytokines such as tumor necrosis factor (TNF) and other early virus gene products are able to interfere with these pathways.

The proliferative T-cell responses in humans are mediated by CD4$^+$ T cells, and structural proteins appear to be important targets. In addition, proliferative responses to the uncommon adenovirus type 35 (Ad35) have been found in individuals without serological evidence of previous Ad35 infection. These findings suggest that CD4$^+$ cells recognize conserved antigens and that this may play a role in modulating infections with a range of serotypes. The mechanisms of the cellular and humoral immune responses have been of intense interest following the development of recombinant adenovirus constructs as vehicles for gene therapy. However, expression of the correct gene is quite often only transient and this seems to be associated with the development of an effective host immune response. For a review of the characteristics of early gene products and adenovirus vectors see Russell 2000.

Diagnosis

Human adenovirus infections are ideally diagnosed by isolation of virus from appropriate clinical samples in a variety of sensitive indicator cell cultures such as HeLa, HEp-2, KB, or A549. The use of the 293 line of adenovirus-transformed cells (Graham et al. 1977) also facilitates the isolation of the enteric adenoviruses 40 and 41. Rounding and aggregation of cells appear after incubation for 1–4 weeks. The culture fluids containing virus and soluble antigens can be used to characterize the virus further by neutralization and by hemagglutination inhibition assay (see Table 22.1).

More sensitive and rapid tests have been introduced over the last few years and have found a place in many diagnostic laboratories. They include, for example, enzyme immunoassays and immunoelectron microscopy. Characterization of serotypes by restriction enzyme mapping has also been of significant value (see above). However, the most sensitive technique for virus recognition is the polymerase chain reaction (PCR) using primers based on those base sequences that are common to the genus. A number of different primers have been utilized. This technique can be exquisitely sensitive and be used where cellular techniques have not been successful (e.g. in blood and urine samples) (Echavarria et al. 1998). PCR has also been utilized successfully for environmental detection using air filters (Echavarria et al. 2000).

Current developments are using 'real-time' PCR to obtain more semiquantitative data (Houng et al. 2002). The advent of automatic sequencing has added yet another dimension to diagnosis and should assist in more precise characterization of isolates.

Control

Vaccination has been used with some success to control epidemics of adenovirus infection in military recruits and in bovines. Both inactivated and live adenovirus vaccines have been used in military recruits but live vaccines proved more effective in reducing the incidence of disease. Initial development concentrated on type 4 serotype; unattenuated virus was fed to volunteers in enteric-coated capsules to establish an asymptomatic infection in the lower alimentary tract. The virus induced moderate amounts of neutralizing antibody and, more importantly, did not spread to susceptible contacts. The type 4 vaccines grown in human diploid cells have been given to several hundred thousand military recruits with no untoward side-effects and with a significant reduction in morbidity. A triple vaccine incorporating types 4, 7, and 21 was also successful (Takafuji et al. 1979). Vaccine production ceased in 1995 and by 1999 the supplies had been exhausted and, not surprisingly, adenovirus respiratory diseases are again becoming a problem in military recruits. Vaccines have not, in general, been considered for use in the general population since the cost of development, production, and control would be quite substantial and would appear not to be commensurate with the risk of clinically significant infection. However, this position may change with the increasing use of transplantation therapies.

There has been one report of the use of normal human immunoglobulin for combating disseminated adenovirus infection (Munoz et al. 1998) and also one report of the successful use of ribavirin (Arav-Boger et al. 2000) but, as yet, there have been no other signs of a substantiated effective antiviral chemotherapy.

REFERENCES

Arav-Boger, R., Echavarria, M., et al. 2000. Clearance of adenoviral hepatitis with ribavirin therapy in a pediatric liver transplant recipient. *Pediatr Infect Dis J*, **19**, 1097–100.

Arnberg, N., Pring-Akerblom, P. and Wadell, G. 2002. Adenovirus type 37 uses sialic acid as a cellular receptor on chang C cells. *J Virol*, **76**, 8834–41.

Benko, M., Harrach, B. and Russell, W.C. 2000. Family *Adenoviridae*. In: van Regenmortel, M.H.V., Fauquet, C.M., et al. (eds), *Virus Taxonomy – 7th Report of ITCV*. New York/San Diego: Academic Press, 227–38.

Benko, M., Elo, P., et al. 2002. First molecular evidence for the existence of distinct fish and snake adenoviruses. *J Virol*, **76**, 10056–9.

Bergelson, J.M., Cunningham, J.A., et al. 1997. Isolation of a common receptor for Coxsackie B viruses and adenoviruses 2 and 5. *Science*, **275**, 1320–3.

De Jong, J.C., Wermenbol, A.G., et al. 1999. Adenoviruses from human immunodeficiency virus-infected individuals, including two strains that represent new candidate serotypes Ad50 and Ad51 of species B1 and D, respectively. *J Clin Microbiol*, **37**, 3940–5.

Dixit, V. and Mak, T.W. 2002. NF-kappaB signaling. Many roads lead to Madrid. *Cell*, **111**, 615–19.

Echavarria, M., Forman, M., et al. 1998. PCR method for detection of adenovirus in urine of healthy and human immunodeficiency virus-infected individuals. *J Clin Microbiol*, **36**, 3323–6.

Echavarria, M., Kolavic, S.A., et al. 2000. Detection of adenoviruses (AdV) in culture-negative environmental samples by PCR during an AdV-associated respiratory disease outbreak. *J Clin Microbiol*, **38**, 2982–4.

Enders, J.F., Bell, J.A., et al. 1956. 'Adenovirus' – a group name proposed for new respiratory tract viruses. *Science*, **124**, 119–20.

Fredman, J.N. and Engler, J.A. 1993. Adenovirus precursor to terminal protein interacts with the nuclear matrix in vivo and in vitro. *J Virol*, **67**, 3384–95.

Ginsberg, H.S. 1999. The life and times of adenoviruses. *Adv Virus Res*, **54**, 1–13.

Graham, F.L., Smiley, J., et al. 1977. Characteristics of a human cell line transformed by DNA from human adenovirus type 5. *J Gen Virol*, **36**, 59–74.

Greber, U.F., Webster, P., et al. 1996. The role of the adenovirus protease on virus entry into cells. *EMBO J*, **15**, 1766–77.

Hierholzer, J.C. 1992. Adenoviruses in the immunocompromised host. *Clin Microbiol Rev*, **5**, 262–74.

Hilleman, M.R. and Werner, J.R. 1954. Recovery of a new agent from patients with acute respiratory illness. *Proc Soc Exp Biol Med*, **85**, 183–8.

Horwitz, M.S. 1990. *Adenoviridae* and their replication. In: Fields, B.H. and Krupe, D.M. (eds), *Virology*, 2nd edn. New York: Raven Press, 1679–721.

Houng, H.S., Liang, S., et al. 2002. Rapid type-specific diagnosis of adenovirus type 4 infection using a hexon-based quantitative fluorogenic PCR. *Diagn Microbiol Infect Dis*, **42**, 227–36.

Kajon, A.E., Mistchenko, A.S., et al. 1996. Molecular epidemiology of adenovirus acute lower respiratory infections of children in the south cone of South America (1991–1994). *J Med Virol*, **48**, 151–6.

Liu, H., Naismith, J.H. and Hay, R.T. 2003. Adenovirus DNA replication. In: Doerfler, W. and Bohm, P. (eds), *Adenoviruses*. Heidelberg: Springer Verlag, 131–64.

Ljungman, M. 2000. Dial 9-1-1 for p53: mechanisms of p53 activation by cellular stress. *Neoplasia*, **2**, 208–25.

Lukashok, S.A. and Horwitz, M.S. 1998. New perspectives in adenoviruses. *Curr Clin Top Infect Dis*, **18**, 286–305.

Matthews, D.A. and Russell, W.C. 1995. Adenovirus protein–protein interactions: molecular parameters governing the binding of protein VI to hexon and the activation of the adenovirus 23K protease. *J Gen Virol*, **76**, 1959–69.

Munoz, F.M., Piedra, P.A. and Demmler, G.J. 1998. Disseminated adenovirus disease in immunocompromised and immunocompetent children. *Clin Infect Dis*, **27**, 1194–200.

Rowe, W.P., Huebner, R.J., et al. 1953. Isolation of a cytopathic agent from human adenoids undergoing spontaneous degeneration in tissue culture. *Proc Soc Exp Biol Med*, **84**, 570–3.

Russell, W.C. 2000. Update on adenovirus and its vectors. *J Gen Virol*, **81**, 2573–604.

Russell, W.C. and Benko, M. 1998. Animal adenoviruses. In: Granoff, A. and Webster, R. (eds), *Encyclopedia of virology*, 2nd edn. London: Academic Press, 14–21.

Russell, W.C. and Matthews, D.A. 2003. Nuclear perturbations following adenovirus infection. In: Doerfler, W. and Bohm, P. (eds), *Adenoviruses*. Heidelberg: Springer Verlag, 399–413.

Russell, W.C., Valentine, R.C. and Pereira, H.G. 1967. The effect of heat on the anatomy of the adenovirus. *J Gen Virol*, **1**, 509–22.

Schnurr, D. and Dondero, M.E. 1993. Two new candidate adenovirus serotypes. *Intervirology*, **36**, 79–83.

Stewart, P.L. and Burnett, R.M. 1995. Adenovirus structure by X-ray crystallography and electron microscopy. *Curr Top Microbiol Immunol*, **199**, 25–38.

Stewart, P.L., Fuller, D. and Burnett, R. 1993. Difference imaging of adenovirus: bridging the restriction gap between X-ray crystallography and electron microscopy. *EMBO J*, **12**, 2589–99.

Takafuji, E.T., Gaydos, J.C., et al. 1979. Simultaneous administration of live, enteric-coated adenovirus types 4, 7 and 21 vaccines: safety and immunogenicity. *J Infect Dis*, **140**, 48–53.

Tollefson, A.E., Ryerse, J.S., et al. 1996. The E3-11.6-kDa adenovirus death protein (ADP) is required for efficient cell death: characterization of cells infected with adp mutants. *Virology*, **220**, 152–62.

Trentin, J.J., Yabe, Y. and Taylor, G. 1962. The quest for human cancer viruses. *Science*, **137**, 835–41.

van Raaij, M.J., Louis, N., et al. 1999. Structure of the human adenovirus serotype 2 fiber head domain at 1.5 Å resolution. *Virology* , **262**, 333–43.

Wadell, G. 2000. Adenoviruses. In: Zuckerman, A.J., Banatvala, J.E. and Pattison, J.E. (eds), *Principles and practice of clinical virology*. Chichester: John Wiley and Sons Ltd.

Watson, G., Burdon, M.G. and Russell, W.C. 1988. An antigenic analysis of the adenovirus type 2 fibre polypeptide. *J Gen Virol*, **69**, 525–35.

Webster, A., Russell, S., et al. 1989. Characterization of the adenovirus proteinase: substrate specificity. *J Gen Virol*, **70**, 3225–3234.

Webster, A., Hay, R.T. and Kemp, G. 1993. The adenovirus protease is activated by a virus-coded disulphide-linked peptide. *Cell*, **72**, 97–104.

Zhang, W., Low, J.A., et al. 2001. Role for the adenovirus IVa2 protein in packaging of viral DNA. *J Virol*, **75**, 10446–54.

23

Papillomaviruses

MARGARET STANLEY AND MARK PETT

BACKGROUND

Papillomaviruses are small double-stranded DNA viruses that induce warts on cutaneous and mucosal surfaces in many vertebrates, including humans. The infectious nature of warts was shown unequivocally in 1907 by the Italian physician Ciuffo, who demonstrated person-to-person transmission of lesions by cell-free wart filtrates. Seminal aspects of the biology and, in particular, the oncogenic potential of this group of viruses were demonstrated by Richard Shope in the 1930s, when he showed that the cottontail rabbit papillomavirus (CRPV) was the etiologic agent in cutaneous papillomatosis in the rabbit. The use of the electron microscope as a research tool in biology in the 1950s revealed papillomaviruses to be the infectious agent for human warts, but although the viruses were known in 1964 to have a genome consisting of circular double-stranded DNA, biochemical characterization of their proteins was slow because no tissue culture system for virus growth was available. Virus particles had to be obtained from clinical lesions, and the amount of virus in warts was highly variable; thus virions were abundant in plantar warts but sparse in laryngeal and genital warts. These handicaps severely limited immunologic and virologic studies, and until the mid-1970s the general view was that there was only one human papillomavirus (HPV), and that tissue location rather than

virus type dictated the morphology and behavior of the clinical lesions at a specific epithelial surface.

The advent of molecular cloning and recombinant DNA technologies in the 1970s resulted in a complete reversal of this view, revealing an astonishing plurality of both animal and human papillomaviruses. Papillomaviruses (PV), it emerged, were absolutely species specific, such that human PVs could only infect humans, rabbit PV's only rabbits, and so on. They were also exquisitely tissue trophic, and the different clinical lesions were distinct diseases caused by infection with specific groups of HPV types. It became clear that within a species the individual viruses showed a predilection for either skin or internal squamous mucosae, and that within the groups of skin or mucosal viruses they could be separated into high- or low-risk types, depending upon their oncogenic potential. This was shown dramatically in the genital tract. Genital warts were shown to be associated predominantly with HPV-6 and -11 (low-risk human papillomavirus (LR-HPV)) – viruses that were almost never detected in carcinomas, whereas HPV-16, -18, and their close relatives (high-risk human papillomavirus (HR-HPV)) were associated with intraepithelial lesions, particularly in the cervix, and were detected in more than 99 percent of cervical cancers. This association with premalignant and malignant disease in humans dramatically broadened the spectrum of HPV pathogenicity, revealing these viruses to be not just the cause of cosmetic nuisances but also important human pathogens causing life-threatening diseases.

CLASSIFICATION

The papillomaviruses are widespread in nature, infecting a wide range of species (Stanley et al. 1997). Those viruses infecting ungulates are a distinctive group in that they induce fibropapillomas with a distinctive fibroproliferative component in addition to the epithelial wart. The best studied of this group is bovine papillomavirus type 1 (BPV-1), a virus that can infect rodent cells in vitro and induce morphologic transformation, providing a biological assay with which to analyze those viral functions necessary for the induction of cell proliferation. Papillomaviruses are classified according to the species of origin and the degree of relatedness of the viral genomes according to their sequence homology. The virus types are therefore genotypes, not serotypes. PVs have been divided into five clades or supergroups, designated A–E (Chan et al. 1995) (Figure 23.1). The association of specific HPV types and human cancers has focused attention very much on the human viruses. Initially HPV types were distinguished from each other on the basis of molecular hybridization in liquid medium: 50 percent or less homology with a known HPV type defined a new virus type. At the 1995 meeting of the International Papillomavirus Workshop it was agreed that classification be based on the *L1* gene, and that to be classified as a new type there should be 10 percent or more sequence dissimilarity in *L1* compared to all known types. To date, more than 80 HPV types have been fully sequenced, and in addition many more partially characterized types, based on

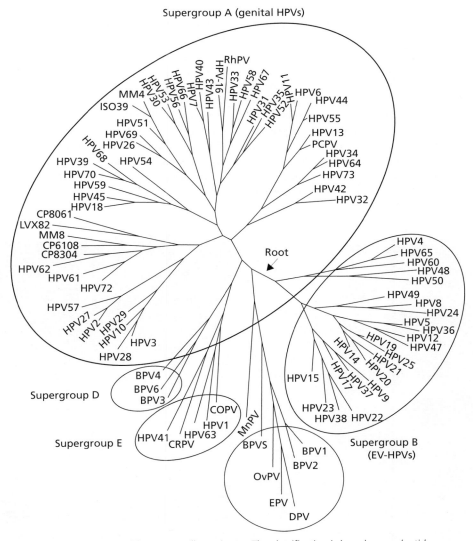

Figure 23.1 *Phylogenetic tree of animal and human papillomaviruses. The classification is based on nucleotide sequence comparisons using a 291-bp segment of L1. Redrawn from Chan et al. 1995, with permission.*

the *L1* open reading frame (ORF) only, have been identified (see the 'HPV sequence database' at www.stdgen.lanl.gov/stdgen/virus/hpv). Phylogenetic relationships between HPV types based on genome sequence variation indicate how these viruses have evolved and their relationship to each other. Interestingly, the clinical distinctions between skin and mucosal warts and benign and malignant lesions correlate with the virus phylogenetic tree.

BIOLOGY OF PAPILLOMAVIRUSES

Viral structure

PV particles are approximately 55 nm in diameter, harboring a single molecule of circular dsDNA of approximately 7.9 kb contained within a spherical icosahedral capsid composed of 72 pentameric capsomeres arranged on a T = 7 surface lattice. The capsomeres exist in two states, one capable of making contact with five neighbors in the 12 pentavalent capsomers, and the other capable of making contact with six neighbors in the 60 hexavalent capsomers (Baker et al. 1991) (Figure 23.2). The capsid is composed of the two structural proteins, the major capsid protein L1 and the minor L2. L1 is about 55 kDa in size and represents about 80 percent of the total viral protein. Expression of L1, either alone or with L2 via mammalian expression systems, results in the formation of virus-like particles (VLP) (Figure 23.2) that are morphologically identical to intact virus particles (Zhou et al. 1991; Kirnbauer et al. 1992; Rose et al. 1993). L1 VLPs are highly immunogenic, generating serum neutralizing antibodies (Christensen et al. 1994), and it is thought that the major neutralizing epitope is within L1. L2 is about 70 kDa, and although not essential for assembly its presence increases the efficiency of VLP production and stability of the VLPs (Hagensee et al. 1993; Kirnbauer et al. 1993; Zhou et al. 1993).

Genome organization of the papillomaviruses

The papillomaviruses exhibit a high degree of conservation of genomic organization (Figure 23.3). The genome can be divided into three domains: a noncoding upstream regulatory region (URR) (also known as the 'long control region'), an 'early' region comprising the ORF E6, E7, E1, E2, E4, and E5 that encode proteins required for regulation of viral DNA replication and viral gene expression, and a 'late' region encoding the L1 and L2 viral capsid proteins. The prefix 'E' or 'L' relates to the position of the ORFs within the genome, and also the timing of expression relative to vegetative viral replication. Only one strand of the dsDNA serves as the template for viral gene expression, coding for a number of polycistronic mRNA transcripts. Transcription is regulated by enhancer sequences located in the URR, which are bound by a number of cellular factors as well as the viral E2 product. The transcription start sites of viral promoters differ depending on the virus type, but in all types promoter usage is differentiation dependent. Figure 23.4 gives a detailed outline of the genomic organization and transcription map of HPV-16.

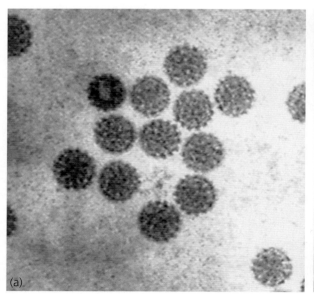
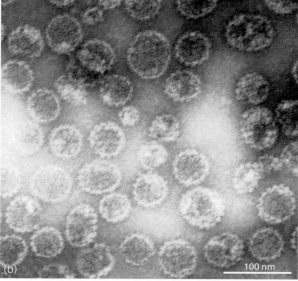

Figure 23.2 *Virus morphology.* **(a)** *Electron micrograph of negatively stained canine oral papillomavirus particles. The virions are about 55 nm in diameter.* **(b)** *HPV 16 L1 virus-like particles (VLPs) produced by expressing L1, the major capsid protein, in a baculovirus expression system. Scale bar = 100 nm.*

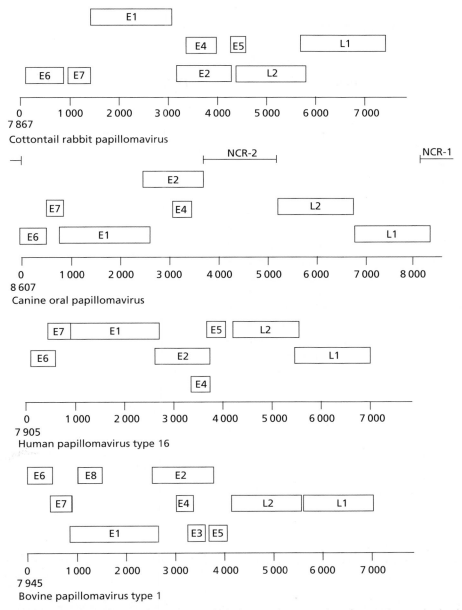

Figure 23.3 *The genomic structure of four papillomaviruses. A high degree of conservation of genomic organization is evident.*

THE INFECTIOUS CYCLE

The virus lifecycle is the key to understanding the pathogenesis of papillomavirus-associated disease. These viruses have an absolutely restricted host range and tissue specificity; in the natural infection papillomaviruses, with the exception of the supergroup C viruses, only infect human keratinocytes or cells with the potential for squamous maturation, such as the reserve cells of the uterine cervix. There is no tissue culture system that supports a complete infectious cycle, i.e. infection of cells in culture with virus and the subsequent generation and release of new infectious virus particles. It is unlikely that the cellular receptor for the virus defines the epithelial tropism, as virions and VLPs will bind to and enter mouse fibroblasts. The nature of the receptor(s) is unclear. The evidence that the $\alpha 6 \beta 4$ integrin is the primary receptor (Evander et al. 1997) has not been supported in all studies (Sibbet et al. 2000), and although there is good evidence that papillomaviruses can bind heparin and cell surface glycoproteins (Joyce et al. 1999) on keratinocytes, such binding is characteristic of many viruses.

The complete infectious cycle is absolutely dependent upon the differentiation program of the keratinocyte. Virus infects keratinocytes in the basal layer of the epithelium, but only in terminally differentiated keratinocytes are viral capsid proteins and virus particles

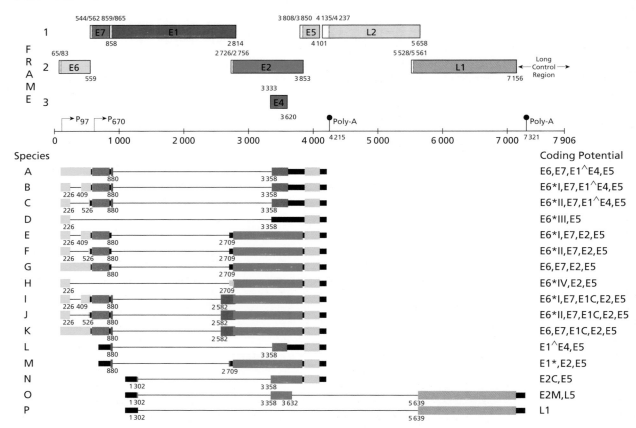

Figure 23.4 *Genomic organization and transcription map of HPV-16. Organization of the linearized HPV-16 genome is presented, illustrating ORFs of functional significance, well-characterized promoters (P97 and P670) and poly(A) signals. The lower panel illustrates previously characterized polycistronic mRNA species coded by the virus. These have been isolated from transfected cells and a variety of tumor cell lines and lesions. Thin black lines and colored bars represent introns and exons, respectively, and the coding potential of each species is indicated to the right. The P97 promoter is active in monolayer culture as well as systems permitting keratinocyte differentiation, and hence is the best characterized.*

assembled (Figure 23.5). Squamous epithelia are usually composed of 20–30 layers of cells exhibiting a coordinated pattern of gene expression concurrent with differentiation. It is thought that HPV infections occur via microwounds, which expose basal cells to viral entry. Despite the lack of unequivocal evidence, the current hypothesis is that the specific target cell for infection is the keratinocyte stem cell that resides within the hair follicle and the basal layer of squamous epithelium (Stanley 2001a). Following infection, viral genomes are established as stable episomes within the host nucleus by amplifying to approximately 20–100 copies per cell: these subsequently replicate coordinately with cellular DNA replication in a phase of plasmid maintenance.

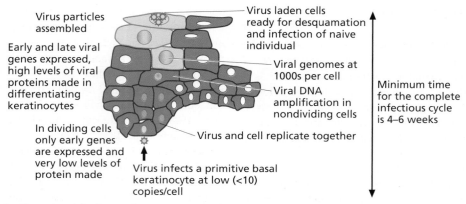

Figure 23.5 *The* Papillomavirus *infectious cycle*

As infected cells migrate up from the basal region and undergo differentiation, cellular replication ceases and, coordinate with the expression of differentiation-specific markers such as filaggrin, activation of differentiation-dependent late gene expression and viral capsid assembly occurs, along with amplification of viral DNA to thousands of copies per cell (Stanley 1994; Stanley et al. 1989). Koilocytes, the pathognomonic cells of papillomavirus infections, are the location of viral DNA amplification, late gene expression, and viral assembly. Productive infection only slightly alters the normal differentiation programme, with the most significant change being the retention of nuclei throughout all layers.

Our knowledge of the temporal and spatial patterns of viral gene expression comes mainly from animal models such as the dog, cow, and rabbit, and the rodent xenograft system first described by Kreider and colleagues (Kreider et al. 1987), which is permissive for vegetative growth of some HPVs. These studies show that in the first 3–4 weeks after infection with large amounts of virus, viral DNA cannot be detected in the epithelium by in situ hybridization (Stoler et al. 1990; Nicholls et al. 1999). At 4–5 weeks viral DNA can be detected in the lower layers of the epithelium and transcripts for the early genes are present. At 5–8 weeks strong signals for viral DNA are detected in the middle to upper layers of the epithelium, and in some cells viral copy number can be of the order of 1 000 or more per cell. E6 and E7 mRNAs are present at low levels in the lower dividing epithelial layers but are highly abundant in the upper differentiating layers. At about 8 weeks post-infection L1 and L2 capsid protein expression can be detected in the most superficial cells of the epithelium. The sequence of events for one of these experimental models, the canine oral papillomavirus (COPV), a low-risk mucosal virus infecting the oropharynx of dogs, is shown in Figure 23.6. There are variations in this spatial and temporal expression pattern and these have recently been elegantly outlined (Peh et al. 2002). Importantly, the high-risk genital HPVs (16, 18, etc.) show a similar spatial and temporal pattern of gene expression, but the regulation of the early genes *E6* and *E7* is under very tight control in the proliferating compartment of the epithelium, with very low levels of mRNA expression in these cells. E6 and E7 mRNAs are expressed abundantly only in the upper stratum spinosum and granulosum (Durst et al. 1992; Higgins et al. 1992).

TARGET CELL FOR INFECTION AND VIRAL LATENCY

The dependence upon the keratinocyte lineage for viral gene expression extends to the target cell for infection. In experimental CRPV infections, viral gene transcription is detected first in the hair follicle, in cells that have the characteristics of stem cells (Schmitt et al. 1996) This is also true in COPV, where viral DNA amplification and early gene transcription are first detected at the extreme tips of the rete ridges, thought to be the site of interfollicular keratinocyte stem cells (Figure 23.6). If the target cell for infection is the stem cell then this does offer an explanation for some interesting aspects of papillomavirus biology. There is, for example, the phenomenon of the lag phase between infection and the first detection of viral DNA and early gene expression. The length of this lag in experimental models such as the rabbit, the dog, and rodent xenografts of HPV 11, is consistently between 3 and 5 weeks. Anecdotal evidence in humans suggests a similar time lag for genital warts (Oriel 1971). One attractive explanation for this is that the virus infects a stem cell in the G_0 phase of the cell cycle. The 3–5-week delay before viral gene expression is detectable would then reflect the time for the stem cell to enter G_1, divide, and for committed daughter cells to enter the transit amplifying population of basal and parabasal cells permissive for viral gene expression.

Dependence upon the stem cell milieu for infection and immediate early viral gene expression would also partly explain the phenomenon of latency. HPV is frequently present as a latent infection in the female genital tract (Toon et al. 1986), and the frequent lesion recurrence observed in respiratory papillomatosis is generally believed to reflect reactivation of latent infection, rather than reinfection (Abramson et al. 1987). This is supported by the observation that histologically normal, but HPV positive, laryngeal tissues express low-abundance transcripts coding for E1 and E2 (Maran et al. 1995). Similarly, in the rabbit, low doses of CRPV lead to viral persistence and expression of truncated E1 and E2 transcripts, but no lesion unless – and until – reactivation is induced by skin irritation (Amella et al. 1994). Furthermore, CRPV can persist at the site of regressed papillomas in 60 percent of cases (Selvakumar et al. 1997) with occasional lesion recurrence, and similar phenomena are seen in BPV (Campo et al. 1994) and COPV infections (Moore et al. 2002). Latency is a poorly understood aspect of papillomavirus biology but clearly of importance for therapeutic and prophylactic intervention strategies.

REGULATION OF GENE EXPRESSION

Papillomavirus transcription is complex owing to the presence of multiple promoters and the differential production of mRNA species in different cells; viral gene expression is regulated both temporally and spatially. Transcription has been most extensively analysed for BPV-1 (Baker 1993), but information is available for the high-risk genital HPVs (Doorbar et al.

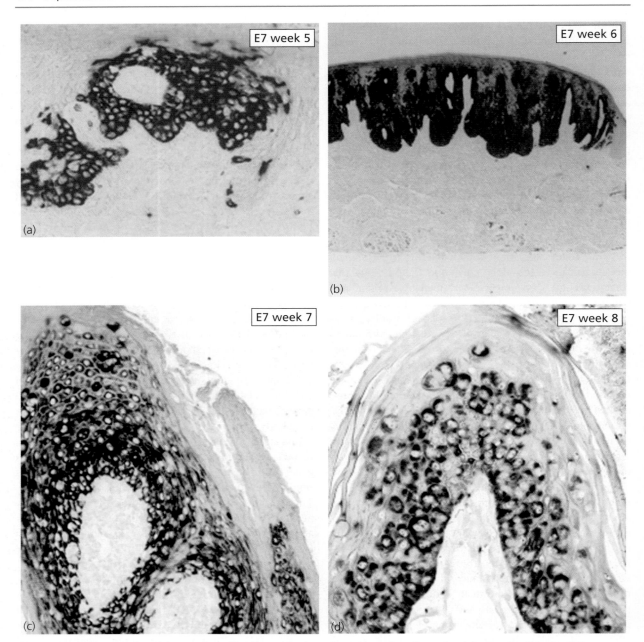

Figure 23.6 *Temporal and spatial expression of Papillomavirus genes in canine oral papillomavirus infection.* **(a–d)** *In situ RNA hybridization of experimental COPV lesions with digoxigenin-labeled E7 probe. Abundant transcripts in detected in early lesions. At week 6 there are abundant basal layer and some suprabasal transcripts persisting through to week 8. (Continued over)*

1990; Stubenrauch and Laimins 1999) and the following discussion concentrates on these.

Early gene expression

Early gene expression of genital HPVs is positively and negatively modulated by a complex interplay between a variety of cellular transcription factors and the viral E2 protein. Early polycistronic transcripts of the HR-HPVs are initiated at the early promoter upstream of the E6 ORF and terminate at a polyadenylation site at the end of the early region (Figure 23.3). The promoter, known as P97 in HPV-16 and HPV-31, and P105 in HPV-18 by virtue of the nucleotide from which transcription is initiated, comprises binding sites (Desaintes and Demeret 1996) for a number of cellular factors that are essential for viral transcription (see Figure 23.4). Binding sites for the viral E2 protein are also located within the early promoter. These allow E2 to exert its function as a transcriptional regulator.

Early gene transcription is further regulated by a *cis*-acting transcriptional enhancer located in the central

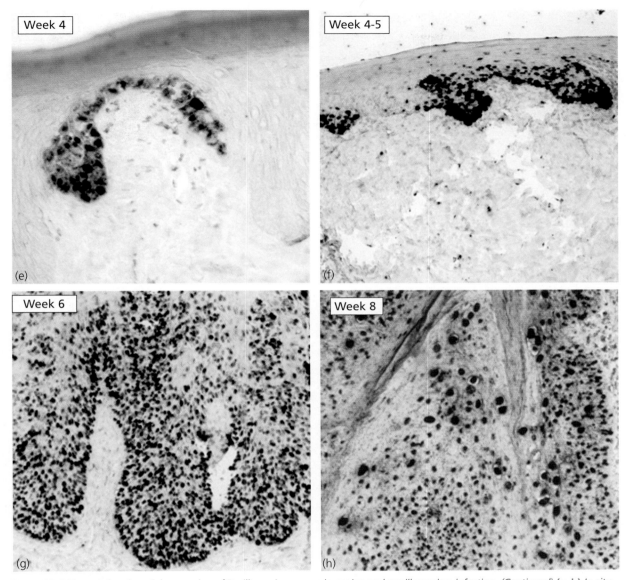

Figure 23.6 *Temporal and spatial expression of* Papillomavirus *genes in canine oral papillomavirus infection. (Continued)* **(e–h)** *In situ DNA hybridization of experimental COPV lesions with a digoxigenin-labeled genomic COPV probe. Viral DNA was undetectable from weeks 1 to 3 post infection. By week 4, viral DNA was found in multiple clusters each arising from a rete ridge. By 6 weeks almost all basal cells and a majority of suprabasal cells were positive for viral DNA. At week 8 sporadic cells in the more superficial epithelium had the strongest signal, together with vacuolated cytoplasm typical of koilocytes. (Continued over)*

region of the URR. This is a major determinant of HPV epithelial tropism, as it is only active in epithelial cells. The epithelial specificity of action appears to be conferred not through the action of keratinocyte-specific activators, but rather through the combinatorial action of multiple ubiquitous cellular transcription factors (Desaintes and Demeret 1996). Although the binding elements for these factors, as well as their spatial organization, vary according to viral type, organization of the enhancer appears quite conserved among the genital HPVs (O'Connor et al. 1995). In the case of the HPV-16 enhancer (see Figure 23.7), identified binding sites that have also been shown to regulate

a number of other genital HPVs include those for NF1 (Apt et al. 1993), AP-1 (Chan et al. 1990), Oct-1 (O'Connor and Bernard 1995; Sibbet and Campo 1990), TEF-1 (Ishiji et al. 1992), and YY1 (O'Connor et al. 1996). Activity of the early promoter is differentiation dependent, with extremely low levels of early transcripts being detected in basal cells of infected epithelium, and expression increasing in the intermediate layers (Durst et al. 1992; Higgins et al. 1992; Stoler et al. 1992; Cheng et al. 1995).

There is an important difference in the expression of the E6 and E7 mRNAs of the HR-HPVs and the LR-HPVs. The HR-HPVs are expressed from a single

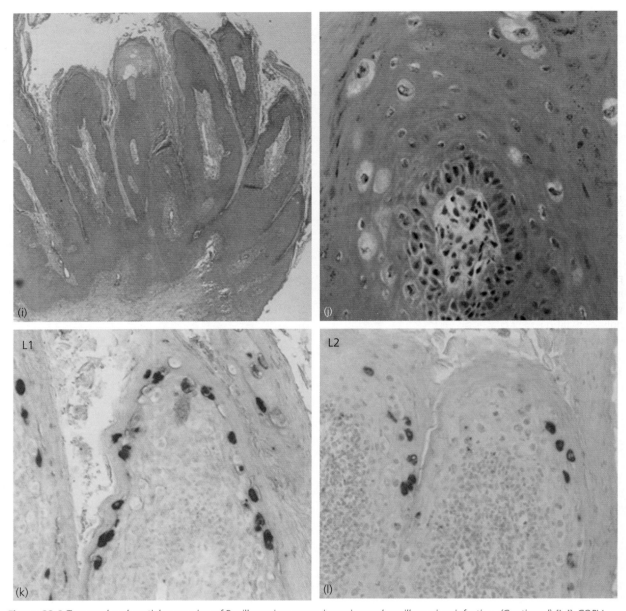

Figure 23.6 *Temporal and spatial expression of* Papillomavirus *genes in canine oral papillomavirus infection. (Continued)* **(i–l)** *COPV wart morphology at week 8 post infection showing the elongated filiform papillae typical of mature warts* **(i–j)**. *Koilocytes were present in the papillae by week 7* **(k–l)**. *Probes for transcripts from L1 and L2 both detected occasional positive superficial cells at 7 weeks, and abundant positive superficial cells by 8 weeks.*

promoter that directs the expression of mRNAs for E6 and E7 with splices in the *E6* gene. The mRNAs with spliced E6 splice to the 5′ end of the E6 ORF (E6*) to a transition frame with a stop codon allowing sufficient spacing for translation reinitiation of the E7 ORF. In contrast, the *E6* and *E7* of the LR-HPVs are expressed from two independent promoters (Chow and Broker 1997).

Late gene expression

The application of in vitro systems, such as organotypic raft cultures (Asselineau et al. 1986), that induce stratifi-

cation and terminal differentiation of keratinocytes has permitted analysis of late gene expression (Wilson et al. 1992). The raft culture system can fully support the late stages of the virus lifecycle (Bedell et al. 1991; Stanley 1994). In genital HPVs a differentiation-dependent promoter has been detected that has a transcription start site within the E7 ORF (see Figure 23.4) (Grassmann et al. 1996; Hummel et al. 1992). Most polycistronic late transcripts initiated from this promoter have coding potential for the E1–E4 fusion protein (Hummel et al. 1995). More recently, it has been shown that transcripts encoding E1 and E2 are also generated from the late

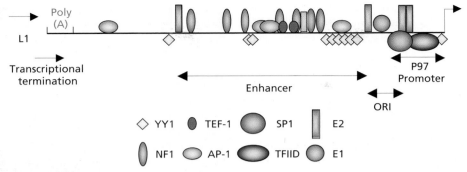

Figure 23.7 *Schematic representation of the HPV-16 URR (O'Connor et al., 1996). The E2 binding sites divide the URR into three functional distinct regions referred to as the 5', central, and 3' segments. The 5' segment of the URR contains a transcription termination signal (poly(A)), the central segment contains the epithelial cell-specific enhancer comprising the majority of the transcription factor binding sites, and the 3' segment contains the origin of replication (ORI), the E1 binding site, and the P97 promoter. Shown are the binding sites for a number of transcription factors with a role in transcriptional control of all genital HPVs.*

promoter (Klumpp and Laimins 1999). Also generated are transcripts coding for the L1 and L2 capsid proteins, which are translated from mRNAs that utilize the late polyadenylation signal located within the URR (Terhune et al. 1999). Importantly, the organotypic culture systems show clearly that the induction of late gene expression requires that the viral genomes be maintained as extrachromosomal elements, and that the induction of terminal differentiation alone is insufficient (Frattini et al. 1996).

REGULATION OF HPV REPLICATION

Viral replication is dependent on the action of viral proteins and components of the cellular replication machinery, including DNA polymerase α-primase, DNA polymerase δ, replication protein A (RPA), replication protein C (RPC), proliferating cell nuclear antigen (PCNA), and topoisomerases I and II (Desaintes and Demeret 1996). These are not present normally in differentiating cells and are induced as a consequence of the viral E7 protein. In transient replication assays (Chiang et al. 1992; Del Vecchio et al. 1992; Ustav et al. 1991) and in cell-free systems (Kuo et al. 1994) the viral proteins E1 and E2 are required for efficient replication of viral origin of replication (ORI)-containing plasmids. However, in certain transient replication studies low-level replication of ORI-containing plasmids has been observed if E1 alone is expressed (Gopalakrishnan and Khan 1994; Sakai et al. 1996), indicating that E2 has an auxiliary function in viral replication and that E1 is the principal replication protein. E2 is considered a specificity factor, directing the replication initiator E1 preferentially to viral DNA to initiate highly efficient virus-specific replication. However, E2 mediates interaction of PV genomes with host chromosomes, suggesting that during plasmid maintenance E2 ensures that viral genomes are segregated to daughter cells in approximately equal numbers (Skiadopoulos and McBride 1998).

PROPERTIES AND FUNCTIONS OF VIRAL ORFS

Many biochemical properties and functions of PV ORFs were originally elucidated using BPV-1 as a model system. Many of these functions have proved applicable to HPVs.

E1 ORF

The product of the E1 ORF is a 600–650 amino acid nuclear phosphoprotein with structural and sequence similarities to regions of the simian virus 40 (SV40) large T antigen required for viral replication initiation. Consistent with a replication initiator role for the E1 protein, it binds the viral origin ORI and exhibits ATPase and ATP-dependent helicase activities (Desaintes and Demeret 1996). Hence, together with the product of the E2 ORF, expression of *E1* is critical for efficient viral DNA replication and thus plays an essential role in maintenance of episomal viral genomes during the HPV lifecycle. *E1* is the most conserved of all the PV genes, and hence *E1* gene products of different PVs are expected to be comparable in terms of both structure and function.

E1 forms complexes with E2 in solution (Blitz and Laimins 1991; Frattini and Laimins 1994; Mohr et al. 1990). Although E1 alone can bind with low affinity to the A/T-rich sequence in the viral ORI (Frattini and Laimins 1994), E1:E2 complexes bind the ORI with higher affinity and specificity (Kuo et al. 1994), which is attributable to the presence of E2-binding sites flanking the single E1-binding site in the viral ORI (see Figure 23.2). E2 acts as a specificity factor to promote highly efficient virus-specific replication. In the current model, the E1:E2:ORI complex constitutes the inactive preinitiation complex. This serves as a precursor for the recruitment of additional E1 molecules and the formation of a multimeric E1 complex bound to the ORI

(Lusky et al. 1994). In vitro, this is accompanied by displacement of E2 from the origin (Lusky et al. 1994). E1 assembles into hexameric structures, with hexamer formation concomitant with ATPase activity and DNA unwinding (Sedman and Stenlund 1998). Thus, the hexameric form of E1 is the enzymatically active ATP-dependent helicase required during the elongation phase of replication to unwind DNA ahead of the replication fork (Hughes and Romanos 1993).

E1 also interacts with host replication factors that are required for viral replication. For example, it interacts with DNA polymerase α-primase and brings it to the viral ORI in order to initiate replication (Masterson et al. 1998). Thus the combination of the multimeric E1:ORI complex and recruited cellular factors constitutes the active replication 'initiation' complex.

E2 ORF

The product of the E2 ORF is a regulator of both viral transcription and replication. E2 is a nuclear phosphoprotein comprising an N-terminal transactivation domain and a C-terminal DNA-binding domain, both highly conserved among all PVs, separated by a nonconserved 'hinge' region of variable length. E2 binds to DNA as a dimer, with α-helices from each monomer forming specific contacts with DNA. The consensus E2-binding site is the palindromic sequence ACCGNNNCGGT, of which there are four in the viral URR of genital HPVs (see Figure 23.7). The role of E2, together with E1, in viral replication has been discussed above.

Most experiments have demonstrated that, unlike BPV-1 E2, the E2 proteins of mucosal HPVs act as transcriptional repressors of the early viral promoter (Bernard et al. 1989). Repression depends on the interaction between E2 and its promoter proximal binding sites at the transcriptional control region, and this is proposed to hinder assembly of the transcription initiation complex (Dong et al. 1994). However, it has also been demonstrated that E2 can *trans*-activate gene expression from the early promoter when specific E2-binding sites are mutated (Thierry and Howley 1991) One model suggests that at low concentration E2 binds the high-affinity promoter distal E2-binding site and *trans*-activates the early promoter, whereas at higher concentrations the promoter proximal sites are bound and transcription is repressed (Steger and Corbach 1997). The E2 of both high- and low-risk genital HPVs can also influence transcription of host genes, and can downregulate the promoter of the reverse transcriptase component of telomerase (Lee et al. 2002).

E4 ORF

The most abundant mRNA species detected in productive HPV infection initiates from the late promoter,

splices a short 5′ sequence of the E1 ORF to the E4 ORF, and codes for the major product of the E4 ORF, the E1–E4 fusion protein (referred to hereafter as E4) (Desaintes and Demeret 1996). E4 proteins of cutaneous and mucosal HPVs vary greatly in terms of sequence homology and biological properties. The E4 of the mucosal PVs is a cytoplasmic phosphoprotein of around 90 amino acids that can self-associate to form multimeric species (Bryan et al. 1998). It comprises relatively conserved N-terminal and C-terminal regions, separated by a highly variable region. Although E4 is located in the early gene region, transcripts with coding potential for E4 are expressed at a high level late in the productive lifecycle through activation of the differentiation-dependent late promoter located in the E7 ORF. The function of E4 is poorly understood, but current hypotheses suggest that it may function at the level of control of viral replication and/or release of infectious virions.

In cultured human keratinocytes E4 has been shown to associate with the keratin intermediate filament (IF) network and, in the case of HPV-16, to cause its collapse (Doorbar et al. 1991; Roberts et al. 1993). A leucine-rich N-terminal motif was a crucial determinant in mediating cytoplasmic localization of E4, whereas C-terminal residues mediated self-association, association with the keratin IF network, and efficient disruption of the keratin IF network (Bryan et al. 1998; Roberts et al. 1997). Because of the observed cytopathic effect, it has been hypothesized that E4 may enhance the release of infectious virions in superficial layers by promoting cell lysis (Doorbar et al. 1991). However, although colocalization of E4 with the keratin IF network was demonstrated within HPV-infected epithelium, collapse of the network was not (Sterling et al. 1993; Pray and Laimins 1995). More recently, it has been shown that E4 binds and disrupts specific components of the cornified cell envelope (CCE), contributing to its altered physical characteristics of HPV-11-infected epithelium (Brown and Bryan 2000; Bryan and Brown 2000). Given that one of these is increased cell fragility, the hypothesis that E4 may enhance virion release may hold true, via disruption of the CCE and/or collapse of the keratin IF network.

Expression of HPV-16 *E4* in SiHa cells results in arrest of the cell cycle at G2 and colocalization of the Cdc2/cyclin B mitosis-promoting complex with E4 at the keratin IF network (Davy et al. 2002). Because nuclear localization of this complex is required for entry into mitosis, cytoplasmic sequestration would account for the observed G2 arrest. Thus, it has been suggested that E4-induced G2 arrest, combined with the viral oncogene cell cycle progression out of G_1 phase, creates a 'pseudo S-phase' environment ideal for replication of the viral genome.

E5 ORF

The contribution of the E5 protein to the HPV lifecycle is poorly understood. However, given that it is among the most abundant transcripts in low-grade intra-epithelial lesions, its cellular effects are likely to be important in productive HPV infections. HPV-16 E5 is a small hydrophobic protein of approximately 90 amino acids in length. Apart from its overall hydrophobic sequence, it does not share significant sequence homology with BPV-1 E5 (DiMaio and Mattoon 2001). Like BPV-1 E5, HPV-16 E5 localizes to the Golgi apparatus, endoplasmic reticulum, and nuclear membranes (Conrad et al. 1993), but unlike its bovine counterpart has only weak transforming activity (DiMaio and Mattoon 2001). The transforming capacity of HPV16 E5 correlates with its ability to inhibit downregulation of the EGF receptor in human keratinocytes (Straight et al. 1993). This is consistent with the enhanced transforming capacity of E5 in the presence of EGF (Bouvard et al. 1994). It has been shown that E5 interacts with the 16 kDa component of the vacuolar proton ATPase (Conrad et al. 1993). This impairs its function in acid-ification of endosomes, which is essential for their proteolytic functions (Conrad et al. 1993; Straight et al. 1995). Hence, the current model is that HR-HPV E5 transforms cells by increasing their sensitivity to extra-cellular EGF levels by increasing receptor recycling to the membrane (DiMaio and Mattoon 2001).

E6 ORF

The viral oncoproteins E6 and E7 are the major trans-forming and immortalizing proteins of the oncogenic or HR-HPVs. The transforming and immortalizing capacity of the oncoproteins of specific HPV types correlates with viral oncogenicity in vivo. Thus, the association of HR-HPVs, but not LR-HPVs, with the development of cervical carcinoma is attributable to differences in the activity of the E6 and E7 proteins. However, the proper-ties of these proteins must be viewed primarily in terms of their function in the virus lifecycle, as it is in this context that they have evolved.

STRUCTURE AND LOCALIZATION OF E6

The HPV E6 protein is a polypeptide of approximately 150 amino acids. Although there is sequence variation of E6 in different HPV types, all retain strict conservation of four C–X–X–C motifs that allow the formation of two zinc fingers (Barbosa et al. 1989; Grossman and Laimins 1989). Owing to low levels of endogenous E6, detection of its intracellular location has been difficult. However, induction of high-level E6 expression with a baculovirus vector reveals localization to the nucleus, and also to nonnuclear membranes (Grossman et al. 1989), consis-tent with the notion that E6 protein is multifunctional.

INTERACTION BETWEEN E6 AND P53

A large number of cellular targets of HR-HPV E6 have been defined, although the best studied is the interaction

with the tumor suppressor gene (TSG) *TP53*. The E6 protein of HR-HPVs has been shown to bind in vitro translated p53 (Werness et al. 1990), resulting in degra-dation of the p53 via the ATP-dependent ubiquitin pathway (Scheffner et al. 1990). This is consistent with the observation that low levels of wildtype p53 are detected in HR-HPV-positive cervical cancer cell lines and E6-immortalized human mammary epithelial cells (Band et al. 1991; Hubbert et al. 1992; Scheffner et al. 1991). There are conflicting reports as to whether E6 of LR-HPV can bind p53 (Crook et al. 1991; Lechner and Laimins 1994; Werness et al. 1990). However, this is a low-affinity interaction compared to that of HR-HPV E6, and does not induce degradation of p53. Thus, the oncogenicity of HPVs correlates with an ability to bind and induce the degradation of p53. Indeed, the demon-stration that HR-HPV E6-expressing cells do not gener-ally undergo cell cycle arrest in response to DNA damage shows that the HR-HPV E6/TP53 interaction can abrogate the normal function of this TSG (Kessis et al. 1993).

The induction of degradation of p53 by E6 is medi-ated by a cellular protein E6-associated protein (E6-AP) which can bind E6 of HR-HPVs, but not the E6 of LR-HPVs, in the absence of p53 (Huibregtse et al. 1991; Scheffner et al. 1993). E6 recruits E6-AP to prevent the accumulation of p53.

ADDITIONAL CELLULAR TARGETS OF E6

E6 has binding partners apart from p53 (zur Hausen 2000) (Table 23.1). The consequences of these various protein/protein-binding reactions with regard to E6 oncogenicity are not currently understood, but they do involve key aspects of cellular function and behavior in the maintenance of tissue architecture, the disruption of which accompanies carcinogenic progression. However, given the low levels of E6 expressed in HPV-positive lesions, it is uncertain which interactions take place in an infected cell during permissive viral growth.

FUNCTION OF E6 IN THE VIRUS LIFE CYCLE

Viral DNA amplification occurs in terminally differ-entiated postmitotic cells and, because the virus requires the host DNA replication machinery to achieve this, a central role of the E7 protein is to induce S-phase entry. However, one response of a normal cell to the induction of inappropriate DNA replication – for example during differentiation, at confluence, or upon growth factor withdrawal – is growth arrest or apoptosis via induction of p53. Indeed, E7-expressing primary keratinocytes show an increase in p53 levels (Demers et al. 1994). Through its ability to bind and degrade p53, the E6 protein mediates inhibition of apoptosis, a function elegantly demonstrated in transgenic mice expressing the HPV-16 oncoproteins in the ocular lens. The expression

Table 23.1 *Additional cellular targets and properties of the E6 oncoprotein*

Cellular binding protein or property	Notes	References
ERC-55	Calcium-binding protein of unknown function. The mouse homologue is the vitamin D receptor-associated factor that transduces the growth-suppressive effects of vitamin D. Thus, the association with E6 may inhibit these growth-suppressing signals	Imai et al. 1991
Paxillin	Focal adhesion protein that transduces signals from the plasma membrane to focal adhesions and the actin cytoskeleton. The association of E6 possibly disrupts growth-inhibitory signals from cell–cell contact	Turner 2000
hDLG	Membrane-associated PDZ motif containing protein that is the human homologue of *Drosophila* discs large TSG. Binds APC and negatively regulates cell-cycle progression. E6 induces proteasome-mediated degradation and could inhibit the inhibitory hDLG/APC interaction and also cell–cell contact	Gardiol et al. 1999
MCM7	Required for formation of the DNA replication licensing system, which allows initiation of cellular DNA replication and restricts it to a single round per cell cycle. The E6 association may be a normal requirement for the viral lifecycle	Kukimoto et al. 1998
Interferon regulatory factor (IRF-3)	Activated in response to virus infection to induce expression of the antiviral type I interferon (IFN) IFN-β. The E6 interaction does not cause degradation of IRF-3, but reduces expression of IFN-β. This is likely to be of significance in the normal viral lifecycle	Ronco et al. 1998
Enhanced degradation of MYC and BAC	BAK is a proapoptotic member of the BCL-2 family, expressed in differentiated epithelial cells. MYC can also induce apoptosis if proliferation is unscheduled. The E6-induced degradation of MYC and BAK may partly explain the TP53-independent inhibition of apoptosis by E6. This may also be of significance in the normal viral lifecycle	Thomas and Banks 1999
Induction of hTERT expression	Retrovirally delivered E6 can induce high levels of telomerase activity in preimmortal keratinocytes. This is mediated by activation of the hTERT promoter. The mechanism of activation is poorly understood, but as upregulation of the hTERT promoter correlates with the ability of E6 to bind E6-AP, it is possible that E6 targets a negative regulator of expression for degradation	Klingelhutz et al. 1996

of E7 alone induced cellular proliferation in spatially inappropriate regions and apoptosis of these cells before differentiation could occur. The expression of E6 alone inhibited the apoptosis that was observed in the lenses of nontransgenic embryos, whereas co-expression of E6 and E7 resulted in abrogation of the E7-induced apoptosis, and led to tumor formation in 40 percent of adult mice (Griep et al. 1993; Pan and Griep 1994). The ability of E6 to bind and degrade BAK and MYC (see Table 23.2) is consistent with inhibition of p53-independent apoptosis.

THE E6* PROTEIN

A number of early transcripts of high-risk, but not low-risk, HPVs utilize a splice donor site within the E6 ORF to yield coding potential for a number of nontransforming truncated E6 proteins known as E6* (Schwarz et al. 1985). It has been shown that E6* is capable of interacting with both the full-length E6 protein and E6-AP in vitro, blocking the association of E6 with TP53 (Pim et al. 1997). As a consequence, E6*

proteins can inhibit the E6-induced degradation of TP53 (Pim et al. 1997; Shally et al. 1996). The role of E6* in the viral lifecycle remains unclear, however.

E7 ORF

STRUCTURE AND LOCALIZATION OF E7

The HPV E7 protein is a phosphoprotein of approximately 100 amino acids. Consistent with its multifunctional nature, E7 has been detected at a variety of locations within the cell, including the cytoplasm, nucleus, and nucleoli (Greenfield et al. 1991; Smotkin and Wettstein 1987). The N-terminal region of E7 comprises two regions known as conserved domains 1 and 2 (CD1 and CD2). CD2 contains a 'pocket protein'-binding L–X–C–X–E motif, and also a consensus phosphorylation site for casein kinase II (CK II). A third conserved region, CD3, resides at the C terminus and comprises two C–X–X–C motifs with the ability to bind zinc and form a zinc finger (Barbosa et al. 1989; McIntyre et al. 1993). This domain confers the ability of

Table 23.2 *Additional cellular targets of the E7 oncoprotein*

Cellular binding protein	Notes	References
p21$^{WAF1/CIP1}$ and p27^{KIP1}	Inhibitors of cyclin A/E-dependent kinases, with a role in cell-cycle arrest, differentiation, and apoptosis. Association with E7 abrogates these activities. Effects on terminal differentiation-associated growth arrest may possibly play a role in the viral life cycle	Funk et al. 1997
TATA box-binding protein	Component of the TFIID transcription factor complex. Interaction of E7 may control expression of genes related to E7-associated transformation	Massimi et al. 1997
JUN	Member of the AP-1 family of transcription factors. The E7 interaction can induce transcription from JUN-responsive promoters. However, JUN also binds RB and induces activation of AP-1-regulated genes in differentiated keratinocytes. The interaction of E7 with JUN inhibits this activation. Thus, E7 can act as both a positive and negative regulator of JUN-responsive promoters	Antinore et al. 1996
M2 pyruvate kinase (M2-PK)	This is the first example of a cytoplasmic, noncell cycle-associated target of E7. In its tetrameric form, M2-PK promotes flux of metabolites through the glycolytic pathway. Binding of E7 converts M2-PK to a dimeric form, which decreases this flux. This increases the pool of metabolites available for biosynthesis of nucleic acids. Thus, this interaction may play an important role in the viral lifecycle by increasing the pool of nucleic acids available for viral replication	Zwerschke et al. 1999

E7 to form homodimers, and mutational analysis has shown that it also contributes to the transforming potential of the HR-HPV E7 proteins (Edmonds and Vousden 1989; McIntyre et al. 1993).

INTERACTION OF E7 WITH RB AND OTHER POCKET PROTEINS

The best-characterized interaction of HPV E7 is with the TSG RB. A significant breakthrough regarding the molecular basis of transformation by HPV E7 was the demonstration that HPV-16 E7 can bind pRB both in vitro and in vivo (Munger et al. 1989). Furthermore, the affinity of this association is greater for HR-HPV than for LR-HPV E7 (Munger et al. 1989), suggesting that this property is likely to contribute to the oncogenic potential of HR-HPVs. Indeed, mutational analysis has demonstrated that E7-induced transformation is impaired if the pRB/E7 association is disrupted (Barbosa et al. 1990; Edmonds and Vousden 1989; Watanabe et al. 1990). E7 preferentially binds the hypophosphorylated form of pRB (Imai et al. 1991), disrupting the pRB/E2F association and thus inducing the expression of E2F-dependent genes required for G$_1$–S progression (Chellappan et al. 1992). It has also been shown that HR-HPV E7 induces degradation of pRB via the ubiquitin-mediated proteasomal pathway (Boyer et al. 1996). Thus, efficient abrogation of pRB function by E7 is mediated by protein degradation as well as binding and, consistent with this, the transforming capacity of E7 mutants correlates more closely with their ability to degrade pRB rather than just bind it (Jones and Munger 1996).

E7 also binds the pRB-related pocket proteins p107 and p130 (Dyson et al. 1992), which are also involved in cell-cycle regulation via association with E2F proteins. However, given that similar sequences of E7 are required to mediate interactions with all the pocket proteins, it is difficult to determine which of these are the most functionally significant targets of E7 using mutational analysis.

ADDITIONAL CELLULAR TARGETS OF E7

Mutational studies have shown that the E7/pRB interaction is necessary, but not sufficient, for cellular transformation (Edmonds and Vousden 1989; Phelps et al. 1992). Consistent with this, a number of additional cellular targets of E7 are now recognized (Table 23.2). These are likely to contribute to the ability of E7 to modulate the cell cycle as well as other cellular activities. As with E6, a number of these targets are more efficiently abrogated by E7 from HR-HPVs, and thus may further contribute to the oncogenic potential of HR-HPVs. However, the low level of E7 protein detected in clinical lesions raises the issue of which of these interactions are relevant in permissive infection.

FUNCTION OF E7 IN THE VIRUS LIFECYCLE

Because they do not encode a unique DNA polymerase, papillomaviruses are completely dependent upon the host DNA replication machinery for generation of progeny virions. Given that viral vegetative DNA replication occurs in postmitotic differentiated cells, this presents a problem for the virus. In a usual differentiation program, as postmitotic differentiated cells migrate up the epithelium their nuclei are gradually degraded and no longer active. Thus, an important role of the virus is to maintain suprabasal cells in a replication-competent state and reactivate the host DNA replication machinery while preserving the differentiation process to allow late gene expression.

It has been shown that the E7 of HR-HPVs and, to a lesser extent, LR-HPVs under the control of the homologous URR, is sufficient to induce expression of proliferating cell nuclear antigen (PCNA) and induce cellular DNA synthesis within suprabasal cells (Cheng et al. 1995). Thus, induction of entry into S-phase and the activation of host DNA replication machinery is a crucial role of the E7 protein. Unscheduled exit from G_1 can lead to apoptosis, and this is overcome by the viral oncoprotein E6. The cellular targets of E7 are consistent with this function. Through its interaction with members of the RB family of pocket proteins, E7 can induce the activity of the E2F family of transcription factors that control the expression of genes required for entry into S-phase.

Abrogation of the effects of cyclin-dependent kinase inhibitors (CDKI) such as p21$^{WAF1/CIP1}$ and p27^{KIP1} is another important role of E7 in the viral lifecycle. CDKIs have roles both in cell-cycle regulation and in keratinocyte differentiation (Missero et al. 1995; Di Cunto et al. 1998) In vitro studies have shown that E7 inhibits the cell-cycle arrest function of both p21$^{WAF1/CIP1}$ and p27^{KIP1} when E7-expressing keratinocytes are induced to differentiate (Jones et al. 1997; Ruesch and Laimins 1998); PCNA is induced within these cells, and markers of terminal of differentiation are expressed. The abrogation by E7 of keratinocyte differentiation-associated CDKIs (Missero et al. 1995, 1996; Di Cunto et al. 1998) may be associated with its ability to maintain a replication-competent state while permitting the development of a differentiated environment compatible with viral late functions.

L1 and L2 ORFs

The products of the L1 and L2 ORFs are expressed in only the most terminally differentiated keratinocytes and form the viral capsid. The capsid comprises 360 molecules of L1, arranged as 72 capsomers, in an icosahedral surface lattice. Recombinant HPV11 L1 with cysteine-to-glycine mutations forms capsomeres but cannot assemble into capsid-like structures, suggesting that disulphide bonds mediate capsomere binding in the papillomavirus capsid (Li et al. 1998). Cryo-electron microscopy indicates that the L2 protein is situated at the center of pentameric capsomeres in mature virions (Trus et al. 1997).

A number of studies have demonstrated that L2 is required for encapsidation of viral genomes into infectious virions (Roden et al. 1996; Stauffer et al. 1998;

Zhou et al. 1993). In the model for L2-mediated assembly of papillomavirus virions, L2 localization to subnuclear domains causes the subsequent recruitment of E2 with bound viral genome and L1 (Okun et al. 2001). This L2–L1–E2-genome association confers an appropriate environment and/or concentration of components for virion assembly. The E2-binding capacity of L2 is important to confer selective encapsidation of PV DNA, and hence this is another possible function of E2-binding sites within the viral genome. Given that virions containing E2 protein have not been detected, it is proposed that E2 acts catalytically in the process of DNA encapsidation during virion assembly.

CLINICAL ASPECTS OF HPV INFECTION

Nongenital skin warts

These are common benign proliferations that occur most frequently in children and young adults. The classification of cutaneous warts includes verruca vulgaris (common warts; Figure 23.8) verruca plana (plane warts), verruca plantaris (deep plantar warts), mosaic plantar warts, butchers' warts, and erythrodysplasia verruciformis. Although not absolute, each classification is associated with specific HPV types, clinical and histologic appearance, and prognostic features (Moore and

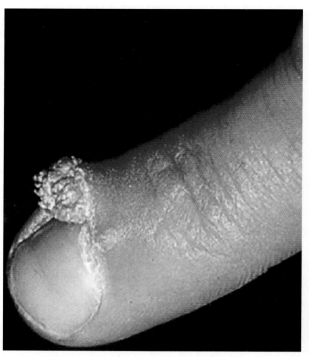

Figure 23.8 *Common wart showing the characteristic appearance of a rough keratotic papule. Lesions may be multiple or single on cutaneous surfaces, with the most common sites being the dorsal aspects of hands and fingers. Photograph courtesy of Dr Libby Edwards.*

Tyring 2001). Butchers and meat handlers have an unusually high prevalence of hand warts, most of which are caused by HPV-7 and attributed to the combination of maceration and trauma to which these workers are subjected. Studies of warts in children show that spontaneous regression will occur within 2 years in about 60 percent of cases; the remaining third show a spectrum of responses, but eventually most lesions resolve (Massing and Epstein 1963). Immunosuppression as a consequence of transplantation, malignant, or infectious disease (HIV) increases the incidence of skin warts. These lesions are larger, more persistent, and refractory to treatment than in immunocompetent individuals, and HPV types usually identified in Epidermodysplasia verruciformis (EV) (Table 23.3) are frequently detected in addition to the common cutaneous HPVs.

Epidermodysplasia verruciformis

EV is a genodermatosis and is an HPV-associated, lifelong, genetic disease (for review see (Majewski and Jablonska 2001). The warts appear in early childhood, become widespread, tend not to regress, and invasive cancers can develop from them (Figure 23.9). EV is an autosomal recessive condition and is associated with specific HPV types (Orth et al. 2001) (Table 23.3) that persist for life, generating clinical lesions that are

Table 23.3 *Clinical lesions associated with HPV*

Lesion	HPV Types	
	Frequent association	**Infrequent association**
Skin warts		
Plantar warts	1	2, 4, 63
Common warts	2, 27	1, 4, 7, 26, 28, 29, 57, 60, 65
Flat warts	3, 10	2, 26, 27, 28, 29, 41, 49
Erythrodysplasia verruciformis-specific skin lesions	5, 8, 17, 20	9, 12, 14, 15, 19, 21–25, 36, 38, 46, 46, 47, 50
Malignant and premalignant skin lesions		
Bowens disease of the skin	2, 16, 34	
Skin cancers in patients with Erythrodysplasia verruciformis	5, 8	14, 17, 20, 47
Skin cancers in renal transplant patients	1–6, 8, 10, 11, 14–16, 18–20, 23-25, 27, 29, 36, 38, 41, 47, 48	
SCC of the finger	16	
Benign head and neck lesions		
Oral papillomas and leukoplakias	2, 6, 11, 16	7
Focal epithelial hyperplasia	13, 32	
Laryngeal papillomas (RRP patients)	6, 11	
Conjunctival papillomas	6, 11	
Nasal papillomas		6, 11, 57
Malignant head and neck lesions		
Laryngeal cancer		6, 11, 16, 18, 35
Oral cancer		3, 6, 11, 16, 18, 57
Tonsillar/pharyngeal cancer		16, 18, 33
Esophageal cancer		6, 11, 16, 18
Nasal cancer		16, 57
Benign anogenital lesions		
Condyloma acuminata	6, 11	30, 34, 33, 40, 41, 42, 44, 42, 44, 45, 54, 55, 61
Malignant and premalignant anogenital lesions		
CIN, VAIN, VIN, PAIN, PIN	6, 11, 16, 18, 31	30, 34, 35, 39, 40, 42–45, 51, 52, 56–59, 61, 62, 64, 66, 67, 69
Cervical cancer	16, 18, 31, 45	6, 10, 11, 26, 33, 35, 39, 51, 52, 5, 56, 58, 59, 66, 68, plus unclassified types
Buschke–Löwenstein tumors	6, 11	

Abbreviations CIN, cervical intraepithelial neoplasia; PAIN, perianal intraepithelial neoplasia; PIN, penile intraepithelial neoplasia; RRP, recurrent respiratory papillomatosis; SCC, squamous cell carcinoma; VAIN, vaginal intraepithelial neoplasia; VIN, vulval intraepithelial neoplasia.

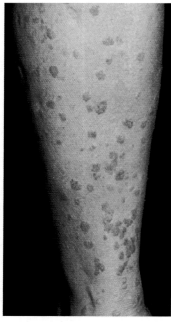

Figure 23.9 *Erythropdysplasia verruciformis characterized by flat wart-like lesions or reddish macules, mainly on the face, trunk, and extensor surfaces of arms and legs (Gross et al. 1997 with permission).*

refractory to treatment. In the immunocompetent host, EV HPV types are present in a latent form in the skin but do not manifest themselves clinically unless the individual is immunosuppressed, in which case EV types can be identified in cutaneous neoplasms. Overall, the evidence indicates that the defect in EV is an inadequate cell-mediated immune response to the EV HPV subset. Consistent with this notion is the fact that cutaneous responses to contact sensitizers such as dinitrochlorobenzene (DNCB) are absent in EV patients. An important feature of the carcinomas in EV is that they develop on sun-exposed surfaces, suggesting that UV light is a cofactor in EV HPV viral oncogenesis.

Nonmelanoma skin cancer

Nonmelanoma skin cancer (NMSC) (basal cell carcinoma (BCC) and squamous cell carcinoma (SCC)) are the most prevalent malignancies in fair-skinned individuals worldwide. Epidemiologic studies have implicated HPVs in these cancers, particularly in those arising in immunosuppressed individuals (for review see Harwood and Proby 2002). Depending on the sensitivity of the assays HPV DNA can be detected in up to 80–90 percent of SCCs arising in transplant patients. EV HPV types predominate, but no specific HPV is associated with malignancy (Harwood and Proby 2002). The prevalence of HPV DNA in premalignant lesions such as keratoacanthomas, actinic keratoses, and carcinoma in situ in transplant patients can be as high as in SCCs. The same HPV types predominate in these lesions and

in BCCs, although HPV prevalence is lower in the latter (Berkhout et al. 2000).

NMSCs in immunocompetent individuals also harbor HPV DNA but the prevalence is lower (0–50 percent for SCC, 31–44 percent for BCC). However, HPV DNA can be detected in normal skin biopsies in 30–35 percent of individuals, and EV HPV types predominate (Berkhout et al. 2000). Importantly, EV HPVs have been detected in benign hyperproliferative skin disorders such as psoriasis, where 90 percent of lesional skin biopsies contain HPV, particularly HPV-5 and HPV-36 (Favre et al. 2000). This raises the possibility that these associations are not causal but represent reactivation of latent HPV genomes in proliferating keratinocytes, and at present the evidence that HPV is the initiating factor in NMSC is inconclusive.

Aerodigestive tract

Papillomatosis can occur anywhere in the aerodigestive tract – the oral cavity, nasal sinuses, hypopharynx, larynx, bronchial tree, and esophagus. In the oral cavity HPV infection is associated with a range of benign proliferative lesions (Table 23.4), of which squamous papilloma caused by HPV-6 or -11 is the most common (Figure 23.10). HR-HPV types are detected in dysplasias and squamous cell carcinomas, but these types are also present in normal oral mucosa and the etiologic role of HPV in oral cancer is questionable. However, the high prevalence of HPV-16 and HPV-33 in tonsillar carcinomas does imply a causal role for HPV in these cancers, and there are some laboratory data to support this (Snijders et al. 1994).

Papilloma is one of the most common benign laryngeal tumors, but its prevalence is difficult to estimate. The incidence of recurrent respiratory papillomatosis (RRP) in children is estimated at 4.3/100 000, and among adults 1.8/100 000 (Derkay 1995). HPVs are the causal agent, with HPV-11 infections predominating followed by HPV-6, -16, and -18 (Dickens et al. 1991). Mixed infections are common. Histologically the lesions are benign, but morbidity is significant as recurrence and/or dissemination affect the patency of the airways. Clinical behavior is variable, and lesions may regress, persist, or progress to malignancy. The latter is cofactor dependent and smoking is a significant risk factor here. Treatment is usually endoscopic excision under magnification. The frequent recurrence and often confluent spread of these lesions make treatment difficult, and patients usually require multiple surgical interventions. Noninvasive effective therapies are desperately required for these individuals.

GENITAL TRACT INFECTIONS

HPV infection of the anogenital skin and mucosae results in lesions with two morphologies: anogenital

Table 23.4 *HPV types in benign lesions of the oral mucosa*

Lesion	HPV types found	
	Frequently	Infrequently
Normal mucosa	6, 11, 16, 18	7, 31, 33, 59, 61
Verruca vulgaris	2, 4, 57	1, 6, 11, 16
Squamous papilloma	6, 11	2, 13, 16, 32, 31, 33, 35
Focal epithelial hyperplasia	13, 32	6, 11, 16, 24
Koilocytic dysplasia	16, 18, 31, 33, 35	6, 11
Oral epithelial dysplasia	16, 18	2, 6, 11, 31, 33, 35
Leukoplakia	6, 11	2, 16, 18
Oral warts in HIV+ patients	7, 32	2, 6, 11, 13, 16, 18, 55, 59, 69, 72, 73

warts (condyloma acuminata) and squamous intraepithelial lesions (SIL). Condylomata are associated predominantly, but not exclusively, with infection by LR-HPV types and have a low to negligible risk of malignant progression (Table 23.3). SIL are associated with both low- and high-risk genital HPV types, and high-risk HR-HPV-infected lesions can progress to malignancy. The majority of epidemiologic studies have been focused on HPV infection in the lower genital tract of women, and relatively little is known about nongenital HPV infection and genital HPV infection in men. In women, genital HPV transmission is primarily by sexual contact after the sexual debut, and there is a strong positive trend between prevalence of infection and increasing number of sexual partners (IARC 1996).

Condyloma acuminata

External anogenital warts are the commonest viral sexually transmitted disease (PHLS Communicable Disease Centre 1989). They have been recorded as occurring at an incidence rate of 2.4 cases/1000, with a peak attack rate of 1.2 percent in men and women

aged 20–24 years (Persson et al. 1996). The warts are usually exophytic, often mutiple lesions that can occur anywhere on the external genitalia, but are found mainly the perineum and anus in women (Figure 23.11a) and on the penis and anus in men (Figure 23.11b). Most lesions regress spontaneously over time if left alone, but in a fraction of infected individuals they can persist for years. They are more frequent in the immunosuppressed, and are refractory to treatment in these patients. Most lesions are caused by HPV-6, about 15 percent are attributable to HPV-11, and a tiny fraction to other HPV types, including HPV-16. Current treatments suffer from high recurrence rates, although trials with the immunomodulator Imiquimod report significantly reduced recurrences post-therapy (Edwards et al. 1998). A rare anogenital form of condyloma acuminata is the Buschke–Löwenstein tumor, which is locally invasive but nonmetastasizing. These lesions usually contain HPV-6 or -11, and rarely HPV-16 (Boshart and zur Hausen 1986).

Squamous intraepithelial lesions and anogenital cancers

Squamous intraepithelial lesions (SIL) are classified histologically and form a distinct spectrum of histological atypia. Three grades of cervical intraepithelial neoplasia (CIN) are recognized in the European classification: CIN 1 – mild, CIN 2 – moderate, and CIN 3 – severe. The Bethesda classification for cytology used in the USA recognizes two classes: low-grade squamous intraepithelial lesions (LGSIL) (CIN 1) and high-grade squamous intraepithelial lesions (HGSIL) (CIN 2/3). In the vagina, vulva, penis, and anus a similar but not identical spectrum of changes can be identified – VAIN, VIN, PAIN, and PIN – but the likelihood of progression of these lesions to frank malignancies is still unclear. It is probable, but not unequivocally proven, that the majority of these intraepithelial lesions are a result of HPV infection. LGSIL at any site can be associated with both high- and low-risk HPV types, although high-risk types predominate. HGSIL are associated

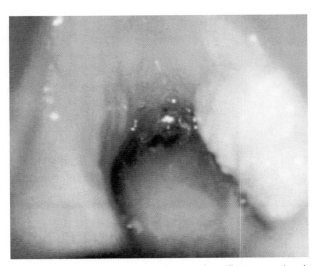

Figure 23.10 *Solitary adult-onset laryngeal papilloma, associated predominantly with HPV-11 (Gross et al. 1997, with permission).*

The epidemiological evidence relating HPV infection to cervical cancer is very strong and the association is considered to be causal (IARC 1996). In all methodologically sound case–control series using reliable HPV DNA detection methods the association between HR-HPVs and cervical carcinoma or the high-grade precursor lesions is very strong with ORs over 15 (reviewed in (Muñoz and Bosch 1996). The strength of this association rules out the possibility of chance, bias, or confounding. Furthermore, the association is consistent, as equally strong associations are found in countries with a high or low incidence of cervical cancer (Muñoz et al. 1992). Reliable large-scale prospective data are available, and it is clear that infection with

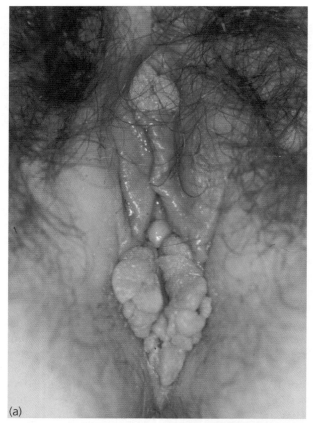

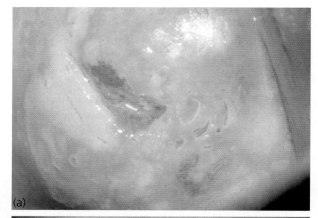

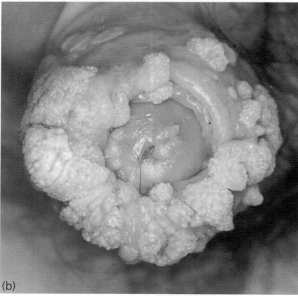

Figure 23.11 *Condyloma acuminata associated principally with HPV 6.* **(a)** *Severe vulval warts in a 35-year-old woman.* **(b)** *Penile and prepuce warts in a 34-year-old HIV-positive man. Immunosuppression is frequently associated with florid condylomata that are refractory to treatment. Photographs courtesy of Dr Colm O'Mahony.*

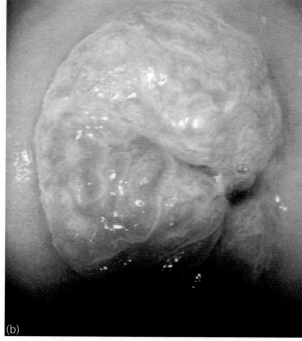

Figure 23.12 *Intraepithelial lesions.* **(a)** *Low-grade cervical intraepithelial neoplasia seen as a raised white area on the posterior lip of the cervix; both low- and high-risk HPVs can be detected in these lesions.* **(b)** *High-grade intraepithelial neoplasia and invasive carcinoma of the cervix, associated with high-risk HPVs, particularly HPV-16 (Gross et al. 1997 with permission).*

almost exclusively with high-risk types. The gross appearance of low- and high-grade cervical SIL is shown in Figure 23.12.

HR-HPV types precedes the development of HGSIL (Schiffman and Brinton 1995). The epidemiological evidence alone indicates that more than 95 percent of cervical cancers are attributable to HPV infection (Walboomers et al. 1999). A summary of the natural history of cervical HPV infection is as follows:

- Transient genital HPV infections are quite common (prevalence about 11–20%) in young sexually active women;
- Most infections are subclinical and resolve. Most lesions are self limiting proliferations (LGSIL) and resolve;
- A minority of women develop persistent infections with focally high levels of DNA;
- Some of these persistent infections with high risk HPVs progress to HGSIL;
- Some HGSIL progress to carcinoma.

Mechanisms of genital HPV oncogenesis

As discussed above, experimental studies show that the E6 and E7 genes of the high-risk genital viruses encode oncoproteins that deregulate key controls in cell proliferation. E7 binds the retinoblastoma protein pRb, effectively blocking the transcriptional repressor function of this protein and overriding the G_1/S checkpoint of the cell cycle. The E6 of the HR-HPVs binds to p53 to form a stable complex which, in combination with E6-AP, undergoes ubiquitin-mediated proteolysis. The ability to form the E6–E6-AP–p53 complex seems to be restricted to the HR-HPVs. This interaction with p53 is crucial, compromising the ability of the cell to effect growth arrest in the face of DNA damage. As a consequence of these interactions cell-cycle checkpoints are bypassed, mutations may be accumulated, and the HPV-infected cell may acquire the immortal phenotype. However, malignant transformation is a rare consequence of infection with HR-HPVs, only a fraction of infected individuals progress to CIN 3, and only 30–50 percent of CIN-3 progress to invasive cancer. In the normal viral infectious cycle viral gene expression is tightly controlled and E6/E7 expression is confined to nondividing differentiated cells, where the oncogenic potential of these genes is not allowed to flourish. HPV oncogenesis requires the deregulation of viral and cellular gene expression so that early genes are inappropriately expressed in dividing cells. In cervical carcinomas and many HGSIL this deregulation is achieved by integration of the HPV genome into host chromosomes (Daniel et al. 1995; Schwarz et al. 1985).

TRANSMISSION

Transmission occurs primarily through person-to-person contact, with shedding of viral particles from the infected individual to microwounds on the skin or mucosa of a naïve recipient. Genital HPVs are transmitted primarily, but not exclusively, via sexual contact. There is evidence for transmission from the fingers in individuals who have genital warts (Strauss et al. 1999) and for vertical transmission of HPV-16 resulting in oral infection (Puranen et al. 1997). A history of genital warts is a risk factor for juvenile recurrent respiratory papillomatosis (Shah et al. 1998), suggesting intrapartum infection.

LABORATORY DIAGNOSIS

HPVs cannot be grown efficiently in tissue culture or in animal models. Diagnosis of HPV infection relies therefore on the direct detection of HPV genomes and/or gene products by molecular hybridization procedures, usually preceded by nucleic acid amplification, in fresh or fixed tissue biopsies, tissue scrapings, and exfoliated cells. HPV detection and typing are tests not routinely available in diagnostic laboratories.

Serology

Individuals infected with HPV do make a type-specific serum antibody response to the major viral capsid protein L1 (Nonnenmacher et al. 1995; Steele and Gallimore 1990). Virions are not available for ELISA, but L1 VLPs have been used widely as the target antigen in ELISA in seroepidemiologic studies (Stanley 1997). Unfortunately, owing to the highly variable interval between infection, lesion development and seroconversion, plus the relatively low sensitivity of the assay, the detection of anticapsid serum antibody is not useful in diagnosis in the individual patient.

IMMUNITY

HPV infections are common, but the immunopathogenesis of these infections is still poorly understood. The majority of studies have focused on genital infections, and it is clear that these are common in young sexually active individuals, the majority of whom apparently clear the infection without overt clinical disease. Those who develop warts or low-grade intraepithelial lesions also in most cases mount an effective cell-mediated immune response and the lesions regress. Nonregressing anogenital warts and LGSIL are not associated with inflammation or histological evidence of immune activity, but regression of anogenital warts is accompanied by a dense mononuclear cell infiltrate dominated by T cells and macrophages and a cytokine expression characteristic of a Th1 cell-mediated immune response (Coleman et al. 1994). Animal models support this and provide evidence that the response is regulated by CD4$^+$ T cell-dependent mechanisms (Nicholls et al. 2001). The central importance of the CD4$^+$ T-cell population in the control of HPV infection is shown by the increased prevalence of HPV infections in individuals immunosuppressed as a consequence of either organ transplantation or HIV infection (Benton and Arends 1996). Although it seems clear that the CD4$^+$ T-cell subset is critical for the induction and regulation of the host response to HPV, the antigenic targets and the nature of the effector response are still not known unequivocally. Evidence from both animal models and human infections indicates that one of the dominant responses is to E2 antigens, but responses to other early proteins E6 and E7 have also been identified (Stanley, 2001b). There is increasing evidence that both NK cells and antigen-specific CTLs are important effectors, but these responses are poorly understood.

Neutralizing antibody to the L1 capsid protein accompanies the induction of successful cell-mediated immunity, and these responses are certainly protective against subsequent viral challenge in natural infections in animals, suggesting that vaccines inducing serum neutralizing antibodies to L1 will be protective (Stanley 1997). Prophylactic immunization with VLP subunit vaccines composed of the major capsid protein L1 of some of the genital HPVs are now in phase III clinical trials. The vaccines are immunogenic, inducing type-specific responses; they are safe and early results indicate efficacy (Koutsky et al. 2002).

If the cell-mediated response fails to induce lesion regression and viral clearance then a persistent viral infection results that is, in part, due to operational immune tolerance. This seems to be reflected by the detection in vitro, in persistently infected individuals, of enhanced cellular and humoral responses to early viral proteins but the failure to clear virus in vivo (de Gruijl et al. 1996a; de Gruijl et al. 1996b). The importance of the MHC in susceptibility to or protection from *Papillomavirus* infection and associated neoplastic disease is supported by data from animal models and clinical studies (Beskow et al. 2001), but this area remains a crucial one for further investigation. The increasing understanding of the mechanisms by which the host responds effectively to HPV infection, and the reasons for the failure of these defense mechanisms in a minority of circumstances, has led to the development of therapeutic immunologically based strategies targeted to both high- and low-risk viruses.

REFERENCES

Abramson, A.L., Steinberg, B.M. and Winkler, B. 1987. Laryngeal papillomatosis: clinical, histopathologic and molecular studies. *Laryngoscope*, **97**, 678–85.

Amella, C.A., Lofgren, L.A., et al. 1994. Latent infection induced with cottontail rabbit papillomavirus: A model for human papillomavirus latency. *Am J Pathol*, **144**, 1167–71.

Antinore, M.J., Birrer, M.J., et al. 1996. The human papillomavirus type 16 E7 gene product interacts with and *trans*-activates the AP1 family of transcription factors. *EMBO J*, **15**, 1950–60.

Apt, D., Chong, T., et al. 1993. Nuclear factor I and epithelial cell specific transcription of human papillomavirus type 16. *J Virol*, **67**, 4455–63.

Asselineau, D., Bernard, B.A., et al. 1986. Human epidermis reconstructed by culture: is it 'normal'? *J Invest Dermatol*, **86**, 181–6.

Baker, C.C. 1993. The genomes of the papillomaviruses. In: O'Brien, S.J. (ed.), *Genetic maps: locus maps of complex genomes*. Cold Spring Harbor: Cold Spring Harbor Press, 134–46.

Baker, T.S., Newcomb, W.W., et al. 1991. Structures of bovine and human papillomaviruses. Analysis by cryoelectron microscopy and three-dimensional image reconstruction. *Biophys J*, **60**, 1445–56.

Band, V., De Caprio, J.A., et al. 1991. Loss of p53 protein in human papillomavirus type 16 E6 immortalized human mammary epithelial cells. *J Virol*, **65**, 6671–6.

Barbosa, M.S., Lowy, D.R. and Schiller, J.T. 1989. Papillomavirus polypeptides E6 and E7 are zinc binding proteins. *J Virol*, **63**, 1404–7.

Barbosa, M.S., Edmonds, C., et al. 1990. The region of the HPV E7 oncoprotein homologous to adenovirus E1a and Sv40 large T antigen contains separate domains for Rb binding and casein kinase II phosphorylation. *EMBO J*, **9**, 153–60.

Bedell, M.A., Hudson, J.B., et al. 1991. Amplification of human papillomavirus genomes in vitro is dependent on epithelial differentiation. *J Virol*, **65**, 2254–60.

Benton, E.C. and Arends, M.J. 1996. Human papillomavirus in the immunosuppressed. In: Lacey, C. (ed.), *Papillomavirus reviews: current research on papillomaviruses*. Leeds: Leeds University Press, 271–9.

Berkhout, R.J., Bouwes Bavinck, J.N. and ter Schegget, J. 2000. Persistence of human papillomavirus DNA in benign and (pre)malignant skin lesions from renal transplant recipients. *J Clin Microbiol*, **38**, 2087–96.

Bernard, B.A., Bailly, C., et al. 1989. The human papillomavirus type 18 (HPV18) E2 gene product is a repressor of the HPV18 regulatory region in human keratinocytes. *J Virol*, **63**, 4317–24.

Beskow, A.H., Josefsson, A.M. and Gyllensten, U.B. 2001. HLA class II alleles associated with infection by HPV16 in cervical cancer in situ. *Int J Cancer*, **93**, 817–22.

Blitz, I.L. and Laimins, L.A. 1991. The 68-kilodalton E1 protein of bovine papillomavirus is a DNA binding phosphoprotein which associates with the E2 transcriptional activator in vitro. *J Virol*, **65**, 649–56.

Boshart, M. and zur Hausen, H. 1986. Human papillomaviruses in Buschke-Löwenstein tumors: physical state of the DNA and identification of a tandem duplication in the noncoding region of a human papillomavirus 6 subtype. *J Virol*, **58**, 963–6.

Bouvard, V., Matlashewski, G., et al. 1994. The human papillomavirus type 16 E5 gene cooperates with the E7 gene to stimulate proliferation of primary cells and increases viral gene expression. *Virology*, **203**, 73–80.

Boyer, S.N., Wazer, D.E. and Band, V. 1996. E7 protein of human papillomavirus type 16 induces degradation of retinoblastoma protein through the ubiquitin-proteasome pathway. *Cancer Res*, **56**, 4620–4.

Brown, D.R. and Bryan, J.T. 2000. Abnormalities of cornified cell envelopes isolated from human papillomavirus type 11-infected genital epithelium. *Virology*, **271**, 65–70.

Bryan, J.T. and Brown, D.R. 2000. Association of the human papillomavirus type 11 E1^E4 protein with cornified cell envelopes derived from infected genital epithelium. *Virology*, **277**, 262–9.

Bryan, J.T., Fife, K.H. and Brown, D.R. 1998. The intracellular expression pattern of the human papillomavirus type 11 E1^E4 protein correlates with its ability to self associate. *Virology*, **241**, 49–60.

Campo, M.S., Jarrett, W.F., et al. 1994. Latent papillomavirus infection in cattle. *Res Vet Sci*, **56**, 151–7.

Chan, S.Y., Delius, H., et al. 1995. Analysis of genomic sequences of 95 papillomavirus types: uniting typing, phylogeny, and taxonomy. *J Virol*, **69**, 3074–83.

Chan, W.K., Chong, T., et al. 1990. Transcription of the transforming genes of the oncogenic human papillomavirus 16 is stimulated by tumor promotors through AP1 binding sites. *Nucleic Acids Res*, **18**, 763–9.

Chellappan, S., Kraus, V.B., et al. 1992. Adenovirus E1A, simian virus 40 tumor antigen, and human papillomavirus E7 protein share the capacity to disrupt the interaction between transcription factor E2F and the retinoblastoma gene product. *Proc Natl Acad Sci USA*, **89**, 4549–53.

Cheng, S., Schmidt Grimminger, D.C., et al. 1995. Differentiation-dependent up-regulation of the human papillomavirus E7 gene reactivates cellular DNA replication in suprabasal differentiated keratinocytes. *Genes Dev*, **9**, 2335–49.

Chiang, C.M., Ustav, M., et al. 1992. Viral E1 and E2 proteins support replication of homologous and heterologous papillomaviral origins. *Proc Natl Acad Sci USA*, **89**, 5799–803.

Chow, L.T. and Broker, T.R. 1997. Small DNA tumor viruses. In: Nathanson , N. (ed.), *Viral pathogenesis*. Philadelphia: Lippincott-Raven, 267–301.

Christensen, N.D., Hopfl, R., et al. 1994. Assembled baculovirus expressed human papillomavirus type 11 L1 capsid protein virus like particles are recognized by neutralizing monoclonal antibodies and induce high titres of neutralizing antibodies. *J Gen Virol*, **75**, 2271–6.

Coleman, N., Birley, H.D., et al. 1994. Immunological events in regressing genital warts. *Am J Clin Pathol*, **102**, 768–74.

Conrad, M., Bubb, V.J. and Schlegel, R. 1993. The human papillomavirus type 6 and 16 E5 proteins are membrane associated proteins which associate with the 16 kilodalton pore forming protein. *J Virol*, **67**, 6170–8.

Crook, T., Tidy, J.A. and Vousden, K.H. 1991. Degradation of p53 can be targeted by HPV E6 sequences distinct from those required for p53 binding and *trans* activation. *Cell*, **67**, 547–56.

Daniel, B., Mukherjee, G., et al. 1995. Changes in the physical state and expression of human papillomavirus type 16 in the progression of cervical intraepithelial neoplasia lesions analysed by PCR. *J Gen Virol*, **76**, 2589–93.

Davy, C.E., Jackson, D.J., et al. 2002. Identification of a G(2) arrest domain in the E1 wedge E4 protein of human papillomavirus type 16. *J Virol*, **76**, 9806–18.

de Gruijl, T.D., Bontkes, H.J., et al. 1996a. T cell proliferative responses against human papillomavirus type 16 E7 oncoprotein are most prominent in cervical intraepithelial neoplasia patients with persistent viral infection. *J Gen Virol*, **77**, 2183–91.

de Gruijl, T.D. and Bontkes, H.J. 1996b. Analysis of IgG reactivity against human papillomavirus type-16 E7 in patients with cervical intraepithelial neoplasia indicates an association with clearance of viral infection: results of a prospective study. *Int J Cancer*, **68**, 731–8.

Del Vecchio, A.M., Romanczuk, H., et al. 1992. Transient replication of human papillomavirus DNAs. *J Virol*, **66**, 5949–58.

Demers, G.W., Halbert, C.L. and Galloway, D.A. 1994. Elevated wild type p53 protein levels in human epithelial cell lines immortalized by the human papillomavirus type 16 E7 gene. *Virology*, **198**, 169–74.

Derkay, C.S. 1995. Task force on recurrent respiratory papillomas. A preliminary report. *Arch Otolaryngol Head Neck Surg*, **121**, 1386–91.

Desaintes, C. and Demeret, C. 1996. Control of papillomavirus DNA replication and transcription. *Semin Cancer Biol*, **7**, 339–47.

Dickens, P., Srivastava, G., et al. 1991. Human papillomavirus 6, 11, and 16 in laryngeal papillomas. *J Pathol*, **165**, 243–6.

Di Cunto, F., Topley, G., et al. 1998. Inhibitory function of p21Cip1/WAF1 in differentiation of primary mouse keratinocytes independent of cell cycle control. *Science*, **280**, 1069–72.

DiMaio, D. and Mattoon, D. 2001. Mechanisms of cell transformation by papillomavirus E5 proteins. *Oncogene*, **20**, 7866–73.

Dong, G., Broker, T.R. and Chow, L.T. 1994. Human papillomavirus type 11 E2 proteins repress the homologous E6 promoter by interfering with the binding of host transcription factors to adjacent elements. *J Virol*, **68**, 1115–27.

Doorbar, J., Parton, A., et al. 1990. Detection of novel splicing patterns in a HPV16 containing keratinocyte cell line. *Virology*, **178**, 254–62.

Doorbar, J., Ely, S., et al. 1991. Specific interaction between HPV 16 E1 E4 and cytokeratins results in collapse of the epithelial cell intermediate filament network. *Nature*, **352**, 824–7.

Durst, M., Glitz, D., et al. 1992. Human papillomavirus type 16 (HPV 16) gene expression and DNA replication in cervical neoplasia: analysis by in situ hybridization. *Virology*, **189**, 132–40.

Dyson, N., Guida, P., et al. 1992. Homologous sequences in adenovirus E1A and human papillomavirus E7 proteins mediate interaction with the same set of cellular proteins. *J Virol*, **66**, 6893–902.

Edmonds, C. and Vousden, K.H. 1989. A point mutational analysis of human papillomavirus type 16 E7 protein. *J Virol*, **63**, 2650–6.

Edwards, L., Ferenczy, A., et al. 1998. Self-administered topical 5% imiquimod cream for external anogenital warts. HPV Study Group. Human papilloma virus. *Arch Dermatol*, **134**, 25–30.

Evander, M., Frazer, I.H., et al. 1997. Identification of the alpha 6 integrin as the candidate receptor for papillomaviruses. *J Virol*, **71**, 2449–56.

Favre, M., Majewski, S., et al. 2000. Antibodies to human papillomavirus type 5 are generated in epidermal repair processes. *J Invest Dermatol*, **114**, 403–7.

Frattini, M.G. and Laimins, L.A. 1994. The role of the E1 and E2 proteins in the replication of human papillomavirus type 31b. *Virology*, **204**, 799–804.

Frattini, M.G., Lim, H.B. and Laimins, L.A. 1996. In vitro synthesis of oncogenic human papillomaviruses requires episomal genomes for differentiation dependent late expression. *Proc Natl Acad Sci USA*, **93**, 3062–7.

Funk, J.O., Waga, S., et al. 1997. Inhibition of CDK activity and PCNA-dependent DNA replication by p21 is blocked by interaction with the HPV-16 E7 oncoprotein. *Genes Dev*, **11**, 2090–100.

Gardiol, D., Kuhne, C., et al. 1999. Oncogenic human papillomavirus E6 proteins target the discs large tumour suppressor for proteasome-mediated degradation. *Oncogene*, **18**, 5487–96.

Gopalakrishnan, V. and Khan, S.A. 1994. E1 protein of human papillomavirus type 1a is sufficient for initiation of viral DNA replication. *Proc Natl Acad Sci USA*, **91**, 9597–601.

Grassmann, K., Rapp, B., et al. 1996. Identification of a differentiation-inducible promoter in the E7 open reading frame of human papillomavirus type 16 (HPV-16) in raft cultures of a new cell line containing high copy numbers of episomal HPV-16 DNA. *J Virol*, **70**, 2339–49.

Greenfield, I., Nickerson, J., et al. 1991. Human papillomavirus 16 E7 protein is associated with the nuclear matrix. *Proc Natl Acad Sci USA*, **88**, 11217–21.

Griep, A.E., Herber, R., et al. 1993. Tumorigenicity by human papillomavirus type 16 E6 and E7 in transgenic mice correlates with alterations in epithelial cell growth and differentiation. *J Virol*, **67**, 1373–84.

Gross, G.E., Jablonska, S. and Hugel, H. 1997. Skin: diagnosis. In: Gross, G.E. and Barrasso, R. (eds), *Human papillomavirus infection. A clinical atlas*. Berlin: Ullstein Mosby, 107.

Grossman, S.R. and Laimins, L.A. 1989. E6 protein of human papillomavirus type 18 binds zinc. *Oncogene*, **4**, 1089–93.

Grossman, S.R., Mora, R. and Laimins, L.A. 1989. Intracellular localization and DNA binding properties of human papillomavirus type 18 E6 protein expressed with a baculovirus vector. *J Virol*, **63**, 366–74.

Hagensee, M.E., Yaegashi, N. and Galloway, D.A. 1993. Self assembly of human papillomavirus type 1 capsids by expression of the L1 protein alone or by coexpression of the L1 and L2 capsid proteins. *J Virol*, **67**, 315–22.

Harwood, C.A. and Proby, C.M. 2002. Human papillomaviruses and nonmelanoma skin cancer. *Curr Opin Infect Dis*, **15**, 101–14.

Higgins, G.D., Uzelin, D.M., et al. 1992. Transcription patterns of human papillomavirus type 16 in genital intraepithelial neoplasia: evidence for promoter usage within the E7 open reading frame during epithelial differentiation. *J Gen Virol*, **73**, 2047–57.

Hubbert, N.L., Sedman, S.A. and Schiller, J.T. 1992. Human papillomavirus type 16 E6 increases the degradation rate of p53 in human keratinocytes. *J Virol*, **66**, 6237–41.

Hughes, F.J. and Romanos, M.A. 1993. E1 protein of human papillomavirus is a DNA helicase/ATPase. *Nucleic Acids Res*, **21**, 5817–23.

Huibregtse, J.M., Scheffner, M. and Howley, P.M. 1991. A cellular protein mediates association of p53 with the E6 oncoprotein of human papillomavirus types 16 or 18. *EMBO J*, **10**, 4129–35.

Hummel, M., Hudson, J.B. and Laimins, L.A. 1992. Differentiation induced and constitutive transcription of human papillomavirus type 31b in cell lines containing viral episomes. *J Virol*, **66**, 6070–80.

Hummel, M., Lim, H.B. and Laimins, L.A. 1995. Human papillomavirus type 31b late gene expression is regulated through protein kinase C mediated changes in RNA processing. *J Virol*, **69**, 3381–8.

IARC Monographs on the Evaluation of Carcinogen Risks to Humans. (1996) Vol. 64, *Human Papillomaviruses*. Lyon, France:World Health Organization International Agency for Research on Cancer, 1995 (Meeting of IARC Working Group on 6–13 June 1995).

Imai, Y., Matsushima, Y., et al. 1991. Purification and characterization of human papillomavirus type 16 E7 protein with preferential binding capacity to the underphosphorylated form of retinoblastoma gene product. *J Virol*, **65**, 4966–72.

Ishiji, T., Lace, M.J., et al. 1992. Transcriptional enhancer factor (TEF) 1 and its cell-specific co-activator activate human papillomavirus 16 E6 and E7 oncogene transcription in keratinocytes and cervical carcinoma cells. *EMBO J*, **11**, 2271–81.

Jones, D.L. and Munger, K. 1996. Interactions of the human papillomavirus E7 protein with cell cycle regulators. *Semin Cancer Biol*, **7**, 327–37.

Jones, D.L., Alani, R.M. and Munger, K. 1997. The human papillomavirus E7 oncoprotein can uncouple cellular differentiation and proliferation in human keratinocytes by abrogating p21Cip1-mediated inhibition of cdk2. *Genes Dev*, **11**, 2101–11.

Joyce, J.G., Tung, J.S., et al. 1999. The L1 major capsid protein of human papillomavirus type 11 recombinant virus-like particles interacts with heparin and cell-surface glycosaminoglycans on human keratinocytes. *J Biol Chem*, **274**, 5810–22.

Kessis, T.D., Slebos, R.J., et al. 1993. Human papillomavirus 16 E6 expression disrupts the p53 mediated cellular response to DNA damage. *Proc Natl Acad Sci USA*, **90**, 3988–92.

Kirnbauer, R., Booy, F., et al. 1992. Papillomavirus L1 major capsid protein self-assembles into virus-like particles that are highly immunogenic. *Proc Natl Acad Sci USA*, **89**, 12180–4.

Kirnbauer, R., Taub, J., et al. 1993. Efficient self assembly of human papillomavirus type 16 L1 and L1 L2 into virus like particles. *J Virol*, **67**, 6929–36.

Klingelhutz, A.J., Foster, S.A. and McDougall, J.K. 1996. Telomerase activation by the E6 gene product of human papillomavirus type 16. *Nature*, **380**, 79–82.

Klumpp, D.J. and Laimins, L.A. 1999. Differentiation-induced changes in promoter usage for transcripts encoding the human papillomavirus type 31 replication protein E1. *Virology*, **257**, 239–46.

Koutsky, L.A., Ault, K.A., et al. 2002. A controlled trial of a human papillomavirus type 16 vaccine. *N Engl J Med*, **347**, 1645–51.

Kreider, J.W., Howett, M.K., et al. 1987. Laboratory production in vivo of infectious human papillomavirus type 11. *J Virol*, **61**, 590–3.

Kukimoto, I., Aihara, S., et al. 1998. Human papillomavirus oncoprotein E6 binds to the C-terminal region of human minichromosome maintenance 7 protein. *Biochem Biophys Res Commun*, **249**, 258–62.

Kuo, S.R., Liu, J.S., et al. 1994. Cell free replication of the human papillomavirus DNA with homologous viral E1 and E2 proteins and human cell extracts. *J Biol Chem*, **269**, 24058–65.

Lechner, M.S. and Laimins, L.A. 1994. Inhibition of p53 DNA binding by human papillomavirus E6 proteins. *J Virol*, **68**, 4262–73.

Lee, D., Kim, H.Z., et al. 2002. Human papillomavirus E2 down-regulates the human telomerase reverse transcriptase promoter. *J Biol Chem*, **277**, 27748–56.

Li, M., Beard, P., et al. 1998. Intercapsomeric disulfide bonds in papillomavirus assembly and disassembly. *J Virol*, **72**, 2160–7.

Lusky, M., Hurwitz, J. and Seo, Y.S. 1994. The bovine papillomavirus E2 protein modulates the assembly of but is not stably maintained in a replication-competent multimeric E1-replication origin complex. *Proc Natl Acad Sci USA*, **91**, 8895–9.

Majewski, S. and Jablonska, S. 2001. Epidermodysplasia verruciformis. In: Sterling, J.C. and Tyring, S.K. (eds), *Human papillomaviruses: clinical and scientific advances*. London: Arnold, 90–101.

Maran, A., Amella, C.A., et al. 1995. Human papillomavirus type 11 transcripts are present at low abundance in latently infected respiratory tissues. *Virology*, **212**, 285–94.

Massimi, P., Pim, D. and Banks, L. 1997. Human papillomavirus type 16 E7 binds to the conserved carboxy-terminal region of the TATA box binding protein and this contributes to E7 transforming activity. *J Gen Virol*, **78**, 2607–13.

Massing, A.M. and Epstein, W.L. 1963. Natural history of warts: a two year study. *Arch Dermatol*, **87**, 306.

Masterson, P.J., Stanley, M.A., et al. 1998. A C-terminal helicase domain of the human papillomavirus E1 protein binds E2 and the DNA polymerase alpha-primase p68 subunit. *J Virol*, **72**, 7407–19.

McIntyre, M.C., Frattini, M.G., et al. 1993. Human papillomavirus type 18 E7 protein requires intact Cys-X-X-Cys motifs for zinc binding, dimerization, and transformation but not for Rb binding. *J Virol*, **67**, 3142–50.

Missero, C., Calautti, E., et al. 1995. Involvement of the cell cycle inhibitor Cip1/WAF1 and the E1A associated p300 protein in terminal differentiation. *Proc Natl Acad Sci USA*, **92**, 5451–5.

Missero, C., Di Cunto, F., et al. 1996. The absence of p21Cip1/WAF1 alters keratinocyte growth and differentiation and promotes *ras* tumor progression. *Genes Dev*, **10**, 3065–75.

Mohr, I.J., Clark, R., et al. 1990. Targeting the E1 replication protein to the papillomavirus origin of replication by complex formation with the E2 transactivator. *Science*, **250**, 1694–9.

Moore, A.Y. and Tyring, S.K. 2001. Cutaneous warts. In: Sterling, J.C. and Tyring, S.K. (eds), *Human papillomaviruses: clinical and scientific advances*. London: Arnold, 52–9.

Moore, R.A., Nicholls, P.K., et al. 2002. COPV DNA absence following prophylactic L1 PMID vaccination. *J Gen Virol*, **83**, 2299–301.

Munger, K., Werness, B.A., et al. 1989. Complex formation of human papillomavirus E7 proteins with the retinoblastoma tumor suppressor gene product. *EMBO J*, **8**, 4099–105.

Muñoz, N. and Bosch, F.X. 1996. Critical views on the epidemiology of HPV and cervical cancer. In: Lacey, C. (ed.), *Papillomavirus reviews: current research on papillomaviruses*. Leeds: Leeds University Press, 227–37.

Muñoz, N., Bosch, F.X., et al. 1992. The causal link between human papillomavirus and invasive cervical cancer: a population based case control study in Colombia and Spain. *Int J Cancer*, **52**, 743–9.

Nicholls, P.K., Klaunberg, B.A., et al. 1999. Naturally occurring nonregressing canine oral papillomavirus infection: host immunity, virus characterization, and experimental infection. *Virology*, **265**, 365–74.

Nicholls, P.K., Moore, P.F., et al. 2001. Regression of canine oral papillomas is associated with infiltration of CD4+ and CD8+ lymphocytes. *Virology*, **283**, 31–9.

Nonnenmacher, B., Hubbert, N.L., et al. 1995. Serologic response to human papillomavirus type 16 (HPV 16) virus like particles in HPV 16 DNA positive invasive cervical cancer and cervical intraepithelial neoplasia grade III patients and controls from Colombia and Spain. *J Infect Dis*, **172**, 19–24.

O'Connor, M. and Bernard, H.U. 1995. Oct 1 activates the epithelial specific enhancer of human papillomavirus type 16 via a synergistic interaction with NFI at a conserved composite regulatory element. *Virology*, **207**, 77–88.

O'Connor, M., Chan, S.Y. and Bernard, H.U. 1995. Transcription factor binding sites in the long control region of genital HPVs. In: Myers, G., Bernard, H.U., et al. (eds), *Human papillomaviruses*. Los Alamos: University of California, 21–40.

O'Connor, M.J., Tan, C.H., et al. 1996. YY1 represses human papillomavirus type 16 transcription by quenching AP-1 activity. *J Virol*, **70**, 6529–39.

Okun, M.M., Day, P.M., et al. 2001. L1 interaction domains of papillomavirus l2 necessary for viral genome encapsidation. *J Virol*, **75**, 4332–42.

Oriel, J.D. 1971. Natural history of genital warts. *Br J Venereal Dis*, **47**, 1–13.

Orth, G., Favre, M., et al. 2001. Epidermodysplasia verruciformis defines a subset of cutaneous human papillomaviruses. *J Virol*, **75**, 4952–3.

Pan, H. and Griep, A.E. 1994. Altered cell cycle regulation in the lens of HPV 16 E6 or E7 transgenic mice: implications for tumor suppressor gene function in development. *Genes Dev*, **8**, 1285–99.

Peh, W.L., Middleton, K., et al. 2002. Life cycle heterogeneity in animal models of human papillomavirus-associated disease. *J Virol*, **76**, 10401–16.

Persson, G., Andersson, K. and Krantz, I. 1996. Symptomatic genital papillomavirus infection in a community. Incidence and clinical picture. *Acta Obstet Gynecol Scand*, **75**, 287–90.

Phelps, W.C., Munger, K., et al. 1992. Structure/function analysis of the human papillomavirus type 16 E7 oncoprotein. *J Virol*, **66**, 2418–27.

PHLS Communicable Disease Centre, 1989. Sexually transmitted disease in Britain 1985–1986. *Genitourinary Med*, **65**, 117–21.

Pim, D., Massimi, P. and Banks, L. 1997. Alternatively spliced HPV-18 E6* protein inhibits E6 mediated degradation of p53 and suppresses transformed cell growth. *Oncogene*, **15**, 257–64.

Pray, T.R. and Laimins, L.A. 1995. Differentiation-dependent expression of E1–E4 proteins in cell lines maintaining episomes of human papillomavirus type 31b. *Virology*, **206**, 679–85.

Puranen, M.H., Yliskoski, M.H., et al. 1997. Exposure of an infant to cervical human papillomavirus infection of the mother is common. *Am J Obstet Gynecol*, **176**, 1039–45.

Roberts, S., Ashmole, I., et al. 1993. Cutaneous and mucosal human papillomavirus E4 proteins form intermediate filament like structures in epithelial cells. *Virology*, **197**, 176–87.

Roberts, S., Ashmole, I., et al. 1997. Mutational analysis of the human papillomavirus type 16 E1–E4 protein shows that the C terminus is dispensable for keratin cytoskeleton association but is involved in inducing disruption of the keratin filaments. *J Virol*, **71**, 3554–62.

Roden, R.B., Greenstone, H.L., et al. 1996. In vitro generation and type-specific neutralization of a human papillomavirus type 16 virion pseudotype. *J Virol*, **70**, 5875–83.

Ronco, L.V., Karpova, A.Y., et al. 1998. Human papillomavirus 16 E6 oncoprotein binds to interferon regulatory factor-3 and inhibits its transcriptional activity. *Genes Dev*, **12**, 2061–72.

Rose, R.C., Bonnez, W., et al. 1993. Expression of human papillomavirus type 11 L1 protein in insect cells: in vivo and in vitro assembly of viruslike particles. *J Virol*, **67**, 1936–44.

Ruesch, M.N. and Laimins, L.A. 1998. Human papillomavirus oncoproteins alter differentiation-dependent cell cycle exit on suspension in semisolid medium. *Virology*, **250**, 19–29.

Sakai, H., Yasugi, T., et al. 1996. Targeted mutagenesis of the human papillomavirus type 16 E2 transactivation domain reveals separable transcriptional activation and DNA replication functions. *J Virol*, **70**, 1602–11.

Scheffner, M., Werness, B.A., et al. 1990. The E6 oncoprotein encoded by human papillomavirus types 16 and 18 promotes the degradation of p53. *Cell*, **63**, 1129–36.

Scheffner, M., Munger, K., et al. 1991. The state of the p53 and retinoblastoma genes in human cervical carcinoma cell lines. *Proc Natl Acad Sci USA*, **88**, 5523–7.

Scheffner, M., Huibregtse, J., et al. 1993. The HPV 16 E6 and E6 AP complex functions as a ubiquitin protein ligase in the ubiquitination of p53. *Cell*, **75**, 495–505.

Schiffman, M.H. and Brinton, L.A. 1995. The epidemiology of cervical carcinogenesis. *Cancer*, **76**, 1888–901.

Schmitt, A., Rochat, A., et al. 1996. The primary target cells of the high-risk cottontail rabbit papillomavirus colocalize with hair follicle stem cells. *J Virol*, **70**, 1912–22.

Schwarz, E., Freese, U.K., et al. 1985. Structure and transcription of human papillomavirus sequences in cervical carcinoma cells. *Nature*, **314**, 111–14.

Sedman, J. and Stenlund, A. 1998. The papillomavirus E1 protein forms a DNA-dependent hexameric complex with ATPase and DNA helicase activities. *J Virol*, **72**, 6893–7.

Selvakumar, R., Schmitt, A., et al. 1997. Regression of papillomas induced by cotton tail rabbit papillomavirus is associated with infiltration of CD8$^+$ cells and persistence of viral DNA after regression. *J Virol*, **71**, 5540–8.

Shah, K.V., Stern, W.F., et al. 1998. Risk factors for juvenile onset recurrent respiratory papillomatosis. *Pediatr Infect Dis J*, **17**, 372–6.

Shally, M., Alloul, N., et al. 1996. The E6 variant proteins E6I-E6IV of human papillomavirus 16: expression in cell free systems and bacteria and study of their interaction with p53. *Virus Res*, **42**, 81–96.

Sibbet, G.J. and Campo, M.S. 1990. Multiple interactions between cellular factors and the non coding region of human papillomavirus type 16. *J Gen Virol*, **71**, 2699–707.

Sibbet, G., Romero Graillet, C., et al. 2000. α6 integrin is not the obligatory cell receptor for bovine papillomavirus type 4. *J Gen Virol*, **81**, 327–34.

Skiadopoulos, M.H. and McBride, A.A. 1998. Bovine papillomavirus type 1 genomes and the E2 transactivator protein are closely associated with mitotic chromatin. *J Virol*, **72**, 2079–88.

Smotkin, D. and Wettstein, F.O. 1987. The major human papillomavirus protein in cervical cancers is a cytoplasmic phosphoprotein. *J Virol*, **61**, 1686–9.

Snijders, P.J., Van Den Brule, A.J., et al. 1994. Papillomaviruses and cancer of the upper digestive and respiratory tracts. *Curr Topics Microbiol Immunol*, **186**, 177–98.

Stanley, M.A. 1994. Replication of human papillomaviruses in cell culture. *Antiviral Res*, **24**, 1–15.

Stanley, M.A. 1997. Genital papillomaviruses – prospects for vaccination. *Curr Opin Infect Dis*, **10**, 55–61.

Stanley, M.A. 2001a. Pathobiology of human papillomaviruses. In: Grand, R.A. (ed.), *Viruses, cell transformation and cancer*. Amsterdam: Elsevier, 129–44.

Stanley, M.A. 2001b. Immune responses to human papillomaviruses. In: Sterling, J.C. and Tyring, S.K. (eds), *Human papillomaviruses. Clinical and scientific advances*. London: Arnold, 38–49.

Stanley, M.A., Browne, H.M., et al. 1989. Properties of a non tumorigenic human cervical keratinocyte cell line. *Int J Cancer*, **43**, 672–6.

Stanley, M.A., Masterson, P.J. and Nicholls, P.K. 1997. In vitro and animal models for antiviral therapy for papillomavirus infections. *Antivir Chem Chemother*, **8**, 381–400.

Stauffer, Y., Raj, K., et al. 1998. Infectious human papillomavirus type 18 pseudovirions. *J Mol Biol*, **283**, 529–36.

Steele, J.C. and Gallimore, P.H. 1990. Humoral assays of human sera to disrupted and nondisrupted epitopes of human papillomavirus type 1. *Virology*, **174**, 388–98.

Steger, G. and Corbach, S. 1997. Dose-dependent regulation of the early promoter of human papillomavirus type 18 by the viral E2 protein. *J Virol*, **71**, 50–8.

Sterling, J.C., Skepper, J.N. and Stanley, M.A. 1993. Immunoelectron microscopical localization of human papillomavirus type 16 L1 and E4 proteins in cervical keratinocytes cultured in vivo. *J Invest Dermatol.*, **100**, 154–8.

Stoler, M.H., Rhodes, C.R., et al. 1992. Human papillomavirus type 16 and 18 gene expression in cervical neoplasias. *Hum Pathol*, **23**, 117–28.

Stoler, M.H., Whitbeck, A., et al. 1990. Infectious cycle of human papillomavirus type 11 in human foreskin xenografts in nude mice. *J Virol*, **64**, 3310–18.

Straight, S.W., Hinkle, P.M., et al. 1993. The E5 oncoprotein of human papillomavirus type 16 transforms fibroblasts and effects the downregulation of the epidermal growth factor receptor in keratinocytes. *J Virol*, **67**, 4521–32.

Straight, S.W., Herman, B. and McCance, D.J. 1995. The E5 oncoprotein of human papillomavirus type 16 inhibits the acidification of endosomes in human keratinocytes. *J Virol*, **69**, 3185–92.

Strauss, S., Jordens, J.Z., et al. 1999. Detection and typing of human papillomavirus DNA in paired urine and cervical scrapes. *Eur J Epidemiol*, **15**, 537–43.

Stubenrauch, F. and Laimins, L.A. 1999. Human papillomavirus life cycle: active and latent phases. *Semin Cancer Biol*, **9**, 379–86.

Terhune, S.S., Milcarek, C. and Laimins, L.A. 1999. Regulation of human papillomavirus type 31 polyadenylation during the differentiation-dependent life cycle. *J Virol*, **73**, 7185–92.

Thierry, F. and Howley, P.M. 1991. Functional analysis of E2 mediated repression of the HPV18 P105 promoter. *New Biol*, **3**, 90–100.

Thomas, M. and Banks, L. 1999. Human papillomavirus (HPV) E6 interactions with Bak are conserved amongst E6 proteins from high and low risk HPV types. *J Gen Virol*, **80**, 1513–17.

Toon, P.G., Arrand, J.R., et al. 1986. Human papillomavirus infection of the uterine cervix of women without cytological signs of neoplasia. *Br Med J Clin Res*, **293**, 1261–4.

Trus, B.L., Roden, R.B., et al. 1997. Novel structural features of bovine papillomavirus capsid protein revealed by a three-dimensional reconstruction to 9 Å resolution. *Nature Struct Biol*, **4**, 413–20.

Turner, C.E. 2000. Paxillin and focal adhesion signalling. *Nature Cell Biol*, **2**, E231–236.

Ustav, M., Ustav, E., et al. 1991. Identification of the origin of replication of bovine papillomavirus and characterization of the viral origin recognition factor E1. *EMBO J*, **10**, 4321–9.

Walboomers, J.M., Jacobs, M.V., et al. 1999. Human papillomavirus is a necessary cause of invasive cervical cancer worldwide. *J Pathol*, **189**, 12–19.

Watanabe, S., Kanda, T., et al. 1990. Mutational analysis of human papillomavirus type 16 E7 functions. *J Virol*, **64**, 207–14.

Werness, B.A., Levine, A.J. and Howley, P.M. 1990. Association of human papillomavirus types 16 and 18 E6 proteins with p53. *Science*, **248**, 76–9.

Wilson, J.L., Dollard, S.C., et al. 1992. Epithelial specific gene expression during differentiation of stratified primary human keratinocyte cultures. *Cell Growth Differ*, **3**, 471–83.

Zhou, J., Sun, X.Y., et al. 1991. Expression of vaccinia recombinant HPV 16 L1 and L2 ORF proteins in epithelial cells is sufficient for assembly of HPV virion like particles. *Virology*, **185**, 251–7.

Zhou, J., Sun, X.Y. and Frazer, I.H. 1993. Glycosylation of human papillomavirus type 16 L1 protein. *Virology*, **194**, 210–18.

zur Hausen, H. 2000. Papillomaviruses causing cancer: evasion from host-cell control in early events in carcinogenesis. *J Natl Cancer Inst*, **92**, 690–8.

Zwerschke, W., Mazurek, S., et al. 1999. Modulation of type M2 pyruvate kinase activity by the human papillomavirus type 16 E7 oncoprotein. *Proc Natl Acad Sci USA*, **96**, 1291–6.

24

Polyomaviruses

JESSICA OTTE, MAHMUT SAFAK, AND KAMEL KHALILI

INTRODUCTION

During the last 30 years polyomaviruses, in particular SV40, have been extensively utilized by molecular biologists to decipher complicated biological events including gene transcription, RNA processing, control of RNA translation, and DNA replication in eukaryotic cells. In recent years, these viruses have received special attention in the field of biomedical science due to their involvement and association with diseases in humans, ranging from demyelinating disorders and nephropathy to various types of cancers including brain tumors, lung malignancy, and lymphomas. These new developments have encouraged many biomedical and basic scientists to employ a variety of approaches and techniques to unravel the interaction of polyomaviruses with their specific host cells, and decipher the pathogenesis of the diseases associated with polyomaviral infection. Here, we have provided an overview highlighting the general features of polyomaviruses that include their structural organization, gene regulation, and replication prior to focusing our attention on three members of this group of viruses, JCV, BKV, and SV40, due to their increasing importance in the clinical setting. We further emphasize JCV due to its established association with the fatal demyelinating disease of the brain and its association with neural and nonneural malignancies.

GENERAL DESCRIPTION

Polyomaviruses have been isolated from a number of species including monkeys, rodents, and birds, as well as humans. The common feature of the members of the family *Polyomaviridae* rests on their unique morphology which includes a 45-nm icosahedral particle comprised of three capsid proteins, and their genome which consists of double-stranded circular DNA of approximately 5 000 nucleotides in size.

While productive infection with polyomaviruses is generally species-specific, expression of the viral genome appears to be less restricted and occurs in a broad range of species. Nevertheless, transcription activation of the viral promoter is tissue-specific for some members of the polyomavirus family. Humans are the established host for BKV and JCV, while primates, including rhesus monkeys, African green monkeys, baboons, and stump-tailed macaques are the hosts for simian virus 40 (SV40), lymphotropic papovavirus (LPV), simian agent 12 (SA12), and stump-tailed macaque virus (STMV), respectively. Detection of SV40 in several human tumors in recent years has raised the possibility of humans as co-hosts for this virus. Mice are the host for polyomavirus (PYV), while rabbits and hamsters are considered the hosts for rabbit kidney vacuolating virus (RKV), and hamster polyomavirus (HaPyV), respectively. Bovine polyomavirus (BPyV) and budgerigar fledgling polyomavirus (BFPyV) target cattle and birds, respectively. In general, polyomaviruses possess an oncogenic potential in several experimental animals and it is believed that the viral early protein plays a role in the oncogenicity of the virus.

In permissive hosts, lytic infection of the cells with polyomaviruses begins by binding of the virion to the cell surface proteins. For example, the association of SV40 with class I major histocompatibility complex is an early event for infection of monkey kidney cells with the virus. Human polyomaviruses, such as JCV, however, appear to employ different cell surface receptors, most probably *N*-linked glycoprotein containing terminal α (2–6) linked sialic acid for its attachment to permissive cells (Atwood 2001). In either case, it is believed that the major capsid protein, VP1, plays a critical role in binding of the virus to its cell surface receptor. Once attached to the cell membrane, the virus internalizes through the process of endocytosis, and after uncoating, viral DNA appears in the nucleus. The viral DNA is present in a chromatin-like structure associated with cellular histone protein H2A, H2B, H3, and H4. The genome of the polyomavirus is divided into early and late regions on the basis of whether they are expressed before or after DNA replication. Viral proteins are encoded on both DNA strands and are transcribed divergently from a central regulatory region. The early genes encode the large and small tumor antigens, multifunctional proteins that regulate progression of the viral lytic cycle, and deregulate several important pathways in host cells. The small t- and large T-antigens have a common amino terminus and arise from alternatively spliced transcripts. In more recent studies, an altered isoform of T-antigen, named T′, has been detected in JCV infected cells (Frisque 2001). In SV40, a third protein named SELP, whose open reading frame is located in the leader of some early DNA species, has been reported yet its function remains unknown (Khalili et al. 1987b). Other polyomaviruses, including JCV and BKV, also possess an early leader open reading frame which exhibits greater than 50 percent homology with SELP. The late genes encode structural components of the viral capsid proteins, VP1, VP2, and VP3. VP1 is encoded by the 3′ end of the late region and is translated from a distinct mRNA in a different reading frame than the other two capsid proteins, VP2 and VP3. Both VP2 and VP3 are encoded in the 5′ end of the late region and are translated from a common mRNA. The VP1 mRNA leader sequence codes for a small protein named 'Agnoprotein' which is found only in SV40, JCV, and BKV polyoma species.

The full lytic infection cycle of polyomaviruses can be divided into two phases: the early phase occurs prior to viral DNA replication and the late phase, which includes all events such as viral DNA replication, expression of the viral late genes, assembly of progeny viral particles, and viral release. During the early phase, the virus attaches to the cell surface, enters the cell through endocytosis, transports to the cell nucleus and after uncoating, the viral early gene begins to transcribe and synthesize viral early RNA, and after translocation, the early proteins, T-antigen, and its various isoforms. Once T-antigen is accumulated in the nucleus of the cells, it cooperates with cellular DNA replication factors to stimulate viral DNA replication, and at the same time enhances the level of viral late gene expression. The products of the late genes including the capsid proteins,

VP1, VP2, and VP3, enter the nucleus and participate in the assembly of viral progeny through the association of the viral capsid proteins with the newly synthesized viral DNA. One of the most intense areas of research on polyomaviruses has been on the regulation of viral gene transcription, cell type-specific activation of the viral genome, and the control of viral DNA replication. The DNA regulatory sequence which is responsible for transcription and replication of the viral genome spans the 400–500 nucleotides which are positioned between the viral early and late genomes.

This region is composed of many *cis*-acting regulatory motifs that provide targets for binding of cellular transcription factors. Of note, the transcription of polyomaviruses is dependent on the host transcriptional machinery. The association of the proper transcriptional factors with the viral DNA sequence potentiates RNA polymerase II and its subunits to initiate viral early gene transcription. Lengthy studies on the identification of cellular factors that stimulate the SV40 promoter led to the identification of several important proteins, such as Sp1 and the AP1 family, which exhibit a broad spectrum of regulatory functions upon eukaryotic gene transcription. It was also noted that the interaction of cellular proteins with the viral DNA sequence may not be sufficient for stimulation of viral promoters, suggesting that cross-communication and indirect interaction may play a critical role in viral gene expression.

HUMAN POLYOMAVIRUSES

JCV

The infection process of JCV, as of any nonenveloped small DNA virus, begins with the attachment of the viral particles to the cell surface receptors. Recent reports indicate that JCV enters the susceptible cells through clathrin-dependent endocytosis and α(2–3)-linked sialic acid appears to be critical in this process (Atwood 2001; Liu et al. 1998a,b; Pho et al. 2000). Subsequently, the viral genome is targeted into the nucleus by an unknown mechanism. Infectious virions are formed after DNA replication and expression of capsid proteins and finally, viral particles are released upon cell death.

The nucleotide sequence analysis of JCV genome has revealed that it is composed of three functional regions including the viral early coding region, the viral late coding region, and the viral noncoding regulatory region (Frisque et al. 1984) (Figure 24.1). Comparison of JCV sequences with two other closely related polyomaviruses, BK virus and SV40, has revealed that it exhibits extensive sequence homology in coding regions to its counterparts. However, the sequences within the regulatory region of JCV show the greatest degree of divergence from those of BK virus and SV40. Studies over the years have shown that the regulatory region of

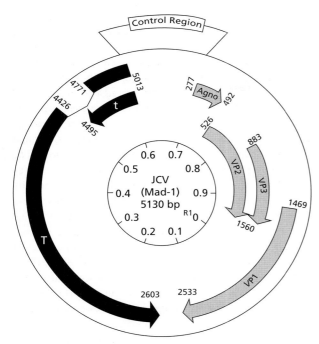

Figure 24.1 *Circular map of the JCV genome. Schematic representation of the JCV genome. Directions of the early and late coding regions are depicted with arrows. Early genes encode small t- and large T-antigens. Late genes encode the viral capsid proteins, VP1, VP2, and VP3, and Agnoprotein. The regulatory region is located between the two coding regions.*

JCV confers, at least in part, the tissue specificity of JCV gene expression (Ahmed et al. 1990a; Amemiya et al. 1989, 1992; Chowdhury et al. 1990, 1992, 1993; Khalili et al. 1988; Tada and Khalili 1992; Tada et al. 1989, 1991).

The regulatory region of JCV is composed of the origin of DNA replication, promoter elements for both early and late genes and *cis*-acting enhancer elements (Figure 24.2). The JCV origin of DNA replication is a 98-bp element located between the NF-κB motif and the first tandem repeat of JCV Mad-1 strain. It shows

extensive homology to the SV40 origin (Frisque and White 1992; Kim et al. 2001). The enhancer elements are composed of two complete 98-bp tandem repeats (Mad-1 strain), each of which contains its own TATA box located in the early site of individual repeat. The first TATA box with respect to the origin of DNA replication is involved in the positioning of the transcription start sites for viral early genes (Frisque and White 1992; Kim et al. 2001; Lynch and Frisque 1990, 1991). The second TATA box does not appear to have a similar function for the viral late genes. The remaining regions within the 98-bp repeats have been shown to confer crucial *cis*-acting elements which were shown to serve as binding sites for several transcription factors (Frisque and White 1992; Kim et al. 2001; Major et al. 1992; Raj and Khalili 1995).

The regulatory region of JCV appears to be hypervariable in nature (Vaz et al. 2000; Yogo et al. 2001; Zoltick et al. 1995). Comparison of the regulatory sequences among a number of JCV isolates revealed that the hypervariability is mostly confined to 98 base pair tandem repeat region (Figure 24.2). Based on the variations including deletions and duplications, JCV isolates are classified into two classes or groups (Frisque and White 1992; Vaz et al. 2000; Yogo et al. 2001; Zoltick et al. 1995). The class I viruses are characterized by the presence of the 98-bp tandem repeat within its regulatory region. The Mad-1 strain of JCV belongs to class I. The class II viruses contain strains that exhibit variations from the regulatory region of the class I with deletions and insertions. Ninety-eight base pair repeats appear to vary in size and the distal repeat with respect to the origin of DNA replication lacks the TATA box sequences. There tends to be a full length or partial duplication of the 23-bp sequence element usually occurring at nucleotide 36 of the first tandem repeat (Frisque and White 1992). Although the mechanism by which these deletions and duplications occur and give rise to new strains of JCV remains unknown, it is generally

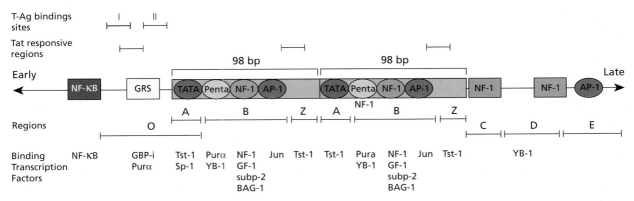

Figure 24.2 *Multiple transcription factor binding sites in the enhancer/promoter region of Mad-1. Transcription factors that have been shown to bind to the promoters are illustrated at the bottom of the schematic. Cis-acting elements are depicted in the boxes or circles in the schematic of the promoter. T-antigen binding sites and Tat responsive elements are indicated. Arbitrary subregions including A, B, Z, C, D, E, and O are indicated.*

accepted that both classes are derived from a common ancestral form of the JCV archetype strain which is mainly detected in the kidney (Gardner et al. 1971). It is postulated that alterations within the regulatory region of the JCV archetype strain can result in novel regulatory rearrangements of the virus with altered features. The new virus is then capable of replicating in new cells and tissues (Frisque and White 1992).

The Mad-1 strain of JCV has been used for most of the replication and transcriptional studies of JCV. As a result, the descriptions of the viral promoter-enhancer elements and the participation of these elements in viral gene transcription and DNA replication will be discussed with respect to Mad-1. In addition to containing the NF-κB motif and origin of DNA replication, the regulatory region of Mad-1 also confers two exact 98-bp tandem repeats (Figure 24.2) (Frisque and White 1992), which dictate the transcription of early and late genes in opposite directions. The *cis*-acting elements present within and around the 98-bp repeats were shown to be targets for tissue-specific and ubiquitous transcription factors (Figure 24.2). In addition to these cellular factors, the viral regulatory proteins, including large T-antigen and Agnoprotein, were also shown to regulate expression of the viral promoters (Raj et al. 1996; Safak et al. 2001, 2002). As stated earlier large T-antigen is a multifunctional phosphoprotein involved in both viral early and late gene expression, as well as in T-antigen-dependent viral DNA replication. Together with the cellular factors which are required for DNA replication, T-antigen binds to the viral origin of DNA replication, unwinds it and initiates replication bidirectionally (Lynch and Frisque 1990; Tavis and Frisque 1991). T-antigen regulates its own transcription via an autoregulatory loop, and plays a major role in the transcriptional switch from viral early to late gene expression (Khalili et al. 1987a; Lashgari et al. 1989).

The regulatory region of JCV is subdivided into arbitrary regions for the sake of simple transcriptional analysis (Figure 24.2). The cellular factors that interact with B region for example are extensively studied and include a 45 kDa protein (Khalili et al. 1988; Raj et al. 1998), GF-1 (Kerr and Khalili 1991), YB-1 (Raj et al. 1996), Purα (Chen et al. 1995), and AP-1 (Amemiya et al. 1992; Sadowska et al. 2003), Subp-2 (Fukita et al. 1993; Kerr and Khalili 1991), and BAG-1 (Devireddy et al. 2000). Computer-aided experimental analysis of the regulatory region have revealed the presence of multiple NF-1 binding sites included in the B, C, and D regions (Raj and Khalili 1995). The NF-1 transcription factor was shown to be involved in both viral transcription and replication (Kumar et al. 1993; Sock et al. 1993; Tamura et al. 1988, 1990). GF-1 is a partial recombinant protein cloned by Kerr and Khalili (1991) from a human fetal brain expression library and represents a human homologue of the cloned murine Sμbp-2 protein (Fukita et al. 1993). Its binding specificity is similar to that of

NF-1. GF-1 was found to *trans*-activate viral early and late promoters (Kerr and Khalili 1991). YB-1 and Purα were shown to interact with this region. Recently, a novel Bcl-1-interacting protein, BAG-1, was cloned from p19 embryonic carcinoma cells using the JCV NF-1-binding site as a probe. It is expressed ubiquitously and regulates JCV early and late promoters through the NF-1 binding site (Devireddy et al. 2000). Another cellular factor that interacts with the B region is c-Jun, a member of the AP-1 family of transcription factors. The members of this family are known as the immediate–early inducible proto-oncogenes. Its binding activity to the B region appears to be modulated by NF-1 transcription factor which binds to adjacent NF-1-like sequences (Amemiya et al. 1992). It has been demonstrated recently that it interacts directly with its target sequences and activates transcription from the JCV promoters (Amemiya et al. 1992; Sadowska et al. 2003). Like AP-1, NF-κB, and GBP-i represent inducible cellular factors that modulate gene expression from viral early and late promoters. NF-κB represents a large family of transcription factors which are inducible in response to a wide variety of extracellular stimuli including the presence of phorbol esters and cytokines. The NF-κB family of proteins was shown to play a role in determining the basal and induced levels of transcription from viral early and late promoters (Ranganathan and Khalili 1993). While constitutively expressed subunits p50 and p52 activate transcription from the D domain (Raj et al. 1996), subunit p65 activates transcription from the NF-κB motif (Ranganathan and Khalili 1993). p50/p65 were also shown to indirectly influence JCV gene transcription through a 23-bp element present within the regulatory regions of many JCV variants (Safak et al. 1999). GBP-i interacts with GRS sequences and suppresses viral late promoter activity (Raj and Khalili 1994). Another regulator of viral early and late gene expression is the transcription factor Tst-1, a member of the well-characterized tissue-specific and developmentally regulated POU family of transcription factors. It was found to have distinct binding sites at A and Z regions. Tst-1 regulates viral early and late gene promoters by interacting with the A region (Renner et al. 1994; Wegner et al. 1993). In addition, the physical interaction of Tst-1 with JCV T-antigen was shown to lead to synergistic activation from both promoters (Renner et al. 1994). Even though a potential binding site for a ubiquitously expressed transcription factor, Sp-1, exists within the regulatory region of JCV, its function in the viral transcription is largely unknown. However, a polymerase chain reaction (PCR)-amplified variant of JCV was recently shown to confer a functional Sp-1 binding site. Transcriptional studies using Sp-1 as a *trans*-activator revealed that Sp1 stimulates transcription from the viral early promoter (Henson et al. 1992; Henson 1994). In addition to its own regulatory proteins, the JCV genome was also shown to be cross-regulated by the regulatory proteins encoded by other viruses outside the polyomavirus family, including the HIV-1 Tat protein and the cytomegalovirus (CMV) immediate–early *trans*-activator protein 2 (IE2) (Tada et al. 1990; Winklhofer et al. 2000).

Compared to its counterpart, SV40, JCV exhibits a relatively long and inefficient lytic cycle which does not appear to conform with the progression of the viral illness, progressive multifocal leukoencephalopathy (PML). However, there is now experimental evidence to account for this discrepancy. In addition to its transcriptional regulation by a number of cellular factors and its own large T antigen, the JCV promoter has also been shown to be regulated by additional factors including cytokines, growth factors associated with immunosuppression, helper viruses such as human immunodeficiency virus type 1 (HIV-1) (Atwood et al. 1995; Tada et al. 1990), and cytomegalovirus (Heilbronn et al. 1993; Winklhofer et al. 2000). Growth factors and cytokines appear to mediate direct or indirect effects on viral promoters by induction of transcription factors, including GBP-i, NF-κB, and c-Jun (Raj and Khalili 1994; Ranganathan and Khalili 1993; Sadowska et al. 2003). An HIV-1-encoded transregulatory protein, Tat, was shown to transactivate the JCV promoter by interacting with two distinct regions within the viral regulatory region (Chowdhury et al. 1990, 1992, 1993; Tada et al. 1990).

NEUROTROPIC FEATURES OF THE JCV GENOME

Observations from both promoter-swapping experiments and somatic cell hybridization studies have indicated that the *cis*-acting promoter/enhancer elements of JCV and tissue specific cellular factors are the two main determinants that contribute to the narrow host range and neurotropism of JCV. The promoter/enhancer swapping experiments between SV40 and JCV in transgenic mice (Feigenbaum et al. 1992) and transfection studies in tissue culture indicated that narrow host range and cell specificity of JCV may be largely attributed to the JCV promoter/enhancer elements, as well as to the unique characteristics of JCV T antigen (Feigenbaum et al. 1987; Frisque and White 1992; Lashgari et al. 1989; Lynch et al. 1994; Tada et al. 1989). Reporter gene experiments using the regulatory region of JCV in in vivo and in vitro transcription assays (Ahmed et al. 1990a,b) indicated that expression of the viral early promoter is substantially higher in glial cells than nonglial cells, pointing to the importance of tissue-specific factors in JCV neurotropism (Ahmed et al. 1990b). However, JCV DNA replication and late gene expression can occur when large T-antigen is provided in nonglial cells (Lashgari et al. 1989). Somatic cell hybridization studies between transformed hamster glial cells expressing viral T antigen and mouse fibroblast cells supported the finding from transfection studies and

suggested the presence of positive regulatory factors in glial cells and negative regulatory factors in nonglial cells (Beggs et al. 1988).

DISEASES ASSOCIATED WITH JCV INFECTIONS
Progressive multifocal leukoencephalopathy

PML is a white matter disease of the central nervous system resulting from the lytic infection of oligodendrocytes by JCV (Berger and Concha 1995; Major et al. 1992; Walker et al. 1973). The JCV archetype strain initially causes a latent infection in the kidneys. Immunosuppression of the host system due to an underlying disease, such as Hodgkin's lymphoma, lymphoproliferative disease, or acquired immune deficiency syndrome (AIDS) leads to the reactivation of the JCV archetype strain. During this reactivation period, the virus undergoes rearrangement in its regulatory region resulting in the Mad strains. The Mad strains then travel to the brain by an unknown mechanism, perhaps through B lymphocytes, and infect the myelin-producing cells of the central nervous system, the oligodendrocytes. Infection of oligodendrocytes results in the destruction of myelin, creating sporadic plaques of demyelination in the brain. Hence, demyelination occurs as a multifocal process, rarely unifocal, and develops in the white matter of the cortex, though plaques may also occur in any region of the central nervous system (CNS) including the brainstem and cerebellum, but excluding the spinal cord (Brooks and Walker 1984; Thomson and Jones 1968). Clinically, visual deficits are a common sign and symptom of PML at the time of presentation, accounting for 35 to 45 percent of cases, while motor weakness accounts for 25 to 33 percent of cases, and mental deficits (emotional liability, difficulty in memory, and dementia), account for 33 percent of cases at presentation (Berger and Concha 1995). PML usually progresses to death within 4–6 months. In occasional cases, clinical signs and symptoms appear to remain stable for a long period of time (Berger and Concha 1995; Major et al. 1992; Zoltick et al. 1995).

Historically, PML-like pathological cases were described by German pathologist Hallervorden as early as 1930 (Hallervorden, 1930) in a monograph entitled *Unique and non-classifiable processes*. However, the term PML was not crystallized as a distinct entity until the late 1950s. Astrom et al. described the illness in 1958 on the basis of its unique pathological features: demyelination, abnormal oligodendroglial nuclei, and giant astrocytes (Astrom et al. 1958). Descriptions made by these investigators were consistent with the development of a multifocal distribution of small or confluent white matter lesions in the cerebellum, basal ganglia, thalamus, and brain stem. Although the cause of these lesions was not known at that time, involvement of a virus in the pathogenesis of PML was suspected when inclusion bodies were seen in the nuclei of damaged oligodendrocytes (Cavanaugh et al. 1959). Several years later, the use of electron microscopy for the identification of the suspected particles revealed that these particles resembled a polyomavirus in the enlarged nuclei of oligodendrocytes (Zu Rhein 1969; Zu Rhein and Chou 1965). Several attempts were made to isolate the suspect virus without success because of its unrecognized and unique biological properties, such as narrow host range and tissue specificity. In 1971, when Padgett and colleagues used brain tissue from a patient with PML as a source of innoculum in cell cultures derived from human fetal brain, they were successful in isolating a human polyomavirus from long-term cultures mainly consisting of glial cells (Padgett et al. 1971). This was the first direct evidence suggesting that a neurotropic viral agent was associated with the occurrence of PML. It was a coincidence that a virus similar in structure found in the urine of a patient who underwent a renal transplantation was also isolated at the same time (Gardner et al. 1971). Both viruses were associated with immunosuppressive states and named with the initials of donors, JC virus (JCV) for the patient with PML and BK virus (BKV) for the patient undergoing a renal transplantation.

Lytic infection of oligodendrocytes by JCV results in the destruction of the myelin-producing cells. The primary function of these glial cells is to myelinate the axons that project from the neuronal cell bodies of the overlying cortex. Destruction of these cells initially leads to microscopic lesions (Berger 2000; Major et al. 1992) (Figure 24.3b), but as the disease progresses, demyelinated areas become enlarged and eventually may coalesce, making them visible upon gross examination of cut sections (Astrom et al. 1958) (Figure 24.3a). In most cases astrocytes, the other component of glial cells, are also affected by infection exhibiting enlarged, lobulated, and bizarre looking nuclear structures (Major et al. 1992; Walker et al. 1973) (Figure 24.3b). Lipid-laden macrophages are frequently found in the areas of demyelination. Perhaps they are recruited into the CNS as a result of immune reactivation to phagocytize the myelin breakdown products. In most cases, due to the association of PML with AIDS, large numbers of HIV-infected macrophages are also found in extremely extensive necrotic lesions (Berger et al. 1987). It is not clear, however, how these immune cells infiltrated the areas of demyelination. One possible explanation is that JCV infection may recruit HIV-infected macrophages into the demyelinated areas or alternatively, uninfected macrophages may become infected by HIV after they are recruited into the nervous system.

Association of JCV with cancer

JCV causes tumors in experimental animals
It is well established that polyomaviruses including JCV, BKV, and SV40 induce a variety of tumors in experimental animals (Krynska et al. 1999a; London et al. 1978, 1983; Varakis et al. 1978; Walker et al. 1973). They have the ability to induce neoplastic cell transformation in tissue culture as well. Shortly after its isolation from a brain tissue sample of a PML patient, JCV, like SV40, was confirmed to have tumorigenic potential in tissues of neuronal origin (Varakis et al. 1978; Walker et al. 1973). In this line of experiments, inoculation of JCV into several experimental animals resulted in a variety of tumors depending on the animal type, age, and site of inoculation. For example, more than 80 percent of newborn Syrian hamsters when inoculated intracerebrally and subcutaneously with the Mad-1 strain of JCV developed medulloblastomas, glioblastomas, and neuroblastomas (Varakis et al. 1978; Walker et al. 1973). In addition, the presence of an entire biologically active JCV genome was demonstrated when cells from these tumors were cocultivated with permissive glial cells (Walker et al. 1973). In another experiment, JCV was inoculated intraocularly into newborn hamsters. Abdominal neuroblastomas were developed in some cases. Metastases occurred to the bone marrow, lymph nodes, and liver (Walker et al. 1973).

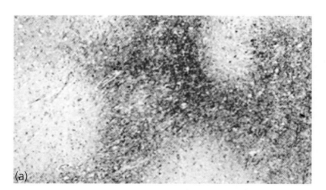
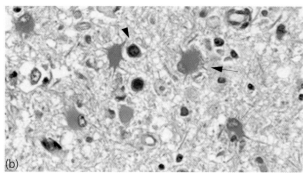

Figure 24.3 *Histopathological examination of a progressive multifocal leukoencephalopathy case.* (a) *A special staining for myelin demonstrates several areas of myelin loss in the white matter (Luxol Fast Blue, original magnification ×40).* (b) *Enlarged transformed astrocytes (arrow), and oligodendrocytes harboring intranuclear inclusion bodies (arrowhead) are present within the demyelinated plaques (hematoxylin-eosin, original magnification ×400).*

Interestingly, unlike the other members of the polyomavirus family (BK virus and SV40), JCV was shown to have the potential to induce tumors in nonhuman primates, i.e. monkeys. In order to mimic a case resembling PML in humans, owl and squirrel monkeys were inoculated with JCV subcutaneously, intraperitoneally, or intracerebrally (London et al. 1978, 1983). After inoculation, animals developed tumors at varying time intervals. For instance, one owl monkey developed a malignant cerebral tumor similar to an astrocytoma seen in humans 16 months after inoculation. Another developed a malignant neuroblastoma 25 months after inoculation.

Transgenic mice were used to mimic the acute demyelination seen in PML-affected brain tissue. In this line of experiments, a transgenic mouse line was created with the regulatory and coding sequences for JCV T-antigen (Small et al. 1986b). Some of the offspring from this transgenic mouse exhibited a mild to severe tremor phenotype. Hypomyelination and dysmyelination were observed in the CNS, but not in the peripheral nervous system. In addition, dysmyelination was further characterized in transgenic mice by Trapp et al. (1988) by examining the expression of JCV T-antigen and myelin-specific genes. Initial examination of brains from transgenic mice revealed that the amount of myelin sheath wrapped around the axons was relatively low. The expression levels of proteolipid protein (PLP), myelin basic protein (MBP), and myelin-associated glycoprotein (MAG) genes appeared to be normal. However, respective protein levels for each gene were shown to be reduced. Although the mechanism by which T-antigen plays a critical role in the reduction of respective protein levels in the brain of transgenic mice remains unknown, several suggestions were made in this regard. T-antigen may exert its function by altering the levels of both proteolipid and myelin basic protein synthesis or by inhibiting the maturation of oligodendrocytes. Additionally, JCV T-antigen may mediate its tumorigenic potential through its interaction with tumor suppressor genes, such as p53 and retinoblastoma gene products, Rb. Consequently their functions appear to be disturbed by the presence of T-antigen in the cell cycle. Coimmunoprecipitation assays using cellular extracts from JCV-transformed glial cells have revealed that JCV T-antigen forms complexes with Rb, p53, and p107 (Monier 1986). Supporting these findings, a report by Rencic et al. (1996) suggests a role for T-antigen in the induction of an oligoastrocytoma in an immunocompetent patient. This group also described the formation of different tumors in tissues derived from neuronal origin in transgenic mouse models (Franks et al. 1996; Gordon et al. 2000; Krynska et al. 1999a). The JCV early gene, large T-antigen, under the control of its own promoter was utilized to create these transgenic animal models. Histological and histochemical analysis of the tumor masses revealed the expression of the JCV oncogenic protein large T-antigen in tumors but not in control tissues. Oddly, transgenic animals created with the early region of JCV archetype strain (Krynska et al. 1999a) did not show any sign of hypomyelination in the central nervous system that is a feature that was seen with a transgenic animal created by Small et al. (1986b). On the contrary, cerebellar tumors which resemble human medulloblastomas were induced in those transgenic animals (Krynska et al. 1999a). In another transgenic line, half of the animals developed large, solid masses within the base of the skull by 1 year of age. Histological evaluation of the tumors by location and immunohistochemical studies demonstrated that these tumors arose from the pituitary gland (Gordon et al. 2000).

Detection of JCV in human tumors In addition to the induction of tumors in experimental animals, the JCV genome has also been detected in a variety of human tumors, which increases the likelihood of the involvement of JCV large T-antigen in tumor formation. In fact, Richardson, who first described PML (Richardson 1961), reported an incidental case of oligodendroglioma in a patient with concomitant chronic lymphatic leukemia and PML. Following this report, several more cases describing the concomitant occurrence of PML with different human tumors were also reported. Sima et al. reported the association of PML with multiple astrocytomas in 1983 (Sima et al. 1983). Similarly, Castaigne et al. (1974) described a case where a patient with a long history of immunodeficiency syndrome, in addition to PML, showed numerous foci of anaplastic astrocytes. Examination of the demyelinating lesions by electron microscopy demonstrated the presence of viral particles in both oligodendrocytes and astrocytes within PML foci, but not in the neoplastic astrocytes (Castaigne et al. 1974). A recent report by Shintaku and colleagues revealed dysplastic ganglion-like cells in a patient with PML (Shintaku et al. 2000). A large number of dysplastic or dysmorphic cells which showed properties of neurons were detected in the cerebral cortex. The expression of JCV large T-antigen, but not the viral capsid proteins, was detected in the infected neurons.

In addition to the cases of concomitant PML and cerebral neoplasm, JCV has been shown to be associated with human brain tumors in the absence of PML lesions. Boldorini et al. reported the detection of JCV DNA in the brain tumors of an immunocompetent patient with a pleomorphic xantoastrocytoma (Boldorini et al. 1998). Detection of JCV viral DNA and expression of large T-antigen were reported by Rencic et al. in tumor tissue from an immunocompetent HIV-negative patient with an oligoastrocytoma (Rencic et al. 1996). These two cases demonstrated the association of JCV in brain tumors of immunocompetent non-PML patients. Such findings further prompted attempts to establish the association of JCV with different types of brain tumors in humans. Analysis of multiple brain tumors for the detection of JCV genome revealed that 57.1 percent of oligodendrogliomas, 83.3 percent of ependymomas, 80 percent of pilocytic astrocytomas, 76.9 percent of astrocytomas, 62.5 percent of oligoastrocytomas, and 66 percent of anaplastic oligodendrogliomas contained JCV early gene sequences (Del Valle et al. 2001, 2002a). Further, the JCV genome has been repeatedly detected in pediatric cerebellum tumors, medulloblastomas, and the viral early protein and the late auxiliary protein, Agnoprotein have been detected in tumor cells (Figure 24.4) (Del Valle et al. 2002b; Krynska et al. 1999b).

JCV genomic DNA has also been detected in tumor tissues that arise from other than neural origin. Recent reports indicate that the JCV genome is detected in the gastrointestinal tract and solid non-neural tumors such as colorectal cancers (Enam et al. 2002; Laghi et al. 1999; Ricciardiello et al. 2000, 2001).

BKV

Similar to JCV, BK virus (BKV) is widespread in the human population. Greater than 80 percent of the world's population is seropositive for viral proteins. The BKV genome is composed of 5 153 nucleotides and has a typical polyomavirus genomic organization. BKV shares greater than 75 percent sequence identity with JCV, with great divergence within the 300–500-bp noncoding regulatory region. The control region of BKV exhibits sequence variation among the various isolates as a result of nucleotide insertions, deletions, and rearrangements. The control region of the BKV archetype spanning a 375-bp sequence is comprised of several regulatory motifs serving as the potential binding site for regulatory proteins such as Sp1, NF-1, NF-κB, c-Jun, AP1, and many others. These elements are scattered within five arbitrarily divided regions named O (142 bp), P (68 bp), Q (39 bp), R (63 bp), and S (163 bp). In a typical BKV serotype 1 Dunlop strain, the control region is comprised of O (142 bp), three imperfect P regions: P (68 bp), P (50 bp), P (64 bp), and S (63 bp). It is postulated that rearrangement in the control region alters the architectural organization of the viral enhancer/promoter permitting efficient expression of the viral genome in the host. Lytic infection of BKV begins with the expression of the early genome whose product, T-antigen, orchestrates viral DNA replication and late gene activation. Similar to JCV, primary infection with BKV is usually asymptomatic and occurs during childhood with the highest incidence of transmission between the ages of 1 and 6 years. While the route of infection has not been well established, the association of mild upper respiratory illness and tonsillitis during exposure to the virus and subsequent seroconversions have led to speculation that the upper respiratory tract is the route of primary infection with BKV. After primary infection, BKV is likely distributed to all organs via peripheral blood cells and establishes a harmless latency, most notably in the kidney. Reactivation of BKV has been observed in the urinary tract under certain physiological conditions such as pregnancy; kidney, bone marrow, and heart transplantation; immunodeficiency disorders; systemic lupus erythematosus; and immunosuppressive therapy. After reactivation of BKV, an inflammatory syndrome affecting several organs has been detected. It is hypothesized that changes in the immune system and other physiological conditions cause dysregulation of cytokines and immunomodulators that lead to potentiation of transcriptional factors and/or suppression of transcriptional inhibitors that are involved in the control of BKV enhancer/promoter activities. Supporting this notion, it was demonstrated that interaction of nuclear factor (NF-1) with its target sequence within the BKV

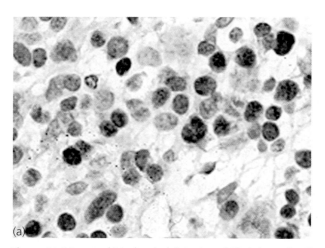
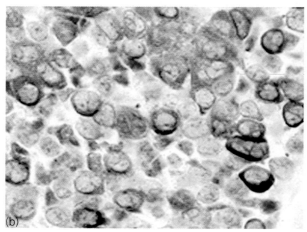

Figure 24.4 *Immunohistochemical detection of JC viral proteins, T-antigen and Agnoprotein in human medulloblastomas: High magnification view of a human medulloblastoma, demonstrates the presence of T-antigen in the nuclei of approximately 60 percent of the neoplastic cells ((a) T-antigen 1:100 dilution, original magnification ×100). When tested with an anti-Agno antibody the cells show a robust cytoplasmic immunoreactivity ((b) Agno 1:2 000 dilution, original magnification ×100).*

promoter results in suppression of viral late transcription. The presence of NF-κB, on the other hand, suggests a role for NF-κB inducible pathways via the p50/p65 transcription factor upon stimulation of cells with various tumor necrosis factors, cytokines, and immunomodulators, such as TNF-α and IL-2. Also, activation of the viral promoter can occur upon hormonal imbalances; the presence of estrogen responsive and glucocorticoid responsive elements suggest activation of BKV gene transcription by estrogen-induced transcription factors. During pregnancy, maximum reactivation of the virus is observed during the third trimester when the levels of estrogen and progesterone are at their highest, pointing to a role for glucocorticoid responsive element (GRE) and estrogen responsive element (ERE) in the induction of BKV gene transcription.

BKV AND HUMAN DISEASES

Hemorrhagic cystitis and nephritis

Reactivation of BKV and its appearance in urine is frequently observed in pregnant women without any sign of illness. Considering the kidney as a primary site for BKV reactivation, much attention has been focused on the role of BKV in renal allograft dysfunction and failure. BKV-associated nephropathy (BKVN) ranges from asymptomatic hematuria to hemorrhagic cystitis in renal graft transplants, as well as in patients with bone marrow transplantation (Andrews et al. 1988; Bedi et al. 1995; Bogdanovic et al. 1998; Chan et al. 1994; Coleman et al. 1973; Vögeli et al. 1999). In addition, BKV-associated ureteric stenosis and tubulointerstitial nephritis has been reported in individuals with renal allograft transplantation (Coleman et al. 1978; Gardner et al. 1971, 1984; Mathur et al. 1997; Nebuloni et al. 1999; Pappo et al. 1996; Purighalla et al. 1995; Smith et al. 1998). Hemorrhagic cystitis associated with BKV has also been seen in AIDS patients (Gluck et al. 1994). It has been speculated that treatment of recipients of renal allograft transplants with immunosuppressive drugs leads to reactivation of latently infected BKV in the donated organs. The reactivation of BKV that is histologically observed by areas of by tubular necrosis is in concurrence with the loss of organs. While there is no direct evidence for the induction of nephropathy by BKV in humans, earlier observations from experimental animals is consistent with the assumption that BKV is able to induce nephropathy in humans. According to that observation, a member of the polyomavirus family named cynomolgus polyomavirus induces interstitial nephritis, ureteritis, and enteritis, the symptoms which are seen in BKVN in immunosuppressed cynomolgus monkey (Van Gorder et al. 1999).

Reactivation of BKV and renal tubular injury has been repeatedly observed among AIDS patients. The clinical symptoms caused by BKV activation in AIDS patients includes meningoencephalitis, retinitis, and nephritis (Bratt et al. 1999; Nebuloni et al. 1999).

While there is no established treatment for patients with BKV-associated renal disease, it is believed that a decrease in the doses of immunosuppressive drugs in patients who undergo kidney allograft transplantation may result in viral clearance.

Association of BKV with cancer

BKV causes tumors in experimental animals Similar to its close family member JCV, BKV is tumorigenic in several experimental animals. For example, intracerebral or intravenous inoculation of BKV in hamster results in the genesis of a broad range of tumors, such as ependymoma, neuroblastoma, pineal gland tumors, fibrosarcoma, osteosarcoma, and tumors of pancreatic islets (Corallini et al. 1977, 1978, 1982; Costa et al. 1976; Dougherty, 1976; Greenlee et al. 1977; Nase et al. 1975; Noss and Stauch 1984; Noss et al. 1981; Shah et al. 1975; Uchida et al. 1976; van der Noordaa 1976). Inoculation of BKV in rats and mice caused formation of fibrosarcoma, liposarcoma, osteosarcoma, glioma, choroid plexus papilloma, and nephroblastoma (Corallini et al. 2001; Noss and Stauch 1984; Noss et al. 1981). It is believed that the oncogenicity of BKV is due to the expression of T-antigen, which has a transforming activity in cell culture. The evidence for the involvement of BKV T-antigen in tumorigenicity of the virus stems from a study in transgenic mice in which the affected animals expressing BKV T-antigen developed renal tumors, lymphoproliferative disease, and hepatocellular carcinoma (Dalrymple and Beemon 1990; Small et al. 1986a). The T-antigen of BKV has the potential to associate with tumor suppressors such as p53 and the pRb family to functionally inactivate these important cell cycle regulatory proteins (Dyson et al. 1989, 1990; Harris et al. 1996; Kang and Folk 1992; Shivakumar and Das 1996). In addition to its role in the deregulation of cell cycle pathways, BKV T-antigen may be involved in genomic instability and random chromosomal abnormalities. While the mechanism whereby BKV T-antigen induces chromosome aberrations remains unknown, several characteristics of the protein, such as the ability of T-antigen to associate with topoisomerase I, p53, and helicase activity may contribute to this event. Indeed, other viral proteins, including small t-antigen and the late regulatory protein, Agnoprotein, may also play a role in the tumorigenicity of BKV, as well as its ability to cause chromosomal damage.

Detection of BKV in human cancer The oncogenic potential of BKV in several experimental animals, the transforming activity of BKV T-antigen in vitro, and its tumorigenicity in transgenic animals prompted many investigators to search for the presence of BKV in various human tumors. Examination of 74 human brains by conventional hybridization techniques revealed the presence of episomal free DNA of BKV in 19 samples (Corallini et al. 1987a). BKV DNA was also detected in significant numbers (44 percent) of tumors in pancreatic islets (Corallini et al. 1987b). In recent years, the search for the presence of BKV DNA in several laboratories using more sensitive assays, i.e. PCR, revealed the presence of BKV DNA in 50 out of 58, 74 out of 83, and 18 out of 18 brain tumors (De Mattei et al. 1995; Flaegstad et al. 1999; Martini et al. 1996). Using the same techniques, other laboratories failed to detect BKV DNA in ten brain tumor samples (Völter et al. 1997). The brain tumors which were studied included ependymomas, meningiomas, glioblastomas, gliomas, neuroblastomas, oligodendrogliomas, spongioblastomas, choroid plexus papillomas (Corallini et al., 1977, 1987b; De Mattei et al. 1994, 1995; Dörries et al. 1987; Negrini et al. 1990). While there is no established role for BKV in human neoplasia, it is evident that studies to establish a correlation between BKV and tumors of the central nervous system and urinary tract are essential.

SV40

SV40 represents the most studied member of the family *Polyomaviridae*. Originally isolated from monkeys, in recent years it has been repeatedly detected in a selected group of human tumors. The control region of SV40, responsible for transcription of the viral early and late genome, is comprised of three 21 base pair GC-rich repeats and two 72-bp tandem repeats with multiple binding sites for DNA binding transcription factors. A TATA box positioned in front of the GC-rich motif provides a site for the formation of a transcription initiation complex. By utilizing the SV40 regulatory sequence as a model for studying regulation of eukaryotic promoters, investigators were able to discover several key general transcription factors such as the families of Sp1, AP1, etc., to decipher complicated events involved in the initiation and elongation of the transcription process. The origin of viral DNA replication is located near the TATA box and contains the core origin and the auxiliary sequences which enhance the efficiency of viral DNA replication. The interaction of the viral early protein, T-antigen, with the sequences surrounding the origin of DNA replication is pivotal for the start of viral DNA replication indicating that expression of the early genome is the first step in the lytic cycle of SV40.

The early genome of SV40 has two transcription units that are transcribed from a region near the origin of DNA replication (Khalili et al. 1986). The early–early (E_E) transcription unit whose RNA is responsible for production of large and small T-antigen predominates at the early times after infection. The late–early (L_E) transcription unit whose RNA start sites are located upstream of the E_E TATA box, have coding sequences for both small t- and large T-antigen, and a small 2–7 kDa protein, the SV40 early leader protein (SELP) (Khalili et al. 1987b). The L_E transcription unit functions at late times after infection, and while the function of SELP remains to be investigated, it is evident that transition of the sites of early RNAs from E_E to L_E position results in the inclusion of two AUGs in the leader of the RNA. These additional AUG decrease the utilization of the AGG which is responsible for T-antigen production, thus bringing additional steps to regulate early gene transcription at the translational level. The large T-antigen of SV40 has a modular structure with several biological activities including ATPase, DNA helicase, DNA-binding, and protein-binding activities. Large T-antigen can undergo post-translational modifications, events that could potentiate its function upon the viral life cycle and/or host-cell behavior.

Replication of viral DNA is a complicated process that requires a functional origin of replication, large T-antigen with its DNA binding and helicase activities, and the host replication machinery. DNA replication usually occurs between 4 and 8 h after infection and is followed by the enhanced transcription of the late region of this virus. Results from a large volume of molecular studies have revealed that direct and indirect association of T-antigen with several cellular transcription factors is involved in the replication of viral late gene expression. Once the viral late proteins are produced, consistent with the general scheme of polyomaviruses, the assembly of the virion occurs in the nuclei of the cells.

SV40 AND HUMAN DISEASE

It is believed that the introduction of SV40 into the human population is related to the development and distribution of poliovaccines. Evidently, the initial preparations of poliovaccines that were inadvertently contaminated with SV40 caused exposure of hundreds of millions of persons to the virus. It is estimated that more than 98 million people in the United States who received poliovaccine between 1955 and 1963 were exposed to SV40 (Shah and Nathanson 1976). Other poliovaccine preparations using adenovirus types 3 and 7, which were utilized between 1961 and 1965, were also contaminated with SV40 (Lewis et al. 1973). In light of cell culture studies showing the transforming ability of SV40 T-antigen and results from animal experiments verifying the oncogenicity of T-antigen, the observed distribution of SV40 in a large population of humans via the poliovaccine has become an important subject in cancer development in humans.

SV40 caused tumors in experimental animals

In 1962, several laboratories demonstrated that SV40 can induce tumors in Syrian hamsters (Eddy et al. 1962; Girardi et al. 1962). The type of tumors induced by

SV40 was dependent on the route of viral inoculation. Systemic inoculation of SV40 resulted in the development of mesotheliomas, osteosarcomas, and lymphomas, while intracranial inoculation of hamsters with SV40 led to the development of brain tumors, such as ependymoma, and subcutaneous inoculation caused soft tissue sarcoma. Transgenic mice containing the SV40 early genome developed choroid plexus papilloma in which T-antigen expression was detected.

SV40 and human tumors

Results from many studies in recent years point to the possible role of SV40 in cancer development in humans (Gazdar et al. 2002). The first evidence of the association of SV40 with human cancer was presented in 1974 (Soriano et al. 1974) in a patient with metastatic malignant melanoma in which viral proteins were present in the lung, liver, and muscle metastases, but not normal tissues. Subsequently, SV40 has been detected by standard Southern blot and gene amplification in adult, as well as pediatric tumors of the brain including choroid plexus, ependymomas, and medulloblastomas (Bergsagel et al. 1992; Huang et al. 1999; Lednicky et al. 1995).

In one study the presence of SV40 DNA sequences has been reported in 32 percent of osteosarcomas and 41 percent of several other tumors (Carbone et al. 1996). Perhaps the most studied cases related to SV40 and cancer are malignant mesotheliomas in which nearly half of the cases contain the viral genome (Bocchetta et al. 2000; Carbone et al. 1994, 2002; Cicala et al. 1993; Rizzo et al. 1999, 2001; Shivapurkar et al. 1999, 2000; Testa et al. 1998; Toyooka et al. 2001). In the most recent studies, the SV40 sequence has been found in non-Hodgkin's lymphomas (Shivapurkar et al. 2002; Vilchez et al. 2002). Continuous detection of SV40 DNA in certain human tumors suggests that this DNA tumor virus has the ability to play a role in human disease. The inactivation of several tumor suppressors, deregulation of the cell cycle, and several other signaling pathways can serve as a potential path for the genesis of cancer by SV40 in experimental animals and perhaps in humans as well.

CONCLUDING REMARKS

The polyomaviruses have a long history of being utilized as a tool to decipher the interaction of viruses with their host cells, and to investigate pathways involved in the regulation of eukaryotic gene expression, mRNA translation, and DNA replication. Further, the polyomavirus early protein, such as SV40 T-antigen in the early years of the 'fight against cancer' has provided critical insight into the mechanism involved in the development of neoplasia. More recent studies from several basic science laboratories along with clinical observations have brought polyomaviruses to center stage in medical virology due to their involvement in various human diseases as outlined in this chapter. It is, therefore, essential to once again pay special attention to these viruses, and by employing more novel approaches and technology, study the various cellular events that can occur upon infection. The outcome will provide a better understanding of the pathogenesis of diseases associated with polyomaviruses. This information will facilitate development of effective antiviral drugs and vaccines for the prevention and treatment of diseases associated with polyomaviruses.

REFERENCES

Ahmed, S., Chowdhury, M. and Khalili, K. 1990a. Regulation of a human neurotropic virus promoter, JCVE: Identification of a novel activator domain located upstream from the 98 bp enhancer promoter region. *Nucleic Acids Res*, **18**, 7417–23.

Ahmed, S., Rappaport, J., et al. 1990b. A nuclear protein derived from brain cells stimulates transcription of the human neurotropic virus promoter, JCVE, in vitro. *J Biol Chem*, **265**, 13899–905.

Amemiya, K., Traub, R., et al. 1989. Interaction of a nuclear factor-1-like protein with the regulatory region of the human polyomavirus JC virus. *J Biol Chem*, **264**, 7025–32.

Amemiya, K., Traub, R., et al. 1992. Adjacent nuclear factor-1 and activator protein binding sites in the enhancer of the neurotropic JC virus. A common characteristic of many brain-specific genes. *J Biol Chem*, **267**, 14204–11.

Andrews, C.A., Shah, K.V., et al. 1988. A serological investigation of BK virus and JC virus infections in recipients of renal allografts. *J Infect Dis*, **158**, 176–81.

Astrom, K.E., Mancall, E.L. and Richardson, E.P. Jr. 1958. Progressive multifocal encephalopathy: A hitherto unrecognized complication of chronic lymphocytic leukemia and lymphoma. *Brain*, **81**, 99–111.

Atwood, W.J. 2001. Cellular receptors for the polyomaviruses. In: Khalili, K. and Stoner, G.L. (eds), *Human polyomaviruses: molecular and clinical perspectives*. New York: Wiley-Liss, Inc, 179–98.

Atwood, W.J., Wang, L., et al. 1995. Evaluation of the role of cytokine activation in the multiplication of JC virus (JCV) in human fetal glial cells. *J Neurovirol*, **1**, 40–9.

Bedi, A., Miller, C.B., et al. 1995. Association of BK virus with failure of prophylaxis against hemorrhagic cystitis following bone marrow transplantation. *J Clin Oncol*, **13**, 1103–9.

Beggs, A.H., Frisque, R.J. and Scangos, G.A. 1988. Extinction of JC virus tumor-antigen expression in glial cell–fibroblast hybrids. *Proc Natl Acad Sci USA*, **85**, 7632–6.

Berger, J.R. 2000. Progressive multifocal leukoencephalopathy. *Curr Treat Option Neurol*, **2**, 361–8.

Berger, J.R. and Concha, M. 1995. Progressive multifocal leukoencephalopathy: The evolution of a disease once considered rare. *J Neurovirol*, **1**, 5–18.

Berger, J.R., Kaszovitz, B., et al. 1987. Progressive multifocal leukoencephalopathy associated with immunodeficiency virus infection. A review of the literature with a report of sixteen cases. *Ann Intern Med*, **107**, 78–87.

Bergsagel, D.J., Finegold, M.J., et al. 1992. DNA sequences similar to those of simian virus 40 in ependymomas and choroid plexus tumors of childhood. *New Engl J Med*, **326**, 988–93.

Bocchetta, M., Di Resta, I., et al. 2000. Human mesothelial cells are unusually susceptible to simian virus 40-mediated transformation and asbestos cocarcinogenicity. *Proc Natl Acad Sci USA*, **97**, 10214–19.

Bogdanovic, G., Priftakis, P., et al. 1998. Primary BK virus (BKV) infection due to possible BKV transmission during bone marrow transplantation is not the major cause of haemorrhagic cystitis in transplanted children. *Pediatr Transplant*, **2**, 288–93.

Boldorini, R., Caldarelli-Stefano, R., et al. 1998. PCR detection of JC virus DNA in the brain tissue of a 9-year-old child with pleomorphic xanthoastrocytoma. *J Neurovirol*, **4**, 24.

Bratt, G., Hammarin, A.L., et al. 1999. BK virus as the cause of meningoencephalitis, retinitis and nephritis in a patient with AIDS. *AIDS*, **13**, 1071–5.

Brooks, B.R. and Walker, D.L. 1984. Progressive multifocal encephalopathy. *Neurol Clin*, **2**, 299–313.

Carbone, M., Pass, H.I., et al. 1994. Simian virus 40-like DNA sequences in human pleural mesothelioma. *Oncogene*, **9**, 1781–90.

Carbone, M., Rizzo, P., et al. 1996. SV40-like sequences in human bone tumors. *Oncogene*, **13**, 527–35.

Carbone, M., Kratzke, R.A. and Testa, J.R. 2002. The pathogenesis of mesothelioma. *Semin Oncol*, **29**, 2–17.

Castaigne, P.R., Rondot, P., et al. 1974. Progressive multifocal leukoencephalopathy and multiple gliomas. *Rev Neuro Paris*, **130**, 379–92.

Cavanaugh, J.B., Greenbaum, D., et al. 1959. Cerebral demyelination associated with disorder of the reticuloendothelial system. *Lancet*, **ii**, 524–9.

Chan, P.K., Ip, K.W., et al. 1994. Association between polyomavirus and microscopic haematuria in bone marrow transplant patients. *J Infect*, **29**, 139–46.

Chen, N.N., Chang, C.F., et al. 1995. Cooperative action of cellular proteins YB-1 and Pur alpha with the tumor antigen of the human JC polyomavirus determines their interaction with the viral lytic control element. *Proc Natl Acad Sci USA*, **92**, 1087–91.

Chowdhury, M., Taylor, J.P., et al. 1990. Regulation of the human neurotropic virus promoter by JCV-T antigen and HIV-1 tat protein. *Oncogene*, **5**, 1737–42.

Chowdhury, M., Taylor, J.P., et al. 1992. Evidence that a sequence similar to TAR is important for induction of the JC virus late promoter by human immunodeficiency virus type 1 Tat. *J Virol*, **66**, 7355–61.

Chowdhury, M., Kundu, M. and Khalili, K. 1993. GA/GC-rich sequence confers Tat responsiveness to human neurotropic virus promoter, JCVL, in cells derived from central nervous system. *Oncogene*, **8**, 887–92.

Cicala, C., Pompetti, F. and Carbone, M. 1993. SV40 induces mesotheliomas in hamsters. *Am J Pathol*, **142**, 1524–33.

Coleman, D.V., Gardner, S.D. and Field, A.M. 1973. Human polyomavirus infection in renal allograft recipients. *Br Med J*, **3**, 371–5.

Coleman, D.V., Mackenzie, E.F.D., et al. 1978. Human polyomavirus (BK) infection and ureteric stenosis in renal allograft recipients. *J Clin Pathol*, **31**, 338–47.

Corallini, A., Barbanti-Brodano, G., et al. 1977. High incidence of ependymomas induced by BK virus, a human papovavirus. *J Natl Cancer Inst*, **59**, 1561–3.

Corallini, A., Altavilla, G., et al. 1978. Ependymomas, malignant tumors of pancreatic islets and osteosarcomas induced in hamsters by BK virus, a human papovavirus. *J Natl Cancer Inst*, **61**, 875–83.

Corallini, A., Altavilla, G., et al. 1982. Oncogenicity of BK virus for immunosuppressed hamsters. *Arch Virol*, **73**, 243–53.

Corallini, A., Pagnani, M., et al. 1987a. Induction of malignant subcutaneous sarcomas in hamsters by a recombinant DNA containing BK virus early region and the activated human c-Harvey-ras oncogene. *Cancer Res*, **47**, 6671–7.

Corallini, A., Pagnani, M., et al. 1987b. Association of BK virus with human brain tumors and tumors of pancreatic islets. *Int J Cancer*, **39**, 60–7.

Corallini, A., Tognon, M., et al. 2001. Evidence for BK virus as a human tumor virus. In: Khalili, K. and Stoner, G.L. (eds), *Human polyomaviruses: molecular and clinical perspectives*. New York: Wiley-Liss, 431–60.

Costa, T., Yee, C., et al. 1976. Hamster ependymomas produced by intracerebral inoculation of human papovavirus (MMV). *J Natl Cancer Inst*, **56**, 863–4.

Dalrymple, S.A. and Beemon, K.L. 1990. BK virus T antigen induces kidney carcinomas and thymoproliferative disorders in transgenic mice. *J Virol*, **64**, 1182–91.

Del Valle, L., Gordon, J., et al. 2001. Detection of JC virus DNA sequences and expression of the viral regulatory protein T-antigen in tumors of the central nervous system. *Cancer Res*, **61**, 4287–93.

Del Valle, L., Delbue, S., et al. 2002a. Expression of JC virus T-antigen in a patient with MS and glioblastoma multiforme. *Neurology*, **58**, 895–900.

Del Valle, L., Gordon, J., et al. 2002b. Expression of human neurotropic polyomavirus JCV late gene product AGNO protein in human medulloblastoma. *J Natl Cancer Inst*, **94**, 267–73.

De Mattei, M., Martini, F., et al. 1994. Polyomavirus latency and human tumors. *J Infect Dis*, **169**, 1175–6.

De Mattei, M., Martini, F., et al. 1995. High incidence of BK virus large T-antigen-coding sequences in normal human tissues and tumors of different histotypes. *Int J Cancer*, **61**, 756–60.

Devireddy, L.R., Kumar, K.U., et al. 2000. BAG-1, a novel Bcl-2-interacting protein, activates expression of human JC virus. *J Gen Virol*, **81**, 351–7.

Dougherty, R.M. 1976. Induction of tumors in Syrian hamster by a human renal papovavirus, RF strain. *J Natl Cancer Inst*, **57**, 395–400.

Dörries, K., Leober, G. and Meixenberger, J. 1987. Association of polyomavirus JC, SV40 and BK with human brain tumors. *Virology*, **160**, 268–70.

Dyson, N., Buchkovich, K., et al. 1989. The cellular 107K protein that binds to adenovirus E1A also associates with the large T antigen of SV40 and JC virus. *Cell*, **58**, 249–55.

Dyson, N., Bernards, R., et al. 1990. Large T antigens of many polyomaviruses are able to form complexes with the retinoblastoma protein. *J Virol*, **64**, 1353–6.

Eddy, B.E., Borman, G.S., et al. 1962. Identification of the oncogenic substance in rhesus monkey cell cultures as simian virus 40. *Virology*, **17**, 65–75.

Enam, S., Del Valle, L., et al. 2002. Association of human polyomavirus JCV with colon cancer: evidence for interaction of viral T-antigen and beta-catenin. *Cancer Res*, **62**, 7093–101.

Feigenbaum, L., Khalili, K., et al. 1987. Regulation of the host range of human papovavirus JCV. *Proc Natl Acad Sci USA*, **84**, 3695–8.

Feigenbaum, L., Hinrichs, S.H. and Jay, G. 1992. JC virus and simian virus 40 enhancers and transforming proteins: role in determining tissue specificity and pathogenicity in transgenic mice. *J Virol*, **66**, 1176–82.

Flaegstad, T., Andresen, P.A., et al. 1999. A possible contributory role of BK virus infection in neuroblastoma. *Cancer Res*, **59**, 1160–3.

Franks, R.R., Rencic, A., et al. 1996. Formation of undifferentiated mesenteric tumors in transgenic mice expressing human neurotropic polymavirus early protein. *Oncogene*, **12**, 2573–8.

Frisque, R.J. 2001. Structure and function of JC virus T proteins. *J Neurovirol*, **7**, 293–7.

Frisque, R.J. and White, F.A. 1992. The molecular biology of JC virus, causative agent of progressive multifocal leukoencephalopathy. In: Roos, E.R.P. (ed.), *Molecular neurovirology: pathogenesis of viral CNS infections*. Totowa, NJ: Humana Press, 25–158.

Frisque, R.J., Bream, G.L. and Cannella, M.T. 1984. Human polyomavirus JC virus genome. *J Virol*, **51**, 458–69.

Fukita, Y., Mizuta, T.R., et al. 1993. The human Smu bp-2, a DNA-binding protein specific to the single-stranded guanine-rich sequence related to the immunoglobulin mu chain switch region. *J Biol Chem*, **268**, 17463–70.

Gardner, S.D., Feild, A.M., et al. 1971. New human papovavirus (BK) isolated from urine after renal transplantation. *Lancet*, **I**, 1253–7.

Gardner, S.D., Mackenzie, E.F., et al. 1984. Prospective study of the human polyomaviruses BK and JVC and cytomegalovirus in renal transplant recipients. *J Clin Pathol*, **37**, 578–86.

Gazdar, A.F., Butel, J.S. and Carbone, M. 2002. SV40 and human tumours: myth, association, or causality. *Nature Cancer Rev*, **2**, 957–64.

Girardi, A.J., Sweet, B.H., et al. 1962. Development of tumors in hamsters inoculated in the neonatal period with vacuolating virus, SV40. *Proc Soc Exp Biol Med*, **109**, 649–60.

Gluck, T.A., Knowles, W.A., et al. 1994. BK virus-associated haemorrhagic cystitis in an HIV-infected man. *AIDS*, **8**, 391–2.

Gordon, J., Del Valle, L., et al. 2000. Pituitary neoplasia induced by expression of human neurotropic polyomavirus, JCV, early genome in transgenic mice. *Oncogene*, **19**, 4840–6.

Greenlee, J.E., Narayan, O., et al. 1977. Induction of brain tumors in hamsters with BK virus, a human papovavirus. *Lab Invest*, **36**, 636–42.

Hallervorden, J. 1930. Eigennartige und nicht rubrizierbare Prozesse. In: Bumke, O. (ed.), *Die Anatomie der Psychosen. Handbuch der Geiteskrankeiten*, Vol. 2. Berlin: Springer, 1063–107.

Harris, K.F., Christensen, J.B. and Imperiale, M.J. 1996. BK virus large T antigen: interactions with the retinoblastoma family of tumor suppressor proteins and effects on cellular growth control. *J Virol*, **70**, 2378–86.

Heilbronn, R., Albrecht, I., et al. 1993. Human cytomegalovirus induces JC virus DNA replication in human fibroblasts. *Proc Natl Acad Sci USA*, **90**, 11406–10.

Henson, J.W. 1994. Regulation of the glial-specific JC virus early promoter by the transcription factor Sp1. *J Biol Chem*, **269**, 1046–10450.

Henson, J., Saffer, J. and Furneaux, H. 1992. The transcription factor Sp1 binds to the JC virus promoter and is selectively expressed in glial cells in human brain. *Ann Neurol*, **32**, 72–7.

Huang, H., Reis, R., et al. 1999. Identification in human brain tumors of DNA sequences specific for SV40 large T antigen. *Brain Pathol*, **9**, 33–42.

Kang, S. and Folk, W.R. 1992. Lymphotropic papovavirus transforms hamster cells without altering the amount or stability of p53. *Virology*, **191**, 754–64.

Kerr, D. and Khalili, K. 1991. A recombinant cDNA derived from human brain encodes a DNA binding protein that stimulates transcription of the human neurotropic virus JCV. *J Biol Chem*, **266**, 15876–81.

Khalili, K., Khoury, G. and Brady, J. 1986. Spacing between SV40 early transcriptional control sequences is important for regulation of early RNA synthesis and gene expression. *J Virol*, **60**, 935–42.

Khalili, K., Feigenbaum, L. and Khoury, G. 1987a. Evidence for a shift in 5′-termini of early viral RNA during the lytic cycle of JC virus. *Virology*, **158**, 469–72.

Khalili, K., Brady, J. and Khoury, G. 1987b. Translational regulation of SV40 early mRNA defines a new viral protein. *Cell*, **48**, 639–45.

Khalili, K., Rappaport, J. and Khoury, G. 1988. Nuclear factors in human brain cells bind specifically to the JCV regulatory region. *EMBO J*, **7**, 1205–10.

Kim, H.-S., Henson, J.W. and Frisque, R.J. 2001. Transcription and replication in the human polyomaviruses. In: Khalili, K. and Stoner, G.L. (eds), *Human polyomaviruses: molecular and clinical perspectives*. New York: Wiley-Liss, 73–126.

Krynska, B., Otte, J., et al. 1999a. Human ubiquitous JCV(CY) T-antigen gene induces brain tumors in experimental animals. *Oncogene*, **18**, 39–46.

Krynska, B., Del Valle, L., et al. 1999b. Detection of human neurotropic JC virus DNA sequence and expression of the viral oncogenic protein in pediatric medulloblastomas. *Proc Natl Acad Sci USA*, **96**, 11519–24.

Kumar, K.U., Pater, A. and Pater, M.M. 1993. Human JC virus perfect palindromic nuclear factor 1-binding sequences important for glial cell-specific expression in differentiating embryonal carcinoma cells. *J Virol*, **67**, 572–6.

Laghi, L., Randolph, A.E., et al. 1999. JC virus DNA is present in the mucosa of the human colon and in colorectal cancers. *Proc Natl Acad Sci USA*, **96**, 7484–9.

Lashgari, M.S., Tada, H., et al. 1989. Regulation of JCVL promoter function: transactivation of JCVL promoter by JCV and SV40 early proteins. *Virology*, **170**, 292–5.

Lednicky, J.A., Garcea, R.L., et al. 1995. Natural simian virus 40 strains are present in human choroid plexus and ependymoma tumors. *Virology*, **212**, 710–7171.

Lewis, A.M. Jr., Levine, A.S., et al. 1973. Studies of nondefective adenovirus 2-simian virus 40 hybrid viruses. V. Isolation of additional hybrids which differ in their simian virus 40-specific biological properties. *J Virol*, **11**, 655–64.

Liu, C.K., Hope, A.P. and Atwood, W.J. 1998a. The human polyomavirus, JCV, does not share receptor specificity with SV40 on human glial cells. *J Neurovirol*, **4**, 49–58.

Liu, C.K., Wei, G. and Atwood, W.J. 1998b. Infection of glial cells by the human polyomavirus JC is mediated by an N-linked glycoprotein containing terminal alpha(2-6)-linked sialic acids. *J Virol*, **72**, 4643–9.

London, W.T., Houff, S.A., et al. 1978. Brain tumors in owl monkeys inoculated with a human polyomavirus (JC virus). *Science*, **201**, 1246–9.

London, W.T., Houff, S.A., et al. 1983. Viral-induced astrocytomas in squirrel monkeys. *Prog Clin Biol Res*, **105**, 227–37.

Lynch, K.J. and Frisque, R.J. 1990. Identification of critical elements within the JC virus DNA replication origin. *J Virol*, **64**, 5812–22.

Lynch, K.J. and Frisque, R.J. 1991. Factors contributing to the restricted DNA replicating activity of JC virus. *Virology*, **180**, 306–17.

Lynch, K.J., Haggerty, S. and Frisque, R.J. 1994. DNA replication of chimeric JC virus-simian virus 40 genomes. *Virology*, **204**, 819–22.

Major, E.O., Amemiya, K., et al. 1992. Pathogenesis and molecular biology of progressive multifocal leukoencephalopathy, the JC virus-induced demyelinating disease of the human brain. *Clin Microbiol Rev*, **5**, 49–73.

Martini, F., Iaccheri, L., et al. 1996. SV40 early region and large T-antigen in human brain tumors, peripheral blood cells, and sperm fluids from healthy individuals. *Cancer Res*, **56**, 4820–5.

Mathur, V.S., Olson, J.L., et al. 1997. Polyomavirus-induced interstitial nephritis in two renal transplant recipients: case report and review of the literature. *Am J Kidney Dis*, **29**, 754–8.

Monier, R. 1986. Transformation by SV40 and polyomaviruses. In: Salzman, N.P. (ed.), *The polyomaviruses*, Vol. 1. New York: Plenum Press.

Nase, L.M., Karkkaiven, M. and Matyjarvi, R.A. 1975. Transplantable hamster tumors induced with the BK virus. *Acta Pathol Microbiol Scand*, **83**, 347–52.

Nebuloni, M., Osoni, A., et al. 1999. BK virus renal infection in a patient with the acquired immunodeficiency syndrome. *Arch Pathol Lab Med*, **123**, 807–11.

Negrini, M., Remessi, P., et al. 1990. Characterization of BK virus variants rescued from human tumors and tumor cell lines. *J Gen Virol*, **71**, 2731–6.

Noss, G. and Stauch, G. 1984. Oncogenic activity of the BK type of human papovavirus in inbred rat strains. *Arch Virol*, **81**, 41–50.

Noss, G., Stauch, G., et al. 1981. Oncogenic activity of the BK type of human papovavirus in newborn Wistar rats. *Arch Virol*, **69**, 239–51.

Padgett, B.L., Zu Rhein, G.M., et al. 1971. Cultivation of papova-like virus from human brain with progressive multifocal leukoencephalopathy. *Lancet*, **i**, 1257–60.

Pappo, O., Demetris, A.J., et al. 1996. Human polyomavirus infection of renal allografts: histopathologic diagnosis, clinical significance, and literataure review. *Mod Pathol*, **9**, 105–9.

Pho, M.T., Ashok, A. and Atwood, W.J. 2000. JC virus enters human glial cells by clathrin-dependent receptor-mediated endocytosis. *J Virol*, **74**, 2288–92.

Purighalla, R., Shapiro, R., et al. 1995. BK virus infection in a kidney allograft diagnosed by needle biopsy. *Am J Kidney Dis*, **26**, 671–3.

Raj, G.V. and Khalili, K. 1994. Identification and characterization of a novel GGA/C-binding protein, GBP-i, that is rapidly inducible by cytokines. *Mol Cell Biol*, **14**, 7770–81.

Raj, G.V. and Khalili, K. 1995. Transcriptional regulation: lessons from the human neurotropic polyomavirus, JCV. *Virology*, **213**, 283–91.

Raj, G.V., Safak, M., et al. 1996. Transcriptional regulation of human polyomavirus JC: evidence for a functional interaction between RelA (p65) and the Y-box-binding protein, YB-1. *J Virol*, **70**, 5944–53.

Raj, G.V., Gallia, G.L. et al. 1998. T-antigen-dependent transcriptional initiation and its role in the regulation of human neurotropic JC virus late gene expression. *J Gen Virol*, **79**, 2147–55.

Ranganathan, P.N. and Khalili, K. 1993. The transcriptional enhancer element, kappa B, regulates promoter activity of the human neurotropic virus, JCV, in cells derived from the CNS. *Nucleic Acids Res*, **21**, 1959–64.

Rencic, A., Gordon, J., et al. 1996. Detection of JC virus DNA sequence and expression of the viral oncoprotein, tumor antigen, in brain of immunocompetent patient with oligoastrocytoma. *Proc Natl Acad Sci USA*, **93**, 7352–7.

Renner, K., Leger, H. and Wegner, M. 1994. The POU domain protein Tst-1 and papovaviral large tumor antigen function synergistically to stimulate glia-specific gene expression of JC virus. *Proc Natl Acad Sci USA*, **91**, 6433–7.

Ricciardiello, L., Laghi, L., et al. 2000. JC virus DNA sequences are frequently present in the human upper and lower gastrointestinal tract. *Gastroenterology*, **119**, 1228–35.

Ricciardiello, L., Chang, D.K., et al. 2001. Mad-1 is the exclusive JC virus strain present in the human colon, and its transcriptional control region has a deleted 98-base-pair sequence in colon cancer tissues. *J Virol*, **75**, 1996–2001.

Richardson, E.P. 1961. Progressive multifocal encephalopathy. *New Engl J Med*, **265**, 815–23.

Rizzo, P., Carbone, M., et al. 1999. Simian virus 40 is present in most United States human mesotheliomas, but it is rarely present in non-Hodgkin's lymphoma. *Chest*, **116**, 470S–3S.

Rizzo, P., Bocchetta, M., et al. 2001. SV40 and the pathogenesis of mesothelioma. *Semin Cancer Biol*, **11**, 63–71.

Sadowska, B., Barrucco, R., et al. 2003. Regulation of human polyomavirus, JC virus, gene transcription by AP-1 in glial cells. *J Virol*, **77**, 665–72.

Safak, M., Gallia, G.L. and Khalili, K. 1999. A 23-bp sequence element from human neurotropic JC virus is responsive to NF-kappa B subunits. *Virology*, **262**, 178–89.

Safak, M., Barrucco, R., et al. 2001. Interaction of JC virus agno protein with T antigen modulates transcription and replication of the viral genome in glial cells. *J Virol*, **75**, 1476–86.

Safak, M., Sadowska, B., et al. 2002. Functional interaction between JC virus late regulatory agnoprotein and cellular Y-box binding transcription factor, YB-1. *J Virol*, **76**, 3828–38.

Shah, K. and Nathanson, N. 1976. Human exposure to SV40: review and comment. *Am J Epidemiol*, **103**, 1–12.

Shah, K.V., Daniel, R.W. and Strandberg, J. 1975. Sarcoma in a hamster inoculated with BK virus, a human papovavirus. *J Natl Cancer Inst*, **54**, 945–9.

Shintaku, M., Matsumoto, R., et al. 2000. Infection with JC virus and possible dysplastic ganglion-like transformation of the cerebral cortical neurons in a case of progressive multifocal leukoencephalopathy. *J Neuropathol Exp Neurol*, **59**, 921–9.

Shivakumar, C.V. and Das, G.C. 1996. Interaction of human polyomavirus BK with the tumor suppressor protein p53. *Oncogene*, **13**, 323–32.

Shivapurkar, N., Wiethege, T., et al. 1999. Presence of simian virus 40 sequences in malignant mesotheliomas and mesothelial cell proliferations. *J Cell Biochem*, **76**, 181–8.

Shivapurkar, N., Wiethege, T., et al. 2000. Presence of simian virus 40 sequences in malignant pleural, peritoneal, and noninvasive mesotheliomas. *Int J Cancer*, **85**, 743–5.

Shivapurkar, N., Harada, K., et al. 2002. Presence of simian virus 40 DNA sequences in human lymphomas. *Lancet*, **359**, 851–2.

Sima, A.A., Finkelstein, S.D. and McLachlan, D.R. 1983. Multiple malignant astrocytomas in a patient with spontaneous progressive multifocal leukoencephalopathy. *Ann Neurol*, **14**, 183–8.

Small, J.A., Khoury, G., et al. 1986a. Early regions of JC virus and BK virus induce distinct and tissue-specific tumors in transgenic mice. *Proc Natl Acad Sci USA*, **83**, 8288–92.

Small, J.A., Scangos, G.A., et al. 1986b. The early region of human papovavirus JC induces dysmyelination in transgenic mice. *Cell*, **46**, 13–18.

Smith, R.D., Galla, J.H., et al. 1998. Tubulointerstitial nephritis due to mutant polyomavirus BK virus strain, BKV(Cin), causing end-stage renal disease. *J Clin Microbiol*, **36**, 1660–5.

Sock, E., Wegner, M., et al. 1993. Large T-antigen and sequences within the regulatory region of JC virus both contribute to the features of JC virus DNA replication. *Virology*, **197**, 537–48.

Soriano, F., Shelburne, C.E. and Gokcen, M. 1974. Simian virus 40 in a human cancer. *Nature*, **249**, 421–4.

Tada, H. and Khalili, K. 1992. A novel sequence-specific DNA-binding protein, LCP-1, interacts with single-stranded DNA and differentially regulates early gene expression of the human neurotropic JC virus. *J Virol*, **66**, 6885–92.

Tada, H., Lashgari, M., et al. 1989. Cell type-specific expression of JC virus early promoter is determined by positive and negative regulation. *J Virol*, **63**, 463–6.

Tada, H., Rappaport, J., et al. 1990. Trans-activation of the JC virus late promoter by the tat protein of type 1 human immunodeficiency virus in glial cells. *Proc Natl Acad Sci USA*, **87**, 3479–83.

Tada, H., Lashgari, M.S. and Khalili, K. 1991. Regulation of JCVL promoter function: evidence that a pentanucleotide 'silencer' repeat sequence AGGGAAGGGA down-regulates transcription of the JC virus late promoter. *Virology*, **180**, 327–38.

Tamura, T., Miura, M., et al. 1988. Analysis of transcription control elements of the mouse myelin basic protein gene in HeLa cell extracts: demonstration of a strong NFI- binding motif in the upstream region. *Nucleic Acids Res*, **16**, 11441–59.

Tamura, T., Aoyama, A., et al. 1990. A new transcription element in the JC virus enhancer. *J Gen Virol*, **71**, 1829–33.

Tavis, J.E. and Frisque, R.J. 1991. Altered DNA binding and replication activities of JC virus T-antigen mutants. *Virology*, **183**, 239–50.

Testa, J.R., Carbone, M., et al. 1998. A multi-institutional study confirms the presence and expression of simian virus 40 in human malignant mesotheliomas. *Cancer Res*, **58**, 4505–9.

Thomson, R.A. and Jones, M. 1968. Remission in progressive multifocal leukoencephalopathy. *Neurology*, **18**, 308.

Toyooka, S., Pass, H.I., et al. 2001. Aberrant methylation and simian virus 40 tag sequences in malignant mesothelioma. *Cancer Res*, **61**, 5727–30.

Trapp, B.D., Small, J.A., et al. 1988. Dysmyelination in transgenic mice containing JC virus early region. *Ann Neurol*, **23**, 38–48.

Uchida, S., Watanabe, S., et al. 1976. Induction of papillary ependymomas and insulinomas in the Syrian golden hamster by BK virus, a human papovavirus. *Gann*, **67**, 857–65.

van der Nordaa, J. 1976. Infectivity, oncogenity, and transforming ability of BK virus and BK virus DNA. *J Gen Virol*, **30**, 371–3.

Van Gorder, M.A., Pelle, P.D., et al. 1999. Cynomolgus polyoma virus infection. A new member of the polyomavirus family causes interstitial nephritis, ureteritis, and enteritis in immunosuppressed cynomolgus monkeys. *Am J Pathol*, **154**, 1273–84.

Varakis, J., Zu Rhein, G.M., et al. 1978. Induction of peripheral neuroblastomas in Syrian hamsters after injection as neonates with JC virus, a human polyoma virus. *Cancer Res*, **38**, 1718–22.

Vaz, B., Cinque, P., et al. 2000. Analysis of the transcriptional control region in progressive multifocal leukoencephalopathy. *J Neurovirol*, **6**, 398–409.

Vilchez, R.A., Madden, C.R., et al. 2002. Association between simian virus 40 and non-Hodgkin lymphoma. *Lancet*, **359**, 817–23.

Vögeli, T.A., Peinemann, F., et al. 1999. Urological treatment and clinical course of BK polyomavirus-associated hemorrhagic cystitis in children after bone marrow transplantation. *Eur Urol*, **36**, 252–7.

Völter, C., Zur Hausen, H., et al. 1997. Screening human tumor samples with a broad-spectrum polymerase chain reaction method for the detection of polyomaviruses. *Virology*, **237**, 389–96.

Walker, D.L., Padgett, B.L., et al. 1973. Human papovavirus (JC): induction of brain tumors in hamsters. *Science*, **181**, 674–6.

Wegner, M., Drolet, D.W. and Rosenfeld, M.G. 1993. Regulation of JC virus by the POU-domain transcription factor Tst-1: implications for progressive multifocal leukoencephalopathy. *Proc Natl Acad Sci USA*, **90**, 4743–7.

Winklhofer, K.F., Albrecht, I., et al. 2000. Human cytomegalovirus immediate–early gene 2 expression leads to JCV replication in nonpermissive cells via transcriptional activation of JCV T antigen. *Virology*, **275**, 323–34.

Yogo, Y., Matsushima-Ohno, T., et al. 2001. JC virus regulatory region rearrangements in the brain of a long surviving patient with progressive multifocal leukoencephalopathy. *J Neurol Neurosurg Psychiatry*, **71**, 397–400.

Zoltick, P.W., Mayreddy, R.P., et al. 1995. Isolation and characterization of a type II JC virus from a brain biopsy of a patient with PML. *J Neurovirol*, **1**, 307–15.

Zu Rhein, G.M. 1969. Association of papovavirions with a human demyelination disease (progressive multifocal leukoencephalopathy). *Prog Med Virol*, **11**, 185–24.

Zu Rhein, G.M. and Chou, S.M. 1965. Particles resembling papovavirus in human cerebral demyelinating disease. *Science*, **148**, 1477–9.

25

Herpesviruses: general properties

ANDREW J. DAVISON AND J. BARKLIE CLEMENTS

INTRODUCTION

The involvement of herpesviruses in a range of prominent medical or veterinary diseases makes them one of the most important virus families. Their ubiquitous occurrence, genetic complexity, evolutionary diversity, and widely differing biological properties have motivated great research effort worldwide, so that our understanding of these agents is now considerable. This is particularly apparent in the area of molecular genetics, and we can expect the knowledge gained to be applied increasingly to key questions about herpesvirus biology and to the development of effective therapies.

In this overview, we have focused on the best characterized member of the family, herpes simplex virus type 1 (HSV-1). Although a number of properties are shared by herpesviruses, many are not. For this reason, we have included pertinent information on the other human herpesviruses and, in a few cases, herpesviruses with nonhuman hosts. In this review, it is impossible to develop a comprehensive bibliography for such a vast area of research. Consequently, we have chosen to describe the accepted picture without extensive citation, instead referring to reviews and a limited selection of seminal or recent research papers.

CLASSIFICATION

The family *Herpesviridae*

The family *Herpesviridae* comprises over 120 viruses that infect a wide range of vertebrates, including fish,

amphibians, reptiles, birds, marsupials, and other mammals including humans, and at least one invertebrate, the oyster (Minson et al. 2000). These viruses are ubiquitous and highly successful parasites, but each is usually restricted in natural infection to a single species and spreads from host to host by direct contact or by the respiratory route. Herpesviruses have large enveloped virions containing double-stranded linear DNA genomes that exhibit considerable diversity of size and structure. They vary greatly in their pathology and biology, but one common feature is their ability, following primary infection, to establish lifelong latent infections that can recrudesce to cause a second round, or even recurrent rounds, of disease. Herpesviruses are well adapted to their hosts, and it is not uncommon for primary or recurring latent infections to be inapparent or trivial in the natural setting. Under certain conditions, however, particularly those resulting in a degree of immune suppression, herpesviruses can be life-threatening. Several herpesviruses have also been implicated in various types of cancer.

On the criteria of host range, duration of reproductive cycle, cytopathology, and characteristics of latent infection, mammalian and avian herpesviruses have been divided into three subfamilies: the *Alpha-*, *Beta-* and *Gammaherpesvirinae*. Each subfamily is subdivided: for example, subfamily *Gammaherpesvirinae* comprises the *Lymphocryptovirus* and *Rhadinovirus* genera. In this review, however, we have also employed a simplified terminology used widely in the literature; for example, using α-herpesvirus (subfamily) and α_1-herpesvirus (genus) instead of *Alphaherpesvirinae* and *Simplexvirus*.

The herpesvirus nomenclature recommended by the International Committee on Taxonomy of Viruses (ICTV) uses the taxonomic unit to which the natural host belongs followed by a number. This rational scheme is used for many herpesviruses, but most human herpesviruses are generally known by their common names.

Alphaherpesvirinae exhibit a variable host range in cell culture, have a short growth cycle, spread rapidly with efficient destruction of infected cells and are neurotropic in that they have the capacity to establish latent infections primarily in sensory ganglia. *Betaherpesvirinae* are typified by a narrow host range and a long reproductive cycle in cell culture with slow virus spread. Infected cells frequently become enlarged and carrier cultures may be established. Viruses may become latent in secretory glands and lymphoreticular cells. *Gammaherpesvirinae* are associated with lymphoproliferative diseases in their natural hosts, and infect lymphoblastoid cells in vitro. Some cause lytic infections in certain epithelial and fibroblastoid cell lines. Viruses are specific for B or T lymphocytes, in which infection is frequently arrested without production of infectious progeny, and latent virus may be found in lymphoid tissue. The term 'lymphotropic' has been used to describe these viruses, but this is arguably a misleading term as lymphocytes are at best semipermissive.

This classification scheme, which is based predominantly on biological features, has been largely vindicated by studies of genetic relationships deduced from analyses of DNA sequence data. Genetic data have now superseded biological properties for classifying herpesviruses.

Human herpesviruses

To date, eight different herpesviruses have been identified whose natural host is humans (Table 25.1), all but two of which (HSV-2 and HHV-8) are ubiquitous in human populations. Three of these viruses have been discovered within the last 20 years. HHV-6 was first isolated from patients with a variety of lymphoproliferative and immunosuppressive disorders (Salahuddin et al. 1986), and exists in two closely related forms (Ablashi et al. 1993), one of which (HHV-6B) has been implicated as a causative agent of exanthem subitum (or roseola infantum), a common disease of infancy (Yamanishi et al. 1988). HHV-7 was first isolated from activated $CD4^+$ cells from a healthy person (Frenkel et al. 1990), and has also been implicated in exanthem subitum (Tanaka et al. 1994). HHV-8 was discovered by the detection of DNA sequences in Kaposi's sarcoma (KS) tissue from acquired immunodeficiency syndrome (AIDS) patients, but not in normal tissue (Chang et al. 1994). These sequences were subsequently detected in KS tissue from patients displaying the classic or endemic African forms of the disease and, often in association with Epstein–Barr virus (EBV), in AIDS-related primary effusion lymphomas. HHV-8 is now accepted as a causal agent of KS and, as a human tumor virus, is the subject of extensive research effort (Schulz 1998; Moore and Chang 2001a). Studies of HHV-8 counterparts in nonhuman primates have indicated that a ninth human herpesvirus species related to HHV-8 might exist (Schultz et al. 2000). To date, however, evidence has not been forthcoming.

Genome sequences for all known human herpesviruses are now available. Consequently, we know a great deal about how the genes are organized and what their functions are. Relating this type of information to general and particular aspects of herpesvirus pathogenesis presents an exciting challenge and has as an objective the control or prevention of infection.

Table 25.1 *Human herpesviruses*

Virus	Abbreviation	Genus	ICTV species name	G+C content (mol%)	Genome size (bp)
Herpes simplex virus type 1	HSV-1	α_1	Human herpesvirus 1	67	152 261
Herpes simplex virus type 2	HSV-2	α_1	Human herpesvirus 2	69	154 746
Varicella-zoster virus	VZV	α_2	Human herpesvirus 3	46	124 884
Epstein–Barr virus	EBV	γ_1	Human herpesvirus 4	60	171 823
Human cytomegalovirus	HCMV	β_1	Human herpesvirus 5	57	230 283[a]
Human herpesvirus 6[b]	HHV-6	β_2	Human herpesvirus 6	43	159 321
					161 573
					162 114
Human herpesvirus 7[b]	HHV-7	β_2	Human herpesvirus 7	40	144 861
					153 080
Kaposi's sarcoma-associated herpesvirus[b]	HHV-8 (KSHV)	γ_2	Human herpesvirus 8	54	~140 500/801[c]

a) Laboratory strain (AD169; 229 354 bp) plus a 929 bp region deleted from a clone sequenced originally. Clinical isolates are approximately 5 kbp larger.
b) More than one strain has been sequenced.
c) Expressed as size of unique region/size of terminal repeat. Sequence at right end of unique region is unknown for the two sequenced isolates.

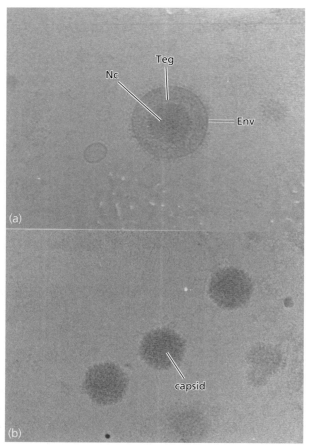

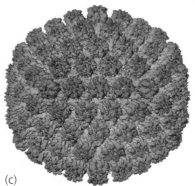

(c)

Figure 25.1 (a) *Electron cryomicrographs of* **(a)** *virions and* **(b)** *capsids of HSV-1. Visible in* **(a)** *are the capsid (Nc), tegument (Teg) and envelope (Env) with associated glycoprotein spikes (courtesy of Dr. F.J. Rixon);* **(c)** *three-dimensional reconstruction of the HSV-1 capsid surface structure. The view is along the two-fold axis. The hexons, pentons, and triplexes are shown in blue, red, and green, respectively (courtesy of Drs. H. Zhou and W. Chiu).*

MORPHOLOGY AND STRUCTURE

Morphology is the main factor in assigning viruses to the family *Herpesviridae*. Virions are comprised of four distinct structural elements: envelope, tegument, capsid, and core (Dargan 1986; Figure 25.1). The virion and capsid have diameters of 200–250 nm and 125 nm, respectively.

The lipid envelope is visible in negatively stained preparations as a pleomorphic structure with many short glycoprotein spikes. Contained within the envelope is the characteristic icosadeltahedral capsid, which in negatively stained preparations appears as an orderly array of stain-penetrated capsomers. Forming the icosahedron are 12 pentavalent capsomers at the vertices, 60 hexavalent capsomers at the 20 faces, and 90 hexavalent capsomers along the 30 edges – a total of 162 capsomers (Wildy et al. 1960). Electron-dense material is clearly present between the envelope and capsid, and the term 'tegument' has been used to describe this poorly understood region, which contains more than 20 viral proteins. Electron cryomicroscopy has been used to study frozen, hydrated herpesviruses, particularly capsids (Zhou et al. 2000). This approach allows direct examination of the three-dimensional structure without the use of stain or fixative. When combined with computer-assisted image enhancement, considerable surface detail is visible (Figure 25.1). Electron cryomicroscopic studies have also shown that the densely staining spherical core inside the capsid consists of the viral DNA packed at high density apparently without internal protein associations. Descriptions of toroidal structures detected in the core in earlier studies (e.g. Furlong et al. 1972) persist into the modern literature but are now accepted as artifacts of negative staining techniques.

REPLICATION

The replication cycle has been studied most fully with HSV-1, and this is the basis of the brief account given here. Fuller accounts of specific aspects of this subject are given in subsequent sections. An outline of the events that occur during HSV-1 replication is shown in Figure 25.2.

General aspects of the HSV-1 replication cycle are identical for HSV-2, but for other human herpesviruses less information is available, largely because of difficulties in propagating the viruses. No truly permissive cell culture system exists for EBV or HHV-8, and studies have been largely restricted to examination of latently infected cell lines. The diverse nature of human herpesviruses implies that details of their patterns of replication will vary. Nevertheless, replication cycles are all consistent with a sequential order of three major regulated phases of transcription and protein synthesis (Roizman and Knipe 2001).

The external glycoproteins of the virion have important roles in adsorption of virus to cells and subsequent penetration (Spear et al. 2000). Fusion of the virus envelope with the plasma membrane occurs at the cell surface rather than in internalized vesicles. Capsids are transferred to the nucleus via microtubules (Dohner et al. 2002), and viral DNA and at least some tegument proteins enter the nucleus, where transcription,

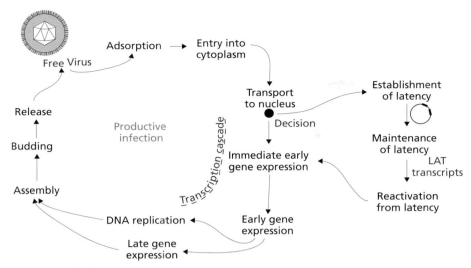

Figure 25.2 *The replication cycle of HSV-1*

replication of viral DNA and capsid assembly take place.

Viral DNA is transcribed into mRNA throughout infection by host RNA polymerase II, with various viral factors participating at all stages (Wagner 1985). Initially, a series of immediate–early (IE), or α genes is expressed whose transcription is independent of viral protein synthesis and is greatly enhanced by a tegument protein (O'Hare 1993). Certain IE proteins are *trans*-acting regulators of virus genes, and initiate a cascade of expression of early (or β) and late (or γ) genes (Honess and Roizman 1974). The products of early genes, defined as the subset expressed in the presence of functional IE products and before the onset of DNA replication, include several enzymes involved in DNA replication and nucleotide metabolism and a subset of glycoproteins. Late genes are dependent on functional IE proteins for expression, and in addition full levels of late protein synthesis require DNA replication. They encode mainly virion proteins. Small noncoding RNAs characteristic of γ-herpesvirus genomes are probably transcribed by RNA polymerase III.

A subset of viral genes is involved in DNA replication and packaging of DNA into capsids. DNA synthesis is initiated from one or more origins of DNA replication, generating head-to-tail concatemeric genomes apparently by a rolling circle mechanism (Boehmer and Lehman 1997). Concatemers are then cleaved and packaged into preformed capsids.

The process by which virion maturation occurs has long been controversial, but it is known that several genes are involved in directing envelopment and egress. The following scheme is probably correct (Elliott and O'Hare 1999; Skepper et al. 2001; Mettenleiter 2002). Capsids gain certain tegument proteins in the nucleus and then a membrane upon budding into the space between the two nuclear membranes. The membrane is lost on transit to the cytoplasm, where additional tegument proteins are added. Tegumented capsids then gain their envelope by budding into a component of the Golgi apparatus, or vesicles derived therefrom, and are released from the infected cell by reverse endocytosis.

The effects of these processes on host cells vary with the different viruses, and for an individual virus, depend on the cell type. The time taken for the cytopathic effect to become evident may range from hours to days, and cells may lyze, round up, or fuse. Also, the proportions of particles that are released from infected cells and the fraction that are enveloped are very variable.

Infection with HSV-1 leads to a rapid inhibition of host macromolecular synthesis. The initial phase of host shutoff is mediated by a virion component. Reduction of the functional half-lives of both infected cell and viral mRNAs by the virion shutoff component could promote rapid changes in viral gene expression in response to alterations at the level of transcription.

During infection, viral proteins interact with each other and with cellular proteins, and an increasing number of methods are available to detect such interactions. However, demonstrating physiological significance is often not straightforward and demands particular rigor. The great majority of studies of the replication cycle are carried out in vitro on infected tissue culture cells. Investigations of the replication cycle in vivo are revealing fresh insights and new gene functions. For example, analysis of the neural circuit-specific spread of α-herpesviruses (Enquist 2002). In addition to a lytic cycle of infection, all herpesviruses examined to date are able to undergo a latent cycle, discovering the molecular mechanisms of which presents further challenges to researchers (see Chapter 26, Alphaherpesviruses: herpes simplex and varicella-zoster).

GENOME STRUCTURE

Types of structure

Herpesvirus genomes range in size from 125 to 245 kbp and nucleotide compositions from 32 to 74 percent G + C (Honess 1984). The γ-herpesviruses exhibit a global deficit in the 5′-CG dinucleotide, presumably as an evolutionary result of latency in dividing cells (Honess et al. 1989). The genome structures of many herpesviruses are known, but the majority of viruses in this family have not been examined at this level. Figure 25.3 illustrates the six types of genome arrangement that have been characterized thus far. A common characteristic is the presence of repeated regions at the ends of, or internally within, the genome. Similar genome structures have arisen independently during herpesvirus evolution, implying that this feature is not a reliable taxonomic tool in the absence of other data.

The simplest genome arrangement is that of group 1, which consists of a unique sequence flanked by a direct repeat. It was first described for channel catfish virus (CCV), and has since been found for equine herpesvirus 2 (EHV-2; γ₂-herpesvirus), and HHV-6. The genome of murine cytomegalovirus (MCMV; β₁-herpesvirus), also has this arrangement, but the direct repeats are much smaller.

Group 2 genomes contain a short sequence repeated a variable number of times at the termini instead of a

single direct repeat, and are found among the γ₂-herpesviruses, such as HHV-8. The addition of a variable number of the terminal repeats in inverse orientation internally results in the group 3 genome structure, which has been described for cottontail rabbit herpesvirus, also a γ₂-herpesvirus. This genome exists in four equimolar isomers in virion DNA, since inversion of the two unique regions can occur by recombination between inverted repeats. The group 4 structure results from the presence of an internal set of direct repeats unrelated to the terminal set and is typified by EBV. The two unique regions do not invert in such a structure because of lack of homology between internal and terminal repeats.

In the group 5 structure, two unique regions (U_L and U_S) are each flanked by unrelated inverted repeats (TR_L/IR_L and TR_S/IR_S). The two orientations of U_S are present in equimolar amounts in virion DNA, but U_L is found predominantly or completely in a single orientation. Group 5 genomes are characteristic of α₂-herpesviruses, such as varicella zoster virus (VZV), but a separately evolved example is present in a fish herpesvirus, salmonid herpesvirus 1.

The group 6 structure is the most complex, although it was the first type to be described, for HSV-1 (Sheldrick and Berthelot 1974). It is similar to that of group 5, except that TR_L/IR_L is much larger, and the two orientations of U_L, as well as those of U_S, are present in equimolar amounts in virion DNA. HSV-2 and bovine herpesvirus 2, also an α₁-herpesvirus, and HCMV share this structure. Unlike group 5 genomes, group 6 genomes are terminally redundant, possessing a short sequence (termed the a sequence, some 400 bp in HSV-1) that is repeated directly at the genome termini and inversely at the IR_L–IR_S junction (Wagner and Summers 1978).

Human herpesviruses

Figure 25.4 shows a scale representation of human herpesvirus genome structures. The HSV-1 and HSV-2 genomes exhibit a group 6 structure and are essentially colinear. Preparations of virion DNA from both viruses contain equivalent amounts of four isomers that differ in the relative orientations of U_L and U_S (Hayward et al. 1975), a phenomenon termed genome isomerization. These isomers appear to be functionally equivalent, and one has been chosen arbitrarily to serve as a prototype for depicting restriction endonuclease sites and the gene arrangement. As the a sequence contains signals for cleavage and packaging concatemeric DNA generated during viral DNA replication, the presence of internal copies as alternative sites, in combination with homologous recombination events between TR_L and IR_L or TR_S and IR_S, provides a means for generating the genome isomers.

The VZV genome, as an example of a group 5 structure, is not terminally redundant although sequences

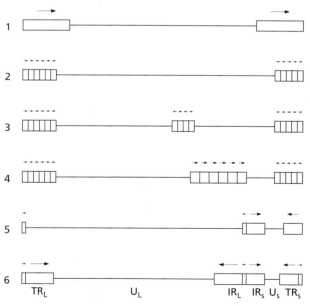

Figure 25.3 *Types of herpesvirus genome structure. The genomes are not drawn to scale. Unique and repeat regions are shown as horizontal lines and rectangles, respectively. The orientations of repeats are shown by arrows. The nomenclature used to designate regions of the HSV-1 genome are shown at the foot of the figure (from Davison and McGeoch 1995, courtesy of Cambridge University Press).*

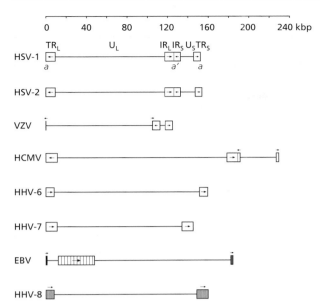

Figure 25.4 *Sizes and structures of human herpesvirus genome shown to scale. Unique and repeat regions are shown as horizontal lines and rectangles, respectively. The orientations of repeats are shown by arrows. The nomenclature used to designate regions of the HSV-1 genome is shown at the top of the figure. The sequence that is directly repeated at the genome termini and also present in inverse orientation is shown as a and a', respectively.*

involved in cleavage and packaging of replicated DNA are present at the genome termini. U_L is flanked by a small inverted repeat of 88 bp that results in 5 percent of virions containing genomes with U_L inverted, and U_S is found equally in both orientations.

The general arrangement of the HCMV genome resembles that of HSV-1, with a similar arrangement of unique and repeated elements and the presence of four equimolar genome isomers, although it is 60 percent larger. TR_L/IR_L is much smaller in clinical isolates than in the sequenced laboratory strain (Prichard et al. 2001). Phylogenetic studies indicate that the genome structures of HSV-1 and HCMV developed independently. HHV-6 and HHV-7 are the only known β_2-herpesviruses. Although genetically related to HCMV, they share the distinct group 1 genome structure.

EBV DNA displays a linear, noninverting structure. The terminal regions consist of up to 12 copies of a tandem repeat (523 or 538 bp), and the internal repeat region comprises between six and 12 tandemly reiterated copies of a 3072 bp sequence. The HHV-8 genome is typical of that of γ_2-herpesviruses, consisting of a unique region flanked by a variable number of copies of an 801 bp terminal repeat.

In addition to large scale repeats, most human herpesvirus genomes contain several regions consisting of tandem reiterations of short sequence elements. The presence of the repeated elements in variable copy numbers results in genome size heterogeneity. These sequences may be coding or noncoding; in the former

case, they exist as multiples of 3 bp and encode repeated amino acid sequences. A further type of genome heterogeneity is represented by the loss or gain of restriction endonuclease sites and is presumably due to differences in individual nucleotides. The DNA cleavage patterns of epidemiologically unrelated HSV-1 or HSV-2 isolates are not identical, and are stable when viruses are passed in cell culture. This characteristic has an important diagnostic use and has been employed to examine modes of transmission and epidemiology of HSV-1 and HSV-2 in human populations (Umene and Sakaoka 1999). Sequence data are being employed increasingly in studies of this type.

GENETIC CONTENT

Arrangement and expression

The complete (or almost complete) DNA sequences of 29 herpesviruses have been published to date, several for more than one strain. These are listed in Table 25.2. In addition, a substantial amount of data is available for parts of other herpesvirus genomes. Analyses of these sequences have given a detailed view of genetic content and usually form the starting point for experimental studies on particular genes.

The number of protein-coding genes estimated from sequence analyses ranges from about 70 in smaller genomes (e.g. HSV-1 and VZV) to over 160 in the larger (e.g. HCMV). In general, the great majority of the DNA is protein-coding, and genes are arranged about equally between the two strands. Regions of overlap between genes in different reading frames on the same strand or on opposing strands are infrequent and usually not extensive. Most genes are expressed as single exons from their own promoters, but it is common for families of genes arranged tandemly on the same strand to share a polyadenylation site downstream from the most 3' member (Wagner 1985). Few α-herpesvirus genes specify spliced mRNAs, but splicing is more common in the β- and γ-herpesviruses. Most splicing in EBV specifically involves genes expressed during latency (Kieff and Rickinson 2001), particularly a family of genes distributed over 100 kbp that is expressed by differential splicing of transcripts from a common promoter. Complete transcript maps are not available for any herpesvirus, but transcriptome analyses have been derived from oligonucleotide microarray data for several, such as HSV-1 (Stingley et al. 2000). Microarray technology has also been used to investigate changes in cellular gene expression during infection with herpesviruses, such as HCMV (Zhu et al. 1998).

HSV-1

HSV-1 is the best characterized herpesvirus at the molecular level. The genome is considered to contain 74

Table 25.2 *Herpesvirus genome sequences*

Virus	Genome (bp)	GenBank accession	Primary reference
Alphaherpesvirinae			
Simplexvirus (α_1)			
Herpes simplex virus type 1	152261	X14112	McGeoch et al. (1988)
Herpes simplex virus type 2	154746	Z86099	Dolan et al. (1998)
Varicellovirus (α_2)			
Varicella-zoster virus	124884	X04370	Davison and Scott (1986)
Simian varicella virus	124138	AF275348	Gray et al. (2001)
Equine herpesvirus 1	150224	M86664	Telford et al. (1992)
Equine herpesvirus 4	145597	AF030027	Telford et al. (1998)
Bovine herpesvirus 1	135301	AJ004801	Schwyzer and Ackermann (1996)
Mardivirus (α_3)			
Marek's disease virus type 1	177874	AF243438	Tulman et al. (2000)
Marek's disease virus type 2	164270	AB049735	Izumiya et al. (2001)
Turkey herpesvirus	159160	AF291866	Afonso et al. (2001)
Betaherpesvirinae			
Cytomegalovirus (β_1)			
Human cytomegalovirus[a]	230285	X17403	Chee et al. (1990)
Chimpanzee cytomegalovirus	241087	AF480884	Davison et al. (2003)
Muromegalovirus			
Murine cytomegalovirus	230278	U68299	Rawlinson et al. (1996)
Rat cytomegalovirus	230138	AF232689	Vink et al. (2000)
Roseolovirus (β_2)			
Human herpesvirus 6	159321	X83413	Gompels et al. (1995)
	161573	AB021506	Isegawa et al. (1999)
	162114	AF157706	Dominguez et al. (1999)
Human herpesvirus 7	144861	U43400	Nicholas (1996)
	153080	AF037218	Megaw et al. (1998)
Unassigned			
Tupaiid herpesvirus	195859	AF281817	Bahr and Darai (2001)
Gammaherpesvirinae			
Lymphocryptovirus (γ_1)			
Epstein–Barr virus	184113	M35547	
		V01555	Baer et al. (1984)
		M80517	Parker et al. (1990)
	171823	AH507799[b]	Unpublished
Marmoset lymphocryptovirus	149696	AF319782	Rivailler et al. (2002a)
Rhesus lymphocryptovirus	171096	AY037858	Rivailler et al. (2002b)
Rhadinovirus (γ_2)[c]			
Herpesvirus saimiri	112930/1444	X64346	Albrecht et al. (1992)
Herpesvirus ateles	108409/1582	AF083424	Albrecht (2000)
Alcelaphine herpesvirus 1	130608/1113	AF005370	Ensser et al. (1997)
Human herpesvirus 8	~140500/801	U75698	Russo et al. (1996)
		U93872	Neipel et al. (1997)
Rhesus rhadinovirus	131364/~2100	AF083501	Searles et al. (1999)
	130733/?	AF210726	Alexander et al. (2000)
Murine herpesvirus 68	118237/1213	U97553	Virgin et al. (1997)
	118311/1239	AF105037	Nash et al. (2001)
Bovine herpesvirus 4	108873/2267	AF318573	Zimmermann et al. (2001)
Equine herpesvirus 2	184427	U20824	Telford et al. (1995)
Undefined subfamily			
Ictalurivirus			
Channel catfish virus	134226	M75136	Davison (1992b)

?, not known

a) See footnote (a) in Table 25.1.

b) Updated version of previous accession numbers.

c) Except for EHV-2, expressed as size of unique region/size of terminal repeat. Sequence at right end of unique region is unknown in the two HHV-8 isolates.

different genes, three of them present twice in the inverted repeats. The gene arrangement is shown in Figure 25.5. Data continue to accumulate on the properties and functions of the proteins encoded by these genes, and the current state of knowledge is summarized in Table 25.3. Several other potential protein-coding regions have been identified that overlap extensively with recognized genes, but their functional significance remains dubious (McGeoch and Davison 1999).

Overall, in excess of 85 percent of the DNA is protein-coding, and genes are tightly packed with about equal numbers oriented rightwards and leftwards. Several examples of two or more genes specifying mRNAs that share a 3' terminus are visible in Figure 25.5. Larger mRNAs within these nested families contain more than one reading frame, and conventional wisdom suggests that translation initiates at the AUG codon proximal to the mRNA 5' end. Owing to this nested arrangement, promoter sequences for certain internal mRNAs lie within the protein-coding sequences of overlapping mRNAs. HSV-1 has four genes that are expressed as spliced mRNAs, two (UL15 and RL2) with introns in protein-coding regions, and two (US1 and US12) with a common spliced 5' noncoding leader in TR_S/IR_S. In addition, the HSV-1 latency-associated transcripts (LAT), which probably do not encode proteins, are also spliced. The LATs are the only transcripts expressed during latency (see Chapter 26, Alphaherpes-viruses: herpes simplex and varicella-zoster).

Presumably, all the genes present in a herpesvirus genome are required for natural growth and transmission of the virus. However, over half of the genes present in HSV-1 are 'nonessential', in that each of them may be removed individually without eliminating viral growth in cell culture (Roizman and Knipe 2001; see Table 25.3). Many of these mutants are attenuated when assayed in animal models.

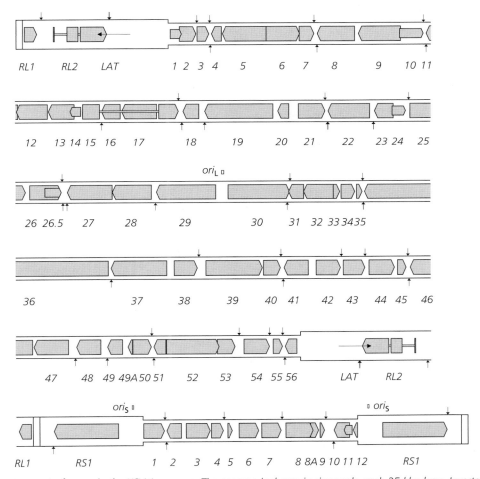

Figure 25.5 Arrangement of genes in the HSV-1 genome. The genome is shown in six panels, each 25 kbp long. Inverted repeats are denoted by the thicker parts of the genome outline, and protein-coding regions are shown as shaded horizontal arrows. For the sake of clarity, the prefixes 'UL' (58 genes) and 'US' (13 genes) have been omitted from the gene nomenclature given below the genome; see Figure 25.4 for the locations of these regions. The major LAT RNA, presumed to be derived from a stable intron generated from a larger transcript, is also indicated by a horizontal arrow. Introns in genes RL2 and UL15 are shown as narrow bars; genes US1 and US12 are also spliced, but the intron is not shown because the 5' exon is noncoding. Possible polyadenylation sites for mRNAs are indicated by vertical arrows above and below the genome for right and left oriented genes, respectively. The locations of ori_S and ori_L are shown by white rectangles above the genome (adapted from Davison (1992a), by courtesy of R&W Publications).

Table 25.3 *Properties of HSV-1 proteins*

Gene	Predicted mass	Status	Function or properties
RL1	26194	NE	Neurovirulence factor (ICP34.5); inhibits host-controlled shutoff of protein synthesis
RL2	78452	NE	IE protein (ICP0; Vmw110); promiscuous transcriptional activator; role in ubiquitin-proteosome pathway
UL1	24932	E	Envelope glycoprotein L; complexes with glycoprotein H (UL22)
UL2	36326	NE	Uracil-DNA glycosylase
UL3	25607	NE	Nucleolar phosphoprotein
UL4	21516	NE	Nuclear protein
UL5	98710	E	Component of DNA helicase–primase complex; possesses helicase motifs
UL6	74087	E	Minor capsid protein; role in DNA packaging; putative portal protein
UL7	33057	NE	Tegument protein
UL8	79921	E	Component of DNA helicase-primase complex
UL9	94246	E	Binds to origins of DNA synthesis; possesses helicase motifs
UL10	51389	NE	Envelope glycoprotein M; disulfide-linked to UL49A protein
UL11	10486	NE	Myristylated tegument protein; role in virion envelopment
UL12	67503	(E)	Deoxyribonuclease; role in maturation/packaging of DNA
UL13	57193	NE	Tegument protein; probable serine-threonine protein kinase
UL14	23454	NE	Tegument protein; role in egress
UL15	80918	E	Role in DNA packaging; putative ATPase subunit of terminase; complexes with UL28 protein
UL16	40440	NE	Tegument protein
UL17	74577	E	Tegument protein; role in DNA packaging
UL18	34268	E	Capsid protein (VP23); component of intercapsomeric triplex
UL19	149075	E	Major capsid protein (VP5); forms hexons and pentons
UL20	24229	E/NE	Integral membrane protein; role in egress of nascent virions; host range phenotype
UL21	57638	NE	Tegument protein
UL22	90361	E	Envelope glycoprotein H; complexes with glycoprotein L (UL1); role in cell entry
UL23	40918	NE	Deoxypyrimidine kinase (dPyK or TK)
UL24	29474	NE	Nuclear protein
UL25	62664	E	Capsid-associated tegument protein
UL26	62466	E	Autocatalytically cleaved by N-terminal protease domain to give capsid protein (VP24) from N terminus and minor scaffold protein (VP21) of immature capsids
UL26.5	33758	(E)	Cleaved by UL26 protein to give major scaffold protein (VP22a) of immature capsids
UL27	100287	E	Envelope glycoprotein B; role in cell entry
UL28	85573	E	Role in DNA packaging; complexes with UL15 protein
UL29	128342	E	Single-stranded DNA-binding protein
UL30	136413	E	Catalytic subunit of replicative DNA polymerase; complexes with UL42 protein
UL31	33951	(E)	Nuclear matrix phosphoprotein involved in nuclear egress; complexes with UL34 protein
UL32	63946	E	Role in DNA packaging
UL33	14436	E	Role in DNA packaging
UL34	29788	(E)	Type II nuclear membrane protein involved in nuclear egress; complexes with UL31 protein
UL35	12095	NE	Capsid protein (VP26); located on tips of hexons
UL36	335841	E	Very large tegument protein
UL37	120549	E	Tegument protein
UL38	50260	E	Capsid protein (VP19C); component of intercapsomeric triplex
UL39	124043	E/NE	Ribonucleotide reductase large subunit (RR1)
UL40	38017	E/NE	Ribonucleotide reductase small subunit (RR2)
UL41	54914	NE	Tegument protein; virion host shutoff factor; RNase component
UL42	51156	E	Processivity subunit of replicative DNA polymerase; complexes with UL30 protein
UL43	44905	NE	Probable integral membrane protein
UL44	54995	NE	Envelope glycoprotein C; role in cell entry

(Continued over)

Table 25.3 *Properties of HSV-1 proteins (Continued)*

Gene	Predicted mass	Status	Function or properties
UL45	18178	NE	Type II membrane protein associated with envelope/tegument
UL46	78239	NE	Tegument protein; modulates IE gene transactivation VP16
UL47	73812	NE	Tegument protein; modulates IE gene transactivation by VP16
UL48	54342	E	Tegument protein (VP16; α-TIF; Vmw65); transactivates IE genes
UL49	32252	NE?	Tegument protein (VP22); capable of intercellular transport to uninfected cell nuclei; bundles microtubules
UL49A	9201	NE	Envelope protein disulfide-linked to glycoprotein M; glycosylated in some herpesviruses
UL50	39125	NE	Deoxyuridine triphosphatase (dUTPase)
UL51	25468	NE	Tegument protein
UL52	114416	E	Component of DNA helicase-primase complex
UL53	37570	(E)	Glycoprotein K; role in egress
UL54	55249	E	IE protein (ICP27; Vmw63); post-transcriptional regulator of gene expression
UL55	20491	NE	Nuclear protein
UL56	25319	NE	Membrane protein
RS1	132835	E	IE protein (ICP4; Vmw175); transcriptional regulator
US1	46521	E/NE	IE protein (ICP22; Vmw68); host range determinant
US2	32468	NE	Virion protein; interacts with cytokeratin 18
US3	52831	NE	Probably serine-threonine protein kinase; anti-apoptotic role; involved in nuclear egress
US4	25236	NE	Envelope glycoprotein G
US5	9555	NE	Envelope glycoprotein J; anti-apoptotic role
US6	43344	E	Envelope glycoprotein D; role in cell entry
US7	41366	NE	Envelope glycoprotein I; complexed with glycoprotein E in Fc receptor
US8	59090	NE	Envelope glycoprotein E; complexed with glycoprotein I in Fc receptor
US8A	16801	NE	Nucleolar phosphoprotein
US9	10026	NE	Type II membrane protein associated with envelope/tegument; role in axonal localization of viral membrane proteins
US10	34053	NE	Tegument protein
US11	17756	NE	Virion protein; double-stranded RNA-binding protein; prevents cellular PKR activation
US12	9792	NE	IE protein (ICP47; Vmw12); interferes with maturation of MHC class I molecules

Developed from Davison and Scott (1986), McGeoch et al. (1988), (1993), McGeoch (1989), McGeoch and Schaffer (1993), Davison (1993), Ward and Roizman (1994), and Davison (2000).

Genes in bold type are thought to have been inherited from the ancestor of the α-, β-, and γ-herpesviruses, and all but *UL9*, *UL23*, and *UL40* are conserved in each subfamily. The status of each gene in cell culture is indicated: E, essential; NE, non-essential; NE?, probably essential; (E), a mutant is viable, but very disabled; E/NE, non-essential under certain conditions.

Other herpesviruses

Comparisons of amino acid sequences predicted from DNA sequence data have shown that, despite substantial differences in nucleotide composition or genome structure, members of the same subfamily share the great majority of genes in a very similar layout. For example, all but six VZV genes have counterparts at equivalent locations in the HSV-1 genome. The utility of comparing a less well understood genome (e.g. VZV) with a better characterized one (HSV-1) depends on this genetic correspondence. When viruses in the three subfamilies are compared, however, divergence is much greater, with a set of 'core' genes conserved in blocks that have been rearranged during evolution. These genes number

43 and were inherited from the common ancestor of the α-, β-, and γ-herpesviruses. They are indicated in bold type in Table 25.3, and presumably function in processes that are central to growth and survival. Three core genes are found in only two of the three subfamilies, and this probably reflects genetic loss from one lineage. Genes encoding thymidine kinase and the small subunit of ribonucleotide reductase, for example, are not present in the β-herpesviruses. The 'noncore' genes are characteristic of each subfamily, and some are unique to one or a few very closely related viruses. Many are involved in aspects of pathogenesis that contribute to survival of the virus in its particular ecological niche. Most genes involved in control processes and latency also fall into this category.

Herpesvirus evolution

Analyses of the genetic relationships between α-, β-, and γ-herpesviruses implies that they have evolved from a common ancestor by processes including substitution, deletion, and insertion of nucleotides to modify genes or produce genes de novo and recombination processes resulting in gene duplication and divergence, capture of host genes, and gene rearrangement (McGeoch and Davison 1999). The results of phylogenetic studies (McGeoch et al. 1995, 2000) are in general accord with the notion that herpesviruses have generally (but not universally) coevolved with their hosts, and this has allowed a timescale to be proposed for the evolution of mammalian herpesviruses (Figure 25.6). These studies provide a firm basis for herpesvirus classification based on genetic relationships rather than on phenotypic properties.

Herpesviruses of birds and reptiles are similar to those of mammals, grouping with the α-herpesviruses. The family also contains two other major clades: fish and amphibian herpesviruses, and invertebrate herpesviruses (McGeoch and Davison 1999). The fish herpesviruses, exemplified by CCV, are only marginally related to herpesviruses that infect mammals or birds (Davison 1992b). However, evidence relating to capsid structure and assembly indicates that these herpesviruses share a common ancestor presumably dating from the time when the lineages leading to fish and other vertebrates separated (approximately 400 million years ago). The two viral lineages seem to have diverged so far that their shared inheritance is no longer discernible by amino acid sequence comparisons. The single known herpesvirus of an invertebrate, which infects several bivalve species including oysters, is very tenuously related to both fish and mammalian herpesviruses. The common ancestor of

modern invertebrate and vertebrate herpesviruses is proposed as having existed about a billion years ago.

GENE FUNCTION

Determination of function

Computer-aided comparisons of predicted amino acid sequences have facilitated the identification of some herpesvirus gene functions, but the majority of evidence has come from direct genetic and biochemical experimentation based on sequence information. Most information has been gained for HSV-1, and derived functions of core genes have been imputed to homologous genes in other herpesviruses. Considerable progress has also been made with noncore genes, including those of HCMV, EBV, and HHV-8. The major categories of gene functions are described below.

Control

Some proteins are involved in control processes, the most intensively studied acting directly or indirectly at the level of transcription to regulate gene expression during the infectious cycle. One such, the HSV-1 virion transactivator (Campbell et al. 1984), an essential structural component of the tegument termed VP16 (Vmw65 or α-TIF; gene *UL48*), acts to stimulate selective transcription of IE genes. Although the transactivation function of VP16 is not essential for virus growth, mutants in the appropriate domain initiate replication inefficiently at low multiplicities of infection and are avirulent in some animal model systems. Induction of HSV-1 IE genes may determine aspects of cell tropism and could play a role in reactivation from latency. Transactivation by a related protein may also occur in other α-herpesviruses, but it is not clear that the mechanism is the same. An unrelated virion protein transactivates HCMV promoters (Liu and Stinski 1992).

Coordinate induction of HSV-1 IE genes requires a consensus DNA signal (TAATGARAT) that is well conserved upstream of all five IE genes. This positive regulation of IE transcription acts through the cellular Oct-1 DNA-binding protein, and studies of VP16 function have shed light on the assembly of multicomponent transcriptional complexes (O'Hare 1993). Four IE proteins are involved in regulation of early and late virus genes (Everett 1987). Two, ICP4 (Vmw175; gene *RS1*) and ICP27 (Vmw63; gene *UL54*) are essential for replication, but precisely how these two proteins function remains obscure. ICP4 is required throughout productive infection (Watson and Clements 1980), and acts at the transcriptional level exhibiting nonspecific DNA-binding. ICP27 is a multifunctional protein that regulates transcriptional and post-transcriptional processes (Phelan

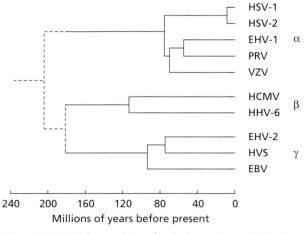

Figure 25.6 *A phylogenetic tree for the herpesviruses derived from sequence comparisons, with a time-scale based on the hypothesis that viruses cospeciate with their hosts. Broken lines indicate regions of lower confidence. PRV, pseudorabies virus (from McGeoch et al. 1995, with permission from Elsevier).*

and Clements 1998). Among its post-transcriptional effects are inhibition of splicing of viral and cellular transcripts and promotion of nuclear export of viral RNAs (Koffa et al. 2001). ICP0 (Vmw110; gene *RL2*) is not absolutely required for HSV-1 replication, but is required for reactivation from latency. It has a role in overcoming suppression of viral genomes by degrading a number of cellular proteins via the ubiquitin-proteosome pathway (Everett 2000), and acts as a ubiquitin ligase in vitro (Boutell et al. 2002). Mutants of ICP22 (Vmw68; gene *US1*) are viable, but affected in host range in cell culture. The functions of this protein are not yet understood.

Considerable information is available on regulation of β-herpesvirus gene expression, largely from HCMV studies, particularly on gene functions that promote the regulated cascade of gene expression and on the viral *cis*-acting DNA sequences involved (Mocarski and Tan Courcelle 2001). Similarly, EBV and HHV-8 have been well studied both in terms of gene expression during latent infection of B-lymphocytes, and of lytic gene expression occurring following treatment of latently infected cell lines with various inducers (Kieff and Rickinson 2001; Moore and Chang 2001b).

These studies have shown that all herpesviruses examined encode strong transcriptional regulators that are expressed in the IE replication phase. However, the relevant genes appear to have developed separately in the herpesvirus lineages. This diversity is also shown by the DNA sequences that regulate synthesis of these proteins. Perhaps a similarity in tertiary structure enables these proteins to act in similar ways; alternatively, they may exert their effects by interaction with different host cell factors.

Other virus proteins modulate replicative processes in the infected cell. Amongst the α-herpesviruses, two protein kinases (encoded by genes *UL13* and *US3*, the former conserved in β- and γ-herpesviruses) are likely to act in this way. Numerous viral and cellular targets have been identified, but their physiological relevance, and hence the true roles of the enzymes, remain to be identified. The virion host shutoff function encoded by gene *UL41* is a component of an RNase that reduces the cytoplasmic stability of both cellular and viral mRNAs and serves to switch off synthesis of host cell proteins (Lu et al. 2001). This activity may also contribute to the downregulation of early viral gene expression. Viruses in each subfamily also have sophisticated genetic mechanisms for suppressing the host's immune response.

Nucleotide metabolism

Herpesviruses specify several enzymes involved in nucleotide metabolism or DNA repair (Morrison 1991). It is likely that the genes encoding these enzymes were captured at various times from the cell. Virus-specified enzyme activities generally have biochemical properties that differ from their cellular counterparts, and this is an important feature for specific targeting of certain antiviral compounds (Coen 1992).

Two HSV-1 enzymes catalyze reactions in the biosynthesis of DNA precursors: thymidine kinase (TK) and ribonucleotide reductase (RR). HSV-1 TK (gene *UL23*) appears to be evolutionarily derived from cellular deoxyribonucleoside kinase, which is known in humans as mitochondrial thymidine kinase 2 (Johansson et al. 1999). In being able to phosphorylate thymidine and deoxycytidine, the viral enzyme is more accurately described as a deoxypyrimidine kinase. HSV-1 TK activity is important for the inhibitory action of nucleoside analogs, such as acyclovir, which are phosphorylated to their monophosphate forms by the viral enzyme and subsequently to the di- and tri-phosphate forms by cellular enzymes. HSV-1 TK is not essential for viral replication in actively growing cells, but is required for growth in resting cells. The pathogenicity of TK-deficient viruses is reduced in animal models, presumably because TK activity is required to raise dTTP levels in targeting nondividing cells. As might be expected, the enzymatic properties of TK enzymes specified by different herpesviruses differ, for example in their relative ability to phosphorylate thymidine and deoxycytidine. The TK gene is not ubiquitous: the α- and γ-herpesviruses (and even CCV) contain TK genes, but the β-herpesviruses such as HCMV and HHV-6, do not, presumably because of gene loss in that lineage.

RR catalyzes the reduction of nucleoside diphosphates to deoxynucleoside diphosphates, and comprises a large (RR1) and a small (RR2) subunit encoded by genes *UL39* and *UL40*, respectively (Connor et al. 1994). It occupies a central role in metabolic routes for the supply of DNA precursors, and is required for efficient growth of virus in cell culture. RR-deficient viruses grow slowly and are nonpathogenic. Kinetic experiments have shown that RR2 is one of the earliest HSV-1 gene functions to be expressed. The genes encoding both subunits of RR are present in α- and γ-herpesvirus genomes. However, only RR1 is encoded by β-herpesviruses, and the absence of active site residues indicates that it is probably inactive. CCV lacks both genes. Interest has focused on the intersubunit interaction as a target for antiviral compounds, and this in turn has turned attention on essential interactions between other herpesvirus proteins, such as those involved in DNA replication, capsid assembly and DNA packaging (Marsden 1992).

HSV-1 encodes a deoxyuridine triphosphatase (dUTPase; gene *UL50*), which is not essential for growth in cell culture. This enzyme catalyses conversion of dUTP to dUMP, which can then be methylated to dTMP by cellular thymidylate synthase. The important function of viral dUTPase in infected cells, however, may be to reduce misincorporation of uracil during

DNA synthesis. A dUTPase gene is present in all herpesviruses studied to date, and appears to have developed in the α-, β-, and γ-herpesviruses by capture of the gene, followed by gene duplication and fusion of the two protein-coding regions. An analysis of conserved motifs casts strong doubt, however, on whether the β-herpesvirus gene is a functional dUTPase.

HSV-1 gene *UL2* encodes a uracil-DNA glycosylase, which is likely to function in removing spontaneously deaminated cytosine and misincorporated uracil residues from viral DNA and thus reduce mutations. This gene is highly conserved in the α-, β-, and γ-herpesviruses (not CCV), but is not essential for growth of HSV-1 in cell culture.

Other enzymes with roles or potential roles in nucleotide supply have been characterized in certain herpesviruses. Thymidylate synthase (TS), which catalyzes methylation of dUMP to dTMP, is encoded by VZV and certain γ_2-herpesviruses, such as HHV-8. Dihydrofolate reductase, which catalyses reduction of dihydrofolate to tetrahydrofolate, an essential step in purine synthesis and in the action of TS, is also specified by certain γ_2-herpesviruses. γ-Herpesviruses contain one or more copies of genes derived from cellular phosphoribosylformylglycinamidine synthase, which is involved in purine biosythesis. CCV possesses duplicated deoxynucleoside monophosphate kinase genes apparently captured from a bacteriophage.

DNA replication

Seven HSV-1 proteins constitute essential components of the DNA synthesis machinery, including a replicative DNA polymerase comprising two subunits, a single-stranded DNA-binding protein, three constituents of a helicase–primase complex and a protein that recognizes the origins of viral DNA replication (Challberg 1991). There has been significant progress in understanding the roles of these proteins, and several interactions in the replication complex have been characterized (Stow 2000). The possible involvement of cellular proteins, however, has not been investigated in any detail, and no origin-dependent in vitro DNA replication system has been developed. The replicative machinery of α-, β-, and γ-herpesviruses is in broad outline the same, since counterparts of six of the seven proteins are present in all mammalian herpesviruses. However, each subfamily utilizes a different means of directing the replication complex to viral DNA, and this is reflected in the lack of conservation of the α-herpesvirus origin-binding protein in the other subfamilies (except the β_2-herpesviruses) and the observation that each subfamily uses a different type of origin of replication. These differences have presumably arisen as a result of evolutionary pressures exerted on each virus during the lytic and latent cycles of infection.

HSV-1 has an origin of replication (ori$_S$) which, being located in TR$_S$/IR$_S$, is present in two copies in the genome (Figure 25.5). In addition, a related origin (ori$_L$) is located near the center of U$_L$. Other α-herpesviruses also possess ori$_S$ at an equivalent location. Most have ori$_L$, in some cases at a different location in U$_L$, but VZV lacks this origin of replication. Both copies of ori$_S$ or the single copy of ori$_L$ may be deleted from the HSV-1 genome without affecting viability. Ori$_S$ and ori$_L$ are related in sequence and consist of an AT-rich palindrome flanked by short sequences that are recognized by the origin-binding protein, and both probably function during lytic replication. EBV also has two unrelated origins of DNA replication but, in contrast to HSV-1, these function at different stages of the life cycle (Hammerschmidt and Mankertz 1991). Ori$_P$ is required for maintaining genome copy number in dividing cells, and is recognized by an EBV-encoded protein, EBNA-1. Ori$_{Lyt}$, which is required for lytic amplification of EBV genomes, consists of a much more extended region than HSV-1 ori$_S$ or ori$_L$, and contains several important sequence elements. Ori$_{Lyt}$ has also been identified in the HCMV and HHV-8 genomes (Hamzeh et al. 1990; AuCoin et al. 2002), and ori$_P$ in the HHV-8 genome (Garber et al. 2001).

DNA polymerase has been well characterized at the genetic and biochemical levels. The catalytic subunit (gene *UL30*) is the target of antiviral agents, such as phosphonoformic and phosphonoacetic acids, which mimic dNTPs, and is the site of genetic resistance to such compounds. The associated, smaller subunit of DNA polymerase (gene *UL42*) increases the processivity of the holoenzyme. Two of the components of the helicase-primase complex (genes *UL5* and *UL52*) are essential for both enzyme activities; the UL5 protein contains a helicase domain. The third component (gene *UL8*) has an auxiliary function, and also interacts with the origin-binding protein. The origin-binding protein (UL9) consists of a homodimer, with each subunit comprising a domain that binds to the origin of replication and a helicase domain that may function in unwinding the origin to allow access to the replication complex. The single-stranded DNA-binding protein (gene *UL29*) also interacts with the origin-binding protein.

DNA packaging

The events that occur during packaging of viral DNA into immature capsids are not well understood. As with capsid assembly, this area attracts interest because of the possibility of antiviral intervention in essential herpesvirus-specific processes. Indeed, it is encouraging that one class of compound (benzimidazole ribonucleosides) has been shown to inhibit the machinery involved in DNA packaging (Underwood et al. 1998).

Eight HSV-1 genes have thus far been identified from their phenotypic effects on mutant viruses as having roles in DNA packaging (*UL6*, *UL12*, *UL15*, *UL17*, *UL25*, *UL28*, *UL32*, and *UL33*). It is unlikely that the products of these genes are all central to the packaging mechanism. The UL6, UL25, and UL17 proteins are virion components. The UL6 protein is exclusively part of the capsid and is thought to form the portal for entry of DNA (Newcomb et al. 2001). At least a proportion of the UL25 protein is capsid-associated, and the UL17 protein is in the tegument. The UL15 protein is of interest because it bears sequence similarity to ATPases and to the large subunit of the bacteriophage T4 terminase, which is responsible for energy-driven insertion of DNA into the capsid. This observation suggests that some aspects of HSV-1 DNA packaging might find parallels in bacteriophage T4, and supports the speculative view that herpesviruses and T4 may share a common, but very ancient, evolutionary origin. The *UL15* gene is unusual in that has highly conserved counterparts in all herpesviruses and is expressed as a spliced mRNA in the vertebrate viruses. The UL15 protein interacts with the UL28 protein. UL12 encodes an alkaline exonuclease, which may be responsible for resolving DNA structures produced during replication.

Virion structure

DEGREE OF COMPLEXITY

About half of the total number of HSV-1 genes specify components of the viral particle. These proteins include eight capsid constituents, at least 20 tegument components, and more than ten proteins, most glycosylated, in the envelope. The proteins making up the capsid are better characterized than those in the envelope or tegument. Capsid proteins can be envisaged as providing a robust, self-assembling container for the viral genome, tegument proteins as ancillary factors responsible for enhancing viral infection, and envelope proteins as molecules involved in allowing infecting virions to enter cells efficiently and facilitating mature virions to exit the infected cell.

CAPSID

The proteins that make up HSV-1 capsids are conserved in other herpesviruses, and the capsid structures of widely diverged members (such as HSV-1 and CCV) are similar. Thus, it is likely that the same basic mechanism for capsid maturation is fundamental to all herpesviruses. The proteins that make up the HSV-1 capsid have undergone extensive characterization (Homa and Brown 1997), and the structure of the capsid has been analyzed in some detail by electron cryomicroscopy. A single protein, VP5 (gene *UL19*), makes up the hexameric and pentameric capsomers of the HSV-1 capsid, and the intercapsomeric regions are composed of a complex (known as a triplex) of two copies of VP23 (gene *UL18*) plus a single copy of VP19C (gene *UL38*). The external tips of hexameric capsomers are decorated with a small protein, VP26 (gene *UL35*). The capsid also contains a protease, VP24 (gene *UL26*). The protein encoded by gene *UL6* is present in a small number of copies per capsid.

The steps that occur during capsid formation are reminiscent of those that take place during maturation of certain DNA-containing bacteriophages, such as T4, in that replicated DNA enters preformed immature capsids containing a core of scaffolding proteins, which are expelled in a process involving specific proteolytic events. The HSV-1 scaffold proteins are encoded by the overlapping genes *UL26* and *UL26.5* (Liu and Roizman 1991; Figure 25.5). The UL26.5 protein is identical to the C-terminal portion of the UL26 protein. Proteolytic action of the N-terminal domain of the UL26 protein on the UL26 protein itself at two locations, one central and one near the C terminus, and on the UL26.5 protein at the site near the C terminus generates VP24 (the protease) and VP21 (the minor scaffold protein) from the UL26 protein, and VP22a (the major scaffold protein) from the UL26.5 protein. During DNA packaging, VP21 and VP22a are expelled from the capsid interior, but VP24 is retained.

The molecular events that occur during capsid maturation have been unraveled with the aid of a system in which the HSV-1 proteins are expressed from baculovirus recombinants (Thomsen et al. 1994; Tatman et al. 1994), and, more recently, with purified proteins (Newcomb et al. 1999). VP5, VP23, VP19C are essential for capsid assembly, plus either the gene UL26.5 protein which gives rise to VP22a or, at a reduced efficiency, the gene UL26 protein which gives rise to VP21 and VP24. The proteolytic function of the UL26 protein is thus not essential in this system, but its requirement for virus production during HSV-1 infection indicates that it is involved in removal of the scaffold proteins during DNA packaging. It appears that the immediate product of capsid assembly is a spherical 'procapsid' which angularizes to a capsid during DNA packaging (Trus et al. 1996).

TEGUMENT

The tegument has a complex composition, and demonstrates icosahedral structure only in the region immediately adjacent to the capsid surface (Chen et al. 1999). It is a feature of all members of the family but, in contrast to capsid proteins, most components of the tegument are specific to a particular subfamily or genus and are therefore likely to have important roles in modulating the virus–host interaction, rather than as passive structural components of the virion. Examples of such roles for HSV-1 tegument proteins are the virion host shutoff factor (gene *UL41*), VP16 (gene *UL48*) and the UL13 protein kinase. It is likely that additional functions for tegument proteins will emerge as this area of research develops.

ENVELOPE

At least 11 HSV-1 genes encode membrane-associated glycoproteins, and most of these are present in the virion envelope. The glycoproteins are located in membranes by virtue of one or several hydrophobic domains, and thus are exposed on the exterior of infected cells or virions. Also, some are functionally associated with initial virus–host interactions (Shukla and Spear 2001) and are therefore likely to be of considerable importance for pathogenicity. For this reason, and because of their utility in vaccine development, herpesvirus glycoproteins have been the subject of intense scrutiny.

Many glycoproteins are specific to genera or subfamilies. For example, three HSV-1 glycoproteins lack counterparts in VZV (gD, gG, gJ). Only gB, gH, gL, gM, and gN (which is not glycosylated in some herpesviruses, including HSV-1) have counterparts across the α-, β-, and γ-herpesviruses. HCMV contains extensive families of related glycoprotein genes that appear to have been generated by gene duplication and divergence (Chee et al. 1990), and thus represent a striking evolutionary experiment in generating genetic diversity.

The initial interaction of HSV-1 with cells involves the binding of gC or gB to heparan sulfate proteoglycans present on the cell surface (Spear et al. 2000). gD then binds to one of several receptors in the TNF-receptor family or immunoglobulin superfamily or to specific forms of heparan sulfate. The viral and cellular membranes fuse in a process that requires gB, gD, gH, gL, and the gD receptor, and the capsid and tegument are released into the cytoplasm. Like HSV, HCMV uses heparan sulfate as a cell surface receptor for the initial binding of virus. EBV, however, binds to cells in a different manner. The EBV virion glycoprotein gp350/220, which lacks sequence counterparts in the α- and β-herpesviruses, binds the cellular receptor CD21 that is found on B-lymphocytes (Kieff and Rickinson 2001). The nature of the receptor for EBV on epithelial cells remains unresolved. HHV-8 appears to enter cells via heparan sulfate and an integrin receptor (Akula et al. 2002).

Of the HSV-1 glycoproteins that are not required for growth of virus in cell culture, three interact with key elements of the immune system: gC binds to the C3b component of the complement system and gE and gI form a complex that can bind the Fc constant region of immunoglobulin G. Of the essential glycoproteins, gH and gL associate during maturation in endoplasmic reticulum and are present as a heterodimer in virions. Also, gM is disulfide-linked to gN. HSV-1 is unusual in that gB in other herpesviruses is processed by a trypsin-like cleavage into a disulfide-linked dimer.

Pathogenesis

Some viral proteins have specific roles in disease processes, including latency. These proteins help to fit a virus to an ecological niche and are usually specific to a subfamily or genus. They may have little effect on the growth of virus in cell culture, but may profoundly influence virus virulence in vivo. Functional analyses of such genes are fundamental to our understanding of herpesviruses as infectious agents. This information is crucial for the design of safe and effective herpesvirus vectors for gene replacement and tumor therapy and for the development of live vaccines. The mechanisms used by herpesviruses to control the processes of natural infection are steadily being elucidated, and the knowledge gained is likely to lead to novel therapies. Herpesviruses are seen increasingly as sophisticated manipulators of various cellular mechanisms and defenses in sophisticated ways, including the cell cycle, apoptosis and various aspects of the immune response (Roizman and Knipe 2001; Hengel et al. 1998).

Herpesvirus genes that modulate the immune response appear to be more numerous in the β- and γ-herpesviruses (Johnson and Hill 1998; Reddehase 2000; Neipel et al. 1997). Among the α-herpesviruses, in addition to gC, gE, and gI which can interact with the immune system, a gene specific to HSV-1 and HSV-2 (gene *US12*) encodes an IE protein (ICP47 or Vmw12) which interferes with maturation of MHC class I proteins in infected cells by interacting with the TAP peptide transporter complex (York et al. 1994). The product of gene *RL1* (ICP34.5) is specific to HSV-1 and HSV-2 and related to proteins implicated in cell differentiation, and has a profound effect on neuropathogenicity (Chou et al. 1990). It appears to function by promoting dephosphorylation of eIF-2α and thereby inhibits host-controlled shutoff of protein synthesis (He et al. 1997). RL1 null mutant viruses are not neurovirulent in vivo, and exhibit limited replication at peripheral sites, but fail to replicate in neurons of the peripheral nervous system. These viruses can, however, establish latent infections from which they can be reactivated. RL1 mutants are currently being evaluated for their possible utility in human tumor therapy (Markert et al. 2001).

REFERENCES

Ablashi, D., Agut, H., et al. 1993. Human herpesvirus-6 strain groups: a nomenclature. *Arch Virol*, **129**, 363–6.

Afonso, C.L., Tulman, E.R., et al. 2001. The genome of turkey herpesvirus. *J Virol*, **75**, 971–8.

Akula, S.M., Pramod, N.P., et al. 2002. Integrin α3β1 (CD 49c/29) is a cellular receptor for Kaposi's sarcoma-associated herpesvirus (KSHV/HHV-8) entry into the target cells. *Cell*, **108**, 407–19.

Albrecht, J.-C. 2000. Primary structure of the *Herpesvirus ateles* genome. *J Virol*, **74**, 1033–7.

Albrecht, J.-C., Nicholas, J., et al. 1992. Primary structure of the herpesvirus saimiri genome. *Virology*, **66**, 5047–58.

Alexander, L., Denekamp, L., et al. 2000. The primary sequence of rhesus monkey rhadinovirus isolate 26–95: sequence similarities to Kaposi's sarcoma-associated herpesvirus and rhesus monkey rhadinovirus isolate 17577. *J Virol*, **74**, 3388–98.

AuCoin, D.P., Colletti, K.S., et al. 2002. Kaposi's sarcoma-associated herpesvirus (human herpesvirus 8) contains two functional lytic origins of DNA replication. *J Virol*, **76**, 7890–6.

Baer, R., Bankier, A.T., et al. 1984. DNA sequence and expression of the B95-8 Epstein–Barr virus genome. *Nature*, **310**, 207–11.

Bahr, U. and Darai, G.J. 2001. Analysis and characterization of the complete genome of tupaia (tree shrew) herpesvirus. *Virology*, **75**, 4854–70.

Boehmer, P.E. and Lehman, I.R. 1997. Herpes simplex virus DNA replication. *Ann Rev Biochem*, **66**, 347–84.

Boutell, C., Sadis, S. and Everett, R.D. 2002. Herpes simplex virus type 1 immediate–early protein ICP0 and its isolated RING finger domain act as ubiquitin E3 ligases in vitro. *J Virol*, **76**, 841–50.

Campbell, M.E.M., Palfreyman, J.W. and Preston, C.M. 1984. Identification of herpes simplex virus DNA sequences which encode a *trans*-acting polypeptide responsible for stimulation of immediate early transcription. *J Mol Biol*, **180**, 1–19.

Challberg, M.D. 1991. Herpes simplex virus DNA replication. *Semin Virol*, **2**, 247–56.

Chang, Y., Cesarman, E., et al. 1994. Identification of herpesvirus-like DNA sequences in AIDS-associated Kaposi's sarcoma. *Science*, **266**, 1865–9.

Chee, M.S., Bankier, A.T., et al. 1990. Analysis of the protein-coding content of the sequence of human cytomegalovirus strain AD169. *Curr Top Microbiol Immunol*, **154**, 125–69.

Chen, D.H., Jiang, H., et al. 1999. Three-dimensional visualization of tegument/capsid interactions in the intact human cytomegalovirus. *Virology*, **260**, 10–16.

Chou, J., Kern, E.R., et al. 1990. Mapping of herpes simplex virus-1 neurovirulence to γ₁34.5, a gene nonessential for growth in culture. *Science*, **250**, 1262–5.

Coen, D.M. 1992. Molecular aspects of anti-herpesvirus drugs. *Semin Virol*, **3**, 3–12.

Connor, J., Marsden, H. and Clements, J.B. 1994. Ribonucleotide reductase of herpesviruses. *Semin Virol*, **4**, 25–34.

Dargan, D.J. 1986. The structure and assembly of herpesviruses. In: Harris, J.R. and Horne, R.W. (eds), *Electron microscopy of proteins*. Vol. 5. London: Academic Press, 359–436.

Davison, A.J. 1992a. Genetic structure and content of herpesviruses. In: Plowright, W., Rossdale, P.D. and Wade, J.F. (eds), *Equine infectious diseases VI*. Newmarket: R&W Publications Ltd, 165–74.

Davison, A.J. 1992b. Channel catfish virus: a new type of herpesvirus. *Virology*, **186**, 9–14.

Davison, A.J. 1993. Herpesvirus genes. *Rev Med Virol*, **3**, 237–44.

Davison, A.J. 2000. Molecular evolution of alphaherpesviruses. In: Arvin, A.M. and Gershon, A.A. (eds), *Varicella-zoster virus*. Cambridge: Cambridge University Press, 25–50.

Davison, A.J. and Scott, J.E. 1986. The complete DNA sequence of varicella-zoster virus. *J Gen Virol*, **67**, 1759–816.

Davison, A.J., Dolan, A., et al. 2003. The human cytomegalovirus genome revisited: comparison with the chimpanzee cytomegalovirus genome. *J Gen Virol*, **84**, 17–28.

Davison, A.J. and McGeoch, D.J. 1995. Herpesviridae. In: Gibbs, A.J., Callisher, C.H. and García-Arenal, F. (eds), *Molecular basis of virus evolution*. Cambridge: Cambridge University Press, 290–309.

Dohner, K., Wolfstein, A., et al. 2002. Function of dynein and dynactin in herpes simplex virus capsid transport. *Mol Biol Cell*, **13**, 2795–809.

Dolan, A., Jamieson, F.E., et al. 1998. The genome sequence of herpes simplex virus type 2. *J Virol*, **72**, 2010–21.

Dominguez, G., Dambaugh, T.R., et al. 1999. Human herpesvirus 6B genome sequence: coding content and comparison with human herpesvirus 6A. *J Virol*, **73**, 8040–52.

Elliott, G. and O'Hare, P. 1999. Live-cell analysis of a green fluorescent protein-tagged herpes simplex virus infection. *J Virol*, **73**, 4110–19.

Enquist, L.W. 2002. Exploiting circuit-specific spread of pseudorabies virus in the central nervous system: insights to pathogenesis and circuit tracers. *J Infect Dis*, **186**, Suppl. 2, S209–14.

Ensser, A., Pflanz, R. and Fleckenstein, B. 1997. Primary structure of the alcelaphine herpesvirus 1 genome. *J Virol*, **71**, 6517–25.

Everett, R.D. 1987. The regulation of transcription of viral and cellular genes by herpesvirus immediate–early gene products. *Anticancer Res*, **7**, 589–604.

Everett, R.D. 2000. ICP0, a regulator of herpes simplex virus during lytic and latent infection. *Bioessays*, **22**, 761–70.

Frenkel, N., Schirmer, E.C., et al. 1990. Isolation of a new herpesvirus from human CD4⁺ T cells. *Proc Natl Acad Sci USA*, **87**, 748–52.

Furlong, D., Swift, H. and Roizman, B. 1972. Arrangement of herpesvirus deoxyribonucleic acid in the core. *J Virol*, **10**, 1071–4.

Garber, A.C., Shu, M.A., et al. 2001. DNA binding and modulation of gene expression by the latency-associated nuclear antigen of Kaposi's sarcoma-associated herpesvirus. *J Virol*, **75**, 7882–92.

Gray, W.L., Starnes, B., et al. 2001. The DNA sequence of the simian varicella virus genome. *Virology*, **284**, 123–30.

Gompels, U.A., Nicholas, J., et al. 1995. DNA sequence of human herpesvirus 6: structure, coding content, and genome evolution. *Virology*, **209**, 29–51.

Hammerschmidt, W. and Mankertz, J. 1991. Herpesviral DNA replication: between the known and unknown. *Semin Virol*, **2**, 257–69.

Hamzeh, F.M., Lietman, P.S., et al. 1990. Identification of the lytic origin of DNA replication in human cytomegalovirus by a novel approach utilizing ganciclovir-induced chain termination. *J Virol*, **64**, 6184–95.

Hayward, G.S., Jacob, R.J., et al. 1975. Anatomy of herpes simplex virus DNA: evidence for four populations that differ in the relative orientations of their long and short components. *Proc Natl Acad Sci USA*, **72**, 4243–7.

He, B., Gross, M. and Roizman, B. 1997. The γ₁34.5 protein of herpes simplex virus 1 complexes with protein phosphatase 1α to dephosphorylate the α subunit of eukaryotic translation initiation factor 2 and preclude the shutoff of protein synthesis by double-stranded RNA-activated protein kinase. *Proc Natl Acad Sci USA*, **94**, 843–8.

Hengel, H., Brune, W. and Koszinowski, U.H. 1998. Immune evasion by cytomegalovirus-survival strategies of a highly adapted opportunist. *Trend Microbiol*, **6**, 190–7.

Homa, F.L. and Brown, J.C. 1997. Capsid assembly and DNA packaging in herpes simplex virus. *Rev Med Virol*, **7**, 107–22.

Honess, R.W. 1984. Herpes simplex and 'the herpes complex': diverse observations and a unifying hypothesis. *J Gen Virol*, **65**, 2077–107.

Honess, R.W. and Roizman, B. 1974. Regulation of herpesvirus macromolecular synthesis. I. Cascade regulation of the synthesis of three groups of viral proteins. *J Virol*, **14**, 8–19.

Honess, R.W., Gompels, U.A., et al. 1989. Deviations from expected frequencies of CpG dinucleotides in herpesvirus DNAs may be diagnostic of differences in the states of their latent genomes. *J Gen Virol*, **70**, 837–55.

Isegawa, Y., Mukai, T., et al. 1999. Comparison of the complete DNA sequences of human herpesvirus 6 variants A and B. *J Virol*, **73**, 8053–63.

Izumiya, Y., Jang, H., et al. 2001. A complete genomic DNA sequence of Marek's disease virus type 2, strain HPRS24. *Curr Top Microbiol Immunol*, **255**, 191–221.

Johansson, M., van Rompay, A.R., et al. 1999. Cloning and characterization of the multisubstrate deoxyribonucleoside kinase of *Drosophila melanogaster*. *J Biol Chem*, **274**, 23814–19.

Johnson, D.C. and Hill, A.B. 1998. Herpesvirus evasion of the immune system. *Curr Top Microbiol Immunol*, **232**, 149–77.

Kieff, E. and Rickinson, A.B. 2001. Epstein–Barr virus and its replication. In: Knipe, D.M. and Howley, P.M. (eds), *Fields' Virology*, 4th edn. Philadelphia: Lippincott Williams and Wilkins, 2511–73.

Koffa, M.D., Clements, J.B., et al. 2001. Herpes simplex virus ICP27 protein provides viral mRNAs with access to the cellular mRNA export pathway. *EMBO J*, **20**, 5769–78.

Liu, B. and Stinski, M.F. 1992. Human cytomegalovirus contains a tegument protein that enhances transcription from promoters with upstream ATF and AP-1-*cis*-acting elements. *J Virol*, **66**, 4434–44.

Liu, F. and Roizman, B. 1991. The promoter, transcriptional unit, and coding sequence of the herpes simplex virus 1 family 35 proteins are contained within and in frame with the U$_L$26 open reading frame. *J Virol*, **65**, 206–12.

Lu, P., Jones, F.E., et al. 2001. Herpes simplex virus virion host shutoff protein requires a mammalian factor for efficient in vitro endoribonuclease activity. *J Virol*, **75**, 1172–85.

Markert, J.M., Parker, J.N., et al. 2001. Genetically engineered human herpes simplex virus in the treatment of brain tumours. *Herpes*, **8**, 17–22.

Marsden, H.S. 1992. Disruption of protein–subunit interactions. *Semin Virol*, **3**, 67–75.

McGeoch, D.J. 1989. The genomes of the human herpesviruses: contents, relationships and evolution. *Ann Rev Microbiol*, **43**, 235–65.

McGeoch, D.J. and Davison, A.J. 1999. The molecular evolutionary history of the herpesviruses. In: Domingo, E., Webster, R. and Holland, J. (eds), *Origin and evolution of viruses*. London: Academic Press, 441–65.

McGeoch, D.J. and Schaffer, P.A. 1993. Herpes simplex virus. In: O'Brien, S. (ed.), *Genetic maps*, Vol. 1. 6th edn. New York: Cold Spring Harbor Press, 147–56.

McGeoch, D.J., Dalrymple, M.A., et al. 1988. The complete DNA sequence of the long unique region in the genome of herpes simplex virus type 1. *J Gen Virol*, **69**, 1531–74.

McGeoch, D.J., Barnett, B.C. and MacLean, C.A. 1993. Emerging functions of alphaherpesvirus genes. *Semin Virol*, **4**, 125–44.

McGeoch, D.J., Cook, S., et al. 1995. Molecular phylogeny and evolutionary timescale for the family of mammalian herpesviruses. *J Mol Biol*, **247**, 443–58.

McGeoch, D.J., Dolan, A. and Ralph, A.C. 2000. Toward a comprehensive phylogeny for mammalian and avian herpesviruses. *J Virol*, **74**, 10401–6.

Megaw, A.G., Rapaport, D., et al. 1998. The DNA sequence of the RK strain of human herpesvirus 7. *Virology*, **244**, 119–32.

Mettenleiter, T.C. 2002. Herpesvirus assembly and egress. *J Virol*, **76**, 1537–47.

Minson, A.C., Davison, A., et al. 2000. Family *Herpesviridae*. In: Van Regenmortel, M.H.V., Fauquet, C.M. and Bishop, D.H.L. (eds), *Virus taxonomy*. San Diego: Academic Press, 203–25.

Mocarski, E.S. and Tan Courcelle, C. 2001. Cytomegaloviruses and their replication. In: Knipe, D.M. and Howley, P.M. (eds), *Fields' Virology*, 4th edn. Philadelphia: Lippincott Williams and Wilkins, 2629–73.

Moore, P.S. and Chang, Y. 2001a. Molecular virology of Kaposi's sarcoma-associated herpesvirus. *Phil Trans R Soc Lond, Ser B, Biol Sci*, **356**, 499–516.

Moore, P.S. and Chang, Y. 2001b. Kaposi's sarcoma-associated herpesvirus. In: Knipe, D.M. and Howley, P.M. (eds), *Fields' Virology*, 4th edn. Philadelphia: Lippincott Williams and Wilkins, 2803–33.

Morrison, J.M. 1991. *Virus induced enzymes*. Chichester: Wiley.

Nash, A.A., Dutia, B.M., et al. 2001. Natural history of murine gammaherpesvirus infection. *Phil Trans R Soc Lond, Ser B, Biol Sci*, **356**, 569–79.

Neipel, F., Albrecht, J.C. and Fleckenstein, B. 1997. Cell-homologous genes in the Kaposi's sarcoma-associated rhadinovirus human herpesvirus 8: determinants of its pathogenicity? *J Virol*, **71**, 4187–92.

Newcomb, W.W., Homa, F.L., et al. 1999. Assembly of the herpes simplex virus procapsid from purified components and identification of

small complexes containing the major capsid and scaffolding proteins. *J Virol*, **73**, 4239–50.

Newcomb, W.W., Juhas, R.M., et al. 2001. The UL6 gene product forms the portal for entry of DNA into the herpes simplex virus capsid. *J Virol*, **75**, 10923–32.

Nicholas, J. 1996. Determination and analysis of the complete nucleotide sequence of human herpesvirus 7. *J Virol*, **70**, 5975–89.

O'Hare, P. 1993. The virion transactivator of herpes simplex virus. *Semin Virol*, **4**, 145–55.

Parker, B.D., Bankier, A., et al. 1990. Sequence and transcription of Raji Epstein–Barr virus DNA spanning the B95-8 deletion region. *Virology*, **179**, 339–46.

Phelan, A. and Clements, J.B. 1998. Posttranscriptional regulation in herpes simplex virus. *Semin Virol*, **8**, 309–18.

Prichard, M.N., Penfold, M.E., et al. 2001. A review of genetic differences between limited and extensively passaged human cytomegalovirus strains. *Rev Med Virol*, **11**, 191–200.

Rawlinson, W.D., Farrell, H.E. and Barrell, B.G. 1996. Analysis of the complete DNA sequence of murine cytomegalovirus. *J Virol*, **70**, 8833–49.

Reddehase, M.J. 2000. The immunogenicity of human and murine cytomegaloviruses. *Curr Opin Immunol*, **12**, 390–6.

Rivailler, P., Cho, Y.G. and Wang, F. 2002a. Complete genomic sequence of an Epstein–Barr virus-related herpesvirus naturally infecting a new world primate: a defining point in the evolution of oncogenic lymphocryptoviruses. *J Virol*, **76**, 12055–68.

Rivailler, P., Jiang, H., et al. 2002b. Complete nucleotide sequence of the rhesus lymphocryptovirus: genetic validation for an Epstein–Barr virus animal model. *J Virol*, **76**, 421–6.

Roizman, B. and Knipe, D.M. 2001. Herpes simplex viruses and their replication. In: Knipe, D.M. and Howley, P.M. (eds), *Fields' Virology*, 4th edn. Philadelphia: Lippincott Williams and Wilkins, 2399–459.

Russo, J.J., Bohenzky, R.A., et al. 1996. Nucleotide sequence of the Kaposi sarcoma-associated herpesvirus (HHV8). *Proc Natl Acad Sci USA*, **93**, 14862–7.

Salahuddin, S.Z., Ablashi, D.V., et al. 1986. Isolation of a new virus, HBLV, in patients with lymphoproliferative disorders. *Science*, **234**, 596–601.

Schultz, E.R., Rankin, G.W. Jr., et al. 2000. Characterization of two divergent lineages of macaque rhadinoviruses related to Kaposi's sarcoma-associated herpesvirus. *J Virol*, **74**, 4919–28.

Schulz, T.F. 1998. Kaposi's sarcoma-associated herpesvirus (human herpesvirus-8). *J Gen Virol*, **79**, 1573–91.

Schwyzer, M. and Ackermann, M. 1996. Molecular virology of ruminant herpesviruses. *Vet Microbiol*, **53**, 17–29.

Searles, R.P., Bergquam, E.P., et al. 1999. Sequence and genomic analysis of a rhesus macaque rhadinovirus with similarity to Kaposi's sarcoma-associated herpesvirus/human herpesvirus 8. *J Virol*, **73**, 3040–53.

Sheldrick, P. and Berthelot, N. 1974. Inverted repetitions in the chromosome of herpes simplex virus. *Cold Spring Symp Quant Biol*, **39**, 667–78.

Shukla, D. and Spear, P.G. 2001. Herpesviruses and heparan sulfate: an intimate relationship in aid of viral entry. *J Clin Invest*, **108**, 503–10.

Skepper, J.N., Whiteley, A., et al. 2001. Herpes simplex virus nucleocapsids mature to progeny virions by an envelopment → deenvelopment → reenvelopment pathway. *J Virol*, **75**, 5697–702.

Spear, P.G., Eisenberg, R.J. and Cohen, G.H. 2000. Three classes of cell surface receptors for alphaherpesvirus entry. *Virology*, **275**, 1–8.

Stingley, S.W., Ramirez, J.J., et al. 2000. Global analysis of herpes simplex virus type 1 transcription using an oligonucleotide-based DNA microarray. *J Virol*, **74**, 9916–27.

Stow, N.D. 2000. Molecular interactions in herpes simplex virus DNA replication. In: Cann, A.J. (ed.), *Frontiers in molecular biology: DNA virus replication*. Oxford: Oxford University Press, 66–104.

Tanaka, K., Kondo, T., et al. 1994. Human herpesvirus 7: another causal agent for roseola (exanthem subitum). *J Pediatr*, **125**, 1–5.

Tatman, J.D., Preston, V.G., et al. 1994. Assembly of herpes simplex virus type 1 capsids using a panel of recombinant baculoviruses. *J Gen Virol*, **75**, 1101–13.

Telford, E.A.R., Watson, M.S., et al. 1992. The DNA sequence of equine herpesvirus-1. *Virology*, **189**, 304–16.

Telford, E.A.R., Watson, M.S., et al. 1995. The DNA sequence of equine herpesvirus 2. *J Mol Biol*, **249**, 520–8.

Telford, E.A.R., Watson, M.S., et al. 1998. The DNA sequence of equine herpesvirus 4. *J Gen Virol*, **79**, 1197–203.

Thomsen, D.R., Roof, L.L. and Homa, F.L. 1994. Assembly of herpes simplex virus (HSV) intermediate capsids in insect cells infected with recombinant baculoviruses expressing HSV capsid proteins. *J Virol*, **68**, 2442–57.

Trus, B.L., Booy, F.P., et al. 1996. The herpes simplex virus procapsid: structure, conformational changes upon maturation, and roles of the triplex proteins VP19c and VP23 in assembly. *J Mol Biol*, **263**, 447–62.

Tulman, E.R., Afonso, C.L., et al. 2000. The genome of a very virulent Marek's disease virus. *J Virol*, **74**, 7980–8.

Underwood, M.R., Harvey, R.J., et al. 1998. Inhibition of human cytomegalovirus DNA maturation by a benzimidazole ribonucleoside is mediated through the UL89 gene product. *J Virol*, **72**, 717–25.

Umene, K. and Sakaoka, H. 1999. Evolution of herpes simplex virus type 1 under herpesviral evolutionary processes. *Arch Virol*, **144**, 637–56.

Vink, C., Beuken, E. and Bruggeman, C.A. 2000. Complete DNA sequence of the rat cytomegalovirus genome. *J Virol*, **74**, 7656–65.

Virgin, H.W., Latreille, P., et al. 1997. Complete sequence and genomic analysis of murine gammaherpesvirus 68. *J Virol*, **71**, 5894–904.

Wagner, E.K. 1985. Individual HSV transcripts. In: Roizman, B. (ed.), *The herpesviruses*. Vol. 3. New York: Plenum Press, 45–104.

Wagner, M.J. and Summers, W.C. 1978. Structures of the joint region and the termini of the DNA of herpes simplex virus type 1. *J Virol*, **27**, 374–87.

Ward, P.L. and Roizman, B. 1994. *Herpes simplex* genes: the blueprint of a successful human pathogen. *Trend Genet*, **10**, 267–74.

Watson, R.J. and Clements, J.B. 1980. A herpes simplex virus type 1 function continuously required for early and late virus RNA synthesis. *Nature*, **285**, 329–30.

Wildy, P., Russell, W.C. and Horne, R.W. 1960. The morphology of herpesvirus. *Virology*, **12**, 204–22.

Yamanishi, K., Okuno, T., et al. 1988. Identification of human herpesvirus-6 as a causal agent for exanthem subitum. *Lancet*, **1**, 1065–7.

York, I.A., Roop, C., et al. 1994. A cytosolic herpes simplex protein inhibits antigen presentation to CD8[+] T lymphocytes. *Cell*, **77**, 525–35.

Zhou, Z.H., Dougherty, M., et al. 2000. Seeing the herpesvirus capsid at 8.5 Å. *Science*, **288**, 877–80.

Zhu, H., Cong, J.P., et al. 1998. Cellular gene expression altered by human cytomegalovirus: global monitoring with oligonucleotide arrays. *Proc Natl Acad Sci USA*, **95**, 14470–5.

Zimmermann, W., Broll, H., et al. 2001. Genome sequence of bovine herpesvirus 4, a bovine *Rhadinovirus*, and identification of an origin of DNA replication. *J Virol*, **75**, 1186–94.

26

Alphaherpesviruses: herpes simplex and varicella-zoster

ANTHONY C. MINSON

Herpes simplex virus (HSV) types 1 and 2 (HSV-1 and HSV-2) and varicella-zoster virus (VZV) are alpha herpesviruses that are related in their genetic and biological properties. Their genomes are composed of homologous sets of genes organized in a co-linear fashion; they cause productive cytolytic infection of epithelial cells, and establish life-long latent infections in sensory nerve ganglia. There are, however, important biological differences:

- VZV infection has a viremic phase whereas HSV infectivity is usually limited to the epithelium and sensory nerves at the infection site
- HSV is transmitted only by contact whereas VZV is airborne and contagious
- VZV is highly species-specific whereas HSV can infect, experimentally, a wide range of species.

Indeed, our knowledge of HSV pathogenesis and immunity derives largely from studies of the virus in rodents. HSV-1 and HSV-2 are closely related: they crossreact antigenically, exhibit extensive nucleotide sequence homology and their genes are functionally homologous because stable intertypic recombinants can be generated readily in tissue culture. However, despite the fact that HSV-1 and HSV-2 can infect similar sites in humans, recombination between these viruses does not appear to occur in vivo, and genetic comparison suggests that the two subtypes have evolved independently for more than 5 million years (McGeoch and Cook 1994).

HERPES SIMPLEX VIRUS

Clinical manifestations

HSV infects mucosal epithelium or damaged cutaneous epithelium, and infection can therefore occur at a variety of sites, but oral and genital infections are most common. HSV-2 is predominantly responsible for genital infection but HSV-1 contributes significantly, representing 30–50 percent of genital isolates in some studies (Buckmaster et al. 1984; Ross et al. 1993). By contrast, HSV-2 is rarely isolated from oral lesions. The basis of this preference for different mucosal surfaces by the two virus types is unknown but the predominance of HSV-2 'below the waist' and HSV-1 'above the waist' extends to other sites. Thus anal lesions, cutaneous lesions of the thighs and buttocks, and infections of the neonate during birth are more frequently caused by HSV-2 whilst eye infections and cutaneous lesions of the head and neck are usually caused by HSV-1. Regardless of the site of infection or the virus type, HSV enters sensory nerve endings during primary infection and is transported to the neuronal cell body where latent infection is established. Since oral and genital infections are by far the most common, the trigeminal and sacral ganglia are the usual sites of latent infection by HSV-1 and HSV-2, respectively. The majority of the adult population is latently infected with HSV, but it is clear that infection rates greatly exceed clinical disease rates and many, perhaps most, individuals who are latently infected with HSV have no recollection of primary infection and do not suffer recurrent lesions.

Primary oral infection presents as an acute gingivostomatitis comprising painful ulcers in the mouth, which resolve within a few weeks, often accompanied by fever and enlargement of local lymph nodes. A significant proportion of sore throats is also thought to be caused by primary oral HSV, and this may be the most common manifestation of primary infection. During the course of primary infection the virus establishes a lifelong latent infection in neurons of the trigeminal ganglia, and 'reactivation' results in the reseeding of virus into the oral epithelium and shedding in saliva. A minority of seropositive people suffer periodic clinical recurrences, the classic 'cold sores,' crops of vesicles on the mucocutaneous junctions of the mouth and nose which ulcerate, crust, and heal within 4–7 days (Figure 26.1). Some of these individuals recognize a prodromal tingling or burning sensation which heralds the development of the recurrent lesion. Recurrences are provoked by a variety of stimuli, including sunlight, physical trauma, stress, respiratory infections, and hormonal change, but it is not known whether these stimuli act by a common pathway. The development of a cold sore requires reactivation of the latent virus in the ganglia followed by the establishment of a focus of epithelial infection; a provoking stimulus might operate either by triggering a reactivation in the ganglia or by modifying the susceptibility of the relevant epithelium such that a ganglionic reactivation, which would otherwise have been silent, results in a clinical recurrence.

Genital herpes consists of painful vesicles on the genitalia or anal region. Aseptic meningitis has been reported as a complication of primary infection, and proctitis has been reported in homosexual men. HSV-2 appears to be almost exclusively responsible for these complications. As with oral infection, many primary genital infections are inapparent and the first indication of infection may be a recurrence, an episode that has been termed 'initial infection' to distinguish it from the primary infection (Corey et al. 1983). Genital herpes infections recur at a higher frequency than oral infections, and genital HSV-2 infections recur more frequently than genital HSV-1 infections (Lafferty et al. 1987). The frequency and severity of recurrent episodes usually decrease with time but recurrent genital herpes is a painful and distressing disease, and many patients suffer frequent recurrences for many years. Reactivation of latent virus and shedding in genital secretions occur at a much higher rate than clinical disease.

Infection of the skin, manifest as a crop of classic herpetic vesicles, can occur on any part of the body, most commonly the head or neck, and probably always results from the contamination of damaged skin by virus in saliva or genital secretions. Infection may result from intimacy or activities likely to cause abrasion, such as wrestling (herpes gladiatorum) or rugby (scrum pox). Lesions on the fingers (herpetic whitlows) are an occupational hazard for healthcare workers. A particularly severe disease results from infection of eczematous skin (eczema herpeticum), in which the virus spreads widely, causing large areas of ulceration.

Herpes infections of the eye are second only to oral and genital infections in frequency. Primary infections are associated with keratoconjunctivitis and are often bilateral whereas recurrences are usually unilateral and result in dendritic ulcers or stromal involvement. Repeated recurrences may lead to scarring and opacification of the cornea, and consequent sight impairment.

Invasion of the central nervous system (CNS) is manifest as herpes encephalitis, a cytolytic infection, primarily of neurons, with a propensity to focus in the temporal lobes (see Chapter 62, Infections of the central nervous system). Untreated, the disease has a mortality of >70 percent and most survivors are neurologically impaired. All age groups are susceptible but the disease is rare; about one case per million population is reported each year in the UK and the USA. Symptoms generally begin with fever and headache, rapidly followed by disorientation and progressive deterioration in consciousness, but the symptoms are not diagnostic and can be confused with other syndromes. Predisposing factors are unknown. Herpes encephalitis can apparently result from primary or recurrent infection (Nahmias et al. 1982; Whitley et al. 1982), but the route to the CNS is uncertain. A focal encephalitis, similar to that observed in humans, results from infection of mice by the olfactory route (Anderson and Field 1983). Aciclovir therapy has greatly reduced the morbidity and mortality of herpes encephalitis but effective treatment depends on prompt diagnosis.

The neonate is highly susceptible to HSV infection, and neonatal infection is frequently fatal. The disease presents classically as a generalized infection affecting multiple organs, including the lung, liver, adrenals, CNS, and skin, but in some cases the infection is more limited, involving the skin or the CNS or both. The prognosis is very poor for those with disseminated or CNS infection.

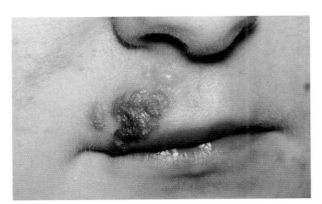

Figure 26.1 *Vesicular cold sores due to recurrent herpes simplex. (Photograph courtesy of Dr. Jane Sterling, Addenbrooke's Hospital, Cambridge, UK: Copyright Addenbrooke's NHS Trust.)*

In the USA neonatal herpes is estimated to occur with an incidence of 1 per 2 000–5 000 deliveries and is perceived as a major public health problem, but in the UK the disease is rare (Sullivan-Bolyai et al. 1983; PHLS Report 1987), an unexplained discrepancy that cannot be accounted for by differences in the overall frequency of genital herpes in the two populations. The infection is most commonly acquired during birth from a genital infection of the mother but infections in utero and in the immediate postnatal period have also been documented and probably represent a significant proportion of the total. Primary infection in the mother close to term presents a much higher risk to the neonate than does recurrent infection (Prober et al. 1987), probably owing to the higher virus titers present during primary infection and perhaps to the protective effect of maternal antibody present in the neonate exposed to recurrent infection. Delivery by cesarean section is usually recommended when genital lesions are present at term. Superficial damage to the skin by fetal scalp monitors is thought to provide the virus with a route of entry, and the use of scalp monitors is contraindicated if the mother has a history of recurrent genital infection.

Not surprisingly, the immunocompromised patient has an increased susceptibility to HSV infection. The most common manifestation is a reduced capacity to control recurrent oral lesions which occur more frequently and spread more widely on the head and neck and to the respiratory tract (e.g. Smyth et al. 1990). These infections resolve slowly, if at all, in the absence of therapy. Although these infections can be very severe, they are nevertheless limited to the skin and mucosa, even in profoundly immunosuppressed patients. Disseminated, generalized infection, as seen in the neonate, has been reported in adults very rarely.

Epidemiology

A wide range of mammalian species can be infected experimentally with HSV but there is no evidence that this occurs naturally. Humans are the only natural host, and latent virus in trigeminal and sacral ganglia is the reservoir. The source of transmitted virus is oral or genital secretions, and transmission requires contact. There is no seasonal variation in disease incidence. Because HSV-2 is primarily a sexually transmitted disease and occurs only rarely as an oral infection, evidence of HSV-2 infection is found almost exclusively in adolescents and adults, whereas HSV-1 is a common infection of childhood. Despite this straightforward picture, which emerges from a large number of sero-epidemiological and virological studies, precise data on the incidence of HSV-1 and HSV-2 infections in different study populations have been difficult to obtain because of the high proportion of asymptomatic infections and problems in distinguishing antibodies to the two subtypes.

In many populations, virtually all children are infected with HSV-1 during the first 5 years of life, but sero-conversion rates vary greatly with geographical area and socioeconomic group. In higher socioeconomic groups in industrialized countries, seroconversion may be as low as 20 percent during the first 5 years, rising to 40–60 percent during adolescence and early adulthood. Young children secrete virus asymptomatically more frequently and for much more prolonged periods than seropositive adults; this, together with higher levels of contact activity, probably accounts for the high attack rates in this group. Seroepidemiological surveys emphasize the view that HSV-2 is transmitted primarily by the sexual route: antibodies specific for HSV-2 are virtually nonexistent in nuns but are found in the majority of prostitutes, and the appearance of HSV-2 antibodies correlates with the onset of sexual activity. The reported overall incidence of HSV-2 antibodies in the adult population varies in different studies, and many historical surveys suffer from technical problems associated with the serological crossreactivity of HSV-1 and HSV-2. More recent studies estimate that 15–25 percent of the adult US population is infected with HSV-2, and broadly similar data have been obtained in the UK (Ades et al. 1989), though prevalence rates vary significantly among different ethnic groups. As noted above, HSV-1 can also be transmitted by the sexual route, and in some studies nearly 50 percent of genital isolates were of this type (Ross et al. 1993). It is supposed, though not proven, that the large number of HSV-1 genital infections and the occasional HSV-2 oral infection result from orogenital sex.

Pathology and pathogenesis

The portal of entry in primary infection is the damaged skin or mucosa and the classic lesion is a vesicle beneath the keratinized squamous epithelial cells (Figure 26.2).

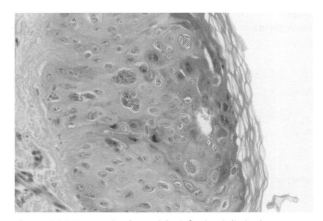

Figure 26.2 *Herpes simplex vesicle: infection is limited to epithelial cells, which become disorganized and exhibit characteristic nuclear inclusions. Multinuclear cells result from cell fusion. The lesion shown is at a relatively early state and contains very few inflammatory cells. (Photograph courtesy of Dr. Jane Sterling, Addenbrooke's Hospital, Cambridge, UK.)*

The infection of epithelial cells is cytolytic; the cells lose adhesion, occasionally become multinucleate as a result of virus-induced cell fusion and contain Cowdry type A nuclear inclusions. The vesicle drains and the lesion crusts before healing occurs, sometimes with residual scarring, and draining lymph nodes are commonly enlarged during this process. Recurrent lesions are morphologically and histologically similar but are usually less extensive, and lymph node swelling is inapparent. In the immune competent patient the lesion resolves within 7–10 days of its appearance.

LATENCY AND REACTIVATION

During primary infection of the skin or mucosa the virus enters sensory nerve endings and is transported by fast retrograde axonal flow to the neuronal bodies of the dorsal root ganglia innervating the site of infection. In animal models this is followed by a period of limited virus replication in the ganglia, during which virus antigen can be detected in a small number of neurons. Within about 10 days, no infectious virus can be detected in the ganglia or at the site of inoculation, but the presence of latent virus can be detected for the lifetime of the infected animal by dissection and in vitro culture of the relevant sensory ganglia (Stevens and Cook 1971; Hill et al. 1975). Similarly, 'in vitro reactivation' of latent virus can be achieved by culture of trigeminal ganglia from cadavers of HSV-1 seropositive humans.

Many lines of evidence show that HSV establishes a true latent infection rather than a low level chronic infection. Mutant viruses that are incapable of replicating at the internal temperature of the mouse establish and maintain latency (McLennan and Darby 1980). Long-term treatment of infected mice or humans with aciclovir does not cure latency (Fife et al. 1994); the state of the viral genome in latent infection is unique. HSV DNA within virus particles is a linear molecule whereas viral DNA in latently infected ganglia is endless and is thought to be present as a circular episome (Mellerick and Fraser 1987). The latently infected ganglion contains a unique set of transcripts, the 'latency-associated transcripts' (LAT) synthesized from a single promoter (the LAT promoter) situated in the repeat sequences flanking the unique long region of the viral genome (Stevens et al. 1987). These transcripts are readily detected by in situ hybridization in latently infected human trigeminal ganglia or in ganglia from experimental animals, and they are found exclusively in neurons (Figure 26.3) – consistent with other evidence that this cell type is the site of latent infection. The function of the latency-associated transcripts is uncertain. Mutations that modify the transcripts, or abolish their synthesis, do not prevent the virus from establishing or maintaining latent infection in animal models. Indeed, despite extensive study, no HSV gene has been identified that is essential for latent

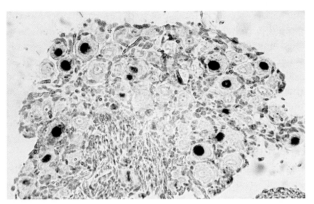

Figure 26.3 *Virus-specific transcripts in a sensory ganglion from a mouse latently infected with HSV-1. LATs are detected by hybridization in situ within the nuclei of a minority of sensory neurons. No viral antigens, productive cycle transcripts or virus particles are detectable. Latent infection of the tissue can be demonstrated by explant culture. (Photograph courtesy of Dr. R Lachmann, Department of Pathology, University of Cambridge.)*

infection, and one view is that latency requires no gene function but occurs by default if the productive cycle fails. On this supposition the transcriptional machinery of the neuron is the key factor in latency and reactivation: if the neuron fails to transcribe the viral immediate–early genes (see Chapter 25, Herpesviruses: general properties), the productive cycle cannot be initiated and the viral genome is latent by default, but at some later time perturbation of the sensory nerve may change the transcriptional program of the neuron. The viral immediate–early genes may then be expressed, the productive cycle is initiated, and the latent virus reactivates. The evidence for this mechanism is largely negative but is consistent with the characteristics of an in vitro latency model in which the level of expression of one of the immediate–early genes appears to be a key factor in determining whether the virus enters the lytic cycle or remains latent (Preston 2000). Evidence is accumulating that the LAT has anti-apoptotic functions and this protects the neuron during establishment of latency and during reactivation. This would account for the fact that HSV mutants unable to synthesize LATs are capable of establishing latency but do so with reduced frequency and reactivate less efficiently (Jones 2003).

Perturbation of the sensory nerve can induce HSV reactivation, an observation first made by Cushing (1905), who noted the frequent appearance of cold sores after sectioning the posterior sensory root of the trigeminal ganglion, a result that has been confirmed in animal models. Furthermore, virus in latently infected rat sympathetic ganglia cultured in vitro reactivates after withdrawal of nerve growth factor (Wilcox et al. 1990). Nevertheless, the specific neuronal changes that lead to reactivation are unknown. A wide variety of stimuli provoke clinical recurrence but, as noted earlier, many of these stimuli may act to enhance virus replication at the periphery rather than to induce reactivation in the ganglion. What is certain is that reactivation and virus shedding are much more common than clinical recurrence. The fate of the neuron in which reactivation occurs is also unknown. It is axiomatic of HSV infection that the productive cycle is cytolytic, yet reactivation and seeding of epithelium with infectious particles must require productive infection in the neuron. There is no evidence of sensory loss, even in patients who suffer frequent recurrences over a very long period, and it is uncertain whether reactivation results in the loss of the neuron or if, unlike other cell types, the neuron can survive virus replication.

Immune response

HSV infection in humans induces a vigorous humoral and cell-mediated response, but studies of the details are confounded by the very large number of antigens specified by the virus (>70) and by the technical problem of examining the response to primary infection. Most studies in humans have been of the response to latent infection or recurrent disease, whereas much information on the primary response derives from experiments in inbred mice.

Infection is followed within a few days by the appearance of IgM antibodies, closely followed by IgG and IgA. IgG persists indefinitely and antibodies against at least 30 different viral polypeptides have been identified. The surface glycoproteins of the virus (of which there are at least 10) are among the most immunogenic and these are also the targets for complement-dependent and complement-independent antibody-mediated neutralization. Glycoprotein D, delivered as a subunit protein or using live vectors, is probably the most potent inducer of neutralizing antibody and, in humans, anti-gD titers correlate with serum neutralizing titers. The role of antibody in infection is, however, uncertain. High levels of passive antibody protect mice from infection and modulate infection (Simmons and Nash 1985) but B-cell-deficient mice recover more or less normally from infection and agammaglobulinemic patients do not suffer particularly severe HSV infections (Corey and Spear 1986; Simmons and Nash 1987). While antibody can protect against infection, at least in mice, the cell-mediated responses are of central importance in controlling an established infection since, in humans and in mice, T-cell deficiencies result in severe disease and inefficient clearance of virus. The importance of different T-cell subsets and of innate cellular defense mechanisms varies in mice, depending on the strain and infection route. Nevertheless, CD4$^+$ T cells predominate in clearance of infection from the skin and mucosa (Nash and Gell 1983; Schmid 1988), whereas classic major histocompatibility complex (MHC) class I-restricted cytotoxic T cells are readily detected in mice but difficult to detect in humans. There is evidence that CD8$^+$ T cells

control HSV in the nervous system but by a cytokine-mediated mechanism rather than by direct cytotoxicity (Simmons and Tscharke 1992). Innate defenses are also likely to be of central importance. HSV has a very broad cell tropism yet systemic generalized disease is found almost exclusively in the neonate and not in profoundly immunosuppressed children or adults. In mice, interferon responses, NK cell activity, and macrophage function have all been shown to control HSV infection, and deficiencies in these defenses may contribute to the susceptibility of the neonate (Cunningham and Merigan 1983; Lopez 1985; Wu and Morahan 1992). Severe HSV infection in a child with an NK-cell deficiency has been reported (Biron et al. 1989) but there are conflicting data on the importance of NK cells in controlling HSV (Bukowski and Welsh 1986).

It is worth reiterating that studies of the response to HSV in the mouse are almost exclusively concerned with primary infections. Recurrent infections do not occur in inbred mice, and in guinea pigs and rabbits, which exhibit recurrent disease, the immune response is not amenable to detailed analysis. In humans, recurrent episodes are not usually accompanied by significant changes in antibody levels but changes in T-cell proliferative responses have been reported. Comparisons of immune responses in seropositive patients with and without recurrent disease have given no indication of a consistent quantitative or qualitative difference in response in these two groups, and it may be that other factors, such as latent virus load, rather than the immune response, determine recurrence frequency. Nevertheless, the fact that recurrences usually decrease in frequency with time and that immunocompromised patients suffer more recurrent episodes suggests that recurrences can be suppressed by an acquired immune response. This is an issue of some consequence because the identification of the key elements of the response might allow the development of immunotherapeutic approaches to the prevention of recurrent disease. Immune responses to HSV infection have been reviewed by Daheshia et al. (1998) and Nash (2000).

HSV has evolved a number of mechanisms to evade the immune response. Glycoprotein C binds to the C3b complement component and inhibits the complement cascade (Fries et al. 1986). The glycoprotein E/glycoprotein I complex binds to Fc regions of IgG and inhibits Fc-mediated effector mechanisms (Frank and Friedman 1989; Bell et al. 1990). The US12 gene product binds the transporter associated with antigen processing (TAP) and prevents antigen presentation on MHC class I molecules (York et al. 1994; Hill et al. 1995). None of these evasion mechanisms operates efficiently in mice, and there is good reason to doubt, therefore, whether immune control of HSV in mice precisely mimics events in humans.

Diagnosis

HSV infection is usually diagnosed by virus culture or by polymerase chain reaction (PCR). The virus is labile and sensitive to desiccation, so swabs should be kept in transport medium and cultured as soon as possible. HSV grows rapidly in a variety of fibroblasts and epithelial cell types, causing a characteristic cell rounding or 'ballooning' which develops within a few days and spreads rapidly. Unlike laboratory-passaged strains, which are often syncytial, fresh isolates cause little, if any, cell fusion. In combination with clinical presentation, the development of characteristic cytopathic effect (CPE) in culture is usually sufficient for confident diagnosis, but if necessary this can be confirmed by a variety of immunocytochemical or antigen capture tests. The sensitivity of these tests allows diagnosis within 24 hours of culture, before extensive CPE develops, and also allows distinction between HSV-1 and HSV-2 isolates with type-specific reagents. Primary infections can also be diagnosed serologically by the detection of virus-specific IgM or by the rising IgG titer. A variety of tests are available but enzyme-linked immunosorbent assay (ELISA) is the most widely used. The diagnosis of herpes encephalitis presents a special problem and rapid diagnosis is of importance because of the urgency of appropriate treatment. Diagnosis used to require the identification of virus or virus antigen in brain biopsies, but is now achieved by detection of viral DNA in the cerebrospinal fluid using PCR (Lakeman et al. 1995). The sample must, however, be taken before aciclovir therapy is begun.

The distinction between serum antibodies to HSV-1 and HSV-2 is rarely of clinical relevance but is crucial in seroepidemiological surveys of infection incidence. Serum against either virus reacts with both types in all assays, and historical methods of measuring type-specific antibody such as cross-adsorption and kinetic neutralization were time-consuming and unreliable. More recent methods are based on the observation that glycoprotein G of HSV-1 and HSV-2 is highly immunogenic and shows very little antigenic cross-reaction. Glycoprotein G, purified from infected cells or prepared as a recombinant protein, can therefore be used as a target for type-specific antibody detection using standard enzyme-linked assays (Lee et al. 1986; Sanchez-Martinez et al. 1991; Ho et al. 1992). Although these methods are clearly an improvement on previous approaches, discrepant results have been reported when compared with western blot assays, which are generally regarded as well validated but relatively tedious (Ashley et al. 1988; Safrin et al. 1992).

Control

Like other nonepidemic diseases transmitted by contact, HSV infection cannot be controlled by public health measures. Reduction in sexual transmission can be attempted by public education on the risks of unprotected sex. Despite education campaigns aimed at reducing the spread of the human immunodeficiency virus (HIV), the reported incidence of genital herpes has risen in the UK (Barton 1995), though it is questionable whether this represents a real increase in transmission frequency.

VACCINATION

No licensed vaccine is currently available for prophylaxis against HSV. Indeed, the fact that reinfection is possible and that restimulation of the response by a recurrence does not prevent further recurrences has been used to argue that the development of a successful vaccine is impossible. Two lines of evidence suggest that this is not so. First, infection by HSV-1 decreases the incidence and severity of subsequent HSV-2 genital infections (Mertz et al. 1992). Second, a variety of immunogens, including killed virus, glycoprotein subunits, viral antigens expressed by live vectors, and attenuated or disabled HSV, will all protect mice and guinea pigs from challenge infection. As noted previously, the virus has evolved immune evasion mechanisms that do not operate efficiently in rodents, and data obtained from animal models must be treated with caution. Nevertheless, these results suggest that a protective response can be mounted, and the successful development of attenuated vaccines against other human and animal alphaherpesviruses gives some confidence in the principle of vaccination against HSV. Many candidate vaccines have been developed based on the production of immunogenic subunits or the construction of rationally attenuated or disabled live HSV. A number of candidates have been studied in clinical trials, though most trials tested therapeutic benefit against established recurrent infection rather than prophylactic efficacy. The difficulty of conducting a fully controlled prophylactic trial, and in particular of monitoring subclinical infection in participants, is illustrated by the study conducted by Mertz et al. (1990). Progress and prospects in the development of HSV vaccines has been reviewed by Whitley and Roizman (2002) and Koelle and Corey (2003).

CHEMOTHERAPY

HSV, together with other human herpesviruses, is among the most studied targets for antiviral chemotherapy, a subject covered in detail elsewhere (see Chapter 67, Immunoprophylaxis of viral diseases). Nucleoside analogues such as idoxuridine, trifluorodeoxyuridine, and adenine arabinoside were used for many years to inhibit viral DNA replication, but these analogues lacked selectivity and their cytotoxicity limited their use to topical treatment in all but the most life-threatening circumstances. The development of aciclovir transformed the treatment of HSV infections. Aciclovir is a guanosine analogue in which the sugar is replaced by an acyclic ring lacking the 2′ and 3′ carbons. The analogue is converted to the 5′-monophosphate by the HSV-specific thymidine kinase (TK) and then to the triphosphate by cellular kinases. The viral DNA polymerase incorporates the triphosphate into the growing viral DNA where it acts as a chain terminator. The inability of host-cell kinases to convert aciclovir into its monophosphate accounts primarily for its selective action against HSV-infected cells and its nontoxicity, although, in addition, the viral DNA polymerase has a higher affinity than its cellular counterpart for the triphosphate. Aciclovir is available in a number of formulations and can be administered topically, orally, or intravenously. Its oral bioavailability is 15–30 percent and plasma half-life about 2–3 hours, so relatively frequent doses are required to maintain therapeutic concentration. The route of administration depends on the site and severity of infection: topical application is used for eye infections and oral lesions, oral administration for severe genital infections and intravenous administration for encephalitis and life-threatening infection of immunocompromised patients. A cream formulation is available without a prescription ('over the counter') in the UK for cold sore treatment, but not in the USA.

Mutants of HSV resistant to aciclovir arise readily in culture, almost invariably due to loss of a functional virus TK gene. This gene function is irrelevant for virus growth in vitro but its loss results in severe attenuation in vivo. Alternative routes to resistance are point mutations in the TK gene or DNA polymerase gene that reduce enzyme affinity for aciclovir and aciclovir triphosphate, respectively (Furman et al. 1981; Larder et al. 1983; Larder and Darby 1984). Resistance to therapy has been observed most frequently in immunocompromised patients receiving long-term therapy. The mutants isolated from these patients include those with altered TK or DNA polymerase enzymes, but the most frequent finding is of a heterogeneous population of viruses with a range of TK activities from entirely deficient to almost normal. The basis of this form of resistance is uncertain, but it is known that TK-negative viruses can be complemented, in vivo, by a wild-type virus (Efstathiou et al. 1989) and it appears that aciclovir selective pressure, particularly in the immunocompromised, can maintain a dynamic mixture of TK-kinase-positive and -negative viruses.

During the past 10 years, a second generation of anti-herpes drugs based on aciclovir, with the same mechanism of action, has been developed (famciclovir, valaciclovir). A second class of analogues with anti-HSV activity are pyrophosphate analogues which act as inhibitors of HSV DNA polymerase. Foscarnet is the sole example in clinical use. Topical application is well tolerated but intravenous administration can cause nephrotoxicity and severe nausea. Foscarnet has no advantage over aciclovir but is of value in treating aciclovir-resistant infections.

Finally, anti-herpes chemotherapy suppresses virus growth but has no apparent effect on latent infection. Patients who have been treated with aciclovir continuously for as long as 6 years experience recurrences after drug withdrawal (Fife et al. 1994).

VARICELLA-ZOSTER VIRUS

It has been recognized for many years that varicella (chickenpox) and zoster (shingles) are caused by the same virus and that zoster results from the reactivation of an endogenous virus acquired during primary varicella. Our understanding of the pathogenesis of VZV derives almost entirely from clinical studies. The virus is highly species-specific in vivo, though it has been adapted to grow in guinea-pig cells and isolates thus adapted will cause a varicella-like disease in guinea pigs (Pavan-Langston and Dunkel 1989). A closely related virus, simian varicella virus, has been isolated from Old World monkeys (Soike et al. 1984; Padovan and Cantrell 1986).

Clinical manifestations

VARICELLA

Chickenpox is one of the common childhood exanthems, affecting most children during their early school years. The incubation period is about 2 weeks, after which the characteristic rash appears, composed of macules which rapidly develop into fluid-filled vesicles. These vesicles crust within a few days and heal, usually without scarring, within a few weeks. The lesions appear in crops, so any one area will contain macules, vesicles, and crusted lesions (Figure 26.4). The rash tends to be centripetal and is variable in severity; a high density of vesicles is present on all parts of the skin and on mucosal membranes of the mouth and genitalia in some cases,

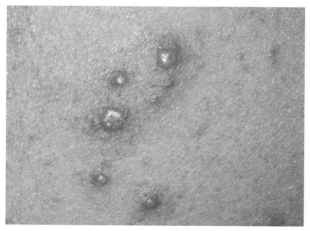

Figure 26.4 *Chickenpox macules and vesicles. (Photograph courtesy of Dr. Jane Sterling, Addenbrooke's Hospital, Cambridge, UK: Copyright Addenbrooke's NHS Trust.)*

while at the other extreme the number of vesicles may be very small or the infection inapparent. The accompanying fever is usually low grade, but reflects the severity of the rash and persists as long as new lesions continue to appear. The incidence of complications in normal children is low, the most common problem being secondary infection of lesions and consequent scarring, a problem that can usually be solved by antibiotic treatment. Central nervous system involvement is rare and may take the form of an invasive encephalitis or a transient ataxia, or may be a prelude to Reye's syndrome. Although primary varicella is usually a benign disease of the normal child, infection of malnourished children is much more severe (Salomon et al. 1966). The main groups in which complications occur are, however, the adult, the neonate, and the immunocompromised.

Infection of adults (Figure 26.5) is generally more severe than in children; the vesicles heal more slowly, secondary bacterial infection and scarring are more common, and the accompanying fever is higher and more prolonged. The most serious complication is varicella pneumonia which appears a few days after onset of the rash and usually resolves in the immunocompetent patient, though there may be residual nodular calcification. Pregnant women are thought to be particularly prone to varicella pneumonia, symptomatic pneumonia being reported in as many as 10 percent of primary varicella cases, with occasional mortality, though some studies report much lower frequencies of morbidity and mortality (Brunell 1992).

Primary varicella during pregnancy places the fetus at risk from two routes: infection in utero and neonatal infection. Infection in utero can result in congenital malformations which include limb hypoplasia, cicatrizing skin lesions, and sensory and motor deficiencies. These conditions are associated with maternal infection during the first 20 weeks of pregnancy. Primary varicella in the mother close to term is associated with severe disease in the neonate: symptoms appear in the infant about 7 days after birth and include pneumonia and visceral involvement, particularly of the liver. A full account of maternal, fetal and neonatal infections with VZV is given in Chapter 63, Infections of the fetus and neonate, other than rubella.

Varicella is severe and often life-threatening in immunocompromised patients. Leukemic children form a major risk group but patients undergoing chemotherapy or steroid treatment or who have any acquired or inborn immune deficiency are at risk. The most common complications are varicella pneumonia, visceral involvement, and CNS infection, but also include hemorrhagic varicella ranging from bleeding into lesions to purpura fulminans (Feldman et al. 1975).

HERPES ZOSTER

Like HSV, VZV establishes a life-long latent infection of sensory dorsal root ganglia, but, because VZV is disseminated, latency is established in multiple ganglia. Reactivation and recurrences take the form of a unilateral rash, herpes zoster, limited to a single dermatome, the area of skin innervated by a single sensory ganglion. The rash appears most commonly in the thoracic dermatomes (Figure 26.6), reflecting the high density of vesicles in this area during primary varicella, but also occurs (in about 10 percent of cases) as cranial zoster, often with eye involvement and may, in rare instances, appear on almost any part of the skin or mucosa (Figure 26.7). In healthy people zoster is relatively uncommon; many people never experience it and few have more than one or two episodes, although it is common to suffer an episode in old age.

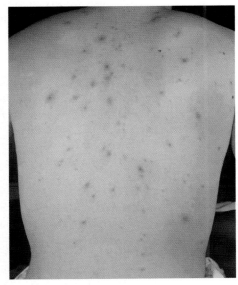

Figure 26.5 *Adult with chickenpox: slow healing and resolution of vesicles. (Photograph courtesy of Dr. Jane Sterling, Addenbrooke's Hospital, Cambridge, UK: Copyright Addenbrooke's NHS Trust.)*

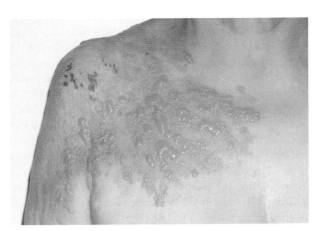

Figure 26.6 *Thoracic zoster. (Photograph courtesy of Dr. Jane Sterling, Addenbrooke's Hospital, Cambridge, UK: Copyright Addenbrooke's NHS Trust.)*

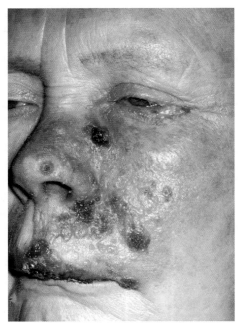

Figure 26.7 *Mandibular zoster. (Photograph courtesy of Dr. Jane Sterling, Addenbrooke's Hospital, Cambridge, UK: Copyright Addenbrooke's NHS Trust.)*

The rash of herpes zoster is usually preceded by pain in the involved dermatome, which begins a few days before the rash appears and remains during its development. The rash is composed of varicella-like vesicles but often so densely packed as to appear as a continuous area of eruption (Figure 26.6). The rash develops over the course of about a week and usually crusts and heals in 2–3 weeks, but the course is variable and, particularly in the elderly, the symptoms are often more severe and prolonged. Unlike oral HSV recurrences, no stimuli have been identified that provoke zoster. The susceptibility of the elderly to zoster has been interpreted to reflect a waning immunity, a view consistent with the increased frequency of zoster in the immunocompromised patient, but it is probable that the immune system controls reactivated virus rather than prevents reactivation. The detection of VZV DNA fragments in circulating mononuclear cells of healthy patients (Gilden et al. 1983) implies that reactivation of latent virus may be much more common than clinical zoster. *Zoster sine herpete* is the term applied to a syndrome in which a typical zoster prodrome is unaccompanied by the subsequent development of a zoster rash (Easton 1970; Gilden et al. 1992a).

Complications associated with zoster are uncommon in children and young adults but occur frequently in the elderly and the immunocompromised. Post-herpetic neuralgia is the most common complication and is defined as pain lasting longer than 1 month after lesions heal. It is rare in patients under 40 years of age but occurs in 50 percent of patients over 60 and, although the pain usually resolves in a few months, it can last for a year or more and is a major cause of morbidity in the elderly. It is most frequently associated with zoster of the ophthalmic branch of the trigeminal (cranial zoster), and cases of sufficient severity and protraction may require surgical ablation of the ganglion. In some instances, anesthesia of the involved dermatome occurs and may result in residual palsy. The pathogenesis of post-herpetic neuralgia is unknown.

Other complications of zoster usually reflect underlying immunological defects. Zoster occurs with high frequency in immunocompromised patients and is unusually severe. Failure to control the recurrences is often illustrated by the spread of vesicles beyond the dermatome in which the initial rash occurs. The disease may become widely disseminated and correspond to severe varicella with involvement of the lungs or CNS. In these circumstances zoster may be fatal, most commonly as a result of pneumonia.

Epidemiology

VZV infects only humans. The reservoir is latent virus in sensory ganglia. Primary infection causes varicella, a common disease of childhood. Only a small minority of young adults remain uninfected but by late middle age infection and immunity are virtually universal in industrial societies. Infection is usually accompanied by the characteristic syndrome; asymptomatic infection does occur, but the proportion of subclinical infections is difficult to estimate and is based largely on patient recall. The disease occurs in epidemics which, in temperate zones, usually appear in late winter every 2 or 3 years in young schoolchildren. Airborne spread has been demonstrated (Gustafson et al. 1982) and the attack rate is high: more than 60 percent within households, and 20 percent in society as a whole (Yorke and London 1973), a rate lower than observed for measles. However, data collected before the advent of measles vaccination revealed that more young adults had been infected with VZV than with measles, a reflection of the fact that measles infection occurs almost exclusively during epidemics whereas varicella infection often occurs in unrecorded 'mini-epidemics' or as isolated cases resulting from contact with zoster. The risk of varicella infection through contact with zoster within a household has been estimated to be about threefold lower than through contact with varicella (Hope-Simpson 1965).

Zoster exhibits no seasonal incidence, and is not correlated with outbreaks of varicella. Despite reports of 'outbreaks' of zoster, all evidence favors the view that zoster is the reactivation of latent virus rather than a transmissible syndrome and reports of 'outbreaks' almost certainly refer to statistical anomalies. In immunocompetent people the incidence of zoster correlates only with age, the disease incidence being approximately proportional to the age of the study group.

Pathogenesis and pathology

Like other relatively benign diseases of humans, varicella pathogenesis cannot be studied in detail in the
normal host. Our understanding of VZV pathogenesis
derives, at least in part, from studies of severe or fatal
disease and by analogy with other, better studied, exanthems. The route of entry is probably the upper respiratory tract or oropharynx where replication in epithelial
cells occurs. During the incubation period of about 2
weeks, cell-associated virus can be detected in the
bloodstream, primarily in mononuclear cells, and skin
lesions are then initiated by infection of capillary endothelial cells. Whether the systemic amplification of virus
is limited to circulating cells and capillary endothelium
in the normal individual is unknown. In fatal varicella of
the newborn or immunosuppressed, productive lesions
can be found on all mucosal surfaces and in the
parenchyma of almost every organ, and it is probable
that limited replication at these sites contributes to the
viremia in normal benign infection. The cutaneous vesicles of varicella are histologically similar to those of
herpes simplex. Vesicles on mucosal surfaces rapidly
develop into shallow ulcers. The vesicle contains large
numbers of free virus particles, suggesting that replication in epithelial cells results in secretion of free virus,
whereas in most cell types VZV is strongly cell associated. The production of free virus in the oral cavity
and upper respiratory tract is the probable major source
of transmission. The patient is infectious for a few days
before lesions appear until a few days after new lesions
cease to appear.

The virus establishes latent infection in sensory
ganglia. VZV DNA can be detected in the thoracic
ganglia of seropositive cadavers, and similar results have
been obtained with simian varicella virus (Gilden et al.
1983; Mahalingham et al. 1991). By analogy with HSV,
access to the ganglia is assumed to be from the skin via
sensory nerve endings, but a hematogenous route cannot
be excluded. VZV latency is poorly understood by
comparison with HSV latency. The virus has not been
reactivated from human ganglia by culture in vitro, the
physical state of the viral genome has not been ascer-
tained, and the pattern of transcription during latency, in
contrast to HSV, appears to involve the immediate–
early productive cycle genes (reviewed by Gilden et al.
1992b). Indeed, there is some disagreement as to the cell
type in which latent infection is established, and true
latency, as opposed to chronic infection, is not proven
(Gilden et al. 1987; Croen et al. 1988). Recurrent infection with herpes zoster, is, by analogy with HSV,
assumed to result from reactivation of latent virus in a
sensory ganglion and seeding of infectious virions into
epithelium via sensory nerve endings, a view entirely
consistent with the appearance of zoster within a single
dermatome. The details of these events are uncertain.

As noted earlier (see section on Herpes zoster), clinical
zoster is an infrequent event and most triggering conditions, such as cytotoxic drug treatment, lymphoma, or
heavy metal poisoning, are immunosuppressive, suggesting
a failure to control reactivated virus rather than stimulating reactivation. The frequency of reactivation rather
than recurrence is unknown. The pain associated with
zoster and the frequency and prolonged nature of post-
herpetic neuralgia distinguish VZV recurrences from
those of HSV, and it is proposed that these features
reflect more widespread growth and consequent inflammation in sensory ganglia during VZV recurrence. This
plausible explanation implies a quantitative difference
between VZV and HSV recurrence but fundamental
differences in the nature of latency, reactivation, and
recurrence of the two viruses cannot be excluded.

Immune response

Primary infection results in life-long immunity to
exogenous reinfection. Humoral response, T-cell proliferative responses and cytotoxic T-cell responses are all
detectable soon after symptoms appear, rise during
convalescence, and remain detectable throughout life.
Recurrence is accompanied by a pronounced anamnestic
response, an observation in contrast to HSV recurrence.
Antibodies to at least 35 different VZV antigens have
been identified in convalescent sera, including neutralizing antibodies directed against viral glycoproteins, but,
despite the use of passive immunoglobulin in therapy,
there is little evidence that humoral responses are
important in controlling infection. No correlation has
been found between titer or spectrum of VZV-specific
antibodies and severity of varicella or the recurrence or
severity of zoster (Brunell et al. 1987). Agammaglobulinemic patients do not suffer from unusually severe
varicella or from frequent or severe zoster. By contrast,
many studies have demonstrated a correlation with deficiencies in cell-mediated immunity and the severity of
varicella infection and the frequency and severity of
zoster. T-cell proliferative responses, cytotoxic T-cell
responses and interferon responses are all detected in
human infection and in animal models (Arvin 1992;
Rotbart et al. 1993). Responses to individual virus antigens, both structural and immediate early nonstructural
proteins, have been found, but the importance of particular responses to individual antigens has yet to be
determined. The decline in cell-mediated responses to
VZV in the elderly is thought to be responsible for the
increased frequency of zoster in this group (Miller 1980;
Berger et al. 1981), and is consistent with the occurrence
of zoster in immunocompromised patients. The maintenance of adequate levels of cell-mediated immunity to
varicella in the population is therefore important but it
is uncertain whether restimulation of the response
occurs primarily through subclinical reactivation or

results from re-exposure to varicella. Evidence exists for both mechanisms (Meyers et al. 1980; Arvin et al. 1983), but their relative contribution is of importance in predicting the possible consequences of mass vaccination and the need to vaccinate seropositive people carrying wild VZV.

Diagnosis

Virus particles are present at high concentrations in vesicular fluid and can be cultured in a variety of human and primate cell lines. The cytopathic effect is focal and develops slowly with typical cell 'ballooning' and fusion. Immunofluorescence of infected cultures with specific antibody confirms the presence of VZV and allows more rapid diagnosis. The virus in culture is very strongly cell-associated and efficient storage of isolates requires freezing of viable infected cells. Electron microscopic examination of vesicular fluid reveals the presence of large numbers of herpesvirus particles, a method used historically to allow a rapid distinction between chickenpox and smallpox but which cannot distinguish VZV and HSV. Detection of VZV DNA by PCR is now widely used, particularly for diagnosis of severe disease where rapid differential diagnosis is required.

A wide range of serological tests for VZV-specific IgG have been described, including complement fixation, latex agglutination, radioimmunoassay, and ELISA. ELISAs for VZV-specific IgG and IgM are commercially available. A suspect rash can be confirmed as varicella by the presence of IgM or by a rising IgG titer. Zoster can be similarly confirmed because, in contrast to HSV, recurrence is usually associated with a significant rise in antibody titer. A skin test for cell-mediated immunity has been described (Kamiya et al. 1977; Takahashi et al. 1992) and is thought to provide a relevant measure of immunity to zoster.

Control

EPIDEMIOLOGICAL CONTROL

No attempt is made to limit the spread of varicella in the general population because, as a rule, acquisition of the virus early in life is preferable to infection as an adult. Within hospitals, however, VZV infection has serious consequences for high-risk groups such as premature babies, leukemic children and transplant recipients, and patient isolation may be necessary to protect these groups. Healthcare staff can be monitored for immunity to VZV, and seronegative staff who suspect they have contracted varicella or staff suffering a zoster recurrence should avoid contact with high-risk patients.

VACCINE

A live attenuated vaccine was developed in Japan by passage of the Oka strain in guinea pig cells and its effi-

cacy was first reported by Takahashi et al. (1974). Since then the vaccine has been used extensively in normal and immunocompromised children and adults. The vaccine is licensed as a childhood vaccine in the USA and has recently been licensed in the UK for particular risk groups. Japanese and US experience with the vaccine is broadly similar (reviewed by Gershon et al. 1992 and Arvin 2001). A single vaccine dose gives >90 percent seroconversion and an 85 percent protection against subsequent varicella, which, when they occur, are mild. Both humoral and cell-mediated immunity are long-lasting but it is uncertain whether this is due to subclinical challenge with circulating virus. Vaccination of leukemic children provides similar levels of protection but vaccination of adults results in somewhat lower protection rates. There are few side effects of the vaccine in healthy children, some 5 percent suffering a mild rash occasionally accompanied by fever, but in leukemic children side effects are more noticeable, about half the vaccinees developing a rash, in some cases resembling typical varicella. Nevertheless, the vaccine-related reactions in these patients are benign compared with the risk of varicella infection. Vaccination of seropositive adults results in an enhancement of cell-mediated immunity and may therefore be of value in protecting the elderly against zoster (Berger et al. 1984; Takahashi et al. 1992).

It is not certain whether the vaccine establishes latent infection in all recipients. A few leukemic vaccinees have experienced zoster due to recurrence of the vaccine strain but these individuals suffered a varicella rash following vaccination, consistent with the expectation that latency and recurrence are related to virus load in the skin during primary infection. Because most healthy vaccinees have no rash, it is reasonable to suppose that they will not suffer recurrence, and to date this is the case. In view of its safety and efficacy, the Oka strain has been proposed for universal vaccination of children. It has been used successfully in combination with measles, mumps, and rubella vaccinations.

PASSIVE ANTIBODY

Passive immunization with specific zoster immunoglobulin (ZIG) (derived from donors with high anti-VZV titers) has been used to prevent or modify infection in high-risk patients who are thought to have come into contact with varicella or zoster (Gershon et al. 1974; Zaia et al. 1983; Berger et al. 1984; Takahashi et al. 1992). Examples include non-immune pregnant women, immunocompromised patients, premature babies in special care units, and neonates born to mothers with varicella at term.

CHEMOTHERAPY

VZV, like HSV and other alphaherpesviruses, specifies a TK and is sensitive to aciclovir. VZV is considerably less sensitive than HSV, however, and much higher doses are required to achieve therapeutic benefit. Nevertheless, aciclovir is now widely used in the treatment of varicella and zoster (Whitley 1992, reviewed by Griffiths 1995). Treatment of uncomplicated varicella in children with oral aciclovir within 24 hours of the onset of the rash resulted in fewer skin lesions and reduced fever but the benefit is relatively small. Similar treatment of adults, who suffer more severe varicella, achieved essentially similar results but the benefit was more pronounced. Oral aciclovir is used both prophylactically and therapeutically in immunocompromised patients at risk from or suffering from varicella. Because of the relatively poor oral bioavailability of the drug, hospitalized patients with severe varicella are treated intravenously.

Oral aciclovir reduces pain and duration of the rash in zoster patients but has little or no effect on post-herpetic neuralgia. Two pro-drug derivatives of aciclovir, famciclovir, and valacilovir, with similar modes of action but different pharmacokinetic properties are now licensed for use against zoster. Their greater bioavailability offers advantages in some clinical settings (Carrington 1994; Murray 1995) (see also Chapter 69, Antiviral chemotherapy).

REFERENCES

Ades, A.E., Peckham, C.S., et al. 1989. Prevalence of antibodies to herpes simplex virus type 1 and 2 in pregnant women and estimated rates of infection. *J Epidemiol Community Health*, **43**, 53–60.

Anderson, J.R. and Field, H.J. 1983. The distribution of herpes simplex type 1 antigen in the mouse central nervous system after different routes of inoculation. *J Neurol Sci*, **60**, 181–95.

Arvin, A.M. 1992. Cell mediated immunity to varicella zoster virus. *J Infect Dis*, **166**, Suppl 1, 35–41.

Arvin, A.M. 2001. Varicella vaccine – the first six years. *N Engl J Med*, **344**, 1007–8.

Arvin, A.M., Koropchak, C.M. and Wittek, A.E. 1983. Immunologic evidence of reinfection with varicella-zoster virus. *J Infect Dis*, **148**, 200–5.

Ashley, R., Millitoni, J., et al. 1988. Comparison of western blot (immunoblot) and glycoprotein-G specific immunodot enzyme assays for detecting antibodies to herpes simplex virus types 1 and 2 in human sera. *J Clin Microbiol*, **26**, 662–7.

Barton, S.E. 1995. Current issues in the management of genital herpes. *Antiviral Chem Chemother*, **6**, Suppl 1, 3–6.

Bell, S., Cranage, M., et al. 1990. Induction of immunoglobulin G Fc receptors by recombinant vaccinia viruses expressing glycoproteins E and I of herpes simplex virus type 1. *J Virol*, **64**, 2181–6.

Berger, R., Florent, G. and Just, M. 1981. Decrease of the lymphoproliferative response to varicella zoster virus antigen in the aged. *Infect Immun*, **32**, 24–7.

Berger, R., Luescher, D. and Just, M. 1984. Enhancement of varicella-zoster specific immune responses in the elderly by boosting with varicella vaccine. *J Infect Dis*, **149**, 647.

Biron, C.A., Byron, H.S. and Sullivan, J.L. 1989. Severe herpes virus infections in an adolescent without natural killer cells. *N Engl J Med*, **320**, 1731–5.

Brunell, P.A. 1992. Varicella in pregnancy, the fetus and the newborn: problems in management. *J Infect Dis*, **166**, Suppl 1, 42–7.

Brunell, P.A., Novelli, V.M., et al. 1987. Antibodies to the three major glycoproteins of varicella-zoster virus: search for the relevant host immune response. *J Infect Dis*, **156**, 430–5.

Buckmaster, E.A., Cranage, M.P., et al. 1984. The use of monoclonal antibodies to differentiate isolates of herpes simplex virus types 1 and 2 by neutralisation and reverse passive haemagglutination tests. *J Med Virol*, **13**, 193–202.

Bukowski, J.F. and Welsh, R.M. 1986. The role of natural killer cells and interferon in resistance to acute infection of mice with herpes simplex virus type 1. *J Immunol*, **136**, 3481–5.

Carrington, D. 1994. Prospects for improved efficacy with antiviral prodrugs: will valaciclovir and famciclovir meet the clinical challenge? *Int Antivir News*, **2**, 50–3.

Corey, L. and Spear, P.G. 1986. Infections with herpes simplex viruses. *N Engl J Med*, **314**, 686–91.

Corey, L., Adams, H.G., et al. 1983. Genital herpes simplex virus infections: clinical manifestations, course and complications. *Ann Intern Med*, **98**, 958–72.

Croen, K.D., Ostrove, J.M., et al. 1988. Patterns of gene expression and sites of latency in human nerve ganglia are different for varicella zoster and herpes simplex viruses. *Proc Natl Acad Sci U S A*, **85**, 9773–7.

Cunningham, A.L. and Merigan, T.C. 1983. Gamma interferon production appears to predict time of recurrence of herpes labialis. *J Immunol*, **130**, 2397–400.

Cushing, H. 1905. Surgical aspects of major neuralgia of the trigeminal nerve: report of 20 cases of operation upon the gasserian ganglion with anatomic and physiologic notes on the consequences of its removal. *JAMA*, **44**, 1002–8.

Daheshia, M., Feldman, L.T. and Rouse, B.T. 1998. Herpes simplex virus latency and the immune response. *Curr Opin Microbiol*, **1**, 430–5.

Easton, H.G. 1970. Zoster sine herpete causing acute trigeminal neuralgia. *Lancet*, **2**, 1065–6.

Efstathiou, S., Kemp, S., et al. 1989. The role of herpes simplex virus type 1 thymidine kinase in pathogenesis. *J Gen Virol*, **70**, 869–79.

Feldman, S., Hughes, W.T. and Daniel, C.B. 1975. Varicella in children with cancer: seventy seven cases. *Pediatrics*, **56**, 388–97.

Fife, K.H., Crumpacker, C.S., et al. 1994. Recurrence and resistance patterns of herpes simplex virus following cessation of >6 years of chronic suppression with acyclovir. *J Infect Dis*, **169**, 1338–41.

Frank, I. and Friedman, H.M. 1989. A novel function of the herpes simplex virus Fc receptor: participation in bi-polar bridging of antiviral immunoglobulin G. *J Virol*, **63**, 4479–88.

Fries, L.F., Friedman, H.M., et al. 1986. Glycoprotein C of herpes simplex virus type 1 is an inhibitor of the complement cascade. *J Immunol*, **137**, 1636–42.

Furman, P.A., Coen, D.M., et al. 1981. Acyclovir resistant mutants of herpes simplex virus type 1 express altered DNA polymerase or reduced acyclovir phosphorylating activity. *J Virol*, **40**, 936–41.

Gershon, A.A., Stainberg, S. and Brunell, P.A. 1974. Zoster immune globulin: a further assessment. *N Engl J Med*, **290**, 243–5.

Gershon, A.A., La Russa, P., et al. 1992. Varicella vaccine: the American experience. *J Infect Dis*, **166**, Suppl 1, 63–8.

Gilden, D.H., Vafai, A., et al. 1983. Varicella-zoster virus DNA in human sensory ganglia. *Nature (Lond)*, **306**, 478–80.

Gilden, D.H., Rosemann, Y., et al. 1987. Detection of varicella zoster virus nucleic acid in neurons of normal human thoracic ganglia. *Ann Neurol*, **22**, 377–80.

Gilden, D.H., Dueland, A.N., et al. 1992a. Varicella zoster virus reactivation without rash. *J Infect Dis*, **166**, Suppl 1, 30–4.

Gilden, D.H., Mahalingham, R., et al. 1992b. Herpes zoster: pathogenesis and latency. *Progr Med Virol*, **39**, 19–75.

Griffiths, P.D. 1995. Progress in the clinical management of herpesvirus infections. *Antivir Chem Chemother*, **6**, 191–209.

Gustafson, T.L., Lavely, G.B., et al. 1982. An outbreak of airborne nosocomial varicella. *Pediatrics*, **70**, 550–6.

Hill, A., Jugovic, P., et al. 1995. Herpes simplex virus turns off the TAP to evade host immunity. *Nature (Lond)*, **375**, 411–15.

Hill, T.J., Field, H.J. and Blyth, W.A. 1975. Acute and recurrent infection with herpes simplex virus in the mouse: a model for studying latency and recurrent disease. *J Gen Virol*, **28**, 341–53.

Ho, D.W.T., Field, P.R., et al. 1992. Indirect ELISA for the detection of HSV-2 specific IgG and IgM antibodies with glycoprotein G (gG-2). *J Virol Methods*, **36**, 249–64.

Hope-Simpson, R.E. 1965. The nature of herpes zoster: a long-term study and a new hypothesis. *Proc R Soc Med*, **58**, 9–20.

Jones, C. 2003. Herpes simplex virus type 1 and bovine herpesvirus 1 latency. *Clin Microbiol Rev*, **16**, 79–95.

Kamiya, H., Ihara, T., et al. 1977. Diagnostic skin test reactions with varicella virus antigen and clinical applications of the test. *J Infect Dis*, **136**, 784–8.

Koelle, D.M. and Corey, L. 2003. Recent progress in herpes simplex virus immunobiology and vaccine research. *Clin Microbiol Rev*, **16**, 96–113.

Lafferty, W.E., Coombs, R.W., et al. 1987. Recurrences after oral and genital herpes simplex virus infection. Influence of site of infection and viral type. *N Engl J Med*, **316**, 1444–9.

Lakeman, F.D., Whitley, R.J., et al. 1995. Diagnosis of herpes simplex encephalitis: application of polymerase chain reaction to cerebrospinal fluid from brain-biopsied patients and correlation with disease. *J Infect Dis*, **171**, 857–63.

Larder, B.A. and Darby, G. 1984. Virus drug resistance: mechanisms and consequences. *Antivir Res*, **4**, 1–42.

Larder, B.A., Derse, D., et al. 1983. Properties of purified enzymes induced by pathogenic drug resistant mutants of herpes simplex virus. Evidence for variants expressing normal DNA polymerase and altered thymidine kinase. *J Biol Chem*, **258**, 2027–33.

Lee, F.K., Pereira, L., et al. 1986. A novel glycoprotein for detection of herpes simplex virus type 1 specific antibodies. *J Virol Methods*, **14**, 111–18.

Lopez, C. 1985. Natural resistance mechanisms in herpes simplex virus infections. In: Roizman, B. and Lopez, C. (eds), *The Herpesviruses*, vol. 4. New York: Plenum Press, 37–68.

Mahalingham, R., Smith, D., et al. 1991. Simian varicella virus DNA in dorsal root ganglia. *Proc Natl Acad Sci U S A*, **88**, 2750–2.

McGeoch, D.J. and Cook, S. 1994. Molecular phylogeny of the alphaherpesvirus subfamily and a proposed evolutionary timescale. *J Mol Biol*, **238**, 9–22.

McLennan, J.L. and Darby, G. 1980. Herpes simplex virus latency: the cellular location of virus in dorsal root ganglia and the fate of the infected cell following virus reactivation. *J Gen Virol*, **51**, 233–43.

Mellerick, D.M. and Fraser, N.W. 1987. Physical state of the latent herpes simplex virus genome in a mouse model system: evidence suggesting an episomal state. *Virology*, **158**, 265–75.

Mertz, G.J., Ashley, R., et al. 1990. Double-blind placebo controlled trial of a herpes simplex virus type 2 glycoprotein vaccine in persons at high risk for genital herpes infection. *J Infect Dis*, **161**, 653–60.

Mertz, GJ., Benedetti, J., et al. 1992. Risk factors for the sexual transmission of genital herpes. *Ann Intern Med*, **116**, 197–202.

Meyers, J.D., Flournoy, N. and Thomas, E.D. 1980. Cell mediated immunity to varicella zoster virus after allogenic marrow transplant. *J Infect Dis*, **141**, 479–87.

Miller, A.E. 1980. Selective decline in cellular immune response to varicella zoster in the elderly. *Neurology*, **30**, 582–7.

Murray, A.B. 1995. Valaciclovir – an improvement over aciclovir for the treatment of zoster. *Antiviral Chem Chemother*, **6**, Suppl 1, 34–8.

Nahmias, A.J., Whitley, R.J., et al. 1982. Herpes simplex encephalitis: laboratory evaluations and their diagnostic significance. *J Infect Dis*, **145**, 829–6.

Nash, A.A. 2000. T cells and the regulation of herpes simplex virus latency and reactivation. *J Exp Med*, **191**, 1455–7.

Nash, A.A. and Gell, P.G.H. 1983. Membrane phenotype of murine effector and suppressor T cells involved in delayed hypersensitivity and protective immunity to herpes simplex virus. *Cell Immunol*, **75**, 348–55.

Padovan, D. and Cantrell, C.A. 1986. Varicella-like herpesvirus infections of non-human primates. *Lab Anim Sci*, **36**, 7–13.

Pavan-Langston, D. and Dunkel, E.C. 1989. Ocular varicella zoster virus infection in the guinea pig. *Arch Ophthalmol*, **107**, 1068–72.

PHLS Report. 1987. Report from the PHLS Communicable Disease Surveillance Centre. *Br Med J*, **294**, 361–2.

Preston, C.M. 2000. Repression of viral transcription during herpes simplex virus latency. *J Gen Virol*, **81**, 1–19.

Prober, C.G., Sullender, W.M., et al. 1987. Low risk of herpes simplex virus infections in neonates exposed to the virus at the time of vaginal delivery to mothers with recurrent genital herpes simplex virus infection. *N Engl J Med*, **316**, 240–4.

Ross, J.D.C., Smith, I.W. and Elton, R.A. 1993. The epidemiology of herpes simplex types 1 and 2 infection of the genital tract in Edinburgh, 1978–1991. *Genitourin Med*, **69**, 381–3.

Rotbart, H.A., Levin, M.J. and Hayward, A.R. 1993. Immune responses to varicella zoster virus infections in healthy children. *J Infect Dis*, **167**, 195–9.

Safrin, S., Arvin, A., et al. 1992. Comparison of the western immunoblot assay and a glycoprotein G enzyme immunoassay for detection of serum antibodies to herpes simplex virus type 2 in patients with AIDS. *J Clin Microbiol*, **30**, 1312–14.

Salomon, J.B., Gordon, J.E. and Scrimshaw, N.S. 1966. Studies of diarrheal disease in Central America. X. Associated chickenpox, diarrhea and kwashiorkor in a highland Guatemalan village. *Am J Trop Med Hyg*, **15**, 997–1002.

Sanchez-Martinez, D., Schmid, D.S., et al. 1991. Evaluation of a test based on baculovirus-expressed glycoprotein G for detection of herpes simplex virus type-specific antibodies. *J Infect Dis*, **164**, 1196–9.

Schmid, D.S. 1988. The human MHC-restricted cellular response to herpes simplex virus type 1 is mediated by CD4+, CD8– T cells and is restricted to the DR region of the MHC complex. *J Immunol*, **140**, 3610–16.

Simmons, A. and Nash, A.A. 1985. The role of antibody in primary and recurrent herpes simplex virus infection. *J Virol*, **53**, 944–8.

Simmons, A. and Nash, A.A. 1987. Effect of B cell suppression on primary and reinfection of mice with herpes simplex virus. *J Infect Dis*, **13**, 108–14.

Simmons, A. and Tscharke, D.C. 1992. Anti-CD8 impairs clearance of HSV from the nervous system: implications for the rate of virally infected neurones. *J Exp Med*, **175**, 1337–44.

Smyth, R.L., Higenbottam, T.W., et al. 1990. Herpes simplex virus infection in heart–lung transplant recipients. *Transplantation*, **49**, 735–9.

Soike, K.F., Rangan, S.R.S. and Gerone, P.J. 1984. Viral disease models in primates. *Adv Vet Sci Comp Med*, **28**, 151–99.

Stevens, J.G. and Cook, M.L. 1971. Latent herpes simplex virus in sensory ganglia. *Science*, **173**, 843–5.

Stevens, J.G., Wagner, E.K., et al. 1987. RNA complementary to a herpes alpha gene mRNA is prominent in latently infected neurones. *Science*, **235**, 1056–9.

Sullivan-Bolyai, J., Hull, H.F., et al. 1983. Neonatal herpes simplex virus infection in King County, Washington: increasing incidence and epidemiological correlates. *JAMA*, **250**, 3059–62.

Takahashi, M., Otsuka, T., et al. 1974. Live vaccine used to prevent the spread of varicella in children in hospital. *Lancet*, **2**, 1288–90.

Takahashi, M., Ikatani, T., et al. 1992. Immunisation of the elderly and patients with collagen vascular disease with live varicella vaccine and use of varicella skin antigen. *J Infect Dis*, **166**, Suppl 1, 58–62.

Whitley, R.J. 1992. Therapeutic approaches to varicella-zoster virus infections. *J Infect Dis*, **166**, Suppl 1, 51–7.

Whitley, R.J. and Roizman, B. 2002. Herpes simplex viruses: is a vaccine tenable? *J Clin Invest*, **110**, 145–51.

Whitley, R.J., Lakeman, A.D., et al. 1982. DNA restriction enzyme analysis of herpes simplex virus isolates obtained from patients with encephalitis. *N Engl J Med*, **307**, 1060–2.

Wilcox, C.L., Smith, R.L., et al. 1990. Nerve growth factor dependence of herpes simplex virus latency in peripheral sympathetic and sensory neurones in vitro. *J Neurosci*, **10**, 1268–75.

Wu, L. and Morahan, P.S. 1992. Macrophages and other non-specific defenses: role in modulating resistance against herpes simplex virus. *Curr Top Microbiol Immunol*, **179**, 89–110.

York, I.A., Roop, C., et al. 1994. A cytosolic herpes simplex virus protein inhibits antigen presentation to CD8+ lymphocytes. *Cell*, **77**, 525–35.

Yorke, J.A. and London, W.P. 1973. Recurrent outbreaks of measles, chickenpox and mumps. II. Systemic differences in contact rates and stochastic effects. *Am J Epidemiol*, **98**, 469–82.

Zaia, J.A., Levin, M.J., et al. 1983. Evaluation of varicella zoster immune globulin: protection of immunosuppressed children after household exposure to varicella. *J Infect Dis*, **147**, 737–43.

27

Betaherpesviruses: cytomegalovirus, human herpesviruses 6 and 7

WILLIAM BRITT

Betaherpesviruses that infect humans include human cytomegalovirus (CMV), human herpesvirus 5, human herpesvirus 6 (HHV-6), and human herpesvirus 7 (HHV-7). These viruses share many common biological characteristics, including restricted in vivo and in vitro cell tropism and an extended replicative cycle. Furthermore, productive virus replication, including the production of progeny virus is restricted to cells of host origin, suggesting that these viruses co-evolved with their animal hosts. This is perhaps best illustrated by cytomegaloviruses, a group of viruses with common replication strategies and conserved blocks of genes, but viruses from each mammalian species also encode additional viral genes unique to their species of origin. This observation suggests that these viruses have developed strategies and captured host genes that favor their replication and persistence in their specific host. Similarly, the in vitro and in vivo replication of betaherpesviruses is highly restricted to specific cell types and cells at particular stages of differentiation. They are also characteristically highly cell associated and replicate slowly as compared with alphaherpesviruses. The genome of betaherpesviruses range in size from the largest of all human herpesviruses, human CMV with a genome of nearly 260 kb pair to HHV-6 with a genome of 180 kb pairs. Of the well-studied betaherpesviruses, only human CMV and the closely related chimpanzee CMV contain repeated sequences at the termini of a unique long and short component of its genome, thereby permitting these components to be arranged in four isomeric forms, similar to the genomic organization of herpes simplex virus (Mocarski and Tan Courcelle 2001; Davison et al.

2003). The remaining members of this group of viruses have only a single genomic structure with repeats at the junction of the long and short regions of the genome. There are antigenic cross-reactivities between conserved structural and nonstructural proteins encoded by these viruses (Adler et al. 1993; Loh et al. 1994). Finally, infections caused by betaherpesviruses are usually subclinical and acquired at an early age in most populations. Life- or organ-threatening disease following infection is usually limited to immunocompromised hosts. More recently, chronic persistent infection with these viruses has been suggested to contribute to chronic inflammatory and proliferative diseases such as atherosclerosis and multiple sclerosis, and perhaps human cancers. The spectrum of disease associated with persistent infections caused by these viruses remains far from being fully defined.

CYTOMEGALOVIRUS

Infection with CMV is common in all human populations and infrequently associated with symptomatic illness in normal hosts. In contrast, it is a major cause of multi-organ disease in immunocompromised patients, the severity of disease being related to the degree of immunosuppression. Permissive infection in tissue culture is restricted to a very limited number of cell types, and then only in cells of human origin. CMV infections in susceptible hosts are widespread with involvement of all organ systems. Although most investigators believe that CMV can establish a persistent infection and early studies utilizing murine CMV demonstrated a latent infection, only relatively recently have investigators demonstrated a true latent infection with human CMV (Jordan 1983; Soderberg-Naucler et al. 1997). The role of latent infection in the transmission of CMVs by blood or during allograft transplantation is well accepted; however, the importance of latent versus a persistent productive infection in the maintenance of the virus in the individual and a population remains unclear. Finally, it is of some interest that human CMV can be found in tissue from a variety of inflammatory and neoplastic diseases, raising the possibility that this virus may directly or indirectly contribute to chronic inflammatory disease and cancer.

Clinical manifestations

Although CMV rarely causes symptomatic infection in normal hosts, it has been estimated to cause between 20 and 50 percent of cases of heterophile-negative infectious mononucleosis (Klemola et al. 1970). A characteristic syndrome of fever, hepatitis, and atypical lymphocytosis following administration of blood products for cardiac surgery (postperfusion syndrome) has been attributed to CMV and represents virus transmission from blood products (Perillie and Glenn 1962; Reyman 1966). Other disease states including rheumatological diseases have been linked to CMV, although the biological and epidemiological relevance of these associations remains unclear. Recent studies have renewed interest in a possible role of CMV in the development of atherosclerotic coronary artery disease and animal models of disease have been developed which support a potentially important role of this virus in atherosclerotic heart disease (Adam et al. 1987; Petrie et al. 1988; Speir et al. 1994; Zhou et al. 1996; Zhu et al. 1999; Streblow et al. 2001; Libby 2002). Similarly, CMV gene products and nucleic acids have been detected in autopsy tissue from human brain and colon tumors and have raised the possibility that this large DNA virus could contribute to the pathogenesis of cancer (Cobbs et al. 2002; Harkins et al. 2002). Although these findings are provocative, it is unclear whether these findings represent an association between CMV and cancer or merely represent the detection of a CMV as a passenger in these tissues.

Three groups of patients are at risk for invasive acute CMV disease: (1) newborn infants infected in utero, (2) immunocompromised allograft recipients and (3) patients with AIDS. Infants infected in utero may be born with subclinical infections or may have a constellation of clinical abnormalities characteristic of what has been termed cytomegalic inclusion disease (CID) of the newborn (Jesionek and Kiolemenoglou 1904). Clinical findings include hepatosplenomegaly, jaundice, thrombocytopenia, purpura, microcephaly, chorioretinitis and, rarely, pneumonia in approximately 10 percent of congenitally infected infants (Table 27.1) (McCracken et al. 1969; Boppana et al. 1992). Mortality rates range from 11 to 20 percent in symptomatic infection, and up to 50 percent of long-term survivors of symptomatic infections will have deficits in perceptual and cognitive functions (McCracken et al. 1969; Alford 1984; Boppana et al. 1992; Boppana et al. 1999). A significant number of infants with asymptomatic infections are also at risk of developmental abnormalities, hearing loss being the most common (Yow et al. 1988; Fowler et al. 1992, 1997). Persistent infection with prolonged viral shedding is nearly universal in infants with either symptomatic or asymptomatic congenital infection (Stagno et al. 1975; Alford 1984).

CMV infections in the post-transplant period are a major cause of morbidity and mortality in allograft recipients. Infections can develop following reactivation of persistent or latent virus in the previously infected recipient, as the result of reinfection by virus present in the transplanted organ, or less frequently following transfusion of blood from a CMV-infected donor. The severity of infection depends on several characteristics but the two most consistently observed risk factors for severe infection are: (1) transplantation of an organ from a previously infected donor into a CMV non-immune host and (2) significant immunosuppression, including that caused by specific therapies directed at T-lymphocyte function (Singh et al. 1988; Weir et al. 1988; Fishman and Rubin 1998; Rubin 2002). Several studies using quantita-

Table 27.1 Clinical manifestations of CMV infection in different patient populations

Population	Clinical manifestations	
	Acute infection	Long term
Immunocompetent	Subclinical infection, mononucleosis syndrome	Prolonged virus shedding; inflammatory vascular disease
Immunocompromised:		
Fetuses	Hepatitis, encephalitis, retinitis, thrombocytopenia microcephaly	Hearing loss, cognitive dysfunction, developmental delay, prolonged virus shedding
Allograft recipients	Fever, hepatitis, pneumonitis, hematological abnormalities	Graft dysfunction/loss, excessive long-term mortality; transplant vasculopathy
AIDS	Retinitis, encephalitis, colitis, oesophagitis	Vision loss, wasting syndrome, decreased survival time, encephalopathy

tive measures of CMV DNA in blood have demonstrated that the viral burden of an individual patient, regardless of assignment of risk based on donor and recipient serological status, has significant predictive value of invasive CMV disease (Cope et al. 1997; Emery et al. 2000). More recent studies in hematopoietic transplant recipients have been consistent with earlier observations suggesting that the use of steroids in the post-transplant period were associated with an increased risk invasive CMV disease, presumably as a result of lymphotoxic activity of these reagents, including their activity against natural killer cells. CMV infection in allograft recipients can range from asymptomatic excretion to fulminant multi-organ disease. The most common clinical syndrome associated with CMV infection in the post-transplant period is fever, leucopenia, and mild to inapparent hepatic dysfunction (Table 27.1). Pneumonia attributed to CMV in the post-transplant population continues to carry a significant mortality rate. Infection of the central nervous system (CNS), including the retina, is rare in transplant patients. Long-term effects of chronic infection in allograft recipients, especially cardiac allograft recipients, include a characteristic vasculopathy described as transplant vascular sclerosis or transplant vasculopathy (Grattan et al. 1989; Koskinen et al. 1999; Streblow et al. 2001). This disease has been faithfully recapitulated in rodent models and disease appears directly related to CMV infection and virus-gene expression in the endothelium of the allograft (Lemstrom et al. 1997; De La Melena et al. 2001; Streblow et al. 2003). The vascular disease in the allograft has been proposed to represent an accelerated variant of atherosclerotic coronary heart disease in the normal host and may offer clues to the mechanism of virus-induced vascular disease.

In certain HIV-infected populations, the incidence of CMV infection is extraordinarily high with rates exceeding 95 percent (Drew et al. 1981; Collier et al. 1987). Prior to the widespread introduction of effective antiretroviral therapy (ART) for the control of HIV replication, CMV was the most common cause of clinically important opportunistic infection in long-lived AIDS patients in the USA (Gallant et al. 1992; Pertel et al. 1992). Although numerous reports documented CMV infection in every organ system in this patient population, the gastrointestinal tract, retina and brain represent the more commonly described sites of CMV disease (Jacobson and Mills 1988; Francis et al. 1989; Schmidbauer et al. 1989; Vinters et al. 1989; Pertel et al. 1992). Colitis, persistent diarrhea with wasting, vision-threatening retinitis, and encephalopathy are common manifestations of CMV infection in patients with end-stage HIV infections (Table 27.1). With the advent of multidrug therapy for the control of HIV replication, the incidence of invasive CMV disease has fallen dramatically, such that new cases of retinitis in many study populations are very infrequent and develop only in patients who either present to medical care with invasive CMV disease or fail ART.

Epidemiology

The epidemiology of CMV infections can be most readily understood by examining the sources of virus, identifying populations at risk for exposure to infectious virus, and defining patients with deficits in immunity who are at risk of severe CMV infections. CMV can be cultured from most body fluids for extended periods following primary infection with significant amounts of infectious virus being found in urine, genital secretions (including semen), saliva, and breast milk. Virus is also readily transmitted by cellular elements in blood products, especially leucocytes, and by solid organs during transplantation (Prince et al. 1971; Ho et al. 1975; Gnann et al. 1988; Bowden 1991). Periodic reactivation or persistent low-level shedding from these sites is also a characteristic of CMV-infected hosts. In fact, it could be argued that, for the human host, persistent infection in the form of continuous low level replication is likely to be more frequent than periodic reactivation from latency. Sources of infection in normal hosts include exposure to virus-infected body fluids, such as occurs in crowded living conditions in developing countries and in child-care centers in developed societies. In both situations there is frequent infection of children and of susceptible child carers (Murph et al. 1986; Pass et al. 1987; Adler 1989; Murph et al. 1998). An additional source of virus exposure in infancy is breast feeding with transmission occurring in 30–70 percent of infants breast fed by mothers with serological evidence of previous infection (Dworsky et al. 1983). In adolescents and adults, CMV infection is acquired commonly through sexual exposure (Chandler et al. 1985; Handsfield et al. 1985; Chandler et al. 1987; Collier et al. 1987; Fowler and Pass 1991). Overall, it has been estimated that the rate of infection after childhood is ca. 1 percent per year (Stagno et al. 1984). Reinfections with genetically different strains of virus has been well documented in normal hosts, including children in day care and women attending sexually transmitted disease clinics (Chandler et al. 1985; Handsfield et al. 1985; Murph et al. 1986; Collier et al. 1989; Bale et al. 1996; Boppana et al. 2001). Finally, it is also likely that normal individuals can be infected with several genetically unique strains of CMV, raising questions about the definition of protective immune reactivity in patients following an acute infection.

Clinically significant infections develop in patients with deficits in immunity resulting from pharmacological immunosuppression, acquired deficits in immunity such as HIV infection or developmental immaturity of the immune system. The natural history of CMV infection in transplant recipients suggests that infection is nearly universal in those exposed, but that clinical disease is dependent on specific risk factors. In all but bone marrow allograft recipients, a major and perhaps the most important risk factor, is the transplantation of an organ from a donor with previous infection into a CMV non-immune recipient (Ho 1991; Rubin 2002). Disease rates as high as 70 percent in renal allograft recipients following CMV mismatched donor–recipient transplantation have been reported (Rubin 2002). In the past, mortality rates in excess of 50 percent in cardiac/lung transplants limited CMV mismatched donor–recipient transplantation in some centers (Smyth et al. 1991). As the intensity of immunosuppression increases, so does the severity of CMV infections, as illustrated by the often fatal CMV infections that occur in bone marrow allograft recipients (Meyers et al. 1982; Winston et al. 1990; Schmidt et al. 1991; Zaia 2002; Boeckh et al. 2003). More recent findings have suggested that mismatched donor: recipients loci encoding natural killer (NK) cell recognition: activation antigens may also lead to significant CMV infections in the post-transplant period. If confirmed, this finding would argue for a critical role of innate immunity in resistance to CMV disease in these patients.

The natural history of CMV infections in AIDS patients has been most closely related to the depletion of $CD4^+$ lymphocytes. Several prospective studies documented high rates of CMV shedding in almost all AIDS patients, but invasive disease was more commonly observed in patients with <50 $CD4^+$ lymphocytes/mm^3 (Gallant et al. 1992). Reinfection is common and isolation of multiple strains of virus from individual patients has been reported (Drew et al. 1984; Spector et al. 1984; Chern et al. 1998). Characteristics of CMV infection that lead to severe disease and specific organ involvement are not understood, but evidence has been presented that residual virus-specific immunity may modulate disease progression (Boppana et al. 1995; Autran et al. 1997; Komanduri et al. 1998; Alberola et al. 2000; Alberola et al. 2001).

Congenital CMV infection is the most common viral infection of the human fetus (Alford 1984). In the USA the incidence of congenital CMV infection is ca. 1 percent in live births (Fowler et al. 1993; Britt and Alford 1996). In the developing world, rates of congenital infections as high as 2–3 percent have been described, suggesting that immunity does not prevent intrauterine infection (Yamamoto et al. 2001). An estimated 10 percent of infected infants will have significant infections that result in long lasting CNS sequelae (Alford; Fowler et al. 1993; Britt and Alford 1996; Boppana et al. 1999). The characteristics of the maternal infection have been claimed to be of paramount importance to the outcome of fetal infection; pre-existing maternal immunity can limit damage to the fetus, a situation analogous to that in allograft patients (Fowler et al. 1993). Primary gestational infection with CMV results in a 35–50 percent fetal transmission rate, whereas gestational reactivation or reinfection in women with preconceptional immunity is associated with a fetal infection rate of between 1–3 percent (Alford 1984; Britt and Alford 1996). Furthermore, it is estimated that fetal infection following primary maternal infection during pregnancy results in damage three times more often than infection that follows reactivation or reinfection in women with preconceptional immunity (Fowler et al. 1993). More recent findings have challenged these claims. These data include the finding that maternal reinfections with a genetically different strain of CMV do occur at a significant rate (10–12 percent) and that maternal reinfections can lead to damaging congenital infection (Ahlfors et al. 1999; Boppana et al. 2001). Furthermore, at least two different groups of investigators have reported that congenital infections following non-primary maternal infections can result in a similar incidence of long term sequelae as observed in infants infected as a result of primary maternal infections during pregnancy (Ahlfors et al. 1999, 2001; Boppana et al. 1999). Naturally acquired intrapartum or postnatal CMV infection in normal newborn infants has not been associated with severe infections and the permanent sequelae characteristic of infants infected in utero (see Table 27.2) (Alford 1984; Britt and Alford 1996).

Pathogenesis

In the context of currently available information, the pathogenesis of CMV infection must be viewed as a lytic viral infection resulting from a failure of host immunity to control effectively viral replication and spread. This model of CMV pathogenesis is accurately reflected by the virus burden as measured by polymerase chain reaction (PCR) or virus isolation during acute infection (Lockridge et al. 1999; Emery et al. 2000; Humar et al. 2002). However, it is almost a certainty that CMV exerts its pathogenetic potential through nonlytic mechanisms as well. These may include modulation of normal host cell functions by limited expression of its genome, and perhaps by affecting neighboring cellular functions through the induction of chemokine and cytokine production. Other pathways of host-cell damage may include the generation of host-derived immunopathological responses that result in significant organ damage, a mechanism that would explain the association of CMV with diseases such as atherosclerosis (Grattan et al. 1989; Epstein et al. 1999; Streblow et al. 2001; Libby 2002; Streblow et al. 2003). Such a mechanism has also been offered as an explanation of the severe pneumonia associated with CMV infection in bone allograft recipients and would be consistent with very early descriptions of this disease that indicated that only a few areas of the lung were infected with CMV (Myerson et al. 1984; Grundy et al. 1987). Perhaps the most convincing evidence of the importance of nonlytic mechanisms leading to disease have been provided by animal models of CMV infection leading to allograft disease, specifically transplant vascular sclerosis (Lemstrom et al. 1997;

Table 27.2 *Acquisitions of CMV infection in different populations*

Community acquired		Hospital acquired	
Age	**Mode of acquisition**	**Sources of CMV infections**	**Risks associated with virus transmission**
Perinatal	Intrauterine fetal infection (congenital)	Blood products	Blood products from seropositive donors
	Intrapartum		Multiple transfusions
	Breast milk acquired		White blood cell containing blood products
Infancy and childhood	Exposure to saliva and other body fluids	Allografts	Allograft from seropositive donors
			Graft rejection
Adolescence and adulthood	Sexually transmitted		
	Exposure to young children		

Koskinen et al. 1999; Streblow et al. 2003). Experimental systems including animal models have illustrated the role for virus-induced amplification of host inflammatory functions such as expression of adhesions molecules, induction of chemokine expression, and activation of transcriptional factors such as NF-κB that are central to the host inflammatory responses to virus infected cells. Such mechanisms could explain the association between CMV infection, virus gene expression in inflammatory diseases as exemplified by allograft dysfunction, and graft loss.

Pathological findings in CMV infection include evidence of virus infection in almost all organ systems (Becroft 1981; Britt and Alford 1996). Histological findings include large refractile cells (cytomegalic) with so-called owl's eye intranuclear inclusions. In some instances, organ dysfunction exceeds what would be expected from the number of infected cells detected by routine histopathological techniques. This discrepancy was initially confirmed using more sensitive techniques for demonstration of CMV (Myerson et al. 1984). Thus, the pathogenic mechanisms which account for end organ disease associated with CMV replication are unclear, as has been stated above and will likely not be explained by qualitative measures of virus within involved tissue.

Immune responses

Protective immune responses against CMV have not been definitely identified, and may not be the same in different populations. Both cellular and antibody responses to CMV participate in the immune responses that are thought to resolve infection in normal hosts (Rasmussen 1990; Walter et al. 1995; Britt and Alford 1996; Alberola et al. 2000, 2001). Most investigators who have suggested a dominant role for one arm of the immune system in protective immune responses against CMV have based these claims on findings from transplant recipients and patients with AIDS (Reusser et al. 1991; Walter et al.

1995; Autran et al. 1997; Komanduri et al. 1998; Aubert et al. 2001; Boeckh et al. 2003). In these patients, disease was associated with a decrease in either antibody or cellular responses to CMV as a result of immunosuppressive drug therapy or HIV infection. However, it must be noted that components of protective immunity in normal individuals have yet to be fully defined and that the clinical outcome in the post-transplant period that was previously attributed cellular immune effecter functions can also be related to the presence of virus neutralizing antibodies (Snydman 1993; Schoppel et al. 1997; Alberola et al. 2000). In fact, recent studies in a simian model of CMV infection in a rhesus macaques infected with a simian immunodeficiency virus have argued for a role of virus neutralizing antibodies and disease control (Kaur et al. 2003). Lastly, the importance of NK cells responses in control of murine CMV is well documented and further demonstrated by the presence of viral genes that specifically blunt the NK response (Krmpotic et al. 2002). Very recent findings would argue for a similar role of NK cells in the control of CMV infections in transplant recipients. Thus, a precise role for specific effector functions of the immune system in control of virus replication in infected host remains undefined.

In both solid organ and bone marrow transplant recipients, decreased cellular responses, especially CMV-specific CD8[+], MHC-restricted T lymphocyte responses, have been correlated with more severe CMV infections in the post-transplant period (Reusser et al. 1991). Reconstitution of these responses with in vitro expanded CMV-specific cytotoxic T lymphocytes has been shown to reduce post-transplant mortality secondary to CMV (Gavin et al. 1993; Walter et al. 1995). However, several studies from this same institution have shown a similar correlation of survival with the presence of virus-specific CD4[+]-specific lymphocyte responses, especially in the late (>100 days) post-transplant period (Li et al. 1994; Walter et al. 1995; Boeckh et al. 2003). The advent of effective antiviral therapy has altered the natural history of CMV in the transplant population such that CMV disease more commonly occurs late (180 days) in the post-transplant period (Boeckh et al. 2003). Thus, the value of a transient CD8[+] antiviral response provided by transferred antiviral T cells could require reassessment, particularly in light of recent experimental findings that have demonstrated the critical importance of antigen-specific CD4[+] responses in the maintenance of CD8[+] responses to infectious agents (Sun and Bevan 2003). As noted above, studies in patients with AIDS have clearly demonstrated that protective immune effector functions correlate with the restoration of CMV-specific CD4[+] responses (Autran et al. 1997; Komanduri et al. 1998). Findings from pregnant women have also suggested a correlation of cellular responses to CMV and intrauterine transmission, but these studies remain controversial (Gehrz et al. 1981). In AIDS patients with invasive CMV disease, cellular responses are absent because of lymphocyte depletion, yet recent improvements in the analysis of these responses have permitted the detection of CMV-specific responses in AIDS patients with severe depletion of peripheral CD4[+] lymphocyte numbers, indicating that only limited residual cellular immunity is required for control of CMV replication (Autran et al. 1997; Waldrop et al. 1997; Komanduri et al. 1998; O'Sullivan et al. 1999). Cellular immune responses appear to be directed primarily at the protein components of virion tegument, the products of the UL83 open reading frame (ORF), phosphoprotein 65 (pp65), and the UL32 ORF, phosphoprotein 150 (pp150). Although other CMV-encoded proteins such as the products of the IE-1 gene elicit cellular responses, responder cell frequency analysis has indicated that these two proteins represent dominant targets of cellular immunity (Kern et al. 1999; Kern et al. 2002; Gallez-Hawkins et al. 2003). The role of cytokines in cellular responses against CMV is unknown; however, in animal models of human CMV disease, interferon (IFN)-γ has been shown to have significant antiviral activity. Finally, it has been reported that CMV infections are associated both with decreased cellular immune responses in normal individuals and with decreased CMV-specific responses in congenitally infected children (Gehrz et al. 1977; Pass et al. 1983). More recent studies using sensitive techniques such as intracellular cytokine staining following antigen exposure have demonstrated that congenitally infected infants do indeed have cellular immune responses to CMV. Depression in cellular immune responses may also contribute to superinfection with fungal pathogens in transplant recipients infected with CMV. This clinical association remains unproven but is widely held by transplant physicians.

ANTIBODY RESPONSES

Serological responses to CMV are complex because of the large number of virus proteins. Several studies have documented responses to a number of the more immunogenic proteins of CMV in both normal and immunocompromised hosts (Zaia et al. 1986; Hayes et al. 1987; Landini et al. 1988, 1993; Britt et al. 1995; Schoppel et al. 1997). These studies have provided important clues for identification of viral-encoded proteins that induce protective antibody responses as well as antibody responses which could be used in the diagnosis of acute and past CMV infections. The only well-characterized in vitro assay of antibody activity that correlates with patient outcome is virus neutralizing antibody (Adler et al. 1995; Boppana and Britt 1995; Schoppel et al. 1997). Virus-neutralizing serological responses are limited to antibodies against virus-encoded glycoproteins, as these represent the only class of viral proteins that are surface exposed in a native form. The majority of virus-neutralizing antibodies are directed against the products of the UL55 (gB), UL75 (gH), and UL73/UL100 (gM/gN) ORFs (Britt et al. 1990; Rasmussen et al. 1991). Studies have suggested that immunization with these proteins can induce neutralizing antibodies as well as antibodies reactive with the surface of virus-infected cells (Rasmussen 1990; Britt et al. 1995; Pass et al. 1999). The identification of intense and durable antibody responses to components of the viral tegument, both pp65 and pp150, has provided a rationale for including these proteins in a recombinant protein based diagnostic assay for serological reactivity to CMV (Landini 1993). Conversely, the presence of significant IgM responses to a nonstructural protein, pp50 (UL44), has led to its use as a serological target for detection of IgM and, therefore, recent infection (Landini 1993; Lazzarotto et al. 1998).

Diagnosis

The diagnosis of CMV relies either on demonstration of the agent (virus, viral proteins, nucleic acids) in body fluids, and/or tissue or on serological responses in a patient with clinical findings consistent with CMV infection. Because of the ubiquitous nature of CMV, it is important that a distinction be made between the detection of CMV and demonstration of CMV in the context of an infectious syndrome compatible with CMV. Multiple methods of recovering virus have been employed, including culture on permissive cells such as primary human fibroblasts and centrifugation enhanced culture followed by early antigen detection with monoclonal antibodies. This latter technique is widely used and can provide positive results within 24 h. In contrast, conventional tube culture may require up to 4 weeks to reveal cytopathology (Pass et al. 1995; Revello and Gerna 2002).

Techniques of viral antigen detection have been relatively limited with the exception of the antigenemia assay (van der Bij et al. 1988; Gerna et al. 1991; Miller et al. 1991; Boeckh and Bowden 1995), which uses the immunological detection of the virus structural protein pp65 within polymorphonuclear leucocytes. Because this assay can be quantified relatively easily, it has been used to predict the likelihood of invasive disease in transplant patients and patients with AIDS (van der Bij et al. 1988; van den Berg et al. 1989). It is a widely used assay in many transplant centers and seems to be of practical value for the management of transplant patients. It is less sensitive than PCR but this may offer some advantage, including a greater positive predictive value for presence of disease because the increased sensitivity of PCR has limited its predictive value in many circumstances.

Detection of viral nucleic acids has been used extensively to document CMV infections. Dot-blot hybridization, in situ hybridization, and PCR have all been applied to clinical specimens. PCR is the most widely used assay and in certain clinical situations, such as screening newborn urine for CMV, is a highly sensitive method of diagnosis. PCR of plasma and peripheral blood buffy coat cells has been used to detect significant infection in transplant recipients and AIDS patients (Spector et al. 1992; Boeckh et al. 1997; Cope et al. 1997; Razonable et al. 2002). More recent modifications of the PCR, including real-time PCR, that permit quantitation of viral burden has provided significant new information relevant to our understanding of CMV infections in the immunocompromised patient. Spector and colleagues were one of the first groups to demonstrate that the viral burden was predictive of the likelihood of an individual patient developing invasive disease (Spector et al. 1996). Several additional reports have also demonstrated the value of this approach (Cope et al. 1997; Emery et al. 2000; Zaia 2002). Real-time PCR with extended linear ranges of nucleic acid detection have permitted rapid and accurate measurement of virus burden in a variety of patient specimens.

Serological assays of antibody reactivity to CMV include nearly every imaginable technology. Detection of IgG is straightforward and seropositivity is evidence of infection only, and relative titers are usually of little clinical value. Seropositivity does not indicate active virus shedding, but should be taken as evidence of the potential infectivity of blood or organs from the individual. The measurement of CMV-specific IgM responses offers the possibility of distinguishing between acute infection and past infection (Stagno et al. 1985; Kropff et al. 1993). Unfortunately, this assay is often associated with low sensitivity and, occasionally, low specificity (Stagno et al. 1985; Landini 1993; Revello and Gerna 2002). Furthermore, the presence of rheumatoid factors may lead to false positive IgM results (Griffiths et al. 1982). Lastly, IgM antibodies are not present in the absence of IgG reactivity, so competition for antigenic sites between IgG and IgM antibodies is possible. IgM antibodies can persist for significant periods of time post acute infection and in some patients can persist for extended periods of time. The use of IgM reactivity to establish the chronicity of an infection is controversial and up to 40 percent of patients with past infection will have IgM anti-CMV antibodies (Revello and Gerna 2002) More recently, several laboratories have demonstrated that the measurement of anti-CMV IgG avidity can help distinguish between recent and past infection with CMV (Lazzarotto et al. 1998, 1999; Revello and Gerna 2002) This approach has been incorporated into an algorithm for the diagnosis and management of CMV infections during pregnancy (Bodeus et al. 2002; Revello and Gerna 2002).

Control

ANTIVIRAL THERAPY

Two agents with activity against CMV, ganciclovir and foscarnet are in current clinical use (Coen 1992). Both have significant toxicity, and resistant isolates have developed during treatment. Their use in AIDS patients is problematic since neither is virucidal and, when treatment is interrupted, virus replication resumes. Two additional compounds have recently been licensed for treatment of CMV infections in AIDS patients, specifically retinitis – Cidofovir and Fomivirsen.

Ganciclovir is a nucleoside analogue that inhibits chain elongation both by its activity as a chain terminator and through direct inhibition of the viral DNA polymerase (Sullivan et al. 1992, 1993). It is inactive until phosphorylated by the phosphotransferase activity of the UL97 ORF (Sullivan et al. 1992). It has been used to treat invasive infections in transplant recipients, retinitis and colitis in AIDS patients, and as part of a protocol to examine its efficacy in limiting sequelae in infants with congenital CMV infections (Meyers 1991; Spector et al. 1993) (Kimberlin et al. 2003). It also has some value as an antiviral prophylaxis in bone marrow transplant recipients (Goodrich et al. 1993; Seu et al. 1997; Ljungman 2001). Ganciclovir treatment causes primarily bone marrow toxicity with neutropenia as a major adverse effect. Ganciclovir is very poorly absorbed when given orally but dosing with sufficient drug can achieve similar serum levels as an intravenously given drug and similar therapeutic efficacy (Paya et al. 2002). However, its valine ester, valganciclovir, is readily absorbed and equivalent serum levels can be achieved with standard oral dosing regimens (Gane et al. 1997; Miller et al. 1997; Pescovitz et al. 2000; Curran and Noble 2001). This formulation of ganciclovir has been licensed for treatment of CMV infections in patients with AIDS following the demonstration of similar efficacy and safety profile of the oral valganciclovir when compared to intravenous ganciclovir for the treatment of CMV retinitis (Lalezari et al. 2002; Martin et al. 2002). Debate continues over the use of ganciclovir as prophylaxis or as treatment when virus replication is detected (preemptive therapy). Both approaches have been shown to modify CMV disease in the post-transplant period (Emery 2001; Ljungman 2001; Singh 2001).

Foscarnet is an inhibitor of CMV DNA polymerases (Snoeck et al. 1993). It is also active against a wide variety of viral polymerases. This agent has been used extensively in AIDS patients and has demonstrated efficacy in CMV retinitis (Palestine et al. 1991). It causes significant renal toxicity, thus limiting its use under certain situations arising transplant recipients. This agent has been used extensively in patients who fail ganciclovir therapy.

Cidofovir and Fomivirsen are two compounds that were licensed for the treatment of CMV retinitis in AIDS patients. Cidofovir is a nucleoside analogue and inhibits CMV DNA replication in much the same manner as ganciclovir, with the exception that it does not require phosphorylation (De Clercq 1998). This latter property makes it useful for the treatment of patients who fail ganciclovir therapy secondary to mutations in the UL97 ORF (De Clercq 1998). Unfortunately, this agent has significant nephrotoxicity that has limited its use in almost all patient populations. Fomivirsen (ISIS 2922) is the first antisense RNA compound licensed for treatment of a human disease and is active against CMV in vivo and in vitro. The clinical experience with this compound is limited because of the changing natural history of opportunistic infections in AIDS patients which has followed HAART, but injection of this compound into the eye appears to be effective therapy for HCMV retinitis.

VACCINES

Past and recent epidemiological studies have argued that CMV is a vaccine-modifiable disease (Fowler et al. 1993; Fowler et al. 2003). Previous and current approaches for vaccine development have focused on replicating live viral vaccines. These have been referred to as attenuated viruses; however, as CMV does not exhibit identifiable virulence markers, this claim remains contentious. Vaccination of renal allograft recipients with one of these candidate viruses, the Towne strain of CMV, provided some evidence that it could induce protective responses (Plotkin et al. 1991). In a recent study, this vaccine failed to protect normal women from reinfection following exposure to children in a group care setting (Adler et al. 1995). Thus, it is unclear whether this vaccine in its current formulation is sufficiently immunogenic to induce protective immunity. Clinical trials are currently underway using a recombinant glycoprotein B combined with an adjuvant as an alternative approach. Although this vaccine appears to induce antibodies, including virus neutralizing antibodies, the durability of this response appears to be limited. It should be noted that recent studies have indicated that reinfection of previously immune women with genetically different strains of virus are relatively common in some populations, raising questions about the nature of protective immunity and therefore current vaccine strategies that attempt to recapitulate natural immunity (Boppana et al. 2001).

HUMAN HERPESVIRUSES 6 AND 7

HHV-6 and HHV-7 are two relatively recently described human viruses whose clinical importance remains to be fully defined. Isolation of HHV-6 from AIDS patients initially prompted speculation that it was an important cofactor in this disease (Salahuddin et al. 1986). This initial excitement was subsequently tempered by findings which demonstrated that infection with HHV-6 was common in all populations and that persistent shedding was characteristic of the biology of this virus. A second lymphotrophic betaherpesvirus, HHV-7, was isolated from $CD4^+$ T lymphocytes of normal individuals (Frenkel et al. 1990). Both viruses are acquired at an early age and seroprevalence is in excess of 60–80 percent by adulthood in most populations. Genetically, these viruses are closely related to CMV and exhibit genetic homology with CMV over an estimated two-thirds of their genomes (Lawrence et al. 1990; Inoue et al. 1993; Gompels et al. 1995; Megaw et al. 1998). A single serotype of HHV-7 has been described, whereas HHV-6 can be divided into two groups, A and B, based on biology, serological reactivity, and genetic composition (Ablashi et al. 1991; Schirmer et al. 1991). HHV-7 utilizes $CD4^+$ as its receptor whereas the receptor for HHV-6 is CD46, the same receptor utilized by measles virus (Lusso et al. 1994; Santoro et al. 1999). Subsequent studies have indicated that the CXC chemokine receptor 4 is not a coreceptor for HHV-7 as was initially proposed (Zhang et al. 2000).

Clinical manifestations

Recognizable clinical syndromes associated with HHV-6 and HHV-7 infection and confirmed by virological studies have been limited to primary infections in children. HHV-6 is the etiological agent of exanthem subitum (roseola), a common febrile illness of early childhood (Yamanishi et al. 1988). The clinical findings of this illness include high fevers ($>39°C$) of 3–5 days duration, nonspecific findings such as pharyngeal injection and diarrhea, and, perhaps most characteristically, rapid defervescence followed nearly coincidentally by the appearance of a generalized maculopapular rash (Okada et al. 1993; Asano et al. 1994; Hall et al. 1994; Suga et al. 1997; Caserta et al. 1998, 2001; Clark 2000). In contrast to this classical presentation, other studies have suggested that only about 10 percent of infants with primary HHV-6 infection exhibit the full spectrum of exanthem subitum (Pruksananonda et al. 1992; Caserta et al. 2001). Interestingly, only the HHV-6B variant has been associated with exanthema subitum (Dewhurst et al. 1993). Symptoms including irritability, bulging anterior fontanelle, and seizures in a significant percentage of infants with roseola have been suggested as evidence of CNS infection (Kondo et al. 1993; Asano et al. 1994; Hall et al. 1994; Yoshikawa and Asano 2000). It has been suggested that primary infection with HHV-6 (strain B) and invasion of the CNS may predispose to the development and recurrence of febrile seizures (Kondo et al. 1993; Caserta et al. 1994; Yoshikawa and Asano 2000). Consistent with a direct role of HHV-6 in the development of seizures, other studies have documented the presence of HHV-6 nucleic acids in the cerebrospinal fluid (CSF) from patients with acute HHV-6 infection and also in the brain tissue from both immunocompetent and immunocompromised patients (Yoshikawa et al. 1992; Suga et al. 1993; Luppi et al. 1994; Ohashi et al. 2002). From these and other studies it appears that HHV-6 is neurotropic. HHV-6, and possibly HHV-7, are important causes of acute febrile illnesses in childhood, accounting for nearly 20 percent of hospital emergency room visits in the USA (Hall et al. 1994). Primary infection with HHV-7 is less well described but appears to cause a clinical syndrome very similar to that reported for HHV-6 with a possible difference being that primary HHV-7 infection occurs at an older age (Tanaka et al. 1994; Asano et al. 1995; Torigoe et al. 1995; Caserta et al. 1998). At least one report suggested that HHV-7 may be associated with the common childhood exanthem, pityriasis rosea, while other reports have failed to confirm this association (Drago et al. 1997; Kosuge et al. 2000). Clinically apparent infections in normal adults with either virus have been infrequently reported but, when diagnosed, resemble infectious mononucleosis (Steeper et al. 1990; Akashi et al. 1993). Reactivation of HHV-6, and possibly of HHV-7, often follows febrile illnesses, and reactivation of HHV-6 follows HHV-7 infection in vitro and in vivo (Kusuhara et al. 1991; Frenkel and Wyatt 1992; Asano et al. 1995). HHV-6 has also been associated with several rare disorders, including sinus histocytosis syndrome or Rosai–Dorfman disease (Foucar et al. 1990; Levine et al. 1992). It has been argued that HHV-6, and possibly HHV-6 infection, are associated with chronic fatigue syndrome; however, several studies have failed to demonstrate an increased incidence of infection with either of these viruses and this syndrome (Braun et al. 1995; Reeves et al. 2000). Clinical reports have linked HHV-6 with multiple sclerosis (MS) based on increased immunological responses to HHV-6, including HHV-6 specific IgG and IgM antibodies in patients with MS (Soldan et al. 2000). The experimental findings linking HHV-6 with the chronic demyelinating disease include: (1) detection of HHV-6 DNA by PCR in CSF from patients with MS at a higher frequency

than controls; (2) detection of HHV-6 sequences in oligodendrocytes adjacent to plaques in the brain tissue from patients with MS but not control patients; (3) HHV-6-specific immunohistochemical staining of oligodendrocytes from plaques obtained from patients with MS but not control patients (Wilborn et al. 1994b; Challoner et al. 1995; Friedman et al. 1999; Akhyani et al. 2000; Knox et al. 2000; Tejada-Simon et al. 2002). In contrast, other studies have not reproduced these early findings (Hebart et al. 1997; Coates and Bell 1998; Mirandola et al. 1999). To date, definitive evidence of causality has not been presented but the association between HHV-6 and MS is intriguing and mandate additional studies to define this relationship.

Infection with HHV-6 can result in severe organ involvement, especially in immunocompromised hosts. It has been associated with a variety of specific clinical entities, including encephalitis, pneumonitis, hepatitis, and bone marrow dysfunction (Asano et al. 1990; Tajiri et al. 1990; Carrigan et al. 1991; Yoshikawa et al. 1992; Cone et al. 1993; Knox and Carrigan 1994; Singh 2000). This latter disorder may result from HHV-6 infection of hematopoietic progenitor cells, contributing to graft dysfunction in bone marrow transplant recipients (Knox and Carrigan 1992; Carrigan and Knox 1994). The proposed mechanisms responsible for bone marrow suppression in the bone marrow recipient have included both HHV-6 mediated cytolysis of progenitor cells and/ or suppression of colony forming units through stimulation of cytokine production (Knox and Carrigan 1992; Drobyski et al. 1993). However, it should also be noted that 30–45 percent of hematopoietic cell allograft recipients develop HHV-6 viremia or HHV-6 DNAemia (Imbert-Marcille et al. 2000; Caserta et al. 2001; Yoshikawa et al. 2002; Boutolleau et al. 2003). Thus, it has been difficult to ascribe specific disease syndromes to HHV-6 infection/reactivation in these patients because the majority of allograft recipients with HHV-6 do not have symptoms attributable to this virus. The importance of HHV-6 in the solid organ allograft recipients is also unclear even though up to 50–60 percent of transplant recipients will reactivate the virus in the posttransplant period (Schmidt et al. 1996; Griffiths et al. 1999; Griffiths et al. 2000). Perhaps more interesting is the association between the reactivation of HHV-6 and CMV in the post-transplant period and the association between severe CMV disease and concomitant HHV-6 infection (Dockrell et al. 1997; Lowance et al. 1999; Humar et al. 2000; Kidd et al. 2000; DesJardin et al. 2001). As noted above, several studies have suggested that HHV-6 (or HHV-7) may play a role in graft dysfunction in the post-transplant period, including graft rejection; however, these findings must be interpreted in the context of the use of potent immunosuppressive agents to maintain graft function and the reactivation of a variety of herpesviruses including HCMV (Okuno et al. 1990; Griffiths et al. 1999).

Although numerous case reports have linked HHV-6 infection to specific organ damage in the post-transplant period, it remains to be determined whether HHV-6 is a major cause of morbidity in this patient population because many of the patients in these studies were also infected with other agents such as HCMV. Alternatively, it has been argued that the success of antivirals in limiting post-transplant complications associated with CMV replication may also be explained by the activity of these compounds against HHV-6. Similarly, in patients with AIDS, HHV-6 and HHV-7 have been associated with a variety of clinical findings but their role, if any, in AIDS pathogenesis is unclear. In vitro studies have shown that HHV-6 can activate CD4$^+$ expression in CD4$^-$ cells raising the possibility that HHV-6 could increase the number of target cells for HIV infection in the HIV infected host (Lusso et al. 1991; Flamand et al. 1998). In contrast, other studies have suggested that HHV-6 infection can suppress HIV replication in dendritic cells and that HHV-6 can down-regulate the HIV coreceptor, CXC chemokine receptor 4 (CXCR4), in CD4$^+$ lymphocytes (Asada et al. 1999; Hasegawa et al. 2001). In clinical studies, there appears to be no quantitative relationship between the level of HHV-6 in peripheral blood mononuclear cell (PBMC) and CD4$^+$ lymphocyte counts in patients with AIDS, although HHV-6 dissemination appears to be more widespread in AIDS patients than controls (Fairfax et al. 1994; Clark et al. 1996; Fabio et al. 1997). In contrast, primary HHV-6 infection has been associated with more rapid progression of HIV disease in children (Kosita-nont et al. 1999). Whilst some investigators have suggested that HHV-6 and HHV-7 may function as cofactors in the development of the immune deficiency associated with HIV infection, there is currently little definitive information to support this hypothesis.

Epidemiology

The seroprevalence of HHV-6 increases rapidly through early childhood such that over 90 percent of infants in developed countries will be seropositive by the age of 2 years (Saxinger et al. 1988; Balachandra et al., 1989; Okuno et al. 1989). Serological reactivity in adults is also nearly universal. The vast majority of newborn infants are antibody positive, presumably because of trans-placentally acquired maternal antibody, but become seronegative by 6 months of age (Balachandra et al. 1989; Yanagi et al. 1990). Approximately 10 percent of infants less than 1 month old can have detectable HHV-6 DNA in peripheral blood mononuclear cells, suggesting that in a minority of cases HHV-6 is acquired in the perinatal period (Hall et al. 1994). Because the rate of infection as measured by seroconversion increases rapidly during the interval between 6 and 12 months with a peak age of virus acquisition between 6–9

months of age, it has been hypothesized that maternal antibody may provide protective immunity early in infancy. In North America, HHV-6B is almost always associated with primary infection in infancy in contrast to the epidemiology in Zambia in which the majority of infections in infancy are associated with HHV-6A (Dewhurst et al. 1993; Kasolo et al. 1997). Co-infection with HHV-6A and 6B is common (Cone et al. 1996). In contrast, the seroprevalence of HHV-7 increases steadily throughout childhood and by 10 years of age almost all individuals are seropositive (Wyatt et al. 1991). Furthermore, the prevalence of HHV-7 antibody reactivity in different geographical locations is more variable than that reported for HHV-6 (Wyatt et al. 1991; Yoshikawa et al. 1993; Ablashi et al. 1994). Serological reactivity for HHV-6 does not prevent infection with HHV-7 as evidenced by the later age of acquisition of HHV-7 as compared to HHV-6 and the frequent occurrence of HHV-6 and HHV-7 infection in older patients. Reactivation of HHV-6 occurs in about 40 percent of seropositive women during pregnancy and HHV-6 DNA was reported in about 1 percent of cord blood (Dahl et al. 1999). Other reports have suggested that intrauterine transmission of either virus is exceedingly rare (Bala-chandra et al. 1989; Yanagi et al. 1990; Aubin et al. 1992). Furthermore, HHV-6 can be found in the cervix but perinatal transmission appears infrequent (Okuno et al. 1989; Leach et al. 1993).

HHV-6 and HHV-7 can be readily isolated in the early post-transplant period from both solid organ and bone marrow allograft recipients. Increases in sero-logical responses and viremia, as measured by culture and/or PCR, are commonly detected in up to 80 percent of transplant recipients in the first 3 months after transplantation (Okuno et al. 1990; Wilborn et al. 1994b; Chan et al. 1997; Imbert-Marcille et al. 2000; Yoshikawa et al. 2002; Boutolleau et al. 2003). More recent studies have indicated that HHV-7 was isolated in the post-transplant period as often as HHV-6 in HCMV-infected patients and when HHV-7 DNA was assayed by PCR, HHV-7 was detected more frequently than in HHV-6 in the post-transplant period (Kidd et al. 2000; Mendez et al. 2001; Lautenschlager et al. 2002; Boutolleau et al. 2003). In addition, HHV-6 antigens can be detected in up to 60 percent of renal allograft biopsies, a finding consistent with the proposed role of HHV-6 in graft rejection (Hoshino et al. 1995; Griffiths et al. 1999). However, as noted previously, the contribution of HHV-6 (and presumably HHV-7) to post-transplant morbidity and mortality remains uncertain and recent studies have demonstrated a significantly lower incidence of HHV-6 reactivation than HCMV in heart-lung transplant recipients (Michaelides et al. 2002). Furthermore, HHV-6 DNA could be detected in lung tissue in patients, both bone marrow transplant recipients and controls, who were HHV-6 seropositive (Cone et al. 1993). Similarly, the rate of HHV-7 detection in a group of stem cell transplant recipients was nearly equivalent in peripheral blood specimens analyzed pre- and post-transplant (Boutolleau et al. 2003). Thus, it remains difficult to assign causality to HHV-6 and/or HHV-7 in post-transplant syndromes such as pneumonitis because of the near universal recovery of HHV-6 and the frequent presence of other agents such as HCMV or adenovirus in the same biopsy tissue from transplant patients.

Sources of virus include exposure to saliva, genital secretions, and PBMC (Levy et al. 1990a; Wyatt and Frenkel 1992; Black et al. 1993; Cone et al. 1994; Leach et al. 1994). Although breast milk would seem to be a likely source of HHV-6 and HHV-7, current understanding of the natural history of these infections suggests that breast milk is not a common mode of transmission. There appear to be no significant differences in the rate or age of acquisition of HHV-6 between breast-fed and nonbreast-fed infants (Takahashi et al. 1988). This epidemiologic observation is consistent with at least one study indicating that HHV-6 could not be detected in breast milk (Dunne and Jevon 1993). Limited studies in families have suggested that exposure to respiratory secretions is the most likely mode of intrafamilial spread of HHV-6 (Mukai et al. 1994). HHV-6 and HHV-7 are persistently excreted in the saliva following primary infection and in individuals with past infections, although it appears that HHV-7 is more frequently detected in saliva than HHV-6 (Levy et al. 1990b; Wyatt and Frenkel 1992; Black et al. 1993; Mukai et al. 1994; Kidd et al. 1996; Lucht et al. 1998). HHV-7 has been isolated from saliva in 60–80 percent of seropositive adults (Black et al. 1993; Hidaka et al. 1993; Black and Pellett 1999). Both viruses can be detected in PBMC from seropositive individuals using PCR, suggesting that blood may be an important source of virus transmission in hospitalized patients (Cone et al. 1994; Kidd et al. 1996).

The biological behavior of the virus in tissue culture, including such characteristics as the cellular tropism of the different HHV-6 variants and the virus yield from cord blood lymphocytes, initially suggested the possibility of variants of HHV-6 (Wyatt et al. 1990; Ablashi et al. 1993; Gompels et al. 1993). Additional studies have documented the presence of two genetically and serologically distinct variants of HHV-6, type A and type B (Ablashi et al. 1991; Schirmer et al. 1991). Comparison of the genomes from prototypic HHV-6A and HHV-6B viruses have revealed identical nucleotide sequence over 75–97 percent of the genome, depending on the region of the genome analyzed (Gompels et al. 1995). Overall, there is approximately 95 percent identity for most genes found in conserved gene blocks, but only 75 percent conservation in genes found in HHV-6 and not in other betaherpesviruses. Interestingly, recombination between variants occurs uncommonly, if at all. These variants are also associated with specific diseases as illustrated by the finding that over 95 percent of cases

of roseola in the USA are caused by group B viruses (Dewhurst et al. 1993). Furthermore, HHV-6B, but not HHV-6A, has been shown to replicate in salivary glands as evidenced by its isolation from saliva (Harnett et al. 1990; Levy et al. 1990a; French et al. 1999). Studies from several different transplant centers have also documented that the B variant is more frequently associated with infections in the post-transplant period (Frenkel et al. 1994; Wilborn et al. 1994a; Boutolleau et al. 2003). The basis for the association between the B variant of HHV-6 and specific clinical syndromes remains unexplained. Together, these findings have been used by some investigators to suggest that HHV-6a and HHV-6b are distinct betaherpesviruses and not merely variants of one another.

Pathogenesis

Little is known about the pathogenesis of HHV-6 and HHV-7 infections; however, it must be assumed that, as the majority of infections are subclinical, normal host responses can effectively limit virus-induced cellular damage. In addition, there are no consistent and specific histopathological changes in target organs that suggest direct virus mediated cytopathology (Kurata et al. 1990). Because the severity of roseola can be related to the level of HHV-6 viremia, viral load may be an important determinant of this disease, and presumably of organ damage (Asano et al. 1991). Recent findings in transplant patients infected with HHV-6 also argue for a correlation between virus load and clinical disease (Ljungman 2002; Zerr et al. 2002; Boutolleau et al. 2003) The pathogenetic mechanism(s) leading to the clinical syndrome of roseola are unknown, but the lymphocyte tropism of the virus suggests that cytokines could contribute to the symptoms associated with this infection. HHV-6 infection of lymphocytes induces production of a variety of lymphokines, including TNF, IL-1β, IL-10, IL-12, and interferons (Flamand et al. 1991; Flamand et al. 1996; Campadelli-Fiume et al. 1999). Furthermore, HHV-6 encodes at least two chemokine receptor (UL12, UL51), of which at least one, UL12, is a functional receptor (Isegawa et al. 1999). Together with its lymphotropic behavior, it is almost certain that many of the clinical findings associated with primary infection with HHV-6 can be related to host derived inflammatory responses and not virus-induced cytopathology. Using techniques that detect viral nucleic acids or viral antigens in the absence of histopathological changes, HHV-6 has been demonstrated in alveolar macrophages from transplant patients with pneumonitis, hepatocytes from patients with hepatitis, and brain tissue from patients with encephalitis (Asano et al. 1990; Carrigan et al. 1991; Carrigan and Knox 1994; Cone et al. 1994). It has also been suggested that HHV-6 infection in bone marrow transplant recipients may contribute to more severe graft-versus-host disease (Wilborn et al. 1994a).

As noted previously, the possible role of HHV-6 in the pathogenesis of end organ diseases in transplant recipients is controversial because of the presence of other opportunistic pathogens and the near universal presence of HHV-6 and HHV-7 in the adult population (Cone et al. 1994, 1999; Black and Pellett 1999).

If the relationship between HHV-6 infection and disease can be considered to be incompletely defined, the relationship between specific syndromes and clinical disease and HHV-7 infection is unknown. HHV-7 infection is associated with reactivation of HHV-6 and, therefore, the assignment of the relative contribution of each virus to a clinical illness is impossible. However, the later age of HHV-7 acquisition and the lack of definable syndromes associated with HHV-7 infection suggest that its potential to cause disease in the normal host is limited. In the immunocompromised host however, HHV-7 has been proposed to be an important cofactor in the severity of disease associated with human cytomegalovirus infection in the post-transplant period (Kidd et al. 2000; Tong et al. 2000; Mendez et al. 2001). An interesting finding in these studies was that disease association between these viruses was only demonstrated when the quantity of virus in blood was measured and not just the qualitative presence or absence of either virus. Thus, it would appear that clinically significant interactions between these viruses require increased viral loads, a feature unique to patients with more significant immune dysfunction. In vitro, HHV-7 has been shown to induce CD4$^+$ lymphocyte death by both direct cytolysis and apoptosis, raising the possibility that active HHV-7 replication could contribute to the immune suppression in the post-transplant period (Secchiero et al. 1997). Perhaps this or a related mechanism could explain the role of HHV-7 in severe HCMV infection in the post-transplant period.

The association of HHV-6 infection with central nervous dysfunction, most commonly manifest as seizure activity, is particularly intriguing. Roseola is frequently associated with irritability and a bulging anterior fontanelle, two nonspecific findings of CNS involvement in this childhood infection. Case reports have provided evidence of CNS infection by HHV-6, including detection of HHV-6 nucleic acids in the CSF and in brain tissue from fatal cases (Asano et al. 1990; Ishiguro et al. 1990; Yoshikawa et al. 1992; Yoshikawa and Asano 2000). Virus could also be demonstrated in endothelial cells in the brain of fatal cases of HHV-6 encephalitis, suggesting the possibility of vasculitis as a cause for CNS disease (Yoshikawa and Asano 2000). HHV-6 has also been detected in a variety of cell types in brain tissue from HHV-6 infected patients with AIDS, including astrocytes, oligodendrocytes, microglia, and neurons (Ohashi et al. 2002). Other studies have also demonstrated, by PCR, viral nucleic acid in the CSF (Kondo et al. 1993; Suga et al. 1993; Achim et al. 1994; Caserta et al. 1994; Wilborn et al. 1994a). Interestingly, in

several of these studies, including the largest in terms of number of patients, virus could not be isolated from the CSF (Hall et al. 1994). Because of the propensity of HHV-6 to reactivate after a febrile illness, including HHV-7 infection, the demonstration of viral nucleic acid in the CSF without additional evidence of tissue invasion or local replication of virus, suggests only an association between HHV-6 and CNS dysfunction and not causality. Although HHV-6 nucleic acids have been detected in normal hosts with encephalitis and compelling arguments can be made for this virus as a cause of sporadic encephalitis, definitive evidence for a direct role in childhood seizures associated with primary infection is lacking (Yoshikawa et al. 1991). Similarly, primary HHV-7 infection has been associated with the development of seizure activity (Torigoe et al. 1995; Caserta et al. 1998). It has been suggested that primary HHV-7 infection is more frequently associated with seizures in young infants, but little definitive evidence is available to support a direct role for this virus in CNS dysfunction in the normal host.

Since their discovery, HHV-6 and HHV-7 have been suspected to have a role in the pathogenesis of HIV infection. Several biological characteristics support this suspicion. These include: (1) growth in T lymphocytes in vivo and in vitro, (2) the use of CD4 as a cellular receptor by HHV-7, (3) induction of CD4 expression after infection of lymphocytes, and (4) transactivation of the HIV long terminal repeat (Ensoli et al. 1989; Takahashi et al. 1989; Ablashi et al. 1991; Lusso et al. 1991, 1994; Martin et al. 1991; Kashanchi et al. 1994; Wang et al. 1994; Zhou et al. 1994; Lusso and Gallo 1995). However, epidemiological studies have provided little definitive evidence suggesting that either HHV-6 or HHV-7 plays an important role in the progression to AIDS in HIV-infected individuals (Fox et al. 1988; Spira et al. 1990; Fairfax et al. 1994; Lusso et al. 1994). Furthermore, HHV-6 has been shown to inhibit the replication of HIV in vitro (Levy et al. 1990b). In contrast to this early finding, other studies have suggested that co-infection of HIV-infected cells with lower inocula of HHV-6 may actually lead to enhanced HIV replication (Lusso et al. 1994). Thus, it remains to be determined whether co-infection with HHV-6 or HHV-7 contributes to the progression of HIV infections.

Immunity

Immunological responses in normal hosts are sufficient to limit the replication and spread of HHV-6 and HHV-7 as evidenced by the infrequent development of symptomatic infection and the self-limited nature of the infection. The natural history of HHV-6 infection suggests that passively acquired immunity in early infancy is sufficient to prevent infection. It is unclear what role maternal immunity plays in the natural history of HHV-7. Host immune responses that limit reactivation in normal hosts and curtail invasive infection in immuno-compromised hosts are unknown, but, if analogous to other herpesvirus infections, are probably virus-specific cellular responses. The frequent shedding of both viruses in patients undergoing immunosuppressive therapy or individuals with HIV is consistent with a critical role for cellular immunological effector functions in limiting virus replication.

CELLULAR IMMUNE RESPONSES

HHV-6 infection can induce the production of antiviral cytokines, including interferons. NK cell activity and interferon-α levels have also been reported to be elevated in acute HHV-6 infection and in vitro studies have suggested that these activities may play a role in controlling HHV-6 in replication in vivo (Kikuta et al. 1990; Takahashi et al. 1992). Analysis of $CD4^+$ lympho-cyte clones derived from infected individuals has revealed that, although most were specific for HHV-6, about 10 percent responded to both HHV-6 and HHV-7 and an even smaller number were cross-reactive with HHV-6, HHV-7, and CMV (Yasukawa et al. 1993). Group A and B variants of HHV-6 could be distinguished by reactivity of 7 percent of the clones. MHC-restricted cytotoxic T cell clones specific for HHV-6 infected cells have also been isolated (Yakushijin et al. 1992). The antigen specificity of the cellular responses against HHV-6 and HHV-7 remains to be defined.

ANTIBODY RESPONSES

The serological responses to HHV-6 and HHV-7 are extraordinarily complex. In the case of HHV-6, IgM antibodies specific for HHV-6 appear 5–7 days after the onset of clinical symptoms and peak around 2–3 weeks (Suga et al. 1993). The IgG antibody response to HHV-6 can first be detected 7–10 days after resolution of clinical symptoms and remain detectable for the life of the host (Ueda et al. 1989). The serological reactivity to HHV-7 appears to have similar kinetics (Yoshida et al. 2002). A large number of virus-encoded proteins are recognized by convalescent sera, but to date the antibody components of protective immunity have not been defined. Immune precipitation of radiolabelled virus-infected cell proteins with convalescent serum revealed over 20 different proteins could be precipitated (Bala-chandran et al. 1991). At least five glycoproteins were precipitated from infected cells (Balachandran et al. 1991). More recent studies have identified specific viral proteins that are targets of antibody responses including the gB and gH HHV-6 homologues (Ellinger et al. 1993; Liu et al. 1993; Qian et al. 1993). In addition, the major glycoprotein complex of the A variant of HHV-6, gp82-105, has been shown to be a target of neutralizing antibodies (Pfeiffer et al. 1993). A major antigenic protein of HHV-6, designated p100, is the homologue of CMV pp150 (UL32) and probably represents a dominant

target of virus-specific antibodies (Neipel et al. 1992). Cross-reactivity exists between conserved structural proteins such as the major capsid protein and the nonstructural protein CD41 (homologue of CMV pp50 (UL44)) (Loh et al. 1994). Interestingly, cross-reactivity has also been shown between the major envelope glyco-protein of CMV (gB) and HHV-6 (Adler et al. 1993). The serological response to HHV-7 is equally complex, with over 15 radiolabelled infected cell proteins demonstrable by immune precipitation (Foa-Tomasi et al. 1994). Several HHV-7 encoded proteins have been shown to be recognized by immune human serum, including an 80 kDa glycoprotein which probably represents the HHV-7 homologue of gH, the gB homologue, an immunogenic tegument protein of estimated mass of 85 kDa (U14), and p86 (U11) (Foa-Tomasi et al. 1996; Nakagawa et al. 1997; Stefan et al. 1997; Stefan et al. 1999; Franti et al. 2002). Antigenic cross-reactivity between HHV-6 and HHV-7 encoded proteins has also been demonstrated and likely is an explanation for the confusion that surrounds the interpretation of seropreva-lence studies (Foa-Tomasi et al. 1994, 1996; Black and Pellett 1999). Currently, routine serological assays cannot distinguish between the two variants of HHV-6.

Diagnosis

The diagnosis of HHV-6 and/or HHV-7 infection requires the detection of virus, viral antigens or viral nucleic acids in an appropriate specimen from a patient with a clinical syndrome compatible with infection by either of these viruses. HHV-6 and HHV-7 can be recovered with a reasonable degree of success from children in the early phase of exanthem subitum by cocultivation of peripheral blood lymphocytes with umbilical cord lymphocytes. Both HHV-6 and HHV-7 can also be recovered from saliva, although less consistently than from lymphocytes. Other cells suitable for virus isolation include phytohemagglutinin-stimulated PBMC. Cell lines such as HSB2, Sup T1, and Molt-3 have been used to propagate HHV-6, although tropism for specific cell lines may vary (Osman et al. 1993). Isolation of HHV-6 remains a reliable method for the diagnosis of active HHV-6 infection (Carrigan and Knox 2000). Cell lines permissive for HHV-7 have not been described. Viral antigens within infected cells can be readily detected by immunological assays that incorporate HHV-6 or HHV-7 specific monoclonal antibodies (Yamamoto et al. 1990; Ablashi et al. 1993; Parker and Weber 1993). Mono-clonal antibodies can be used to distinguish between HHV-6A and HHV-6B (Foa-Tomasi et al. 1994). Perhaps the most useful assays for HHV-6 and HHV-7 are PCR amplification of specific regions of the viruses. These can be carried out on a number different clinical specimens, including PBMC, saliva, and plasma. The judicious selection of primers allows HHV-7 and the two variants of HHV-6 to be distinguished from one another

(Aubin et al. 1994; Yamamoto et al. 1994; Secchiero et al. 1995). Quantitative PCR assays aid in distinguishing between asymptomatic shedding of HHV-6 and/or HHV-7 and invasive disease (Clark et al. 1996; Kidd et al. 1996; Kidd et al. 2000). Finally, an antigenemia assay similar to the widely employed HCMV antigenemia assay has been used to identify active HHV-6 infection in transplant recipients (Lautenschlager et al. 2002).

Serological assays have yet to be rigorously standardized and, because of significant cross-reactivity between HHV-6 variants and HHV-7, confirmatory testing including absorption with heterologous viral antigens should be considered (Braun et al. 1995; Ward et al. 2001). Antibody avidity assays have been reported that can distinguish between primary HHV-6 and HHV-7 infections (Ward et al. 2001). With the identification of specific viral proteins and their corresponding ORFs, recombinant antigen-based serological assays could overcome issues of cross-reactivity and the high seroprevalence rates in the population.

Control

Although ganciclovir and foscarnet are virustatic for both HHV-6 and HHV-7, current in vitro testing of antiviral susceptibility of these viruses is poorly standardized (Williams 1992). As an example, reports have indicated that some strains of HHV-6 may be relatively resistant to ganciclovir whereas others are susceptible (Akesson-Johansson et al. 1990). Therefore, it is unclear whether adequate in vivo concentrations of drug can be achieved; however, a study in hemapoietic stem cell transplants suggested that ganciclovir treatment resulted in a significant fall in HHV-6 viral burden (Zerr et al. 2002). The HCMV UL97 homologue in HHV-6 (UL69) has been assigned to orf UL69 based on its expression in a recombinant insect virus and its capacity to phosphorylate ganciclovir (Ansari and Emery 1999). Consistent with this finding, some isolates have exhibited drug sensitivities comparable to those reported for CMV. Clinical indications for antiviral therapy will most likely be limited to immunocompromised patients with significant end organ disease; end organ disease such as pneumonitis, in which biopsy tissue could be used to confirm a clinical diagnosis, could be one group that may benefit from antiviral therapy.

REFERENCES

Ablashi, D.V., Balachandran, N., et al. 1991. Genomic polymorphism, growth properties, and immunologic variations in human herpesvirus-6 isolates. *Virology*, **184**, 545–52.

Ablashi, D., Agut, H., et al. 1993. Human herpesvirus-6 strain groups: a nomenclature. *Arch Virol*, **129**, 363–6.

Ablashi, D.V., Berneman, Z.N., et al. 1994. Human herpesvirus-7 (HHV-7). *In Vivo*, **8**, 549–54.

Achim, C.L., Wang, R., et al. 1994. Brain viral burden in HIV infection. *J Neuropathol Exp Neurol*, **53**, 284–93.

Adam, E., Melnick, J.L., et al. 1987. High levels of cytomegalovirus antibody in patients requiring vascular surgery for atherosclerosis. *Lancet*, **2**, 8554, 291–3.

Adler, S.P. 1989. Cytomegalovirus and child day care. Evidence for an increased infection rate among day-care workers. *New Engl J Med*, **321**, 1290–6.

Adler, S.P., McVoy, M., et al. 1993. Antibodies induced by a primary cytomegalovirus infection react with human herpes virus 6 proteins. *J Infect Dis*, **168**, 1119–26.

Adler, S.P., Starr, S.E., et al. 1995. Immunity induced by primary human cytomegalovirus infection protects against secondary infection among women of childbearing age. *J Infect Dis*, **171**, 26–32.

Ahlfors, K., Ivarsson, S.A., et al. 1999. Report on a long-term study of maternal and congenital cytomegalovirus infection in Sweden. Review of prospective studies available in the literature. *Scand J Infect Dis*, **31**, 443–57.

Ahlfors, K., Ivarsson, S.A., et al. 2001. Secondary maternal cytomegalovirus infection – a significant cause of congenital disease. *Pediatrics*, **107**, 5, 1227–8.

Akashi, K., Eizuru, Y., et al. 1993. Brief report: severe infectious mononucleosis-like syndrome and primary human herpesvirus 6 infection in an adult. *New Engl J Med*, **329**, 168–71.

Akesson-Johansson, A., Harmenberg, J., et al. 1990. Inhibition of human herpesvirus 6 replication by 9-[4-hydroxy-2-(hydroxymethyl)butyl]guanine (2HM-HBG) and other antiviral compounds. *Antimicrob Agents Chemother*, **34**, 2417–19.

Akhyani, N., Berti, R., et al. 2000. Tissue distribution and variant characterization of human herpesvirus (HHV)-6: increased prevalence of HHV-6A in patients with multiple sclerosis. *J Infect Dis*, **182**, 5, 1321–5.

Alberola, J., Tamarit, A., et al. 2000. Early neutralizing and glycoprotein B (gB)-specific antibody responses to human cytomegalovirus (HCMV) in immunocompetent individuals with distinct clinical presentations of primary HCMV infection. *J Clin Virol*, **16**, 2, 113–22.

Alberola, J., Tamarit, A., et al. 2001. Longitudinal analysis of human cytomegalovirus glycoprotein B (gB)-specific and neutralizing antibodies in AIDS patients either with or without cytomegalovirus end-organ disease. *J Med Virol*, **64**, 1, 35–41.

Alford, C.A. 1984. Chronic intrauterine and perinatal infections. In: Galasso, G.J., Merigan, T.C. and Buchanan, R.A. (eds), *Antiviral agents and viral diseases of man*, 2nd edn. New York: Raven Press, 433–86.

Ansari, A. and Emery, V.C. 1999. The U69 gene of human herpesvirus 6 encodes a protein kinase which can confer ganciclovir sensitivity to baculoviruses. *J Virol*, **73**, 4, 3284–91.

Asada, H., Klaus-Kovtun, V., et al. 1999. Human herpesvirus 6 infects dendritic cells and suppresses human immunodeficiency virus type 1 replication in coinfected cultures. *J Virol*, **73**, 5, 4019–28.

Asano, Y., Yoshikawa, T., et al. 1990. Fatal fulminant hepatitis in an infant with human herpesvirus 6 infection. *Lancet*, **335**, 862–3.

Asano, Y., Nakashima, T., et al. 1991. Severity of human herpesvirus-6 viremia and clinical findings in infants with exanthem subitum. *J Pediatr*, **118**, 891–5.

Asano, Y., Yoshikawa, T., et al. 1994. Clinical features of infants with primary human herpesvirus 6 infection (exanthem subitum, roeola infantum). *Pediatrics*, **93**, 104–8.

Asano, Y., Suga, S., et al. 1995. Clinical features and viral excretion in an infant with primary human herpesvirus 7 infection. *Pediatrics*, **95**, 187.

Aubert, G., Hassan-Walker, A.F., et al. 2001. Cytomegalovirus-specific cellular immune responses and viremia in recipients of allogeneic stem cell transplants. *J Infect Dis*, **184**, 8, 955–63.

Aubin, J.T., Poirel, L., et al. 1992. Intrauterine transmission of human herpesvirus 6. *Lancet*, **340**, 482–3.

Aubin, J.T., Poirel, L., et al. 1994. Identification of human herpesvirus 6 variants A and B by amplimer hybridization with variant-specific olignonucleotides and amplification with variant-specific primers. *J Clin Microbiol*, **32**, 2434–40.

Autran, B., Carcelain, G., et al. 1997. Positive effects of combined antiretroviral therapy on CD4+ T cell homeostasis and function in advanced HIV disease. *Science*, **277**, 5322, 112–16.

Balachandra, K., Ayuthaya, P.I., et al. 1989. Prevalence of antibody to human herpesvirus 6 in women and children. *Microbiol Immunol*, **33**, 515–18.

Balachandran, N., Tirawatnapong, S., et al. 1991. Electrophoretic analysis of human herpesvirus 6 polypeptides immunoprecipitated from infected cells with human sera. *J Infect Dis*, **163**, 29–34.

Bale, J.F. Jr., Petheram, S.J., et al. 1996. Cytomegalovirus reinfection in young children. *J Pediatr*, **128**, 3, 347–52.

Becroft, D.M.O. 1981. Prenatal cytomegalovirus infection: epidemiology, pathology, and pathogenesis. In: Rosenberg, H.S. and Bernstein, J. (eds), *Perspective in pediatric pathology*, Vol. 6. . New York: Masson Press, 203–41.

Black, J.B., Inoue, N., et al. 1993. Frequent isolation of human herpesvirus 7 from saliva. *Virus Res*, **29**, 91–8.

Black, J.B. and Pellett, P.E. 1999. Human herpesvirus 7. *Rev Med Virol*, **9**, 4, 245–62.

Bodeus, M., Van Ranst, M., et al. 2002. Anti-cytomegalovirus IgG avidity in pregnancy: a 2-year prospective study. *Fetal Diagn Ther*, **17**, 6, 362–6.

Boeckh, M. and Bowden, R. 1995. Cytomegalovirus infection in marrow transplantation. In: Buckner, C.D. (ed.), *Technical and biological components of marrow transplantation*. Boston: Kluwer Academic Publishers, 97–136.

Boeckh, M., Gallez-Hawkins, G.M., et al. 1997. Plasma polymerase chain reaction for cytomegalovirus DNA after allogeneic marrow transplantation: comparison with polymerase chain reaction using peripheral blood leukocytes, pp65 antigenemia, and viral culture. *Transplantation*, **64**, 1, 108–13.

Boeckh, M., Leisenring, W., et al. 2003. Late cytomegalovirus disease and mortality in recipients of allogeneic hematopoietic stem cell transplants: importance of viral load and T-cell immunity. *Blood*, **101**, 2, 407–14.

Boppana, S.B. and Britt, W.J. 1995. Antiviral antibody responses and intrauterine transmission after primary maternal cytomegalovirus infection. *J Infect Dis*, **171**, 1115–21.

Boppana, S.B., Pass, R.F., et al. 1992. Symptomatic congenital cytomegalovirus infection: neonatal morbidity and mortality. *Pediatr Infect Dis J*, **11**, 93–9.

Boppana, S.B., Polis, M.A., et al. 1995. Virus specific antibody responses to human cytomegalovirus (HCMV) in human immunodeficiency virus type 1-infected individuals with HCMV retinitis. *J Infect Dis*, **171**, 182–5.

Boppana, S.B., Fowler, K.B., et al. 1999. Symptomatic congenital cytomegalovirus infection in infants born to mothers with preexisting immunity to cytomegalovirus. *Pediatrics*, **104**, 55–60.

Boppana, S.B., Rivera, L.B., et al. 2001. Intrauterine transmission of cytomegalovirus to infants of women with preconceptional immunity. *New Engl J Med*, **344**, 18, 1366–71.

Boutolleau, D., Fernandez, C., et al. 2003. Human herpesvirus (HHV)-6 and HHV-7: two closely related viruses with different infection profiles in stem cell transplantation recipients. *J Infect Dis*, **187**, 2, 179–86.

Bowden, R.A. 1991. Cytomegalovirus infections in transplant patients: methods of prevention of primary cytomegalovirus. *Transplant Proc*, **23**, 136–8.

Braun, D.K., Pellett, P.E., et al. 1995. Presence and expression of human herpesvirus 6 in peripheral blood mononuclear cells of S100-positive, T cell chronic lymphoproliferative disease. *J Infect Dis*, **171**, 1351–5.

Britt, W., Fay, J., et al. 1995. Formulation of an immunogenic human cytomegalovirus vaccine: responses in experimental animals. *J Infect Dis*, **171**, 18–25.

Britt, W.J. and Alford, C.A. 1996. Cytomegalovirus. In: Fields, B.N., Knipe, D.M. and Howley, P.M. (eds), *Fields virology*. New York: Raven Press, 2493–523.

Britt, W.J., Vugler, L., et al. 1990. Cell surface expression of human cytomegalovirus (HCMV) gp55-116 (gB): use of HCMV-vaccinia recombinant virus infected cells in analysis of the human neutralizing antibody response. *J Virol*, **64**, 1079–85.

Campadelli-Fiume, G., Mirandola, P., et al. 1999. Human herpesvirus 6: An emerging pathogen. *Emerg Infect Dis*, **5**, 3, 353–66.

Carrigan, D.R., Drobyski, W.R., et al. 1991. Interstitial pneumonitis associated with human herpesvirus-6 infection after marrow transplantation. *Lancet*, **338**, 147–9.

Carrigan, D.R. and Knox, K.K. 1994. Human herpesvirus 6 (HHV-6) isolation from bone marrow: HHV-6-associated bone marrow suppression in bone marrow transplant patients. *Blood*, **84**, 3307–10.

Carrigan, D.R. and Knox, K.K. 2000. Human herpesvirus 6: diagnosis of active infection. *Am Clin Lab*, **19**, 7, 12.

Caserta, M.T., Hall, C.B., et al. 1994. Neuroinvasion and persistence of human herpesvirus 6 in children. *J Infect Dis*, **170**, 1586–9.

Caserta, M.T., Hall, C.B., et al. 1998. Primary human herpesvirus 7 infection: a comparison of human herpesvirus 7 and human herpesvirus 6 infections in children. *J Pediatr*, **133**, 3, 386–9.

Caserta, M.T., Mock, D.J., et al. 2001. Human herpesvirus 6. *Clin Infect Dis*, **33**, 6, 829–33.

Challoner, P.B., Smith, K.T., et al. 1995. Plaque-associated expression of human herpesvirus 6 in multiple sclerosis. *Proc Natl Acad Sci USA*, **92**, 7440–4.

Chan, P.K., Peiris, J.S., et al. 1997. Human herpesvirus 6 and human herpesvirus 7 infections in bone marrow transplant recipients. *J Med Virol*, **53**, 3, 295–305.

Chandler, S.H., Holmes, K.K., et al. 1985. The epidemiology of cytomegaloviral infection in women attending a sexually transmitted disease clinic. *J Infect Dis*, **152**, 597–605.

Chandler, S.H., Handsfield, H.H., et al. 1987. Isolation of multiple strains of cytomegalovirus from women attending a clinic for sexually transmitted disease. *J Infect Dis*, **155**, 4, 655–60.

Chern, K.C., Chandler, D.B., et al. 1998. Glycoprotein B subtyping of cytomegalovirus (CMV) in the vitreous of patients with AIDS and CMV retinitis. *J Infect Dis*, **178**, 4, 1149–53.

Clark, D.A. 2000. Human herpesvirus 6. *Rev Med Virol*, **10**, 3, 155–73.

Clark, D.A., Ait-Khaled, M., et al. 1996. Quantification of human herpesvirus 6 in immunocompetent persons and post-mortem tissues from AIDS patients by PCR. *J Gen Virol*, **77**, 2271–5.

Coates, A.R. and Bell, J. 1998. HHV-6 and multiple sclerosis. *Nature Med*, **4**, 5, 537–8.

Cobbs, C.S., Harkins, L., et al. 2002. Human cytomegalovirus infection and expression in human malignant glioma. *Cancer Res*, **62**, 12, 3347–50.

Coen, D.M. 1992. Molecular aspects of anti-herpesvirus drugs. *Sem Virol*, **3**, 3–12.

Collier, A.C., Meyers, J.D., et al. 1987. Cytomegalovirus infection in homosexual men. Relationship to sexual practices, antibody to human immunodeficiency virus, and cell-mediated immunity. *Am J Med*, **23**, 593–601.

Collier, A.C., Chandler, S.H., et al. 1989. Identification of multiple strains of cytomegalovirus in homosexual men. *J Infect Dis*, **159**, 1, 123–6.

Cone, R.W., Hackman, R.C., et al. 1993. Human herpesvirus 6 in lung tissues from patients with pneumonitis after bone marrow transplantation. *New Engl J Med*, **329**, 156–61.

Cone, R.W., Huang, M.L., et al. 1994. Human herpesvirus 6 and pneumonia. *Leuk Lymphoma*, **15**, 235–41.

Cone, R.W., Huang, M.L., et al. 1996. Coinfection with human herpesvirus 6 variants A and B in lung tissue. *J Clin Microbiol*, **34**, 4, 877–81.

Cone, R.W., Huang, M.L., et al. 1999. Human herpesvirus 6 infections after bone marrow transplantation: clinical and virologic manifestations. *J Infect Dis*, **179**, 2, 311–18.

Cope, A.V., Sabin, C., et al. 1997. Interrelationships among quantity of human cytomegalovirus (HCMV) DNA in blood, donor-recipient serostatus, and administration of methylprednisolone as risk factors for HCMV disease following liver transplantation. *J Infect Dis*, **176**, 1484–90.

Curran, M. and Noble, S. 2001. Valganciclovir. *Drugs*, **61**, 1145–50, discussion 1151–2.

Dahl, H., Fjaertoft, G., et al. 1999. Reactivation of human herpesvirus 6 during pregnancy. *J Infect Dis*, **180**, 2035–8.

Davison, A.J., Dolan, A., et al. 2003. The human cytomegalovirus genome revisited: comparison with the chimpanzee cytomegalovirus genome. *J Gen Virol*, **84**, 17–28, [erratum appears in *J Gen Virol*, **84**, 1053.

De Clercq, E. 1998. Antiviral agents that are active against CMV: potential of Cidofovir for the treatment of CMV and other virus infections. In: Scholz, M., Rabenau, H.F., et al. (eds), *CMV-Related immunopathology*. Basel: S. Karger, 193–214.

De La Melena, V.T., Kreklywich, C.N., et al. 2001. Kinetics and development of CMV-accelerated transplant vascular sclerosis in rat cardiac allografts is linked to early increase in chemokine expression and presence of virus. *Transplant Proc*, **33**, 1822–3.

DesJardin, J.A., Cho, E., et al. 2001. Association of human herpesvirus 6 reactivation with severe cytomegalovirus-associated disease in orthotopic liver transplant recipients. *Clin Infect Dis*, **33**, 1358–62.

Dewhurst, S., McIntyre, K., et al. 1993. Human herpesvirus 6 (HHV-6) variant B accounts for the majority of symptomatic primary HHV-6 infections in a population of US infants. *J Clin Microbiol*, **31**, 416–18.

Dockrell, D.H., Prada, J., et al. 1997. Seroconversion to human herpesvirus 6 following liver transplantation is a marker of cytomegalovirus disease. *J Infect Dis*, **176**, 1135–40.

Drago, F., Ranieri, E., et al. 1997. Human herpesvirus 7 in patients with pityriasis rosea. Electron microscopy investigations and polymerase chain reaction in mononuclear cells, plasma, and skin. *Dermatology*, **195**, 374–8.

Drew, W.L., Mintz, L., et al. 1981. Prevalence of cytomegalovirus infection in homosexual men. *J Infect Dis*, **143**, 188–92.

Drew, W.L., Sweet, E.S., et al. 1984. Multiple infections by cytomegalovirus in patients with acquired immune deficiency syndrome: documentation by Southern blot hybridization. *J Infect Dis*, **150**, 952–3.

Drobyski, W.R., Eberle, M., et al. 1993. Prevalence of human herpesvirus 6 variant A and B infections in bone marrow transplant recipients as determined by polymerase chain reaction and sequence-specific oligonucleotide probe hybridization. *J Clin Microbiol*, **31**, 1515–20.

Dunne, W.M. Jr. and Jevon, M. 1993. Examination of human breast milk for evidence of human herpesvirus 6 by polymerase chain reaction. *J Infect Dis*, **168**, 250.

Dworsky, M., Yow, M., et al. 1983. Cytomegalovirus infection of breast milk and transmission in infancy. *Pediatrics*, **72**, 295–9.

Ellinger, K., Neipel, F., et al. 1993. The glycoprotein B homologue of human herpesvirus 6. *J Gen Virol*, **74**, 495–500.

Emery, V.C. 2001. Prophylaxis for CMV should not now replace pre-emptive therapy in solid organ transplantation [comment]. *Rev Med Virol*, **11**, 83–6.

Emery, V.C., Sabin, C.A., et al. 2000. Application of viral-load kinetics to identify patients who develop cytomegalovirus disease after transplantation [comment]. *Lancet*, **355**, 2032–6.

Ensoli, B., Lusso, P., et al. 1989. Human herpesvirus-6 increases HIV-1 expression in co-infected T cells via nuclear factors binding to the HIV-1 enhancer. *EMBO J*, **8**, 3019–27.

Epstein, S.E., Zhou, Y.F., et al. 1999. Infection and atherosclerosis: emerging mechanistic paradigms. *Circulation*, **100**, e20–28.

Fabio, G., Knight, S.N., et al. 1997. Prospective study of human herpesvirus 6, human herpesvirus 7, and cytomegalovirus infections in human immunodeficiency virus-positive patients. *J Clin Microbiol*, **35**, 2657–9.

Fairfax, M.R., Schacker, T., et al. 1994. Human herpesvirus 6 DNA in blood cells of human immunodeficiency virus-infected men: correlation of high levels with high CD4 cell counts. *J Infect Dis*, **169**, 1342–5.

Fishman, J.A. and Rubin, R.H. 1998. Infection in organ-transplant recipients [comment]. *New Engl J Med*, **338**, 1741–51.

Flamand, L., Gosselin, J., et al. 1991. Human herpesvirus 6 induces interleukin-1 beta and tumor necrosis factor alpha, but not interleukin-6, in peripheral blood mononuclear cell cultures. *J Virol*, **65**, 5105–10.

Flamand, L., Stefanescu, I., et al. 1996. Human herpesvirus-6 enhances natural killer cell cytotoxicity via IL-15. *J Clin Invest*, **97**, 1373–81.

Flamand, L., Romerio, F., et al. 1998. CD4 promoter transactivation by human herpesvirus 6. *J Virol*, **72**, 8797–805.

Foa-Tomasi, L., Avitabile, E., et al. 1994. Polyvalent and monoclonal antibodies identify major immunogenic proteins specific for human herpesvirus 7-infected cells and have weak cross-reactivity with human herpesvirus 6. *J Gen Virol*, **75**, 2719–27.

Foa-Tomasi, L., Fiorilli, M.P., et al. 1996. Identification of an kDa phosphoprotein as an immunodominant protein specific for human herpesvirus 7-infected cells. *J Gen Virol*, **77**, 511–18.

Foucar, E., Rosai, J., et al. 1990. Sinus histiocytosis with massive lymphadenopathy (Rosai–Dorfman disease): review of the entity. *Semin Diagn Pathol*, **7**, 19–73.

Fowler, K.B. and Pass, R.F. 1991. Sexually transmitted diseases in mothers of neonates with congenital cytomegalovirus infection. *J Infect Dis*, **164**, 259–64.

Fowler, K.B., Stagno, S., et al. 1992. The outcome of congenital cytomegalovirus infection in relation to maternal antibody status. *New Engl J Med*, **326**, 663–7.

Fowler, K.B., Stagno, S., et al. 1993. Maternal age and congenital cytomegalovirus infection: screening of two diverse newborn populations, 1980–1990. *J Infect Dis*, **168**, 552–6.

Fowler, K.B., McCollister, F.P., et al. 1997. Progressive and fluctuating sensorineural hearing loss in children with asymptomatic congenital cytomegalovirus infection. *J Pediatr*, **130**, 624–30.

Fowler, K.B., Stagno, S., et al. 2003. Maternal immunity and prevention of congenital cytomegalovirus infection. *JAMA*, **289**, 1008–11.

Fox, J., Briggs, M., et al. 1988. Antibody to human herpesvirus 6 in HIV-1 positive and negative homosexual men. *Lancet*, **2**, 396–7.

Francis, N.D., Boylston, A.W., et al. 1989. Cytomegalovirus infection in gastrointestinal tracts of patients infected with HIV-1 or AIDS. *J Clin Pathol*, **42**, 1055–64.

Franti, M., Aubin, J.T., et al. 2002. Immune reactivity of human sera to the glycoprotein B of human herpesvirus 7. *J Clin Microbiol*, **40**, 44–51.

French, C., Menegazzi, P., et al. 1999. Novel, nonconsensus cellular splicing regulates expression of a gene encoding a chemokine-like protein that shows high variation and is specific for human herpesvirus 6. *Virology*, **262**, 139–51.

Frenkel, N. and Wyatt, L.S. 1992. HHV-6 and HHV-7 as exogenous agents in human lymphocytes. *Dev Biol Standard*, **76**, 259–65.

Frenkel, N., Schirmer, E.C., et al. 1990. Isolation of a new herpesvirus from human CD4+ T cells. *Proc Natl Acad Sci USA*, **87**, 748–52.

Frenkel, N., Katsafanas, G.C., et al. 1994. Bone marrow transplant recipients harbor the B variant of human herpesvirus 6. *Bone Marrow Transplant*, **14**, 839–43.

Friedman, J.E., Lyons, M.J., et al. 1999. The association of the human herpesvirus-6 and MS. *Multiple Sclerosis*, **5**, 355–62.

Gallant, J.E., Moore, R.D., et al. 1992. Incidence and natural history of cytomegalovirus disease in patients with advanced human immunodeficiency virus disease treated with zidovudine. *J Infect Dis*, **166**, 1223–7.

Gallez-Hawkins, G., Villacres, M.C., et al. 2003. Use of transgenic HLA A*0201/Kb and HHD II mice to evaluate frequency of cytomegalovirus IE1-derived peptide usage in eliciting human CD8 cytokine response. *J Virol*, **77**, 4457–62.

Gane, E., Saliba, F., et al. 1997. Randomised trial of efficacy and safety of oral ganciclovir in the prevention of cytomegalovirus disease in liver-transplant recipients. *Lancet*, **350**, 1729–33.

Gavin, M.A., Gilbert, M.J., et al. 1993. Alkali hydrolysis of recombinant proteins allows for the rapid identification of class I MHC-restricted CTL epitopes. *J Immunol*, **151**, 3971–80.

Gehrz, R.C., Marker, S.C., et al. 1977. Specific cell-mediated immune defect in active cytomegalovirus infection of young children and their mothers. *Lancet*, **2**, 844–7.

Gehrz, R.C., Christianson, W.R., et al. 1981. Cytomegalovirus specific humoral and cellular immune responses in human pregnancy. *J Infect Dis*, **143**, 391–5.

Gerna, G., Zipeto, D., et al. 1991. Early virus isolation, early structural antigen detection and DNA amplification by the polymerase chain reaction in polymorphonuclear leukocytes from AIDS patients with human cytomegalovirus viraemia. *Mol Cell Probes*, **5**, 365–74.

Gnann, J.W. Jr., Ahlmen, J., et al. 1988. Inflammatory cells in transplanted kidneys are infected by human cytomegalovirus. *Am J Pathol*, **132**, 239–48.

Gompels, U.A., Carrigan, D.R., et al. 1993. Two groups of human herpesvirus 6 identified by sequence analyses of laboratory strains and variants from Hodgkin's lymphoma and bone marrow transplant patients. *J Gen Virol*, **74**, 613–22.

Gompels, U.A., Nicholas, J., et al. 1995. The DNA sequence of human herpesvirus 6: structure, coding content, and genome evolution. *Virology*, **209**, 29–51.

Goodrich, J.M., Bowden, R.A., et al. 1993. Ganciclovir prophylaxis to prevent cytomegalovirus disease after allogeneic marrow transplant. *Ann Intern Med*, **118**, 173–8.

Grattan, M.T., Moreno-Cabral, C.E., et al. 1989. Cytomegalovirus infection is associated with cardiac allograft rejection and atherosclerosis. *JAMA*, **261**, 3561–6.

Griffiths, P.D., Stagno, S., et al. 1982. Infection with cytomegalovirus during pregnancy: specific IgM antibodies as a marker of recent primary infection. *J Infect Dis*, **145**, 647–53.

Griffiths, P.D., Ait-Khaled, M., et al. 1999. Human herpesviruses 6 and 7 as potential pathogens after liver transplant: prospective comparison with the effect of cytomegalovirus. *J Med Virol*, **59**, 496–501.

Griffiths, P.D., Clark, D.A., et al. 2000. Betaherpesviruses in transplant recipients. *J Antimicrob Chemother*, **45**, Suppl T3, 29–34.

Grundy, J.E., Shanley, J.D., et al. 1987. Is cytomegalovirus interstitial pneumonitis in transplant recipients an immunopathological condition? *Lancet*, **2**, 996–9.

Hall, C.B., Long, C.E., et al. 1994. Human herpesvirus-6 infection in children. A prospective study of complications and reactivation. *New Engl J Med*, **331**, 432–8.

Handsfield, H.H., Chandler, S.H., et al. 1985. Cytomegalovirus infection in sex partners: evidence for sexual transmission. *J Infect Dis*, **151**, 344–8.

Harkins, L., Volk, A.L., et al. 2002. Specific localisation of human cytomegalovirus nucleic acids and proteins in human colorectal cancer. *Lancet*, **360**, 1557–63.

Harnett, G.B., Farr, T.J., et al. 1990. Frequent shedding of human herpesvirus 6 in saliva. *J Med Virol*, **30**, 128–30.

Hasegawa, A., Yasukawa, M., et al. 2001. Transcriptional down-regulation of CXC chemokine receptor 4 induced by impaired association of transcription regulator YY1 with c-Myc in human herpesvirus 6-infected cells. *J Immunol*, **166**, 1125–31.

Hayes, K., Alford, C.A., et al. 1987. Antibody response to virus-encoded proteins after cytomegalovirus mononucleosis. *J Infect Dis*, **156**, 615–21.

Hebart, H., Schroder, A., et al. 1997. Cytomegalovirus monitoring by polymerase chain reaction of whole blood samples from patients undergoing autologous bone marrow or peripheral blood progenitor cell transplantation. *J Infect Dis*, **175**, 1490–3.

Hidaka, Y., Liu, Y., et al. 1993. Frequent isolation of human herpesvirus 7 from saliva samples. *J Med Virol*, **40**, 343–6.

Ho, M. (ed.) 1991. *Cytomegalovirus biology and infection*. New York: Plenum Press.

Ho, M., Suwansirikul, S., et al. 1975. The transplanted kidney as a source of cytomegalovirus infections. *New Engl J Med*, **293**, 1109–12.

Hoshino, K., Nishi, T., et al. 1995. Human herpesvirus 6 infection in renal allografts: retrospective immunohistochemical study in Japanese recipients. *Transplant Int*, **8**, 169–73.

Humar, A., Malkan, G., et al. 2000. Human herpesvirus-6 is associated with cytomegalovirus reactivation in liver transplant recipients. *J Infect Dis*, **181**, 1450–3.

Humar, A., Kumar, D., et al. 2002. Cytomegalovirus (CMV) virus load kinetics to predict recurrent disease in solid-organ transplant patients with CMV disease. *J Infect Dis*, **186**, 829–33.

Imbert-Marcille, B.M., Tang, X.W., et al. 2000. Human herpesvirus 6 infection after autologous or allogeneic stem cell transplantation: a single-center prospective longitudinal study of 92 patients. *Clin Infect Dis*, **31**, 881–6.

Inoue, N., Dambaugh, T.R., et al. 1993. Molecular biology of human herpesvirus 6A and 6B. *Infect Agent Dis*, **2**, 343–60.

Isegawa, Y., Mukai, T., et al. 1999. Comparison of the complete DNA sequences of human herpesvirus 6 variants A and B. *J Virol*, **73**, 8053–63.

Ishiguro, N., Yamada, S., et al. 1990. Meningo-encephalitis associated with HHV-6 related exanthem subitum. *Acta Paediatr Scand*, **79**, 987–9.

Jacobson, M.A. and Mills, J. 1988. Serious cytomegalovirus disease in the acquired immunodeficiency syndrome (AIDS). *Ann Intern Med*, **108**, 585–94.

Jesionek, A. and Kiolemenoglou, B. 1904. Uber einen befund von protozoenartigen gebilden in den organen eines heriditarluetischen fotus. *Munch Med Wochenschr*, **51**, 1905–7.

Jordan, M.C. 1983. Latent infection and the elusive cytomegalovirus. *Rev Infect Dis*, **5**, 205–15.

Kashanchi, F., Thompson, J., et al. 1994. Transcriptional activation of minimal HIV-1 promoter by ORF-1 protein expressed from the Sall-L fragment of human herpesvirus-6. *Virology*, **201**, 95–106.

Kasolo, F.C., Mpabalwani, E., et al. 1997. Infection with AIDS-related herpesviruses in human immunodeficiency virus-negative infants and endemic childhood Kaposi's sarcoma in Africa. *J Gen Virol*, **78**, 847–55.

Kaur, A., Kassis, N., et al. 2003. Direct relationship between suppression of virus-specific immunity and emergence of cytomegalovirus disease in simian AIDS. *J Virol*, **77**, 5749–58.

Kern, F., Surel, I.P., et al. 1999. Target structures of the CD8[+]-T-cell response to human cytomegalovirus: the 72-kilodalton major immediate-early protein revisited. *J Virol*, **73**, 8179–84.

Kern, F., Bunde, T., et al. 2002. Cytomegalovirus (CMV) phosphoprotein 65 makes a large contribution to shaping the T cell repertoire in CMV-exposed individuals. *J Infect Dis*, **185**, 1709–16.

Kidd, I.M., Clark, D.A., et al. 1996. Measurement of human herpesvirus 7 load in peripheral blood and saliva of healthy subjects by quantitative polymerase chain reaction. *J Infect Dis*, **174**, 396–401.

Kidd, I.M., Clark, D.A., et al. 2000. Prospective study of human betaherpesviruses after renal transplantation: association of human herpesvirus 7 and cytomegalovirus co-infection with cytomegalovirus disease and increased rejection. *Transplantation*, **69**, 2400–4.

Kikuta, H., Nakane, A., et al. 1990. Interferon induction by human herpesvirus 6 in human mononuclear cells. *J Infect Dis*, **162**, 35–8.

Kimberlin, D.W., Lin, C.Y., et al. 2003. Effect of ganciclovir therapy on hearing in symptomatic congenital cytomegalovirus disease involving the central nervous system: a randomized, controlled trial. *J Pediatr*, **143**, 16–25.

Klemola, E., Von Essen, R., et al. 1970. Infectious mononucleosis-like disease with negative heterophil agglutination test. Clinical features in relation to Epstein-Barr virus and cytomegalovirus antibodies. *J Infect Dis*, **121**, 608–14.

Knox, K.K., Brewer, J.H., et al. 2000. Human herpesvirus 6 and multiple sclerosis: systemic active infections in patients with early disease. *Clin Infect Dis*, **31**, 894–903.

Knox, K.K. and Carrigan, D.R. 1992. In vitro suppression of bone marrow progenitor cell differentiation by human herpesvirus 6 infection. *J Infect Dis*, **165**, 925–9.

Knox, K.K. and Carrigan, D.R. 1994. Disseminated active HHV-6 infections in patients with AIDS. *Lancet*, **343**, 577–8.

Komanduri, K.V., Viswanathan, M.N., et al. 1998. Restoration of cytomegalovirus-specific CD4+ T-lymphocyte responses after ganciclovir and highly active antiretroviral therapy in individuals infected with HIV-1. *Nature Med*, **4**, 953–6.

Kondo, K., Nagafuji, H., et al. 1993. Association of human herpesvirus 6 infection of the central nervous system with recurrence of febrile convulsions. *J Infect Dis*, **167**, 1197–200.

Kositanont, U., Wasi, C., et al. 1999. Primary infection of human herpesvirus 6 in children with vertical infection of human immunodeficiency virus type 1. *J Infect Dis*, **180**, 50–5.

Koskinen, P.K., Kallio, E.A., et al. 1999. Cytomegalovirus infection and cardiac allograft vasculopathy. *Transplant Infect Dis*, **1**, 115–26.

Kosuge, H., Tanaka-Taya, K., et al. 2000. Epidemiological study of human herpesvirus-6 and human herpesvirus-7 in pityriasis rosea [comment]. *Br J Dermatol*, **143**, 795–8.

Krmpotic, A., Busch, D.H., et al. 2002. MCMV glycoprotein gp40 confers virus resistance to CD8+ T cells and NK cells in vivo [comment]. *Nature Immunol*, **3**, 529–35.

Kropff, B., Landini, M.P., et al. 1993. An ELISA using recombinant proteins for the detection of neutralizing antibodies against human cytomegalovirus. *J Med Virol*, **39**, 187–95.

Kurata, T., Kwasaki, T., et al. 1990. Viral pathology of human herpesvirus 6 infection. In: Lopez, C., Mori, R., et al. (eds), *Immunobiology and prophylaxis of human herpesvirus infections*. New York: Plenum Press, 39–47.

Kusuhara, K., Ueda, K., et al. 1991. Do second attacks of exanthema subitum result from human herpesvirus 6 reactivation or reinfection? *Pediatr Infect Dis J*, **10**, 468–70.

Lalezari, J., Lindley, J., et al. 2002. A safety study of oral valganciclovir maintenance treatment of cytomegalovirus retinitis. *J Acquir Immune Defic Syndr*, **30**, 392–400.

Landini, M.P. 1993. New approaches and perspectives in cytomegalovirus diagnosis. *Prog Med Virol*, **40**, 157–77.

Landini, M.P., Baldassarri, B., et al. 1988. Reactivity of cytomegalovirus structural polypeptides with different subclasses of IgG present in human serum. *J Infect Dis*, **16**, 163–7.

Lautenschlager, I., Lappalainen, M., et al. 2002. CMV infection is usually associated with concurrent HHV-6 and HHV-7 antigenemia in liver transplant patients. *J Clin Virol*, **25**, Suppl 2, S57–61.

Lawrence, G.L., Chee, M., et al. 1990. Human herpesvirus 6 is closely related to human cytomegalovirus. *J Virol*, **64**, 287.

Lazzarotto, T., Ripalti, A., et al. 1998. Development of a new cytomegalovirus (CMV) immunoglobulin M (IgM) immunoblot for detection of CMV-specific IGM. *J Clin Microbiol*, **36**, 3337–41.

Lazzarotto, T., Spezzacatena, P., et al. 1999. Anticytomegalovirus (anti-CMV) immunoglobulin G avidity in identification of pregnant women at risk of transmitting congenital CMV infection. *Clin Diag Lab Immunol*, **6**, 127–9.

Leach, C.T., Cherry, J.D., et al. 1993. The relationship between T-cell levels and CMV infection in asymptomatic HIV-1 antibody-positive homosexual men. *J Acquir Immune Defic Syndr*, **6**, 407–13.

Leach, C.T., Newton, E.R., et al. 1994. Human herpesvirus 6 infection for the female genital tract. *J Infect Dis*, **169**, 1281–3.

Lemstrom, K., Sihvola, R., et al. 1997. Cytomegalovirus infection-enhanced cardiac allograft vasculopathy is abolished by DHPG prophylaxis in the rat. *Circulation*, **95**, 2614–16.

Levine, P.H., Jahan, N., et al. 1992. Detection of human herpesvirus 6 in tissues involved by sinus histiocytosis with massive lymphadenopathy (Rosai-Dorfman disease). *J Infect Dis*, **166**, 291–5.

Levy, J.A., Ferro, F., et al. 1990a. Frequent isolation of HHV-6 from saliva and high seroprevalence of the virus in the population. *Lancet*, **335**, 1047–50.

Levy, J.A., Landay, A., et al. 1990b. Human herpesvirus 6 inhibits human immunodeficiency virus type 1 replication in cell culture. *J Clin Microbiol*, **28**, 2362–4.

Li, C.R., Greenberg, P.D., et al. 1994. Recovery of HLA-restricted cytomegalovirus (CMV)-specific T-cell responses after allogeneic bone marrow transplant: correlation with CMV disease and effect of ganciclovir prophylaxis. *Blood*, **83**, 1971–9.

Libby, P. 2002. Inflammation in atherosclerosis. *Nature*, **420**, 868–74.

Liu, D.X., Gompels, U.A., et al. 1993. Identification and expression of the human herpesvirus 6 glycoprotein H and interaction with an accessory 40k glycoprotein. *J Gen Virol*, **74**, 1847–57.

Ljungman, P. 2001. Prophylaxis against herpesvirus infections in transplant recipients. *Drugs*, **61**, 187–96.

Ljungman, P. 2002. Beta-herpesvirus challenges in the transplant recipient. *J Infect Dis*, **186**, Suppl 1, S99–S109.

Lockridge, K.M., Sequar, G., et al. 1999. Pathogenesis of experimental rhesus cytomegalovirus infection. *J Virol*, **73**, 9576–83.

Loh, L.C., Britt, W.J., et al. 1994. Sequence analysis and expression of the murine cytomegalovirus phosphoprotein pp50, a homolog of the human cytomegalovirus UL44 gene product. *Virology*, **200**, 413–27.

Lowance, D., Neumayer, H.H., et al. 1999. Valacyclovir for the prevention of cytomegalovirus disease after renal transplantation. International Valacyclovir Cytomegalovirus Prophylaxis Transplantation Study Group. *New Engl J Med*, **340**, 1462–70.

Lucht, E., Brytting, M., et al. 1998. Shedding of cytomegalovirus and herpesvirus 6, 7, and 8 in saliva of human immunodeficiency virus type 1-infected patients and healthy controls. *Clin Infect Dis*, **27**, 137–41.

Luppi, M., Barozzi, P., et al. 1994. Human herpesvirus 6 infection in normal human brain tissue. *J Infect Dis*, **169**, 943–4.

Lusso, P. and Gallo, R.C. 1995. Human herpesvirus 6 in AIDS. *Immunol Today*, **16**, 67–71.

Lusso, P., De Maria, A., et al. 1991. Induction of CD4 and susceptibility to HIV-1 infection in human CD8+ T lymphocytes by human herpesvirus 6. *Nature*, **349**, 533–5.

Lusso, P., Secchiero, P., et al. 1994. CD4 is a critical component of the receptor for human herpesvirus 7: interference with human immunodeficiency virus. *Proc Natl Acad Sci USA*, **91**, 3872–6.

Martin, D.F., Sierra-Madero, J., et al. 2002. A controlled trial of valganciclovir as induction therapy for cytomegalovirus retinitis. *New Engl J Med*, **346**, 1119–26, [erratum appears in *New Engl J Med* 2002 **347**, 862.

Martin, M.E.D., Thomson, B.J., et al. 1991. The genome of human herpesvirus 6: maps of unit-length and concatemeric genomes for nine restriction endonucleases. *J Gen Virol*, **72**, 157–68.

McCracken, G.J., Shinefield, H.R., et al. 1969. Congenital cytomegalic inclusion disease. A longitudinal study of 20 patients. *Am J Dis Child*, **117**, 522–39.

Megaw, A.G., Rapaport, D., et al. 1998. The DNA sequence of the RK strain of human herpesvirus 7. *Virology*, **244**, 119–32.

Mendez, J.C., Dockrell, D.H., et al. 2001. Human beta-herpesvirus interactions in solid organ transplant recipients. *J Infect Dis*, **183**, 179–84.

Meyers, J.D. 1991. Critical evaluation of agents used in the treatment and prevention of cytomegalovirus infection in immunocompromised patients. *Transplant Proc*, **23**, 139–43.

Meyers, J.D., Flournoy, N., et al. 1982. Nonbacterial pneumonia after allogeneic marrow transplantation: a review of ten years' experience. *Rev Infect Dis*, **4**, 1119–32.

Michaelides, A., Glare, E.M., et al. 2002. beta-Herpesvirus (human cytomegalovirus and human herpesvirus 6) reactivation in at-risk lung transplant recipients and in human immunodeficiency virus-infected patients. *J Infect Dis*, **186**, 173–80.

Miller, E., Waight, P., et al. 1997. The epidemiology of rubella in England and Wales before and after the 1994 measles and rubella vaccination campaign: fourth joint report from the PHLS and the National Congenital Rubella Surveillance Programme. Communicable Disease Report. *CDR Rev*, **7**, R26–32.

Miller, H., Rossier, E., et al. 1991. Prospective study of cytomegalovirus antigenemia in allograft recipients. *J Clin Microbiol*, **29**, 1054–5.

Mirandola, P., Stefan, A., et al. 1999. Absence of human herpesvirus 6 and 7 from spinal fluid and serum of multiple sclerosis patients. *Neurology*, **53**, 1367–8.

Mocarski, E.S. and Tan Courcelle, C. 2001. Cytomegaloviruses and their replication. In: Knipe, D.M., Howley, P.M., et al. (eds), *Fields virology*, Vol. 2. Philadelphia: Lippincott Williams and Wilkins, 2629–73.

Mukai, T., Yamamoto, T., et al. 1994. Molecular epidemiological studies of human herpesvirus 6 in families. *J Med Virol*, **42**, 224–7.

Murph, J.R., Bale, J.F., et al. 1986. Cytomegalovirus transmission in a Midwest day care center: possible relationship to child care practices. *J Pediatr*, **109**, 35–9.

Murph, J.R., Souza, I.E., et al. 1998. Epidemiology of congenital cytomegalovirus infection: maternal risk factors and molecular analysis of cytomegalovirus strains. *Am J Epidemiol*, **147**, 940–7.

Myerson, D., Hackman, R.C., et al. 1984. Widespread presence of histologically occult cytomegalovirus. *Hum Pathol*, **15**, 430–9.

Nakagawa, N., Mukai, T., et al. 1997. Antigenic analysis of human herpesvirus 7 (HHV-7) and HHV-6 using immune sera and monoclonal antibodies against HHV-7. *J Gen Virol*, **78**, 1131–7.

Neipel, F., Ellinger, K., et al. 1992. Gene for the major antigenic structural protein (p100) of human herpesvirus 6. *J Virol*, **66**, 3918–24.

Ohashi, M., Yoshikawa, T., et al. 2002. Reactivation of human herpesvirus 6 and 7 in pregnant women. *J Med Virol.*, **67**, 354–8.

Okada, K., Ueda, K., et al. 1993. Exanthema subitum and human herpesvirus 6 infection: clinical observations in fifty-seven cases. *Pediatr Infect Dis J*, **12**, 204–8.

Okuno, T., Takahashi, K., et al. 1989. Seroepidemiology of human herpesvirus 6 infection in normal children and adults. *J Clin Microbiol*, **27**, 651–3.

Okuno, T., Higashi, K., et al. 1990. Human herpesvirus 6 infection in renal transplantation. *Transplantation*, **49**, 519–22.

Osman, H.K., Wells, C., et al. 1993. Growth characteristics of human herpesvirus-6: comparison of antigen production in two cell lines. *J Med Virol*, **39**, 303–11.

O'Sullivan, C.E., Drew, W.L., et al. 1999. Decrease of cytomegalovirus replication in human immunodeficiency virus infected-patients after treatment with highly active antiretroviral therapy [comment]. *J Infect Dis*, **180**, 847–9.

Palestine, A.G., Polis, M.A., et al. 1991. A randomized, controlled trial of foscarnet in the treatment of cytomegalovirus retinitis in patients with AIDS. *Ann Intern Med*, **115**, 665–73.

Parker, C.A. and Weber, J.M. 1993. An enzyme-linked immunosorbent assay for the detection of IgG and IgM antibodies to human herpesvirus type 6. *J Virol Meth*, **41**, 265–75.

Pass, R.F., Britt, W.J., et al. 1995. Cytomegalovirus. In: Lennette, E.H., Lennette, D.A. and Lennette, E.T. (eds), *Diagnostic procedures for viral, rickettsial and chlamydial infections*, 7th edn. Washington, DC: APHA, 253–71.

Pass, R.F., Duliege, A.M., et al. 1999. A subunit cytomegalovirus vaccine based on recombinant envelope glycoprotein B and a new adjuvant. *J Infect Dis*, **180**, 970–5.

Pass, R.F., Stagno, S., et al. 1983. Specific cell mediated immunity and the natural history of congenital infection with cytomegalovirus. *J Infect Dis*, **148**, 953–61.

Pass, R.F., Little, E.A., et al. 1987. Young children as a probable source of maternal and congenital cytomegalovirus infection. *New Engl J Med*, **316**, 1366–70.

Paya, C.V., Wilson, J.A., et al. 2002. Preemptive use of oral ganciclovir to prevent cytomegalovirus infection in liver transplant patients: a randomized, placebo-controlled trial. *J Infect Dis*, **185**, 854–60.

Perillie, P.E. and Glenn, W.W.L. 1962. Fever, splenomegaly and eosinophilia: a new postpericardiotomy syndrome. *Yale J Biol Med*, **34**, 625–8.

Pertel, P., Hirschtick, R., et al. 1992. Risk of developing cytomegalovirus retinitis in persons infected with the human immunodeficiency virus. *J Acquir Immune Defic Syndr*, **5**, 1069–74.

Pescovitz, M.D., Rabkin, J., et al. 2000. Valganciclovir results in improved oral absorption of ganciclovir in liver transplant recipients. *Antimicrob Agents Chemother*, **44**, 2811–15.

Petrie, B.L., Adam, E., et al. 1988. Association of herpesvirus/ cytomegalovirus infections with human atherosclerosis. *Prog Med Virol*, **35**, 21–42.

Pfeiffer, B., Berneman, Z.N., et al. 1993. Identification and mapping of the gene encoding the glycoprotein complex gp82-gp105 of human herpesvirus 6 and mapping of the neutralizing epitope recognized by monoclonal antibodies. *J Virol*, **67**, 4611–20.

Plotkin, S.A., Starr, S.E., et al. 1991. Effect of Towne live virus vaccine on cytomegalovirus disease after renal transplant. A controlled trial. *Ann Intern Med*, **114**, 525–31.

Prince, A.M., Szumuness, W., et al. 1971. A serologic study of cytomegalovirus infections associated with blood transfusions. *New Engl J Med*, **284**, 1125–31.

Pruksananonda, P., Hall, C.B., et al. 1992. Primary human herpesvirus 6 infection in young children. *New Engl J Med*, **326**, 1445–50.

Qian, G., Wood, C., et al. 1993. Identification and characterization of glycoprotein gH of human herpesvirus-6. *Virology*, **194**, 380–6.

Rasmussen, L. 1990. Immune response to human cytomegalovirus infection. *Curr Top Microbiol Immunol*, **154**, 222–54.

Rasmussen, L., Matkin, C., et al. 1991. Antibody response to human cytomegalovirus glycoproteins gB and gH after natural infection in humans. *J Infect Dis*, **164**, 835–42.

Razonable, R.R., Brown, R.A., et al. 2002. The clinical use of various blood compartments for cytomegalovirus (CMV) DNA quantitation in transplant recipients with CMV disease. *Transplantation*, **73**, 968–73.

Reeves, W.C., Stamey, F.R., et al. 2000. Human herpesviruses 6 and 7 in chronic fatigue syndrome: a case-control study. *Clin Infect Dis*, **31**, 48–52.

Reusser, P., Riddell, S.R., et al. 1991. Cytotoxic T-lymphocyte response to cytomegalovirus after human allogeneic bone marrow transplantation: pattern of recovery and correlation with cytomegalovirus infection and disease. *Blood*, **78**, 1373–80.

Revello, M.G. and Gerna, G. 2002. Diagnosis and management of human cytomegalovirus infection in the mother, fetus, and newborn infant. *Clin Microbiol Rev*, **15**, 680–715.

Reyman, T.A. 1966. Postperfusion syndrome: a review and report of 21 cases. *Am Heart J*, **72**, 116–23.

Rubin, R. 2002. Clinical approach to infection in the compromised host. In: Rubin, R. and Young, L.S. (eds), *Infection in the organ transplant recipient*. New York: Kluwer Academic Press, 573–679.

Salahuddin, S.Z., Ablashi, D.V., et al. 1986. Isolation of a new virus, HBLV, in patients with lymphoproliferative disorders. *Science*, **234**, 596–600.

Santoro, F., Kennedy, P.E., et al. 1999. CD46 is a cellular receptor for human herpesvirus 6. *Cell*, **99**, 817–27.

Saxinger, C., Polesky, H., et al. 1988. Antibody reactivity with HBLV (HHV-6) in US populations. *J Virol Method*, **21**, 199–208.

Schirmer, E.C., Wyatt, L.S., et al. 1991. Differentiation between two distinct classes of viruses now classified as human herpesvirus 6. *Proc Natl Acad Sci USA*, **88**, 5922–6.

Schmidbauer, M., Budka, H., et al. 1989. Cytomegalovirus (CMV) disease of the brain in AIDS and connatal infection: a comparative study by histology, immunocytochemistry and in situ DNA hybridization. *Acta Neuropathol (Berl)*, **79**, 286–93.

Schmidt, C.A., Wilbron, F., et al. 1996. A prospective study of human herpesvirus type 6 detected by polymerase chain reaction after liver transplantation. *Transplantation*, **61**, 662–4.

Schmidt, G.M., Horak, D.A., et al. 1991. A randomized, controlled trial of prophylactic ganciclovir for cytomegalovirus pulmonary infection in recipients of allogeneic bone marrow transplants. *New Engl J Med*, **324**, 1005–11.

Schoppel, K., Kropff, B., et al. 1997. The humoral immune response against human cytomegalovirus is characterized by a delayed synthesis of glycoprotein-specific antibodies. *J Infect Dis*, **175**, 533–44.

Secchiero, P., Carrigan, D.R., et al. 1995. Detection of human herpesvirus 6 in plasma of children with primary infection and immunosuppressed patients by polymerase chain reaction. *J Infect Dis*, **171**, 273–80.

Secchiero, P., Flamand, L., et al. 1997. Human herpesvirus 7 induced CD4⁺ T-cell death by two distinct mechanisms: necrotic lysis in productively infected cells and apoptosis in uninfected or nonproductively infected cells. *Blood*, **90**, 4502–12.

Seu, P., Winston, D.J., et al. 1997. Long-term ganciclovir prophylaxis for successful prevention of primary cytomegalovirus (CMV) disease in CMV-seronegative liver transplant recipients with CMV-seropositive donors. *Transplantation*, **64**, 1614–17.

Singh, N. 2000. Human herpesviruses-6, -7 and -8 in organ transplant recipients. *Clin Microbiol Infect*, **6**, 453–9.

Singh, N. 2001. Preemptive therapy versus universal prophylaxis with ganciclovir for cytomegalovirus in solid organ transplant recipients. *Clin Infect Dis*, **32**, 742–51.

Singh, N., Dummer, J.S., et al. 1988. Infections with cytomegalovirus and other herpesviruses in 121 liver transplant recipients: transmission by donated organ and the effect of OKT3 antibodies. *J Infect Dis*, **158**, 124–31.

Smyth, R.L., Scott, J.P., et al. 1991. Cytomegalovirus infection in heart-lung transplant recipients: risk factors, clinical associations, and response to treatment. *J Infect Dis*, **164**, 1045–50.

Snoeck, R., Neyts, J., et al. 1993. Strategies for the treatment of cytomegalovirus infections. In: Michelson, S. and Plotkin, S.A. (eds), *Multidisciplinary approach to understanding cytomegalovirus disease*. Amsterdam: Elsevier Science Publishers, 269–78.

Snydman, D.R. 1993. Review of the efficacy of cytomegalovirus immune globulin in the prophylaxis of CMV disease in renal transplant recipients. *Transplant Proc*, **25**, Suppl 4, 25–6.

Soderberg-Naucler, C., Fish, K.N., et al. 1997. Reactivation of latent human cytomegalovirus by allogeneic stimulation of blood cells from healthy donors. *Cell*, **91**, 119–26.

Soldan, S.S., Leist, T.P., et al. 2000. Increased lymphoproliferative response to human herpesvirus type 6A variant in multiple sclerosis patients. *Ann Neurol*, **47**, 306–13.

Spector, S.A., Hirata, K.K., et al. 1984. Identification of multiple cytomegalovirus strains in homosexual men with acquired immunodeficiency syndrome. *J Infect Dis*, **150**, 953–6.

Spector, S.A., Merrill, R., et al. 1992. Detection of human cytomegalovirus in plasma of AIDS patients during acute visceral disease by DNA amplification. *J Clin Microbiol*, **30**, 2359–65.

Spector, S.A., Weingeist, T., et al. 1993. A randomized, controlled study of intravenous ganciclovir therapy for cytomegalovirus peripheral retinitis in patients with AIDS. AIDS Clinical Trials Group and Cytomegalovirus Cooperative Study Group. *J Infect Dis*, **168**, 557–63.

Spector, S.A., McKinley, G.F., et al. 1996. Oral ganciclovir for the prevention of cytomegalovirus disease in persons with AIDS. *New Engl J Med*, **334**, 1491–7.

Speir, E., Modali, R., et al. 1994. Potential role of human cytomegalovirus and p53 interaction in coronary restenosis. *Science*, **265**, 391–4.

Spira, T.J., Bozeman, L.H., et al. 1990. Lack of correlation between human herpesvirus-6 infection and the course of human immunodeficiency virus infection. *J Infect Dis*, **161**, 567–70.

Stagno, S., Reynolds, D.W., et al. 1975. Comparative serial virologic and serologic studies of symptomatic and subclinical congenitally and natally acquired cytomegalovirus infections. *J Infect Dis*, **132**, 568–77.

Stagno, S., Cloud, G., et al. 1984. Factors associated with primary cytomegalovirus infection during pregnancy. *J Med Virol*, **13**, 347–53.

Stagno, S., Tinker, M.K., et al. 1985. Immunoglobulin M antibodies detected by enzyme-linked immunosorbent assay and radioimmunoassay in the diagnosis of cytomegalovirus infections in pregnant women and newborn infants. *J Clin Microbiol*, **21**, 930–5.

Steeper, T.A., Horwitz, C.A., et al. 1990. The spectrum of clinical and laboratory findings resulting from human herpesvirus-6 in patients with mononucleosis-like illnesses not resulting from Epstein–Barr virus or cytomegalovirus. *Am J Clin Pathol*, **93**, 776–83.

Stefan, A., Secchiero, P., et al. 1997. The 85-kilodalton phosphoprotein (pp85) of human herpesvirus 7 is encoded by open reading frame U14

and localizes to a tegument substructure in virion particles. *J Virol*, **71**, 5758–63.

Stefan, A., De Lillo, M., et al. 1999. Development of recombinant diagnostic reagents based on pp85(U14) and p86(U11) proteins to detect the human immune response to human herpesvirus 7 infection. *J Clin Microbiol*, **37**, 3980–5.

Streblow, D.N., Orloff, S.L., et al. 2001. Do pathogens accelerate atherosclerosis? *J Nutr*, **131**, 2798S–804S.

Streblow, D.N., Kreklywich, C., et al. 2003. Cytomegalovirus-mediated upregulation of chemokine expression correlates with the acceleration of chronic rejection in rat heart transplants. *J Virol.*, **77**, 2182–94.

Suga, S., Yoshikawa, T., et al. 1993. Clinical and virological analyses of 21 infants with exanthem subitum and central nervous system complications. *Ann Neurol*, **33**, 597–603.

Suga, S., Yoshikawa, T., et al. 1997. Clinical features and virological findings in children with primary human herpesvirus 7 infection. *Pediatrics*, **99**, E4.

Sullivan, V., Talarico, C.L., et al. 1992. A protein kinase homologue controls phosphorylation of ganciclovir in human cytomegalovirus-infected cells. *Nature*, **358**, 162–4.

Sullivan, V., Biron, K.K., et al. 1993. A point mutation in the human cytomegalovirus DNA polymerase gene confers resistance to ganciclovir and phosphonylmethoxyalkyl derivatives. *Antimicrob Agents Chemother*, **37**, 19–25.

Sun, J.C. and Bevan, M.J. 2003. Defective CD8 T cell memory following acute infection without CD4 T cell help. *Science*, **300**, 339–42.

Tajiri, H., Nose, O., et al. 1990. Human herpesvirus-6 infection with liver injury in neonatal hepatitis. *Lancet*, **335**, 863.

Takahashi, K., Sonoda, S., et al. 1988. Human herpesvirus 6 and exanthem subitum. *Lancet*, **i**, 1463.

Takahashi, K., Sonoda, S., et al. 1989. Predominant CD4 T-lymphocyte tropism of human herpesvirus 6-related virus. *J Virol*, **63**, 3161–3.

Takahashi, K., Segal, E., et al. 1992. Interferon and natural killer cell activity in patients with exanthem subitum. *Pediatr Infect Dis J*, **11**, 369–73.

Tanaka, K., Kondo, T., et al. 1994. Human herpesvirus 7: another causal agent for roseola. *J Pediatr*, **125**, 1–5.

Tejada-Simon, M.V., Zang, Y.C., et al. 2002. Detection of viral DNA and immune responses to the human herpesvirus 6 101-kilodalton virion protein in patients with multiple sclerosis and in controls. *J Virol*, **76**, 6147–54.

Tong, C.Y., Bakran, A., et al. 2000. Association of human herpesvirus 7 with cytomegalovirus disease in renal transplant recipients. *Transplantation*, **70**, 213–16.

Torigoe, S., Kumamoto, T., et al. 1995. Clinical manifestations associated with human herpesvirus 7 infection. *Arch Dis Child*, **72**, 518–19.

Ueda, K., Kusuhara, K., et al. 1989. Exanthem subitum and antibody to human herpesvirus-6. *J Infect Dis*, **159**, 750–2.

van den Berg, A.P., van der Bij, W., et al. 1989. Cytomegalovirus antigenemia as a useful marker of symptomatic cytomegalovirus infection after renal transplantation: a report of 130 consecutive patients. *Transplantation*, **48**, 991–5.

van der Bij, W., Torensma, R., et al. 1988. Rapid immunodiagnosis of active cytomegalovirus infection by monoclonal antibody staining of blood leucocytes. *J Med Virol*, **25**, 179–88.

Vinters, H.V., Kwok, M.K., et al. 1989. Cytomegalovirus in the nervous system of patients with the acquired immune deficiency syndrome. *Brain*, **112**, 245–68.

Waldrop, S.L., Pitcher, C.J., et al. 1997. Determination of antigen-specific memory/effector CD4+ T cell frequencies by flow cytometry. Evidence for a novel, antigen-specific homeostatic mechanism in HIV-associated immunodeficiency. *J Clin Invest*, **99**, 1739–50.

Walter, E.A., Greenberg, P.D., et al. 1995. Reconstitution of cellular immunity against cytomegalovirus in recipients of allogeneic bone marrow by transfer of T-cell clones from the donor. *New Engl J Med*, **333**, 1038–44.

Wang, J., Jones, C., et al. 1994. Identification and characterization of a human herpesvirus 6 gene segment capable of transactivating the human immunodeficiency virus type 1 long terminal repeat in an Sp1 binding site-dependent manner. *J Virol*, **68**, 1706–13.

Ward, K.N., Turner, D.J., et al. 2001. Use of immunoglobulin G antibody avidity for differentiation of primary human herpesvirus 6 and 7 infections. *J Clin Microbiol*, **39**, 959–63.

Weir, M.R., Henry, M.L., et al. 1988. Incidence and morbidity of cytomegalovirus disease associated with a seronegative recipient receiving seropositive donor-specific transfusion and living related donor transplantation: a multicenter evaluation. *Transplantation*, **45**, 111–16.

Wilborn, F., Brinkmann, V., et al. 1994a. Herpesvirus type 6 in patients undergoing bone marrow transplantation: serologic features and detection by polymerase chain reaction. *Blood*, **83**, 3052–8.

Wilborn, F., Schmidt, C.A., et al. 1994b. A potential role for human herpesvirus type 6 in nervous system disease. *J Neuroimmunol*, **49**, 213–14.

Williams, M.V. 1992. HHV-6: response to antiviral agents. In: Ablashi, D.V., Krueger, G.R.F. and Salahuddin, S.Z. (eds), *Human herpesvirus-6: Epidemiology, molecular biology, and clinical pathology*. Amsterdam: Elsevier Biomedical Press, 317–35.

Winston, D.J., Ho, W.G., et al. 1990. Cytomegalovirus infections after bone marrow transplantation. *Rev Infect Dis*, **12**, S776–92.

Wyatt, L.S. and Frenkel, N. 1992. Human herpesvirus 7 is a constitutive inhabitant of adult human saliva. *J Virol*, **66**, 3206–9.

Wyatt, L.S., Balachandran, N., et al. 1990. Variations in the replication and antigenic properties of human herpesvirus 6 strains. *J Infect Dis*, **162**, 852–7.

Wyatt, L.S., Rodriguez, W.J., et al. 1991. Human herpesvirus 7: antigenic properties and prevalence in children and adults. *J Virol*, **65**, 6260–5.

Yakushijin, Y., Yasukawa, M., et al. 1992. Establishment and functional characterization of human herpesvirus 6-specific CD4+ human T-cell clones. *J Virol*, **66**, 2773–9.

Yamamoto, M., Black, J.B., et al. 1990. Identification of a nucleocapsid protein as a specific serological marker of human herpesvirus 6 infection. *J Clin Microbiol*, **28**, 1957–62.

Yamamoto, T., Mukai, T., et al. 1994. Variation of DNA sequence in immediate-early gene of human herpesvirus 6 and variant identification by PCR. *J Clin Microbiol*, **32**, 473–6.

Yamamoto, A.P., Mussi-Pinhata, M.M., et al. 2001. Congenital cytomegalovirus infection in preterm and full-term newborn infants from a population with a high seroprevalence rate. *Pediatr Infect Dis J*, **20**, 188–92.

Yamanishi, K., Okuno, T., et al. 1988. Identification of human herpesvirus 6 as causal agent for exanthem subitum. *Lancet*, **1**, 1065–7.

Yanagi, K., Harada, S., et al. 1990. High prevalence of antibody to human herpesvirus 6 and decrease in titer in age in Japan. *J Infect Dis*, **161**, 153–4.

Yasukawa, M., Yakushijin, Y., et al. 1993. Specificity analysis of human CD4+ T-cell clones directed against human herpesvirus 6 (HHV-6), HHV-7, and human cytomegalovirus. *J Virol*, **67**, 6259–64.

Yoshida, M., Torigoe, S., et al. 2002. Neutralizing antibody responses to human herpesviruses 6 and 7 do not cross-react with each other, and maternal neutralizing antibodies contribute to sequential infection with these viruses in childhood. *Clin Diagn Lab Immunol*, **9**, 388–93.

Yoshikawa, T. and Asano, Y. 2000. Central nervous system complications in human herpesvirus-6 infection. *Brain Dev*, **22**, 307–14.

Yoshikawa, T., Suga, S., et al. 1991. Human herpesvirus-6 infection in bone marrow transplantation. *Blood*, **78**, 1381–4.

Yoshikawa, T., Nakashima, T., et al. 1992. Human herpesvirus-6 DNA in cerebrospinal fluid of a child with exanthem subitum and meningoencephalitis. *Pediatrics*, **89**, 888–90.

Yoshikawa, T., Asano, Y., et al. 1993. Seroepidemiology of human herpesvirus 7 in healthy children and adults in Japan. *J Med Virol*, **41**, 319–23.

Yoshikawa, T., Asano, Y., et al. 2002. Human herpesvirus 6 viremia in bone marrow transplant recipients: clinical features and risk factors. *J Infect Dis*, **185**, 847–53.

Yow, M.D., Williamson, D.W., et al. 1988. Epidemiologic characteristics of cytomegalovirus infection in mothers and their infants. *Am J Obstet Gynecol*, **158**, 1189–95.

Zaia, J.A. 2002. Prevention and management of CMV-related problems after hematopoietic stem cell transplantation. *Bone Marrow Transplant*, **29**, 633–8.

Zaia, J.A., Forman, S.J., et al. 1986. Polypeptide-specific antibody response to human cytomegalovirus after infection in bone marrow transplant recipients. *J Infect Dis*, **153**, 780–7.

Zerr, D.M., Gupta, D., et al. 2002. Effect of antivirals on human herpesvirus 6 replication in hematopoietic stem cell transplant recipients. *Clin Infect Dis*, **34**, 309–17.

Zhang, Y., Hatse, S., et al. 2000. CXC-chemokine receptor 4 is not a coreceptor for human herpesvirus 7 entry into CD4+ T cells. *J Virol*, **74**, 2011–16.

Zhou, Y., Chang, C.K., et al. 1994. *trans*-activation of the HIV promoter by a cDNA and its genomic clones of human herpesvirus-6. *Virology*, **199**, 311–22.

Zhou, Y.F., Leon, M.B., et al. 1996. Association between prior cytomegalovirus infection and the risk of restenosis after coronary atherectomy [comment]. *New Engl J Med*, **335**, 624–30.

Zhu, J., Quyyumi, A.A., et al. 1999. Cytomegalovirus in the pathogenesis of atherosclerosis: the role of inflammation as reflected by elevated C-reactive protein levels. *J Am Coll Cardiol*, **34**, 1738–43.

28

Human herpesvirus 8

BERNHARD FLECKENSTEIN AND FRANK NEIPEL

PROPERTIES OF THE VIRUS

DISCOVERY OF THE VIRUS

Kaposi's sarcoma (KS), first described in 1872 by the Viennese dermatologist Moriz Kaposi (Kaposi 1872) in the classic form, has since been known as a peculiar semi-malignant tumor of the skin. It afflicted mainly elderly men of southern or east European descent. The frequent appearance of an unusually aggressive form of KS in young homosexual men was one of the observations marking the advent of the acquired immune deficiency syndrome (AIDS) epidemic in developed countries (Friedman Kien et al. 1982). The uneven distribution of KS amongst different transmission groups for the human immunodeficiency virus (HIV) resulted in the hypothesis that an environmental factor or a transmissible agent other than HIV is involved in KS pathogenesis (Beral et al. 1990). Most notably, whereas more than 20 percent of homosexual and bisexual AIDS patients developed KS, only 1 percent of age- and sex-matched men with hemophilia suffered from this uncommon tumor, suggesting – amongst others – transmission of a KS-related virus by sexual practice. Application of representational difference analysis (Lisitsyn et al. 1993) a polymerase chain reaction (PCR)-based method, resulted in the identification of two short DNA fragments from a new herpesvirus (Chang et al. 1994). The virus is now termed human herpesvirus 8 (HHV-8) or Kaposi's sarcoma-associated herpesvirus (KSHV). The latter name reflects a finding that was previously claimed in the paper describing the identification of HHV-8 (Chang et al. 1994). HHV-8 DNA is regularly found in KS tissues, but not in uninvolved skin or the vast majority of other malignancies. These include most solid tumors as well as various lymphomas. The few notable exceptions identified to date are two types of B-cell lymphoma or lymphoproliferative lesion, namely primary effusion lymphoma (PEL), and the plasma-cell-rich variant of multifocal Castleman disease (MCD). Similar to KS, HHV-8 DNA is almost always present in PEL and in the majority of MCD cases, suggesting a causative role of the virus in oncogenesis.

CLASSIFICATION

HHV-8 is the first and only known human member of the genus *Rhadinovirus* or γ_2-herpesvirus. This classification is based on DNA homology between the HHV-8 genome and that of other γ_2-herpesviruses (McGeoch 2001).

Related primate rhadinoviruses

Rhadinoviruses have been known for many years as animal viruses infecting primates (Fleckenstein and Desrosiers 1982; Fleckenstein et al. 1978), rodents and ungulates (Table 28.1). These viruses are usually widespread and generally apathogenic in their natural host. However, upon infection of closely related but distinct species, several animal rhadinoviruses are known to induce diseases, such as malignant catarrhal fever in

Table 28.1 *The genus* Rhadinovirus

Virus type	Natural host	Pathogenicity in natural host	Foreign hosts	Pathogenic properties in foreign hosts
Human herpesvirus type 8	Human	Kaposi's sarcoma, MCD, PEL		
Herpesvirus saimiri	Squirrel monkey		Marmosets, etc.	Polyclonal malignant T-cell lymphomas
Herpesvirus ateles	Spider monkey		Marmosets, etc.	Polyclonal malignant T-cell lymphomas
Rhesus monkey rhadinovirus	Rhesus monkey	Lymphadenopathy		
Retroperitoneal fibromatosis-associated herpesvirus of *Macaca mulatta*/*Macaca nemestrina*	*Macaca mulatta*/*Macaca nemestrina*	Retroperitoneal fibromatosis?		?
Pan troglotydes rhadinovirus-1	Chimpanzee	?	?	?
Gorilla rhadinovirus-1	Gorilla	?	?	?
Alcelaphine herpesvirus type 1	Wildebeest		Cattle, buffalo	Malignant catarrhal fever
Ovine herpesvirus type 2	Sheep		Cattle	Malignant catarrhal fever
Bovine herpesvirus type 4	Cattle			
Equine herpesvirus type 2	Horse	Transient immunosuppression in foals		
Herpesvirus sylvilagus	Cottontail rabbit	(Benign) lymphoproliferative syndrome		
Murine herpesvirus-68	Wood mouse		Mouse	Benign splenomegaly

Various primate- and nonprimate rhadinoviruses, their natural host and, if applicable, foreign hosts as well as pathogenic properties in a foreign host are given. Please note that in the case of Pan troglotydes rhadinovirus-1, Gorilla rhadinovirus-1, and the retroperitoneal fibromatosis-associated rhadinoviruses, the complete virus has not thus far been isolated. Only fragments from the DNA polymerase gene could be amplified and sequenced using a degenerate PCR approach.

cattle or T-cell lymphoma in certain neotropical primates (Table 28.1).

HERPESVIRUS SAIMIRI

Herpesvirus saimiri is a well-studied example of this group (Fickenscher and Fleckenstein 2001). Herpesvirus saimiri is apathogenic in its natural host, the squirrel monkey *Saimiri sciureus*. However, closely related new world primates like the marmoset succumb with highly malignant T-cell proliferation upon experimental infection with herpesvirus saimiri. Certain strains of herpesvirus saimiri effectively transform cultured human T-lymphocytes (Biesinger et al. 1992). The genes responsible for growth transformation are essentially known, and nontransforming deletion mutants have been generated. In contrast to HHV-8, the closely related herpesvirus saimiri can be effectively propagated in cell culture. It has thus been used as a model system for HHV-8 (Lee et al. 1998; Jung et al. 1999).

RHESUS RHADINOVIRUS

The discovery of HHV-8/KSHV as the first human rhadinovirus in 1994 stimulated the search for rhadinoviruses in other Old World primates. Serological studies using HHV-8-derived antigens indicated that a herpesvirus closely related to HHV-8 may exist in rhesus monkeys. Co-cultivation of lymphocytes from seropositive rhesus monkeys with fibroblasts resulted in the isolation of a novel rhesus rhadinovirus (RRV) (Desrosiers et al. 1997). The complete genomic sequences from two independent RRV isolates are available (Alexander et al. 2000; Searles et al. 1999). This revealed that RRV is indeed more closely related to HHV-8 than the prototypic rhadinovirus herpesvirus saimiri (HVS). The genomes of RRV and HHV-8 are essentially colinear. RRV contains (at least) 84 genes, 80 of which are homologous to genes found in HHV-8. Thus, at this point in time RRV is the closest known relative of HHV-8 which has been fully sequenced. RRV seems to be very widespread amongst monkeys kept in captivity. No clear disease association has been identified for RRV in otherwise healthy macaques as yet. However, inoculation with RRV resulted in the development of a multifocal lymphoproliferative disease when rhesus macaques were immunosuppressed as a consequence of infection with simian immunodeficiency virus (Alexander et al. 2000; Wong et al. 1999). In contrast to HHV-8, RRV can be readily propagated in cell culture.

RETROPERITONEAL FIBROSIS RHADINOVIRUSES

In a second approach targeted at the identification of Old World primate rhadinoviruses, Rose and co-workers studied tissue specimens from simian retroperitoneal fibromatosis (RF). RF has been identified as an infrequent disease syndrome occurring in immunosuppressed macaques (Giddens et al. 1985). RF lesions consist of an aggressively proliferating fibrous tissue with a high degree of vascularization and thus remotely resemble KS. Transmission studies indicated that an infectious agent may be involved in RF pathogenesis (Giddens et al. 1985). By using a degenerated PCR technique, fragments of a herpesvirus DNA polymerase gene were identified in RF tissues from two macaque species, *Macaca nemestrina* and *Macaca mulatta* (Rose et al. 1997). Sequence comparisons indicated that at least the DNA polymerase genes of these two novel rhadinoviruses, tentatively termed RFHVMm and RFHVMn, are more closely related to KSHV than the DNA polymerase genes of RRV. However, attempts to isolate these viruses on cultured cells or to obtain additional sequence information have not been successful so far.

HHV-8 VIRION MORPHOLOGY

The morphology of the enveloped HHV-8 virion is comparable to other herpesviruses. The three-dimensional structure of the human herpesvirus 8 capsid has been determined by cryo-electronmicroscopy using viral particles produced from cultured primary effusion lymphoma (PEL) cells at a resolution of 22–24 Å (Trus et al. 2001; Wu et al. 2000). The HHV-8 capsid is similar to those of other herpesviruses, especially herpes simplex virus-1. The icosahedral capsid shell is composed of 162 capsomers (12 pentons, 150 hexons).

MOLECULAR BIOLOGY

Genome structure

The HHV-8 genome is a linear, double-stranded DNA of approximately 160 kbp and has the overall structure typical for rhadinoviruses (Figure 28.1). A complete rhadinovirus genome is usually termed M genome, as it is of inter*m*ediate density (M-DNA). The γ2-herpesviruses were termed rhadinoviruses utilizing the ancient Greek word for fragile, because this M-DNA tends to split into two fractions of DNA molecules with highly different density, the L-DNA containing genes (low density, low G+C content) and the terminal repetitive H-DNA (high density, high G+C content). The latter is, as far as currently known, without coding capacity. The almost complete nucleotide sequence of HHV-8 was determined from both a PEL cell line (Russo et al. 1996) and from a KS biopsy specimen (Neipel et al. 1997b). The central low-GC (53.3 percent G+C, L-DNA) coding fragment is flanked by numerous tandem repeats of high GC content (84.5 percent G+C, H-DNA). The L-DNA contains at least 89 open reading frames, 67 of which have homologues in the closely related γ2-herpesvirus prototype herpesvirus saimiri (Figure 28.1). The overall amino acid sequence identity of these 67 HHV-8 reading frames to homologues identified in herpesvirus saimiri ranges from

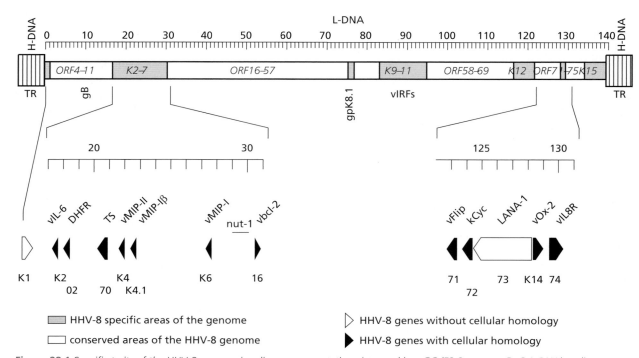

Figure 28.1 *Specific traits of the HHV-8 genome in a linear representation. A central low-GC (53.3 percent G+C, L-DNA) coding fragment is flanked by numerous tandem repeats (TR) of high G+C content (84.5 percent G+C, H-DNA). The L-DNA contains at least 89 open reading frames, most of which have homologues in other herpesviruses. These blocks of conserved herpesvirus genes are symbolized by open boxes in the upper half of the figure. They are interrupted by nonconserved areas shown in light gray. Most of the HHV-8 genes thought to be directly involved in pathogenesis – either by direct growth transformation or through paraendocrine mechanisms – are located within these HHV-8-specific areas. They are shown enlarged in the lower part of the figure. Black arrows indicate HHV-8 genes with homology to cellular genes. HHV-8 genes without known homology to cellular genes are shown as open arrows. HHV-8 reading frames that share homology with herpesvirus saimiri were assigned the corresponding reading frame numbers following the nomenclature by Albrecht et al. (1992). HHV-8 genes without recognizable homologues in herpesvirus saimiri were numbered separately and given the prefix K (K1–K15) (Russo et al. 1996). DHFR, dihydrofolate reductase; gB, glycoprotein B; gpK8.1, glycoprotein K8.1; kCyc, HHV-8 cyclin-D homologue; nut-1, nuclear tRNA-like transcript; TS, thymidylate syntase; vbcl-2, viral bcl-2; vFlip, viral FLICE inhibitory protein; vIL-6, viral interleukin-6; vIL8R, viral interleukin-8 receptor; vIRFs, viral interferon response factor homologue; vMIP-I/II, viral macrophage inflammatory protein-I/II; vMIP-1β, open reading frame with homology to macrophage inflammatory protein-1β or macrophage chemoattractant protein; vOx-2, viral Ox-2 homologous gene.*

22.4 to 66 percent (average, 42 percent). Conserved genes are usually found in a comparable genomic position and orientation. Thus, HHV-8 genes that share homology with herpesvirus saimiri are numbered from left to right according to their position on the herpesvirus saimiri genome. Open reading frames which do not share recognizable amino acid homology with genes in herpesvirus saimiri are numbered with the prefix K (Figure 28.1). To date, 19 genes have been identified which are not clearly homologous to genes identified in herpesvirus saimiri (K1–K15, K4.1, K4.2, K8.1, K10.5). Frequently, these 'K'-genes are strikingly homologous to known cellular genes. They code for proteins interfering with the immune system, for enzymes of the nucleotide metabolism, and for putative regulators of cell growth (Figure 28.1).

Virus-coded proteins

Human herpesvirus-8 DNA is present in the vast majority of KS spindle cells and primary effusion

lymphoma B cells. The virus establishes a latent infection in these cells: virus progeny is not produced and only a limited set of viral genes is expressed. Whereas the HHV-8 genome is quickly lost from cultured KS spindle cells, cultured PEL cells maintain the viral genome. The full lytic program is spontaneously activated in only a few cells of a PEL culture (<1 percent). However, lytic replication can be induced in up to 5–40 percent of PEL cells by the addition of phorbol esters and/or sodium butyrate (Renne et al. 1996). Genes expressed during the HHV-8 lytic replication cycle have been essentially studied on cultured PEL cells treated with such agents. Most of these genes have pronounced homology to those of other herpesviruses. Although de novo infection of cultured cells has not been studied extensively, HHV-8 lytic genes have been divided into immediate–early, early, and late depending on their temporal expression following reactivation from latently infected, cultured cells: (1) transcription of immediate–early genes is inducible by TPA/butyrate even in the presence of agents blocking protein biosynthesis; (2)

expression of early genes requires the presence of immediate–early protein, but takes place in the absence of DNA replication; (3) transcription of late viral genes does not take place when DNA replication is inhibited. This temporal gene expression pattern where one set of genes is activated by genes expressed earlier during the lytic cycle was initially defined using herpes simplex virus and de novo infection of cultured cells. The situation in HHV-8 is different so far, as most data on temporal gene regulation were derived from latently infected PEL cells where lytic replication of the virus is activated by phorbol esters or sodium butyrate. In an alternative classification, HHV-8 transcripts were divided into three groups according to their inducibility by tetradecanoylphorbol acetate (TPA) (Sarid et al. 1998). Class I genes were transcribed constitutively, i.e. under standard growth conditions without the addition of stimulating agents like TPA; their expression did not increase when the lytic cycle was induced by TPA. Class I genes were mapped to a region close to the right end of the L-DNA encoding ORF73 (latent nuclear antigen 1, LANA), ORF72 (viral cyclin-D, vCyclin) and ORF71 (viral flice inhibitory protein, vFLIP). They constitute bona fide latently expressed genes. Class II transcripts were detectable without TPA treatment, but clearly induced to higher transcription by the addition of TPA. Essentially, immediate–early and early genes belong to this intermediate class. Until today, three immediate–early transcripts have been identified in HHV-8: ORF4.2, ORF45, and ORF50 (Zhu et al. 1999). Class III transcripts were not detectable without stimulation of cultured PEL cells by TPA or butyrate. Essentially, they comprise the late, structural proteins of HHV-8.

Lytic regulatory proteins

The lytic regulatory proteins of HHV-8 studied so far include open reading frame 50, also termed replication and transcription activator (RTA), Lyta (lytic transactivator) or ART (activator or replication and transcription), K8 (also termed K-bZip), and ORF45. As in vitro transmission of the virus is still laborious and inefficient, most data were obtained from PEL cells or transfection studies using permanent cell lines.

ORF50 codes for the key immediate–early regulator protein required for the switch from latent to lytic infection. ORF45 seems to be involved in counteracting the interferon response very early in infection. K8 protein is expressed with early kinetics and plays a role in HHV-8 DNA replication.

ORF50/K-RTA

ORF50 is translated from a 3.6-kb spliced mRNA that also contains the reading frames coding for K8. Due to an additional 5′ exon, the whole ORF50 protein comprises 691 amino acids with a calculated molecular weight of 73.7 kDa. It shares limited homology with the R-*trans*-activator of EBV (16 percent amino acid identity, 30 percent similarity), and was hence initially termed K-RTA. It is well established that RTA or ART of HHV-8 is the key immediate–early regulator protein of HHV-8. In cultured PEL cells, RTA is both sufficient and required for the switch from latent infection to lytic replication (Lukac et al. 1998, 1999). It *trans*-activates the expression of several early and delayed-early genes of HHV-8, including K8, ORF57 (Byun et al. 2002), and ORF59. In addition, RTA of HHV-8 interacts with CREB binding protein (CBP) and thus represses transcriptional activity of p53 and p53-induced apoptosis (Hwang et al. 2001). By direct interaction with cellular STAT3, ORF50 mediates STAT3 nuclear translocation, dimerization, and activation of STAT3-dependent transcription without prior phosphorylation of STAT3 (Byun et al. 2002).

ORF45-PROTEIN

A second immediate–early transcript of 1.7 kb was mapped to the ORF45 locus. ORF45 has the capacity to encode a protein of 407 amino acids and 43.3 kDa. Genes homologous to ORF45 of HHV-8 are conserved amongst the γ-herpesviruses. HHV-8 ORF45 seems to interact with cellular interferon-regulatory factor 7 (IRF-7) (Zhu et al. 2002). It inhibits IRF-7 phosphorylation and accumulation in the nucleus. Phosphorylation and nuclear translocation of IRF-7 normally results in activation of type I interferon genes. Thus, ORF45 could inhibit the activation of interferon very early in viral infection by blocking phosphorylation of IRF-7.

K8/K-BZIP

K-bZip is a 237 amino acid early nuclear protein. It includes a basic leucine zipper motif (K-bZIP), and is distantly related to the EBV lytic-cycle Z *trans*-activator (ZTA) protein. However, in HHV-8 the lytic cycle is induced by ORF50, and the role of HHV-8 K8 seems to be distinct. A 1.3-kb transcript that is not detectable until delayed early in the HHV-8 infectious cycle seems to contribute largely to K8/K-bZip protein synthesis (Saveliev et al. 2002). More compatible with the delayed early expression of K8 is its role as a negative regulator of ORF50 expression (Izumiya et al. 2003) and its function in DNA replication. Both in infected cells and in transfection assays, K-bZip is recruited into viral DNA replication compartments (Wu et al. 2001). Recent data indicate that K8, which also locates to the POD/ND10 domains, mediates arrest of the cell cycle in G1 phase (Wu et al. 2002). There is increasing evidence that herpesviral DNA replication takes place preferentially in G1 arrested cells to avoid competition with host-cell DNA replication (Flemington 2001). Thus, in contrast to its distant relative ZTA in EBV, the K-bZip of HHV-8 plays an important role in DNA replication and is hence also termed RAP (replication associated protein).

Virion proteins

VIRAL CAPSID PROTEINS

Detailed study of HHV-8 proteins forming the viral nucleocapsid has been hindered by the lack of an efficient lytic cell culture system. The major capsid protein is encoded by ORF25. Triplex proteins are encoded by ORF62 and ORF26, also termed minor capsid protein. The immunogenic ORF65 protein is also part of the nucleocapsid (Trus et al. 2001).

GLYCOPROTEINS

As in other herpesviruses, HHV-8 envelope glycoproteins play a crucial role in target cell recognition and entry. HHV-8 encodes at least five envelope glycoproteins, four of which (gB, gH, gL, gM) are conserved throughout the *Herpesviridae*. The function of two glycoproteins, gB and the HHV-8-specific K8.1, has been studied in more detail. Both are involved in binding of HHV-8 to its cellular attachment or entry receptors, heparan sulfate, and integrin $\alpha_3\beta_1$, respectively.

Glycoprotein K8.1

The gene encoding glycoprotein K8.1 (gpK8.1) is located approximately in the middle of the HHV-8 genome (Figure 28.1) within a block of conserved genes. However, as the designation as gpK8.1 indicates, it does not share recognizable homology with genes present in any other herpesvirus. gpK8.1 is translated from alternatively spliced messages giving rise to two variants, gpK8.1A and gpK8.1B, the larger A form being predominant. gpK8.1 is a major target for the humoral immunoresponse, and the glycoprotein is thus frequently a component of serological assays for HHV-8 (Chandran et al. 1998; Raab et al. 1998). gpK8.1 is part of the virion envelope and involved in attachment to target cells by binding to cell surface heparan sulfate (Birkmann et al. 2001).

Glycoprotein B

The conserved herpesvirus glycoprotein B (gB) is encoded close to the left end of the HHV-8 L-DNA (Figure 28.1). Like gpK8.1, gB has been shown to be part of the virion envelope. It binds to cell surface glycosaminoglycans (Akula et al. 2001). In addition, gB binds to integrin $\alpha_3\beta_1$, and this interaction seems to be involved in the entry of HHV-8 into target cells (Akula et al. 2002). The use of integrins as an entry receptor suggest that HHV-8 enters the cell by endocytotic pathways. This, however, is rather unusual for a herpesvirus. Although endocytosis of virions has been shown to occur with other herpesviruses, especially herpes simplex virus (Nicola et al. 2003), the biologically relevant way of infection by a herpesvirus is usually fusion of the virion envelope with the cytoplasma membrane at neutral pH.

Latent proteins

It is a common feature of oncogenic viruses that lytic replication is turned off in the vast majority of transformed cells. Essentially, this holds true for HHV-8. At least in Kaposi's sarcoma lesions and primary effusion lymphoma cells, expression of HHV-8 structural proteins is observed in only few cells (Figure 28.2a, b), whereas the viral genome is present in almost all tumor cells in a latent state with only few genes being expressed (Figure 28.2c, d). Although this observation does clearly not exclude that the lytic cycle genes play a role in HHV-8 pathogenesis, the few latent genes expressed by the vast majority of cells are particularly important for understanding HHV-8 biology and pathogenesis. Unfortunately, known latently expressed genes of EBV and, with few exceptions, HVS are not conserved in KSHV. Until recently, latent transcripts have been identified from only three loci of the HHV-8 genome. The major latency locus was found close to the right end of the genome (Figure 28.1). It comprises genes encoding the latency associated nuclear antigen 1 (LANA-1), a viral cyclin D homologue (k-cyclin, Figure 28.2d), and the viral anti-apoptotic flice inhibitory protein (v-Flip). Several transcripts of K12 (Kaposin) are also detectable both in KS and PEL. The third locus maps to the middle of the genome where various genes with homology to the interferon-regulatory protein family of transcription factors can be found. At least in PEL cells, two of these transcripts can be detected in latent infection.

LATENT NUCLEAR ANTIGEN 1 (LANA-1, LNA-1)

An area close to the right end of the HHV-8 L-DNA was consistently found to be transcriptionally active in latency. It comprises *orf71/vFLIP*, *orf72/k-cyclin*, and *orf73/LANA-1*. LANA-1 (LNA-1) was initially identified as the major antigen detected by KS patient sera in latently infected PEL cells (Gao et al. 1996a; Rainbow et al. 1997). It is now clear that LANA-1 is important for maintenance of the episomal HHV-8 genome in latently infected cells (Ballestas et al. 1999; Ballestas and Kaye 2001). It can therefore be seen as a functional analog of the Epstein–Barr virus nuclear antigen 1, which mediates maintenance of the latent EBV-episome by binding to the plasmid origin of replication, oriP. However, the *cis*-sequence required for HHV-8 LANA-1 to fulfil its function seems to be located within the high-density terminal repeats (Hu et al. 2002). Due to their high GC-content, the H-DNA differs clearly

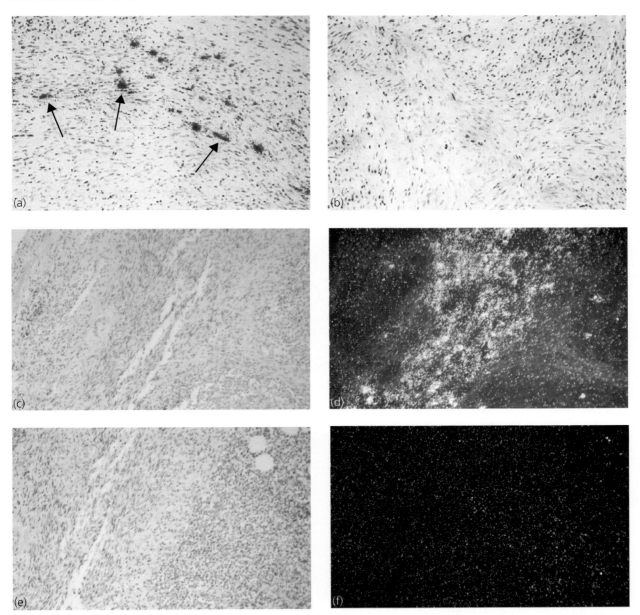

Figure 28.2 *Expression of HHV-8 genes in Kaposi's sarcoma. Lytic cycle genes like the minor capsid protein are detectable in only a few cells in a KS lesion* **(a)**. *The majority of spindle cells carry the HHV-8 genome in a latent state, and transcripts mapping to the k-cyclin locus are detectable* **(d)**. **(a)** *Productively HHV-8-infected cells in KS tumors were identified by in situ hybridization with strand-specific radiolabeled RNA probes directed against the mRNA coding for the HHV-8 minor capsid protein (VP23) Signals can be seen overlying single cells* **(a)**, *which are arranged in clusters between the KS spindle cells. HHV-8-positive cells are marked by arrows. Their distribution suggests that at least part of the positive cells are monocytes. Magnification, ×3 500.* **(b)** *Control hybridization. No staining was observed when a surplus of the unlabeled sense-strand RNA probe was applied to the tissue sections simultaneously with the radiolabeled antisense RNA probe. Magnification ×3 500.* **(c,d)** *Prominent signals in the majority of KS spindle cells were obtained when a probe against k-cyclin was used (c, bright field; d, dark field). A consecutive section of the same KS tissue specimen was hybridized with a HHV-8 minor capsid protein probe (VP23; e, bright field; d, dark field). The VP23 gene was not expressed in this section, indicating a more predominantly latent infection than in the sample shown in* **(a)** *(modified from Stürzl et al. (1999) and Blasig et al. (1997) with permission).*

from oriP or other eukaryotic origins of DNA replication. In addition to its well established function in maintenance of the viral genome, LANA-1 has been described to inhibit p53 and to provide protection from cell death (Friborg et al. 1999; Radkov et al. 2000). Recent data indicate that LANA stimulates S-phase entry by stabilizing β-catenin (Fujimuro et al. 2003). In summary, the latency-associated nuclear antigen 1 of HHV-8 is a multifunctional protein involved in maintenance episomal DNA, transcription regulation, and cell cycle control possibly contributing to cell transformation.

VFLIP

The viral FLIP (FLICE/caspase-8 inhibiting protein) is homologous to a cellular apoptosis inhibitor. Bi-cistronic transcripts comprising both the viral cyclin-D homologue and vFlip are detectable in latently infected cells (Figure 28.2b). It may play an important role in HHV-8 pathogenesis by blocking apoptosis induced by antiviral cytotoxic T cells (Thome et al. 1997) or growth factor withdrawal (Sun et al. 2003).

K-CYCLIN

Transcription of the HHV-8 encoded cyclin D homologue (k-cyclin) is driven from the same latent promoter as transcription of ORF73/LANA. It is the first gene on a bi-cistronic message also encoding vFLIP. k-Cyclin has been shown to associate with the catalytic subunit cdk6 to form an active holoenzyme (Li et al. 1997; Godden-Kent et al. 1997). This complex is able to phosphorylate retinoblastoma protein and to stimulate cell cycle progression from G1 to S in quiescent fibroblasts. It is especially important that the activity of the k-cyclin/cdk6 holoenzyme was resistant to inhibition by CDK inhibitory proteins $p21^{cip1}$ and $p27^{Kip1}$ (Swanton et al. 1997). These distinctive features of k-cyclin biochemistry were expanded by two papers published later (Ellis et al. 1999; Mann et al. 1999). Not only is the k-cyclin/cdk6 complex resistant to inhibition by $p27^{kip1}$, it also has a broader substrate range including $p27^{kip1}$ and substrates of cdk2. Phosphorylation of $p27^{kip1}$ results in the proteolytic degradation of this CDK-inhibitor and progression of cells arrested in G1 to S (Ellis et al. 1999; Mann et al. 1999). Deregulation of the G1/S restriction point is a feature shared by many tumor cells and DNA tumor viruses (reviewed by Pines (1995)). It is therefore intriguing to speculate that k-cyclin is involved in HHV-8 pathogenesis. However, it must be noted that at present there is no direct, experimental evidence for a transforming ability of the cyclin D homologue encoded by HHV-8, and the viral cyclin homologue has been shown to be dispensable for oncogenic transformation by the closely related herpesvirus saimiri (Ensser et al. 2001).

K12

A HHV-8 transcript of 0.7 kb (T0.7) was originally described as being abundantly expressed in nonstimulated PEL cells. T0.7 mRNA, which contains the putative open reading frame K12, is also detectable in the majority of KS spindle cells. The oncogenic potential of K12 in rodent fibroblast transformation assays was not very pronounced (Muralidhar et al. 1998) and the data remain controversial. It is therefore not yet possible to assess the oncogenic potential of K12 or T0.7 with certainty.

VIRAL INTERFERON REGULATORY FACTORS

The HHV-8 genome contains four genes with homology to cellular interferon regulatory factors (vIRFs), termed K9, K10, K10.5, and K11. At least one of these transcription factors, K10.5, is expressed in latently infected PEL cells. Whereas the vIRF-1 encoded by K9 has been shown to antagonize the action of class I interferons, the function of the latently expressed K10.5 is less clear as yet. It is interesting, however, to note that its closest cellular homologues are IRF-4 and the interferon consensus sequence binding protein, ICSBP. Expression of both IRFs is restricted to lymphoid cells. IRF-4 is clearly important for differentiation and proliferation of B-lymphocytes (Pernis 2002).

Inflammatory cytokines and related genes encoded by HHV-8

HHV-8 codes for several proteins which are not generally conserved amongst the different herpesvirus families, but which share striking homology with genes of the host cell. It is very likely that these genes have been captured from the host cell during evolution (Table 28.2). Interestingly, whereas the cellular genes usually consist of several exons, their viral homologous are usually translated from nonspliced messenger RNA. It is thus likely that these genes have been acquired from cellular mRNAs after reverse transcription. With the few exceptions discussed above (k-cyclin, vFlip, K10.5), these virus-cell homologous genes are not expressed in latently infected cells, but seem to be active early in the lytic replication cycle. Typically, they are coding for proteins interfering with the immune system, for enzymes of the nucleotide metabolism, and for putative regulators of cell growth. Thus, their main function seems to be to provide an environment suitable for replication of the virus by counteracting early immune responses (IRFs, anti-apoptotic proteins like vbcl-2, complement regulatory protein homologue CCPH), providing sufficient pools of nucleotides for viral replication or to increase the number of target cells for HHV-8 infection (macrophage inflammatory protein homologues, viral interleukin-8 receptor, interleukin-6). It seems to be a 'rule of thumb,' that such viral genes encode proteins which are usual functional agonists of their cellular counterparts. However, they frequently escape from the usual regulatory mechanisms. Examples are receptors with constitutive activity (e.g. the viral interleukin-8 receptor), a viral cyclinD homologue that escapes from control by cyclin inhibitory proteins, or cytokines like the viral interleukin-6 that are able to bind to a cellular receptor without additional molecules. It is possible that HHV-8 encoded cytokines or cytokine receptors are involved in KS or PEL pathogenesis by para-endocrine mechanisms. Although the HHV-8 genome is present in a latent state in the vast majority of tumor cells, a few cells in a lesion express HHV-8 lytic cycle genes.

VIRAL INTERLEUKIN-6

The open reading frame K2 of HHV-8 encodes viral IL-6 (vIL-6), a protein with moderate yet significant

Table 28.2 HHV-8 genes putatively involved in pathogenesis

ORF	Gene product	Suggested function in pathogenesis	Experimental evidence
K1	Nonconserved transmembrane glycoprotein	Positional and (possibly) functional analogue to other rhadinoviral oncoproteins	Transformation of Rat1 cells; recombinant herpesvirus saimiri: lymphocyte immortalization, lymphoma induction (Lee et al. 1998)
K2	Viral IL-6	Paracrine growth stimulation independent of gp80	Proliferation of B cells; IL-6Rα chain not required (Chatterjee et al. 2002; Burger et al. 1998; Molden et al. 1997)
vMIPs (K4, K4.1, K5)	Viral macrophage inflammatory proteins	Angiogenesis; attraction of Th2 lymphocytes	Binding to both CC and CXC receptors; induction of angiogenesis (Boshoff et al. 1997)
K9, K10, K10.5, K11	Interferon response factor homologues	Interfering with the antiproliferative action of IRF-1	K9: antagonistic to IRF-1, transformation of 3T3 cells (Li et al. 1998)
K12	Kaposin A	Transformation	Transformation of Rat-3 cells; increased cellular adhesion
ORF16	vbcl-2	Stabilizing productively infected cells	Anti-apoptotic activity
ORF71	vFLIP	Stabilizing latently infected cells	In situ: increased expression correlates with reduced apoptosis
ORF72	k-Cyclin	Dysregulated cell cycle progression, inhibits cell cycle arrest by p53	Activates cdk6, evades inhibition by CDK-inhibitors, destabilizes p27 (Swanton et al. 1997)
ORF73	LANA-1	Maintains latent viral infection	Mediates HHV-8 DNA persistence (Ballestas et al. 1999)
ORF74	vIL-8R	Angiogenesis, transformation of endothelial cells	Constitutively active; induces VEGF secretion, transforms rodent fibroblasts; KS-like lesions in transgenic mice (Bais et al. 1998; Yang et al. 2000)
K15	Integral membrane protein reminiscent of EBV LMP-2	Differentiation and proliferation of B lymphocytes	

EBV, Epstein–Barr virus; IL-6, interleukin-6; IL-6Rα, interleukin-6 receptor α-chain (gp80); IRF, interferon regulatory factor; k-cylin, KSHV-encoded cyclin D homologue; LANA-1, latent nuclear antigen-1; LMP-2, latent membrane protein-2 of Epstein–Barr virus; ORF, open reading frame; VEGF, vascular endothelial cell growth factor; vFLIP, viral FLICE inhibitory protein; vIL-8R, viral interleukin-8 receptor homologue.

homology to the multifunctional human cytokine IL-6 (hIL-6) (Neipel et al. 1997a). The vIL-6 cytokine is functional and supports the proliferation of both murine and human IL-6-dependent cells (Burger et al. 1998). Both human and viral IL-6 are produced in KS lesions and the proliferation of cultured spindle cells can be stimulated with oncostatin M and hIL-6 (Masood et al. 1994; Miles et al. 1992). Nevertheless, the relevance of IL-6 for KS pathogenesis has been questioned as some groups were not able to detect expression of the IL-6 receptor α-chain (IL-6Rα) by KS spindle cells (Murakami Mori et al. 1995). The IL-6R consists of two chains. The β-chain, also termed gp130, is almost ubiquitously expressed. It is responsible for ligand-dependent signal transduction and is shared by several receptors of four-helical cytokines such as IL-6, IL-11, ciliary neurotrophic factor, cardiotrophin-1, oncostatin M, and leukemia inhibitory factor. The β-chain alone is not sufficient for hIL-6 binding. hIL-6 first needs to bind to the second chain (IL-6Rα), and this complex then associates with gp130. There is compelling evidence that IL-6Rα is not required for binding of vIL-6 to the signal transducer gp130 (Chow et al. 2001; Li et al. 2001; Molden et al. 1997). Thus, vIL-6 can induce gp130 signal transduction on almost any cell. This may be important for autocrine growth stimulation of HHV-8 infected cells, as expression of the gp80 chain is reduced by interferon-α. By producing vIL-6 which is not dependent on gp80, HHV-8 infected cells escape from one of the mechanisms of growth control by interferon-α (Chatterjee et al. 2002).

CHEMOKINES ENCODED BY HHV-8

Three genes with homology to the family of CC chemokines are located in the same nonconserved region of the HHV-8 genome as vIL-6 (Figure 28.1, Table 28.2). The proteins encoded by the open reading frames K4 and K6 are homologous to the macrophage inflammatory protein 1α (MIP-1α). They have been termed vMIP-II and vMIP-I, respectively (Nicholas et al. 1997; Russo et al. 1996). The amino acid sequence identity of these viral proteins to their cellular counterpart is only about 30 percent, but 48 percent of the viral sequences are identical to each other. This could indicate a gene duplication event that occurred in the evolution of the genes rather than independent acquisition from the host cell genome. Another HHV-8 reading frame, K4.1, is also homologous to the CC chemokine family, with similarity to both MIP-1β and macrophage chemoattractant protein. Functional data are available for vMIP-I (K6) and vMIP-II (K4). vMIP-II binds efficiently to the CC-chemokine receptor CCR3 (Boshoff et al. 1997). In contrast to cellular MIP-1α, it does also bind to CXC-chemokine receptors such as CXCR4, albeit with lower affinity. The CC-chemokine receptor CCR3 is known to be relevant for the chemoattraction of both eosinophil

granulocytes and Th2 lymphocytes. Correspondingly, a potent chemoattractive effect of vMIP-II on eosinophils was described (Boshoff et al. 1997). In contrast to cellular MIP-1α and to the CC-chemokine RANTES, both vMIP-I and vMIP-II were highly angiogenic in the chorioallantoic assay (Boshoff et al. 1997). The chemokine homologues encoded by HHV-8 could thus contribute to two features of KS histology: the presence of inflammatory infiltrates containing Th2 lymphocytes, and the prominent angiohyperplasy.

VGPCR/VIL-8R

Similarly to most other rhadinoviruses, HHV-8 encodes a protein with homology to the family of G-protein coupled receptors (GPCR) with seven transmembrane regions (Table 28.2). The HHV-8 gene is most homologous to the human IL-8R and hence termed vIL-8R. This viral receptor is capable of activating the protein kinase C pathway, regardless of whether a suitable chemokine is present or not. This constitutive activity was sufficient to enhance the proliferation of transfected primary rat fibroblasts (Arvanitakis et al. 1997). Moreover, the transfection of vIL-8R induced focus formation in fibroblasts with an efficiency comparable to the m1 muscarinic receptor, but independently of an extracellular ligand. vIL-8R transformed cells efficiently formed tumors in nude mice (Bais et al. 1998). Transgenic mice were generated that expressed vIL-8R under control of the CD2 promoter on lymphoid cells. Interestingly, this resulted in angioproliferative lesions in multiple organs. Histologically, these lesions strikingly resembled KS (Yang et al. 2000). Thus, the constitutively signaling viral IL-8R homologue is another potential HHV-8-encoded oncogene.

CLINICAL AND PATHOLOGICAL ASPECTS

INTRODUCTION

Extensive studies on HHV-8 molecular epidemiology have shown that, although not discovered until 1994, HHV-8 has most likely been present in the human population for at least 35 000–60 000 years (Hayward 1999). Thus, HHV-8 is a typical herpesvirus which has evolved to stay precisely balanced with its host organism. As a consequence, HHV-8 infection is usually benign and often asymptomatic. Nevertheless, persistent HHV-8 infection is clearly associated with three diseases: Kaposi's sarcoma, multifocal Castleman's disease, and primary effusion lymphoma, which represent a spectrum from a hyperproliferative process (Kaposi's sarcoma) to true monoclonal lymphoma (primary effusion lymphoma). All three diseases occur more frequently in immunosuppressed patients, especially in HIV-infected patients.

EPIDEMIOLOGY

HHV-8 DNA is almost invariably detectable in all epidemiological forms of Kaposi's sarcoma, in primary effusion lymphomas, and most cases of multifocal Castleman's disease. In contrast, attempts to amplify HHV-8 DNA from various other malignant and non-malignant diseases, as well as healthy individuals were either unsuccessful or difficult to reproduce. Thus, it appears that at least amongst populations of the northern hemisphere, the detection of HHV-8 DNA is restricted to KS, PEL, and MCD, where it is regularly found. Most human tumor viruses are relatively wide-spread when compared to the frequency of the malignancy they cause. This is true for Epstein–Barr virus, the human herpesvirus most closely related to HHV-8, and for human papillomaviruses. The epidemiology of AIDS-associated KS in the metropolitan areas of the northern hemisphere suggested that a relatively infrequent, sexually transmitted agent is involved in KS pathogenesis (Figure 28.3). This poses three important epidemiological questions: firstly, is the HHV-8 prevalence significantly increased in KS risk groups, as compared to the general population? Second, does the infection precede KS development? Third, are the modes of transmission compatible with the claimed transmissible agent? Nucleic acid detection is not sufficient to answer these questions, as the high level of viral replication found in immunosuppressed patients makes detection of viral genomes much more likely in this group. Serological studies are more suitable. The first serological studies were solely based on immuno-fluorescence techniques using HHV-8-positive cell lines derived from primary effusion lymphomas (Cesarman et al. 1995b). In the meantime, enzyme linked immuno-sorbent assays utilizing purified virus, recombinant

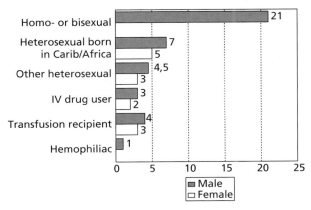

Figure 28.3 *Percentage of AIDS patients with Kaposi's sarcoma by HIV transmission group. The data are taken from Beral et al. (1990). A total of 90 990 persons with AIDS were included in the study. Whereas 21 percent of the HIV-infected patients in the homo- or bisexual transmission group developed KS, only 1 to 4 percent of patients infected via blood or blood products suffered from this tumor.*

antigen, or synthetic peptides are also available. The validity of these assays, especially when it comes to the crucial question of seroprevalence in persons not at risk for KS, is still under debate (Pellett et al. 2003). This is essentially due to the high interassay variability observed with low-titered sera from non-KS patients. However, as justified as it may be, this debate should not obscure three important findings: firstly, the prevalence of (high) anti-KS antibody titers correlates very well with KS. This is true both when various AIDS-transmission groups are compared within one geographic area, and when areas of low KS prevalence (e.g. Northern Europe or the United States) are compared with regions where KS is endemic, e.g. Mediterranean Europe or parts of Africa (Gao et al. 1996b; Kedes et al. 1996; Miller et al. 1996; Simpson et al. 1996). HHV-8 seroprevalence is in the range from 0 to 5 percent in the general population of northern Europe and the United States. The increased incidence of Kaposi sarcoma in Italy is reflected by a higher HHV-8 seroprevalence, especially in southern parts of Italy, including Sicily and Sardinia. Depending on the geographic area, HHV-8 seroprevalence in Italy can be as high as 45 percent (Santarelli et al. 2001), with an average of about 12 percent in Mediterranean countries. In sub-Saharan Africa, however, where KS has been described as the most frequent malignancy even before the beginning of the AIDS epidemic, HHV-8 seroprevalence is usually above 60 percent. Second, HHV-8 seroconversion or at least a marked increase in anti-HHV-8 antibody titer precedes KS development in homosexual AIDS patients (Gao et al. 1996a; Martin et al. 1998). Third, high anti-HHV-8 antibody titers were also associated with the number of homosexual partners and a history of other sexually transmitted diseases (Martin et al. 1998). In summary, serological data largely agree that the titer of anti-HHV-8 antibodies reflects KS or the risk of KS development. Although some uncertainty still remains with the current serological assays and reactivation of HHV-8 cannot be excluded as the reason for the markedly increased anti-HHV-8 titers in KS patients, the high levels of antibodies in groups at risk of KS and seroconversion preceding the onset of the disease clearly hint at a pathogenetic role of HHV-8 infection in KS.

CLINICAL MANIFESTATIONS

Primary infection

Like other herpesviruses, HHV-8 is usually entirely benign under normal conditions. Nonsexual transmission is most likely predominant in areas of high HHV-8 prevalence, e.g. southern European and African countries, and the virus has been detected in the saliva of children seropositive for HHV-8, making it likely that transmission via saliva is a main route in this age group.

However, modes and routes of transmission in areas of low HHV-8 prevalence are less clear. The epidemiology of AIDS-associated KS in these areas suggests transmission in the context of sexual activity. Among men, HHV-8 seroprevalence correlates with the number of homosexual partners and is a risk factor for KS development (Martin et al. 1998). Primary infection is usually asymptomatic but may be associated with a febrile illness and maculopapular rash in children (Andreoni et al. 2002). After primary infection, life-long latency is likely established in memory B cells which becomes only manifest as a disease if the virus–host balance is severely disturbed, e.g. by immunosuppression. In the latter case, three malignant diseases are clearly associated with HHV-8 infection: Kaposi's sarcoma, primary effusion lymphoma, and multifocal Castleman disease.

Kaposi's sarcoma

EPIDEMIOLOGY

Kaposi's sarcoma occurs in four epidemiological variants. The classical form afflicts mainly elderly men of southeastern European descent. It was described in 1872 by Moriz Kaposi as 'sarcoma idiopathicum multiplex hemorrhagicum.' The incidence of classic KS in northern Europe is less then 1/100 000 total population, and about ten-fold higher in endemic regions of southern Europe. The male/female ratio of classical KS is about 10/1. African endemic KS had already been described before the advent of the human immunodeficiency virus. The prevalence of African endemic KS is as high as 12 percent in certain areas of sub-Saharan Africa (Wabinga et al. 2000). Iatrogenic KS occurs in therapeutically immunosuppressed patients. The incidence of post-transplant KS correlates with the general HHV-8 seroprevalence. It is thus more frequent in southern Europe and the Arabian peninsula, where as much as 5 percent of kidney transplant recipients may develop KS (Lesnoni La Parola et al. 1997; Qunibi et al. 1988). The unusual distribution of AIDS-associated KS, the fourth epidemiological form, triggered the search for an infectious agent other than HIV in KS (Beral et al. 1990). At the beginning of the AIDS epidemic, up to 30 percent of male homosexual HIV patients developed this unusually aggressive form of KS, in contrast to only 1 percent of age- and sex-matched HIV-infected patients with hemophilia.

SYMPTOMS AND SIGNS

Initially, KS lesions present as pink or red macular eruptions that progress to plaques and nodules, which subsequently frequently ulcerate. The lesions are often accompanied by lymphedema, which, especially at the nodular and ulcerating stage, cause discomfort and pain. From the very beginning, the clinical presentation of all forms of KS is characterized by a multifocal, often symmetric distribution of the lesions. The most important predilection site is the skin, especially the skin of the lower limbs. However, lymph nodes and viscera are involved in at least 50 percent of cases, even in the more benign classic KS. The disease may afflict any organ with the apparent exception of the central nervous system. The progression from patch to plaque and nodule may take several years in classic KS, and single lesions may even disappear spontaneously. Classic KS is a chronic disease that progresses slowly over many years. Mean survival time of classic KS is 10–15 years and many patients die of an unrelated cause. Other forms of KS, however, are much more aggressive and may progress quickly, often within a few month. This holds particularly true for AIDS-associated KS (Figure 28.4). A standardized staging system for KS has been developed by the AIDS Clinical Trial Group (Krown et al. 1997). African endemic KS occurs in at least three different clinical pictures: a more slowly progressing form in young adults that resembles European classic KS, an aggressive cutaneous form with frequent visceral involvement that is fatal within 5–7 years, and a very aggressive lymphadenopathic form that occurs in young children (mean age, 3 years; male/female ratio, 3/1).

PATHOLOGY

Although Kaposi's sarcoma occurs in four distinct epidemiological forms which also differ in clinical course and prognosis, all forms share the same histopathology (Figure 28.2) and can be considered one disease entity. At least in its early stages, KS is not a typical sarcoma. It develops in a polyclonal fashion. Multiple lesions appear simultaneously, often with an almost symmetrical distribution which is not compatible with metastatic tumor growth. In contrast to other sarcomas, classic KS may wax and wane over decades, and single lesions may disappear completely. This was also observed for the more aggressive AIDS-associated form of KS, where complete remissions were seen during antiretroviral combination therapy (Lebbe et al. 1998). Although molecular data on the clonality of several KS lesions in a single patient are conflicting, it appears that, at least in its early stages, KS is not a monoclonal tumor (Delabesse et al. 1997; Gill et al. 1997). However, late nodular lesions may eventually progress to true sarcoma as indicated by clonality (Gill et al. 1998; Rabkin et al. 1997). The histological picture of (early) KS lesions is not typical for other sarcomas. The lesions contain many different cell types. The so-called KS spindle cells are considered the tumor-defining, malignant cell type of the disease. KS spindle cells are thought to be derived from lymphatic endothelial cells (Weninger et al. 1999). However, they are not the dominant cell type until late stage disease. KS lesions begin as subtle neovascularization (Ruszczak et al. 1987a), and the pathognomonic spindle cells are not yet detectable. In addition, KS

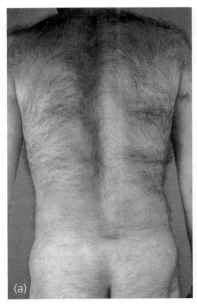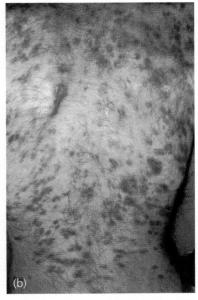

Figure 28.4 *AIDS-associated Kaposi's sarcoma. One of the first AIDS patients seen in New York in 1981. Initially, the 36-year-old man presented with only a few macular KS lesions on his face and oral mucosa, and there were no lesions seen on his back* (a). *A follow-up photograph of the same patient was taken 6 months later* (b). *It illustrates the rapid development of disseminated Kaposi's sarcoma plaques in immunosuppressed patients (from Friedman-Kien,* Color atlas of AIDS, *with permission).*

lesions contain infiltrating inflammatory cells and multi-centrically arising vascular endothelia forming capillaries and other vessels (Ruszczak et al. 1987b). The proliferation of cultured spindle cells is highly dependent on inflammatory cytokines and, with a few exceptions, KS spindle cells are not tumorigenic in nude mice (Nakamura et al. 1988; Salahuddin et al. 1988).

THERAPY

Treatment of Kaposi's sarcoma depends not only on the extent of the tumor and organ involvement, but especially on the type of KS (Hengge et al. 2002). A staging system has been provided by the AIDS Clinical Trials Group (Krown et al. 1997). Classic KS is initially treated with local therapy (excision of single lesions, radiation, intralesional and topical chemotherapy using vinblastine or vincristine). However, the lesions usually reappear. Systemic chemotherapy is used when classic KS is more advanced, disseminated, and symptomatic. The more aggressive forms of African KS (except lymphadenopathic KS in children) also respond well to systemic chemotherapy. Cytotoxic agents used in KS chemotherapy include liposomal doxorubicin, bleomycin, vinca alcaloids, and paclitaxel. Since it is known that HHV-8 is most likely required albeit not sufficient to cause KS, specific antiviral treatment has also been used in KS therapy. HHV-8 replication can be inhibited with foscarnet and ganciclovir in cell culture systems. In one study, a 75 percent reduction in the rate of new KS was seen after high-dose ganciclovir treatment for cytomegalovirus retinitis (Martin et al. 1999). However, data on the treatment of pre-existing KS lesions with

ganciclovir or foscarnet are less consistent. The use of interferon-α seems to be more promising. A reduction in up to 30 percent of individuals has been reported following the therapy with high doses of interferon-α (Krown 2001). The therapeutic efficacy of interferon-α is not only due to its antiviral activity. Class I interferons have also been shown to reduce cell proliferation and angiogenesis. Iatrogenic KS usually regresses after reduction of immunosuppressive therapy. However, when immunsuppressive therapy is reinitiated, KS lesions often reappear. Thus, chemotherapy is often used in more disseminated disease. Local or systemic therapy does not increase the survival time of patients with AIDS-KS. The most effective treatment for AIDS-KS is highly active antiretroviral therapy (HAART) (Cattelan et al. 2002). Reconstitution of the immune system by HAART frequently results in complete remission of AIDS-KS.

PRIMARY EFFUSION LYMPHOMA

Primary effusion lymphoma is a rare non-Hodgkin B-cell lymphoma which is primarily seen in immunosuppressed patients. In contrast to KS, which has features of both a hyperproliferative inflammatory lesion and malignant neoplasia, PEL represents a more typical, monoclonal neoplastic process. The name primary effusion lymphoma or body-cavity-based lymphoma (BCBL) indicates that the disease manifests by pleural, pericardial, or peritoneal effusion, often without a solid tumor. Primary effusion lymphomas regularly contain HHV-8, and 50 percent of the cases are also positive for Epstein–Barr virus. Whereas HHV-8 is invariably present in PEL, it has not been found in any other lymphoma (Cesarman et al. 1995a). PEL cells do not express B- or T-cell antigens. It is indicated by immunoglobulin rearrangement, lack of Bcl-6 expression, and expression of syndecan-1 that PEL cells are derived from post-germinal B cells. AIDS-associated PEL is usually highly aggressive with a mean survival from diagnosis of 5 to 7 months. Several permanent cell lines have been established from PEL cases. The HHV-8 genome is maintained in cultured PEL cells in a latent state with only a few genes being expressed. However, lytic replication can be induced in cultured PEL cells by chemicals such as tetra-phorbol acetate or sodium butyrate. Thus, cell lines derived from PEL are at present an invaluable tool in KS research.

MULTIFOCAL CASTLEMAN'S DISEASE

Multifocal or multicentric Castleman's disease is an atypical lymphoproliferative disorder. The plasma cell type, but not the hyaline vascular type, of MCD is associated with HHV-8 infection and epidemiologically related with both AIDS-associated and classic KS. However, in contrast to both KS and PEL, even the plasma cell type of MCD is not invariably positive for HHV-8. This may indicate that MCD represents a diverse group of lesions. Clinically, MCD is characterized by generalized lymphadenopathy, hypergammaglobulinemia, and fever. Histological examination of affected lymph nodes reveals large follicles, expanded germinal centers separated by vascular lymphoid tissue. HHV-8 harboring cells in MCD resemble immunoblasts which reside in the mantle zone of B-cell follicles. These isolated immunoblasts may eventually form monoclonal, microscopic lymphomas (Dupin et al. 2000), and monoclonal plasmablastic lymphoma may develop in MCD patients. The plasmablastic, HHV-8 associated variant of MCD is frequently resistant to systemic chemotherapy and lethal. Systemic symptoms of MCD have ben shown to correlate with increased serum levels of interleukin-6. Treatment with both anti-IL-6 antibodies, as well as an antibody directed against the interleukin-6 receptor efficiently reduces fever, fatigue, and lymphadenopathy. Whereas HAART has clearly reduced the incidence of KS and PEL, an increase in fatal MCD has been observed following highly active antiretroviral therapy (Zietz et al. 1999).

MODELS OF PATHOGENESIS

Consistent detection of viral DNA in tumor tissue is not sufficient to prove that a virus is involved in oncogenesis. In theory, different roles are possible for HHV-8 in KS pathogenesis (Neipel et al. 1997c), ranging from a mere 'passenger model,' where HHV-8 would be an innocent bystander, to the role of a directly transforming virus. Several lines of evidence strongly suggest that HHV-8 plays an essential role in KS pathogenesis: the

virus is invariably present in KS, HHV-8 infection precedes KS development, the virus is present in the tumor cells themselves, and it is rather infrequently found outside the population at risk of KS. Moreover, HHV-8 belongs to a group of herpesviruses known to be oncogenic. It is difficult, however, to assess the pathogenic potential of HHV-8 more reliably without identification of the genes and mechanism involved in pathogenesis. Research on HHV-8 pathogenesis is hampered by the lack of a cell culture system for transformation as it exists for EBV or herpesvirus saimiri. In addition, several attempts have been made to establish animal models for HHV-8 proliferative diseases. Unfortunately, infections of various primates did not result in overt disease. Studies using rodents transgenic for single HHV-8 genes were more successful. However, results from such experiments must be interpreted with great caution, no matter how tempting the resemblance of lesions in mice transgenic for vIL8R to KS may be (Yang et al. 2000). In summary, several genes with oncogenic potential have been identified in cell culture transformation assays or transgenic animals, and various models were developed. However, statements on their relevance in KS, PEL, and MCD remain speculative to date.

At least two concurring models exist for the role of HHV-8 in KS pathogenesis. The 'cytokine model' emphasizes the role of inflammatory cytokines induced or produced by HHV-8. A closer look at the clinical course and histopathology of KS raises doubts about the relevance of 'classical,' transforming genes for the pathogenesis of this peculiar tumor. The peculiar pathology of KS hints at a more complex, indirect mechanism of pathogenesis. Based on clinical observations and data derived from cell culture systems, models of KS pathogenesis were developed before HHV-8 was discovered. Several groups agreed upon the notion that KS develops as an interplay of inflammatory cytokines and angiogenic factors (Ensoli and Stürzl 1998; Samaniego et al. 1998), although the cytokines focused on various different reports. Amongst them are basic fibroblast growth factor, vascular endothelial growth factor (VEGF), IL-6, tumor necrosis factor (TNF)α and β, and oncostatin M. Interestingly, HHV-8 encodes or induces several cytokines with intriguing similarity to the cellular factors shown to be required for in vitro models of KS. An example is VEGF, which is secreted by cells expressing the constitutively active vIL-8R. This leads to a model of KS pathogenesis, where increased secretion of both viral and cellular cytokines, the latter in part induced by HHV-8, promote inflammatory infiltrates (vMIP, vIL-6), angiogenesis (vMIP, vIL-8R), and enhance spindle cell proliferation (vIL-6, vIL-8R via VEGF). The reliable presence of HHV-8 in the spindle cells points to additional factors beyond those induced through the 1–3 percent productively infected cells, voting for a role more compatible with a typical 'oncogenic transformation' model by latently expressed viral genes.

Starting from the close relationship to EBV and herpesvirus saimiri, it is intriguing to assume that transmembrane proteins mimicking constitutively active receptors mechanisms – similar to those identified in EBV and herpesvirus saimiri – might be relevant for HHV-8 pathogenesis. At first sight, HHV-8 genes K1 and K15 might fall into this category. However, attempts to detect expression of these genes in latently infected tumor cells remained unsuccessful, voting against a role of K1 and K15 in transformation. Only few viral genes were found expressed in latently infected cells. These include the viral interferon regulatory factor K10.5, LANA-1, the viral cyclin D homologue, and possibly vFLIP. Although clearly not considered a common rhadinoviral oncogene (Ensser et al. 2001), the viral k-cyclin may be such a factor in KS. It is transcribed in the majority of latently infected tumor cells, and deregulation of the G1/S checkpoint is a feature common to various malignancies and human tumor viruses. k-Cyclin has been shown to overcome arrest in G1 and to force progression of the cell cycle. One physiological function of the restriction point in G1/S is to block cell division in the case of DNA damage. This is usually achieved through the activation of p53 which in turn results in an increased synthesis of cdk inhibitors such as p21. However, the k-cyclin/cdk6 complex is resistant to inhibition by several cdk inhibitors (Swanton et al. 1997). Thus, k-cyclin may not only be responsible for increased proliferation of HHV-8-infected endothelial and spindle cells, but sustained expression of k-cyclin may also result in the unrestricted acquisition of somatic mutations, eventually resulting in the malignant phenotype and monoclonality associated with advanced stage disease. As described above, LANA-1 seems to be a multifunctional protein. It is not only required for maintenance of the viral episome, but also in transcription regulation and cell cycle control possibly contributing to cell transformation. The role of K10.5 remains speculative. Its similarity to the cellular genes IRF-4 and interferon consensus sequence binding protein suggests that it may play a role in lymphocyte development.

Thus, KS may result from a complex interplay of both viral and cellular cytokines and angiogenic factors, induced by a sustained inflammatory reaction initiated by up to 3 percent productively infected cells. The viral cyclin and perhaps other latency-associated proteins, such as LANA-1, might further enhance the proliferation of KS cells and favor the development of truly malignant cells by indirect means, e.g. the reduced control of accidental DNA damage. As KS is an unusual malignancy, resembling hyperplastic, angioproliferative inflammatory changes rather than true sarcoma, such a multistep/multifactorial model might be more compatible with KS pathogenesis than classical transformation

models by viral oncogenes (Stürzl et al. 2001), as described for EBV, herpesvirus saimiri, and possibly for HHV-8-associated B-cell malignancies (PEL).

REFERENCES

Akula, S.M., Pramod, N.P., et al. 2001. Human herpesvirus 8 envelope-associated glycoprotein B interacts with heparan sulfate-like moieties. *Virology*, **284**, 2, 235–49.

Akula, S.M., Pramod, N.P., et al. 2002. Integrin alpha3beta1 (CD 49c/29) is a cellular receptor for Kaposi's sarcoma-associated herpesvirus (KSHV/HHV-8) entry into the target cells. *Cell*, **108**, 3, 407–19.

Albrecht, J.C., Nicholas, J., et al. 1992. Primary structure of the herpesvirus saimiri genome. *J Virol*, **66**, 5047–58.

Alexander, L., Denekamp, L., et al. 2000. The primary sequence of rhesus monkey rhadinovirus isolate 26-95: sequence similarities to Kaposi's sarcoma-associated herpesvirus and rhesus monkey rhadinovirus isolate 17577. *J Virol*, **74**, 7, 3388–98.

Andreoni, M., Sarmati, L., et al. 2002. Primary human herpesvirus 8 infection in immunocompetent children. *JAMA*, **287**, 10, 1295–300.

Arvanitakis, L., Geras Raaka, E., et al. 1997. Human herpesvirus KSHV encodes a constitutively active G-protein-coupled receptor linked to cell proliferation. *Nature*, **385**, 6614, 347–50.

Bais, C., Santomasso, B., et al. 1998. G-protein-coupled receptor of Kaposi's sarcoma-associated herpesvirus is a viral oncogene and angiogenesis activator. *Nature*, **391**, 6662, 86–9.

Ballestas, M.E., Chatis, P.A. and Kaye, K.M. 1999. Efficient persistence of extrachromosomal KSHV DNA mediated by latency- associated nuclear antigen. *Science*, **284**, 5414, 641–4.

Ballestas, M.E. and Kaye, K.M. 2001. Kaposi's sarcoma-associated herpesvirus latency-associated nuclear antigen 1 mediates episome persistence through cis-acting terminal repeat (TR) sequence and specifically binds TR DNA. *J Virol*, **75**, 7, 3250–8.

Beral, V., Peterman, T.A., et al. 1990. Kaposi's sarcoma among persons with AIDS: a sexually transmitted infection? *Lancet*, **335**, 123–8.

Biesinger, B., Müller-Fleckenstein, I., et al. 1992. Stable growth transformation of human T lymphocytes by Herpesvirus saimiri. *Proc Natl Acad Sci USA*, **89**, 7, 3116–19.

Birkmann, A., Mahr, K., et al. 2001. Cell surface heparan sulfate is a receptor for human herpesvirus 8 and interacts with envelope glycoprotein K8.1. *J Virol*, **75**, 23, 11583–93.

Blasig, C., Zietz, C., et al. 1997. Monocytes in Kaposi's sarcoma lesions are productively infected by human herpesvirus 8. *J Virol*, **71**, 10, 7963–8.

Boshoff, C., Endo, Y., et al. 1997. Angiogenic and HIV-inhibitory functions of KSHV-encoded chemokines. *Science*, **278**, 5336, 290–4.

Burger, R., Neipel, F., et al. 1998. Human herpesvirus type 8 interleukin-6 homologue is functionally active on human myeloma cells. *Blood*, **91**, 6, 1858–63.

Byun, H., Gwack, Y., et al. 2002. Kaposi's sarcoma-associated herpesvirus open reading frame (ORF) 50 transactivates K8 and ORF57 promoters via heterogeneous response elements. *Mol Cell*, **14**, 2, 185–91.

Cattelan, A.M., Trevenzoli, M. and Aversa, S.M. 2002. Recent advances in the treatment of AIDS-related Kaposi's sarcoma. *Am J Clin Dermatol*, **3**, 7, 451–62.

Cesarman, E., Chang, Y., et al. 1995a. Kaposi's sarcoma-associated herpesvirus-like DNA sequences in AIDS-related body-cavity-based lymphomas. *New Engl J Med*, **332**, 1186–91.

Cesarman, E., Moore, P.S., et al. 1995b. In vitro establishment and characterization of two acquired immunodeficiency syndrome-related lymphoma cell lines (BC-1 and BC-2) containing Kaposi's sarcoma-associated herpesvirus-like (KSHV) DNA sequences. *Blood*, **86**, 2708–14.

Chandran, B., Bloomer, C., et al. 1998. Human herpesvirus-8 ORF K8.1 gene encodes immunogenic glycoproteins generated by spliced transcripts. *Virology*, **249**, 1, 140–9.

Chang, Y., Cesarman, E., et al. 1994. Identification of herpesvirus-like DNA sequences in AIDS-associated Kaposi's sarcoma. *Science*, **266**, 1865–9.

Chatterjee, M., Osborne, J., et al. 2002. Viral IL-6-induced cell proliferation and immune evasion of interferon activity. *Science*, **298**, 5597, 1432–5.

Chow, D., He, X., et al. 2001. Structure of an extracellular gp130 cytokine receptor signaling complex. *Science*, **291**, 5511, 2150–5.

Delabesse, E., Oksenhendler, E., et al. 1997. Molecular analysis of clonality in Kaposi's sarcoma. *J Clin Pathol*, **50**, 8, 664–8.

Desrosiers, R.C., Sasseville, V.G., et al. 1997. A herpesvirus of rhesus monkeys related to the human Kaposi's sarcoma-associated herpesvirus. *J Virol*, **71**, 12, 9764–9.

Dupin, N., Diss, T.L., et al. 2000. HHV-8 is associated with a plasmablastic variant of Castleman disease that is linked to HHV-8-positive plasmablastic lymphoma. *Blood*, **95**, 4, 1406–12.

Ellis, M., Chew, Y.P., et al. 1999. Degradation of p27(Kip) cdk inhibitor triggered by Kaposi's sarcoma virus cyclin-cdk6 complex. *EMBO J*, **18**, 3, 644–53.

Ensoli, B. and Stürzl, M. 1998. Kaposi's sarcoma: a result of the interplay among inflammatory cytokines, angiogenic factors and viral agents. *Cytokine Growth Factor Rev*, **9**, 1, 63–83.

Ensser, A., Glykofrydes, D., et al. 2001. Independence of herpesvirus-induced T cell lymphoma from viral cyclin D homologue. *J Exp Med*, **193**, 5, 637–42.

Fickenscher, H. and Fleckenstein, B. 2001. Herpesvirus saimiri. *Phil Trans R Soc Lond B Biol Sci*, **356**, 1408, 545–67.

Fleckenstein, B. and Desrosiers, R.C. 1982. Herpesvirus saimiri and Herpesvirus ateles. In: Roizman, B. (ed.), *The herpesviruses*, Vol. 1. New York: Plenum Press, 253–331.

Fleckenstein, B., Bornkamm, G.W., et al. 1978. Herpesvirus ateles DNA and its homology with herpesvirus saimiri nucleic acid. *J Virol*, **25**, 1, 361–73.

Flemington, E.K. 2001. Herpesvirus lytic replication and the cell cycle: arresting new developments. *J Virol*, **75**, 10, 4475–81.

Friborg, J. Jr., Kong, W., et al. 1999. p53 inhibition by the LANA protein of KSHV protects against cell death. *Nature*, **402**, 6764, 889–94.

Friedman Kien, A.E., Laubenstein, L.J., et al. 1982. Disseminated Kaposi's sarcoma in homosexual men. *Ann Intern Med*, **96**, 6 Pt 1, 693–700.

Fujimuro, M., Wu, F.Y., et al. 2003. A novel viral mechanism for dysregulation of beta-catenin in Kaposi's sarcoma-associated herpesvirus latency. *Nat Med*, **9**, 3, 300–6.

Gao, S.J., Kingsley, L., et al. 1996a. Seroconversion to antibodies against Kaposi's sarcoma-associated herpesvirus-related latent nuclear antigens before the development of Kaposi's sarcoma. *New Engl J Med*, **335**, 233–41.

Gao, S.J., Kingsley, L., et al. 1996b. KSHV antibodies among Americans, Italians and Ugandans with and without Kaposi's sarcoma. *Nat Med*, **2**, 925–8.

Giddens, W.E. Jr., Tsai, C.C., et al. 1985. Retroperitoneal fibromatosis and acquired immunodeficiency syndrome in macaques. Pathologic observations and transmission studies. *Am J Pathol*, **119**, 2, 253–63.

Gill, P., Tsai, Y., et al. 1997. Clonality in Kaposi's sarcoma. *New Engl J Med*, **337**, 8, 570–1.

Gill, P.S., Tsai, Y.C., et al. 1998. Evidence for multiclonality in multicentric Kaposi's sarcoma. *Proc Natl Acad Sci USA*, **95**, 14, 8257–61.

Godden-Kent, D., Talbot, S.J., et al. 1997. The cyclin encoded by Kaposi's sarcoma-associated herpesvirus stimulates cdk6 to phosphorylate the retinoblastoma protein and histone H1. *J Virol*, **71**, 6, 4193–8.

Hayward, G.S. 1999. KSHV strains: the origins and global spread of the virus. *Semin Cancer Biol*, **9**, 3, 187–99.

Hengge, U.R., Ruzicka, T., et al. 2002. Update on Kaposi's sarcoma and other HHV8 associated diseases. Part 1: epidemiology, environmental predispositions, clinical manifestations, and therapy. *Lancet Infect Dis*, **2**, 5, 281–92.

Hu, J., Garber, A.C. and Renne, R. 2002. The latency-associated nuclear antigen of Kaposi's sarcoma-associated herpesvirus supports latent DNA replication in dividing cells. *J Virol*, **76**, 22, 11677.

Hwang, S., Gwack, Y., et al. 2001. The Kaposi's sarcoma-associated herpesvirus K8 protein interacts with CREB-binding protein (CBP) and represses CBP-mediated transcription. *J Virol*, **75**, 19, 9509–16.

Izumiya, Y., Lin, S.F., et al. 2003. Kaposi's sarcoma-associated herpesvirus K-bZIP is a coregulator of K-Rta: Physical association and promoter-dependent transcriptional repression. *J Virol*, **77**, 2, 1441–51.

Jung, J.U., Choi, J.K., et al. 1999. Herpesvirus saimiri as a model for gammaherpesvirus oncogenesis. *Semin Cancer Biol*, **9**, 3, 231–9.

Kaposi, M. 1872. Idiopathisches multiples Pigment-Sarcom der Haut. *Arch Dermatol Syph*, **4**, 265–73.

Kedes, D., Operalski, E., et al. 1996. The seroepidemiology of human herpesvirus 8 (Kaposi's sarcoma-associated herpesvirus): Distribution of infection in KS risk groups and evidence for sexual transmission. *Nat Med*, **2**, 8, 918–24.

Krown, S.E. 2001. Management of Kaposi sarcoma: The role of interferon and thalidomide. *Curr Opin Oncol*, **13**, 5, 374–81.

Krown, S.E., Testa, M.A. and Huang, J. AIDS Clinical Trials Group Oncology Committee, 1997. AIDS-related Kaposi's sarcoma: prospective validation of the AIDS Clinical Trials Group staging classification. *J Clin Oncol*, **15**, 9, 3085–92.

Lebbe, C., Blum, L., et al. 1998. Clinical and biological impact of antiretroviral therapy with protease inhibitors on HIV-related Kaposi's sarcoma. *AIDS*, **12**, 7, F45–9.

Lee, H., Veazey, R., et al. 1998. Deregulation of cell growth by the K1 gene of Kaposi's sarcoma-associated herpesvirus. *Nat Med*, **4**, 4, 435–40.

Lesnoni La Parola, I., Masini, C., et al. 1997. Kaposi's sarcoma in renal-transplant recipients: experience at the Catholic University in Rome, 1988–1996. *Dermatology*, **194**, 3, 229–33.

Li, H., Wang, H. and Nicholas, J. 2001. Detection of direct binding of human herpesvirus 8-encoded interleukin-6 (vIL-6) to both gp130 and IL-6 receptor (IL-6R) and identification of amino acid residues of vIL-6 important for IL-6R-dependent and -independent signaling. *J Virol*, **75**, 7, 3325–34.

Li, M., Lee, H., et al. 1998. Kaposi's sarcoma-associated herpesvirus viral interferon regulatory factor. *J Virol*, **72**, 7, 5433–40.

Li, M., Lee, H., et al. 1997. Kaposi's sarcoma-associated herpesvirus encodes a functional cyclin. *J Virol*, **71**, 3, 1984–91.

Lisitsyn, N.A., Lisitsyn, N. and Wigler, M. 1993. Cloning the differences between two complex genomes. *Science*, **259**, 5097, 946–51.

Lukac, D.M., Renne, R., et al. 1998. Reactivation of Kaposi's sarcoma-associated herpesvirus infection from latency by expression of the ORF 50 transactivator, a homolog of the EBV R protein. *Virology*, **252**, 2, 304–12.

Lukac, D.M., Kirshner, J.R. and Ganem, D. 1999. Transcriptional activation by the product of open reading frame 50 of Kaposi's sarcoma-associated herpesvirus is required for lytic viral reactivation in B cells. *J Virol*, **73**, 11, 9348–61.

Mann, D.J., Child, E.S., et al. 1999. Modulation of p27(Kip1) levels by the cyclin encoded by Kaposi's sarcoma-associated herpesvirus. *EMBO J*, **18**, 3, 654–63.

Martin, D.F., Kuppermann, B.D., Roche Ganciclovir Study Group, et al. 1999. Oral ganciclovir for patients with cytomegalovirus retinitis treated with a ganciclovir implant. *N Engl J Med*, **340**, 14, 1063–70.

Martin, J.N., Ganem, D.E., et al. 1998. Sexual transmission and the natural history of human herpesvirus 8 infection. *New Engl J Med*, **338**, 14, 948–54.

Masood, R., Lunardi Iskandar, Y., et al. 1994. Inhibition of AIDS-associated Kaposi's sarcoma cell growth by DAB389-interleukin 6. *AIDS Res Hum Retrovir*, **10**, 969–75.

McGeoch, D.J. 2001. Molecular evolution of the gamma-Herpesvirinae. *Phil Trans R Soc Lond B Biol Sci*, **356**, 1408, 421–35.

Miles, S.A., Martinez Maza, O., et al. 1992. Oncostatin M as a potent mitogen for AIDS-Kaposi's sarcoma-derived cells. *Science*, **255**, 1432–4.

Miller, G., Rigsby, M.O., et al. 1996. Antibodies to butyrate-inducible antigens of Kaposi's sarcoma-associated herpesvirus inpatients with HIV-1 infection. *New Engl J Med*, **334**, 1292–7.

Molden, J., Chang, Y., et al. 1997. A Kaposi's sarcoma-associated herpesvirus-encoded cytokine homolog (vIL-6) activates signaling through the shared gp130 receptor subunit. *J Biol Chem*, **272**, 31, 19625–31.

Murakami Mori, K., Taga, T., et al. 1995. AIDS-associated Kaposi's sarcoma (KS) cells express oncostatin M (OM)-specific receptor but not leukemia inhibitory factor/OM receptor or interleukin-6 receptor. Complete block of OM-induced KS cell growth and OM binding by anti-gp130 antibodies. *J Clin Invest*, **96**, 1319–27.

Muralidhar, S., Pumfery, A.M., et al. 1998. Identification of kaposin (open reading frame K12) as a human herpesvirus 8 (Kaposi's sarcoma-associated herpesvirus) transforming gene. *J Virol*, **72**, 6, 4980–8.

Nakamura, S., Salahuddin, S.Z., et al. 1988. Kaposi's sarcoma cells: long-term culture with growth factor from retrovirus-infected CD4+ T cells. *Science*, **242**, 4877, 426–30.

Neipel, F., Albrecht, J.C., et al. 1997a. Human herpesvirus 8 encodes a homolog of interleukin-6. *J Virol*, **71**, 1, 839–42.

Neipel, F., Albrecht, J.C. et al. 1997b. Primary structure of the Kaposi's sarcoma associated human herpesvirus 8. Genbank accession no. KSU75698.

Neipel, F., Albrecht, J.C. and Fleckenstein, B. 1997c. Cell-homologous genes in the Kaposi's sarcoma-associated rhadinovirus human herpesvirus 8: determinants of its pathogenicity? *J Virol*, **71**, 6, 4187–2.

Nicholas, J., Ruvolo, V.R., et al. 1997. Kaposi's sarcoma-associated human herpesvirus-8 encodes homologues of macrophage inflammatory protein-1 and interleukin-6. *Nat Med*, **3**, 3, 287–92.

Nicola, A.V., McEvoy, A.M. and Straus, S.E. 2003. Roles for endocytosis and low pH in herpes simplex virus entry into HeLa and Chinese hamster ovary cells. *J Virol*, **77**, 9, 5324.

Pellett, P.E., Wright, D.J., et al. 2003. Multicenter comparison of serologic assays and estimation of *Human herpesvirus 8* seroprevalence among US blood donors. *Transfusion*, **43**, 9, 1260–8.

Pernis, A.B. 2002. The role of IRF-4 in B and T cell activation and differentiation. *J Interferon Cytokine Res*, **22**, 1, 111–20.

Pines, J. 1995. Cyclins, CDKs and cancer. *Semin Cancer Biol*, **6**, 2, 63–72.

Qunibi, W., Akhtar, M., et al. 1988. Kaposi's sarcoma: the most common tumor after renal transplantation in Saudi Arabia. *Am J Med*, **84**, 2, 225–32.

Raab, M.S., Albrecht, J.C., et al. 1998. The immunogenic glycoprotein gp35-37 of human herpesvirus 8 is encoded by open reading frame K8.1. *J Virol*, **72**, 8, 6725–31.

Rabkin, C.S., Janz, S., et al. 1997. Monoclonal origin of multicentric Kaposi's sarcoma lesions. *New Engl J Med*, **336**, 14, 988–93.

Radkov, S.A., Kellam, P. and Boshoff, C. 2000. The latent nuclear antigen of kaposi sarcoma-associated herpesvirus targets the retinoblastoma-E2F pathway and with the oncogene Hras transforms primary rat cells. *Nat Med*, **6**, 10, 1121–7.

Rainbow, L., Platt, G.M., et al. 1997. The 222- to 234-kilodalton latent nuclear protein (LNA) of Kaposi's sarcoma-associated herpesvirus (human herpesvirus 8) is encoded by orf73 and is a component of the latency-associated nuclear antigen. *J Virol*, **71**, 8, 5915–21.

Renne, R., Zhong, W., et al. 1996. Lytic growth of Kaposi's sarcoma-associated herpesvirus (human herpesvirus 8) in culture. *Nat Med*, **2**, 2, 342–6.

Rose, T.M., Strand, K.B., et al. 1997. Identification of two homologs of the Kaposi's sarcoma-associated herpesvirus (human herpesvirus 8) in retroperitoneal fibromatosis of different macaque species. *J Virol*, **71**, 5, 4138–44.

Russo, J.J., Bohenzky, R.A., et al. 1996. Nucleotide sequence of the Kaposi's sarcoma-accociated herpesvirus (HHV8). *Proc Natl Acad Sci USA*, **93**, 14862–7.

Ruszczak, Z., Mayer-Da, S.A. and Orfanos, C.E. 1987a. Kaposi's sarcoma in AIDS. Multicentric angioneoplasia in early skin lesions. *Am J Dermatopathol*, **9**, 5, 388–98.

Ruszczak, Z., Mayer, D.S. and Orfanos, C.E. 1987b. Angioproliferative changes in clinically noninvolved, perilesional skin in AIDS-associated Kaposi's sarcoma. *Dermatologica*, **175**, 6, 270–9.

Salahuddin, S.Z., Nakamura, S., et al. 1988. Angiogenic properties of Kaposi's sarcoma-derived cells after long-term culture in vitro. *Science*, **242**, 4877, 430–3.

Samaniego, F., Markham, P.D., et al. 1998. Vascular endothelial growth factor and basic fibroblast growth factor present in Kaposi's sarcoma (KS) are induced by inflammatory cytokines and synergize to promote vascular permeability and KS lesion development. *Am J Pathol*, **152**, 6, 1433–43.

Santarelli, R., De Marco, R., et al. 2001. Direct correlation between human herpesvirus-8 seroprevalence and classic Kaposi's sarcoma incidence in northern Sardinia. *J Med Virol*, **65**, 2, 368–72.

Sarid, R., Flore, O., et al. 1998. Transcription mapping of the Kaposi's sarcoma-associated herpesvirus (human herpesvirus 8) genome in a body cavity-based lymphoma cell line (BC-1). *J Virol*, **72**, 2, 1005–12.

Saveliev, A., Zhu, F. and Yuan, Y. 2002. Transcription mapping and expression patterns of genes in the major immediate–early region of Kaposi's sarcoma-associated herpesvirus. *Virology*, **299**, 2, 301–14.

Searles, R.P., Bergquam, E.P., et al. 1999. Sequence and genomic analysis of a rhesus macaque rhadinovirus with similarity to Kaposi's sarcoma-associated Herpesvirus/Human herpesvirus 8. *J Virol*, **73**, 4, 3040–53.

Simpson, G.R., Schulz, T.F., et al. 1996. Prevalence of Kaposi's sarcoma associated herpesvirus infection measured by antibodies to recombinant capsid protein and latent immunofluorescence antigen. *Lancet*, **348**, 9035, 1133–8.

Stürzl, M., Wunderlich, A., et al. 1999. Human herpesvirus-8 (HHV-8) gene expression in Kaposi's sarcoma (KS) primary lesions: an in situ hybridization study. *Leukemia*, **13**, Suppl. 1, S110–12.

Stürzl, M., Zietz, C., et al. 2001. Human herpesvirus-8 and Kaposi's sarcoma: relationship with the multistep concept of tumorigenesis. *Adv Cancer Res*, **81**, 125–59.

Sun, Q., Matta, H. and Chaudhary, P.M. 2003. The human herpes virus 8-encoded viral FLICE inhibitory protein protects against growth factor withdrawal-induced apoptosis via NF-kappa B activation. *Blood*, **101**, 5, 1956.

Swanton, C., Mann, D.J., et al. 1997. Herpes viral cyclin/cdk6 complexes evade inhibition by cdk inhibitor proteins. *Nature*, **390**, 6656, 184–7.

Thome, M., Schneider, P., et al. 1997. Viral FLICE-inhibitory proteins (FLIPs) prevent apoptosis induced by death receptors. *Nature*, **386**, 6624, 517–21.

Trus, B.L., Heymann, J.B., et al. 2001. Capsid structure of Kaposi's sarcoma-associated herpesvirus, a gammaherpesvirus, compared to those of an alphaherpesvirus, herpes simplex virus type 1, and a betaherpesvirus, cytomegalovirus. *J Virol*, **75**, 6, 2879–90.

Wabinga, H.R., Parkin, D.M., et al. 2000. Trends in cancer incidence zin Kyadondo County, Uganda, 1960–1997. *Br J Cancer*, **82**, 9, 1585–92.

Weninger, W., Partanen, T.A., et al. 1999. Expression of vascular endothelial growth factor receptor-3 and podoplanin suggests a lymphatic endothelial cell origin of Kaposi's sarcoma tumor cells. *Lab Invest*, **79**, 2, 243–51.

Wong, S.W., Bergquam, E.P., et al. 1999. Induction of B cell hyperplasia in simian immunodeficiency virus-infected rhesus macaques with the simian homologue of Kaposi's sarcoma-associated herpesvirus. *J Exp Med*, **190**, 6, 827–40.

Wu, F.Y., Ahn, J.H., et al. 2001. Origin-independent assembly of Kaposi's sarcoma-associated herpesvirus DNA replication compartments in transient cotransfection assays and association with the ORF-K8 protein and cellular PML. *J Virol*, **75**, 3, 1487–506.

Wu, F.Y., Tang, Q.Q., et al. 2002. Lytic replication-associated protein (RAP) encoded by Kaposi sarcoma-associated herpesvirus causes p21CIP-1-mediated G1 cell cycle arrest through CCAAT/enhancer-binding protein-alpha. *Proc Natl Acad Sci USA*, **99**, 16, 10683–8.

Wu, L., Lo, P., et al. 2000. Three-dimensional structure of the human herpesvirus 8 capsid. *J Virol*, **74**, 20, 9646–54.

Yang, B.T., Chen, S.C., et al. 2000. Transgenic expression of the chemokine receptor encoded by human herpesvirus 8 induces an angioproliferative disease resembling Kaposi's sarcoma. *J Exp Med*, **191**, 3, 445–54.

Zhu, F.X., Cusano, T. and Yuan, Y. 1999. Identification of the immediate–early transcripts of Kaposi's sarcoma-associated herpesvirus. *J Virol*, **73**, 7, 5556–67.

Zhu, F.X., King, S.M., et al. 2002. A Kaposi's sarcoma-associated herpesviral protein inhibits virus-mediated induction of type I interferon by blocking IRF-7 phosphorylation and nuclear accumulation. *Proc Natl Acad Sci USA*, **99**, 8, 5573–8.

Zietz, C., Bogner, J.R., et al. 1999. An unusual cluster of cases of Castleman's disease during highly active antiretroviral therapy for AIDS. *New Engl J Med*, **340**, 24, 1923–4, letter.

29

Gammaherpesviruses: Epstein–Barr virus

M. ANTHONY EPSTEIN AND DOROTHY H. CRAWFORD

PROPERTIES OF THE VIRUS

INTRODUCTION

The Epstein–Barr virus (EBV) was discovered in 1964 (Epstein et al. 1964) in the course of a sustained search (Epstein 1999) for a possible causative virus in tumor samples from cases of endemic (African) Burkitt's lymphoma (BL). EBV is a very ancient parasite of humans. The fact that EBV-like herpesviruses have been known for many years in Old World apes and monkeys (Deinhardt and Deinhardt 1979) and have now recently been found in New World monkeys (Cho et al. 2001, Wang et al. 2001) indicates that such viruses were already infecting early primates some time before the Old World/New World evolutionary split took place, about 35 Myr ago based on palaeontology (McGeogh and Cook 1994) or 45 Myr ago based on more recent DNA sequence data (Kumar and Hedges 1998). EBV infects almost all of the world's adult population and, like all human herpesviruses, establishes lifelong persistence. However, despite the trivial nature of the infection in most individuals, the virus is the most potent immortalizing agent for mammalian B cells in vitro, is associated with a spectrum of human malignant proliferations in vivo, and causes rapidly fatal malignant tumors on experimental injection in cottontop tamarins.

EBV has a restricted host range, with humans as its natural host, but certain nonhuman primates can be infected experimentally. The virus is B lymphotropic in vivo and readily infects B lymphocytes in vitro (Pattengale et al. 1973), resulting in B-cell immortalization and the generation of continuously proliferating lymphoblastoid cell lines (LCL) (Pope et al. 1968). EBV also infects squamous epithelial cells in certain pathological conditions in vivo (see later under Nasopharyngeal carcinoma and Oral hairy leukoplakia), and such cells can support full virus replication. However, in vitro infection of primary epithelial cells is problematic, and thus no fully permissive system is available for the study of individual replicative gene functions, in contrast to latent infection, which has been extensively investigated because of the ease with which immortalization of B cells can be brought about.

CLASSIFICATION

EBV is a member of the *Herpesviridae* and is in the *Gammaherpesvirinae* subfamily, genus *Lymphocryptovirus*. This classification is based on DNA homology between the EBV genome and that of other gammaherpesviruses, the G+C content of the genome and the lymphotropism of the virus.

MORPHOLOGY AND PARTICLE STRUCTURE

Like other herpesviruses, EBV has a protein core containing DNA, a nucleocapsid composed of 162 capsomers that forms an icosahedral protein shell, and an outer envelope derived from cellular membranes and containing virus-coded glycoprotein spikes.

MOLECULAR BIOLOGY

Genome structure and function

The EBV genome is a linear molecule of double-stranded DNA that contains 184 kb (www.med.ic.ac.uk/ludwig/EBV.htm) and has coding potential for about 70 proteins. EBV DNA contains several internal repeats interspersed with unique sequences and flanked by two terminal repeat sequences (Figure 29.1). EBV was the first herpesvirus to be cloned (Dambaugh et al. 1980) and sequenced (Baer et al. 1984). The nomenclature for the promoters and open reading frames within the viral genome has been assigned using the abbreviated name of the *Bam*HI restriction fragment: for example, BARF1 is the first, rightward open reading frame in the *Bam*HI A fragment of the EBV genome.

Two types of EBV exist, 1 and 2 (also called A and B) (Dambaugh et al. 1986), with an overall DNA sequence homology of 70–85 percent (Sample et al. 1990). They differ in the regions of the viral genome coding for the Epstein–Barr virus nuclear antigens (EBNA) 2, 3A, B, C (Rowe et al. 1989) and the Epstein–Barr virus-encoded small RNAs (EBER) (Arrand et al. 1989). These differences are reflected in biological diversity, type 1 viruses being more efficient than type 2 at immortalization of B lymphocytes in vitro (Rickinson et al. 1987). Type 1 EBV predominates worldwide. Type 2 is rare in western societies but more common in African communities. Dual infection may occur in individuals with immunosuppression (Zimber et al. 1986; Sculley et al. 1990). However, no type-specific disease associations have been noted. In addition to EBV type variation, individual viral isolates differ in the number of tandem repeats in their internal DNA repeat sequences. This heterogeneity can be used to define individual EBV isolates (Falk et al. 1995).

Latent infection of a B lymphocyte is associated with circularization of the EBV genome to form an episome (Lindahl et al. 1976), which later amplifies to give multiple copies. Genome circularization is achieved by covalent linkage of the terminal repeat elements, and the number of repeat sequences varies with different circularization events. Thus, when the viral episome is passed from one latently infected cell to a daughter cell (without linearizing) the number remains the same, indicating viral clonality. Estimation of the terminal repeats can therefore be used to determine whether virus infection of cells occurred before or after cell proliferation in tumor samples (Raab-Traub and Flynn 1986).

Virus-coded proteins

On infection of B lymphocytes in vitro, EBV establishes a latent type of infection with the expression of a restricted number of viral genes (latent genes) and continued cell survival and division without the production of viral progeny. The characteristics of these latent genes and their products are described below and listed with their alternative names in Table 29.1; the locations of their open reading frames are shown in Figure 29.1. This type of infection can be switched to a lytic infection with new virus production and cell death by certain stimuli that induce B-cell activation/differentiation and thereby cause the cell to become permissive for viral replication (Crawford and Ando 1986).

LATENT PROTEINS

The latent gene products include six EBNAs (1, 2, 3A,B,C leader protein (LP)) and three membrane proteins (latent membrane proteins (LMP) 1, 2A, B). In addition, two small RNAs (EBERs 1 and 2) are transcribed by RNA polymerase III but are not translated. The EBNAs initiate from promoters in either the W or the C fragments of the genome as long polycistronic messages which are subsequently spliced to give indivi-

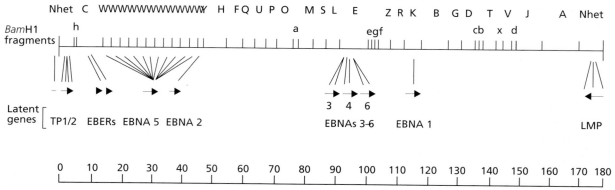

Figure 29.1 *Linear representation of the Epstein–Barr virus genome. Bam*HI *fragments are shown above and the location of the latent gene open reading frames is shown below. The arrows indicate the direction of transcription. The scale is in kilobases. EBERS, EB-coded small RNAs; EBNA, EB viral nuclear antigen; LMP, latent membrane protein.*

Table 29.1 *EBV latent genes*

Open reading frame[a]	Gene product	Alternative nomenclature	Mol. wt (kDa)	Cellular location	Required for immortalization	Suggested functions/ properties
BKRF1	EBNA1	–	65–85	Nucleus	+	Plasmid maintenance
BYRF1	EBNA2	–	86	Nucleus	+	Viral oncogene, transactivator of viral and cellular genes
BLRF3–BERF1	EBNA3A	EBNA 3	140–157	Nucleus	+	Viral oncogene, transcriptional regulator
BERF2a–BERF2b	EBNA3B	EBNA 4	148–180	Nucleus	-	NK
BERF3-BERF4	EBNA3C	EBNA 6	160	Nucleus	+	Viral oncogene, transcriptional regulator
BRWF1	EBNA (LP)	EBNA 5	20–130	Nucleus	+/-	Co-activates EBNA2 responsive genes. Increases efficiency of immortalization
BNLF1	LMP1	LMP	58–63	Membrane	+	Viral oncogene, transactivates cellular genes, mimics ligation of CD40
BARF1/ BNRF1	LMP2A	Terminal protein (TP)1	53	Membrane	-	Mimics BCR to enhance B-cell survival, inhibit B-cell activation and entry into lytic cycle
BNRF1	LMP2B	TP2	40	Membrane	-	NK
BCRF1	EBER1, 2	–	–	Cytoplasm/ nucleus	-	Regulation of PKR activity, inhibits apoptosis
BARF0	*Bam*HI A transcripts		–	Cytoplasm	-	NK

BCR, B-cell receptor; EBNA, EB virus nuclear antigen; LMP, latent membrane protein; LP. leader protein; NK, not known; PKR, double-stranded RNA protein kinase.
a) Abbreviated using the *Bam*HI(B) fragment (A–Z) LF or RF for left- or rightward open reading frame (ORF) followed by the number of the gene in a particular ORF.

dual mRNAs. In contrast, the LMPs each initiate from their own promoters. EBNAs 2, 3A,C and LMP1 have been shown by analysis of recombinant mutant viruses to be essential for immortalization, whereas EBNA3B and LP, LMP2A, B and EBERs 1 and 2 are not (for a review see Bornkamm and Hammerschmidt 2001). In addition to these proteins, complex transcripts arising from the *Bam*HI A open reading frame have been demonstrated in latently infected B cells, some of which may be translated into proteins, but their role in the life-cycle of EBV remains unclear (Smith 2001).

EBNA1

EBNA1 is a highly stable, DNA-binding nuclear phosphoprotein that is coded for by the BKRF1 open reading frame. It has a molecular weight ranging from 65 to 85 kDa, the variation being due to the different lengths of the repeat sequences in the molecule. EBNA1 protein consists of about 641 amino acids, is proline-rich, and contains a glycine–alanine repeat sequence; it binds to a specific DNA sequence by the carboxy terminus domain, which is rich in acidic and basic residues. Multiple EBNA1-binding sites occur in the latent viral

origin of replication (*oriP*) domain, where the binding of EBNA1 is the only viral factor required for maintenance of the viral episome (Yates et al. 1985). This binding also enhances transcription of EBNA1 and other latent viral genes because it activates the *oriP* enhancer, which regulates the EBNA promoter, Cp, and the LMP promoter (Gahn and Sugden 1995).

EBNA1 binds nonspecifically to metaphase chromosomes, thereby ensuring the equal partitioning of the viral episomes into the two daughter cells at mitosis. Thus EBNA1 expression is a requirement not only for the maintenance of the viral episome in latently infected cells, but also for the synchronization of virus genome replication with cell division.

Mice expressing EBNA1 as a transgene in B cells develop B-cell lymphoma, suggesting a direct role for EBNA1 in B-cell oncogenesis; however, the mechanism involved in this process is unknown (Wilson et al. 1996).

The glycine–alanine domain of EBNA1 inhibits proteosome-mediated degradation of EBNA1 and thereby prevents EBNA1 peptides being displayed on the cell surface bound to MHC class 1 molecules. Thus EBNA1-expressing cells are not recognized by CD8[+] cytotoxic T cells (Levitskaya et al. 1995).

EBNA2

EBNA2 is an acidic, nuclear phosphoprotein with a molecular weight of 86 kDa and is coded for by the BYRF1 open reading frame. The protein is a transactivator of viral and cellular genes and is essential for the immortalization of B lymphocytes in vitro (Cohen et al. 1989). EBNA2 does not bind directly to DNA, but interacts with a variety of cellular factors to induce B-cell activation. Three domains of EBNA2 have been identified as essential for immortalization. The acidic activator domain near the carboxy terminus (amino acids 420–464) recruits basal and activating transcription factors (TF) IIB, CBP/p300, TBP, TAF40, and TFIIH, causing transcriptional activation (Johannsen et al. 1995). The second essential domain between amino acids 180 and 337 interacts with the DNA-binding proteins RBP-Jk (also called CBF1), which is ubiquitous, and PU1, which is expressed in a restricted number of hemopoietic cell types, including B cells (Ling et al. 1994; Johannsen et al. 1995). As a result of these interactions EBNA2 transactivates the latent viral genes LMP1, 2A, 2B and the Cp promoter, which gives rise to EBNAs 1, LP, 2, 3A, B, C transcripts. A number of cellular genes, including the oncogenes c-*fgr* and c-*myc* and the B-cell activation molecules CD21 and CD23, are also upregulated by EBNA2. RBP-Jk naturally interacts with the evolutionarily conserved Notch protein signaling pathways, and EBNA2 appears to exploit these in the immortalization process (Hsieh et al. 1997). The third essential domain in EBNA2 is within the most conserved regions of the gene at the amino and carboxy termini, only one of which is required for immortalization. These regions aid the formation of the homotypic and heterotypic associations necessary for EBNA2 to recruit multiple transcription factors (Tsui and Schubach 1994).

The *EBNA2* gene shows considerable DNA sequence diversity between type 1 and 2 EBV, with an overall homology of about 55 percent.

EBNA3A, B, C

These three hydrophilic nuclear proteins are coded for by the BERF open reading frames and clearly arise from a common origin. Their molecular weights range from 140 to 180 kDa, owing to the variable repeat sequences present in each protein. Expression of EBNA3A and C is required for immortalization, whereas that of EBNA3B is not (Tomkinson et al. 1993). All three proteins are transcriptional regulators and bind to RBP-Jk, effectively competing with EBNA2 binding and thereby regulating its function (Zhao et al. 1996). EBNA3A and 3C can repress transcription when targeted to DNA, and have oncogenic activity in cooperation with mutant *ras* (Touitou et al. 2001; Hickabottom et al. 2002).

EBNA-LP

EBNA-LP is a nuclear phosphoprotein that is encoded by the BWRF1 open reading frame, which forms either the leader sequence of the EBNA mRNAs or, by alternative splicing, EBNA-LP mRNA. Because of the DNA repeats in this part of the genome, EBNA-LP protein consists of multiple repeat sequences of 22 and 44 amino acids flanked by unique amino and carboxy termini. Because the DNA repeat sequences vary in number in different virus isolates, the size of EBNA-LP protein varies accordingly. Immunoblotting of EBNA-LP in electrophoretically separated proteins from EBV-infected B cells reveals a ladder of bands differing by 6–8 kDa and corresponding to products of 20–130 kDa, an effect that is probably due to differential splicing of the mRNA.

The function of EBNA-LP is unknown and it is not strictly essential for immortalization, although it increases growth efficiency of infected B cells (Hammerschmidt and Sugden 1989). The protein contains a domain which coactivates gene transcription with EBNA2, and another that inhibits this effect. However, overall EBNA-LP has an activating role which is essential for efficient immortalization.

LMP1

LMP1 is a cytoplasmic and membrane protein that is coded for by the BNLF1 open reading frame. It has a molecular weight of 58–63 kDa and is phosphorylated on serine and threonine residues. The protein associates with the cytoskeleton in the plasma membrane, appearing as discrete patches on staining. LMP1 mRNA is the most abundant viral transcript found in latently infected B cells. The primary amino acid sequence of LMP1 suggests an integral membrane protein with a short 23 amino acid cytoplasmic amino terminus, a large 200 amino acid cytoplasmic carboxy terminus, and six hydrophobic transmembrane segments forming three external loops. A smaller LMP1 mRNA also exists, coding for a protein that lacks the amino terminus of the full-length protein, is expressed in lytically infected cells, and is present in the virus particle.

Full-length LMP1 is a classic viral oncoprotein that is essential for B-cell immortalization (Kaye et al. 1993). Transfection studies using the *LMP1* gene under a heterologous promoter have shown that it induces loss of contact inhibition and anchorage dependence, altered cell morphology, and tumorigenic potential in rodent fibroblasts (Wang et al. 1985). In human EBV-negative B-cell lines and primary B cells, LMP1 induces the changes associated with immortalization. These include an increase in cell size and steady-state calcium levels, upregulation of cell activation and cell adhesion molecule (CAM) expression, as well as upregulation of the cytoskeletal protein vimentin, CD54, and interleukin-6

(IL-6) (Wang et al. 1988). LMP1 expression protects B cells from cell death, probably through induction of the anti-apoptotic protein A20. LMP1 induces cellular genes by activation of the transcription factor NFκB (Hammarskjold and Simurdo 1992) via an interaction with tumor necrosis factor (TNF)-associated cell cytoplasmic factors (TRAFs). Cell activation by this pathway is similar to that of the B-cell surface molecule CD40, which mediates activation on B-cell-receptor engagement by antigen, and LMP1 can partially mimic this function in CD40 knockout mice (Uchida et al. 1999). Studies with LMP1 deletion mutants show that these effects are mediated by the amino terminus of LMP1. Sequencing studies on *LMP*1 genes from EBV isolates from different geographical locations have identified a common 30-bp deletion in the C terminus of LMP1 as well as several point mutations compared to the prototype B95.8 sequence (Hu et al. 1991). This deletion confers increased tumorigenicity in rodent fibroblasts and epithelial cells (Hu et al. 1993), and has been suggested to be more commonly associated with lympholiferative disorders and nasopharyngeal carcinoma than the undeleted form. However, more recent studies show that the incidence of the deletion in tumors reflects the incidence in the general population in each geographical location (Khanim et al. 1996).

LMP2A, 2B

The sequences that make up the LMP2 open reading frame are located at the two ends of the linear EBV genome in BARF1/BNRF1 and are completed only when the genome has circularized to form an episome (Laux et al. 1988). LMP2A and B are produced by alternative splicing of the mRNA, giving rise to proteins of 53 and 40 kDa, respectively. Neither is essential for immortalization of B cells in vitro. Both are hydrophobic membrane proteins with 12 transmembrane segments and 27 amino acid carboxy termini, but whereas LMP2A has 119 amino acids in the amino terminus domain LMP2B has only three. Both LMP2A and B localize to patches in the plasma membrane, and LMP2A colocalizes with LMP1. The amino terminus of LMP2A contains an immunoreceptor tyrosine-based activation motif (ITAM) similar to that found in the B-cell receptor (BCR) molecule, where the phosphorylated motif plays a central role in activation and differentiation processes through its interaction with src and Syk protein tyrosine kinases (PTK). LMP2A associates with these PTKs through its ITAM (Longnecker et al. 1991), and this interaction inhibits calcium mobilization following BCR stimulation of B lymphocytes latently infected with EBV. In this way LMP2A may prevent fortuitous activation of the viral lytic cycle (Miller et al. 1994). LMP2A transgenic mice show abnormal B-cell development, with survival of immunoglobulin negative B cells in peripheral lymphoid tissue (Caldwell et al.

1998). Thus it seems possible that LMP2A can promote B-cell proliferation and survival in the absence of BCR signals, and thereby promote long-term EBV latency in B cells.

The function of LMP2B is not known, but it may play a role in regulating LMP2A function.

EBERs 1 and 2

These two small nonpolyadenylated RNA molecules are coded for by the BCRF1 open reading frame and are the most abundant RNAs in latently infected B cells (10^4–10^5 copies per cell). They are localized mainly in the nucleus, where they bind to the La protein and the large ribosomal subunit protein L22 (Clemens 1994). Although the significance of this complex formation is not known, EBERs show sequence homology to the VA1 and 2 RNAs of adenovirus, which also bind La and are thought to be involved in RNA splicing. EBERs are not required for the in vitro immortalization process or for virus replication (Swaminathan et al. 1991) but, like VA1, bind to and regulate the activity of the protein kinase PKR. This interaction may inhibit the antiviral and antiproliferative effects of interferon, because PKR is induced by, and mediates, interferon activity (Clemens 1994).

Recently EBER expression has been shown to increase the tumorigenicity of Burkitt's lymphoma cell lines by upregulating the expression of Bcl-2 (Komano et al. 1999), but the significance of this finding to BL pathogenesis has not so far been elucidated.

LYTIC PROTEINS

Genes expressed during the EBV lytic cycle have been characterized in LCL that have been induced by various agents (zur Hausen et al. 1978; Luka et al. 1979; Tovey et al. 1978); such genes have extensive homology with those of other herpesviruses. Like other herpesviruses they follow an orderly sequence of expression, each set being activated by the previous set. Lytic genes can be divided into immediate–early genes which are transcribed prior to viral protein synthesis; early genes which are transcribed in the absence of viral DNA synthesis; and late genes which represent the structural proteins and are expressed only after viral DNA synthesis. However, EBV is unique among herpesviruses in possessing a set of latent genes that are already transcribed in infected B cells and may therefore influence subsequent lytic gene expression, although a viral transactivator of the immediate early genes has not been identified among them.

Immediate–early gene products

EBV possesses two genes that can be classified as immediate–early genes: *BZLF1* (Z) and *BRLF1* (R). These two genes code for nuclear proteins which are

DNA sequence specific acidic transactivators and are derived from three mRNA species, one of which contains both R and Z sequences. R and Z coordinately upregulate expression of the early genes by binding to specific sites in the promoter regions. The early promoter elements in the duplication left (DL) and right (DR) regions of the EBV genome, which also include the origin of lytic viral DNA replication (orilyt), contain multiple Z binding sites, and code many early transcripts, including *BHRF1* and *BHLF1* mRNAs.

Z is a DNA-binding protein that shows homology to the DNA-binding domain of the c-*jun* oncogene and binds to AP-1 sites (Farrell et al. 1989). The Z and R promoters (Zp, Rp) contain AP-1 sites and so Z transactivates its own activity as well as that of R. Z interacts with NF-κB and p53 in vivo (Gutsch et al. 1994), and these interactions are thought to inhibit p53-mediated apoptosis during lytic replication and prevent toxic levels of Z accumulating late in the lytic cycle.

Two of the early EBV nuclear proteins (BSMLF1 and BMRF1) may also cooperate in the transactivation of the early genes.

Early gene products

First identified by the staining pattern of sera containing antibodies to EBV when applied to the Raji cell line, which lacks expression of the late genes, the early gene products (early antigens (EA)) were characterized as diffuse (D) (nuclear and cytoplasmic staining) and restricted (R) (nuclear staining) (Henle et al. 1971). It is now known that these complexes consist of approximately 30 proteins, most of which have enzymic func-

tions required for viral DNA replication. Many of these were identified by their homology with early genes from other herpesviruses (Table 29.2).

Late gene products

Viral capsid proteins This antigen complex (VCA) consists of the nonglycosylated viral structural proteins. They have not yet been analyzed in detail because of the lack of a fully lytic system for EBV in vitro. The major capsid protein is coded for by the BCLF1 open reading frame, other components possibly arising from BNRF1 and BXRF1.

BCRF1 is a gene expressed only late in the lytic cycle that shows ca. 90 percent amino acid sequence homology with the human *IL-10* gene. The protein has been shown to have similar properties to human IL-10, and probably acts to reduce T- and NK-cell responses on initial infection and reactivation in vivo.

EBV glycoproteins The EBV-coded glycoproteins are involved in viral infectivity and spread and show extensive homology with herpes simplex glycoproteins (Table 29.3). Ten have been identified, most of which are inserted into the membranes of the infected cell, and several become components of the viral envelope (membrane antigens (MA)).

The major viral envelope glycoprotein, gp340/220, is coded for by the BLLF1 open reading frame. The two forms of the protein (molecular weights 340 and 220 kDa) are created by alternative splicing of the mRNA. The protein is found in the Golgi apparatus as well as the plasma membrane of infected cells. The

Table 29.2 *Early proteins involved in EBV replication*

Open reading frame	Mol. wt (kDa)	Cellular localization	Herpes simplex virus homology/ putative function
BMLF5	–	–	DNA polymerase
BALF5	–	–	DNA polymerase
BXLF1	–	–	Thymidine kinase
BGLF5	–	–	Alkaline exonuclease
BORF1	140	–	Ribonucleotide reductase
BARF1	38	–	Ribonucleotide reductase
BMRF1	47	Nucleus	DNA polymerase-associated protein
BALF2	135	–	Single-strand DNA-binding protein
BBLF4	–	–	Helicase/primase
BSLF1	–	–	Helicase/primase
BCRF2/3	–	–	Helicase/primase
BHRF1	18	Nuclear and cytoplasmic membrane	*bcl*-2 homologue
BKRF3	–	–	Uracil DNA glycosylase
BMLF1	–	Nucleus	Transactivator
BBLF2/3	–	–	Spliced primase–helicase complex component

Table 29.3 *EBV glycoproteins*

Open reading frame	Mol. wt (kDa)	Putative function	Present in viral envelope
BLLF1	340/220	Receptor (CR2) binding. HSV gC functional homologue	Yes
BALF4	110.0	Virulence factor. HSV gB homologue	No
BXLF2	85	Fusion of viral and cellular membranes. Complexes with gp42 and gp25. HSV gH homologue	Yes
BZLF2	42	Binds MHC class II – viral penetration. Complexes with gp85 and gp25. Functional HSV gD homologue	Yes
BKRF2	25	Complexes with gp85 and gp42. HSV gL homologue	Yes
BILF2	78/55	–	Yes
BDLF3	150	–	Yes

HSV, herpes simplex virus.

mature protein is heavily *N*- and *O*-glycosylated, about 50 percent of the molecule being carbohydrate. Gp340/220 mediates virus attachment to the B-cell surface by binding to the EBV receptor CR2 (also called CD21) (Nemerow et al. 1987). Thus both naturally occurring and experimentally induced antibodies to gp340/220 prevent infection by blocking attachment.

Gp85 is coded for by the BXLF2 open reading frame and has homology to the herpes simplex virus glycoprotein gH. Gp25 is required for the correct folding, transport to the cell surface and function of gp85. These proteins are localized to the plasma membrane and viral envelope, where they form a trimolecular complex with gp42. Gp42 is coded for by the BZLF2 open reading frame and is involved in penetration of the virus through the cell membrane during B-cell infection by its binding to HLA class II molecules on the B-cell surface. This glycoprotein is not required for viral entry into epithelial cells that are HLA class II negative (Borza and Hutt-Fletcher 2002).

Gp110 is coded for by the BALF4 open reading frame and has homology with the herpes simplex virus glycoprotein gB. It is *O*- and *N*-glycosylated and is localized to the nuclear and cytoplasmic membranes of infected cells. Gp110 has an important role as a virulence factor; high levels of expression can determine infection of cells other than B lymphocytes (Neuhierl et al. 2002).

Immortalization

Binding of EBV to B lymphocytes occurs through a ligand–receptor interaction between the major viral envelope glycoprotein gp340/220 and the cell surface complement receptor molecule CR2 (CD21) (Nemerow et al. 1987). CR2 is a member of the immunoglobulin superfamily and is expressed on all mature circulating B lymphocytes. It forms part of a signal transduction complex including CD19, TAPA1, and Leu-13 (Bradbury et al. 1992); it is postulated that the binding of EBV to CR2 induces initial B-cell-activating signals, but these have not yet been clearly defined. Once bound, the trimolecular complex of gp85, 42, and 25 on the viral envelope initiate fusion with the cell membrane, releasing the capsid into the cytoplasm. The viral genome rapidly enters the cell nucleus where it circularizes to form an episome, which later amplifies to give multiple copies per cell.

EBNAs 2 and LP, originating from the W promoter (Wp), are the first virus-coded proteins to be detected, at around 12–15 h post infection. EBNA2 protein then generally initiates a promoter switch from Wp to Cp (Woisetschlaeger et al. 1991) by complexing with RBP-Jk at the EBNA2 response element upstream of Cp, thereby allowing expression of all the EBNA proteins by 24 h. EBNA and LP also upregulate the LMP promoters, so that full latent viral gene expression is achieved by 48 h post infection.

Cell enlargement and activation with the expression of the B-cell activation marker CD23 occur at around 48 h post infection and can be attributed mainly to the action of LMP1 (Wang et al. 1990). By 72 h some cells have progressed through the G_1, S, and G_2 phases of the cell cycle and are entering mitosis. The cells then continue to cycle indefinitely, giving rise to an immortalized LCL. The phenotype of cells in an LCL is similar to that of antigen-stimulated lymphoblasts, with the expression of the B-cell-activation markers typical of this stage of B-cell differentiation (e.g. CD23, CD39, CD30, CD70, ki24) as well as the CAMs, CD11a, CD54, and CD58.

A few cells in an LCL (0–5 percent) enter the lytic cycle, a switch that seems to be triggered by physiological stimuli such as differentiation of the cell (Crawford and Ando 1986), and which can be induced by B-cell-activating agents such as phorbol esters (zur Hausen et al. 1978), sodium butyrate (Luka et al. 1979), and anti-immunoglobulin (Tovey et al. 1978). Cells of LCLs are immortal but cytogenetically normal. They are not, by definition, transformed cells because they do not form colonies in soft agar or give rise to tumors in nude mice (Nilsson et al. 1971). These characteristics differ from those of EBV-carrying cell lines derived from BL biopsy material (see EBV gene expression).

EBV replication

The induction of the lytic cycle in B lymphocytes or squamous epithelial cells infected in vitro is associated with differentiation of the cell (Crawford and Ando 1986; Kirimi et al. 1995), suggesting that the availability of cellular transcription factors determines the outcome of infection. In addition, the lytic cycle can be activated by transfection of the *BZLF1* gene or superinfection with the P3HR1 strain of virus, which contains defective virus in which *BZLF1* is adjacent to Wp (Miller et al. 1984).

Replication of EBV DNA begins at the origin of lytic replication, which is 1.4 kb in length and contains many inverted repeat sequences (Hammerschmidt and Sugden 1988). *ori*lyt acts as an amplicon, giving rise to many linear concatemers of the genome by the rolling circle method, and EBV-coded DNA polymerase is required for this process. The terminal repeat elements are required for cleaving and packaging the newly formed virions.

EBV gene expression

Infection of B lymphocytes in vitro leads to initiation of transcription of the polycistronic EBNA mRNA from Wp with an EBNA2-induced switch to Cp after 48–72 h (Woisetschlaeger et al. 1991). This results in expression of all the EBNA proteins as well as expression of the three latent membrane proteins from their own promoters. In addition, EBERs and *Bam*H1 A transcripts are detectable, and this gene expression pattern is termed full latent gene expression, or latency type III (Rowe et al. 1992). However, in vivo, other patterns of viral gene expression have been identified. In BL cells, which are small, nonactivated cells expressing the cellular markers of a germinal centre B cell (CD10, CD77), only

EBNA1 protein, EBERs and *Bam*H1 A transcripts are detected (latency type I) (Rowe et al. 1986). The EBNA1 mRNA initiates from a promoter in the Q region of the genome (Qp). Wp and Cp are silent and have been shown to be methylated (Masucci et al. 1989). However, when BL cells are cultured, demethylation often occurs, associated with a drift to full latent viral gene expression and a lymphoblastoid phenotype (Rowe et al. 1987).

An alternative pattern of transcription (latency type II) is seen in Reed–Sternberg cells in EBV-positive Hodgkin's disease (Deacon et al. 1993) and the malignant epithelial cells of nasopharyngeal carcinoma (Brooks et al. 1992). Here EBNA1 is expressed from Qp, and LMP1 and 2 are also expressed in the absence of the EBNAs. EBERs and the *Bam*H1 A transcripts are again detectable (Table 29.4).

Viral gene expression in circulating latently infected memory B cells in vivo is a controversial issue, as RT-PCR is the only technique with sufficient sensitivity to detect these rare cells. This technique does not give an indication of the genes expressed in individual cells or determine whether translation to protein occurs; however, the most regularly detected transcripts are EBERs and LMP2.

CLINICAL AND PATHOLOGICAL ASPECTS

INTRODUCTION

As a very ancient parasite of humans, EBV has established a delicately balanced relationship with its host that is almost entirely benign under normal conditions. Natural primary infection is usually inapparent, and is always followed by a lifelong, silent carrier state that becomes manifest as disease only if the virus–host balance is disturbed (Table 29.5).

EPIDEMIOLOGY

EBV is found in all human populations and, under natural conditions, primary infection occurs in early

Table 29.4 *Latent viral gene expression in EBV-associated tumors*

| Tumor | EBNA | | | | | | LMP | | | EBERs | EBNA promoter usage |
	1	2	3A	3B	3C	LP	1	2A	2B		
Burkitt's lymphoma	+	–	–	–	–	–	–	–	–	+	Qp
B lymphoproliferative disease	+	+	+	+	+	+	+	+	+	+	Cp/Wp
Nasopharyngeal carcinoma	+	–	–	–	–	–	+/–	+	+/–	+	Qp
Hodgkin's lymphoma	+	–	–	–	–	–	++	+	+	+	Qp

EBNA, EB viral nuclear antigen; EBERs, EB virus-coded small RNAs; LMP, latent membrane protein; LP, leader protein.

Table 29.5 *Conditions associated with EBV infection in humans*

Condition	Occurrence
Clinically silent childhood primary infection	Universal in developing countries; common in developed countries
Delayed primary infection (teenagers/young adults)	Seen in developed countries: ca. 50% are clinically silent, as in childhood, ca. 50% have acute infectious mononucleosis – usually resolves; may become chronic
Primary infection with fatal outcome	Very rare familial X-linked lymphoproliferative disease (Duncan syndrome)
Lymphomas in immunodepression	In organ graft recipients
	In AIDS patients
Oral hairy leucoplakia	In AIDS patients and other T-cell immunodeficiencies
Endemic Burkitt's lymphoma	Common in children where falciparum malaria is hyperendemic
Nasopharyngeal carcinoma	Common in south Chinese and Inuit adults
Hodgkin's disease	Developed countries: ca. 50% are EBV associated. Developing countries: <90% EBV associated
Tumors with tenuous or suspected links to EBV infection	Some T-cell lymphomas, leiomyosarcomas, salivary gland cancers, undifferentiated carcinoma of the stomach

childhood; thus, in developing countries, 99.9 percent of all children are infected by 2–4 years of age, depending on geographical region. However, in industrialized countries with high standards of hygiene a considerable number of people do not become infected as young children, the percentage of each age group remaining free of infection as teenagers or young adults depending in western societies on socioeconomic status: the higher the standard of living, the greater the percentage (Henle and Henle 1979b). Among the very affluent as many as 50 percent of young adults may never have been infected.

Primary infection in early childhood is symptom-free and leads only to the generation of antibodies to the viral and virus-determined antigens (Henle and Henle 1979b) and to the development of specific cytotoxic T lymphocytes (Murray et al. 1992). These humoral and cellular immunological responses are maintained continuously thereafter and are responsible for keeping the lifelong EBV infection in check; the virus persists as a latent infection in a few circulating B lymphocytes (Lewin et al. 1987) and as a productive infection somewhere in the mouth and pharynx, the urogenital tract and, perhaps, the salivary glands. EBV is shed into the buccal fluid in readily detectable amounts in about 20 percent of those who have been infected, and in small amounts from time to time in many of the remainder (Yao et al. 1985); the virus has also been detected in genital secretions (Sixbey et al. 1986; Israele et al. 1991). The nature of the permissive cells producing infectious virions in the oro- and nasopharynx was for long a continuing controversy (Allday and Crawford 1988; Niedobitek and Young 1994): was the virus coming from squamous epithelial cells or from intraepithelial B lymphocytes? Evidence suggesting that it might only be the latter has recently emerged because in the absence of lymphocytes, as occurs in patients with X-linked agammaglobulinemia, EBV infection does not seem to take place (Faulkner et al. 1999). However, even if this

observation appears to indicate that EBV does not normally infect and replicate in squamous epithelial cells of the mouth and pharynx, doubts and problems remain; squamous epithelial cells become infected in several conditions and an explanation of how and why the virus infects them is still required. Furthermore, such cells are capable of virus production; the latent EBV infection always carried by the malignant epithelial cells of nasopharyngeal carcinoma can be activated in vitro into a replicative cycle (Trumper et al. 1976), with release of infectious virus (Trumper et al. 1977), and virions are regularly produced in the squamous epithelial cells of oral 'hairy' leukoplakia (Greenspan et al. 1985).

Nevertheless, it has been clear for a great many years that virus in the buccal fluid is the main source of transmission of the infection in the population, by droplets and casually contaminated objects in the case of young children, and by direct salivary transfer during kissing among the sexually active (Hoagland 1955).

Those who miss the clinically silent natural primary infection in childhood are likely, sooner or later, to undergo delayed primary infection. Although 50 percent of such delayed infections are symptom-free, as in childhood, the other 50 percent are accompanied by disease: classic infectious mononucleosis (IM) (Sawyer et al. 1971; Hallee et al. 1974).

CLINICAL MANIFESTATIONS

Infectious mononucleosis

The fact that it is the teenagers and young adults in the upper classes of western countries who tend to escape silent infection as children makes IM predominantly a disease of the most affluent groups, and causes it to be exceptionally rare in developing countries. Although most cases of IM occur in adolescents and young adults, older children and the middle-aged may occasionally develop the disease as a consequence of primary EBV infection, and rarely also the elderly. IM has long been known to be associated with kissing among young people (Hoagland 1955), and the pattern of acquisition results from a healthy carrier who is shedding virus in his or her saliva passing this during close buccal contact directly into the oropharynx of a partner who has not been primarily infected in the usual way as a child. This method of spread explains why case-to-case infection and epidemics are not seen with IM, and why the incubation period – perhaps 30–50 days – is difficult to calculate. Primary EBV infection giving IM-like symptoms may also be transmitted by blood transfusion (Gerber et al. 1969) or organ grafting (Haque et al. 1996) from an infected donor to a previously uninfected recipient.

SYMPTOMS AND SIGNS

There may be vague prodromal indisposition or an abrupt onset with sore throat, fever and sweating, anorexia, headache, and marked malaise. Brief dysphagia and orbital edema may be noticed. Severe edema of the tonsils and pharynx can sometimes cause pharyngeal obstruction. Erythematous rashes occur in a small number of untreated patients, but affect most of those who have been taking ampicillin. The pharynx, fauces, soft palate, and uvula are red and swollen, and may develop a greyish exudate. Generalized lymphadenopathy is almost invariable, most marked in the cervical region, with symmetrical, discrete, slightly tender glands; splenomegaly is seen in 60 percent of cases, an enlarged liver in 10 percent, and actual jaundice in about 8 percent. Crops of palatal petechiae are found in about one-third of patients. If mild, IM may resolve in days, but usually continues for 1–2 weeks, and is often followed by a period of marked lethargy before complete recovery. The length of convalescence may be influenced by psychological factors, but about one case in 2 000 continues in a truly chronic or recurrent form for several months or even years; exhaustive investigation of such patients has sometimes revealed minor immunological defects (Virelizier et al. 1978).

In contrast, an extremely rare genetically determined, X-linked lymphoproliferative condition (XLP disease or Duncan syndrome) first described by Bar et al. (1974) is due to a specific inability to respond normally to EBV during primary infection, and the affected young males of certain kindred die from IM owing to progressive destruction of vital organs and multisystem failure (Gaspar et al. 2002). The gene for XLP syndrome has now been cloned (Coffey et al. 1998; Sayos et al. 1998); it lies on the long arm of the X chromosome and codes for a protein responsible for controlling normal T-cell activation. Because the gene is mutated in XLP syndrome cases, failure of this control probably permits the cytotoxic T cells generated by primary EBV infec-

tion to extend their action from the true targets provided by EBV-infected B cells to include the destruction of normal cells of the patient's vital organs (Howie et al. 2000).

COMPLICATIONS

Serious but rare complications include secondary bacterial throat infections, traumatic rupture of the enlarged spleen, asphyxia from pharyngeal edema, massive hepatic necrosis, Guillain–Barré syndrome, and autoimmune manifestations such as thrombocytopenia and hemolytic anemia (Finch 1969).

PATHOGENESIS

The very long evolutionary association of EBV with its human host (more than 35–45 Myr) has ensured that it can establish an inapparent infection in early childhood which thereafter persists for life (Henle and Henle 1979b). When delayed primary infection occurs as a result of the high living standards of modern western countries, young adults encounter the virus for the first time at an age when the mode of infection and size of infecting dose are different from those in children: children come into contact with saliva from a shedder as airborne droplets or contamination on some sucked object, and thus receive a much smaller amount of virus than a young person taking in large quantities of virus-containing saliva from such a carrier during mouth-to-mouth kissing (Hoagland 1955). An exaggerated immunological response to a very large infecting dose of EBV fits well with the changes of IM: large numbers of activated $CD8^+$ T cells stimulated by a mass of infected B cells (expressing all the known latent viral genes) in the circulation, in lymph nodes, tonsils, lymphoid tissue of the mouth and pharynx, spleen, liver, and elsewhere. These T cells kill EBV-infected target cells (Callan et al. 1998), secrete multiple lymphokines (Foss et al. 1994), and are thus the cause, by immunopathological mechanisms, of the sore throat, fever, malaise, lymphadenopathy, and hepatosplenomegaly.

IMMUNE RESPONSES AND DIAGNOSIS

During acute IM, serum IgM and IgG antibodies to VCA and IgG anti-EA antibodies appear early, whereas anti-EBNA1 antibodies are not usually detectable until convalescence (Henle and Henle 1979b). On recovery, IgM anti-VCA and IgG anti-EA disappear but IgG antibodies to VCA and EBNA1 are maintained for life (Figure 29.2) (Henle and Henle 1979a).

Because it is not usually possible to document seroconversion, the presence of IgM antibodies to viral capsid antigen provides the most reliable diagnostic test. This may be corroborated by finding anti-EA antibodies (usually of D type) or the absence of antibodies to EBNA1, or both (Henle and Henle 1979a). These tests

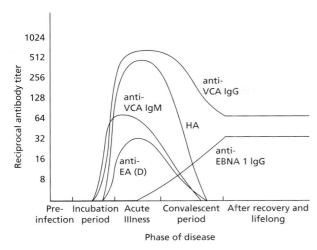

Figure 29.2 *Epstein–Barr virus-specific antibody response in infectious mononucleosis. Typical serum antibody titers as assessed by indirect immunofluorescence are indicated. EA (D), early antigen (diffuse); EBNA, EB viral nuclear antigen; HA, heterophile antibody; VCA, viral capsid antigen.*

depend on immunofluorescence staining of B-cell lines expressing viral antigens, are time-consuming, and are usually carried out only in larger laboratories. A number of commercial ELISAs are available but they lack the sensitivity of immunostaining. The rapid screening Monospot test is more widely used; this has been adapted from the earlier Paul–Bunnell test for IgM heterophil antibodies which agglutinate red cells from nonhuman sources. Although the heterophil antibodies are not directed against viral-coded antigens they are present in up to 85 percent of IM sera, but it must be remembered that cases of Monospot-negative IM are frequent outside the classic 15–25-year age range, and false positives may occur in pregnancy and autoimmune disease (Okano et al. 1988). An additional diagnostic feature of IM is the presence of a lymphocytosis of up to $15 \times 10^9/l$, most cells having an 'atypical' morphology. The clinical and hematological findings and a positive Monospot test give a reliable diagnosis, but if the latter is negative, tests for IgM anti-VCA antibodies must be done. Retrospective diagnosis may be possible if suitable samples are available to allow seroconversion to, or a rising titer of, EBNA1 IgG antibody to be detected.

Endemic ('African') Burkitt's lymphoma

Classic BL (Burkitt 1963) is a B-cell tumor found in parts of Africa and Papua New Guinea, where the temperature does not fall below 16.5°C or the annual rainfall below 55 cm (Burkitt 1970a). BL is overwhelmingly a disease of children, and is extremely rare over the age of 14 years. In endemic areas it is more common than all other childhood cancers added together. There is no evidence in the tumor belt for any tribal or racial susceptibility (Burkitt 1963). Endemic BL

is distinct from the 'Burkitt-like' tumors (sometimes called 'American' or 'sporadic' BL) seen sporadically everywhere in the world, which have a different age incidence, anatomical distribution and response to therapy. The term 'Burkitt type' is sometimes also applied to certain leukemias because of morphological resemblances of the malignant cells.

Some 97 percent of endemic BL carries the EBV genome, whereas only 12–25 percent of the sporadic tumors are EBV-positive (Ziegler et al. 1976); it would seem that the 3 percent of EBV-negative BLs occurring in endemic areas are in fact sporadic BLs that occur at low incidence worldwide.

The association between EBV and endemic BL is so close that it is now generally accepted that the virus is a necessary (albeit not solely sufficient) element in causation of the disease. It is an essential link, together with cofactors, in a complicated chain of events that leads to the malignant change (Epstein and Achong 1979). BL cells contain the EBV genome, but only EBNA 1 is expressed. Hyperendemic falciparum malaria is an important cofactor, and its spread by anopheline mosquitoes that require warmth and moisture explains the climate dependence of the tumor (Burkitt 1969).

SYMPTOMS AND SIGNS

The tumor is usually multifocal, occurs in a variety of sites, and the symptoms depend on the anatomical location of the lesions (Burkitt 1963). Tumors in the maxilla or mandible are present in 70 percent of patients and are the presenting feature of most of these (Figure 29.3). They may be multiple in two, three or even all four

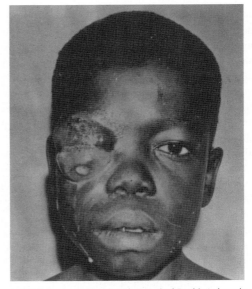

Figure 29.3 *A 9-year-old girl with a typical Burkitt's lymphoma of the right upper maxilla presenting through the orbit. The Epstein–Barr virus was first identified in cultured malignant lymphoblasts from this tumor.*

quadrants of the jaws, and are almost always accompanied by tumors elsewhere. A rapidly growing mass, loosening of teeth, and exophthalmos due to orbital spread are the main consequences. Abdominal tumors are also common, involving retroperitoneal nodes, liver, ovaries, intestine, and kidneys. BL may present in the thyroid, the adolescent female breast, the testicles, the salivary glands, and the skeleton. Extradural spinal tumors cause paraplegia of rapid onset. An unusual and characteristic feature of this lymphoma is its failure to involve the spleen and the peripheral lymph nodes.

Clinically, the tumors are firm, very rapidly growing, and painless; even when large, they cause minimal constitutional disturbance. The clinical signs are determined by the tumor sites, but wherever these may be BL grows relentlessly and, in the absence of treatment, death ensues within a few months (Burkitt 1963).

PATHOGENESIS

Molecular biological investigations are successfully unraveling the sequence of EBV gene expression that enables the virus to immortalize normal human B lymphocytes in vitro into continuously growing cell lines. Explanations are also beginning to emerge as to how the viral genes, in combination with cofactors, can bring about the malignant change leading to BL. There are currently two possibilities:

- EBV infection in the presence of the impaired immunological control brought about by hyperendemic malaria leads to a high level of EBV-driven B-cell proliferation, perhaps by similar mechanisms to in vitro immortalization; this proliferation in turn increases the chances of one or another of three BL-specific chromosomal translocations (t8:14; t8:22; t2:8) occurring, each of which can deregulate the c-*myc* oncogene on chromosome 8 by bringing it under the influence of an immunoglobulin gene promoter on chromosomes 14, 22, or 2. This deregulation causes malignant change in the affected cell and the rapid outgrowth of a clone of tumor cells (Klein 1987).
- The chronic immunological stimulation of hyperendemic malaria generates a high turnover of pre-B cells in the bone marrow; one or more of these early lymphocytes acquires one of the three chromosomal translocations involving c-*myc* deregulation by an error occurring during immunoglobulin gene rearrangement, and this renders the affected cell responsive to growth signals; infection of such a cell by EBV finally provides viral functions conferring malignancy and a tumor clone grows out (Lenoir and Bornkamm 1987).

However, with either possibility the virus–host balance is disturbed by hyperendemic malaria, and additional molecular explanations continue to emerge (Farrell et al. 1991, Kelly et al. 2002).

IMMUNE RESPONSES AND DIAGNOSIS

In the appropriate geographical regions endemic BL can often be diagnosed on clinical grounds, but this should be confirmed by histological examination of a biopsy specimen. In addition, antibodies to EBV antigens have a unique pattern in BL: titres rise as the disease progresses and fall as tumors regress in response to treatment. These changes may be used to assess disease outcome. IgG antibodies to VCA are found at 8–10 times higher geometric mean titers than in healthy controls matched for age, gender, and residence. IgG antibodies to EA-R and MA are also detectable (Henle et al. 1969), and likewise vary with disease progression; successful treatment causes a rise in anti-MA and a fall in anti-EA-R, whereas the reversal of this pattern usually heralds a recurrence of the tumor.

THERAPY

Surgery and radiotherapy are not effective, but excellent results are obtainable with moderate courses of chemotherapy (Burkitt 1970b). Cyclophosphamide is the drug of choice, and dramatic and sustained resolution is not uncommon when tumors are small.

Lymphomas in immunosuppressed individuals

The lifelong EBV infection present in all normal seropositive individuals is controlled by cell-mediated immune mechanisms. In primary and secondary suppression of cellular immunity this control of persisting EBV infection is lost, leading to increased virus replication in the oral cavity, increased numbers of virus-carrying B lymphocytes in the circulation, and increased levels of serum antibodies to lytic-cycle EBV antigens (VCA, EA). When this occurs it is sometimes described as a 'reactivated infection', although the condition is clinically silent. However, on occasions the loss of control results in EBV-associated lymphoproliferative disease. This type of disease also occurs when immunosuppressed individuals undergo primary infection and fail to mount the normal immunological response to the virus (Thomas et al. 1991).

ORGAN GRAFT RECIPIENTS

It has long been known that organ graft recipients who receive lifelong immunosuppressive drugs to prevent graft rejection have an increased risk of developing lymphoproliferative disease and lymphoma (28–100 times that of normal controls) (Penn 1983). Most of these conditions, known as post-transplant lymphoproliferative disease (PTLD), are of B-cell origin, contain the EBV genome, and express viral antigens in their cells. Lymphoproliferative disease has two forms of clinical presentation. In about 50 percent of cases it occurs within the first year after transplantation, in a young age group, has IM-like symptoms, and is associated with primary EBV infection in patients who were seronegative at the time of grafting. The second type of presentation occurs in older patients late after transplantation, and takes the form of a localized mass, commonly in the gut, central nervous system, or transplanted organ (Hanto et al. 1981, 1985). Biopsy of the lesion reveals large-cell lymphoma, which is usually monoclonal in origin, although progression from a polyclonal B-cell proliferation probably occurs early in the disease (Frizzera et al. 1981, Frizzera 1987). The fact that all the EBV latent viral genes are expressed in these lymphoproliferative diseases, just as with lymphoblastoid cell lines immortalized by the virus in vitro, suggests that EBV is of prime importance in the etiology of the lesions (Thomas et al. 1990), although other events – perhaps cytogenetic abnormalities – may be necessary to cause the monoclonal growth.

Reduction of immunosuppressive drugs, with or without acyclovir therapy, has caused complete and often sustained regression of the tumors in many cases (Starzl et al. 1984). This has therefore become the first line of treatment, cytotoxic drugs and/or radiotherapy being used only when there is no response or after recurrence. EBV-specific cytotoxic T cells grown in vitro have been given after bone marrow transplantation to protect against such EBV-driven lymphoproliferation prior to regeneration of the immune system (Rooney et al. 1995), and to treat PTLD in bone marrow and solid organ transplant recipients (Haque et al. 2002).

AIDS PATIENTS

Two types of lymphoma are seen with increasing frequency in AIDS patients: large-cell lymphoma and Burkitt's lymphoma. Both of these may be associated with EBV (Kalter et al. 1985).

Large-cell lymphomas similar to those seen in organ graft recipients occur in severely immunocompromised AIDS patients; their distribution is extranodal and involves many unusual sites, the most common being the central nervous system. These lymphomas have a strong association with EBV, which reaches 100 percent in cerebral tumors (Herndier et al. 1994). The clinical presentation depends on the site involved, but the progression is rapid, with a mean survival time from diagnosis of 3–4 months. The treatment of choice is radiotherapy, although the results are disappointing, mainly because patients in the terminal stages of the underlying AIDS are in such poor general condition.

Burkitt's lymphoma occurs earlier in the course of human immunodeficiency virus (HIV) disease, while the immune system is still relatively intact, and is therefore more amenable to treatment. About 50 percent of these lymphomas contain EBV DNA.

Hodgkin's disease

There has long been a suspicion that EBV may play some part in the induction of Hodgkin's disease (HD) because of the similar socioeconomic epidemiology of HD and IM, and because of the well established fact that within 5 years of IM there is a four- to sixfold increase in the likelihood of developing HD (Mueller et al. 1989). In recent years, evidence has been obtained that about 60 percent of HD is EBV associated, and this mainly involves the mixed cellularity type. However, surprisingly, the majority of EBV-associated mixed cellularity HD cases do not occur in the post-IM age group (Jarrett 2002).

In EBV-associated HD EBV DNA is carried and viral proteins expressed (latency II) in Reed–Sternberg and the tumor reticulum cells (Weiss et al. 1989; Herbst and Niedobitek 1994), and both these cell types are now known to be of germinal center B-cell origin (Marafioti et al. 2000). These intriguing findings appear to implicate EBV in certain types of HD.

T-cell lymphomas

EBV DNA has been detected with varying frequency in different types of T-cell lymphoma. Detection rates of up to 97 percent have been recorded in angioimmunoblastic lymphadenopathy (Ott et al. 1992), 84 percent in nasal lymphoma (previously called midline granuloma) (Harabuchi et al. 1990), and in 46 percent of peripheral T-cell lymphoma (Jones et al. 1988). In addition, sporadic cases of EBV-positive angiocentric T-cell lymphoma and of T-cell lymphoma related to immunosuppression and chronic EBV infection also occur. In these lesions the cell phenotype is usually that of clonal, mature T cells, which more often express the CD4 than the CD8 marker. The EBV gene expression is usually of the latency II type, but the latency III pattern has also been recorded.

Although it is now clear that EBV can infect T cells under certain conditions, the involvement of the virus in the pathogenesis of T-cell lymphoma remains to be elucidated.

Various other malignancies

Recent reports have linked EBV to various cancers, including some thymic epithelial tumors (Leyvraz et al. 1985; Wu and Kuo 1993), some undifferentiated salivary gland carcinomas (Hamilton-Dutoit et al. 1991) and, more regularly, to several types of gastric carcinoma (Takada 2000); surprisingly, smooth muscle tumors carrying EBV have also been reported in immunosuppressed children (Lee et al. 1995; McClain et al. 1995). Little is known about the EBV gene expression in any of these tumors, and further work is required before a definite association can be established.

Nasopharyngeal carcinoma

Nasopharyngeal carcinoma (NPC) arises from the squamous epithelial cells of the postnasal space; primary tumors are not found outside this well-defined anatomical site. About 70 percent of NPC are undifferentiated in type; the remainder show squamous differentiation. The tumor occurs rarely throughout the world, but has a very high incidence in southern Chinese wherever they live, and in the Inuit and related races of North America and Greenland. Among populations with a high incidence, NPC is the most common cancer of men and the second most common of women. There is also a high incidence of NPC in Malays, Dyaks, Indonesians, Filipinos, and Vietnamese, and a moderately raised incidence in a belt across North Africa, down through the Sudan and into the Kenyan Highlands. Comprehensive reviews have been given by Shanmugaratnam (1971, 1978). The tumor is usually a disease of middle or old age, except that in medium–high incidence areas of Africa it has bimodal age peaks, the first involving children and young people under 20 years of age (Cammoun et al. 1974), and a second affecting much older people. The tumor cells of undifferentiated NPC always carry the EBV genome (Klein 1979; Niedobitek et al. 1991), and most authorities agree that the virus plays a role in causation as a necessary but not the sole element in the etiological complex.

SYMPTOMS AND SIGNS

About two-thirds of patients present with one or more symptoms caused by the local effects of the tumor: nasal obstruction, discharge or bleeding; deafness, tinnitus, or earache; ocular paresis from tumor spread to affect cranial nerves. The remaining third complain only of cervical lymph node enlargement due to metastatic spread from a primary tumor that is frequently occult. The signs result either from local tumor spread, causing soft tissue distortion around the postnasal space or cranial nerve palsies, or as a consequence of lymphatic spread to cervical and later supraclavicular lymph glands, which become hard and fixed. Bloodborne metastases may be in any organ but are frequent in bones, liver, and lungs, the signs depending on the organ involved (Shanmugaratnam 1971).

PATHOGENESIS

Little is known of EBV gene function in normal infected epithelial cells, but viral gene expression in the malignant cells of NPC is well characterized; although restricted, it is less so than in BL cells with EBNA1 detected in every tumor cell of undifferentiated NPC and LMP1 in a variable proportion (latency type II) (Young et al. 1988). In addition to the virus, racial predisposition plays a role, and, among southern Chinese, a modest genetic predisposition has also been demonstrated (Simons et al. 1974; Chan et al. 1983). Environmental cofactors associated with the Chinese way of life have emerged from studies on migrants (Buell 1974; Henderson 1974), and two likely candidates have been identified:

- Traditional herbal remedies (taken as snuff) made from dried plants of the *Euphorbiaceae* and *Thymeliaceae* families, which contain tumor-promoting phorbol esters (Hirayama and Ito 1981).
- Traditional salt fish dishes, which contain carcinogenic nitrosamines (Huang et al. 1978).

Because EBV replicates in the nasopharynx of all carriers, and because southern Chinese always undergo primary infection as very young children (Henle and Henle 1979b), the taking of snuffs containing phorbol esters is significant because these chemicals are also powerful activators of EBV replication (zur Hausen et al. 1979) as well as having tumor-promoting effects. Thus, if virus production is greatly increased in people with a genetic predisposition to NPC, there will be an unusually large pool of EBV-infected cells that might progress to malignancy, perhaps through a combination of EBV *LMP1* oncogene function with nitrosamine carcinogenicity and phorbol ester tumor-promoting effects.

IMMUNE RESPONSES AND DIAGNOSIS

The diagnosis of NPC is usually made histologically on a biopsy sample from the primary tumor or from an enlarged cervical lymph gland. In addition, serum antibody titers show a characteristic and specific pattern of reaction, regardless of geographical location, and can therefore be used for diagnosis; IgG and IgA antibodies to VCA and EA-D are raised, and IgA against these antigens can be found in the saliva (Klein 1979). In the high incidence areas of southern China, mass screening of susceptible populations for serum IgA antibodies to VCA has been successful in detecting very early cases of NPC (Zeng et al. 1982), an important achievement because such early lesions usually respond very well to treatment.

THERAPY

The treatment of choice is radiotherapy, which gives 5-year survival rates of 60 percent or more in the earliest stages of the disease. Of those who survive, 70 percent remain permanently free of relapse (Ho et al. 1983). More advanced stages have correspondingly worse prognoses.

Oral hairy leukoplakia

This unusual condition is seen fairly frequently in HIV-positive homosexual men, often before AIDS develops, but sometimes heralding or accompanying the onset of clinical AIDS. Painless white patches occur on the tongue and/or the lateral buccal mucosa; the lesions are usually multiple, measure up to 3 cm in diameter, are slightly raised, and have a 'hairy' or corrugated surface (Greenspan et al. 1985).

The squamous epithelial cells affected by this condition contain large amounts of actively replicating EBV (Greenspan et al. 1985). Acyclovir arrests the virus replication and the lesions regress, but only for the period during which drug treatment is continued.

VACCINES AGAINST EBV

In the mid-1970s evidence linking EBV to some causative role in endemic BL and NPC was sufficiently strong to warrant the suggestion that vaccine prevention of the virus infection might be a way of decreasing the incidence of the associated cancers in high-risk populations (Epstein 1976). Although BL is of outstanding importance as a model for human viral carcinogenesis, and is exceedingly common in endemic areas, in terms of world cancer it is insignificant; however, NPC is a major oncological problem for very large populations, justifying efforts to control it through the development of a vaccine against EBV. Vaccine protection against IM would also be useful.

An extended program of work on an MA-based anti-EBV vaccine (Epstein 1986, 1994) succeeded in establishing that the purified gp340 component of MA induced virus-neutralizing antibodies, and indeed cytotoxic T-cell responses (Wilson et al. 1999), on injection into cottontop tamarins. Furthermore, the latter – the only animal known to respond with lesions to experimental EBV infection – when immunized in this way were protected against a 100 percent carcinogenic challenge dose of virus (Epstein 1986, 1994). Recently, gp340 purified from cultures of mammalian cells into which the *gp340* gene had been engineered (Jackman et al. 1999) was used in a successful phase I trial in human volunteers (Gilbert 1999). A phase II trial subsequently conducted for a major pharmaceutical company in a larger group of volunteers has given preliminary results that show some encouraging protective effects (Bollen 2002); a phase II placebo-controlled trial is currently in progress.

Other approaches are also going forward. Recombinant vaccinia viruses expressing gp340 have been made, and a small scale vaccination experiment using this in nine Chinese children has given some evidence of protection (Gu et al. 1995), but a wildtype strain of vaccinia was employed for the construct which would not be acceptable for general application. A quite different project has sought to induce specific cytotoxic T-cell immunity, not antibodies: selected EBV epitopes have been fused together in a synthetic polyepitope protein for injection, not to prevent infection, but to limit EBV replication after infection by destruction of virus-producing cells by the stimulated T cells, and thereby perhaps decrease disease manifestations. Preliminary trials to explore this technique in volunteers have begun (Khanna et al. 1999).

REFERENCES

Allday, M.J. and Crawford, D.H. 1988. Role of epithelium in EBV persistence and pathogenesis of B cell tumours. *Lancet*, **1**, 855–7.

Arrand, J.R., Young, L.S. and Tugwood, J.D. 1989. Two families of sequences in the small RNA-encoding region of Epstein–Barr virus (EBV) correlate with EBV types A and B. *J Virol*, **63**, 983–6.

Baer, R., Bankier, A.T., et al. 1984. DNA sequence and expression of the B95-8 Epstein–Barr virus genome. *Nature (London)*, **310**, 207–11.

Bar, R.S., Delor, C.J., et al. 1974. Fatal infectious mononucleosis in a family. *N Engl J Med*, **290**, 363–7.

Bollen, A. 2002. Encouraging results from Epstein-Barr vaccine Phase II trial, Henogen Press Release, 3 October. Belgium: Charleroi.

Bornkamm, G.W. and Hammerschmidt, W. 2001. Molecular virology of Epstein-Barr virus. In: Epstein, M.A., Rickinson, A.B. and Weiss, R.A. (eds), *Oncogenic γ-herpesviruses: an expanding family. Phil Trans Roy Soc Lond B Biol Sci*, **356**, 437–59.

Borza, C.M. and Hutt-Fletcher, L.M. 2002. Alternate replication in B cells and epithelial cells switches tropism of Epstein–Barr virus. *Nature Med*, **8**, 594–9.

Bradbury, L.E., Kansas, G.S., et al. 1992. The CD19/CD21 signal transducing complex of human B lymphocytes includes the target of antiproliferative antibody-1 and Leu-13 molecules. *J Immunol*, **149**, 2841–50.

Brooks, L., Yao, Q.Y., et al. 1992. Epstein–Barr virus latent gene transcription in nasopharyngeal carcinoma cells: coexpression of EBNA1 LMP1, and LMP2 transcripts. *J Virol*, **66**, 2689–97.

Buell, P. 1974. The effect of migration on the risk of nasopharyngeal carcinoma among Chinese. *Cancer Res*, **34**, 1189–91.

Burkitt, D. 1963. A lymphoma syndrome in tropical Africa. In: Richter, G.W. and Epstein, M.A. (eds), *International review of experimental pathology 2*. New York: Academic Press, 67–138.

Burkitt, D.P. 1969. Etiology of Burkitt's lymphoma – an alternative hypothesis to a vectored virus. *J Natl Cancer Inst*, **42**, 19–28.

Burkitt, D.P. 1970a. Geographical distribution. In: Burkitt, D.P. and Wright, D.H. (eds), *Burkitt's lymphoma*. Edinburgh: E & S Livingstone, 186–97.

Burkitt, D.P. 1970b. Treatment: general features. In: Burkitt, D.P. and Wright, D.H. (eds), *Burkitt's lymphoma*. Edinburgh: E & S Livingstone, 43–51.

Caldwell, R.G., Wilson, J.B., et al. 1998. Epstein–Barr virus LMP2A drives B cell development and survival in the absence of normal B cell receptor signals. *Immunity*, **9**, 405–11.

Callan, M.F.C., Tan, L., et al. 1998. Direct visualization of antigen-specific CD8[+] T cells during the primary immune response to Epstein–Barr virus in vivo. *J Exp Med*, **187**, 1395–402.

Cammoun, M., Hoerner, G.V. and Mourali, N. 1974. Tumors of the nasopharynx in Tunisia: an anatomic and clinical study based on 143 cases. *Cancer*, **33**, 184–92.

Chan, S.H., Wee, G.B., et al. 1983. HLA locus B and DR antigen associations in Chinese NPC patients and controls. In: Prasad, U., Ablashi, D.V., et al. (eds), *Nasopharyngeal carcinoma: current concepts*. Kuala Lumpur: University of Malaya Press, 307–12.

Cho, Y., Ramer, J., et al. 2001. Epstein–Barr related herpesvirus from marmoset lymphomas. *Proc Natl Acad Sci USA*, **98**, 1224–9.

Clemens, M.J. 1994. Functional significance of the Epstein-Barr virus-encoded small RNAs. *Epstein–Barr Virus Rep*, **1**, 107–12.

Coffey, A.J., Brooksbank, R.A., et al. 1998. Host response to EBV infection in X-linked lymphoproliferative disease results from mutations in an SH2-domain encoding gene. *Nature Genet*, **20**, 129–35.

Cohen, J.I., Wang, F., et al. 1989. Epstein–Barr virus nuclear protein 2 is a key determinant of lymphocyte transformation. *Proc Natl Acad Sci USA*, **86**, 9558–62.

Crawford, D.H. and Ando, I. 1986. EB virus induction is associated with B cell maturation. *Immunology*, **59**, 405–9.

Dambaugh, T., Beisel, C., et al. 1980. EBV DNA. VII. Molecular cloning and detailed mapping of EBV (B95-8) DNA. *Proc Natl Acad Sci USA*, **77**, 2999–3003.

Dambaugh, T., Wang, F., et al. 1986. Expression of the Epstein–Barr virus nuclear protein 2 in rodent cells. *J Virol*, **59**, 453–62.

Deacon, E.M., Pallesen, G., et al. 1993. Epstein–Barr virus and Hodgkin's disease: transcriptional analysis of virus latency in the malignant cells. *J Exp Med*, **177**, 339–49.

Deinhardt, F. and Deinhardt, J. 1979. Comparative aspects: oncogenic animal herpesviruses. In: Epstein, M.A. and Achong, B.G. (eds), *The Epstein–Barr virus*. Berlin: Springer-Verlag, 373–415.

Epstein, M.A. 1976. Epstein–Barr virus – is it time to develop a vaccine program? *J Natl Cancer Inst*, **56**, 697–700.

Epstein, M.A. 1986. Vaccination against Epstein–Barr virus: current progress and future strategies. *Lancet*, **1**, 1425–7.

Epstein, M.A. 1994. Le programme de vaccination pour la prévention des cancers associés au virus d'Epstein-Barr chez l'homme. *CR Acad Sci Sér Gen*, **11**, 11–18.

Epstein, M.A. 1999. On the discovery of Epstein–Barr virus: a memoir. *Epstein–Barr Virus Report*, **6**, 58–63.

Epstein, M.A. and Achong, B.G. 1979. The relationship of the virus to Burkitt's lymphoma. In: Epstein, M.A. and Achong, B.G. (eds), *The Epstein–Barr virus*. Berlin: Springer-Verlag, 321–37.

Epstein, M.A., Achong, B.G. and Barr, Y.M. 1964. Virus particles in cultured lymphoblasts from Burkitt's lymphoma. *Lancet*, **1**, 702–3.

Falk, K., Gratama, J.W., et al. 1995. The role of repetitive DNA sequences in the size of Epstein-Barr virus (EBV) nuclear antigens and the identification of different EBV isolates using RFLP and PCR analysis. *J Gen Virol*, **76**, 779–90.

Farrell, P., Rowe, D., et al. 1989. Epstein–Barr virus, BZLF-1 trans-activator specifically binds to consensus AP-1 sites and is related to c-*fos*. *EMBO J*, **8**, 127–32.

Farrell, P.J., Allan, G.J., et al. 1991. p53 is frequently mutated in Burkitt's lymphoma cell lines. *EMBO J*, **10**, 2879–87.

Faulkner, G.C., Burrows, S.R., et al. 1999. X-linked agammaglobulinaemia patients are not infected with Epstein–Barr virus. *J Virol*, **73**, 1555–64.

Finch, S.C. 1969. Clinical symptoms and signs of infectious mononucleosis. In: Carter, R.L. and Penman, H.G. (eds), *Infectious mononucleosis*. Oxford: Blackwell Scientific, 19–46.

Foss, H-D, Herbst, H., et al. 1994. Patterns of cytokine gene expression in infectious mononucleosis. *Blood*, **83**, 707–12.

Frizzera, G. 1987. The clinico-pathological expressions of Epstein–Barr virus infection in lymphoid tissues. *Virchows Arch B*, **53**, 1–12.

Frizzera, G., Hanto, D.W., et al. 1981. Polymorphic diffuse B-cell hyperplasias and lymphomas in renal transplant recipients. *Cancer Res*, **41**, 4262–79.

Gahn, T.A. and Sugden, B. 1995. An EBNA-1-dependent enhancer acts from a distance of 10 kilobase pairs to increase expression of the Epstein–Barr virus LMP gene. *J Virol*, **69**, 2633–6.

Gaspar, H.B., Sharifi, R., et al. 2002. X-linked lymphoproliferative disease: clinical diagnostic and molecular perspective. *Br J Haematol*, **119**, 585–95.

Gerber, P., Walsh, J.H., et al. 1969. Association of EB-virus infection with the post-perfusion syndrome. *Lancet*, **1**, 593–5.

Gilbert, K. 1999. Results of Phase I clinical trial for Epstein-Barr virus vaccine. *Aviron Press Release*, 11 August, California, USA: Mountain View.

Greenspan, J.S., Greenspan, D., et al. 1985. Replication of Epstein–Barr virus within the epithelial cells of oral 'hairy' leukoplakia, an AIDS-associated lesion. *N Engl J Med*, **313**, 1564–71.

Gu, S.Y., Huang, T.M., et al. 1995. First EBV vaccine trial in humans using recombinant vaccinia expressing the major membrane antigen. *Dev Biol Stand*, **84**, 171–7.

Gutsch, D.E., Holley-Guthrie, E.A., et al. 1994. The bZIP transactivator of Epstein-Barr virus, BZLF1, functionally and physically interacts with the p65 subunit of NF-kappa B. *Mol Cell Biol*, **14**, 182–95.

Hallee, T.J., Evans, A.S., et al. 1974. Infectious mononucleosis at the United States Military Academy. A prospective study of a single class over four years. *Yale J Biol Med*, **47**, 182–95.

Hamilton-Dutoit, S.J., Therkildsen, M.H., et al. 1991. Undifferentiated carcinoma of the salivary gland in Greenland Eskimos: demonstration of Epstein–Barr virus DNA by in situ nucleic acid hybridization. *Hum Pathol*, **22**, 811–15.

Hammarskjold, M-L and Simurdo, M.C. 1992. Epstein–Barr virus latent membrane protein transactivates the human immunodeficiency virus type I long terminal repeat through induction of NF-κB activity. *J Virol*, **66**, 6496–501.

Hammerschmidt, W. and Sugden, B. 1988. Identification and characterization of oriLyt, a lytic orgin of DNA replication of Epstein–Barr virus. *Cell*, **55**, 427–33.

Hammerschmidt, W. and Sugden, B. 1989. Genetic analysis of immortalising functions of Epstein-Barr virus in human B lymphocytes. *Nature (Lond)*, **340**, 393–7.

Hanto, D.W., Frizzera, G., et al. 1981. Clinical spectrum of lymphoproliferative disorders in renal transplant recipients and evidence for the role of Epstein–Barr virus. *Cancer Res*, **41**, 4253–61.

Hanto, D.W., Frizzera, G., et al. 1985. Epstein–Barr virus, immunodeficiency and B cell lymphoproliferation. *Transplantation*, **39**, 461–72.

Haque, T., Thomas, J.A., et al. 1996. Transmission of donor Epstein–Barr virus (EBV) in transplanted organs causes lymphoproliferative disease in recipients. *J Gen Virol*, **77**, 1169–72.

Haque, T., Wilkie, G.M., et al. 2002. Treatment of Epstein–Barr virus-positive post transplant lymphoproliferative disease using partially HLA-matched allogeneic cytotoxic T cells. *Lancet*, **360**, 436–42.

Harabuchi, Y., Yamanaka, N., et al. 1990. Epstein–Barr virus in nasal T-cell lymphomas in patients with midline granuloma. *Lancet*, **1**, 128–30.

Henderson, B.E. 1974. Nasopharyngeal carcinoma: present status of knowledge. *Cancer Res*, **34**, 1187–8.

Henle, G. and Henle, W. 1979a. The virus as the etiologic agent of infectious mononucleosis. In: Epstein, M.A. and Achong, B.G. (eds), *The Epstein–Barr virus*. Berlin: Springer-Verlag, 279–320.

Henle, W. and Henle, G. 1979b. Seroepidemiology of the virus. In: Epstein, M.A. and Achong, B.G. (eds), *The Epstein-Barr virus*. Berlin: Springer-Verlag, 61–78.

Henle, G., Henle, W., et al. 1969. Antibodies to EBV in BL and control groups. *J Natl Cancer Inst*, **43**, 1147–57.

Henle, G., Henle, W., et al. 1971. Demonstration of two distinct components in the early antigen complex of Epstein–Barr virus-infected cell. *Int J Cancer*, **8**, 272–82.

Herbst, H. and Niedobitek, G. 1994. Epstein–Barr virus in Hodgkin's disease. *Epstein–Barr Virus Rep*, **1**, 31–5.

Herndier, B.G., Kaplan, L.D. and McGrath, M.S. 1994. Pathogenesis of AIDS lymphoma. *AIDS*, **8**, 1025–49.

Hickabottom, M., Parker, G.A., et al. 2002. Two nonconsensus sites in the Epstein–Barr virus oncoprotein EBNA3A cooperate to bind the co-repressor carboxyl-terminal-binding protein (CtBP). *J Biol Chem*, **277**, 47197–204.

Hirayama, T. and Ito, Y. 1981. A new view of the etiology of nasopharyngeal carcinoma. *Prev Med*, **10**, 614–22.

Ho, J.H.C., Lau, W.H. and Fong, M. 1983. Treatment of nasopharyngeal carcinoma: current status. In: Prasad, U., Ablashi, D.V., et al. (eds), *Nasopharyngeal carcinoma: current concepts*. Kuala Lumpur: University of Malaya Press, 389–95.

Hoagland, R.J. 1955. The transmission of infectious mononucleosis. *Am J Med Sci*, **229**, 262–72.

Howie, D., Sayos, J. and Morra, M. 2000. The gene defective in X-linked lymphoproliferative disease controls T-cell dependent immune surveillance against Epstein–Barr virus. *Curr Opin Immunol*, **12**, 474–8.

Hsieh, J.J.D., Nofziger, D.E., et al. 1997. Epstein–Barr virus immortalization: Notch2 interacts with CBF1 and blocks differentiation. *J Virol*, **71**, 1938–45.

Hu, L.F., Zabarovsky, E.R. and Chen, F. 1991. Isolation and sequencing of the Epstein–Barr virus BNLF-1 (LMP1) from a Chinese nasopharyngeal carcinoma. *J Gen Virol*, **72**, 2399–409.

Hu, L.F., Chen, F., et al. 1993. Clonability and tumorigenicity of human epithelial cells expressing the EBV encoded membrane protein LMP1. *Oncogene*, **8**, 1575–83.

Huang, D.P., Ho, J.C.H. and Gough, T.A. 1978. Analysis for volatile nitrosomines in salt preserved foodstuffs traditionally consumed by southern Chinese. In: de Thé, G., Ito, Y. and Davis, W. (eds), *Nasopharyngeal carcinoma: etiology and control*. Lyon: International Agency for Research on Cancer, 309–14.

Israele, V., Shirley, P. and Sixbey, J.W. 1991. Excretion of the Epstein–Barr virus from the genital tract of men. *J Infect Dis*, **163**, 1341–3.

Jackman, W.T., Mann, K.A., et al. 1999. Expression of Epstein–Barr virus gp350 as a single chain glycoprotein for an EBV subunit vaccine. *Vaccine*, **17**, 660–8.

Jarrett, R.F. 2002. Viruses and Hodgkin's lymphoma. *Ann Oncol*, **13**, 23–9.

Johannsen, E., Koh, E., et al. 1995. Epstein–Barr virus nuclear protein 2 transactivation of the latent membrane protein 1 promotor is mediated by Jk and PU1. *J Virol*, **69**, 253–62.

Jones, J.F., Shurin, S., et al. 1988. T cell lymphomas containing Epstein–Barr viral DNA in patients with chronic Epstein–Barr virus infections. *N Engl J Med*, **318**, 733–41.

Kalter, S.P., Riggs, S.A., et al. 1985. Aggressive non-Hodgkin's lymphoma in immunocompromised homosexual males. *Blood*, **66**, 655–9.

Kaye, K.M., Izumi, K.M. and Kieff, E. 1993. Epstein–Barr virus latent membrane protein 1 is essential for B lymphocyte growth transformation. *Proc Natl Acad Sci USA*, **90**, 9150–4.

Kelly, G., Bell, A. and Rickinson, A. 2002. Epstein–Barr virus-associated Burkitt lymphomagenesis selects for downregulation of the nuclear antigen EBNA2. *Nature Med*, **8**, 1098–104.

Khanim, F., Yao, Q-Y, et al. 1996. Analysis of Epstein–Barr virus gene polymorphisms in normal donors and in virus-associated tumors from different geographical locations. *Blood*, **88**, 3491–501.

Khanna, R., Moss, D.J. and Burrows, S.R. 1999. Vaccine strategies against EBV-associated diseases: lessons from studies on cytotoxic T-cell mediated immune regulation. *Immunol Rev*, **170**, 49–64.

Kirimi, L., Crawford, D.H. and Nicholson, L.J. 1995. Identification of an epithelial cell differentiation responsive region within the BZLF1 promoter of the Epstein–Barr virus. *J Gen Virol*, **76**, 759–65.

Klein, G. 1979. The relationship of the virus to nasopharyngeal carcinoma. In: Epstein, M.A. and Achong, B.G. (eds), *The Epstein–Barr virus*. Berlin: Springer-Verlag, 339–50.

Klein, G. 1987. In defense of the 'old' Burkitt lymphoma scenario. In: Klein, G. (ed.), *Advances in viral oncology*, 7. New York: Raven Press, 207–11.

Komano, J., Maruo, S., et al. 1999. Oncogenic role for Epstein–Barr virus-encoded RNAs I Burkitt's lymphoma cell line Akata. *J Virol*, **73**, 9827–31.

Kumar, S. and Hedges, S.B. 1998. A molecular timescale for vertebrate evolution. *Nature*, **392**, 417–20.

Laux, G., Perricaudet, M. and Farrell, P.J. 1988. A spliced Epstein–Barr virus gene expressed in immortalized lymphocytes is created by circularization of the linear viral genome. *EMBO J*, **7**, 769–74.

Lee, E.S., Locker, M., et al. 1995. The association of Epstein–Barr virus with smooth muscle tumors occurring after organ transplantation. *N Engl J Med*, **332**, 19–25.

Lenoir, G.M. and Bornkamm, G.W. 1987. Burkitt's lymphoma: a human cancer model for the study of the multistep development of cancer; proposal for a new scenario. In: Klein, G. (ed.), *Advances in viral oncology 7*. New York: Raven Press, 173–206.

Lewin, N., Åman, P., et al. 1987. Characterization of EBV-carrying B cell populations in healthy seropositive individuals with regard to density, release of transforming virus, and spontaneous outgrowth. *Int J Cancer*, **39**, 472–6.

Levitskaya, J., Cerran, M., et al. 1995. Inhibition of antigen processing by the internal repeat region of the Epstein–Barr virus nuclear antigen-1. *Nature*, **375**, 685–8.

Leyvraz, S., Henle, W., et al. 1985. Association of Epstein–Barr virus with thymic carcinoma. *N Engl J Med*, **213**, 1296–9.

Lindahl, T., Adams, A., et al. 1976. Covalently closed circular duplex DNA of EBV in a human lymphoid cell line. *J Mol Biol*, **102**, 511–30.

Ling, P.D., Hsieh, JJ-D, et al. 1994. EBNA-2 upregulation of Epstein–Barr virus latency promoters and the cellular CD23 promoter utilize a common targeting intermediate, CBF1. *J Virol*, **68**, 5375–83.

Longnecker, R., Druker, B., et al. 1991. An Epstein–Barr virus protein associated with cell growth transformation interacts with a tyrosine kinase. *J Virol*, **65**, 3681–92.

Luka, J., Kallin, B. and Klein, G. 1979. Induction of the Epstein–Barr virus (EBV) cycle in latently infected cells by *n*-butyrate. *Virology*, **94**, 228–31.

McClain, K.L., Leach, C.T., et al. 1995. Association of Epstein–Barr virus with leiomyosarcomas in children with AIDS. *N Engl J Med*, **332**, 12–18.

McGeogh, D.J. and Cook, S. 1994. Molecular phylogeny of the Alphaherpesvirus family and a proposed evolutionary timescale. *J Mol Biol*, **238**, 9–22.

Marafioti, T., Hummel, M., et al. 2000. Hodgkin and Reed–Sternberg cells represent an expansion of a single clone originating from a germinal center B-cell with immunoglobulin rearrangements but defective immunoglobulin transcription. *Blood*, **95**, 1443–50.

Masucci, M.G., Contreras-Salazar, B., et al. 1989. 5-Azacytidine upregulates the expression of Epstein–Barr virus nuclear antigen 2 (EBNA2) through EBNA6 and latent membrane protein in the Burkitt's lymphoma line Rael. *J Virol*, **63**, 3135–41.

Miller, G., Heston, L. and Countryman, J. 1984. P3HR-1 EBV with heterogeneous DNA disrupts latency. *J Virol*, **50**, 174–82.

Miller, C.L., Lee, J.H., et al. 1994. An integral membrane protein (LMP2) blocks reactivation of Epstein–Barr virus from latency following surface immunoglobulin crosslinking. *Proc Natl Acad Sci USA*, **91**, 772–6.

Mueller, N., Evans, A., et al. 1989. Hodgkin's disease and EBV: altered antibody pattern before diagnosis. *N Engl J Med*, **320**, 696–701.

Murray, R.J., Kurilla, M.G., et al. 1992. Identification of target antigens for the human cytotoxic T cell response to Epstein–Barr virus (EBV): implication for the immune control of EBV-positive malignancies. *J Exp Med*, **176**, 157–68.

Nemerow, G.R., Mold, C., et al. 1987. Identification of gp350 as the viral glycoprotein mediating attachment of Epstein–Barr virus (EBV) to the EBV/C3d receptor of B cells: sequence homology of gp350 and C3 complement fragment C3d. *J Virol*, **61**, 1416–20.

Neuhierl, B., Hammerschmidt, W. and Delecluse, H.J. 2002. Glycoprotein gp110 of Epstein-Barr virus determines viral tropism and efficiency of infection. *Proc Natl Acad Sci USA*, **99**, 10536–41.

Niedobitek, G. and Young, L.S. 1994. Epstein–Barr virus persistence and virus associated tumours. *Lancet*, **343**, 333–5.

Niedobitek, G., Hansmann, M.L., et al. 1991. Epstein–Barr virus and carcinomas: undifferentiated carcinomas but not squamous cell carcinomas of the nasopharynx are regularly associated with the virus. *J Pathol*, **165**, 17–24.

Nilsson, K., Klein, G., et al. 1971. The establishment of lymphoblastoid lines from adult and foetal human lymphoid cells and its dependence on EBV. *Int J Cancer*, **8**, 443–50.

Okano, M., Thiele, G.M., et al. 1988. Epstein–Barr virus and human diseases: recent advances in diagnosis. *Clin Microbiol Rev*, **1**, 300–12.

Ott, G., Ott, M.M., et al. 1992. Prevalence of Epstein–Barr virus DNA in different T-cell lymphoma entities in a European population. *Int J Cancer*, **51**, 562–7.

Pattengale, P.K., Smith, R.W. and Gerber, P. 1973. Selective transformation of B lymphocytes by EB virus. *Lancet*, **2**, 93–4.

Penn, I. 1983. Lymphomas complicating organ transplantation. *Transplant Proc*, **15**, suppl 1, 2790–7.

Pope, J.H., Horne, M.K. and Scott, W. 1968. Transformation of foetal human leucocytes in vitro by filtrates of a human leukaemia cell line containing herpes-like virus. *Int J Cancer*, **3**, 857–66.

Raab-Traub, N. and Flynn, K. 1986. The structure of the termini of the Epstein–Barr virus as a marker of clonal cellular proliferation. *Cell*, **47**, 883–9.

Rickinson, A.B., Young, L.S. and Rowe, M. 1987. Influence of the Epstein–Barr virus nuclear antigen EBNA2 on the growth phenotype of virus-transformed B cells. *J Virol*, **61**, 1310–17.

Rooney, C.M., Smith, C.A., et al. 1995. Use of gene-modified virus-specific T lymphocytes to control Epstein–Barr virus-related lymphoproliferation. *Lancet*, **345**, 9–12.

Rowe, D.T., Rowe, M., et al. 1986. Restricted expression of EBV latent genes and T-lymphocyte-detected membrane antigen in Burkitt's lymphoma cells. *EMBO J*, **5**, 2599–608.

Rowe, M., Rowe, D.T., et al. 1987. Differences in B cell growth phenotype reflect novel patterns of Epstein–Barr virus latent gene expression in Burkitt's lymphoma cells. *EMBO J*, **6**, 2743–51.

Rowe, M., Young, L.S., et al. 1989. Distinction between Epstein–Barr virus type A (EBNA 2A) and type B (EBNA 2B) isolates extends to the EBNA 3 family of nuclear proteins. *J Virol*, **63**, 1031–9.

Rowe, M., Lear, A.L., et al. 1992. Three pathways of Epstein–Barr virus gene activation from EBNA1-positive latency in B lymphocytes. *J Virol*, **66**, 122–31.

Sample, J., Young, L., et al. 1990. Epstein–Barr virus types 1 and 2 differ in their EBNA-3A, EBNA-3B, and EBNA-3C genes. *J Virol*, **64**, 4084–92.

Sawyer, R.N., Evans, A.S., et al. 1971. Prospective studies of a group of Yale University freshmen. I. Occurrence of infectious mononucleosis. *J Infect Dis*, **123**, 263–70.

Sayos, J., Wu, C., et al. 1998. The X-linked lymphoproliferative gene product SAP regulates signals induced through the co-receptor SLAM. *Nature*, **395**, 462–9.

Sculley, T.B., Apolloni, A., et al. 1990. Coinfection with A- and B-type Epstein–Barr virus in human immunodeficiency virus-positive subjects. *J Infect Dis*, **162**, 643–8.

Shanmugaratnam, K. 1971. Studies on the etiology of nasopharyngeal carcinoma. In: Richter, R.W. and Epstein, M.A. (eds), *International review of experimental pathology*, 10. New York: Academic Press, 361–413.

Shanmugaratnam, K. 1978. Histological typing of nasopharyngeal carcinoma. In: de Thé, G., Ito, Y. and Davis, W. (eds), *Nasopharyngeal carcinoma: etiology and control*. Lyon: International Agency for Research on Cancer, 3–12.

Simons, M.J., Wee, G.B., et al. 1974. Immunogenetic aspects of nasopharyngeal carcinoma. I. Differences in HL-A antigen profiles between patients and control groups. *Int J Cancer*, **13**, 122–34.

Sixbey, J.W., Lemon, S.M. and Pagano, J.S. 1986. A second site for Epstein–Barr virus shedding: the uterine cervix. *Lancet*, **2**, 1122–4.

Smith, P.R. 2001. Epstein–Barr virus complementary strand transcripts (CSTs/BARTs) and cancer. *Semin Cancer Biol*, **11**, 469–76.

Starzl, T.E., Porter, K.A., et al. 1984. Reversibility of lymphomas and lymphoproliferative lesions developing under cyclosporin-steroid therapy. *Lancet*, **1**, 583–7.

Swaminathan, S., Tomkinson, B. and Kieff, E. 1991. Recombinant Epstein–Barr virus with small RNA (EBER) genes deleted transforms lymphocytes and replicates in vitro. *Proc Natl Acad Sci USA*, **88**, 1546–50.

Takada, K. 2000. EBV and gastric carcinoma. *Mol Pathol*, **53**, 255–61.

Thomas, J.A., Hotchin, N., et al. 1990. Immunohistology of Epstein–Barr virus associated antigens in B cell disorders from immunocompromised individuals. *Transplantation*, **49**, 944–53.

Thomas, J.A., Allday, M.J. and Crawford, D.H. 1991. Epstein-Barr virus-associated lymphoproliferative disorders in immunocompromised individuals. *Adv Cancer Res*, **57**, 329–80.

Tomkinson, B., Robertson, E. and Kieff, E. 1993. Epstein–Barr virus nuclear proteins EBNA-3A and EBNA-3C are essential for B-lymphocyte growth transformation. *J Virol*, **67**, 2014–25.

Touitou, R., Hickabottom, M., et al. 2001. Physical and functional interactions between the corepressor CtBP and the Epstein–Barr virus nuclear antigen EBNA3C. *J Virol*, **75**, 7749–55.

Tovey, M.G., Lenoir, G. and Begon-Lours, J. 1978. Activation of latent Epstein–Barr virus by antibody to human IgM. *Nature (Lond)*, **276**, 270–2.

Trumper, P.A., Epstein, M.A. and Giovanella, B.C. 1976. Activation in vitro by BudR of a productive EB virus infection in the epithelial cells of nasopharyngeal carcinoma. *Int J Cancer*, **17**, 578–87.

Trumper, P.A., Epstein, M.A., et al. 1977. Isolation of infectious EB virus from the epithelial tumour cells of nasopharyngeal carcinoma. *Int J Cancer*, **20**, 655–62.

Tsui, S. and Schubach, W.H. 1994. Epstein–Barr virus nuclear protein 2A forms oligomers in vitro and in vivo through a region required for B-cell transformation. *J Virol*, **68**, 4287–94.

Uchida, J., Yasui, T., et al. 1999. Mimicry of CD40 signals by Epstein–Barr virus LMP1 in B lymphocyte responses. *Science*, **286**, 300–3.

Virelizier, J.L., Lenoir, G. and Griscelli, C. 1978. Persistent Epstein–Barr virus infection in a child with hypergammaglobulinaemia and immunoblastic proliferation associated with a selective defect in immune interferon secretion. *Lancet*, **2**, 231–4.

Wang, D., Liebowitz, D. and Kieff, E. 1985. An EBV membrane protein expressed in immortalized lymphocytes transforms established rodent cells. *Cell*, **43**, 831–40.

Wang, D., Liebowitz, D., et al. 1988. Epstein–Barr virus latent infection membrane protein alters the human B-lymphocyte phenotype: deletion of the amino terminus abolishes activity. *J Virol*, **62**, 4137–84.

Wang, F., Gregory, C., et al. 1990. Epstein–Barr virus latent membrane protein (LMP1) and nuclear proteins 2 and 3C are effectors of phenotypic changes in B lymphocytes: EBNA-2 and LMP1 cooperatively induce CD23. *J Virol*, **64**, 2309–18.

Wang, F., Rivailler, P., et al. 2001. Simian homologues of Epstein-Barr virus. In: Epstein, M.A., Rickinson, A.B., Weiss, R.A. (eds), *Oncogenic γ-herpesviruses: an expanding family*. *Phil Trans RS B*, **353**, 489–97.

Weiss, L.M., Movahed, A.M., et al. 1989. Detection of Epstein–Barr viral genomes in Reed–Sternberg cells of Hodgkin's disease. *N Engl J Med*, **320**, 502–6.

Wilson, A.D., Lövgren-Bengtsson, K., et al. 1999. The major Epstein–Barr virus (EBV) envelope glycoprotein gp340 when incorporated into Iscoms primes cytotoxic T-cell responses directed against EBV lymphoblastoid cell lines. *Vaccine*, **17**, 1282–90.

Wilson, J.B., Bell, J.L., et al. 1996. Expression of Epstein–Barr virus nuclear antigen-1 induces B cell neoplasia in transgenic mice. *EMBO J*, **15**, 3117–26.

Woisetschlaeger, M., Jin, X.W., et al. 1991. Role for the Epstein–Barr virus nuclear antigen 2 in viral promoter switching during initial stages of infection. *Proc Natl Acad Sci USA*, **88**, 3942–6.

Wu, T-C and Kuo, T-T 1993. Study of Epstein–Barr virus early RNA1 (EBER1) expression by in situ hybridization in thymic epithelial tumours of Chinese patients in Taiwan. *Hum Pathol*, **24**, 235–8.

Yao, Q.Y., Rickinson, A.B. and Epstein, M.A. 1985. A re-examination of the Epstein–Barr virus carrier state in healthy seropositive individuals. *Int J Cancer*, **35**, 35–42.

Yates, J.L., Warren, N. and Sugden, B. 1985. Stable replication of plasmids derived from Epstein–Barr virus in mammalian cells. *Nature (Lond)*, **313**, 812–15.

Young, L.S., Dawson, C.W., et al. 1988. Epstein–Barr virus gene expression in nasopharyngeal carcinoma. *J Gen Virol*, **69**, 1051–65.

Zeng, Y., Zhang, L.G., et al. 1982. Serological mass survey for early detection of nasopharyngeal carcinoma in Wuzhou City, China. *Int J Cancer*, **29**, 139–41.

Zhao, B., Marshall, D.R. and Sample, C.E. 1996. A conserved domain of the Epstein–Barr virus nuclear antigens 3A and 3C binds to a discrete domain of Jkappa. *J Virol*, **70**, 4228–36.

Ziegler, J.L., Andersson, M., et al. 1976. Detection of Epstein–Barr virus DNA in American Burkitt's lymphoma. *Int J Cancer*, **17**, 701–6.

Zimber, U., Adldinger, H.K., et al. 1986. Geographical prevalence of two types of Epstein–Barr virus. *Virology*, **154**, 56–66.

zur Hausen, H., O'Neill, F.J., et al. 1978. Persisting oncogenic herpesvirus induced by the tumour promoter TPA. *Nature (Lond)*, **272**, 373–5.

zur Hausen, H., Bornkamm, G.W., et al. 1979. Tumor initiators and promoters in induction of Epstein–Barr virus. *Proc Natl Acad Sci USA*, **76**, 782–5.

30

Poxviruses

GEOFFREY L. SMITH

INTRODUCTION

The molecular aspects of poxvirus replication are considered in Chapter 31, Poxvirus replication. This chapter considers the origin of vaccinia virus and its use to eradicate smallpox, the classification and phylogenetic relationships of poxviruses, how these viruses are transmitted and cause disease in their hosts and how they may be controlled. Lastly, the potential use of poxviruses in bioterrorism is discussed.

WHAT IS A POXVIRUS?

Poxviruses are large viruses that have double-stranded DNA genomes ⩾135 kb. The virions are large and complex, are surrounded by a lipid envelope and lack icosahedral or helical symmetry. Unlike most DNA viruses, poxviruses replicate in the cell cytoplasm and therefore encode the great majority of the proteins needed for their transcription and DNA replication. Poxviruses also encode many virulence factors that are nonessential for virus replication in cell culture, but help the virus to survive in its particular host(s). These viruses infect a wide range of vertebrate and invertebrate species, although this chapter is very largely restricted to poxviruses of chordates. Some poxviruses cause severe disease such as smallpox, camelpox, or

myxomatosis, but equally poxviruses may cause only asymptomatic infections. Historically, these viruses have played important roles in human medicine and biomedical science. The most serious human poxvirus, variola virus, caused the disease smallpox. This disease was eradicated in 1977 but, remarkably, the origin of the smallpox vaccine (vaccinia virus) remains an enigma of virology. For reviews of poxvirus properties see Chapter 31, Poxvirus replication, as well as Fenner (1996) and Moss (2001).

HISTORICAL ROLES OF POXVIRUSES

Poxviruses have played important roles in human history, medicine, and biological science. Smallpox was a devastating disease that killed up to 40 percent of those infected and has influenced the history of mankind (Hopkins 1983; Fenner et al. 1988; Glynn and Glynn 2004). It is likely that this disease became prevalent after *Homo sapiens* adopted intensive agriculture rather than living as a hunter-gatherer. This profound change in our behavior took place between 5 000 and 10 000 BC and enabled human population densities to increase so that diseases such as smallpox and measles could remain endemic. It has been estimated that populations of at least 300 000 are needed for measles to survive in mankind. In populations smaller than this, an epidemic would leave too few nonimmune hosts for the virus to be transmitted and so it could not persist in the population. Smallpox is less easily transmitted from person to person than measles, and so the population needed for smallpox to remain endemic was smaller and might be closer to 100 000. It is uncertain exactly when smallpox appeared in man, but examination of the mummified corpse of the Egyptian pharaoh Ramses V, who died in 1160 BC, revealed characteristic dermal pocks, suggesting he may have died from the disease. Smallpox probably existed in man for many centuries previously, although there is no proof of this.

Smallpox was caused by Variola virus, a member of the genus *Orthopoxvirus* (Table 30.1). When this disease was introduced into hitherto naive populations the effect was devastating. For instance, the introduction of smallpox into Central America in the early sixteenth century decimated the local American Indian population and helped the Spanish invaders to conquer the Aztec nation with 500 soldiers. Smallpox had a profound effect on the population of Europe and it is estimated to have killed between 200 000 and 600 000 people annually during the sixteenth and seventeenth centuries. Even during the twentieth century, smallpox was a major cause of premature mortality. In 1967 there were 131 418 cases of smallpox reported from 44 countries, but due to under-reporting the real number of cases may have been nearer to 10 million (Henderson 1976). For reviews of smallpox in history, the reader is referred to excellent texts on this topic (Hopkins 1983; Fenner et al. 1988; Glynn and Glynn 2004).

THE ERADICATION OF SMALLPOX

The eradication of smallpox has been described in a monumental book *Smallpox and its eradication* (Fenner et al. 1988) and only an outline is given here. Before Edward Jenner introduced vaccination in 1796, the only means of preventing smallpox was variolation (also called inoculation). This involved the deliberate inoculation of infectious variola virus into the skin (usually the upper arm) of the patient brave enough to be infected. The matter inoculated came directly from a patient with smallpox, or was taken from such a patient and stored in dry form until use. Introduction of the virus into the skin gave a less serious disease than that following natural infection via the respiratory tract. Nevertheless, variolation could, and did, cause serious disease and approximately 1 percent of variolated patients developed smallpox and died. Moreover, both these patients and those who survived the infection were able to transmit the infection to others and start epidemics. So variolation was a dangerous practice and was tolerated only because of the tremendous fear of contracting smallpox naturally.

Jenner himself was a variolator and was well aware of the risks and perhaps this contributed to his search for an alternative and safer way to prevent smallpox. Jenner noticed that milkmaids who sometimes became infected on their hands with cowpox virus derived from the cows they milked were spared from smallpox when an epidemic would rage through the community. They were also resistant to variolation. Although Jenner was not the first to notice these facts, he was the first to test systematically the hypothesis that it was the prior

Table 30.1 Poxviridae

Subfamily	Genus	Species[a]
Chordopoxvirinae	Orthopoxvirus	**Vaccinia virus**[b], *Variola virus*[c], *Cowpox virus*[d], *Camelpox virus, Monkeypox virus, Ectromelia virus, Raccoonpox virus, Volepox virus, Taterapox (gerbil) virus*
	Parapoxvirus	**Orf virus** (contagious pustular dermatitis), *Pseudocowpox virus, Bovine papular stomatitis virus*
	Capripoxvirus	**Sheeppox virus**, *Goatpox virus, Lumpy skin disease virus*
	Leporipoxvirus	**Myxoma virus**, rabbit (Shope) fibroma virus, *Hare fibroma virus, Squirrel fibroma virus, Rabbit fibroma virus*
	Suipoxvirus	**Swinepox virus**
	Molluscipoxvirus	*Molluscum contagiosum virus*
	Yatapoxvirus	**Yaba monkey tumor virus**, Yaba-like disease virus, *Tanapox virus*
	Avipoxvirus	**Fowlpox virus**, *Canarypox virus, Turkeypox virus, Pigeonpox virus*
Entomopoxvirinae	A	
	B	Amsacta moorei, Melanoplus sanguinipes
	C	

a) Type species in bold.
b) Includes buffalopox virus and rabbitpox virus as subspecies.
c) Includes variola major and variola minor (alastrim).
d) Includes isolates from felines and captive exotic species.

infection with cowpox virus that caused immunity to smallpox. For this he rightly deserved the accolade for the discovery of vaccination. On 14 May 1796, Jenner vaccinated a boy, James Phipps, with material taken from the hand of a milkmaid, Sarah Nelmes, who had been infected from her cow, Blossom. Subsequently, Jenner demonstrated that Phipps was resistant to variolation. His work was submitted to the Royal Society of London, but not accepted. After being unable to publish his discovery, Jenner performed more vaccinations to obtain additional data in support of his theory. He showed by challenging some of these vaccinees that they too were resistant to variolation (Figure 30.1). In 1798, he wrote his famous article *An enquiry into the causes and effects of variolae vaccinae, a disease discovered in some of the western countries of England, particularly Gloucestershire, and known by the name of Cowpox* and published this privately (Jenner 1798). The success of vaccination was evident rapidly and enabled Jenner to predict in 1801, that 'the annihilation of the smallpox, the most dreadful scourge of the human species, must be the final result of this practice' (Jenner 1801). This prophecy was correct but took another 176 years to be fulfilled. Jenner's discovery of vaccination was not patented and he did not seek financial reward from it. Perhaps partly in view of this, in 1802 the British Parliament debated his discovery and awarded him a sum of £10 000, a princely sum in the early nineteenth century. In the same year, the American president, Thomas Jefferson, said of vaccination and Jenner, 'Medicine has never before produced any single improvement of such utility. You have erased from the calendar of human afflictions one of its greatest.' Five years later the British

Parliament awarded Jenner another £20 000. In view of the success of vaccination and the dangers inherent in variolation, the latter practice was banned in the UK by Act of Parliament in 1840.

Given that vaccination was so effective in preventing smallpox, why did eradication take so long? Factors that contributed to this were the shortage of vaccine, loss of vaccine potency, and the refusal of some people to be vaccinated due to fear of vaccination or prejudice. From Jenner's discovery until the third quarter of the twentieth century, the vaccine supply was inadequate. Cowpox was a relatively rare disease and even though vaccine was also derived from horses, where it caused a disease called 'the grease,' vaccine shortage was a frequent problem. To overcome this, virus was passaged in humans by arm-to-arm transfer, indeed Jenner himself did this in the second series of vaccinations described in the enquiry (Figure 30.1). This method was used to disseminate the vaccine throughout Europe and the Spanish adopted it to transfer the vaccine to Central America in 1803. Twenty-two orphan children were taken on a voyage across the Atlantic Ocean and groups of children were vaccinated regularly en route so that virus was still growing on one or more children when the ship reached the Americas.

The process of arm-to-arm transfer provided an increased supply of vaccine but was also dangerous because it disseminated other pathogens and both measles and syphilis were transmitted in this way. Consequently, arm-to-arm transfer was banned in the UK by the Vaccination Act of 1898, but not before several epidemics of other diseases had been started. In 1885, in a shipyard in Bremen, Germany, an outbreak of

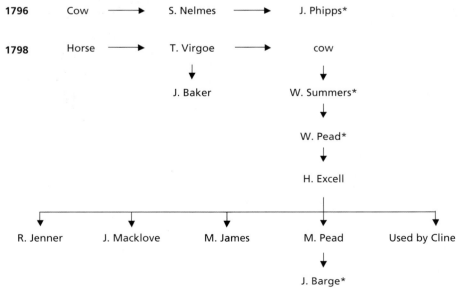

Figure 30.1 *The series of vaccinations performed by Jenner (1798). Nelmes and Virgoe were infected accidentally from a cow and a horse, respectively. An asterisk indicates that this person was resistant to subsequent variolation (redrawn from Baxby (1981) with permission).*

infectious hepatitis, very likely caused by hepatitis B virus, was blamed on a contaminated batch of smallpox vaccine composed of human lymph. This represented the first documented epidemic of infectious hepatitis B virus (Lurman 1885).

From the 1880s onwards, vaccine was produced on the skin of calves and became known as calf lymph vaccine. This was more plentiful, more easily standardized and free from some other human pathogens. Its proper use led to the containment of smallpox in parts of the world, but in many places the disease remained endemic. This was due partly to inadequate control of vaccine potency and this was a particular problem in tropical regions. In the early 1950s this problem was overcome by Leslie Collier and co-workers at the Lister Institute in London who developed a method to freeze-dry the vaccine such that it was stable at ambient temperature for long periods (Collier 1954, 1955). In fact the vaccine prepared in this way has remarkable stability and can resist incubation at 37°C for 3 months or even 100°C for 1 h. This was a very major advance, for now the vaccine could be used throughout the world and reconstituted under field conditions without loss of potency.

In 1959, the Soviet Union proposed to the World Health Organization that smallpox should be eradicated from the world. This proposal was endorsed enthusiastically, but despite the availability of stable vaccine there was relatively little progress during the next decade and, as mentioned above, smallpox was still endemic in at least 44 countries in 1967. After 1967, the vaccination policy was modified. Hitherto the objective was to vaccinate everyone, but obtaining blanket vaccination was virtually impossible. After 1967, ring vaccination was adopted and was more effective. This relied upon surveillance, quarantine, and vaccination. Photographs of smallpox patients were distributed widely and those identifying a case of smallpox were rewarded financially. Once identified, the patient was quarantined and all contacts were traced and vaccinated. These contacts were observed and if they developed fever, they were quarantined, and their contacts were traced and vaccinated. By this method, the spread of infection was halted and the focus of infection snuffed out. This was highly effective so that by 1975 the last case of smallpox occurred in the Indian subcontinent and the last naturally occurring case of smallpox was recorded in October 1977 near Mogadishu in Somalia.

Sadly, this was not the last case of smallpox and there was an outbreak in Birmingham, UK in 1978 following the escape of variola virus from a laboratory. In this outbreak one person died. Notably this fatality occurred despite the patient having been vaccinated twice previously, once as a child and once 12 years before contracting the disease. So immunity is not lifelong and this was recognized by the World Health Organization who recommended that those working in areas where smallpox was endemic should be vaccinated every 3 years. Of all the claims made by Jenner in 1798 about vaccination, nearly everything was correct except his belief that vaccination provided lifelong immunity.

It is largely because of the tragedy in Birmingham in 1978 that today the stocks of variola virus are held in only two locations in the world, in the Centers for Disease Control and Prevention, Atlanta, USA and in Vector, Novosobirsk, Russia. These stocks are stored in maximum security (BSL4) laboratories and all work with live virus requires prior approval by the World Health Organization which also inspects these laboratories regularly. The chance of an escape of virus from these sites is at best remote, but the concern about the potential use of variola virus in bioterrorism (see below) derives not so much from these virus repositories but from the possibility that the virus is held elsewhere illegally.

THE ORIGIN OF VACCINIA VIRUS

The virus used by Jenner in 1796 as the first human vaccine may have been cowpox virus, although this is uncertain because the original virus is not available for characterization. We know only that the virus was taken from the hand of Sarah Nelmes, who presumably was infected from her cow, and this virus was used to immunize James Phipps (Jenner 1798). However, vaccine was not only acquired from cows. In the series of vaccinations in 1798, described in Jenner's Enquiry, it is stated that Thomas Virgoe was infected from a horse and from Virgoe the virus was used to vaccinate a 5-year-old boy, John Baker (Figure 30.1). In addition, in 1813 and 1817, Jenner sent vaccine derived from horses to the National Vaccine Establishment, which was set up in England to provide smallpox vaccine. Vaccines were therefore derived from both cows and horses.

In 1939 in Liverpool, UK, Alan W. Downie showed that all the vaccines used to prevent smallpox in the twentieth century formed a homogeneous group that was distinct from both cowpox virus and variola virus and represented a distinct species of Orthopoxvirus that became known as vaccinia virus (Downie 1939a, b). If Jenner had used cowpox virus in 1796, sometime between then and 1939 this was replaced by vaccinia virus. Exactly when this took place is uncertain, but it is likely to have been early during the nineteenth century. Several anecdotes support his conclusion. First, the smallpox vaccine that was taken to the USA in 1856, was passed serially thereafter and became the New York City Board of Health vaccine, is vaccinia virus and not cowpox virus. Second, pathologists from the late nineteenth century who studied the cytopathic effect induced by the smallpox vaccine, noted the eosinophilic B type inclusion bodies that are made by both vaccinia virus and cowpox virus, but did not report the more obvious A type inclusion bodies that are made by cowpox virus and not vaccinia virus. Lastly, the drawings made of lesions induced by the vaccine used by Jenner are similar to those induced by the vaccine in use today. So it is possible that Jenner used vaccinia virus, or cowpox virus, or both, but at different times. Both these viruses have a broad host range and may infect many species.

This origin of vaccinia virus was reviewed by Baxby (1981) and he suggested that it might be horsepox virus. If so, perhaps our language is wrong; for the name of the smallpox vaccine should be equinia virus (not vaccinia virus), and we use equines (not vaccines) to equinate people by the process of equination! It is remarkable that vaccinia virus is the only vaccine to have eradicated a human disease and yet its origin and natural host remain an enigma. It is also remarkable, in comparison with the regulatory paperwork needed today before any clinical trial may be undertaken, that for smallpox:

- there was no ethical or safety evaluation given to the first use of the vaccine, or the challenge of vaccinated subjects;
- the paper reporting the use of the vaccine to prevent smallpox did not survive peer-review;
- there was no properly controlled clinical trial to demonstrate the efficacy of the vaccine;
- there was (and is) no understanding of how the vaccine worked.

Yet there was anecdotal evidence that the vaccine worked: namely the global eradication of smallpox.

OTHER CONTRIBUTIONS OF VACCINIA VIRUS TO BIOMEDICAL SCIENCE

Despite its uncertain origin, vaccinia virus has played several seminal roles in biological science and medicine. In addition to its use to eradicate smallpox, vaccinia virus was the first mammalian virus to be purified, analyzed chemically, and titrated accurately. Work with vaccinia virus in the 1960s discovered the first virus-encoded nucleic acid polymerase (Munyon et al. 1967) and this discovery prompted the search for polymerases in other viruses. The study of vaccinia virus enzymes that catalyze the addition of a methylated cap structure at the 5′ end (Martin and Moss 1975) and a poly(A) tail at the 3′ end of mRNAs (Brown et al. 1973) have been informative for the study of these cellular processes. In 1982, genetically engineered vaccinia viruses were constructed that expressed genes derived from other organisms (Mackett et al. 1982; Panicali and Paoletti 1982) and such recombinant viruses were shown to have potential as vaccines against other infectious agents (Panicali et al. 1983; Smith et al. 1983a,b). This concept pioneered the development of genetically engineered viruses as live vaccines, a concept applied subsequently to other viruses and micro-organisms. More recently, studies of poxvirus virulence have revealed a wide range of proteins that inhibit specific components of the host immune response to infection (Seet et al. 2003). Lastly, studies of the interaction of vaccinia virus with the host

cell have discovered how these viruses exploit cell biology to enable their entry into, movement within, and exit from the cell (Smith et al. 2003). Although smallpox has been eradicated and poxviruses now cause little human disease, there are compelling reasons to continue to study these viruses.

CLASSIFICATION

The *Poxviridae* is divided into the *Entomopoxvirinae* and *Chordopoxvirinae* subfamilies that infect insects and chordates, respectively (Table 30.1). The entomopoxviruses are subdivided into three genera (A, B, and C), although genome sequence data from two members of group B (Melanoplus sanguinipes and Amsacta moorei) have revealed considerable diversity suggesting that these viruses might be reclassified in different genera (Afonso et al. 1999; Bawden et al. 2000). The genomes of these entomopoxviruses are rich in adenine and thymine (A+T), 81.5 and 81.7 percent. These viruses are not considered further here and the reader is referred to other reviews of this topic (Moyer 1994, 1999).

The chordopoxviruses are now considered in greater detail. This subfamily is divided into eight genera: *Orthopoxvirus*, *Leporipoxvirus*, *Molluscipoxvirus*, *Avipoxvirus*, *Yatapoxvirus*, *Suipoxvirus*, *Capripoxvirus*, and *Parapoxvirus* (see Table 30.1). Within each genus there are distinct species and often there are multiple strains of each species. For instance, the genus *Orthopoxvirus* contains several members, one of which is *Vaccinia virus* and there are a score or so different *Vaccinia virus* strains. Historically, the definition of a genus is that its members are immunologically cross-reactive and cross-protective, whereas viruses of different genera are neither cross-reactive nor cross-protective. This has been a reasonable method of classification and is largely supported by the analysis of virus genome sequences that are becoming available.

Sequencing of additional poxviruses from divergent species may cause an increase in the number of genera. For instance, poxviruses have been isolated from north American deer (Afonso et al. 2002), Finnish reindeer (Tikkanen et al. 2004), farmed Nile crocodiles (Horner 1988), Mongolian horses (Tulman et al. 2002a), South African sea lions (Wilson and Poglayen-Newall 1971), lizards (Stauber and Gogolewski 1990), kangaroos (Bagnall and Wilson 1974), squirrels (Thomas et al. 2003), South American rodents (Ueda et al. 1978; Esposito et al. 1980), and chameleons (Jacobson and Telford 1990). In addition, orthopoxviruses that resemble vaccinia virus strains were isolated from buffaloes in India (Dumbell and Richardson 1993), and cattle (de Souza Trindade et al. 2003) and rodents (Fonseca et al. 1998; da Fonseca et al., 2002) in South America. Possibly these viruses became endemic after transmission from man following widespread use of vaccinia virus as the smallpox vaccine.

IDENTIFICATION OF POXVIRUSES

Traditionally, the identification of poxviruses has been based upon biological observations, such as species of origin, growth properties in animal tissue or on the chorioallantoic membrane of the fertile hen's egg, reactivity with specific sera, and electron microscopy. These observations remain useful, but the rapid identification of a new virus as a poxvirus is now usually done by electron microscopy, polymerase chain reaction (PCR) (Meyer et al. 1994; Ropp et al. 1995; Heine et al. 1999), and genome sequencing. PCR shows great sensitivity, speed, and specificity. For instance, using specific sets of oligonucleotide primers it is possible to say not only that a new isolate is an orthopoxvirus, but which species it is. This was useful for the identification of the agent causing fever and generalized rash in humans in the midwest of USA during 2003 as monkeypox virus (Reed et al. 2004). PCR-based detection methods have been developed, validated, and deployed to detect variola virus that might be deliberately released by bioterrorists (see below) (Sofi Ibrahim et al. 2003).

PHYLOGENETIC RELATIONSHIPS

Genomes of representative members of all *Chordopoxvirus* genera have been sequenced (see http://www.poxvirus.org for details) and all except the parapoxviruses (that were sequenced most recently) have been used in phylogenetic comparisons (McLysaght et al. 2003; Upton et al. 2003; Gubser et al. 2004). These genomes range in size from 135 kb (Yaba monkey tumor virus) (Brunetti et al. 2003) to 288 kb (a pathogenic strain of fowlpox virus from the Animal Health Inspection Service Center for Veterinary Biologics, Ames, IA, USA) (Afonso et al. 2000) and from 36 percent A+T in genus *Parapoxvirus* to 75 percent A+T in capripoxvirus. All these genomes share a similar overall arrangement. In the central region (approximately 100 kb) the genes are conserved and many of these encode proteins that are essential for virus transcription, DNA replication, or assembly of new virions (Figure 30.2). In this region there are 90 genes that are conserved in all sequenced chordopoxviruses, but this number decreases to 49 when the entomopoxviruses are included, reflecting the greater diversity of the latter group. Genes in the terminal regions of the chordopoxvirus genomes are more variable and most are nonessential for virus replication in cell culture. Indeed, outside the central conserved region there is no gene that is conserved in all sequenced chordopoxviruses. These nonessential genes encode luxury functions that aid the virus in vivo and may function to inhibit aspects of the host immune response to infection, or influence host range and virulence (Smith and McFadden 2002). The types of genes that are present here reflect the different life styles that these viruses have evolved with their hosts.

A phylogenetic comparison of the chordopoxviruses (excluding parapoxviruses) using 17 of the 49 genes that are conserved in all poxviruses revealed that the sequenced *Chordopoxvirus* genera fall into four groups (Gubser et al. 2004) (Figure 30.3). An analysis using a different collection of genes reached a very similar conclusion (McLysaght et al. 2003). The most divergent group is the *Avipoxvirus* genus represented by *Fowlpox virus* (FPV). This avian virus has the largest genome (288 kb), the greatest number of genes that are unique to any genus (113), and the most divergent genome organization. Whereas genomes of all the other *Chordopoxvirus* genera have a consistent order and orientation of genes within the conserved, central region, FPV differs in that there are genome inversions and translocations (Figure 30.2).

The next most divergent group is the genus *Molluscipox virus*. This contains a single member, *Molluscum contagiosum virus*, of which there are two types, that infects only man. This virus also has many (70) unique genes that are not found in other *Chordopoxvirus* genera. It also lacks many genes found in other poxviruses such as those involved in immune regulation and instead has its own unique set of immunoregulators (Senkevich et al. 1996, 1997).

The third group includes the genera *Leporipoxvirus*, *Suipoxvirus*, *Yatapoxvirus*, and *Capripoxvirus*. These genomes are all smaller than those of the *Orthopoxvirus* genus and have several common features. For instance, the counterpart of *Vaccinia virus* strain Copenhagen gene *C7L* is present in these genera in the central region of the genome rather than being near the left end in members of the genus *Orthopoxvirus* (Figure 30.2).

The last group is represented by genus *Orthopoxvirus*. Orthopoxviruses have genomes of approximately 200 kb that are rich in adenine and thymine (67 percent) and form a tight cluster. They are distinguished from other chordopoxviruses by the presence of genes corresponding to *Vaccinia virus* strain Copenhagen genes *F14L*, *E7L*, and *O2L* within the central conserved region. Orthopoxviruses have been of greatest importance to man and most members of this genus have been sequenced. In addition to *Variola virus*, this genus includes *Vaccinia virus*, *Cowpox virus*, *Ectromelia virus*, the cause of mousepox, *Monkeypox virus*, and *Camelpox virus* (Table 30.1). Some of the names of these species are misnomers; for instance, neither *Cowpox virus* nor *Monkeypox virus* are naturally resident in cows or monkeys, instead they have rodent or squirrel reservoirs and may be transmitted to cows, monkeys, man, and other species as zoonoses (Khodakevich et al. 1987a; Crouch et al. 1995; Kulesh et al. 2004).

Although the parapoxviruses were not included in the above analysis, the genomes of orf virus and *Bovine papular stomatitis virus* were sequenced recently (Delhon

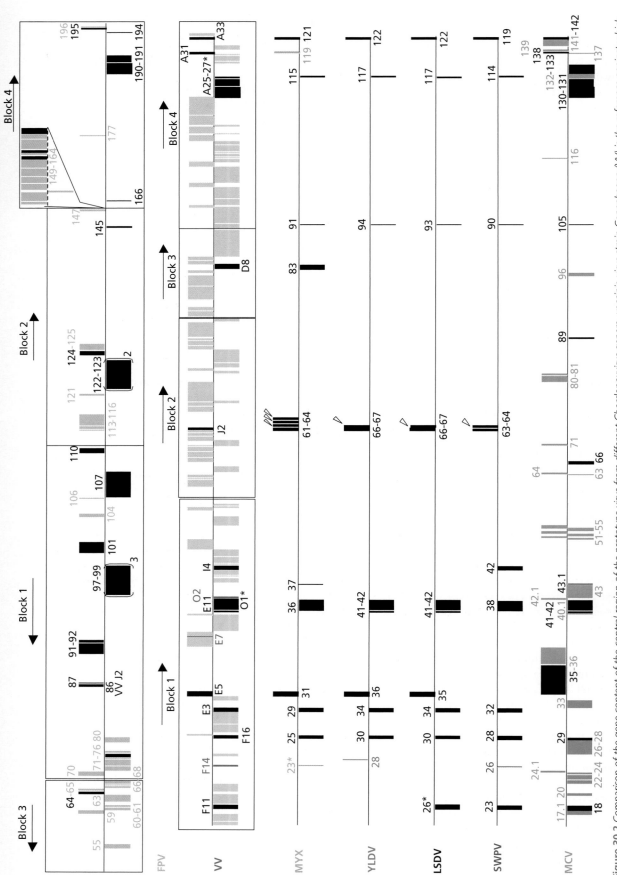

Figure 30.2 Comparison of the gene content of the central region of the prototype virus from different Chordopoxvirus genera. vaccinia virus strain Copenhagen (VV) is the reference against which the other viruses (FPV, fowlpox virus; MYX, myxoma virus; LSDV, lumpy skin disease virus; YLDV, Yaba-like disease virus; SWPV, swinepox virus; MCV, Molluscum contagiosum disease virus) are compared. For each virus, genes (vertical bars) that are transcribed rightwards or leftwards are shown above or below the horizontal line, respectively. The 90 genes that are conserved in all sequenced chordopoxviruses are shown in gray for vaccinia virus. Genes conserved between two or more viruses from the different genera (but not one of the 90 conserved genes) are shown in black and genes that are unique to one genus are represented in the same color as the virus name. Genes that are present in only some members of a specific genus, but are fragmented or absent in other members of that genus, are indicated with an asterix. Block 1, counterparts of vaccinia virus strain Copenhagen F9L–G4L; block 2, counterparts of vaccinia virus strain Copenhagen G5R–D2L;

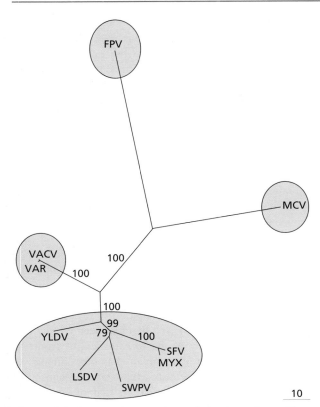

Figure 30.3 *Phyogenetic comparisons of chordopoxviruses. The amino acid sequence of 17 poxvirus proteins (corresponding to vaccinia virus strain Copenhagen E9L, I7L, I8R, G9R, J3R, J6R, H2R, H4L, H6R, D1R, D5R, D6R, D11L, D13L, A7L, A16L, and A24R) were aligned and an unrooted maximum-likelihood tree was obtained using the program ProML from the Phylip package version 3.0. The bootstrap values from 1 000 replica samplings and the divergence scale (substitutions/site) are indicated. Abbreviations as in Figure 30.2. Redrawn with modifications from Gubser et al.(2004) with permission.*

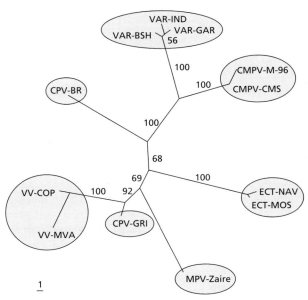

Figure 30.4 *Unrooted maximum likelihood phylogenetic tree showing the relationships of 12 orthopoxviruses. The amino acid sequences of proteins corresponding to vaccinia virus strain Copenhagen C6L, C7L, N1L, K2L, F2L, F4L, F6L, F8L, A56R, B1R, B5R, B15R (all encoded in the terminal regions of the genomes) were aligned and used to generate the tree using the program ProML. The bootstrap values from 1 000 replica samplings and the divergence scale (substitutions/site) are indicated. VAR-IND, variola virus strain India 1967; VAR-BSH, variola virus strain Bangladesh 1975; VAR-GAR, variola virus strain Garcia 1966; CPV-BR, cowpox virus Brighton Red; CPV-GRI, cowpox virus GRI-90; CMPV-CMS, camelpox virus strain CMS; CMPV-M-96; camelpox virus M-96; ECT-Nav, Ectromelia virus strain Naval; ECT-MOS, Ectromelia virus strain Moscow; VV-COP vaccinia virus strain Copenhagen; VV-MVA, vaccinia virus strain modified virus Ankara; MPV-Zaire, monkeypox virus strain Zaire. Redrawn with modifications from Gubser et al. (2004) with permission.*

et al. 2004), and phylogenetic trees including these viruses or sequences from other parapoxviruses (Tikkanen et al. 2004) showed that parapoxviruses are quite separate from other *Chordopoxvirus* genera, and the nearest genus is *Molluscipoxvirus*. The parapoxviruses share with molluscipoxviruses a high GC content and lack several genes encoding enzymes for nucleotide metabolism that are found in other chordopoxviruses.

A phylogenetic comparison of the orthopoxviruses using 12 genes that are conserved in the terminal regions of these genomes (Figure 30.4) showed that *Variola virus* and *Camelpox virus* are closely related (Gubser and Smith 2002), but *Monkeypox virus* is one of the most divergent viruses of this genus despite causing a disease in man similar to smallpox (Gubser et al. 2004). Another study using a different collection of genes conserved in these viruses came to a similar conclusion (McLysaght et al. 2003). These observations imply that one or more of these viruses have jumped species during their evolution; for *Variola virus*, a human virus, is closer to a virus that infects only camels than to

Monkeypox virus that infects man, primates, and other species. Different strains of most *Orthopoxvirus* species form a tight cluster, consistent with their classification, however, with *Cowpox virus* the two sequenced members, Brighton Red (BR) and GRI-90 (Shchelkunov et al. 1998), are sufficiently divergent to justify their reclassification as separate species (Gubser et al. 2004). It will be interesting to compare the sequences of *Vaccinia virus* and *Cowpox virus* strains with the geographical site of isolation. Another interesting conclusion from the phylogenetic study of McLysaght et al. (2003) was that the rate of gene acquisition by the orthopoxviruses has been greater than that for *Leporipoxvirus*, *Suipoxvirus*, *Capripoxvirus*, and *Yatapoxvirus*.

There has also been significant gene loss during the evolution of the orthopoxviruses from the immediate ancestor of this group. This was shown by several genes being disrupted by mutation in one of more virus, but intact in at least one other (Aguado et al. 1992; Gubser and Smith 2002). An example is a gene encoding a soluble binding protein for interleukin (IL)-1β in many strains of *Vaccinia virus* and *Cowpox virus* (Alcami and

Smith 1992, 1996; Spriggs et al. 1992), but the disruption of this gene in all sequenced strains of variola virus. Similarly, a gene in *Vaccinia virus* that encodes an enzyme that synthesizes steroid hormones (Moore and Smith 1992) is disrupted in *Variola virus* strains into small fragments (Aguado et al. 1992; Shchelkunov et al. 1995).

There has also been recombination between *Orthopoxvirus* genomes during the evolution of these viruses. Evidence for this came from comparing the sequences of genes from the terminal regions of *Cowpox virus* strain BR and *Ectromelia virus* strain Naval with the corresponding genes from (1) the *Variola virus*/*Camelpox virus* subgroup; and (2) the *Vaccinia virus* subgroup (Gubser et al. 2004). This revealed that genes from the left end of *Cowpox virus* BR were closer to the *Vaccinia virus* subgroup than to the *Variola virus*/*Camelpox virus* subgroup. However, genes from the right end of *Cowpox virus* BR had the opposite relationship. Conversely, genes taken from the right end of *Ectromelia virus* Naval were closer to the *Vaccinia virus* subgroup, whereas genes from the left end were roughly equidistant from either group (Gubser et al. 2004).

VIRION STRUCTURE

This topic has been the subject of much debate and disagreement and is considered in detail in Chapter 31, Poxvirus replication. It is mentioned briefly here because the conclusion of this author differs from that of Moyer and Condit. Using vaccinia virus as the model poxvirus, there is general agreement that there are two forms of infectious virus produced from each infected cell, the intracellular mature virus (IMV) and extracellular enveloped virus (EEV), for review see Smith et al. (2002). There is also agreement that EEV contains one more membrane than IMV, but the number of membranes around IMV, how this (these) are formed and how each form of virus enters cells have been disputed. Originally, IMV was proposed to be surrounded by a single membrane that was synthesized de novo (Dales and Siminovitch 1961). Later, this model was challenged by workers who claimed there were two closed apposed membranes derived from the intermediate compartment of the cell, although it was acknowledged by these authors that 'the membranes of this cisterna are so tightly apposed that it is often difficult to distinguish the two bilayers' (Sodeik et al. 1993). Subsequently, measurement of the thickness of the IMV membrane structure found only a single lipid bilayer of 5 nm (equivalent to the thickness of cell membranes) and no continuity was detected with cell membranes (Hollinshead et al. 1999). Moreover, clear images were presented showing continuity between a single IMV membrane and the plasma membrane during IMV entry and no other membranes were visible (Armstrong et al. 1973; Chang and Metz 1976). Taken together, these data

are interpreted by this author as unequivocal evidence that IMV has only a single membrane and therefore EEV has two. The challenge for the future is to elucidate how a single membrane is formed in the cytoplasm.

DISEASES CAUSED BY POXVIRUSES

Smallpox

Smallpox was a disease of man only and was a life-threatening systemic infection that spread through the body in several phases. Its impact on human health and its influence on our history can hardly be overstated. Even today, 25 years after the eradication of this disease, it has an impact as a potential bioterror weapon and has forced responses from governments around the world (see below).

Infection by variola virus was initiated by inhalation of virions released from the respiratory tract of infected patients or from scab material that had been ground into dust. A detailed study of the spread of virus from the respiratory system to other organs has been impossible in man for obvious reasons, but the mechanism of spread is believed to be similar to that of Ectromelia virus in mice, which causes the systemic disease mousepox (Buller and Palumbo 1991; Fenner 1992). With Ectromelia virus, infection spreads from the epithelium to the local lymph nodes where the virus replicates and is released into the blood stream (primary viremia) as free virions or within infected white cells. From here the virus causes an extensive infection of the reticuloendothelial system and higher levels of virus are released into the bloodstream (secondary viremia). Finally, the virus reaches the dermis where it induces formation of the characteristic skin lesions. With smallpox, there was a long incubation period before the patient became ill (8–14 days, average 11). Illness started with malaise, fever, aches, and prostration. The skin lesions progressed from papules to macules to blisters with a clear fluid containing virus. Eventually the lesions dried forming scabs that detached leaving a local scar. Once all scabs had detached from the body, the patient was no longer infectious. Smallpox lesions had a characteristic centrifugal distribution that was helpful in its diagnosis and distinction from chickenpox caused by a herpes virus, varicella-zoster virus. Smallpox lesions were abundant on the face, hands, and feet and less so on the trunk. In contrast, lesions caused by chickenpox are more abundant on the trunk than the periphery.

The mortality resulting from infection by variola virus depended upon whether infection was caused by variola major or variola minor and whether there was existing immunity. Infection by variola major in unvaccinated patients or immunologically naive populations caused up to 40 percent mortality, whereas with variola minor (also called alastrim) mortality was approximately 1 percent

(Fenner et al. 1988). Factors that predisposed to greater disease severity were immunological deficiency and pregnancy. The degree of protection provided by existing immunity depended on the time since vaccination, for epidemiological evidence showed that immunological protection does not endure for life. Those immunized long ago do have residual humoral or cell-mediated immunity or both (Hammarlund et al. 2003; Terajima et al. 2003), but it is uncertain if this will prevent infection or disease. Existing immunity may protect against mortality in most cases, but those infected might still transmit virus to others. Despite the sequencing of the genomes of minor and major strains of variola virus, it has not been possible to elucidate the basis for this large difference in virulence (Shchelkunov et al. 2000).

Monkeypox

This disease is caused by monkeypox virus, so called because it was isolated first from captive monkeys in Copenhagen in 1958, but its natural host is probably rodents and or squirrels in central and west Africa (Khodakevich et al. 1987a, b; Jezek and Fenner 1988; Kulesh et al. 2004). Monkeypox virus causes a disease in man that is clinically similar to smallpox and, until 2003, outbreaks were associated with significant mortality (1–10 percent). One important difference between monkeypox and smallpox is that the former is transmitted less efficiently from human to human and so outbreaks of monkeypox in man have tended to be isolated index cases or with very short chains of human transmission. The recognition of monkeypox as a human disease during the latter stages of the smallpox eradication campaign was of concern to the World Health Organization because it was feared that this virus might mutate into a variola-like virus and cause increased human-to-human transmission. Worse, if this virus retained its broad host range and became endemic in nonhuman hosts, it might be introduced repeatedly into man from an animal reservoir. However, these fears were largely dispelled by the sequencing of the monkeypox virus genome that showed that, within the *Orthopoxvirus* genus, monkeypox virus is one of the more divergent viruses from variola virus (Shchelkunov et al. 2001) and so evolution into a variola-like virus seems unlikely by passage and mutation.

In 2003, there was an outbreak of monkeypox in the USA that was caused by the importation of Gambian rodents (Di Giulio and Eckburg 2004; Reed et al. 2004). These rodents carried monkeypox virus without overt signs of illness, but transmitted the virus to American rodents, including prairie dogs, when cohoused in pet shops. The infected prairie dogs became ill and, as household pets, transmitted infection to man by close bodily contact, skin abrasions, or bites. Of the 81 humans infected, many became seriously ill, but there were no fatalities. Human infection was attributed to contact with infected animals rather than human-to-human transmission.

The epidemic outbreak of a febrile illness associated with a pustular rash caused concerns in USA that smallpox had re-emerged, and this fear was increased when the cause of the disease was diagnosed by electron microscopy as a poxvirus. However, these fears were allayed promptly when monkeypox virus was identified by PCR. Genome sequencing showed that the isolates from man and prairie dogs were very closely linked and were distinct from the strain of monkeypox virus that was sequenced from central Africa (Zaire) (Shchelkunov et al. 2001). This difference may explain the lack of mortality during the USA epidemic, compared with outbreaks in central Africa where mortality was up to 10 percent. Alternatively, the infected populations might have different inherent susceptibility to the disease or the disease outcome was affected by different quality of health care.

The episode of monkeypox in USA in 2003 has caused legislation banning the importation of exotic animals to be enacted and importation must now be subject to careful screening and quarantine.

Cowpox virus

Cowpox virus, like monkeypox virus, is a misnomer as the virus is not naturally resident in cows and its reservoir is probably rodents (Baxby et al. 1994; Crouch et al. 1995; Chantrey et al. 1999). However, cowpox virus has a broad host range and has infected many animals including rodents, large felines, domestic cats, cows, man, and elephants. In man, cowpox virus infections are usually single lesions (sometimes with satellites) on the hands that were acquired by handling infected animals. These can be painful and take weeks to resolve fully, but usually heal without lasting adverse effects, except for a local scar. The sequences of two cowpox virus strains (Brighton Red and GRI-90) showed that these viruses are quite diverse (see above) (Gubser et al. 2004); however, among the orthopoxviruses, the cowpox virus genomes have the greatest number of intact genes and the fewest number of broken genes fragments. This led to the suggestion that cowpox virus was closest to the ancestral poxvirus from which the other orthopoxviruses evolved (Shchelkunov et al. 1998).

Molluscum contagiosum virus

Molluscum contagiosum virus (MCV) is a strictly human virus that causes benign skin proliferations (often in children) that may persist for a year or more but then resolve. In patients with immunodeficiency caused, for instance, by infection with human immunodeficiency virus (HIV), MCV infections are more severe and a greater problem. MCV cannot be cultivated in cell culture and its genome has diverged significantly from other chordopoxviruses (Senkevich et al. 1996). Seventy out of the 182 MCV genes are not found in other poxviruses, and some of these encode immunomodulatory proteins unique to MCV (Senkevich et al. 1997). A notable feature of MCV lesions is the walling off of the lesion from the underlying tissue and the restricted infiltration of inflammatory cells into the lesion itself. This is likely to be due to one or more of the immunomodulatory proteins encoded by MCV. The center of the MCV lesion is often packed with new virions that are shed from the lesion surface into the environment. Transmission is by close contact with virus shed form the skin surface.

Parapoxvirus

The genus *Parapoxvirus* includes viruses that infect sheep, goats, and deer (Table 30.1) and two members of this genus have been sequenced (Delhon et al. 2004). The disease caused by Orf virus has been called contagious pustular dermatitis or scabby mouth and causes significant economic loss in sheep due to the painful lesions on lips and teats that discourage feeding. Virus is shed into the environment and can be transmitted to new stock from infected pasture, or by direct animal to animal contact. A notable feature of orf infections is that animals can be reinfected indicating that prior infection does not induce solid immunity. For a review of *Parapoxvirus* biology, see Robinson and Lyttle (1992). Orf virus lesions have a peculiar pathology and lesions are highly vascularized and this may be due in part to expression of a virus-encoded vascular endothelial growth factor (Lyttle et al. 1994). The gene encoding this protein is nonessential for growth in cell culture but influences the outcome of infection in vivo (Savory et al. 2000). Orf infection can be transmitted to man where it causes dermal skin lesions that can be painful.

Other parapoxviruses include pseudocowpox virus, viruses that infect seals, and a virus of reindeer (Tikkanen et al. 2004). Historically, confusion between cowpox virus and pseudocowpox virus caused Jenner's claim about the efficacy of vaccination against smallpox to be challenged. The use of pseudocowpox virus, which was also obtained from the teats of cows, provided no protection against smallpox because the virus belongs to a different genus, and this caused some to state that Jenner was incorrect.

In cases where the genomes of members of this genus have been analyzed, the genomes are rich in guanosine and cytosine (G+C) (64 percent for Orf virus), but despite this, these viruses have a gene content and genome organization that is conserved with other chordopoxviruses. Overall, they are closest to the genus *Molluscipoxvirus*, and share some features with MCV, such as a G+C-rich genome and few genes for nucleotide metabolism (Delhon et al. 2004).

Leporipoxvirus

The leporipoxviruses infect rabbits. myxoma virus was isolated from its natural host in South America (*Sylvilagus* spp.) in which it does not cause severe disease, but in the European rabbit (*Oryctolagus cuniculus*) it causes the disease myxomatosis (McFadden 1988). Myxoma virus was used in the 1950s to control the huge population of European rabbits that had built up in Australia and its release and adaptation to its host provides an excellent example of how virus and host co-evolve (Fenner and Ratcliffe 1965). Initially, after the release of virulent virus most of the rabbits died and only virulent virus was isolated from the field. Subsequently, the virus strains present in the rabbit population were of more modest virulence, and the surviving rabbits became more resistant to the original virus. This demonstrates that evolution favors the emergence of pathogens of modest virulence. The basis for the changes in virulence of the myxoma viruses isolated from Australia is not understood.

The genome sequences of myxoma virus (Cameron et al. 1999) and Shope fibroma virus (Willer et al. 1999) showed more diversity exists between these leporipoxviruses than between members of genus *Orthopoxvirus*. But like the orthopoxviruses, the terminal regions of the leporipoxvirus genomes encode a diverse range of immunomodulatory proteins that inhibit aspects of the immune response to infection and that have been subject to genetic manipulation and functional characterization (Nash et al. 1999). The virulence of myxoma virus has been assessed largely in the European rabbit where it causes a fatal disease rather than in its natural host where the asymptomatic nature of the infection makes study of pathogenesis more difficult.

Capripoxvirus

The capripoxviruses infect sheep, goats, and cattle in parts of Africa and Asia and are a cause of significant mortality, morbidity, and economic loss. Transmission of infection can be via direct contact and entry through skin abrasions, close airborne transmission, or via arthropod vectors. Comparisons of the genomes (Gershon and Black 1988) and antigenicity (Kitching et al. 1986) of these viruses indicated that they are closely related; nonetheless, these viruses vary considerably in virulence and attenuated strains have been used as live vaccines. The genomes of lumpy skin disease virus and several sheeppox and goatpox viruses have been sequenced and compared (Tulman et al. 2001, 2002b). These studies identified some differences between virulent and attenuated strains near the genome termini, but which changes are responsible for attenuation is unknown. Like other chordopoxviruses, these viruses contain many genes encoding immunomodulators near the genome termini and several of these are unique to the genus *Capripoxvirus*.

Avipoxvirus

The genus *Avipoxvirus* includes a wide range of viruses that are distributed worldwide. Some of these viruses may cause severe disease and are a cause of economic loss in the poultry industry. Respiratory infection is usually more severe than dermal infection. The sequence of the prototype avipoxvirus, fowlpox virus, shows that genus *Avipoxvirus* is the most divergent genus of the *Chordopoxvirus* genera and has the largest genome and the greatest number of genes unique to this genus (see above). A notable feature of some strains of fowlpox virus was the presence of the provirus genome of an avian retrovirus, reticuloendotheliosis virus, integrated into the avipoxvirus genome (Hertig et al. 1997). Although there was no evidence of reverse transcriptase activity in fowlpox virus-infected cells, the integrated retrovirus is infectious because transfection of isolated virus DNA into uninfected cells yielded infectious retrovirus. Comparison of the genome sequences of a virulent (Afonso et al. 2000) and attenuated fowlpox virus genomes (Laidlaw and Skinner 2004) have identified many changes and the basis for attenuation is likely to be multifactorial.

Yatapoxvirus

The genus *Yatapoxirus* (Table 30.1) contains three members, tanapox virus, yaba monkey tumor virus (YMTV), and yaba-like disease virus (YLDV) and the genomes of the latter two viruses have been sequenced (Lee et al. 2001; Brunetti et al. 2003). *Tanapox virus* was first isolated in East Africa where it caused a febrile illness associated with one or more poxviruslike lesions, but the virus has also been isolated in Zaire and may be present across tropical Africa. The natural host is uncertain but the ability to cause disease only in monkeys would be consistent with a simian origin. Serological evidence of infection in African monkeys (Tsuchiya and Tagaya 1971; Downie 1974) established that these animals may be infected, but it remains unclear if monkeys are the natural host, or whether infections in monkeys are zoonoses after transmission from another reservoir. Human infections were more common close to rivers or following periods of flooding suggesting transmission by a biting arthropod. YMTV causes histiocytomas in rhesus monkeys and man (Niven et al. 1961).

POXVIRUSES AND BIOTERRORISM

The terrorist attacks in Washington DC and New York in 2001 and the subsequent release of anthrax spores in the USA prompted an urgent evaluation of whether there was adequate preparation against microbial pathogens that might be used in bioterrorism. If terrorists were prepared to commit suicide and mass murder by flying aeroplanes into civilian populations, it seemed probable that they might also be willing to obtain, grow, and release pathogenic micro-organisms. Top of the list of potential bioterror agents was variola virus. At the end of 2001, the preparedness for a smallpox epidemic was far from adequate. Smallpox vaccination had been discontinued for approximately 30 years and so roughly 40 percent of the population was immunologically naive for orthopoxviruses. Furthermore, it was uncertain if those vaccinated several decades previously had retained sufficient immunity to provide protection against variola virus. The stocks of vaccine were both old and limited. Indeed, during the 1990s, the World Health Organization (WHO) had ordered the destruction of millions of doses of vaccine that were deemed no longer required. The release of variola virus in a densely populated public place, perhaps a center of public transportation, might cause infection of many citizens. Given that smallpox takes an average of 11 days to develop following infection, those infected might have traveled far and wide and disseminated the infection to others before the outbreak was realized. Faced with this situation, health authorities would have an immensely challenging task of identifying all those exposed initially and all the contacts of those exposed. It was likely that the supply of vaccine would rapidly become exhausted.

Faced with this scenario, several governments initiated programs to replenish their stocks of smallpox vaccine, to increase surveillance for smallpox and to vaccinate some of their citizens. The US Government purchased sufficient vaccine to immunize each of its citizens and vaccination programs were initiated to protect approximately 500 000 first-line responders during the first quarter of 2003, approximately 11 million by the end of 2003 and, possibly, the whole population thereafter. In other western countries, the response was less radical. The UK Government vaccinated only 350 healthcare workers (www.doh.gov.uk) and bought sufficient vaccine to immunize the population if there were an outbreak. Elsewhere in Europe, some governments simply purchased vaccine, but did not vaccinate their citizens.

The decision not to vaccinate large fractions of the population was driven mostly by the fears of complications with the existing smallpox vaccines. During mass smallpox immunizations, it was recognized that immunization could cause complications such as progressive vaccinia, eczema vaccinatum, and neurological conditions with a death rate of approximately 1–5 per million vaccinees (Lane et al. 1969; Feery 1977). Those with immunological deficiency or eczema were more susceptible and pregnancy was also a condition that increased the risk of complications or their severity (Fenner et al. 1988). Today, the frequency of complications would probably be greater because a significant fraction of the population is immunosuppressed due to HIV infection and more people have eczema. In view of this, and to minimize the risk of complications, potential vaccinees (and their close contacts) were screened carefully for contraindications to vaccination and vaccinees were monitored after vaccination. Despite this, complications occurred in the USA and the vaccination program has largely halted after approximately 500 000 vaccinations. An unexpectedly frequent complication was myocarditis (Cassimatis et al. 2004) that had been reported more rarely during previous smallpox vaccination programs (Feery 1977).

The strain of vaccine to be used in the new vaccination programs and to be stockpiled for national reserves was a source of contention. The smallpox vaccines strains that were widely used to achieve global eradication were Lister and New York City Board of Health (Wyeth) and these were effective at preventing smallpox by all strains of variola virus. Although, these vaccines were known to be effective, they were also known to have an imperfect safety record (Lane et al. 1969; Feery 1977). These vaccines had similar rates of complication, although precise comparisons are difficult because of differing populations in which these vaccines were used and different methods of assessing complication rates. Alternative vaccines based upon more attenuated strains of vaccinia virus such as LC18m8 in Japan (Hashizume et al. 1985) and modified virus Ankara (MVA) in Germany (Stickl et al. 1974) had been developed and shown to be safer in man, but their effectiveness at preventing smallpox was unproven because those immunized were never exposed naturally to variola virus. Faced with the choice of using an established vaccine that worked but caused complications, or a safer vaccine that was not proven to be effective, most governments bought the old vaccine. However, these new stocks of vaccine stocks were manufactured under modern good manufacturing practice conditions (in some cases after plaque purification) in sterile tissue culture and with rigorous screening for exogenous pathogens. In contrast, the old smallpox vaccines had been grown on the side of sheep or cattle and contained significant bacteriological contamination.

In countries where a cohort of first-line responders has been vaccinated, who would be able to treat smallpox patients without contracting and spreading the disease, there will be a need to maintain vaccination for as long as the perceived threat of smallpox remains. WHO recommended revaccination every 3 years for those in areas where smallpox was endemic.

ANTI-POXVIRUS DRUGS

The availability of an effective vaccine against smallpox was a disincentive for the development of effective drugs for combating smallpox or other poxvirus infections. However, the worries of bioterrorism and the potential to enhance the virulence of pathogenic poxviruses by genetic engineering (Jackson et al. 2001) have increased the need for effective drugs. Recent drug screening programs have identified several potentially useful drugs. The first of these is cidofovir, a licensed anti-herpes virus drug used to combat human cytomegalovirus infections. Cidofovir prevents replication of many orthopoxviruses (including variola virus) in cell culture and can protect against orthopoxvirus infection in animal models (Bray et al. 2000). There are some disadvantages to cidofovir, however, such as renal toxicity and the need for the drug to be administered by intravenous injection. These difficulties are being overcome by the development of chemically modified versions of cidofovir. These can be taken orally, have enhanced activity against poxviruses, and, importantly, are no longer toxic for kidneys (Ciesla et al. 2003) but accumulate in the respiratory system, the site of primary infection by variola virus. Preliminary animal experiments show that the drug can protect against orthopoxviruses in vivo (Buller et al. 2004).

Cidofovir's mode of action is by inhibition of the virus DNA polymerase, but other virus proteins that are essential for virus replication are also being considered as targets for antipoxvirus drugs. These include dUTPase, topoisomerase, and proteins critical for virus morphogenesis. With all of these new drugs, although it will be possible to determine if they can protect against orthopoxviruses in animal models, it will be impossible to demonstrate efficacy against smallpox in man. This poses a regulatory problem for licensing.

IMMUNE RESPONSE TO SMALLPOX VACCINATION

During the smallpox eradication campaign, the immune response to vaccination had been evaluated with techniques that by today's standards were primitive. Moreover, the importance of immunity to the antigens specific to the EEV had not been fully appreciated and the immune response was evaluated predominantly against IMV. Tests such as hemagglutination inhibition (HAI), complement fixation, and plaque neutralization were employed, although the latter test was almost invariably performed against IMV. However, it was known that although vaccines composed of inactivated IMV induced very good levels of neutralizing antibody to IMV in man or animals, they failed to confer protection because they did not induce immune response to EEV antigens, for reviews see (Boulter and Appleyard 1973; Smith et al. 2002). Overall, there was only a rudimentary understanding of the immunological responses to smallpox vaccination and there was no clear benchmark that correlated with protection from smallpox. Instead a recent vaccination scar (within 3 years) was considered the best evidence.

Against this background, the recent smallpox vaccination programs in the USA and UK have provided an opportunity to evaluate the response to smallpox vaccination using modern immunological techniques. These have included measurement of both cell-mediated and humoral immunity and have analyzed the antibody responses to IMV, EEV, and specific antigens from either virion. This is providing a benchmark against which the immunity remaining in individuals immunized decades previously or the immune response induced by new smallpox vaccines can be compared. An encouraging finding is that the immunological responses to vaccination are retained for several decades (Hammarlund et al. 2003; Terajima et al. 2003), although there must be caution in interpreting this as evidence of protection against smallpox.

The continuing worry about smallpox and bioterrorism, and the inadequate safety profile of traditional smallpox vaccines is prompting more research to develop safer vaccines. Strains LC16m8 and MVA are both being evaluated. MVA, in particular, shows promise. It was established that primary infection with MVA is safe in man and that this primary vaccination would cause the response to a subsequent vaccination with conventional vaccine to be modified, indicating existing immunity. MVA can also induce protection against challenge with other orthopoxviruses, such as vaccinia or monkeypox in rodent and animal models (Drexler et al. 2003; Earl et al. 2004). However, its efficacy in man remains unproven and a recent report showed that two immunizations with MVA induced inferior protection against monkeypox virus challenge than a single immunization with a conventional vaccine (DRYVAX) (Earl et al. 2004).

LC16m8 also has a good safety record in man and primary vaccination induced less severe reactions than those induced by the Lister strain from which LC16m8 was derived (Hashizume et al. 1985). However, a potential difficulty with LC16m8 is a mutation in the B5R gene that prevents expression of the B5R protein (Takahashi-Nishimaki et al. 1991). As well as being required to make a normal plaque size, B5R has been identified as the only EEV-specific protein that is the target for antibodies that neutralize EEV infectivity (Galmiche et al. 1999; Law and Smith 2001; Hooper et al. 2003). Given that responses to EEV are important for protection against orthopoxviruses, the omission of *B5R* is a potential problem for this vaccine. It would seem logical in the design of new smallpox vaccines to include this antigen.

REFERENCES

Afonso, C.L., Tulman, E.R., et al. 1999. The genome of *Melanoplus sanguinipes* entomopoxvirus. *J Virol*, **73**, 533–52.

Afonso, C.L., Tulman, E.R., et al. 2000. The genome of fowlpox virus. *J Virol*, **74**, 3815–31.

Afonso, C.L., Tulman, E.R., et al. 2002. The genome of deerpox virus. In Niles, E.G. (ed.), *XIV International Poxvirus and Iridovirus Conference*, Lake Placid, NY, USA, p. 5.

Aguado, B., Selmes, I.P. and Smith, G.L. 1992. Nucleotide sequence of 21.8 kbp of variola major virus strain Harvey and comparison with vaccinia virus. *J Gen Virol*, **73**, 2887–902.

Alcami, A. and Smith, G.L. 1992. A soluble receptor for interleukin-1 beta encoded by vaccinia virus: a novel mechanism of virus modulation of the host response to infection. *Cell*, **71**, 153–67.

Alcami, A. and Smith, G.L. 1996. A mechanism for the inhibition of fever by a virus. *Proc Natl Acad Sci USA*, **93**, 11029–34.

Armstrong, J.A., Metz, D.H. and Young, M.R. 1973. The mode of entry of vaccinia virus into L cells. *J Gen Virol*, **21**, 533–7.

Bagnall, B.G. and Wilson, G.R. 1974. *Molluscum contagiosum* in a red kangaroo. *Aust J Derm*, **15**, 115–20.

Bawden, A.L., Glassberg, K.J., et al. 2000. Complete genomic sequence of the *Amsacta moorei* entomopoxvirus: analysis and comparison with other poxviruses. *Virology*, **274**, 120–39.

Baxby, D. 1981. *Jenner's smallpox vaccine. The riddle of the origin of vaccinia virus*. London: Heinemann.

Baxby, D., Bennett, M. and Getty, B. 1994. Human cowpox 1969–93: a review based on 54 cases. *Br J Dermatol*, **131**, 598–607.

Boulter, E.A. and Appleyard, G. 1973. Differences between extracellular and intracellular forms of poxvirus and their implications. *Prog Med Virol*, **16**, 86–108.

Bray, M., Martinez, M., et al. 2000. Cidofovir protects mice against lethal aerosol or intranasal cowpox virus challenge. *J Infect Dis*, **181**, 10–19.

Brown, M., Dorson, J.W. and Bollum, F.J. 1973. Terminal riboadenylate transferase: a poly A polymerase in purified vaccinia virus. *J Virol*, **12**, 203–8.

Brunetti, C.R., Amano, H., et al. 2003. Complete genomic sequence and comparative analysis of the tumorigenic poxvirus Yaba monkey tumor virus. *J Virol*, **77**, 13335–47.

Buller, R.M. and Palumbo, G.J. 1991. Poxvirus pathogenesis. *Microbiol Rev*, **55**, 80–122.

Buller, R.M., Owens, G., et al. 2004. Efficacy of oral active ether lipid analogs of cidofovir in a lethal mousepox model. *Virology*, **318**, 474–81.

Cameron, C., Hota-Mitchell, S., et al. 1999. The complete DNA sequence of myxoma virus. *Virology*, **264**, 298–318.

Cassimatis, D.C., Atwood, J.E., et al. 2004. Smallpox vaccination and myopericarditis: a clinical review. *J Am Coll Cardiol*, **43**, 1503–10.

Chang, A. and Metz, D.H. 1976. Further investigations on the mode of entry of vaccinia virus into cells. *J Gen Virol*, **32**, 275–82.

Chantrey, J., Meyer, H., et al. 1999. Cowpox: reservoir hosts and geographic range. *Epidemiol Infect*, **122**, 455–60.

Ciesla, S.L., Trahan, J., et al. 2003. Esterification of cidofovir with alkoxyalkanols increases oral bioavailability and diminishes drug accumulation in kidney. *Antiviral Res*, **59**, 163–71.

Collier, L.H. 1954. The preservation of vaccinia virus. *Bacteriol Rev*, **18**, 74.

Collier, L.H. 1955. The development of a stable smallpox vaccine. *J Hyg*, **53**, 76.

Crouch, A.C., Baxby, D., et al. 1995. Serological evidence for the reservoir hosts of cowpox virus in British wildlife. *Epidemiol Infect*, **115**, 185–91.

da Fonseca, F.G., Trindade, G.S., et al. 2002. Characterization of a vaccinia-like virus isolated in a Brazilian forest. *J Gen Virol*, **83**, 223–8.

Dales, S. and Siminovitch, L. 1961. The development of vaccinia virus in Earle's L strain cells as examined by electron microscopy. *J Biophys Biochem Cytol*, **10**, 475–503.

de Souza Trindade, G., da Fonseca, F.G., et al. 2003. Aracatuba virus: a vaccinia-like virus associated with infection in humans and cattle. *Emerg Infect Dis*, **9**, 155–60.

Delhon, G., Tulman, E.R., et al. 2004. Genomes of the parapoxviruses ORF virus and bovine papular stomatitis virus. *J Virol*, **78**, 168–77.

Di Giulio, D.B. and Eckburg, P.B. 2004. Human monkeypox: an emerging zoonosis. *Lancet Infect Dis*, **4**, 15–25.

Downie, A.W. 1974. Serological evidence of infection with Tana and Yaba poxviruses among several species of monkey. *J Hyg (Lond)*, **72**, 245–50.

Downie, A.W. 1939a. Immunological relationship of the virus of spontaneous cowpox to vaccinia virus. *Br J Exp Pathol*, **20**, 158–76.

Downie, A.W. 1939b. A study of the lesions produced experimentally by cowpox virus. *J Pathol Bacteriol*, **48**, 361–79.

Drexler, I., Staib, C., et al. 2003. Identification of vaccinia virus epitope-specific HLA-A*0201-restricted T cells and comparative analysis of smallpox vaccines. *Proc Natl Acad Sci USA*, **100**, 217–22.

Dumbell, K. and Richardson, M. 1993. Virological investigations of specimens from buffaloes affected by buffalopox in Maharashtra State, India between 1985 and 1987. *Arch Virol*, **128**, 257–67.

Earl, P.L., Americo, J.L., et al. 2004. Immunogenicity of a highly attenuated MVA smallpox vaccine and protection against monkeypox. *Nature*, **428**, 182–5.

Esposito, J.J., Palmer, E.L., et al. 1980. Studies on the poxvirus Cotia. *J Gen Virol*, **47**, 37–46.

Feery, B.J. 1977. Adverse reactions after smallpox vaccination. *Med J Aust*, **2**, 180–3.

Fenner, F. 1992. Vaccinia virus as a vaccine, and poxvirus pathogenesis. In: Binns, M.M. and Smith, G.L. (eds), *Recombinant poxviruses*. Boca Raton, FL: CRC Press, 1–43.

Fenner, F. 1996. Poxviruses. In: Fields, B.N. and Howley, P.M. (eds), *Fields virology*, 3rd edn. Philadelphia: Lippincott-Raven Publishers, 2673–702.

Fenner, F. and Ratcliffe, F.N. 1965. *Myxomatosis*. Cambridge: Cambridge University Press.

Fenner, F., Henderson, D.A., et al. 1988. *Smallpox and its eradication*. Geneva: World Health Organization.

Fonseca, F.G., Lanna, M.C., et al. 1998. Morphological and molecular characterization of the poxvirus BeAn 58058. *Arch Virol*, **143**, 1171–86.

Galmiche, M.C., Goenaga, J., et al. 1999. Neutralizing and protective antibodies directed against vaccinia virus envelope antigens. *Virology*, **254**, 71–80.

Gershon, P.D. and Black, D.N. 1988. A comparison of the genomes of capripoxvirus isolates of sheep, goats and cattle. *Virology*, **164**, 341–9.

Glynn, I. and Glynn, J. 2004. *The life and death of smallpox*. London: Profile Books.

Gubser, C. and Smith, G.L. 2002. The sequence of camelpox virus shows it is most closely related to variola virus, the cause of smallpox. *J Gen Virol*, **83**, 855–72.

Gubser, C., Hué, S., et al. 2004. Poxvirus genomes: a phylogenetic analysis. *J Gen Virol*, **85**, 105–17.

Hammarlund, E., Lewis, M.W., et al. 2003. Duration of antiviral immunity after smallpox vaccination. *Nat Med*, **9**, 1131–7.

Hashizume, S., Yoshizawa, H., et al. 1985. Properties of attenuated mutant of vaccinia virus, LC16m8, derived from Lister strain. In: Quinnan, G.V. (ed.), *Vaccinia viruses as vectors for vaccine antigens*. New York: Elsevier Science, 87–99.

Heine, H.G., Stevens, M.P., et al. 1999. A capripoxvirus detection PCR and antibody ELISA based on the major antigen P32, the homolog of the vaccinia virus H3L gene. *J Immunol Meth*, **227**, 187–96.

Henderson, D.A. 1976. The eradication of smallpox. *Sci Am*, **235**, 25–33.

Hertig, C., Coupar, B.E., et al. 1997. Field and vaccine strains of fowlpox virus carry integrated sequences from the avian retrovirus, reticuloendotheliosis virus. *Virology*, **235**, 367–76.

Hollinshead, M., Vanderplasschen, A., et al. 1999. Vaccinia virus intracellular mature virions contain only one lipid membrane. *J Virol*, **73**, 1503–17.

Hooper, J.W., Custer, D.M. and Thompson, E. 2003. Four-gene-combination DNA vaccine protects mice against a lethal vaccinia virus challenge and elicits appropriate antibody responses in nonhuman primates. *Virology*, **306**, 181–95.

Hopkins, D.A. 1983. *Princes and peasants. Smallpox in history*. London: University of Chicago Press, pp. 380.

Horner, R.F. 1988. Poxvirus in farmed Nile crocodiles. *Vet Rec*, **122**, 459–62.

Jackson, R.J., Ramsay, A.J., et al. 2001. Expression of mouse IL-4 by a recombinant ectromelia virus suppresses cytolytic lymphocyte responses and overcomes genetic resistance to mousepox. *J Virol*, **75**, 1205–10.

Jacobson, E.R. and Telford, S.R. 1990. Chlamydial and poxvirus infections of circulating monocytes of a flap-necked chameleon (*Chamaeleo dilepsis*). *J Wildl Dis*, **26**, 572–7.

Jenner, E. 1798. An enquiry into the causes and effects of variolae vaccinae, a disease discovered in some western counties of England, particularly Gloucestershire, and known by the name of cow pox. Reprinted by Cassell, 1896, London.

Jenner, E. 1801. *The origin of the vaccine inoculation*. London: D.N. Shury.

Jezek, Z. and Fenner, F. 1988. Human monkeypox. In Melnick, J.L. (ed.), *Monographs in virology*. Basel: Karger.

Khodakevich, L., Szczeniowski, M., et al. 1987a. The role of squirrels in sustaining monkeypox virus transmission. *Trop Geogr Med*, **39**, 115–22.

Khodakevich, L., Szczeniowski, M., et al. 1987b. Monkeypox virus in relation to the ecological features surrounding human settlements in Bumba zone, Zaire. *Trop Geogr Med*, **39**, 56–63.

Kitching, R.P., Hammond, J.M. and Black, D.N. 1986. Studies on the major common precipitating antigen of capripoxviruses. *J Gen Virol*, **67**, 139–48.

Kulesh, D.A., Loveless, B.M., et al. 2004. Monkeypox virus detection in rodents using real-time 3′-minor groove binder TaqMan® assays on the Roche LightCycler. *Lab Invest*, **84**, 1200–8.

Laidlaw, S.M. and Skinner, M.A. 2004. Comparison of the genome sequence of FP9, an attenuated, tissue culture-adapted European strain of fowlpox virus, with those of virulent American and European viruses. *J Gen Virol*, **85**, 305–22.

Lane, J.M., Ruben, F.L., et al. 1969. Complications of smallpox vaccination, 1968. National surveillance in the United States. *New Engl J Med*, **281**, 1201–8.

Law, M. and Smith, G.L. 2001. Antibody neutralization of the extracellular enveloped form of vaccinia virus. *Virology*, **280**, 132–42.

Lee, H.J., Essani, K. and Smith, G.L. 2001. The genome sequence of Yaba-like disease virus, a yatapoxvirus. *Virology*, **281**, 170–92.

Lurman, A. 1885. Eine icterusepidermie. *Berlin Klin Wschr*, **22**, 20.

Lyttle, D.J., Fraser, K.M., et al. 1994. Homologs of vascular endothelial growth factor are encoded by the poxvirus orf virus. *J Virol*, **68**, 84–92.

Mackett, M., Smith, G.L. and Moss, B. 1982. Vaccinia virus: a selectable eukaryotic cloning and expression vector. *Proc Natl Acad Sci USA*, **79**, 7415–19.

Martin, S.A. and Moss, B. 1975. Modification of RNA by mRNA guanylyltransferase and mRNA (guanine-7-)methyltransferase from vaccinia virions. *J Biol Chem*, **250**, 9330–5.

McFadden, G. 1988. Poxviruses of rabbits. In: Desai, G. (ed.), *Virus diseases in laboratory and captive animals*. New York: Kluwer Academic, 37–62.

McLysaght, A., Baldi, P.F. and Gaut, B.S. 2003. Extensive gene gain associated with adaptive evolution of poxviruses. *Proc Natl Acad Sci USA*, **100**, 15655–60.

Meyer, H., Pfeffer, M. and Rziha, H.J. 1994. Sequence alterations within and downstream of the A-type inclusion protein genes allow differentiation of Orthopoxvirus species by polymerase chain reaction. *J Gen Virol*, **75**, 1975–81.

Moore, J.B. and Smith, G.L. 1992. Steroid hormone synthesis by a vaccinia enzyme: a new type of virus virulence factor. *EMBO J*, **11**, 1973–80.

Moss, B. 2001. Poxviridae: the viruses and their replication. In: Fields, B.N., Knipe, B.N., et al. (eds), *Virology*, 4th edn. Philadelphia: Lippincott-Raven, 2849–83.

Moyer, R.W. 1994. Entomopoxviruses. In: Webster, R.G. and Granoff, A. (eds), *Encyclopedia of virology*. Orlando, FL: Academic Press, 392–8.

Moyer, R.W. 1999. Entomopoxviruses (Poxviridae). In: Webster, R.G. and Granoff, A. (eds), *Encyclopedia of virology*. London: Academic Press, 474–81.

Munyon, W., Paoletti, E. and Grace, J.T. Jr. 1967. RNA polymerase activity in purified infectious vaccinia virus. *Proc Natl Acad Sci USA*, **58**, 2280–7.

Nash, P., Barrett, J., et al. 1999. Immunomodulation by viruses: the myxoma virus story. *Immunol Rev*, **168**, 103–20.

Niven, J.S.F., Armstrong, J.A., et al. 1961. Subcutaneous growths in monkeys produced by a poxvirus. *J Pathol Bacteriol*, **81**, 1–14.

Panicali, D. and Paoletti, E. 1982. Construction of poxviruses as cloning vectors: insertion of the thymidine kinase gene from herpes simplex virus into the DNA of infectious vaccinia virus. *Proc Natl Acad Sci USA*, **79**, 4927–31.

Panicali, D., Davis, S.W., et al. 1983. Construction of live vaccines by using genetically engineered poxviruses: biological activity of recombinant vaccinia virus expressing influenza virus hemagglutinin. *Proc Natl Acad Sci USA*, **80**, 5364–8.

Reed, K.D., Melski, J.W., et al. 2004. The detection of monkeypox in humans in the western hemisphere. *N Engl J Med*, **350**, 342–50.

Robinson, A.J. and Lyttle, D.J. 1992. Parapoxviruses: their biology and potential as recombinant vaccines. In: Binns, M.M. and Smith, G.L. (eds), *Recombinant poxviruses*. Boca Raton, FL: CRC Press, 285–327.

Ropp, S.L., Jin, Q., et al. 1995. PCR strategy for identification and differentiation of small pox and other orthopoxviruses. *J Clin Microbiol*, **33**, 2069–76.

Savory, L.J., Stacker, S.A., et al. 2000. Viral vascular endothelial growth factor plays a critical role in orf virus infection. *J Virol*, **74**, 10699–706.

Seet, B.T., Johnston, J.B., et al. 2003. Poxviruses and immune evasion. *Annu Rev Immunol*, **21**, 377–423.

Senkevich, T.G., Bugert, J.J., et al. 1996. Genome sequence of a human tumorigenic poxvirus: prediction of specific host response–evasion genes. *Science*, **273**, 813–16.

Senkevich, T.G., Koonin, E.V., et al. 1997. The genome of molluscum contagiosum virus: analysis and comparison with other poxviruses. *Virology*, **233**, 19–42.

Shchelkunov, S.N., Massung, R.F. and Esposito, J.J. 1995. Comparison of the genome DNA sequences of Bangladesh-1975 and India-1967 variola viruses. *Virus Res*, **36**, 107–18.

Shchelkunov, S.N., Safronov, P.F., et al. 1998. The genomic sequence analysis of the left and right species-specific terminal region of a cowpox virus strain reveals unique sequences and a cluster of intact ORFs for immunomodulatory and host range proteins. *Virology*, **243**, 432–60.

Shchelkunov, S.N., Totmenin, A.V., et al. 2000. Alastrim smallpox variola minor virus genome DNA sequences. *Virology*, **266**, 361–86.

Shchelkunov, S.N., Totmenin, A.V., et al. 2001. Human monkeypox and smallpox viruses: genomic comparison. *FEBS Lett*, **509**, 66–70.

Smith, G.L. and McFadden, G. 2002. Smallpox, anything to declare? *Nat Immunol Rev*, **2**, 521–7.

Smith, G.L., Mackett, M. and Moss, B. 1983a. Infectious vaccinia virus recombinants that express hepatitis B virus surface antigen. *Nature*, **302**, 490–5.

Smith, G.L., Murphy, B.R. and Moss, B. 1983b. Construction and characterization of an infectious vaccinia virus recombinant that expresses the influenza hemagglutinin gene and induces resistance to influenza virus infection in hamsters. *Proc Natl Acad Sci USA*, **80**, 7155–9.

Smith, G.L., Vanderplasschen, A. and Law, M. 2002. The formation and function of extracellular enveloped vaccinia virus. *J Gen Virol*, **83**, 2915–31.

Smith, G.L., Murphy, B.J. and Law, M. 2003. Vaccinia virus motility. *Annu Rev Microbiol*, **57**, 323–42.

Sodeik, B., Doms, R.W., et al. 1993. Assembly of vaccinia virus: role of the intermediate compartment between the endoplasmic reticulum and the Golgi stacks. *J Cell Biol*, **121**, 521–41.

Sofi Ibrahim, M., Kulesh, D.A., et al. 2003. Real-time PCR assay to detect smallpox virus. *J Clin Microbiol*, **41**, 3835–9.

Spriggs, M.K., Hruby, D.E., et al. 1992. Vaccinia and cowpox viruses encode a novel secreted interleukin-1-binding protein. *Cell*, **71**, 145–52.

Stauber, E. and Gogolewski, R. 1990. Poxvirus dermatitis in a tegu lizard (*Tupinambis teguixin*). *J Zoo Wildl Med*, **21**, 228–30.

Stickl, H., Hochstein Mintzel, V., et al. 1974. [MVA vaccination against smallpox: clinical tests with an attenuated live vaccinia virus strain (MVA) (author's transl)]. *Dtsch Med Wochenschr*, **99**, 2386–92.

Takahashi-Nishimaki, F., Funahashi, S.-I., et al. 1991. Regulation of plaque size and host range by a vaccinia virus gene related to complement system proteins. *Virology*, **181**, 158–64.

Terajima, M., Cruz, J., et al. 2003. Quantitation of CD8+ T cell responses to newly identified HLA-A*0201-restricted T cell epitopes conserved among vaccinia and variola (smallpox) viruses. *J Exp Med*, **197**, 927–32.

Thomas, K., Tompkins, D.M., et al. 2003. A novel poxvirus lethal to red squirrels (*Sciurus vulgaris*). *J Gen Virol*, **84**, 3337–41.

Tikkanen, M.K., McInnes, C.J., et al. 2004. Recent isolates of parapoxvirus of Finnish reindeer (*Rangifer tarandus tarandus*) are closely related to bovine pseudocowpox virus. *J Gen Virol*, **85**, 1413–18.

Tsuchiya, Y. and Tagaya, L. 1971. Sero-epidemiological survey on Yaba and 1211 virus infections among several species of monkey. *J Hyg (Lond)*, **69**, 445–51.

Tulman, E.R., Afonso, C.L., et al. 2001. Genome of lumpy skin disease virus. *J Virol*, **75**, 7122–30.

Tulman, E.R., Afonso, C.L., et al. 2002a. The genome of horsepox virus. In Niles, E.G. (ed.), *XIV International Poxvirus and Iridovirus Conference,* Lake Placid, NY, USA.

Tulman, E.R., Afonso, C.L., et al. 2002b. The genomes of sheeppox and goatpox viruses. *J Virol*, **76**, 6054–61.

Ueda, Y., Dumbell, K.R., et al. 1978. Studies on Cotia virus – an unclassified poxvirus. *J Gen Virol*, **40**, 263–76.

Upton, C., Slack, S., et al. 2003. Poxvirus orthologous clusters: towards defining the minimum essential poxvirus genome. *J Virol*, **77**, 7590–600.

Willer, D.O., McFadden, G. and Evans, D.H. 1999. The complete genome sequence of Shope (rabbit) fibroma virus. *Virology*, **264**, 319–43.

Wilson, T.M. and Poglayen-Newall, I. 1971. Pox in South American sea lions (*Otaria byronia*). *Can J Comp Med*, **35**, 174–7.

31

Poxvirus replication

RICHARD C. CONDIT AND RICHARD W. MOYER

POXVIRUS CLASSIFICATION AND VIRION STRUCTURE

Poxviruses are one of the most complex DNA-containing virus families. The strategy for growth and reproduction of this family of viruses is sufficiently robust and adaptable to have become established in a variety of eukaryotic hosts from insects, birds, and reptiles to higher vertebrates including man. Taxonomically, the *Poxviridae* family comprises two subfamilies: the *Chordopoxvirinae* (viruses of vertebrates) and the *Entomopoxvirinae* (viruses of insects) (Moyer et al. 2000) (Table 31.1). There are eight *Chordopoxvirinae* genera: *orthopoxvirus*, *Parapoxvirus*, *Avipoxvirus*, *Capripoxvirus*, *Leporipoxvirus*, *Suipoxvirus*, *Molluscipoxvirus*, and *Yatapoxvirus*, of which four (*orthopoxvirus*, *Parapoxvirus*, *Yatapoxvirus*, and *Molluscipoxvirus*) can cause human infections. Of these, the most clinically significant diseases are those caused by the orthopoxvirus *Variola virus* (VARV) (smallpox) and *Monkeypox virus* (MPXV), and the molluscipoxvirus *Molluscum contagiosum virus* (MOCV) (Esposito and Fenner 2001). There are three genera of entomopoxviruses, designated A, B, and C, based mainly on host range. Many entomopoxviruses await further classification.

Poxvirus family members share a number of unique features including:

- a large complex enveloped virion that appears as an enveloped, brick-shaped structure and is of sufficient size to be visualized under a light microscope
- the packaging in virions of a variety of enzymes including all those required to carry out transcription of poxvirus early genes from the DNA contained within the virus
- a cytoplasmic site of replication
- a double-stranded genomic DNA which can range in size from approximately 144 kb (Yaba-like disease virus, Lee et al. 2001) to nearly 300 kb (*Fowlpox virus*, Afonso et al. 2000) and up to nearly 400 kb for some entomopoxviruses (Moyer et al. 2000)
- a hairpin loop of DNA comprised of imperfectly paired heteroduplex DNA present at both termini of the genome
- a complex mechanism for assembly of infectious virions.

The overall virus growth cycle is depicted in Figure 31.1 p. 596 and will be expanded upon throughout this chapter.

Vertebrate poxviruses also share a co-linear core of conserved genes located within the central-most region of the genome (Figure 31.2 p. 596). These core genes comprise about 60 percent of the coding capacity of the virus. They are generally required for virus growth and are thus associated with essential virus functions such as transcription and DNA replication. On the other hand, the 'variable regions,' comprising the remainder of the genome extending to both termini, contain genes many of which are not essential for growth, including those devoted to control of host range as well as the responses of the cell or animal host to infection. While entomopoxviruses also contain most genes of the common

Table 31.1 *Family* Poxviridae *taxonomy*

Subfamilies	Genera	Member viruses	Features
Chordopoxvirinae	Orthopoxvirus	Camelpox,[c] cowpox,[c] ectromelia,[c] MPXV,[c] raccoonpox, skunkpox, Uasin Gishu,[a] vaccinia,[b,c] variola,[c] volepox	Brick-shaped virion, DNA ca. 200 kbp, G+C ca. 36%, wide to narrow host range, variola (smallpox), vaccinia (smallpox vaccine)
	Parapoxvirus	Auzduk disease,[a] chamois contagious ecthyma,[a] orf,[b] pseudocowpox, parapox of deer, sealpox[a]	Ovoid virion, DNA ca. 140 kbp, G+C ca. 64%
	Avipoxvirus	Canarypox, fowlpox,[b,c] juncopox, mynahpox, pigeonpox, psittacinepox, quailpox, peacockpox,[a] penguinpox,[a] sparrowpox, starlingpox, turkeypox	Brick-shaped virion, DNA ca. 260 kbp, G+C ca. 35%, birds, arthropod transmission
	Capripoxvirus	Goatpox, lumpy skin disease, sheeppox[b]	Brick-shaped virion, DNA ca. 150 kbp, ungulates, arthropod transmission
	Leporipoxvirus	Hare fibroma, myxoma,[b,c] rabbit fibroma,[c] squirrel fibroma	Brick-shaped virion, DNA ca. 160 kbp, G+C ca. 40%, leoporids and squirrels
	Suipoxvirus	Swinepox[c]	Brick-shaped virion, DNA ca. 170 kbp, narrow host range
	Molluscipoxvirus	MOCV	Brick-shaped virion, DNA ca. 180 kbp, G+C ca. 60%, human host, localized tumors, contact spread
	Yatapoxvirus	Tanapox, Yaba monkey tumor[b]	Brick-shaped virion, DNA ca. 145 kbp, G+C ca. 33%, primates and ? rodents
Entomopoxvirinae	Entomopoxvirus A	Melontha melontha[b]	Ovoid virion, DNA ca. 260–370 kbp, Coleoptera
	Entomopoxvirus B	Amsacta moorei[b,c]	Ovoid, DNA ca. 236 kbp, G+C ca. 18%, Lepidoptera and Orthoptera
	Entomopoxvirus C	Chrionimus luridus[b]	Brick-shaped virion, DNA ca. 250–380 kbp, Diptera
	Unclassified	Melanoplus sanguinipes[c]	

a) Probable member of genus.
b) Prototypal member.
c) Completely sequenced.

vertebrate poxvirus core, the genes are not conserved in the typical co-linear vertebrate virus core fashion, but rather are dispersed throughout the genome. The significance, if any, of the altered organization pattern in entomopoxviruses is not clear.

In the case of vertebrate viruses, while the diseases caused by individual viruses can vary greatly, the molecular events which govern basic functions such as transcription, DNA synthesis, and morphogenesis are quite similar. What distinguishes individual viruses physiologically, and is likely responsible at least in part for the distinct clinical syndromes, are the genes associated with host range and the different sets of immunomodulatory genes, found mainly in the variable regions of the genome. Much of what we know about *orthopoxvirus* genes of this nature has been derived from studies with Vaccinia virus. We will discuss some of these host range and immunomodulatory genes later in this chapter.

Some comment on the poxvirus gene nomenclature used for this chapter is in order. The first poxvirus genome to be sequenced in its entirety was vaccinia Copenhagen (Goebel et al. 1990). The open reading frame (ORF) designations adopted for the Copenhagen sequence were based on the *Hin*dIII restriction map of the genome and the direction of transcription. For example, the viral DNA topoisomerase was designated as H6R, the sixth ORF from the left end of the *Hin*dIII H DNA fragment, transcribed in a rightward direction. Because it was the first complete vaccinia sequence available, the Copenhagen nomenclature became the standard in the field. However, the vaccinia strain WR has been the de facto strain used for experimentation for more than 30 years, even though the complete WR genome sequence only recently became available. Recent nomenclature rules adopted by the International Committee on Taxonomy of Viruses (ICTV) and applied to the more recently sequenced poxvirus genomes uses a linear designation beginning at the left-hand end of the genome and continuing to the right end of the genome. Using the newer nomenclature, the WR ortholog of the vaccinia Copenhagen *H6R* gene is

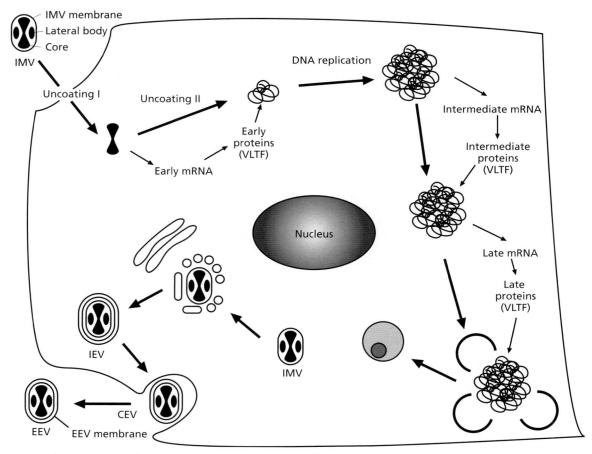

Figure 31.1 *The poxvirus growth cycle. Features of growth shared by all poxviruses include a temporal pattern of gene expression, a cytoplasmic site of development. Orthopoxviruses, such as variola virus and vaccinia virus, produce two distinct forms of virions. Initially, IMV is the first infectious virus formed. A small portion of that virus is wrapped within two additional layers of Golgi-derived membranes to form IEV. IEV is externalized by fusion of the outermost membrane of IEV with the plasma membrane of the cell to form CEV. CEV released from the cell surface produces free EEV. CEV, cell-associated enveloped virus; EEV, extracellular enveloped virus; IEV, intracellular enveloped virus; IMV, intracellular mature virus; VETF, viral early transcription factors; VITF, viral intermediate transcription factors; VLTF, viral late transcription factors.*

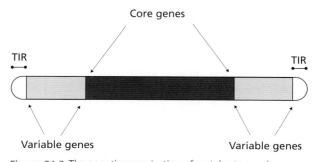

Figure 31.2 *The genetic organization of vertebrate poxviruses. The poxvirus is comprised of double-stranded DNA but is variable, ranging from 130 to 330 kb in individual viruses. The central-most region of the viral chromosome contains a generally conserved linear core of genes, most of which are shared by all vertebrate poxviruses. Genes within the regions to the left and right of the core gene region are the most variable and serve to distinguish the individual members of the family. Genes within this region tend to be virus-specific. The termini of the genome are highlighted by imperfectly paired TIRs. The two DNA strands are linked, resistant to exonuclease digestion, and thus form a loop or hairpin.*

designated as *VACV-WR_104*. So while acknowledging the history of the field and the use of Copenhagen nomenclature in much of the literature to date, yet mindful that vaccinia WR is the prototypic vaccinia strain and that nomenclature procedures have been changed, we have designated ORFs by both the original Copenhagen and the newer vaccinia WR designations where possible.

Virions and virion structure

The poxvirus virion structure is both unique and unconventional compared to other viruses. In general, poxvirus virions bear none of the classical features of a helical or icosahedral nucleocapsid, and while they are enveloped, the structure and biogenesis of the envelope is unusual.

Mature poxvirus virions exist in four forms which differ in the number of membranes and hence surface antigens surrounding the particle (reviewed by Smith et al. 2002). The four forms are designated intracellular mature virus (IMV), intracellular enveloped virus (IEV), cell-associated enveloped virus (CEV), and extracellular enveloped virus (EEV) (Figures 31.1 and 31.11). IMV, the first assembled and simplest infectious form of virus, is a membraned particle that, as the name implies, remains inside cells following virus maturation (Boulter and Appleyard 1973). IEV is an intermediate in the formation of CEV and EEV, these latter two being infectious extracellular forms of virus. IEV is essentially IMV that has acquired two additional membranes via wrapping in Golgi-derived cisternae (Ichihashi et al. 1971). CEV is derived from IEV by fusion of the outermost IEV membrane with the plasma membrane (Blasco and Moss 1992). CEV is thus essentially an IMV particle that is wrapped in one additional lipid bilayer and that remains attached to the outer surface of the cell. EEV is CEV that has been released from the surface of the cell (Boulter and Appleyard 1973). IEV contains an additional seven membrane proteins not found in IMV, while CEV and EEV each contain five of these seven proteins (Smith et al. 2002). Although it is a membraned particle, IMV is extraordinarily stable, and therefore presumably provides the virus with a mechanism for maintaining infectivity in the environment between hosts over long periods of time. EEV and CEV are thought to be critical for cell-to-cell spread during infection. Thus, collectively, the multiple forms of poxviruses encompass all of the advantages of both enveloped and non-enveloped viruses.

EEV is experimentally distinguished from IMV based on antigenic differences due to the presence of different surface components, and by the fact that the extra lipid envelope confers a lighter buoyant density to the EEV particle compared to IMV (reviewed by Smith et al. 2002). The distinction between the various forms of virus is also clinically significant. It has been proposed that prevention of disease caused by orthopoxviruses is primarily related to EEV particles rather than IMV. For example, during the smallpox eradication program, some vaccines were prepared from inactivated virus obtained following disruption of infected cells (IMV). These vaccines were largely ineffective in preventing orthopoxvirus infections in humans (Kaplan 1962; Kaplan et al. 1962, 1965). Indeed, the relative efficacy of anti-IMV and EEV antisera to prevent spread of the IMV-induced infections in animals has clearly shown that anti-EEV antibodies are of much greater benefit even when there is a subsequent virus challenge (Boulter et al. 1971; Boulter and Appleyard 1973). Although EEV production is typically low compared to IMV, there are two experimental methods by which to assay and verify the presence of EEV. The first is the test for 'comets' (Law et al. 2002) where strains that produce high levels of EEV, such as vaccinia strain IHD (International Health Division) or rabbitpox virus (RPV), are allowed to grow on cell monolayers in the absence of the typical agar overlay. Such strains will generate 'comet-shaped' rather than spherical plaques, resulting from

release of EEV from the primary plaque and spread of the infection to distant sites on the monolayer. Comets are inhibited by antisera to EEV but not IMV. The second method represents a modified neutralization assay in which EEV is pretreated with antibody against inactivated IMV. EEV escapes neutralization by this antibody and will produce a plaque when titered.

The structure of intact IMV, the simplest and predominant form of the virus, has been extensively studied by electron microscopy (EM). Analysis of whole virions by cryo-electron microscopy, which is thought to preserve best the natural surface features of the virion, reveals a rectangular structure with dimensions of 350×270 nm, including a 30 nm thick 'surface domain' which is less electron dense relative to the inner domain of the particle (Figure 31.3) (Dubochet et al. 1994; Griffiths et al. 2001b). By contrast, conventional EM of negatively stained, dehydrated samples of purified IMV reveal numerous rodlike protrusions, called surface tubule elements (STE), on or near the surface of the virion (Figure 31.3) (Wilton et al. 1995). Cross-sections of IMV reveal four distinct virion substructures: the envelope, the lateral bodies, the core wall, and the core (Figure 31.3) (Dales and Pogo 1981; Ichihashi et al. 1984; Griffiths et al. 2001a, 2001b). In many sections, the core and its wall possess a biconcave dumbbell or peanut shape; however, in many sections the core appears round, rectangular, or even somewhat irregularly shaped, ultimately suggesting a three-dimensional structure similar to an elongated biconcave disk. The core wall is a bilaminar structure, with an inner smooth layer approximately 5 nm thick and an outer layer, sometimes referred to as the 'palisade layer,' made up of regularly arranged projections approximately 10 nm in length and 5 nm in diameter (Easterbrook 1966). The lateral bodies are uniform in electron density and fill the space between the concavities in the core and the envelope. The envelope, which contains the lipid outer membrane, is also a bilaminar structure, with an inner layer approximately 5 nm thick and an outer layer approximately 9 nm thick (Hollinshead et al. 1999).

IMV substructure

The precise biochemical make-up of the poxvirus virion has been investigated by controlled degradation of purified virions coupled with deductions made from studies of virus assembly. Virions contain as many as 100 proteins, most, if not all, of which are virus coded (Essani and Dales 1979; Jensen et al. 1996). The precise substructure of the virion envelope is controversial: while some studies conclude that the envelope contains a single lipid bilayer, others conclude that it contains two tightly apposed bilayers (Hollinshead et al. 1999; Sodeik and Krijnse-Locker 2002) (see section on Poxvirus morphogenesis: IV and IMV membrane formation, below).

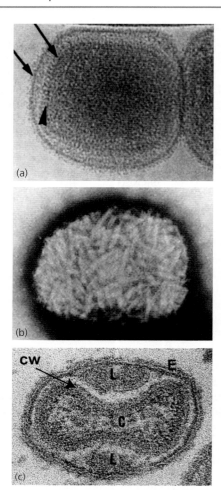

Figure 31.3 *Vaccinia virion structure.* **(a)** *Cryo-election microscopy of positively stained isolated particles. Two layers are evident (arrows) that are separated by a spike or spicule layer (arrowhead).* **(b)** *Negatively stained isolated particles showing surface tubule elements.* **(c)** *Thin section of a vaccinia virion showing envelope (E), lateral bodies (L), and the core (C) surrounded by the core wall (CW).* **(a)** *is reproduced from Griffiths et al. 2001b;* **(b)** *from Wilton et al. 1995;* **(c)** *from Pogo and Dales 1969.*

Treatment of virus with neutral detergent and a reducing agent solubilizes the envelope and as many as a dozen envelope-associated proteins (Easterbrook 1966; Ichihashi et al. 1984; Jensen et al. 1996). Under appropriate conditions, some of these solubilized proteins are contained in tubular structures which may be equivalent to the STEs seen in dehydrated, negatively stained intact IMV (Wilton et al. 1995). Several of the IMV envelope proteins exist in a disulfide-bonded complex (Rodriguez et al. 1997). Upon solubilization of the outer envelope, the virion core, which now assumes a more rectangular or brick-shaped structure, can be isolated with the lateral bodies still attached (Easterbrook 1966). The lateral bodies can be removed with controlled trypsin treatment and therefore are proteinaceous in nature. The exact chemical composition of the core wall is unclear. While some investigators contend that the core wall contains a

true lipid bilayer (or two tightly apposed bilayers), others argue that it contains no lipid (Wilton et al. 1995; Griffiths et al. 2001b). At least one of the major virion structural proteins, 4b, localizes to the outer surface of the core wall (Ichihashi et al. 1984; Wilton et al. 1995). Within the core resides the viral DNA complexed with several virus-coded DNA-binding proteins (Ichihashi et al. 1984).

Because poxviruses initiate infection and thereafter express information from a DNA molecule in the cell cytoplasm, the virions contain the full complement of enzymes required for synthesis of early viral mRNA. Virion cores are thus a rich source of the viral enzymes necessary for viral transcription and modification (Kates and McAuslan 1967; Kates and Beeson 1970a; Shuman and Moss 1990) (Table 31.2). The subviral core is capable of synthesizing authentic early viral mRNAs in vitro which are capped, methylated, and polyadenylated (Kates and Beeson 1970b; Wei and Moss 1975; Bossart et al. 1978; Pelham et al. 1978). The enzymology of viral mRNA metabolism is discussed in detail below (see section on Poxvirus transcription and regulation of viral gene expression). The precise localization and organization of viral enzymes within the core is not known. Presumably, as the virus particle transverses the cellular membrane during the entry process, partial uncoating of the intact IMV must occur, thereby creating the transcriptionally active core (Pedersen et al. 2000).

In addition to the enzymes and factors listed in Table 31.2, which have an obvious direct role in RNA metabolism, the virion contains other enzymes with activities suggesting roles in nucleic acid or protein modification (Table 31.3). These include a topoisomerase (H6R/VACV-WR_104), an RNA helicase (I8R/VACV-WR_077), two protein kinases (F10L/VACV-WR_049 and B1R/VACV-WR_183), a protein phosphatase (H1L/VACV-WR_099), a glutaredoxin (O2L/VACV-WR_069), and three thiol oxidoreductases (G4L/VACV-COP_099, E10R/VACV-COP_082, and A2.5L/VACV-WR_121). Mutants in the RNA helicase are defective in the virus core-directed in vitro transcription reaction in a fashion which suggests that the RNA helicase may play a role in transporting newly synthesized early viral mRNA out of the core particle (Gross and Shuman 1996). For reasons unknown, mutants in the H1L phosphatase are also defective in early viral transcription (Liu et al. 1995). The F10L protein kinase seems to play a role in regulation of virion morphogenesis via phosphorylation, discussed in more detail below (see section on Poxvirus morphogenesis: IV and IMV membrane formation) (Traktman et al. 1995). The B1R kinase plays an essential role in viral DNA replication, discussed in more detail below (see section on The structure and replication of poxvirus DNA: The enzymology of DNA replication) (Rempel and Traktman 1992). While the O2L glutaredoxin is nonessential, the G4L, E10R, and A2.5L thiol reductases form a complex which comprises a complete disulfide-bonding pathway which targets at least two other vaccinia

Table 31.2 *Virus-coded mRNA metabolism enzymes and factors*

Function/Enzyme or factor[a]/Encoding gene(s) (common/Copenhagen/WR)[b]	Mol mass (kDa)	Virion[c]	Homologies; alternate functions	Reference[d]
RNA polymerization				
RNA polymerase				
RPO 147/J6R/VACV-WR_098	147	Yes	Homology to eucaryotic RNA polymerase	Broyles and Moss 1986
RPO 132/A24R/VACV-WR_144	133	Yes	Homology to eukaryotic RNA polymerase	Amegadzie et al. 1991b
RAP 94/H4L/VACV-WR_102	94	Yes	Early promoter specificity; early termination	Ahn et al. 1994
RPO 35/A29L/VACV-WR_152	35	Yes		Amegadzie et al. 1991a
RPO 30/E4L/VACV-WR_060	30	Yes	TFIIS homology; VITF-1	Ahn et al. 1990a
RPO 22/J4R/VACV-WR_096	21	Yes		Broyles and Moss 1986
RPO 19/A5R/VACV-WR_124	19	Yes		Ahn et al. 1992
RPO 18/D7R/VACV-WR_112	18	Yes		Ahn et al. 1990b
RPO 7/G5.5R/VACV-WR_083	7	Yes	Homology to eukaryotic RNA polymerase	Amegadzie et al. 1992
mRNA capping				
Capping enzyme				
DIR/VACV-WR_106	97	Yes	Early termination, intermediate transcription	Morgan et al. 1984
D12L/VACV-WR_117	33	Yes	Early termination, intermediate transcription	Niles et al. 1989
(Nucleoside-2′-O-)-methyltransferase				
VP39/J3R/VACV-WR_095	39	Yes	Poly(A) polymerase subunit; intermediate/late elongation	Schnierle et al. 1992
mRNA polyadenylation				
Poly(A) polymerase				
VP55/VACV-WR_057	55	Yes		Gershon et al. 1991
VP39/J3R/VACV-WR_095	39	Yes	mRNA cap methylation; intermediate/late elongation	Gershon et al. 1991
Early transcription factors				
VETF				
A7L/VACV-WR_126	82	Yes		Gershon and Moss 1990
D6R/VACV-WR_111	73	Yes		Gershon and Moss 1990
Early termination factors				
VTF				
D1R/VACV-WR_106	97	Yes	mRNA capping, intermediate transcription	Shuman et al. 1987
D12L/VACV-WR_117	33	Yes	mRNA capping, intermediate transcription	Shuman et al. 1987
Nucleoside phosphohydrolase I				
D11L/VACV-WR_116	72	Yes		Deng and Shuman 1998

(Continued over)

Table 31.2 *Virus-coded mRNA metabolism enzymes and factors (Continued)*

Function/Enzyme or factor[a]/Encoding gene(s) (common/Copenhagen/WR)[b]	Mol mass (kDa)	Virion[c]	Homologies; alternate functions	Reference[d]
H4L				
RAP 94/H4L/VACV-WR_102	94	Yes	RNA polymerase subunit; early promoter specificity	Mohamed and Niles 2001
Intermediate transcription factors				
Capping enzyme				
D1R/ VACV-WR_106	97	Yes	Early termination, mRNA capping	Vos et al. 1991
D12L/ VACV-WR_117	33	Yes	Early termination, mRNA capping	Vos et al. 1991
VITF-1				
RPO 30/E4L/VACV-WR_060	30	Yes	RNA polymerase subunit; TFIIS homology	Rosales et al. 1994a
VITF-3				
A23R/VACV-WR_143	44	No		Sanz and Moss 1999
A8R/VACV-WR_127	33	No		Sanz and Moss 1999
Late transcription factors				
VLTF-1				
G8R/VACV-WR_086	30	No		Keck et al. 1990
VLTF-2				
A1L/VACV-WR_119	17	No		Keck et al. 1990
VLTF-3				
A2L/VACV-WR_120	26	No		Keck et al. 1990
VLTF-4				
H5R/VACV-WR_103	22	No		
Intermediate/late elongation factors				
Negative elongation/RNA release factor				
A18R/VACV-WR_138	57	Yes		Lackner and Condit 2000
Positive elongation factor				
G2R/VACV-WR_080	26	No		Black and Condit 1996
VP39/J3R/VACV-WR_095	39	Yes	mRNA cap methylation; poly(A) polymerase	Latner et al. 2000

a) Multiple genes indented under a single enzyme/factor designates a multisubunit enzyme/factor.
b) See text for description of nomenclature. Many genes do not have a 'common' name, thus only the Copenhagen and WR designations are used.
c) Designates whether or not the gene product is packaged in virions.
d) A single reference is given that identifies the gene or assigns an alternative function. See text for additional references.

structural proteins and is essential for successful virion morphogenesis (Senkevich et al. 2002). While the biochemistry of the topoisomerase is understood in exquisite detail, the role of this enzyme in poxvirus replication is not known because no virus mutants in the *H6R* gene have been isolated (Tian et al. 2003).

THE STRUCTURE AND REPLICATION OF POXVIRUS DNA

The structure of poxvirus DNA

There are several observations and structural features relevant to poxvirus DNA replication which must be considered within the context of replication. First is the rather unusual structure of the viral DNA, which is comprised of linear double-stranded DNA, terminating in inverted repeats linked through an imperfectly paired DNA 'loop' or 'hairpin' (Figures 31.2 and 31.4a). Second, during the process of replication, concatemeric intermediates are formed, necessitating the need to excise functional monomeric molecules as well as to recreate the terminal hairpins or loops at the end of the genome. Third, consistent with the cytoplasmic nature of these viruses, DNA replication does not occur within the nucleus, which demands that the virus encode a variety of replicative enzymes whose cellular equivalents are confined to the nucleus.

Table 31.3 *Vaccinia virion enzymes[a]*

Function/Enzyme or factor[b]/Encoding gene(s) (common/Copenhagen/WR)[c]	Mol. mass (kDa)	Comment	Reference[d]
Protein modification			
F10L ser/thr kinase *F10L/VACV-WR_049*	52	Required for virion morphogenesis	Traktman et al. 1995
B1R ser/thr kinase *B1R/VACV-WR_183*	34	Required for DNA replication	Rempel and Traktman 1992
Tyr/Ser protein phosphatase *VH1/H1L/VACV-WR_099*	20	Required for early transcription	Guan et al. 1991
Thiol oxidoreductase *E10R/VACV-COP_082*	11	Required for virion morphogenesis	Senkevich et al. 2002
G4L/VACV-COP_099	14	Required for virion morphogenesis	Senkevich et al. 2002
A2.5L/VACV-WR_121	9	Required for virion morphogenesis	Senkevich et al. 2002
Glutaredoxin *O2L/VACV-WR_069*	12	Non-essential	Rajagopal et al. 1995
Nucleic acid topology			
Topoisomerase *H6R/VACV-WR_104*	37	Function unknown	Cheng et al. 1998
RNA helicase *I8R/VACV-WR_077*	78	Required for early transcription	Gross and Shuman 1996

a) Enzymes in this table are those that have not been shown to play a direct role in transcription. See Table 31.2 for virion transcription enzymes.
b) Multiple genes indented under a single enzyme/factor designates a multisubunit enzyme/factor.
c) See text for description of nomenclature. Many genes do not have a 'common' name; thus only the Copenhagen and WR designations are used.
d) A single reference is given which identifies the gene or assigns a function. See text for additional references.

The terminal most region of DNA comprising the hairpin or loop abuts a series of tandem repeats of various sizes (Figure 31.4b). The DNA within the hairpin or loop per se that 'caps' the larger terminal inverted sequence region (TIR) serves to link the two complementary strands and creates a telomere comprised of an imperfectly paired A+T-rich region of DNA (Figure 31.4b, c). The hairpins exist in two forms, sometimes call 'flip' and 'flop,' which are perfect inverse complements of each other, such that when base paired with each other they form a perfect duplex (Figure 31.4c, d). The duplexed flip and flop hairpins form the junction between concatemers (Figure 31.4d), and have important implications in the mechanism of DNA replication described below. Following and next to each terminal hairpin, the TIRs present at both the left and right extremes of the molecule continue inward. The total length of TIRs can vary from as little as 58 bp in variola virus (Shchelkunov et al. 1995) to more than 12 kb in Shope fibroma virus, a *Leporipoxvirus* (Willer et al. 1999). Indeed, there is at least one example where the TIRs have been shown to exhibit marked variation in size and sequence (up to 30 kb) from different plaque isolates of one virus (Figure 31.5) (Moyer and Graves 1981). A possible mechanism for the generation of variable TIRs is discussed later in the chapter. Because the TIR sequences are by definition repeated at both termini of the genome,

ORFs contained within the TIRs are diploid. The sequences at the very left or right extremes of the TIRs nearest the hairpin which contain the series of small tandem, conserved repeats also contain a sequence which serves as a 'nicking site' to initiate the DNA replication process. This nicking site may also be involved in the maturation of mature length molecules from replicative DNA concatemeric intermediates (Moyer and Graves 1981). Viral DNA concatemers are not only a key feature and intermediate in poxvirus genome replication but they also allow for rapid evolution, adaptation, and diversity at the terminal extremes of the molecule which in turn constitute the primary genetic distinctions among individual poxviruses.

Several additional features of the general organization of individual poxvirus genes are noteworthy. All genes are uninterrupted, linear, and without introns. Generally, there is little overlap between individual genes. While transcription of genes can occur in either direction, genes at the termini of the viral chromosome tend to be transcribed predominantly towards the end of the chromosome.

The mechanism of DNA replication

DNA replication not only serves to provide DNA for progeny virus but also provides a functional template for the temporal expression of intermediate and late

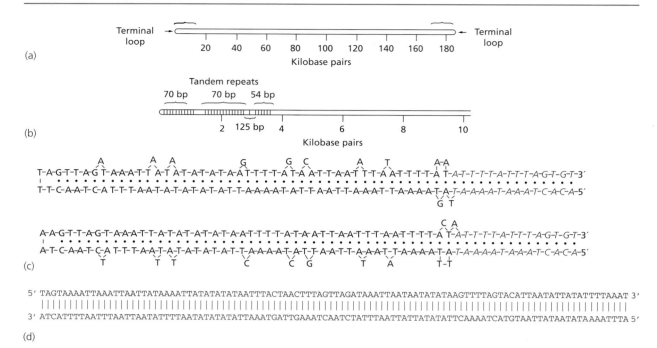

Figure 31.4 *Structural features of the vaccinia virus genome. From the top down is shown:* **(a)** *a unit length genome emphasizing size, inverted terminal repetition, and hairpin (terminal) loops;* **(b)** *an enlargement of the inverted terminal repeat, emphasizing the tandem repeats within the terminal repeat;* **(c)** *the two hairpin loops (non-italic font) as they are joined to the terminal repeats (italic font);* **(d)** *the duplex structure formed at a concatemer junction, consisting of the unfolded hairpins base paired to each other. (Modified from Moss 2001)*

viral genes. Synthesis of DNA occurs within the cytoplasm and is readily visualized by electron microscopy as electron-dense bodies or 'factories' which serve as the site of initiation for the assembly of mature virions. The mechanism of DNA synthesis takes into consideration the following features of viral DNA already discussed: the TIRs, the terminal DNA hairpin loops, and the generation of replicative concatemeric DNA.

The onset of replication is heralded by introduction of a nick within one or both inverted terminal repeats (ITR), most likely within 200 bp of the end of the molecule (Du and Traktman 1996). The nicking can occur at either or both termini, but for simplicity is only shown at one end (Figure 31.6). Strand extension at the 3′ terminus of the nick with concomitant strand displacement allows the terminal nucleotides to be copied. Hybridization of the newly synthesized terminal-most nucleotides to the parental strand leads to formation of flip and flop hairpins (Figure 31.4c; Baroudy et al. 1982). Thereafter polymerization continues, eventually giving rise to concatemers comprising complete genomic units of fused head-to-head or tail-to-tail genome length monomers (Moyer and Graves 1981). Additional complexity can be conferred to replicating DNA through either strand invasion by other molecules, by initiating a second replication cycle on molecules actively replicating or through recombination. There are a number of biochemical studies consistent with the proposed mechanism.

Concatemeric DNA must be resolved and unit length genomes excised in order to assemble mature virus. A graphic illustration of a possible mechanism for this process is shown in Figure 31.7, p. 605, in which resolution is initiated by a sequence-specific nick. The detailed requirements for concatemer resolution include a small recognition cleavage sequence (Delange et al. 1986; Merchlinsky and Moss 1986, 1989) present as an inverted repeat on both sides of the fused RR or LL hairpin loop contained within the L–RR–LL–R head-to-head or tail-to-tail concatemers that results from the replication process. It has been proposed that resolution may also occur via site-specific recombination and oriented branch migration (Merchlinsky 1990), or by nicking and sealing of extruded cruciform, holiday-like structures (McFadden et al. 2003).

It is possible for concatemers to exist as large cruciform structures and deletions can readily occur within such structures. During genome maturation, such deletion events allow for expansion and contraction of the terminal regions of the chromosome and creation of TIRs of varying length as described (Figure 31.8, p. 606). The terminal variability is theoretically limited only by the need to retain the essential genes in or at the conserved core and the *cis*-sequences required for replication (Moyer et al. 1980; Moyer and Graves 1981) and provides a mechanism for rapid evolution of genes within this region. The documented ability of terminal regions of the virus to expand and contract implies that

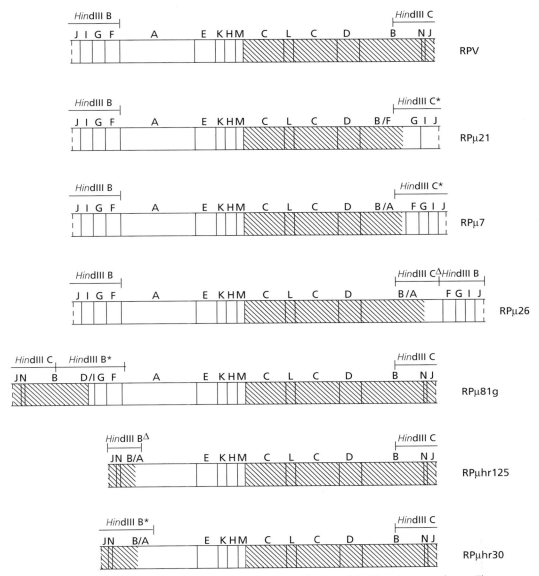

Figure 31.5 *Variation in size of poxvirus terminal repeats. The XhoI maps of RPV and six TIR variants are shown. The genome of RPV and all variants are sized to scale. Genome sizes are drawn to scale. The right and left halves of the parental RPV genome are distinguished by shading. The mutants RPμ21, RPμ7, and RPμ26 have expanded terminal repeats derived from the left region of wild-type RPV. The TIRs of RPμ26 are sufficiently large to contain many functional genes. The mutants RPμ81g, RPμhr125, and RPμhr30 likewise have expanded terminal repeats compared to wild-type RPV (from Moyer and Graves 1981). The generation of expanded TIRs through duplication and transposition of either left or right regions of the genome is likely a consequence of replication (see text).*

the amount of DNA packaged within a virion is not fixed and is determined by the location of the concatemer resolution sequences rather than the amount of DNA within a given chromosome. Indeed, it has been shown the amount of DNA packaged can be far larger than the minimum genome normally associated with a given virus and the entire bacteriophage lambda chromosome can be stably maintained within vaccinia virus (Smith and Moss 1983). This genomic plasticity has been exploited in the creation of a wide variety of recombinant poxviruses with large inserts of foreign DNA for a variety of applications.

The enzymology of DNA replication

Although poxviruses encode many enzymes associated with aspects of DNA synthesis, those that are conserved among many members are likely to constitute the 'basic' or core replication machinery (Table 31.4, p. 607). A subset of these conserved proteins, have been shown through the study of mutants, to exhibit defects in DNA synthesis (Table 31.4, top). The role of other conserved genes is in post-synthetic steps of DNA maturation or is unknown. The subset of proteins known to be involved in DNA synthesis include a DNA polymerase (ORF

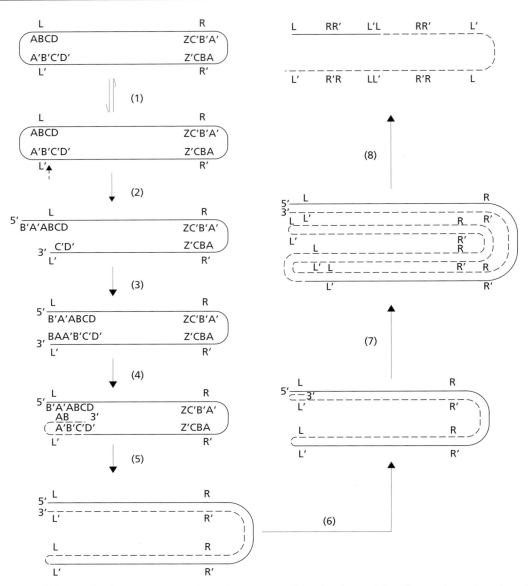

Figure 31.6 *The replication of Orthopoxvirus DNA. The viral genome is indicated at the top left with 'L' and 'R' orientation of the molecule as indicated. Replication begins with introduction of a nick near one or both termini of the genome (indicated schematically by arrow between B' and C') followed by strand extension. Parental DNA is indicated by solid lines, newly synthesized DNA by dashed lines. Following strand extension, self-primed replication creates a new hairpin, replication of the genome, and creation of a concatemeric genomic dimer. See text for details. (From Moyer and Graves 1981)*

E9L,VACWR 065) (McDonald and Traktman 1994), a uracil DNA glycosylase (ORF D4R, VACWR 109) (Stuart et al. 1993; Upton et al. 1993; Millns et al. 1994), a serine/threonine protein kinase (ORF B1R, VACWR 183) (Banham and Smith 1992), an NTPase (ORF D5R, VACWR 110), (Evans and Traktman 1992; Evans et al. 1995), and ORF A20, VACWR 141, a processivity factor (Ishii and Moss 2001a); (Punjabi et al. 2001) which acts in concert with the E9L DNA polymerase. The single known exception to the universal conservation of these proteins is B1R, which is absent from MCV. Inactivation of any of these proteins leads to a DNA negative phenotype and is lethal to the virus.

The DNA polymerase is a 110 kDa protein with a 3'-exonuclease proofreading activity and is a target of several antiviral drugs such as aphidicolin (DeFilippes 1984), cytosine arabinoside, and phosphonoacetic acid (Traktman et al. 1989; Taddie and Traktman 1993). Recently, A20R has been shown to function as a processivity factor for the DNA polymerase and to interact with the D4R and D5R proteins as well (McCraith et al. 2000; Ishii and Moss 2001a; Klemperer et al. 2001; Punjabi et al. 2001; Ishii and Moss 2002). Temperature-sensitive mutants in either protein lead to rapid inhibition of DNA synthesis (Sridhar and Condit 1983; Punjabi et al. 2001).

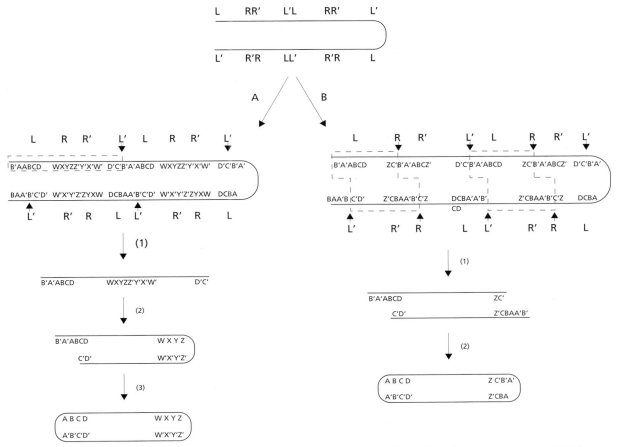

Figure 31.7 *Generation of mature poxvirus virion DNA from replicative concatamers. Generation of monomeric genomic DNA is initiated by single-stranded nicking (B'C') as indicated by the arrow. Genomic DNA can be derived either in a cis (left) or trans (right) fashion from the concatemer as indicated by the red boxes. The designations L and R serve to orient the left and right termini of the molecules and where L' and R' are sequences complementary to those of L and R, respectively. (From Moyer and Graves 1981)*

The uracil DNA glycosylase is a small 25 kDa protein and in most systems typically functions as a repair enzyme, excising from DNA uracil residues which arise from misincorporation of dUMP by the DNA polymerase or by deamination of cytosine. The ultimate result of this activity is to leave a gap that is filled by the DNA polymerase. Therefore, the discovery that this protein is absolutely required for the replication of poxvirus DNA (Stuart et al. 1993; Millns et al. 1994; Ellison et al. 1996) was somewhat surprising. Recently, the conserved reactive site of the glycosylase was mutated, eliminating the enzymatic activity which excises uracil from DNA, yet the protein could still function in the process of DNA replication (De Silva and Moss, 2003). Therefore, while the D4R protein is required for DNA replication, the uracil DNA glycosylase activity per se is not. Interestingly, virus containing the enzymatically inactive glycosylase gene, while normal for DNA replication, is attenuated when the virus was used to infect mice.

The NTPase is a 785 amino acid protein which exhibits DNA-independent hydrolysis of both ribo- and deoxy-NTPs. Temperature-sensitive mutants in the protein exhibit a 'fast stop' inhibition of DNA synthesis at nonpermissive temperatures (Evans et al. 1995) as well as being impaired in homologous recombination (Evans and Traktman 1992). As might be expected at nonpermissive temperatures, intermediate and late gene expression is severely affected (Diaz-Guerra and Esteban 1993).

The B1R serine/threonine protein kinase is a 34 kDa protein. When a virus containing thermosensitive mutations in this gene are incubated at nonpermissive temperatures, DNA synthesis ceases. This protein is expressed early in infection but is packaged into mature virions (Banham and Smith 1992; Lin et al. 1992; Rempel and Traktman 1992). One substrate of the B1R kinase is the *H5R* gene (Beaud et al. 1995), which also forms a complex with B1R (McCraith et al. 2000). However, the role of the H5R phosphoprotein is complex and appears to be involved both in the transcription of late viral genes (Kovacs and Moss 1996) as well as morphogenesis (Demasi and Traktman 2000).

The *A50R/VACV-WR_176* gene, encodes a 63 kDa DNA ligase (Kerr and Smith 1991; Parks et al. 1994,

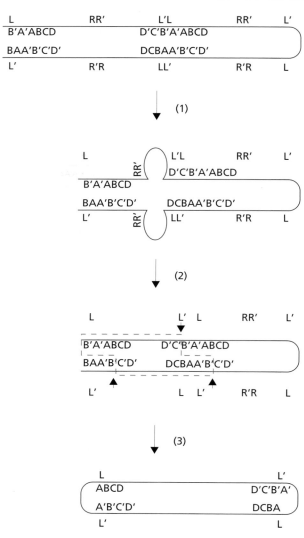

Figure 31.8 *Mechanism for expansion and contraction of TIR regions. A replicative, concatemeric DNA intermediate is shown. Deletion from within the array (step 1) followed by molecular excision is governed by the hypothetical concatemeric resolution signal (B'C') and indicated by the red box. Limits of the deletion are theoretical determined by viability of the deleted genomic molecule. In the example shown, the TIR is expanded by addition of sequences from the left end of wild-type molecule. (From Moyer and Graves 1981)*

1998). Disruptions of the DNA ligase lead to a cell-line-dependent phenotype. In some cell lines, there is poor growth of virus accompanied by a two- to tenfold decrease in DNA synthesis. In other cell lines, there is little if any effect (Parks et al. 1998). This difference may be due to the levels of available host DNA ligase present in the cytoplasm.

A number of the other conserved proteins are assumed to be required for later steps in the replicative process but direct genetic evidence is lacking for most of them. Mutations in these genes would be predicted to not lead to defects in DNA synthesis per se, but rather

to defects in maturation of the newly synthesized DNA which in turn leads to inhibition of progeny virus formation. The *A22R/VACV-WR_142* gene encodes a resolvase and has been shown by the use of conditional, inducible mutants to be required for resolution of concatemeric DNA into monomers (Garcia et al. 2000; Garcia and Moss 2001).

The function of two of these conserved genes is not yet clear. The *H6R/VACV-WR_104* gene encodes a 314 amino acid type 1 topoisomerase (Shuman and Moss 1987; Shuman et al. 1989), which is the smallest known topoisomerase. Attempts to isolate mutant virus deleted for this gene were unsuccessful, suggesting the gene is essential for growth (Shuman et al. 1989). Furthermore, no conditional lethal mutant has yet been isolated so the precise function of the topoisomerase in virus growth remains to be elucidated. The 34 kDa *I3L/VACV-WR_072* gene encodes a single-stranded DNA-binding protein (Rochester and Traktman 1998; Tseng et al. 1999). The I3L protein has been found localized to virosomes or factories during DNA replication (Rochester and Traktman 1998). When DNA synthesis is blocked, the protein is found in distinct foci within the cytoplasm (Domi and Beaud 2000). It has been suggested that these cytoplasmic spots are specialized sites where DNA release from incoming virus cores accumulates (Welsch et al. 2003). Elucidation of the precise role of both the *H6R* and *I3L* genes in the replicative process awaits isolation of conditional lethal mutants.

Recombination is an essential feature of DNA replication. Indeed, recombination between genetically marked viruses or transfected plasmids and viral DNA is rampant, which in practice facilitates generation of genetically engineered viruses. The processes of recombination and replication are linked and mutations which impair recombination are also impaired in DNA replication (Merchlinsky 1989; Colinas et al. 1990; Evans and Traktman 1992).

Finally, there are a number of poxvirus genes devoted to the purpose of maintaining intracellular nucleotide pools which serve as substrates for DNA synthesis. These enzymes, many of which are not absolutely essential for growth include:

- the 177 amino acid *J2R/VACV-WR_094*) which encodes a thymidine kinase (Hruby and Ball 1982) active as a tetramer (Black and Hruby 1990)
- the *A48R/VACV-WR_178* protein, a 204 amino acid thymidylate kinase (Hughes et al. 1991)
- a 147 amino acid dUTPase, the product of gene *F2L/VACV-WR_041* (Broyles 1993)
- the heterodimeric ribonucleotide reductase comprising the 771 amino acid *I4L/VACV-WR_073* and the 319 amino acid *F4L/VACV-WR_043* subunits (Slabaugh and Mathews 1986; Slabaugh et al. 1988; Tengelsen et al. 1988; Rajagopal et al. 1995).

Table 31.4 *Poxvirus genes involved in DNA replication*

VACCOP ORF	VACWR ORF	Size (aa)	Description
Orthopoxvirus proteins required for DNA synthesis			
A20R	141	49.1 kDa (426)	DNA polymerase processivity factor
B1R	183	34 kDa (300)	Serine/Threonine phosphokinase
D4R	109	25 kDa (218)	Uracil DNA glycosylase
D5R	110	90 kDa (785)	Nucleoside triphosphatase
E9L	065	116 kDa (1 006)	DNA polymerase
Orthopoxvirus proteins required for other aspects of DNA replication			
A22R	142	22 kDa (187)	Holliday junction resolvase
H6R	104	36 kDa (314)	DNA topisomerase
I3L	072	24 kDa (269)	ssDNA-binding protein
A50R	176	63 kDa (552)	DNA ligase
D5R	110	90 kDa (785)	Nucleotide phosphatase

Poxvirus genes involved in DNA replication are divided into two groups: viral genes directly involved in the synthesis of DNA for which genetic evidence (*ts* mutants exist) (top) or those genes involved in replication and/or post-replicative events for which genetic evidence needed to conclude these genes are essential for replication is generally lacking.

POXVIRUS TRANSCRIPTION AND REGULATION OF VIRAL GENE EXPRESSION

Overview

Gene expression during poxvirus infection occurs in a tightly regulated temporal cascade featuring sequential synthesis of early, intermediate, and late gene (the latter two are termed postreplicative) products. The regulation of poxviral gene expression is most dramatically and elegantly revealed in a simple protein metabolic labeling experiment in which infected cells are pulse labeled with a radioactive amino acid at varying times after infection and the proteins synthesized during each pulse are visualized by gel electrophoresis and autoradiography (Figure 31.9). Typically this experiment reveals a rapid shutoff of host protein synthesis within the first 4 hours of infection, a burst of early protein synthesis which peaks at 2 hours post-infection and disappears by 6 hours post-infection, synthesis of intermediate proteins which peaks by 4 hours post-infection and decays thereafter, followed by synthesis of late proteins which peaks by 6 hours post-infection and persists through at least 16 hours of infection. Importantly, viral DNA replication initiates with the peak of early protein synthesis, and is a prerequisite for intermediate and late protein synthesis (Pennington 1974).

Mechanistically, gene expression is regulated at the level of transcription (reviewed by Condit and Niles 2002; Broyles 2003). The early, intermediate, and late gene classes are distinguished by class-specific transcriptional promoters and cognate *trans*-acting factors. In general, each gene class encodes factors required for transcription of the succeeding gene class, resulting in the observed temporal cascade of gene expression (Kovacs et al. 1994). Thus, early mRNAs, transcribed by enzymes packaged within infecting virions, encode intermediate gene transcription factors; intermediate genes encode late gene transcription factors; late genes encode early gene transcription factors which are packaged into virions together with RNA polymerase and other RNA metabolism enzymes for the next round of infection. As noted above, both intermediate and late transcription are coupled to DNA replication, that is, inhibitors of DNA replication prevent synthesis of intermediate and late RNAs (Oda and Joklik 1967; Vos and Stunnenberg 1988; Baldick and Moss 1993). Transcription of intermediate and late genes also requires the synthesis of new RNA polymerase, which is synthesized early during infection (Hooda-Dhingra et al. 1989).

All poxvirus genes apparently contain their own promoters; polycistronic mRNAs with internal ribosome entry sites have not been described, and poxviral mRNAs are not spliced. Regardless of gene class, poxvirus promoters are relatively simple and are contained entirely within approximately 30 nt upstream from the transcription initiation site (Davison and Moss 1989a, 1989b; Baldick et al. 1992). Importantly, several genes have been described which contain compound promoters and are therefore expressed at multiple stages of infection (Wittek et al. 1980; Broyles and Pennington 1990).

As stated previously, because poxviruses replicate in the cytoplasm of infected cells, the virus encodes virtually all of the enzymes required for regulated synthesis and modification of mRNAs suitable for translation in a eukaryotic environment. Thus at least 23 virus genes

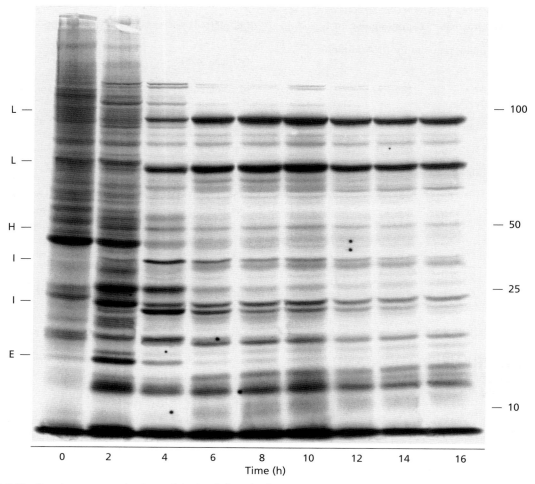

Figure 31.9 *Kinetics of gene expression in vaccinia virus-infected cells. Cells were infected with vaccinia virus at a multiplicity of infection of 10 plaque-forming units/cell, and metabolically pulse labeled with [^{35}S]methionine for 15 minutes at 2-hour intervals following infection. Proteins were separated by SDS-PAGE. An autoradiograph of the dried gel is shown. Each lane on the autoradiogram reveals the proteins that were being synthesized at the time after infection that the radiolabel was present, indicated under each lane. Molecular mass markers are shown at the right of the autoradiogram. At the left is indicated the migration of selected late (L), intermediate (I), and early (E) viral proteins, and a host (H) protein.*

have been described which play a direct role in viral mRNA synthesis and modification (Table 31.2). Interestingly, viral transcription may not be completely independent of the host; a limited number of host proteins have also been identified which may play a role in virus transcription (Rosales et al. 1994b; Broyles et al. 1999; Wright et al. 2001).

In the paragraphs below, we first describe the enzymes and reactions common to synthesis and modification of all classes of poxviral mRNA, and then focus in detail on differences in the expression of each gene class.

RNA polymerase

The virus-encoded RNA polymerase is a multisubunit enzyme which exists in two forms, one specific for early genes and one specific for intermediate and late genes (Table 31.2). The two forms of the enzyme contain eight subunits in common; the only difference between the two forms of the enzyme is that the early gene-specific enzyme contains one additional subunit, RAP94 (H4L/VACV-WR_102) (Nevins and Joklik 1977; Baroudy and Moss 1980; Ahn et al. 1994). Among the eight common subunits, the two largest, RPO147 (J6R/VACV-WR_098) and RPO132 (A24R/VACV-WR_144), share extensive homology with the largest subunits of both eukaryotic and prokaryotic multisubunit RNA polymerases (Broyles and Moss 1986; Patel and Pickup 1989; Amegadzie et al. 1991b). Another subunit, RPO30 (E4L/VACV-WR_060), also shows homology with the eukaryotic transcription elongation factor TFIIS (Ahn et al. 1990a). Interestingly, this subunit also serves as an intermediate gene transcription factor (Rosales et al. 1994a). The smallest vaccinia RNA polymerase subunit, RPO7 (G5.5R/VACV-WR_083), shows homology to the smallest subunit of eukaryotic RNA polymerase II

(Amegadzie et al. 1992). Neither of the remaining four common subunits nor RAP94 show significant homology to other eukaryotic or prokaryotic proteins.

Both forms of the viral RNA polymerase, RAP94+ and RAP94−, are found in virions as well as in the cytoplasm of infected cells. The activities of these enzymes are mutually exclusive, that is, the RAP94+ enzyme transcribes only early viral genes and not postreplicative genes, whereas the RAP94− enzyme transcribes only postreplicative genes and not early genes (Wright and Coroneos 1995). Importantly, this means that the RNA polymerase which transcribes either early or postreplicative genes retains a memory of the class of promoter at which transcription was initiated. This impacts significantly on termination of transcription, which occurs differently on early and postreplicative genes, as described in more detail below.

mRNA capping

All classes of poxviral mRNAs contain a 5′ cap-1 structure, in which the first transcribed nucleotide is modified by addition of a 7-methylguanine in a 5′– 5′ triphosphate linkage, and is also methylated on the 2′-hydroxyl group of the ribose moiety (Wei and Moss 1975). The entire process comprises four reactions carried out by two virus-coded enzymes (Table 31.4). The first three reactions are carried out by the mRNA capping enzyme, a heterodimer composed of the 97 kDa *D1R* gene product (*D1R/VACV-WR_106*) and the 33 kDa *D12L* gene product (*D12L/VACV-WR_117*) (Martin et al. 1975; Morgan et al. 1984; Niles et al. 1989). The capping enzyme first removes the gamma phosphate from a nascent, triphosphorylated mRNA, then adds a GMP in a 5′–5′ linkage, and finally methylates the added guanine in the 7 position to yield a cap-0 structure. The triphosphatase and guanylyltransferase active sites are located on the large D1R subunit of the enzyme, whereas the guanine methyltransferase active site is located on the small, D12L subunit of the enzyme (Shuman and Morham 1990; Higman et al. 1994; Mao and Shuman 1994). Methylation of the ribose on the first transcribed nucleotide requires the cap-0 RNA (guanylylated and methylated on the cap guanine base, but not ribose methylated) as a substrate, and is catalyzed by a monomeric (nucleoside-2′-*O*-)-methyltransferase, the 39 kDa product of the *J3R* gene (*J3R/VACV-WR_095*), to yield a cap-1 structure (Barbosa and Moss 1978a; Barbosa and Moss 1978b; Schnierle et al. 1992). Interestingly, both the capping enzyme and the (nucleoside-2′-*O*-)-methyltransferase are multifunctional enzymes. The D1R/D12L capping enzyme also participates in early gene transcription termination, intermediate gene transcription initiation, and may also play a role in telomere resolution during processing of replicated viral DNA concatemers to monomeric genomes

(Shuman et al. 1987; Carpenter and DeLange 1991; Vos et al. 1991; Hassett et al. 1997). In addition to its role in mRNA capping, the J3R (nucleoside-2′-*O*-)-methyltransferase serves as a stimulatory subunit for the viral poly(A) polymerase, and also as a transcription elongation factor for postreplicative genes (Gershon et al. 1991; Latner et al. 2002). All three genes involved in the capping reactions are essential virus genes; however, the phenotypes of mutants in these genes do not obviously relate to the capping reaction per se. Specifically, temperature-sensitive mutants in either of the mRNA capping enzyme subunit genes (*D1R* or *D12L*) are unaffected in viral gene expression but defective in telomere resolution and morphogenesis (Carpenter and DeLange 1991; Hassett et al. 1997). Formation of the cap-0 structure is presumed to be essential for mRNA stability and translation during virus infection, but this has never been demonstrated in poxviruses directly. The J3R protein is essential only for its transcription elongation function; selective inactivation of the (nucleoside-2′-*O*-)-methyltransferase activity of the J3R protein to produce a virus which synthesizes only cap-0 mRNAs has no apparent effect on virus growth (Latner et al. 2002).

Polyadenylation

All classes of poxviral mRNAs are polyadenylated by a virus-coded heterodimeric enzyme consisting of the 55 kDa *E1L* gene product (*E1L/VACV-WR_057*) and the 39 kDa *J3R* gene product (*J3R/VACV-WR_095*) (reviewed by Gershon 1998) (Table 31.2). The catalytic site for polyadenylation resides in the E1L protein; however, the E1L protein on its own can processively add only approximately 35 adenylate residues to an RNA 3′ end (Gershon and Moss 1992). In the presence of the J3R subunit, full length poly(A) tails averaging 100 nt in length are synthesized; thus the J3R protein is described as the stimulatory or processivity subunit of the poly(A) polymerase (Gershon and Moss 1993a). The poly(A) polymerase is relatively promiscuous and will polyadenylate virtually any available RNA 3′ end providing it contains uridylate residues positioned at specific sites near the RNA 3′ end (Gershon and Moss 1993b). The poly(A) stimulatory and ribose methyltransferase activities of the J3R protein are independent of one another, and occupy opposite faces of an oblate sphere (Hodel et al. 1996; Gershon et al. 1998).

Early gene transcription

Early vaccinia genes are transcribed in the cell cytoplasm from partially uncoated virion cores. Early transcripts are detectable within 20 minutes following infection, they reach a peak of synthesis by 100 minutes following infection, and decline thereafter with a half-life of approximately 30 minutes (Baldick and

Moss 1993). Early gene products number at least 50, representing at least 25 percent of the coding capacity of the vaccinia genome, and include enzymes required for DNA replication, new viral RNA polymerase and capping enzyme, host defense functions, plus intermediate gene-specific transcription factors (viral intermediate transcription factors (VITF)) required for transcription from intermediate transcriptional promoters.

Mutational analysis demonstrates that poxvirus early transcriptional promoters contain an A/T rich critical core region located between −13 and −27 relative to the RNA start site (Davison and Moss 1989a). Transcription usually starts with a purine residue, but otherwise the residues between −1 and −12, described as a 'spacer' region, are insensitive to substitution mutation. Early transcription start sites are usually located approximately 5–30 nt upstream of the ATG translation initiation codon for a given gene; however, early mRNA 5′ untranslated regions of up to 600 nt in length have been reported (Lee-Chen et al. 1988; Pacha et al. 1990; Meis and Condit 1991).

The viral early transcription factor (VETF) is a heterodimeric promoter-binding ATPase composed of the 82 kDa *A7L* gene product (*A7L/VACV-WR_126*) and the 74 kDa *D6R* gene product (*D6R/VACV-WR_111*) (Broyles and Fesler 1990; Gershon and Moss 1990) (Table 31.2). VETF is the only member of the poxvirus transcription factors that has been shown to bind directly and specifically to its cognate promoter. VETF makes sequence-specific contacts with the promoter core region, and also makes DNA contacts in a nonsequence-specific fashion directly downstream of the initiator (Broyles et al. 1991; Cassetti and Moss 1996). Upon binding to the promoter, VETF recruits RNA polymerase to the promoter and then dissociates, hydrolyzing ATP in the process (Broyles 1991). As noted above, the RAP94 subunit of the RNA polymerase is also required for initiation at early promoters.

Termination of early gene transcription is an energy-dependent, sequence-specific event requiring virus-coded *trans*-acting factors (reviewed by Condit and Niles 2002). The sequence which triggers early gene transcription termination is UUUUUNU, occurring in the nascent RNA (Yuen and Moss 1987; Shuman and Moss 1988). Termination occurs 30–50 nt downstream from this sequence. Three viral proteins are required for early termination, the capping enzyme (called the viral termination factor (VTF) in the context of termination), the RAP94 early RNA polymerase subunit, and a 72 kDa DNA-dependent ATPase, called NPH I, the product of gene *D11L* (*D11L/VACV-WR_116*) (Shuman et al. 1987; Christen et al. 1998; Deng and Shuman 1998; Mohamed and Niles 2001) (Table 31.2). NPH I provides the energy required for termination, and directly contacts RAP94 (Mohamed and Niles 2000). The activity of the capping enzyme in termination is independent of its mRNA

capping activity (Luo et al. 1995; Yu and Shuman 1996). Otherwise, the precise roles of these three proteins in early gene termination and the mechanism of sequence recognition remain to be determined.

Intermediate gene transcription

Intermediate transcription is triggered by the synthesis of intermediate gene transcription factors coupled with the initiation of viral DNA replication (Vos and Stunnenberg 1988). Intermediate mRNAs are detectable by 100 minutes post-infection and peak by 120 minutes post-infection, declining thereafter with a 30 minute half-life (Baldick and Moss 1993).

The identification of intermediate genes from among postreplicative genes is not straightforward and requires one or more specific in vivo or in vitro tests. For example, individual candidate genes may be tested for expression in vivo after infection with a temperature-sensitive mutant virus which is specifically defective in a late transcription factor (Carpenter and DeLange 1992). Only seven intermediate genes have so far been positively identified, and these encode a variety of functions including some host defense functions, DNA and RNA metabolism functions, and, importantly, viral late transcription factors (VLTF) which are required for recognition of late viral transcriptional promoters (Keck et al. 1990; Zhang et al. 1992; Xiang et al. 1998). Many of the postreplicative genes which are now classified as late will probably ultimately prove to be intermediate when subjected to appropriate tests for expression.

Intermediate gene promoters consist of two critical elements, an initiator region, TAAA, located at −1 to +3 relative to the RNA start site, and an A/T rich core element located at −13 to −26 (Baldick et al. 1992). The spacer region from −2 to −12 is insensitive to substitution mutation. The TAAA initiator motif may be located directly upstream from or even incorporate the translation initiating ATG. When initiating at intermediate promoters, RNA polymerase apparently retranscribes the AAA sequence of the initiator multiple times, slipping upstream between transcription events without releasing the nascent RNA, resulting in synthesis of a 30 nt nontemplated 5′ 'poly(A) head' (Bertholet et al. 1987; Schwer et al. 1987; Baldick and Moss 1993). (Because of this slippage reaction, the +1 nucleotide cannot be unambiguously assigned; it is arbitrarily and logically designated as the upstream A in the TAAA initiator motif.) No function for the poly(A) head has been demonstrated; however, it would provide a 5′ untranslated region for mRNAs transcribed from genes in which the promoter is directly abutted to the translation initiation ATG.

Four factors have been identified which are required for maximal expression of intermediate genes in vitro (Table 31.2). These include the heterodimeric D1R/D12L mRNA capping enzyme, and three intermediate transcription factors, VITF 1, VITF 2, and VITF 3 (Vos et al. 1991; Rosales et al. 1994a, 1994b; Sanz and Moss 1999). (Earlier, independent experiments identified the mRNA capping enzyme and one additional intermediate gene transcription factor, VITF-B; the relationship between VITF-B and VITF 1–3 has not been determined; Vos et al. 1991.) VITF 1 and 3 are virus-coded, and VITF 2 is a cellular protein. VITF 1 is identical to the 30 kDa RNA polymerase subunit RPO30, the product of the *E4L* gene (*E4L/VACV-WR_060*). VITF 3 is a heterodimer comprising the 34 kDa *A8R* gene product (*A8R/VACV-WR_127*) and the 45 kDa *A23R* gene product (*A23R/VACV-WR_143*). The cellular protein remains to be identified. The precise mechanism of action of these proteins in intermediate gene transcription remains to be determined. In addition to these four factors, evidence suggests that the cellular transcription factor YY1 may play a role in transcription of some intermediate genes (Broyles et al. 1999; Broyles 2003). Specifically, YY1 is mobilized from the cell nucleus into the cytoplasm following poxvirus infection, and binds in vitro to intermediate promoters containing the sequence TAAATGG.

Termination of intermediate and late gene transcription occurs by a similar mechanism and is fundamentally different from termination of early gene transcription (reviewed by Condit and Niles 2002). During transcription of intermediate genes, the early transcription termination signal, UUUUUNU, is ignored, presumably because the RNA polymerase which transcribes intermediate genes lacks RAP94 (Condit et al. 1996a). Instead, RNA polymerase transcribing intermediate genes apparently terminates inefficiently at multiple sites, such that each intermediate gene is transcribed to yield an extremely 3'-end heterogeneous family of transcripts ranging in size from 1 to 4 kb, regardless of the size of the gene being transcribed (Mahr and Roberts 1984). Genetic and biochemical experiments have identified three virus-coded factors which influence the length of intermediate transcripts, and therefore play a role in intermediate gene transcription elongation or termination (Table 31.2). Specifically, genetic inactivation of the *A18R* gene (*A18R/VACV-WR_138*) results in the synthesis of longer than normal intermediate mRNAs, while conversely, genetic inactivation of either the *G2R* (*G2R/VACV-WR_080*) or *J3R* (*J3R/VACV-WR_095*) genes results in the synthesis of 3'-truncated mRNAs (Black and Condit 1996; Xiang et al. 1998; Latner et al. 2000). The complementary phenotypes of these mutants is reinforced by the fact that mutations in either *G2R* or *J3R* will suppress mutations in *A18R* (Condit et al. 1996b; Latner et al. 2000). The 56 kDa *A18R* gene product is a DNA-dependent ATPase and a 3'–5' DNA helicase, and will catalyze release of RNA from a transcription elongation complex in an energy-dependent fashion in vitro (Bayliss and Condit 1995; Simpson and Condit 1995; Lackner and

Condit 2000). The A18R protein is therefore likely to be a transcription termination factor, consistent with the phenotype of A18R-deficient mutants in vivo. As described above, the J3R protein also serves as the mRNA cap (nucleoside-2'-*O*-)-methyltransferase, and the poly(A) polymerase stimulatory factor. The transcription elongation activity of J3R is genetically separable from and therefore functionally independent from its other two activities (Latner et al. 2002). The 26 kDa G2R protein has no significant homology to other characterized proteins. In vitro assays for the transcription elongation functions of J3R and G2R have yet to be developed.

Late gene transcription

Late viral mRNAs are detectable by 140 minutes post-infection, and continue to be synthesized throughout infection (Baldick and Moss 1993). Genes currently classified as late genes may comprise as much as 75 percent of the vaccinia genome; however, some of these are likely to be intermediate genes as discussed above. Late mRNAs encode the majority of virus structural and assembly functions and virion enzymes, including the VETF which is packaged into newly assembled virions along with RNA polymerase and RNA modification enzymes for use in the next round of infection.

Late transcriptional promoters are very similar to intermediate transcriptional promoters. Late promoters consist of an AT-rich core located at −11 to −16 relative to the RNA start site, and a TAAAT initiator motif located between −1 and +4 (Davison and Moss 1989b; Broyles 2003). The similarity between late and intermediate promoters is illustrated by the observation that mutation of an ACA trinucleotide to CCC at positions −15 to −17 in the gene *I3L* intermediate promoter changes the promoter to a late promoter (Hirschmann et al. 1990). Like intermediate transcripts, late gene mRNAs contain a 5' poly(A) head, synthesized via RNA polymerase slippage at the TAAAT initiator motif (Patel and Pickup 1987; Ahn and Moss 1989).

Genetic and biochemical experiments have identified at least five VLTFs which are required for maximal transcription from late promoters (Table 31.2). VLTF 1–4 are virus-coded factors. VLTF 1–3, identified through genetic experiments, are the products of the intermediate genes *G8R* (*G8R/VACV-WR_086*, 30 kDa), *A1L* (*A1L/VACV-WR_119*, 17 kDa), and *A2L* (*A2L/VACV-WR_120*, 26 kDa), respectively. VLTF 4 is the product of gene *H5R* (*H5R/VACV-WR_103*), a 22 kD early phosphoprotein which stimulates late transcription in vitro. A fifth cellular factor, VLTF-X, which stimulates transcription from late vaccinia promoters in vitro, has recently been identified as consisting of the heterogeneous nuclear ribonucleoproteins A2/B1 and RBM3 (Wright et al. 2001). The specific roles of each of the late transcription factors has yet to be determined.

Elongation and termination of late mRNAs appears to occur by mechanisms identical to intermediate mRNAs. Specifically, late mRNAs are 3'-end heterogeneous, and their length is regulated by the products of genes *A18R*, *G2R*, and *J3R* (Condit and Niles 2002).

Interestingly, a few late poxvirus mRNAs possess homogeneous 3' ends, and in the case of the cowpox virus *ATI* gene, it has been determined that the homogeneous 3' end is generated by a sequence-specific, posttranscriptional endoribonuclease cleavage reaction catalyzed by a virus-induced enzyme (Howard et al. 1999). Whether this cleavage reaction is limited to just a few mRNAs or plays a broader role in infection remains to be determined.

Additional regulation: host shutoff and RNA turnover

Sequential synthesis of transcription initiation factors accounts only for the onset of synthesis of successive classes of poxvirus gene products; additional mechanisms must regulate the shutoff of host gene expression and the decay in expression of early and intermediate genes as infection progresses. One factor which clearly plays a role in the decay of cellular and viral gene expression is a global reduction in stability of mRNA induced by poxvirus infection. For example, β-actin mRNA, which normally has a half-life of 10 hours in uninfected cells, is rapidly degraded upon vaccinia infection (Rice and Roberts 1983). In general, late viral mRNAs have a half-life of less than 60 minutes (Oda and Joklik 1967). In addition, host-gene expression may be altered by virus infection both by inhibition of cellular RNA polymerase and by inhibition of translation of cellular mRNA (Puckett and Moss 1983; Cacoullos and Bablanian 1993) .

POXVIRUS MORPHOGENESIS

Overview

Electron microscopic examination of poxvirus-infected cells reveals discrete stages of virus morphogenesis with characteristic intermediate structures associated with each stage (Dales and Pogo 1981; Griffiths et al. 2001a, 2001b; Risco et al. 2002; Sodeik and Krijnse-Locker 2002). The earliest evidence of poxvirus infection is the appearance in the cytoplasm of discrete granular foci which are largely devoid of normal cellular organelles. These foci, called 'viroplasm' or 'viral factories,' contain replicating viral DNA and are often surrounded by cellular membranes derived from the endoplasmic reticulum (Tolonen et al. 2001). As the infection progresses, viral factories increase in size. The first evidence of virion morphogenesis is the appearance within the viroplasm of rigid, crescent-shaped membrane structures

(cupules in three dimensions) which are precursors to the IMV membrane (Figure 31.10). The origin of these viral membranes is discussed in more detail below. Crescents evolve into circles (spheres in three dimensions), called immature virions (IV), which enclose relatively dense viroplasm (Figure 31.10). Some IV contain internal 'nucleoids,' which are unbounded, extremely electron-dense, DNA-containing structures presumed to be precursors to the virion core (Figure 31.10). Formation of these nucleoid-containing IV (IVN) is associated with viral DNA packaging, described in more detail below. IVN then mature to IMV containing the classical biconcave core, core envelope, lateral bodies, and outer membrane (Figure 31.11). Maturation of IV to IMV is essentially a metamorphosis which is presumed to take place via rearrangement of the contents of IVN; while structures which are thought to be intermediates in the IVN to IMV transition have been observed, they are

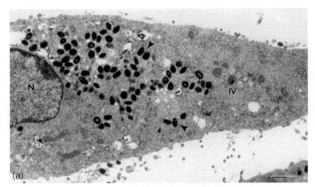

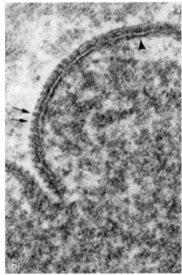

Figure 31.10 *Electron microscopy of vaccinia virus-infected cells.* **(a)** *Low-magnification field of infected HeLa cells 24 hours postinfection, showing the characteristic accumulation of spherical IV and IVN (marked IV), and dense brick-shaped mature viruses (arrowheads).* **(b)** *High-magnification field showing viral crescents. Arrow head indicates the crescent internal membrane. Arrows indicate spikes typical of crescents. (From Risco et al. 2002)*

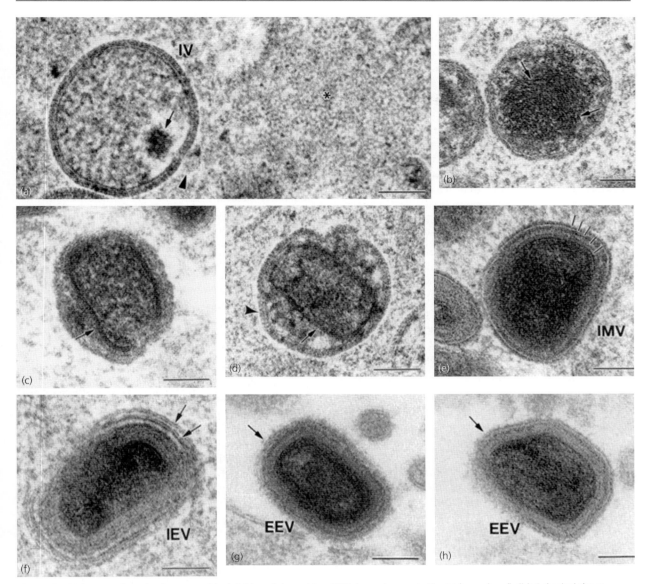

Figure 31.11 *Intermediates in virus assembly.* **(a)** *IV particle packing DNA (arrow); pore in the IV (arrowhead).* **(b)** *Spherical dense particles with fibrous, DNA-like, internal material (arrows).* **(c)** *and* **(d)***. Potential intermediate maturation stages in the construction of the internal viral core (arrows) and the IMV.* **(e)** *IMV.* **(f)** *IEV with the additional double membrane (arrows).* **(g)** *and* **(h)** *Two different section planes of EEV, which have an external fuzzy coat (arrows). Bars, 100 nm. (From Risco et al. 2002)*

relatively rare and therefore the process of IMV matura-tion is probably rapid (Figure 31.11). Maturation from IVN to IMV is accompanied by proteolysis of several major virion structural proteins; mutation of one of the viral proteases involved in virion protein cleavage inter-rupts morphogenesis at the IVN to IMV transition (Ericsson et al. 1995; Byrd et al. 2002). Maturation from IVN to IMV is also accompanied by microtubule-mediated migration of the particles from viroplasm toward the periphery of the cell (Sanderson et al. 2000). More than 90 percent of virus does not mature past the IMV stage; a small percentage matures further to eventually be exported from the cell as EEV (Boulter and Appleyard 1973). As described earlier, EEV formation involves first the formation of IEV. IEV

consists of IMV surrounded by two additional membranes, acquired via wrapping of IMV in trans-Golgi-network-derived cisternae which have been modified by the incorporation of specific virus proteins (Figure 31.11) (Schmelz et al. 1994). IEV are mobi-lized to the undersurface of the plasma membrane on microtubules, where the outermost IEV mem-brane fuses with the plasma membrane to form CEV (Blasco and Moss 1992; Hollinshead et al. 2001). CEV thus consists of IMV wrapped in one additional membrane, and remains attached to the external surface of the plasma membrane. Actin filament bundles then form beneath CEV pushing outward, resulting even-tually in the formation of long, specialized actin-containing microvilli, each of which contains a single

CEV perched at the tip (Stokes 1976; Cudmore et al. 1996). CEV is eventually released from the surface of the cell to become EEV, which, like CEV, consists of IMV surrounded by one additional membrane. Both CEV and EEV mediate short-range and long-range cell-to-cell spread of virus, respectively (Blasco and Moss 1992; Law et al. 2002).

Some poxviruses, including certain strains of cowpox, ectromelia, raccoonpox, fowlpox, and canarypox, also produce an occluded form of virus. These viruses encode an A-type inclusion protein which is produced in large amounts late in infection and which condenses into large, electron dense aggregates in the cell cytoplasm (McKelvey et al. 2002). A-type inclusions are embedded with numerous IMV (Figure 31.12). While no function for A-type inclusions has been proven, it seems reasonable to assume that they would provide increased environmental stability for the embedded IMV.

Over the past decade, information regarding the contribution of individual virus genes to virus morphogenesis has been gathered by studying virus assembly following infection with mutants in at least 32 different virion proteins. The mutants which have been characterized can be roughly staged into six categories corresponding to the major intermediates in virus assembly (one recent representative reference is provided for each class):

- mutants defective in viral membrane synthesis which accumulate viroplasm devoid of crescents (Demasi and Traktman 2000)
- mutants defective in IV synthesis which accumulate viroplasm containing crescent membranes but no complete IV (Chiu and Chang 2002)

- mutants defective in IVN synthesis which accumulate viroplasm containing IV (Yeh et al. 2000)
- mutants defective in IMV synthesis which accumulate viroplasm containing IV and IVN but no IMV (Garcia and Moss 2001)
- mutants which accumulate normal looking IMV which are not infectious (Liu et al. 1995)
- mutants defective in EEV synthesis which accumulate IMV (Sanderson et al. 2000).

Mutants in several of these categories accumulate structures which are not normally seen during wild-type virus infections; such structures may be either normal intermediates in virus assembly or dead-end defective products. Logically, mutants in several IMV membrane proteins are defective in crescent or IV formation (Rodriguez et al. 1995, 1998; Wolffe et al. 1996; Traktman et al. 2000), mutants in several core proteins are defective in maturation of IV to IMV (Klemperer et al. 1997; Williams et al. 1999), and mutants in several EEV membrane proteins are defective in maturation of IMV to EEV (Blasco and Moss 1991; Engelstad and Smith 1993; Wolffe et al. 1993). However, it is also true that mutants in several core proteins and enzymes affect viral membrane formation (Wang and Shuman 1995; Demasi and Traktman 2000), and conversely that mutants in some membrane proteins affect the transition from IV to IMV (Ravanello and Hruby 1994). These genetic studies have also revealed that poxviruses encode a complete pathway for disulfide bond formation which is required for formation of at least some of the disulfide bonds critical for virus structure and assembly (Senkevich et al. 2002). Mutation of any of the genes in the pathway interrupts morphogenesis at the IV to IVN stage.

IV and IMV membrane formation

Two distinct models have been proposed to describe the origin and structure of viral crescents and the IMV membrane. One model proposes that the crescent membranes comprise a single lipid bilayer which arises de novo, that is without continuity with any other intracellular membrane structure (Dales and Mosbach 1968; Hollinshead et al. 1999). This de novo model is based on the observation that, using conventional EM techniques, the crescents and the IMV membrane have dimensions consistent with a single lipid bilayer, and that in most standard EM preparations of virus-infected cells, no convincing connection can be observed between the crescents and any other intracellular membrane system. The notion of de novo biogenesis of a lipid bilayer membrane with free ends and two cytoplasmic surfaces is unprecedented in cell biology. An alternative model which is more consistent with established cell biology principles is that the crescents are formed from membrane cisternae derived from the endoplasmic reticulum–Golgi intermediate

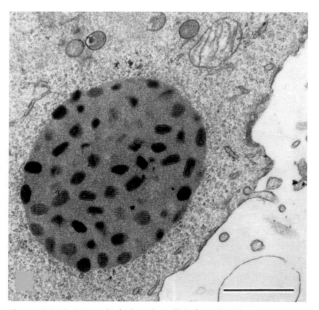

Figure 31.12 *A-type inclusions in cells infected with cowpox virus. The inclusion contains multiple IMV. Note the IV and IVN immature particles above the inclusion. Bar, 1 000 nm. (From McKelvey et al. 2002)*

compartment (ERGIC), which, through incorporation of viral proteins, collapse into rigid crescents, such that the crescents and IMV membranes actually comprise two tightly apposed lipid bilayers (Sodeik and Krijnse-Locker 2002). This 'double membrane' model is supported by EM images of IV prepared by freeze substitution, and by EM examination of thin cryosections of infected cells, which under some circumstances reveal apparent localized separation of two membranes within a crescent. In addition, cryosections stained with antibodies to both cellular and viral proteins show labeling of ERGIC membranes with viral proteins, and continuity between crescents and cell-derived ERGIC membrane cisternae (Sodeik et al. 1993; Salmons et al. 1997; Rodriguez et al. 1997; Risco et al. 2002). The double-membrane model is further supported by the clear demonstration of a remarkably similar mechanism of virion membrane biogenesis during maturation of another cytoplasmic DNA virus, African swine fever virus (Andres et al. 1998). Interestingly, infection with mutants in either of the poxvirus IMV membrane proteins A17L or A14L results in aberrant or deficient synthesis of crescents, and accumulation of numerous small vesicles containing viral membrane proteins (Rodriguez et al. 1995, 1998; Wolffe et al. 1996; Traktman et al. 2000). It has been proposed that these vesicles may normally be intermediates in crescent formation (Traktman et al. 2000). The vesicles could be shed from the ERGIC, and would normally be short lived. Crescents formed by fusion and collapse of these vesicles would comprise tightly apposed double membranes, but consistent continuity with the intermediate compartment would be rare, thus explaining the apparent de novo evolution of viral membrane crescents. A similar model of viral membrane formation proposes that the IV membrane is formed by the fusion of ERGIC-derived, viral protein-modified tubules (Risco et al. 2002). Phosphorylation may play a critical role in regulating viral membrane formation, since both the A17L and A14L membrane proteins are phosphorylated by the virus-coded F10L kinase, and mutational inactivation of the F10L kinase abrogates crescent formation (Traktman et al. 1995; Betakova et al. 1999; Derrien et al. 1999).

Viral DNA packaging

The mechanism by which viral DNA is packaged into virions is incompletely understood. Viral DNA concatemers are resolved to unit length genomes during infection with virus mutants that are incapable of forming even the earliest crescent membranes; therefore the final stages of viral DNA processing do not seem to be coupled to morphogenesis (Demasi and Traktman 2000). In theory, unit length viral DNA genomes could be incorporated into IV during membrane synthesis and subsequently condense into nucleoids. However, several investigators have observed IV which are incompletely

sealed and which possess a chromatin- or nucleoidlike material positioned across a small opening or pore in the IV, sometimes apparently continuous with the internal nucleoid (Figure 31.11) (Morgan 1976; Ericsson et al. 1995; Risco et al. 2002). These images are interpreted to mean that DNA is specifically packaged late during IV assembly to form IVN. Interestingly, mutation of the viral gene A32L, which contains a predicted ATP/GTP-binding site 'P loop' motif, interrupts virus assembly at the IV to IVN transition, resulting in the accumulation of reduced amounts of IVN and large amounts of a novel, electron-dense spherical particle which does not contain DNA (Cassetti et al. 1998). These observations are consistent with a late DNA packaging model and suggest that the A32L gene product may mediate DNA packaging.

One group has proposed recently that viral DNA is packaged through an association of DNA with ERGIC and a second infolding of the DNA-membrane complex into the IV membrane during IVN morphogenesis (Griffiths et al. 2001a, 2001b). This model predicts that the core wall is in fact a double membrane similar to the proposed double-membrane structure for the IV and IMV membrane. Further research is required to substantiate this model.

POXVIRUS GENETICS

Overview

Genetic manipulation of poxviruses has had a broad impact on both poxvirology in particular and biomedical science in general. The influence of poxvirus genetics can be broken down into three specific areas:

- construction of virus mutants for use in determining the function of individual poxvirus genes
- use of recombinant poxviruses for protein over-expression
- use of recombinant poxviruses as vaccine vectors.

Genetic manipulation of poxviruses has taken liberal advantage of both classical 'forward' genetic techniques and modern 'reverse' genetic techniques. Classical forward genetics consists of chemical mutagenesis and random isolation of temperature-sensitive, host-range, drug-resistant, and drug-dependent mutants, followed by employment of genetic mapping procedures to determine which genes have been affected. Modern reverse genetics consists of site-specific engineering of the viral genome, from alteration of existing poxvirus genes in situ to introduction of foreign genes and heterologous transcriptional operons into the poxvirus genome.

Regardless of the application, reverse genetic engineering of poxvirus genomes follows the same fundamental 'in vivo recombination' protocol (Nakano et al. 1982). Specifically, if cells are first infected with a poxvirus and then transfected with a DNA molecule which has homology with the infecting poxvirus genome, the transfecting DNA molecule will undergo homologous recombination with the infecting genome. A simple example of this principle is marker rescue mapping of temperature-sensitive mutants of vaccinia virus (Thompson and Condit 1986). In this example, cells are infected with mutant virus and transfected with candidate DNA molecules derived from wild-type virus. Homologous recombination between the mutant genome and a transfected DNA molecule which contains the wild-type allele of the gene will generate wild-type virus, thus mapping the temperature-sensitive lesion to a specific rescuing DNA fragment. Several variations on the basic in vivo recombination scheme have been derived which improve the efficiency of the procedure and/or enhance selection for recombinant genomes (Chakrabarti et al. 1985; Franke et al. 1985; Fathi et al. 1986; Falkner and Moss 1990; Merchlinsky and Moss 1992; Scheiflinger et al. 1992). In general, poxvirus recombination is efficient and the genome contains numerous nonessential insertion sites and can accommodate large amounts of foreign DNA, so that almost any recombinant that can be imagined can be constructed. Recently, a novel engineering scheme has been developed in which the entire vaccinia genome is contained in a bacterial artificial chromosome, where it can be engineered and subsequently reactivated by infection of cells infected with a nonreplicating helper fowlpox virus (Domi and Moss 2002).

In the sections that follow, we consider briefly the principles and practice of each of the specific areas of poxvirus genetics described above.

Construction of virus mutants for use in determining the function of individual poxvirus genes

Several laboratories have used classical forward genetic methods to assemble collections of conditional lethal mutants to be used for the study of the function of individual poxvirus genes (reviewed by Condit and Niles 1990). Recently, a complete complementation analysis combining two independent mutant collections has been conducted, resulting in a combined collection of 138 temperature-sensitive mutants comprising 53 complementation groups (Lackner et al. 2003). These temperature-sensitive mutants, along with numerous drug-resistant, drug-dependent, and host-range mutants, have been and will continue to be a powerful resource for determining poxvirus gene function. However, given that the poxvirus genome contains approximately 200 genes, and assuming that approximately 150 of these genes are essential for virus growth in culture, even this combined collection provides only about one-third coverage of the genome. With this in mind, two alternative methods for

reverse genetic engineering of mutants in specific poxviral genes have been developed.

One reverse genetic method for creating conditional lethal poxvirus mutants involves regulating transcription of the poxvirus gene of interest using elements from a bacterial operon (Fuerst et al. 1989; Rodriguez and Smith 1990; Traktman et al. 2000). In its simplest form this involves construction of a recombinant poxvirus which constitutively expresses a bacterial repressor protein, for example the lac repressor, and which also contains a cognate operator (that is a repressor-binding site) between the transcriptional promoter and the coding sequence of the target gene to be regulated. In such a recombinant the expression of the gene can be controlled by use of an inducer molecule during virus infection, for example IPTG in the case of lac repressor control. Appropriate regulation of the target gene sometimes requires more baroque constructions. For example, recombinants can be constructed which contain bacteriophage T7 RNA polymerase under lac repressor control, and in which the target gene is regulated by both a T7 RNA polymerase promoter and a lac operator (Ward et al. 1995). Numerous inducible recombinant poxviruses have been constructed which have proven invaluable for the study of individual poxvirus genes. One drawback of this approach is that some poxviral genes, most notably early genes, cannot be cleanly regulated.

An alternative approach to creating conditional lethal poxvirus mutants is the construction of temperature-sensitive mutants using clustered charge to alanine scanning mutagenesis (Hassett and Condit 1994). Clusters of charged residues are identified within the linear amino acid sequence of a given target gene, and all of the charged residues in a given cluster are changed to alanine in a cloned copy of the gene. Individual clustered charge to alanine mutants are then recombined into the viral genome and recombinant viruses are tested for temperature sensitivity. Empirically, approximately 30 percent of clustered charge to alanine mutants prove to be temperature-sensitive, theoretically because the charge clusters normally reside on the surface of a protein, and the genetic neutralization of the charge weakens protein–protein interactions. Useful clustered charge to alanine temperature-sensitive mutants have been created in several vaccinia genes which were inaccessible via bacterial operon regulation (Hassett et al. 1997; Demasi and Traktman 2000; Ishii and Moss 2001b; Punjabi et al. 2001).

Use of recombinant poxviruses for protein overexpression

The technical foundation for use of poxviruses to overexpress proteins is a recombinant poxvirus which constitutively expresses the bacteriophage T7 RNA polymerase (called here vvT7) and a target gene which is expressed from a bacteriophage T7 transcriptional promoter (Fuerst et al. 1986). Depending on the goal of the expression, the target gene may be presented in one of three different forms. The target gene may be contained on a plasmid, in which case expression is achieved by infection with the vvT7 and transfection with the target plasmid. The target gene may be recombined into another poxvirus, in which case expression is achieved by coinfection with vvT7 and the target gene-containing virus. Lastly, the target gene may be recombined into vvT7 itself as described above, providing that the system is under inducible control of a bacterial operon system.

Overexpression of proteins from poxvirus vectors has three principal uses (Moss 1996). First, the system can provide for eukaryotic expression of large quantities of protein for purification and use in biochemical studies (Bayliss and Condit 1995). Second, the system can be used for transient expression of proteins in eukaryotic cells in order to study protein function, for example function of paramyxovirus replication proteins (Smallwood et al. 2002). Third, the system has been used to launch synthesis of viral genomes and viral gene products for construction of recombinant viruses, for example rhabdoviruses (Roberts and Rose 1998).

Use of recombinant poxviruses as vaccine vectors

Infection of animals or humans with recombinant poxviruses which express foreign antigens under the control of poxvirus transcriptional promoters can result in a robust humoral and cellular immune response to the foreign antigen (Paoletti 1996). This strategy has potential for providing immunization against organisms for which conventional vaccines are lacking. Recombinant poxvirus vaccines have been used with clinical success in animals; for example, a vaccinia recombinant that expresses the rabies glycoprotein has been used in the wild to control the spread of rabies virus (Pastoret and Brochier 1996). While recombinant poxvirus vaccines would undoubtedly be effective in humans, none is currently licensed for human use, primarily because of safety concerns associated with the poxvirus vector. Vaccinia vectors with increased safety features have been created by deleting numerous genes nonessential for growth in culture, and alternative poxvirus vectors have been developed, most notably attenuated vaccinia virus strains (Modified Vaccinia Ankara) and avipoxvirus vectors such as canarypox (Paoletti et al. 1995).

POXVIRUS GENES RESPONSIBLE FOR IMMUNE EVASION, HOST RANGE, AND CONTROL OF APOPTOSIS

Poxviruses adopt a wide variety of strategies to ensure survival. These strategies include the shutoff of host transcription, synthesis of different forms of infectious virus particles with differing surface components that facilitate cell spread and viremia, and assembly of virus particles into environmentally resistant inclusion bodies. In addition, as the virus family evolved and became established in different vertebrate hosts or sites within a host, poxviruses developed the means to capture essential host genes which then evolved to target critical aspects of host defenses such as host range, inflammation, and other immunomodulatory mechanisms which serve to enhance virus survival. As described previously, many of these modulatory genes are located within the variable or noncore region of the poxvirus genome and are non-essential for virus growth in cell culture. There has been much speculation as to how poxviruses which develop in the cytoplasm might capture cellular genes. One clue is suggested by the finding that strains of fowlpox virus have incorporated a reticuloendotheliosis virus (a retrovirus) within the fowlpox virus genome (Hertig et al. 1997). It is possible that the reverse transcriptase encoded by a retrovirus might reverse transcribe cellular transcripts which might subsequently be incorporated into the poxvirus genome.

Many of the poxvirus-encoded immune modulatory genes are shared by a number of poxviruses, particularly those that cause similar diseases even though the viruses belong to different genera. However, these genes can also be quite different in the case where two viruses cause very dissimilar disease, as is the case if one compares one of the orthopoxviruses such as vaccinia virus or variola virus to MCV. Both these viruses employ the same basic molecular strategies of replication, transcription, contain the same central core of conserved genes and have a similar genome size. However, variola virus is associated with a severe, generalized disseminated infection with high morbidity and mortality whereas the disease caused by MCV in normal individuals is typically rather benign, albeit persistent, and consists of single or multiple 2–5 mm non-inflammatory, painless, papular, dermal lesions, which can arise on various parts of the body. These lesions may persist for months or longer and frequently resolve without treatment. In immunocompromised individuals, the disease is frequently more severe and causes severe discomfort and disfiguration (Esposito and Fenner 2001) (see Chapter 64, Virus infections in immunocompromised patients).

It is likely that the genes contained within the variable regions of these two viruses play a major role in the disease process. In the case of MCV, these genes would be consistent with virus growth restricted to the dermis and be particularly effective against the host immune defenses operative at that site. On the other hand, vaccinia virus or variola virus might be expected to encode an entirely different coterie of genes best suited to overcome immune and host responses directed against an overt generalized infection. While cautioning against oversimplification, this is a useful model to consider. These genes are summarized in Table 31.5.

In the discussion that follows, we focus our attention on vaccinia virus, much of which extrapolates to variola virus and to a lesser extent MCV because these are the most significant from the point of view of human disease. Much of what we know about virus-encoded immune modulatory genes encoded by poxviruses causing general, disseminated infections is derived from studies on the prototype orthopoxvirus vaccinia virus and from other poxviruses, most notably leporipoxvirus myxoma virus, and thus must be extrapolated to variola virus. We take note of the fact that there is some data to suggest that variola orthologs of vaccinia virus genes may be particularly attuned to human hosts (Rosengard et al. 2002) in much the same way as myxoma virus immunomodulatory genes tend to be particularly effective within rabbits. In the case of MCV, the virus can not be grown in cell culture so that study of MCV genes must be done either on the expressed and purified protein or following cloning of the MCV gene into a surrogate virus, typically vaccinia virus. There are at least five excellent, comprehensive reviews of poxvirus immunomodulatory proteins (Moss et al. 2000; Moss and Shisler 2001; Shisler and Moss 2001a; Alcami 2003; Seet et al. 2003). The following discussion draws from all these reviews.

General considerations of poxvirus-mediated control of the host response to infection

Generally, the initial exposure of a given host to viruses, including poxviruses, involves macrophage and lympho-cytes and leads to inflammation in response to tissue damage and to the production of interferon. Interferon in turn stimulates natural killer (NK) cells which can kill virus-infected cells as a first line of defense in a non-specific fashion independent of the more sophisticated, adaptive immune response. Similarly, the activation of the complement cascade also functions as a first line of defense. Synthesis of antigenic virus proteins are then processed by antigen-producing cells such as dendritic cells and macrophages. This processing generates peptides which then complex with the major histo-compatibility complex (MHC) and are presented by these antigen-presenting cells to lymphocytes. There are

Table 31.5 *Poxvirus immunomodulatory, anti-apoptotic and host range genes*

Virus	Gene		Protein	Description
Molluscum contagiosum virus	**MCV ORF**		Size (aa)	**Cellular homolog**
	080R		395	MHC class I α-chain homolog
	033L		579	Thymocyte antigen? CDIc T-cell surface antigen?
	066L		220	Glutathione peroxidase
	159R		241	Caspase-8 and FADD apoptosis-like inhibitor
	148R		104	Chemokine homolog
	054		235	IL-18 binding protein
Vaccinia virus	**VVCOP ORF**	**VACWR ORF**	Size (aa)	**Description**
	C3L	*025*	263	Complement control protein
	K3L	*034*	88	elf2-α homolog
	E3L	*059*	190	dsRNA binding protein
	B8R	*190*	272	IFN-α receptor decoy
	B19R	*200*	353	IFN-α/β binding protein
	Absent	*013*	126	IL-18 binding protein
	B13/14R	*195*	345	Serpin (SPI-/crmA)
	A46R	*172*	240	TIR-like
	A52R	*178*	190	TIR-like
	A53R	*179*	103	TNF-like receptor*
	C22L/B28R	*004, 215*	122	Soluble TNFR
	A41L	*166*	219	Chemokine-binding protein, unknown ligand, anti-inflammatory
	A38L	*162*	277	CD47-like protein
	K2L	*033*	369	Serpin (SPI-3)
	A39R	*163*	295	Semaphorin
	A44L	*170*	346	Hydroxysteroid dehydrogenase
	C23L (B29R)	*218*	244	Type II chemokine-binding protein
	B16R	*197*	326	IL-1β binding protein
	C12L/B22R	*205*	353	Serpin (SPI-1)
	K1L	*032*	284	Host range, ankyrin repeat protein
	C7L	*021*	150	Host range, ankyrin repeat protein

a number of lymphocytes including CD8[+] T lymphocytes (CTL) that expand to clear infected cells and that comprises the basis of cell-mediated immunity (CMI). There are two types of T-helper cells that contribute to CTL activity. Type I CD4[+] helper T lymphocytes are involved in inducing longlasting CTL activity and the type 2 CD4[+] helper T lymphocytes interact with B cells to produce neutralizing antibodies, which prevent newly released virus from initiating subsequent infection (humoral immunity). CTLs recognize antigen in conjunction with class I MHC, whereas CD4[+] helper cells recognize antigen presented in conjunction with MHC class II (Esposito and Fenner 2001).

Orthopoxviruses have genes designed to neutralize both the interferon and complement responses. There is no evidence to suggest that MCV controls the complement response nor is involved in the control of interferons to anywhere the same degree as the orthopoxviruses. Following the innate response, in a naive host, the CTL response occurs and is primarily responsible for clearing an infection (Buller and Palumbo 1991; Palumbo et al. 1994; Ada and Blanden 1994; Barry and Bleackley 2002). However, antibodies formed soon thereafter may be instrumental in preventing newly synthesized particles from accessing sites not readily accessible to adaptive CTLs such as the skin. Therefore, it is reasonable to assume that virus-coded genes that deflect host responses would be designed not only to interfere with antigen presentation in the context of class I and II MHC but also to interfere with the consequences of that antigen presentation, namely virus clearance and ultimately immunological memory. There is some evidence to suggest that MCV controls the MHC but little evidence to suggest that orthopoxviruses do so directly.

However, a significant and general effort is mounted by all poxviruses against cytokines and chemokines, which are involved in both innate and adaptive immunity. The virus-mediated deflection of these responses serves to mask the infection by various means and 'buy time' during which the infection becomes established. orthopoxvirus-encoded proteins include those that interfere with complement, various cytokines (tumor necrosis factor (TNF), interferons (IFN)-α, β, and γ, interleukins (IL)-1β and IL-18), and Toll-like receptors (TLR) (Table 31.5). There are also poxvirus proteins designed to bind to and interfere with cellular chemokines as well as poxvirus-encoded chemokine-like molecules. Some of these and additional proteins interfere with aspects of inflammation, apoptosis, and host range. The repertoire of MCV appears to be more limited. As mentioned, it is likely that MCV controls the MHC system. MCV proteins that inhibit apoptosis, an IL-18 binding protein and a chemokine homologue have been identified. Each of these activities is described in more detail below. The orthopoxvirus ORF designation uses the dual nomenclature of vaccinia virus Copenhagen for convenience

but cross-referencing to the ortholog in vaccinia WR is shown in Table 31.5.

Control of the MHC by MCV (MC080 and MC033)

A striking feature of MCV infections is the absence of inflammation at the sites of replication even in immunocompetent individuals (Heng et al. 1989). Also, lesion areas are devoid of NK, Langerhans, and T cells and no longer display β$_2$-macrogobulin reactivity (Viac and Chardonnet 1990). There are two MCV proteins which could potentially interact with or replace components of the MHC class I system. The *MC080R* gene of MCV encodes an MHC class I (α-) heavy chain homologue, which theoretically could compromise normal MHC class I function. However, the function of the MC080R protein is unclear because complexes of MC080R and β$_2$-macroglobulin form only at high concentrations of MC080R and are not detected on the surface of cells (Senkevich and Moss 1998). It is also noteworthy that even when complexes were detected under conditions when MC080R was overexpressed, HLA-A2 appears to successfully compete with the MC080R protein for binding to β$_2$-microglobulin (Senkevich and Moss 1998). Hence the mechanism by which MC080R acts is unclear. The *MC033L* ORF has some homology to thymocyte antigen and to the CD1c T-cell surface glycoprotein but the mechanism of action is unknown.

Myxoma virus, like vaccinia virus, causes a generalized disseminated infection and down-regulates class I MHC epitopes (Boshkov et al. 1992) through the M153R protein. The M153R protein contains a leukemia-associated protein (LAP) domain and localizes to the endoplasmic reticulum and is believed to target β$_2$-macroglobulin-associated MHC I molecules both at the cell surface and in the post-Golgi compartment for retention and subsequent lysosomal degradation (Guerin et al. 2002). There is little evidence to suggest direct control of the MHC by vaccinia virus. In fact, were MHC presentation significantly affected by vaccinia virus, vaccinia would not be nearly as effective as a vaccine vector as it appears to be (Nash et al. 1999; Moss 2001).

Complement (ORF C3L)

The complement control protein (VCP) was one of the first poxvirus anti-host defense genes discovered (Kotwal and Moss 1988; Kotwal et al. 1990). The protein is characterized by short consensus repeat sequences (SCR) characteristic of complement regulatory proteins (Kotwal and Moss 1988). VCP inhibits both the classical and alternative activation of complement by inhibiting C3b and C4b proteins, which are key in the formation of active complement (Kotwal et al. 1990). VCP also inhibits the antibody-dependent, complement-mediated neutralization of IMV. Deletion of the *VCP* gene from vaccinia virus leads to production of smaller lesions in infected animals (Isaacs et al. 1992). It is interesting to note that the corresponding variola virus gene is much more efficient than the vaccinia VCP in inhibiting human complement (Rosengard et al. 2002). Another orthopoxvirus protein that contains SCRs, is the *B5R/VACV-WR_187* gene product (Takahashi-Nishimaki et al. 1991; Engelstad et al. 1992). B5R is a component of EEV membranes but is not found in IMV (Herrera et al. 1998). Despite the presence of SCRs, B5R does not appear to exert any effects on complement.

Interferons (IFN) (ORFs B8R, E3L, and K3L)

IFN-γ

The role of IFNs in controlling virus infections is well known. IFNs regulate a number of intracellular signaling pathways through kinase activation and these pathways are targeted in some fashion by both the orthopoxviruses and MCV, albeit differently. IFN-γ acts to up-regulate the double-stranded RNA-dependent protein kinase, phosphokinase R (PKR), a key component in cellular signaling pathways. In the case of orthopoxviruses, IFN-γ action is regulated both intracellularly by the *K3L* and *E3L* genes and extracellularly by a soluble, secreted type II IFN receptor (B8R).

The orthopoxvirus-secreted IFN-γ receptor (B8R) serves as an IFN-γ decoy binding protein, which acts to sequester IFN-γ and to prevent productive binding of the cytokine to cellular receptors. This decoy protein, typical of many 'viroceptors,' contains sequences similar to the cytokine-binding domain but lacks the transmembrane and cytoplasmic signaling sequences. While the vaccinia IFN-γ receptor decoy binds IFN-γ from many species, a similar protein isolated from myxoma virus binds only rabbit IFN-γ, indicative of adaptation to the rabbit host (Mossman et al. 1995) and the comparable gene of ectromelia virus is specific for mouse IFN-γ (Smith and Alcami 2002). Deletion of the IFN-γ receptor from vaccinia virus leads to attenuation of the virus in mouse models (Verardi et al. 2001).

The proteins E3L and K3L are involved in anti-host defense strategies that regulate the IFN responses through accessory cellular proteins including PKR, a protein induced by IFN, and the enzyme 2′,5′-oligoadenylate synthetase (OAS) (Sen 2001). Both E3L and K3L can effectively prevent PKR-mediated inhibition of protein synthesis at the level of RNA or translation, respectively. The intracellular *K3L* gene, which resembles the protein translation factor eIF2α, acts as a nonfunctional substate for PKR, which is induced by IFN-γ (Davies et al. 1993). The *E3L* gene encodes a double-stranded RNA-binding protein of either 20 or 25 kDa. Hence, by binding double-stranded RNA, the E3L protein prevents double-stranded RNA activation of PRK (Chang and Jacobs 1993; Yuwen et al. 1993). There is also some evidence to suggest that E3L can interact directly with PKR to form an inactive heterodimer (Romano et al. 1998). The binding of E3L to dsRNA also serves to abrogate activation of OAS. Initially synthesized as an inactive enzyme, OAS requires dsRNA for activation, a step also prevented by the binding of E3L to dsRNA. Once activated, OAS synthesizes 2′–5′-linked oligoadenylate which serves as a cofactor for ribonuclease L. Ribonuclease L cleaves both ribosomal and mRNA, leading to inhibition of protein synthesis at the RNA level. Deletion of the *E3L* gene has a major effect on virulence and deletion of either gene leads to a reduced host range of the virus which is discussed further under poxvirus genes that affect host range.

As is discussed below, like IFN-γ, IL-β is also controlled in an intra- and extracellular fashion. The dual means by which the virus acts to prevent the action of these cytokines suggests that the pathways controlled by these cytokines are very important in counteracting the virus infection.

IFN-α/β

Orthopoxviruses, including variola virus, encode a type I interferon binding protein (ORF B19R) which binds both IFN-α and β (Symons et al. 1995). Unlike the IFN-γ soluble receptor just described, this protein has little or no similarity to the cellular counterpart. A folding of the immunoglobulin domains contained in the viral IFN-α/β binding protein and the fibronectin type III domains of the cellular receptor have been proposed to account for their interaction with the same ligands (Alcami 2003). The protein binds to and inhibits the type I interferons IFN-α,β as well as IFN-δ and ω (Symons et al. 1995; Liptakova et al. 1997; Vancova et al. 1998; Smith and Alcami 2002). Deletion of the gene leads to attenuation of the virus (Verardi et al. 2001).

Interleukin (IL)-18-binding proteins (VACV-WR_013, MC054)

The IFN pathway is targeted indirectly by proteins which bind to and functionally eliminate IL-18, a potent inducer of IFN-γ. An IL-18-binding protein is encoded by some but not all strains of vaccinia virus and is absent in strain Copenhagen (Symons et al. 2002). This protein also has little or no sequence similarity to the cellular IL-18-binding protein. An equivalent protein is encoded by MCV. Originally, IL-18 was identified as a powerful inducer of IFN-γ, but also induces the synthesis of a number of the cytokines and chemokines, which in turn can influence the Th1 or Th2 cellular response and influence activation of NK and cytotoxic T cells

(Nakanishi et al. 2001). Deletion of the IL-18-binding protein encoded by vaccinia virus WR results in attenuated infections (Symons et al. 2002). Deletion of the IL-18-binding protein gene encoded by ectromelia virus, a pathogen of mice, also resulted in virus attenuation (Born et al. 2000).

The MCV genomic sequence indicates that none of the plethora of soluble cytokine-receptor or cytokine-binding proteins or decoy receptors found in the orthopoxviruses are encoded by MCV. However, as stated above, the virus does encode an IL-18-binding protein (MC054) (Xiang and Moss 1999). Strong binding of IL-18 has been observed with MC054 (Xiang and Moss 1999). Two additional MCV proteins encoded by ORFs, MC051 and MC053, are related to MC054, but these two proteins lack conserved residues associated with high-affinity binding to IL-18. Therefore, it is likely these two proteins bind other ligands (Xiang and Moss 2001). Unlike the orthopoxvirus IL-18-binding proteins, the MC054 protein contains a long C-terminal extension. The C-terminal tail binds with high-affinity to glycosaminoglycans and hence to cell surfaces (Xiang and Moss 2003). MC054 contains a furin cleavage site which separates the glycosaminoglycan-binding C-terminal tail of the molecule from the IL-18-binding portion of the protein (Xiang and Moss 2003). This allows for a secreted as well as cell-bound form of the IL-18-binding protein. It has been proposed that the C-terminal tail may function to alter the half-life of the IL-18-binding protein and serve to concentrate the protein in the vicinity of MCV-infected cells where it is most needed. The cleaved form may allow IL-18 binding and sequestration activity to leave the site of infection for activity at distal sites.

Interleukin (IL)-1β (ORFs B16R, B13R/B14R, A46R, and A52R)

Vaccinia virus encodes a secreted IL-1β-decoy receptor (ORF B16R), (Alcami and Smith 1992; Spriggs et al. 1992) but interestingly, the gene is present but inactive in all variola virus strains examined to date. This decoy receptor binds IL-1β but not IL-1α or the host IL-1 receptor antagonist (Alcami and Smith 1992; Spriggs et al. 1992; Smith and Alcami 2000). Deletion of this gene from vaccinia virus suggested that IL-1β serves to control fever during poxvirus infections (Alcami and Smith 1996). Virus lacking a functional B16R is attenuated when animals are infected via the intracranial route (Spriggs et al. 1992) but exhibits enhanced virulence during intranasal infections (Alcami and Smith 1992).

IL-1β, like IFN-γ, is also regulated both intracellularly as well as extracellularly. In the case of IL-β, intracellular regulation is mediated by one of the three virus-encoded serpins, crmA/SPI-2 (ORF B13R/B14R).

The protein encoded by crmA/SPI-2 is a potent inhibitor of caspases-1 and 8 and perhaps 10 as well as granzyme B. Hence this protein has the unusual property of inhibiting both serine (granzyme B) and thiol proteases (caspases). Caspase-1 is responsible for synthesis of active, proinflammatory IL-1β from the inactive precursor proIL-1β (Ray et al. 1992) as well as activating IL-18 from proIL-18 (Gu et al. 1997). Therefore, crmA/SPI-2 can influence the levels of both IL-β and IL-18. The ability to inhibit caspase-8 can serve to block apoptosis via several pathways including not only extrinsically induced apoptosis induced by Fas/Fas ligand and granzyme B, but also apoptosis intrinsically mediated by caspase-8. However, deletion of this gene from vaccinia virus or cowpox virus leads to only modest attenuation (Tscharke et al. 2002).

Finally, IL-β can potentially be regulated intracellularly in one additional way. After ligand engagement, IL-1β receptor-mediated signaling can be disrupted by poxvirus proteins that contain signaling components of Toll-like receptors (TLR). TLRs are important in innate immunity and serve as pattern recognition receptors on cells of the innate immune system (O'Neill 2000). Variola virus encodes one such gene, vaccinia virus two (A46R and A52R). Each of these proteins contains a Toll/IL-1 receptor (TIR) domain motif within the cytoplasmic portion of the molecule which allows for interaction with adaptor molecules to prevent intracellular signaling downstream of the IL-1 receptor (Bowie et al. 2000). Of the two vaccinia proteins, A52R appears the more effective in inhibiting activation of NF-κB, a transcription factor involved in cytokine expression (Bowie et al. 2000). As might be anticipated, proteins such as A52R appear to endow the virus with the ability to inhibit a number of signaling pathways which are initiated from TIR domain-containing cell surface receptors such as TLRs and IL-1R (Harte et al. 2003). Deletion of A52R from vaccinia virus has no effect on growth or plaque size but the virus is attenuated in intranasally infected mice as evidenced by milder signs of illness and less weight loss (Harte et al. 2003).

Tumor necrosis factor (TNF) (ORFs C22L, B28R)

TNFs are potent proinflammatory cytokines secreted by macrophages and activated T cells comprise a family of powerful proinflammatory cytokines (Smith et al. 1994). There are at least three classes of TNFs: TNF, lymphotoxin (LT)-α and LT-β. All are active as trimers that recognize two members of the superfamily of TNF receptors (TNFR), TNFRI (p55) and TNFRII (p75). The main effect of host-encoded TNF is to induce an antiviral state that controls lysis of infected cells (Locksley et al. 2001). Poxviruses encode a number of homologues of the TNFR and some viruses, for example cowpox virus, encode four (Hu et al. 1994; Smith et al. 1996; Loparev et al. 1998; Saraiva and Alcami 2001) designated as CrmB, CrmC, CrmD and CrmE (Cunnion 1999; Saraiva and Alcami 2001). Variola virus also encodes a TNFR homologue as does vaccinia virus strain Lister; however, many vaccinia strains lack any TNF receptor homologue (Alcami et al. 1999). Vaccinia virus strain Copenhagen encodes an inactive gene, which, because it is located in the TIR of the genome, is present in two copies (C22L, B28R). These virus-coded TNFRs have sequence similarity to extracellular domains of both p55 and p75 of the host cell but lack the anchoring C-terminal transmembrane domain that anchors the cellular protein on the cell surface (Smith et al. 1991; Upton et al. 1991; Schreiber et al. 1996; Loparev et al. 1998). These molecules function as decoy TNF-binding proteins, binding TNF to prevent TNF from interacting with the appropriate cellular receptor (Cunnion 1999; Xu et al. 2000). Another member of this family of proteins, found in cowpox virus, is a protein called VD30, which resembles cellular CD30 and binds to the cognate cellular target CD153 (Panus et al. 2002). In the case of myxoma virus, deletion of the viral TNFR homologue gene leads to a strong attenuation of the virus (Upton et al. 1991).

Regulation of chemokines (ORFs C23R, B29R, and MC148R)

Chemokines are small molecules generally involved in attracting leukocytes to the site of damage produced in response to various cellular insults including infection. However, within the context of virus infection, there are numerous possibilities for the possible function of virus-encoded chemokines and chemokine receptors (Alcami 2003). Chemokine agonists might attract leukocytes capable of supporting virus infection or induce migration of Th2 cells and thereby alter the immune response to infection. Chemokine agonists might also induce angiogenesis and/or contribute to infection pathology. Virus-encoded antagonists might prevent migration of immune cells (Th1 cells) that lead to an antiviral response. The regulation of chemokines may also alter critical signaling pathways in such a way as to promote virus infection. Viral-encoded chemokine receptors could lower the concentration of critical cytokines at localized sites of infection and could down-regulate the production of the chemokine itself, which would allow for immune evasion. Cellular-bound chemokine receptors could, in response to the appropriate chemokine, lead to migration of the particular cell leading to spread of the viral infection. Finally, the receptors could induce expression of chemokines and thereby modulate the immune response or contribute to immunopathology. The poxviruses have the potential to regulate these responses by encoding chemokine-binding proteins, chemokine receptors, or chemokine ligand mimics (Kotwal 2000;

Lalani et al. 2000; Mahalingam and Karupiah 2000; Mahalingam et al. 2000; Murphy 2001). Binding proteins have been grouped into low-affinity (type I) and high-affinity chemokine-binding proteins (type II). Orthopoxviruses encode a high-affinity (type II) binding protein found in two copies within the ITRs in vaccinia virus (C23R, B29R) but only one copy in variola virus, which has far smaller ITRs. This protein, also called vCCI or CBR II, binds CC chemokines but not CXC or C chemokines. The binding to CC chemokines serves to prevent binding of the CC chemokines to the appropriate G-protein-coupled receptor (Graham et al. 1997; Smith et al. 1997; Alcami et al. 1998; Smith and Alcami 2000). The orthopoxvirus protein binds to a large variety but not all CC chemokines (Burns et al. 2002). Despite the ability to bind to a wide spectrum of CC chemokines, disruption of the gene in vaccinia virus leads to only modest attenuation but an increased leukocyte infiltration (Martinez-Pomares et al. 1995; Graham et al. 1997; Lalani et al. 1999).

Rather than encode chemokine-soluble receptors or binding proteins, MCV encodes a chemokine homologue (MC148R) (Senkevich et al. 1996). The protein is a secreted 104 amino acid protein related to the CC-chemokine family (Bugert et al. 1998) but contains an N-terminal deletion which precedes a dicysteine motif that is critical for activation of receptors. Therefore, the protein can engage or titrate receptors in a nonproductive fashion and function as an antagonist. Indeed, the protein inhibits binding, signaling, and chemotaxis of leukocytes to various CC and CXC chemokines (Krathwohl et al. 1997; Damon et al. 1998). While the protein has only been studied in the context of vaccinia virus recombinants, or as a purified protein, it can be argued that MC148R exhibits anti-inflammatory effects because it can inhibit allograft rejection in transgenic mice (DeBruyne et al. 2000).

3β-Hydroxysteroid dehydrogenase (ORF A44L)

The A44L protein catalyzes the synthesis of immunosuppressive steroids and is capable of converting pregnenolone to the steroid hormone progesterone (Moore and Smith 1992). Deletion of this gene from vaccinia virus leads to somewhat smaller dermal lesions and attenuation (Moore and Smith 1992; Sroller et al. 1998; Tscharke et al. 2002).

Semaphorin (A39R)

Semaphorins are a highly conserved family of regulatory proteins defined by the presence of a SEMA domain and an extracellular component that determines receptor-binding specificity. Semaphorins can be anchored to membranes, occur as transmembrane components, or be secreted (Spriggs and Sher 1999; Tamagnone and Comoglio 2000). Semaphorins originally were not associated with the immune system; they serve as axonal guidance clues in the developing nervous sytem. However, they also serve as chemoattractants or chemorepellants in the immune system. Recent evidence suggests additional roles for semaphorins in regulating the immune response. The semaphorin SEMA4D (CD100) SEMA4D (CD100), expressed constitutively by T cells, enhances the activation of B cells and dendritic cells (DC) through its cell-surface receptor, CD72. SEMA4A, when expressed by DCs, is involved in the activation of T cells through interactions with TIM2. Emerging evidence indicates that additional semaphorins and related molecules are involved in T-cell antigen-presenting cell (APC) interactions (Kikutani and Kumanogoh 2003). The vaccinia virus protein (A39R) encodes a 55 kDa protein with 25 percent homology to cellular semaphorins (Kolodkin et al. 1993; Comeau et al. 1998). It is believed that the A39R protein interacts with an appropriate semaphorin protein receptor, VESPR (also referred to as CD232 or plexin C1) to induce production of the cytokines IL-6 and IL-8 to control inflammation (Comeau et al. 1998). Deletion of the gene from vaccinia virus led to increased size and prolonged persistence of skin lesions but in a virus-strain-dependent manner (Gardner et al. 2001). It has been suggested that the protein has direct or indirect proinflammatory effects (Gardner et al. 2001).

Serpins

Orthopoxviruses encode three serpins (serine proteinase inhibitors) designated as SPI-1 (C12L), SPI-2/crmA (B13R/B14R), and SPI-3 (K2L). The leporipoxviruses also encode three serpins, designated SERP1, SERP2, and SERP3. The number of serpins encoded by an individual virus can vary. The avipoxviruses can encode five or more. The serpin most universally distributed appears by sequence to be an ortholog of SPI-2/crmA. SPI-2/crmA is functionally very similar to SERP2 and SPI-3 is very similar to SERP1. MCV encodes no serpins.

SPI-3

SPI-3 (K2L, VACWR033) and SERP1 of myxoma virus are biochemically very similar. The proteinases inhibited by SERP1 include plasmin, tissue plasminogen activator, urokinase, and thrombin (Lomas et al. 1993; Nash et al. 1998). These proteases are the same as those inhibited by the SPI-3 protein even though the two proteins are only 29 percent identical (Turner et al. 2000). Nevertheless, SPI-3 can not replace SERP1 to maintain virulence in myxoma virus (Wang et al. 2000) and deletion of SPI-3 from vaccinia virus or cowpox virus leads to little if any attenuation of the virus in animals. SPI-3 inhibits orthopoxvirus-infected cell fusion, a property

absent in SERP1 (Wang et al. 2000). The myxoma virus SERP1 is an extremely powerful anti-inflammatory protein (Upton et al. 1990; Macen et al. 1993) which when deleted leads to increased inflammation and a marked attenuation and more rapid clearance of myxoma virus in rabbits (Upton et al. 1990; Macen et al. 1993). Purified SERP1 has been shown to prevent inflammation following balloon angioplasty (Lucas et al. 1996; Liu et al. 2000) and allograft and xenograft transplant rejection in animal models (Miller et al. 2000).

SPI-2/CRMA

The SPI-2 gene (B13R/B14R in vaccinia virus), was originally discovered in cowpox virus where the gene was designated as crmA. The role of this protein in regulating IL-1β and IL-18 has been discussed earlier in this chapter. In addition to being an effective inhibitor of caspase-1, it is also an effective inhibitor of caspase-8 and perhaps caspase-10. Inhibition of caspases-8 and/or 10 targets key apical caspases in the pathways of apoptosis, initiated by caspase-8, TNF- or Fas-ligands (Enari et al. 1995; Tewari and Dixit 1995; Dobbelstein and Shenk 1996; Kettle et al. 1997). This serpin can also inhibit the serine protease granzyme B, a product of NK and cytotoxic T cells, delivered to target cells to initiate perforin-dependent apoptotic killing (Quan et al. 1995; Tewari et al. 1995). Therefore SPI-2/crmA is referred to as a cross-class inhibitor because of activity against both thiol and serine proteases. This cross-class specificity is shared by the myxoma virus SERP2 protein (Turner et al. 1999). Deletion of SERP2 from myxoma virus leads to attenuation, increased inflammation, and apoptosis of lymphoid cells (Petit et al. 1996; Messud-Petit et al. 1998). Despite the overt functional similarities between SERP2 and the orthopoxvirus SPI-2/crmA, deletion of the gene from vaccinia virus (Kettle et al. 1995) or cowpox virus (Thompson et al. 1993) leads to little if any attenuation of intranasal virus infection of animals. However, when virus is introduced into the ear pinnae of the mouse, deletion of the SPI-2/crmA gene leads to enhanced virulence (Tscharke et al. 2002). In addition to serpin-mediated inhibition of apoptosis, a second activity, as yet unidentified, also directly modulates the mitochondrial apoptotic pathway by influencing the permeability transition core (Wasilenko et al. 2001).

SPI-1

Although grouped for simplicity with the other serpins, the SPI-1 gene is best known as a host-range gene and is discussed below.

Host-range genes

SPI-1 (ORF C12L/B22R)

The orthopoxvirus serpin SPI-1 inhibits cathepsin G, a major constituent of neutrophils (Moon et al. 1999) and deletion of the gene leads to loss of the ability of the virus to grow on human and swine cells (Ali et al. 1994). The phenotype conferred on infected cells appears perhaps to be virus dependent. In the case of RPV, infection of nonpermissive human cells leads to viral DNA replication and full expression of viral proteins and an apoptoticlike phenotype (Brooks et al. 1995) but with vaccinia virus, the nonpermissive infection was characterized by very low levels of intermediate and late viral mRNAs (Shisler et al. 1999). Deletion of the gene from the virus has only modest effects on virulence (Blake et al. 1995).

K3L AND E3L

The orthopoxvirus genes K3L and E3L have been previously discussed in the context of their involvement in controlling the interferon response. They are also required for broad virus host range. The E3L gene product, which binds double-stranded RNA, is required for replication in HeLa cells, but not BHK cells. The K3L gene functions as a competitive inhibitor for eIF2α phosphorylation. BHK cells are believed to contain relatively low levels of PKR. It is believed that during infection of BHK cells, there are sufficient levels of K3L, even in the absence of E3L, to prevent activation of PKR, thus offering an explanation for why K3L is required for replication in BHK cells. The reverse situation exists for HeLa cells where E3L is required. In this situation, the levels of E3L are sufficient to sequester all virus-induced dsRNA, alleviating the need for K3L (Langland and Jacobs 2002). Infection of nonpermissive cells with virus deleted for E3L also leads to apoptosis and the virus is profoundly attenuated when used to infect mice either intracranially or intranasally (Brandt and Jacobs 2001). Infection of nonpermissive cells with virus deleted for K3L also leads to apoptosis but the virus has not yet been tested in mice (B. Jacobs, personal communication).

CHOHR (CP77), K1L, AND C7L

Three orthopoxvirus host-range genes have been identified. All three gene products contain ankyrin repeats. The genes are dissimilar in size and sequence but are functionally related. The CP77 gene of cowpox virus encodes a 77 kDa protein that confers on the virus the ability to grow on Chinese hamster ovary (CHO) cells (Spehner et al. 1988). The corresponding gene is present intact in variola virus (D6L, Garcia strain) but is truncated and nonfunctional in vaccinia virus strain WR (B24L) and deleted in vaccinia virus Copenhagen. Vaccinia can not grow on CHO cells. The K1L and C7L genes which encode 30 and 17 kDa proteins, respectively, and the CP77 gene are under certain conditions functionally interchangeable and somewhat hierarchical in terms of control of host range. Each will allow growth of virus in porcine or human cells. Similarly, the K1L

and CP77 genes are interchangeable in that both allow virus growth in RK13 cells. Defects in K1L (Ink et al. 1995; Chung et al. 1997) have been linked to induction of apoptosis during infection of the respective nonpermissive cells, but apoptosis is likely not the primary cause of the abortive infection. When virus defective in K1L is used to infect nonpermissive RK13 cells, early transcripts are synthesized but early protein synthesis is arrested (Ramsey-Ewing and Moss 1996; Chung et al. 1997). Vaccinia virus infection of CHO cells is characterized by a block in the translation of intermediate mRNAs which prevents synthesis of late mRNAs (Ramsey-Ewing and Moss 1995). There appears to be no effect of either the the K1L or CP77 gene in animal models (Chen et al. 1992, 1993). Less is known about the function of the C7L gene (Oguiura et al. 1993).

Inhibition of apoptosis

A number of the genes previously discussed control apoptosis. These include the orthopoxvirus caspase and granzyme B inhibitor SPI-2/crmA. Viral proteins which target the IFN response pathway, such as the decoy receptors and the E3L and K3L genes, can also be viewed as inhibitors of apoptosis because induction of both PKR and OAS which are intimately controlled by these viral proteins also induce apoptosis by activating caspase-8 (Gil and Esteban 2000). MCV encodes some unique regulators of apoptosis.

MC66

The MC66 ORF encodes an inhibitor of ultraviolet- or peroxide-mediated apoptosis (Shisler et al. 1998). The protein has homology to human glutathione peroxidase and is a member of the class of selenocysteine-containing proteins (Moss et al. 2000) that can be considered to function as an antioxidants. This MCV selenoprotein protects human keratinocytes against the cytotoxic effects of ultraviolet irradiation and hydrogen peroxide, providing a mechanism for a virus to defend itself against environmental stress. Enzymes such as these convert hydrogen peroxide into water and oxygen, which together with catalase and superoxide dismutase reduce levels of oxygen-reactive metabolites, which if left unchecked, would damage the cellular environment or induce apoptosis.

MC159R

Both MC159R and the related protein M160R each contain two death effector domains (DED) (Senkevich et al. 1997), which are critical motifs involved in regulating apoptosis. MC159 binds to Fas-associated death domain (FADD) as well as procaspase-8 and acts to protect transfected cells against death effector filament formation and apoptosis induced by either Fas ligand or TNF-α (Bertin et al. 1997; Hu et al. 1997; Thome et al. 1997; Tsukumo and Yonehara 1999). Proteins such as this are referred to as viral FLICE inhibitory proteins (vFLIP) because of their ability to complex with procaspase-8 or FADD to prevent activation of procaspase-8 to active caspase-8. The function of MC160R, despite having two DED domains, is less clear. While the MC160R protein does have some anti-apoptotic activity, it is weak (Hu et al. 1997). Furthermore, the protein undergoes degradation by caspases in the absence of MC159R, indicating that one role of MC159R is to stabilize MC160R (Shisler and Moss 2001b).

REFERENCES

Ada, G.L. and Blanden, R.V. 1994. CTL immunity and cytokine regulation in viral infection. *Res Immunol*, **145**, 625–8.

Afonso, C.L., Tulman, E.R., et al. 2000. The genome of fowlpox virus. *J Virol*, **74**, 3815–31.

Ahn, B.Y. and Moss, B. 1989. Capped poly(A) leaders of variable lengths at the 5′ ends of vaccinia virus late mRNAs. *J Virol*, **63**, 226–32.

Ahn, B.Y., Gershon, P.D., et al. 1990a. Identification of *rpo30*, a vaccinia virus RNA polymerase gene with structural similarity to a eucaryotic transcription elongation factor. *Mol Cell Biol*, **10**, 5433–41.

Ahn, B.Y., Jones, E.V. and Moss, B. 1990b. Identification of the vaccinia virus gene encoding an 18-kilodalton subunit of RNA polymerase and demonstration of a 5′ poly(A) leader on its early transcript. *J Virol*, **64**, 3019–24.

Ahn, B.Y., Rosel, J., et al. 1992. Identification and expression of *rpo19*, a vaccinia virus gene encoding a 19-kilodalton DNA-dependent RNA polymerase subunit. *J Virol*, **66**, 971–82.

Ahn, B.Y., Gershon, P.D. and Moss, B. 1994. RNA polymerase-associated protein Rap94 confers promoter specificity for initiating transcription of vaccinia virus early stage genes. *J Biol Chem*, **269**, 7552–7.

Alcami, A. 2003. Viral mimicry of cytokines, chemokines and their receptors. *Nat Rev Immunol*, **3**, 36–50.

Alcami, A. and Smith, G.L. 1992. A soluble receptor for interleukin-1β encoded by vaccinia virus: a novel mechanism of virus modulation of the host response to infection. *Cell*, **71**, 153–67.

Alcami, A. and Smith, G.L. 1996. A mechanism for the inhibition of fever by a virus. *Proc Natl Acad Sci U S A*, **93**, 11029–34.

Alcami, A., Symons, J.A., et al. 1998. Blockade of chemokine activity by a soluble chemokine binding protein from vaccinia virus. *J Immunol*, **160**, 624–33.

Alcami, A., Khanna, A., et al. 1999. Vaccinia virus strains Lister, USSR and Evans express soluble and cell-surface tumour necrosis factor receptors. *J Gen Virol*, **80**, 949–59.

Ali, A.N., Turner, P.C., et al. 1994. The *SPI-1* gene of rabbitpox virus determines host range and is required for hemorrhagic pock formation. *Virology*, **202**, 306–14.

Amegadzie, B.Y., Ahn, B.Y. and Moss, B. 1991a. Identification, sequence, and expression of the gene encoding a Mr 35,000 subunit of the vaccinia virus DNA-dependent RNA polymerase. *J Biol Chem*, **266**, 13712–18.

Amegadzie, B.Y., Holmes, M.H., et al. 1991b. Identification, sequence, and expression of the gene encoding the second-largest subunit of the vaccinia virus DNA-dependent RNA polymerase. *Virology*, **180**, 88–98.

Amegadzie, B.Y., Ahn, B.Y. and Moss, B. 1992. Characterization of a 7-kilodalton subunit of vaccinia virus DNA-dependent RNA polymerase with structural similarities to the smallest subunit of eukaryotic RNA polymerase II. *J Virol*, **66**, 3003–10.

Andres, G., Garcia-Escudero, R., et al. 1998. African swine fever virus is enveloped by a two-membraned collapsed cisterna derived from the endoplasmic reticulum. *J Virol*, **72**, 8988–9001.

Baldick, C.J.J. and Moss, B. 1993. Characterization and temporal regulation of mRNAs encoded by vaccinia virus intermediate-stage genes. *J Virol*, **67**, 3515–27.

Banham, A.H. and Smith, G.L. 1992. Vaccinia virus gene *B1R* encodes a 34-kDa serine/threonine protein kinase that localizes in cytoplasmic factories and is packaged into virions. *Virology*, **191**, 803–12.

Baldick, C.J.J., Keck, J.G. and Moss, B. 1992. Mutational analysis of the core, spacer, and initiator regions of vaccinia virus intermediate-class promoters. *J Virol*, **66**, 4710–19.

Barbosa, E. and Moss, B. 1978a. mRNA(nucleoside-2′-)-methyltransferase from vaccinia virus. Characteristics and substrate specificity. *J Biol Chem*, **253**, 7698–702.

Barbosa, E. and Moss, B. 1978b. mRNA(nucleoside-2′-)-methyltransferase from vaccinia virus. Purification and physical properties. *J Biol Chem*, **253**, 7692–7.

Baroudy, B.M. and Moss, B. 1980. Purification and characterization of a DNA-dependent RNA polymerase from vaccinia virions. *J Biol Chem*, **255**, 4372–80.

Baroudy, B.M., Venkatesan, S. and Moss, B. 1982. Incompletely base-paired flip-flop terminal loops link the two DNA strands of the vaccinia virus genome into one uninterrupted polynucleotide chain. *Cell*, **28**, 315–24.

Barry, M. and Bleackley, R.C. 2002. Cytotoxic T lymphocytes: all roads lead to death. *Nat Rev Immunol*, **2**, 401–9.

Bayliss, C.D. and Condit, R.C. 1995. The vaccinia virus *A18R* gene product is a DNA-dependent ATPase. *J Biol Chem*, **270**, 1550–6.

Beaud, G., Beaud, R. and Leader, D.P. 1995. Vaccinia virus gene *H5R* encodes a protein that is phosphorylated by the multisubstrate vaccinia virus B1R protein kinase. *J Virol*, **69**, 1819–26.

Bertholet, C., Van Meir, E., et al. 1987. Vaccinia virus produces late mRNAs by discontinuous synthesis. *Cell*, **50**, 153–62.

Bertin, J., Armstrong, R.C., et al. 1997. Death effector domain-containing herpesvirus and poxvirus proteins inhibit both Fas- and TNFR1-induced apoptosis. *Proc Natl Acad Sci U S A*, **94**, 1172–6.

Betakova, T., Wolffe, E.J. and Moss, B. 1999. Regulation of vaccinia virus morphogenesis: phosphorylation of the A14L and A17L membrane proteins and C-terminal truncation of the A17L protein are dependent on the F10L kinase. *J Virol*, **73**, 3534–43.

Black, E.P. and Condit, R.C. 1996. Phenotypic characterization of mutants in vaccinia virus gene *G2R*, a putative transcription elongation factor. *J Virol*, **70**, 47–54.

Black, M.E. and Hruby, D.E. 1990. Quaternary structure of vaccinia virus thymidine kinase. *Biochem Biophys Res Commun*, **169**, 1080–6.

Blake, N.W., Kettle, S., et al. 1995. Vaccinia virus serpins B13R and B22R do not inhibit antigen presentation to class I-restricted cytotoxic T lymphocytes. *J Gen Virol*, **76**, 2393–8.

Blasco, R. and Moss, B. 1991. Extracellular vaccinia virus formation and cell-to-cell virus transmission are prevented by deletion of the gene encoding the 37,000-Dalton outer envelope protein. *J Virol*, **65**, 5910–20.

Blasco, R. and Moss, B. 1992. Role of cell-associated enveloped vaccinia virus in cell-to-cell spread. *J Virol*, **66**, 4170–9.

Born, T.L., Morrison, L.A., et al. 2000. A poxvirus protein that binds to and inactivates IL-18, and inhibits NK cell response. *J Immunol*, **164**, 3246–54.

Boshkov, L.K., Macen, J.L. and McFadden, G. 1992. Virus-induced loss of class I MHC antigens from the surface of cells infected with myxoma virus and malignant rabbit fibroma virus. *J Immunol*, **148**, 881–7.

Bossart, W., Nuss, D.L. and Paoletti, E. 1978. Effect of UV irradiation on the expression of vaccinia virus gene products synthesized in a cell-free system coupling transcription and translation. *J Virol*, **26**, 673–80.

Boulter, E.A. and Appleyard, G. 1973. Differences between extracellular and intracellular forms of poxvirus and their implications. *Prog Med Virol*, **16**, 86–108.

Boulter, E.A., Zwartouw, H.T., et al. 1971. The nature of the immune state produced by inactivated vaccinia virus in rabbits. *Am J Epidemiol*, **94**, 612–20.

Bowie, A., Kiss-Toth, E., et al. 2000. A46R and A52R from vaccinia virus are antagonists of host IL-1 and toll- like receptor signaling. *Proc Natl Acad Sci U S A*, **97**, 10162–7.

Brandt, T.A. and Jacobs, B.L. 2001. Both carboxy- and amino-terminal domains of the vaccinia virus interferon resistance gene, *E3L*, are required for pathogenesis in a mouse model. *J Virol*, **75**, 850–6.

Brooks, M.A., Ali, A.N., et al. 1995. A rabbitpox virus serpin gene controls host range by inhibiting apoptosis in restrictive cells. *J Virol*, **12**, 7688–98.

Broyles, S.S. 1991. A role for ATP hydrolysis in vaccinia virus early gene transcription. Dissociation of the early transcription factor-promoter complex. *J Biol Chem*, **266**, 15545–8.

Broyles, S.S. 1993. Vaccinia virus encodes a functional dUTPase. *Virology*, **195**, 863–5.

Broyles, S.S. 2003. Vaccinia virus transcription. *J Gen Virol*, **84**, 2293–303.

Broyles, S.S. and Fesler, B.S. 1990. Vaccinia virus gene encoding a component of the viral early transcription factor. *J Virol*, **64**, 1523–9.

Broyles, S.S. and Moss, B. 1986. Homology between RNA polymerases of poxviruses, prokaryotes, and eukaryotes: nucleotide sequence and transcriptional analysis of vaccinia virus genes encoding 147-kDa and 22-kDa subunits. *Proc Natl Acad Sci U S A*, **83**, 3141–5.

Broyles, S.S. and Pennington, M.J. 1990. Vaccinia virus gene encoding a 30-kilodalton subunit of the viral DNA- dependent RNA polymerase. *J Virol*, **64**, 5376–82.

Broyles, S.S., Li, J. and Moss, B. 1991. Promoter DNA contacts made by the vaccinia virus early transcription factor. *J Biol Chem*, **266**, 15539–44.

Broyles, S.S., Liu, X., et al. 1999. Transcription factor YY1 is a vaccinia virus late promoter activator. *J Biol Chem*, **274**, 35662–7.

Bugert, J.J., Lohmuller, C., et al. 1998. Chemokine homolog of molluscum contagiosum virus: sequence conservation and expression. *Virology*, **242**, 51–9.

Buller, R.M. and Palumbo, G.J. 1991. Poxvirus pathogenesis. *Microbiol Rev*, **55**, 80–122.

Burns, J.M., Dairaghi, D.J., et al. 2002. Comprehensive mapping of poxvirus vCCI chemokine-binding protein – expanded range of ligand interactions and unusual dissociation kinetics. *J Biol Chem*, **277**, 2785–9.

Byrd, C.M., Bolken, T.C. and Hruby, D.E. 2002. The vaccinia virus *I7L* gene product is the core protein proteinase. *J Virol*, **76**, 8973–6.

Cacoullos, N. and Bablanian, R. 1993. Role of polyadenylated RNA sequences (POLADS) in vaccinia virus infection: correlation between accumulation of POLADS and extent of shut-off in infected cells. *Cell Mol Biol Res*, **39**, 657–64.

Carpenter, M.S. and DeLange, A.M. 1991. A temperature-sensitive lesion in the small subunit of the vaccinia virus-encoded mRNA capping enzyme causes a defect in viral telomere resolution. *J Virol*, **65**, 4042–50.

Carpenter, M.S. and DeLange, A.M. 1992. Identification of a temperature-sensitive mutant of vaccinia virus defective in late but not intermediate gene expression. *Virology*, **188**, 233–44.

Cassetti, M.A. and Moss, B. 1996. Interaction of the 82-kDa subunit of the vaccinia virus early transcription factor heterodimer with the promoter core sequence directs downstream DNA binding of the 70-kDa subunit. *Proc Natl Acad Sci U S A*, **93**, 7540–5.

Cassetti, M.C., Merchlinsky, M., et al. 1998. DNA packaging mutant: repression of the vaccinia virus *A32* gene results in noninfectious, DNA-deficient, spherical, enveloped particles. *J Virol*, **72**, 5769–80.

Chakrabarti, S., Brechling, K. and Moss, B. 1985. Vaccinia virus expression vector: coexpression of beta-galactosidase provides visual screening of recombinant virus plaques. *Mol Cell Biol*, **5**, 3403–9.

Chang, H.W. and Jacobs, B.L. 1993. Identification of a conserved motif that is necessary for binding of the vaccinia virus *E3L* gene products to double-stranded RNA. *Virology*, **194**, 537–47.

Chen, W., Drillien, R., et al. 1992. Restricted replication of ectromelia virus in cell culture correlates with mutations in virus-encoded host range gene. *Virology*, **187**, 433–42.

Chen, W., Drillien, R., et al. 1993. In vitro and in vivo study of ectromelia virus homolog of the vaccinia virus *K1L* host range gene. *Virology*, **196**, 682–93.

Cheng, C., Kussie, P., et al. 1998. Conservation of structure and mechanism between eukaryotic topoisomerase I and site-specific recombinases. *Cell*, **92**, 841–50.

Chiu, W.L. and Chang, W. 2002. Vaccinia virus J1R protein: a viral membrane protein that is essential for virion morphogenesis. *J Virol*, **76**, 9575–87.

Christen, L.M., Sanders, M., et al. 1998. Vaccinia virus nucleoside triphosphate phosphohydrolase I is an essential viral early gene transcription termination factor. *Virology*, **245**, 360–71.

Chung, C.S., Vasilevskaya, I.A., et al. 1997. Apoptosis and host restriction of vaccinia virus in RK13 cells. *Virus Res*, **52**, 121–32.

Colinas, R.J., Condit, R.C. and Paoletti, E. 1990. Extrachromosomal recombination in vaccinia-infected cells requires a functional DNA polymerase participating at a level other than DNA replication. *Virus Res*, **18**, 49–70.

Comeau, M.R., Johnson, R., et al. 1998. A poxvirus-encoded semaphorin induces cytokine production from monocytes and binds to a novel cellular semaphorin receptor, VESPR. *Immunity*, **8**, 473–82.

Condit, R.C. and Niles, E.G. 1990. Orthopoxvirus genetics. *Curr Top Microbiol Immunol*, **163**, 1–39.

Condit, R.C. and Niles, E.G. 2002. Regulation of viral transcription elongation and termination during vaccinia virus infection. *Biochim Biophys Acta*, **1577**, 325–36.

Condit, R.C., Lewis, J.I., et al. 1996a. Use of lysolecithin-permeabilized infected-cell extracts to investigate the in vitro biochemical phenotypes of poxvirus ts mutations altered in viral transcription activity. *Virology*, **218**, 169–80.

Condit, R.C., Xiang, Y. and Lewis, J.I. 1996b. Mutation of vaccinia virus gene *G2R* causes suppression of gene *A18R ts* mutants: implications for control of transcription. *Virology*, **220**, 10–19.

Cudmore, S., Reckmann, I., et al. 1996. Vaccinia virus: a model system for actin-membrane interactions. *J Cell Sci*, **109**, 1739–47.

Cunnion, K.M. 1999. Tumor necrosis factor receptors encoded by poxviruses. *Mol Genet Metab*, **67**, 278–82.

Dales, S. and Mosbach, E.H. 1968. Vaccinia as a model for membrane biogenesis. *Virology*, **35**, 564–83.

Dales, S. and Pogo, B.G. 1981. Biology of poxviruses. *Virol Monogr*, **18**, 1–109.

Damon, I., Murphy, P.M. and Moss, B. 1998. Broad spectrum chemokine antagonistic activity of a human poxvirus chemokine homolog. *Proc Natl Acad Sci U S A*, **95**, 6403–7.

Davies, M.V., Chang, H.W., et al. 1993. The *E3L* and *K3L* vaccinia virus gene products stimulate translation through inhibition of the double-stranded RNA-dependent protein kinase by different mechanisms. *J Virol*, **67**, 1688–92.

Davison, A.J. and Moss, B. 1989a. Structure of vaccinia virus early promoters. *J Mol Biol*, **210**, 749–69.

Davison, A.J. and Moss, B. 1989b. Structure of vaccinia virus late promoters. *J Mol Biol*, **210**, 771–84.

DeBruyne, L.A., Li, K., et al. 2000. Gene transfer of virally encoded chemokine antagonists vMIP-II and MC148 prolongs cardiac allograft survival and inhibits donor-specific immunity. *Gene Ther*, **7**, 575–82.

DeFilippes, F.M. 1984. Effect of aphidicolin on vaccinia virus: isolation of an aphidicolin-resistant mutant. *J Virol*, **52**, 474–82.

Delange, A.M., Reddy, M., et al. 1986. Replication and resolution of cloned poxvirus telomeres in vivo generates linear minichromosomes with intact viral hairpin termini. *J Virol*, **59**, 249–59.

DeMasi, J. and Traktman, P. 2000. Clustered charge-to-alanine mutagenesis of the vaccinia virus *H5* gene: isolation of a dominant, temperature-sensitive mutant with a profound defect in morphogenesis. *J Virol*, **74**, 2393–405.

Deng, L. and Shuman, S. 1998. Vaccinia NPH-I, a DExH-box ATPase, is the energy coupling factor for mRNA transcription termination. *Genes Dev*, **12**, 538–46.

Derrien, M., Punjabi, A., et al. 1999. Tyrosine phosphorylation of *A17* during vaccinia virus infection: involvement of the H1 phosphatase and the F10 kinase. *J Virol*, **73**, 7287–96.

De Silva, F.S. and Moss, B. 2003. Vaccinia virus uracil DNA glycosylase has an essential role in DNA synthesis that is independent of its glycosylase activity: catalytic site mutations reduce virulence but not virus replication in cultured cells. *J Virol*, **77**, 159–66.

Diaz-Guerra, M. and Esteban, M. 1993. Vaccinia virus nucleoside triphosphate phosphohydrolase I controls early and late gene expression by regulating the rate of transcription. *J Virol*, **67**, 7561–72.

Dobbelstein, M. and Shenk, T. 1996. Protection against apoptosis by the vaccinia virus *SPI-2* (*B13R*) gene product. *J Virol*, **70**, 6479–85.

Domi, A. and Beaud, G. 2000. The punctate sites of accumulation of vaccinia virus early proteins are precursors of sites of viral DNA synthesis. *J Gen Virol*, **81**, 1231–5.

Domi, A. and Moss, B. 2002. Cloning the vaccinia virus genome as a bacterial artificial chromosome in *Escherichia coli* and recovery of infectious virus in mammalian cells. *Proc Natl Acad Sci U S A*, **99**, 12415–20.

Du, S. and Traktman, P. 1996. Vaccinia virus DNA replication: two hundred base pairs of telomeric sequence confer optimal replication efficiency on minichromosome templates. *Proc Natl Acad Sci U S A*, **93**, 9693–8.

Dubochet, J., Adrian, M., et al. 1994. Structure of intracellular mature vaccinia virus observed by cryoelectron microscopy. *J Virol*, **68**, 1935–41.

Easterbrook, K.B. 1966. Controlled degradation of vaccinia virions in vitro: an electron microscopic study. *J Ultrastruct Res*, **14**, 484–96.

Ellison, K.S., Peng, W. and McFadden, G. 1996. Mutations in active-site residues of the uracil-DNA glycosylase encoded by vaccinia virus are incompatible with virus viability. *J Virol*, **70**, 7965–73.

Enari, M., Hug, H. and Nagata, S. 1995. Involvement of an ICE-like protease in Fas-mediated apoptosis. *Nature*, **375**, 78–81.

Engelstad, M. and Smith, G.L. 1993. The vaccinia virus 42-kDa envelope protein is required for the envelopment and egress of extracellular virus and for virus virulence. *Virology*, **194**, 627–37.

Engelstad, M., Howard, S.T. and Smith, G.L. 1992. A constitutively expressed vaccinia gene encodes a 42-kDa glycoprotein related to complement control factors that forms part of the extracellular virus envelope. *Virology*, **188**, 801–10.

Ericsson, M., Cudmore, S., et al. 1995. Characterization of ts 16, a temperature-sensitive mutant of vaccinia virus. *J Virol*, **69**, 7072–86.

Esposito, J. and Fenner, F. 2001. Poxviruses. In: Knipe, D.E. and Howley, P.M. (eds), *Fields virology*. New York: Lippincott Williams and Wilkins, 2885–922.

Essani, K. and Dales, S. 1979. Biogenesis of vaccinia: evidence for more than 100 polypeptides in the virion. *Virology*, **95**, 385–94.

Evans, E. and Traktman, P. 1992. Characterization of vaccinia virus DNA replication mutants with lesions in the *D5* gene. *Chromosoma*, **102**, S72–82.

Evans, E., Klemperer, N., et al. 1995. The vaccinia virus D5 protein, which is required for DNA replication, is a nucleic acid-independent nucleoside triphosphatase. *J Virol*, **69**, 5353–61.

Falkner, F.G. and Moss, B. 1990. Transient dominant selection of recombinant vaccinia viruses. *J Virol*, **64**, 3108–11.

Fathi, Z., Sridhar, P., et al. 1986. Efficient targeted insertion of an unselected marker into the vaccinia virus genome. *Virology*, **155**, 97–105.

Franke, C.A., Rice, C.M., et al. 1985. Neomycin resistance as a dominant selectable marker for selection and isolation of vaccinia virus recombinants. *Mol Cell Biol*, **5**, 1918–24.

Fuerst, T.R., Niles, E.G., et al. 1986. Eukaryotic transient-expression system based on recombinant vaccinia virus that synthesizes bacteriophage T7 RNA polymerase. *Proc Natl Acad Sci U S A*, **83**, 8122–6.

Fuerst, T.R., Fernandez, M.P. and Moss, B. 1989. Transfer of the inducible lac repressor/operator system from *Escherichia coli* to a vaccinia virus expression vector. *Proc Natl Acad Sci U S A*, **86**, 2549–53.

Garcia, A.D. and Moss, B. 2001. Repression of vaccinia virus Holliday junction resolvase inhibits processing of viral DNA into unit-length genomes. *J Virol*, **75**, 6460–71.

Garcia, A.D., Aravind, L., et al. 2000. Bacterial-type DNA Holliday junction resolvases in eukaryotic viruses. *Proc Natl Acad Sci U S A*, **97**, 8926–31.

Gardner, J.D., Tscharke, D.C., et al. 2001. Vaccinia virus semaphorin A39R is a 50–55 kDa secreted glycoprotein that affects the outcome of infection in a murine intradermal model. *J Gen Virol*, **82**, 2083–93.

Gershon, P.D. 1998. mRNA 3′ end formation by vaccinia virus: mechanism of action of a heterodimeric poly(A) polymerase. *Semin Virol*, **8**, 343–50.

Gershon, P.D. and Moss, B. 1990. Early transcription factor subunits are encoded by vaccinia virus late genes. *Proc Natl Acad Sci U S A*, **87**, 4401–5.

Gershon, P.D. and Moss, B. 1992. Transition from rapid processive to slow nonprocessive polyadenylation by vaccinia virus poly(A) polymerase catalytic subunit is regulated by the net length of the poly(A) tail. *Genes Dev*, **6**, 1575–86.

Gershon, P.D. and Moss, B. 1993a. Stimulation of poly(A) tail elongation by the VP39 subunit of the vaccinia virus-encoded poly(A) polymerase. *J Biol Chem*, **268**, 2203–10.

Gershon, P.D. and Moss, B. 1993b. Uridylate-containing RNA sequences determine specificity for binding and polyadenylation by the catalytic subunit of vaccinia virus poly(A) polymerase. *EMBO J*, **12**, 4705–14.

Gershon, P.D., Ahn, B.Y., et al. 1991. Poly(A) polymerase and a dissociable polyadenylation stimulatory factor encoded by vaccinia virus. *Cell*, **66**, 1269–78.

Gershon, P.D., Shi, X. and Hodel, A.E. 1998. Evidence that the RNA methylation and poly(A) polymerase stimulatory activities of vaccinia virus protein VP39 do not impinge upon one another. *Virology*, **246**, 253–65.

Gil, J. and Esteban, M. 2000. Induction of apoptosis by the dsRNA-dependent protein kinase (PKR): Mechanism of action. *Apoptosis*, **5**, 107–14.

Goebel, S.J., Johnson, G.P., et al. 1990. The complete DNA sequence of vaccinia virus. *Virology*, **179**, 247-266, 517–63.

Graham, K.A., Lalani, A.S., et al. 1997. The T1/35kDa family of poxvirus secreted proteins bind chemokines and modulate leukocyte influx into virus infected tissues. *Virology*, **229**, 12–24.

Griffiths, G., Roos, N., et al. 2001a. Structure and assembly of intracellular mature vaccinia virus: thin-section analyses. *J Virol*, **75**, 11056–70.

Griffiths, G., Wepf, R., et al. 2001b. Structure and assembly of intracellular mature vaccinia virus: isolated-particle analysis. *J Virol*, **75**, 11034–55.

Gross, C.H. and Shuman, S. 1996. Vaccinia virions lacking the RNA helicase nucleoside triphosphate phosphohydrolase II are defective in early transcription. *J Virol*, **70**, 8549–57.

Gu, Y., Kuida, K., et al. 1997. Activation of interferon-gamma inducing factor mediated by interleukin-1beta converting enzyme. *Science*, **275**, 206–9.

Guan, K.L., Broyles, S.S. and Dixon, J.E. 1991. A Tyr/Ser protein phosphatase encoded by vaccinia virus. *Nature*, **350**, 359–62.

Guerin, J.L., Gelfi, J., et al. 2002. Myxoma virus leukemia-associated protein is responsible for major histocompatibility complex class I and Fas-CD95 down-regulation and defines scrapins, a new group of surface cellular receptor abductor proteins. *J Virol*, **76**, 2912–23.

Harte, M.T., Haga, I.R., et al. 2003. The poxvirus protein A52R targets Toll-like receptor signaling complexes to suppress host defense. *J Exp Med*, **197**, 343–51.

Hassett, D.E. and Condit, R.C. 1994. Targeted construction of temperature-sensitive mutations in vaccinia virus by replacing clustered charged residues with alanine. *Proc Natl Acad Sci U S A*, **91**, 4554–8.

Hassett, D.E., Lewis, J.I., et al. 1997. Analysis of a temperature-sensitive vaccinia virus mutant in the viral mRNA capping enzyme isolated by clustered charge-to-alanine mutagenesis and transient dominant selection. *Virology*, **238**, 391–409.

Heng, M.C., Steuer, M.E., et al. 1989. Lack of host cellular immune response in eruptive molluscum contagiosum. *Am J Dermatopathol*, **11**, 248–54.

Herrera, E., Lorenzo, M.D., et al. 1998. Functional analysis of vaccinia virus B5R protein: essential role in virus envelopment is independent of a large portion of the extracellular domain. *J Virol*, **72**, 294–302.

Hertig, C., Coupar, B.E.H., et al. 1997. Field and vaccine strains of fowlpox virus carry integrated sequences from the avian retrovirus, reticuloendotheliosis virus. *Virology*, **235**, 367–76.

Higman, M.A., Christen, L.A. and Niles, E.G. 1994. The mRNA (guanine-7-)methyltransferase domain of the vaccinia virus mRNA capping enzyme. Expression in *Escherichia coli* and structural and kinetic comparison to the intact capping enzyme. *J Biol Chem*, **269**, 14974–81.

Hirschmann, P., Vos, J.C. and Stunnenberg, H.G. 1990. Mutational analysis of a vaccinia virus intermediate promoter in vivo and in vitro. *J Virol*, **64**, 6063–9.

Hodel, A.E., Gershon, P.D., et al. 1996. The 1.85 A structure of vaccinia protein VP39: a bifunctional enzyme that participates in the modification of both mRNA ends. *Cell*, **85**, 247–56.

Hollinshead, M., Vanderplasschen, A., et al. 1999. Vaccinia virus intracellular mature virions contain only one lipid membrane. *J Virol*, **73**, 1503–17.

Hollinshead, M., Rodger, G., et al. 2001. Vaccinia virus utilizes microtubules for movement to the cell surface. *J Cell Biol*, **154**, 389–402.

Hooda-Dhingra, U., Thompson, C.L. and Condit, R.C. 1989. Detailed phenotypic characterization of five temperature-sensitive mutants in the 22- and 147-kilodalton subunits of vaccinia virus DNA-dependent RNA polymerase. *J Virol*, **63**, 714–29.

Howard, S.T., Ray, C.A., et al. 1999. A 43-nucleotide RNA cis-acting element governs the site-specific formation of the 3′ end of a poxvirus late mRNA. *Virology*, **255**, 190–204.

Hruby, D.E. and Ball, L.A. 1982. Mapping and identification of the vaccinia virus thymidine kinase gene. *J Virol*, **43**, 403–9.

Hu, F.Q., Smith, C.A. and Pickup, D.J. 1994. Cowpox virus contains two copies of an early gene encoding a soluble secreted form of the type II TNF receptor. *Virology*, **204**, 343–56.

Hu, S., Vincenz, C., et al. 1997. A novel family of viral death effector domain-containing molecules that inhibit both CD-95- and tumor necrosis factor receptor-1-induced apoptosis. *J Biol Chem*, **272**, 9621–9624.

Hughes, S.J., Johnston, L.H., et al. 1991. Vaccinia virus encodes an active thymidylate kinase that complements a *cdc8* mutant of *Saccharomyces cerevisiae*. *J Biol Chem*, **266**, 20103–9.

Ichihashi, Y., Matsumoto, S. and Dales, S. 1971. Biogenesis of poxviruses: role of A-type inclusions and host cell membranes in virus dissemination. *Virology*, **46**, 507–32.

Ichihashi, Y., Oie, M. and Tsuruhara, T. 1984. Location of DNA-binding proteins and disulfide-linked proteins in vaccinia virus structural elements. *J Virol*, **50**, 929–38.

Ink, B.S., Gilbert, C.S. and Evan, G.I. 1995. Delay of vaccinia virus-induced apoptosis in nonpermissive Chinese hamster ovary cells by the cowpox virus *CHOhr* and adenovirus *E1B* 19K genes. *J Virol*, **69**, 661–8.

Isaacs, S.N., Kotwal, G.J. and Moss, B. 1992. Vaccinia virus complement-control protein prevents antibody-dependent complement-enhanced neutralization of infectivity and contributes to virulence. *Proc Natl Acad Sci U S A*, **89**, 628–32.

Ishii, K. and Moss, B. 2001a. Role of vaccinia virus A20R protein in DNA replication: construction and characterization of temperature-sensitive mutants. *J Virol*, **75**, 1656–63.

Ishii, K. and Moss, B. 2001b. Role of vaccinia virus A20R protein in DNA replication: construction and characterization of temperature-sensitive mutants. *J Virol*, **75**, 1656–63.

Ishii, K. and Moss, B. 2002. Mapping interaction sites of the A20R protein component of the vaccinia virus DNA replication complex. *Virology*, **303**, 232–9.

Jensen, O.N., Houthaeve, T., et al. 1996. Identification of the major membrane and core proteins of vaccinia virus by two-dimensional electrophoresis. *J Virol*, **70**, 7485–97.

Kaplan, C. 1962. A non-infectious smallpox vaccine. *Lancet*, **2**, 1027–8.

Kaplan, C., McClean, D. and Vallet, L. 1962. A note on the immunogenicity of ultra-violet irradiated vaccinia virus in man. *J Hyg (Camb)*, **60**, 79–83.

Kaplan, C., Benson, P.F. and Butler, N.R. 1965. Immunogenicity of ultraviolet-irradiated non-infectious vaccinia-virus vaccine in infants and young children. *Lancet*, **1**, 573–4.

Kates, J. and Beeson, J. 1970a. Ribonucleic acid synthesis in vaccinia virus. I. The mechanism of synthesis and release of RNA in vaccinia cores. *J Mol Biol*, **50**, 1–18.

Kates, J. and Beeson, J. 1970b. Ribonucleic acid synthesis in vaccinia virus. II. Synthesis of polyriboadenylic acid. *J Mol Biol*, **50**, 19–33.

Kates, J.R. and McAuslan, B.R. 1967. Poxvirus DNA-dependent RNA polymerase. *Proc Natl Acad Sci U S A*, **58**, 134–41.

Keck, J.G., Baldick, C.J.J. and Moss, B. 1990. Role of DNA replication in vaccinia virus gene expression: a naked template is required for transcription of three late trans-activator genes. *Cell*, **61**, 801–9.

Kerr, S.M. and Smith, G.L. 1991. Vaccinia virus DNA ligase is nonessential for virus replication: recovery of plasmids from virus-infected cells. *Virology*, **180**, 625–32.

Kettle, S., Blake, N.W., et al. 1995. Vaccinia virus serpins B13R (SPI-2) and B22R (SPI-1) encode M(r) 38.5 and 40K, intracellular polypeptides that do not affect virus virulence in a murine intranasal model. *Virology*, **206**, 136–47.

Kettle, S., Alcami, A., et al. 1997. Vaccinia virus serpin B13R (SPI-2) inhibits interleukin-1 beta- converting enzyme and protects virus-infected cells from TNF- and Fas-mediated apoptosis, but does not prevent IL-1 beta-induced fever. *J Gen Virol*, **78**, 677–85.

Kikutani, H. and Kumanogoh, A. 2003. Semaphorins in interactions between T cells and antigen-presenting cells. *Nat Rev Immunol*, **3**, 159–67.

Klemperer, N., Ward, J., et al. 1997. The vaccinia virus I1 protein is essential for the assembly of mature virions. *J Virol*, **71**, 9285–94.

Klemperer, N., McDonald, W., et al. 2001. The A20R protein Is a stoichiometric component of the processive form of vaccinia virus DNA polymerase. *J Virol*, **75**, 12298–307.

Kolodkin, A.L., Matthes, D.J. and Goodman, C.S. 1993. The semaphorin genes encode a family of transmembrane and secreted growth cone guidance molecules. *Cell*, **75**, 1389–99.

Kotwal, G.J. 2000. Poxviral mimicry of complement and chemokine system components: what's the end game? *Immunol Today*, **21**, 242–8.

Kotwal, G.J. and Moss, B. 1988. Vaccinia virus encodes a secretory polypeptide structurally related to complement control proteins. *Nature*, **335**, 176–8.

Kotwal, G.J., Isaacs, S.N., et al. 1990. Inhibition of the complement cascade by the major secretory protein of vaccinia virus. *Science*, **250**, 827–30.

Kovacs, G.R. and Moss, B. 1996. The vaccinia virus *H5R* gene encodes late gene transcription factor 4: purification, cloning, and overexpression. *J Virol*, **70**, 6796–802.

Kovacs, G.R., Rosales, R., et al. 1994. Modification of the cascade model for regulation of vaccinia virus gene expression: purification of a prereplicative, late-stage-specific transcription factor. *J Virol*, **68**, 3443–7.

Krathwohl, M.D., Hromas, R., et al. 1997. Functional characterization of the C–C chemokine-like molecules encoded by molluscum contagiosum virus types 1 and 2. *Proc Natl Acad Sci U S A*, **94**, 9875–80.

Lackner, C.A. and Condit, R.C. 2000. Vaccinia virus gene *A18R* DNA helicase is a transcript release factor. *J Biol Chem*, **275**, 1485–94.

Lackner, C.A., D'Costa, S.M., et al. 2003. Complementation analysis of the dales collection of vaccinia virus temperature-sensitive mutants. *Virology*, **305**, 240–59.

Lalani, A.S., Masters, J., et al. 1999. Role of the myxoma virus soluble CC-chemokine inhibitor glycoprotein, M-T1, during myxoma virus pathogenesis. *Virology*, **256**, 233–45.

Lalani, A.S., Barrett, J.W. and McFadden, G. 2000. Modulating chemokines: more lessons from viruses. *Immunol Today*, **21**, 100–6.

Langland, J.O. and Jacobs, B.L. 2002. The role of the PKR-inhibitory genes, *E3L* and *K3L*, in determining vaccinia virus host range. *Virology*, **299**, 133–41.

Latner, D.R., Xiang, Y., et al. 2000. The vaccinia virus bifunctional gene *J3* (nucleoside-2′-O-)- methyltransferase and poly(A) polymerase stimulatory factor is implicated as a positive transcription elongation factor by two genetic approaches. *Virology*, **269**, 345–55.

Latner, D.R., Thompson, J.M., et al. 2002. The positive transcription elongation factor activity of the vaccinia virus J3 protein is independent from its (nucleoside-2′-O-) methyltransferase and poly(A) polymerase stimulatory functions. *Virology*, **301**, 64–80.

Law, M., Hollinshead, R. and Smith, G.L. 2002. Antibody-sensitive and antibody-resistant cell-to-cell spread by vaccinia virus: role of the A33R protein in antibody-resistant spread. *J Gen Virol*, **83**, 209–22.

Lee, H.J., Essani, K. and Smith, G.L. 2001. The genome sequence of yaba-like disease virus, a yatapoxvirus. *Virology*, **281**, 170–92.

Lee-Chen, G.J., Bourgeois, N., et al. 1988. Structure of the transcription initiation and termination sequences of seven early genes in the vaccinia virus *Hin*dIII D fragment. *Virology*, **163**, 64–79.

Lin, S., Chen, W. and Broyles, S.S. 1992. The vaccinia virus *B1R* gene product is a serine/threonine protein kinase. *J Virol*, **66**, 2717–23.

Liptakova, H., Kontsekova, E., et al. 1997. Analysis of an interaction between the soluble vaccinia virus-coded type I interferon (IFN)-receptor and human IFN-alpha 1 and IFN-alpha 2. *Virology*, **232**, 86–90.

Liu, K., Lemon, B. and Traktman, P. 1995. The dual-specificity phosphatase encoded by vaccinia virus, *VH1*, is essential for viral transcription in vivo and in vitro. *J Virol*, **69**, 7823–34.

Liu, L.Y., Lalani, A., et al. 2000. The viral anti-inflammatory chemokine-binding protein M-T7 reduces intimal hyperplasia after vascular injury. *J Clin Invest*, **105**, 1613–21.

Locksley, R.M., Killeen, N. and Lenardo, M.J. 2001. The TNF and TNF receptor superfamilies: integrating mammalian biology. *Cell*, **104**, 487–501.

Lomas, D.A., Evans, D.L., et al. 1993. Inhibition of plasmin, urokinase, tissue plasminogen activator and C1S by a myxoma virus serine proteinase inhibitor. *J Biol Chem*, **268**, 516–21.

Loparev, V.N., Parsons, J.M., et al. 1998. A third distinct tumor necrosis factor receptor of orthopoxviruses. *Proc Natl Acad Sci U S A*, **95**, 3786–91.

Lucas, A., Liu, L.Y., et al. 1996. Virus-encoded serine proteinase inhibitor SERP-1 inhibits atherosclerotic plaque development after balloon angioplasty. *Circulation*, **94**, 2890–900.

Luo, Y., Mao, X., et al. 1995. The D1 and D12 subunits are both essential for the transcription termination factor activity of vaccinia virus capping enzyme. *J Virol*, **69**, 3852–6.

Macen, J.L., Upton, C., et al. 1993. SERP1, a serine proteinase inhibitor encoded by myxoma virus, is a secreted glycoprotein that interferes with inflammation. *Virology*, **195**, 348–63.

Mahalingam, S. and Karupiah, G. 2000. Modulation of chemokines by poxvirus infections. *Curr Opin Immunol*, **12**, 409–12.

Mahalingam, S., Foster, P.S., et al. 2000. Interferon-inducible chemokines and immunity to poxvirus infections. *Immunol Rev*, **177**, 127–33.

Mahr, A. and Roberts, B.E. 1984. Arrangement of late RNAs transcribed from a 7.1-kilobase *Eco*RI vaccinia virus DNA fragment. *J Virol*, **49**, 510–20.

Mao, X. and Shuman, S. 1994. Intrinsic RNA (guanine-7) methyltransferase activity of the vaccinia virus capping enzyme D1 subunit is stimulated by the D12 subunit. Identification of amino acid residues in the D1 protein required for subunit association and methyl group transfer. *J Biol Chem*, **269**, 24472–9.

Martin, S.A., Paoletti, E. and Moss, B. 1975. Purification of mRNA guanylyltransferase and mRNA (guanine-7-)methyltransferase from vaccinia virions. *J Biol Chem*, **250**, 9322–9.

Martinez-Pomares, L., Thompson, J.P. and Moyer, R.W. 1995. Mapping and investigation of the role in pathogenesis of the major unique secreted 35-kDa protein of rabbitpox virus. *Virology*, **206**, 591–600.

McCraith, S., Holtzman, T., et al. 2000. Genome-wide analysis of vaccinia virus protein–protein interactions. *Proc Natl Acad Sci U S A*, **97**, 4879–84.

McDonald, W.F. and Traktman, P. 1994. Vaccinia virus DNA polymerase. In vitro analysis of parameters affecting processivity. *J Biol Chem*, **269**, 31190–7.

McFadden, G., Stuart, D., et al. 2003. Replication and resolution of poxvirus telomeres. *Cancer Cells*, **6**, 77–85.

McKelvey, T.A., Andrews, S.C., et al. 2002. Identification of the orthopoxvirus *p4c* gene, which encodes a structural protein that directs intracellular mature virus particles into A-type inclusions. *J Virol*, **76**, 11216–25.

Meis, R.J. and Condit, R.C. 1991. Genetic and molecular biological characterization of a vaccinia virus gene which renders the virus dependent on isatin-beta-thiosemicarbazone (IBT). *Virology*, **182**, 442–54.

Merchlinsky, M. 1989. Intramolecular homologous recombination in cells infected with temperature-sensitive mutants of vaccinia virus. *J Virol*, **63**, 2030–5.

Merchlinsky, M. 1990. Resolution of poxvirus telomeres: processing of vaccinia virus concatemer junctions by conservative strand exchange. *J Virol*, **64**, 3437–46.

Merchlinsky, M. and Moss, B. 1986. Resolution of linear minichromosomes with hairpin ends from circular plasmids containing vaccinia virus concatemer junctions. *Cell*, **45**, 879–84.

Merchlinsky, M. and Moss, B. 1989. Nucleotide sequence required for resolution of the concatemer junction of vaccinia virus DNA. *J Virol*, **63**, 4354–61.

Merchlinsky, M. and Moss, B. 1992. Introduction of foreign DNA into the vaccinia virus genome by in vitro ligation: recombination-independent selectable cloning vectors. *Virology*, **190**, 522–6, published erratum appears in *Virology* 1993; **192**: 717.

Messud-Petit, F., Gelfi, J., et al. 1998. Serp2, an inhibitor of the interleukin-1 beta-converting enzyme, is critical in the pathobiology of myxoma virus. *J Virol*, **72**, 7830–9.

Miller, L.W., Dai, E., et al. 2000. Inhibition of transplant vasculopathy in a rat aortic allograft model after infusion of anti-inflammatory viral serpin. *Circulation*, **101**, 1598–605.

Millns, A.K., Carpenter, M.S. and Delange, A.M. 1994. The vaccinia virus-encoded uracil DNA glycosylase has an essential role in viral DNA replication. *Virology*, **198**, 504–13.

Mohamed, M.R. and Niles, E.G. 2000. Interaction between nucleoside triphosphate phosphohydrolase I and the H4L subunit of the viral

RNA polymerase is required for vaccinia virus early gene transcript release. *J Biol Chem*, **275**, 25798–804.

Mohamed, M.R. and Niles, E.G. 2001. The viral RNA polymerase H4L subunit is required for vaccinia virus early gene transcription termination. *J Biol Chem*, **276**, 20758–65.

Moon, K.B., Turner, P.C. and Moyer, R.W. 1999. SPI-1-dependent host range of rabbitpox virus and complex formation with cathepsin G is associated with serpin motifs. *J Virol*, **73**, 8999–9010.

Moore, J.B. and Smith, G.L. 1992. Steroid hormone synthesis by a vaccinia enzyme: a new type of virus virulence factor. *EMBO J*, **11**, 1973–80.

Morgan, C. 1976. The insertion of DNA into vaccinia virus. *Science*, **193**, 591–2.

Morgan, J.R., Cohen, L.K. and Roberts, B.E. 1984. Identification of the DNA sequences encoding the large subunit of the mRNA-capping enzyme of vaccinia virus. *J Virol*, **52**, 206–14.

Moss, B. 1996. Genetically engineered poxviruses for recombinant gene expression, vaccination, and safety. *Proc Natl Acad Sci U S A*, **93**, 11341–8.

Moss, B. 2001. *Poxviridae*: the viruses and their replication. In: Knipe, D.E. and Howley, P.M. (eds), *Fields virology*, vol. 2. . New York: Lippincott Williams and Wilkins, 2849–84.

Moss, B. and Shisler, J.L. 2001. Immunology 101 at poxvirus U: immune evasion genes. *Semin Immunol*, **13**, 59–66.

Moss, B., Shisler, J.L., et al. 2000. Immune-defense molecules of molluscum contagiosum virus, a human poxvirus. *Trends Microbiol*, **8**, 473–7.

Mossman, K., Upton, C. and McFadden, G. 1995. The myxoma virus-soluble interferon-gamma receptor homolog, M-T7, inhibits interferon-gamma in a species-specific manner. *J Biol Chem*, **270**, 3031–8.

Moyer, R.W. and Graves, R.L. 1981. The mechanism of cytoplasmic orthopoxvirus DNA replication. *Cell*, **27**, 391–401.

Moyer, R.W., Graves, R.L. and Rothe, C.T. 1980. The white pock (mu) mutants of rabbit poxvirus. III. Terminal DNA sequence duplication and transposition in rabbit poxvirus. *Cell*, **22**, 545–53.

Moyer, R.W., Arif, B., et al. 2000. Family *Poxviridae*. In: van Regenmortel, M.H.V., Fauquet, C.M., et al. (eds), *Virus taxonomy*. San Diego: Academic Press, 137–47.

Murphy, P.M. 2001. Viral exploitation and subversion of the immune system through chemokine mimicry. *Nat Immunol*, **2**, 116–22.

Nakanishi, K., Yoshimoto, T., et al. 2001. Interleukin-18 regulates both Th1 and Th2 responses. *Annu Rev Immunol*, **19**, 423–74.

Nakano, E., Panicali, D. and Paoletti, E. 1982. Molecular genetics of vaccinia virus: demonstration of marker rescue. *Proc Natl Acad Sci U S A*, **79**, 1593–6.

Nash, P., Whitty, A., et al. 1998. Inhibitory specificity of the anti-inflammatory myxoma virus serpin, SERP-1. *J Biol Chem*, **273**, 20982–91.

Nash, P., Barrett, J., et al. 1999. Immunomodulation by viruses: the myxoma virus story. *Immunol Rev*, **168**, 103–20.

Nevins, J.R. and Joklik, W.K. 1977. Isolation and properties of the vaccinia virus DNA-dependent RNA polymerase. *J Biol Chem*, **252**, 6930–8.

Niles, E.G., Lee-Chen, G.J., et al. 1989. Vaccinia virus gene *D12L* encodes the small subunit of the viral mRNA capping enzyme. *Virology*, **172**, 513–22.

Oda, K.I. and Joklik, W.K. 1967. Hybridization and sedimentation studies on 'early' and 'late' vaccinia messenger RNA. *J Mol Biol*, **27**, 395–419.

Oguiura, N., Spehner, D. and Drillien, R. 1993. Detection of a protein encoded by the vaccinia virus C7L open reading frame and study of its effect on virus multiplication in different cell lines. *J Gen Virol*, **74**, 1409–13.

O'Neill, L. 2000. The Toll/interleukin-1 receptor domain: a molecular switch for inflammation and host defence. *Biochem Soc Trans*, **28**, 557–63.

Pacha, R.F., Meis, R.J. and Condit, R.C. 1990. Structure and expression of the vaccinia virus gene which prevents virus-induced breakdown of RNA. *J Virol*, **64**, 3853–63.

Palumbo, G.J., Buller, R.M. and Glasgow, W.C. 1994. Multigenic evasion of inflammation by poxviruses. *J Virol*, **68**, 1737–49.

Panus, J.F., Smith, C.A., et al. 2002. Cowpox virus encodes a fifth member of the tumor necrosis factor receptor family: a soluble, secreted CD30 homologue. *Proc Natl Acad Sci U S A*, **99**, 8348–53.

Paoletti, E. 1996. Applications of pox virus vectors to vaccination: an update. *Proc Natl Acad Sci U S A*, **93**, 11349–53.

Paoletti, E., Taylor, J., et al. 1995. Highly attenuated poxvirus vectors: NYVAC, ALVAC and TROVAC. *Dev Biol Stand*, **84**, 159–63.

Parks, R.J., Lichty, B.D., et al. 1994. Characterization of the Shope fibroma virus DNA ligase gene. *Virology*, **202**, 642–50.

Parks, R.J., Winchcombe-Forhan, C., et al. 1998. DNA ligase gene disruptions can depress viral growth and replication in poxvirus-infected cells. *Virus Res*, **56**, 135–47.

Pastoret, P.P. and Brochier, B. 1996. The development and use of a vaccinia-rabies recombinant oral vaccine for the control of wildlife rabies; a link between Jenner and Pasteur. *Epidemiol Infect*, **116**, 235–40.

Patel, D.D. and Pickup, D.J. 1987. Messenger RNAs of a strongly-expressed late gene of cowpox virus contain 5′-terminal poly(A) sequences. *EMBO J*, **6**, 3787–94.

Patel, D.D. and Pickup, D.J. 1989. The second-largest subunit of the poxvirus RNA polymerase is similar to the corresponding subunits of procaryotic and eucaryotic RNA polymerases. *J Virol*, **63**, 1076–86.

Pedersen, K., Snijder, E.J., et al. 2000. Characterization of vaccinia virus intracellular cores: implications for viral uncoating and core structure. *J Virol*, **74**, 3525–36.

Pelham, H.R., Sykes, J.M. and Hunt, T. 1978. Characteristics of a coupled cell-free transcription and translation system directed by vaccinia cores. *Eur J Biochem*, **82**, 199–209.

Pennington, T.H. 1974. Vaccinia virus polypeptide synthesis: sequential appearance and stability of pre- and post-replicative polypeptides. *J Gen Virol*, **25**, 433–44.

Petit, F., Bergagnoli, S., et al. 1996. Characterization of a myxoma virus-encoded serpin-like protein with activity against interleukin-1β converting enzyme. *J Virol*, **70**, 5860–6.

Pogo, B.G. and Dales, S. 1969. Two deoxyribonuclease activities within purified vaccinia virus. *Proc Natl Acad Sci U S A*, **63**, 820–7.

Puckett, C. and Moss, B. 1983. Selective transcription of vaccinia virus genes in template dependent soluble extracts of infected cells. *Cell*, **35**, 441–8.

Punjabi, A., Boyle, K., et al. 2001. Clustered charge-to-alanine mutagenesis of the vaccinia virus *A20* gene: temperature-sensitive mutants have a DNA-minus phenotype and are defective in the production of processive DNA polymerase activity. *J Virol*, **75**, 12308–18.

Quan, L.T., Caputo, A., et al. 1995. Granzyme B is inhibited by the cowpox virus serpin cytokine response modifier A. *J Biol Chem*, **270**, 10377–9.

Rajagopal, I., Ahn, B.Y., et al. 1995. Roles of vaccinia virus ribonucleotide reductase and glutaredoxin in DNA precursor biosynthesis. *J Biol Chem*, **270**, 27415–18.

Ramsey-Ewing, A. and Moss, B. 1995. Restriction of vaccinia virus replication in CHO cells occurs at the stage of viral intermediate protein synthesis. *Virology*, **206**, 984–93.

Ramsey-Ewing, A.L. and Moss, B. 1996. Complementation of a vaccinia virus host-range *K1L* gene deletion by the nonhomologous *CP77* gene. *Virology*, **222**, 75–86.

Ravanello, M.P. and Hruby, D.E. 1994. Conditional lethal expression of the vaccinia virus L1R myristylated protein reveals a role in virion assembly. *J Virol*, **68**, 6401–10.

Ray, C.A., Black, R.A., et al. 1992. Viral inhibition of inflammation: cowpox virus encodes an inhibitor of the interleukin-1 beta converting enzyme. *Cell*, **69**, 597–604.

Rempel, R.E. and Traktman, P. 1992. Vaccinia virus B1 kinase: phenotypic analysis of temperature-sensitive mutants and enzymatic characterization of recombinant proteins. *J Virol*, **66**, 4413–26.

Rice, A.P. and Roberts, B.E. 1983. Vaccinia virus induces cellular mRNA degradation. *J Virol*, **47**, 529–39.

Risco, C., Rodriguez, J.R., et al. 2002. Endoplasmic reticulum-Golgi intermediate compartment membranes and vimentin filaments participate in vaccinia virus assembly. *J Virol*, **76**, 1839–55.

Roberts, A. and Rose, J.K. 1998. Recovery of negative-strand RNA viruses from plasmid DNAs: a positive approach revitalizes a negative field. *Virology*, **247**, 1–6.

Rochester, S.C. and Traktman, P. 1998. Characterization of the single-stranded DNA binding protein encoded by the vaccinia virus *I3* gene. *J Virol*, **72**, 2917–26.

Rodriguez, D., Esteban, M. and Rodriguez, J.R. 1995. Vaccinia virus *A17L* gene product is essential for an early step in virion morphogenesis. *J Virol*, **69**, 4640–8.

Rodriguez, J.F. and Smith, G.L. 1990. Inducible gene expression from vaccinia virus vectors. *Virology*, **177**, 239–50.

Rodriguez, J.R., Risco, C., et al. 1997. Characterization of early stages in vaccinia virus membrane biogenesis: implications of the 21-kilodalton protein and a newly identified 15-kilodalton envelope protein. *J Virol*, **71**, 1821–33.

Rodriguez, J.R., Risco, C., et al. 1998. Vaccinia virus 15-kilodalton (A14L) protein is essential for assembly and attachment of viral crescents to virosomes. *J Virol*, **72**, 1287–96.

Romano, P.R., Zhang, F., et al. 1998. Inhibition of double-stranded RNA-dependent protein kinase PKR by vaccinia virus E3: role of complex formation and the E3 N-terminal domain. *Mol Cell Biol*, **18**, 7304–16.

Rosales, R., Harris, N., et al. 1994a. Purification and identification of a vaccinia virus-encoded intermediate stage promoter-specific transcription factor that has homology to eukaryotic transcription factor SII (TFIIS) and an additional role as a viral RNA polymerase subunit. *J Biol Chem*, **269**, 14260–7.

Rosales, R., Sutter, G. and Moss, B. 1994b. A cellular factor is required for transcription of vaccinia viral intermediate-stage genes. *Proc Natl Acad Sci U S A*, **91**, 3794–8.

Rosengard, A.M., Liu, Y., et al. 2002. Variola virus immune evasion design: expression of a highly efficient inhibitor of human complement. *Proc Natl Acad Sci U S A*, **99**, 8808–13.

Salmons, T., Kuhn, A., et al. 1997. Vaccinia virus membrane proteins p8 and p16 are cotranslationally inserted into the rough endoplasmic reticulum and retained in the intermediate compartment. *J Virol*, **71**, 7404–20.

Sanderson, C.M., Hollinshead, M. and Smith, G.L. 2000. The vaccinia virus A27L protein is needed for the microtubule-dependent transport of intracellular mature virus particles. *J Gen Virol*, **81**, 47–58.

Sanz, P. and Moss, B. 1999. Identification of a transcription factor, encoded by two vaccinia virus early genes, that regulates the intermediate stage of viral gene expression. *Proc Natl Acad Sci U S A*, **96**, 2692–7.

Saraiva, M. and Alcami, A. 2001. CrmE, a novel soluble tumor necrosis factor receptor encoded by poxviruses. *J Virol*, **75**, 226–33.

Scheiflinger, F., Dorner, F. and Falkner, F.G. 1992. Construction of chimeric vaccinia viruses by molecular cloning and packaging. *Proc Natl Acad Sci U S A*, **89**, 9977–81.

Schmelz, M., Sodeik, B., et al. 1994. Assembly of vaccinia virus: the second wrapping cisterna is derived from the trans Golgi network. *J Virol*, **68**, 130–47.

Schnierle, B.S., Gershon, P.D. and Moss, B. 1992. Cap-specific mRNA (nucleoside-$O^{2'}$-)-methyltransferase and poly(A) polymerase stimulatory activities of vaccinia virus are mediated by a single protein. *Proc Natl Acad Sci U S A*, **89**, 2897–901.

Schreiber, M., Rajarathnam, K. and McFadden, G. 1996. Myxoma virus T2 protein, a tumor necrosis factor (TNF) receptor homolog, is secreted as a monomer and dimer that each bind rabbit TNFalpha, but the dimer is a more potent TNF inhibitor. *J Biol Chem*, **271**, 13333–41.

Schwer, B., Visca, P., et al. 1987. Discontinuous transcription or RNA processing of vaccinia virus late messengers results in a 5′ poly(A) leader. *Cell*, **50**, 163–9.

Seet, B.T., Johnston, J.B., et al. 2003. Poxviruses and immune evasion. *Annu Rev Immunol*, **21**, 377–423.

Sen, G.C. 2001. Viruses and interferons. *Annu Rev Microbiol*, **55**, 255–81.

Senkevich, T.G. and Moss, B. 1998. Domain structure, intracellular trafficking, and beta 2-microglobulin binding of a major histocompatibility complex class I homolog encoded by molluscum contagiosum virus. *Virology*, **250**, 397–407.

Senkevich, T.G., Bugert, J.J., et al. 1996. Genome sequence of a human tumorigenic poxvirus: prediction of specific host response-evasion genes. *Science*, **273**, 813–16.

Senkevich, T.G., Koonin, E.V., et al. 1997. The genome of molluscum contagiosum virus: analysis and comparison with other poxviruses. *Virology*, **233**, 19–42.

Senkevich, T.G., White, C.L., et al. 2002. Complete pathway for protein disulfide bond formation encoded by poxviruses. *Proc Natl Acad Sci U S A*, **99**, 6667–72.

Shchelkunov, S.N., Massung, R.F. and Esposito, J.J. 1995. Comparison of the genome DNA sequences of Bangladesh-1975 and India-1967 variola viruses. *Virus Res*, **36**, 107–18.

Shisler, J.L. and Moss, B. 2001a. Immunology 102 at poxvirus U: avoiding apoptosis. *Semin Immunol*, **13**, 67–72.

Shisler, J.L. and Moss, B. 2001b. Molluscum contagiosum virus inhibitors of apoptosis: the MC159 v-FLIP protein blocks Fas-induced activation of procaspases and degradation of the related MC160 protein. *Virology*, **282**, 14–25.

Shisler, J.L., Senkevich, T.G., et al. 1998. Ultraviolet-induced cell death blocked by a selenoprotein from a human dermatotropic poxvirus. *Science*, **279**, 102–5.

Shisler, J.L., Isaacs, S.N. and Moss, B. 1999. Vaccinia virus serpin-1 deletion mutant exhibits a host range defect characterized by low levels of Intermediate and late mRNAs. *Virology*, **262**, 298–311.

Shuman, S. and Morham, S.G. 1990. Domain structure of vaccinia virus mRNA capping enzyme. Activity of the Mr 95,000 subunit expressed in *Escherichia coli*. *J Biol Chem*, **265**, 11967–72.

Shuman, S. and Moss, B. 1987. Identification of a vaccinia virus gene encoding a type I DNA topoisomerase. *Proc Natl Acad Sci U S A*, **84**, 7478–82.

Shuman, S. and Moss, B. 1988. Factor-dependent transcription termination by vaccinia virus RNA polymerase. Evidence that the *cis*-acting termination signal is in nascent RNA. *J Biol Chem*, **263**, 6220–5.

Shuman, S. and Moss, B. 1990. Purification and use of vaccinia virus messenger RNA capping enzyme. *Methods Enzymol*, **181**, 170–80.

Shuman, S., Broyles, S.S. and Moss, B. 1987. Purification and characterization of a transcription termination factor from vaccinia virions. *J Biol Chem*, **262**, 12372–80.

Shuman, S., Golder, M. and Moss, B. 1989. Insertional mutagenesis of the vaccinia virus gene encoding a type I DNA topoisomerase: evidence that the gene is essential for virus growth. *Virology*, **170**, 302–6.

Simpson, D.A. and Condit, R.C. 1995. Vaccinia virus gene *A18R* encodes an essential DNA helicase. *J Virol*, **69**, 6131–9.

Slabaugh, M.B. and Mathews, C.K. 1986. Hydroxyurea-resistant vaccinia virus: overproduction of ribonucleotide reductase. *J Virol*, **60**, 506–14.

Slabaugh, M., Roseman, N., et al. 1988. Vaccinia virus-encoded ribonucleotide reductase: sequence conservation of the gene for the small subunit and its amplification in hydroxyurea-resistant mutants. *J Virol*, **62**, 519–27.

Smallwood, S., Cevik, B. and Moyer, S.A. 2002. Intragenic complementation and oligomerization of the L subunit of the sendai virus RNA polymerase. *Virology*, **304**, 235–45.

Smith, C.A., Davis, T., et al. 1991. T2 open reading frame from the Shope fibroma virus encodes a soluble form of the TNF receptor. *Biochem Biophys Res Commun*, **176**, 335–42.

Smith, C.A., Farrah, T. and Goodwin, R.G. 1994. The TNF receptor superfamily of cellular and viral proteins: Activation, costimulation, and death. *Cell*, **76**, 959–62.

Smith, C.A., Hu, F.Q., et al. 1996. Cowpox virus genome encodes a second soluble homologue of cellular TNF receptors, distinct from CrmB, that binds TNF but not LT alpha. *Virology*, **223**, 132–47.

Smith, C.A., Smith, T.D., et al. 1997. Poxvirus genomes encode a secreted, soluble protein that preferentially inhibits beta chemokine activity yet lacks sequence homology to known chemokine receptors. *Virology*, **236**, 316–27.

Smith, G.L. and Moss, B. 1983. Infectious poxvirus vectors have capacity for at least 25,000 base pairs of foreign DNA. *Gene*, **25**, 21–8.

Smith, G.L., Vanderplasschen, A. and Law, M. 2002. The formation and function of extracellular enveloped vaccinia virus. *J Gen Virol*, **83**, 2915–31.

Smith, V.P. and Alcami, A. 2000. Expression of secreted cytokine and chemokine inhibitors by ectromelia virus. *J Virol*, **74**, 8460–71.

Smith, V.P. and Alcami, A. 2002. Inhibition of interferons by ectromelia virus. *J Virol*, **76**, 1124–34.

Sodeik, B. and Krijnse-Locker, J. 2002. Assembly of vaccinia virus revisited: de novo membrane synthesis or acquisition from the host? *Trends Microbiol*, **10**, 15–24.

Sodeik, B., Doms, R.W., et al. 1993. Assembly of vaccinia virus: role of the intermediate compartment between the endoplasmic reticulum and the Golgi stacks. *J Cell Biol*, **121**, 521–41.

Spehner, D., Gillard, S., et al. 1988. A cowpox virus gene required for multiplication in Chinese hamster ovary cells. *J Virol*, **62**, 1297–304.

Spriggs, M.K. and Sher, A. 1999. New lessons for immunology at the host–pathogen interface. *Curr Opin Immunol*, **11**, 363–4.

Spriggs, M.K., Hruby, D.E., et al. 1992. Vaccinia and Cowpox viruses encode a novel secreted interleukin-1 binding protein. *Cell*, **71**, 145–52.

Sridhar, P. and Condit, R.C. 1983. Selection for temperature-sensitive mutations in specific vaccinia virus genes: isolation and characterization of a virus mutant which encodes a phosphonoacetic acid-resistant, temperature-sensitive DNA polymerase. *Virology*, **128**, 444–57.

Sroller, V., Kutinova, L., et al. 1998. Effect of 3-beta-hydroxysteroid dehydrogenase gene deletion on virulence and immunogenicity of different vaccinia viruses and their recombinants. *Arch Virol*, **143**, 1311–20.

Stokes, G.V. 1976. High-voltage electron microscope study of the release of vaccinia virus from whole cells. *J Virol*, **18**, 636–43.

Stuart, D.T., Upton, C., et al. 1993. A poxvirus-encoded uracil DNA glycosylase is essential for virus viability. *J Virol*, **67**, 2503–12.

Symons, J.A., Alcami, A. and Smith, G.L. 1995. Vaccinia virus encodes a soluble type I interferon receptor of novel structure and broad species specificity. *Cell*, **81**, 551–60.

Symons, J.A., Adams, E., et al. 2002. The vaccinia virus C12L protein inhibits mouse IL-18 and promotes virus virulence in the murine intranasal model. *J Gen Virol*, **83**, 2833–44.

Taddie, J.A. and Traktman, P. 1993. Genetic characterization of the vaccinia virus DNA polymerase: cytosine arabinoside resistance requires a variable lesion conferring phosphonoacetate resistance in conjunction with an invariant mutation localized to the 3′–5′ exonuclease domain. *J Virol*, **67**, 4323–36.

Takahashi Nishimaki, F., Funahashi, S., et al. 1991. Regulation of plaque size and host range by a vaccinia virus gene related to complement system proteins. *Virology*, **181**, 158–64.

Tamagnone, L. and Comoglio, P.M. 2000. Signalling by semaphorin receptors: cell guidance and beyond. *Trends Cell Biol*, **10**, 377–83.

Tengelsen, L.A., Slabaugh, M.B., et al. 1988. Nucleotide sequence and molecular genetic analysis of the large subunit of ribonucleotide reductase encoded by vaccinia virus. *Virology*, **164**, 121–31.

Tewari, M. and Dixit, V.M. 1995. Fas- and tumor necrosis factor-induced apoptosis is inhibited by the poxvirus *crmA* gene product. *J Biol Chem*, **270**, 3255–60.

Tewari, M., Telford, W.G., et al. 1995. CrmA, a poxvirus-encoded serpin, inhibits cytotoxic T-lymphocyte-mediated apoptosis. *J Biol Chem*, **270**, 22705–8.

Thome, M., Schneider, P., et al. 1997. Viral FLICE-inhibitory proteins (FLIPs) prevent apoptosis induced by death receptors. *Nature*, **386**, 517–21.

Thompson, C.L. and Condit, R.C. 1986. Marker rescue mapping of vaccinia virus temperature-sensitive mutants using overlapping cosmid clones representing the entire virus genome. *Virology*, **150**, 10–20.

Thompson, J.P., Turner, P.C., et al. 1993. The effects of serpin gene mutations on the distinctive pathobiology of cowpox and rabbitpox virus following intranasal inoculation of Balb/c mice. *Virology*, **197**, 328–38.

Tian, L., Sayer, J.M., et al. 2003. Benzo[a]pyrene-dG adduct interference illuminates the interface of vaccinia topoisomerase with the DNA minor groove. *J Biol Chem*, **278**, 9905–11.

Tolonen, N., Doglio, L., et al. 2001. Vaccinia virus DNA replication occurs in endoplasmic reticulum-enclosed cytoplasmic mini-nuclei. *Mol Biol Cell*, **12**, 2031–46.

Traktman, P., Kelvin, M. and Pacheco, S. 1989. Molecular genetic analysis of vaccinia virus DNA polymerase mutants. *J Virol*, **63**, 841–6.

Traktman, P., Caligiuri, A., et al. 1995. Temperature-sensitive mutants with lesions in the vaccinia virus F10 kinase undergo arrest at the earliest stage of virion morphogenesis. *J Virol*, **69**, 6581–7.

Traktman, P., Liu, K., et al. 2000. Elucidating the essential role of the A14 phosphoprotein in vaccinia virus morphogenesis: construction and characterization of a tetracycline-inducible recombinant. *J Virol*, **74**, 3682–95.

Tscharke, D.C., Reading, P.C. and Smith, G.L. 2002. Dermal infection with vaccinia virus reveals roles for virus proteins not seen using other inoculation routes. *J Gen Virol*, **83**, 1977–86.

Tseng, M., Palaniyar, N., et al. 1999. DNA binding and aggregation properties of the vaccinia virus *I3L* gene product. *J Biol Chem*, **274**, 21637–44.

Tsukumo, S.I. and Yonehara, S. 1999. Requirement of cooperative functions of two repeated death effector domains in caspase-8 and in MC159 for induction and inhibition of apoptosis, respectively. *Genes Cells*, **4**, 541–9.

Turner, P.C., Sancho, M.C., et al. 1999. Myxoma virus Serp2 is a weak inhibitor of granzyme B and interleukin-1 beta-converting enzyme in vitro and unlike CrmA cannot block apoptosis in cowpox virus-infected cells. *J Virol*, **73**, 6394–404.

Turner, P.C., Baquero, M.T., et al. 2000. The cowpox virus serpin SPI-3 complexes with and inhibits urokinase-type and tissue-type plasminogen activators and plasmin. *Virology*, **272**, 267–80.

Upton, C., Macen, J.L., et al. 1990. Myxoma virus and malignant rabbit fibroma virus encode a serpin-like protein important for virus virulence. *Virology*, **179**, 618–31.

Upton, C., Macen, J.L., et al. 1991. Myxoma virus expresses a secreted protein with homology to the tumor necrosis factor receptor gene family that contributes to viral virulence. *Virology*, **184**, 370–82.

Upton, C., Stuart, D.T. and McFadden, G. 1993. Identification of a poxvirus gene encoding a uracil DNA glycosylase. *Proc Natl Acad Sci U S A*, **90**, 4518–22.

Vancova, I., La Bonnardiere, C. and Kontsek, P. 1998. Vaccinia virus protein B18R inhibits the activity and cellular binding of the novel type interferon-delta. *J Gen Virol*, **79**, 1647–9.

Verardi, P.H., Jones, L.A., et al. 2001. Vaccinia virus vectors with an inactivated gamma interferon receptor homolog gene (*B8R*) are attenuated in vivo without a concomitant reduction in immunogenicity. *J Virol*, **75**, 11–18.

Viac, J. and Chardonnet, Y. 1990. Immunocompetent cells and epithelial cell modifications in molluscum contagiosum. *J Cutaneous Pathol*, **17**, 202–5.

Vos, J.C. and Stunnenberg, H.G. 1988. Derepression of a novel class of vaccinia virus genes upon DNA replication. *EMBO J*, **7**, 3487–92.

Vos, J.C., Sasker, M. and Stunnenberg, H.G. 1991. Vaccinia virus capping enzyme is a transcription initiation factor. *EMBO J*, **10**, 2553–8.

Wang, S. and Shuman, S. 1995. Vaccinia virus morphogenesis is blocked by temperature-sensitive mutations in the *F10* gene, which encodes protein kinase 2. *J Virol*, **69**, 6376–88.

Wang, Y.X., Turner, P.C., et al. 2000. The cowpox virus SPI-3 and myxoma virus SERP1 serpins are not functionally interchangeable despite their similar proteinase inhibition profiles in vitro. *Virology*, **272**, 281–92.

Ward, G.A., Stover, C.K., et al. 1995. Stringent chemical and thermal regulation of recombinant gene expression by vaccinia virus vectors in mammalian cells. *Proc Natl Acad Sci U S A*, **92**, 6773–7.

Wasilenko, S.T., Meyers, A.F., et al. 2001. Vaccinia virus infection disarms the mitochondrion-mediated pathway of the apoptotic cascade by modulating the permeability transition pore. *J Virol*, **75**, 11437–48.

Wei, C.M. and Moss, B. 1975. Methylated nucleotides block 5′-terminus of vaccinia virus messenger RNA. *Proc Natl Acad Sci U S A*, **72**, 318–22.

Welsch, S., Doglio, L., et al. 2003. The vaccinia virus *I3L* gene product is localized to a complex endoplasmic reticulum-associated structure that contains the viral parental DNA. *J Virol*, **77**, 6014–28.

Willer, D.O., McFadden, G. and Evans, D.H. 1999. The complete genome sequence of shope (rabbit) fibroma virus. *Virology*, **264**, 319–43.

Williams, O., Wolffe, E.J., et al. 1999. Vaccinia virus WR gene *A5L* is required for morphogenesis of mature virions. *J Virol*, **73**, 4590–9.

Wilton, S., Mohandas, A.R. and Dales, S. 1995. Organization of the vaccinia envelope and relationship to the structure of intracellular mature virions. *Virology*, **214**, 503–11.

Wittek, R., Cooper, J.A., et al. 1980. Expression of the vaccinia virus genome: analysis and mapping of mRNAs encoded within the inverted terminal repetition. *Cell*, **21**, 487–93.

Wolffe, E.J., Isaacs, S.N. and Moss, B. 1993. Deletion of the vaccinia virus *B5R* gene encoding a 42-kilodalton membrane glycoprotein inhibits extracellular virus envelope formation and dissemination. *J Virol*, **67**, 4732–41.

Wolffe, E.J., Moore, D.M., et al. 1996. Vaccinia virus A17L open reading frame encodes an essential component of nascent viral membranes that is required to initiate morphogenesis. *J Virol*, **70**, 2797–808.

Wright, C.F. and Coroneos, A.M. 1995. The H4 subunit of vaccinia virus RNA polymerase is not required for transcription initiation at a viral late promoter. *J Virol*, **69**, 2602–4.

Wright, C.F., Oswald, B.W. and Dellis, S. 2001. Vaccinia virus late transcription is activated in vitro by cellular heterogeneous nuclear ribonucleoproteins. *J Biol Chem*, **276**, 40680–6.

Xiang, Y. and Moss, B. 1999. IL-18 binding and inhibition of interferon gamma induction by human poxvirus-encoded proteins. *Proc Natl Acad Sci U S A*, **96**, 11537–42.

Xiang, Y. and Moss, B. 2001. Correspondence of the functional epitopes of poxvirus and human interleukin-18-binding proteins. *J Virol*, **75**, 9947–54.

Xiang, Y. and Moss, B. 2003. Molluscum contagiosum virus interleukin-18 (IL-18) binding protein is secreted as a full-length form that binds cell surface glycosaminoglycans through the C-terminal tail and a furin-cleaved form with only the IL-18 binding domain. *J Virol*, **77**, 2623–30.

Xiang, Y., Simpson, D.A., et al. 1998. The vaccinia virus A18R DNA helicase is a postreplicative negative transcription elongation factor. *J Virol*, **72**, 7012–23.

Xu, X.M., Nash, P. and McFadden, G. 2000. Myxoma virus expresses a TNF receptor homolog with two distinct functions. *Virus Genes*, **21**, 97–109.

Yeh, W.W., Moss, B. and Wolffe, E.J. 2000. The vaccinia virus *A9L* gene encodes a membrane protein required for an early step in virion morphogenesis. *J Virol*, **74**, 9701–11.

Yu, L. and Shuman, S. 1996. Mutational analysis of the RNA triphosphatase component of vaccinia virus mRNA capping enzyme. *J Virol*, **70**, 6162–8.

Yuen, L. and Moss, B. 1987. Oligonucleotide sequence signaling transcriptional termination of vaccinia virus early genes. *Proc Natl Acad Sci U S A*, **84**, 6417–21.

Yuwen, H., Cox, J.H., et al. 1993. Nuclear localization of a double-stranded RNA-binding protein encoded by the vaccinia virus *E3L* gene. *Virology*, **195**, 732–44.

Zhang, Y., Keck, J.G. and Moss, B. 1992. Transcription of viral late genes is dependent on expression of the viral intermediate gene *G8R* in cells infected with an inducible conditional-lethal mutant vaccinia virus. *J Virol*, **66**, 6470–9.

32

Orthomyxoviruses: influenza

NANCY J. COX, GABRIELE NEUMANN, RUBEN O. DONIS, AND YOSHIHIRO KAWAOKA

INTRODUCTION

Influenza viruses are unique in their ability to cause recurrent seasonal epidemics of varying severity, as well as global pandemics during which acute febrile respiratory disease occurs explosively in all age groups. Excess hospitalization and death often accompany less serious but widespread morbidity during both seasonal epidemics and pandemics of influenza.

Two features of influenza virus replication and evolution account for much of the epidemiological success of these viruses. First, there is the ability of novel influenza A viruses that circulate naturally in avian reservoirs to emerge unpredictably, either through genetic reassortment or through direct transmission, and spread in a naïve human population to cause an influenza pandemic. Second, there is the relatively rapid and unpredictable antigenic change that accompanies the evolution of influenza viruses once they have become established in humans. Although influenza viruses have been studied intensively for more than 70 years and have often been used as a research model for other pathogens, much remains to be learned about influenza virus replication, pathogenicity, epidemiology, immunology, and the factors that lead to the development of influenza pandemics.

Historical record

Influenza has probably existed from antiquity, although the lack of specific pathognomonic signs makes this assertion less definite than in the case of smallpox or cholera (Kilbourne 1987). Even so, historical records of rapidly spreading 'catarrhal fevers' in Great Britain (Table 32.1) suggest that major influenza epidemics affected human populations as early as the sixteenth century. Pandemic outbreaks are probably a more recent development, paralleling the increases in the world population and the growth of mass transportation systems. Animals may have played a leading role in past influenza epidemics. In the eighteenth and nineteenth centuries, for example, outbreaks of respiratory disease among horses were recorded concurrently with outbreaks in humans (Table 32.1). Although direct evidence for horse-to-human transmission of influenza viruses is lacking, the sizeable concentrations of these animals near previous centers of human population makes them attractive candidates as disease intermediaries (Hirsch 1883). In modern times, pigs have been accorded a prominent role in the generation of major influenza outbreaks (Goldfield et al. 1977; Scholtissek et al. 1985) (see 'Ecology of influenza'). Until recently, direct avian-to-human transmission associated with fatal outcome in infected individuals was believed not to occur. This changed in 1997 when 18 individuals – six of whom died – were infected with H5N1 avian viruses in Hong Kong (Claas et al. 1998a, b; Subbarao et al. 1998). Since then, direct avian-to-human transmission has been reported in several other incidents, such as human infection with H7N7 avian virus in the Netherlands in 2003 (Fouchier et al. 2004; Koopmans et al.

Table 32.1 *Influenza: a summary of major epidemics affecting Great Britain and other regions of the world, 1510–1890*

Epidemic year(s)	Season	Prevalence[a]	Temporally associated animal disease	Anomalous symptoms
1510	...	Pandemic	Murrain in cattle	'Gastrodynia'
1557	Autumn	Pandemic	...	Double tertian fever
1580	Autumn	European	Murrain in beasts (Kent)	Parotid swelling
1658	Spring	Britain, Europe	...	'Cephalic affection'
1675	Autumn	Britain, Europe	...	...
1688	...	Dublin	'Nasal defluxin' in horses	...
1693	Autumn	Britain, Europe	Antecedent nasal discharge in horses	...
1710	Spring	Britain, Europe	...	'Quick pulse'
1729	Winter	England, Europe	...	...
1732/3	Spring to winter	Pandemic	Cough in horses	Parotid swelling
1737/8	Autumn	England, Europe, North America	'Disease among horses'	...
1743	Spring	Britain, Europe	'Cough among horses'	...
1758	Autumn	North America, Europe, Britain	...	...
1762	Autumn	Britain, Europe	Antecedent 'horse colds' (1760)	Variable mortality
1767	Summer	Britain, Europe, North America	Dogs and horses, horse cold	...
1775	Autumn	Pandemic	Disease in dogs and horses	Prurigo, erysipelas, pustules
1782	Spring	Pandemic	...	...
1802/3	Spring	Britain, Europe	Cattle and domestic animals	'Interchanging with scarlatina'
1833	Spring	Pandemic	Concurrent disease in horses	...
1836/7	Winter	Pandemic	...	...
1847/8	Autumn	Pandemic	...	...
1889/90	Winter	Pandemic	...	Increased mortality age 20–60 (Jan. 1890)

From Kilbourne (1987).
a) Pandemic implies historical evidence of involvement of more than two continents.

2004) or H5N1 avian viruses in Hong Kong in 2003 (Peiris et al. 2004) and in Vietnam and Thailand where 42 cases and 30 deaths were reported through September of 2004 (Tran et al. 2004) (www.who.int/en/). Although only limited human-to-human transmission occurred, these episodes clearly emphasize the crucial role of avian species in influenza virus epidemiology.

Seroarcheology

Testing of sera from older adults for influenza virus antibodies (so-called seroarcheology) had suggested that the influenza in humans between 1889 and 1898 was caused by influenza A(H2N2) viruses (see Classification section), whereas epidemics or pandemics occurring in 1899–1917 and in 1918–1957 were the result of H3N8 and H1N1 viruses, respectively (Masurel and Marine 1973; Masurel and Heijtink 1983; Mulder et al. 1958; Noble 1982; Rekart et al. 1982). A more recent careful analysis of data from these earlier publications, using the clearly documented emergence of H1 viruses in 1918 as a model, indicates that the H3 subtype is linked to the pandemic of 1889–91, not that of 1900 as often quoted,

and that the H2 subtype was unlikely to have caused a pandemic in the late 1800s (Dowdle 1999). Recent pandemic strains share the hemagglutinin (HA) and neuraminidase (NA) subtypes of these earlier strains; however, they are probably not direct descendants, as they show a close relationship to avian viruses (Scholtissek et al. 1978c; Webster and Laver 1972). Thus, the similarity of the HAs and NAs of recently circulating human viruses to those of the past may reflect certain properties of the surface molecules that favor viral replication in human hosts. Indeed, of the many HA and NA subtypes maintained in nature, only three had become established in humans: H1N1, H2N2, and H3N2 subtypes. However, a reassortant H1N2 virus emerged in the human population in 2001 (Gregory et al. 2002), and has since become established (Figure 32.1).

Virus isolation

The historical record of influenza viruses remained sparse until technological advances permitted their isolation. In 1901, a 'filterable agent' was isolated from chickens suffering from fowl plague (it was later classified by

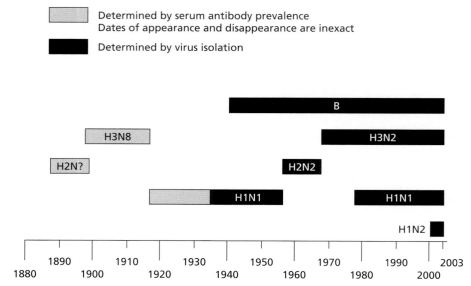

Figure 32.1 *Eras of prevalence of influenza A and B viruses. The periods designated in black were defined by virus isolation while the periods designated in gray were approximated by determining serum antibody prevalence in retrospective serological studies.*

Schäfer (1955) as an influenza A virus). Smith et al. (1933) inoculated ferrets intranasally with human nasopharyngeal washes, which produced a form of influenza that spread to the animals' cage mates. The human virus [A/Wilson-Smith(WS)/33(H1N1)] was transmitted from an infected ferret to a junior investigator on the project (later Sir Charles Stuart-Harris), from whom it was subsequently re-isolated. An antigenically distinct virus, isolated by Francis (1940), was classified as a type B strain (B/Lee/40) to distinguish it from the 1933 isolate. The third major type of influenza virus, influenza C, was first isolated in 1947 by Taylor (1949).

Major research advances

Influenza research gained enormous momentum when it was shown that the virus could be isolated by inoculating samples into the chorioallantoic membrane of fertilized hens' eggs (Burnet 1940; Francis and Magill 1937). Hirst (1941) and McClelland and Hare (1941) discovered that influenza virus particles agglutinate the erythrocytes of fowl as well as of other animal species. This advance established the concept of hemagglutinin inhibition in the detection of specific serum antibodies, making it possible to distinguish between viruses of the same type. Hirst (1950) further demonstrated the presence of a receptor-destroying enzyme, now known as neuraminidase. Later biochemical work (Gottschalk 1957) revealed that influenza viruses contain the HA and NA as major structural and antigenic components of the virus particle.

Subsequent advances included identification of the segmented nature of the RNA genome and assignment of corresponding protein products (McGeoch et al. 1976;

Palese 1977); discovery of the antiviral compound amantadine (Davies et al. 1964); introduction of 'split' and subunit vaccines (Webster and Laver 1966); experimental work on cold-adapted vaccines; and elucidation of influenza gene replication (Inglis et al. 1979; Krug et al. 1979; Lamb and Choppin 1979). More recently, the viral genome has been completely sequenced; the three-dimensional structures of the HA (Wilson et al. 1981) and the NA (Varghese et al. 1983) have been resolved by X-ray crystallography; or the ion channel activity of the M2 protein discovered (Pinto et al. 1992; Sugrue et al. 1990b).

The establishment of reverse genetics techniques that allow the artificial generation of virus from cloned cDNA provided perhaps the most significant stimulus to influenza research in the past two decades. In 1989, a virus was generated that contained a viral RNA segment derived from cloned cDNA (Luytjes et al. 1989), followed by the generation of influenza A virus entirely from plasmids in 1999 (Fodor et al. 1999; Neumann et al. 1999). These techniques facilitated studies of the role of influenza virus proteins in the viral life cycle, identification of the determinants of viral pathogenicity, development of influenza virus vaccines, and exploration of influenza virus as a vaccine vector.

Despite this progress, much remains to be learned about influenza viruses, particularly the molecular mechanism of influenza pathogenesis, interaction between viral and host gene products, and the mechanisms giving rise to new pandemic strains.

CLASSIFICATION

The *Orthomyxoviridae* family consists of five genera: *Influenzavirus A*, *Influenzavirus B*, *Influenzavirus C*,

Thogotovirus, which includes the *Thogoto virus* and *Dhori virus*, and *Isavirus*, which includes infectious salmon anemia virus (ISAV) (Klenk et al. 1995; van Regenmortel 2000). Orthomyxoviruses (Greek: orthos, straight or correct; myxa, mucus) contain segmented, linear, and negative-sense (complementary to mRNA) single-stranded RNA. The number of RNA segments differs among the genera: eight for influenza A, B and ISAV, seven for influenza C, six for *Thogoto virus*, and probably seven for *Dhori virus*. Accordingly, influenza A and B viruses contain HA and NA activities in different glycoproteins, whereas influenza C viruses lack NA, containing instead a hemagglutinin–esterase fusion (HEF) protein. *Thogoto virus* and *Dhori virus* possess a single glycoprotein (GP) that is not related to any known influenza virus protein but is related to the gp64 glycoprotein of baculoviruses (Morse et al. 1992). The virion has a molecular weight of 250 000 kDa and buoyant density in aqueous sucrose of 1.19 g/cm^3. Virions are sensitive to heat, lipid solvents, non-ionic detergents, formaldehyde, irradiation, and oxidizing agents.

Influenza A viruses are further classified into subtypes based on the antigenicity of their HA and NA molecules. Currently, there are 16 recognized HA subtypes (Fouchier et al. 2005) (H1, H2, etc.) and nine NA subtypes (N1, N2, etc.). The full nomenclature (WHO Memorandum 1980) for each new isolate includes the type of virus, the host of origin (except for human), geographical site of isolation, strain number, and year of isolation. The antigenic description of the HA and NA is given in parentheses. For example, a type A virus isolated in Memphis, Tennessee, from a mallard duck in 1995 with a strain number of 123 and an H3N8 subtype, would be designated A/mallard/Memphis/123/95 (H3N8). So far, no antigenic subtypes have been identified among the influenza B and C viruses. *Thogoto virus* and *Dhori virus* do not cross-react antigenically.

MORPHOLOGY AND STRUCTURE

All influenza viruses have a segmented negative-sense RNA core surrounded by a lipid envelope (Figure 32.2). The A and B types are distinguished by two integral membrane glycoproteins, HA and NA, that protrude from the virion surface. Influenza C virus, by contrast, contains only one type of membrane glycoprotein, HEF. A third transmembrane protein, encoded by the *M2* gene of influenza A viruses and the *BM2* gene of influenza B viruses, serves as an ion channel. Within the lipid envelope exists the matrix (M1) protein. The RNA segments are associated with nucleoprotein (NP) and

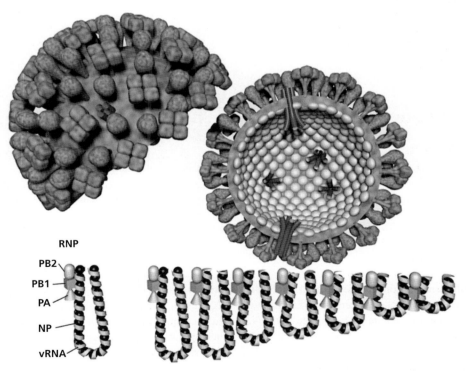

Figure 32.2 *Schematic diagram of an influenza A virion. The virion contains hemagglutinin (HA) and neuraminidase (NA) spikes in addition to a third membrane protein, M2. Within the viral envelope one finds ribonucleoprotein (RNP) consisting of RNA segments associated with nucleoprotein (NP), and the PA, PB1, and PB2 polymerase proteins. Three polymerase proteins are associated with the ends of vRNAs (insert). The precise location of M1 in virions is unknown, although it is associated with virion envelope, RNP, and NS2. (Courtesy of Yuko Kawaoka).*

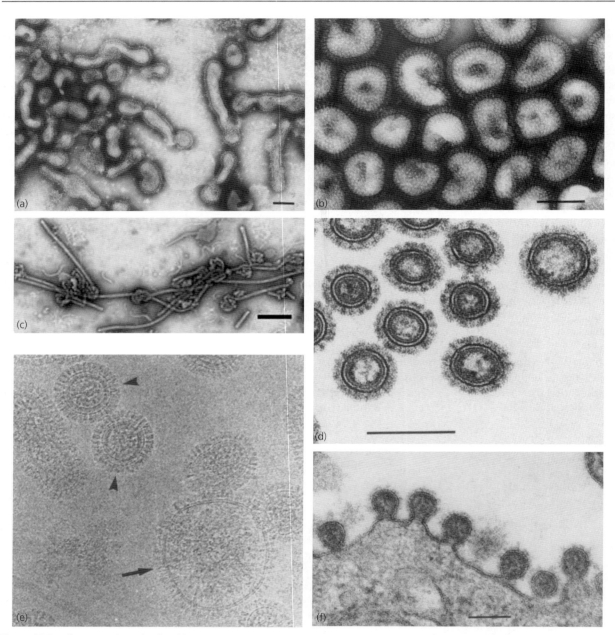

Figure 32.3 *Influenza A virus visualized by transmission electron microscopy. Two types of negatively stained virions are apparent:*
(a) *filamentous and pleomorphic and* **(b)** *largely spherical. Bar = 100 nm. (Courtesy of Dr. K.G. Murti) (Murti and Webster 1986).*
(c) *Filamentous A/Udorn/72 virus. (Courtesy of Dr. T. Noda.)* **(d)** *Sectioned virions with internal structures exposed. Bar = 100 nm.*
(e) *High-resolution electron micrograph of influenza virus. Note the two distinct types of virions: those with thick membranes*
(arrowhead) and those with typical thin lipid bilayers (arrow). The former group possesses more M1 protein than does the latter.
(Courtesy of Dr. Y. Fujiyoshi) (Fujiyoshi et al. 1994). **(f)** *Virus budding from plasma membrane. Bar = 100 nm.*

three large polymerase proteins, designated PA, PB1, and PB2 on the basis of their overall acidic or basic amino acid composition, that are responsible for RNA replication and transcription (Krug et al. 1989).

Influenza virus particles are pleomorphic (Hoyle 1968) with spherical or filamentous morphology, or a mixture of both (Figure 32.3). Among clinical isolates that have undergone a limited number of passages in eggs or tissue culture, there are more filamentous than spherical particles, whereas extensively passaged laboratory strains consist almost exclusively of spherical virions (80–120 nm in diameter). Despite their distinctive shape, the filamentous virions possess many of the serological, hemagglutinating, and enzymatic characteristics of the spherical particles. The morphology of influenza virions seems to be primarily determined by the *M* gene (Bourmakina and Garcia-Sastre 2003; Roberts and Compans 1998), although both the *HA* and *NP* genes likely contribute (Jin et al. 1997; Mitnaul et al. 1996; Smirnov et al. 1991).

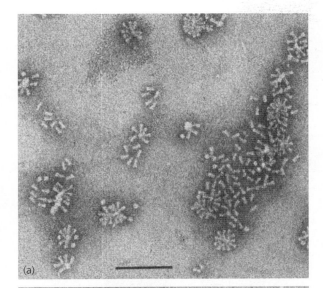

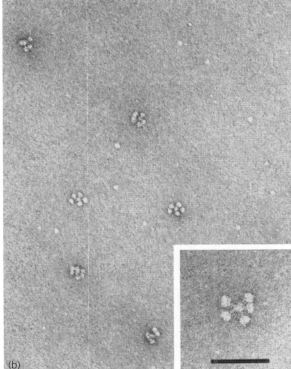

Figure 32.4 (a) *Hemagglutinin (HA) (bar = 100 nm) and* **(b)** *neuraminidase (NA) (bar = 50 nm) proteins isolated from detergent-disrupted virus. The molecules associate by hydrophobic C- (HA) and N- (NA) terminal sequences after the detergent has been removed. (Courtesy of Dr. K.G. Murti.) (Murti and Webster 1986).*

The HA and NA molecules that stud the surface of influenza A and B viruses range from 10 to 12 nm in length. The mean ratio of HA to NA spikes is ca. 5:1. The HA spikes are rod-shaped, whereas the NA spikes resemble mushrooms with slender stalks (Figure 32.4). They are not distinguishable by electron microscopy unless either the HA or NA is removed from the virion

surface with a protease or rosettes of the HA and NA are formed after virions are treated with detergent. The NA distribution on virions remains uncertain. If the HA is removed with trypsin, the NA seems to be evenly distributed (Erickson and Kilbourne 1980); however, by immunoelectron microscopy with monoclonal antibodies, but not polyclonal antibodies, it seems to be clustered (Amano et al. 1992; Murti and Webster 1986). The HEF glycoproteins on influenza C viruses (8–10 nm long) are organized as hexagonal arrays of latticelike structures on the virion surface (Flewett and Apostolov 1967; Hewat et al. 1984) (Figure 32.5).

Within the lipid envelope, the viral RNA is associated with NP and three polymerase proteins, PA, PB1, and PB2. The organization of this ribonucleoprotein (RNP) complex within virions remains unclear. Electron microscopy has revealed helical structures in spontaneously lysed virions and in those partially disrupted with detergent (Figure 32.6). Similar structures can be made only with use of purified M1 protein (Ruigrok et al. 1989), indicating a significant role for this component in the generation of the RNP complex, with which M1 is known to associate (Hara et al. 2003; Kawakami and Ishihama 1983). Isolated RNP forms rod-shaped, right-handed helices that vary in length from 50 to 150 nm (Compans et al. 1972). Three-dimensional reconstitution of artificially generated viral RNPs reveal a circular shape composed of nine NP monomers, two of which form contacts with the polymerase complex (Martin-Benito et al. 2001). Each NP monomer interacts with approximately 24 nucleotides (Ortega et al. 2000) without apparent sequence specificity, and exposes the bases to the solvent (Baudin et al. 1994; Klumpp et al. 1997). The 5′ and 3′ terminal ends of viral RNA, which are complementary to each other, form a panhandle-like structure (Hsu et al. 1987).

The M1 protein is the primary determinant of virus budding (Gomez-Puertas et al. 2000; Latham and Galarza 2001) and its role in this process may be similar to that of Ebola matrix or retroviral gag proteins (Edbauer and Naso 1984; Harris et al. 1999; Jasenosky et al. 2001). Immunogold labeling with monoclonal antibodies to M1 failed to decorate the protein in virions unless they were first treated with a protease or a detergent (Murti et al. 1992). Recent cryo-electron microscopic studies suggest that M1 can modify the lipid bilayer, causing thickening of the viral envelope (Fujiyoshi et al. 1994) (see Figure 32.3e).

GENOME STRUCTURE AND FUNCTION

Influenza A and B viruses possess eight single-stranded RNA segments, each encoding at least one protein, whereas influenza C viruses contain only seven segments. Genome lengths differ widely among the three types of influenza viruses, some variations also being found among strains within the same type. Type B

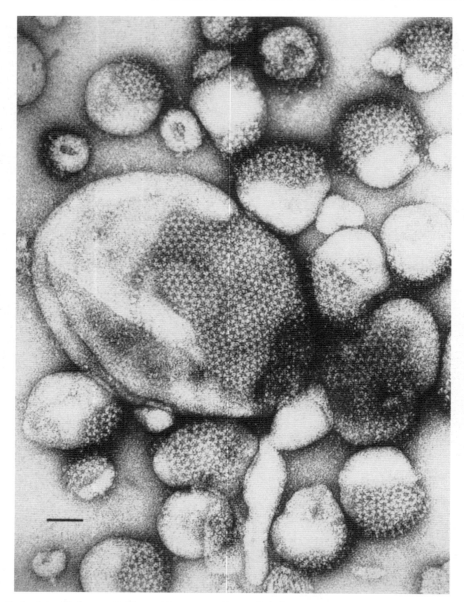

Figure 32.5 *Negatively stained influenza C virions with an array of extended glycoproteins. Bar = 50 nm. (Courtesy of Dr. R.W.H. Ruigrok.) (Hewat et al. 1984).*

viruses have the longest genome (ca. 14 600 nt) followed by A (ca. 13 600 nt) and then C (ca. 12 900 nt). Within each type, the lengths of genes other than the HA and NA (for A and B viruses) and the HEF (for C viruses) are highly conserved. The viral genome constitutes 2 percent of the mass of the virion.

In each of the eight RNA segments of all influenza A viruses, the first 12 nucleotides at the 3′ end and the last 13 at the 5′ end are highly conserved and contain promoter activity (Fodor et al. 1994; Fodor et al. 1995; Li and Palese 1992; Neumann and Hobom 1995; Parvin et al. 1989; Piccone et al. 1993; Seong and Brownlee 1992a; Seong and Brownlee 1992b; Yamanaka et al. 1991b) (Figure 32.7). Similar structures have been identified in the RNA segments of influenza B (conserved

sequence: 5′ AGUAG(A/U)AACAA and 3′ UCGU-CUUCGC) and C (conserved sequence: 5′ AGCA-GUAGCAA and 3′ UCGU(U/C)UUCGUCC) viruses as well. The promoter regions of influenza A and B virus RNAs are interchangeable (Crescenzo-Chaigne et al. 1999; Muster et al. 1991), although the chimeric virus resulting from such modification is attenuated (Muster et al. 1991). The partially complementary 5′ and 3′ ends of the vRNA or cRNA, respectively, were thought to form a panhandle structure (Hsu et al. 1987). However, extensive characterization of promoter mutants indicated that the promoter region adopts a so-called 'cork-screw' structure characterized by intrastrand – rather than interstrand – base-pairing between the 5′ and 3′ terminal nucleotides (Flick et al. 1996; Flick and Hobom

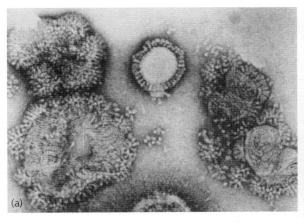
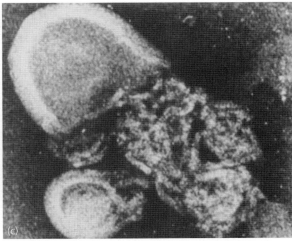
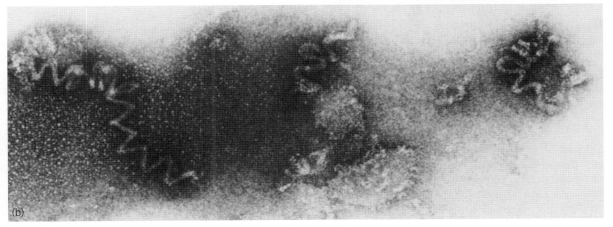

Figure 32.6 *Electron micrograph of the internal structure of an influenza virus.* **(a)** *Naturally disrupted virions.* **(b)** *Extended coil structures resulting from detergent treatment of virus.* **(c)** *M1 protein reconstituted into liposomes. (Courtesy of Dr. R.W.H. Ruigrok, Ruigrok et al. 1989.)*

1999). Similar promoter structures have been identified for influenza C virus (Crescenzo-Chaigne and van der Werf, 2001) and Thogotovirus (Weber et al. 1997).

Most viral genes encode a single protein (Table 32.2); the exceptions are the *M* and nonstructural (*NS*) genes of all influenza viruses and the *NA* gene of type B virus, that encode two proteins each (Lamb and Horvath 1991). The *NS* gene of type A virus encodes both a 26-kDa (NS1) protein translated from unspliced mRNA and a 14-kDa (NS2) protein translated from spliced mRNA (Inglis et al. 1979; Lamb and Choppin 1979) (Figure 32.8a), which share the same AUG initiation codon and nine subsequent amino acids. A similar protein-coding strategy is employed by the type B and C influenza viruses. Some influenza A virus *PB1* genes encode a second polypeptide, termed PB1-F2, which is encoded in the +1 reading frame (W. Chen et al. 2001) (Figure 32.8c).

By contrast, each type of influenza virus possesses a different mechanism for expression of *M* gene products. The *M* gene of type A viruses generates an unspliced transcript encoding the M1 protein, as well as two other alternatively spliced RNAs, designated M2 and mRNA3, which differ in their use of 5' splice sites (Inglis and Brown 1981; Lamb et al. 1981) (Figure 32.8b). However, a translation product of mRNA3 has not been found in vivo. The leader sequence of the M2 mRNA contains the AUG initiation codon and codons for eight subsequent residues that are shared with the M1 protein; this region is followed by a sequence encoding 88 residues in the +1 reading frame. The nine amino acid peptide encoded by mRNA3 has not been detected in infected cells. By binding to the 5' end of the viral M1 mRNA in a sequence-specific, cap-dependent manner, the viral polymerase complex promotes splicing at the M2 mRNA 5' site over the mRNA3 5' site (Shih et al. 1995). The *M* gene of influenza B viruses also encodes two proteins, M1 and BM2, which are translated via a termination-reinitiation scheme of tandem cistrons; a pentanucleotide sequence, UAAUG, contains the termination codon for the M1 and the initiation codon for the BM2 (Horvath et al. 1990) (Figure 32.8d). Finally, in contrast to the scheme employed by influenza A viruses, type C viruses rely on spliced transcripts to produce M1 protein

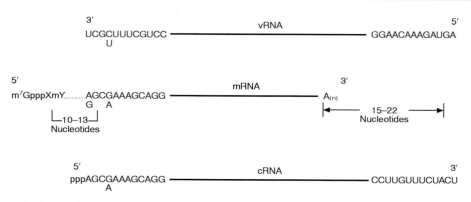

Figure 32.7 *Schematic diagram illustrating the differences between influenza virus virion RNA (vRNA) segments, mRNAs, and full-length cRNA (template for vRNA). The conserved 12 nucleotides at the 3′ end and 13 nucleotides at the 5′ end of each of the influenza A virus vRNA segments are indicated. Similar conserved sequences are found at the 3′ and 5′ ends of the influenza B and C virus RNA segments.*

(Yamashita et al. 1988) (Figure 32.8f). Splicing of the primary transcript introduces a translational termination codon, resulting in the synthesis of the M1 protein of 242 amino acids. The unspliced mRNA has the coding capacity for a 374 amino acid protein (P42) which is proteolytically cleaved to yield CM2 and M1′ (Hongo et al. 1999; Pekosz and Lamb 1998). CM2 is composed of 115 amino acids corresponding to the carboxy-terminal region of the primary transcript (Hongo et al. 1994) and has biochemical properties similar to those of the influenza A virus M2 protein (Hongo et al. 1997).

Still another mechanism of viral protein expression is represented by the influenza B virus *NA* gene, which gives rise to a bicistronic mRNA containing two initiating AUG codons that are separated by four nucleotides (Figure 32.8e). The 100 amino acid NB protein is translated from the 5′ AUG codon, while the 466 amino acid NA protein is translated from the second AUG codon. Even though the NA initiation codon is positioned downstream of the NB initiation site, greater amounts of NA protein (1:0.6) accumulate in cells (Williams and Lamb 1989).

Replication

The replication cycle of influenza viruses has been studied most extensively with type A strains; therefore, unless otherwise noted, the processes described below refer to viruses of that type (Figure 32.9).

ATTACHMENT TO UNCOATING

An influenza virus infects cells through binding of its HA or HEF protein to the cell's sialyloligosaccharide receptor. After binding, the attached virion undergoes endocytosis (White et al. 1983). The low pH of the late endocytotic vesicle triggers a conformational change in the cleavage-activated HA (Skehel et al. 1982), initiating fusion of the viral and vesicular membranes. Fusion

releases the contents of the virion into the cytoplasm of the cell (uncoating). Before fusion, M2 proteins (BM2 protein for type B viruses, and possibly NB for type B viruses), by ion channeling, introduce protons into the inside of the virion, exposing the core to low pH (Hay 1992; Helenius 1992; Pinto et al. 1992; Sugrue et al. 1990b) (Figure 32.10). Such an event is thought to promote dissociation of the M1 from the RNP by disrupting the low pH-sensitive interaction between these molecules (Zhirnov 1990), allowing the RNP to migrate to the nucleus through the nuclear pore in an ATP-dependent manner (Kemler et al. 1994; Martin and Helenius 1991). Exposure of the viral core to low pH, however, is not required for dissociation of M1 from RNP in type C viruses (Zhirnov and Grigoriev 1994).

TRANSCRIPTION AND TRANSLATION

Once the RNP migrates into the host-cell nucleus, the associated polymerase complexes (PA, PB1, and PB2) begin primary transcription of mRNA (Krug et al. 1979), which requires cooperation with ongoing transcription by cellular RNA polymerase II. The reason for this requirement is that initiation of influenza virus mRNA synthesis depends on m⁷GpppXm-containing capped primers (10–13 nt long, containing 5′-GCA-3′ at their 3′ proximal ends) that are generated from host cell RNAs by an influenza virus-encoded, cap-dependent endonuclease (Krug et al. 1989; Plotch et al. 1981). The endonuclease activity resides in the PB1 subunit (M.L. Li et al. 2001) and requires the presence of influenza viral RNA (Hagen et al. 1994); however, the requirement of both the 5′ and 3′ ends of vRNA remains controversial and may depend on the experimental parameters (Cianci et al. 1995; Li et al. 1998; Rao et al. 2003).

mRNA synthesis begins with incorporation of a G residue complementary to the penultimate C residue on the vRNAs (Beaton and Krug 1981; Kawakami and Ishihama 1983). Chain elongation is carried out by the PB1 subunit, which contains four consensus motifs for nucleic

Table 32.2 *Influenza A virus genome RNA and protein coding assignments*

Segment	Length (nucleotides)[a]	Encoded polypeptide	Nascent polypeptide length (amino acids)	Experimentally determined mol. wt (kDa) of polypeptides	Carbohydrates	Approx. copy no. per virion	Remarks
1	2 341	PB2	759	87	–	30–60	Component of RNA transcriptase complex Host-cell capped mRNA recognition and binding
2	2 341	PB1	757	96	–	30–60	Component of RNA transcriptase complex RNA-dependent RNA polymerase activity; capped mRNA endonuclease activity
		PB1-F2[b]	87	10.5	–	2 650	Induction of apoptosis
3	2 233	PA	716	85	–	30–60	Component of RNA transcriptase complex Required for replication; possible role in transcription
4	1 778	HA	566	63	+	500	Surface trimer glycoprotein Cleaved into HA1 and HA2 Major antigenic determinant Functions in virus binding to cell surface receptors and fusion
5	1 565	NP	498	56	–	1 000	Associated with RNA segments to form ribonucleoprotein
6	1 413	NA	454	60	+	100	Surface tetramer glycoprotein; neuraminidase activity Functions in virus release; target of neuraminidase inhibitors
7	1 027	M1	252	27	–	3 000	Major virion component; involved in RNP transport out of nucleus
		M2	97	14	–	20–60	Coded from spliced mRNA; ion channel activity; target of adamantanes
8	890	NS1	230	26	–	NA	Nonstructural protein; inhibits mRNA transport from nucleus; interferon antagonist
		NS2(= NEP)	121	14	–	130–200	Coded from spliced mRNA; viral nuclear export protein

a) The lengths of the *HA* and *NA* genes differ among the strains.
b) Not encoded by all influenza A viruses; NA, not applicable.

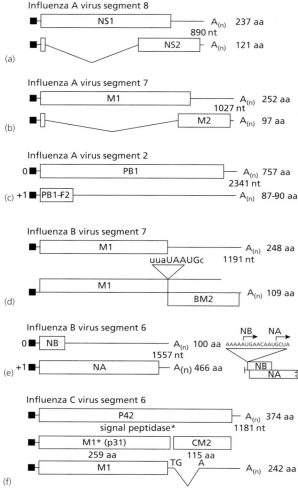

Figure 32.8 *Coding strategies of influenza virus genes.* **(a)** *Influenza A virus NS1 and NS2 mRNAs and their coding regions. NS1 and NS2 share ten amino-terminal residues, including the initiating methionine. The reading frame of NS2 mRNA (nucleotide positions 529–861) differs from that of NS1.* **(b)** *Influenza A virus M1 and M2 mRNAs and their coding regions. M1 and M2 share nine amino-terminal residues, including the initiating methionine; however, the reading frame of M2 mRNA (nucleotide positions 740–1 004) differs from that of M1.* **(c)** *Influenza A virus PB1 segment coding regions. Based on Kozak's rule, PB1 translation initiation may be inefficient, thereby allowing translation initiation of the PB1-F2 open reading frame by ribosomal scanning.* **(d)** *Influenza B virus RNA segment 7 open reading frames and the organization of the open reading frames used to translate the M1 and BM2 proteins. The stop–start pentanucleotide is also illustrated.* **(e)** *Open reading frames in influenza B virus RNA segment 6, illustrating the overlapping reading frames of NB and neuraminidase (NA). Nucleotide sequence surrounding the two AUG initiation codons, in mRNA sense, is shown to the right.* **(f)** *Influenza C virus mRNAs derived from RNA segment 6. The unspliced and spliced mRNAs encode P42 and M1, respectively. Cleavage of P42 by a signal peptidase yields M1' (p31) and CM2. Thin lines at the 5' and 3' termini of the mRNAs represent untranslated regions. Introns in the mRNAs are shown by V-shaped lines; filled rectangles at the 5' ends of mRNAs represent heterogeneous nucleotides derived from cellular RNAs that are covalently linked to viral sequences (Virus Taxonomy 2005).*

acid polymerases (Argos 1988; Biswas and Nayak 1994; Ishihama and Barbier 1994; Poch et al. 1989) as well as nucleotide binding sites (Asano et al. 1995; Asano and Ishihama 1997; Romanos and Hay 1984). Transcription continues until it reaches the poly(A) addition site, located 15–22 nt from the 5' end of the vRNA. Three elements are critical for polyadenylation: a stretch of uridines near the 5' end of the virion RNA (optimal with 5–7 residues and 16 nt from the 5' end), which serves as the poly(A) signal (Li and Palese 1994; Luo et al. 1991; Poon et al. 1999; Zheng et al. 1999); the RNA duplex of the promoter structure; and specific nucleotides near the 5' end of the vRNA (Pritlove et al. 1999). The current model predicts threading of the vRNA through the polymerase complex which is stably bound to the 5' end of the vRNA throughout transcription (Fodor et al. 1994; Hagen et al. 1994). In this model, the polymerase complex bound to the promoter region would serve as a physical barrier that causes reiterative copying at the neighboring uridine stretch. The primary transcripts are then used in the production of viral proteins by the cell's cytoplasmic translation machinery. Three polymerase proteins (PA, PB1, and PB2), as well as NP, NS1, and NS2 proteins, are transported to the nucleus. The negative-strand genomic segment and the positive-strand antigenomic segments, but not viral mRNA, are coated with NP. NS1 inhibits the transport of cellular mRNA to the cytoplasm by binding to the poly(A) region (Qiu and Krug 1994) and maximizing the availability of capped primers for viral mRNA synthesis. The products of viral mRNA synthesis change as infection proceeds, indicating a temporal form of regulation (Hatada et al. 1989; Hay et al. 1977). Early in infection, the synthesis of mRNAs encoding NP and NS1 dominates; later the production of mRNAs for HA, NA, and M1 increases, while transcripts for the polymerase proteins are relatively low throughout the infection cycle, except at the earliest time. The relative amounts of mRNAs correlate with the amounts of their corresponding proteins, indicating that viral gene expression is regulated at the transcriptional level, in addition to the temporal control mechanisms governing the translational efficiency of viral mRNA (Yamanaka et al. 1988, 1991a). The production of full-length viral complementary RNA (cRNA) was believed to be delayed until viral protein had been synthesized. In this model, newly synthesized NP promoted 'read-through' of the poly(A) site, allowing the synthesis of cRNA transcripts (Beaton and Krug 1986; Shapiro and Krug 1988) which in turn serve as templates for the production of vRNA. Recent findings, however, suggest that cRNA synthesis occurs early in infection as well; at this time point, cRNA may be degraded rapidly by cellular nucleases, while increasing amounts of polymerase proteins may protect the cRNA later in infection (Vreede et al. 2004). Equimolar quantities of cRNA are synthesized throughout

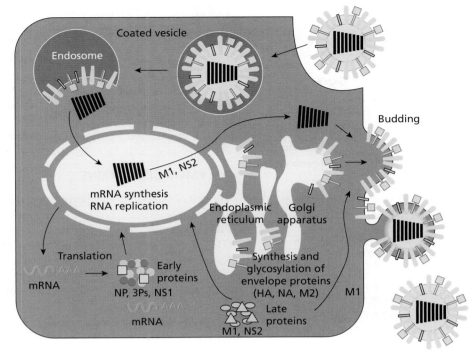

Figure 32.9 *Replication cycle of influenza A virus, from binding of the virus to the host cell surface to its exit from the plasma membrane. Ps, polymerase proteins. (Lamb et al. 1994.)*

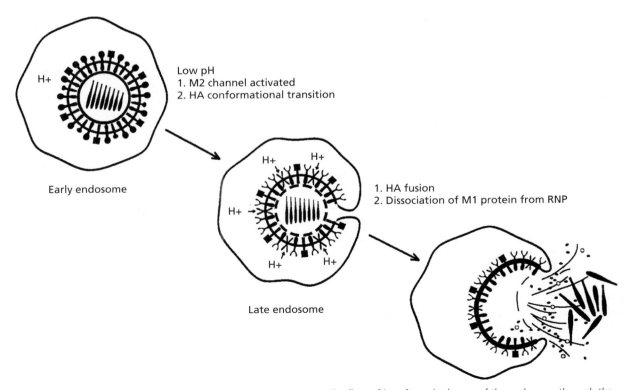

Figure 32.10 *Ion channel activity of the M2 protein upon virus entry. The flow of ions from the lumen of the endosome through the M2 channel into the virion interior allows the dissociation of protein–protein interactions between M1 and RNP, facilitating RNP transport to the nucleus. (Lamb et al. 1994; © Mary K. Bryson.)*

infection (Hay et al. 1977), indicating a lack of regulation of this process.

After their translation in the endoplasmic reticulum (ER), viral membrane proteins – HA, NA, and M2 for the type A viruses, NB for type B and HEF for type C – are translocated into the lumen of the ER, where they undergo oligomerization prior to their transport to the Golgi apparatus (Doms et al. 1993) and subsequent transport to the plasma membrane. The proteins are glycosylated in the ER (high mannose type), and then processed further in the Golgi to contain oligosaccharide of the complex type.

VIRION MORPHOGENESIS AND BUDDING

Nuclear export of vRNP complexes is mediated by the NS2 protein (Neumann et al. 2000; O'Neill et al. 1998) now also referred to as nuclear export protein (NEP), which interacts with the cellular export factor CRM1 (Neumann et al. 2000). In addition, the M1 protein is also required for nuclear export of vRNP complexes (Bui et al. 2000; Huang et al. 2001; Martin and Helenius 1991; Whittaker et al. 1995) and may execute its function by bridging viral ribonucleoprotein complexes and NS2 (NEP) (Sakaguchi et al. 2003). Electron microscopy of influenza virus-infected cells has not identified viral core structures, nor has an association of RNP with the plasma membrane been found; rather, RNP seems to associate with viral membrane proteins only when the virion is beginning to assume its shape (Patterson et al. 1988). Segment-specific virion incorporation signals have been identified on viral RNAs (Fujii et al. 2003; Watanabe et al. 2003) that promote their efficient incorporation into virions. These signals are located in the nontranslated regions at both ends of the vRNAs and extend into the translated regions, thereby conferring segment specificity. Although influenza virus can accommodate more than eight viral segments (Enami et al. 1991; Scholtissek et al. 1978b) – a finding that suggested random incorporation of vRNAs – efficient packaging relies on cis-acting signals that govern the incorporation of eight viral RNA segments into virions. The mechanism for selective vRNA virion incorporation remains to be determined. Few details of the final assembly process are known. Presumably, RNP buds outward through the cell membrane. Substantial amounts of M1 are found in the cytoplasm throughout the infection period. M1 interacts with cellular membranes (Bucher et al. 1980; Gregoriades and Frangione 1981; Hay 1974; Kretzschmar et al. 1996), and induces the formation of viruslike particles (Gomez-Puertas et al. 2000; Latham and Galarza 2001). Because at least a fraction of M1 is associated with RNP in the virion (Kawakami and Ishihama 1983; Rees and Dimmock 1981), this protein possibly serves as a molecular 'glue', interacting with RNP on the one hand and with HA, NA, or M2 on the other (Ali et al. 2000; Barman et al. 2001; Hara et al. 2003). Such interactions may function as a budding signal.

Polypeptides: nonstructural and structural

Influenza A virus comprises nine structural and one nonstructural protein (see Table 32.2), compared with nine structural and two nonstructural proteins in influenza B virus, and six structural and three nonstructural proteins in influenza C virus. For some influenza A viruses, an additional polypeptide is expressed from the *PB1* gene (see Table 32.2 and below).

POLYMERASE PROTEINS

The exact nature of the polymerase complex remains under investigation. Trimeric complexes composed of PB2, PB1, and PA are formed in virus-infected cells (Detjen et al. 1987; Honda et al. 1990; Kato et al. 1985; Kawakami and Ishihama 1983) and in transfected cells expressing all components of vRNP complexes (Digard et al. 1989; Honda et al. 2002; Hwang et al. 2000). Functional studies suggest that dimeric complexes consisting of PB1–PB2 or PB1–PA have transcriptase or replicase activity, respectively (Honda and Ishihama 1997; Honda et al. 2002; Lee et al. 2002); however, all three polymerase subunits may be required for efficient replication and transcription (Fodor et al. 2002; Perales and Ortin 1997). The polymerase complex recognizes the influenza virus promoter structure in a sequence-specific manner (Honda et al. 1987; Tiley et al. 1994) and also interacts with NP (Biswas et al. 1998). PB1 forms the structural backbone of the polymerase complex by interacting with both PB2 and PA (Honda and Ishihama 1997; Ishihama 1996; Ohtsu et al. 2002; Perez and Donis 2001; Toyoda et al. 1996). Artificially assembled vRNP complexes allowed the determination of a three-dimensional structure that revealed a compact polymerase complex with points of interaction with NP (Area et al. 2004) (Figure 32.11). The three polymerase proteins are highly conserved among type A viruses (Gorman et al. 1990b; Kawaoka and Webster 1989; Okazaki et al. 1989).

PB1

This protein is required for the initiation and elongation of newly synthesized viral RNA (Braam et al. 1983). Conserved PB1 residues Ser444–Asp445–Asp446 of type A viruses (443–445 for type B and 445–447 for type C), which resemble the signature sequences of other viral RNA polymerases, may form the core of the transcriptase/replicase activity (Biswas and Nayak 1994). Binding of PB1 to the viral promoter structure (Gonzalez and Ortin 1999a, b) activates the protein's capped mRNA endonuclease activity (Cianci et al. 1995; Gonzalez and Ortin 1999a, b; Li et al. 1998; M.L. Li et al. 2001; Rao et al. 2003). PB1 contains two discontinuous regions, both essential for nuclear localization (Nath and Nayak 1990).

Some influenza A virus *PB1* genes contain a second open reading frame yielding the so-called PB1-F2 polypep-

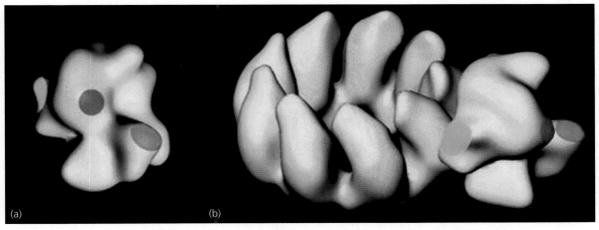

Figure 32.11 *Three-dimensional model for the influenza virus polymerase complex based on electron microscopic images. The colored areas depict the location of subunit domains: N-terminal region of PB2 (red), C-terminal region of PA (blue), C-terminal region of PB1 (green).* **(a)** *Polymerase model;* **(b)** *position of the polymerase subunits relative to the ringlike RNP structure. (Courtesy of Dr. J. Ortin; Area et al. 2004.)*

tide (W. Chen et al. 2001). The 87 amino acid peptide localizes to mitochondria where it induces apoptosis (D. Chen et al. 2001; Gibbs et al. 2003). The absence of this open reading frame from some animal (particularly swine) virus isolates leaves in question the overall contribution of this peptide to influenza virus pathogenesis.

PB2

PB2 is crucial for recognizing and binding to type I cap structures of cellular mRNAs (Blaas et al. 1982; Plotch et al. 1981; Ulmanen et al. 1983). Several amino acids/amino acid stretches at position 242–282 (Honda et al. 1999), 533–564 (M.L. Li et al. 2001), and/or 363 and 404 (Fechter et al. 2003) have been identified as critical for cap-binding. PB2 is essential for viral mRNA synthesis, although its requirement for replication remains controversial (Gastaminza et al. 2003; Nakagawa et al. 1995). Two signals mediate nuclear localization of influenza A PB2 protein, one of which is involved in PB2 perinuclear binding (Mukaigawa and Nayak 1991).

PB2 plays a role in host range restriction (Almond 1977; Subbarao et al. 1993; Yao et al. 2001). In 1997, H5N1 avian influenza viruses infected humans in Hong Kong, resulting in fatal outcomes in several individuals. Reverse genetics experiments demonstrated a critical role of amino acid 627 of PB2 for efficient replication in mice (Hatta et al. 2001); a mutation from glutamic acid (found in avian isolates at this position) to lysine (found in all human influenza viruses) enhances viral replication in mice (and likely in humans), leading to increased virulence. This finding was substantiated by the identification of the same Glu-to-Lys replacement in an H7N7 influenza virus isolated from a Dutch veterinarian who succumbed to influenza virus infection in 2003 (Fouchier et al. 2004), and in H5N1 viruses isolated from Vietnamese influenza virus victims in 2004 (K.S. Li et al. 2004). This replacement affects the level of viral RNA tran-

scription/replication (Crescenzo-Chaigne et al. 2002; Massin et al. 2001; Naffakh et al. 2000; Shinya et al. 2004). However, in the ferret model, increased virulence has not been associated with this change (Zitzow et al. 2002) and viruses without this mutation have been isolated from severe and fatal human cases of influenza (Shaw et al. 2002; Ruben Donis unpublished).

PA

The PA protein is an essential component of the viral polymerase complex; however, its exact role in replication or transcription is less well defined than those of PB2 or PB1. PA is required for viral RNA replication (Honda and Ishihama 1997; Honda et al. 2002; Krug et al. 1989; Lee et al. 2002), possibly by acting as an elongation factor (Fodor et al. 2003) or by facilitating the binding of PB1 to viral RNA (Lee et al. 2002). It has also been implicated in transcription (Fodor et al. 2002). PA reduces the half-lives of co-expressed proteins (Sanz-Ezquerro et al. 1995, 1996) but the significance of this proteolytic activity remains obscure (Naffakh et al. 2001; Perales et al. 2000). In addition, a serine protease activity has been described for this protein (Hara et al. 2001) which is not critical for viral replication in cell culture (Fodor et al. 2002), but does support efficient viral growth (Toyoda et al. 2003). Expression of PA does not result in complete nuclear localization, which can only be achieved after coexpression of PB1 or NS1 (Nieto et al. 1992).

HEMAGGLUTININ

Encoded by the fourth largest RNA segment, the HA accounts for about 25 percent of viral protein and is distributed evenly on the surface of virions. It is responsible for the attachment and subsequent penetration of viruses into cells. The HA spikes, approximately 14 × 4 nm, protrude from the virion surface (Laver and

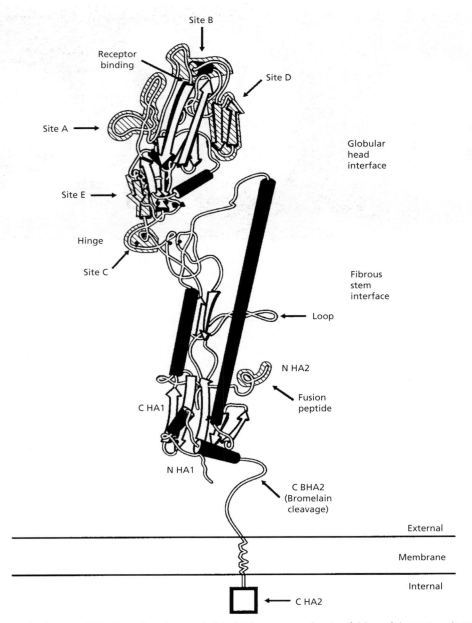

Figure 32.12 *Schematic diagram of the Hong Kong hemagglutinin (HA) monomer, showing folding of the HA1 and HA2 polypeptides. The shaded areas show the putative locations of the five independent antigenic areas (sites A–E). Note that the fusion peptide is also buried in the intact molecule and is exposed only after a conformational change at low pH (Bullough et al. 1994; Wilson et al. 1981).*

Valentine 1969) (Figure 32.12, and see Figure 32.3). The HA homotrimer (Wiley et al. 1977) is synthesized as a single polypeptide chain (HA0) that undergoes post-translational cleavage by cellular proteases (Klenk et al. 1975; Lazarowitz and Choppin 1975). The resulting HA1 and HA2 subunits (36 and 27 kDa) are covalently attached by a disulfide bond, while the 'two-chain' monomers are associated noncovalently to form trimers. An N-terminal signal sequence is removed. HA cleavage is required for infectivity (Klenk et al. 1975; Lazarowitz and Choppin 1975) to expose the hydrophobic amino terminus of HA2, which mediates fusion between the viral envelope and the endosomal membrane (White 1992).

Three-dimensional structure

For the ectodomain of human H3N2 virus, X-ray crystallographic structures have been determined for three different conformations: Bromelain-cleaved soluble HA (BHA) of A/Aichi/2/68(H3N2) (Wiley et al. 1981; Wilson et al. 1981; Wilson and Cox 1990) which represents the conformation of cleaved HA, the uncleaved HA0 precursor (Chen et al. 1998), and fragments of low pH-treated BHA (Bizebard et al. 1995; Bullough et al. 1994). Furthermore, the HA structures of the 1918 pandemic virus (Stevens et al. 2004), of H3 and H5 avian viruses, and an H9 swine virus have been determined (Ha et al. 2001; Ha et al. 2003). The BHA is 13.5 nm long and 1.4–4 nm in triangular cross-section, and contains all of the HA1 and the first 175 of the 221 amino acids of the HA2 subunit; it lacks only the hydrophobic membrane-anchoring peptide (Brand and Skehel 1972). The HA is folded into two structurally distinct domains, a globular head and a fibrous stalk. The globular head is entirely composed of HA1 residues and contains an eight-stranded antiparallel β-sheet. This framework supports the receptor-binding site, which is surrounded by highly variable antigenic loop structures. The fibrous stalk region, more proximal to the viral membrane, consists of residues from both HA1 and HA2. The cleavage site between HA1 and HA2 is located in the middle of the stalk. The trimeric structure is principally stabilized by the fibrous stem regions with a rather loose association of the globular heads. HA0 and cleaved HA1+HA2 are superimposable except for the region spanning the cleavage site. In uncleaved HA, the cleavage site forms a prominent surface loop in the middle of the stalk. A cavity is located next to the cleavage site that is partially filled by the carboxy terminus of HA1. Upon cleavage, the carboxy terminus of HA1 becomes exposed on the trimer surface, ca. 2.2 nm from the terminus of HA2, indicating significant rearrangement and conformational change after cleavage of the HA0. The hydrophobic amino terminus of the HA2 (fusion peptide) becomes buried in the trimeric structure, filling the cavity. The cleaved HA is presumed to be metastable.

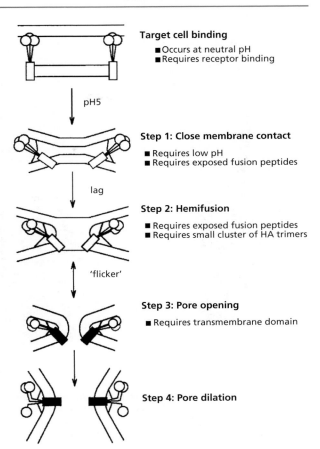

Figure 32.13 *Steps in HA-mediated membrane fusion. Processes described in the diagram occur after virus attachment to a cell membrane (White 1994).*

Fusion

The fusion of influenza viruses to the endosomal membrane is mediated by the HA (White 1992) (Figures 32.13 and 32.14). Under conditions of neutral pH, the fusion peptide, which forms a small part of the amino terminus of the HA2, is located in the fibrous stem of the molecule (ca. 3.5 nm away from the viral membrane and, hence, 10 nm from the target endosomal membrane), and is well integrated into the subunit interface by a network of hydrogen bonds. The importance of the peptide in HA-mediated fusion is evident from the ability of mutations in this region that alter (Daniels et al. 1987) or abolish (Gething et al. 1986b) fusion activity. When the pH is ca. 5 (late endosomal pH), the tertiary structure of the HA is altered (Skehel et al. 1982; White and Wilson 1987) (Figure 32.14). This change is critical for fusion of the viral and endosomal membranes (Skehel et al. 1982; Stegmann et al. 1990; White and Wilson 1987). The three-dimensional structure of the HA1 globular head remains largely unaltered (Bizebard et al. 1995), although partial dissociation of the globular heads may occur (Godley et al. 1992). By contrast, HA2 undergoes a refolding event in which the fusion peptide is relocated more than 100 Å toward the target membrane. At neutral pH, HA2 amino acid residues 38 to 55 form a short α-helix, followed by an extended loop (residues 56–75) and a long α-helix (residues 76–126) (Wilson et al. 1981). By contrast, the X-ray crystallographic structure of proteolytic fragments of the low pH-induced form of HA2 (Bullough et al. 1994; Carr and Kim 1993; Chen et al. 1999b) reveals a triple stranded α-helical coiled-coil formed by residues 40–105. Residues 106 to 112 form a loop that connects to a shorter α-helix (residues 113 to 129) that runs antiparallel to the long α-helix. The amino- and carboxy-terminal amino acids of HA2 are connected through numerous interactions that hold these residues in place at the 'tip' of the structure. The conformational states of the HA after exposure to low pH may differ among different subtypes of the molecules (Melikyan et al. 1999; Puri et al. 1990).

The exact mechanism of membrane fusion is the subject of intensive investigation and is currently believed to involve the following steps (discussed in detail in Bentz and Mittal (2003), Skehel and Wiley (2000), and Stegmann (2000), (Figure 32.13). Fusion is initiated by low pH that triggers a conformational change to expose the fusion peptide, which becomes inserted into the target membrane. Next, the outer leaf-

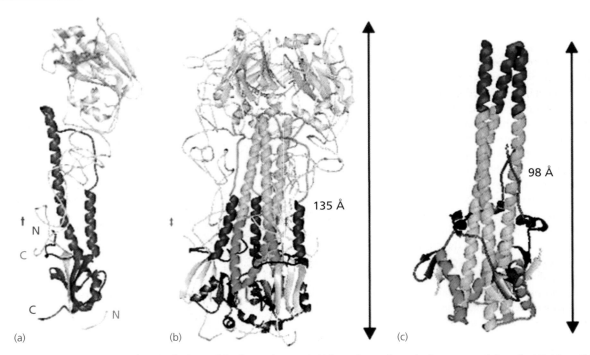

Figure 32.14 *Ribbon diagram of HA in the bromelain-digested neutral pH form shown for a single monomer* **(a)** *or the HA trimer* **(b)***; ribbon diagram of the low pH, trimeric fragment composed of amino acids 38–175 of HA2 which are linked through disulphide bonds to residues 1–27 of the HA1 subunit* **(c)***. In* **(a)***, HA1 and HA2 are depicted in gray and red, respectively, while the receptor-binding residues are shown in green. In* **(b)** *and* **(c)***, the helices/coils shown in red (amino acids 38–55), blue (amino acids 56–75), green (residues 106–129), and dark gray (amino acids 130–175) undergo a conformational change upon exposure to low pH, while amino acids 76–105 (yellow) maintain their conformation. In* **(b)***, the fusion peptides of the individual monomers are depicted in magenta (courtesy of Dr. I. Bahar) (Isin et al. 2002).*

lets of the membrane bilayer fuse (hemifusion), followed by fusion of the inner monolayer. Further observations suggest that oligosaccharides in the stem stabilize HA in a conformation prone to undergo structural changes that are necessary for fusion (Ohuchi et al. 1997). The length of the HA cytoplasmic tail affects fusion activity (Ohuchi et al. 1998) and the transmembrane region of HA has an important, though still undefined, role in the fusion process, as glycosylphosphatidylinositol-anchored HA is impaired in its ability to form pores (Armstrong et al. 2000; Kemble et al. 1994; Markosyan et al. 2000; Nussler et al. 1997).

Folding, assembly, and intracellular transport

During its synthesis in the ER, the HA interacts transiently with the BiP/GRP78 protein (Gething et al. 1986a; Hurtley et al. 1989) and calnexin (Chen et al. 1995; Hammond et al. 1994) before acquiring high mannose-type oligosaccharide and forming trimers, a prerequisite for its transport out of the ER (Doms et al. 1993). Through interaction with *N*-linked glycans in the HA, lectin chaperones such as calnexin and calreticulin regulate and facilitate HA folding (Daniels et al. 2003). Cysteine residues in the ectodomain are essential both for efficient folding and for stabilization of the folded molecule (Segal et al. 1992). Disulfide bond formation

occurs co-translationally. In the Golgi apparatus, the oligosaccharides of the HA are further processed to the complex type. The HAs of virulent avian H5 and H7 viruses are cleaved in the trans-Golgi or trans-Golgi network by ubiquitous proteases (see below). In polarized cells, the final step of HA maturation is transport to the apical cell surface (Roth et al. 1983); its transport from the trans-Golgi network is energy-dependent (Gravotta et al. 1990). The proteolipid MAL, a non-glycosylated integral membrane protein that is a component of the apical transport pathway, is required for HA apical transport (Puertollano et al. 1999). Signals responsible for apical transport reside in the transmembrane and/or cytoplasmic domains (Brewer and Roth 1991; Lin et al. 1998). The generation of basolateral-sorting signals in the HA cytoplasmic tail directed 50–60 percent of the mutant HAs to the basolateral membrane; however, the mutant virus budded almost exclusively from the apical surface, indicating that factors other than the HA-sorting signal contribute to virus budding (Barman et al. 2003; Mora et al. 2002). The transmembrane and cytoplasmic domains contain signals for specific incorporation of the HA into virions in studies with a complementation assay (Naim and Roth 1993), although an HA tail-less mutant replicated almost as well as its parent (Jin et al. 1994).

Lipid rafts are sphingomyelin- and cholesterol-enriched microdomains in the cellular membrane. They are believed to provide platforms for the assembly and budding of viruses, likely by increasing the local concentration of viral structural proteins. HA associates with rafts through its transmembrane domain (Scheiffele et al. 1997; Shvartsman et al. 2003; Takeda et al. 2003); however, deletion of the HA cytoplasmic tail affects raft association as well (Zhang et al. 2000). Wild-type HA forms clusters at the surface of infected cells; by contrast, a mutant that lost the ability to associate with rafts was distributed randomly (Takeda et al. 2003). A mutant virus containing the 'nonraft' HA was characterized by reduced budding and fusion activity (Takeda et al. 2003).

HA cleavage

A link between HA cleavability and virulence is well established in avian influenza A viruses (Horimoto and Kawaoka 2001; Klenk and Rott 1988; Steinhauer et al. 1991; Webster and Rott 1987). In virulent H5 and H7 avian viruses, the HAs contain multiple basic amino acids at the cleavage site, which are cleaved intracellularly by endogenous proteases. By contrast, in avirulent avian viruses as well as non-avian influenza A viruses, with the exception of H7N7 equine viruses (Kawaoka 1991), the HAs lack a series of basic residues and are not subject to cleavage by such proteases (Bosch et al. 1979; Bosch et al. 1981). Thus, the tissue tropism of viruses may be determined by the availability of proteases responsible for the cleavage of different HAs, leading to differences in virulence.

Two groups of proteases seem to be responsible for HA cleavage. One includes enzymes recognizing a single arginine and able to cleave 'avirulent'-type HAs, such as plasmin (Lazarowitz et al. 1973), blood-clotting factor X-like protease (Gotoh et al. 1990), tryptase Clara (Kido et al. 1992), and bacterial proteases (Tashiro et al. 1987). The second group, which remains to be identified in vivo, comprises ubiquitous intracellular subtilisin-related proteases, furin, and PC6, which cleave virulent-type HAs with multiple basic residues at the cleavage site (Horimoto and Kawaoka 1994; Stieneke-Grober et al. 1992). Studies with HA cleavage mutants have demonstrated that the number of basic amino acids at the cleavage site and the presence or absence of a nearby carbohydrate affect HA cleavability by intracellular proteases in an interrelated manner (Kawaoka et al. 1984; Kawaoka and Webster 1988, 1989; Ohuchi et al. 1989; Vey et al. 1992). The proposed sequence requirement for HA cleavage by intracellular proteases, in the absence of a nearby carbohydrate (at residue 11 in H5 numbering) is Q–R/K–X–R/K–R (X = non-basic residue). If the carbohydrate moiety is present, virulence is maintained only if two basic amino acids are inserted (Q–X–X–R/K–X–R/K–R), or if the conserved glutamine

at position –5 or the proline at position –6 is altered (i.e. B(X)–X(B)–R/K–X–R/K–R (B = basic residue)). In addition, the amino acid immediately downstream of the cleavage site (the amino terminal residue of the HA2) affects HA cleavage by intracellular proteases (Horimoto and Kawaoka 1995). The HA cleavage enzyme seems to be located in either the trans-Golgi or the trans-Golgi network, to be calcium-dependent, and to have an acidic pH optimum (Klenk et al. 1974, 1984; Walker et al. 1992). HA cleavage can be augmented by the ability of the A/WSN/33 (H1N1) NA protein to sequester plasminogen (Goto and Kawaoka 1998), hence increasing the local concentration of this ubiquitous protease precursor. This NA function relies on the presence of a carboxy-terminal lysine residue and the absence of an oligosaccharide side chain at position 146 (N2 numbering).

Oligosaccharide side-chains

The location and number of glycosylation sites are not conserved among HAs of different strains and subtypes (Goto and Kawaoka 1998; Nobusawa et al. 1991). Rather, these sites are scattered throughout the HA, although they tend to cluster around the antigenic sites on the globular heads. The HAs of individual virus strains contain from 5 to 11 sites, with the glycosylation sequence around residues 20–22 conserved in type A strains, except in some virulent avian strains in which the HA is cleaved by intracellular proteases (corresponding to residue 11 in the H5 numbering system; see section on HA cleavage). Some 17–20 percent of the total protein surface of the H3 HA could be covered by carbohydrate. The presence or absence of oligosaccharide side-chains in the HA (reviewed in Schulze (1997), affects antibody (Skehel et al. 1984) and CD4$^+$ T cell (Jackson et al. 1994) recognition of the molecule, calnexin/calreticulin binding (Hebert et al. 1996), receptor binding affinity and/or specificity (Gambaryan et al. 1998; Gunther et al. 1993; Matrosovich et al. 1999; Ohuchi et al. 1997; Tsuchiya et al. 2002), virulence (Hartley et al. 1997; Naeve et al. 1984), replication (Wagner et al. 2002), host range (Romanova et al. 2003), and fusion activity (Ohuchi et al. 1997). Reverse genetics studies demonstrated that growth restriction due to the lack of HA glycosylation site(s) can be partially overcome by the introduction of an NA of a different subtype (Baigent and McCauley 2001; Wagner et al. 2000), indicating that a functional balance between HA and NA is critical for efficient virus replication. Moreover, in H3 (Gallagher et al. 1992) and H7 (Roberts et al. 1993) HAs, no particular oligosaccharide side-chain is required for folding, intracellular transport or function of the molecule; however, at least two or three oligosaccharide chains (depending on the source of the HA) must be present to ensure transport of the molecule to the cell surface.

Acylation

The three cysteine residues in the carboxyl-terminal region of HA2 are acylated with palmitic (Schmidt 1982) by a thioester linkage (Veit et al. 1990). The lack of HA acylation affects HAs differently depending on the subtype. For instance, loss of palmitic acid does not impede the fusion activity of H3 (Steinhauer et al. 1991) or H7 HA (Philipp et al. 1995; Veit et al. 1991), but does affect syncytial formation of the latter (Fischer et al. 1998). An H3 virus with deletion of the HA cytoplasmic tail, which contains the acylation site, was generated by reverse genetics and replicates almost as well as its parent (Jin et al. 1994). On the other hand, a virus with a substitution at the carboxy-terminal cysteine of HA (Cys563 in WSN HA numbering) was not generated by reverse genetics, possibly because of structural constraints rather than the altered palmitylation (Zurcher et al. 1994). For H1 HA, replacement of the conserved cysteine residue did not affect hemifusion but restricted fusion pore formation, suggesting that palmitic acids facilitate the transition from hemifusion to fusion pore formation (Sakai et al. 2002). Results for the H2 HAs are more controversial. One report stresses the importance of each of the cysteine residues for fusion activity (Naeve and Williams 1990), while another indicates the absence of such an effect (Naim et al. 1992).

Receptor binding

Influenza A and B virus HAs bind to oligosaccharide-containing terminal sialic acids, including (α2,6)sialyl-actose, N-acetylneuraminic acid-α2,6-galactose-(Neu Acα2,6Galβ1),4Glc and (α2,3)sialyllactose, NeuAcα2,3Galβ1,4Glc. Topologically, the binding site is a depression. The amino acid residues that contact the terminal sialic acids (Weis et al. 1988, 1990) are highly conserved among the different HA subtypes (Nobusawa et al. 1991). The hydroxy groups at C7 and C8 of the glycerol side-chain and the N-acetyl group, but not the hydroxy group of C9, are important for recognition by the HA (Kelm et al. 1992; Matrosovich et al. 1992). A second ligand-binding site, for which the affinity of sialyllactose is four times weaker than that for the primary site, has been identified in the HA (Sauter et al. 1992). The biological significance of the secondary ligand binding site is unknown.

The receptor specificity of the HA differs among influenza A viruses: most avian and equine influenza viruses bind preferentially the NeuAcα2,3Gal linkage, whereas human and classic H1N1 swine influenza viruses preferentially bind the NeuAcα2,6Gal linkage on the cell surface sialyloligosaccharides (Rogers and Paulson 1983; Rogers et al. 1983b; Rogers and D'Souza 1989). Early studies suggested that epithelial cells in human trachea contain sialic acid (SA) α2,6Gal but not SAα2,3Gal sialyloligosaccharides on the cell surface (Baum and Paulson 1990), and that virus with NeuAcα2,6Gal specificity binds epithelial cells lining human trachea, whereas those with NeuAcα2,3Gal specificity do not (Couceiro et al. 1993). Recent findings using cultures of differentiated human airway epithelial cells indicate that SAα2,6Gal sialyloligosaccharides are expressed on nonciliated epithelial cells, whereas ciliated cells (which represent a minor cell population of the epithelium) express SAα2,3Gal sialyloligosaccharides (Matrosovich et al. 2004). In accordance with this finding, human viruses infect preferentially nonciliated cells, while avian viruses infect ciliated cells. These results support recent documentation of human infection by avian viruses (Claas et al., 1998a, b; Fouchier et al. 2004; K.S. Li et al. 2004). However, it remains unknown whether the prevalence of different cell types in this in vitro system correlates with that in a natural setting (i.e. human respiratory tract). Thus, it has yet to be established whether the relative inefficiency of human infection by avian viruses (Beare and Webster 1991) is due to a limited number of cells susceptible to avian viruses in human airway or other unknown restrictions.

Epithelial cells in duck intestine (the replication site of avian influenza viruses) and those in horse trachea contain SAcα2,3Gal but not SAα2,6Gal sialyloligosaccharides (Ito et al. 1997; Ito and Kawaoka 2000). It is interesting that epithelial cells in pig trachea contain both types of sialyloligosaccharides (Ito et al. 1998) which explains why both human and avian viruses replicate efficiently in pigs (Kida et al. 1994). Thus, the receptor specificities of the viruses correspond to the presence of the receptor at the replication site of the virus (reviewed in Ito and Kawaoka (2000)). The HAs of influenza B viruses also preferentially recognize NeuAcα2,6Gal linkages (Xu et al. 1994). However, an avian H5N1 virus isolated from an individual in Hong Kong in 1997 bound to NeuAcα2,3Gal-containing receptors but not to those containing an α2,6-linkage (Matrosovich et al. 1999), indicating that receptor specificity (while being an important determinant of host range restriction) does not prohibit avian-to-human transmission.

Human H1 viruses from the 1918 and 1957 pandemic period seem to recognize both SAα2,6Gal- and SAα2,3Gal-containing receptors, while those isolated after 1977 have human-like receptor binding specificity (Rogers and D'Souza 1989). X-ray crystallographic studies of the pandemic 1918 HA (H1 subtype) and related human and swine HAs suggest that a combination of (minor) structural modifications allowed the 1918 HA to bind to human receptors, despite its avian-like amino acid sequence (Gamblin et al. 2004; Stevens et al. 2004).

In addition to the importance of linkage specificity between sialic acid and galactose (i.e. α2,3 vs α2,6 linkage), the sialic acid species (i.e. N-acetyl vs N-glycolyl sialic acid) is also involved in host range restriction of influenza viruses. Influenza viruses differ in their recognition of *N*-acetyl vs *N*-glycolyl sialic acid (Higa et al. 1985); correspondingly, the prevalence of sialic acid species differs among animal species. *N*-glycolyl sialic acid linked to galactose by α2,3 linkages (NeuGcα2,3Gal) is prevalent in epithelial cells of horse trachea, allowing replication of viruses recognizing this glycoconjugate moiety but not of those recognizing *N*-acetyl sialic acid (Suzuki et al. 2000). Likewise, NeuGcα2,3Gal is a determinant of host range restriction in ducks (Ito et al. 2000).

Receptor specificity is largely determined by the nature of the amino acids at position 226 and 228. For human H2 and H3 viruses, substitution of Gln-226 with Leu and Gly-228 with Ser shifts receptor specificity from avian to human receptor binding (Connor et al. 1994; Naeve et al. 1984; Rogers et al. 1983a). Human H3 virus replication in ducks depends on the presence of avian-like amino acids at these positions (Hinshaw et al. 1983b; Naeve et al. 1983, 1984; Vines et al. 1998). In addition to these positions, substitution of residues at position 136, 190, 195, or 225, affect receptor binding affinity or specificity to various extents (Martin et al. 1998; Matrosovich et al. 2000; Nobusawa et al. 2000).

Host-cell-mediated selection of antigenic variants

The HA antigenicity of human influenza A and B viruses grown in embryonated hens' eggs differs from that of viruses isolated and passaged in a variety of cell cultures, including chicken embryo fibroblasts (Katz et al. 1987; Katz and Webster 1992; Robertson et al. 1987; Schild et al. 1983); even so, minor egg isolates contain the same antigenic phenotype as the tissue culture-grown viruses (Oxford et al. 1991). A similar phenomenon was discovered by Burnet and Clarke (1942) as 'O (as original)–D (as derived)' variation during passages of human viruses in eggs; O form virus agglutinated human or guinea-pig erythrocytes in preference to fowl erythrocytes, while D form viruses agglutinated them equally. Because tissue culture-grown viruses contain the same amino acid sequences of the HA as those replicating in humans, mutants are selected during replication in eggs (Katz et al. 1990; Rajakumar et al. 1990; Robertson et al. 1990). This finding is supported by the greater efficiency of primary isolation of human virus in cell culture than in eggs (Dumitrescu et al. 1981; Monto et al. 1981). Comparison of the HA sequence among viruses recently isolated in eggs or cell culture revealed mutations around the receptor binding pocket. Growth of human isolates in the allantois of eggs leads to the selection of receptor-binding variants (Ito et al. 1997; Mochalova et al. 2003; Smirnov et al. 2000) and results in enhanced receptor-binding affinity (Gambaryan et al. 1999). A/Hong Kong/156/97 virus grown in cell culture was significantly more pathogenic in mice than its egg-grown counterpart (Hiromoto et al. 2000); sequence analysis revealed amino acid changes in HA, PB1, PA, NP, and NS1. Inactivated vaccines prepared from tissue culture-grown viruses induce better protective immunity than do those from egg-grown viruses in animal models (Katz and Webster 1992; Newman et al. 1993; Wood et al. 1989) as well as in humans (Newman et al. 1993), although differences were not found when animals were immunized with vaccinia viruses that expressed the HAs of viruses grown in eggs or tissue culture (Rota et al. 1987, 1989).

NP

The NP (reviewed in Portela and Digard (2002)), the most abundant component of RNP, is a type-specific antigen associated with viral RNA. It covers 20–24 nucleotides (Compans et al. 1972; Duesberg 1969; Jennings et al. 1983; Ortega et al. 2000), exposing the bases to the outside and inducing melting of the secondary structure (Baudin et al. 1994; Klumpp et al. 1997). Thus, vRNA wraps around the NP scaffold. The RNA-binding region of the NP of influenza A virus has been mapped between residues 91 and 188 (Albo et al. 1995; Kobayashi et al. 1994). By electron microscopy, purified NP has a rodlike shape with dimensions of 6.2×3.5 nm and mostly exists in polymeric forms, ranging from trimers to large structures that resemble intact viral RNP (Ruigrok et al. 1989) (Figure 32.15). However, the formation of helical structures similar in conformation and density to intact viral RNP requires the presence of vRNA and M1 (Huang et al. 2001).

NP may undergo several stages of maturation, in which early disulfide-linked NPs are converted into disulfide-free NP which forms noncovalently stabilized oligomers (Elton et al. 1999; Prokudina et al. 2004; Zhao et al. 1998). It possesses several signals that regulate its nuclear import early in infection, but cytoplasmic accumulation late in infection (Bullido et al. 2000; Davey et al. 1985; Neumann et al. 1997; O'Neil and Palese 1995; Wang et al. 1997; Weber et al. 1998). Migration back to the cytoplasm presumably occurs as a component of RNP (Martin and Helenius 1991; Rey and Nayak 1992) and cytoplasmic accumulation requires interaction of NP with actin filaments (Digard et al. 1999). These transport processes are regulated by phosphorylation (Bui et al. 2002; Bullido et al. 2000; Neumann et al. 1997). NP also interacts with CRM1 (Elton et al. 2001), a cellular nuclear export factor; however, the significance of this finding for virus replication is not yet known. Free NP is needed for vRNA synthesis (Beaton and Krug 1986) and NP mutants have been identified that lead to defects in RNA replication, presumably by affecting the protein's ability to interact with the polymerase complex (Biswas et al. 1998; Mena et al. 1999). NP is also thought to play a role in host range restriction, as indicated by successful, host-dependent rescue of the ts phenotype (Scholtissek et al. 1985) and restriction of avian–human influenza A virus reassortants for replication in primates (Clements et al. 1992; Murphy and Clements 1989; Snyder et al. 1987). This evidence notwithstanding, direct support for this role of NP is lacking.

NA

The tetrameric NA protein of influenza A viruses (Figure 32.16), a type II glycoprotein with its amino terminus inside the cell and its carboxyl terminus outside (Air and Laver 1989), is one of two major glycoproteins on the virus surface. It has an uncleaved amino-terminal signal/anchor domain and a six amino-acid tail (Blok and Air 1982b; Fields et al. 1981). Although the precise location of the amino-terminal six polar residues is unknown, they are presumed to be exposed to the cytoplasm. The NA has a box-shaped head (10 × 10 × 6 nm) comprising four co-planar and roughly spherical subunits and contains the enzyme-active center and major antigenic sites (Colman et al. 1983; Varghese et al. 1983) (Figure 32.17). The stalk is centrally attached to the head with a hydrophobic region by which the stalk is embedded in the viral membrane (Blok and Air 1982b; Fields et al. 1981). The stalk region is flexible in length and sequence. In contrast to the remainder of the NA, the six amino-acid cytoplasmic tail is highly conserved among all NA subtypes of influenza A virus (Blok and Air 1982a, b). This region is important for incorporation of the NA into virions but is not essential for virus replication (Bilsel et al. 1993; Garcia-Sastre and Palese 1995; Jin et al. 1994). Although deletion of five of these residues (leaving the initiating methionine) does not affect the viability of viruses, it causes attenuation because of the reduction in virion

NA molecules. Mutant viruses lacking the NA or NA and HA cytoplasmic tails contain more filamentous than spherical particles (Jin et al. 1997; Mitnaul et al. 1996). An HA/NA-tail-less mutant had reduced vRNA-to-protein content (Zhang et al. 2000), suggesting an interaction of the NA and/or HA cytoplasmic tails with other viral or cellular components during vRNA virion incorporation and virion formation.

Reverse genetics experiments demonstrated that the NA stalk can be deleted almost completely or be extended by 58 amino acids to accommodate a variety of foreign sequences (Castrucci and Kawaoka 1993; Castrucci et al. 1994; Luo et al. 1993). In addition to laboratory isolates, avian viruses, especially those circulating in land-based birds (e.g. chickens) contain deletions in the NA stalk region (Banks et al. 2001; Bender et al. 1999; Blok and Air 1982b; Blok et al. 1982; Matrosovich et al. 1999; Spackman et al. 2003). 'Short-NA-stalk' viruses are characterized by mutations in HA1 which could affect receptor binding (Baigent and McCauley 2001; Banks et al. 2001; Bender et al. 1999; Matrosovich et al. 1999; Mitnaul et al. 2000; Spackman et al. 2003); these mutations likely compensate for a decreased ability to release viruses with shortened stalks. The occurrence of interrelated mutations indicates that the balance between HA and NA functions is critical for efficient influenza virus replication (reviewed in Wagner et al. (2002)).

A recombinant virus expressing reduced levels of NA was attenuated in mice (Solorzano et al. 2000). NA-deficient viruses, generated by repeated passage in the presence of bacterial NA and antibodies to viral NA, replicate in cell culture when a bacterial NA is added exogenously, as well as in animals (Hughes et al. 2000; Liu and Air 1993; Liu et al. 1995). These viruses possess

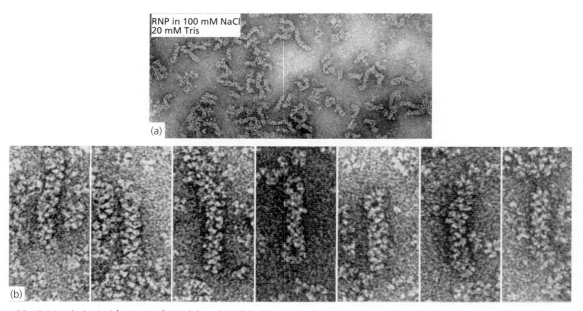

RNP in 100 mM NaCl
20 mM Tris

(a)

(b)

Figure 32.15 *Morphological features of RNP* **(a)** *and NP* **(b)***. (Courtesy of Dr. Rob W.H. Ruigrok) (Ruigrok and Baudin 1995)*

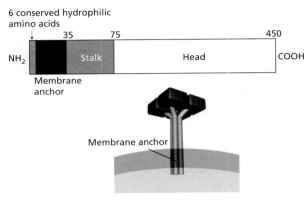

6 conserved hydrophilic amino acids

Figure 32.16 *Schematic diagram of the neuraminidase molecule. (Courtesy of Yuko Kawaoka) (Webster et al. 1984).*

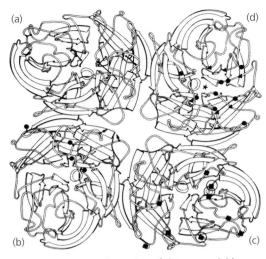

Figure 32.17 *Schematic illustration of the neuraminidase tetramer viewed from above, down the symmetry axis. The four subunits highlight different features of the structure:* **(a)** *disulfide bonds;* **(b)** *carbohydrate attachment sites at positions 86, 146, 200, and 234 (circle), and metal ligands Asp-113 and Asp-114 (arrows);* **(c)** *residues that change in N2 (squares) and N9 (black circles) variants selected with monoclonal antibodies;* **(d)** *conserved acidic (circles) and basic (triangles) residues in influenza A and B neuraminidase and the sialic acid binding site (star). (Courtesy of Dr. G.M. Air) (Air and Laver 1989).*

internal deletions of 800–900 nt, leaving regions encoding the cytoplasmic and transmembrane domains and part of the stalk. Whether the truncated NA molecule exists in infected cells remains unknown. With the identification of segment-specific virion incorporation signals at the 5' and 3' ends of viral RNAs (Fujii et al. 2003), it seems more likely that the terminal NA sequences are maintained to ensure efficient virion incorporation. Analysis of NA-deficient viruses revealed mutations around the HA receptor-binding pocket (Hughes et al. 2000), further emphasizing the importance of a balance between HA and NA functions.

The NA plays a role in host range restriction (Hinshaw et al. 1983b). While the sialidase activity of most human and pig isolates becomes undetectable below pH 4.5, duck isolates retain their enzymatic activity under these conditions (Takahashi et al. 2001), consistent with virus propagation in the acid environment of the digestive tract. NA is also important for plaque formation by A/WSN/33(H1N1) in Madin–Darby bovine kidney (MDBK) cells and for the neurovirulence of this virus (Nakajima and Sugiura 1980; Schulman and Palese 1977; Sugiura and Ueda 1980). These phenotypes were characterized by loss of the oligosaccharide side-chain from the WSN NA, which is conserved among the NAs of all other influenza A viruses (Li et al. 1993). This observation is now explained by HA cleavage promoted by plasminogen-binding activity of WSN NA (see HA cleavage section) (Goto and Kawaoka 1998). In addition, NA seems to induce apoptosis (Mohsin et al. 2002; Morris et al. 2002), likely through the activation of transforming growth factor beta (TGF-β) (Schultz-Cherry and Hinshaw 1996), although the significance of this finding for influenza pathogenesis is not known.

Three-dimensional structure

The NA three-dimensional structure has been solved in both type A and B viruses. Despite the 28 percent homology between these two types of viruses, the overall folding patterns of their NAs are almost identical

(Burmeister et al. 1992; Colman et al. 1983; Janakiraman et al. 1994; Varghese et al. 1983), and type B NA can functionally replace the type A enzyme (Ghate and Air 1999). The tetrameric NA protein has circular four-fold symmetry stabilized by calcium. The polypeptide chain folds into six topologically identical four-stranded anti-parallel β-sheets arranged like propeller blades (Figure 32.17). The product of catalysis, sialic acid, is bound in a large pocket on the distal surface, flanked and surrounded by nine acidic residues, six basic residues and three hydrophobic residues – each of which is strictly conserved in all known influenza viral NA sequences. Alteration of more than half of these residues results in molecules deficient in enzyme activity (Lentz et al. 1987). The three-dimensional structure of the NA led to the synthesis of a potent sialidase inhibitor, 4-guanidino-2,4-dideoxy-2,3-dehydro-*N*-acetylneuraminic acid (von Itzstein et al. 1993), which inhibits the NA activity of both type A and B viruses (inhibition constants, 10^{-9}–10^{-10} m). The structures of NA complexed with the inhibitor 2,3-didehydro-2-deoxy-n:-acetylneuraminic acid (DANA) (Smith et al. 2001) and of a mutant NA (E119G) that is resistant to the inhibitor 4-guanidino-Neu5Ac2en (4-GuDANA) (Colacino et al. 1997) have been solved. The latter structure suggests that the E119G replacement destabilizes the NA tetramer.

Sialidase activity

The NA catalyzes the cleavage of the α-ketosidic linkage between a terminal sialic acid and an adjacent sugar residue (Gottschalk 1957). The pH optimum of the enzyme ranges from 5.8 to 6.6, with an apparent K_m of 0.4 mm with use of N-acetylneuraminyllactose (Drzeniek and Kaluza 1972; Mountford et al. 1982). Removal of sialic acid residues by the NA promotes both entry and release of virus from infected cells (Palese et al. 1974). Avian NAs cleave NeuAcα2,3Gal in preference to NeuAcα2,6Gal. For human N2 NAs, a shift from NeuAcα2,3Gal to NeuAcα2,6Gal linkages has been observed since their introduction into the human population (Baum and Paulson 1991), presumably corresponding to the preferential recognition of the latter linkages by the HA molecule. The NA substrate specificity is determined by the nature of the amino acid at position 275 (Kobasa et al. 1999). In addition to substrate specificity, the specific activity of NA is also critical for the adaptation of avian viruses to growth in humans (Kobasa et al. 2001).

Folding, assembly, and intracellular transport

Synthesized as a monomer in the ER and translocated into the lumen of that structure, the NA rapidly forms a disulfide-linked dimer, which then non-covalently associates to form a tetramer ($t_{1/2}$ ca. 1.5–2 min). After transiently associating with the BiP/GRP78 ($t_{1/2}$ ca. 5 min), the NA is transported through the Golgi apparatus, where it acquires complex carbohydrates, rendering it resistant to endo H ($t_{1/2}$ ca. 25 min), and finally to the cell surface (Hogue and Nayak 1992; Saito et al. 1994). The mature NA contains signals for apical transport in its cytoplasmic and transmembrane domains (Barman and Nayak 2000; Kundu and Nayak 1994; Zhang et al. 2000). The transmembrane domain also contains a signal for raft association which does not overlap the apical sorting signal (Barman and Nayak 2000).

HA activity

All avian virus NAs possess HA activity (Hausmann et al. 1995; Kobasa et al. 1997; Laver et al. 1984). The HA activity can be transferred to NAs lacking this activity by altering amino acid residues that are located apart from the sialidase-active site (Nuss and Air 1991), indicating discrete HA- and NA-active sites in the NA molecule. A mutant virus with an altered HA-binding site displayed a significantly reduced hemadsorption activity and a reduction in NA enzymatic activity, but was not impaired in its ability to replicate in an avian host (Kobasa et al. 1997); thus, the biological significance of the HA activity in NA remains unknown.

NB

The dimeric, type II integral membrane protein NB (Williams and Lamb 1986) is unique to type B viruses. It is abundantly expressed in infected cells and incorporated into virions (Brassard et al. 1996). NB is composed of an 18 amino acid ectodomain, a 22 amino acid transmembrane domain, and a 60 amino-acid cytoplasmic tail (Brassard et al. 1996; Williams and Lamb 1988). Structural similarity with the M2 protein and ion channel activity (Sunstrom et al. 1996) led to the speculation that NB is the equivalent of the type A M2 protein. However, reverse genetics experiments demonstrated that NB is not critical for virus replication in vitro (Hatta and Kawaoka 2003). The role of this protein in viral replication remains obscure.

M1

The most abundant virion protein and a type-specific antigen of influenza viruses, the M1 has long been thought to be located underneath and adds to the rigidity of the lipid bilayer, although direct evidence for such a role is lacking. Immunogold labeling with anti-M1 monoclonal antibodies failed to decorate the M1 in virions unless they were first treated with a protease or a detergent (Murti et al. 1992). Cryo-electron microscopic studies suggested that the M1 can modify the lipid bilayer, causing the viral envelope to thicken (Fujiyoshi et al. 1994) (see Figure 32.3e). M1 is the primary determinant of virus budding and assembles into viruslike particles that are released into the medium (Gomez-Puertas et al. 2000). Furthermore, it determines the morphology of influenza virions (Bourmakina and Garcia-Sastre 2003; Roberts and Compans 1998), although other gene products may contribute (Jin et al. 1997; Mitnaul et al. 1996; Smirnov et al. 1991). Crystal structures of the N-terminal domain (amino acids 1–162) at neutral or acidic pH show a long ribbon of stacked dimers at neutral pH, while dimers were rotated in relation to each other at acidic pH (Harris et al. 2001; Sha and Luo 1997).

Located in both the nucleus and the cytoplasm (Patterson et al. 1988; Smith et al. 1987), this protein contains a karyophilic signal at residues 101–105 (RKLKR) (Ye et al. 1995). Depending on the nature of the replacement, mutations in this region have different outcomes on virus replication (Hui et al. 2003; Liu and Ye 2002). Replacement of residues 100–104 with the 'late domain' motifs PTAP or YPDL yielded virus with wild-type phenotypes (Hui et al. 2003), suggesting that this region of M1 may have a function similar to the late domains of Ebola virus or retrovirus matrix proteins. Structural similarities between M1 and human immunodeficiency virus (HIV) matrix and capsid proteins substantiate this assumption (Harris et al. 1999). In accordance with its proposed role, M1 has multiple lipid-binding regions (Bucher et al. 1980; Gregoriades and Frangione 1981; Hay 1974; Kretzschmar et al. 1996). In the cytoplasm, it is associated with cytoskeletal elements (Avalos et al. 1997).

M1 is required for nuclear export of vRNP complexes (Huang et al. 2001; Martin and Helenius 1991;

Whittaker et al. 1995), a function that relies on the association of M1 with vRNP complexes (Sakaguchi et al. 2003). M1 may therefore bridge the viral nuclear export factor NS2(NEP) and components of vRNP complexes such as PA (Hara et al. 2003).

The M1 proteins of influenza A and B viruses have a 'zinc finger' motif (Wakefield and Brownlee 1989), and purified virions contain zinc (Elster et al. 1994); however, the amount of zinc is not correlated with the RNA-binding activity of the protein and replacement of the conserved cysteine and histidine residues in the zinc finger motif did not significantly impair virus replication in cell culture (Hui et al. 2003; Liu and Ye 2002). Although serine residues between amino acids 108 and 126 of A/WSN/33(H1N1) M1 are phosphorylated (Gregoriades et al. 1990), the role of this property in viral replication is unknown; it may be important for viral replication involving intracellular movement of the protein (Whittaker et al. 1995). The influenza B M1 protein is also phosphorylated. M1 also inhibits RNP transcription activity (Perez and Donis 1998; Ye et al. 1989; Zvonarjev and Ghendon 1980), and thus is considered to serve as a molecular switch that initiates the final step of virus assembly. Furthermore, M1 contains RNA-binding domains (Eister et al. 1997; Ye et al. 1989, 1999), which have been mapped between residues 90–109 and 129–164.

One of the *M* gene products (most likely M1) contributes to the dominance phenotype shown by cold-adapted A/Ann Arbor/6/60(H2N2) in coinfection studies with other strains, both in vitro and in vivo (Whitaker-Dowling et al. 1990, 1991; Youngner et al. 1994). M1 may also be linked to rapid virus growth (Baez et al. 1980; Yasuda et al. 1994), presumably defined by the strength of its association with vRNP complexes (Liu and Ye 2002).

M2

The integral homotetrameric M2 membrane protein (Holsinger and Lamb 1991; Lamb et al. 1985; Panayotov and Schlesinger 1992; Sugrue and Hay 1991), abundantly expressed at the surface of virus-infected cells, is, nevertheless, a relatively minor component of virions (Zebedee and Lamb 1988). Sharing eight amino-terminal residues with M1, the M2 protein comprises 97 amino acids: 24 as the ecto-, 19 as the transmembrane, and 54 as the cytoplasmic domain. M2 functions as a pH-activated ion channel that permits protons to enter the virion during uncoating (Pinto et al. 1992; Sugrue et al. 1990b) and that modulates the pH of intracellular compartments, an essential function for the prevention of acid-induced conformational changes of intracellularly cleaved HAs (H5 and H7 HA subtypes of virulent avian influenza A virus) in the trans-Golgi network (Ohuchi et al. 1994; Sugrue et al. 1990b; Takeuchi and Lamb 1994). Both the imidazole ring of His-37 and the indole

moiety of Trp-41 are critical for the activation and regulation of the ion channel (Okada et al. 2001; Smondyrev and Voth 2002; Tang et al. 2002; Zhong et al. 2000). The activity of the M2 ion channel is blocked by the anti-influenza drug amantadine hydrochloride (see Chemotherapy section). The M2-associated ion channel activity resides in the transmembrane region (Duff and Ashley 1992), the primary site of mutations (residues 27, 30, 31, and 34) in amantadine-resistant mutants (Hay et al. 1985). Amantadine presumably blocks the ion channel activity of M2 by steric hindrance, resulting from insertion of the active drug between Val-27 and Ser-31 of the M2 molecule (Duff et al. 1994). Reverse genetics allowed for testing of viruses with mutations or deletions in the transmembrane region of M2 (Takeda et al. 2002; Watabe et al. 2001). While such viruses are viable, they are impaired in their growth. These findings indicate that influenza A virus can undergo limited replication in cell culture without M2 ion channel activity; this activity, however, is required for efficient viral replication.

The functional role of the M2 cytoplasmic region, the longest among the influenza viral membrane proteins, is unknown but is important for virus replication (Castrucci and Kawaoka 1995). M2 co-precipitates with the RNP core prepared from purified virus (Bron et al. 1993), indicating its high affinity for this protein, a property that presumably involves the M2 cytoplasmic tail. The M2 protein forms a homotetramer by non-covalent association of M2 dimers disulfide-linked at Cys-17 or -19, or both (Holsinger and Lamb 1991; Panayotov and Schlesinger 1992; Sugrue and Hay 1991). None of the cysteine residues in the M2 is essential for viral replication (Castrucci et al. 1997), although disulfide bond formation stabilizes the M2 tetramer (Holsinger and Lamb 1991). M2 proteins are palmitylated at Cys-50 with the exception of those in H3N8 equine viruses, but are not essential for virus replication (Sugrue et al. 1990b; Veit et al. 1991). The protein is also phosphorylated, mainly at Ser-64 (85 percent), but also at Ser-82, -89, and -93 (Holsinger et al. 1995); however, replacement of Ser-64 did not affect virus replication in vitro or in vivo (Thomas et al. 1998). The M2 ectodomain may play a role in virion incorporation (Park et al. 1998).

OTHER *M* GENE PRODUCTS OF TYPE B AND C VIRUSES

BM2, encoded by the *M* gene of type B virus (Horvath et al. 1990), is expressed in large amounts late in infection and has been detected in virions (Odagiri et al. 1999). It has no obvious structural similarities with type A M2 protein (Briedis et al. 1982); however, it is an oligomeric – most likely tetrameric – integral membrane protein, and its transmembrane domain contains histidine and tryptophane residues at the same relative location and spacing as those critical for the ion channel activity of type A M2 protein (Paterson et al. 2003). In fact, BM2 possesses ion channel activity and prevents co-expressed HA from adopting the low pH-induced conformation during transport to the cell surface (Horvath et al. 1990). These findings, together with reverse genetics studies demonstrating that BM2 is critical for the viral life cycle (Hatta et al. 2004; Jackson et al. 2004), indicate that BM2 is the equivalent of the type A M2 protein.

CM2, which resides in infected cells (Hongo et al. 1994), is generated by proteolytical cleavage of a precursor protein translated from unspliced transcripts of the *M* gene (Hongo et al. 1999; Pekosz and Lamb 1998). It is composed of 115 amino acids corresponding to the carboxy-terminal region of the precursor protein and has biochemical properties similar to the influenza A virus M2 protein (Paterson et al. 2003; Pekosz and Lamb 1997). The protein is palmitylated and phosphorylated, and the latter modification seems to accelerate tetramer formation (Z.N. Li et al. 2001; Tada et al. 1998). While these findings suggest a role of CM2 as the type C ion channel protein, direct experimental evidence is missing.

NS1

The only nonstructural protein of influenza A virus, NS1 is made in abundance during early infection. It is encoded by a co-linear mRNA, consists of 202–238 amino acids, is phosphorylated (Pekosz and Lamb 1998), and contains two karyophilic signals (Greenspan et al. 1988) as well as a latent nuclear export signal (Li et al. 1998).

The major function of NS1 is the inhibition of the cellular, anti-viral interferon (IFN) response (Garcia-Sastre et al. 1998) (reviewed in Garcia-Sastre (2001) and Katze et al. (2002)) to ensure efficient viral replication in IFN-competent hosts. In virus-infected cells, double-stranded RNA (dsRNA) is believed to trigger the activation of transcription factors such as ATF-2/c-Jun, NF-κB, or IFN-regulatory factors (IRF) that regulate IFN-β production. Similarly, IFN-α is also induced in response to virus infection. IFN induces the phosphorylation of STAT1 and STAT2, which, after dimerization and recruitment of IRF-9, activate the transcription of IFN-stimulated genes (ISG). ISGs comprise a large number of genes that establish an antiviral state in cells, including those encoding dsRNA-activated protein kinase (PKR) (PKR), Mx proteins, or proteins responsible for mRNA degradation such as 2′–5′-oligoadenylate synthetase (OAS) and RNase L. NS1 seems to interfere with these pathways by inhibiting the activation of transcription factors (Ludwig et al. 2002; Smith et al. 2001; Talon et al. 2000; Wang et al. 2000) and PKR (Bergmann et al. 2000; Hatada et al. 1999; Lu et al. 1995). It may execute its function by binding to dsRNA; however, direct protein–protein interactions between NS1 and components of the IFN system cannot be ruled out. The H5N1 avian viruses isolated in Hong Kong in 1997 induce high levels of proinflammatory cytokines, particularly tumor necrosis factor (TNF)-α and IFN-β (Cheung et al. 2002), while being resistant to the antiviral effects of these cytokines (Seo et al. 2002). These properties have been linked to the *NS* gene or NS1 protein, respectively, further emphasizing the protein's contribution to virulence (Cheung et al. 2002; Seo et al. 2002).

Besides its role in the regulation of the cellular IFN response, NS1 acts as a post-transcriptional regulator by inhibiting mRNA splicing and the nuclear export of cellular mRNA (Alonso-Caplen et al. 1992; Chen and Krug 2000; Krug et al. 2003; Lu et al. 1994; Qian et al. 1994), thereby maximizing the availability of substrate for capped primers and promoting viral mRNA synthesis. Interaction of NS1 and the cellular poly(A)-binding protein II (PABII) with the 30-kd subunit of cleavage and polyadenylation specificity factor (CPSF) blocks the binding of this protein to the AAUAAA sequence of some cellular pre-mRNAs, hence inhibiting their polyadenylation (Nemeroff et al. 1998). For some cellular mRNAs, short poly(A)-stretches have been detected whose elongation is blocked by the interaction of NS1 with PABII (Chen et al. 1999a). Both species – non-polyadenylated mRNAs and mRNAs with short poly(A) tails – remain in the nucleus where they become substrates for the endonucleolytic activity of the polymerase complex. In vitro, inhibition of splicing of mRNAs is mediated by binding of NS1 to a stem-bulge in U6snRNA (Wang and Krug 1998), which plays a critical role in the assembly/activity of spliceosomes. By contrast, in vivo, inhibition of splicing is brought about by binding of NS1 to the 30-kd subunit of CPSF (Y. Li et al. 2001). The interaction of NS1 with the 30-kd subunit of CPSF also induces the transcription of antiviral genes in an IFN-independent manner (Kim et al. 2002; Noah et al. 2003).

Two functional domains have been identified for NS1. The amino-terminal 73 amino acids constitute the RNA-binding domain and are sufficient for dimerization, as shown by structural analysis and experimental findings (Chien et al. 1997; Liu et al. 1997; Wang et al. 1999). Although mutational analysis suggested that amino acids 134–161 form the 'effector' domain that is required for the inhibition of nuclear export of poly(A)-containing cellular mRNAs (Qian et al. 1994), the entire carboxy-terminal half of the protein (amino acids 74–237) might be necessary.

NS1 induces apoptosis in infected cells (Schultz-Cherry et al. 2001), a phenotype that relies on the RNA-binding/multimerization, but not the effector, domain. However, mutations in the RNA-binding/multimerization domain are not sufficient to inhibit the induction of apoptosis, indicating that other viral proteins such as NA (Morris et al. 1999; Schultz-Cherry and Hinshaw 1996) also contribute to the induction of apoptosis.

NS2(NEP)

Encoded by a spliced mRNA (Inglis et al. 1979; Lamb and Choppin 1979), the NS2(NEP) protein comprises 121 amino acids (Lamb and Lai 1980), is phosphorylated, localizes to both the nucleus and cytoplasm of infected cells, and is incorporated into virions (Richardson and Akkina 1991). NS2(NEP) contains a classical nuclear export signal (NES) in its amino-terminal region (O'Neill et al. 1998) and interacts with the cellular nuclear export factor CRM1 (Neumann et al. 2000), which mediates export of proteins containing classical NESs. In cells infected with viruslike particles lacking NS2(NEP), viral RNP complexes are retained in the nucleus. Likely, NS2(NEP) functions by connecting the cellular export machinery with vRNPs through M1 (Akarsu et al. 2003; Yasuda et al. 1993). Based on its role as the viral nuclear export protein, NS2 is now also referred to as NEP.

The NS2 proteins of type A viruses are more conserved than the NS1 protein (76.9 percent vs 64.3 percent); however, neither product is conserved to the extent of other internal proteins (Buonagurio et al. 1986; Kawaoka et al. 1998; Ludwig et al. 1991; Nakajima et al. 1990a, b; Suarez and Perdue 1998).

HEF

The HEF protein of influenza C virus, which is synthesized as a single polypeptide with subsequent trimer formation and then cleaved into two disulfide-linked subunits, HEF1 and HEF2 (Formanowski and Meier-Ewert 1988; Herrler et al. 1979; Herrler and Klenk 1991; Hewat et al. 1984), exists on the virion surface as projections and has a reticular structure consisting mainly of hexagons (Flewett and Apostolov 1967) (see Figure 32.5). Its structure has been determined by X-ray crystallography (Rosenthal et al. 1998; Zhang et al. 1999). The HEF is composed of an extended, membrane proximal stalklike domain (composed of both HEF1 and HEF2 amino acids) and a membrane distal globular head that consists of HEF1 residues. The head region contains the receptor binding site which is situated on top of the protein. Two regions of significant sequence difference in HEF1, when compared to HA1 (residues 41–73 and 311–366), form the esterase domain which is located under the receptor-binding site. This confirms earlier findings that suggested separate esterase and receptor-binding sites, as di-isopropyl fluorophosphate inhibits only the esterase activity (Muchmore and Varki 1987). Calcium ion is essential for maintenance of the HEF structure. The HEF facilitates binding of influenza C virus to its cell surface receptor, an oligosaccharide containing a terminal 9-O-acetyl-N-acetylneuraminic acid (Herrler et al. 1985; Rogers et al. 1986).

The receptor-destroying enzyme (esterase) contains the 'catalytic triad' of a serine (position 57), a histidine (position 355), and an aspartic acid residue (position 352) (Rosenthal et al. 1998) that are characteristic for the active sites of esterases. The 9-O-acetyl group is critical for the binding of HEF, which does not recognize N-acetyl or N-glycolyl sialic acid (Rogers et al. 1986; Suzuki et al. 1992). Unlike the NA of type A and B viruses, HEF does not catalyze the cleavage of the α-ketosidic linkage between terminal sialic acid and an adjacent sugar residue, but instead catalyzes the cleavage of the 9-O-acetyl group of 9-O-acetyl-N-acetylneuraminic acid (Herrler et al. 1985; Vlasak et al. 1987). The protein also possesses fusion activity, which requires a low pH optimum (between 5.0 and 5.7) (Herrler et al. 1988; Ohuchi et al. 1982). The acetylesterase activity may be required for entry of the C virus into target cells (Strobl and Vlasak 1993), but not for hemolysis (Herrler et al. 1992). The host cell-dependent variant selection also occurs in influenza C viruses with mutations in the HEF protein (Umetsu et al. 1992). HEF is also acylated, but with stearic acid instead of palmitic acid, as in type A and B HAs (Veit et al. 1990).

Reverse genetics

A major research advance occurred when Palese and colleagues established a system which allows one to generate influenza viruses containing genes derived from cloned cDNA (Enami et al. 1990; Luytjes et al. 1989). While this system allowed, for the first time, modification of the influenza viral genome, it was limited by its low efficiency and the requirement for selection systems (reviewed in Neumann and Kawaoka (1999, 2001, 2002) and Neumann et al. (2002)). In 1999, a system was established for the de novo generation of influenza A virus from plasmids (Neumann et al. 1999) (Figure 32.18). This system relies on the cellular enzyme RNA polymerase I for intracellular synthesis of influenza viral RNA. Artificial virus generation therefore requires fusion of cDNAs encoding all eight influenza viral genes to RNA polymerase I promoter and terminator sequences, and transfection of these transcription units into eukaryotic cells. Viral RNA synthesized by cellular RNA polymerase I is then replicated and transcribed by the viral polymerase and NP proteins that are provided from RNA polymerase II-driven protein expression plasmids. Although this approach requires cotransfection of cells with 12 different plasmids, it routinely yields 10^8 infectious viruses per ml of supernatant derived from transfected cells. Modifications include the use of ribozymes for the generation of vRNA 3′ ends (Fodor et al. 1999), or – through the combination of RNA polymerase I and II promoters on one plasmid – the synthesis of vRNA and mRNA from one template, thereby reducing the number of plasmids required for rescue to eight (Hoffmann et al. 2000). These approaches also allow the artificial generation of influenza B virus (Hoffmann et al. 2002; Jackson et al. 2002) and Thogotovirus

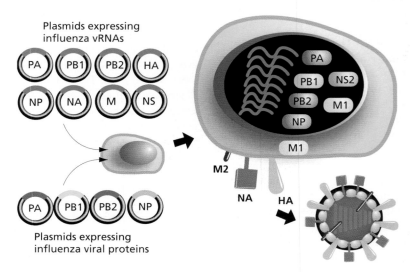

Figure 32.18 *Reverse genetics procedure. Influenza viral cDNAs are cloned in negative-sense orientation between RNA polymerase I promoter and terminator sequences. In plasmid-transfected cells, all eight influenza vRNAs are transcribed by the cellular enzyme RNA polymerase I. The three polymerase proteins and NP are provided from RNA polymerase II-driven protein expression plasmids. (Courtesy of Yuko Kawaoka.)*

(another member of the *Orthomyxoviridae* family) (Wagner et al. 2001).

The ability to modify the viral genome in any way desired has promoted research in the field tremendously. Current advances attributable to reverse genetics include the identification of factors determining viral pathogenicity (Hatta et al. 2001; Seo et al. 2002), the ongoing reconstruction of the 1918 pandemic virus (Basler et al. 2001; Reid et al. 1999, 2000, 2002; Tumpey et al. 2004), the re-assignment of functions encoded by the influenza B virus BM2 and NB proteins (Hatta and Kawaoka 2003; Hatta et al. 2004; Jackson et al. 2004), and the characterization of influenza viral proteins (Barman et al. 2003, 2004; Bourmakina and Garcia-Sastre 2003; Cross et al. 2001; Elleman and Barclay 2004; Hatta et al. 2001, 2002; Hui et al. 2003; Liu and Ye 2002; Neumann et al. 2000; Wagner et al. 2000; Yao et al. 2001). Moreover, reverse genetics is expected to have an enormous impact on public health by allowing the design and/or characterization of conventional (inactivated) or live attenuated vaccine viruses (de Wit et al. 2004; Hoffmann et al. 2002; Jin et al. 2003, 2004; M. Liu et al. 2003; Ozaki et al. 2004; Schickli et al. 2001; Subbarao et al. 2003; Watanabe et al. 2002; Webby et al. 2004), replication-incompetent virus-like particles (Neumann et al. 2000; Watanabe et al. 2002), or by exploring the potential of influenza virus as a vaccine vector (Shinya et al. 2004; Watanabe et al. 2003).

CLINICAL MANIFESTATIONS AND PATHOGENESIS

The spectrum of symptoms occurring during influenza virus infections is highly variable, ranging from mild respiratory disease with rhinitis or pharyngitis to primary viral pneumonia with a fatal outcome. Rates of asymptomatic infection may be nearly as high as those for symptomatic infection during some epidemics (Foy et al. 1976; Hayslett et al. 1962; Noble 1982). Often a physician's diagnosis is based on the patient's symptoms and the knowledge that influenza activity is occurring in the community. The presence of fever and cough along with sudden onset help distinguish influenza from other respiratory infections caused by other co-circulating respiratory pathogens; however, the physical signs and symptoms of influenza are not distinct enough from those of other respiratory infections to make a definitive clinical diagnosis without laboratory confirmation. In addition, symptoms in certain populations, notably babies, young children, and elderly people, may be atypical. However, during times when influenza is known to be circulating in a community, physicians participating in various studies have been able to diagnose influenza among adults with fever and cough with reported sensitivities and specificities of between 63 and 78 percent and 55 and 71 percent, respectively, compared with viral culture (Boivin et al. 2000; Monto et al. 2000).

Adults

Early symptoms in adults typically include fever, chills, headache, sore throat, dry cough, myalgias, anorexia, and malaise. A fever of 38–40°C that peaks within 24 h of onset is common, but peaks as high as 41°C can also occur. Pyrexia typically lasts 3 days but may last from 1 to 5 days or longer. Other symptoms that occur less frequently include substernal soreness, photophobia and other ocular symptoms, nausea, abdominal pain, and diarrhea (Douglas 1975; Nicholson 1992). Although most symptoms typically resolve within a week, cough and malaise may persist for 1 or more weeks after fever has subsided. Type A influenza viruses of the H1N1, H2N2, and H3N2 subtypes as well as type B influenza viruses cause a similar spectrum of illness (Frank et al. 1985; Nicholson 1992; Spelman and McHardy 1985). However, in general, the frequency of severe infections requiring hospital admission or causing death is lower for influenza B than for influenza A(H3N2) viruses (Thompson et al. 2003, 2004). Elderly, debilitated people may have signs and symptoms that are not immediately recognized as influenza. Symptoms in uncomplicated disease in this group include lassitude, anorexia, cough, rhinitis, unexplained fever, general malaise, and confusion.

Infants and children

Influenza A and B viruses are significant causes of both upper and lower respiratory tract illness in children (Glezen 1980; Glezen et al. 1980a; Kim et al. 1979). In children, symptoms are similar to those in adults, but gastrointestinal symptoms such as vomiting, abdominal pain, and diarrhea are seen more frequently. Maximum temperatures also tend to be higher in children than in adults, and febrile convulsions can occur. In addition, myositis, croup, and otitis media occur more frequently in children. Influenza infection of neonates can be life-threatening and may be manifest only as an unexplained febrile illness (Meibalane et al. 1977). Hospitalization rates for infants and young children may increase during influenza outbreaks (Glezen et al. 1980b; Kim et al. 1979).

Complications

Complications of the upper respiratory tract after influenza infection include bacterial sinusitis and otitis media. Lower respiratory tract complications include exacerbation of chronic obstructive pulmonary disease and chronic congestive heart failure, croup, bronchitis, bronchiolitis, wheezing attacks in asthmatics, and pneumonia (primary viral pneumonia, secondary bacterial pneumonia or combined bacterial and viral pneumonia) (Betts 1995; Nicholson 1992).

Primary influenza pneumonia, which often develops abruptly and progresses rapidly, was described in detail during the 1957/8 Asian influenza pandemic (Hers et al. 1957; Louria et al. 1959). This type of pneumonia is uncommon, and occurs mainly among those at increased risk for complications of influenza. Rapid respiration rate, tachycardia, cyanosis, high fever, and hypotension are frequent symptoms. Diffuse pulmonary infiltrates and acute respiratory failure with a high mortality rate are also features of this disease. Combined viral and bacterial pneumonia is more common than primary viral pneumonia and may be clinically indistinguishable from it.

Secondary bacterial infections typically occur 5–10 days after initial onset of influenza symptoms and are responsible for most pneumonias during influenza epidemics. Productive cough, pleuritic chest pain, and chills are common symptoms of this type of pneumonia. *Streptococcus pneumoniae*, *Staphylococcus aureus*, and *Hemophilus influenzae* are the organisms most commonly involved (Schwarzmann et al. 1971). These illnesses respond to appropriate antimicrobial agents and have a lower case fatality rate than primary viral pneumonia.

Other reported but less frequent complications of influenza include myositis, myocarditis and pericarditis, acute renal failure, encephalopathy, encephalitis, transverse myelitis, Guillain–Barré syndrome and a range of other neurological complications, Reye's syndrome, and toxic shock syndrome (Betts 1995; Noble 1982).

Higher rates of spontaneous abortion, stillbirths, and premature births were reported among pregnant women during the major pandemics of 1918/19 and 1957/8 (Bland 1919; Hardy et al. 1961; Woolston and Conley 1918); increased maternal risk for death following influenza infection was also documented (Eickhoff et al. 1961; Greenberg et al. 1958). In addition, case reports (Irving et al. 2000; Schoenbaum and Weinstein 1979; Shahab and Glezen 1994) and a retrospective study during 17 interpandemic influenza seasons demonstrated an increased risk for influenza-related hospitalization for women in their second or third trimesters of pregnancy (CDC 2004).

Serious complications of influenza most often occur in people 65 years of age and older, in the very young, and in those of any age with underlying chronic cardiac, pulmonary, or metabolic disease (Barker and Mullooly 1980). Complications in elderly people, particularly among those with pulmonary, cardiovascular, or other chronic diseases, account for most of the mortality in influenza epidemics (Eickhoff et al. 1961). The highest rates of hospitalization and death following influenza infection occur in those at opposite ends of the age spectrum, i.e. less than two or 65 years and older. Recent studies have shown that otherwise healthy children aged 6–23 months of age are at a substantially increased risk for influenza-related hospitalization, compared to older healthy children and healthy adults (Izurieta et al. 2000; Neuzil et al. 2000). In general, hospital admissions are 10–20 times higher than the mortality rate in the elderly (Barker and Mullooly 1980; Glezen et al. 1987), but are an order of magnitude higher for children under 5 years of age (Thompson et al. 2004).

Pathogenesis

Much remains to be learned about the pathogenesis of influenza virus replication and its relationship to the clinical manifestations and complications of the infection.

Many studies to investigate the pathogenesis of influenza infections were conducted during the 1957/8 pandemic of Asian influenza (Hers and Mulder 1961; Walsh et al. 1961). These studies demonstrated that the principal site of replication is the columnar epithelial cells, but histological studies indicate that viral replication can occur throughout the respiratory tract. Infected ciliated columnar cells become vacuolated and lose their cilia, and infected mucosal and ciliated epithelial cells become necrotic and desquamate. In studies in which bronchoscopy was conducted on, or nasal and bronchial biopsy specimens were taken from, individuals with uncomplicated acute influenza infections, inflammation of the larynx, trachea, and bronchi, and desquamation of ciliated columnar epithelium into the lumen of the bronchus were observed. Regeneration of the respiratory epithelial cells takes ca. 3–4 weeks, during which time pulmonary function abnormalities may persist (Hall et al. 1976). In these typical cases of influenza in which infection is confined to the respiratory tract, prostration, fever, and myalgia often seem to be disproportionate to objective clinical signs or observed pathological changes.

Lungs from fatal cases of primary viral pneumonia most notably show hyaline membrane coverage of alveolar walls together with extensive intra-alveolar edema and hemorrhage. Tracheitis and bronchitis are also observed (Hers and Mulder 1961; Martin et al. 1959). Patients with secondary bacterial pneumonia have changes characteristic of bacterial pneumonia in addition to the tracheobronchial findings of influenza.

The occurrence of systemic illness and fever suggests dissemination of virus via the blood stream, but systematic studies (Kilbourne 1959; Minuse et al. 1962) and limited case reports (Lehmann and Gust 1971; Naficy 1963) suggest that viremia is detected only rarely.

Apoptosis

Influenza A and B viruses induce apoptosis in both permissive (MDCK) and non-permissive cells (Takizawa et al. 1993; Hinshaw et al. 1994), which can be blocked by the *bcl*-2 product (Hinshaw et al. 1994). Apoptosis induced by influenza virus infection seems to involve activation of the Fas antigen-encoding gene (Takizawa et al. 1995) as well as the PKR, and IFN type I secretion. The latter sensitizes cells to apoptosis signaling through FADD/caspase-8 activation (Balachandran et al. 2000). The role of apoptosis in the clinical signs and symptoms of influenza is controversial. Indirect evidence indicates that programmed cell death could help reduce viral load and pathology (inflammation and tissue damage), yet others have found that activation of caspase 3, a critical enzyme involved in apoptosis, enhances influenza replication (Wurzer et al. 2003). The PB1-F2 protein induces apoptosis in various cell types, including human monocytic cells, leading to the hypothesis that this protein

functions to kill host immune cells responding to influenza virus infection (Chen et al. 2001). Influenza virus-infected cells undergoing apoptosis are readily engulfed by macrophages (Shiratsuchi et al. 2000). Infection of macrophages but not dendritic cells can trigger apoptosis (Bender 1998). It has also been reported that specific types of differentiated airway cells may undergo necrotic cell death, promoting inflammatory damage in the airway (Brydon et al. 2003).

MX PROTEIN

The pathogenesis of influenza virus infection is modulated by parameters specified by both the virus and the host. Although the available evidence suggests that numerous host genes have antiviral functions, most of them have not been identified and characterized. One exception is the Mx family of proteins, which mediate inhibition of orthomyxovirus replication (Staeheli 1990). This family of proteins is induced directly by viral infection as well as by type I interferons and may act either in the cytoplasm, as in the case of the human MxA protein, or in the nucleus, as in the case of the mouse Mx1 protein (Pavlovic et al. 1992; Noah et al. 2003). The Mx proteins belong to the dynamin superfamily of large GTPases (reviewed in Haller and Kochs 2002). The Mx GTPases seem to constitute an intracellular surveillance system that monitors the cell for viral infection by sensing viral nucleocapsids or viral ribonucleoprotein complexes. These viral components are thought to be derailed in their intracellular traffic and rendered inactive by sequestration. Specifically, MxA inhibits viral protein synthesis and genome amplification, suggesting that MxA protein interfered with either transcription, intracytoplasmic transport of viral mRNAs, viral protein synthesis, or translocation of newly synthesized viral proteins to the cell nucleus (Horisberger 1992; Turan et al. 2004; reviewed in Haller and Kochs 2002).

Immune response

INNATE IMMUNITY

During primary infection with influenza, the early host protective response involves the immediate action of cells such as phagocytes, natural killer (NK) cells, and B cells, as well as soluble factors including complement, IFN, cytokines, and chemokines. Cells and soluble factors converge to reduce the permissiveness of cells and tissues for the replication and spread of the invading virus (Kase et al. 1999; Kaufmann et al. 2001; Medzhitov and Janeway 2000; Siren et al. 2004). This early host response is triggered by receptors which recognize nonspecific alarm signals of viral infection (Coccia et al. 2004; Ehrhardt et al. 2004; Lund et al. 2004; Yoneyama et al. 2004). These receptor molecules are expressed in the germline of the host. In contrast, the receptors and effectors of the adaptive immune system (antibodies and

T cell receptors) result from gene rearrangements and are pathogen-specific, leading to the establishment of immunological memory. Germline immune receptors such as the Toll-like receptors (TLR) are expressed in a variety of cells such as macrophages, dendritic cells, and intestinal epithelium. TLR-3 and TLR-7 are involved in the recognition of viral dsRNA and ssRNA respectively, promoting dendritic cell maturation and activation of IFN production (Lund et al. 2004). Viral dsRNA is also involved in the activation of proteins with antiviral activity such as the kinase PKR, which inhibits protein translation and may trigger apoptosis (Katze et al. 1988). The cellular response to infection has been studied using DNA microarray techniques that allow the analysis of the gene expression changes in cultured infected cells (Geiss et al. 2001, 2002). Using this approach, it was noted that influenza infection causes profound changes in the expression of a large number of cellular genes involved in interferon production and signaling, apoptosis, and oxidative stress. Influenza-infected patients trigger the activation of antiviral genes and production of cytokines, such as interleukin (IL)-6 and IFN-alpha which reach their highest concentration in nasal fluids within 48 h of infection, correlating with the onset of fever (Hayden et al. 1998). Other cytokines, such as TNF-alpha and IL-8 reach maximum levels 4–5 days after infection. IL-8 is temporally correlated with lower respiratory tract involvement. Influenza viruses have evolved mechanisms to counter the innate antiviral responses of the host. The viral NS1 protein antagonizes interferon production and the activation of PKR in influenza-infected cells (Garcia-Sastre et al. 1998; Lu et al. 1995; Wang et al. 2000).

Besides its importance in the early arrest of viral replication, the innate immune responses to influenza interface with and condition the acquired cellular immune response. IFN and certain cytokines induced by viral infection, such as IL-12, have a powerful influence on the nature of the adaptive immune response (Janeway and Medzhitov 2002). Evidence from a murine model of influenza shows that type I IFN plays a critical role coordinating the immune response to viral infection, by reducing inflammation (Durbin et al. 2000). The enhanced pathology that was observed in mice that lacked IFN production was not attributable to the absence of the antiviral activity of IFN but to the excess of pro-inflammatory mediators.

A new type of innate antiviral mechanism, termed RNA interference (RNAi), may also play a role in controlling influenza replication during the early stages of infection. This system involves the formation of a ribonucleoprotein complex that targets viral RNA for degradation in a sequence specific manner. Experimental studies in tissue culture and in laboratory animals showed that RNAi can cause a marked reduction of influenza virus replication. The influenza virus NS1 protein was found to antagonize RNAi activity,

suggesting that this innate immune mechanism may be functional in vivo. It is not known if this antiviral mechanism is functional in human influenza infection (Ge et al. 2003, 2004; W.X. Li et al. 2004; Tompkins et al. 2004).

ADAPTIVE IMMUNITY

Antigen-nonspecific innate immune mechanisms generally inhibit, but do not eliminate, viral infection. They restrict viral replication until the more effective adaptive response is fully engaged. The adaptive immune response to infection with influenza viruses leads to induction of both virus-specific B- and T-cell immune responses to clear infection and generate long-lasting specific immunologic memory. Antibodies are made against the viral external glycoproteins HA and NA as well as the internal type-specific proteins NP and M1 (see section on Antigens). Neutralizing antibody directed against the HA is the primary immune mediator of protection from infection and clinical illness due to influenza viruses. Both mucosal and systemic immunity contribute to resistance to infection and disease (Clements et al. 1983, 1986). Influenza-specific lymphocytes have been detected in blood and lower respiratory tract secretions of infected subjects (Jurgensen et al. 1973; Yewdell and Hackett 1989). The primary cytotoxic T-cell response is detectable in blood after 1–2 weeks but is relatively short lived (Ennis et al. 1981). Evidence from animal models indicates that cytotoxic T-cell responses at mucosal surfaces play an important role in host protection (B. Liu et al. 2003a).

HUMORAL IMMUNE RESPONSE

Antibody to HA mediates neutralization of virus, complement fixation, prevention of virus attachment, and antibody-dependent cellular cytotoxicity. Resistance to infection is correlated with serum anti-HA antibody levels (Dowdle et al. 1973; Hobson et al. 1972) and can be demonstrated by protection against challenge after passive transfer of immune serum in a mouse model (Virelizier 1975). More recent studies have shown that protection from live virus challenge is associated with local neutralizing antibody and secretory IgA as well as serum anti-HA antibody (Clements et al. 1986; Johnson et al. 1986). Although antibodies to NA are inefficient in neutralizing influenza viruses, they restrict virus release from infected cells, reduce the intensity of infection and enhance recovery (see section on Antigens).

Serum antibody to HA can persist for decades and retrospective serosurveys suggest that a limited number of influenza subtypes have recycled (Masurel and Marine 1973). Decade-long persistence of immunity was demonstrated dramatically when influenza A (H1N1) strains, similar to viruses that had circulated in 1950, spread throughout the world during 1977/8. Little disease occurred in individuals born before 1950, indicating that substantial immunity remained after almost 30 years. Disease occurred in people <20 years old, however, irrespective of whether they were infected by influenza viruses of the H3N2 subtype. This and numerous observations during the pandemics of 1957 and 1968 suggest that intersubtypic immunity is weak in humans. In contrast, intrasubtypic immunity to influenza A (H3N2) viruses in adults can last for 4–7 years and include two or more variants of the same subtype, depending on the extent of antigenic drift (Couch and Kasel 1983).

The fact that a repeat infection with an antigenically related strain boosts the antibody response to the first virus encountered was originally described in 1953 by Davenport and colleagues (1953). This phenomenon, known as 'original antigenic sin,' is believed to be a selective anamnestic response orientated toward both the HA and the NA antigens experienced during the original infection. Thus, cross-reactive epitopes will stimulate a predominant secondary antibody response whereas new epitopes in the reinfecting variant induce a primary response. The precise importance of this phenomenon to immunity induced by infection or vaccination is unknown, but observations on original antigenic sin suggest that induced immunity during sequential infections may be biased toward older, less relevant strains rather than the current infecting strain.

Sequence analysis of the HA genes of monoclonal antibody escape variants, along with field isolates and location of amino acid changes on the three-dimensional structure of the HA, have defined five antibody-combining sites. The relationship of these sites to antibodies produced via natural infection has yet to be determined precisely, but the specificity of the antibody response to HA seems to be limited in humans and may vary from individual to individual (Natali et al. 1981; Wang et al. 1986). A limited range of specificities of anti-HA antibodies in individual mice and rabbits have also been demonstrated (Lambkin et al. 1994; Lambkin and Dimmock 1995). These findings may have implications for antigenic drift and the epidemiological success of influenza viruses in humans.

Among children with no previous exposure to influenza viruses, vaccination with live-attenuated influenza viruses results in the appearance of serum anti-HA IgM, IgG, and IgA antibodies within 2 weeks. IgM and IgA antibodies decline after this time, but the IgG response peaks after ca. 6 weeks, declines over the next 6 months or so, and then remains relatively stable for 2–3 years (Murphy and Webster 1996; Murphy et al. 1982). Antiviral IgA, IgG, and IgM responses can be detected in nasal secretions in most individuals and persist for several months (Murphy and Clements 1989; Wright et al. 1983). A secondary response to infection in primed young adults results in serum IgG and IgA and mucosal IgA in most cases. Serum hemagglutination inhibition (HAI) responses decline initially after infection, but may

then remain quite stable for years (Ada and Jones 1986). Serum antibodies to NA are rarely induced in primary infection and generally occur after re-exposure to NA of the same subtype. Antibodies to type-specific NP and M1 proteins are boosted via reinfection and may help diagnose a recent exposure to virus.

T-CELL RESPONSES

Antibodies and T cells play complementary roles in clearing the infection and promoting recovery. CD4$^+$ (Th1 and Th2) and CD8$^+$ T-cell responses to influenza are type-specific and are largely cross-reactive among influenza A viruses of different subtypes. T-cell recognition of antigen is restricted by the major histocompatibility complex (MHC) molecules, and the ability to respond to a given viral epitope depends on the HLA phenotype of an individual, a fact that complicates various T-cell vaccine approaches to vaccination against influenza. In naturally infected humans the CD4$^+$ cell response recognizes epitopes on the internal proteins NP and M1 as well as the surface proteins NA and HA.

CD4$^+$ T cells provide help for the activation of CD8$^+$ T cells by virtue of their ability to activate antigen presenting cells (dendritic cells, macrophages, etc.) primarily via CD40–CD40L interactions. Activated antigen presenting cells are essential for CD28 signaling to CD8$^+$ T cells leading to vigorous protective cytotoxic cell response to influenza infection (Prilliman et al. 2002; Schoenberger et al. 1998). The CD4$^+$ T cells are indispensable for an effective B cell antibody response to influenza. CD4$^+$ T cells can also enhance the proliferation of virus-specific CD8$^+$ T cells and maintaining CD8$^+$ T-cell memory capacity (Doherty et al. 1997).

The CD8$^+$ cytotoxic T lymphocyte response is directed to multiple surface and internal influenza proteins, in which many epitopes are potentially recognized, as determined by their binding to class I MHC molecules (Gianfrani et al. 2000; Gotch et al. 1987; Jameson et al. 1998; Robbins et al. 1997; Yewdell and Hackett 1989). However, a limited subset of immunodominant epitopes is recognized by lymphocytes primed by influenza infection (Belz et al. 2000; Yewdell and Bennink 1999).

Cytolytic CD8$^+$ effector cells fall into two subpopulations based on cytokine secretion. Both subpopulations lyse targets by production of perforin or Fas. Type 1 CD8$^+$ T cells (Tc1) secrete IFN-γ, whereas type 2 CD8$^+$ T cells (Tc2) secrete IL-4 and IL-5. Influenza virus infections elicit both Tc1 and Tc2 cells specific for class I-restricted epitopes. Tc1 cells are thought to contribute to the protective antiviral response, whereas the Tc2 component may act to limit the lung-associated pathology associated with influenza virus infection. Recent animal model studies have shown that both CD4$^+$ and CD8$^+$ T cells can contribute to immunity to influenza viruses. Animals that are deficient in both

CD4$^+$ and CD8$^+$ T cells do not survive influenza infection, but animals deficient in only CD4$^+$ or CD8$^+$ T cells are able to clear virus (Eichelberger et al. 1991a, b; Flynn et al. 1998; Lightman et al. 1987). The increased severity of influenza infections in geriatric patients has been correlated with a combination of functional impairments in their T-cell responses to influenza (Deng et al. 2004; Katz et al. 2004; Po et al. 2002).

The emergence of viral variants with altered surface antigens is a hallmark of influenza biology. Selection of antigenic variants is not limited to mutations in the HA and NA which allow escape from antibody neutralization. Evidence from influenza infections in humans and experimental animals shows that T-cell responses can select escape viruses with amino acid changes in the T-cell epitopes of the viral proteins (Boon et al. 2002; Price et al. 2000).

ANTIGENS

Polymerase proteins

There is no detectable antibody response to the polymerase proteins in convalescent sera. Their extremely low abundance in infected cells may contribute to this observation. These proteins have not been examined extensively for antigenic variants, although monoclonal antibodies to PA and PB2 are now available (Barcena et al. 1994). Cytotoxic T lymphocytes can recognize each of the three polymerase proteins (Bastin et al. 1987b; Bennink et al. 1984, 1987; Reay et al. 1989). Some viral strains produce an additional polypeptide, termed PB1-F2, encoded by the *PB1* gene segment (W. Chen et al. 2001). The PB1-F2 protein is translated from a downstream AUG initiation codon in an alternative reading frame. PB1-F2 is a mitochondria-targeted pro-apoptotic protein that has been associated with some emerging pandemic strains. This polypeptide induces CD8 T-cell responses in mice.

HA

The HA antigen is the major inducer of protective immunity to influenza viruses. Influenza A virus HAs show subtype specificity and are thought to possess five antigenic sites in the three-dimensional structure (Wiley et al. 1981; Wiley and Skehel 1987), although some subdivision and overlap of these areas have been noted (Caton et al. 1982; Daniels et al. 1983). For H3 virus strains (Wiley et al. 1981; Wiley and Skehel 1987), the sites are A, B, C, D, and E, and for the H1 strains they are Ca1, Ca2, Cb, Sa, and Sb (Caton et al. 1982). Each of these sites was derived from amino acid sequence changes in antigenic variants selected with monoclonal antibodies, as well as in natural variants. Monoclonal antibodies to each of the five sites neutralize the infectivity of the virus (Wiley and Skehel 1987). Mutations

that result in gain or loss of N-linked glycosylation sites in the HA can result in major changes in the antigenic structure of the virus (Skehel et al. 1984).

Helper T lymphocytes recognize several distinct regions of the HA1 and HA2 subunits located either on the surface or the interior of the intact molecule, as well as conformational determinants on the HA (Yewdell and Hackett 1989). Helper T lymphocyte recognition includes specificity for determinants on the variable regions of the molecule to which antibodies are also directed (Hackett et al. 1983; Mills et al. 1988). The immunodominant peptide most readily recognized by both subtype-specific and cross-reactive helper T lymphocyte clones is HA1 306–328 (H3 numbering system). Most memory T-cell clones recognize sites B, C, and E (HA1 56–76; H3 numbering) (Barnett et al. 1989; Graham et al. 1989). Residues important in antibody recognition affect T-cell recognition (Barnett et al. 1989; Graham et al. 1989), indicating that both B and T cells may recognize similar sites on the HA and hence that both systems may provide selective immune pressure. Cytotoxic T cells recognize both the HA1 and HA2 subunits (Wabuke-Bunoti and Fan 1983; Wabuke-Bunoti et al. 1984).

NP

Although a type-specific protein, the NP of influenza A viruses shows antigenic variation (Herlocher et al. 1992). It contains at least three non-overlapping antibody-binding areas (Van Wyke et al. 1980), one of which is highly conserved. Monoclonal antibody binding to this site inhibits transcription of viral RNA in vitro (Van Wyke et al. 1981). The NP epitopes recognized by dominant helper T lymphocytes in humans are located in residues 206–229, whereas those of mice are found in residues 260–283, with the distinct specificity of these regions depending on haplotypes. As a major antigen recognized by cytotoxic T lymphocytes, the NP possesses several T cell-specific epitopes that are conserved among human influenza A viruses (Bastin et al. 1987a; Bodmer et al. 1988; Yewdell and Hackett 1989). Transfer of cytotoxic T lymphocytes specific to NP protects mice from lethal influenza challenge (Taylor and Askonas 1986). The protective role of HLA-restricted cytotoxic T lymphocytes that recognize NP epitopes is evidenced by the identification of virus variants with altered NP epitopes which emerged in sequential chronological order with the cognate CTL; indicative of escape from CTL immunity (Boon et al. 2002).

NA

The subtype-specific influenza A virus NA has four antigenic sites, each consisting of multiple epitopes

(Webster et al. 1984). These antigenic sites differ in that antibodies to some, but not other, sites inhibit enzyme activity. Amino acids that change during antigenic drift cluster mainly in the distal surface loops connecting the various strands of β-sheets (Air et al. 1985).

Antigenic structures of the N9 NA have been extensively studied. Analysis of the crystal structure of a complex of N9 NA from A/tern/Australia/G75 with the Fab fragment of monoclonal antibody NC41 (Colman et al. 1987; Tulip et al. 1992) shows that the antibody contacts the NA over a surface area of 900 Å^2, comprising 19 amino acid residues localized on five polypeptide loops surrounding the enzyme active site. Site-specific mutagenesis indicates that, of the 19 amino acids in this epitope, only a few provide the critical contacts required for antibody recognition (Nuss et al. 1993). These findings support the observation of limited sites of sequence changes and local changes to the structure in escape mutants (Tulip et al. 1991; Varghese et al. 1988; Webster et al. 1987), implying (1) that antibody escape mutants are selected only when they contain changes at critical sites, or changes that introduce bulky side-chains capable of sterically preventing antibody attachment, and (2) that the other contact residues are providing 'passive surface complementarity' (Nuss et al. 1993). Antibodies to NA are inefficient in neutralizing the virus, but reduce plaque sizes in cell culture (Jahiel and Kilbourne 1966; Kilbourne et al. 1968; Rott et al. 1974). In agreement with these findings, immunity to NA in natural infection has only a small role in influenza protection as exemplified by the 1968 pandemic, whose causative agent possessed the NA from a previously circulating human virus; the immunity to the NA that existed in the human population did not protect humans from pandemic influenza (Cockburn et al. 1969). However, in experimental infections in animal models, passive transfer of monoclonal antibodies to NA or immunization with the vaccinia virus expressing the NA protected animals against lethal challenge (Webster et al. 1988) or reduced virus titers (Rott et al. 1974; Schulman et al. 1968). Helper and cytotoxic T lymphocyte responses to NA were found in influenza virus-infected mice, but were limited compared with responses to the HA, NP, and M1 (Caton and Gerhard 1992; Hurwitz et al. 1985; Reay et al. 1989; Wysocka and Hackett 1990).

M1

Even though this protein is considered a highly conserved type-specific antigen, some variations have been found among influenza A strains studied with a panel of monoclonal antibodies (Herlocher et al. 1992; Van Wyke et al. 1984). Helper T lymphocytes specific for the M1 protein are cross-reactive between viruses of different subtypes (Hurwitz et al. 1985). M1 is also

recognized by cytotoxic T lymphocytes (Gotch et al. 1987). A CTL epitope in the M1 protein that is recognized by human CD8 T cells was shown to mediate protection in transgenic mice expressing the cognate human HLA molecule (Plotnicky et al. 2003).

M2

Antibodies to the M2 protein have been found in humans infected with influenza A virus (Black et al. 1993). Passively transferred monoclonal antibodies reduced virus replication in mice (Treanor et al. 1990), and it has recently been shown that M2 protein plays a role in recovery from infection in mice (Slepushkin et al. 1995). Some antigenic variation can be found among the M2s as a result of amino acid changes in the ectodomain (Zebedee and Lamb 1988). However, antibodies elicited by M2 have been shown to mediate protection against different virus subtypes in animal models (Neirynck et al. 1999). Cytotoxic T lymphocytes specific for M2 have been isolated from convalescent mice and humans (Gianfrani et al. 2000; Jameson et al. 1998).

NS1

The influenza A virus NS1 proteins from different animal species cross-react with polyclonal antibodies. Although a panel of monoclonal antibodies distinguishes avian virus NS1 from those of human, swine, and equine strains, there is no evidence of antigenic variations among the latter group of proteins (Brown et al. 1983). Cytotoxic T lymphocytes recognizing NS1 are highly cross-reactive (Bennink and Yewdell 1988).

NS2

The antigenic properties of NS2 are poorly understood; however, mouse cytotoxic T lymphocytes specific for this protein have been found (Yewdell and Hackett 1989).

Host range restriction

Multiple genetic factors affect host range restriction for influenza viruses. Changes in host range can parallel changes in pathogenicity. At present, more is known about how particular amino acid changes at positions in or near the receptor-binding pocket of the hemagglutinin confer different receptor specificities and thus different host ranges. These receptor-binding specificities correspond to the composition of the receptor at the replication site in the host (see section on Receptor binding).

There is also indirect evidence that other genes, particularly the *NP* and *NA* genes, play a role in host range restriction. For example, replacement of the *NP* gene of an avian virus with the *NP* gene of a human virus alters host range (Scholtissek et al. 1978a), and phylogenetic analyses of *NP* gene sequences have shown that there are five distinct host-specific lineages (Gammelin et al. 1990; Gorman et al. 1990a). Other internal genes of influenza A viruses also apparently play a role in host range and virulence (Klenk and Rott 1988). The PB2 subunit of the polymerase complex plays a role in the restriction of avian influenza viruses for certain mammalian species (Subbarao et al. 1993). Recent studies revealed that amino acid 627 of PB2 modulates the replication efficiency of avian influenza viruses in mice (Hatta et al. 2001).

EPIDEMIOLOGY

Although human type A and B influenza viruses were not isolated until 1933 and 1940, respectively, descriptions of epidemics and pandemics of respiratory disease with characteristics suggestive of influenza have been recorded for over four centuries (see section on Historical record). Certain well documented epidemiological features of modern epidemics of influenza also emerge from the early accounts. Epidemics of varying severity occurred at irregular intervals, caused the highest mortality in elderly people, and were thought to have spread from Asia. These records detail epidemics of cough, fever, chills, and muscle aches that affected many people of different ages within a short time.

An epidemic of influenza is an outbreak of disease in a circumscribed location, which may affect a town, a city, or an entire country. Localized epidemics within a community often have a characteristic pattern in which the epidemic begins abruptly, peaks within 2–3 weeks and has a total duration of 5–8 weeks (Glezen and Couch 1978). The spread of influenza virus through a community typically causes large increases in medical visits for febrile respiratory disease (Glezen 1982). Absence from school due to influenza often occurs early in the epidemic, and school children are believed to be important in disseminating the virus in the community. Although reports of increased numbers of children with febrile respiratory illness are often the first indication that influenza is circulating in a community, it is not uncommon for a laboratory-confirmed outbreak in a nursing home to be the first report that influenza is present. Absence from work, hospitalization for pneumonia, and other complications of influenza, and death due to pneumonia and influenza and its complications all tend to peak later during an epidemic.

The size of outbreaks and epidemics that occur during the interpandemic intervals is quite variable, but are almost always smaller than those that occur following the introduction of a new virus subtype. The size of epidemics and their impact reflect the interplay between the extent of antigenic variation of the virus, the extent of immunity in the population and the population groups that are most affected in a given year.

A pandemic of influenza is an epidemic of disease that involves most if not all age groups on several continents. Influenza experts agree that at least three true pandemics of influenza have occurred during the past century: Spanish influenza in 1918, Asian influenza A(H2N2) in 1957 and Hong Kong influenza A(H3N2) in 1968. Human infections with highly pathogenic avian influenza A(H5N1) viruses have raised the specter of the emergence of another influenza pandemic due to unprecedented human exposure to these viruses causing epizootics in several Asian countries in 2004.

Current epidemiology

The simultaneous circulation of two subtypes of influenza A together with influenza B viruses since 1977 has made the current epidemiology of influenza unusually complex. Influenza B viruses have circulated continuously in humans since their first isolation in 1940, whereas influenza A(H3N2) viruses have been present since their emergence in pandemic form in 1968. Unlike the situation in 1957 and again in 1968 when new pandemic strains totally replaced the previously circulating influenza A strains, the influenza A(H1N1) viruses that emerged in 1977 were unable to supplant viruses of the A(H3N2) subtype. Instead, two distinct subtypes of influenza A viruses have co-circulated worldwide since then (see Figure 32.1).

Prevalence of these three groups of viruses may vary temporally and geographically within a country (Chapman et al. 1993) and between countries and continents during a given influenza season (World Health Organization 1996). In the USA the circulation of influenza A(H3N2) viruses has, in recent years, been associated most often with excess pneumonia and influenza (P and I) mortality. Major peaks of excess P and I mortality were documented by the US 121 Cities Mortality Reporting System during the 1989/90 and 1993/4 influenza seasons, during which influenza A(H3N2) viruses accounted for over 98 percent of the viruses reported.

Transmission and seasonality

It is generally accepted that influenza viruses are spread primarily by aerosols of virus-laden respiratory secretions that are expelled into the air during coughing, sneezing, or talking by an infected person (Betts 1995; Moser et al. 1979). Spread by direct contact is, however, also possible. The incubation period for influenza is relatively short (1–4 days), and the explosive nature of influenza epidemics and pandemics and simultaneous onset in many people suggest that a single infected person can transmit the virus to a relatively large number of susceptible individuals.

It is also generally accepted that influenza viruses are maintained in humans only by direct person-to-person spread, as there is no firm evidence for reintroduction from latently or persistently infected individuals. This is supported by evidence from local and global surveillance of influenza viruses, which has shown that antigenic variation and the consequent epidemiological behavior of influenza viruses follow a relatively uniform pattern, each successive antigenic variant replacing the previously circulating one in such a way that the co-circulation of distinct antigenic variants of a given subtype occurs for relatively short periods (Stuart-Harris et al. 1985; Cox and Bender 1995; Smith et al. 2004). These data have shown that consecutive epidemics in a community are caused by the reintroduction of anti-genically drifted, genetically distinct influenza viruses. Intensive community-wide surveillance in large popula-tion centers has shown that influenza activity can often be detected during the summer months (Fox et al. 1982; Monto and Kioumehr 1975). Global influenza surveil-lance also indicates that influenza viruses are generally isolated every month from humans somewhere in the world (Noble 1982; World Health Organization 1996).

The seasonality of influenza activity has been well documented in many countries with temperate climates in Europe, North America, and Asia. In these countries, influenza epidemics generally occur from December to March. Evidence that survival of influenza viruses in an aerosol is favored by low relative humidity and low temperature (Hemmes et al. 1960; Schaffer et al. 1976) is often cited as an explanation for winter seasonality of influenza in temperate climates. Seasonality in tropical or subtropical climates is less well studied; however, influenza viruses may be isolated throughout the year, with peaks of activity often occurring in the summer months (Reichelderfer et al. 1989). Other reports have suggested that peak influenza activity in tropical and subtropical areas may follow changes in weather such as the onset of the rainy season (Rao et al. 1982). The environmental and epidemiological factors responsible for these observations remain to be elucidated.

Antigenic drift and its impact

The epidemiological success of influenza viruses is largely due to the two types of antigenic variation that occur in the HA and the NA. Antigenic variation renders an individual susceptible to new strains – despite previous experience with other influenza viruses. The first kind of variation, called antigenic drift, occurs with both influenza A and B viruses, and is the gradual alteration of the structure of the protein by single amino acid substitutions (mutation) in the HA and NA within type B influenza viruses or within a given subtype of influenza A viruses. This kind of variation is the result of positive selection of spontaneous mutants by neutra-

lizing antibodies (Bush et al. 1999; Plotkin and Dushoff 2003). The amino acid changes result in the inability of antibody to previous strains to neutralize the mutant virus. Variations in the amino acid sequences of the HA and NA occur at a rate of <1 percent per year during antigenic drift.

Antigenic drift variants are responsible for periodic epidemics that occur between pandemics. Thus, influ-enza among humans is caused by distinguishable anti-genic variant strains of influenza A and B viruses that emerge and become predominant over a period of 2–5 years, only to be replaced by the subsequently successful antigenic variant.

Phylogenetic analyses have revealed that *HA* genes of human influenza A and B viruses have a regular rela-tionship between the isolation date and their position on the evolutionary tree. When evolutionary rates are esti-mated by regression of the year of isolation against the number of nucleotide or amino acid substitutions from a common ancestor (A/Puerto Rico/8/34, A/USSR/90/77, A/Aichi/2/68, and B/Lee/40 for the old A(H1N1), contemporary A(H1N1), A(H3N2), and B viruses, respectively), it is apparent that the *HA* genes of human influenza A viruses of the H1N1 and H3N2 subtypes evolve at about the same rates, whereas *HA* genes of influenza B viruses evolve more slowly (Table 32.3). Recent phylogenetic analyses have also shown that, although co-circulating lineages of *HA* genes of influ-enza B viruses can co-exist longer than for influenza A *HA* genes, the overall patterns and the rates of evolu-tion of the *HA* genes of these two types of influenza viruses are more similar than was previously believed (Cox and Bender 1995).

When amino acid changes in the HAs of field strains of influenza A(H3N2) viruses are plotted on the three-dimensional structure of the HA, it is apparent that much of the surface of the molecule has been altered by amino acid substitutions during the circulation of these viruses since 1968 (Figure 32.19). At least four changes that can be assigned to at least two antigenic sites have been observed between major epidemic strains of human influenza A viruses (Wilson and Cox 1990). Thus, the HA molecule seems to have a vast potential for antigenic change within a subtype as well as between subtypes without jeopardizing its function. This feature along with the apparent extensive nature of the anti-genic regions in the HA molecule (Caton et al. 1982; Wilson and Cox 1990) make it extremely difficult to predict future antigenic variants of influenza before they arise.

MORBIDITY

Quantifying morbidity due to influenza is difficult. The spectrum of symptoms occurring during influenza virus infections is quite variable. In addition, many other respiratory pathogens cause influenza-like illness, so

Table 32.3 *Evolutionary rates for the HA1 portion of the HA gene and protein*

Virus	Period	Number	Nucleotide changes per nucleotide site per year	Amino acid changes per amino acid site per year
H1N1	1934–1957	24	3.9×10^{-3}	5.3×10^{-3}
H1N1	1977–1996	146	2.7×10^{-3}	4.2×10^{-3}
H3N2	1968–1996	340	3.7×10^{-3}	4.1×10^{-3}
B	1940–1996	168	1.2×10^{-3}	1.1×10^{-3}

parallel laboratory studies are essential to define influenza-related morbidity. Many methods have been used for estimating the impact of influenza illnesses in a community or country, including prospective surveillance of illnesses and influenza infections in all members of a defined population. Regular interviews of a randomly selected population to detect all symptomatic respiratory illnesses, coupled with laboratory studies to detect symptomatic and asymptomatic influenza infections, provide the most precise measurement of age-specific influenza morbidity and rates of asymptomatic infection. A number of these community- and family-based studies have been carried out during pandemic and interpandemic influenza outbreaks (Foy et al. 1976; Hall et al. 1971, 1973; Jennings and Miles 1978; Jordan et al. 1958; Monto and Ullman 1974; Philip and Bell 1961). These studies have shown that influenza epidemics disrupt school attendance and work productivity, place heavy demands on health care systems, and result in morbidity and mortality among high-risk populations almost every year.

During average epidemics overall infection rates are estimated to be 10–20 percent, but in selected populations or age groups, attack rates of 40–50 percent are not unusual. It is apparent from studies conducted during both pandemic years and interpandemic periods that age-specific attack rates are highest in school children (Glezen 1996). This correlates well with the observation that school absenteeism is followed by employee absenteeism during influenza epidemics. Elderly people are often admitted to hospital during the latter part of the epidemic. Both type A and B influenza viruses are important causes of respiratory infection within nursing homes and other long-term care facilities.

MORTALITY

One of the hallmarks of influenza is the increase in mortality during pandemics and many epidemics. William Farr (1885) is credited with developing the concept of 'excess mortality', i.e. the number of deaths observed during an epidemic of influenza-like illness in excess of the number expected. Estimating influenza-associated excess mortality provides one of the most objective measures of the severity of influenza epidemics and pandemics. Methods for determining the baseline or expected number of deaths for the winter season in the absence of an influenza epidemic have changed over the

years. Various statistical approaches, ranging from a moving average to cyclical regression models and autoregressive integrated moving average (ARIMA) time series analyses have been used to calculate the baseline and threshold values (Choi and Thacker 1982; Collins and Lehmann 1951; Lui and Kendal 1987; Simonsen et al. 1997; Thompson et al. 2003).

Increased influenza mortality results not only from pneumonia and influenza (P and I) but also from cardiopulmonary and other chronic diseases that can be exacerbated by influenza (Collins and Lehmann 1951; Eickhoff et al. 1961). Quantification of deaths caused by influenza is complicated by the fact that information recorded on death certificates may fail to indicate that influenza was a cause of death because a laboratory diagnosis was not made or because influenza was not listed as a primary underlying or contributory cause of death. Therefore, calculations of influenza-associated excess mortality are based both on excess deaths from P and I as well as from all causes. Although excess mortality occurs primarily in elderly people, it can occur in all age groups, particularly among individuals who are at increased risk for complications of influenza. Excess mortality has been documented during circulation of both type A and B influenza viruses, but has been associated most often with circulation of influenza A subtypes H2N2 and H3N2. Since 1986, excess mortality in the USA has been associated most frequently with the circulation of influenza A(H3N2) viruses; ca. 90 percent of these influenza-associated excess deaths have occurred in individuals 65 or more years of age (CDC 2004).

It is estimated that >20 000 influenza-associated excess deaths occurred in the USA during each of nine different epidemics between 1972 and 1991; >40 000 influenza-associated deaths occurred during each of three of these epidemics (Simonsen et al. 1997) (Table 32.4).

ANTIGENIC SHIFT AND ITS IMPACT

Only influenza A viruses exhibit the second, more dramatic, kind of antigenic variation, called antigenic shift. Antigenic shift is the appearance in the human population of a new subtype of influenza A viruses containing a novel HA or a novel HA and NA immunologically distinct from isolates circulating previously. When antigenic shift occurs, the HA of the new strain

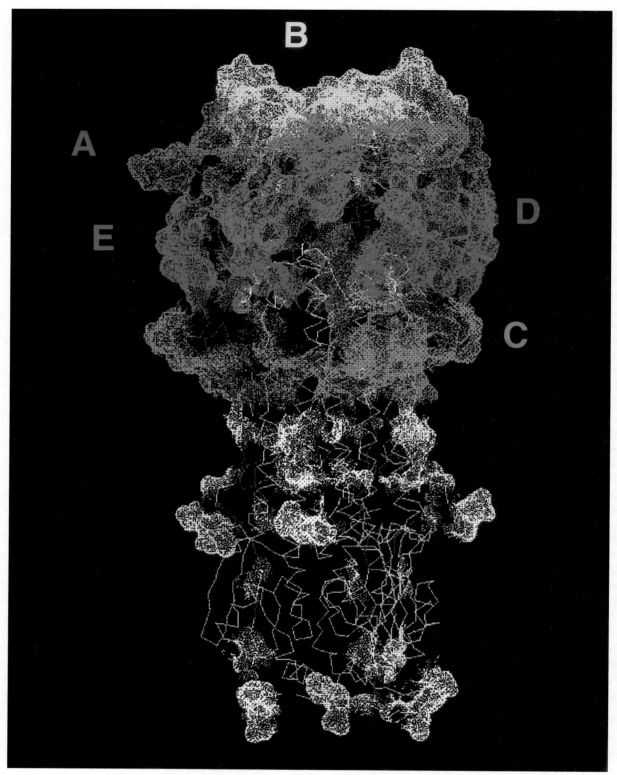

Figure 32.19 *Natural antigenic variation in the hemagglutinin (HA) of the H3 subtype of influenza A viruses circulating between 1968 and 1996. The HA trimer is depicted with the HA polypeptide backbone represented by an α-carbon trace in violet for the HA1 domain and in yellow for the HA2 domain. The solvent-accessible surface of residues that have changed during this period are represented by a dot surface. Antigenic regions are color coded and designated A (red), B (yellow), C (magenta), D (blue), and E (green). Amino acid residues shown in white are surface accessible but not assigned to antibody-combining sites. This graphic representation demonstrates that most of the surface-accessible amino acids in the globular head region of the HA have changed during this 28-year period of circulation in humans of influenza A(H3N2) viruses.*

Table 32.4 *Influenza excess mortality*

Period	Excess deaths
'Spanish' influenza	
September 1918 to April 1919	500 000
'Asian' influenza	
September 1957 to March 1969	69 800
'Hong Kong' influenza	
September 1968 to March 1969	33 800
Total	603 600
Interpandemic years	
1957–1990	600 800

would be expected to vary at the amino acid level 20–50 percent from the corresponding protein of previously circulating strains. Antigenic shift is responsible for worldwide pandemics, which occur at irregular and unpredictable intervals.

Although 16 subtypes of influenza HA have been identified in avian species, epidemics and pandemics of influenza among humans during this century seem to have been caused by viruses with HAs of only three different subtypes: H1, H2, and H3 (see Figure 32.1). The most severe recorded pandemic of influenza was that of Spanish influenza in 1918–1919.

Retrospective serological and genetic evidence suggests that this pandemic was caused by viruses closely related to classic swine influenza A(H1N1) virus, but its origin is unknown (Reid et al. 2004). Outbreaks of disease occurred almost simultaneously in North America, Europe, and Africa during the spring and early summer of 1918 (Crosby 1989). During the autumn of 1918 a second, more serious, wave of disease occurred. This wave peaked by the end of October but was followed by yet another wave of disease in mid-winter. Illness rates of nearly 40 percent occurred among school children during the autumn wave in the USA (Frost 1920). The differentiating features of this pandemic are the large numbers of cases with pneumonia and the unusually high case fatality rates, particularly in young healthy adults between the ages of 20 and 40 (Frost 1919). The social and medical consequences of the Spanish influenza pandemic are difficult to imagine today. About half of the 2 billion people living at that time were infected and at least 20 million of them died (Noble 1982). Hospitals were overflowing and there was a general shortage of medical services and vast disruption of community life.

Records indicate that the 1957/8 pandemic of Asian influenza A(H2N2) began in February in the southern Chinese province of Guizhou, spreading during March to Yunan province and during April to Singapore and Hong Kong (Stuart-Harris et al. 1985). The first virus isolates were obtained in Japan during May. This pandemic strain possessed completely different HA and NA antigens from the formerly circulating H1N1 viruses

and spread rapidly worldwide by November 1957. Although H2N2 viruses were first isolated in the UK and the USA in June or July of 1957, peak incidence of the disease did not occur until October. This first wave of disease in both countries was followed by a second in January 1958; both waves were accompanied by excess mortality, primarily in the elderly. The timetable of key events for the pandemic of Asian influenza shown in Table 32.5 illustrates the short time frame for response to this pandemic and the missed opportunities for immunization after the first wave of disease. The highest attack rates during this pandemic were >50 percent in children aged 5–19 (Glezen 1996). Total influenza-associated excess mortality in the USA during this pandemic was estimated to be 69 800 (Noble 1982).

Viruses causing the Hong Kong H3N2 pandemic were first isolated in Hong Kong in July 1968. These viruses had a different HA antigen but shared the N2 NA antigen with the previously circulating Asian viruses. Widespread disease with increased excess mortality was observed in the USA during the winter of 1968/9, but in many other countries, including the UK, this did not happen until the winter of 1969/70 (Stuart-Harris et al. 1985). Total influenza-associated excess mortality in the USA for this pandemic was estimated to be 33 800 (Noble 1982).

In May 1977 the first outbreaks of disease caused by re-emerging influenza A(H1N1) viruses were observed in Tientsin, China (Kung et al. 1978). The H1N1 virus spread to other parts of Asia and reached Russia by November. Spread to Europe, North America, and the southern hemisphere followed. Illness occurred almost exclusively among people less than 20 years of age and the highest attack rates of >50 percent were among school children. These viruses were antigenically and genetically similar to H1N1 viruses that had circulated widely during the early 1950s (Kendal et al. 1978; Nakajima et al. 1978). The absence of morbidity in people over 20 years of age has been explained by the fact that they were infected with similar viruses during the 1950s. Some experts have suggested that these H1N1 viruses may have been 'genetically frozen' in nature, while others have speculated that these viruses may have accidentally escaped from a laboratory; the source remains unknown.

Although antigenic shift seems to have been a requirement for the appearance of true pandemic influenza, the emergence of influenza A viruses of a new subtype in humans does not necessarily result in a pandemic (Dowdle and Millar 1978).

Ecology of influenza

The term influenza was used to describe a variety of acute respiratory and other diseases of a number of animal species, especially horses (see section on Histor-

Table 32.5 *Timetable of events for the Asian influenza pandemic of 1957/58*

Date	Event
February 1957	Outbreaks of influenzalike illness in Guizhou Province, China
Early March 1957	Outbreaks of influenzalike illness in Yunan Province, China
Mid March 1957	Outbreaks widespread in China
April 1957	Outbreaks in Hong Kong, Singapore, and Taiwan
Mid May 1957	Virus isolated in Japan
June/July 1957	Virus first isolated in the USA. Outbreaks reported
September 1957	Widespread occurrence of influenza begun in the USA
October 1957	Peak incidence of disease occurred in the USA. Attack rates were highest among school children and young adults
November 1957	Incidence of disease declined in the USA. First peak of pneumonia and influenza-related deaths observed
Early December 1957	Cumulative total of 60 million doses of vaccine released in the USA; much of the vaccine was unused
January/February 1958	Second peak of pneumonia and influenza-related mortality observed with a higher proportion than usual of deaths in the elderly. It was recognized retrospectively that a second wave of disease occurred in older adults and the elderly

ical record), for many years. However, influenza A viruses have been isolated only from humans, swine, horses, cats, dogs, a variety of sea mammals, and a wide variety of both domestic and wild birds, including ducks, geese, terns, shearwaters, gulls, turkeys, chickens, quail, and pheasants (Easterday 1975; Hinshaw et al. 1980; Webster et al. 1992; Dubovi et al. 2004; Keawcharoen et al. 2004).

Studies in Asia, Australia, Europe, and North America have revealed that viruses with all 16 subtypes of HA and nine subtypes of NA have been isolated from ducks and other feral water birds (Easterday 1975; Rohm et al. 1996; Webster et al. 1992) (Table 32.6), an observation suggesting that avian species serve as the primary reservoir for the emergence of new pandemic strains (Webster et al. 1992). These studies have also suggested that aquatic birds are likely to be the only source for influenza viruses in other species. Infections in avian species by most influenza viruses are asymptomatic, virus replicating preferentially in cells lining the intestinal tract (Webster et al. 1978). High titers of these viruses are excreted into their water habitat by asymptomatic birds. Avirulent influenza infections in birds may be the result of influenza viruses adapting to the host over many centuries. However, a few members of the H5 and H7 subtypes can cause a lethal systemic infection owing to the susceptibility of the HAs of these viruses to cleavage in many host tissues. The large reservoir for the 16 subtypes of influenza A viruses ensures their perpetuation in nature. The avian origin of strains of influenza in humans, cats, seals, whales, pigs, horses, and domestic poultry has been documented (Webster et al. 1992; Webster and Kawaoka 1994; Li et al. 2004).

Phylogenetic studies have revealed clues that have changed our thinking about the ecology and origins of influenza A viruses of different subtypes. There are species-specific lineages of viral genes (Bean et al. 1992;

Gorman et al., 1990a, b; Ito et al. 1991; Kawaoka et al. 1989), and it appears that all mammalian influenza viruses originate from the avian reservoir (Shortridge 1992; Webster and Kawaoka 1994). Besides the phylogenetic evidence supporting an avian ancestry of mammalian viruses, there is evidence from antigenic and structural studies in support of this hypothesis. Antigenic analyses of the earliest human isolate available (A/PR/8/34) suggested a direct descent from the avian-like H1N1 pandemic strain of 1918 (Brownlee and Fodor 2001). The atomic structure of the HA from the 1918 pandemic virus, A/South Carolina/1/18, has clearly revealed that the sialic acid binding pocket is very similar to that of avian influenza HA, suggesting an avian origin of this gene (Stevens et al. 2004).

Poultry, especially chickens, quail, and geese, are playing an increasingly significant role in the ecology of influenza. They are susceptible to infection with a variety of influenza subtypes from migratory waterfowl. Viral circulation in flocks, initially without causing substantial pathology, leads to the adaptation to the new species. The process of adaptation of influenza strains of the H5 and H7 subtypes to terrestrial poultry often results in acquisition of mutations at the cleavage site of the HA. These changes render the HA highly cleavable by ubiquitous proteases throughout the body which allows the virus to spread systemically. Consequently, these viruses are lethal for many bird species. The closeness of domestic poultry to human habitats and retail sales of infected live poultry have resulted in the transmission of these highly pathogenic avian viruses to humans, leading to several fatal infections in healthy children and adults (K.S. Li et al. 2004; Peiris et al. 2004; Subbarao et al. 1998).

Avian influenza H9N2 caused illness in three people in Hong Kong in 1991 and 2003, but retrospective sero-surveys detected subclinical infections in the general

Table 32.6 *Influenza A viruses isolated from avian species, examples of HA and NA subtypes*

HA subtype designation	NA subtype designation	Avian influenza A viruses
H1	N1	A/duck/Alberta/35/76(H1N1)[a]
	N8	A/duck/Alberta/97/77(H1N8)
H2	N9	A/duck/Germany/1/72(H2N9)[a]
	N9	A/duck/Germany/1/72(H2N9)
H3	N8	A/duck/Ukraine/1/63(H3N8)[a]
	N8	A/duck/England/62(H3N8)
	N2	A/turkey/England/69(H3N2)
H4	N6	A/duck/Czechoslovakia/56(H4N6)[a]
	N3	A/duck/Alberta/300/77(H4N3)
H5	N3	A/tern/South Africa/61(H5N3)[a]
	N9	A/turkey/Ontario/7732/66(H5N9)
	N1	A/chick/Scotland/59(H5N1)
H6	N2	A/turkey/Massachusetts/3740/65(H6N2)[a]
	N8	A/turkey/Canada/63(H6N8)
	N5	A/shearwater/Australia/72(H6N5)
	N1	A/duck/Germany/1868/68(H6N1)
H7	N7	A/fowl plague virus/Dutch/27(H7N7)[a]
	N1	A/chick/Brescia/1902(H7N1)
	N3	A/turkey/England/63(H7N3)
	N1	A/fowl plague virus/Rostock/34(H7N1)
H8	N4	A/turkey/Ontario/6118/68(H8N4)[a]
H9	N2	A/turkey/Wisconsin/1/66(H9N2)[a]
	N6	A/duck/Hong Kong/147/77(H9N6)
H10	N7	A/chick/Germany/N/49(H10N7)[a]
	N8	A/quail/Italy/1117/65(H10N8)
H11	N6	A/duck/England/56(H11N6)[a]
	N9	A/duck/Memphis/546/74(H11N9)
H12	N5	A/duck/Alberta/60/76(H12N5)[a]
H13	N6	A/gull/Maryland/704/77(H13N6)[a]
H14	N4	A/duck/Gurjev/263/83(H14N4)[a]
H15	N8	A/duck/Australia/341/83(H15N8)[a]
	N9	A/shearwater/Australia/2576/83(H15N9)
H16	N3	A/black-headed gull/Sweden/5/99

a) Reference strains

population (Peiris et al. 1999). The H9N2 viruses have also circulated extensively in swine herds in Asia and elsewhere. Because H9N2 viruses can readily bind sialic acid receptors present in airway epithelium of humans and other mammals, they constitute potential pandemic candidates to be monitored in surveillance programs (Matrosovich et al. 2001).

SWINE INFLUENZA

Koen (1919) reported the occurrence of an epizootic of respiratory disease among swine in Iowa, which seemed to be a new clinical entity and which co-incided with the start of the 1918 pandemic of influenza in the Midwest of the USA. Because the clinical symptoms of the disease were similar to those occurring in humans, the disease was called swine influenza. Shope (1931) demonstrated the viral cause of swine influenza in 1930, 3 years

before it was shown that influenza is a viral infection in people. Retrospective serological studies in humans (Davenport et al. 1953) and subsequent investigations (reviewed by Stuart-Harris et al. (1985)) provided strong circumstantial evidence that the Shope strain was antigenically close to the virus responsible for the 1918 pandemic of Spanish influenza.

The North American Swine influenza A subtype H1N1 viruses spread from the US to Europe in 1976 (Nardelli et al. 1978). This lineage was replaced in 1979 by another H1N1 virus that had been introduced from birds into pigs (Pensaert et al. 1981). Swine influenza strains are enzootic in pig populations in many parts of the world and have also infected turkeys in the USA (Hinshaw et al. 1983a).

A number of cases or outbreaks attributable to swine H1N1 virus transmission from ill swine to people have been documented, and each is connected with concern stemming from the association of swine disease and antibodies to swine influenza viruses with the 1918 Spanish influenza pandemic. This concern is best exemplified by the swine influenza immunization campaign that was begun in the USA after a swine influenza virus (A/New Jersey/8/76) was isolated from a young military recruit who died of pneumonia (Goldfield et al. 1977).

Serological evidence suggested that this virus was antigenically similar to the viruses believed to have caused the 1918 pandemic and that the virus had spread to other recruits (Dowdle and Millar 1978). Since that time, additional fatal cases of swine H1N1 influenza in humans have been documented, but these viruses have so far shown a limited capacity to spread in humans.

Swine influenza virus is one of the most common causes of respiratory disease in swine, and serological surveys in the USA have indicated that nearly half of the herds have antibody against this virus. Clinical evidence indicates that influenza A strains vary in the severity of disease that they cause in infected swine. The relative prevalence of different influenza A viruses in swine varies throughout the world, but it is clear that a large reservoir of influenza A viruses exists in pigs worldwide.

Critical to the hypothesis that pigs may play a crucial role in the emergence of new pandemic strains of influenza is the observation that swine are susceptible to infection by swine, avian, and human influenza viruses (see section on Receptor binding). This susceptibility to a variety of subtypes of influenza viruses provides the opportunity for genetic reassortment in swine. These findings underscore the possible role of swine as a 'mixing vessel' for the emergence of novel influenza strains (Scholtissek et al. 1985). Furthermore, classic A(H1N1) swine viruses, avian A(H1N1) viruses, and human A(H1N1) (H3N2), and type C influenza viruses have all been isolated from naturally infected swine. Avian–swine influenza reassortants were first detected in Europe in 1979 (Scholtissek et al. 1983) and continue to circulate in pigs in that part of the world. Human–avian H3N2 viruses emerged between 1983 and 1985 in Italy and have been isolated repeatedly from pigs in Europe (Webster et al. 1992).

Human H3N2 influenza entered the North American swine herds around 1995 and gave rise to double-reassortants with classical swine influenza genes in which the surface and PB1 protein genes are of human origin. These reassortants later acquired two avian internal protein genes (PA and PB2) in addition to the human and swine genes seen in the double reassortant (Zhou et al. 1999). These triple reassortants became widespread in 1998 and have circulated widely in the pig population since then (Webby et al. 2000). Experimental infection of pigs with avian viruses representing 13 of the 16 HA subtypes has also been reported (Kida et al. 1994).

DIAGNOSIS

A number of techniques have been developed for the diagnosis of influenza virus infections. Virus isolation in cultured cells or in fertilized hens' eggs or demonstration of a four-fold or greater rise in specific antibodies between acute and convalescent sera are techniques that have been used for many years. More recently, detection of viral antigens directly in clinical specimens by immunological methods and detection of viral nucleic acids by hybridization or using polymerase chain reaction (PCR) has greatly increased the speed of laboratory diagnosis.

Virus isolation and propagation

Embryonated hens' eggs, a number of primary tissue culture systems and continuous cell lines such as Madin–Darby canine kidney (MDCK; American Type Culture Collection, Rockville MD) cells can be used to isolate and grow influenza viruses for identification or research purposes. Recognition that proteolytic cleavage of the HA is necessary for viral infectivity and that inclusion of trypsin in the tissue culture fluid cleaves the HA expanded the culture systems available for influenza isolation and propagation. Replication of influenza viruses in all of its laboratory hosts is often detected by agglutination of erythrocytes added to culture fluid or by hemadsorption of erythrocytes to infected cells. On initial passage in eggs or tissue culture, some influenza viruses preferentially agglutinate guinea-pig over chicken erythrocytes, but on continued passage the viruses may preferentially agglutinate erythrocytes from chickens (Burnet and Bull 1943).

ISOLATION IN EMBRYONATED EGGS

Soon after the first identification of human influenza A viruses, Burnet (1936) reported that embryonated hens' eggs could serve as a host system for their propagation. This host system is still used for vaccine production and for generating large quantities of influenza virus that are occasionally necessary for research. To isolate both type A and type B influenza viruses, clinical samples are inoculated into the amniotic and allantoic cavities of 10–11-day-old embryonated hens' eggs. The eggs are usually incubated at 33–34°C for 2–3 days before the virus is harvested. Most type A and B influenza viruses that are originally isolated in eggs will grow well in the allantoic cavity after one or two passages. Type C influenza viruses, on the other hand, grow only in the amniotic cavity and are best propagated in 7–8-day-old embryonated hens' eggs after 5 days' incubation.

ISOLATION IN TISSUE CULTURE

Primary cynomolgus or rhesus monkey kidney cells (PMKC) are susceptible to a variety of respiratory viruses, including influenza viruses. Disadvantages with these cells include their cost and the presence of spuma-viruses. Influenza A, B, and C viruses can also be isolated in the MDCK cell line in the presence of trypsin. Primary monkey kidney and MDCK cells are most often used for the primary isolation of influenza viruses from humans.

Influenza virus isolation is still used in many laboratories worldwide. When performed correctly with properly collected specimens along with good quality laboratory cells and reagents, this method is highly sensitive. The shell vial tissue culture isolation method combines rapid detection of virus in the inoculated cells after 48–72 h, increased sensitivity being obtained by centrifugation of specimens onto the cells. Monoclonal antibodies are often used for immunofluorescent detection of viral antigens in the inoculated cells (Kalin and Grandien 1993). Obtaining isolates for further antigenic and genetic characterization is an essential part of worldwide surveillance for the emergence of significant antigenic variants of influenza. Detection of these new variants may signal the need to revise the formulation of the influenza vaccine or to recommend other measures for public health control.

Serology

Serology may establish that infection by influenza viruses has occurred when the virus is not detected by any other method. Serological tests include complement fixation (CF), hemagglutination inhibition (HAI), neutralization, and enzyme immunoassays (EIA). These techniques are the fundamental tools in epidemiological and immunological studies as well as in the evaluation of the immunogenic properties of the vaccine.

The CF test measures antibodies against the NP and thus allows type-specific detection of antibodies to type A and B influenza viruses rather than a subtype- or strain-specific diagnosis. This test is relatively insensitive in detecting rises in pairs of serum titers from individuals with a recent infection, but can be used when more specific reagents are not available. HAI and neutralization are more sensitive and measure antibodies against subtype- and strain-specific antigens. EIA tests can be configured according to the nature of the antigens and the isotype of immunoglobulin chosen for the assay (Ziegler et al. 1995).

The HAI test is the serological test most often applied to influenza viruses (Figure 32.20). Because of the instability of HA, the dilution of antigen used must be precisely determined by HA titration each time the HAI test is performed. The test is also complicated by the presence in sera of several species of nonspecific inhibitors of hemagglutination. These inhibitors interact with the HA molecule and prevent the agglutination of erythrocytes, even in the absence of specific antibodies. The non-specific inhibitors fall into three classes: α

inhibitors, which are present in human serum and are heat-stable sialylated glycoproteins that inhibit hemagglutination but do not neutralize viral infectivity; β inhibitors, which are also present in human serum and but are heat-labile and have neutralizing activity; and γ inhibitors, which are present in horse serum and are heat-stable sialylated sialoproteins with neutralizing activity. The α and γ inhibitors function as receptor analogues by competing with red cell receptors for binding to HA. Removal of nonspecific inhibitors from sera by using receptor-destroying enzyme or periodate is an essential step in the HAI test (Kendal et al. 1982). In addition, interference by antineuraminidase antibody and variability of viruses in avidity for red cells and antibody can influence the test results.

Rapid virus diagnosis

POINT-OF-CARE TESTS

The availability of influenza antiviral drugs has increased both physician and patient demand for rapid diagnosis. Rapid EIAs for influenza A and influenza B viruses which produce a result in 15 to 20 min are commercially available (Johnston and Bloy 1993; Ryan-Poirier et al. 1992; Todd et al. 1995; Waner et al. 1991). A positive result can be obtained with as few as 20 influenza virus-infected cells or 2 000 infectious virus particles. There currently are many commercially available point-of-care tests that rely on antigen detection in clinical specimens. Most of the tests use an immunoassay method to detect viral NP antigen, while one uses an enzyme-based chromogenic indicator to detect the presence of viral NA. These tests have a sensitivity of 50 to 100 percent and a specificity of 50 to 100 percent according to the manufacturers. Variation in sensitivity and specificity may depend on the study design, the type of sample collected, the timing of sample collection, the age of the patient, and other factors. Such tests show promise in certain clinical settings; however, the sensitivity and specificity of these tests under field conditions may be lower than reported in the published controlled studies. Furthermore, the positive predictive value of these tests may be quite low early in the influenza season, when influenza infections are relatively rare. All of these tests are less sensitive and specific than more traditional laboratory diagnostic methods such as virus isolation and serological diagnosis by the HI test, but they allow a test result to be obtained in time to treat the patient. These tests are useful in clinical laboratories of hospitals and nursing homes to detect institutional influenza outbreaks. However, because both false-positive and false-negative results are reported frequently for these point-of-care rapid tests, it is important to test multiple samples from the same outbreak before making decisions about treatment or prophylaxis for institutionalized patients.

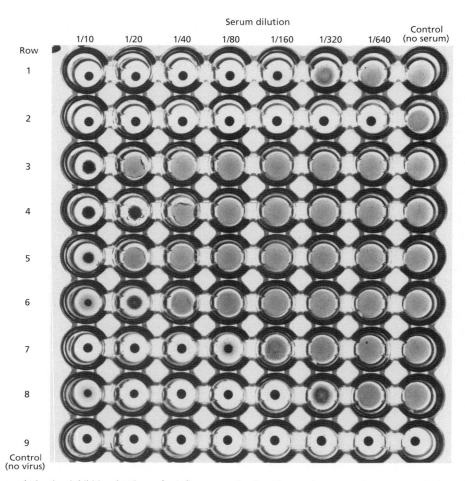

Figure 32.20 *Hemagglutination inhibition (HAI) test for influenza antibodies. The HAI is a competitive test in which antibodies present in an immune serum compete with red blood cells to bind the viral hemagglutinin. Row 1 shows results when antibodies are present and virus-induced hemagglutination of erythrocytes is inhibited with a consequent formation of erythrocyte 'buttons.' Row 3 shows results obtained when antibody is not present to inhibit viral hemagglutination.*

MOLECULAR METHODS

Molecular methods are being applied more widely in the diagnosis of influenza virus infections as well as in the characterization of influenza virus isolates. Molecular techniques are likely to supplant virus culture as the 'gold standard' for virus detection because they are more sensitive and offer advantages of speed and more precise characterization over other, more traditional laboratory methods. Abundant sequence data derived from isolates collected over several decades and from many geographic regions are available for selecting conserved target sequences to allow the identification of all isolates within a subtype, to discriminate between subtypes, and to distinguish between strains within a subtype. The genetic analysis of a large number of influenza viruses isolated throughout the world each year provides information for a timely update of vaccine strains and of molecular reagents for diagnosis. With currently available technology, updating molecular probes is more rapid and practical than updating MAbs on a regular basis.

For reverse transcriptase polymerase chain reaction (RT-PCR), viral nucleic acids are extracted from clinical specimens, allantoic fluid of embryonated hen eggs, or cell culture material by using the guanidium thiocyanate method (Boom et al. 1990) or commercial kits. cDNA is synthesized by in vitro reverse transcription of viral RNA primed either by specific synthetic oligonucleotides matching known nucleotide sequences on the viral genes or by random hexamers. This cDNA is amplified with specific primers and DNA polymerase. Finally, the amplified product is detected by any of numerous methods developed for this purpose.

Use of RT-PCR amplification of influenza virus RNA to diagnose influenza has been reported by Zhang and Evans (1991), Claas et al. (1992, 1993), Ellis et al. (1997a), Stockton et al. (1998), and Wright et al. (1995). Wright and colleagues developed a multiplex RT-PCR for type- and subtype-specific identification of currently circulating human influenza viruses. Three sets of oligonucleotide primers were used to identify the *NP* gene of influenza A viruses, the *NS* gene of influenza B viruses, the *HA* genes of influenza A subtypes H1 and H3, and the *NA* gene of influenza A subtypes N1 and N2. A type- and subtype-specific multiplex nested RT-PCR format was evaluated on 619 specimens collected during the 1995 to 1996 influenza season in England (Ellis et al. 1997a).

The superiority of RT-PCR over virus culture recently has been reported in several studies (Boivin et al. 2001; Cherian et al. 1994; Ellis et al. 1997a; Herrmann et al. 2001; Kehl et al. 2001; Plakokefalos et al. 2000; Zambon et al. 2001). Nested RT-PCR and similar primers were used for most of these studies. Conserved matrix gene primers were used for typing samples as influenza A or B virus, and primers designed for detecting the HA and NA genes were used for subtyping influenza A virus specimens. In the largest of these studies, data were available for 1 033 patients; of these, 730 patients were positive by RT-PCR, 629 were positive by serological testing, and 579 were positive by virus culture (Zambon et al. 2001). RT-PCR is a useful method for rapidly processing large numbers of clinical isolates for influenza diagnosis in centralized laboratories that have sufficient resources and expertise.

A new approach to influenza diagnosis is to use DNA microarrays containing nucleic acid probes for typing and subtyping influenza viruses and to identify common respiratory viral pathogens such as influenza A, B, and C viruses, respiratory syncytial virus, parainfluenza viruses, and adenoviruses. One study demonstrated that a model microarray containing multiple probes derived from cloned PCR-amplified fragments of influenza A and B virus matrix, HA, and NA genes correctly identified complementary influenza virus-specific DNA (J. Li et al. 2001). Although more extensive studies are needed, microarray technology appears to hold future promise for rapid and accurate diagnosis and large-scale surveillance.

PCR combined with endonuclease restriction analysis has been applied to the genetic characterization of influenza viruses. For this technique, oligonucleotide primers are designed to amplify a product that contains unique restriction enzyme cleavage sites. This method can discriminate between two lineages of influenza A (H3N2) viruses which circulated simultaneously during an influenza season (Ellis et al. 1997b; Zou 1997); can determine the genetic stability of cold-adapted, reassortant live vaccine strains (Klimov and Cox 1995); and allows the rapid identification of drug-resistant influenza virus isolates (Klimov et al. 1995).

CONTROL

The morbidity and mortality caused by influenza virus infections and the disruptive effects of epidemics and pandemics on the community justify strenuous efforts to prevent this disease. Two measures are currently available to reduce the impact of influenza: immunoprophy-laxis with influenza vaccines and chemoprophylaxis, or therapy with the antiviral drugs. Research to develop additional influenza vaccines and antiviral agents may result in additional products for the prevention and control of influenza.

Immunization

Vaccination is currently the most effective measure for reducing the impact of influenza. Immunization is focused mainly on individuals at increased risk of complications of influenza infection and on individuals who might transmit influenza to such people (CDC 2004; Fedson et al. 1995; Nicholson et al. 1995). For example, influenza vaccine is currently strongly recommended in the USA for anyone $\geqslant$6 months of age who, because of age or an underlying medical condition, is at increased risk for complications of influenza. They include people $\geqslant$65 years of age; people in residential or nursing homes; those with chronic disorders of the pulmonary or cardio-vascular systems, including children with asthma; children aged 6–23 months; women who will be pregnant during the influenza season; anyone who has required regular medical follow-up or hospitalization during the preceding year because of chronic metabolic diseases (including diabetes mellitus), renal dysfunction, hemo-globinopathies, or immunosuppression (including immuno-suppression caused by medications); and children and teenagers (6 months to 18 years of age) who are taking aspirin in the long term and may be at risk of developing Reye syndrome after influenza. People who should receive vaccination to reduce the likelihood of transmission to high-risk groups include: physicians, nurses, and other personnel in both hospital and outpatient care settings; staff, visitors, and volunteers in residential and nursing homes; providers of home care to individuals at high risk and household members (including children) of such people.

Vaccination is generally considered safe for anyone who can eat foods containing egg. Hypersensitivity to hens' eggs, the substrate for vaccine production, is the only contraindication. Desensitization to eggs followed by vaccination can be considered for individuals in high-risk groups.

VACCINE FORMULATION

Each February the World Health Organization makes recommendations concerning the antigenic properties of the strains of influenza that are to be used in vaccines during the following influenza season. These recommendations are based on data gathered by the four World Health Organization (WHO) Collaborating Centers (Atlanta, USA; London, UK; Melbourne, Australia; and Tokyo, Japan) together with data gathered by many national WHO collaborating laboratories. The objective

Table 32.7 *Influenza vaccine strains recommended by WHO, 1987/8 to 2004/5 for the northern hemisphere*

Year	H1N1	H3N2	B
1987/8	A/Singapore/06/86-like[a]	A/Leningrad/360/86-like	B/Ann Arbor/1/86-like
1988/9	A/Singapore/06/86-like[a]	A/Sichuan/02/87-like	B/Beijing/1/87-like
1989/90	A/Singapore/06/86-like[a]	A/Shanghai/11/87-like	B/Yamagata/16/88-like
1990/1	A/Singapore/06/86-like[a]	A/Guizhou/54/89-like[c]	B/Yamagata/16/88-like
1991/2	A/Singapore/06/86-like[a]	A/Beijing/353/89-like	Either B/Yamagata/16/88-like or B/Panama/45/90-like
1992/3	A/Singapore/06/86-like[a]	A/Beijing/353/89-like	Either B /Yamagata/16/88-like or B/Panama/45/90-like
1993/4	A/Singapore/06/86-like[a]	A/Beijing/32/92-like	B/Panama/45/90-like
1994/5	A/Singapore/06/86-like[b]	A/Shangdong/09/93-like	B/Panama/45/90-like
1995/6	A/Singapore/06/86-like[b]	A/Johannesburg/33/94-like	B/Beijing/184/93-like[e]
1996/7	A/Singapore/06/86-like[b]	A/Wuhan/359/95-like[d]	B/Beijing/184/93-like[e]
1997/8	A/Johannesburg/82/96-like	A/Wuhan/359/95-like[d]	B/Beijing/184/93-like[e]
1998/9	A/Beijing/262/95-like	A/Sydney/5/97-like	B/Beijing/184/93-like[e]
1999/00	A/New Caledonia/20/99-like	A/Sydney/5/97-like	B/Beijing/184/93-like virus or B/Shangdong/7/97-like[f]
2000/01	A/New Caledonia/20/99-like	A/Moscow/10/99-like[g]	B/Sichuan/379/99-like
2001/02	A/New Caledonia/20/99-like	A/Moscow/10/99-like[g]	B/Sichuan/379/99-like
2002/03	A/New Caledonia/20/99-like	A/Moscow/10/99-like[g]	B/Hong Kong/330/2001-like
2003/04	A/New Caledonia/20/99-like	A/Moscow/110/99-like[g]	B/Hong Kong/330/2001-like
2004/2005	A/New Caledonia/20/99-like	A/Fujian/411/2002-like	B/Shanghai/361/2002-like[h]

a) Most countries used the antigenically equivalent A/Taiwan/1/86 virus.
b) Most countries used the antigenically equivalent A/Texas/36/91 virus.
c) Most countries used the antigenically equivalent A/Shanghai/16/89 virus.
d) Most countries used the antigenically equivalent A/Nanchang/33/95 virus.
e) Most countries used the antigenically equivalent B/Harbin/7/94 virus.
f) Most countries used the antigenically equivalent B/Yamanashi/166/98 virus.
g) Most countries used the antigenically equivalent A/Panama/2007/99 virus.
h) Most countries used the antigenically equivalent B/Jiangsu/10/2003 or B/Jilin/20/2003 virus.
i) Most countries used the antigenically equivalent A/Wyoming.

is to match the antigenic properties of the HA and NA of the recommended vaccine strains as closely as possible with those of strains that are emerging and are likely to circulate the following winter.

Three types of data are used to make the WHO influenza vaccine strain recommendations each year. First, data are obtained from reference antigenic and genetic analyses of influenza viruses isolated through WHO's global influenza surveillance network. These data are used to detect new antigenic variants that might have emerged since the previous recommendations were issued and to determine how these variants are genetically and antigenically related to other circulating strains. Second, epidemiological and virological data are combined to determine whether newly identified variants are detected in association with outbreaks of disease in multiple locations or are associated only with a single case or a few sporadic cases. Third, the ability of the existing vaccine strains to induce an antibody response in humans to the newly detected variants is examined. These three types of data are combined to determine what new antigenic variants are circulating, whether these variants are associated with significant disease, and whether immunization with the existing vaccine could protect against disease caused by the new variants.

Influenza vaccines in recent years have been trivalent, containing strains of the two influenza A subtypes that are circulating along with a representative type B strain (Table 32.7). Viruses used by vaccine manufacturers for the type B component of the vaccine are naturally occurring virus strains that replicate to relatively high titers in the allantoic cavity of embryonated hens' eggs. The strains most often used for the type A components are high-growth reassortant viruses that contain internal genes that specify the property of high growth in eggs derived from the A/PR/8/34(H1N1) laboratory adapted strain together with the surface glycoproteins, HA and NA, from the recommended field strain. Vaccine strains are grown individually in the allantoic cavity of embryonated hens' eggs and then purified and concentrated by zonal centrifugation or column chromatography and finally inactivated with formalin or other chemicals. Vaccines are routinely standardized by means of single radial diffusion tests (Wood et al. 1981) to contain 15 µg HA per virus strain per dose; the quantity of NA is not standardized and may vary between vaccines.

Influenza vaccines currently in use are live-attenuated vaccines or inactivated subvirion (SV), or surface antigen vaccines. Live-attenuated vaccine contains avirulent replicating virus; SV vaccine contains detergent-disrupted inactivated virus; surface antigen vaccines contain isolated HA and NA proteins (CDC 2004). Although current viruses are still produced by growing viruses in the allantoic sac of embryonated hens' eggs, numerous refinements have improved the immunogenicity and reactogenicity of current inactivated vaccines; they include the use of zonal centrifugation, the use of ether or other lipid solvents to disrupt the virus, the introduction of high-yield reassortants to improve yields, and the development of better methods to quantify the amount of viral antigens present in the vaccines. Thus modern influenza vaccines are associated with minimal side effects. Up to one-third of inactivated vaccine recipients may feel some discomfort at the vaccination site for up to 2 days after vaccination; only about 1–2 percent have fever, malaise, myalgia, or other systemic reaction, which may begin 6–12 h after vaccination and persists for 1–2 days (Betts 1995; CDC 2004).

EFFECTIVENESS OF INACTIVATED INFLUENZA VACCINES

Inactivated parenterally administered influenza vaccines have been in use since the 1940s. A large number of trials in both military and civilian populations have demonstrated the efficacy of inactivated vaccines in the prevention of naturally occurring outbreaks of influenza A(H1H1), (H2N2), and (H3N2) viruses (Ada et al. 1987; Couch et al. 1986; Dowdle 1981; Monto and Terpenning 1996). The large variations in vaccine efficacy and clinical effectiveness reported in the literature are due to differences in the ages and immunocompetence of the vaccine recipients, the degree of antigenic similarity between the vaccine and circulating virus strains, the vaccine potency, the extent and intensity of transmission of influenza, and other respiratory viruses circulating during the study period, as well as the surveillance and laboratory methods used for the studies. Current inactivated vaccines protect 70–90 percent of normal healthy adult recipients against naturally occurring disease when the antigens of the vaccine and those of the circulating influenza viruses are closely related. In people >65 years of age (a group that is a primary target of vaccination programmes in a number of countries), the antibody response to HA is reduced and clinical effectiveness of vaccine is lower. This is probably a reflection of reduced immunocompetence (Ershler et al. 1984). For older people living in the community, the effectiveness of influenza vaccine in preventing hospitalization for P and I ranges from 30 percent to 70 percent. Among elderly people living in nursing homes, inactivated vaccines confer less protection against illness than in younger healthy individuals; they are more effective in preventing severe illness or secondary complications requiring hospitalization (50–60 percent) and death (80 percent) than in protecting against disease (30–40 percent) (CDC 2004).

Chemotherapy

The chemically related drugs amantadine and rimantadine hydrochloride interfere with the replication cycle of all subtypes of type A but not type B influenza viruses (Hayden 1996; Van Voris and Newell 1992). Amantadine and rimantadine, its α-methyl derivative, share mechanisms of action, antiviral spectrums, oral bioavailability, prolonged plasma half-life, and clinical efficacy. Both drugs inhibit the replication of influenza A viruses at low, clinically achievable concentrations of <1 µg/ml (Tominack and Hayden 1987), but concerns about side-effects involving the central nervous system have limited the use of amantadine.

Amantadine and rimantadine are 70–90 percent effective in preventing illness caused by naturally occurring strains of type A influenza viruses when administered prophylactically to healthy adults or children when influenza viruses are circulating. These drugs can also reduce the severity and duration of illness caused by influenza A viruses when administered within 48 h of onset of symptoms.

The antiviral activity of both of these compounds is exerted through interference with two different ion channel functions of the viral M2 protein (see section entitled M2). The first involves inhibition of the acid-mediated dissociation of the matrix protein from the RNP complex within endosomes early in replication; this dissociation is essential for initiating viral replication (Pinto et al. 1992; Sugrue et al. 1990a). A second effect on virus maturation relating to a low pH-mediated alteration of the HA protein during its transport to the cell surface occurs during the replication of certain avian influenza viruses (Ohuchi et al. 1994; Sugrue et al. 1990a; Takeuchi and Lamb 1994).

Influenza A viruses are cross-susceptible and cross-resistant to amantadine and rimantadine. Viral strains responsible for pandemics and epidemics in recent years have all been drug-sensitive (Hayden 1996), but resistance to these compounds is readily selected by growth in the presence of these drugs either in vivo or in vitro. Resistance is associated with single nucleotide changes in RNA segment 7 and corresponding amino acid substitutions at one of four sites (amino acids 26, 27, 30, and 31 for human influenza A viruses) in the transmembrane region of the M2 protein (Hay 1992). Resistant viruses can emerge when either of these drugs is administered for treatment in adults or children. Although the frequency of the emergence of resistance is not firmly established, resistant variants have been recovered from ca. 30 percent of treated children or adults (Hall et al. 1987; Hayden et al. 1989). Nevertheless, treated individuals who shed resistant viruses recover rapidly and the duration of shedding is relatively short, so the clinical significance of the emergence of resistance in an individual is unclear. Apparent transmission of resistant virus associated with failure of drug prophylaxis has been documented in nursing home residents receiving amantadine and in household contacts of rimantadine-treated individuals (Degelau et al. 1992; Hayden et al. 1989; Houck et al. 1995; Mast et al. 1991). Resistant viruses seem to be pathogenic and can cause typical influenza, but resistant viruses are no more transmissible or virulent than strains sensitive to amantadine and rimantadine (Hayden 1996).

Neuraminidase inhibitors

Multi-cycle replication of influenza virus in the host requires an active neuraminidase on the virus particles (see Table 32.2 and NA section). Zanamivir and oseltamivir are chemically related drugs known as neuraminidase inhibitors that have antiviral activity against both influenza A and B viruses (Hayden 1999, 2000). Both zanamivir and oseltamivir are approved for treating uncomplicated influenza infections. Zanamivir is approved for persons aged ≥ 7 years, and oseltamivir is approved for patients aged ≥ 1 year. Oseltamivir is administered orally, whereas zanamivir is for inhalation. When administered within 2 days of illness onset to otherwise healthy adults, zanamivir and oseltamivir can reduce the duration of uncomplicated influenza A and B illness by approximately 1 day, compared with placebo (Hayden et al. 1997; Makela et al. 2000; Demichelli et al. 2000). The course of oseltamivir therapy for persons with influenza A illness is 5 days. Oseltamivir is the only drug that has been approved for prophylactic use, being restricted to persons aged ≥ 13 years (Monto et al. 2002). Up to 82 percent of febrile, laboratory-confirmed influenza illnesses were prevented by oseltaminvir prophylaxis (Hayden et al. 1999; Monto et al. 1999). Besides their traditional use for the currently circulating strains of influenza A and B, neuraminidase inhibitors could prove critical to protect the health of the population at risk of infection by an emerging pandemic strain of influenza virus, until a suitable vaccine becomes available.

Emergence zanamivir and oseltamivir-resistant variants can be induced in influenza A and B viruses in vitro, but induction of resistance requires multiple passages in cell culture (Gubareva et al. 1997). Development of viral resistance to zanamivir and oseltamivir during treatment has been identified but does not appear to be frequent, with children providing a higher yield of resistant variants (Kiso et al. 2004; McKimm-Breschkin 2003). Available diagnostic tests are not optimal for detecting clinical resistance to the neuraminidase inhibitor antiviral drugs, but new diagnostic tests may revert this situation (McSharry et al. 2004). Coordinated surveillance activities that have been conducted since 1999 to detect the emergence of neuraminidase resistant variants provide the necessary information regarding the continuity of drug efficacy (Zambon and Hayden 2001).

REFERENCES

Ada, G.L. and Jones, P.D. 1986. The immune response to influenza infection. *Curr Top Microbiol Immunol*, **128**, 1–54.

Ada, G.L., Alexandrova, G., et al. 1987. Progress in the development of influenza vaccines: memorandum from a WHO meeting. *Bull WHO*, **65**, 289–93.

Air, G.M. and Laver, W.G. 1989. The neuraminidase of influenza virus proteins: structure, function, and genetics. *Proteins*, **6**, 341–56.

Air, G.M., Els, M.C., et al. 1985. Location of antigenic sites on the three-dimensional structure of the influenza N2 virus neuraminidase. *Virology*, **145**, 237–48.

Akarsu, H., Burmeister, W.P., et al. 2003. Crystal structure of the M1 protein-binding domain of the influenza A virus nuclear export protein (NEP/NS2). *EMBO J*, **22**, 4646–55.

Albo, C., Valencia, A. and Portela, A. 1995. Identification of an RNA binding region within the N-terminal third of the influenza A virus nucleoprotein. *J Virol*, **69**, 3799–806.

Ali, A., Avalos, R.T., et al. 2000. Influenza virus assembly: effect of influenza virus glycoproteins on the membrane association of M1 protein. *J Virol*, **74**, 8709–19.

Almond, J.W. 1977. A single gene determines the host range of influenza virus. *Nature*, **270**, 617–18.

Alonso-Caplen, F.V., Nemeroff, M.E., et al. 1992. Nucleocytoplasmic transport: the influenza virus NS1 protein regulates the transport of spliced NS2 mRNA and its precursor NS1 mRNA. *Genes Dev*, **6**, 255–67.

Amano, H., Uemoto, H., et al. 1992. Immunoelectron microscopy of influenza A virus neuraminidase glycoprotein topography. *J Gen Virol*, **73**, Pt 8, 1969–75.

Area, E., Martin-Benito, J., et al. 2004. 3D structure of the influenza virus polymerase complex: localization of subunit domains. *Proc Natl Acad Sci USA*, **101**, 308–13.

Argos, P. 1988. A sequence motif in many polymerases. *Nucleic Acids Res*, **16**, 9909–16.

Armstrong, R.T., Kushnir, A.S. and White, J.M. 2000. The transmembrane domain of influenza hemagglutinin exhibits a stringent length requirement to support the hemifusion to fusion transition. *J Cell Biol*, **151**, 425–37.

Asano, Y. and Ishihama, A. 1997. Identification of two nucleotide-binding domains on the PB1 subunit of influenza virus RNA polymerase. *J Biochem (Tokyo)*, **122**, 627–34.

Asano, Y., Mizumoto, K., et al. 1995. Photoaffinity labeling of influenza virus RNA polymerase PB1 subunit with 8-azido GTP. *J Biochem (Tokyo)*, **117**, 677–82.

Avalos, R.T., Yu, Z. and Nayak, D.P. 1997. Association of influenza virus NP and M1 proteins with cellular cytoskeletal elements in influenza virus-infected cells. *J Virol*, **71**, 2947–58.

Baez, M., Palese, P. and Kilbourne, E.D. 1980. Gene composition of high-yielding influenza vaccine strains obtained by recombination. *J Infect Dis*, **141**, 362–5.

Baigent, S.J. and McCauley, J.W. 2001. Glycosylation of haemagglutinin and stalk-length of neuraminidase combine to regulate the growth of avian influenza viruses in tissue culture. *Virus Res*, **79**, 177–85.

Balachandran, S., Roberts, P.C., et al. 2000. Alpha/beta interferons potentiate virus-induced apoptosis through activation of the FADD/Caspase-8 death signaling pathway. *J Virol*, **74**, 1513–23.

Banks, J., Speidel, E.S., et al. 2001. Changes in the haemagglutinin and the neuraminidase genes prior to the emergence of highly pathogenic H7N1 avian influenza viruses in Italy. *Arch Virol*, **146**, 963–73.

Barcena, J., de la Ochoa, M., et al. 1994. Monoclonal antibodies against influenza virus PB2 and NP polypeptides interfere with the initiation step of viral mRNA synthesis in vitro. *J Virol*, **68**, 6900–9.

Barker, W.H. and Mullooly, J.P. 1980. Impact of epidemic type A influenza in a defined adult population. *Am J Epidemiol*, **112**, 798–811.

Barman, S. and Nayak, D.P. 2000. Analysis of the transmembrane domain of influenza virus neuraminidase, a type II transmembrane glycoprotein, for apical sorting and raft association. *J Virol*, **74**, 6538–45.

Barman, S., Ali, A., et al. 2001. Transport of viral proteins to the apical membranes and interaction of matrix protein with glycoproteins in the assembly of influenza viruses. *Virus Res*, **77**, 61–9.

Barman, S., Adhikary, L., et al. 2003. Influenza A virus hemagglutinin containing basolateral localization signal does not alter the apical budding of a recombinant influenza A virus in polarized MDCK cells. *Virology*, **305**, 138–52.

Barman, S., Adhikary, L., et al. 2004. Role of transmembrane domain and cytoplasmic tail amino acid sequences of influenza a virus neuraminidase in raft association and virus budding. *J Virol*, **78**, 5258–69.

Barnett, B.C., Graham, C.M., et al. 1989. The immune response of BALB/c mice to influenza hemagglutinin: commonality of the B cell and T cell repertoires and their relevance to antigenic drift. *Eur J Immunol*, **19**, 515–21.

Basler, C.F., Reid, A.H., et al. 2001. Sequence of the 1918 pandemic influenza virus nonstructural gene (NS) segment and characterization of recombinant viruses bearing the 1918 NS genes. *Proc Natl Acad Sci USA*, **98**, 2746–51.

Bastin, J., Rothbard, J., et al. 1987a. Use of synthetic peptides of influenza nucleoprotein to define epitopes recognized by class I-restricted cytotoxic T lymphocytes. *J Exp Med*, **165**, 1508–23.

Bastin, J.M., Townsend, A.R. and McMichael, A.J. 1987b. Specific recognition of influenza virus polymerase protein (PB1) by a murine cytotoxic T-cell clone. *Virology*, **160**, 278–80.

Baudin, F., Bach, C., et al. 1994. Structure of influenza virus RNP. I. Influenza virus nucleoprotein melts secondary structure in panhandle RNA and exposes the bases to the solvent. *EMBO J*, **13**, 3158–65.

Baum, L.G. and Paulson, J.C. 1990. Sialyloligosaccharides of the respiratory epithelium in the selection of human influenza virus receptor specificity. *Acta Histochem*, **40**, 35–8.

Baum, L.G. and Paulson, J.C. 1991. The N2 neuraminidase of human influenza virus has acquired a substrate specificity complementary to the hemagglutinin receptor specificity. *Virology*, **180**, 10–15.

Bean, W.J., Schell, M., et al. 1992. Evolution of the H3 influenza virus hemagglutinin from human and nonhuman hosts. *J Virol*, **66**, 1129–38.

Beare, A.S. and Webster, R.G. 1991. Replication of avian influenza viruses in humans. *Arch Virol*, **119**, 37–42.

Beaton, A.R. and Krug, R.M. 1981. Selected host cell capped RNA fragments prime influenza viral RNA transcription in vivo. *Nucleic Acids Res*, **9**, 4423–36.

Beaton, A.R. and Krug, R.M. 1986. Transcription antitermination during influenza viral template RNA synthesis requires the nucleocapsid protein and the absence of a 5′ capped end. *Proc Natl Acad Sci USA*, **83**, 6282–6.

Belz, G.T., Xie, W., et al. 2000. A previously unrecognized H-2D(b)-restricted peptide prominent in the primary influenza A virus-specific CD8+ T-cell response is much less apparent following secondary challenge. *J Virol*, **74**, 3486–93.

Bender, A., Albert, M., et al. 1998. The distinctive features of influenza virus infection of dendritic cells. *Immunobiology*, **198**, 552–67.

Bender, C., Hall, H., et al. 1999. Characterization of the surface proteins of influenza A (H5N1) viruses isolated from humans in 1997-1998. *Virology*, **254**, 115–23.

Bennink, J.R. and Yewdell, J.W. 1988. Murine cytotoxic T lymphocyte recognition of individual influenza virus proteins. High frequency of nonresponder MHC class I alleles. *J Exp Med*, **168**, 1935–9.

Bennink, J.R., Yewdell, J.W., et al. 1984. Recombinant vaccinia virus primes and stimulates influenza haemagglutinin-specific cytotoxic T cells. *Nature*, **311**, 578–9.

Bennink, J.R., Yewdell, J.W., et al. 1987. Anti-influenza virus cytotoxic T lymphocytes recognize the three viral polymerases and a nonstructural protein: responsiveness to individual viral antigens is major histocompatibility complex controlled. *J Virol*, **61**, 1098–102.

Bentz, J. and Mittal, A. 2003. Architecture of the influenza hemagglutinin membrane fusion site. *Biochim Biophys Acta*, **1614**, 24–35.

Bergmann, M., Garcia-Sastre, A., et al. 2000. Influenza virus NS1 protein counteracts PKR-mediated inhibition of replication. *J Virol*, **74**, 6203–6.

Betts, R.F. 1995. Influenza virus. In: Mandell, G.L., Bennett, J.E. and Dolin, R. (eds), *Mandell, Douglas and Bennett's principles and practice of infectious diseases*. New York, Edinburgh, London, Melbourne, Tokyo: Churchill Livingston, 1546–67.

Bilsel, P., Castrucci, M.R. and Kawaoka, Y. 1993. Mutations in the cytoplasmic tail of influenza A virus neuraminidase affect incorporation into virions. *J Virol*, **67**, 6762–7.

Biswas, S.K. and Nayak, D.P. 1994. Mutational analysis of the conserved motifs of influenza A virus polymerase basic protein 1. *J Virol*, **68**, 1819–26.

Biswas, S.K., Boutz, P.L. and Nayak, D.P. 1998. Influenza virus nucleoprotein interacts with influenza virus polymerase proteins. *J Virol*, **72**, 5493–501.

Bizebard, T., Gigant, B., et al. 1995. Structure of influenza virus haemagglutinin complexed with a neutralizing antibody. *Nature*, **376**, 92–4.

Blaas, D., Patzelt, E. and Kuechler, E. 1982. Identification of the cap binding protein of influenza virus. *Nucleic Acids Res*, **10**, 4803–12.

Black, R.A., Rota, P.A., et al. 1993. Antibody response to the M2 protein of influenza A virus expressed in insect cells. *J Gen Virol*, **74**, Pt 1, 143–6.

Bland, P.B. 1919. Influenza in its relation to pregnancy and labor. *Am J Obstet Gynecol*, **79**, 184.

Blok, J. and Air, G.M. 1982a. Sequence variation at the 3′ end of the neuraminidase gene from 39 influenza type A viruses. *Virology*, **121**, 211–29.

Blok, J. and Air, G.M. 1982b. Variation in the membrane-insertion and stalk sequences in eight subtypes of influenza type A virus neuraminidase. *Biochemistry*, **21**, 4001–7.

Blok, J., Air, G.M., et al. 1982. Studies on the size, chemical composition, and partial sequence of the neuraminidase (NA) from type A influenza viruses show that the N-terminal region of the NA is not processed and serves to anchor the NA in the viral membrane. *Virology*, **119**, 109–21.

Bodmer, H.C., Pemberton, R.M., et al. 1988. Enhanced recognition of a modified peptide antigen by cytotoxic T cells specific for influenza nucleoprotein. *Cell*, **52**, 253–8.

Boivin, G., Hardy, I., et al. 2000. Predicting influenza infections during epidemics with use of a clinical case definition. *Clin Infect Dis*, **31**, 1166–9.

Boivin, G., Hardy, I. and Kress, A. 2001. Evaluation of a Rapid Optical Immunoassay for Influenza Viruses (FLU OIA Test) in comparison with cell culture and reverse transcription-PCR. *J Clin Microbiol*, **39**, 730–2.

Boom, R., Sol, C.J., et al. 1990. Rapid and simple method for purification of nucleic acids. *J Clin Microbiol*, **28**, 495–503.

Boon, A.C., de Mutsert, G., et al. 2002. Sequence variation in a newly identified HLA-B35-restricted epitope in the influenza A virus nucleoprotein associated with escape from cytotoxic T lymphocytes. *J Virol*, **76**, 2567–72.

Bosch, F.X., Orlich, M., et al. 1979. The structure of the hemagglutinin, a determinant for the pathogenicity of influenza viruses. *Virology*, **95**, 197–207.

Bosch, F.X., Garten, W., et al. 1981. Proteolytic cleavage of influenza virus hemagglutinins: primary structure of the connecting peptide between HA1 and HA2 determines proteolytic cleavability and pathogenicity of Avian influenza viruses. *Virology*, **113**, 725–35.

Bourmakina, S.V. and Garcia-Sastre, A. 2003. Reverse genetics studies on the filamentous morphology of influenza A virus. *J Gen Virol*, **84**, 517–27.

Braam, J., Ulmanen, I. and Krug, R.M. 1983. Molecular model of a eucaryotic transcription complex: functions and movements of influenza P proteins during capped RNA-primed transcription. *Cell*, **34**, 609–18.

Brand, C.M. and Skehel, J.J. 1972. Crystalline antigen from the influenza virus envelope. *Nat New Biol*, **238**, 145–7.

Brassard, D.L., Leser, G.P. and Lamb, R.A. 1996. Influenza B virus NB glycoprotein is a component of the virion. *Virology*, **220**, 350–60.

Brewer, C.B. and Roth, M.G. 1991. A single amino acid change in the cytoplasmic domain alters the polarized delivery of influenza virus hemagglutinin. *J Cell Biol*, **114**, 413–21.

Briedis, D.J., Lamb, R.A. and Choppin, P.W. 1982. Sequence of RNA segment 7 of the influenza B virus genome: partial amino acid homology between the membrane proteins (M1) of influenza A and B viruses and conservation of a second open reading frame. *Virology*, **116**, 581–8.

Bron, R., Kendal, A.P., et al. 1993. Role of the M2 protein in influenza virus membrane fusion: effects of amantadine and monensin on fusion kinetics. *Virology*, **195**, 808–11.

Brown, L.E., Hinshaw, V.S. and Webster, R.G. 1983. Antigenic variation in the influenza A virus nonstructural protein, NS1. *Virology*, **130**, 134–43.

Brownlee, G.G. and Fodor, E. 2001. The predicted antigenicity of the haemagglutinin of the 1918 Spanish influenza pandemic suggests an avian origin. *Phil Trans R Soc Lond B Biol Sci*, **356**, 1871–6.

Brydon, E.W., Smith, H. and Sweet, C. 2003. Influenza A virus-induced apoptosis in bronchiolar epithelial (NCI-H292) cells limits pro-inflammatory cytokine release. *J Gen Virol*, **84**, 2389–400.

Bucher, D.J., Kharitonenkov, I.G., et al. 1980. Incorporation of influenza virus M-protein into liposomes. *J Virol*, **36**, 586–90.

Bui, M., Wills, E.G., et al. 2000. Role of the influenza virus M1 protein in nuclear export of viral ribonucleoproteins. *J Virol*, **74**, 1781–6.

Bui, M., Myers, J.E. and Whittaker, G.R. 2002. Nucleo-cytoplasmic localization of influenza virus nucleoprotein depends on cell density and phosphorylation. *Virus Res*, **84**, 37–44.

Bullido, R., Gomez-Puertas, P., et al. 2000. Several protein regions contribute to determine the nuclear and cytoplasmic localization of the influenza A virus nucleoprotein. *J Gen Virol*, **81**, 135–42.

Bullough, P.A., Hughson, F.M., et al. 1994. Structure of influenza haemagglutinin at the pH of membrane fusion. *Nature*, **371**, 37–43.

Buonagurio, D.A., Nakada, S., et al. 1986. Evolution of human influenza A viruses over 50 years: rapid, uniform rate of change in NS gene. *Science*, **232**, 980–2.

Burmeister, W.P., Ruigrok, R.W. and Cusack, S. 1992. The 2.2 Å resolution crystal structure of influenza B neuraminidase and its complex with sialic acid. *EMBO J*, **11**, 49–56.

Burnet, F.M. 1936. Influenza virus on the developing egg. I. Changes associated with the development of an egg-passage strain of virus. *Br J Exp Pathol*, **17**, 282–93.

Burnet, F.M. 1940. Influenza virus infections of the chick embryo lung. *Br J Exp Pathol*, **21**, 147–53.

Burnet, F.M. and Bull, R.D. 1943. Changes in influenza virus associated with adaption to passage in chick embryos. *Aust J Exp Biol Med Sci*, **21**, 55–69.

Burnet, F.M. and Clarke, E. 1942. A survey of the last 50 years in the light of modern work on the virus of epidemic influenza. *Monogr Res Med*, **4**, 1–118.

Bush, R.M., Bender, C.A., et al. 1999. Predicting the evolution of human influenza A. *Science*, **286**, 1921–5.

Carr, C.M. and Kim, P.S. 1993. A spring-loaded mechanism for the conformational change of influenza hemagglutinin. *Cell*, **73**, 823–32.

Castrucci, M.R. and Kawaoka, Y. 1993. Biologic importance of neuraminidase stalk length in influenza A virus. *J Virol*, **67**, 759–64.

Castrucci, M.R. and Kawaoka, Y. 1995. Reverse genetics system for generation of an influenza A virus mutant containing a deletion of the carboxyl-terminal residue of M2 protein. *J Virol*, **69**, 2725–8.

Castrucci, M.R., Hou, S., et al. 1994. Protection against lethal lymphocytic choriomeningitis virus (LCMV) infection by immunization of mice with an influenza virus containing an LCMV epitope recognized by cytotoxic T lymphocytes. *J Virol*, **68**, 3486–90.

Castrucci, M.R., Hughes, M., et al. 1997. The cysteine residues of the M2 protein are not required for influenza A virus replication. *Virology*, **238**, 128–34.

Caton, A.J. and Gerhard, W. 1992. The diversity of the CD4+ T cell response in influenza. *Semin Immunol*, **4**, 85–90.

Caton, A.J., Brownlee, G.G., et al. 1982. The antigenic structure of the influenza virus A/PR/8/34 hemagglutinin (H1 subtype). *Cell*, **31**, 417–27.

CDC, 2004. Prevention and control of influenza: recommendations of the Advisory Committee on Immunization Practices (ACIP). *MMWR Recomm Rep*, **53**, 1–40.

Chapman, L.E., Tipple, M.A., et al. 1993. Influenza – United States, 1988–89. *MMWR CDC Surveill Summ*, **42**, 9–22.

Chen, D., Periwal, S.B., et al. 2001. Serum and mucosal immune responses to an inactivated influenza virus vaccine induced by epidermal powder immunization. *J Virol*, **75**, 7956–65.

Chen, J., Lee, K.H., et al. 1998. Structure of the hemagglutinin precursor cleavage site, a determinant of influenza pathogenicity and the origin of the labile conformation. *Cell*, **95**, 409–17.

Chen, W., Helenius, J., et al. 1995. Cotranslational folding and calnexin binding during glycoprotein synthesis. *Proc Natl Acad Sci USA*, **92**, 6229–33.

Chen, W., Calvo, P.A., et al. 2001. A novel influenza A virus mitochondrial protein that induces cell death. *Nat Med*, **7**, 1306–12.

Chen, W., Calvo, P.A., et al. 2001. A novel influenza A virus mitochondrial protein that induces cell death. *Nat Med*, **7**, 1306–12.

Chen, Z. and Krug, R.M. 2000. Selective nuclear export of viral mRNAs in influenza-virus-infected cells. *Trends Microbiol*, **8**, 376–83.

Chen, Z., Li, Y. and Krug, R.M. 1999a. Influenza A virus NS1 protein targets poly(A)-binding protein II of the cellular 3′-end processing machinery. *EMBO J*, **18**, 2273–83.

Chen, Z., Matsuo, K., et al. 1999b. Enhanced protection against a lethal influenza virus challenge by immunization with both hemagglutinin- and neuraminidase-expressing DNAs. *Vaccine*, **17**, 653–9.

Cherian, T., Bobo, L., et al. 1994. Use of PCR-enzyme immunoassay for identification of influenza A virus matrix RNA in clinical samples negative for cultivable virus. *J Clin Microbiol*, **32**, 623–8.

Cheung, C.Y., Poon, L.L., et al. 2002. Induction of proinflammatory cytokines in human macrophages by influenza A (H5N1) viruses: a mechanism for the unusual severity of human disease? *Lancet*, **360**, 1831–7.

Chien, C.Y., Tejero, R., et al. 1997. A novel RNA-binding motif in influenza A virus non-structural protein 1. *Nat Struct Biol*, **4**, 891–5.

Choi, K. and Thacker, S.B. 1982. Mortality during influenza epidemics in the United States, 1967–1978. *Am J Public Health*, **72**, 1280–3.

Cianci, C., Tiley, L. and Krystal, M. 1995. Differential activation of the influenza virus polymerase via template RNA binding. *J Virol*, **69**, 3995–9.

Claas, E.C., Sprenger, M.J., et al. 1992. Type-specific identification of influenza viruses A, B and C by the polymerase chain reaction. *J Virol Methods*, **39**, 1–13.

Claas, E.C., van Milaan, A.J., et al. 1993. Prospective application of reverse transcriptase polymerase chain reaction for diagnosing influenza infections in respiratory samples from a children's hospital. *J Clin Microbiol*, **31**, 2218–21.

Claas, E.C., de Jong, J.C., et al. 1998a. Human influenza virus A/HongKong/156/97 (H5N1) infection. *Vaccine*, **16**, 977–8.

Claas, E.C., Osterhaus, A.D., et al. 1998b. Human influenza A H5N1 virus related to a highly pathogenic avian influenza virus. *Lancet*, **351**, 472–7.

Clements, M.L., O'Donnell, S., et al. 1983. Dose response of A/Alaska/6/77 (H3N2) cold-adapted reassortant vaccine virus in adult volunteers: role of local antibody in resistance to infection with vaccine virus. *Infect Immun*, **40**, 1044–51.

Clements, M.L., Betts, R.F., et al. 1986. Serum and nasal wash antibodies associated with resistance to experimental challenge with influenza A wild-type virus. *J Clin Microbiol*, **24**, 157–60.

Clements, M.L., Subbarao, E.K., et al. 1992. Use of single-gene reassortant viruses to study the role of avian influenza A virus genes in attenuation of wild-type human influenza A virus for squirrel monkeys and adult human volunteers. *J Clin Microbiol*, **30**, 655–62.

Coccia, E.M., Severa, M., et al. 2004. Viral infection and Toll-like receptor agonists induce a differential expression of type I and lambda interferons in human plasmacytoid and monocyte-derived dendritic cells. *Eur J Immunol*, **34**, 796–805.

Cockburn, W.C., Delon, P.J. and Ferreira, W. 1969. Origin and progress of the 1968–69 Hong Kong influenza epidemic. *Bull World Health Organ*, **41**, 345–8.

Colacino, J.M., Laver, W.G. and Air, G.M. 1997. Selection of influenza A and B viruses for resistance to 4-guanidino-Neu5Ac2en in cell culture. *J Infect Dis*, **176**, Suppl 1, S66–8.

Collins, S.D. and Lehmann, J. 1951. Trends and epidemics of influenza and pneumonia 1918–1951. *Public Hlth Rpt*, **66**, 1487–516.

Colman, P.M., Varghese, J.N. and Laver, W.G. 1983. Structure of the catalytic and antigenic sites in influenza virus neuraminidase. *Nature*, **303**, 41–4.

Colman, P.M., Laver, W.G., et al. 1987. Three-dimensional structure of a complex of antibody with influenza virus neuraminidase. *Nature*, **326**, 358–63.

Compans, R.W., Content, J. and Duesberg, P.H. 1972. Structure of the ribonucleoprotein of influenza virus. *J Virol*, **10**, 795–800.

Connor, R.J., Kawaoka, Y., et al. 1994. Receptor specificity in human, avian, and equine H2 and H3 influenza virus isolates. *Virology*, **205**, 17–23.

Couceiro, J.N., Paulson, J.C. and Baum, L.G. 1993. Influenza virus strains selectively recognize sialyloligosaccharides on human respiratory epithelium; the role of the host cell in selection of hemagglutinin receptor specificity. *Virus Res*, **29**, 155–65.

Couch, R.B. and Kasel, J.A. 1983. Immunity to influenza in man. *Annu Rev Microbiol*, **37**, 529–49.

Couch, R.B., Kasel, J.A., et al. 1986. Influenza: its control in persons and populations. *J Infect Dis*, **153**, 431–40.

Cox, N.J. and Bender, C.A. 1995. The molecular epidemiology of influenza viruses. *Sem Virol*, **6**, 359–70.

Crescenzo-Chaigne, B. and van der Werf, W.S. 2001. Nucleotides at the extremities of the viral RNA of influenza C virus are involved in type-specific interactions with the polymerase complex. *J Gen Virol*, **82**, 1075–83.

Crescenzo-Chaigne, B., Naffakh, N. and van der Werf, W.S. 1999. Comparative analysis of the ability of the polymerase complexes of influenza viruses type A, B and C to assemble into functional RNPs that allow expression and replication of heterotypic model RNA templates in vivo. *Virology*, **265**, 342–53.

Crescenzo-Chaigne, B., van der Werf, W.S. and Naffakh, N. 2002. Differential effect of nucleotide substitutions in the 3′ arm of the influenza A virus vRNA promoter on transcription/replication by avian and human polymerase complexes is related to the nature of PB2 amino acid 627. *Virology*, **303**, 240–52.

Crosby, A.W. 1989. *America's forgotten pandemic: the influenza of 1919*. Cambridge: Cambridge University Press.

Cross, K.J., Wharton, S.A., et al. 2001. Studies on influenza haemagglutinin fusion peptide mutants generated by reverse genetics. *EMBO J*, **20**, 4432–42.

Daniels, P.S., Jeffries, S., et al. 1987. The receptor-binding and membrane-fusion properties of influenza virus variants selected using anti-haemagglutinin monoclonal antibodies. *EMBO J*, **6**, 1459–65.

Daniels, R., Kurowski, B., et al. 2003. N-linked glycans direct the cotranslational folding pathway of influenza hemagglutinin. *Mol Cell*, **11**, 79–90.

Daniels, R.S., Douglas, A.R., et al. 1983. Analyses of the antigenicity of influenza haemagglutinin at the pH optimum for virus-mediated membrane fusion. *J Gen Virol*, **64**, 1657–62.

Davenport, F.M., Hennessy, A.V. and Francis, T. Jr. 1953. Epidemiologic and immunologic significance of age distribution of antibody to antigenic variants of influenza virus. *J Exp Med*, **98**, 641–56.

Davey, J., Dimmock, N.J. and Colman, A. 1985. Identification of the sequence responsible for the nuclear accumulation of the influenza virus nucleoprotein in Xenopus oocytes. *Cell*, **40**, 667–75.

Davies, W.L., Grunert, N.J., et al. 1964. Antiviral activity of 1-adamantanamine (Amantadine). *Science*, **144**, 862–3.

Degelau, J., Somani, S.K., et al. 1992. Amantadine-resistant influenza A in a nursing facility. *Arch Intern Med*, **152**, 390–2.

Demicheli, V., Jefferson, T., et al. 2000. Prevention and early treatment of influenza in healthy adults. *Vaccine*, **18**, 957–1030.

Deng, Y., Jing, Y., et al. 2004. Age-related impaired type 1 T cell responses to influenza: reduced activation ex vivo, decreased expansion in CTL culture in vitro, and blunted response to influenza vaccination in vivo in the elderly. *J Immunol*, **172**, 3437–46.

Detjen, B.M., St Angelo, C., et al. 1987. The three influenza virus polymerase (P) proteins not associated with viral nucleocapsids in the infected cell are in the form of a complex. *J Virol*, **61**, 16–22.

de Wit, E., Spronken, M.I., et al. 2004. Efficient generation and growth of influenza virus A/PR/8/34 from eight cDNA fragments. *Virus Res*, **103**, 155–61.

Digard, P., Blok, V.C. and Inglis, S.C. 1989. Complex formation between influenza virus polymerase proteins expressed in Xenopus oocytes. *Virology*, **171**, 162–9.

Digard, P., Elton, D., et al. 1999. Modulation of nuclear localization of the influenza virus nucleoprotein through interaction with actin filaments. *J Virol*, **73**, 2222–31.

Doherty, P.C., Topham, D.J., et al. 1997. Effector CD4+ and CD8+ T-cell mechanisms in the control of respiratory virus infections. *Immunol Rev*, **159**, 105–17.

Doms, R.W., Lamb, R.A., et al. 1993. Folding and assembly of viral membrane proteins. *Virology*, **193**, 545–62.

Douglas, R.G. 1975. Influenza in man. In: Kilbourne, E.D. (ed.), *Influenza viruses and influenza*. New York: Academic Press, Inc, 395–418.

Dowdle, W.R. 1981. Influenza immunoprophylaxis after 30 years' experience. In: Academic Press, I. (ed.), *Genetic variation among influenza viruses*. New York: Academic Press, Inc, 525–34.

Dowdle, W.R. 1999. Influenza A virus recycling revisited. *Bull World Health Organ*, **77**, 820–8.

Dowdle, W.R. and Millar, J.D. 1978. Swine influenza: lessons learned. *Med Clin North Am*, **62**, 1047–57.

Dowdle, W.R., Coleman, M.T., et al. 1973. Inactivated influenza vaccines. 2. Laboratory indices of protection. *Postgrad Med J*, **49**, 159–63.

Drzeniek, R. and Kaluza, G. 1972. Enzymes as markers in virus preparations. *Z Naturforsch*, **27**, 424–6.

Dubovi, E.J., Crawford, P.C. et al. 2004. Abstract 47th Meeting of American Association of Veterinary Laboratory Diagnosticians, Greensboro, NC.

Duesberg, P.H. 1969. Distinct subunits of the ribonucleoprotein of influenza virus. *J Mol Biol*, **42**, 485–99.

Duff, K.C. and Ashley, R.H. 1992. The transmembrane domain of influenza A M2 protein forms amantadine- sensitive proton channels in planar lipid bilayers. *Virology*, **190**, 485–9.

Duff, K.C., Gilchrist, P.J., et al. 1994. Neutron diffraction reveals the site of amantadine blockade in the influenza A M2 ion channel. *Virology*, **202**, 287–93.

Dumitrescu, M.R., Grobnicu, M., et al. 1981. A three years experience in using MDCK cell line for influenza virus isolation (1979–1981). *Arch Roum Pathol Exp Microbiol*, **40**, 313–16.

Durbin, J.E., Fernandez-Sesma, A., et al. 2000. Type I IFN modulates innate and specific antiviral immunity. *J Immunol*, **164**, 4220–8.

Easterday, B.C. 1975. Animal influenza. In: Kilbourne, E.D. (ed.), *The influenza viruses and influenza*. New York: Academic Press, 449–81.

Edbauer, C.A. and Naso, R.B. 1984. Cytoskeleton-associated Pr65gag and assembly of retrovirus temperature-sensitive mutants in chronically infected cells. *Virology*, **134**, 389–97.

Ehrhardt, C., Kardinal, C., et al. 2004. Rac1 and PAK1 are upstream of IKK-epsilon and TBK-1 in the viral activation of interferon regulatory factor-3. *FEBS Lett*, **567**, 230–8.

Eichelberger, M., Allan, W., et al. 1991a. Clearance of influenza virus respiratory infection in mice lacking class I major histocompatibility complex-restricted CD8+ T cells. *J Exp Med*, **174**, 875–80.

Eichelberger, M.C., Wang, M.L., et al. 1991b. Influenza virus RNA in the lung and lymphoid tissue of immunologically intact and CD4-depleted mice. *J Gen Virol*, **72**, 1695–8.

Eickhoff, T.C., Sherman, I.L. and Serfling, R.E. 1961. Observations on excess mortality associated with epidemic influenza. *JAMA*, **176**, 776–82.

Eister, C., Larsen, K., et al. 1997. Influenza virus M1 protein binds to RNA through its nuclear localization signal. *J Gen Virol*, **78**, 1589–96.

Elleman, C.J. and Barclay, W.S. 2004. The M1 matrix protein controls the filamentous phenotype of influenza A virus. *Virology*, **321**, 144–53.

Ellis, J.S., Fleming, D.M. and Zambon, M.C. 1997a. Multiplex reverse transcription-PCR for surveillance of influenza A and B viruses in England and Wales in 1995 and 1996. *J Clin Microbiol*, **35**, 2076–82.

Ellis, J.S., Sadler, C.J., et al. 1997b. Analysis of influenza A H3N2 strains isolated in England during 1995–1996 using polymerase chain reaction restriction. *J Med Virol*, **51**, 234–41.

Elster, C., Fourest, E., et al. 1994. A small percentage of influenza virus M1 protein contains zinc but zinc does not influence in vitro M1-RNA interaction. *J Gen Virol*, **75**, 37–42.

Elton, D., Medcalf, L., et al. 1999. Identification of amino acid residues of influenza virus nucleoprotein essential for RNA binding. *J Virol*, **73**, 7357–67.

Elton, D., Simpson-Holley, M., et al. 2001. Interaction of the influenza virus nucleoprotein with the cellular CRM1-mediated nuclear export pathway. *J Virol*, **75**, 408–19.

Enami, M., Luytjes, W., et al. 1990. Introduction of site-specific mutations into the genome of influenza virus. *Proc Natl Acad Sci USA*, **87**, 3802–5.

Enami, M., Sharma, G., et al. 1991. An influenza virus containing nine different RNA segments. *Virology*, **185**, 291–8.

Ennis, F.A., Rook, A.H., et al. 1981. HLA restricted virus-specific cytotoxic T-lymphocyte responses to live and inactivated influenza vaccines. *Lancet*, **2**, 887–91.

Erickson, A.H. and Kilbourne, E.D. 1980. Mutation in the hemagglutinin of A/N-WS/33 influenza virus recombinants influencing sensitivity to trypsin and antigenic reactivity. *Virology*, **107**, 320–30.

Ershler, W.B., Moore, A.L. and Socinski, M.A. 1984. Influenza and aging: age-related changes and the effects of thymosin on the antibody response to influenza vaccine. *J Clin Immunol*, **4**, 445–54.

Farr, W. 1885. Vital Statistics: Memorial volume of selections from the writings of William Farr. N. Humphrey (ed.) London: Sanitary Institute of Great Britain, p. 330.

Fechter, P., Mingay, L., et al. 2003. Two aromatic residues in the PB2 subunit of influenza A RNA polymerase are crucial for cap binding. *J Biol Chem*, **278**, 20381–8.

Fedson, D.S., Hannoun, C., et al. 1995. Influenza vaccination in 18 developed countries, 1980–1992. *Vaccine*, **13**, 623–7.

Fields, S., Winter, G. and Brownlee, G.G. 1981. Structure of the neuraminidase gene in human influenza virus A/PR/8/34. *Nature*, **290**, 213–17.

Fischer, C., Schroth-Diez, B., et al. 1998. Acylation of the influenza hemagglutinin modulates fusion activity. *Virology*, **248**, 284–94.

Flewett, T.H. and Apostolov, K. 1967. A reticular structure in the wall of influenza C virus. *J Gen Virol*, **1**, 297–304.

Flick, R. and Hobom, G. 1999. Interaction of influenza virus polymerase with viral RNA in the 'corkscrew' conformation. *J Gen Virol*, **80**, 2565–72.

Flick, R., Neumann, G., et al. 1996. Promoter elements in the influenza vRNA terminal structure. *RNA*, **2**, 1046–57.

Flynn, K.J., Belz, G.T., et al. 1998. Virus-specific CD8+ T cells in primary and secondary influenza pneumonia. *Immunity*, **8**, 683–91.

Fodor, E., Pritlove, D.C. and Brownlee, G.G. 1994. The influenza virus panhandle is involved in the initiation of transcription. *J Virol*, **68**, 4092–6.

Fodor, E., Pritlove, D.C. and Brownlee, G.G. 1995. Characterization of the RNA-fork model of virion RNA in the initiation of transcription in influenza A virus. *J Virol*, **69**, 4012–19.

Fodor, E., Devenish, L., et al. 1999. Rescue of influenza A virus from recombinant DNA. *J Virol*, **73**, 9679–82.

Fodor, E., Crow, M., et al. 2002. A single amino acid mutation in the PA subunit of the influenza virus RNA polymerase inhibits endonucleolytic cleavage of capped RNAs. *J Virol*, **76**, 8989–9001.

Fodor, E., Mingay, L.J., et al. 2003. A single amino acid mutation in the PA subunit of the influenza virus RNA polymerase promotes the generation of defective interfering RNAs. *J Virol*, **77**, 5017–20.

Formanowski, F. and Meier-Ewert, H. 1988. Isolation of the influenza C virus glycoprotein in a soluble form by bromelain digestion. *Virus Res*, **10**, 177–91.

Fouchier, R.A., Schneeberger, P.M., et al. 2004. Avian influenza A virus (H7N7) associated with human conjunctivitis and a fatal case of acute respiratory distress syndrome. *Proc Natl Acad Sci USA*, **101**, 1356–61.

Fouchier, R.A., Munster, V., et al. 2005. Characterization of a novel hemagglutinin subtye (H16) obtained from black-headed gulls. *J Virol*, **79**, 2814–22.

Fox, J.P., Hall, C.E., et al. 1982. Influenzavirus infections in Seattle families, 1975–1979. I. Study design, methods and the occurrence of infections by time and age. *Am J Epidemiol*, **116**, 212–27.

Foy, H.M., Cooney, M.K. and Allan, I. 1976. Longitudinal studies of types A and B influenza among Seattle schoolchildren and families, 1968–74. *J Infect Dis*, **134**, 362–9.

Francis, T. 1940. A new type of virus from epidemic influenza. *Science*, **91**, 405–8.

Francis, T. and Magill, T.P. 1937. Direct isolation of human influenza virus in tissue cultures and in egg membranes. *Proc Soc Exp Biol*, **36**, 134–5.

Frank, A.L., Taber, L.H. and Wells, J.M. 1985. Comparison of infection rates and severity of illness for influenza A subtypes H1N1 and H3N2. *J Infect Dis*, **151**, 73–80.

Frost, W.H. 1919. The epidemiology of influenza. *JAMA*, **73**, 313–18.

Frost, W.H. 1920. Statistics of influenza morbidity: with special reference to certain factors in case incidence. *Pub Health Rep*, **35**, 584–97.

Fujii, Y., Goto, H., et al. 2003. Selective incorporation of influenza virus RNA segments into virions. *Proc Natl Acad Sci USA*, **100**, 2002–7.

Fujiyoshi, Y., Kume, N.P., et al. 1994. Fine structure of influenza A virus observed by electron cryo-microscopy. *EMBO J*, **13**, 318–26.

Gallagher, P.J., Henneberry, J.M., et al. 1992. Glycosylation requirements for intracellular transport and function of the hemagglutinin of influenza A virus. *J Virol*, **66**, 7136–45.

Gambaryan, A.S., Matrosovich, M.N., et al. 1998. Differences in the biological phenotype of low-yielding (L) and high- yielding (H) variants of swine influenza virus A/NJ/11/76 are associated with their different receptor-binding activity. *Virology*, **247**, 223–31.

Gambaryan, A.S., Robertson, J.S. and Matrosovich, M.N. 1999. Effects of egg-adaptation on the receptor-binding properties of human influenza A and B viruses. *Virology*, **258**, 232–9.

Gamblin, S.J., Haire, L.F., et al. 2004. The structure and receptor-binding properties of the 1918 influenza hemagglutinin. *Science*, **303**, 1838–42.

Gammelin, M., Altmuller, A., et al. 1990. Phylogenetic analysis of nucleoproteins suggests that human influenza A viruses emerged from a 19th-century avian ancestor. *Mol Biol Evol*, **7**, 194–200.

Garcia-Sastre, A. 2001. Inhibition of interferon-mediated antiviral responses by influenza A viruses and other negative-strand RNA viruses. *Virology*, **279**, 375–84.

Garcia-Sastre, A. and Palese, P. 1995. The cytoplasmic tail of the neuraminidase protein of influenza A virus does not play an important role in the packaging of this protein into viral envelopes. *Virus Res*, **37**, 37–47.

Garcia-Sastre, A., Egorov, A., et al. 1998. Influenza A virus lacking the NS1 gene replicates in interferon-deficient systems. *Virology*, **252**, 324–30.

Gastaminza, P., Perales, B., et al. 2003. Mutations in the N-terminal region of influenza virus PB2 protein affect virus RNA replication but not transcription. *J Virol*, **77**, 5098–108.

Ge, Q., McManus, M.T., et al. 2003. RNA interference of influenza virus production by directly targeting mRNA for degradation and indirectly inhibiting all viral RNA transcription. *Proc Natl Acad Sci USA*, **100**, 2718–23.

Ge, Q., Filip, L., et al. 2004. Inhibition of influenza virus production in virus-infected mice by RNA interference. *Proc Natl Acad Sci USA*, **101**, 8676–81.

Geiss, G.K., An, M.C., et al. 2001. Global impact of influenza virus on cellular pathways is mediated by both replication-dependent and -independent events. *J Virol*, **75**, 4321–31.

Geiss, G.K., Salvatore, M., et al. 2002. Cellular transcriptional profiling in influenza A virus-infected lung epithelial cells: The role of the nonstructural NS1 protein in the evasion of the host innate defense and its potential contribution to pandemic influenza. *Proc Natl Acad Sci USA*, **99**, 10736–41.

Gething, M.J., Doms, R.W., et al. 1986a. Studies on the mechanism of membrane fusion: site-specific mutagenesis of the hemagglutinin of influenza virus. *J Cell Biol*, **102**, 11–23.

Gething, M.J., McCammon, K. and Sambrook, J. 1986b. Expression of wild-type and mutant forms of influenza hemagglutinin: the role of folding in intracellular transport. *Cell*, **46**, 939–50.

Ghate, A.A. and Air, G.M. 1999. Influenza type B neuraminidase can replace the function of type A neuraminidase. *Virology*, **264**, 265–77.

Gianfrani, C., Oseroff, C., et al. 2000. Human memory CTL response specific for influenza A virus is broad and multispecific. *Hum Immunol*, **61**, 438–52.

Gibbs, J.S., Malide, D., et al. 2003. The influenza A virus PB1-F2 protein targets the inner mitochondrial membrane via a predicted basic amphipathic helix that disrupts mitochondrial function. *J Virol*, **77**, 7214–24.

Glezen, W.P. 1980. Consideration of the risk of influenza in children and indications for prophylaxis. *Rev Infect Dis*, **2**, 408–20.

Glezen, W.P. 1982. Serious morbidity and mortality associated with influenza epidemics. *Epidemiol Rev*, **4**, 25–44.

Glezen, W.P. 1996. Emerging infections: pandemic influenza. *Epidemiol Rev*, **18**, 64–76.

Glezen, W.P. and Couch, R.B. 1978. Interpandemic influenza in the Houston area, 1974–76. *N Engl J Med*, **298**, 587–92.

Glezen, W.P., Couch, R.B., et al. 1980a. Epidemiologic observations of influenza B virus infections in Houston, Texas, 1976–1977. *Am J Epidemiol*, **111**, 13–22.

Glezen, W.P., Paredes, A. and Taber, L.H. 1980b. Influenza in children. Relationship to other respiratory agents. *JAMA*, **243**, 1345–9.

Glezen, W.P., Decker, M. and Perrotta, D.M. 1987. Survey of underlying conditions of persons hospitalized with acute respiratory disease during influenza epidemics in Houston, 1978–1981. *Am Rev Respir Dis*, **136**, 550–5.

Godley, L., Pfeifer, J., et al. 1992. Introduction of intersubunit disulfide bonds in the membrane-distal region of the influenza hemagglutinin abolishes membrane fusion activity. *Cell*, **68**, 635–45.

Goldfield, M., Bartley, J.D., et al. 1977. Influenza in New Jersey in 1976: isolations of influenza A/New Jersey/76 virus at Fort Dix. *J Infect Dis*, **136**, Suppl, S347–55.

Gomez-Puertas, P., Leahy, M.B., et al. 2000. Rescue of synthetic RNAs into thogoto and influenza A virus particles using core proteins purified from Thogoto virus. *Virus Res*, **67**, 41–8.

Gonzalez, S. and Ortin, J. 1999a. Characterization of influenza virus PB1 protein binding to viral RNA: two separate regions of the protein contribute to the interaction domain. *J Virol*, **73**, 631–7.

Gonzalez, S. and Ortin, J. 1999b. Distinct regions of influenza virus PB1 polymerase subunit recognize vRNA and cRNA templates. *EMBO J*, **18**, 3767–75.

Gorman, O.T., Bean, W.J., et al. 1990a. Evolution of the nucleoprotein gene of influenza A virus. *J Virol*, **64**, 1487–97.

Gorman, O.T., Donis, R.O., et al. 1990b. Evolution of influenza A virus PB2 genes: implications for evolution of the ribonucleoprotein complex and origin of human influenza A virus. *J Virol*, **64**, 4893–902.

Gotch, F., McMichael, A., et al. 1987. Identification of viral molecules recognized by influenza-specific human cytotoxic T lymphocytes. *J Exp Med*, **165**, 408–16.

Goto, H. and Kawaoka, Y. 1998. A novel mechanism for the acquisition of virulence by a human influenza A virus. *Proc Natl Acad Sci USA*, **95**, 10224–8.

Gotoh, B., Ogasawara, T., et al. 1990. An endoprotease homologous to the blood clotting factor X as a determinant of viral tropism in chick embryo. *EMBO J*, **9**, 4189–95.

Gottschalk, A. 1957. Neuraminidase: the specific enzyme of influenza virus and Vibrio cholerae. *Biochim Biophys Acta*, **23**, 645–6.

Graham, C.M., Barnett, B.C., et al. 1989. The structural requirements for class II (I-Ad)-restricted T cell recognition of influenza hemagglutinin: B cell epitopes define T cell epitopes. *Eur J Immunol*, **19**, 523–8.

Gravotta, D., Adesnik, M. and Sabatini, D.D. 1990. Transport of influenza HA from the trans-Golgi network to the apical surface of MDCK cells permeabilized in their basolateral plasma membranes: energy dependence and involvement of GTP-binding proteins. *J Cell Biol*, **111**, 2893–908.

Greenberg, M., Jacobziner, H., et al. 1958. Maternal mortality in the epidemic of Asian Influenza, New York City, 1957. *Am J Obstet Gynecol*, **76**, 897–902.

Greenspan, D., Palese, P. and Krystal, M. 1988. Two nuclear location signals in the influenza virus NS1 nonstructural protein. *J Virol*, **62**, 3020–6.

Gregoriades, A. and Frangione, B. 1981. Insertion of influenza M protein into the viral lipid bilayer and localization of site of insertion. *J Virol*, **40**, 323–8.

Gregoriades, A., Guzman, G.G. and Paoletti, E. 1990. The phosphorylation of the integral membrane (M1) protein of influenza virus. *Virus Res*, **16**, 27–41.

Gregory, V., Bennett, M., et al. 2002. Emergence of influenza A H1N2 reassortant viruses in the human population during 2001. *Virology*, **300**, 1–7.

Gubareva, L.V., Robinson, M.J., et al. 1997. Catalytic and framework mutations in the neuraminidase active site of influenza viruses that are resistant to 4-guanidino-Neu5Ac2en. *J Virol*, **71**, 3385–90.

Gunther, I., Glatthaar, B., et al. 1993. A H1 hemagglutinin of a human influenza A virus with a carbohydrate-modulated receptor binding site and an unusual cleavage site. *Virus Res*, **27**, 147–60.

Ha, Y., Stevens, D.J., et al. 2001. X-ray structures of H5 avian and H9 swine influenza virus hemagglutinins bound to avian and human receptor analogs. *Proc Natl Acad Sci USA*, **98**, 11181–6.

Ha, Y., Stevens, D.J., et al. 2003. X-ray structure of the hemagglutinin of a potential H3 avian progenitor of the 1968 Hong Kong pandemic influenza virus. *Virology*, **309**, 209–18.

Hackett, C.J., Dietzschold, B., et al. 1983. Influenza virus site recognized by a murine helper T cell specific for H1 strains. Localization to a nine amino acid sequence in the hemagglutinin molecule. *J Exp Med*, **158**, 294–302.

Hagen, M., Chung, T.D., et al. 1994. Recombinant influenza virus polymerase: requirement of both 5′ and 3′ viral ends for endonuclease activity. *J Virol*, **68**, 1509–15.

Hall, C.B., Dolin, R., et al. 1987. Children with influenza A infection: treatment with rimantadine. *Pediatrics*, **80**, 275–82.

Hall, C.E., Brandt, C.D., et al. 1971. The virus watch program: a continuing surveillance of viral infections in metropolitan New York families. IX. A comparison of infections with several respiratory pathogens in New York and New Orleans families. *Am J Epidemiol*, **94**, 367–85.

Hall, C.E., Cooney, M.K. and Fox, J.P. 1973. The Seattle virus watch. IV. Comparative epidemiologic observations of infections with influenza A and B viruses, 1965–1969, in families with young children. *Am J Epidemiol*, **98**, 365–80.

Hall, W.J., Douglas, R.G., et al. 1976. Pulmonary mechanics after uncomplicated influenza A infection. *Am Rev Respir Dis*, **113**, 141–8.

Hammond, C., Braakman, I. and Helenius, A. 1994. Role of N-linked oligosaccharide recognition, glucose trimming, and calnexin in glycoprotein folding and quality control. *Proc Natl Acad Sci USA*, **91**, 913–17.

Haller, O. and Kochs, G. 2002. Interferon-induced mx proteins: dynamin-like GTPases with antiviral activity. *Traffic*, **3**, 710–17.

Hara, K., Shiota, M., et al. 2001. Influenza virus RNA polymerase PA subunit is a novel serine protease with Ser624 at the active site. *Genes Cells*, **6**, 87–97.

Hara, K., Shiota, M., et al. 2003. Inhibition of the protease activity of influenza virus RNA polymerase PA subunit by viral matrix protein. *Microbiol Immunol*, **47**, 521–6.

Hardy, J.M., Azarowicz, E.N., et al. 1961. The effect of Asian influenza on the outcome of pregnancy, Baltimore, 1957–1958. *Am J Public Health*, **51**, 1182–8.

Harris, A., Sha, B. and Luo, M. 1999. Structural similarities between influenza virus matrix protein M1 and human immunodeficiency virus matrix and capsid proteins: an evolutionary link between negative-stranded RNA viruses and retroviruses. *J Gen Virol*, **80**, 863–9.

Harris, A., Forouhar, F., et al. 2001. The crystal structure of the influenza matrix protein M1 at neutral pH: M1-M1 protein interfaces can rotate in the oligomeric structures of M1. *Virology*, **289**, 34–44.

Hartley, C.A., Reading, P.C., et al. 1997. Changes in the hemagglutinin molecule of influenza type A (H3N2) virus associated with increased virulence for mice. *Arch Virol*, **142**, 75–88.

Hatada, E., Hasegawa, M., et al. 1989. Control of influenza virus gene expression: quantitative analysis of each viral RNA species in infected cells. *J Biochem (Tokyo)*, **105**, 537–46.

Hatada, E., Saito, S. and Fukuda, R. 1999. Mutant influenza viruses with a defective NS1 protein cannot block the activation of PKR in infected cells. *J Virol*, **73**, 2425–33.

Hatta, M. and Kawaoka, Y. 2003. The NB protein of influenza B virus is not necessary for virus replication in vitro. *J Virol*, **77**, 6050–4.

Hatta, M., Gao, P., et al. 2001. Molecular basis for high virulence of Hong Kong H5N1 influenza A viruses. *Science*, **293**, 1840–2.

Hatta, M., Halfmann, P., et al. 2002. Human influenza A viral genes responsible for the restriction of its replication in duck intestine. *Virology*, **295**, 250–5.

Hatta, M., Goto, H. and Kawaoka, Y. 2004. Influenza B virus requires BM2 protein for replication. *J Virol*, **78**, 5576–83.

Hausmann, J., Kretzschmar, E., et al. 1995. N1 neuraminidase of influenza virus A/FPV/Rostock/34 has haemadsorbing activity. *J Gen Virol*, **76**, 1719–28.

Hay, A.J. 1974. Studies on the formation of the influenza virus envelope. *Virology*, **60**, 398–418.

Hay, A.J. 1992. The action of adamantanamines against influenza A viruses: inhibition of the M2 ion channel protein. *Semin Virol*, **3**, 21–30.

Hay, A.J., Lomniczi, B., et al. 1977. Transcription of the influenza virus genome. *Virology*, **83**, 337–55.

Hay, A.J., Wolstenholme, A.J., et al. 1985. The molecular basis of the specific anti-influenza action of amantadine. *EMBO J*, **4**, 3021–4.

Hayden, F.G. 1996. Amantadine and rimantadine – clinical aspects. In: Richman, D.D. (ed.), *Antiviral drug resistance*. New York: John Wiley & Sons Ltd, 59–77.

Hayden, F.G., Belshe, R.B., et al. 1989. Emergence and apparent transmission of rimantadine-resistant influenza A virus in families. *N Engl J Med*, **321**, 1696–702.

Hayden, F.G., Osterhaus, A.D., et al. 1997. Efficacy and safety of the neuraminidase inhibitor zanamivir in the treatment of influenzavirus infections. GG167 Influenza Study Group. *N Engl J Med*, **337**, 874–80.

Hayden, F.G., Fritz, R., et al. 1998. Local and systemic cytokine responses during experimental human influenza A virus infection.

Relation to symptom formation and host defense. *J Clin Invest*, **101**, 643–9.

Hayden, F.G., Atmar, R.L., et al. 1999. Use of the selective oral neuraminidase inhibitor oseltamivir to prevent influenza. *N Engl J Med*, **341**, 1336–43.

Hayden, F.G., Jennings, L., et al. 2000. Oral oseltamivir in human experimental influenza B infection. *Antivir Ther*, **5**, 205–13.

Hayslett, J., McCarroll, J., et al. 1962. Endemic influenza I. Serologic evidence of continuing and subclinical infection in disparate populations in the post-pandemic period. *Am Rev Resp Dis*, **85**, 1–8.

Hebert, D.N., Foellmer, B. and Helenius, A. 1996. Calnexin and calreticulin promote folding, delay oligomerization and suppress degradation of influenza hemagglutinin in microsomes. *EMBO J*, **15**, 2961–8.

Helenius, A. 1992. Unpacking the incoming influenza virus. *Cell*, **69**, 577–8.

Hemmes, J.H., Winkler, K.C. and Kool, S.M. 1960. Virus survival as a seasonal factor in influenza and polimyelitis. *Nature*, **188**, 430–1.

Herlocher, M.L., Bucher, D. and Webster, R.G. 1992. Host range determination and functional mapping of the nucleoprotein and matrix genes of influenza viruses using monoclonal antibodies. *Virus Res*, **22**, 281–93.

Herrler, G. and Klenk, H.D. 1991. Structure and function of the HEF glycoprotein of influenza C virus. *Adv Virus Res*, **40**, 213–34.

Herrler, G., Compans, R.W. and Meier-Ewert, H. 1979. A precursor glycoprotein in influenza C virus. *Virology*, **99**, 49–56.

Herrler, G., Rott, R., et al. 1985. The receptor-destroying enzyme of influenza C virus is neuraminate-O-acetylesterase. *EMBO J*, **4**, 1503–6.

Herrler, G., Durkop, I., et al. 1988. The glycoprotein of influenza C virus is the haemagglutinin, esterase and fusion factor. *J Gen Virol*, **69**, 839–46.

Herrler, G., Gross, H.J., et al. 1992. A synthetic sialic acid analogue is recognized by influenza C virus as a receptor determinant but is resistant to the receptor-destroying enzyme. *J Biol Chem*, **267**, 12501–5.

Herrmann, B., Larsson, C. and Zweygberg, B.W. 2001. Simultaneous detection and typing of influenza viruses A and B by a nested reverse transcription-PCR: comparison to virus isolation and antigen detection by immunofluorescence and optical immunoassay (FLU OIA). *J Clin Microbiol*, **39**, 134–8.

Hers, J.F. and Mulder, J. 1961. Broad aspects of the pathology and pathogenesis of human influenza. *Am Rev Respir Dis*, **83**, 84–97.

Hers, J.F., Goslings, W.R., et al. 1957. Death from Asiatic influenza in the Netherlands. *Lancet*, **273**, 1164–5.

Hewat, E.A., Cusack, S., et al. 1984. Low resolution structure of the influenza C glycoprotein determined by electron microscopy. *J Mol Biol*, **175**, 175–93.

Higa, H.H., Rogers, G.N. and Paulson, J.C. 1985. Influenza virus hemagglutinins differentiate between receptor determinants bearing N-acetyl-, N-glycolyl- and N, O-diacetylneuraminic acids. *Virology*, **144**, 279–82.

Hinshaw, V.S., Webster, R.G. and Turner, B. 1980. The perpetuation of orthomyxoviruses and paramyxoviruses in Canadian waterfowl. *Can J Microbiol*, **26**, 622–9.

Hinshaw, V.S., Webster, R.G., et al. 1983a. Swine influenza-like viruses in turkeys: potential source of virus for humans? *Science*, **220**, 206–8.

Hinshaw, V.S., Webster, R.G., et al. 1983b. Altered tissue tropism of human-avian reassortant influenza viruses. *Virology*, **128**, 260–3.

Hinshaw, V.S., Olsen, C.W., et al. 1994. Apoptosis: a mechanism of cell killing by influenza A and B viruses. *J Virol*, **68**, 3667–73.

Hiromoto, Y., Saito, T., et al. 2000. Characterization of low virulent strains of highly pathogenic A/Hong Kong/156/97 (H5N1) virus in mice after passage in embryonated hens' eggs. *Virology*, **272**, 429–37.

Hirsch, A. 1883. *Handbook of geographical and historical pathology*. London: New Sydenham Society.

Hirst, G.K. 1941. Agglutination of red cells by allantoic fluid of chick embryos infected with influenza virus. *Science*, **94**, 22–3.

Hirst, G.K. 1950. Receptor destruction by viruses of the munps-NDV-influenza group. *J Exp Med*, **91**, 161–75.

Hobson, D., Curry, R.L., et al. 1972. The role of serum haemagglutination-inhibiting antibody in protection against challenge infection with influenza A2 and B viruses. *J Hyg (Lond)*, **70**, 767–77.

Hoffmann, E., Neumann, G., et al. 2000. A DNA transfection system for generation of influenza A virus from eight plasmids. *Proc Natl Acad Sci USA*, **97**, 6108–13.

Hoffmann, E., Krauss, S., et al. 2002. Eight-plasmid system for rapid generation of influenza virus vaccines. *Vaccine*, **20**, 3165–70.

Hogue, B.G. and Nayak, D.P. 1992. Synthesis and processing of the influenza virus neuraminidase, a type II transmembrane glycoprotein. *Virology*, **188**, 510–17.

Holsinger, L.J. and Lamb, R.A. 1991. Influenza virus M2 integral membrane protein is a homotetramer stabilized by formation of disulfide bonds. *Virology*, **183**, 32–43.

Holsinger, L.J., Shaughnessy, M.A., et al. 1995. Analysis of the posttranslational modifications of the influenza virus M2 protein. *J Virol*, **69**, 1219–25.

Honda, A. and Ishihama, A. 1997. The molecular anatomy of influenza virus RNA polymerase. *Biol Chem*, **378**, 483–8.

Honda, A., Ueda, K., et al. 1987. Identification of the RNA polymerase-binding site on genome RNA of influenza virus. *J Biochem (Tokyo)*, **102**, 1241–9.

Honda, A., Mukaigawa, J., et al. 1990. Purification and molecular structure of RNA polymerase from influenza virus A/PR8. *J Biochem (Tokyo)*, **107**, 624–8.

Honda, A., Mizumoto, K. and Ishihama, A. 1999. Two separate sequences of PB2 subunit constitute the RNA cap-binding site of influenza virus RNA polymerase. *Genes Cells*, **4**, 475–85.

Honda, A., Mizumoto, K. and Ishihama, A. 2002. Minimum molecular architectures for transcription and replication of the influenza virus. *Proc Natl Acad Sci USA*, **99**, 13166–71.

Hongo, S., Sugawara, K., et al. 1994. Identification of a second protein encoded by influenza C virus RNA segment 6. *J Gen Virol*, **75**, 12, 3503–10.

Hongo, S., Sugawara, K., et al. 1997. Characterization of a second protein (CM2) encoded by RNA segment 6 of influenza C virus. *J Virol*, **71**, 2786–92.

Hongo, S., Sugawara, K., et al. 1999. Influenza C virus CM2 protein is produced from a 374-amino-acid protein (P42) by signal peptidase cleavage. *J Virol*, **73**, 46–50.

Horimoto, T. and Kawaoka, Y. 1994. Reverse genetics provides direct evidence for a correlation of hemagglutinin cleavability and virulence of an avian influenza A virus. *J Virol*, **68**, 3120–8.

Horimoto, T. and Kawaoka, Y. 1995. The hemagglutinin cleavability of a virulent avian influenza virus by subtilisin-like endoproteases is influenced by the amino acid immediately downstream of the cleavage site. *Virology*, **210**, 466–70.

Horimoto, T. and Kawaoka, Y. 2001. Pandemic threat posed by avian influenza A viruses. *Clin Microbiol Rev*, **14**, 129–49.

Horisberger, M.A. 1992. Interferon-induced human protein MxA is a GTPase which binds transiently to cellular proteins. *J Virol*, **66**, 4705–9.

Horvath, C.M., Williams, M.A. and Lamb, R.A. 1990. Eukaryotic coupled translation of tandem cistrons: identification of the influenza B virus BM2 polypeptide. *EMBO J*, **9**, 2639–47.

Houck, P., Hemphill, M., et al. 1995. Amantadine-resistant influenza A in nursing homes. Identification of a resistant virus prior to drug use. *Arch Intern Med*, **155**, 533–7.

Hoyle, L. (1968). Morphology and physical structure. In: *The influenza viruses*. New York: Springer-Verlag, pp. 49–68.

Hsu, M.T., Parvin, J.D., et al. 1987. Genomic RNAs of influenza viruses are held in a circular conformation in virions and in infected cells by a terminal panhandle. *Proc Natl Acad Sci USA*, **84**, 8140–4.

Huang, X., Liu, T., et al. 2001. Effect of influenza virus matrix protein and viral RNA on ribonucleoprotein formation and nuclear export. *Virology*, **287**, 405–16.

Hughes, M.T., Matrosovich, M., et al. 2000. Influenza A viruses lacking sialidase activity can undergo multiple cycles of replication in cell culture, eggs, or mice. *J Virol*, **74**, 5206–12.

Hui, E.K., Barman, S., et al. 2003. Basic residues of the helix six domain of influenza virus M1 involved in nuclear translocation of M1 can be replaced by PTAP and YPDL late assembly domain motifs. *J Virol*, **77**, 7078–92.

Hurtley, S.M., Bole, D.G., et al. 1989. Interactions of misfolded influenza virus hemagglutinin with binding protein (BiP). *J Cell Biol*, **108**, 2117–26.

Hurwitz, J.L., Hackett, C.J., et al. 1985. Murine TH response to influenza virus: recognition of hemagglutinin, neuraminidase, matrix, and nucleoproteins. *J Immunol*, **134**, 1994–8.

Hwang, J.S., Yamada, K., et al. 2000. Expression of functional influenza virus RNA polymerase in the methylotrophic yeast *Pichia pastoris*. *J Virol*, **74**, 4074–84.

Inglis, S.C. and Brown, C.M. 1981. Spliced and unspliced RNAs encoded by virion RNA segment 7 of influenza virus. *Nucleic Acids Res*, **9**, 2727–40.

Inglis, S.C., Barrett, T., et al. 1979. The smallest genome RNA segment of influenza virus contains two genes that may overlap. *Proc Natl Acad Sci USA*, **76**, 3790–4.

Irving, W.L., James, D.K., et al. 2000. Influenza virus infection in the second and third trimesters of pregnancy: a clinical and seroepidemiological study. *BJOG*, **107**, 1282–9.

Ishihama, A. 1996. A multi-functional enzyme with RNA polymerase and RNase activities: molecular anatomy of influenza virus RNA polymerase. *Biochimie*, **78**, 1097–102.

Ishihama, A. and Barbier, P. 1994. Molecular anatomy of viral RNA-directed RNA polymerases. *Arch Virol*, **134**, 235–58.

Isin, B., Doruker, P. and Bahar, I. 2002. Functional motions of influenza virus hemagglutinin: a structure-based analytical approach. *Biophys J*, **82**, 569–81.

Ito, T. and Kawaoka, Y. 2000. Host-range barrier of influenza A viruses. *Vet Microbiol*, **74**, 71–5.

Ito, T., Gorman, O.T., et al. 1991. Evolutionary analysis of the influenza A virus M gene with comparison of the M1 and M2 proteins. *J Virol*, **65**, 5491–8.

Ito, T., Suzuki, Y., et al. 1997. Receptor specificity of influenza A viruses correlates with the agglutination of erythrocytes from different animal species. *Virology*, **227**, 493–9.

Ito, T., Couceiro, J.N., et al. 1998. Molecular basis for the generation in pigs of influenza A viruses with pandemic potential. *J Virol*, **72**, 7367–73.

Ito, T., Suzuki, Y., et al. 2000. Recognition of N-glycolylneuraminic acid linked to galactose by the alpha2,3 linkage is associated with intestinal replication of influenza A virus in ducks. *J Virol*, **74**, 9300–5.

Izurieta, H.S., Thompson, W.W., et al. 2000. Influenza and the rates of hospitalization for respiratory disease among infants and young children. *N Engl J Med*, **342**, 232–9.

Jackson, D., Cadman, A., et al. 2002. A reverse genetics approach for recovery of recombinant influenza B viruses entirely from cDNA. *J Virol*, **76**, 11744–7.

Jackson, D., Zurcher, T. and Barclay, W. 2004. Reduced incorporation of the influenza B virus BM2 protein in virus particles decreases infectivity. *Virology*, **322**, 276–85.

Jackson, D.C., Drummer, H.E., et al. 1994. Glycosylation of a synthetic peptide representing a T-cell determinant of influenza virus hemagglutinin results in loss of recognition by CD4+ T-cell clones. *Virology*, **199**, 422–30.

Jahiel, R.I. and Kilbourne, E.D. 1966. Reduction in plaque size and reduction in plaque number as differing indices of influenza virus-antibody reactions. *J Bacteriol*, **92**, 1521–34.

Jameson, J., Cruz, J. and Ennis, F.A. 1998. Human cytotoxic T-lymphocyte repertoire to influenza A viruses. *J Virol*, **72**, 8682–9.

Janakiraman, M.N., White, C.L., et al. 1994. Structure of influenza virus neuraminidase B/Lee/40 complexed with sialic acid and a dehydro analog at 1.8-A resolution: implications for the catalytic mechanism. *Biochemistry*, **33**, 8172–9.

Janeway, C.A. Jr. and Medzhitov, R. 2002. Innate immune recognition. *Annu Rev Immunol*, **20**, 197–216.

Jasenosky, L.D., Neumann, G., et al. 2001. Ebola virus VP40-induced particle formation and association with the lipid bilayer. *J Virol*, **75**, 5205–14.

Jennings, L.C. and Miles, J.A. 1978. A study of acute respiratory disease in the community of Port Chalmers. II. Influenza A/Port Chalmers/1/73: intrafamilial spread and the effect of antibodies to the surface antigens. *J Hyg (Lond)*, **81**, 67–75.

Jennings, P.A., Finch, J.T., et al. 1983. Does the higher order structure of the influenza virus ribonucleoprotein guide sequence rearrangements in influenza viral RNA? *Cell*, **34**, 619–27.

Jin, H., Leser, G.P. and Lamb, R.A. 1994. The influenza virus hemagglutinin cytoplasmic tail is not essential for virus assembly or infectivity. *EMBO J*, **13**, 5504–15.

Jin, H., Leser, G.P., et al. 1997. Influenza virus hemagglutinin and neuraminidase cytoplasmic tails control particle shape. *EMBO J*, **16**, 1236–47.

Jin, H., Lu, B., et al. 2003. Multiple amino acid residues confer temperature sensitivity to human influenza virus vaccine strains (FluMist) derived from cold-adapted A/Ann Arbor/6/60. *Virology*, **306**, 18–24.

Jin, H., Zhou, H., et al. 2004. Imparting temperature sensitivity and attenuation in ferrets to A/Puerto Rico/8/34 influenza virus by transferring the genetic signature for temperature sensitivity from cold-adapted A/Ann Arbor/6/60. *J Virol*, **78**, 995–8.

Johnson, P.R., Feldman, S., et al. 1986. Immunity to influenza A virus infection in young children: a comparison of natural infection, live cold-adapted vaccine, and inactivated vaccine. *J Infect Dis*, **154**, 121–7.

Johnston, S.L. and Bloy, H. 1993. Evaluation of a rapid enzyme immunoassay for detection of influenza A virus. *J Clin Microbiol*, **31**, 142–3.

Jordan, W.S., Badger, G.F. and Dingle, J. 1958. A study of illness in a group of Cleveland families XVI. The epidemiology of influenza, 1948–1953. *Am J Hyg*, **68**, 169–89.

Jurgensen, P.F., Olsen, G.N., et al. 1973. Immune response of the human respiratory tract. II. Cell-mediated immunity in the lower respiratory tract to tuberculin and mumps and influenza viruses. *J Infect Dis*, **128**, 730–5.

Kalin, M. and Grandien, M. 1993. Rapid diagnostic methods in respiratory infections. *Curr Opin Infect Dis*, **6**, 150–7.

Kase, T., Suzuki, Y., et al. 1999. Human mannan-binding lectin inhibits the infection of influenza A virus without complement. *Immunology*, **97**, 385–92.

Kato, A., Mizumoto, K. and Ishihama, A. 1985. Purification and enzymatic properties of an RNA polymerase-RNA complex from influenza virus. *Virus Res*, **34**, 115–27.

Katz, J.M. and Webster, R.G. 1992. Amino acid sequence identity between the HA1 of influenza A (H3N2) viruses grown in mammalian and primary chick kidney cells. *J Gen Virol*, **73**, 1159–65.

Katz, J.M., Naeve, C.W. and Webster, R.G. 1987. Host cell-mediated variation in H3N2 influenza viruses. *Virology*, **156**, 386–95.

Katz, J.M., Wang, M. and Webster, R.G. 1990. Direct sequencing of the HA gene of influenza (H3N2) virus in original clinical samples reveals sequence identity with mammalian cell-grown virus. *J Virol*, **64**, 1808–11.

Katz, J.M., Plowden, J., et al. 2004. Immunity to influenza: the challenges of protecting an aging population. *Immunol Res*, **29**, 113–24.

Katze, M.G., He, Y. and Gale, M. Jr. 2002. Viruses and interferon: a fight for supremacy. *Nat Rev Immunol*, **2**, 675–87.

Katze, M.G., Tomita, J., et al. 1988. Influenza virus regulates protein synthesis during infection by repressing autophosphorylation and activity of the cellular 68,000-Mr protein kinase. *J Virol*, **62**, 3710–17.

Kaufmann, A., Salentin, R., et al. 2001. Defense against influenza A virus infection: essential role of the chemokine system. *Immunobiology*, **204**, 603–13.

Kawakami, K. and Ishihama, A. 1983. RNA polymerase of influenza virus. III. Isolation of RNA polymerase-RNA complexes from influenza virus PR8. *J Biochem (Tokyo)*, **93**, 989–96.

Kawaoka, Y. 1991. Equine H7N7 influenza A viruses are highly pathogenic in mice without adaptation: potential use as an animal model. *J Virol*, **65**, 3891–4.

Kawaoka, Y. and Webster, R.G. 1988. Sequence requirements for cleavage activation of influenza virus hemagglutinin expressed in mammalian cells. *Proc Natl Acad Sci USA*, **85**, 324–8.

Kawaoka, Y. and Webster, R.G. 1989. Interplay between carbohydrate in the stalk and the length of the connecting peptide determines the cleavability of influenza virus hemagglutinin. *J Virol*, **63**, 3296–300.

Kawaoka, Y., Naeve, C.W. and Webster, R.G. 1984. Is virulence of H5N2 influenza viruses associated with loss of carbohydrate from the hemagglutinin? *Virology*, **139**, 303–16.

Kawaoka, Y., Krauss, S. and Webster, R.G. 1989. Avian-to-human transmission of the PB1 gene of influenza A viruses in the 1957 and 1968 pandemics. *J Virol*, **63**, 4603–8.

Kawaoka, Y., Gorman, O.T., et al. 1998. Influence of host species on the evolution of the nonstructural (NS) gene of influenza A viruses. *Virus Res*, **55**, 143–56.

Keawcharoen, J., Oraveerakul, K., et al. 2004. Avian influenza H5N1 in tigers and leopards. *Emerg Infect Dis*, **12**, 2189–91.

Kehl, S.C., Henrickson, K.J., et al. 2001. Evaluation of the Hexaplex assay for detection of respiratory viruses in children. *J Clin Microbiol*, **39**, 1696–701.

Kelm, S., Paulson, J.C., et al. 1992. Use of sialic acid analogues to define functional groups involved in binding to the influenza virus hemagglutinin. *Eur J Biochem*, **205**, 147–53.

Kemble, G.W., Danieli, T. and White, J.M. 1994. Lipid-anchored influenza hemagglutinin promotes hemifusion, not complete fusion. *Cell*, **76**, 383–91.

Kemler, I., Whittaker, G. and Helenius, A. 1994. Nuclear import of microinjected influenza virus ribonucleoproteins. *Virology*, **202**, 1028–33.

Kendal, A.P., Noble, G.R., et al. 1978. Antigenic similarity of influenza A (H1N1) viruses from epidemics in 1977–1978 to Scandinavian strains isolated in epidemics of 1950–1951. *Virology*, **89**, 632–6.

Kendal, A.P., Skehel, J.J. and Pereira, M.S. 1982. *Concepts and procedures for laboratory-based influenza surveillance*. Centers for Disease Control, US Department of Health and Human Services (Report).

Kida, H., Ito, T., et al. 1994. Potential for transmission of avian influenza viruses to pigs. *J Gen Virol*, **75**, 2183–8.

Kido, H., Yokogoshi, Y., et al. 1992. Isolation and characterization of a novel trypsin-like protease found in rat bronchiolar epithelial Clara cells. A possible activator of the viral fusion glycoprotein. *J Biol Chem*, **267**, 13573–9.

Kilbourne, E.D. 1959. Studies on influenza in the pandemic of 1957–1958. III. Isolation of influenza A (Asian strain) viruses from influenza patients with pulmonary complications; details of virus isolation and characterization of isolates, with quantitative comparison of isolation methods. *J Clin Invest*, **38**, 266–74.

Kilbourne, E.D. (ed.) 1987. History of influenza. In *Influenza*. New York: Plenum Press, 3–22.

Kilbourne, E.D., Laver, W.G., et al. 1968. Antiviral activity of antiserum specific for an influenza virus neuraminidase. *J Virol*, **2**, 281–8.

Kim, H.W., Brandt, C.D., et al. 1979. Influenza A and B virus infection in infants and young children during the years 1957–1976. *Am J Epidemiol*, **109**, 464–79.

Kim, M.J., Latham, A.G. and Krug, R.M. 2002. Human influenza viruses activate an interferon-independent transcription of cellular antiviral genes: Outcome with influenza A virus is unique. *Proc Natl Acad Sci USA*, **99**, 10096–101.

Kiso, M., Mitamura, K., et al. 2004. Resistant influenza A viruses in children treated with oseltamivir: descriptive study. *Lancet*, **364**, 759–65.

Klenk, H.D. and Rott, R. 1988. The molecular biology of influenza virus pathogenicity. *Adv Virus Res*, **34**, 247–81.

Klenk, H.D., Wollert, W., et al. 1974. Association of influenza virus proteins with cytoplasmic fractions. *Virology*, **57**, 28–41.

Klenk, H.D., Rott, R., et al. 1975. Activation of influenza A viruses by trypsin treatment. *Virology*, **68**, 426–39.

Klenk, H.D., Garten, W. and Rott, R. 1984. Inhibition of proteolytic cleavage of the hemagglutinin of influenza virus by the calcium-specific ionophore A23187. *EMBO J*, **3**, 2911–15.

Klenk, H.D., Cox, N.J., et al. 1995. *Orthomyxoviridae*, virus taxonomy. In: Murphy, F.A. and Fauquet, C.M. (eds), *Virus taxonomy*. Vienna: Springer-Verlag, 293–9.

Klimov, A.I. and Cox, N.J. 1995. PCR restriction analysis of genome composition and stability of cold- adapted reassortant live influenza vaccines. *J Virol Methods*, **52**, 41–9.

Klimov, A.I., Rocha, E., et al. 1995. Prolonged shedding of amantadine-resistant influenzae A viruses by immunodeficient patients: detection by polymerase chain reaction- restriction analysis. *J Infect Dis*, **172**, 1352–5.

Klumpp, K., Ruigrok, R.W. and Baudin, F. 1997. Roles of the influenza virus polymerase and nucleoprotein in forming a functional RNP structure. *EMBO J*, **16**, 1248–57.

Kobasa, D., Rodgers, M.E., et al. 1997. Neuraminidase hemadsorption activity, conserved in avian influenza A viruses, does not influence viral replication in ducks. *J Virol*, **71**, 6706–13.

Kobasa, D., Kodihalli, S., et al. 1999. Amino acid residues contributing to the substrate specificity of the influenza A virus neuraminidase. *J Virol*, **73**, 6743–51.

Kobasa, D., Wells, K. and Kawaoka, Y. 2001. Amino acids responsible for the absolute sialidase activity of the influenza A virus neuraminidase: relationship to growth in the duck intestine. *J Virol*, **75**, 11773–80.

Kobayashi, M., Toyoda, T., et al. 1994. Molecular dissection of influenza virus nucleoprotein: deletion mapping of the RNA binding domain. *J Virol*, **68**, 8433–6.

Koen, J.S. 1919. A practical method for field diagnosis of swine diseases. *J Vet Med*, **14**, 468–70.

Koopmans, M., Wilbrink, B., et al. 2004. Transmission of H7N7 avian influenza A virus to human beings during a large outbreak in commercial poultry farms in the Netherlands. *Lancet*, **363**, 587–93.

Kretzschmar, E., Bui, M. and Rose, J.K. 1996. Membrane association of influenza virus matrix protein does not require specific hydrophobic domains or the viral glycoproteins. *Virology*, **220**, 37–45.

Krug, R.M., Broni, B.A. and Bouloy, M. 1979. Are the 5′ ends of influenza viral mRNAs synthesized in vivo donated by host mRNAs? *Cell*, **18**, 329–34.

Krug, R.M., Alonso-Caplen, F.V., et al. 1989. Expression and replication of the influenza virus genome. In: Krug, R.M. (ed.), *The influenza viruses*. New York: Plenum Press, 89–152.

Krug, R.M., Yuan, W., et al. 2003. Intracellular warfare between human influenza viruses and human cells: the roles of the viral NS1 protein. *Virology*, **309**, 181–9.

Kundu, A. and Nayak, D.P. 1994. Analysis of the signals for polarized transport of influenza virus (A/WSN/33) neuraminidase and human transferrin receptor, type II transmembrane proteins. *J Virol*, **68**, 1812–18.

Kung, H.C., Jen, K.F., et al. 1978. Influenza in China in 1977: recurrence of influenzavirus A subtype H1N1. *Bull World Health Organ*, **56**, 913–18.

Lamb, R.A. and Choppin, P.W. 1979. Segment 8 of the influenza virus genome is unique in coding for two polypeptides. *Proc Natl Acad Sci USA*, **76**, 4908–12.

Lamb, R.A. and Horvath, C.M. 1991. Diversity of coding strategies in influenza viruses. *Trends Genet*, **7**, 261–6.

Lamb, R.A. and Lai, C.J. 1980. Sequence of interrupted and uninterrupted mRNAs and cloned DNA coding for the two overlapping nonstructural proteins of influenza virus. *Cell*, **21**, 475–85.

Lamb, R.A., Lai, C.J. and Choppin, P.W. 1981. Sequences of mRNAs derived from genome RNA segment 7 of influenza virus: colinear and interrupted mRNAs code for overlapping proteins. *Proc Natl Acad Sci USA*, **78**, 4170–4.

Lamb, R.A., Zebedee, S.L. and Richardson, C.D. 1985. Influenza virus M2 protein is an integral membrane protein expressed on the infected-cell surface. *Cell*, **40**, 627–33.

Lamb, R.A., Holsinger, L.J. and Pinto, L.H. 1994. The influenza A virus M2 ion channel protein and its role in the influenza virus life cycle. In: Wimmer, E. (ed.), *Cellular receptors of animal viruses*. Cold Spring Harbor, New York: Cold Spring Harbor Laboratory Press, 303–21.

Lambkin, R. and Dimmock, N.J. 1995. All rabbits immunized with type A influenza virions have a serum haemagglutination-inhibition antibody response biased to a single epitope in antigenic site B. *J Gen Virol*, **76**, 889–97.

Lambkin, R., McLain, L., et al. 1994. Neutralization escape mutants of type A influenza virus are readily selected by antisera from mice immunized with whole virus: a possible mechanism for antigenic drift. *J Gen Virol*, **75**, 3493–502.

Latham, T. and Galarza, J.M. 2001. Formation of wild-type and chimeric influenza virus-like particles following simultaneous expression of only four structural proteins. *J Virol*, **75**, 6154–65.

Laver, W.G. and Valentine, R.C. 1969. Morphology of the isolated hemagglutinin and neuraminidase subunits of influenza virus. *Virology*, **38**, 105–19.

Laver, W.G., Colman, P.M., et al. 1984. Influenza virus neuraminidase with hemagglutinin activity. *Virology*, **137**, 314–23.

Lazarowitz, S.G. and Choppin, P.W. 1975. Enhancement of the infectivity of influenza A and B viruses by proteolytic cleavage of the hemagglutinin polypeptide. *Virology*, **68**, 440–54.

Lazarowitz, S.G., Goldberg, A.R. and Choppin, P.W. 1973. Proteolytic cleavage by plasmin of the HA polypeptide of influenza virus: host cell activation of serum plasminogen. *Virology*, **56**, 172–80.

Lee, M.T., Bishop, K., et al. 2002. Definition of the minimal viral components required for the initiation of unprimed RNA synthesis by influenza virus RNA polymerase. *Nucleic Acids Res*, **30**, 429–38.

Lehmann, N.I. and Gust, I.D. 1971. Viraemia in influenza. A report of two cases. *Med J Aust*, **2**, 1166–9.

Lentz, M.R., Webster, R.G. and Air, G.M. 1987. Site-directed mutation of the active site of influenza neuraminidase and implications for the catalytic mechanism. *Biochemistry*, **26**, 5351–8.

Li, J., Chen, S. and Evans, D.H. 2001. Typing and subtyping influenza virus using DNA microarrays and multiplex reverse transcriptase PCR. *J Clin Microbiol*, **39**, 696–704.

Li, K.S., Guan, Y., et al. 2004. Genesis of a highly pathogenic and potentially pandemic H5N1 influenza virus in eastern Asia. *Nature*, **430**, 209–13.

Li, M.L., Ramirez, B.C. and Krug, R.M. 1998. RNA-dependent activation of primer RNA production by influenza virus polymerase: different regions of the same protein subunit constitute the two required RNA-binding sites. *EMBO J*, **17**, 5844–52.

Li, M.L., Rao, P. and Krug, R.M. 2001. The active sites of the influenza cap-dependent endonuclease are on different polymerase subunits. *EMBO J*, **20**, 2078–86.

Li, S., Schulman, J., et al. 1993. Glycosylation of neuraminidase determines the neurovirulence of influenza A/WSN/33 virus. *J Virol*, **67**, 6667–73.

Li, W.X., Li, H., et al. 2004. Interferon antagonist proteins of influenza and vaccinia viruses are suppressors of RNA silencing. *Proc Natl Acad Sci USA*, **101**, 1350–5.

Li, X. and Palese, P. 1992. Mutational analysis of the promoter required for influenza virus virion RNA synthesis. *J Virol*, **66**, 4331–8.

Li, X. and Palese, P. 1994. Characterization of the polyadenylation signal of influenza virus RNA. *J Virol*, **68**, 1245–9.

Li, Y., Chen, Z.Y., et al. 2001. The 3′-end-processing factor CPSF is required for the splicing of single-intron pre-mRNAs in vivo. *RNA*, **7**, 920–31.

Li, Z.N., Hongo, S., et al. 2001. The sites for fatty acylation, phosphorylation and intermolecular disulphide bond formation of influenza C virus CM2 protein. *J Gen Virol*, **82**, 1085–93.

Lightman, S., Cobbold, S., et al. 1987. Do L3T4+ T cells act as effector cells in protection against influenza virus infection? *Immunology*, **62**, 139–44.

Lin, S., Naim, H.Y., et al. 1998. Mutations in the middle of the transmembrane domain reverse the polarity of transport of the influenza virus hemagglutinin in MDCK epithelial cells. *J Cell Biol*, **142**, 51–7.

Liu, B., Mori, I., et al. 2003. Local immune responses to influenza virus infection in mice with a targeted disruption of perforin gene. *Microb Pathog*, **34**, 161–7.

Liu, C. and Air, G.M. 1993. Selection and characterization of a neuraminidase-minus mutant of influenza virus and its rescue by cloned neuraminidase genes. *Virology*, **194**, 403–7.

Liu, C., Eichelberger, M.C., et al. 1995. Influenza type A virus neuraminidase does not play a role in viral entry, replication, assembly, or budding. *J Virol*, **69**, 1099–106.

Liu, J., Lynch, P.A., et al. 1997. Crystal structure of the unique RNA-binding domain of the influenza virus NS1 protein. *Nat Struct Biol*, **4**, 896–9.

Liu, M., Wood, J.M., et al. 2003. Preparation of a standardized, efficacious agricultural H5N3 vaccine by reverse genetics. *Virology*, **314**, 580–90.

Liu, T. and Ye, Z. 2002. Restriction of viral replication by mutation of the influenza virus matrix protein. *J Virol*, **76**, 13055–61.

Louria, D.B., Blumenfeld, H.L., et al. 1959. Studies on influenza in the pandemic of 1957–1958. II. Pulmonary complications of influenza. *J Clin Invest*, **38**, 213–65.

Lu, Y., Qian, X.Y. and Krug, R.M. 1994. The influenza virus NS1 protein: a novel inhibitor of pre-mRNA splicing. *Genes Dev*, **8**, 1817–28.

Lu, Y., Wambach, M., et al. 1995. Binding of the influenza virus NS1 protein to double-stranded RNA inhibits the activation of the protein kinase that phosphorylates the eIF-2 translation initiation factor. *Virology*, **214**, 222–8.

Ludwig, S., Schultz, U., et al. 1991. Phylogenetic relationship of the nonstructural (NS) genes of influenza A viruses. *Virology*, **183**, 566–77.

Ludwig, S., Wang, X., et al. 2002. The influenza A virus NS1 protein inhibits activation of Jun N-terminal kinase and AP-1 transcription factors. *J Virol*, **76**, 11166–71.

Lui, K.J. and Kendal, A.P. 1987. Impact of influenza epidemics on mortality in the United States from October 1972 to May 1985. *Am J Public Health*, **77**, 712–16.

Lund, J.M., Alexopoulou, L., et al. 2004. Recognition of single-stranded RNA viruses by Toll-like receptor 7. *Proc Natl Acad Sci USA*, **101**, 5598–603.

Luo, G., Chung, J. and Palese, P. 1993. Alterations of the stalk of the influenza virus neuraminidase: deletions and insertions. *Virus Res*, **29**, 141–53.

Luo, G.X., Luytjes, W., et al. 1991. The polyadenylation signal of influenza virus RNA involves a stretch of uridines followed by the RNA duplex of the panhandle structure. *J Virol*, **65**, 2861–7.

Luytjes, W., Krystal, M., et al. 1989. Amplification, expression, and packaging of foreign gene by influenza virus. *Cell*, **59**, 1107–13.

Makela, M.J., Pauksens, K., et al. 2000. Clinical efficacy and safety of the orally inhaled neuraminidase inhibitor zanamivir in the treatment of influenza: a randomized, double-blind, placebo-controlled European study. *J Infect*, **40**, 42–8.

Markosyan, R.M., Cohen, F.S. and Melikyan, G.B. 2000. The lipid-anchored ectodomain of influenza virus hemagglutinin (GPI-HA) is capable of inducing nonenlarging fusion pores. *Mol Biol Cell*, **11**, 1143–52.

Martin, C., Kunin, C.M., et al. 1959. Asian influenza A in Boston, 1957–1958. I. Observations in thirty-two influenza-associated fatal cases. *Arch Intern Med*, **103**, 515–31.

Martin, J., Wharton, S.A., et al. 1998. Studies of the binding properties of influenza hemagglutinin receptor-site mutants. *Virology*, **241**, 101–11.

Martin, K. and Helenius, A. 1991. Nuclear transport of influenza virus ribonucleoproteins: the viral matrix protein (M1) promotes export and inhibits import. *Cell*, **67**, 117–30.

Martin-Benito, J., Area, E., et al. 2001. Three-dimensional reconstruction of a recombinant influenza virus ribonucleoprotein particle. *EMBO Rep*, **2**, 313–17.

Massin, P., van der Werf, W.S. and Naffakh, N. 2001. Residue 627 of PB2 is a determinant of cold sensitivity in RNA replication of avian influenza viruses. *J Virol* , **75**, 5398–404.

Mast, E.E., Harmon, M.W., et al. 1991. Emergence and possible transmission of amantadine-resistant viruses during nursing home outbreaks of influenza A (H3N2). *Am J Epidemiol*, **134**, 988–97.

Masurel, N. and Heijtink, R.A. 1983. Recycling of H1N1 influenza A virus in man – a haemagglutinin antibody study. *J Hyg (Lond)*, **90**, 397–402.

Masurel, N. and Marine, W.M. 1973. Recycling of Asian and Hong Kong influenza A virus hemagglutinins in man. *Am J Epidemiol*, **97**, 44–9.

Matrosovich, M.N., Gambaryan, A.S. and Chumakov, M.P. 1992. Influenza viruses differ in recognition of 4-O-acetyl substitution of sialic acid receptor determinant. *Virology*, **188**, 854–8.

Matrosovich, M., Zhou, N., et al. 1999. The surface glycoproteins of H5 influenza viruses isolated from humans, chickens, and wild aquatic birds have distinguishable properties. *J Virol*, **73**, 1146–55.

Matrosovich, M., Tuzikov, A., et al. 2000. Early alterations of the receptor-binding properties of H1, H2 and H3 avian influenza virus hemagglutinins after their introduction into mammals. *J Virol*, **74**, 8502–12.

Matrosovich, M.N., Krauss, S. and Webster, R.G. 2001. H9N2 influenza A viruses from poultry in Asia have human virus-like receptor specificity. *Virology*, **281**, 156–62.

Matrosovich, M.N., Matrosovich, T.Y., et al. 2004. Human and avian influenza viruses target different cell types in cultures of human airway epithelium. *Proc Natl Acad Sci USA*, **101**, 4620–4.

McClelland, L. and Hare, R. 1941. The adsorption of influenza virus by red cells and a new in vitro method of measuring antibodies for influenza virus. *Can J Public Health*, **32**, 530–8.

McGeoch, D., Fellner, P. and Newton, C. 1976. Influenza virus genome consists of eight distinct RNA species. *Proc Natl Acad Sci USA*, **73**, 3045–9.

McKimm-Breschkin, J., Trivedi, T., et al. 2003. Neuraminidase sequence analysis and susceptibilities of influenza virus clinical isolates to zanamivir and oseltamivir. *Antimicrob Agents Chemother*, **47**, 2264–72.

McSharry, J.J., McDonough, A.C., et al. 2004. Phenotypic drug susceptibility assay for influenza virus neuraminidase inhibitors. *Clin Diagn Lab Immunol*, **11**, 21–8.

Medzhitov, R. and Janeway, C. Jr 2000. Innate immunity. *N Engl J Med*, **343**, 338–44.

Meibalane, R., Sedmak, G.V., et al. 1977. Outbreak of influenza in a neonatal intensive care unit. *J Pediatr*, **91**, 974–6.

Melikyan, G.B., Lin, S., et al. 1999. Amino acid sequence requirements of the transmembrane and cytoplasmic domains of influenza virus hemagglutinin for viable membrane fusion. *Mol Biol Cell*, **10**, 1821–36.

Mena, I., Jambrina, E., et al. 1999. Mutational analysis of influenza A virus nucleoprotein: identification of mutations that affect RNA replication. *J Virol*, **73**, 1186–94.

Mills, K.H., Burt, D.S., et al. 1988. Fine specificity of murine class II-restricted T cell clones for synthetic peptides of influenza virus hemagglutinin. Heterogeneity of antigen interaction with the T cell and the Ia molecule. *J Immunol*, **140**, 4083–90.

Minuse, E. and Willis III, P.W. 1962. An attempt to demonstrate viremia in cases of Asian influenza. *J Lab Clin Med*, **59**, 1016–19.

Mitnaul, L.J., Castrucci, M.R., et al. 1996. The cytoplasmic tail of influenza A virus neuraminidase (NA) affects NA incorporation into virions, virion morphology, and virulence in mice but is not essential for virus replication. *J Virol*, **70**, 873–9.

Mitnaul, L.J., Matrosovich, M.N., et al. 2000. Balanced hemagglutinin and neuraminidase activities are critical for efficient replication of influenza A virus. *J Virol*, **74**, 6015–20.

Mochalova, L., Gambaryan, A., et al. 2003. Receptor-binding properties of modern human influenza viruses primarily isolated in Vero and MDCK cells and chicken embryonated eggs. *Virology*, **313**, 473–80.

Mohsin, M.A., Morris, S.J., et al. 2002. Correlation between levels of apoptosis, levels of infection and haemagglutinin receptor binding interaction of various subtypes of influenza virus: does the viral neuraminidase have a role in these associations. *Virus Res*, **85**, 123–31.

Monto, A.S. and Kioumehr, F. 1975. The Tecumseh Study of Respiratory Illness. IX. Occurence of influenza in the community, 1966–1971. *Am J Epidemiol*, **102**, 553–63.

Monto, A.S. and Terpenning, M.S. 1996. The value of influenza and pneumococcal vaccines in the elderly. *Drugs Aging*, **8**, 445–51.

Monto, A.S. and Ullman, B.M. 1974. Acute respiratory illness in an American community: The Tecumseh study. *JAMA*, **227**, 164–9.

Monto, A.S., Maassab, H.F. and Bryan, E.R. 1981. Relative efficacy of embryonated eggs and cell culture for isolation of contemporary influenza viruses. *J Clin Microbiol*, **13**, 233–5.

Monto, A.S., Robinson, D.P., et al. 1999. Zanamivir in the prevention of influenza among healthy adults: a randomized controlled trial. *JAMA*, **282**, 31–5.

Monto, A.S., Gravenstein, S., et al. 2000. Clinical signs and symptoms predicting influenza infection. *Arch Intern Med*, **160**, 3243–7.

Monto, A.S., Pichichero, M.E., et al. 2002. Zanamivir prophylaxis: an effective strategy for the prevention of influenza types A and B within households. *J Infect Dis*, **186**, 1582–8.

Mora, R., Rodriguez-Boulan, E., et al. 2002. Apical budding of a recombinant influenza A virus expressing a hemagglutinin protein with a basolateral localization signal. *J Virol*, **76**, 3544–53.

Morris, S.J., Price, G.E., et al. 1999. Role of neuraminidase in influenza virus-induced apoptosis. *J Gen Virol*, **80**, Pt 1, 137–46.

Morris, S.J., Smith, H. and Sweet, C. 2002. Exploitation of the Herpes simplex virus translocating protein VP22 to carry influenza virus proteins into cells for studies of apoptosis: direct confirmation that neuraminidase induces apoptosis and indications that other proteins may have a role. *Arch Virol*, **147**, 961–79.

Morse, M.A., Marriott, A.C. and Nuttall, P.A. 1992. The glycoprotein of Thogoto virus (a tick-borne orthomyxo-like virus) is related to the baculovirus glycoprotein GP64. *Virology*, **186**, 640–6.

Moser, M.R., Bender, T.R., et al. 1979. An outbreak of influenza aboard a commercial airliner. *Am J Epidemiol*, **110**, 1–6.

Mountford, C.E., Grossman, G., et al. 1982. Effect of monoclonal anti-neuraminidase antibodies on the kinetic behavior of influenza virus neuraminidase. *Mol Immunol*, **19**, 811–16.

Muchmore, E.A. and Varki, A. 1987. Selective inactivation of influenza C esterase: a probe for detecting 9-O-acetylated sialic acids. *Science*, **236**, 1293–5.

Mukaigawa, J. and Nayak, D.P. 1991. Two signals mediate nuclear localization of influenza virus (A/WSN/33) polymerase basic protein 2. *J Virol*, **65**, 245–53.

Mulder, J., Masurel, N. and Webbers, P.J. 1958. Pre-epidemic antibody against 1957 strain of Asiatic influenza in serum of older people living in the Netherlands. *Lancet*, **1**, 810–14.

Murphy, B.R. and Clements, M.L. 1989. The systemic and mucosal immune response of humans to influenza A virus. *Curr Top Microbiol Immunol*, **146**, 107–16.

Murphy, B.R. and Webster, R.G. 1996. Orthomyxoviruses. In: Fields, B.N. and Knipe, D.M. (eds), *Fields virology*, 3rd edn. Philadelphia: Lippincott Raven, 1397–445.

Murphy, B.R., Nelson, D.L., et al. 1982. Secretory and systemic immunological response in children infected with live attenuated influenza A virus vaccines. *Infect Immun*, **36**, 1102–8.

Murti, K.G. and Webster, R.G. 1986. Distribution of hemagglutinin and neuraminidase on influenza virions as revealed by immunoelectron microscopy. *Virology*, **149**, 36–43.

Murti, K.G., Brown, P.S., et al. 1992. Composition of the helical internal components of influenza virus as revealed by immunogold labeling/electron microscopy. *Virology*, **186**, 294–9.

Muster, T., Subbarao, E.K., et al. 1991. An influenza A virus containing influenza B virus 5′ and 3′ noncoding regions on the neuraminidase gene is attenuated in mice. *Proc Natl Acad Sci USA*, **88**, 5177–81.

Naeve, C.W. and Williams, D. 1990. Fatty acids on the A/Japan/305/57 influenza virus hemagglutinin have a role in membrane fusion. *EMBO J*, **9**, 3857–66.

Naeve, C.W., Webster, R.G. and Hinshaw, V.S. 1983. Phenotypic variation in influenza virus reassortants with identical gene constellations. *Virology*, **128**, 331–40.

Naeve, C.W., Hinshaw, V.S. and Webster, R.G. 1984. Mutations in the hemagglutinin receptor-binding site can change the biological properties of an influenza virus. *J Virol*, **51**, 567–9.

Naffakh, N., Massin, P., et al. 2000. Genetic analysis of the compatibility between polymerase proteins from human and avian strains of influenza A viruses. *J Gen Virol*, **81**, 1283–91.

Naffakh, N., Massin, P. and van der Werf, W.S. 2001. The transcription/replication activity of the polymerase of influenza A viruses is not correlated with the level of proteolysis induced by the PA subunit. *Virology*, **285**, 244–52.

Naficy, K. 1963. Human influenza infection with proved viremia. Report of a case. *N Engl J Med*, **269**, 964–6.

Naim, H.Y. and Roth, M.G. 1993. Basis for selective incorporation of glycoproteins into the influenza virus envelope. *J Virol*, **67**, 4831–41.

Naim, H.Y., Amarneh, B., et al. 1992. Effects of altering palmitylation sites on biosynthesis and function of the influenza virus hemagglutinin. *J Virol*, **66**, 7585–8.

Nakagawa, Y., Kimura, N., et al. 1995. The RNA polymerase PB2 subunit is not required for replication of the influenza virus genome but is involved in capped mRNA synthesis. *J Virol*, **69**, 728–33.

Nakajima, K., Desselberger, U. and Palese, P. 1978. Recent human influenza A (H1N1) viruses are closely related genetically to strains isolated in 1950. *Nature*, **274**, 334–9.

Nakajima, K., Nobusawa, E. and Nakajima, S. 1990a. Evolution of the NS genes of the influenza A viruses. II. Characteristics of the amino acid changes in the NS1 proteins of the influenza A viruses. *Virus Genes*, **4**, 15–26.

Nakajima, K., Nobusawa, E., et al. 1990b. Evolution of the NS genes of the influenza A viruses. I. The genetic relatedness of the NS genes of animal influenza viruses. *Virus Genes*, **4**, 5–13.

Nakajima, S. and Sugiura, A. 1980. Neurovirulence of influenza virus in mice. II. Mechanism of virulence as studied in a neuroblastoma cell line. *Virology*, **101**, 450–7.

Nardelli, L., Pascucci, S., et al. 1978. Outbreaks of classical swine influenza in Italy in 1976. *Zentralbl Veterinarmed B*, **25**, 853–7.

Natali, A., Oxford, J.S. and Schild, G.C. 1981. Frequency of naturally occurring antibody to influenza virus antigenic variants selected in vitro with monoclonal antibody. *J Hyg (Lond)*, **87**, 185–90.

Nath, S.T. and Nayak, D.P. 1990. Function of two discrete regions is required for nuclear localization of polymerase basic protein 1 of A/WSN/33 influenza virus (H1 N1). *Mol Cell Biol*, **10**, 4139–45.

Neirynck, S., Deroo, T., et al. 1999. A universal influenza A vaccine based on the extracellular domain of the M2 protein. *Nat Med*, **5**, 1157–63.

Nemeroff, M.E., Barabino, S.M., et al. 1998. Influenza virus NS1 protein interacts with the cellular 30 kDa subunit of CPSF and inhibits 3 end formation of cellular pre-mRNAs. *Mol Cell*, **1**, 991–1000.

Neumann, G. and Hobom, G. 1995. Mutational analysis of influenza virus promoter elements in vivo. *J Gen Virol*, **76**, Pt 7, 1709–17.

Neumann, G. and Kawaoka, Y. 1999. Genetic engineering of influenza and other negative-strand RNA viruses containing segmented genomes. *Adv Virus Res*, **53**, 265–300.

Neumann, G. and Kawaoka, Y. 2001. Reverse genetics of influenza virus. *Virology*, **287**, 243–50.

Neumann, G. and Kawaoka, Y. 2002. Synthesis of influenza virus: new impetus from an old enzyme, RNA polymerase I. *Virus Res*, **82**, 153–8.

Neumann, G., Castrucci, M.R. and Kawaoka, Y. 1997. Nuclear import and export of influenza virus nucleoprotein. *J Virol*, **71**, 9690–700.

Neumann, G., Watanabe, T., et al. 1999. Generation of influenza A viruses entirely from cloned cDNAs. *Proc Natl Acad Sci USA*, **96**, 9345–50.

Neumann, G., Hughes, M.T. and Kawaoka, Y. 2000. Influenza A virus NS2 protein mediates vRNP nuclear export through NES-independent interaction with hCRM1. *EMBO J*, **19**, 6751–8.

Neumann, G., Whitt, M.A. and Kawaoka, Y. 2002. A decade after the generation of a negative-sense RNA virus from cloned cDNA – what have we learned? *J Gen Virol*, **83**, 2635–62.

Neuzil, K.M., Mellen, B.G., et al. 2000. The effect of influenza on hospitalizations, outpatient visits, and courses of antibiotics in children. *N Engl J Med*, **342**, 225–31.

Newman, R.W., Jennings, R., et al. 1993. Immune response of human volunteers and animals to vaccination with egg- grown influenza A (H1N1) virus is influenced by three amino acid substitutions in the haemagglutinin molecule. *Vaccine*, **11**, 400–6.

Nicholson, K.G. 1992. Clinical features of influenza. *Semin Respir Infect*, **7**, 26–37.

Nicholson, K.G., Snacken, R. and Palache, A.M. 1995. Influenza immunization policies in Europe and the United States. *Vaccine*, **13**, 365–9.

Nieto, A., de la Luna, L.S., et al. 1992. Nuclear transport of influenza virus polymerase PA protein. *Virus Res*, **24**, 65–75.

Noah, D.L., Twu, K.Y. and Krug, R.M. 2003. Cellular antiviral responses against influenza A virus are countered at the posttranscriptional level by the viral NS1A protein via its binding to a cellular protein required for the 3′ end processing of cellular pre-mRNAS. *Virology*, **307**, 386–95.

Noble, G.R. 1982. Epidemiological and clinical aspects of influenza. In: Beare, A.S. (ed.), *Basic and applied influenza research*. Boca Raton: CRC Press, 11–50.

Nobusawa, E., Aoyama, T., et al. 1991. Comparison of complete amino acid sequences and receptor-binding properties among 13 serotypes of hemagglutinins of influenza A viruses. *Virology*, **182**, 475–85.

Nobusawa, E., Ishihara, H., et al. 2000. Change in receptor-binding specificity of recent human influenza A viruses (H3N2): A single amino acid change in hemagglutinin altered its recognition of sialyloligosaccharides. *Virology*, **278**, 587–96.

Nuss, J.M. and Air, G.M. 1991. Transfer of the hemagglutinin activity of influenza virus neuraminidase subtype N9 into an N2 neuraminidase background. *Virology*, **183**, 496–504.

Nuss, J.M., Whitaker, P.B. and Air, G.M. 1993. Identification of critical contact residues in the NC41 epitope of a subtype N9 influenza virus neuraminidase. *Proteins*, **15**, 121–32.

Nussler, F., Clague, M.J. and Herrmann, A. 1997. Meta-stability of the hemifusion intermediate induced by glycosylphosphatidylinositol-anchored influenza hemagglutinin. *Biophys J*, **73**, 2280–91.

O'Neil, R.E. and Palese, P. 1995. NPI-1, the human homolog of SRP-1, interacts with influenza virus nucleoprotein. *Virology*, **206**, 116–25.

O'Neill, R.E., Talon, J. and Palese, P. 1998. The influenza virus NEP (NS2 protein) mediates the nuclear export of viral ribonucleoproteins. *EMBO J*, **17**, 288–96.

Odagiri, T., Hong, J. and Ohara, Y. 1999. The BM2 protein of influenza B virus is synthesized in the late phase of infection and incorporated into virions as a subviral component. *J Gen Virol*, **80**, 2573–81.

Ohtsu, Y., Honda, Y., et al. 2002. Fine mapping of the subunit binding sites of influenza virus RNA polymerase. *Microbiol Immunol*, **46**, 167–75.

Ohuchi, M., Ohuchi, R. and Mifune, K. 1982. Demonstration of hemolytic and fusion activities of influenza C virus. *J Virol*, **42**, 1076–9.

Ohuchi, M., Orlich, M., et al. 1989. Mutations at the cleavage site of the hemagglutinin after the pathogenicity of influenza virus A/chick/Penn/83 (H5N2). *Virology*, **168**, 274–80.

Ohuchi, M., Cramer, A., et al. 1994. Rescue of vector-expressed fowl plague virus hemagglutinin in biologically active form by acidotropic agents and coexpressed M2 protein. *J Virol*, **68**, 920–6.

Ohuchi, R., Ohuchi, M., et al. 1997. Oligosaccharides in the stem region maintain the influenza virus hemagglutinin in the metastable form required for fusion activity. *J Virol*, **71**, 3719–25.

Ohuchi, M., Fischer, C., et al. 1998. Elongation of the cytoplasmic tail interferes with the fusion activity of influenza virus hemagglutinin. *J Virol*, **72**, 3554–9.

Okada, A., Miura, T. and Takeuchi, H. 2001. Protonation of histidine and histidine-tryptophan interaction in the activation of the M2 ion channel from influenza a virus. *Biochemistry*, **40**, 6053–60.

Okazaki, K., Kawaoka, Y. and Webster, R.G. 1989. Evolutionary pathways of the PA genes of influenza A viruses. *Virology*, **172**, 601–8.

Ortega, J., Martin-Benito, J., et al. 2000. Ultrastructural and functional analyses of recombinant influenza virus ribonucleoproteins suggest dimerization of nucleoprotein during virus amplification. *J Virol*, **74**, 156–63.

Oxford, J.S., Newman, R., et al. 1991. Direct isolation in eggs of influenza A (H1N1) and B viruses with haemagglutinins of different antigenic and amino acid composition. *J Gen Virol*, **72**, 185–9.

Ozaki, H., Govorkova, E.A., et al. 2004. Generation of high-yielding influenza A viruses in African green monkey kidney (Vero) cells by reverse genetics. *J Virol*, **78**, 1851–7.

Palese, P. 1977. The genes of influenza virus. *Cell*, **10**, 1–10.

Palese, P., Tobita, K., et al. 1974. Characterization of temperature sensitive influenza virus mutants defective in neuraminidase. *Virology*, **61**, 397–410.

Panayotov, P.P. and Schlesinger, R.W. 1992. Oligomeric organization and strain-specific proteolytic modification of the virion M2 protein of influenza A H1N1 viruses. *Virology*, **186**, 352–5.

Park, E.K., Castrucci, M.R., et al. 1998. The M2 ectodomain is important for its incorporation into influenza A virions. *J Virol*, **72**, 2449–55.

Parvin, J.D., Palese, P., et al. 1989. Promoter analysis of influenza virus RNA polymerase. *J Virol*, **63**, 5142–52.

Paterson, R.G., Takeda, M., et al. 2003. Influenza B virus BM2 protein is an oligomeric integral membrane protein expressed at the cell surface. *Virology*, **306**, 7–17.

Patterson, S., Gross, J. and Oxford, J.S. 1988. The intracellular distribution of influenza virus matrix protein and nucleoprotein in infected cells and their relationship to haemagglutinin in the plasma membrane. *J Gen Virol*, **69**, 1859–72.

Pavlovic, J., Haller, O. and Staeheli, P. 1992. Human and mouse Mx proteins inhibit different steps of the influenza virus multiplication cycle. *J Virol*, **66**, 2564–9.

Peiris, J.S., Yu, W.C., et al. 2004. Re-emergence of fatal human influenza A subtype H5N1 disease. *Lancet*, **363**, 617–19.

Peiris, M., Yuen, K.Y., et al. 1999. Human infection with influenza H9N2. *Lancet*, **354**, 916–17.

Pekosz, A. and Lamb, R.A. 1997. The CM2 protein of influenza C virus is an oligomeric integral membrane glycoprotein structurally analogous to influenza A virus M2 and influenza B virus NB proteins. *Virology*, **237**, 439–51.

Pekosz, A. and Lamb, R.A. 1998. Influenza C virus CM2 integral membrane glycoprotein is produced from a polypeptide precursor by cleavage of an internal signal sequence. *Proc Natl Acad Sci USA*, **95**, 13233–8.

Pensaert, M., Ottis, K., et al. 1981. Evidence for the natural transmission of influenza A virus from wild ducks to swine and its potential importance for man. *Bull Wld Hlth Org*, **59**, 75–8.

Perales, B. and Ortin, J. 1997. The influenza A virus PB2 polymerase subunit is required for the replication of viral RNA. *J Virol*, **71**, 1381–5.

Perales, B., Sanz-Ezquerro, J.J., et al. 2000. The replication activity of influenza virus polymerase is linked to the capacity of the PA subunit to induce proteolysis. *J Virol*, **74**, 1307–12.

Perez, D.R. and Donis, R.O. 1998. The matrix 1 protein of influenza A virus inhibits the transcriptase activity of a model influenza reporter genome in vivo. *Virology*, **249**, 52–61.

Perez, D.R. and Donis, R.O. 2001. Functional analysis of PA binding by influenza a virus PB1: effects on polymerase activity and viral infectivity. *J Virol*, **75**, 8127–36.

Philip, R.N. and Bell, J.A. 1961. Epidemiologic studies on influenza in familial and general population groups, 1951–1956. *Am J Hyg*, **73**, 148–63.

Philipp, H.C., Schroth, B., et al. 1995. Assessment of fusogenic properties of influenza virus hemagglutinin deacylated by site-directed mutagenesis and hydroxylamine treatment. *Virology*, **210**, 20–8.

Piccone, M.E., Fernandez-Sesma, A. and Palese, P. 1993. Mutational analysis of the influenza virus vRNA promoter. *Virus Res*, **28**, 99–112.

Pinto, L.H., Holsinger, L.J. and Lamb, R.A. 1992. Influenza virus M2 protein has ion channel activity. *Cell*, **69**, 517–28.

Plakokefalos, E., Markoulatos, P., et al. 2000. A comparative study of immunocapture ELISA and RT-PCR for screening clinical samples from Southern Greece for human influenza virus types A and B. *J Med Microbiol*, **49**, 1037–41.

Plotch, S.J., Bouloy, M., et al. 1981. A unique cap(m7GpppXm)-dependent influenza virion endonuclease cleaves capped RNAs to generate the primers that initiate viral RNA transcription. *Cell*, **23**, 847–58.

Plotkin, J.B. and Dushoff, J. 2003. Codon bias and frequency-dependent selection on the hemagglutinin epitopes of influenza A virus. *Proc Natl Acad Sci USA*, **100**, 7152–7.

Plotnicky, H., Cyblat-Chanal, D., et al. 2003. The immunodominant influenza matrix T cell epitope recognized in human induces influenza protection in HLA-A2/K(b) transgenic mice. *Virology*, **309**, 320–9.

Po, J.L., Gardner, E.M., et al. 2002. Age-associated decrease in virus-specific CD8+ T lymphocytes during primary influenza infection. *Mech Ageing Dev*, **123**, 1167–81.

Poch, O., Sauvaget, I., et al. 1989. Identification of four conserved motifs among the RNA-dependent polymerase encoding elements. *EMBO J*, **8**, 3867–74.

Poon, L.L., Pritlove, D.C., et al. 1999. Direct evidence that the poly(A) tail of influenza A virus mRNA is synthesized by reiterative copying of a U track in the virion RNA template. *J Virol*, **73**, 3473–6.

Portela, A. and Digard, P. 2002. The influenza virus nucleoprotein: a multifunctional RNA-binding protein pivotal to virus replication. *J Gen Virol*, **83**, 723–34.

Price, G.E., Ou, R., et al. 2000. Viral escape by selection of cytotoxic T cell-resistant variants in influenza A virus pneumonia. *J Exp Med*, **191**, 1853–67.

Prilliman, K.R., Lemmens, E.E., et al. 2002. Cutting edge: a crucial role for B7-CD28 in transmitting T help from APC to CTL. *J Immunol*, **169**, 4094–7.

Pritlove, D.C., Poon, L.L., et al. 1999. A hairpin loop at the 5′ end of influenza A virus virion RNA is required for synthesis of poly(A)+ mRNA in vitro. *J Virol*, **73**, 2109–14.

Prokudina, E.N., Semenova, N.P., et al. 2004. Transient disulfide bonds formation in conformational maturation of influenza virus nucleocapsid protein (NP). *Virus Res*, **99**, 169–75.

Puertollano, R., Martin-Belmonte, F., et al. 1999. The MAL proteolipid is necessary for normal apical transport and accurate sorting of the influenza virus hemagglutinin in Madin-Darby canine kidney cells. *J Cell Biol*, **145**, 141–51.

Puri, A., Booy, F.P., et al. 1990. Conformational changes and fusion activity of influenza virus hemagglutinin of the H2 and H3 subtypes: effects of acid pretreatment. *J Virol*, **64**, 3824–32.

Qian, X.Y., Alonso-Caplen, F. and Krug, R.M. 1994. Two functional domains of the influenza virus NS1 protein are required for regulation of nuclear export of mRNA. *J Virol*, **68**, 2433–41.

Qiu, Y. and Krug, R.M. 1994. The influenza virus NS1 protein is a poly(A)-binding protein that inhibits nuclear export of mRNAs containing poly(A). *J Virol*, **68**, 2425–32.

Rajakumar, A., Swierkosz, E.M. and Schulze, I.T. 1990. Sequence of an influenza virus hemagglutinin determined directly from a clinical sample. *Proc Natl Acad Sci USA*, **87**, 4154–8.

Rao, B.L., Kadam, S.S., et al. 1982. Epidemiological, clinical, and virological features of influenza outbreaks in Pune, India, 1980. *Bull. World Health Organ*, **60**, 639–42.

Rao, P., Yuan, W. and Krug, R.M. 2003. Crucial role of CA cleavage sites in the cap-snatching mechanism for initiating viral mRNA synthesis. *EMBO J*, **22**, 1188–98.

Reay, P.A., Jones, I.M., et al. 1989. Recognition of the PB1, neuraminidase, and matrix proteins of influenza virus A/NT/60/68 by cytotoxic T lymphocytes. *Virology*, **170**, 477–85.

Rees, P.J. and Dimmock, N.J. 1981. Electrophoretic separation of influenza virus ribonucleoproteins. *J Gen Virol*, **53**, 125–32.

Reichelderfer, P.S., Kendal, A.P., et al. 1989. Influenza surveillance in the Pacific Basin. In: Chan, Y.C., Doraisingham, S. and Ling, A.E. (eds), *Current topics in medical mycology*. Singapore: World Scientific, 412–44.

Reid, A.H., Fanning, T.G., et al. 1999. Origin and evolution of the 1918 Spanish influenza virus hemagglutinin gene. *Proc Natl Acad Sci USA*, **96**, 1651–6.

Reid, A.H., Fanning, T.G., et al. 2000. Characterization of the 1918 Spanish influenza virus neuraminidase gene. *Proc Natl Acad Sci USA*, **97**, 6785–90.

Reid, A.H., Fanning, T.G., et al. 2002. Characterization of the 1918 Spanish influenza virus matrix gene segment. *J Virol*, **76**, 10717–23.

Reid, A.H., Taubenberger, J.K., et al. 2004. Evidence of an absence: the genetic origins of the 1918 pandemic influenza virus. *Nat Rev Microbiol*, **2**, 909–14.

Rekart, M., Rupnik, K., et al. 1982. Prevalence of hemagglutination inhibition antibody to current strains of the H3N2 and H1N1 subtypes of influenza A virus in sera collected from the elderly in 1976. *Am J Epidemiol*, **115**, 587–97.

Rey, O. and Nayak, D.P. 1992. Nuclear retention of M1 protein in a temperature-sensitive mutant of influenza (A/WSN/33) virus does not affect nuclear export of viral ribonucleoproteins. *J Virol*, **66**, 5815–24.

Richardson, J.C. and Akkina, R.K. 1991. NS2 protein of influenza virus is found in purified virus and phosphorylated in infected cells. *Arch Virol*, **116**, 69–80.

Robbins, P.A., Rota, P.A. and Shapiro, S.Z. 1997. A broad cytotoxic T lymphocyte response to influenza type B virus presented by multiple HLA molecules. *Int Immunol*, **9**, 815–23.

Roberts, P.C. and Compans, R.W. 1998. Host cell dependence of viral morphology. *Proc Natl Acad Sci USA*, **95**, 5746–51.

Roberts, P.C., Garten, W. and Klenk, H.D. 1993. Role of conserved glycosylation sites in maturation and transport of influenza A virus hemagglutinin. *J Virol*, **67**, 3048–60.

Robertson, J.S., Bootman, J.S., et al. 1987. Structural changes in the haemagglutinin which accompany egg adaptation of an influenza A(H1N1) virus. *Virology*, **160**, 31–7.

Robertson, J.S., Bootman, J.S., et al. 1990. The hemagglutinin of influenza B virus present in clinical material is a single species identical to that of mammalian cell-grown virus. *Virology*, **179**, 35–40.

Rogers, G.N. and D'Souza, B.L. 1989. Receptor binding properties of human and animal H1 influenza virus isolates. *Virology*, **173**, 317–22.

Rogers, G.N. and Paulson, J.C. 1983. Receptor determinants of human and animal influenza virus isolates: differences in receptor specificity of the H3 hemagglutinin based on species of origin. *Virology*, **127**, 361–73.

Rogers, G.N., Paulson, J.C., et al. 1983a. Single amino acid substitutions in influenza haemagglutinin change receptor binding specificity. *Nature*, **304**, 76–8.

Rogers, G.N., Pritchett, T.J., et al. 1983b. Differential sensitivity of human, avian, and equine influenza A viruses to a glycoprotein inhibitor of infection: selection of receptor specific variants. *Virology*, **131**, 394–408.

Rogers, G.N., Herrler, G., et al. 1986. Influenza C virus uses 9-O-acetyl-N-acetylneuraminic acid as a high affinity receptor determinant for attachment to cells. *J Biol Chem*, **261**, 5947–51.

Rohm, C., Zhou, N., et al. 1996. Characterization of a novel influenza hemagglutinin, H15: criteria for determination of influenza A subtypes. *Virology*, **217**, 508–16.

Romanos, M.A. and Hay, A.J. 1984. Identification of the influenza virus transcriptase by affinity-labeling with pyridoxal 5′-phosphate. *Virology*, **132**, 110–17.

Romanova, J., Katinger, D., et al. 2003. Distinct host range of influenza H3N2 virus isolates in Vero and MDCK cells is determined by cell specific glycosylation pattern. *Virology*, **307**, 90–7.

Rosenthal, P.B., Zhang, X., et al. 1998. Structure of the haemagglutinin-esterase-fusion glycoprotein of influenza C virus. *Nature*, **396**, 92–6.

Rota, P.A., Shaw, M.W. and Kendal, A.P. 1987. Comparison of the immune response to variant influenza type B hemagglutinins expressed in vaccinia virus. *Virology*, **161**, 269–75.

Rota, P.A., Shaw, M.W. and Kendal, A.P. 1989. Cross-protection against microvariants of influenza virus type B by vaccinia viruses expressing haemagglutinins from egg- or MDCK cell- derived subpopulations of influenza virus type B/England/222/82. *J Gen Virol*, **70**, 1533–7.

Roth, M.G., Compans, R.W., et al. 1983. Influenza virus hemagglutinin expression is polarized in cells infected with recombinant SV40 viruses carrying cloned hemagglutinin DNA. *Cell*, **33**, 435–43.

Rott, R., Becht, H. and Orlich, M. 1974. The significance of influenza virus neuraminidase in immunity. *J Gen Virol*, **22**, 35–41.

Ruigrok, R.W. and Baudin, F. 1995. Structure of influenza virus ribonucleoprotein particles. II. Purified RNA-free influenza virus ribonucleoprotein forms structures that are indistinguishable from the intact influenza virus ribonucleoprotein particles. *J Gen Virol*, **76**, 1009–14.

Ruigrok, R.W., Calder, L.J. and Wharton, S.A. 1989. Electron microscopy of the influenza virus submembranal structure. *Virology*, **173**, 311–16.

Ryan-Poirier, K.A., Katz, J.M., et al. 1992. Application of Directigen FLU-A for the detection of influenza A virus in human and nonhuman specimens. *J Clin Microbiol*, **30**, 1072–5.

Saito, T., Taylor, G., et al. 1994. Antigenicity of the N8 influenza A virus neuraminidase: existence of an epitope at the subunit interface of the neuraminidase. *J Virol*, **68**, 1790–6.

Sakaguchi, A., Hirayama, E., et al. 2003. Nuclear export of influenza viral ribonucleoprotein is temperature-dependently inhibited by dissociation of viral matrix protein. *Virology*, **306**, 244–53.

Sakai, T., Ohuchi, R. and Ohuchi, M. 2002. Fatty acids on the A/USSR/77 influenza virus hemagglutinin facilitate the transition from hemifusion to fusion pore formation. *J Virol*, **76**, 4603–11.

Sanz-Ezquerro, J.J., de la Luna, L.S., et al. 1995. Individual expression of influenza virus PA protein induces degradation of coexpressed proteins. *J Virol*, **69**, 2420–6.

Sanz-Ezquerro, J.J., Zurcher, T., et al. 1996. The amino-terminal one-third of the influenza virus PA protein is responsible for the induction of proteolysis. *J Virol*, **70**, 1905–11.

Sauter, N.K., Glick, G.D., et al. 1992. Crystallographic detection of a second ligand binding site in influenza virus hemagglutinin. *Proc Natl Acad Sci USA*, **89**, 324–8.

Schafer, W. 1955. Sero-immunologic studies on incomplete forms of the virus of classical fowl plague. *Arch Exp Vet Med*, **9**, 218–30.

Schaffer, F.L., Soergel, M.E. and Straube, D.C. 1976. Survival of airborne influenza virus: effects of propagating host, relative humidity, and composition of spray fluids. *Arch Virol*, **51**, 263–73.

Scheiffele, P., Roth, M.G. and Simons, K. 1997. Interaction of influenza virus haemagglutinin with sphingolipid-cholesterol membrane domains via its transmembrane domain. *EMBO J*, **16**, 5501–8.

Schickli, J.H., Flandorfer, A., et al. 2001. Plasmid-only rescue of influenza A virus vaccine candidates. *Philos Trans R Soc Lond B Biol Sci*, **356**, 1965–73.

Schild, G.C., Oxford, J.S., et al. 1983. Evidence for host-cell selection of influenza virus antigenic variants. *Nature*, **303**, 706–9.

Schmidt, M.F. 1982. Acylation of viral spike glycoproteins: a feature of enveloped RNA viruses. *Virology*, **116**, 327–38.

Schoenbaum, S.C. and Weinstein, L. 1979. Respiratory infection in pregnancy. *Clin Obstet Gynecol*, **22**, 293–300.

Schoenberger, S.P., Toes, R.E., et al. 1998. T-cell help for cytotoxic T lymphocytes is mediated by CD40-CD40L interactions. *Nature*, **393**, 480–3.

Scholtissek, C., Koennecke, I. and Rott, R. 1978a. Host range recombinants of fowl plague (influenza A) virus. *Virology*, **91**, 79–85.

Scholtissek, C., Rohde, W., et al. 1978b. A possible partial heterozygote of an influenza A virus. *Virology*, **89**, 506–16.

Scholtissek, C., Rohde, W., et al. 1978c. On the origin of the human influenza virus subtypes H2N2 and H3N2. *Virology*, **87**, 13–20.

Scholtissek, C., Burger, H., et al. 1983. Genetic relatedness of hemagglutinins of the H1 subtype of influenza A viruses isolated from swine and birds. *Virology*, **129**, 521–3.

Scholtissek, C., Burger, H., et al. 1985. The nucleoprotein as a possible major factor in determining host specificity of influenza H3N2 viruses. *Virology*, **147**, 287–94.

Schulman, J.L. and Palese, P. 1977. Virulence factors of influenza A viruses: WSN virus neuraminidase required for plaque production in MDBK cells. *J Virol*, **24**, 170–6.

Schulman, J.L., Khakpour, M. and Kilbourne, E.D. 1968. Protective effects of specific immunity to viral neuraminidase on influenza virus infection of mice. *J Virol*, **2**, 778–86.

Schultz-Cherry, S. and Hinshaw, V.S. 1996. Influenza virus neuraminidase activates latent transforming growth factor beta. *J Virol*, **70**, 8624–9.

Schultz-Cherry, S., Dybdahl-Sissoko, N., et al. 2001. Influenza virus NS1 protein induces apoptosis in cultured cells. *J Virol*, **75**, 7875–81.

Schulze, I.T. 1997. Effects of glycosylation on the properties and functions of influenza virus hemagglutinin. *J Infect Dis*, **176**, Suppl 1, S24–8.

Schwarzmann, S.W., Adler, J.I., et al. 1971. Bacterial pneumonia during the Hong Kong influenza epidemic of 1968–1969. Experience in a city-county hospital. *Arch Intern Med*, **127**, 1037–41.

Segal, M.S., Bye, J.M., et al. 1992. Disulfide bond formation during the folding of influenza virus hemagglutinin. *J Cell Biol*, **118**, 227–44.

Seo, S.H., Hoffmann, E. and Webster, R.G. 2002. Lethal H5N1 influenza viruses escape host anti-viral cytokine responses. *Nat Med*, **8**, 950–4.

Seong, B.L. and Brownlee, G.G. 1992a. A new method for reconstituting influenza polymerase and RNA in vitro: a study of the promoter elements for cRNA and vRNA synthesis in vitro and viral rescue in vivo. *Virology*, **186**, 247–60.

Seong, B.L. and Brownlee, G.G. 1992b. Nucleotides 9 to 11 of the influenza A virion RNA promoter are crucial for activity in vitro. *J Gen Virol*, **73**, 3115–24.

Sha, B. and Luo, M. 1997. Structure of a bifunctional membrane-RNA binding protein, influenza virus matrix protein M1. *Nat Struct Biol*, **4**, 239–44.

Shahab, S.Z. and Glezen, W.P. 1994. Influenza virus. In: Gonik, B. (ed.), *Viral diseases in pregnancy*. New York: Springer-Verlag, 215–23.

Shapiro, G.I. and Krug, R.M. 1988. Influenza virus RNA replication in vitro: synthesis of viral template RNAs and virion RNAs in the absence of an added primer. *J Virol*, **62**, 2285–90.

Shaw, M., Cooper, L., et al. 2002. Molecular changes associated with the transmission of avian influenza a H5N1 and H9N2 viruses to humans. *J Med Virol*, **66**, 107–14.

Shih, S.R., Nemeroff, M.E. and Krug, R.M. 1995. The choice of alternative 5′ splice sites in influenza virus M1 mRNA is regulated by the viral polymerase complex. *Proc Natl Acad Sci USA*, **92**, 6324–8.

Shinya, K., Hamm, S., et al. 2004. PB2 amino acid at position 627 affects replicative efficiency, but not cell tropism, of Hong Kong H5N1 influenza A viruses in mice. *Virology*, **320**, 258–66.

Shiratsuchi, A., Kaido, M., et al. 2000. Phosphatidylserine-mediated phagocytosis of influenza A virus-infected cells by mouse peritoneal macrophages. *J Virol*, **74**, 9240–4.

Shope, R.E. 1931. Swine influenza; experimental transmission and pathology. *J Exp Med*, **54**, 349–59.

Shortridge, K.F. 1992. Pandemic influenza: a zoonosis? *Semin Respir Infect*, **7**, 11–25.

Shvartsman, D.E., Kotler, M., et al. 2003. Differently anchored influenza hemagglutinin mutants display distinct interaction dynamics with mutual rafts. *J Cell Biol*, **163**, 879–88.

Simonsen, L., Clarke, M.J., et al. 1997. The impact of influenza epidemics on mortality: introducing a severity index. *Am J Public Health*, **87**, 1944–50.

Siren, J., Sareneva, T., et al. 2004. Cytokine and contact-dependent activation of natural killer cells by influenza A or Sendai virus-infected macrophages. *J Gen Virol*, **85**, 2357–64.

Skehel, J.J. and Wiley, D.C. 2000. Receptor binding and membrane fusion in virus entry: the influenza hemagglutinin. *Annu Rev Biochem*, **69**, 531–69.

Skehel, J.J., Bayley, P.M., et al. 1982. Changes in the conformation of influenza virus hemagglutinin at the pH optimum of virus-mediated membrane fusion. *Proc Natl Acad Sci USA*, **79**, 968–72.

Skehel, J.J., Stevens, D.J., et al. 1984. A carbohydrate side chain on hemagglutinins of Hong Kong influenza viruses inhibits recognition by a monoclonal antibody. *Proc Natl Acad Sci USA*, **81**, 1779–83.

Slepushkin, V.A., Katz, J.M., et al. 1995. Protection of mice against influenza A virus challenge by vaccination with baculovirus-expressed M2 protein. *Vaccine*, **13**, 1399–402.

Smirnov, Y.A., Lipatov, A.S., et al. 2000. Characterization of adaptation of an avian influenza A (H5N2) virus to a mammalian host. *Acta Virol*, **44**, 1–8.

Smirnov, Y., Kuznetsova, M.A. and Kaverin, N.V. 1991. The genetic aspects of influenza virus filamentous particle formation. *Arch Virol*, **118**, 279–84.

Smith, B.J., Colman, P.M., et al. 2001. Analysis of inhibitor binding in influenza virus neuraminidase. *Protein Sci*, **10**, 689–96.

Smith, D., Lapedes, A., et al. 2004. Mapping the antigenic and genetic evolution of influenza viruses. *Science*, **305**, 371–6.

Smith, G.L., Levin, J.Z., et al. 1987. Synthesis and cellular location of the ten influenza polypeptides individually expressed by recombinant vaccinia viruses. *Virology*, **160**, 336–45.

Smith, W., Andrewes, C.H. and Laidlaw, P.P. 1933. A virus obtained from influenza patients. *Lancet*, **1**, 66–8.

Smondyrev, A.M. and Voth, G.A. 2002. Molecular dynamics simulation of proton transport through the influenza A virus M2 channel. *Biophys J*, **83**, 1987–96.

Snyder, M.H., Buckler-White, A.J., et al. 1987. The avian influenza virus nucleoprotein gene and a specific constellation of avian and human virus polymerase genes each specify attenuation of avian-human influenza A/Pintail/79 reassortant viruses for monkeys. *J Virol*, **61**, 2857–63.

Solorzano, A., Zheng, H., et al. 2000. Reduced levels of neuraminidase of influenza A viruses correlate with attenuated phenotypes in mice. *J Gen Virol*, **81**, 737–42.

Spackman, E., Senne, D.A., et al. 2003. Sequence analysis of recent H7 avian influenza viruses associated with three different outbreaks in commercial poultry in the United States. *J Virol*, **77**, 13399–402.

Spelman, D.W. and McHardy, C.J. 1985. Concurrent outbreaks of influenza A and influenza B. *J Hyg (Lond)*, **94**, 331–9.

Staeheli, P. 1990. Interferon-induced proteins and the antiviral state. *Adv Virus Res*, **38**, 147–200.

Stegmann, T. 2000. Membrane fusion mechanisms: the influenza hemagglutinin paradigm and its implications for intracellular fusion. *Traffic*, **1**, 598–604.

Stegmann, T., White, J.M. and Helenius, A. 1990. Intermediates in influenza induced membrane fusion. *EMBO J*, **9**, 4231–41.

Steinhauer, D.A., Wharton, S.A., et al. 1991. Deacylation of the hemagglutinin of influenza A/Aichi/2/68 has no effect on membrane fusion properties. *Virology*, **184**, 445–8.

Stevens, J., Corper, A.L., et al. 2004. Structure of the uncleaved human H1 hemagglutinin from the extinct 1918 influenza virus. *Science*, **303**, 1866–70.

Stieneke-Grober, A., Vey, M., et al. 1992. Influenza virus hemagglutinin with multibasic cleavage site is activated by furin, a subtilisin-like endoprotease. *EMBO J*, **11**, 2407–14.

Stockton, J., Ellis, J.S., et al. 1998. Multiplex PCR for typing and subtyping influenza and respiratory syncytial viruses. *J Clin Microbiol*, **36**, 2990–5.

Strobl, B. and Vlasak, R. 1993. The receptor-destroying enzyme of influenza C virus is required for entry into target cells. *Virology*, **192**, 679–82.

Stuart-Harris, C.H., Schild, G. and Oxford, J.S. 1985. The epidemiology of influenza. In: Stuart-Harris, C.H. (ed.), *Influenza, the viruses and the disease*. London: Edward Arnold, 118–30.

Suarez, D.L. and Perdue, M.L. 1998. Multiple alignment comparison of the non-structural genes of influenza A viruses. *Virus Res*, **54**, 59–69.

Subbarao, E.K., London, W. and Murphy, B.R. 1993. A single amino acid in the PB2 gene of influenza A virus is a determinant of host range. *J Virol*, **67**, 1761–4.

Subbarao, K., Klimov, A., et al. 1998. Characterization of an avian influenza A (H5N1) virus isolated from a child with a fatal respiratory illness. *Science*, **279**, 393–6.

Subbarao, K., Chen, H., et al. 2003. Evaluation of a genetically modified reassortant H5N1 influenza A virus vaccine candidate generated by plasmid-based reverse genetics. *Virology*, **305**, 192–200.

Sugiura, A. and Ueda, M. 1980. Neurovirulence of influenza virus in mice. I. Neurovirulence of recombinants between virulent and avirulent virus strains. *Virology*, **101**, 440–9.

Sugrue, R.J. and Hay, A.J. 1991. Structural characteristics of the M2 protein of influenza A viruses: evidence that it forms a tetrameric channel. *Virology*, **180**, 617–24.

Sugrue, R.J., Bahadur, G., et al. 1990a. Specific structural alteration of the influenza haemagglutinin by amantadine. *EMBO J*, **9**, 3469–76.

Sugrue, R.J., Belshe, R.B. and Hay, A.J. 1990b. Palmitoylation of the influenza A virus M2 protein. *Virology*, **179**, 51–6.

Sunstrom, N.A., Premkumar, L.S., et al. 1996. Ion channels formed by NB, an influenza B virus protein. *J Membr Biol*, **150**, 127–32.

Suzuki, Y., Nakao, T., et al. 1992. Structural determination of gangliosides that bind to influenza A, B, and C viruses by an improved binding assay: strain-specific receptor epitopes in sialo-sugar chains. *Virology*, **189**, 121–31.

Suzuki, Y., Ito, T., et al. 2000. Sialic acid species as a determinant of the host range of influenza A viruses. *J Virol*, **74**, 11825–31.

Tada, Y., Hongo, S., et al. 1998. Phosphorylation of influenza C virus CM2 protein. *Virus Res*, **58**, 65–72.

Takahashi, T., Suzuki, Y., et al. 2001. Duck and human pandemic influenza A viruses retain sialidase activity under low pH conditions. *J Biochem (Tokyo)*, **130**, 279–83.

Takeda, M., Pekosz, A., et al. 2002. Influenza A virus M2 ion channel activity is essential for efficient replication in tissue culture. *J Virol*, **76**, 1391–9.

Takeda, M., Leser, G.P., et al. 2003. Influenza virus hemagglutinin concentrates in lipid raft microdomains for efficient viral fusion. *Proc Natl Acad Sci USA*, **100**, 14610–17.

Takeuchi, K. and Lamb, R.A. 1994. Influenza virus M2 protein ion channel activity stabilizes the native form of fowl plague virus hemagglutinin during intracellular transport. *J Virol*, **68**, 911–19.

Takizawa, T., Matsukawa, S., et al. 1993. Induction of programmed cell death (apoptosis) by influenza virus infection in tissue culture cells. *J Gen Virol*, **74**, 2347–55.

Takizawa, T., Fukuda, R., et al. 1995. Activation of the apoptotic Fas antigen-encoding gene upon influenza virus infection involving spontaneously produced beta-interferon. *Virology*, **209**, 288–96.

Talon, J., Salvatore, M., et al. 2000. Influenza A and B viruses expressing altered NS1 proteins: A vaccine approach. *Proc Natl Acad Sci USA*, **97**, 4309–14.

Tang, Y., Zaitseva, F., et al. 2002. The gate of the influenza virus M2 proton channel is formed by a single tryptophan residue. *J Biol Chem*, **277**, 39880–6.

Tashiro, M., Ciborowski, P., et al. 1987. Role of Staphylococcus protease in the development of influenza pneumonia. *Nature*, **325**, 536–7.

Taylor, P.M. and Askonas, B.A. 1986. Influenza nucleoprotein-specific cytotoxic T-cell clones are protective in vivo. *Immunology*, **58**, 417–20.

Taylor, R.M. 1949. Studies on survival of influenza virus between epidemics and antigenic variants of the virus. *Am J Pub Hlth*, **39**, 171–8.

Thomas, J.M., Stevens, M.P., et al. 1998. Phosphorylation of the M2 protein of influenza A virus is not essential for virus viability. *Virology*, **252**, 54–64.

Thompson, W.W., Shay, D.K., et al. 2003. Mortality associated with influenza and respiratory syncytial virus in the United States. *JAMA*, **289**, 179–86.

Thompson, W.W., Shay, D.K., et al. 2004. Influenza-associated hospitalizations in the United States. *JAMA*, **292**, 1333–40.

Tiley, L.S., Hagen, M., et al. 1994. Sequence-specific binding of the influenza virus RNA polymerase to sequences located at the 5' ends of the viral RNAs. *J Virol*, **68**, 5108–16.

Todd, S.J., Minnich, L. and Waner, J.L. 1995. Comparison of rapid immunofluorescence procedure with TestPack RSV and Directigen FLU-A for diagnosis of respiratory syncytial virus and influenza A virus. *J Clin Microbiol*, **33**, 1650–1.

Tominack, R.L. and Hayden, F.G. 1987. Rimantadine hydrochloride and amantadine hydrochloride use in influenza A virus infections. *Infect Dis Clin North Am*, **1**, 459–78.

Tompkins, S.M., Lo, C.Y., et al. 2004. Protection against lethal influenza virus challenge by RNA interference in vivo. *Proc Natl Acad Sci USA*, **101**, 8682–6.

Toyoda, T., Adyshev, D.M., et al. 1996. Molecular assembly of the influenza virus RNA polymerase: determination of the subunit-subunit contact sites. *J Gen Virol*, **77**, 2149–57.

Toyoda, T., Hara, K. and Imamura, Y. 2003. Ser624 of the PA subunit of influenza A virus is not essential for viral growth in cells and mice, but required for the maximal viral growth. *Arch Virol*, **148**, 1687–96.

Tran, T.H., Nguyen, T.L., et al. 2004. Avian influenza A (H5N1) in 10 patients in Vietnam. *N Engl J Med*, **350**, 1179–88.

Treanor, J.J., Tierney, E.L., et al. 1990. Passively transferred monoclonal antibody to the M2 protein inhibits influenza A virus replication in mice. *J Virol*, **64**, 1375–7.

Tsuchiya, E., Sugawara, K., et al. 2002. Effect of addition of new oligosaccharide chains to the globular head of influenza A/H2N2 virus haemagglutinin on the intracellular transport and biological activities of the molecule. *J Gen Virol*, **83**, 1137–46.

Tulip, W.R., Varghese, J.N., et al. 1991. Refined atomic structures of N9 subtype influenza virus neuraminidase and escape mutants. *J Mol Biol*, **221**, 487–97.

Tulip, W.R., Varghese, J.N., et al. 1992. Refined crystal structure of the influenza virus N9 neuraminidase-NC41 Fab complex. *J Mol Biol*, **227**, 122–48.

Tumpey, T.M., Garcia-Sastre, A., et al. 2004. Pathogenicity and immunogenicity of influenza viruses with genes from the 1918 pandemic virus. *Proc Natl Acad Sci USA*, **101**, 3166–71.

Turan, K., Mibayashi, M., et al. 2004. Nuclear MxA proteins form a complex with influenza virus NP and inhibit the transcription of the engineered influenza virus genome. *Nucleic Acids Res*, **32**, 643–52.

Ulmanen, I., Broni, B. and Krug, R.M. 1983. Influenza virus temperature-sensitive cap (m7GpppNm)-dependent endonuclease. *J Virol*, **45**, 27–35.

Umetsu, Y., Sugawara, K., et al. 1992. Selection of antigenically distinct variants of influenza C viruses by the host cell. *Virology*, **189**, 740–4.

van Regenmortel, M.H.V. 2000. Virus taxonomy: the classification and nomenclature of viruses. In: *Virus taxonomy*. San Diego: Academic Press, 1167.

Van Voris, L.P. and Newell, P.M. 1992. Antivirals for the chemoprophylaxis and treatment of influenza. *Semin Respir Infect*, **7**, 61–70.

Van Wyke, K.L., Hinshaw, V.S., et al. 1980. Antigenic variation of influenza A virus nucleoprotein detected with monoclonal antibodies. *J Virol*, **35**, 24–30.

Van Wyke, K.L., Bean, W.J. and Webster, R.G. 1981. Monoclonal antibodies to the influenza A virus nucleoprotein affecting RNA transcription. *J Virol*, **39**, 313–17.

Van Wyke, K.L., Yewdell, J.W., et al. 1984. Antigenic characterization of influenza A virus matrix protein with monoclonal antibodies. *J Virol*, **49**, 248–52.

Varghese, J.N., Laver, W.G. and Colman, P.M. 1983. Structure of the influenza virus glycoprotein antigen neuraminidase at 2.9 A resolution. *Nature*, **303**, 35–40.

Varghese, J.N., Webster, R.G., et al. 1988. Structure of an escape mutant of glycoprotein N2 neuraminidase of influenza virus A/Tokyo/3/67 at 3 A. *J Mol Biol*, **200**, 201–3.

Veit, M., Herrler, G., et al. 1990. The hemagglutinating glycoproteins of influenza B and C viruses are acylated with different fatty acids. *Virology*, **177**, 807–11.

Veit, M., Kretzschmar, E., et al. 1991. Site-specific mutagenesis identifies three cysteine residues in the cytoplasmic tail as acylation sites of influenza virus hemagglutinin. *J Virol*, **65**, 2491–500.

Vey, M., Orlich, M., et al. 1992. Hemagglutinin activation of pathogenic avian influenza viruses of serotype H7 requires the protease recognition motif R-X-K/R-R. *Virology*, **188**, 408–13.

Vines, A., Wells, K., et al. 1998. The role of influenza A virus hemagglutinin residues 226 and 228 in receptor specificity and host range restriction. *J Virol*, **72**, 7626–31.

Virelizier, J.L. 1975. Host defenses against influenza virus: the role of anti-hemagglutinin antibody. *J Immunol*, **115**, 434–9.

Virus Taxonomy. 2005. Eighth report of the international committee on taxonomy of viruses. In: Fauquet, C.M., Mayo, M.A., et al. (eds), *Virus taxonomy*. Elsevier/Academic Press, 681–93.

Vlasak, R., Krystal, M., et al. 1987. The influenza C virus glycoprotein (HE) exhibits receptor-binding (hemagglutinin) and receptor-destroying (esterase) activities. *Virology*, **160**, 419–25.

von Itzstein, M., Wu, W.Y., et al. 1993. Rational design of potent sialidase-based inhibitors of influenza virus replication. *Nature*, **363**, 418–23.

Vreede, F.T., Jung, T.E. and Brownlee, G.G. 2004. Model suggesting that replication of influenza virus is regulated by stabilization of replicative intermediates. *J Virol*, **78**, 7568–72.

Wabuke-Bunoti, M.A. and Fan, D.P. 1983. Isolation and characterization of a CNBr cleavage peptide of influenza viral hemagglutinin stimulatory for mouse cytolytic T lymphocytes. *J Immunol*, **130**, 2386–91.

Wabuke-Bunoti, M.A., Taku, A., et al. 1984. Cytolytic T lymphocyte and antibody responses to synthetic peptides of influenza virus hemagglutinin. *J Immunol*, **133**, 2194–201.

Wagner, E., Engelhardt, O.G., et al. 2001. Rescue of recombinant Thogoto virus from cloned cDNA. *J Virol*, **75**, 9282–6.

Wagner, R., Wolff, T., et al. 2000. Interdependence of hemagglutinin glycosylation and neuraminidase as regulators of influenza virus growth: a study by reverse genetics. *J Virol*, **74**, 6316–23.

Wagner, R., Heuer, D., et al. 2002. N-Glycans attached to the stem domain of haemagglutinin efficiently regulate influenza A virus replication. *J Gen Virol*, **83**, 601–9.

Wakefield, L. and Brownlee, G.G. 1989. RNA-binding properties of influenza A virus matrix protein M1. *Nucleic Acids Res*, **17**, 8569–80.

Walker, J.A., Sakaguchi, T., et al. 1992. Location and character of the cellular enzyme that cleaves the hemagglutinin of a virulent avian influenza virus. *Virology*, **190**, 278–87.

Walsh, J.J., Dietlein, L.F., et al. 1961. Bronchotracheal response in human influenza. Type A, Asian strain, as studied by light and electron microscopic examination of bronchoscopic biopsies. *Arch Intern Med*, **108**, 376–88.

Waner, J.L., Todd, S.J., et al. 1991. Comparison of Directigen FLU-A with viral isolation and direct immunofluorescence for the rapid detection and identification of influenza A virus. *J Clin Microbiol*, **29**, 479–82.

Wang, M.L., Skehel, J.J. and Wiley, D.C. 1986. Comparative analyses of the specificities of anti-influenza hemagglutinin antibodies in human sera. *J Virol*, **57**, 124–8.

Wang, P., Palese, P. and O'Neill, R.E. 1997. The NPI-1/NPI-3 (karyopherin alpha) binding site on the influenza a virus nucleoprotein NP is a nonconventional nuclear localization signal. *J Virol*, **71**, 1850–6.

Wang, W. and Krug, R.M. 1998. U6atac snRNA, the highly divergent counterpart of U6 snRNA, is the specific target that mediates inhibition of AT-AC splicing by the influenza virus NS1 protein. *RNA*, **4**, 55–64.

Wang, W., Riedel, K., et al. 1999. RNA binding by the novel helical domain of the influenza virus NS1 protein requires its dimer structure and a small number of specific basic amino acids. *RNA*, **5**, 195–205.

Wang, X., Li, M., et al. 2000. Influenza A virus NS1 protein prevents activation of NF-kappaB and induction of Alpha/Beta interferon. *J Virol*, **74**, 11566–73.

Watabe, S., Xin, K.Q., et al. 2001. Protection against influenza virus challenge by topical application of influenza DNA vaccine. *Vaccine*, **19**, 4434–44.

Watanabe, I., Ross, T.M., et al. 2003. Protection against influenza virus infection by intranasal administration of C3d-fused hemagglutinin. *Vaccine*, **21**, 4532–8.

Watanabe, T., Watanabe, S., et al. 2002. Immunogenicity and protective efficacy of replication-incompetent influenza virus-like particles. *J Virol*, **76**, 767–73.

Webby, R.J., Swenson, S.L., et al. 2000. Evolution of swine H3N2 influenza viruses in the United States. *J Virol*, **74**, 8243–51.

Webby, R.J., Rossow, K., et al. 2004. Multiple lineages of antigenically and genetically diverse influenza A virus co-circulate in the United States swine population. *Virus Res*, **103**, 67–73.

Weber, F., Haller, O. and Kochs, G. 1997. Conserved vRNA end sequences of Thogoto-orthomyxovirus suggest a new panhandle structure. *Arch Virol*, **142**, 1029–33.

Weber, F., Kochs, G., et al. 1998. A classical bipartite nuclear localization signal on Thogoto and influenza A virus nucleoproteins. *Virology*, **250**, 9–18.

Webster, R.G. and Kawaoka, Y. 1994. Influenza – an emerging and re-emerging disease. *Sem Virol*, **5**, 103–11.

Webster, R.G. and Laver, W.G. 1966. Influenza virus subunit vaccines: immunogenicity and lack of toxicity for rabbits of ether- and detergent-disrupted virus. *J Immunol*, **96**, 596–605.

Webster, R.G. and Laver, W.G. 1972. Studies on the origin of pandemic influenza. I. Antigenic analysis of A 2 influenza viruses isolated before and after the appearance of Hong Kong influenza using antisera to the isolated hemagglutinin subunits. *Virology*, **48**, 433–44.

Webster, R.G. and Rott, R. 1987. Influenza virus A pathogenicity: the pivotal role of hemagglutinin. *Cell*, **50**, 665–6.

Webster, R.G., Yakhno, M., et al. 1978. Intestinal influenza: replication and characterization of influenza viruses in ducks. *Virology*, **84**, 268–78.

Webster, R.G., Brown, L.E. and Laver, W.G. 1984. Antigenic and biological characterization of influenza virus neuraminidase (N2) with monoclonal antibodies. *Virology*, **135**, 30–42.

Webster, R.G., Air, G.M., et al. 1987. Antigenic structure and variation in an influenza virus N9 neuraminidase. *J Virol*, **61**, 2910–16.

Webster, R.G., Reay, P.A. and Laver, W.G. 1988. Protection against lethal influenza with neuraminidase. *Virology*, **164**, 230–7.

Webster, R.G., Bean, W.J., et al. 1992. Evolution and ecology of influenza A viruses. *Microbiol Rev*, **56**, 152–79.

Weis, W., Brown, J.H., et al. 1988. Structure of the influenza virus haemagglutinin complexed with its receptor, sialic acid. *Nature*, **333**, 426–31.

Weis, W.I., Cusack, S.C., et al. 1990. The structure of a membrane fusion mutant of the influenza virus haemagglutinin. *EMBO J*, **9**, 17–24.

Whitaker-Dowling, P., Lucas, W. and Youngner, J.S. 1990. Cold-adapted vaccine strains of influenza A virus act as dominant negative mutants

in mixed infections with wild-type influenza A virus. *Virology*, **175**, 358–64.

Whitaker-Dowling, P., Maassab, H.F. and Youngner, J.S. 1991. Dominant-negative mutants as antiviral agents: simultaneous infection with the cold-adapted live-virus vaccine for influenza A protects ferrets from disease produced by wild-type influenza A. *J Infect Dis*, **164**, 1200–2.

White, J., Kielian, M. and Helenius, A. 1983. Membrane fusion proteins of enveloped animal viruses. *Q Rev Biophys*, **16**, 151–95.

White, J.M. 1992. Membrane fusion. *Science*, **258**, 917–24.

White, J.M. 1994. Fusion of influenza virus in endosomes: role of the hemagglutinin. In: Wimmer, E. (ed.), *Cellular receptors for animal viruses*. Cold Spring Harbor NY: Cold Spring Harbor Laboratory Press, 281–301.

White, J.M. and Wilson, I.A. 1987. Anti-peptide antibodies detect steps in a protein conformational change: low-pH activation of the influenza virus hemagglutinin. *J Cell Biol*, **105**, 2887–96.

Whittaker, G., Kemler, I. and Helenius, A. 1995. Hyperphosphorylation of mutant influenza virus matrix protein, M1, causes its retention in the nucleus. *J Virol*, **69**, 439–45.

W.H.O. 1980. A revision of the system of nomenclature for influenza viruses: a WHO memorandum. *Bull World Health Organ*, **58**, 585–91.

Wiley, D.C. and Skehel, J.J. 1987. The structure and function of the hemagglutinin membrane glycoprotein of influenza virus. *Annu. Rev Biochem*, **56**, 365–94.

Wiley, D.C., Skehel, J.J. and Waterfield, M. 1977. Evidence from studies with a cross-linking reagent that the haemagglutinin of influenza virus is a trimer. *Virology*, **79**, 446–8.

Wiley, D.C., Wilson, I.A. and Skehel, J.J. 1981. Structural identification of the antibody-binding sites of Hong Kong influenza haemagglutinin and their involvement in antigenic variation. *Nature*, **289**, 373–8.

Williams, M.A. and Lamb, R.A. 1986. Determination of the orientation of an integral membrane protein and sites of glycosylation by oligonucleotide-directed mutagenesis: influenza B virus NB glycoprotein lacks a cleavable signal sequence and has an extracellular NH2-terminal region. *Mol Cell Biol*, **6**, 4317–28.

Williams, M.A. and Lamb, R.A. 1988. Polylactosaminoglycan modification of a small integral membrane glycoprotein, influenza B virus NB. *Mol Cell Biol*, **8**, 1186–96.

Williams, M.A. and Lamb, R.A. 1989. Effect of mutations and deletions in a bicistronic mRNA on the synthesis of influenza B virus NB and NA glycoproteins. *J Virol*, **63**, 28–35.

Wilson, I.A. and Cox, N.J. 1990. Structural basis of immune recognition of influenza virus hemagglutinin. *Annu Rev Immunol*, **8**, 737–71.

Wilson, I.A., Skehel, J.J. and Wiley, D.C. 1981. Structure of the haemagglutinin membrane glycoprotein of influenza virus at 3 Å resolution. *Nature*, **289**, 366–73.

Wood, J.M., Seagroatt, V., et al. 1981. International collaborative study of single-radial-diffusion and immunoelectrophoresis techniques for the assay of haemagglutinin antigen of influenza virus. *J Biol Stand*, **9**, 317–30.

Wood, J.M., Oxford, J.S., et al. 1989. Influenza A (H1N1) vaccine efficacy in animal models is influenced by two amino acid substitutions in the hemagglutinin molecule. *Virology*, **171**, 214–21.

Woolston, W.J. and Conley, D.O. 1918. Epidemic pneumonia (Spanish influenza) in pregnancy. *JAMA*, **71**, 1898.

World Health Organization, 1996. Influenza in the world. *Weekly Epidemiol Rec*, **71**, 1–7.

Wright, K.E., Wilson, G.A., et al. 1995. Typing and subtyping of influenza viruses in clinical samples by PCR. *J Clin Microbiol*, **33**, 1180–4.

Wright, P.F., Murphy, B.R., et al. 1983. Secretory immunological response after intranasal inactivated influenza A virus vaccinations: evidence for immunoglobulin A memory. *Infect Immun*, **40**, 1092–5.

Wurzer, W.J., Planz, O., et al. 2003. Caspase 3 activation is essential for efficient influenza virus propagation. *Embo J*, **22**, 2717–28.

Wysocka, M. and Hackett, C.J. 1990. Class I H-2d-restricted cytotoxic T lymphocytes recognize the neuraminidase glycoprotein of influenza virus subtype N1. *J Virol*, **64**, 1028–32.

Xu, G., Suzuki, T., et al. 1994. Specificity of sialyl-sugar chain mediated recognition by the hemagglutinin of human influenza B virus isolates. *J Biochem (Tokyo)*, **115**, 202–7.

Yamanaka, K., Ishihama, A. and Nagata, K. 1988. Translational regulation of influenza virus mRNAs. *Virus Genes*, **2**, 19–30.

Yamanaka, K., Nagata, K. and Ishihama, A. 1991a. Temporal control for translation of influenza virus mRNAs. *Arch Virol*, **120**, 33–42.

Yamanaka, K., Ogasawara, N., et al. 1991b. In vivo analysis of the promoter structure of the influenza virus RNA genome using a transfection system with an engineered RNA. *Proc Natl Acad Sci USA*, **88**, 5369–73.

Yamashita, M., Krystal, M. and Palese, P. 1988. Evidence that the matrix protein of influenza C virus is coded for by a spliced mRNA. *J Virol*, **62**, 3348–55.

Yao, Y., Mingay, L.J., et al. 2001. Sequences in influenza A virus PB2 protein that determine productive infection for an avian influenza virus in mouse and human cell lines. *J Virol*, **75**, 5410–15.

Yasuda, J., Nakada, S., et al. 1993. Molecular assembly of influenza virus: association of the NS2 protein with virion matrix. *Virology*, **196**, 249–55.

Yasuda, J., Bucher, D.J. and Ishihama, A. 1994. Growth control of influenza A virus by M1 protein: analysis of transfectant viruses carrying the chimeric M gene. *J Virol*, **68**, 8141–6.

Ye, Z., Robinson, D. and Wagner, R.R. 1995. Nucleus-targeting domain of the matrix protein (M1) of influenza virus. *J Virol*, **69**, 1964–70.

Ye, Z., Liu, T., et al. 1999. Association of influenza virus matrix protein with ribonucleoproteins. *J Virol*, **73**, 7467–73.

Ye, Z.P., Baylor, N.W. and Wagner, R.R. 1989. Transcription-inhibition and RNA-binding domains of influenza A virus matrix protein mapped with anti-idiotypic antibodies and synthetic peptides. *J Virol*, **63**, 3586–94.

Yewdell, J.W. and Bennink, J.R. 1999. Immunodominance in major histocompatibility complex class I-restricted T lymphocyte responses. *Annu Rev Immunol*, **17**, 51–88.

Yewdell, J.W. and Hackett, C. 1989. Specificity and function of T lymphocytes induced by influenza viruses. In: Krug, R. (ed.), *The influenza viruses*. New York: Plenum Press, 361–429.

Yoneyama, M., Kikuchi, M., et al. 2004. The RNA helicase RIG-I has an essential function in double-stranded RNA-induced innate antiviral responses. *Nat Immunol*, **5**, 730–7.

Youngner, J.S., Treanor, J.J., et al. 1994. Effect of simultaneous administration of cold-adapted and wild-type influenza A viruses on experimental wild-type influenza infection in humans. *J Clin Microbiol*, **32**, 750–4.

Zambon, M. and Hayden, F.G. 2001. Position statement: global neuraminidase inhibitor susceptibility network. *Antiviral Res*, **49**, 147–56.

Zambon, M., Hays, J., et al. 2001. Diagnosis of influenza in the community: relationship of clinical diagnosis to confirmed virological, serologic, or molecular detection of influenza. *Arch Intern Med*, **161**, 2116–22.

Zebedee, S.L. and Lamb, R.A. 1988. Influenza A virus M2 protein: monoclonal antibody restriction of virus growth and detection of M2 in virions. *J Virol*, **62**, 2762–72.

Zhang, J., Pekosz, A. and Lamb, R.A. 2000. Influenza virus assembly and lipid raft microdomains: a role for the cytoplasmic tails of the spike glycoproteins. *J Virol*, **74**, 4634–44.

Zhang, W.D. and Evans, D.H. 1991. Detection and identification of human influenza viruses by the polymerase chain reaction. *J Virol Methods*, **33**, 165–89.

Zhang, X., Rosenthal, P.B., et al. 1999. X-ray crystallographic determination of the structure of the influenza C virus haemagglutinin-esterase-fusion glycoprotein. *Acta Crystallogr D Biol Crystallogr.*, **55**, 945–61.

Zhao, H., Ekstrom, M. and Garoff, H. 1998. The M1 and NP proteins of influenza A virus form homo- but not heterooligomeric complexes when coexpressed in BHK-21 cells. *J Gen Virol*, **79**, 2435–46.

Zheng, H., Lee, H.A., et al. 1999. Influenza A virus RNA polymerase has the ability to stutter at the polyadenylation site of a viral RNA template during RNA replication. *J Virol*, **73**, 5240–3.

Zhirnov, O.P. 1990. Solubilization of matrix protein M1/M from virions occurs at different pH for orthomyxo- and paramyxoviruses. *Virology*, **176**, 274–9.

Zhirnov, O.P. and Grigoriev, V.B. 1994. Disassembly of influenza C viruses, distinct from that of influenza A and B viruses requires neutral-alkaline pH. *Virology*, **200**, 284–91.

Zhong, Q., Newns, D.M., et al. 2000. Two possible conducting states of the influenza A virus M2 ion channel. *FEBS Lett*, **473**, 195–8.

Zhou, N.N., Senne, D.A., et al. 1999. Genetic reassortment of avian, swine, and human influenza A viruses in American pigs. *J Virol*, **73**, 8851–6.

Ziegler, T., Hall, H., et al. 1995. Type- and subtype-specific detection of influenza viruses in clinical specimens by rapid culture assay. *J Clin Microbiol*, **33**, 318–21.

Zitzow, L.A., Rowe, T., et al. 2002. Pathogenesis of avian influenza A (H5N1) viruses in ferrets. *J Virol*, **76**, 4420–9.

Zou, S. 1997. A practical approach to genetic screening for influenza virus variants. *J Clin Microbiol*, **35**, 2623–7.

Zurcher, T., Luo, G. and Palese, P. 1994. Mutations at palmitylation sites of the influenza virus hemagglutinin affect virus formation. *J Virol*, **68**, 5748–54.

Zvonarjev, A.Y. and Ghendon, Y.Z. 1980. Influence of membrane (M) protein on influenza A virus virion transcriptase activity in vitro and its susceptibility to rimantadine. *J Virol*, **33**, 583–6.

33

General properties of the paramyxoviruses

PAUL A. ROTA, BETTINA BANKAMP, AND WILLIAM J. BELLINI

This chapter provides a general overview of the structure and replication of viruses in the family *Paramyxoviridae*. Subsequent chapters describe each group of viruses in greater detail including the diseases associated with these viruses.

CLASSIFICATION

The family *Paramyxoviridae* includes several important human pathogens, as well as viruses affecting various species of mammals, birds, and reptiles. Together with the families *Rhabdoviridae* and *Filoviridae* they form the order *Mononegavirales*. Members of this order have a nonsegmented, single-stranded, negative-sense RNA genome, a conserved gene order, and similar replication strategy. Paramxyoviruses are pleomorphic, enveloped viruses that contain helical nucleocapsids and replicate in the cytoplasm of infected cells. The family is divided into two subfamilies, *Paramyxovirinae* and *Pneumovirinae*, which are distinguished by the diameter and pitch of their nucleocapsids, the number of genes and the presence or absence of a modified transcript of their phosphoprotein (*P*) genes. Several new genera have been added to the family over the past few years. At present, the subfamily *Paramyxovirinae* contains five genera, while the *Pneumovirinae* contains two (Mayo 2002). Viruses representing each of the subfamilies and genera are listed in Table 33.1. Members of the same genus share antigenic cross-reactivity and a higher degree of nucleotide sequence similarity. Distinguishing features of the genera in the subfamily *Paramyxovirinae* include the presence or absence of hemagglutination and neuraminidase activity, the length and conservation of intergenic regions, and the organization and coding capacity of the *P* gene. The two genera of the subfamily *Pneumovirinae* are characterized by the presence or absence of the *NS1* and *NS2* genes and their gene order (Table 33.2, Figure 33.1).

A number of new paramyxoviruses have been isolated recently, but have not yet been assigned to a genus. Sixteen paramyxovirus isolates from reptilian species (Ahne et al. 1999) have been described; the archetype is fer-de-lance virus (Kurath et al. 2004), which has been completely sequenced. This virus has a novel gene located between the *N* and *P* gene, which has no counterpart in any of the other viruses of the family. A number of paramyxoviruses has been isolated from rodents, including Nariva virus and Mossman virus (Roos and Wollman 1979; Miller et al. 2003). Tupaia virus was discovered in a cell line derived from tree shrews (Tidona et al. 1999) and Salem virus was isolated from horses (Renshaw et al. 2000). The natural distribution and pathogenic potential of these viruses are mostly unknown.

MORPHOLOGY AND GENERAL PROPERTIES

Paramyxoviridae are pleomorphic viruses with lipid envelopes derived from the plasma membrane of the

Table 33.1 *Genera and representative species of the family* Paramyxoviridae

Genera and representative species
Subfamily *Paramyxovirinae*
Genus *Respirovirus*
Sendai virus[a]
Human parainfluenza viruses, types 1 and 3
Bovine parainfluenza virus type 3
Genus *Rubulavirus*
Mumps virus[a]
Human parainfluenza viruses, types 2, 4a, and 4b
Simian virus 5
Genus *Morbillivirus*
Measles virus[a]
Canine distemper virus
Rinderpest virus
Genus *Henipavirus*
Hendra virus[a]
Nipah virus
Genus *Avulavirus*
Newcastle disease virus[a]
Avian paramyxoviruses 1–9
Subfamily *Pneumovirinae*
Genus *Pneumovirus*
Human respiratory syncytial virus[a]
Bovine respiratory syncytial virus
Genus *Metapneumovirus*
Turkey rhinotracheitis virus[a]
Human metapneumovirus

a) Type species

infected cell (Klenk and Choppin 1969, 1970). Virus particles range from 150 to 400 nm in diameter and are generally spherical, but can also be filamentous. The virions contain two viral transmembrane glycoproteins that appear as spikes of varying length on electron micrographs. The envelope surrounds the nucleocapsid, which consists of the RNA genome encapsidated by the viral nucleoprotein. Nucleocapsids of *Paramyxovirinae* measure 18 nm in diameter, with a pitch of about 5.0 nm. The nucleocapsids of the *Pneumovirinae* are more slender, with a diameter of 13–14 nm and a pitch of 6.5–7.0 nm (Compans and Choppin 1967a,b; Finch and Gibbs 1970).

Paramyxoviruses are transmitted via close contact or the airborne (droplet or aerosol) route. The two transmembrane glycoproteins serve as attachment and fusion proteins. After attachment to a receptor on the surface of the host cell, fusion of the virion envelope and the host-cell membrane takes place at neutral pH. Fusion can also occur between infected and neighboring uninfected cells, resulting in the characteristic cytopathic effect of syncytium formation in cell culture or the appearance of multinucleated giant cells in host tissues. Cell lysis is another common outcome of infection with paramyxoviruses. In addition to the receptor-binding function, the attachment proteins of the genera *Morbillivirus*, *Respirovirus*, *Rubulavirus*, and *Avulavirus* also agglutinate red blood cells, and the attachment proteins of the latter three possess neuraminidase activities (Lamb and Kolakofsky 2001).

The density of the virus particles is 1.18–1.20 g/cm^3. Protein comprises most of the virion composition by weight (69–74 percent), lipid makes up 20–25 percent, and carbohydrate comprises 5–6 percent of the virion weight. The genomes of all paramyxoviruses are composed of single-stranded RNA with a density of approximately 1.3 g/cm^3. Reagents that disrupt lipids, such as organic solvents and detergents, as well as formaldehyde and oxidizing agents, destroy the infectious nature of the viruses. The viruses are also inactivated by ultraviolet light, heating, and drying.

GENOME STRUCTURE AND ORGANIZATION

The complete genomic sequences of representative viruses from every genus of the family are available on Genbank. Genomes of the *Paramyxoviridae* range from 15 000 to more than 18 000 nucleotides in length. Within the subfamily *Paramyxovirinae*, the gene order of *N–P–M–F–H/HN/G–L* is conserved; however, two members of the genus *Rubulavirus* and at least one member of the genus *Avulavirus* possess a gene encoding a small, hydrophobic protein (*SH*) that is located between the *F* and *HN* genes (Figure 33.1).

All members of the subfamily *Pneumoviridae* contain an *SH* and *M2* gene. The positions of the *SH*, *F*, *G*, and *M2* genes differ between the pneumoviruses and the metapneumoviruses (Figure 33.1). Furthermore, the 'normal' gene order of *F* followed by *G* is reversed in the pneumoviruses. The pneumoviruses are also unusual in that they have two additional genes, *NS1* and *NS2*, preceding the *N* gene.

The total length of the genomes (in nucleotides) of all members of the subfamily *Paramyxovirinae* is evenly divisible by six. This 'rule-of-six' proposes that one nucleocapsid protein binds to six nucleotides, and that the position of the nucleotides of certain regulatory elements within a group of six has consequences for their function (Calain and Roux 1993). The rule of six does not appear to apply to the *Pneumovirinae* (Samal and Collins 1996).

The promoters for both transcription and replication lie in the noncoding regions at the genomic termini. The leader sequence at the 3′ terminus of the genome is approximately 50 nucleotides in length for all *Paramyxoviridae* and contains promoter signals for both transcription and replication. The length of the trailer at the 5′ terminus varies between 20 and 114 nucleotides and only contains the complement of a promoter for replication. The terminal 12–13 nucleotides are very well

Table 33.2 *General properties of the genera of the subfamily* Pneumovirinae

Characteristic	Genus	
	Pneumovirus	**Metapneumovirus**
Genome size	15 kb	13 kb
Virion characteristics:		
Hemagglutination	–	–
Neuraminidase	–	–
Spike length	10–12 nm	13–14 nm
Structural proteins (sizes in kDa)[a]:		
Polymerase protein	200	200
Attachment protein	84–90	83
Fusion protein:		
(F0)	68–70	68
(F1)	47	53
(F2)	20	15
Nucleocapsid protein	42	43
Phosphoprotein	34	40
Matrix protein	26	35
Small hydrophobic protein	8–30	19[b]
Nonstructural proteins	NS1, NS2, M2-1, M2-2	M2-1, M2-2

a) Sizes for type species of each genus.
b) Calculated molecular mass.

conserved within a genus and have a high degree of complementarity with each other.

Each gene contains *cis*-acting, noncoding regions preceding and following the open reading frame (ORF). These regions contain conserved transcriptional start and stop signals. The mRNA stop signal includes several U residues, which serve as templates for polyadenylation of the mRNAs. Within most of the genera, the intergenic regions are conserved trinucleotides. However, the rubulaviruses and the viruses in the subfamily *Pneumoviridae* have intergenic regions with lengths varying from one to 90 nucleotides, with no conservation of sequence (Hardy et al. 1999). Finally, in the morbilliviruses, there is a long untranslated region of approximately 1 000 nucleotides between the M ORF and the F ORF. A similar phenomenon is observed in the henipaviruses, where the 5′ and 3′ untranslated regions for most of the genes are longer than in those of the other paramyxoviruses, especially in the *P* gene (Harcourt et al. 2000). The functional significance of these long, noncoding regions is unknown.

REPLICATION

Attachment and penetration

Attachment of virus particles to the host-cell membranes occurs through the viral glycoprotein, which is variably called G, H, or HN, depending on the presence or absence of hemagglutination (H) or neuraminidase activity (N) (Table 33.2; Table 33.3). Respiroviruses and rubulaviruses bind to sialic acid-containing proteins or lipids, while pneumoviruses attach to glycosaminoglycans containing heparin sulfate and chondroitin sulfate (Feldman et al. 1999). In contrast, morbilliviruses bind specific receptor proteins on the cell surface. For measles virus, two receptors have been identified, CD46, a protein involved in the regulation of complement activation (Dorig et al. 1993; Naniche et al. 1993), and signaling lymphocyte activation molecule (SLAM) (Tatsuo et al. 2000). Canine distemper virus

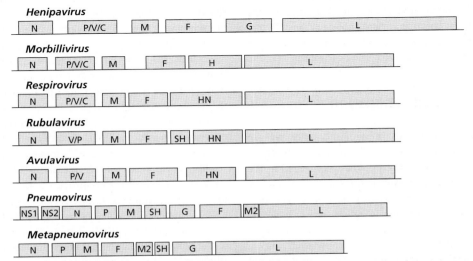

Figure 33.1 *Schematic representations of the genomes of viruses in the family* Paramyxoviridae. *Figure shows representative genome from each genus. Shaded boxes represent individual genes. Thin lines represent noncoding and intergenic regions. C, C protein; F, fusion protein; G, glycoprotein; H, hemagglutinin protein; HN, hemagglutinin-neuraminidase; L, polymerase protein; M, matrix protein; N, nucleoprotein; NS, non-structural protein; P, phosphoprotein; SH, small hydrophobic protein; V, V protein.*

Table 33.3 *General properties of the genera of the subfamily* Paramyxovirinae

Characteristic	Genus				
	Respirovirus	*Rubulavirus*	*Morbillivirus*	*Henipavirus*	*Avulavirus*
Genome size	15–16 kb	15–16 kb	15–16 kb	18–19 kb	15–16 kb
Virion characteristics:					
Hemagglutination	+	+	+	−	+
Neuraminidase	+	+	−	−	+
Spike length	8 nm	8 nm	8 nm	8–17 nm	8–12 nm
Structural proteins (sizes in kDa)[a]:					
Polymerase protein	230	200	200	200	220
Attachment protein	71	79	78	74	74
Fusion protein:					
(F0)	65	74	60	61	66
(F1)	51	61	41	49	53
(F2)	13	16	20	19	10
Nucleocapsid protein	58	72	60	58	56
Phosphoprotein	79	45	72	98	53–56
Matrix protein	38	40	38	42	41
Small hydrophobic protein		6[b]			16[b,c]
V protein		25			
Nonstructural proteins	C, C', Y1, Y2, V, W, X[b]	V, W, I[b]	C, V	C, V, SB[b], W	V, W

a) Sizes for type species of each genus.
b) Some members of the genus only.
c) Calculated molecular mass.

and rinderpest virus bind the canine and bovine homologues of SLAM (Tatsuo et al. 2001). Specific receptors have not yet been identified for other members of the family.

Following attachment, the fusion (F) glycoprotein mediates fusion of the viral envelope with the plasma membrane of the host cell. Fusion occurs at neutral pH and requires the co-operation of the F and G/H/HN proteins. It is postulated that engagement of the receptor triggers conformational changes in F that initiate fusion. As a result of the fusion process, the nucleocapsid is released into the cytoplasm (Lamb 1993).

Transcription and replication

Primary transcription begins immediately after release of the nucleocapsid into the cytoplasm. The viral RNA-dependent RNA polymerase complex is contained in the virion. The nucleocapsid serves as the template for RNA synthesis and does not appear to disassemble. The polymerase complex enters the negative sense genomic template at the promoter region in the 3′ leader to initiate transcription. Each gene is transcribed into a monocistronic mRNA, regulated by the transcriptional start and stop sites at the beginning and end of the gene. The transcripts are capped and methylated at the 5′ terminus and polyadenylated at the 3′ terminus by the

viral polymerase complex. The template for the poly(A) tail is the short poly(U) sequence that is part of the transcription stop signal following each gene. It has been suggested that the polymerase stutters at the stop signals to synthesize poly(A) tails of the mRNAs. While in transcription mode, the polymerase pauses at the gene stop signal, traverses the intergenic region, and reinitiates transcription at the next gene start signal. During this process, some polymerase molecules disengage from the template. Since there is only a single promoter at the 3′ terminus of the genome, the disengaged polymerase molecules can reinitiate transcription only at the 3′ terminus. This process leads to a gradient of transcription, in which the genes located near the 3′ terminus of the genome are more frequently transcribed than the genes at the 5′ terminus. Thus, regulation of viral gene expression is achieved by the establishment of a message gradient (Cattaneo et al. 1987; Homann et al. 1990).

The polymerases of all members of the subfamily *Paramyxovirinae* utilize a process termed RNA editing to insert nontemplated G nucleotides at a specific site to modify some of the mRNAs transcribed from the *P* gene (Thomas et al. 1988). This process results in a shift of the reading frame, beginning at the editing site, in the edited transcripts. The resulting proteins share the same amino terminal sequences as the proteins translated from the unedited transcripts, but have unique carboxyl termini. The protein translated from the unedited transcript is the phosphoprotein (P), while the V protein is encoded by the edited transcript. The exception is found in the rubulaviruses where the unedited transcript codes for the V protein, and the P protein ORF is only accessible through editing. The editing site is highly conserved among the *Paramyxovirinae*. By contrast, all members of the subfamily *Pneumovirinae* produce only the P protein from the *P* gene. An interesting characteristic of the human and bovine respiratory syncytial viruses is that the transcriptional start site for the *L* gene lies within the *M2* gene (Collins et al. 1987).

The translation of primary transcripts leads to the accumulation of viral proteins, and a switch from transcription to replication. In replication mode, the polymerase complex enters the same (or an overlapping) promoter in the 3′ leader sequence, but ignores all transcriptional regulatory signals to transcribe a full-length, positive-sense antigenome. This requires concomitant encapsidation of the nascent strand. It is assumed that the nascent 5′ termini contain specific nucleation sites for encapsidation, although nonspecific encapsidation of nonviral RNA has been reported for several paramyxoviruses. A promoter in the 3′ untranslated region of the new antigenome (the complement to the trailer sequence) serves as a starting point for the synthesis of new, negative-sense genomes. The production of antigenomes and genomes depends on the continuous availability of nucleoprotein. It has long been assumed that the availability of nucleoprotein regulates the switch from transcription to replication; however, there is some evidence that this is not the case (Fearns et al. 1997). New genomes can serve as templates for secondary transcription.

Virus assembly

The assembly of virus particles requires cessation of genome replication, preparation of completed nucleocapsids for packaging, and preparation of regions of the plasma membrane to accept nucleocapsids for budding. The matrix (M) proteins of Sendai virus and measles virus have been shown to inhibit viral transcription in vitro, this function may be involved in the cessation of replication (Suryanarayana et al. 1994; Ogino et al. 2003). Polymerase complexes remain associated with the packaged nucleocapsid and serve to initiate the next cycle of infection. While the nucleocapsid is assembled in the cytoplasm, the glycoproteins are synthesized in the endoplasmic reticulum and undergo maturation during their transport through the Golgi network to the cell membrane. The M protein clearly plays a role in the interaction between the nucleocapsid and the membrane, but it does not appear to be the driving force behind vesicle formation (Schmitt et al. 2002). Budding of virus particles occurs at specialized membrane locations called lipid rafts, which are characterized by a high content of cholesterol and sphingolipids. While viral glycoproteins are concentrated in lipid rafts (Manie et al. 2000), host proteins are excluded from the viral membrane. The cytoplasmic tails of the F and G/H/HN proteins play a role in interaction with the M protein (Ali and Nayak 2000), transport to cell surfaces (Parks and Lamb 1990), and association with rafts (Dolganiuc et al. 2003). The orientation of particle release from the apical membrane may depend on the interaction of M and the cytoplasmic tails of the glycoproteins (Naim et al. 2000). In Sendai virus, interaction of the M protein with the microtubule network is required for apical release of the virus (Tashiro et al. 1993, 1996).

POLYPEPTIDES

Nucleoprotein

As a result of the location of the N gene at or near the 3′ terminus of the genome, the nucleoprotein (N) is the most abundant structural protein in infected cells and virions. N proteins vary in size from 391 to 553 amino acids and play a pivotal role in virus replication. Both genomic and antigenomic RNA must be encapsidated by N to serve as template for transcription or replication. The nucleocapsid binds the polymerase complex, through interaction with the P subunit of that complex. N–N binding sites and separate sites for the interaction of soluble and assembled N with P have been mapped for several members of the family. Structurally, N proteins can be divided into a core, consisting of the amino terminal 80 percent of the protein, and a carboxyl terminal tail. While the core is relatively well conserved among members of a genus, the tail is highly variable, negatively charged and phosphorylated (Hsu and Kingsbury 1982; Curran et al. 1993; Ryan et al. 1993). Presumably the assembled N protein also interacts with the M protein during virion assembly (Coronel et al. 2001). Despite the close association of N with RNA, classic RNA-binding motifs are absent from the predicted amino acid sequences examined (Dreyfuss et al. 1993).

Phosphoprotein

Members of the subfamily *Paramyxovirinae* have evolved unique mechanisms to maximize the available coding capacity of their genes without expanding their overall genome size. These mechanisms include leaky ribosomal scanning, internal ribosomal initiation, and use of non-AUG start codons (Curran and Kolakofsky 1988). Secondly, transcriptional diversity is generated by RNA editing. In contrast, members of the subfamily *Pneumovirinae* encode only a P protein from the cognate gene, thus defining a major difference between the subfamilies.

All *Paramyxovirinae* express a P protein, although the strategy for expression varies among the genera. All genera except for the rubulaviruses express the P from unedited mRNA, while insertion of a single G residue provides access to the V ORF. In rubulaviruses, the unedited transcript codes for the V protein, and the P protein is expressed from an edited message containing an insertion of two G residues. The P proteins are the most variable of the paramyxovirus structural proteins with only 22–40 percent amino acid homology being observed between each genus. The P proteins vary in size from 241 to 709 amino acids and are essential components of the viral polymerase complex.

P proteins are believed to serve as scaffolding proteins by binding both the nucleocapsid and the polymerase (L) proteins. In addition, P proteins act as chaperones for the N protein during nucleocapsid assembly. The active form of P is a tetramer and binding sites for P–P, P–L, P–N, and P–nucleocapsid interactions have been mapped for members of the respiroviruses and morbilliviruses. With the exception of the P–N-binding site, all are located in the unique carboxyl terminal domain. None of the proteins translated from edited mRNAs or alternative reading frames possess these sites. However, the binding site for the soluble N lies within the amino terminus of P and is shared with the V and W proteins (Curran et al. 1995). While information about the P proteins of the *Pneumovirinae* is not as detailed, the available data indicate that the functional domains are similar to those of the *Paramyxovirinae* (Hengst and Kiefer 2000).

The amino terminal domain of the P proteins (and the V proteins) of respiroviruses, morbilliviruses, and henipaviruses is 231–403 amino acids in length, acidic in nature and contains most of the serine and threonine phosphorylation sites. The amino terminal domain of the P proteins of the rubulaviruses and avulaviruses are smaller (134–164 amino acids) and basic in nature. Based on some limited sequence similarity, it has been speculated that the amino terminus of the P and V proteins of rubulaviruses share characteristics with the C proteins found in the other genera of the subfamily *Paramyxovirinae*. In this context, it is interesting that the rubulaviruses are the only genus in the subfamily that does not express a C protein.

V protein and other editing products

Most members of the subfamily *Paramxyovirinae* edit their *P* gene mRNA cotranscriptionally to access additional reading frames. The only exception is human parainfluenzavirus type 1, which has nine stop codons in the V reading frame (Rochat et al. 1992). V proteins are fusion proteins containing the terminal domain of P and a relatively short, conserved cysteine-rich C terminus. As for the P proteins, the amino terminus of the V protein of the rubulaviruses is basic, while the other genera express V proteins with acidic amino termini. The V proteins of the rubulaviruses also differ from those of the other genera by their localization in the nucleus of infected cells, the presence of RNA-binding domains, and the incorporation into virions (Thomas et al. 1988; Takeuchi et al. 1990). V proteins of the other genera are nonstructural proteins and localized in the cytoplasm of infected cells. The seven conserved cysteines in the unique carboxyl terminus of V proteins form zinc-binding domains.

The V proteins of rubulaviruses and morbilliviruses have been shown to interfere with the innate immune system by inhibiting interferon signaling (He et al. 2002; Rodriguez et al. 2002; Palosaari et al. 2003). The inhibition involves sequestering and/or degrading either STAT1 or STAT2 (Parisien et al. 2001). V proteins have been shown to bind a host-cell protein, damage-specific DNA-binding protein (DDB1) (Lin et al. 1998). V proteins inhibit genome replication in a dose-dependent fashion (Curran et al. 1991). Recombinant viruses defective in V expression have been generated for several species, demonstrating that V is dispensable for replication in cell culture. However, all of these viruses are attenuated in animal models, indicating that V proteins are virulence factors, probably due to their role as interferon antagonists (Kato et al. 1997; Schneider et al. 1997; Durbin et al. 1999).

The editing process is not limited to the addition of one G (or two in the rubulaviruses). The number of inserted Gs and relative abundance of edited transcripts vary between viruses. In several viruses, additional proteins have been detected, although their functions have not been determined. The insertion of two nucleotides opens the third reading frame in all genera, except rubulaviruses. These proteins include the W protein of Sendai virus and the D proteins of human parainfluenzavirus 3 and bovine parainfluenzavirus 3. In the rubulaviruses, addition of two Gs accesses the P ORF, but addition of one G leads to the production of the I protein.

C proteins

An overlapping ORF that encodes one or more short (156–215 amino acids), basic proteins can be found near the 5' end of the P mRNA of the respiroviruses, morbilliviruses, and henipaviruses. The respiroviruses express up to four carboxyl coterminal proteins from different start sites in this ORF (C', C, Y1, and Y2) (Curran and Kolakofsky 1989), while the other two genera express only a single C protein. Since the entire ORF is located upstream of the editing site, the C proteins are expressed from both edited and unedited transcripts of the *P* gene. Translation of some of the C related proteins of the respiroviruses start at non-AUG codons (Curran and Kolakofsky 1989). Most of these proteins are nonstructural, although small amounts of the C protein of Sendai virus are found in virions (Yamada et al. 1990).

Several C proteins have been shown to interfere with the interferon response in a manner very similar to that described for V proteins (Gotoh et al. 1999; Shaffer et al. 2003). This function appears to be redundant in at least some viruses that express both C and V proteins. The C proteins of Sendai virus and measles virus have been shown to inhibit replication and transcription (Reutter et al. 2001; Curran et al. 1992), and the C of Sendai may have an additional role in virus assembly (Hasan et al. 2000). Recombinant viruses defective in C expression have been generated for several species, demonstrating that C is dispensable in cell culture (Baron and Barrett 2000; Radecke and Billeter 1996). However, many of these C minus viruses demonstrated altered growth characteristics and attenuation in vitro, and all of them were attenuated in animal models, indicating that C proteins are virulence factors (Valsamakis et al. 1998).

Matrix protein

As noted earlier, the matrix (M) proteins are the most likely candidates for interaction with lipids, the cytoplasmic tails of the glycoproteins (Sanderson et al. 1993) and the newly formed nucleocapsids (Stricker et al. 1994; Yoshida et al. 1986) in preparation for budding (Peeples 1991). The M proteins vary between 245 and 375 amino acid residues in length and are nonglycosylated proteins of an amphipathic nature. They contain both hydrophobic amino acids and basic amino acids. The latter lead to a net positive charge of +14 to +17 at neutral pH (Bellini et al. 1986; Sheshberadaran and Lamb 1990). However, despite the hydrophobic amino acids, M proteins do not contain transmembrane domains. Thus, it is believed that these proteins interact with the inner surfaces of the virion lipid envelope and plasma membrane. The M protein may be involved in the cessation of replication, orientation of particle release from the apical membrane, and interaction with the microtubule network (Tashiro et al. 1993, 1996).

Fusion protein

The F protein promotes fusion between the viral envelope and the plasma membrane of the host cell, as well as fusion between an infected cell and surrounding uninfected cells. These fusion events take place at neutral pH. F proteins are more highly conserved than the attachment proteins and form homotrimers. They are type I integral membrane glycoproteins, which have carboxyl termini extensions into the cytoplasm, while the amino terminus extends into the extracellular milieu. In all paramyxoviruses, F is synthesized as an inactive precursor, F_0. This precursor is proteolytically cleaved into two fragments, F_1 and F_2, which are linked by disulfide bonds and constitute the active form of the molecule. They contain a signal sequence at the amino terminus that is cleaved when the molecule is delivered to the endoplasmic reticular membrane for completion of synthesis. F proteins further contain a hydrophobic domain (known as a stop transfer signal) at the C terminus of F_1 that anchors the protein in the membrane. A short cytoplasmic tail of between 20 and 40 amino acid residues in length extends into the cytoplasm (Figure 33.2). Although regions of extensive amino acid homology are not obvious among the genera, there is similarity in the number and location of cysteine residues suggesting similar folded structures (Morrison and Portner 1991).

Cleavage of F_0 by intracellular or secreted host endoproteases creates two disulfide-linked subunits, F_1 and F_2. The efficiency of cleavage affects the host range and tissue tropism of the virus, such that greater cleavage efficiency is generally associated with disseminated infections and increased virulence, especially in Newcastle disease virus (de Leeuw et al. 2003). The F protein cleavage sites contain either a single or multiple basic amino acids. Viruses that contain a multibasic sequence are cleaved in the trans-Golgi network by a protease with the sequence specificity of R–X–K/R–R. An endoprotease, furin, has been identified as one protease having such properties (Barr 1991; Hosaka et al. 1991; Ortmann et al. 1994). Cleavage sites containing a single basic residue are cleaved by proteases expressed at the cell surface. Several candidate proteases have been identified (Gotoh et al. 1992). The cleavage site of the henipaviruses is unique in having the only F_1 protein that begins with a leucine instead of a phenylalanine (Wang et al. 2001). Most members of the genus *Pneumovirus* have two cleavage sites, both of which are required for activation (van den Hoogen 2004).

The larger subunit, F_1, contains a hydrophobic fusion peptide at its amino terminus (Figure 33.2). The fusion peptide, which is highly conserved among the *Paramyxovirinae*, mediates the fusion of the two membranes. There is less conservation in the fusion peptide within the members of the subfamily *Pneumovirinae*, and very little conservation exists between the fusion peptides of members of the two paramyxovirus subfamilies.

F_1 proteins of the *Paramyxovirinae* contain two heptad repeats (HR) (McGinnes et al. 2001). These are three to four repeats of seven amino acids, with hydrophobic amino acids in positions a and d. It is thought that engagement of the viral attachment protein triggers conformational changes in F that promote fusion (Dutch et al. 2001). The six HR in the F homotrimer form a six-helix bundle that represents the most stable form of the molecule and is required for fusion. HR A occurs adjacent to the fusion peptide and may be involved in the conformational alteration of this peptide that enhances fusion (Chambers et al. 1990). HR B is located adjacent to the transmembrane region. Peptides corresponding to HRs can inhibit fusion (Yao and

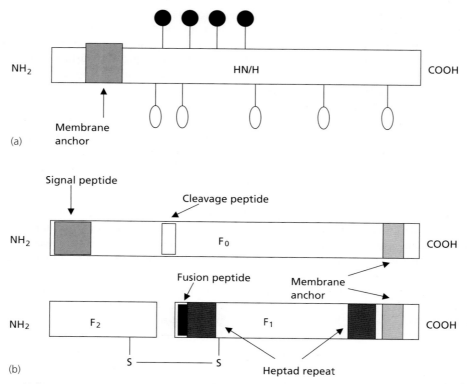

Figure 33.2 *Schematic diagrams depicting the most salient features of the attachment protein and fusion protein of the family Paramyxoviridae.* **(a)** *Figure shows an idealized HN or H attachment type II glycoprotein. The stop transfer or membrane anchor sequences are shown near the amino terminus of the molecule. The lollipop structures in black along the top of the diagram display the clustering of N-linked glycosylation sites observed in the H genes of many morbilliviruses, and the open structures display the more general distribution observed for the HN proteins. The G proteins (not shown) share the same orientation in membrane, contain both N-linked and O-linked glycosylation sites, and are about one-half the size of either HN or H.* **(b)** *The fusion (F) protein is a type I glycoprotein. The uncleaved form of F, F_0, is shown with a signal peptide at the NH2 terminus, which permits entry into the Golgi endoplasmic reticular lumen for membrane-associated protein synthesis. The cleavage peptide, made up of one or more basic residues, is indicated by the open box. Finally, the membrane anchor sequence at the COOH terminus is depicted. Also shown is the cleaved form of F_0 composed of F_1 and F_2 peptides. Note creation of a new NH2 terminus on F_1 containing the fusion peptide. Regions of F1 containing heptad repeats for the Paramyxovirinae subfamily are also clearly labeled. The F protein contains N-linked sugar residues primarily on the F_2 molecule, but often on the F_1 as well. The F_1 and F_2 subunits are covalently linked via a single disulfide bond. (Figure courtesy of K. Sleeman.)*

Compans 1996; Young et al. 1997). The F proteins of paramyxoviruses share important structural features with the fusion proteins of viruses from other families including human immunodeficiency virus, Ebola virus, and influenza A virus. The common features include the structure of the core trimer, proteolytic cleavage requirement, and the position and composition of the HRs (Baker et al. 1999; Lamb et al. 1999).

F proteins of most genera are glycosylated on the F_1 and F_2 subunits except for the morbilliviruses and henipaviruses, in which only the F_2 subunit is glycosylated. Although the attachment proteins are the major targets of neutralizing antibodies, antibodies raised against F proteins are also able to neutralize infections.

Attachment protein

The attachment proteins of the *Paramyxovirinae* are type II integral membrane proteins. Such proteins have

their amino termini extending into the cytoplasm from the inner surface of the plasma membrane and the carboxyl termini extending from the outer surface of the plasma membrane into the extracellular milieu (Figure 33.2). The attachment proteins of the morbilliviruses are referred to as H because they possess hemagglutination activity. The attachment proteins of respiroviruses, rubulaviruses, and avulaviruses have hemagglutination and neuraminidase activities and are abbreviated as HN. Since the attachment proteins of the henipaviruses and the *Pneumovirinae* do not possess hemagglutination nor neuraminidase activities, these proteins are referred to as G. The attachment proteins of the two subfamilies share no sequence homologies and therefore are treated separately in the following paragraphs.

There is considerable sequence homology between the H proteins of morbilliviruses and the HN proteins of the respiroviruses, rubulaviruses, and avulaviruses, while the G proteins of the henipaviruses are quite different. The predicted amino acid sequences of HN proteins range in size from 565 to 582 amino acids, while the H proteins of the morbilliviruses and the G proteins of henipaviruses are larger having 602–617 amino acids. The HN protein of NDV is expressed as an inactive precursor, HN0, which is activated by removal of a carboxyl terminal fragment (Nagai et al. 1989). The HN/H/G proteins are glycosylated with *N*-linked oligosaccharides only, there are between three and eight potential sites per molecule. The general structure of the attachment proteins consists of a cytoplasmic domain, a membrane-spanning region, a stalk region and a globular head. The crystal structure of the NDV HN globular head has been determined (Crennell et al. 2000). Based on these data and extensive computer modeling, the globular head of the attachment proteins of the *Paramyxovirinae* is a propeller-shaped superbarrel of six cyclically arranged beta-sheets, and these proteins are believed to be disulfide-linked homodimers, two of which form noncovalently linked tetramers (Langedijk et al. 1997; Malvoisin and Wild 1993).

The attachment protein promotes fusion, as the ability of the F protein to fuse membranes depends on the presence of the homologous HN/H/G. The exception to this is the *Rubulavirus*, simian virus 5, which does not require the HN protein for fusion. It is believed that HN/H/G positions the membranes for access by the fusion peptide and/or causes a conformational change in F that allows fusion to occur. The fusion-helper function of HN/H/G only occurs with homologous F proteins or those of closely related viruses within the same genus (Bossart et al. 2002).

The HN glycoproteins of the paramyxoviruses and rubulaviruses employ sialic acid-containing cell surface molecules as receptors. The membrane distal globular head region contains the sialic acid-binding site. The HN proteins of respiroviruses proteins contain a conserved amino acid sequence (NRKSKS), similar to the sialic acid-binding site of influenza virus neuraminidase (Morrison and Portner 1991). The neuraminidase activity cleaves sialic acid residues, presumably to prevent budding virions from self-aggregation. Two cellular receptors have been identified for measles virus, CD46, a complement regulatory protein, and human SLAM (Dorig et al. 1993; Naniche et al. 1993; Tatsuo et al. 2000). The canine and bovine homologues of human SLAM serve as receptors for the morbilliviruses, canine distemper virus and rinderpest virus (Tatsuo et al. 2001).

The HN/H is also responsible for the ability of the viruses to bind erythrocytes. Whether there are two separate sites on HN proteins for hemagglutination and neuraminidase activity, or only one, remains unclear. The attachment proteins of the *Paramyxovirinae* are usually highly antigenic and are a major target for neutralizing antibodies.

The G proteins of the subfamily *Pneumovirinae* have little in common with the attachment proteins of the *Paramyxovirinae*, apart from their type II glycoprotein configuration and attachment property. G proteins are about half the size of HN and H proteins, the putative ORF of the G protein of human metapneumovirus is only 263 amino acids long (van den Hoogen 2004). They lack neuraminidase activity, and, with the exception of pneumonia virus of mice, also lack hemagglutination activity. There is little sequence homology even within the subfamily. G proteins probably exist as noncovalently linked trimers or tetramers (Wertz et al. 1989; Collins and Mottet 1992). The major distinguishing feature of the G proteins of the pneumoviruses is the abundance of *O*-linked sugar residues. *O*-linked glycosylation occurs at serine or threonine residues, which comprise 30 percent of the amino acid residues on the G protein of respiratory syncytial virus (Wertz et al. 1989; Collins and Mottet 1992). In addition, there are three to seven potential sites for *N*-linked glycosylation. *N*-linked glycosylation seems to occur co-translationally and is a requirement for the proper folding of the G proteins, as with the attachment proteins of the *Paramyxovirinae*. *O*-linked oligosaccharides are added after the folding is completed. The high carbohydrate content explains the difference between the predicted and apparent molecular weight of the G protein of respiratory syncytial virus (32.6 vs 90 kDa) (Wertz et al. 1985). While it is known that human respiratory syncytial virus attaches to glycosaminoglycans containing heparin sulfate, no specific receptors for this virus or other members of the subfamily have been identified.

Large (polymerase) protein

The gene closest to the 5' terminus of the genome and the least abundant protein is the viral RNA-dependent RNA polymerase or large (L) protein. The protein accounts for 40–50 percent of the coding capacity of the viral genome. The large size of the protein (2 000–2 300 amino acid) reflects the many enzymatic and binding functions ascribed to this protein. The L proteins of the metapneumoviruses are the smallest, with only 2 004 amino acids for avian paramyxovirus (van den Hoogen 2004). The L protein is assumed to carry out all the enzymatic activities of the polymerase complex, namely initiation, elongation, and termination of both mRNA transcription and genome replication. mRNA transcription includes capping and methylation of the 5' end of messages, as well as polyadenylation. The templates for poly(A) tails are the short poly(U) sequences that are part of the transcription termination signals of the genes. It is assumed that the polymerase moves back and forth over these sequences to synthesize poly(A) tails of more than 100 nucleotides. This process has been called 'stuttering.' A similar slippage effect is the basis for the 'editing' of the P mRNAs of the *Paramyxovirinae*. Whether L is involved in phosphorylation of other proteins remains uncertain.

It has recently been shown that the L proteins of respiroviruses form homo oligomers (Smallwood and Moyer 2004). Since P proteins form homo tetramers (Tarbouriech et al. 2000) and the ratio of L to P in the polymerase complex has been shown to be 1:4, the minimal polymerase complex would be L2P8; however, the exact composition is unknown. Since L proteins also interact with C proteins (Horikami et al. 1997; Sweetman et al. 2001; Smallwood and Moyer 2004), they must contain L–L-, L–P-, and L–C-binding sites, several of which have been mapped for morbilliviruses, respiroviruses, and rubulaviruses.

A comparison of the amino acid sequences of the L proteins of several members of the order *Mononegavirales* lead to the identification of six domains, which are characterized by a higher level of similarity (Poch et al. 1990). Within these domains lie shorter regions of even higher conservation that are assumed to be important for polymerase function. Several putative sites for template binding, ATP binding, and nucleotide binding have been identified. A highly conserved GDN motif in domain III may be the catalytic site for phosphodiester bond formation and be analogous to the GDD catalytic site in poliovirus. Interestingly, the amino acids flanking this motif are glutamine (QGDNQ) in all members of the family except in L proteins of the henipaviruses, which have a QGDNE motif (Harcourt et al. 2001).

L proteins are believed to function only in combination with homologous N and P proteins and on templates with homologous termini, although a few exceptions among closely related members of the same genus have been noted (Curran and Kolakofsky 1991). Therefore, binding sites and promoters have co-evolved. Data derived from experimental respiratory syncytial virus and bovine parainfluenzavirus 3 vaccine candidates demonstrate that mutations in L can play a role in viral attenuation (Crowe et al. 1996; Juhasz et al. 1997).

Small hydrophobic proteins

Simian virus 5 and mumps virus (genus *Rubulavirus*), avian paramyxovirus 6 (genus *Avulavirus*), and all members of the subfamily *Pneumovirinae* have genes encoding small hydrophobic proteins (SH). These proteins have little in common beyond the fact that they are integral membrane proteins and they share no sequence homologies. They vary in length from 44 to 183 amino acids. Some are type II membrane proteins (Bukreyev et al. 1997), while others are type I proteins (Takeuchi et al. 1996). The SH proteins of the metapneumoviruses have two potential transmembrane regions (van den Hoogen 2004). The SH proteins of

simian virus 5 and human respiratory syncytial virus are structural proteins; however, this has not been proven for some of the other viruses. Spontaneous deletions of the gene or expression of defective SH proteins have been described for human respiratory syncytial virus and mumps virus strains, and recombinant viruses with deletions of the *SH* gene grow well in cell culture (Takeuchi et al. 1996). However, a recombinant human respiratory syncytial virus with a deletion of the *SH* gene was attenuated in chimpanzees (Bukreyev et al. 1997). The SH protein of simian virus 5 appears to be involved in the suppression of apoptosis (He et al. 2001).

NS1 and NS2 proteins

The members of the genus *Pneumovirus* encode two nonstructural proteins, NS1 and NS2. Their genes are located at the 3′ terminus of the genome, which leads to high levels of transcription. NS1 is 136–139 amino acids long, and NS2 is 124 amino acids in length. NS1 inhibits both transcription and replication in minigenome replication assays and NS2 had a similar, but much less pronounced effect (Atreya et al. 1998). Recombinant viruses with deletions of one or both genes demonstrate that these proteins are dispensable for growth in cell culture; however, the mutants are attenuated both in cell culture and in chimpanzees (Jin et al. 2000). NS1 and NS2 of bovine respiratory syncytial virus and human respiratory syncytial virus have been shown to protect the virus from the effects of interferon-α/β (Schlender et al. 2000; Bossert and Conzelmann 2002). Interestingly, the inhibition of interferon required expression of both proteins, indicating a cooperative action. It appears that the function of the NS proteins may be comparable to that of the C and V proteins of the *Paramyxovirinae*.

M2-1 and M2-2 proteins

All members of the subfamily *Pneumoviridae* have an *M2* gene, which expresses two proteins, M2-1 and M2-2. The M2-1 of human respiratory syncytial virus, also called the 22K protein, is 194 amino acids in length, and is a hydrophilic, phosphorylated, structural protein found associated with the nucleocapsids (Garcia et al. 1993). It acts as a processivity and antitermination factor in transcription (Collins et al. 1996; Hardy and Wertz 1998). The protein is required to transcribe longer genes completely and leads to an increase in read-through transcripts at intergenic junctions. M2-1 has no effect on replication. A C_3H_1 motif near the amino terminus, which may bind zinc, is conserved in all M2-1 proteins and is required for the function of the protein (Hardy and Wertz 2000). M2-1 binds RNA and the N protein (Cuesta et al. 2000). Deletion of the M2-1 ORF does not produce viable virus.

The M2-2 protein is translated from a reading frame that overlaps the end of the M2-1 ORF. The M2-2 protein of human respiratory syncytial virus is 90 amino acids in length and nonstructural. Deletion of the ORF produced a virus viable in cell culture, showing that the gene is dispensable; however, the mutant was attenuated in cell culture and in chimpanzees (Teng et al. 2000). The M2-2 minus mutant was further characterized by a shift from replication to transcription, with increased and continued mRNA production and decreased replication, suggesting that this protein is involved in regulating the balance of transcription and replication (Bermingham and Collins 1999).

ACKNOWLEDGMENTS

This chapter is adapted and expanded from Bellini, W.J., Rota, P.A. and Anderson, L.J. 1998. Paramyxoviruses. In Mahy, B.W.J. and Collier, L. (eds), *Topley & Wilson's microbiology and microbial infections*, 9th edn. Vol. 1, *Virology*. London: Edward Arnold, 435–62.

REFERENCES

Ahne, W., Batts, W.N., et al. 1999. Comparative sequence analyses of sixteen reptilian paramyxoviruses. *Virus Res*, **63**, 65–74.

Ali, A. and Nayak, D.P. 2000. Assembly of Sendai virus, M protein interacts with F and HN proteins and with the cytoplasmic tail and transmembrane domain of F protein. *Virology*, **276**, 289–303.

Atreya, P.L., Peeples, M.E. and Collins, P.L. 1998. The NS1 protein of human respiratory syncytial virus is a potent inhibitor of minigenome transcription and RNA replication. *J Virol*, **72**, 1452–61.

Baker, K.A., Dutch, R.E., et al. 1999. Structural basis for *Paramyxovirus*-mediated membrane fusion. *Mol Cell*, **3**, 309–19.

Baron, M.D. and Barrett, T. 2000. Rinderpest viruses lacking the C and V proteins show specific defects in growth and transcription of viral RNAs. *J Virol*, **74**, 2603–11.

Barr, P.J. 1991. Mammalian subtilisins: the long-sought dibasic processing endoproteases. *Cell*, **66**, 1–3.

Bermingham, A. and Collins, P.L. 1999. The M2-2 protein of human respiratory syncytial virus is a regulatory factor involved in the balance between RNA replication and transcription. *Proc Natl Acad Sci USA*, **96**, 11259–64.

Bellini, W.J., Englund, G., et al. 1986. Matrix genes of measles virus and canine distemper virus: cloning, nucleotide sequences, and deduced amino acid sequences. *J Virol*, **58**, 408–16.

Bossart, K.N., Wang, L.F., et al. 2002. Membrane fusion tropism and heterotypic functional activities of the Nipah virus and Hendra virus envelope glycoproteins. *J Virol*, **76**, 11186–98.

Bossert, B. and Conzelmann, K.K. 2002. Respiratory syncytial virus (RSV) nonstructural (NS) proteins as host range determinants: a chimeric bovine RSV with NS genes from human RSV is attenuated in interferon-competent bovine cells. *J Virol*, **76**, 4287–93.

Bukreyev, A., Whitehead, S.S., et al. 1997. Recombinant respiratory syncytial virus from which the entire SH gene has been deleted grows efficiently in cell culture and exhibits site-specific attenuation in the respiratory tract of the mouse. *J Virol*, **71**, 8973–82.

Calain, P.L. and Roux, L. 1993. The rule of six, a basic feature for efficient replication of Sendai virus defective interfering RNA. *J Virol*, **67**, 4822–30.

Cattaneo, R., Rebmann, G., et al. 1987. Altered transcription of a defective measles virus genome derived from a diseased human brain. *EMBO J*, **6**, 681–8.

Chambers, P., Pringle, C.R. and Easton, A.J. 1990. Heptad repeat sequences are located adjacent to hydrophobic regions in several types of virus fusion glycoproteins. *J Gen Virol*, **71**, 3075–80.

Collins, P.L. and Mottet, G. 1992. Oligomerization and post-translational processing of glycoprotein G of human respiratory syncytial virus: altered O-glycosylation in the presence of brefeldin A. *J Gen Virol*, **73**, 849–63.

Collins, P.L., Olmsted, R.A., et al. 1987. Gene overlap and site-specific attenuation of transcription of the viral polymerase L gene of human respiratory syncytial virus. *Proc Natl Acad Sci USA*, **84**, 5134.

Collins, P.L., Hill, M.G., et al. 1996. Transcription elongation factor of respiratory syncytial virus, a nonsegmented negative-strand RNA virus. *Proc Natl Acad Sci USA*, **93**, 81–5.

Compans, R.W. and Choppin, P.W. 1967a. Isolation and properties of the helical nucleocapsid of the parainfluenza virus simian virus 5. *Proc Natl Acad Sci USA*, **57**, 949–56.

Compans, R.W. and Choppin, P.W. 1967b. The length of the helical nucleocapsid of Newcastle disease virus. *Virology*, **33**, 344–6.

Coronel, E.C., Takimoto, T., et al. 2001. Nucleocapsid incorporation into parainfluenza virus is regulated by specific interaction with matrix protein. *J Virol*, **75**, 1117–23.

Crennell, S., Takimoto, T., et al. 2000. Crystal structure of the multifunctional paramyxovirus hemagglutinin-neuraminidase. *Nat Struct Biol*, **7**, 1068–74.

Crowe, J.E. Jr., Firestone, C.Y., et al. 1996. Acquisition of the ts phenotype by a chemically mutagenized cold-passaged human respiratory syncytial virus vaccine candidate results from the acquisition of a single mutation in the polymerase (L) gene. *Virus Genes*, **13**, 269–73.

Cuesta, I., Geng, X., et al. 2000. Structural phosphoprotein M2-1 of the human respiratory syncytial virus is an RNA binding protein. *J Virol*, **74**, 9858–67.

Curran, J. and Kolakofsky, D. 1988. Ribosomal initiation from an ACG codon in the Sendai virus P/C mRNA. *EMBO J*, **7**, 245.

Curran, J. and Kolakofsky, D. 1989. Scanning independent ribosomal initiation of the Sendai virus Y proteins in vitro and in vivo. *EMBO J*, **8**, 521.

Curran, J.A. and Kolakofsky, D. 1991. Rescue of a Sendai virus DI genome by other parainfluenza viruses: implications for genome replication. *Virology*, **182**, 168–76.

Curran, J.A., Boeck, R. and Kolakofsky, D. 1991. The Sendai virus P gene expresses both an essential protein and an inhibitor of RNA synthesis by shuffling modules via mRNA editing. *EMBO J*, **10**, 3079–85.

Curran, J., Marq, J.B. and Kolakofsky, D. 1992. The Sendai virus nonstructural C proteins specifically inhibit viral mRNA synthesis. *Virology*, **189**, 647–56.

Curran, J.A., Homann, H., et al. 1993. The hypervariable C-terminal tail of the Sendai paramyxovirus nucleocapsid protein is required for template function but not for RNA encapsidation. *J Virol*, **67**, 4358–64.

Curran, J.A., Marq, J.B. and Kolakofsky, D. 1995. An N-terminal domain of the Sendai paramyxovirus P protein acts as a chaperone for the NP protein during the nascent chain assembly step of genome replication. *J Virol*, **69**, 849–55.

de Leeuw, O.S., Hartog, L., et al. 2003. Effect of fusion protein cleavage site mutations on virulence of Newcastle disease virus: non-virulent cleavage site mutants revert to virulence after one passage in chicken brain. *J Gen Virol*, **84**, 475–84.

Dolganiuc, V., McGinnes, L., et al. 2003. Role of the cytoplasmic domain of the Newcastle disease virus fusion protein in association with lipid rafts. *J Virol*, **77**, 12968–79.

Dorig, R.E., Marcil, A., et al. 1993. The human CD46 molecule is a receptor for measles virus (Edmonston strain). *Cell*, **75**, 295–305.

Dreyfuss, G., Matunis, M.J., et al. 1993. hnRNP proteins and the biogenesis of mRNA. *Ann Rev Biochem*, **62**, 289–329.

Durbin, A.P., McAuliffe, J.M., et al. 1999. Mutations in the C, D and V open reading frames of human parainfluenza virus type 3 attenuate replication in rodents and primates. *Virology*, **261**, 319–30.

Dutch, R.E., Hagglund, R.N., et al. 2001. Paramyxovirus fusion (F) protein: a conformational change on cleavage activation. *Virology*, **281**, 138–50.

Fearns, R., Peeples, M.E. and Collins, P.L. 1997. Increased expression of the N protein of respiratory syncytial virus stimulates minigenome replication but does not alter the balance between the synthesis of mRNA and antigenome. *Virology*, **236**, 188–201.

Feldman, S.A., Hendry, R.M. and Beeler, J.A. 1999. Identification of a linear heparin binding domain for human respiratory syncytial virus attachment glycoprotein G. *J Virol*, **73**, 6610–17.

Finch, J.T. and Gibbs, A.J. 1970. Observations on the structure of the nucleocapsids of some paramyxoviruses. *J Gen Virol*, **6**, 141–50.

Gotoh, I., Yamauchi, F., et al. 1992. Isolation of factor Xa from chick embryo as the amniotic endoprotease responsible for paramyxovirus activation. *FEBS Lett*, **296**, 274–8.

Gotoh, I., Takeuchi, K., et al. 1999. Knockout of the Sendai virus C gene eliminates the viral ability to prevent the interferon-alpha/beta-mediated responses. *FEBS Lett*, **459**, 205–10.

Garcia, J., Garcia-Barreno, B., et al. 1993. Cytoplasmic inclusions of respiratory syncytial virus-infected cells: formation of inclusion bodies in transfected cells that coexpress the nucleoprotein, the phosphoprotein, and the 22K protein. *Virology*, **195**, 243.

Harcourt, B.H., Tamin, A., et al. 2000. Molecular characterization of Nipah virus, a newly emergent paramyxovirus. *Virology*, **271**, 334–49.

Harcourt, B.H., Tamin, A., et al. 2001. Molecular characterization of the polymerase gene and genomic termini of Nipah virus. *Virology*, **287**, 192–201.

Hardy, R.W. and Wertz, G.W. 1998. The product of the respiratory syncytial virus M2 gene ORF1 enhances readthrough of intergenic junctions during viral transcription. *J Virol*, **72**, 520–6.

Hardy, R.W. and Wertz, G.W. 2000. The Cys$_3$-His$_1$ motif of the respiratory syncytial virus M2-1 protein is essential for protein function. *J Virol*, **74**, 5880–5.

Hardy, R.W., Harmon, S.B. and Wertz, G.W. 1999. Diverse gene junctions of respiratory syncytial virus modulate the efficiency of transcription termination and respond differently to M2-mediated antitermination. *J Virol*, **73**, 170–6.

Hasan, M.K., Kato, A., et al. 2000. Versatility of the accessory C proteins of Sendai virus: contribution to virus assembly as an additional role. *J Virol*, **74**, 5619–28.

He, B., Lin, G.Y., et al. 2001. The SH integral membrane protein of the paramyxovirus simian virus 5 is required to block apoptosis in MDBK cells. *J Virol*, **75**, 4068–79.

He, B., Paterson, R.G., et al. 2002. Recovery of paramyxovirus simian virus 5 with a V protein lacking the conserved cysteine-rich domain: the multifunctional V protein blocks both interferon-beta induction and interferon signaling. *Virology*, **303**, 15–32.

Hengst, U. and Kiefer, P. 2000. Domains of human respiratory syncytial virus P protein essential for homodimerization and for binding to N and NS1 protein. *Virus Genes*, **20**, 221–5.

Homann, H.E., Hofschneider, P.H. and Neubert, W.J. 1990. Sendai virus expression in lytically and persistently infected cells. *Virology*, **177**, 131–40.

Horikami, S.M., Hector, R.E., et al. 1997. The Sendai virus C protein binds the L polymerase protein to inhibit viral RNA synthesis. *Virology*, **235**, 261–70.

Hosaka, M., Nagahama, M., et al. 1991. Arg-X-Lys/Arg-Arg motif as a signal for precursor cleavage catalyzed by furin within the constitutive secretory pathway. *J Biol Chem*, **266**, 12127–30.

Hsu, C.-H. and Kingsbury, D.W. 1982. Topography of phosphate residues in Sendai virus proteins. *Virology*, **120**, 225–34.

Jin, H., Zhou, H., et al. 2000. Recombinant respiratory syncytial viruses with deletions in the NS1, NS2, SH and M2-2 genes are attenuated in vitro and in vivo. *Virology*, **273**, 210–18.

Juhasz, K., Whitehead, S.S., et al. 1997. The temperature-sensitive (ts) phenotype of a cold-passaged (cp) live attenuated respiratory syncytial virus vaccine candidate, designated cpts530, results from a single amino acid substitution in the L protein. *J Virol*, **71**, 5814–19.

Kato, A., Kiyotani, K., et al. 1997. The paramyxovirus, Sendai virus, V protein encodes a luxury function required for viral pathogenesis. *EMBO J*, **16**, 578–87.

Klenk, H.D. and Choppin, P.W. 1969. Lipids of plasma membranes of monkey and hamster kidney cells and of parainfluenza virions grown in these cells. *Virology*, **38**, 255–68.

Klenk, H.D. and Choppin, P.W. 1970. Plasma membrane lipids and parainfluenza virus assembly. *Virology*, **40**, 939–47.

Kurath, G., Batts, W.N., et al. 2004. Complete genome sequence of Fer-de-Lance virus reveals a novel gene in reptilian paramyxoviruses. *J Virol*, **78**, 2045–56.

Lamb, R.A. 1993. Paramyxovirus fusion: a hypothesis for changes. *Virology*, **197**, 1–11.

Lamb, R.A. and Kolakofsky, D. 2001. Paramyxoviridae: the viruses and their replication. In: Knipe, D.M., Howley, P.M., et al. (eds), *Fields' Virology*, Vol. 1. Philadelphia: Lippincott, Williams & Wilkins, 1305–41, Chapter 41.

Lamb, R.A., Joshi, S.B. and Dutch, R.E. 1999. The paramyxovirus fusion protein forms an extremely stable core trimer: structural parallels to influenza virus haemagglutinin and HIV-1 gp41. *Mol Membr Biol*, **16**, 11–19.

Langedijk, J.P.M., Daus, F.J. and van Oirschot, J.T. 1997. Sequence and structure alignment of *Paramyxoviridae* attachment proteins and discovery of enzymatic activity for a *Morbillivirus* hemagglutinin. *J Virol*, **71**, 6155–67.

Lin, G.Y., Paterson, R.G., et al. 1998. The V protein of the paramyxovirus SV5 interacts with damage-specific DNA binding protein. *Virology*, **249**, 189–200.

Malvoisin, E. and Wild, T.F. 1993. Measles virus glycoproteins: studies on the structure and interaction of the haemagglutinin and fusion proteins. *J Gen Virol*, **74**, Pt 11, 2365.

Manie, S.N., Debreyne, S., et al. 2000. Measles virus structural components are enriched into lipid raft microdomains: a potential cellular location for virus assembly. *J Virol*, **74**, 305–11.

Mayo, M. 2002. A summary of taxonomic changes recently approved by ICTV. *Arch Virol*, **147**, 1655–6.

McGinnes, L.W., Sergel, T., et al. 2001. Mutational analysis of the membrane proximal heptad repeat of the Newcastle disease virus fusion protein. *Virology*, **289**, 343–52.

Miller, P.J., Boyle, D.B., et al. 2003. Full-length genome sequence of Mossman virus, a novel paramyxovirus isolated from rodents in Australia. *Virology*, **317**, 330–44.

Morrison, T. and Portner, A. 1991. Structure, function, and intracellular processing of the glycoproteins of Paramyxoviridae. In: Kingsbury, D.W. (ed.), *The paramyxoviruses*. New York: Plenum Press, 347–82.

Nagai, Y., Hamaguchi, M. and Toyoda, T. 1989. Molecular biology of Newcastle disease virus. *Prog Vet Microbiol Immunol*, **5**, 16–64.

Naim, H.Y., Ehler, E. and Billeter, M.A. 2000. Measles virus matrix protein specifies apical virus release and glycoprotein sorting in epithelial cells. *EMBO J*, **19**, 3576–85.

Naniche, D., Varior-Krishnan, G., et al. 1993. Human membrane cofactor protein (CD46) acts as a cellular receptor for measles virus. *J Virol*, **67**, 6025–32.

Ogino, T., Iwama, M., et al. 2003. Interaction of cellular tubulin with Sendai virus M protein regulates transcription of viral genome. *Biochem Biophys Res Commun*, **311**, 283–93.

Ortmann, D., Ohuchi, M., et al. 1994. Proteolytic cleavage of wild type and mutants of the F protein of human parainfluenza virus type 3 by two subtilisin-like endoproteases, furin and Kex2. *J Virol*, **68**, 2772–6.

Palosaari, H., Parisien, J.P., et al. 2003. STAT protein interference and suppression of cytokine signal transduction by measles virus V protein. *J Virol*, **77**, 7635–44.

Parisien, J.P., Lau, J.F., et al. 2001. The V protein of human parainfluenza virus 2 antagonizes type I interferon responses by destabilizing signal transducer and activator of transcription 2. *Virology*, **283**, 230–9.

Parks, G.D. and Lamb, R.A. 1990. Defective assembly and intracellular transport of mutant paramyxovirus hemagglutinin-neuraminidase proteins containing altered cytoplasmic domains. *J Virol*, **64**, 3605–16.

Peeples, M.E. 1991. Paramyxovirus M proteins: pulling it all together and taking it on the road. In: Kingsbury, D.W. (ed.), *The paramyxoviruses*. New York: Plenum Press, 427–56.

Poch, O., Blumberg, B.M., et al. 1990. Sequence comparison of five polymerases (L proteins) of unsegmented negative-strand RNA viruses: theoretical assignment of functional domains. *J Gen Virol*, **71**, Pt 5, 1153–62.

Radecke, F. and Billeter, M.A. 1996. The nonstructural C protein is not essential for multiplication of Edmonston B strain measles virus in cultured cells. *Virology*, **217**, 418–21.

Renshaw, R.W., Glaser, A.L., et al. 2000. Identification and phylogenetic comparison of Salem virus, a novel paramyxovirus of horses. *Virology*, **270**, 417–29.

Reutter, G.L., Cortese-Grogan, C., et al. 2001. Mutations in the measles virus C protein that up regulate viral RNA synthesis. *Virology*, **285**, 100–9.

Rochat, S., Komada, H. and Kolakofsky, D. 1992. Loss of V protein expression in human parainfluenza virus type 1 is not a recent event. *Virus Res*, **24**, 137–44.

Rodriguez, J.J., Parisien, J.P. and Horvath, C.M. 2002. Nipah virus V protein evades alpha and gamma interferons by preventing STAT1 and STAT2 activation and nuclear accumulation. *J Virol*, **76**, 11476–83.

Roos, R.P. and Wollmann, R. 1979. Non-productive paramyxovirus infection: Nariva virus infection in hamsters. *Arch Virol*, **62**, 229–40.

Ryan, K.W., Portner, A. and Murti, K.G. 1993. Antibodies to paramyxovirus nucleoproteins define regions important for immunogenicity and nucleocapsid assembly. *Virology*, **193**, 376–84.

Samal, S.K. and Collins, P.L. 1996. RNA replication by a respiratory syncytial virus RNA analog does not obey the rule of six. *J Virol*, **70**, 5075–82.

Sanderson, C.M., Wu, H.-H. and Nayak, D.P. 1993. Sendai virus M protein binds independently to either the F or the HN glycoprotein in vivo. *J Virol*, **68**, 69–76.

Schlender, J., Bossert, B., et al. 2000. Bovine respiratory syncytial virus nonstructural proteins NS1 and NS2 cooperatively antagonize alpha/beta interferon-induced antiviral response. *J Virol*, **74**, 8234–42.

Schmitt, A.P., Leser, G.P., et al. 2002. Requirements for budding of paramyxovirus simian virus 5 virus-like particles. *J Virol*, **76**, 3952–64.

Schneider, H., Kaelin, K. and Billeter, M.A. 1997. Recombinant measles viruses defective for RNA editing and V protein synthesis are viable in cultured cells. *Virology*, **227**, 314–22.

Shaffer, J.A., Bellini, W.J. and Rota, P.A. 2003. The C protein of measles virus inhibits the type I interferon response. *Virology*, **315**, 389–97.

Sheshberadaran, H. and Lamb, R.A. 1990. Sequence characterization of the membrane protein gene of paramyxovirus simian virus 5. *Virology*, **176**, 234–43.

Smallwood, S. and Moyer, S.A. 2004. The L polymerase protein of parainfluenza virus 3 forms an oligomer and can interact with the heterologous Sendai virus L, P and C proteins. *Virology*, **318**, 439–50.

Stricker, R., Mottet, G. and Roux, L. 1994. The Sendai virus matrix protein appears to be recruited in the cytoplasm by the viral nucleocapsid to function in viral assembly and budding. *J Gen Virol*, **75**, 1031–42.

Suryanarayana, K., Baczko, K., et al. 1994. Transcription inhibition and other properties of matrix proteins expressed by M genes cloned from measles viruses and diseased human brain tissue. *J Virol*, **68**, 1532–43.

Sweetman, D.A., Miskin, J. and Baron, M.D. 2001. Rinderpest virus C and V proteins interact with the major (L) component of the viral polymerase. *Virology*, **281**, 193–204.

Takeuchi, K., Tanabayashi, K., et al. 1990. Detection and characterization of mumps virus V protein. *Virology*, **178**, 247–53.

Takeuchi, K., Tanabayashi, K., et al. 1996. The mumps virus SH protein is a membrane protein and not essential for virus growth. *Virology*, **225**, 156–62.

Tarbouriech, N., Curran, J., et al. 2000. On the domain structure and the polymerization state of the sendai virus P protein. *Virology*, **266**, 99–109.

Tashiro, M., Seto, J.T., et al. 1993. Possible involvement of microtubule disruption in bipolar budding of a Sendai virus mutant, F1-R, in epithelial MDCK cells. *J Virol*, **67**, 5902–10.

Tashiro, M., McQueen, N.L., et al. 1996. Involvement of the mutated M protein in altered budding polarity of a pantropic mutant, F1-R, of Sendai virus. *J Virol*, **70**, 5990–7.

Tatsuo, H., Ono, N., et al. 2000. SLAM (CDw150) is a cellular receptor for measles virus. *Nature*, **406**, 893–7.

Tatsuo, H., Ono, N. and Yanagi, Y. 2001. Morbilliviruses use signaling lymphocyte activation molecules (CD150) as cellular receptors. *J Virol*, **75**, 5842–50.

Teng, M.N., Whitehead, S.S., et al. 2000. Recombinant respiratory syncytial virus that does not express the NS1 or M2-2 protein is highly attenuated and immunogenic in chimpanzees. *J Virol*, **74**, 9317–21.

Thomas, S.M., Lamb, R.A. and Paterson, R.G. 1988. Two mRNAs that differ from two nontemplated nucleotides encode the amino coterminal proteins P and V of the paramyxovirus simian virus 5. *Cell*, **54**, 891–902.

Tidona, C.A., Kurz, H.W., et al. 1999. Isolation and molecular characterization of a novel cytopathogenic paramyxovirus from tree shrews. *Virology*, **258**, 425–34.

Valsamakis, A., Schneider, H., et al. 1998. Recombinant measles viruses with mutations in the C, V, or F gene have altered growth phenotypes in vivo. *J Virol*, **72**, 7754–61.

van den Hoogen, B.G. 2004. *Human metapneumoviruses*. Rotterdam, The Netherlands: Erasmus University.

Wang, L., Harcourt, B.H., et al. 2001. Molecular biology of Hendra and Nipah viruses. *Microbe Infect*, **3**, 279–87.

Wertz, G.W., Collins, P.L., et al. 1985. Nucleotide sequence of the G protein gene of human respiratory syncytial virus reveals an unusual type of viral membrane protein. *Proc Natl Acad Sci USA*, **82**, 4075–9.

Wertz, G.W., Kreiger, M. and Ball, L.A. 1989. Structure and cell surface alteration of the attachment glycoprotein of human respiratory syncytial virus in a cell line deficient O-glycosylation. *J Virol*, **63**, 4767–76.

Yamada, H., Hayata, S., et al. 1990. Association of the Sendai virus C protein with nucleocapsids. *Arch Virol*, **113**, 245–53.

Yao, Q. and Compans, R.W. 1996. Peptides corresponding to the heptad repeat sequence of human parainfluenza virus fusion protein are potent inhibitors of virus infection. *Virology*, **223**, 103–12.

Yoshida, T., Nakayama, Y., et al. 1986. Inhibition of the assembly of Newcastle disease virus by monensin. *Virus Res*, **4**, 179–95.

Young, J.K., Hicks, R.P., et al. 1997. Analysis of a peptide inhibitor of paramyxovirus (NDV) fusion using biological assays, NMR, and molecular modeling. *Virology*, **238**, 291–304.

34

Morbilliviruses: measles virus

SIBYLLE SCHNEIDER-SCHAULIES AND WILLIAM J. BELLINI

INTRODUCTION

Acute measles is a well-defined clinical entity normally contracted by children and young adults. The causative agent, Measles virus (MeV), is an efficient pathogen, persisting in nature in populations large enough to support it, although it causes an acute infection only once in a lifetime of the individual. The virus is monotypic and antigenically stable, however, several genotypes can be distinguished some of which are inactive, while others are still active and are drifting on a genetic level worldwide. MeV is a highly successful virus, which has efficiently exploited its potential for spread. Although nonhuman primates are susceptible to infection, transmission from animals is not an important means of introducing the disease into a community. The virus may persist on rare occasions in single individuals for years, but these persistent infections are not associated with periodic shedding of infectious virus. A single attack of measles is sufficient to confer long-lasting, probably life-long immunity to re-infection. Consequently, in order to remain endemic in a given community, the virus must rely on the infection of unprotected susceptible individuals, mainly small infants with waning levels of maternal antibodies. The efficiency of this process is documented by the first known report of measles (in Egyptian hieroglyphics), which failed to recognize the infectious nature of the illness, and described it as a normal part of child growth and development.

In the prevaccine era, the maximum incidence of measles was seen in children aged 5–9 years in developed countries. Outbreaks and epidemics centered around elementary schools, while younger children acquired measles as secondary cases from their school-age siblings. By the age of 20, approximately 99 percent of subjects tested had been exposed to the virus. The introduction of the measles vaccine had a significant impact on the age incidence and percentage of measles cases in different age groups. In countries with an optimal vaccine implementation, measles infection has shifted to the teenage group, whereas in areas with inadequate vaccine programs children up to 4 years of age reveal a high primary measles attack rate (Bellini et al. 1994). In contrast, in developing countries, where measles has its greatest incidence in children under 2 years of age, the disease is a serious problem with a high mortality (up to 10 percent), with malnutrition being a precipitating factor for the severity of the disease. Therefore, the pattern of epidemiology observed differs markedly in different parts of the world, and a thorough understanding of this is essential to the development of successful vaccination programs.

CLASSIFICATION

Measles virus (MeV) is a member of the order *Mononegavirales* which includes the families *Rhabdo-*, *Filo-* and *Paramyxoviridae*. As a *Paramyxovirus*, MeV reveals structural and biochemical features associated with this group (see Chapter 33, General properties of the Paramyxoviruses). As it lacks a virion-associated neuraminidase activity and causes formation of intranuclear inclusion bodies, it has been grouped into a separate genus, *Morbillivirus* of which it is the type species. Other members of this genus include *Peste des petits ruminants virus* (PPRV), which infects sheep and goats, *Rinderpest virus* (RPV), which infects cattle, *Canine distemper virus* (CDV), which infects dogs, *Phocine distemper virus* (PDV), which infects seals and sea lions, dolphin morbillivirus (DMV), and porpoise morbillivirus (PMV) (see Chapter 38, Paramyxoviruses of animals). All these viruses exhibit antigenic similarities, and produce similar diseases in their host species. Since MeV most closely resembles RPV, it has been suggested that the virus evolved in an environment in which cattle and humans lived in close proximity. Thus, measles is a relatively new disease of humans and a disease of civilization.

MORPHOLOGY, STRUCTURE, PHYSICOCHEMICAL, AND BIOLOGICAL PROPERTIES

MeV particles consist of a lipid envelope surrounding the viral RNP complex which is composed of genomic RNA associated with proteins (Figure 34.1a). Two transmembrane proteins (fusion (F) and hemagglutinin (H) proteins) project from the envelope surface. Both proteins extend through the virion envelope and appear on its inside surface. The H protein is anchored near its amino terminus (type II glycoprotein), and the F protein near its carboxy terminus (type I glycoprotein). One or both of the cytoplasmic domains functionally and probably physically interact with the matrix (M) protein (Cathomen et al. 1997a; Moll et al. 2001, 2002) which also links the envelope to the RNP core structure. The viral genomic RNA is fully encapsidated by nucleocapsid (N) protein and associated with the polymerase complex, consisting of the phosphoprotein (P) and the large (L) proteins, to form the RNP core structure that resists RNase degradation (Griffin and Bellini 1996). The virions are highly pleomorphic with an average size of 120 to >300 nm and both filamentous and irregular forms are known. The virion shown in an electron micrograph is bounded by a lipid envelope which bears a fringe of spike-like projections (peplomers) 5–8 nm long (Figure 34.2). The membrane below the spikes is 10–20 nm in thickness and the enclosed helical viral RNP core has a diameter of 17 nm and a regular pitch of 5 nm. The cargo space of the particles may vary from

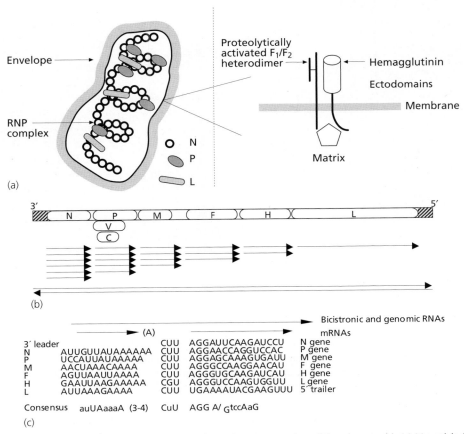

Figure 34.1 *MeV: Structure, genome, and replication.* **(a)** *Schematic representation of the pleomorphic MeV particle (left) and (right) the organization of its membrane proteins.* **(b)** *Genomic organization, open reading frames and representation of monocistronic and genomic transcripts.* **(c)** *Intergenic boundaries separating MeV transcription units and their consensus sequence.*

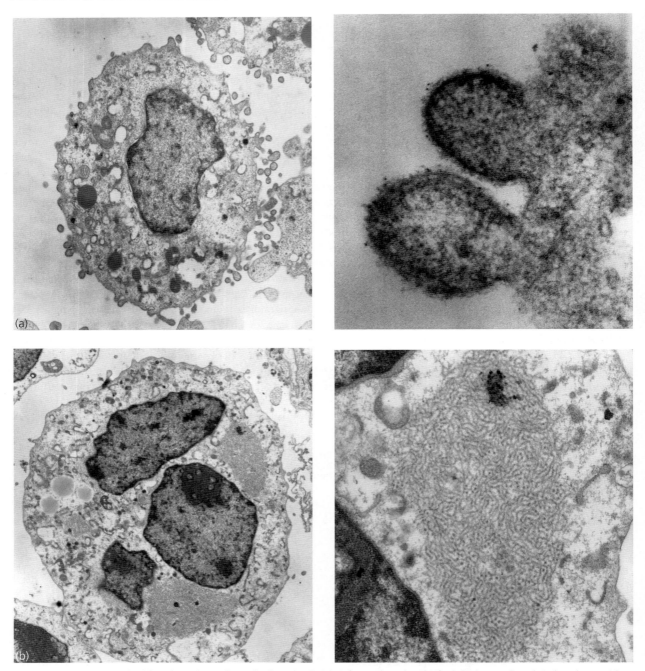

Figure 34.2 *MeV virions budding from the surface of infected cells* **(a)**, *left panel, and magnified, (right panel) and viral nucleocapsids accumulating in large cytoplasmic aggregates* **(b)**, *left panel, and magnified, (right panel) (kindly provided by Jürgen Schneider-Schäulies).*

3×10^5 to $>10^7$ nm^3 and could accommodate >30 genomes. In fact, packaging of multiple genomes within a single particle in vitro has been confirmed (Rager et al. 2002). Immediately below the membrane M proteins appear as a shell of electron dense material. The structure of the virion explains much of the early data concerning the stability of the virus. The integrity of the particle envelope is essential for infectivity which is inactivated by any compound which disrupts this structure,

such as detergents or other lipid solvents including acetone or ether. Particles are acid labile and inactivated below pH 4.5, although they remain infectious between pH 5–9. MeV is thermolabile and has a half-life of 2 h at 37°C. Viability of the virus is maintained for 2 weeks at 4°C, but it is inactivated after 30 min at 56°C. Thermolability is probably due to an effect on the internal structure of the particle, since the hemagglutinin is relatively temperature resistant. The virus can be stored for prolonged periods at $-70°C$ and is amenable to freeze-drying. These properties have important consequences for the transport and storage of the vaccine.

Unlike other members of the morbilliviruses, MeV displays hemagglutination activity. This is easily demonstrated using monkey erythrocytes from rhesus, patas, and African green monkeys and baboons, but not from humans. MeV lacks detectable neuraminidase activity and does not attach to receptors containing sialic acid. Consequently, once attached to a red cell, MeV does not re-elute rapidly. H protein inserted into membranous structures is active in the hemagglutination test (HA). Virus particles separated by isopycnic centrifugation have a buoyant density of 1.23 g/cm^3, where HA activity is also detected. A large amount of hemagglutinating material is also found in the upper regions of the gradient (light hemagglutinin), which most likely represents H protein inserted into empty membranous cell fragments, or defective virus particles. Some lymphotropic MeV wild-type strains have very low hemagglutination activity which may be due to an additional *N*-linked glycosylation site within their H proteins or their low affinity for CD46, the MeV receptor expressed on monkey erythrocytes (see below). H is a major viral immunogen, and H-specific antibodies have hemagglutination-inhibiting (HI) and virus-neutralizing (NT) activities as they block the viral attachment to target cells. These antibodies do not prevent progressive viral cell-to-cell spread mediated by the F protein. The ability to lyze red blood cells once the virus has bound is mediated by the F protein. As with hemagglutination, this property is artificial, but hemolysis (HL) provides a convenient measure of F protein activity which is more sensitive to both pH and temperature than HA, and is optimal at $37°C$ and pH 7.4. The ability of the MeV to fuse at neutral pH accounts for the characteristic cytopathic effect (CPE) induced by these viruses, the formation of giant cells.

Genome structure, function, and replication

The 15 894 bases long viral genome is a nonsegmented RNA molecule of negative polarity that is entirely complexed with N proteins and the rigidity of this interaction is believed to account for the absence of genome recombination in the *Mononegavirales*. Each N protein covers six nucleotides, and this is thought to be the reason why only viral genomes whose number of nucleotides is a multimer of six are efficiently replicated by the viral polymerase. This constraint seems to be essential since in recombinant MeV genomes, hexameric genomic length ensuring accurate RNA encapsidation has been recently found to be actively restored (Rager et al. 2002). As long as the rule of six (Calain and Roux 1993) is maintained, MeV tolerates substantial variations in

total genome length since recombinant genomes carrying foreign genes as diverse as reporter genes, heterologous envelope genes, or growth factors specificity domains displayed on the H protein can be rescued and stably propagated (Schneider et al. 2000). The standard genome is organized into six contiguous, nonoverlapping transcription units that are separated by (except for the M/F gene boundary) short noncoding regions containing signals for transcription termination, polyadenylation, and transcriptional re-initiation (Figure 34.1b, c) (Bellini et al. 1994). The genome is flanked by noncoding 3′ leader and 5′ trailer sequences containing specific encapsidation signals and the viral promoters used for viral transcription and/or replication of genomic and antigenomic RNAs (Horikami and Moyer 1995; Parks et al. 2001) (Figure 34.1c).

During transcription, the polymerase complex enters the genomic RNP at its 3′ end. After synthesis and termination of a short leader RNA, transcription is resumed at the gene start sequence 3′ of the N coding region and pauses at the gene stop sequence where, by a slippage mechanism, a poly(A) stretch is added. After liberation of the N mRNA, transcription of the downstream P mRNA is initiated. By the same stop–restart mechanisms, mRNAs for the other downstream genes are produced. As the polymerase tends to fall off the template at the intergenic boundaries, the probability of transcriptional re-initiation is lower than one, reflected by a decreasing transcriptional efficiency of downstream mRNAs (transcriptional gradient). The differential abundancies of the mRNAs directly translate into the relative amounts of proteins produced. Occasionally, the polymerase complex also ignores the intergenic stop/start signals giving rise to bi- or tricistronic, polyadenylated transcripts. Replication of the genome, or antigenome, respectively, tightly couples elongation and encapsidation. The switch from the transcription to the replication mode of the polymerase complex is thought to be dependent on the availability of N proteins for encapsidation.

From the *P* gene, two nonstructural proteins, C (20 kDa) and V (46 kDa) are expressed. While C protein is encoded within a separate reading frame (Bellini et al. 1985), V protein is translated from cotranscriptionally edited P mRNA. While its amino-terminal domain is identical to that of P, V protein has a unique cysteine-rich domain at the carboxy terminus (Wardrop and Briedis 1991). Editing (nontemplated addition of guanosine (G) ribonucleosides) is an intrinsic activiy of the MeV polymerase and occurs in about 50 percent of the P mRNAs. Additionally, an extremely low abundant protein, termed R, was reported to be expressed from the P mRNA and this required frameshifting (Liston and Briedis 1995). As a pecularity of the morbilliviruses, an approximately 1 kb GC-rich region separates the M and the F ORFs. While several ORFs have been predicted for this region, these could only be accessed by translation from a rare bicistronic transcript via ribosomal reinitiation. None of the putatively encoded proteins has yet been detected in infected cells.

MeV structural and nonstructural proteins

Since its first isolation, dissection of the MeV structure and replication strategy has been greatly aided by the development of tissue culture systems, the availability of monoclonal antibodies and, in particular, the availability of molecular biological approaches and techniques. The definition of MeV protein functions in more detail has long been limited by the lack of a system that allows a reverse genetic approach. As for other members of the *Mononegavirales*, plasmid-based systems to rescue infectious MeV in tissue culture have been developed and allow the introduction of stable alterations into the viral genome (Combredet et al. 2003; Radecke et al. 1995; Schneider et al. 1997; Takeda et al. 2000).

The viral RNP and nonstructural proteins

The N (nucleocapsid) protein (60 kDa; 525 amino acids (aa)), the most abundant of the MeV proteins, fully encapsidates the genomic RNA and this is the unique target for the viral polymerase to initiate transcription and replication. The protein is phosphorylated on serine and threonine residues (Gombart et al. 1995), and possibly tyrosine residues in persistent infections (Segev et al. 1995). It acts to condense the viral leader containing RNAs into a

smaller, more stable, and more readily packaged form. This gives the nucleocapsid its helical form and 'herringbone' appearance in the electron micrograph (Figure 34.2). When expressed in the absence of viral RNA, N proteins, having undergone conformational maturation, aggregate into nuclear and cytoplasmic nucleocapsid-like structures. The N-terminal 398 amino acids are required for self-aggregation (Bankamp et al. 1996; Spehner et al. 1997) (Figure 34.3), while the C-terminal 125 residues are located outside the nucleocapsid. Since it contains a nuclear localization signal, N can be transported into the nucleus. The formation of high affinity protein complexes with the phosphorylated P (for which two noncontiguous domains (aa 4–188 and 304–373) are essential) prevents both nuclear translocation and self-aggregation of N proteins and encapsidation of cellular RNAs during replication of the viral genome (Bankamp et al. 1996; Huber et al. 1991). In addition, there is evidence for the formation of N/V complexes (Tober et al. 1998) (Figure 34.3). N protein also interacts with cellular proteins. A regulatory domain interacting with Hsp72 has been mapped within the C-terminal 24 amino acids of N, and this may be important for the enhancing effect of heat shock on MeV replication (Vasconcelos et al. 1998; Zhang et al. 2002). Moreover, direct interaction of N protein with IRF-3 and an IRF-3-associated virus-activated kinase may be involved in regulating interferon production during infection (Ten Oever et al. 2002) (Figure 34.3).

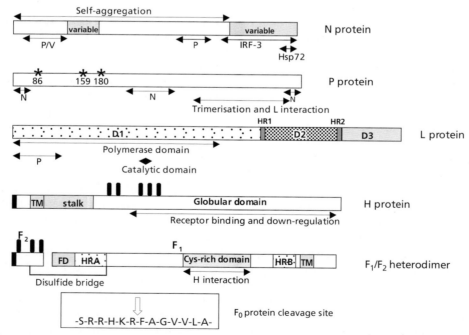

Figure 34.3 *Schematic representation of the major MeV structural proteins. Functional domains or those identified as essential for complex formation with MeV or cellular proteins are indicated by arrows. Phosphorylation sites within the P protein are indicated as asterisks, gylcosylation sites within the F and H proteins are marked. The sequence of the cleavage site within the F_0 protein precursor is indicated at the bottom. D1–D3, domains 1–3 within the L protein; FD, fusion domain; HRA and HRB, heptad repeat domain A and B; HR1, HR2, hinge region 1 and 2 separating domains within the L protein; Hsp72, heat shock protein 72; IRF-3, interferon response factor 3; TM, transmembrane domain.*

The P protein (72 kDa; 507 aa) is abundant in the infected cell, and only small amounts are packaged into virions. The protein is phosphorylated on serine residues 86, 151, and 180 most likely by the cellular casein kinase II (Das et al. 1995). As for the N protein, phosphorylation on tyrosine residues may occur in persistent infection (Ofir et al. 1996). Phosphorylation of P protein is essential for its function as polymerase cofactor. The protein oligomerizes into homotrimers via a predicted coiled-coil region in its carboxy-terminal domain (Curran et al. 1995; Harty and Palese 1995). Domains important for the interaction with the N protein reside in both the amino and carboxy terminus (Harty and Palese 1995), while a small central region (aa 204–321) was also found essential for the ability of P protein to induce N protein redistribution (Huber et al. 1991). Equally important for both transcription and replication, stable complexes between P and L have to be formed, and apparently L protein is stabilized by this interaction. Moreover, P is thought to act as *trans*-activator regulating L protein functions (Horikami and Moyer 1995) (Figure 34.3).

The diffusely distributed cytoplasmic V protein (46 kDa) is expressed from P mRNAs edited by insertion of a nontemplated G residue at position 751 after three genomically encoded Gs (Cattaneo et al. 1989a; Wardrop and Briedis 1991). As V protein shares the aminoterminal 231 amino acids with the P protein, it is also phosphorylated at the very same serine residues and is capable to form complexes via this domain with the N protein, but not to oligomerize or form complexes with the L protein (Liston et al. 1995; Tober et al. 1998). Its 68 amino-acid unique C-terminal domain is cysteine-rich and has zinc-binding properties (Cattaneo et al. 1989a; Liston and Briedis 1994).

The highly basic C protein (28 kDa) is also translated from the P mRNA by usage of a initiator codon 19 nucleotides downstream from that for P (Bellini et al. 1985). There is no evidence for its interaction with other MeV proteins, however both V and C proteins may interact with as yet undefined cellular proteins (Liston et al. 1995). The role of C and V proteins in MeV replication is uncertain. Recombinant MeV in which these reading frames were ablated can be rescued and efficiently amplified in standard cell cultures (Radecke and Billeter 1996; Schneider et al. 1997). These proteins may, however, regulate transcription and/or replication in specialized cell types and in MeV pathogenicity in vivo (Escoffier et al. 1999; Patterson et al. 2000; Tober et al. 1998; Valsamakis et al. 1998). As seen with C and/or V proteins of closely related viruses (Goodbourne et al. 2000), recent studies document that the nonstructural MeV proteins efficiently interfere with signaling via the IFN-α/β, and possibly also the IFN-γ, receptor (Palosaari et al. 2003; Shaffer et al. 2003; Takeuchi et al. 2003; Yokota et al. 2003).

The L protein (220 kDa; 2 183 aa) is expressed at low levels in infected cells and packaged into virions in only catalytic amounts. It is a multifunctional RNP-specific RNA polymerase producing mRNAs, replicative intermediates and progeny viral genomic RNAs (Bankamp et al. 2002). It also has multiple enzymatic activities (see also Chapter 33, General properties of the Paramyxoviruses). Common to RNA polymerases, it contains a conserved duplicated GDDD motif flanked with hydrophobic residues (Bankamp et al. 1999; Blumberg et al. 1988). The polymerases of the *Mononegavirales* may function as multidomain proteins, and three well-conserved domains (D1, D2, and D3) which are linked by two variable hinges (H1 and H2) were defined by sequence alignments (Figure 34.3). Interestingly. D3 apparently enjoys a limited conformational independence from the other domains, since insertion of foreign reading frames into H1, but not H2, abolished replication of recombinant MeV (Duprex et al. 2002). Physical interaction with its co-factor, the P protein, requires the presence of the N-terminal 408 amino acids of the L protein.

The envelope proteins

The RNP core structure is surrounded by a lipid envelope with two glycoproteins on its external surface, the hemagglutinin (H) and the fusion (F) protein that are organized as functional complexes and appear as spikes in the EM. Both proteins are also expressed on the surface of infected cells. The H protein mediates viral attachment to receptors on the surface of target cells and also assists the F protein in causing fusion. Both proteins are protease-sensitive, as virions appear smooth under the EM following protease treatment. They can be isolated by gentle detergent lysis of the virion, although F tends to remain strongly associated with actin filaments. The spikes aggregate, presumably via the hydrophobic tails of both proteins which normally anchor them in the lipid bilayer.

The H protein, a type II glycoprotein, can be isolated as a tetrameric complex from the cell membrane. Analogous with the structure of the NDV HN protein, the ectodomain of the MeV H protein is thought to be organized into a membrane proximal stalk and a membrane distal globular head region composed of a six wing propeller structure (Crennell et al. 2000; Langendijk et al. 1997). It is folded and dimerized in the ER (Plemper et al. 2001a). Amongst the 13 strongly conserved cysteine residues within its ectodomain residues 287, 300, 381, 394, 494, 579, and 583 (all located within the globular domain) were found essential for oligomerization and folding (Hu and Norrby 1995). Moreover, cysteine 154 in the stalk region is essential for the formation of disulfide-linked dimers (Plemper et al. 2000; Santiago et al. 2002). Five potential glycosylation sites, four of which are used, are bunched within a region of 70 amino acids (aa 168–238), and glycosylation was found to be essential for proper folding, export from the Golgi, antigenicity, and hemadsorption, probably by stabilizing the highly complex tertiary structure of the protein (Figure 34.3). Amino acids important for the differential interaction of MeV strains with their cellular MeV receptors, CD46 and CD150, respectively, which include aa 451, 481, 546, and 473–477, also map within the H protein ectodomain (Bartz et al. 1996, 1998; Hsu et al. 1998; Lecouturier et al. 1996; Patterson et al. 1999). In addition to its receptor binding function, H exerts a helper function in F-mediated membrane fusion probably by directing the fusion domain into the optimal distance to the target cell membrane and stabilizing the interaction (Nussbaum et al. 1995). The cytoplasmic domain of the H protein was found to be important for efficient cell surface transport of the molecule and harbors a basolateral sorting signal (Moll et al. 2001, 2002).

The F protein, a type I glycoprotein, is synthesized as inactive precursor (F_0; 60 kDa) from a mRNA which contains an up to 585-nt long 5′ noncoding GC-rich region that is thought to regulate its translational efficiency (Wild and Buckland 1995). The protein is glycosylated, oligomerizes, and is transported to the surface. The precursor is biologically activated by proteolytic cleavage at a conserved multibasic site (aa 108–112) by a subtilisin-like protease resident in the trans-Golgi to yield a disulfide-linked, biologically active F_1 (40kD)/F_2 (18 kDa) heterodimer (Bolt and Pedersen 1999; Sato et al. 1988). Glycosylation of the F_0 precursor is an essential prerequisite for cleavage and transport, and all potential N-glycosylation sites (aa 29, 61, and 67) reside within the F_2 subunit (Wild and Buckland 1995) (Figure 34.3). Because they most likely alter the conformation of this subunit, mutations of any of these sites affect cell surface transport, proteolytic cleavage, stability, and fusogenic activity of the F protein (Hu et al. 1995). The F_1 subunit reveals a topography typical for type I fusion proteins with an amino-terminal stretch of hydrophobic residues (the fusion domain), and two amphipatic α-helical domains, one of which is adjacent to the fusion domain, the other (containing a leucine-zipper motif) N-terminal of the transmembrane region (Bellini et al. 1994; Lambert et al. 1996). A central, cysteine-rich region (aa 337–381) is thought to mediate interaction with the H protein (Fournier et al. 1997; Wild and Buckland 1995) (Figure 34.3). Homo- and hetero-oligomerization of both glycoproteins takes place in the ER (Plemper et al. 2001b), and the strength of the F/H interaction and the fusogenic activity of the complex are also influenced by their cytoplasmic tails, both independent and dependent of their interaction with the M protein (Moll et al. 2001, 2002; Plemper et al. 2001a). Interestingly, the 33-aa long cytoplasmic tail of the F_1 subunit is frequently mutated in persistent infections (Billeter and Cattaneo 1994).

The M protein The M protein (37 kDa), translated from a mRNA with a 400 nt 3′ noncoding region (Bellini

et al. 1986), is found associated with nucleocapsids and the inner layer of the plasma membrane in infected cells (Bellini et al. 1994; Griffin and Bellini 1996). Interaction of M protein with the cytoplasmic domains of one or both MeV glycoproteins has been documented in physical and functional terms (Naim et al. 2000; Plemper et al. 2001b). Thus, M protein was found to modulate the fusogenic activity of the F/H complex (Cathomen et al. 1997a,b) and interactions of M with the glycoprotein cytoplasmic tails allow M-glycoprotein co-segregation from to the apical surface in polarized cells (Naim et al. 2000). Recombinant MeVs carrying deletions of major parts of the M gene bud highly inefficiently thus supporting the initial suggestions that this protein might be essential in this process (Cathomen et al. 1997a). M protein may also negatively regulate MeV transcription when bound to RNPs (Suryanarayana et al. 1994). Mutations within the M reading frame are often found in persistent infections (Billeter and Cattaneo 1994).

THE REPLICATION CYCLE

Receptor interactions and entry

The expression of specific receptors available for the interaction with the MeV H protein on the surface of susceptible target cells is one of the most important determinants of viral tropism. During natural infection, MeV reveals a pronounced tropism for hematopoetic cells, but also enters into and replicates in a variety of cell types as it does in tissue culture. Thus, the receptor should be expressed on most human cells both in vivo and in vitro. This is the case for the first MeV receptor identified CD46 (membrane co-factor protein (MCP)), a member of the 'regulators of complement' (RCA) gene family (Doerig et al. 1993; Naniche et al. 1993) (Figure 34.4 and Table 34.1). CD46 is expressed on all nucleated cells, and is absent from human erythrocytes, which explains why these cannot be agglutinated by MeV H protein. By means of alternative splicing, several isoforms of CD46 are generated from a precursor mRNA in a tissue-specific manner and all of them support MeV uptake (Buchholz et al. 1996a; Johnstone et al. 1993; Manchester et al. 1994). The ectodomain of CD46 consists of four common membrane distal short consensus repeats (SCR 1–4), while the composition of the membrane proximal serine/threonine/proline (STP) segments and the intracellular carboxytermini (Cyt1 and Cyt 2) varies between the CD46 isoforms (Johnstone et al. 1993). CD46 normally binds complement components C3b and C4b via the SCR3 and 4 domains thereby preventing their deposition and formation of an attack complex on the cell surface (Liszewski et al. 1991). In contrast, an extended binding site for MeV H protein maps to SCR 1 and 2 (Casasnovas et al. 1999; Manchester et al. 1995). Glycosylation of these domains is apparently required (Maisner et al. 1994, 1996). The cytoplasmic tail of CD46 is dispensable for its MeV

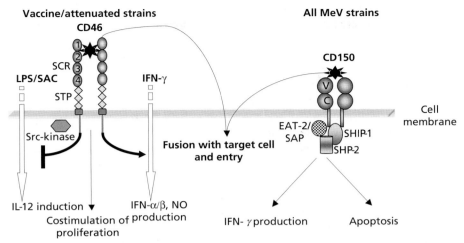

Figure 34.4 *Interaction of measles virus (MeV) with cell-surface receptors and consequences. MeV entry into target cells is supported by CD46 (mainly for attenuated strains) and CD150 (for all MeV strains). Both molecules have signaling properties. Tyrosine phosphorylation of the cytoplasmic domain of CD46 occurs in a Src family kinase-dependent manner, and CD46 ligation by MeV has been linked to enhancement of interferon γ (IFN-γ)-primed release of IFN-α/β and of NO production in CD46-transgenic murine monocytes. CD46-ligation can also suppress lipopolysaccharide (LPS) or* Staphylococcus aureus *Cowan strain I (SAC)-stimulated release of interleukin 12 (IL-12) from monocytes. Ligation of CD150 by specific antibodies triggers its activation, and the subsequent signaling is dependent of the presence of adaptor molecules such as SAP (for signaling lymphocyte activation molecule (SLAM)-associated protein) in T and natural killer (NK) cells and EWS/FLI1- associated transcript 2(EAT-2) in antigen-presenting cells. Triggering of CD150 is involved in recruitment and/or activity of phosphatases with protein (SHP-2; or Src-homology domain 2 (SH2)-domain-containing inositol phosphatase) or dual (SHIP-1; both protein and phospholipid) specificity, and in the induction of IFN-γ or cellular apoptosis. Established consequences of MeV-dependent regulation of signaling by CD150- or CD46-mediated signaling are indicated in plain text and those which have not yet been shown to be exerted by MeV in italics.*

receptor function (Varior-Krishnan et al. 1994), it has, however, signaling properties (Figure 34.4). MeV infection of cells of expression of H protein alone leads to CD46 down-regulation (Bartz et al. 1996; Krantic et al. 1995; Lecouturier et al. 1996; Schneider-Schaulies et al.

1996). Although CD46 was identified as MeV receptor by all criteria in human cells, transgenic expression of this molecule confered susceptibility to MeV infection in only some rodent cell lines and to intracerebral, but not peripheral infection in rodents indicating that as yet

Table 34.1 *Cellular surface molecules interacting with the MeV H protein*

	CD46	CD150	TLR2
Superfamily	Regulators of complement activity	Immunoglobulins	Pattern recognition receptor
Ectodomain	Four short consensus repeats and a variable number of serine–threonine–proline-rich repeats	One variable and one constant Ig-like domain	Repetitive leucine-rich repeats
Tissue distribution	All nucleated human cells	Activated T and B cells, thymocytes, differentiated monocyte/macrophages and dendritic cells	High on professional antigen-presenting cells
Cellular function	Protection from complement mediated lysis	Regulation of lymphocyte function	Activation of antigen-presenting cells
Endogenous ligand	C3b/C4b complement components	Self-ligand	None
MeV interaction			
Interacting MeV	Mostly vaccine and adapted strains	All MeV strains	MeV wild-type strains
Inhibition with specific antibodies	Yes	Yes	Yes
Regulation of host-cell functions	Yes	Yes	Yes
MeV uptake in transfected CHO cells	Yes	Yes	No

poorly defined determinants, including intracellular factors and possibly interferon, restrict MeV replication (Evlashev et al. 2001; Horvat et al. 1996; Mrkic et al. 1998; Naniche et al. 1993; Niewiesk et al. 1997b; Patterson et al. 2002; Vincent et al. 2002). It became, however, clear that the ability to use CD46 as entry receptor is confined to certain MeV strains, mainly vaccine strains and wild-type strains adapted to growth on Vero cells, while most lymphotropic wild-type strains and fresh isolates fail to interact with and to down-regulate CD46 (Bartz et al. 1998; Hsu et al. 1998). These and all other MeV strains tested as yet attach via their H proteins to CD150, a CD2-like molecule of the Ig superfamily (Erlenhoefer et al. 2001, 2002; Hsu et al. 2001; Minagawa et al. 2001; Ono et al., 2001a,b; Tatsuo et al. 2001) (Figure 34.4 and Table 34.1) with H proteins able to interact with both receptors revealing a higher kinetic binding rate for CD46 (Santiago et al. 2002). Amino acids essentially involved in the interaction of CD150 and the H protein have been mapped (Ohno et al. 2003; Vongpunsawad et al. 2004). CD150 is expressed by activated and memory T and B cells, and immature thymocytes, but not on freshly isolated monocytes and immature dendritic cells, but can, however, be induced on these cells upon stimulation (Aversa et al. 1997; Minagawa et al. 2001). For monocytes, this induction is mediated by interaction of the H protein of wild-type MeV strains with Toll-like receptor 2 (TLR2), which per se does not serve as entry receptor (Bieback et al. 2002) (Table 34.1). As for CD46, the most membrane distal portion of CD150, the V domain, is important for MeV binding (Ono et al. 2001b) (Figure 34.4), and the molecule is also down-regulated by MeV infection or H protein interaction (Erlenhoefer et al. 2001). Amino acids determining differential receptor usage of MeV H mainly include aa 481 and aa 546 and 451 (Bartz et al. 1998; Hsu et al. 1998; Lecouturier et al. 1996; Rima et al. 1997; Schneider et al. 2002). Similar to CD46, the cytoplasmic domain of CD150 has signaling properties (Latour et al. 2001; Mikhalap et al. 1999; Morra et al. 2001) (Figure 34.4). The ability of CD150 to confer susceptibility to MeV wild-type infection of lymphocytes, activated monocytes, and dendritic cells is clearly established (Hsu et al. 2001; Minagawa et al. 2001; Ohgimoto et al. 2001; Schneider et al. 2002; Tatsuo et al. 2001). Although CD150 can be induced on monocytes by TLR2 signaling, the question of how lymphotropic strains can enter into these natural target cells in vivo, the mode of MeV entry in CD150-negative cell types such as endothelial, epithelial (during acute measles), and brain cells (as prerequisite for central nervous system (CNS) persistence) is unknown (McQuaid and Cosby 2002). There is evidence for both low affinity interaction of these strains with CD46 and the existence of additional MeV receptors (Manchester et al. 2002; Takeuchi et al. 2002). For viral entry, interaction of the viral glycoproteins with cell surface molecules other than

the known binding receptors may also be required. A role for both substance P receptors and moesin in this context has been suggested but not clarified (Dunster et al. 1994; Harrowe et al. 1992; Schneider-Schäulies et al. 1995b).

The presence of entry receptors is, however, not the sole determinant of tissue tropism and permissivity, as intracellular factors, particularly those associated with cellular maturation and activation, are also essential. Thus, the rodent adapted CAM strains of MeV (by as yet unknown receptors) and the Edmonston vaccine strain (and recombinant derivatives of this strain, by transgenic CD46) enter into and replicate well in neuronal cells of newborn and suckling, but not adult rodents (Duprex et al. 1999a, 2000; Finke and Liebert 1994; Lawrence et al. 1999, 2000; Liebert et al. 1990; Rall et al. 1997) and this is reflected by differential permissivity of maturing neuronal cultures in vitro (Duprex et al. 2000). MeV permissiveness in these systems is confined to the CNS, while intracellular factors restrict viral replication in most rodent cells in vivo and in vitro (see above). In human hematopoetic cells, viral replication is apparently dependent on cellular activation (Fugier-Vivier et al. 1997; Servet-Delprat et al. 2000b).

Intracellular replication, assembly, and budding

As all members of the *Mononegavirales*, MeV replicates exclusively in the cytoplasm of a permissive host cell. MeV transcription is initiated after specific attachment of the polymerase complex to the alleged promoter located within the 3′ end of the genome (Parks et al. 2001) (Figure 34.1b) and progresses to the 5′ end by transcribing monocistronic mRNAs. The tendency of the polymerase complex to disassociate from and reassociate with the template at the gene boundaries is apparently also controlled by host-cell factors, which is reflected by cell type-specific, differential slopes of the transcription gradient (Cattaneo et al. 1987; Griffin and Bellini 1996; Horikami and Moyer 1995; Schneider-Schaulies et al. 1989, 1995c). In the replication mode, the polymerase complex reads through the intergenic boundaries to yield a copy of the entire viral genome, the replicative intermediate. These full-length plus strands are about 100-fold less abundant than those of negative polarity. As replication requires a continuous supply of N protein, it is dependent on protein synthesis. In spite of the ability of the P protein to retain the N protein in the cytoplasm (Huber et al. 1991), intranuclear inclusion bodies consisting of N protein aggregates are typically seen late in infection. Cytoskeletal components may play a role during measles transcription/replication (Moyer and Horikami 1991). It is, however, likely that they are involved in transport of mature intracellular RNPs initially formed in the perinuclear area to the cell membrane (Duprex et al. 2000). They, or associated proteins, could also be involved in the lateral movement of the MeV glycoproteins in the membrane required for patching and subsequent budding (Lydy et al. 1990). This may particularly refer to recruitment of the H protein into lipid rafts which may serve as platforms for MeV assembly. Upon co-expression with the F protein which has the intrinsic ability lo localize in rafts, the H glycoprotein is dragged into the rafts, and assembly of internal MeV proteins into these membrane domains requires the presence of the MeV genome. Synthesis, oligomerization, and maturation of the MeV glycoproteins has been referred to under MeV structural and nonstructural proteins. A sorting signal within their cytoplasmic domains mediates targeting of both MeV F and H proteins to the basolateral membrane in polarized cells, and interactions of M with the glycoprotein cytoplasmic tails allow M-glycoprotein co-segregation to the apical surface, suggesting a vectorial function of M to retarget the glycoproteins for apical virion release (Moll et al. 2001; Naim et al. 2000). The interaction of the cytoplasmic domains of the glycoprotein with M protein also negatively regulates the fusogenic activity of the complex (Cathomen et al. 1997a; Moll et al. 2001, 2002; Naim et al. 2000), and this may be important in viral spread by cell–cell fusion from the basolateral membrane of polarized epithelial cells and in brain tissue (Cathomen et al. 1997a; Ehrengruber et al. 2002; Moll et al. 2002; Naim et al. 2000). Functional inactivation of the M protein reading frame as often seen in persistent brain infections has thus been proposed to favor transneuronal spread in the absence of infectious virus production, which may occur even independent of the H protein (Duprex et al. 1999b, 2000; Ehrengruber et al. 2002; Lawrence et al. 2000; Patterson et al. 2001). Typically for morbilliviruses, the fusogenic activity of the F/H complex requires two conformational changes within the F protein, one of which is induced upon its proteolytic activation, the second after attachment of the H protein to its respective receptor(s) (Baker et al. 1999; Lamb 1993). The mechanism of budding is unclear, but the ability of M protein to aggregate in a crystalline array could confer upon it the capacity to distort the membrane into an outward-facing bulge, and ultimately to bud off the nucleocapsid inside a small vesicular structure. M is thought to act as a trigger in this process, and the absence of functional M protein has been suggested as a crucial element in persistence of MeV. The time taken for MeV replication in a permissive host cell is variable and becomes shorter as the virus adapts to growth in vitro. The growth of the Edmonston strain in Vero cells, is complete within 6–8 h, while for other strains, particularly fresh isolates, replication times of 7–15 days are not uncommon. Similarly, the alterations of host-cell macromolecule synthesis may vary between individual strains and cell types. Cell loss by fusion usually exceeds that caused by infection, and in some cell types, MeV infection induces apoptosis directly (Auwaerter et al. 1996; Grosjean et al. 1997; Okada et al. 2000).

Persistent infections

Persistent MeV infection can be easily established in tissue culture by several methods including passage of virus at high multiplicity with the generation of defective interfering particles, passage of infected cells in the presence of antibody, cultivating cells surviving lytic infection or infection with replication incompetent strains (Griffin and Bellini 1996). A variety of cell types can be persistently infected by one of these methods and factors favoring establishment of persistency include intrinsic or activation/differentiation-dependent regulation of viral RNA or protein synthesis (Schneider-Schaulies et al. 1992, 1993). Heat shock, IFN-inducible or RNA-binding proteins were found to be involved (Leopardi et al. 1993; Ogura et al. 1988) as were increased levels of cyclic AMP which may correlate with restrictions of MeV replication during neuronal differentiation in vitro and in vivo (Duprex et al. 2000; Schneider-Schaulies et al. 1989, 1993; Yoshikawa and Yamanouchi 1984). Moreover, signaling cascades triggered after interaction of MeV H protein with antibodies were found to further down-regulate MeV RNA synthesis in persistently infected neuronal cells (Schneider-Schaulies et al. 1992). There is, however, also evidence that the ability to establish persistent infection may depend on the MeV strain, which, in most cases, is produced in very limited amounts from persistently infected cells (Cattaneo et al. 1988b). In these viruses, mutations within the envelope protein genes lead to production of unstable or functionally impaired proteins (Billeter and Cattaneo 1994; Rima et al. 1995; Schneider-Schaulies et al. 1995c). Cellular protein synthesis is relatively unaffected by persistent MeV infection, although signaling cascades may be altered and specific cellular surface proteins down-regulated (Barrett et al. 1985; Meissner and Koschel 1995; Ofir et al. 1996; Schneider-Schaulies et al. 1992; Segev et al. 1994, 1995). Multinucleated giant cells due to cellular fusion are absent from these cultures, and this is consistent with stable down-regulation of the MeV H receptors from the cell surface (Bartz et al. 1996; Krantic et al. 1995; Schneider-Schaulies et al. 1996).

Measles genotypes

MeV is a serologically monotypic virus. Neutralizing antibody elicited to the Edmonston vaccine strain of measles virus is capable of neutralizing wild-type virus both in vitro and in vivo. With the advent of nucleic acid sequencing methods, regions of genetic variability along the measles genome have been defined (Rima et al. 1995) and exploited for use in what is currently known as 'molecular epidemiology.' The concept is very similar to that used to monitor polio control and eradication efforts. Maximum variability between strains of measles virus was observed within the last 450 nucleotides of the *N* gene, with as much as 12 percent nucleotide variability having been noted. The sequences of this region of the *N* gene and, when finer resolution is necessary, those encoding the entirety of the *H* gene, form the basis of differentiating lineages of wild-type and vaccine strains of MeV (Rota et al. 1996). In 1998, the World Health Organization (WHO) convened a meeting to establish a standard nomenclature for strain assignation. For molecular epidemiologic purposes, the genotype designations are considered the operational taxonomic unit, while related genotypes are grouped by clades (WHO 1998). WHO currently recognizes eight clades designated A, B, C, D, E, F, G, and H. Within these clades, there are 22 recognized genotypes. Genotypes are designated A, B1, B2, B3, C1, C2, D1, D2, D3, D4, D5, D6, D7, D8, D9, E, F, G1, G2, G3, H1, and H2. Some clades contain only a single genotype and, in such cases, the genotype designation is the same as the clade name. Other clades, such as clade D, contain multiple genotypes, and are designated by using the clade letter (in upper case) and genotype number (for example, D1, D2). Several of the genotypes, E, F, G1, D1, appear to be extinct or inactive, and representatives of these have not been isolated for at least 15 years. However, the sequences of the inactive genotypes are maintained in the set of WHO reference sequences for completeness (WHO 2001).

Genetic characterization of measles viruses has proven to be a powerful adjunct to the standard epidemiologic techniques that are used to study the transmission of measles. Genotyping data help suggest or confirm putative sources of virus or suggest a source when one is not obvious from epidemiological data. Genotypic data can also help to establish or to refute putative links between spread cases and outbreaks. Molecular surveillance is most beneficial when it is possible to observe the change in viral genotypes over time in a particular region because this information, when analyzed in conjunction with standard epidemiologic data, has helped to document the interruption of transmission of endemic measles. Thus, molecular characterization of MeVs has provided a valuable tool for measuring the effectiveness of measles control programs (Rota and Bellini 2003; Rota et al. 2004).

Vaccine strains differ from the wild-type isolates, and SSPE-derived sequences are much more similar to those seen in wild-type viruses. Based on these sequence similarities, it has been possible to identify wild-type MeVs having circulated in a given population as likely infectious agents found later in SSPE brain material. These findings resulted in two important conclusions: firstly, SSPE develops after infection with a wild-type MeV and not following vaccination, and secondly, circulating wildtype viruses, and not particular neurotropic strains, initially infect the CNS. So far, evidence indicates that measles is an antigenically stable virus and that the development of complications is not determined solely by the virus. Susceptibility of the host, age, and immune status at the time of infection, and

possibly other factors, are almost certainly more significant than the invading virus. There is, however, no evidence to suggest that the currently used vaccines are not able to control MeV infection with viruses of differing genotypes.

CLINICAL AND PATHOLOGICAL ASPECTS

Acute measles

Measles, an inevitable disease of childhood prior to the vaccine era, has been studied in detail and clinical features are well documented. The course of acute measles is illustrated diagrammatically in Figure 34.5. The virus is acquired via the upper respiratory tract, with tracheal and bronchial epithelial cells being important targets (Sakaguchi et al. 1986). Subsequently the virus reaches the draining lymph nodes from where, after a first round of amplification, it spreads to the rest of the reticuloendothelial system and respiratory tract through the blood (primary viremia). Giant cells containing inclusion bodies (Warthin–Finkeldy cells) are formed in lymphoid tissue and also on the epithelial surfaces of the trachea and bronchi. About 5 days after initial infection, the virus overflows from the compartments in which is has previously been replicating. The viremic spread of MeV to a variety of organs occurs almost completely cell-associated (by infected lymphocytes and monocytes (Esolen et al. 1993; Schneider-Schaulies et al. 1991) with little evidence of plasma viremia (Forthal et al. 1992). Consequently, MeV can be reisolated from the cellular, but usually not the cell-free fraction of blood samples before and at the time of the rash, and this is greatly assisted upon mitogen activation of the cells. MeV spreads to numerous organs (including viscera, bladder, kidney, and skin) where it replicates primarily in endothelial cells, epithelial cells and monocyte/macrophages. Giant cells are formed in all infected tissues, where lymphoid hyperplasia and inflammatory mononuclear cell infiltrates are characteristically seen. Infection of endothelial cells in small vessels is accompanied with vascular dilatation, increased permeability, and inflammation. After about a 10–14 days clinically latent incubation period, the patient enters the prodromal phase which lasts about 2–4 days. Infection-mediated destruction of cells of the thin epithelia of the respiratory tract and conjunctiva lead to the symptoms then observed. These consist of fever, malaise, sneezing, rhinitis, congestion, conjunctivitis, and cough, and a transitory rash can sometimes develop which has an urticarial or macular appearance, which disappears prior to the onset of the typical exanthema. At this time giant cells are present in the sputum, nasopharyngeal secretions, and urinary sediment cells (Katz 1995). Virus is present in blood and secretions, and the patient is

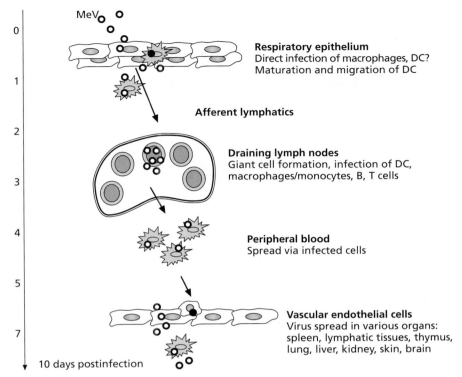

Figure 34.5 *Schematic representation of MeV (indicated by dots) uptake and dissemination.*

highly infectious. During this period Koplik's spots (raised spots with white centers, 1–3 mm, on an erythematous base), the pathognomonic enanthema of measles, appear on the buccal and lower labial mucosa opposite the lower molars. These begin to fade some 2–4 days after the onset of the prodromal phase as the rash develops.

The distinctive maculopapular rash appears about 14 days after exposure and starts behind the ears and on the forehead, then spreads within 3 days to involve the face, neck, trunk, and upper and lower extremities. The rash can become confluent, especially on the upper body and, once the entire body is covered, fades on the 3rd or 4th day. Histologically, the rash is characterized by vascular congestion, edema, epithelial necrosis, and round cell infiltrates. MeV antigen is absent from the spot and rash lesions, but is concentrated near blood vessels and in the endothelial cells of the dermal capillaries. The containment of infection in the skin is thought to be due to the development of cytotoxic T cells and to interferon production. As the rash results from accumulated damage to the vascular walls caused by this DTH reaction, it is often not observed in the immunosuppressed. Respiratory manifestations develop on the basis of diffuse mucosal inflammation in response to widespread MeV infection of epthelial cells and consequent inflammation of the lower respiratory tract. Gastrointestinal symptoms, mainly diarrhea, are common, while electrocardiographic abnormalities seen in about 30 percent of children with uncomplicated measles

usually remain clinically insignificant. Although cerebrospinal fluid (CSF) pleocytosis and EEG changes are frequently seen in uncomplicated measles, neurologic disease in the course of, or after, measles is considered a complication rather than a pathognomonic finding. Once the exanthem has reached its height, the fever usually falls and the conjunctivitis as well as the respiratory symptomatology begins to subside. Antibody titers rise and virus shedding decreases from this point. Normally, the patient shows a rapid improvement. Continuation of clinical symptoms of the respiratory tract or fever suggests complications. On rare occasions, measles follows a hemorrhagic course, and this is characterized by high fever, seizures, delirium, respiratory distress, and hemorrhage into the skin and mucous membranes. In partially immune children, which include those with residual maternal antibodies or individuals who have received immune globulin as post exposure prophylaxis, measles can follow a special course, referred to as modified measles. Occasionally, this infection has also been seen in the course of live vaccine failure. It is usually characterized by a prolonged incubation period, mild prodrome, and sparse, discrete rash of short duration, and mild illness.

Atypical measles

This form of a measles was observed after incomplete measles vaccination prior to the exposure to natural MeV. The majority of reported cases received either several doses of inactivated vaccine or a combination of inactivated vaccine followed by live-attenuated vaccine. The formalin-inactivated vaccine was administered in the United States from 1963 to 1967, and was withdrawn from the market soon after notification of the first cases of atypical measles (Clements and Cutts 1995). Therefore, this disease which was commonly associated with edema of the extremities and frequently with lobular or segmental pneumonia (accompanied by pleural effusion, which results in respiratory distress with dyspnea) is no longer seen. Its pathogenesis is still not fully understood. Hypotheses put forward included abnormally intense cellular immune responses, the inability of the inactivated vaccine to induce local respiratory tract immunity, and lack of production of F-specific antibodies allowing viral spread from cell to cell in the presence of neutralizing antibodies (Merz et al. 1980). As revealed more recently in macaques, the inactivated vaccine fails to induce affinity maturation of complement-fixing antibodies and the disease most likely results from a boosted anamnestic response and is mediated by immune-complex formation and eosinophilia in the presence of fusion-inhibiting antibodies (Polack et al. 1999, 2003).

Complications of measles infection

Complications of acute measles are relatively rare, and the majority results from opportunistic secondary infection of necrotic surfaces, such as those in the respiratory or gastrointestinal tract. Bacteria and other viruses can invade to cause pneumonia or other complications such as otitis media, bronchitis, or severe forms of diarrhea. The most severe complications caused directly by MeV are giant cell pneumonia and measles inclusion body encephalitis (MIBE), both of which occur in the immunocompromised patient, as well as postinfectious encephalitis (PIE) and subacute sclerosing panencephalitis (SSPE) in which no underlying susceptibility factor has been identified. Other unusual manifestations which may complicate acute measles are myocarditis, pericarditis, hepatitis, appendicitis, mesenteric lymphadenitis, and ileocolitis. If measles infection occurs during pregnancy spontaneous abortions or stillbirth may occur as well as an increased rate of low birth-weight infants. Congenital malformations have also been reported.

RESPIRATORY COMPLICATIONS

Symptomatic giant cell pneumonia is seen primarily in the immunocompromised due to unlimited and massive spread of virus to the lower respiratory tract (Breitfeld et al. 1973; Pullan et al. 1976). It is, however, mainly due to secondary bacterial and viral infections that most cases of severe pneumonia complicating measles and leading to chronic pulmonary diseases develop on the

basis of the immunosuppression associated with measles (Gremillion and Crawford 1981; Katz 1995).

NEUROLOGICAL COMPLICATIONS

Postinfectious encephalitis (PIE) and measles inclusion body encephalitis

Transient EEG abnormalities as observed in some patients with acute measles suggests CNS involvement is not uncommon, although it is still a matter of controversy of whether and how MeV may reach this compartment. Acute postinfectious encephalitis (PIE) during the course of measles is a severe complication and is reported in approximately 0.1 percent of cases. In general, about 15 percent of cases are fatal, and 20–40 percent of those who recover are left with lasting neurological sequelae. Encephalitis usually develops when exanthem is still present within a period of 8 days after the onset of measles, but occasionally during the prodromal stage. PIE is characterized by resurgence of fever, headache, vomiting, seizures, cerebellar ataxia, and coma. In common with PIE induced by other viruses, this condition reveals perivascular cuffing, gliosis, and the appearance of fat-laden macrophages near the blood vessel walls and demyelination consistent with immunopathology (Gendelman et al. 1984). CSF findings in measles encephalitis consist usually of mild pleocytosis and absence of measles antibodies. Longterm sequelae include selective brain damage with retardation, recurrent convulsive seizures, hemi-, and paraplegia. Since there is little evidence for MeV RNA or antigen in the brain (Gendelman et al. 1984; Moench et al. 1988), PIE is most likely due to virus-induced autoimmunity to brain antigens (Johnson et al. 1984). In CSF specimens of PIE patients, myelin basic protein (MBP) was detected as a consequence of myelin breakdown and PIE patients and experimentally infected animals may exhibit a proliferative T-lymphocyte response to MBP (Johnson et al. 1984; Liebert et al. 1988). Since PIE is characterized by demyelinating lesions in association with blood vessels as in experimental allergic encephalitis, an MBP-specific lymphoproliferative response in measles infection is considered to be of pathogenetic importance. Mechanisms involved in triggering a T cell-mediated autoimmune response are unknown, and may include molecular mimicry or a deregulation of autoreactive cells occurring secondary to viral infections of lymphocytes.

As measles inclusion body encephalitis (MIBE) only develops in immunosuppressed patients, mainly in children with leukemia undergoing axial radiation therapy (Bitnun et al. 1999; Roos et al. 1981), it can be regarded as an opportunistic MeV CNS infection. In contrast to PIE, viral RNA and antigens are abundant in post mortem brain tissue (Baczko et al. 1988; Bitnun et al. 1999; Roos et al. 1981). The incubation period ranges from a few weeks to 6 months, and the patients often present without a rash. The condition commences with convulsions, mainly myoclonic jerks, and is frequently confused with subacute sclerosing panencephalitis (SSPE). The seizures are often focal and localized to one site. Other findings include hemiplegia, coma, or stupor depending on the localization of the infectious disease process within the CNS. The disease progresses much faster than SSPE and death occurs within weeks or a few months. No or only low titers of MV-specific antibodies are detectable in the CSF.

Subacute sclerosing panencephalitis (SSPE)

SSPE, a fatal, slowly progressing degenerative CNS disease is seen in children and young adults usually 6–8 years after measles, although it can also occur up to 20–30 years after primary infection. Boys are more likely to develop SSPE, but the overall incidence is low (about 2–7 cases per 100 000 of acute measles). Half of the SSPE patients have contracted measles before the age of 2 years, and no unusual features of acute measles have ever been demonstrated. SSPE starts with generalized intellectual deterioration or psychological disturbance which may last for weeks to months and only be recognized as illness until more definite signs appear. These are neurological or motor dysfunctions, such as dyspraxia, generalized convulsions, aphasia, visual disturbances, or mild, repetitive simultaneous myoclonic jerks. The invasion of the retina by MeV leads, in 75 percent of cases, to a chorioretinitis of the macular area followed by blindness. The disease proceeds to progressive cerebral degeneration leading to coma and death within 1–3 years; more rapid forms are, however also known (Katz 1995).

Neuropathologically, a diffuse encephalitis affecting both the white and the gray matter is observed, characterized by perivascular cuffing, diffuse lymphocytic infiltration, and gliosis. Fibrous astrocytes, neurons, and oligodendroglial cells contain massive amounts of intranuclear inclusion bodies (Cowdry bodies), which contain MeV nucleocapsid structures, while giant cell formation or membrane changes consistent with virus maturation or release are not seen (Budka et al. 1982). The lesions lead to characteristic, pathognomonic EEG changes consisting of periodic high-amplitude slow wave complexes, which are synchronous with myoclonic jerks recurring at 3.5–20-s intervals and are remarkably stereotyped. They are bilateral, usually synchronous, symmetrical, consist of two or more delta waves with bi- or polyphasic appearance and may disappear as the disease progresses. Another pathognomonic finding is the state of humoral hyperimmunity against MeV in serum and CSF. The isotypes of MeV-specific antibodies found in CSF include IgG, IgA, and IgD, and in this compartment the immune response is of restricted heterogeneity (Doerries et al. 1988). For diagnostic purposes, determination of measles antibody in the CNS may be sufficient with, if necessary, demonstration of MeV-specific heterogeneity by isoelectric focusing in combination with an immunoblot technique.

OTHER CHRONIC DISEASES

Unlike its clear role in the etiology of the diseases outlined above, MeV has also been implicated in the pathogenesis of Paget's disease (Basle et al. 1986), chronic active hepatitis (Robertson et al. 1987), multiple sclerosis (Allen and Brankin 1993; Haase et al. 1981), and Morbus Crohn (Uhlmann et al. 2002). For each of these diseases an etiological link to measles or measles vaccination is controversial and for none has a definite role for MeV been identified (Birch et al. 1994; Duclos and Ward 1998; Moench et al. 1988).

PATHOGENESIS OF MEASLES AND PERSISTENT MeV CNS INFECTIONS

MeV can replicate in a variety of tissues, including cells of the immune system, and its interaction with the immune system is responsible for some of the key features of the disease. A DTH reaction is implicated in the production of the rash and the ability of the virus to cause a transient, generalized immunosuppression accounts to a major extent for complications associated with acute measles.

The study of MeV pathogenesis in animal models is almost exclusively confined to nonhuman primates which are permissive for intranasal MeV infection and develop disease which shares important features with that seen in humans (van Binnendijk et al. 1995). Attempts to induce measles-like disease in small animals by this route have largely failed (Liebert and Finke 1995). In rodents, MeV replication is impaired due to intracellular restriction as both rats and mice genetically engineered to express CD46, one of the MeV receptors, fail to replicate the virus after peripheral infection (Niewiesk et al. 1997b). Intracerebral infection of small rodents, both transgenic and nontransgenic, has, however, significantly contributed to the understanding of MeV CNS pathogenesis (Liebert and Finke 1995). For unknown reasons, cotton rats reveal a certain permissivity to intranasal MeV infection (Wyde et al. 1992), and, as with acute measles, experimental infection of these animals is accompanied by features compatible with immunosuppression.

Acute measles

MeV receptor interactions in pathogenesis

The usage of cellular receptors, which are discussed under The replication cycle, is an important aspect of MeV pathogenesis. Both CD46 and CD150 are down-regulated from the cell surface after contact with their respective interacting MeV H proteins and after infection (Erlenhoefer et al. 2001; Krantic et al. 1995; Schneider-

Schaulies et al. 1995a). For CD46, at least one consequence of MeV-induced down-regulation is known. Corroborating the 'natural' function of CD46 as a complement regulator, MeV-induced CD46 down-regulation enhances sensitivity to lysis by activated complement of lymphocytes in vitro (Schneider-Schaulies et al. 1996; Schnorr et al. 1995). CD46 can act as a signaling molecule, and ligation of this molecule phosphorylation of tyrosine residues within its cytoplasmic domain 2 occurs in a src family-dependent manner (Wang et al. 2000) (Figure 34.4). Coligation of CD3/CD46 by antibodies enhances T-cell proliferation and activation of signaling molecules, such as by p120[CBL], LAT, CrkL, Vav, Rac, and ERK indicating that CD46 can act as a co-stimulatory molecule (Astier et al. 2000; Zaffran et al. 2001). In CD46 transgenic murine macrophages, MeV-infection induced NO and type I IFN production in the presence of IFN-γ (Katayama et al. 2000) and CD46 ligation by MeV, CD46-specific antibodies or C3b/C4b complement components, interfered with stimulated IL-12 synthesis in monocyte cultures (Figure 34.4) (Karp et al. 1996). Moreover, the ability of CD46-specific antibodies to induce the generation of regulatory T cells in vitro upon CD3 co-ligation has been described (Kemper et al. 2003). Whether this also applies to CD46 ligation by MeV needs to be determined. Consequences of CD150 down-regulation or ligation by MeV remain speculative. Signaling events triggered after ligation of this molecule are complex and can lead to activation but also cellular apoptosis (Mikhalap et al. 1999). Coupling of CD150 to intracellular signaling pathways requires adaptor proteins, such as EAT-2 in antigen-presenting cells (Morra et al. 2001) or SAP in T and NK cells (Latour et al. 2001). In lymphocytes, CD150 ligation by antibodies recruits SHIP-1, a dual specific phosphatase, and thereby regulates recruitment of intracellular signaling molecules (Latour et al. 2001) (Figure 34.4). IFN-γ production from CD4$^+$ T cells can be enhanced upon CD150 ligation (Aversa et al. 1997), and thus it is tempting to speculate that downregulation of this molecule may play a role in impaired Th1 responses as seen in measles (Griffin 1995). Recent evidence, however, suggests that CD150 is more involved in regulating IL-4, rather than IFN-γ, release and thus, consequences of MeV interaction with this molecule remain speculative (Wang et al. 2004).

IMMUNE RESPONSES

MeV induces a marked immune activation as evidenced by spontaneous proliferation of PBMC, polyclonal activation of B cells, expression of activation markers on T cells, and increased plasma levels of cytokines and soluble surface proteins, such as CD4 and IL-2R (Griffin 1995). This activation is co-incident with a generalized immune suppression, and both may continue for many weeks after apparent recovery from measles.

Immune activation

Activation of CD8$^+$ T cells during measles is amply evidenced by proliferation of these cells and the appearance of MeV-specific HLA-restricted CD8$^+$ cytotoxic T lymphocytes in the blood at the time of the rash, some of which develop into CD8 memory cells (van Binnendijk et al. 1990). MeV antigens inducing CD8$^+$ cytotoxic T cells have not been completely identified, however, the F protein is one target for MHC class I-restricted T cells (van Binnendijk et al. 1989). A recent study suggests that the CD8 response plays an important role in the control and clearance of MeV infection (Permar et al. 2003a). CD4$^+$ T cells are also activated in response to MeV infection. Virion protein uptake to an endosomal compartment for subsequent MHC class II-dependent presentation can be triggered by the interaction of H protein with CD46 (Gerlier et al. 1994). CD4$^+$ T cells proliferate during the rash, and classical CD4$^+$ T cell responses such as MeV-antigen-stimulated cytokine production and MHC class II-restricted antigen-specific proliferation are stimulated (Griffin 1995). During the prodrome, plasma levels of IFN-γ, neopterin, and soluble IL-2R rise, followed by elevation of IL-2, soluble CD4, and CD8 at the time of the rash (Griffin et al. 1989, 1992). Subsequently, IL-4 becomes elevated, and this may persist for prolonged periods. This pattern of cytokine production is consistent with an early activation of CD8$^+$ and Th1 CD4$^+$ T cells followed by a predominant Th2 CD4$^+$ T-cell response during recovery (Figure 34.6). Whether or not Th1 responses are less efficiently generated after vaccination has not been entirely resolved (Gans et al. 1999; Griffin and Ward 1993; Schnorr et al. 2001).

Antibodies, which appear at the time of the rash, are initially of the IgM and then switch to IgG1 and IgG4

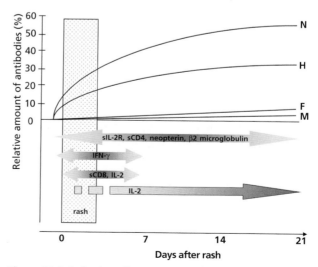

Figure 34.6 *Activation of immune responses during measles. Relative amounts of antibody produced to individual MeV proteins (upper part) and parameters (plasma levels of cytokines and soluble CD4, CD8, IL-2R, and β2 microglobulin, bottom part) in the course of acute measles.*

isotype (Griffin 1995). IgA, IgM, and IgG antibodies are found in secretions. Though antibodies are generated to most viral proteins, the most abundant and rapidly produced antibodies are N-specific (Figure 34.6). Antibodies to the H protein are neutralizing and inhibit agglutination of monkey erythrocytes by MeV by blocking the interaction of H protein with monkey CD46. Antigenicity of the H protein is variable, and up to six major, mainly conformational, epitopes were mapped by competitive binding of monoclonal antibodies (Carter et al. 1983). H-specific antibodies may also inhibit hemolysis, which is, however, a major property of F-specific antibodies. Up to seven linear epitopes within the F protein are recognized by polyclonal sera, and monoclonal F-specific antibodies can cross-react with cellular heat shock proteins (Sheshberadaran and Norrby 1984).

Early nonspecific and innate immunity

Unlike adaptive immunity, the role of early nonspecific and innate immunity in measles is poorly understood. NK-cell activity may be slightly reduced in measles (Griffin and Ward 1990). While production of type I IFN has been documented after vaccination, the production of this cytokine has not been unequivocally observed in patients with measles infections at the time of the rash (Shiozawa et al. 1988). As suggested by recent evidence, MeV vaccine and wild-type strains may also differ in their ability to induce type I IFN and to evade from IFN-mediated control in vitro in PBMC cultures (Naniche et al. 2000). The quality, magnitude, and duration of MeV-specific adaptive immunity is, however, likely to be governed to a major extent by its interaction with professional antigen-presenting cells such as tissue resident macrophages and DCs which reside at or close to its entry sites and fulfill a sentinel, but most likely also a Trojan horse function for MeV transport to the draining lymph nodes. In vitro, both immature and LPS- or CD40-matured DC are infectable with MeV, albeit virus production from pure DC and transmission of virus in DC/T cell co-cultures is very limited (Fugier-Vivier et al. 1997; Grosjean et al. 1997; Klagge et al., 2000; Schnorr et al. 1997b; Servet-Delprat et al. 2000b). There is evidence that wild-type MeV reveal a particular tropism for these cells, which is essentially determined by the interaction of the H protein with CD150 (Ohgimoto et al. 2001; Schnorr et al. 1997b). MeV infection triggers rapid maturation of immature DC as indicated by up-regulation of MHC class II and co-stimulatory molecules, and this again seems to occur more efficiently with certain wild-type strains (Dubois et al. 2001; Klagge et al. 2000; Servet-Delprat et al. 2000b). Cytokines induced in DC as well as in monocytes by MeV infection include IL-1-α/β, IL-1R antagonist, IL-6, TNF-α, type I IFN, and low amounts of IL-12p35 and IL-12p40 (Bieback et al. 2002; Klagge et al. 2000; Schnorr et al. 1997b; Servet-Delprat et al. 2000b),

some of which trigger DC maturation or are directly involved in polarizing ensuing T-cell responses (Figure 34.7a). As outlined under The replication cycle, TLR2 signaling by wildtype MeV is involved in maturation of monocytes (Bieback et al. 2002). Signaling pathways triggered by its activation include the MAP kinases, the Akt kinase, and the NF-κB pathway, and ultimately result in production of proinflammatory cytokines, chemokines, as well as co-stimulatory molecules and CD150 (Aderem and Ulevitch 2000; Bieback et al. 2002). Activation of monocytes and DC is also induced by non-TLR2 agonistic attenuated MeV strains, and this may relate to the ability of intracellular MeV to activate NF-κB directly (Dhib-Jalbut et al. 1999; Hummel et al. 1998). Alternatively, induction of type I IFN does occur particularly with attenuated MeV strains, which, however, again, could be dependent on activation of a TLR, namely TLR3, which recognizes double-stranded RNA (Doyle et al. 2002). Interestingly, TLR3 was found to be up-regulated by laboratory, but not wild-type MeV strains as a consequence of IFN-induction (Tanabe et al. 2003).

MeV-induced immunosuppression

At the same time, when MeV-specific immunity is efficiently generated, a general suppression of responsiveness to other pathogens is established. This was recognized long before the virus was isolated and is the major reason for the constantly high morbidity and mortality rate associated worldwide with acute measles. Typically, patients reveal a marked susceptibility to opportunistic infections and lymphopenia affecting both B and T cells (Okada et al. 2000). The latter is not associated with a decrease in thymic output (Permar et al. 2003b) and may therefore result from lymphocyte depletion due to viral infection, apoptosis or aberrant homing of T cells (Addae et al. 1995; Auwaerter et al. 1996; Nanan et al. 1999; Okada et al., 2000). Immunosuppression, however, is observed up to weeks after the onset of the rash when the lymphocyte counts have returned to normal and MeV-infected cells are, if at all, present with only low frequency (Okada et al. 2001). Key features of MeV-induced immunosuppression are inhibition of DTH responses and a restricted ability of lymphocytes to proliferate in response to recall antigens, as well as polyclonal stimulation (Borrow and Oldstone 1995; Schneider-Schaulies et al. 2001) (Table 34.2). As only a few infected cells are usually detected, several hypotheses have been put forward to explain this finding which include the production of inhibitory factors by infected cells that have not yet been identified (Fujinami et al. 1998). Characteristics of MeV-induced immunosuppression are compatible with deregulation of APC viability and functions, which would be expected to be of significant impact on the induction, efficiency and quality of T-cell responses (Table 34.2). MeV infection causes maturation of immature DC, yet this may be incomplete, and

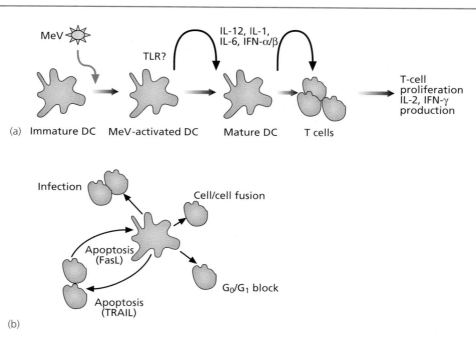

Figure 34.7 *Impact of measles virus (MeV) on dendritic cell (DC) maturation and T-cell activation.* **(a)** *Immature DCs, are activated and mature upon infection or surface interaction with MeV as indicated by up-regulation of MHC and costimulatory molecules and the induction of cytokines, which act as autocrine and paracrine factors further triggering maturation. Both cell–cell contacts and cytokines activate and shape T-cell responses, and this may effectively occur after uptake, processing, and presentation of viral components early after DC infection.* **(b)** *With on-going viral replication, MeV-infected DCs promote DC/T cell fusion and T-cell infection, inhibition of T-cell proliferation by expressing high levels of the MeV glycoprotein complex and T-cell apoptosis by TRAIL expression. DC depletion may result from fusion or FasL-induced apoptosis by T cells.*

Table 34.2 *Characteristic findings related to MeV-induced immuno-suppression*

	Findings
In vivo	Susceptibility to opportunistic infections
	Loss of delayed type hypersensitivity responses
Ex vivo	Leukopenia
	MeV-infected peripheral blood mononuclear cells
	Cytokine imbalance
	Long-term suppression of IL-12 production
	Loss of proliferative responses of lymphocytes
In vitro	
Antigen-presenting cells	Apoptosis and cytotoxicity
	Infection and fusion
	Aberrant terminal maturation
	Suppression of stimulated IL-12 release
B cells	Growth arrest
	Production of inhibitory soluble mediators
T cells	Depletion by aberrant homing and apoptosis
	Production of soluble inhibitory mediators
	Loss of stimulated proliferative responses due to infection or cell-surface signaling by the MeV glycoprotein complex

impaired production of IL-12 from these cells may occur (Atabani et al. 2001; Fugier-Vivier et al. 1997; Servet-Delprat et al. 2000b). The role of IL-12 depletion in MeV-induced immunosuppression is, however, unclear as yet (Hoffman et al. 2003). In MeV-infected DC/T cell cocultures, fusion and apoptosis of both DC and T cells was seen. While the latter has been linked to MeV-mediated upregulation of TRAIL on DC and FasL on T cells (Servet-Delprat et al. 2000a; Vidalain et al. 2000), the first is exerted by the MeV glycoprotein complex expressed on DC at high levels late in infection (Ohgi-moto et al. 2001). It is, however, also evident that MeV-infected DC fail to stimulate allogenic T-cell proliferation and actively inhibit mitogen-stimulated expansion without grossly interfering with the viability of these cells (Fugier-Vivier et al. 1997; Grosjean et al. 1997; Klagge et al. 2000; Schnorr et al. 1997b; Steineur et al. 1998). The inhibitory phenotype of MeV-infected DC has been linked to direct negative signaling to T cells via the MeV glycoproteins rather than to soluble inhibitory mediators (Dubois et al. 2001; Klagge et al. 2000) (Figure 34.7b). Expression of the MeV glycoprotein complex on infected or transfected cells or virions was found necessary and sufficient to induce a state of proliferative unresponsiveness to polyclonal and CD3/CD28 stimulation in lymphocytes (Niewiesk et al. 1997a; Schlender et al. 1996; Schneider-Schaulies et al. 2001).

For this to occur, surface contact of uninfected cells and UV-irradiated virions or cells expressing a complex of H protein and proteolytically activated F protein is required, while soluble inhibitory mediators are not involved (Weidmann et al. 2000a,b) (Figure 34.8a). Contact-mediated inhibition is not associated with the induction of apoptosis, but rather T-cell arrest in the late G_1 phase of the cell cycle as determined by characteristic deregulations in the expression levels and activity of S-phase entry control proteins (Naniche et al. 1999; Niewiesk et al. 1999, 2000; Schnorr et al. 1997a). Not surprisingly, intracellular signaling pathways in T cells are directly targeted by cell surface interaction with MeV. Thus, IL-2- or anti-CD3/CD28-dependent activation of the phosphoinositol-3-kinase/Akt kinase pathway, which is involved in regulating cell cycle control proteins, is disrupted after MeV contact (Avota et al. 2001) (Figure 34.8b). There is evidence that the N protein may also contribute to suppression of lymphocyte functions. It was found to inhibit antibody production in vitro by binding to FcγIIR on B cells (Ravanel et al. 1997), and to induce sustained calcium influx, as well as a G_0/G_1 arrest

of thymic epithelial cells and other cell types (also including lymphocytes) by binding to an unknown, ubiquitously expressed receptor (Laine et al. 2003).

Persistent measles: CNS infections

MEASLES INCLUSION BODY ENCEPHALITIS (MIBE)

As this condition is confined to patients with underlying immunodeficiencies, it is not usually accompanied by intrathecal antibody synthesis. The unprotected cells develop both nuclear and cytoplasmic massive inclusion bodies consisting of virus nucleocapsids (Roos et al. 1981). Infectious virus has only been occasionally isolated by conventional methods from brain tissue, suggesting defects in replication (Baczko et al. 1988, 1993; Ohuchi et al. 1987; Roos et al. 1981). This assumption has been supported by immunohistological and molecular biological studies in MIBE (Baczko et al. 1988). In brain tissue, only N and P, but not the envelope proteins were consistently detected. In

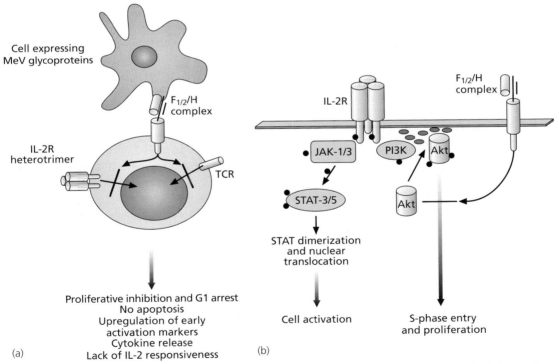

Figure 34.8 *Mechanisms of MeV contact mediated T-cell inhibition and consequences.* **(a)** *The MeV $F_{1/2}$/H complex induces by interaction with an, as yet unknown, receptor proliferative arrest in lymphocytes, which causes their arrest in the G1 phase of the cell cycle. In primary T cells, mitogen-induced expression of activation markers and cytokines is not affected. The IL-2R heterotrimer is expressed to normal levels, yet exogenous IL-2 does restore T-cell proliferation.* **(b)** *Signaling via the interleukin 2 receptor (IL-2R) on T cells involves phosphorylation of the cytoplasmic domains of its β- and γ-subunits. This provides docking sites for the Janus kinases JAK-1/3 which, when autophosphorylated, provide docking sites for and phosphorylate STAT-3 and STAT-5, which then dimerize and translocate to the nucleus. IL-2R signaling also activates phosphatidylinositol 3-kinase (PI3K), which catalyzes phosphorylation of inositol-phosphates. As second messengers, these recruit the Akt kinase to the cell membrane where this kinase is phosphorylated and subsequently regulates the activity of downstream targets. In T cells, this pathway was found to be particularly important for S-phase entry and proliferation. Contact with the MeV $F_{1/2}$/H complex abolishes the IL-2-dependent activation of the PI3K/Akt pathway, but not that of the JAK/STAT pathway.*

contrast, the mRNAs specific for the viral proteins were detectable in brain-derived total RNA samples with the mRNAs for the envelope proteins being under-represented. The latter failed to direct the synthesis of the corresponding proteins in vitro and this restriction was partially explained by a high rate of mutations distributed over the entire MeV genome (Cattaneo et al. 1988a,b; 1989b). Defects in MeV mRNA transcription and envelope protein synthesis apparently did not largely affect the activity of the RNP complex which spread to different areas of the patient's brain. As infectious virus particles may never be formed due to the restriction of the envelope proteins and giant cell formation has never been observed, the spread is thought to occur by microfusion events.

SUBACUTE SCLEROSING PANENCEPHALITIS (SSPE)

MeV was first implicated in the etiology of this disease by immune fluorescence in 1967 and this has since been confirmed by electron microscopy, immunoelectron microscopic (IEM) methods, and finally by the successful rescue of virus by co-cultivation techniques. Despite this, mechanisms underlying the transport of virus into the CNS, establishment and initial maintenance of persistence, and production of disease are still largely unknown. The virus is thought to gain entry to the CNS during viremia in acute measles by infected lymphocytes or infection of cerebral endothelial cells (Kirk et al. 1991; McQuaid and Cosby 2002), but once there, replication most likely proceeds only slowly. It is also not known to what extent virus replication per se is responsible for the development of lesions, or what part is played by the immune system.

Virological aspects

In SSPE, free infectious virus has never been isolated either from the brain or from CSF, and histopathological examinations have consistently failed to reveal the morphological changes associated with virus maturation. As with MIBE, giant cells and thickening of the plasma membrane at points of budding were never seen suggesting the absence of viral glycoproteins. Viral nucleocapsids present in the cytoplasm are randomly scattered and show no sign of regular alignment beneath the plasma membrane. As budding viral particles and infectious virus are not detected, the infection may spread slowly in a strictly cell-associated manner. The ability of MeV to spread transneuronally in the absence of virus production has recently been confirmed in tissue culture and this can occur in the absence of CD46 (Duprex et al. 1999b, 2000; Ehrengruber et al. 2002; Lawrence et al. 2000). Nevertheless, CD46, which is expressed on certain brain cells such as oligodendrocytes and a subset of neurons, is apparently down-regulated

from MeV-positive cells in lesions (McQuaid and Cosby 2002; Ogata et al. 1997).

In SSPE brain sections, only the expression of the MeV N and P proteins and not that of the envelope proteins was consistently detected in infected cells (Liebert et al. 1986). Molecular biological studies on SSPE brain tissue revealed extensive transcriptional and translational alterations affecting mainly MeV envelope-protein specific genes (Baczko et al., 1986, 1988; Cattaneo et al. 1987, 1988b). As in MIBE, mRNAs specific for these genes were detected at only low copy numbers and were highly impaired in directing in vitro protein synthesis. A high rate of mutations was found all over the MeV genome. While the *M* gene was most affected, the *F*, *H*, *P*, and *N* genes were mutated to about the same extent, and the L gene was most conserved (Cattaneo et al. 1988a,b; 1989b). Mutations introduced were either point mutations, or appeared as clustered transitions which are thought to result from the activity of a cellular enzyme complex that actively modifies viral genetic information (Baczko et al. 1993; Cattaneo et al. 1988b). As revealed by detailed analyses, mutated MeV genomes may clonally expand in SSPE (Baczko et al. 1993). As a result of either of these events, translation of viral mRNAs was completely abolished or led to the synthesis of truncated or unstable MeV proteins. With respect to the overall high degree of conservation of the *F* gene within all MeV strains known (Rima et al. 1995), it is remarkable that truncations, mutations or deletions in the cytoplasmic domain of the F protein are almost universal (Billeter and Cattaneo 1994). These findings explain the absence of infectious MeV particles and cell fusion in infected SSPE brain tissue, which both require biologically active MeV envelope proteins. Virus can, however, occasionally be rescued from brain tissue obtained post mortem by cocultivation (Griffin and Bellini 1996). Some of these SSPE isolates have been proven invaluable tools to study virological parameters and specific genetic defects in SSPE, others, however, most likely represent contaminations and are in fact ordinary laboratory MeV strains (Rima et al. 1995). It is still unclear whether true SSPE isolates represent the dominant MeV population in the infected brain or rather small subpopulation of replication/maturation competent viruses or revertants that have been selected by the isolation procedure.

Factors involved in the establishment of persistence by a nondefective MeV in brain tissue are largely unknown. Differential interaction of the M protein with the viral RNP has been suggested for negative regulation of MeV transcription (Suryanarayana et al. 1994). There is, however, evidence that factors intrinsic to the host cell in the brain intimately control and downregulate the efficiency of MeV gene expression. In tissue culture experiments with cells of neural origin and in brain material of experimentally infected animals, evidence has been provided that intracellular factors control the efficiency of

MeV replication (Schneider-Schäulies et al. 1989). These may include unknown factors associated with brain cell differentiation (Schneider-Schäulies et al. 1993; Yoshikawa and Yamanouchi 1984), as well as the type I IFN-inducible MxA protein, which negatively regulates MeV transcription in brain cells, but not in monocytes and fibroblasts (Schneider-Schäulies et al. 1994; Schnorr et al. 1993). In addition, the cellular enzyme activity actively modifying the primary sequence of viral RNAs has been demonstrated in these cells. Thus, intracellular factors present in brain cells act to slow down viral replication after primary infection thereby preventing a rapid host-cell destruction. This may even be enhanced by virus neutralizing antibodies which were found to down-regulate MeV transcription by activating as yet unknown signaling cascades (Schneider-Schaulies et al. 1992; Segev et al. 1994). There is also evidence that MeV may regulate intracellular signaling cascades in a cell type-specific manner since it activates the transcription factor NF-κB in glial, but not neuronal cells (Dhib-Jalbut et al. 1999). Since activation of NF-κB is an essential prerequisite for the induction of most genes associated with cellular defense (such as proinflammatory cytokines), this may interfere with initial control of infection. Differential regulation of cytokines produced in primary and persistently infected glial cells has also been documented (Schneider-Schäulies et al. 1993). Whether these control mechanisms are efficient in establishing and maintaining persistent infection or other factors, such as the introduction of mutations into the viral genome are required, has not been resolved.

Critical components for disease progression and clinical appearance also remain speculative. Infection-induced loss of brain cells is likely to contribute, and this may occur to a certain extent during the asymptomatic phase. Since this is not brought about by giant cell formation, apoptosis as seen in neuronal and macroglial cells both in SSPE brain tissue and experimental CNS infection in mice is likely to be important (Anlar et al. 1999; Manchester et al. 1999). There is, however also evidence from in vitro experimentation that MeV infection does not grossly interfere with brain cell viability, but may specifically target expression of proteins required for luxury functions (Meissner and Koschel 1995).

Immunological aspects

Studies performed in SSPE patients did not reveal any evidence for a global defect in immune responses, which could account for the establishment of a persistent MeV CNS infection. A virus-specific humoral hyperimmune response is pathognomonic for SSPE. There is a significant production of MeV-specific antibodies by plasma cells residing in the CNS leading to marked elevations in the level of CSF immunoglobulin (Connolly et al. 1971). As opposed to the polyclonal response observed in serum, MeV-specific antibodies produced in the CNS are

of restricted heterogeneity leading to the appearance of oligoclonal immunoglobulin bands (Doerries et al. 1988). This suggests that antibody in the CSF is made locally by lymphocytes that have invaded this compartment from the periphery in response to antigens present in the CNS. In serum specimens, antibodies of the IgG and IgD type with specificity to all MeV proteins are present, although recognition of the M protein is low or sometimes absent, whereas antibodies in CSF samples, which are of the IgG, IgA, and IgD types, generally fail completely to detect M protein (Hall et al. 1979). Studies performed on the cellular immunity in SSPE revealed that MeV-specific lymphoproliferation is similar to that of normal measles-seropositive individuals. Similarly, other measures of cellular immunity such as skin test responses to recall antigens and proliferative responses to mitogens are normal (Dhib-Jalbut et al. 1989). The mononuclear inflammatory response in the brain includes CD4+ and CD8+ T cells, monocytes, and Ig-secreting B cells (Nagano et al. 1991). MHC class I and class II expression is increased in the brain, and β2 microglobulin, soluble IL-2R, and soluble CD8 are elevated in CSF (Mehta et al. 1992).

EPIDEMIOLOGY

Measles infections are transmitted via aerosol or droplet exposure generated from a cough or sneeze or via contaminated fomites. The disease is so highly contagious that susceptible individuals who come into close contact with measles patients have a 99 percent probability of acquiring the disease. Measles disease is believed to have emerged as human populations began to organize into larger communities. These communities had sufficient birth cohorts that provided a renewable source of susceptible individuals, thus permitting sustained endemic transmission of the virus within the population. The epidemiology of measles virus differs in unvaccinated versus vaccinated populations. In the prevaccine era, greater than 90 percent of individuals would acquire measles infections before 10 years of age. In unvaccinated populations, measles causes periodic epidemics with interepidemic periods of 2–5 years. These periods decrease as population size and density increase, which is directly related to the availability of susceptible individuals for disease transmission.

In vaccinated populations, the interval between measles outbreaks increases and sufficiently high levels of vaccination can interrupt endemic transmission. With vaccination, the age distribution of cases is determined by which groups are likely to lack vaccine or measles induced immunity. In the United States, an extensive effort to achieve high levels of first dose measles vaccination at 12 to 15 months of age, and addition of a recommended second dose of vaccine in school-aged children has resulted in a decrease in reported measles cases from 400 000 to 500 000 per year in the 1960s to a

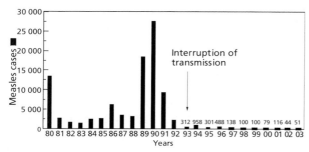

Figure 34.9 *The number of reported cases of measles per year ranging from 1980 to 2003. The arrow indicates the year of interruption of transmission based on no reported cases of measles for a 12-week period in 1993.*

record low of approximately 100 cases per year from 1998 to 2003 (Figure 34.9) (CDC 2004). It is likely that endemic transmission of measles in the United States was interrupted in 1993 and subsequent cases have occurred through periodic introduction of measles from other countries followed by limited spread (Bellini and Rota 1998; Rota et al. 2004). Given widespread international travel, measles will continue to occur even in highly vaccinated populations until global eradication is achieved.

Measles remains a formidable disease of children in many areas of the world. The World Health Organization estimates that over 30 million cases occur annually. Approximately 775 000 measles-associated deaths occur annually worldwide, and about 500 000 deaths occur in Africa alone (WHO 1999). In marked contrast, effective use of available live-attenuated measles vaccines, and a variety of multidose vaccination strategies have combined to eliminate measles in many large geographic regions including the Americas, many Scandinavian countries, and the United Kingdom. The WHO and United Nations Children's Fund have announced a strategic plan aimed at enhancing measles control and reducing global mortality by 50 percent based on the 1999 data by 2005. Most regions of the WHO have established strategic plans and tentative time-lines for measles elimination, but a decision to move to global eradication has not yet been made.

DIAGNOSIS

Before the widespread use of measles-containing vaccines, acute measles was diagnosed on the basis of the distinctive symptoms and laboratory confirmation was seldom necessary. As vaccination programs expand, the diagnostic acumen of many physicians to recognize acute measles has decreased (Helfand et al. 2004). Moreover vaccination itself has led to the emergence of unusual presentations and milder forms of measles. For these reasons and the fact that more patients are either being placed on immunosuppressive regimens, or have immunosuppressive illnesses such as acquired immune deficiency syndrome (AIDS), the need for laboratory diagnosis/confirmation of MeV has increased.

Microscopy

On direct examination, production of multinucleate giant cells with inclusion bodies is pathognomonic for measles during the prodromal phase. Such cells are detectable in the nasopharyngeal secretions (NPS). Clear identification of giant cells and Cowdry inclusion bodies is facilitated if the smear is first fixed in formalin and then stained with hematoxylin or eosin. Both direct and indirect immunofluorescence (IF) have been widely used to stain cells shed in nasal secretions, although it may be necessary to remove antibodies that already coat virus antigens with a low pH buffer. Stained cells include macrophages and ciliated cells, as well as giant cells. Urinary sediment cells have also been examined with a high degree of success. IF-positive cells may be shed in the urine from 2 days before to up to 5 days after the appearance of the rash. This method may therefore be more applicable in later stages than examination of NPS specimens. Such cells may also be present in the urine 4–16 days after vaccination with the live vaccine. IF is useful for the diagnosis of measles in the pre-eruptive phase. Immunoperoxidase histochemical stains have also been used, and the use of monoclonal antibodies has improved sensitivity and reliability of virus detection (Zaki and Bellini 1997).

Serology

In common with other infections, diagnosis of measles may be made if antibody titers rise by more than four-fold between the acute and the convalescent phases or if measles-specific IgM is found. Traditional antibody tests such as hemagglutination inhibition (HI), plaque-reduction neutralization (PRN), and enzyme-linked immunoassay (EIA) have been used extensively in the serologic diagnosis of measles. Because of the availability of sensitive and specific commercial kits, EIA has become the most widely used test format. These tests also have the ability to measure measles-specific IgM, as well as IgG responses and therefore have particular importance in diagnosis as well as measles control programs. Some of the available kits were found to have sensitivities and specificities that compared favorably with plaque reduction neutralization (de Sousa et al. 1991; Ratnam et al. 1995). Most laboratories have trained personnel and are already equipped to run EIA tests.

The recommended laboratory method for the confirmation of clinically diagnosed measles is a serum-based IgM EIA. Several serum-based capture and indirect IgM EIAs are now commercially available for use by public health, clinical, and commercial laboratories and, for the most part, are used worldwide. The network of laboratories within the Pan American Health Organization supported the measles eradication efforts throughout the Americas using EIA as the primary confirmatory assay. The WHO Global Measles Laboratory Network has also recommended the use of the IgM EIA for the laboratory diagnosis of measles. The EIA tests can be done using a single serum specimen, are relatively rapid (2–6 h) and simple to perform, and can be used to diagnose acute measles infection from the time of rash onset until at least 4 weeks after rash onset. Thus, the IgM EIAs fulfill all the basic criteria for the accurate, effective, and efficient diagnosis of measles. Both indirect and IgM capture formats have been used (Erdman et al. 1991; Hummel et al. 1992). Though IgM capture is often regarded as the more sensitive format, studies that have compared the capture and indirect formats found that some of the commercial indirect EIA kits had sensitivities and specificities that equaled those of the capture format (Arista et al. 1995; Ratnam et al. 2000).

Isolation and detection of viral RNA

Until recently, the lack of sensitive cell lines for efficient growth of measles virus made cell culture isolation difficult, even when optimal specimens for virus isolation were available. Previous tissue culture and cell lines, such as primary monkey kidney cells and Vero cells, were considered to be permissive for measles infection. However, it is now recognized that these cells do not possess the appropriate receptor(s) for most wild-type viruses, which explains the low frequency of measles isolation when using these cell types. An Epstein–Barr virus transformed marmoset B lymphocyte cell line (B95a) was demonstrated to be approximately 100 to 1 000 times more sensitive than Vero cells and is currently the cell line of choice for measles virus isolation (Kobune et al. 1990). Attempts at measles isolation indicated that the best success is attained when specimens are collected within 0–5 days of rash onset. Although virus isolation has never been used for routine diagnosis of measles infection, use of the method is encouraged particularly in outbreak settings where there is a requirement for molecular epidemiologic data.

For virus isolation, washings and swabs are collected and mixed with buffered salt solution (pH 7.2) containing antibiotics. Urinary sediment cells are collected by low-speed sedimentation and treated similarly. Measles can be isolated directly from blood, but efficiency is increased if lymphocytes are first separated on a Ficoll gradient and stimulated with mitogen before use. MeV isolated in B95a cells differed in some biological properties from those adapted to Vero cells, suggesting MeV is subject to host cell-mediated selection. It is therefore recommended to include attempts in these cell lines in MeV isolation. Cytopathic effects (CPE) develop usually between 48 h and

15 days, and consist either of a broad syncytium or of a stellate form. Both types reveal inclusion bodies which may be present in both nucleus and cytoplasm. It is not known what governs the different forms of CPE, but the availability of cellular nutrients as well as the type of virus has an effect. Uninoculated identical cultures should also be maintained as controls. If CPE is slow or not clear, it is possible to test whether the cells contain MeV antigens or RNA by appropriate detection methods. RT-PCR-based detection of viral RNA is best applied in specific instances, such as suspected infection of the immunosuppressed in the absence of rash when only limited antiviral immunoglobulins might be expected, developing pneumonia without a rash, or unexplained encephalitis. Finally, both techniques can be attempted as a means of retrospective diagnosis using tissue obtained post mortem. RT-PCR analyses using MeV *N* and/or *F* gene-specific primers are the most commonly performed tests and employ a wide variety of specimens from which RNA is extracted and used as template, including serum, nasopharyngeal aspirates, urine sediment cells. Tissue samples including lung, kidney, skin, and brain are also amenable for testing by RT-PCR following appropriate chaotropic salt treatment and nucleic acid extraction.

Two new approaches show promise in terms of alternatives to specimen collection for the diagnosis of measles: the use of oral fluid and the use of blood spots on filter paper. Oral fluid samples have been used both for detection of measles-specific IgM and IgG, as well as rubella and mumps (Helfand et al. 1996; Perry et al. 1993). This technique is already being used for routine measles surveillance in the UK (Jin et al. 2001). The use of oral fluid samples has appeal because the technique is noninvasive, it can be used for rubella testing, it does not require processing of the sample in the field, and it may be possible to detect not only measles-specific IgM, but measles virus genome for molecular characterization (Riddell et al. 2001). However, oral fluid samples have the disadvantage that the specimens often have heightened background reactivity in commercial assays, or the commercial assays are not sufficiently sensitive when oral fluid specimens are used. Both factors make the use of oral fluid specimens less useful in settings with low measles incidence.

Like oral fluid samples, blood spots collected on filter paper do not require processing in the field, a cold chain does not appear necessary, they can be used to test for rubella as well as for measles (Condorelli et al. 1994, 1998; Helfand et al. 2001), and they can be used for molecular characterization of the measles virus genome (de Swart et al. 2001), although virus isolation would not be possible. In addition, the eluted serum from blood spots can likely be tested in commercially available measles EIA assays without the loss of sensitivity and specificity (de Swart et al. 2001; Helfand et al. 2001), making this technology very attractive for widespread use. Although still considered an invasive technique as a method for sample collection, fingerstick is often more acceptable to parents than phlebotomy (Wassilak et al. 1984).

TREATMENT

Measles is an acute self-limiting disease, which, in the absence of complications, will run its course without the need for specific intervention. Treatment is supportive and there are no proven effective antiviral compounds available. Infection of the undernourished, the immuno-compromised or children suffering from chronic debili-tating diseases is more serious. Such patients as well as children of less than 1 year of age and pregnant women after household contacts can be protected by the admin-istration of human anti-measles gammaglobulin (0.25–0.5 ml/kg). If this is given within the first 3 days after exposure, it is usually effective (CDC 1989). The effec-tiveness is diminished if the globulin is given 4–6 days after exposure, and abolished if more than 6 days have elapsed. Ribavirin has been used to treat pneumonitis and SSPE (Mustafa et al. 1993). Respiratory tract infec-tions cause considerable damage to the ciliated epithe-lium and this may lead to superimposed bacterial infec-tions. In the case of a pneumonia it is sometimes difficult to distinguish between primary viral infections and the superimposed bacterial infection. In any case, treatment with antibiotics is required.

Treatment of acute measles postinfectious encephalitis is only symptomatic and supportive, and does not differ from any other postinfectious encephalitis. Careful attention to fluid and electrolyte balance is essential. Seizure control requires anticonvulsive drugs. Applica-tion of steroids has not been shown to be beneficial. No specific therapy is known for SSPE. A variety of ap-proaches have been attempted, but as yet no convincing results effects have been demonstrated and almost all cases have proved fatal. Evaluation of the effectiveness of treatment is extremely difficult. First, the course of SSPE is highly variable and spontaneous remissions are common. Secondly, SSPE is a rare disease, and clinical trials are therefore inevitably based on a very small number of patients and interpretation is difficult. Isopri-nosine (inosiplex) and interferon (also applied in combi-nation) have been widely used for treatment of SSPE without, however, preventing the lethal outcome of the disease (Gascon 2003). In the case of isoprinosine, it seems likely that treatment may lengthen survival time if given early in the disease.

PREVENTION

Vaccination with measles-containing vaccine is the only effective way to prevent measles infections. The PAHO region of the WHO has effectively eliminated measles using live-attenuated measles vaccine. Although the vaccine strategies in the PAHO member countries markedly varied,

all strategies provided vaccinees with the opportunity to receive two doses of vaccine (de Quadros et al. 2004). Following a resurgence in measles disease between 1989 and 1991, the United States adopted a two dose vaccination schedule (American Academy of Pediatrics 1998). The first dose is administered at 12–15 months of age, and currently the second dose can be given any time between 4 weeks later and school entry. At present, the vaccine coverage in the US is estimated to be 93 percent (Hutchins et al. 2004). As a result of the improved immunization strategy, the number of reported measles cases has dramatically dropped (Figure 34.9) and most of the reported cases can be attrib-uted to importations. In Germany and the UK, where vaccination is not mandatory, philosophical opposition to and distrust of vaccination has led to a lower acceptance rate and less dramatic results have been achieved.

In developing countries, the consequences of MeV infection are most severe. Factors, such as the presence of maternal antibody, underlying infectious diseases, and malnutrition, profoundly interfere and confound vaccine efficacy in age groups most vulnerable to measles. More-over, large influxes of migrating refugees from areas beset by conflict or natural disaster have resulted in the re-introduction of measles into populations that have undergone mass vaccination efforts, thus complicating the assessment of vaccine efficacy. Although the live-attenuated measles-containing vaccines have been successfully used to control and eliminate measles in the Americas and elsewhere (see below), the experience in Africa has led some to consider development of alter-native vaccines, such as high-titered vaccines, DNA-based vaccines with or without adjuvants, thermostable dried powder vaccines, and more. With the exception of the high-titered vaccines, which are no longer recom-mended by the WHO following their association with adverse outcomes (Aaby et al. 1993; Holt et al. 1993), none of the other alternatives have been clinically tested. Nonetheless, any vaccine used in mass vaccina-tion campaigns must be safe, as measles is not normally a life-threatening illness, efficacious, and affordable for mass administration. Its effectiveness should also be long-lasting, if not life-long.

Live vaccine

The first attenuated vaccine strain was the Edmonston B strain produced by serial passage of the virus in human kidney cells, human amnion cells, chick chorioallantoic membrane and, finally, chicken embryo fibroblasts (Rota et al. 1994). This vaccine was administered intramuscu-larly or subcutaneously 12–18 months after the disap-pearance of maternal antibodies. Vaccination resulted in 95 percent seroconversion of recipients, but side-effects of mild measles (fever and rash) were common (5–10 percent). Consequently, the vaccine was administered along with immunoglobulin (Ig) to modify the side-effects (Markowitz and Katz 1994). The side-effects and necessity to provide Ig led to the development of the further attenuated and less reactogenic Schwarz and Moraten strains. These were derived from the Edmonston B vaccine by further passage in the chick embryo at lowered temperature. Further Medical Research Council (UK) trials demonstrated that these were indeed less reactogenic and the incidence of postvaccination febrile convulsions was reduced from 7.7 to 1.9 per 1 000 recipients. Both vaccines produced a 95 percent seroconversion rate, although antibody titers induced by the Schwarz strain declined more rapidly than those produced in response to the Moraten strain but remained at protective levels.

In recent years, the Edmonston B vaccine strain was further passaged in human diploid cells. This vaccine, referred to as Edmonston Zagreb strain, has been shown to produce higher seroconversion rates than the Schwarz vaccine when administered at the same age. Similar observations have been made with the AIK-C vaccine, produced in Japan, but whose lineage stemmed from the Edmonston A virus. All WHO measles vaccines that are currently in use are derived from Edmonston Enders A or B seed stocks. The attenuated strains now in use are so reduced in virulence that encephalitis has only been noted in about one in 1 million vaccine recipients as compared to one per 1 000–5 000 children with natural measles. The measles vaccine is administered subcutaneously usually between the ages of 9 and 20 months for primary vaccination. Humoral immune responses, as defined by HI, NT, and enzyme-linked immunosorbent assay (ELISA), are good and protective as long as the vaccine is given after waning of the maternal antibodies. As with acute measles, the major isotype of MeV-specific antibodies is IgG1. Levels of antibodies induced are generally lower than after natural infection and may decay more rapidly, however, are still measurable in most individuals 30 years after immunization in the absence of boosting infections (Dine et al. 2004). Activation of cell-mediated immunity is generally thought to be similar to that of acute measles in that both MeV-specific $CD4^+$ and $CD8^+$ T cells are stimulated, although CTL-responses after restimulation in vitro are considerably lower than after natural infection. Also similar as with acute measles, administration of live measles vaccine is associated with transient lymphopenia, loss of DTH skin test responses to recall antigen, and decreased in vitro proliferative responses to mitogens. Both leukopenia and atypical lymphocytosis have also been found after revaccination.

Effectiveness of vaccination in the control of measles

In the prevaccine era, an estimated 4–5 million cases occurred annually in the USA and by the age of 15 years 95 percent of the population had seroconverted.

Following the rigorous implementation of the MeV vaccination program in the United States, the case reports fell dramatically from 500 000 annually to 26 000 in 1978 and 1 500 in 1983. From 1984 to 1988 only 3 700 cases were reported (Figure 34.9). As a result of measles vaccination, the mortality and PIE have also declined and the available experience indicates that SSPE can also be prevented by measles vaccination (Halsey 1990). However, in 1989 and 1990 a dramatic increase in acute measles cases was observed in the USA which rose in 1989 to 18 193 and in 1990 to 27 786 cases (Figure 34.9) (Atkinson et al. 1992). The two major causes for this resurgence of measles were the unappreciated low vaccine coverage among preschool-aged children, particularly in urban settings, and vaccine failure (waning immunity) in a low percentage of school-aged children who received only a single dose of vaccine. As a result of this measles epidemic and to address the issue of possible waning immunity, the American Academy of Pediatrics (AAP) and the Immunization Practices Advisory Committee of the USA (ACIP) recommended a change from a one-dose to a two-dose schedule for measles vaccination, as discussed earlier. In 1998, both groups issued a uniform recommendation for a second dose before school entry, and further recommended that all school-aged children receive a second dose of vaccine before 2001 (American Academy of Pediatrics 1998; Watson et al. 1998). The elimination of measles in the USA has taken a strong political and social commitment, uniting the efforts of many professional groups such as the ACIP, AAP, American Academy of Family Physicians (AAFP), state and local governments, and a number of community-based organizations. In 1999, single dose coverage at 2 years and at school entry was 92 and 98 percent, respectively. Seventy percent of school-aged children were estimated to have received two doses of vaccine in 1998 (CDC 2000; Kolasa et al. 2004). The two-dose schedule is only one strategy used to ensure high vaccine coverage in the quest for measles elimination. PAHO has used live-attenuated MeV in a strategy known as keep-up, catch-up, follow-up. This strategy combines routine vaccination (keep-up) with mass vaccination campaigns (catch-up), and 4-year follow-up campaigns (follow-up) (de Quadros et al. 1996). Both this schedule and the two-dose schedule employ the live-attenuated vaccine and are predicated on effective and efficient implementation of routine immunization programs. Furthermore, both strategies provide at least a second immunization opportunity for the vaccinee. Many countries in various regions of the WHO have adopted different variations of the two opportunities for immunization strategy for the interruption of measles transmission with remarkable results (Strebel et al. 2004). When used in conjunction with the two opportunities for measles vaccination, the current live-attenuated measles vaccine has proven to be efficacious, effective, and safe. Initial vaccination can be administered at 6 months of age to children living in high-risk areas (areas with a large inner-city urban population where more than five cases among preschool-aged children occurred during each of the last 5 years or with recent outbreaks among unvaccinated preschool-aged children). Vaccination at ages younger than 12 months is associated with reduced efficacy, thus a second dose of vaccine is critical to ensure protection for those children. In these cases, the second dose should be administered before the determined average age of onset of natural measles for the region/country.

Side-effects of live vaccination, adverse reactions, precautions, and contraindications

The vaccine has an excellent record of safety. Although on rare instances a transient rash or low-grade fever are observed after 5–12 days in some vaccinees, these remain otherwise asymptomatic as for the vast majority of recipients. As with the administration of any agent that can induce fever, some children may have a febrile seizure. Although children with a history of seizures are at increased risk for developing idiopathic epilepsy, febrile seizures following vaccinations do not increase the probability of subsequent epilepsy or neurologic disorders. Most convulsions following measles vaccination are simple febrile seizures, and they affect children without known risk factors. Nevertheless, parents of children who have a personal or family history of seizures should be advised of the small increased risk following measles vaccination which is, however, by far outweighed by the benefits of the protective effects. CNS conditions, such as encephalitis and encephalopathy, have been reported with a frequency of less than one per million doses administered, an incidence which is lower than that of encephalitis of unknown etiology. This finding suggests that the reported severe neurologic disorders temporarily associated with measles vaccination were not caused by the vaccine. Live measles vaccine should not be administered to women who are, or are considering becoming, pregnant within the next 3 months because of the theoretical risk of fetal infection. The decision to administer or delay vaccination because of a current febrile illness depends on the cause of the illness and the severity of symptoms. Hypersensitivity reactions following the administration of live measles vaccine are rare and usually occur at the injection site. Vaccine is contraindicated in persons with a history of anaphylactic reactions to eggs or gelatin following ingestion. Individuals who have experienced anaphylactic reactions to neomycin should not be given the vaccine (Duclos and Ward 1998).

Replication of vaccine viruses can be enhanced in persons with immune-deficiency diseases and in those with immunosuppression, as occurs with leukemia, lymphoma, generalized malignancy, or therapy with alkylating agents, antimetabolites, radiation, or large doses of corticosteroids. Thus, patients with such conditions or therapies (except for HIV infection) should not be given live measles vaccine. Short-term corticosteroid therapy does not contraindicate live measles vaccination. The increasing number of infants and preschoolers with HIV infection in certain countries has directed special attention to the appropriate immunization of these children. Asymptomatic children in need of measles live vaccination should receive it without prior evaluation of HIV infection state. Moreover, vaccination should be considered for all symptomatic HIV-infected children, including those with AIDS, since measles in these children can be severe. Limited data on measles vaccination among both asymptomatic and symptomatic HIV-infected children indicate that the vaccine has not been associated with severe or unusual adverse events, although antibody responses have been unpredictable (Moss et al. 1999, 2003). Exposed symptomatic HIV-infected (as well as other immunocompromised) persons should receive high doses of measles Ig regardless of their previous vaccination status.

REFERENCES

Aaby, P., Knudsen, K., et al. 1993. Long-term survival after Edmonston-Zagreb measles vaccination in Guinea-Bissau: increased female mortality rate. *J Pediatr*, **122**, 904–8.

Addae, M.M., Komada, Y., et al. 1995. Immunological unresponsiveness and apoptotic cell death of T cells in measles virus infection. *Acta Paediat Japan*, **37**, 3, 308–14.

Aderem, A. and Ulevitch, R.J. 2000. Toll-like receptors in the induction of the innate immune response. *Nature*, **406**, 782–7.

Allen, I.V. and Brankin, B. 1993. Pathogenesis of multiple sclerosis: the immune diathesis and the role of viruses. *J Neuropathol Exp Neurol*, **52**, 95–105.

American Academy of Pediatrics. 1998. Age for routine administration of the second dose of measles-mumps-rubella vaccine. *Pediatr* **101**, 129–33.

Anlar, B., Soylemezogulo, F., et al. 1999. Apoptosis in brain biopsies of subacute sclerosing panencephalitis. *J Neuropediatr*, **30**, 239–42.

Arista, S., Ferrano, D., et al. 1995. Detection of IgM antibodies specific for measles virus by capture and indirect enzyme immunoassays. *Res Virol*, **146**, 225–32.

Astier, A., Trescol-Biemont, M.C., et al. 2000. CD46, a new costimulatory molecule for T cells, that induces p120CBL and LAT phosphorylation. *J Immunol*, **164**, 6091–5.

Atabani, S.F., Byrnes, A.A., et al. 2001. Natural measles causes prolonged suppression of interleukin-12 production. *J Infect Dis*, **184**, 1–9.

Atkinson, W.L., Orenstein, W.A. and Krugmann, S. 1992. The resurgence of measles in the United States. *Ann Rev Med*, **43**, 451–63.

Auwaerter, P.G., Kaneshima, H., et al. 1996. Measles virus infection of thymic epithelium in the SCID-hu mouse leads to thymocyte apoptosis. *J Virol*, **70**, 6, 3734–40.

Aversa, G., Chang, C.-C.J., et al. 1997. Engagement of the signalling lymphocytic activation molecule (SLAM) on activated T cells results in IL-2-independent, cyclosporin A-sensitive T cell proliferation and IFN-gamma production. *J Immunol*, **158**, 4036–44.

Avota, E., Avots, A., et al. 2001. Disruption of Akt kinase activation is important for immunosuppression induced by measles virus. *Nature Med*, **7**, 6, 725–31.

Baczko, K., Liebert, U.G., et al. 1986. Expression of defective measles virus genes in brain tissues of patients with subacute sclerosing panencephalitis. *J Virol*, **59**, 472–8.

Baczko, K., Liebert, U.G., et al. 1988. Restriction of measles virus gene expression in measles virus inclusion body encephalitis. *J Infect Dis*, **158**, 144–50.

Baczko, K., Lampe, J., et al. 1993. Clonal expansion of hypermutated measles virus in a SSPE brain. *Virology*, **197**, 188–95.

Baker, K.A., Dutch, R.E., et al. 1999. Structural basis for paramyxovirus mediated membrane fusion. *Mol Cell*, **3**, 309–19.

Bankamp, B., Horikami, S.M., et al. 1996. Domains of the measles virus N protein required for binding to P protein and self-assembly. *Virology*, **216**, 272–7.

Bankamp, B., Bellini, W.J. and Rota, P.A. 1999. Comparison of L proteins of vaccine and wild-type measles viruses. *J Gen Virol*, **80**, 1617–25.

Bankamp, B., Kearney, S.P., et al. 2002. Activity of polymerase proteins of vaccine and wild type measles virus in a minigenome replication assay. *J Virol*, **76**, 7073–81.

Barrett, P.N., Koschel, K., et al. 1985. Effect of measles virus antibodies on a measles SSPE virus persistently infected C6 rat glioma cell line. *J Gen Virol*, **66**, 1411–21.

Bartz, R., Brinckmann, U., et al. 1996. Mapping amino acids of the measles virus hemagglutinin responsible for receptor (CD46) downregulation. *Virology*, **224**, 334–7.

Bartz, R., Firsching, R., et al. 1998. Differential receptor usage by measles virus strains. *J Gen Virol*, **79**, 1015–25.

Basle, M.F., Fournier, J.G., et al. 1986. Measles virus RNA detected in Paget's disease bone tissue by in situ hybridisation. *J Gen Virol*, **67**, 907–13.

Bellini, W.J. and Rota, P.A. 1998. Genetic diversity of wild-type measles viruses: implications for global measles elimination programs. *Emerg Infect Dis*, **4**, 1–7.

Bellini, W.J., Englund, G., et al. 1985. Measles virus P gene codes for two proteins. *J Virol*, **53**, 908–13.

Bellini, W., Englund, G., et al. 1986. Matrix genes of measles virus and canine distemper virus: cloning, nucleotide sequences, and deduced amino acid sequences. *J Virol*, **58**, 408–16.

Bellini, W.J., Rota, J.S. and Rota, P.A. 1994. Virology of measles virus. *J Infect Dis*, **170**, S15–23.

Bieback, K., Lien, E., et al. 2002. The hemagglutinin protein of wildtype measles virus activates Toll-like receptor 2 signaling. *J Virol*, **76**, 8729–36.

Billeter, M.A. and Cattaneo, R. 1994. Generation and properties of measles virus mutations typically associated with subacute sclerosing panencephalitis. *Ann NY Acad Sci*, **724**, 367–77.

Birch, M.A., Taylor, W., et al. 1994. Absence of paramyxovirus RNA in cultures of pagetic bone cells and pagetic bone. *J Bone Miner Res*, **9**, 11–16.

Bitnun, A., Shannon, P., et al. 1999. Measles inclusion body encephalitis caused by the vaccine strain of measles virus. *Clin Infect Dis*, **29**, 855–61.

Blumberg, B.M., Crowley, J.C., et al. 1988. Measles virus L protein evidences elements of ancestral RNA polymerase. *Virology*, **164**, 487–97.

Bolt, G. and Pedersen, I.R. 1999. The role of subtilisin-like proprotein convertases for cleavage of the measles virus fusion glycoprotein in different cell types. *Virology*, **252**, 387–98.

Borrow, P. and Oldstone, M.B.A. 1995. Measles virus- mononuclear cell interactions. In: Billeter, M.A. and ter Meulen, V. (eds), *Measles virus*, Vol. 191. *Curr Top Microbiol Immun*. Berlin, Heidelberg, New York: Springer-Verlag, 85–100.

Breitfeld, V.H.Y., Sherman, F.E., et al. 1973. Fatal measles infection in children with leukemia. *Lab Invest*, **28**, 279–91.

Buchholz, C.J., Gerlier, D., et al. 1996. Selective expression of a subset of measles virus receptor-competent CD46 isoforms in human brain. *Virology*, **217**, 349–55.

Budka, H., Lassmann, H. and Popow-Kraupp, T. 1982. An immunomorphological study stressing dendritic involvement in SSPE. *Acta Neuropath*, **56**, 52–62.

Calain, P. and Roux, L. 1993. The rule of six: a basic feature for efficient replication of Sendai virus defective interfering RNA. *J Virol*, **67**, 4822–30.

Carter, M.J., Willcocks, M.M. and ter Meulen, V. 1983. Defective translation of measles virus matrix protein in a subacute sclerosing panencephalitis cell line. *Nature*, **305**, 153–4.

Casasnovas, J.M., Larvie, M. and Stehle, T. 1999. Crystal structure of two CD46 domains reveals an extended measles virus-binding surface. *EMBO J*, **18**, 2911–22.

Cathomen, T., Mrkic, B., et al. 1997a. A matrix-less measles virus is infectious and elicits extensive cell fusion: consequences for propagation in the brain. *EMBO J*, **17**, 3899–908.

Cathomen, T., Naim, H.Y. and Cattaneo, R. 1997b. Measles viruses with altered envelope protein cytoplasmic tails gain cell fusion competence. *J Virol*, **72**, 1224–34.

Cattaneo, R., Rebmann, G., et al. 1987. Altered transcription of a defective measles virus genome derived from a diseased human brain. *EMBO J*, **6**, 681–7.

Cattaneo, R., Schmid, A., et al. 1988a. Multiple viral mutations rather than host factors cause defective measles virus gene expression in a subacute sclerosing panencephalitis cell line. *J Virol*, **62**, 1388–97.

Cattaneo, R., Schmid, A., et al. 1988b. Biased hypermutation and other genetic changes in defective measles viruses in human brain infections. *Cell*, **55**, 255–65.

Cattaneo, R., Kaelin, K., et al. 1989a. Measles virus editing provides an additional cysteine-rich protein. *Cell*, **56**, 759–64.

Cattaneo, R., Schmid, A., et al. 1989b. Mutated and hypermutated genes of persistent measles viruses which caused lethal human brain diseases. *Virology*, **173**, 415–25.

CDC. 1989. Measles prevention: recommendations of the Immunisation practices advisory committee (ACIP). *MMWR*, **38**, 1–18.

CDC. 2000. Surveillance for vaccination coverage among children and adults – United States. *MMWR*, **49** (SS-9), 1–26.

CDC. 2004. Progress towards measles elimination – regions of the Americas, 2002. *MMWR*, **53** (14), 304–6.

Clements, C.J. and Cutts, F.T. 1995. The epidemiology of measles: thirty years of vaccination. In: Billeter, M.A. and ter Meulen, V. (eds), *Measles virus*, Vol. 191. *Curr Top Microbiol Immun*. Berlin, Heidelberg, New York: Springer-Verlag, 13–34.

Combredet, C., Labrousse, V., et al. 2003. A molecularly cloned Schwarz strain of measles virus vaccine induces strong immune responses in macaques and transgenic mice. *J Virol*, **77**, 11546–54.

Condorelli, F., Scalia, G., et al. 1994. Detection of immunoglobulin G to measles virus, rubella virus and mumps virus in serum samples and in microquantities of whole blood dried filter paper. *J Virol Meth*, **49**, 25–36.

Condorelli, F., Stivala, A., et al. 1998. Use of a microquantity enzyme immunoassay in a large scale study of measles, mumps and rubella immunity in Italy. *Eur J Clin Microbiol Infect Dis*, **17**, 49–52.

Connolly, J.H., Haire, M. and Hadden, D.S. 1971. Measles immunoglobulins in subacute sclerosing panenecephalitis. *Br Med J*, **1**, 23–5.

Crennell, S., Takimoto, T., et al. 2000. Crystal structure of the multifuntional paramyxovirus hemagglutinin-neuraminidase. *Nature Struct Biotechnol*, **7**, 1068–74.

Curran, J., Boeck, R., et al. 1995. Paramyxovirus phosphoproteins form homotrimers as determined by an epitope dilution assay, via predicted coiled coils. *Virology*, **214**, 139–49.

Das, T., Schneider-Schäulies, S., et al. 1995. Cellular casein kinase II phosphorylates measles virus P protein: identification of the sites of phosphorylation. *Virology*, **211**, 218–26.

de Quadros, C.A., Olive, J.M., et al. 1996. Measles elimination in the Americas. Evolving strategies. *JAMA*, **275**, 224–9.

De Quadros, C.A., Izurieta, H., et al. 2004. Measles eradication in the Americas: progress to date. *J Infect Dis*, **189**, Suppl., S227–35.

de Sousa, V.A., Pannuti, C.S., et al. 1991. Enzyme linked immunosorbent assay (ELISA) for measles antibody. A comparison with hemagglutinin inhibition, immunofluorescence and plaque neutralisation tests. *Rev Inst Med Trop Sao Paulo*, **33**, 32–6.

de Swart, R.L., Nur, Y., et al. 2001. Combination of reverse transcriptase PCR analysis and immunoglobulin M detection on filter paper blood samples allows diagnostic and epidemiological studies of measles. *J Clin Microbiol*, **39**, 270–3.

Dhib-Jalbut, S., Jacobsen, S., et al. 1989. Impaired human leukocyte antigen-restricted measles virus-specific cytotoxic T-cell response in subacute sclerosing panencephalitis. *Ann Neurol*, **25**, 272–80.

Dhib-Jalbut, S., Xia, J., et al. 1999. Failure of measles virus to activate nuclear factor-κB in neuronal cells: implications on the immune response to viral infections in the central nervous system. *J Immunol*, **162**, 4024–9.

Dine, M.S., Hutchins, S.S., et al. 2004. Persistence of vaccine induced antibody to measles 26–33 years after vaccination. *J Infect Dis*, **189**, Suppl., 123–30.

Doerig, R.E., Marcil, A., et al. 1993. The human CD46 molecule is a receptor for measles virus (Edmonston strain). *Cell*, **75**, 295–305.

Doerries, R., Liebert, U.G. and ter Meulen, V. 1988. Comparative analysis of virus-specific antibodies and immunoglobulins in serum and cerebrospinal fluid of subacute measles virus-induced encephalomyelitis (SAME) in rats and subacute sclerosing panencephalitis (SSPE). *J Neuroimmunol*, **19**, 339–52.

Doyle, S.E., Vaidya, S.A., et al. 2002. IRF3 mediates a TLR3/TLR4-specific antiviral gene program. *Immunity*, **17**, 251–6.

Dubois, B., Lamy, P.J., et al. 2001. Measles virus exploits dendritic cells to suppress CD4⁺ T cell proliferation via expression of surface viral glycoproteins independently of T-cell *trans*-infection. *Cell Immunol*, **214**, 173–83.

Duclos, P. and Ward, B.J. 1998. Measles vaccines. A review of adverse events. *Drug Exp*, **19**, 435–54.

Dunster, L.M., Schneider-Schäulies, J. and Loeffler, S. 1994. Moesin: a cell membrane protein linked with susceptibility to measles virus infection. *Virology*, **198**, 265–74.

Duprex, P., Duffy, I. and McQuaid, S. 1999a. The H gene of rodent brain-adapted measles virus confers neurovirulence to the Edmonston vaccine strain. *J Virol*, **73**, 6916–22.

Duprex, W.P., McQuaid, S. and Hangartner, L. 1999b. Observation of measles virus cell-to-cell spread in astrocytoma cells by using a green fluorescent protein-expressing recombinant virus. *J Virol*, **73**, 9568–75.

Duprex, W.P., McQuaid, S., et al. 2000. In vitro and in vivo infection of neural cells by a recombinant measles virus expressing enhanced green fluorescent protein. *J Virol*, **74**, 7972–9.

Duprex, W.P., Collins, F.M. and Rima, B.K. 2002. Modulating the function of the measles virus RNA-dependent RNA polymerase by insertion of green fluorescent protein into the open reading frame. *J Virol*, **76**, 7322–8.

Ehrengruber, M.U., Ehler, E., et al. 2002. Measles virus spreads in rat hippocampal neurons by cell-to cell contact and in a polarised fashion. *J Virol*, **76**, 5720–8.

Erdman, D.D., Anderson, L.J., et al. 1991. Evaluation of monoclonal antibody-based capture enzyme immunoassays for detection of specific antibodies to measles virus. *J Clin Microbiol*, **29**, 1466–71.

Erlenhoefer, C., Wurzer, W., et al. 2001. CD150 (SLAM) is a receptor for measles virus but is not involved in contact-mediated proliferation inhibition of lymphocytes. *J Virol*, **75**, 4499–505.

Erlenhoefer, C., Duprex, W.P., et al. 2002. Analysis of the receptor (CD46, CD150) usage by measles virus strains. *J Gen Virol*, **83**, 1431–6.

Escoffier, C., Manie, S., et al. 1999. Nonstructural C protein is required for efficient measles virus replication in human peripheral blood cells. *J Virol*, **73**, 1695–8.

Esolen, L.M., Ward, B.J., et al. 1993. Infection of monocytes during measles. *J Infect Dis*, **168**, 47–52.

Evlashev, A., Valentin, H., et al. 2001. Differential permissivity to measles virus infection of human and CD46 transgenic murine lymphocytes. *J Gen Virol*, **82**, 2125–9.

Finke, D. and Liebert, U.G. 1994. CD4⁺ T cells are essential in overcoming experimental murine measles encephalitis. *Immunol*, **83**, 184–9.

Forthal, D.N., Aarnaes, S., et al. 1992. Degree and length of viremia in adults with measles. *J Infect Dis*, **166**, 421–4.

Fournier, P., Brons, N.H., et al. 1997. Antibodies to a new linear site at the topographical or functional interface between the haemagglutinin and fusion proteins protect against measles encephalitis. *J Gen Virol*, **78**, 1295–302.

Fugier-Vivier, I., Servet-Delprat, C., et al. 1997. Measles virus suppresses cell-mediated immunity by interfering with the survival and fucntion of dendritic cells. *J Exp Med*, **186**, 813–23.

Fujinami, R., Sun, X., et al. 1998. Modulation of immune system function by measles virus infection: role of soluble factor and direct infection. *J Virol*, **72**, 9421–7.

Gans, H.A., Maldonado, Y., et al. 1999. IL-12, IFN-γ and T cell proliferation to measles in immunised infants. *J Immunol*, **162**, 5569–75.

Gascon, G.G. 2003. Randomised treatment study of inosiplex versus combined inosiplex and intraventricular interferon-alpha in subacute sclerosing panencephalitis (SSPE): international multicenter study. *J Child Neurol*, **18**, 819–27.

Gendelman, H.E., Wolinsky, J.S., et al. 1984. Measles encephalomyelitis: lack of evidence of viral invasion of the central nervous system and quantitative study of the nature of demyelination. *Ann Neurol*, **15**, 353–60.

Gerlier, D., Trescol-Biemont, M.C., et al. 1994. Efficient major histocompatibility complex class II-restricted presentation of measles virus relies on hemagglutinin-mediated targeting to its cellular receptor human CD46 expressed by murine B cells. *J Exp Med*, **179**, 353–8.

Gombart, A.F., Hirano, A. and Wong, T.C. 1995. Nucleoprotein phosphorylated on both serine and threonine is preferentially assembled into the nucleocapsids of measles virus. *Virus Res*, **37**, 63–73.

Goodbourne, S., Didcock, L. and Randall, R.E. 2000. Interferons: cell signaling, immune modulation, antiviral responses and virus countermeasures. *J Gen Virol*, **81**, 2341–64.

Gremillion, D.H. and Crawford, D.E. 1981. Measles pneumonia in young adults; an analysis of 106 cases. *Am J Med*, **71**, 539–42.

Griffin, D.E. 1995. Immune responses during measles virus infection. In: Billeter, M.A. and ter Meulen, V. (eds), *Measles virus*, Vol. 191. *Curr Top Microbiol Immunol*. Berlin, Heidelberg, New York: Springer-Verlag, 117–34.

Griffin, D.E. and Bellini, W.J. 1996. Measles virus. In: Fields, B.N., Knipe, D.M. and Howley, P.M. (eds), *Fields Virology*. Philadelphia: Lippincott-Raven Publishers, 1267–312.

Griffin, D.E. and Ward, J.B. 1990. Natural killer cell activity during measles. *Clin Exp Immunol*, **81**, 218–24.

Griffin, D.E. and Ward, J.B. 1993. Differential CD4 T cell activation in measles. *J Infect Dis*, **168**, 275–81.

Griffin, D.E., Ward, B.J., et al. 1989. Immune activation in measles. *N Engl J Med*, **320**, 1667–72.

Griffin, D.E., Ward, B.J., et al. 1992. Immune activation during measles: beta 2-microglobulin in plasma and cerebrospinal fluid in complicated and uncomplicated disease. *J Infect Dis*, **166**, 1170–3.

Grosjean, I., Caux, C., et al. 1997. Measles virus infects human dendritic cells and blocks their allostimulatory properties for CD4⁺ T cells. *J Exp Med*, **186**, 801–12.

Haase, A.T., Ventura, P., et al. 1981. Measles virus nucleotide sequences: detection by in situ hybridisation. *Science*, **212**, 672–5.

Hall, W.W., Lamb, R.A. and Choppin, P.W. 1979. Measles and subacute sclerosing panencephalitis virus proteins: lack of antibodies to the M protein in patients with subacute sclerosing panencephalitis. *Proc Natl Acad Sci USA*, **76**, 2047–51.

Halsey, N. 1990. Risk of subacute sclerosing panencephalitis from measles vaccination. *Infect Dis J*, **9**, 857–8.

Harrowe, G., Sudduth-Klinger, J. and Payan, D.G. 1992. Measles virus–substance P receptor interaction: Jurkat lymphocytes transfected with substance P receptor cDNA enhance measles virus fusion and replication. *Cell Mol Neurobiol*, **12**, 397–409.

Harty, R.N. and Palese, P. 1995. Measles virus phosphoprotein (P) requires the NH2- and COOH-terminal domains for interactions with the nucleoprotein (N) but only the COOH terminus for interactions with itself. *J Gen Virol*, **76**, 2863–7.

Helfand, R.F., Kebede, S., et al. 1996. Comparative detection of measles specific IfM in oral fluid and serum from children by an antibody capture IgM EIA. *J Infect Dis*, **173**, 1470–4.

Helfand, R.F., Keyserling, H.L., et al. 2001. Comparative detection of measles and rubella IgM and IgG derived from filter paper blood and serum samples. *J Med Virol*, **65**, 751–7.

Helfand, R.F., Clubi, T., et al. 2004. Negative impact of clinical misdiagnosis of measles on health workers' confidence in measles vaccine. *Epidemiol Infect*, **132**, 7–10.

Hoffman, S.J., Polack, F.P., et al. 2003. Vaccination of rhesus macaques with a recombinant measles virus expressing interleukin-12 alters humoral and cellular immune responses. *J Infect Dis*, **188**, 1553–61.

Holt, E.A., Moulton, L.H., et al. 1993. Differential mortality by measles vaccine titer and sex. *J Infect Dis*, **168**, 1087–96.

Horikami, S.M. and Moyer, S.A. 1995. Structure, transcription, and replication of measles virus. In: Billeter, M.A. and ter Meulen, V. (eds), *Measles virus*, Vol. 191. *Curr Top Microbiol Immunol*. Berlin, Heidelberg, New York: Springer-Verlag.

Horvat, B., Rivailler, P., et al. 1996. Transgenic mice expressing human measles virus (MV) receptor CD46 provide cells exhibiting different permissivities to MV infections. *J Virol*, **70**, 6673–81.

Hsu, E.C., Sarangi, F., et al. 1998. A single amino acid change in the hemagglutinin protein of measles virus determines its ability to bind CD46 and reveals another receptor on marmoset B cells. *J Virol*, **72**, 2905–16.

Hsu, E.C., Iorio, C., et al. 2001. CDw150 (SLAM) is a receptor for a lymphotropic strain of measles virus and may account for the immunosuppressive properties of this virus. *Virology*, **279**, 9–21.

Hu, A. and Norrby, E. 1995. Role of individual cysteine residues in the processing and antigenicity of measles virus hemagglutinin protein. *J Gen Virol*, **75**, 2173–81.

Hu, A., Cathomen, T., et al. 1995. Influence of N-linked oligosaccharide chains on the processing, cell surface expression and function of the measles virus fusion protein. *J Gen Virol*, **76**, 705–10.

Huber, M., Cattaneo, R., et al. 1991. Measles virus phosphoprotein retains the nucleocapsid protein in the cytoplasm. *Virology*, **185**, 299–308.

Hummel, K.B., Erdman, D.D., et al. 1992. Baculovirus expression of the nucleoprotein gene of measles virus and utility of the recombinant protein in diagnostic enzyme immunoassays. *J Clin Microbiol*, **30**, 2874–80.

Hummel, K., Bellini, W.J. and Offerman, M.K. 1998. Strain-specific differences in LFA-1 induction on measles virus-infected monocytes and adhesion and viral transmission to endothelial cells. *J Virol*, **72**, 8403–7.

Hutchins, S.S., Bellini, W.J., et al. 2004. A population based immunity to measles in the United States, 1999. *J Infect Dis*, **189**, Suppl., S91–7.

Jin, L., Vyse, A. and Brown, D.W. 2001. The role of RT-PCR assay of oral fluid fo diagnosis and surveillance of measles, mumps and rubella. *Bull WHO*, **80**, 76–7.

Johnson, R.T., Griffin, D.E., et al. 1984. Measles encephalomyelitis – clinical and immunologic studies. *N Engl J Med*, **310**, 137–41.

Johnstone, R.W., Russell, S.M., et al. 1993. Polymorphic expression of CD46 protein isoforms due to tissue-specific RNA splicing. *Mol Immunol*, **30**, 1231–41.

Karp, C.L., Wysocka, M., et al. 1996. Mechanism of suppression of cell-mediated immunity by measles virus. *Science*, **273**, 228–31.

Katayama, Y., Hirano, A. and Wong, T.C. 2000. Human receptor for measles virus (CD46) enhances nitric oxide production and restricts virus replication in mouse macrophages by modulating the production of alpha/beta interferon. *J Virol*, **74**, 1252–7.

Katz, M. 1995. Clinical spectrum of measles. In: Billeter, M.A. and ter Meulen, V. (eds), *Measles virus*, Vol. 191. *Curr Top Microbiol Immunol*. Berlin, Heidelberg, New York: Springer-Verlag, 1–12.

Kemper, C., Chan, A.C., et al. 2003. Activation of human CD4⁺ cells with CD3 and CD46 induces a T-regulatory cell 1 phenotype. *Nature*, **421**, 388–92.

Kirk, J., Zhou, A.L., et al. 1991. Cerebral endothelial infection by measles virus in subacute sclerosing panencephalitis: ultrastructural and in situ hybridisation evidence. *Neuropathol Appl Neurobiol*, **17**, 289–97.

Klagge, I.M., ter Meulen, V. and Schneider-Schäulies, S. 2000. Measles virus-induced promotion of dendritic cell maturation by soluble mediators does not overcome the immunosuppressive activity of viral glycoproteins on the cell surface. *Eur J Immunol*, **30**, 2741–50.

Kobune, F., Sakata, H. and Sugiura, A. 1990. Marmoset lymphoblastoid cells as a sensitive host for isolation of measles virus. *J Virol*, **64**, 700–5.

Kolasa, M.S., Klemperer-Johnson, S. and Papania, M.J. 2004. Progress toward implementation of a second dose measles immunisation requirement for all schoolchildren in the United States. *J Infect Dis*, **189**, Suppl., S98–S103.

Krantic, S., Gimenez, C. and Rabourdin-Combe, C. 1995. Cell-to-cell contact via measles virus haemagglutinin–CD46 interaction triggers CD46 downregulation. *J Gen Virol*, **76**, 2793–800.

Laine, D., Trescol-Biemont, M.C., et al. 2003. Measles virus (MV) nucleoprotein binds to a novel cell surface receptor distinct from FcγRII via its C-terminal domain: role in MV-induced immunosuppression. *J Virol*, **77**, 11332–46.

Lamb, R.A. 1993. Paramyxovirus fusion: a hypothesis for changes. *Virology*, **197**, 1–11.

Lambert, D.M., Barney, S., et al. 1996. Peptides from conserved regions of paramyxovirus fusion proteins are potent inhibitors of viral fusion. *Proc Natl Acad Sci USA*, **93**, 2186–91.

Langendijk, J.P.M., Daus, F.J. and van Oirschot, J.T. 1997. Sequence and structure alignment of *Paramyxoviridae* attachment proteins and dicovery of enzymatic activity for a morbillivirus hemagglutinin. *J Virol*, **71**, 6155–67.

Latour, S., Gish, G., et al. 2001. Regulation of SLAM-mediated signal transduction by SAP, the X-linked lymphoproliferative gene product. *Nature Immunol*, **2**, 681–90.

Lawrence, D.M., Vaughn, M.M., et al. 1999. Immune response-mediated protection of adult but not neonatal mice from neuron-restricted measles virus infection and central nervous system disease. *J Virol*, **73**, 1795–801.

Lawrence, D.M.P., Patterson, C.E., et al. 2000. Measles virus spread between neurons requires cell contact but not CD46 expression, syncytium formation, or extracellular virus production. *J Virol*, **74**, 1908–18.

Lecouturier, V., Fayolle, J., et al. 1996. Identification of two amino acids in the hemagglutinin glycoprotein of measles virus (MV) that govern hemadsorption, HeLa cell fusion and CD46 downregulation: phenotypic markers that differentiate vaccine and wild-type MV strains. *J Virol*, **70**, 4200–4.

Leopardi, R., Hukkanen, V., et al. 1993. Cell proteins bind to sites within the 3′ noncoding region and the positive strand leader sequence of measles virus RNA. *J Virol*, **67**, 785–90.

Liebert, U.G. and Finke, D. 1995. Measles infections in rodents. In: Billeter, M.A. and ter Meulen, V. (eds), *Measles virus*, Vol. 191. *Curr Top Microbiol Immunol*. Berlin, Heidelberg, New York: Springer-Verlag, 149–66.

Liebert, U.G., Baczko, K., et al. 1986. Restricted expression of measles virus proteins in brains from cases of subacute sclerosing panencephalitis. *J Gen Virol*, **67**, 2435–44.

Liebert, U.G., Linington, C. and ter Meulen, V. 1988. Induction of autoimmune reactions to myelin basic protein in measles virus encephalitis in Lewis rats. *J Neuroimmunol*, **17**, 103–18.

Liebert, U.G., Schneider-Schäulies, S., et al. 1990. Antibody-induced restriction of viral gene expression in measles encephalitis in rats. *J Virol*, **64**, 706–13.

Liston, P. and Briedis, D.J. 1994. Measles virus V protein binds zinc. *Virology*, **198**, 399–404.

Liston, P. and Briedis, D.J. 1995. Ribosomal frameshifting during translation of measles virus P protein mRNA is capable of directing the synthesis of a unique protein. *J Virol*, **69**, 6742–50.

Liston, P., Di Flumeri, C. and Briedis, D. 1995. Protein interactions entered into by the measles virus P, V and C proteins. *Virus Res*, **38**, 241–59.

Liszewski, K.M., Post, T.W. and Atkinson, J.P. 1991. Membrane cofactor protein (MCP or CD46): newest member of the regulators of complement activation gene cluster. *Ann Rev Immunol*, **9**, 431–55.

Lydy, S.L., Basak, S. and Compans, R.W. 1990. Host cell-dependent lateral mobility of viral glycoproteins. *Microb Pathogen*, **9**, 375–86.

Maisner, A., Schneider-Schäulies, J., et al. 1994. Binding of measles virus to membrane cofactor protein (CD46): importance of disulfide bonds and N-glycans for the receptor function. *J Virol*, **68**, 6299–304.

Maisner, A., Alvarez, J., et al. 1996. The N-glycan of the SCR 2 region is essential for membrane cofactor protein (CD46) to function as a measles virus receptor. *J Virol*, **70**, 4973–7.

Manchester, M., Liszewski, M.K., et al. 1994. Multiple isoforms of CD46 (membrane cofactor protein) serve as receptors for measles virus. *Proc Natl Acad Sci USA*, **91**, 2161–5.

Manchester, M., Valsamakis, A., et al. 1995. Measles virus and C3 binding sites are distinct on membrane cofactor protein (CD46). *Proc Natl Acad Sci USA*, **92**, 2303–7.

Manchester, M., Eto, D.S. and Oldstone, M.B.A. 1999. Characterisation of the inflammatory response during acute measles encephalitis in NSE-CD46 transgenic mice. *J Neuroimmunol*, **96**, 207–17.

Manchester, M., Smith, K.A., et al. 2002. Targeting and hematopoetic suppression of human CD34+ cells by measles virus. *J Virol*, **76**, 6636–42.

Markowitz, L.E. and Katz, S.L. 1994. Measles vaccine. In: Plotkin, S.A. and Mortimer, E.A. (eds), *Vaccines*. Philadelphia, PA: WB Saunders, 229.

McQuaid, S. and Cosby, S.L. 2002. An immunohistochemical study of the distribution of the measles virus receptors, CD46 and SLAM, in normal human tissues and subacute sclerosing panencephalitis. *Lab Invest*, **82**, 403–9.

Mehta, P.D., Kulczycki, J., et al. 1992. Increased levels of beta 2-microglobulin, soluble interleukin-2 receptor, and soluble CD8 in patients with subacute sclerosing panencephalitis. *Clin Immunol Immunopathol*, **65**, 53–9.

Meissner, N.N. and Koschel, K. 1995. Downregulation of endothelin receptor mRNA synthesis in C6 rat astrocytoma cells by persistent measles virus and canine distemper virus infections. *J Virol*, **69**, 5191–4.

Merz, D.C., Scheid, A. and Choppin, P.W. 1980. Importance of antibodies to the fusion glycoprotein of paramyxoviruses in the prevention of infection. *J Exp Med*, **151**, 275–88.

Mikhalap, S.V., Shlapatska, L.M., et al. 1999. CDw150 associates with Src-homology 2-containing inositol phosphatase and modulates CD95-mediated apoptosis. *J Immunol*, **162**, 5719–27.

Minagawa, H., Tanaka, K., et al. 2001. Induction of the measles virus receptor SLAM (CD150) on monocytes. *J Gen Virol*, **82**, 2913–17.

Moench, T.R., Griffin, D.E., et al. 1988. Acute measles in patients with and without clinical neurologic involvement: distribution of measles virus antigen and RNA. *J Infect Dis*, **158**, 433–42.

Moll, M., Klenk, H.D., et al. 2001. A single amino acid change in the cytoplasmic domains of measles glycoproteins H and F alters targeting, endocytosis and cell fusion in polarised Madin-Darby canine kidney cells. *J Biol Chem*, **276**, 17887–94.

Moll, M., Klenk, H.D. and Maisner, A. 2002. Importance of the cytoplasmic tail of the measles virus glycoproteins for fusogenic activity and the generation of recombinant measles viruses. *J Virol*, **76**, 7174–86.

Morra, M., Lu, J., et al. 2001. Structural basis for the interaction of the free SH2 domain of EAT-2 with SLAM receptors in hematopoietic cells. *EMBO J*, **20**, 5840–52.

Moss, W.J., Cutts, F.T. and Griffin, D.E. 1999. Implications of the human immunodeficiency virus epidemic for control and eradication of measles. *Clin Infect Dis*, **29**, 106–12.

Moss, W.J., Clements, C.J. and Halsey, N.A. 2003. Immunisation of children at risk of infection with human immunodeficiency virus. *Bull WHO*, **81**, 61–70.

Moyer, S.A. and Horikami, S.M. 1991. The role of virus and host proteins in paramyxovirus transcription and replication. In: Kingsbury, D.W. (ed.), *The paramyxoviruses*. New York and London: Plenum Press, 249–74.

Mrkic, B., Pavlovic, J., et al. 1998. Measles virus spread and pathogenesis in genetically modified mice. *J Virol*, **72**, 7420–7.

Mustafa, M.M., Weitman, S.D., et al. 1993. Subacute measles encephalitis in the young immunocompromised host: report of two cases diagnosed by polymerase chain reaction and treated with ribavirin and review of the literature. *Clin Infect Dis*, **16**, 654–60.

Nagano, I., Nakamura, S., et al. 1991. Immunohistochemical analysis of the cellular infiltrate in brain lesions in subacute sclerosing panencephalitis. *Neurology*, **41**, 1639–42.

Naim, H.Y., Ehler, E. and Billeter, M.A. 2000. Measles virus matrix protein specifies apical virus release and glycoprotein sorting in epithelial cells. *EMBO J*, **19**, 3576–85.

Nanan, R., Chittka, B., et al. 1999. Measles infection causes transient depletion of activated T cells from peripheral circulation. *J Clin Virol*, **12**, 201–10.

Naniche, D., Varior-Krishnan, G., et al. 1993. Human membrane cofactor protein (CD46) acts as a cellular receptor for measles virus. *J Virol*, **67**, 6025–32.

Naniche, D., Reed, S.I. and Oldstone, M.B.A. 1999. Cell cycle arrest during measles virus infection: a G0-like block leads to suppression of retinoblastoma protein expression. *J Virol*, **73**, 1894–901.

Naniche, D., Yeh, A., et al. 2000. Evasion of host defenses by measles virus: wildtype measles virus infection interferes with induction of alpha/beta interferon production. *J Virol*, **74**, 7478–84.

Niewiesk, S., Eisenhuth, I., et al. 1997a. Measles virus-induced immune suppression in the cotton rat (*Sigmodon hispidus*) model depends on viral glycoproteins. *J Virol*, **71**, 7214–19.

Niewiesk, S., Schneider-Schäulies, J., et al. 1997b. CD46 expression does not overcome the intracellular block of measles virus replication in transgenic rats. *J Virol*, **71**, 7969–73.

Niewiesk, S., Ohnimus, H., et al. 1999. Measles virus-induced immunosuppression in cotton rats is associated with cell cycle retardation in uninfected lymphocytes. *J Gen Virol*, **80**, 2023–9.

Niewiesk, S., Goetzelmann, M. and ter Meulen, V. 2000. Selective suppression of T lymphocyte responses in experimental measles infection. *Proc Natl Acad Sci USA*, **79**, 2695–708.

Nussbaum, O., Broder, C.C., et al. 1995. Functional and structural interactions between measles virus hemagglutinin and CD46. *J Virol*, **69**, 3341–9.

Ofir, R., Weinstein, Y., et al. 1996. Tyrosine phosphorylation of measles virus P phosphoprotein in persistently infected neuroblastoma cells. *Virus Genes*, **13**, 203–10.

Ogata, A., Czub, S., et al. 1997. Absence of measles virus receptor (CD46) in lesions of subacute sclerosing panencephalitis brains. *Acta Neuropathol*, **94**, 444–9.

Ogura, H., Rima, B.K., et al. 1988. Restricted synthesis of the fusion protein of measles virus at elevated temperatures. *J Gen Virol*, **69**, 925–9.

Ohgimoto, S., Ohgimoto, K., et al. 2001. The hemagglutinin protein is an important determinant for measles virus tropism for dendritic cells in vitro and immunosuppression in vivo. *J Gen Virol*, **82**, 1835–44.

Ohno, S., Seki, F., et al. 2003. Histidine at position 61 and its adjacent amino acid residues are critical for SLAM (CD150) to act as a cellular receptor for measles. *J Gen Virol*, **84**, 2381–8.

Ohuchi, M., Ohuchi, R., et al. 1987. Characterization of the measles virus isolated from the brain of a patient with immunosuppressive measles encephalitis. *J Infect Dis*, **156**, 436–41.

Okada, H., Kobune, F., et al. 2000. Extensive leukopenia due to apoptosis of uninfected lymphocytes in acute measles patients. *Arch Virol*, **45**, 905–20.

Okada, H., Sato, T.A., et al. 2001. Comparative analysis of host responses related to immunosuppression between measles patients and vaccine recipients with live attenuated measles vaccines. *Arch Virol*, **146**, 859–74.

Ono, N., Tatsuo, H., et al. 2001a. Measles viruses of throat swabs from measles patients use signaling lymphocytic activation molecule (CDw150) but not 46 as a cellular receptor. *J Virol*, **75**, 4399–401.

Ono, N., Tatsuo, H., et al. 2001b. V domain of human SLAM (CDw150) it essential for its function as a measles receptor. *J Virol*, **75**, 1594–600.

Palosaari, H., Parisien, J.P., et al. 2003. STAT protein interference and suppression of cytokine signal transduction by measles virus V protein. *J Virol*, **77**, 7635–44.

Parks, C.L., Lerch, R.A., et al. 2001. Analysis of the noncoding regions of measles virus strains in the Edmonston vaccine lineage. *J Virol*, **75**, 921–33.

Patterson, C.E., Lawrence, D.M., et al. 2002. Immune-mediated protection from measles virus-induced central nervous system disease is noncytolytic and gamma interferon dependent. *J Virol*, **76**, 4497–506.

Patterson, J.B., Scheiflinger, F., et al. 1999. Structural and functional studies of the measles virus hemagglutinin: identification of a novel site required for CD46 interaction. *Virology*, **256**, 142–51.

Patterson, J.B., Thomas, D., et al. 2000. V and C proteins of measles virus function as virulence factors in vivo. *Virology*, **267**, 80–9.

Patterson, J.B., Carnu, T.I., et al. 2001. Evidence that the hypermutated M protein of a subacute sclerosing panencephalitis virus contributes to the chronic progressive CNS disease. *Virology*, **291**, 215–25.

Permar, S.R., Klumpp, S.A., et al. 2003a. Role of CD8[+] lymphocytes in control and clearance of measles virus infection of rhesus macaques. *J Virol*, **77**, 4396–400.

Permar, S.R., Moss, W.J., et al. 2003b. Increased thymic output during acute measles. *J Virol*, **77**, 7872–9.

Perry, K., Brown, D., et al. 1993. Detection of measles, mumps and rubella antibodies in saliva using antibody capture radioimmunoassay. *J Med Virol*, **40**, 235–40.

Plemper, R.K., Hammond, A.L. and Cattaneo, R. 2000. Characterisation of a region of the measles virus hemagglutinin sufficient for its dimerisation. *J Virol*, **74**, 6485–93.

Plemper, R.K., Hammond, A.L. and Cattaneo, R. 2001a. Measles virus envelope glycoproteins hetero-oligomerise in the endoplasmatic reticulum. *J Biol Chem*, **276**, 44239–46.

Plemper, R.K., Hammond, A.L., et al. 2001b. Strength of envelope protein interaction modulates cytopathogenicity of measles virus. *J Virol*, **76**, 5051–61.

Polack, F.P., Auwaerter, P.G., et al. 1999. Production of atypical measles in rhesus macaques: evidence for disease mediated by immune complex formation and eosinophils in the presence of fusion-inhibiting antibody. *Nature Med*, **5**, 629–34.

Polack, F.P., Hoffman, S.J., et al. 2003. A role for nonprotective complement-fixing antibodies with low avidity for measles virus in atypical measles. *Nature Med*, **9**, 1209–13.

Pullan, C.R., Noble, T.C., et al. 1976. Atypical measles infections in leukemic children on immunosuppressive treatment. *Br Med J*, **1**, 1562–6.

Radecke, F. and Billeter, M.A. 1996. The nonstructural C protein is not essential for multiplication of Edmonston B strain measles virus in cultured cells. *Virology*, **217**, 418–21.

Radecke, F., Spielhofer, P., et al. 1995. Rescue of measles virus from cloned cDNA. *EMBO J*, **14**, 5773–84.

Rager, M., Vongpunsawad, S., et al. 2002. Polyploid measles virus with hexameric genome length. *EMBO J*, **21**, 2364–72.

Rall, G.F., Manchester, M., et al. 1997. A transgenic mouse model for measles virus infection of the brain. *Proc Natl Acad Sci USA*, **94**, 4659–63.

Ratnam, S., Gadag, V., et al. 1995. Comparison of commercial enzyme immunoassay kits with plaque reduction neutralisation test for detection of measles antibody. *J Clin Microbiol*, **33**, 811–15.

Ratnam, S., Tipples, G., et al. 2000. Perfomance of indirect immunoglobulin M (IgM) serology tests and IgM capture assays for laboratory diagnosis of measles. *J Clin Microbiol*, **38**, 99–104.

Ravanel, K., Castelle, C., et al. 1997. Measles virus nucleocapsid protein binds to FcgammaRII and inhibits human B cell antibody production. *J Exp Med*, **186**, 269–78.

Riddell, M.A., Clubo, D., et al. 2001. Investigation of optimal specimen type and sampling time for detection of measles virus RNA during a measles epidemic. *J Clin Microbiol*, **39**, 375–6.

Rima, B.K., Earle, J.A.P., et al. 1995. Measles virus strain variations. In: Billeter, M.A. and ter Meulen, V. (eds), *Measles virus*, Vol. 191. *Curr Top Microbiol Immunol*. Berlin, Heidelberg, New York: Springer-Verlag, 65–84.

Rima, B.K., Earle, J.A.P., et al. 1997. Sequence divergence of measles virus haemagglutinin during natural evolution and adaptation to cell culture. *J Gen Virol*, **78**, 97–106.

Robertson, D.A.F., Guy, E.C., et al. 1987. Persistent measles virus genome in autoimmune chronic active hepatitis. *Lancet*, **4**, 9–11.

Roos, R.P., Graves, M.C., et al. 1981. Immunologic and virologic studies or measles inclusion body encephalitis in an immunosuppressed host: the relationship to subacute sclerosing panencephalitis. *Neurology*, **31**, 1263–70.

Rota, P.A. and Bellini, W.J. 2003. Update on the global distribution of genotypes of wild-type measles viruses. *J Infect Dis*, **187**, Suppl. 1, S270–6.

Rota, J.S., De Wang, Z., et al. 1994. Comparison of sequences of the H, F and N coding genes of measles virus vaccine strains. *Virus Res*, **31**, 317–30.

Rota, J.S., Heath, J.L., et al. 1996. Molecular epidemiology of measles virus: identification of pathways of transmission and implications for measles elimination. *J Infect Dis*, **173**, 32–7.

Rota, P.A., Rota, J.S., et al. 2004. Genetic analysis of measles viruses isolated in the United States between 1989 and 2001: absence of an endemic genotype since 1994. *J Infect Dis*, **189**, Suppl. 1, 160–4.

Sakaguchi, M., Yoshikaww, Y., et al. 1986. Growth of measles virus in epthelial cells and lymphoid tissues of cynomolgous monkeys. *Microb Immunol*, **30**, 1067–73.

Santiago, C., Bjoerling, E., et al. 2002. Distinct kinetics for binding of the CD46 and SLAM receptors to overlapping sites in the measles virus hemagglutinin protein. *J Biol Chem*, **277**, 32294–301.

Sato, T.A., Kohama, T. and Sugiura, A. 1988. Intracellular processing of measles virus fusion protein. *Arch Virol*, **98**, 39–50.

Schlender, J., Schnorr, J.J., et al. 1996. Interaction of measles virus glycoproteins with the surface of uninfected peripheral blood lymphocytes induces immunosuppression in vitro. *Proc Natl Acad Sci USA*, **93**, 13194–9.

Schneider, H., Kaelin, K. and Billeter, M.A. 1997. Recombinant measles viruses defective for RNA editing and V protein synthesis are viable in cultured cells. *Virology*, **227**, 314–22.

Schneider, U., Bullough, F., et al. 2000. Recombinant measles viruses efficiently entering cells through targeted receptors. *J Virol*, **74**, 9928–36.

Schneider, U., von Messling, V., et al. 2002. Efficiency of measles virus entry and dissemination through different receptors. *J Virol*, **76**, 7460–7.

Schneider-Schäulies, S., Liebert, U.G., et al. 1989. Restriction of measles virus gene expression in acute and subacute encephalitis of Lewis rats. *Virology*, **171**, 525–34.

Schneider-Schäulies, S., Kreth, H.W., et al. 1991. Expression of measles virus RNA in peripheral blood mononuclear cells of patients with measles, SSPE, and autoimmune diseases. *Virology*, **182**, 703–11.

Schneider-Schäulies, S., Liebert, U.G., et al. 1992. Antibody-dependent transcriptional regulation of measles virus in persistently infected neural cells. *J Virol*, **66**, 5534–41.

Schneider-Schäulies, S., Schneider-Schäulies, J., et al. 1993. Spontaneous and differentiation-dependent regulation of measles virus gene expression in human glial cells. *J Virol*, **67**, 3375–83.

Schneider-Schäulies, S., Schneider-Schäulies, J., et al. 1994. Cell type-specific MxA-mediated inhibition of measles virus transcription in human brain cells. *J Virol*, **68**, 6910–17.

Schneider-Schäulies, J., Dunster, L.M., et al. 1995a. Differential downregulation of CD46 by measles virus strains. *J Virol*, **69**, 7257–9.

Schneider-Schäulies, J., Dunster, L.M., et al. 1995b. Physical association of moesin and CD46 as a receptor complex for measles virus. *J Virol*, **69**, 2248–56.

Schneider-Schäulies, S., Schneider-Schäulies, J., et al. 1995c. Measles virus gene expression in neural cells. *Curr Top Microbiol Immunol*, **191**, 101–16.

Schneider-Schäulies, J., Schnorr, J.J., et al. 1996. Receptor (CD46) modulation and complement-mediated lysis of uninfected cells after contact with measles virus-infected cells. *J Virol*, **70**, 255–63.

Schneider-Schäulies, S., Niewiesk, S., et al. 2001. Measles virus induced immunosuppression: Targets and effector mechanisms. *Curr Mol Med*, **1**, 163–82.

Schnorr, J.J., Schneider-Schäulies, S., et al. 1993. MxA-dependent inhibition of measles virus glycoprotein synthesis in a stably transfected human monocytic cell line. *J Virol*, **67**, 4760–8.

Schnorr, J.J., Dunster, L.M., et al. 1995. Measles virus-induced down-regulation of CD46 is associated with enhanced sensitivity to complement-mediated lysis of infected cells. *Eur J Immunol*, **25**, 976–84.

Schnorr, J.J., Seufert, M., et al. 1997a. Cell cycle arrest rather than apoptosis is associated with measles virus contact-mediated immunosuppression in vitro. *J Gen Virol*, **78**, 3217–26.

Schnorr, J.J., Xanthakos, S., et al. 1997b. Induction of maturation of human blood dendritic cell precursors by measles virus is associated with immunosuppression. *Proc Natl Acad Sci USA*, **94**, 5326–31.

Schnorr, J.J., Cutts, F.T., et al. 2001. Immune activation after measles vaccination of 6–9 months old Bangladeshi infants. *Vaccine*, **19**, 1503–10.

Segev, Y., Rager-Zisman, B., et al. 1994. Reversal of the measles virus-mediated increase of phosphorylating activity in persistently infected mouse neuroblastoma cells by anti-measles virus antibodies. *J Gen Virol*, **75**, 819–27.

Segev, Y., Ofir, R., et al. 1995. Tyrosine phosphorylation of measles virus nucleocapsid protein in persistently infected neuroblastoma cells. *J Virol*, **69**, 2480–5.

Servet-Delprat, C., Vidalain, O., et al. 2000a. Consequences of Fas-mediated human dendritic cell apoptosis induced by measles virus. *J Virol*, **74**, 4387–93.

Servet-Delprat, C., Vidalain, O., et al. 2000b. Measles virus induces abnormal differentiation of CD40-ligand activated human dendritic cells. *J Immunol*, **164**, 1753–60.

Shaffer, J.A., Bellini, W.J. and Rota, P.A. 2003. The C protein of measles virus inhibits the type I interferon response. *Virology*, **315**, 389–97.

Sheshberadaran, H. and Norrby, E. 1984. Three monoclonal antibodies against measles virus F protein cross-react with cellular stress protein. *J Virol*, **52**, 995–9.

Shiozawa, S.N., Yoshikawa, N., et al. 1988. A sensitive radioimmunoassay for circulating alpha-interferon in the plasma of healthy children and patients with measles virus infection. *Clin Exp Immunol*, **73**, 366–9.

Spehner, D., Drillien, R. and Howley, P.M. 1997. The assembly of measles virus nucleoprotein into nucleocapsid-like particles is modulated by the phosphoprotein. *Virology*, **232**, 260–8.

Steineur, M., Grosjean, I., et al. 1998. Langerhans cells are susceptible to measles virus infection and actively suppress T cell proliferation. *Eur J Dermatol*, **8**, 413–20.

Strebel, P.M., Henao-Restrepo, A.M., et al. 2004. Global measles elimination efforts: the significance of measles elimination in the United States. *J Infect Dis*, **189**, Suppl., S251–257.

Suryanarayana, K., Baczko, K., et al. 1994. Transcription inhibition and other properties of matrix proteins expressed by M genes cloned from measles viruses and diseased human brains. *J Virol*, **68**, 1532–43.

Takeda, M., Takeuchi, K., et al. 2000. Recovery of pathogenic measles virus from cloned cDNA. *J Virol*, **74**, 6643–7.

Takeuchi, K., Takeda, M., et al. 2002. Recombinant wild-type and Edmonston strain measles viruses bearing heterologous H proteins: role of H protein in cell fusion and host cell specificity. *J Virol*, **76**, 4891–900.

Takeuchi, K., Kadota, S.I., et al. 2003. Measles virus V protein blocks interferon (IFN)-alpha/beta but not IFN-gamma signaling by inhibiting STAT1 and STAT2 phosphorylation. *FEBS Lett*, **545**, 177–82.

Tanabe, M., Kurita-Taniguchi, M., et al. 2003. Mechanisms of up-regulation of human Toll-like receptor 3 secondary to infection of measles virus attenuated strains. *Biochem Biophys Res Comm*, **311**, 39–48.

Tatsuo, H., Ono, N. and Yanagi, Y. 2001. Morbilliviruses use signaling lymphocyte activation molecules (CD150) as cellular receptors. *J Virol*, **75**, 5842–50.

Ten Oever, B.R., Servant, M.J., et al. 2002. Recognition of the measles virus nucleocapsid as a mechanism of IRF-3 activation. *J Virol*, **76**, 3659–69.

Tober, C., Seufert, M., et al. 1998. Expression of measles virus V protein is associated with pathogenicity and control of viral RNA synthesis. *J Virol*, **72**, 8124–32.

Uhlmann, V., Martin, C.M., et al. 2002. Potential viral pathogenic mechanism for new variant inflammatory bowel disease. *J Clin Mol Pathol*, **55**, 1–6.

Valsamakis, A., Schneider, H., et al. 1998. Recombinant measles viruses with mutations in the C, V or F reading gene have altered growth phenotypes in vivo. *J Virol*, **72**, 7754–61.

van Binnendijk, R.S., Poelen, M.C.M., et al. 1989. Measles virus-specific human T cell clones: Characterization of specificity and function of CD4 helper/cytotoxic and CD8 cytotoxic T cell clones. *J Immunol*, **142**, 2847–54.

van Binnendijk, R.S., Poelen, M.C.M., et al. 1990. The predominance of CD8 T cells after infection with measles virus suggests a role for CD8 class I MHC-restricted cytotoxic T lymphocytes (CTL) in recovery from measles. *J Immunol*, **144**, 2394–9.

van Binnendijk, R.S., van der Heijden, R.W.J. and Osterhaus, A.D.M.E. 1995. Monkeys in measles research. In: Billeter, M.A. and ter Meulen, V. (eds), *Measles virus*, Vol. 191. *Curr Top Microbiol Immunol*. Berlin, Heidelberg, New York: Springer-Verlag.

Varior-Krishnan, G., Trescol-Biemont, M.C., et al. 1994. Glycosyl-phosphatidylinositol-anchored and transmembrane forms of CD46 display similar measles virus receptor properties: virus binding, fusion, and replication; down-regulation by hemagglutinin; and virus uptake and endocytosis for antigen presentation by major histocompatibility complex class II molecules. *J Virol*, **68**, 7891–9.

Vasconcelos, D., Norrby, E. and Oglesbee, M. 1998. The cellular stress response increases measles virus-induced cytopathic effect. *J Gen Virol*, **79**, 1769–73.

Vidalain, O., Azocar, O., et al. 2000. Measles virus induces functional TRAIL production by human dendritic cells. *J Virol*, **74**, 556–9.

Vincent, S., Tigaud, I., et al. 2002. Restriction of measles virus RNA synthesis by a mouse host cell line: trans-complementation by polymerase components or a human cellular factor(s). *J Virol*, **76**, 6121–30.

Vongpunsawad, S., Oezgun, N., et al. 2004. Selectively receptor-blind measles viruses: idenfication of residues necessary for SLAM- or CD46 induced fusion and their localisation on a new hemagglutinin structural model. *J Virol*, **78**, 302–13.

Wang, G., Liszewski, M.K., et al. 2000. Membrane cofactor protein (MCP; CD46): isoform-specific tyrosine phosphorylation. *J Immunol*, **164**, 1839–46.

Wang, N., Satoskar, A., et al. 2004. The cell surface receptor SLAM controls T cell and macrophage functions. *J Exp Med*, **199**, 1255–64.

Wardrop, E.A. and Briedis, D.J. 1991. Characterization of V protein in measles virus-infected cells. *J Virol*, **65**, 3421–8.

Wassilak, S.F., Bernier, R.H., et al. 1984. Measles seroconfirmation using dried capillary blood specimen in filter paper. *Pediatr Infect Dis*, **3**, 117–21.

Watson, J.C., Hadler, S.C., et al. 1998. Measles, mumps, and rubella – vaccine use and strategies for elimination of measles, mumps and congenital rubella and control of mumps. Recommendations of the Advisory Committee on Immunisation Practices (ACIP). *MMWR*, **47**, RR-S, 1–57.

Weidmann, A., Fischer, C., et al. 2000a. Measles virus-induced immunosuppression in vitro is independent of complex glycosylation of viral glycoproteins and hemifusion. *J Virol*, **74**, 7548–53.

Weidmann, A., Maisner, A., et al. 2000b. Proteolytic cleavage of the fusion protein but not membrane fusion is required for measles virus-induced immunosuppression in vitro. *J Virol*, **74**, 1985–93.

WHO. 1998. Standardization of the nomenclature for describing the genetic characteristics of wild-type measles viruses. *Weekly Epid Rec*, **73**, 265–72.

WHO. 1999. *World health report 1999: making a difference*. Geneva: World Health Organization.

WHO. 2001. Nomenclature for describing the genetic characteristics of wild-type measles viruses (update). *Weekly Epid Rec*, **76**, 421–7.

Wild, T.F. and Buckland, R. 1995. Functional aspects of envelope-associated measles virus proteins. In: Billeter, M.A. and ter Meulen, V. (eds), *Measles virus*. Vol. 191. Berlin, Heidelberg, New York: Springer-Verlag, 51–64.

Wyde, P.R., Ambrosi, M.W., et al. 1992. Measles virus replication in lungs of hispid cotton rats after intranasal inoculation. *Proc Soc Exp Biol Med*, **44**, 80–7.

Yokota, S., Saito, H., et al. 2003. Measles virus suppresses interferon alpha signaling pathway: suppression of Jak1 phosphorylation and association of viral accessory proteins, C and V, with interferon alpha receptor complex. *Virology*, **306**, 135–46.

Yoshikawa, Y. and Yamanouchi, K. 1984. Effect of papaverine treatment on replication of measles virus in human neural and nonneural cells. *J Virol*, **50**, 489–96.

Zaffran, Y., Destaing, O., et al. 2001. CD46/CD3 costimulation induces morphological changes of human T cells and activation of Vav, Rac, and extracellular signal-related kinase mitogen-activated protein kinase. *J Immunol*, **167**, 6780–5.

Zaki, S.R. and Bellini, W.J. 1997. Measles. In: Connor, D.H., Chandler, F.W., et al. (eds), *Pathology of infectious diseases*. Stanford, CT: Appleton and Lange.

Zhang, X., Glendening, C., et al. 2002. Identification and characterisation of a regulatory domain on the caroxyl terminus of the measles virus nucleocapsid protein. *J Virol*, **76**, 8737–46.

35

Rubulavirus: mumps virus

WENDY A. KNOWLES AND LI JIN

IDENTIFICATION OF THE VIRUS AND CLASSIFICATION

As a disease, mumps has been known for centuries (Gordon and Kilham 1949). A population of roughly 200 000 people is needed to sustain mumps infection and this density was first achieved about 4 000 to 5 000 years ago (Carbone and Wolinsky 2001). The first description of a mild epidemic illness with swelling in front of the ear, sometimes accompanied by painful swelling of the testes, is accredited to Hippocrates in the fifth century BC. The name mumps may be derived from the Old English verb meaning 'to sulk' or from the Scottish verb meaning 'to speak indistinctly' (Gershon 1995).

As early as 1908 Granata suggested, from experiments in rabbits, that mumps disease was caused by a filterable agent (Granata, cited in Wollstein 1916). However, it was Johnson and Goodpasture (1934) who first induced parotitis in rhesus monkeys by inoculating fresh saliva from acute mumps cases directly into Stensen's duct, and then passed the infection to further monkeys by inoculation of a sterile parotid gland extract by the same route. A major step forward was the growth of monkey-passaged mumps virus in the yolk sac, amniotic sac, and allantoic sac of developing chick embryos (Habel 1945; Levens and Enders 1945). This was followed by primary isolation from human saliva (Beveridge et al. 1946) and cerebrospinal fluid (CSF) (Henle and McDougall 1947), and eventually the isolation and passage of mumps virus

in cultures of Hela and monkey kidney cells (Henle and Deinhardt 1955).

Mumps virus is classified in the family *Paramyxoviridae*, subfamily *Paramyxovirinae*, genus *Rubulavirus*, based on virus morphology, genome organization, genetic sequences, and the biological activity of viral proteins. Also classified in this genus are the human parainfluenza viruses 2, 4a, and 4b, *Newcastle disease virus*, *Avian paramyxoviruses 2 to 9*, *Simian virus 5*, *Simian virus 41*, *Mapuera virus*, and *Porcine rubulavirus* (van Regenmortel et al. 2000).

PHYSICAL PROPERTIES

Mumps virus morphology

Mumps virions grown in cell culture are heterogeneous in size and shape, and consist of pleomorphic particles measuring between 100 and 600 nm in diameter. There is an outer lipid membrane on the surface of which are glycoprotein projections measuring 8–17 nm. This membrane envelops the nucleocapsid that consists of a coiled helical structure with a mean diameter of 17 nm, a central core of 4–5 nm, a regular periodicity of 5 nm, and a unit length of 1 μm (Figure 35.1). In addition to the roughly spherical virions, filamentous and other bizarre forms commonly occur (Horne et al. 1960; Finch and Gibbs 1970; Kelen and McLeod 1977).

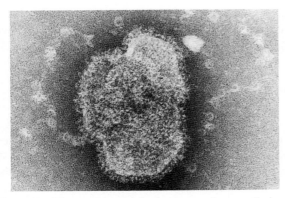

Figure 35.1 *Electron micrograph of a mumps virus negatively stained with phosphotungstic acid. The helical nucleocapsid can be seen extruding through the outer membrane at the bottom right of the virion (×200 000) (courtesy of Dr. H. Appleton).*

Virus stability

Mumps virus infectivity is lost within 3–4 days at room temperature, but may remain for several weeks at 4°C, and for years at −50°C or below. The presence of protein, for example 1 percent bovine albumin, 0.5 percent gelatin, or 2 percent serum, stabilizes the virus which otherwise loses 90–99 percent infectivity within 2 h at 4°C in a protein-free medium. Mumps virus infectivity is destroyed by heat (55°C for 20 min) and by reagents which disrupt lipids such as organic solvents, e.g. ether, acetone, or chloroform, detergents, oxidizing agents, β-propiolactone, 0.2 percent formalin at 4°C for 2 h, low pH, drying, and intense ultraviolet radiation. Mumps virus antigens are not destroyed by these treatments, however (Kelen and McLeod 1977; Hopps and Parkman 1979).

GENOMIC STRUCTURE

Organization of the genome

The mumps virus genome consists of a nonsegmented single-stranded RNA macromolecule of negative polarity that contains 15 384 nucleotides (nt), based on several mumps strains that have been completely sequenced (Elango et al. 1988, 1989a, b; Elliott et al. 1990; Okazaki et al. 1992; Clarke et al. 2000; Jin et al. 2000). There are seven genes coding for six major structural proteins that were identified by many investigators, and a seventh small hydrophobic protein (SH) of uncertain function (Figure 35.2, Table 35.1).

The NP, P, and L proteins

The NP, P, and L proteins are components of the viral nucleocapsid (NC). The nucleocapsid-associated protein (NP) is a major NC associated protein and protects the genomic RNA from cellular proteases. NP contains 549 amino acids (aa) and has an estimated molecular weight of about 61.4 kDa (Tanabayashi et al. 1990a). The NP is susceptible to proteolytic degradation following phosphorylation (McCarthy and Lazzarini 1982). Three antigenic sites have been identified residing within the 74 aa C-terminal region (aa 475–549), between aa 412 and aa 475, and within the N-terminal half of NP (Tanabayashi et al. 1990a). Amino acid substitutions identified in mumps strains are located mainly in the C-terminal half of NP (Jin et al. 2000). The primary structure of NP is well conserved among phenotypically divergent mumps virus strains (Carbone and Wolinsky 2001).

The 1 320 nt phosphoprotein (*P*) gene (including 3′ and 5′ noncoding regions) encodes a protein of 391 aa. The P protein is phosphorylated and has a predicted mass of 41.6 kDa. P is also NC-associated and forms part of the transcriptase complex. The generation of the P protein requires the insertion of two nontemplated guanosine residues into the *P* gene transcript at a G-rich region of the *P* gene. An alternative transcription pathway leading to a 224 aa virion (V) protein is produced in the absence of RNA editing by G-nucleotide insertion (Elliott et al. 1990; Paterson and Lamb 1990; Carbone and Wolinsky 2001). A relative abundance of cysteine residues is present at the C terminus of the V protein, and this feature indicates that the cysteine-rich V protein may have a regulatory function in RNA transcription (Paterson and Lamb 1990).

The large (*L*) gene is 6 925 nt in length excluding the polyA tract, and encodes a putative protein of 2 261 aa with a predicted molecular weight of 256.6 kDa (Okazaki et al. 1992). The L protein is associated with the viral nucleocapsid structure as part of the trancriptase complex. There are important motifs including the active polymerase catalytic site (aa 778–780), an RNA template contact region (aa 555–643) and an ATP binding site (aa 1814–1818) (Okazaki et al. 1992; Tanabayashi et al. 1992).

The HN, F, and M proteins

Two surface glycoproteins, hemagglutinin-neuraminidase (HN) and fusion (F), together with nonglycoprotein M (matrix), form the virus envelope. The putative HN protein consists of 582 aa and has a molecular weight of about 64 kDa. The HN protein mediates adsorption of the virus to the host cell. A hydrophobic domain of 19 residues (aa 35–53) at the N-terminus of HN, which appears to anchor the protein in the viral envelope, is conserved (Waxham et al. 1988). An A for G substitution at nt position 1081 resulting in a change from Glu^{335} to Lys^{335}, which has been suggested as a marker for virulence, was found in some strains (Brown et al. 1996; Brown and Wright 1998), but was not observed in others (Jin et al. 2000). There are nine potential glycosylation

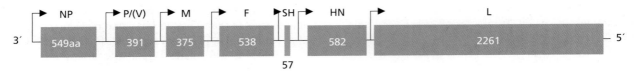

Figure 35.2 *The structure of the mumps virus genome showing the seven coding regions. The numbers in the boxes denote the number of amino acids in each gene product.*

sites and 17 cysteine residues within the putative HN protein, which are important antigen recognition sites.

The *F* gene encodes a 538 aa protein with a calculated molecular weight of about 58.8 kDa (Waxham et al. 1987). The functionally important domains within the *F* gene include the hydrophobic amino terminus domain (aa 20–23) which is presumed to be the region for initiating the fusion process, and the sequence Arg–Arg–His–Lys–Arg (aa 98–102), recognized by a host-cell protease which activates the F protein (Waxham et al. 1987). The mature form of the F protein is a disulfide-linked complex of F_1 and F_2, a sole cysteine in F_2 providing the only disulfide link with the membrane-bound F_1 (Carbone and Wolinsky 2001). Depending on the strain there are six or seven potential glycosylation sites and 14 cysteine residues within the F protein. Serine at position 195 was reported to be responsible for the in vitro cell fusion observed with certain mumps virus strains (Tanabayashi et al. 1993).

The M protein is composed of 375 aa and has an estimated mass of about 41.6 kDa. It plays a critical role in the assembly of mumps virions by mediating the alignment of the nucleocapsid beneath virus-modified areas of the host cell membrane before budding of the virion (Matsumoto 1982). The M sequence of various mumps strains is highly conserved, the aa differences amongst strains ranging between 0.3 and 1.9 percent (Tanabayashi et al. 1990b; Jin et al. 2000).

The SH protein

The small hydrophobic (SH) protein is a putative membrane protein (Takeuchi et al. 1996) of unknown function. SH mRNA is found in mumps virus-infected cells and encodes a 57 aa molecule (Elango et al. 1989b). The *SH* gene is the most variable part of the mumps virus genome and phylogenetic relationships among mumps strains have been determined using SH gene sequences (Afzal et al. 1997a; Wu et al. 1998; Jin et al. 1999). In contrast to other genes, where nt and aa divergence range from 3.2 to 4.0 percent and 0.5 to 3.0 percent, respectively (Jin et al. 2000), variations between strains of up to 20 and 41 percent, respectively, are seen in the *SH* gene (Jin et al. 1999). This confirms that the *SH* gene is the most suitable target for genotyping (Afzal et al. 1997a; Orvell et al. 1997; Wu et al. 1998), and sequence analysis of the *SH* gene has proved to be a useful tool for studying the molecular epidemiology of mumps (Cohen et al. 1999; Jin et al. 1999, 2004).

The 3′ and 5′ noncoding regions

The 3′ and 5′ noncoding regions (NTR) are situated at the start and end of each gene, as well as between each gene (intergenic). These regions are involved in transcript termination and in initiating the addition of the poly(A) tails that are present at the ends of all viral transcripts. A high degree of variation was noted at the intergenic junctions amongst mumps strains (Jin et al. 2000), as well as in other rubulaviruses (Bellini et al. 1998). The terminal RNA regions of the genomic and antigenomic RNAs of the paramyxoviruses are known to contain sequences essential for RNA replication and transcription (Elango et al. 1988; Harty and Palese 1995). The 5′ NTR of the *F* gene is critical for pathogenicity in other paramyxoviruses (Evans et al. 1990;

Table 35.1 *Position and size of mumps virus gene products*

Gene	3′ NTR (number of nts)	ORF position (nt numbers)	5′ NTR (number of nts)	Intergenic sequence (number of nts)
3′ Leader	55	–	–	–
NP	90	146–1 795	111	2
V/P	70	1 979–2 653/3 152	74	1
M	36	3 264–4 391	90	1
F	63	4 546–6 162	48	7
SH	50	6 268–6 441	92	2
HN	78	6 614–8 362	66	1
L	8	8 438–15 223	137	–
5′ Trailer	24	–	–	–

nt, nucleotide; NTR, nontranslated region; ORF, open reading frame.

Valsamakis et al. 1998). However, the significance of variations in the NTR of mumps strains, which may affect biological function, remains unclear.

Strain variation

It is generally believed that RNA viruses are prone to rapid mutation (Domingo et al. 1997), and genetic mutations could accumulate during virus transmission, cell adaptation or in vitro replication. Although mumps virus is serologically monotypic, distinct lineages of wildtype viruses exist and have been observed to cocirculate globally since genetic characterization of viruses became widely available in the 1980s. Genotypes A–J have so far been reported for mumps virus. The strain diversity was identified based on the nucleotide sequence of the most variable gene, the *SH* gene (Afzal et al. 1997a; Orvell et al. 1997; Jin et al. 1999, 2004; Kim et al. 2000; Tecle et al. 2001; Uchida et al. 2001). Studies demonstrating the overall stability of the mumps genome support the use of the *SH* gene, which shows the greatest diversity, for genotyping of mumps virus strains (Jin et al. 2000). Genetic characterization of wild-type viruses has become invaluable for mumps control by identifying the transmission pathways of the viruses (WHO 2001) and oral fluid samples may be used for this purpose (Jin et al. 2004). However, there is insufficient evidence to show that mumps genotypes are associated with particular clinical symptoms or that the current vaccine would not protect against all the genotypes (Yates et al. 1996). Further studies of mumps virus diversity are required to understand its evolution, to define the relationship between strains and to understand the effects of these mutations on biological functions.

BIOLOGICAL PROPERTIES

In vitro replication

Paramyxovirus infection of a susceptible cell includes the steps of adsorption, penetration, internalization of the virion, and uncoating (Galinski and Wechsler 1991). The F and HN proteins mediate fusion of the viral envelope with the plasma membrane, although the cell receptors for mumps virus have not yet been identified. Subsequently, virus nucleocapsids are released into the cytoplasm (Lamb 1993). Viral proteins are synthesized in the cytoplasm of infected cells, and the assembly of virions occurs on the plasma membrane by a budding process. Regions that contain the fully processed and glycosylated HN and activated F proteins are prepared on the plasma membrane to accept the nucleocapsids for budding. The M protein is thought to interact with both the cytoplasmic portions of the glycoproteins and with the nucleocapsids at the budding site. The final assembly

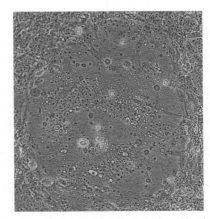

Figure 35.3 *Syncytial cytopathic effect produced by the replication of a* mumps virus *isolate in Vero cell cultures.*

process of mumps virus packaging and bud formation remains unclear (Bellini et al. 1998).

Mumps virus will grow in vitro in the allantoic cavity, amniotic cavity, and yolk sac of fertile hens' eggs, and in a number of primary cell cultures, such as chicken embryo fibroblasts, monkey kidney cells, monkey testicular cells, human embryonic kidney, human amnion, and bovine kidney cells. Many semicontinuous mammalian cell strains and continuous cell lines are also susceptible to mumps virus including Vero, BS-C-1, LLC-MK2, MDBK, MDCK, Hela, Hep-2, KB, B95a, BHK, and human fibroblasts (Shelokov et al. 1958; Hopps and Parkman 1979; Carbone and Wolinsky 2001; Knowles and Cohen 2001). Mumps virus replication has been reported in human fetal pancreatic beta cells (Notkins 1977; Vuorinen et al. 1992) and human leukocyte cultures (Duc-Nguyen and Henle 1966), and persistent mumps virus infection occurred in vitro in synovial cells, although viral antigens were not expressed on the surface of infected cells (Huppertz 1994). Typically a syncytial cytopathic effect (CPE) is seen within 3–7 days after inoculation (Figure 35.3), but vacuoles, spindlelike cells, or cell pyknosis may also occur or CPE may be minimal (Gresser and Enders 1961; McCarthy et al. 1980). Syncytium formation is dependent on cell fusion for which expression of the glycoproteins HN and F on the cell surface are essential, together with the presence of the amino acid serine at position 195 in the fusion protein (Tanabayashi et al. 1993).

Hemagglutination and hemadsorption

Mumps virus hemagglutinates guinea pig erythrocytes at 4–37°C, and also those of chickens, rodents, simians, and humans. However, elution occurs rapidly above 4°C (Beveridge and Lind 1946; Kelen and McLeod 1977). Furthermore, due to the expression of HN on the cell surface, mumps virus-infected cells, with or without CPE, hemadsorb guinea-pig, chicken, rhesus, sheep, and human O red blood cells at 4 and 20°C (Shelokov et al. 1958; Duc-Nguyen 1968; Person et al. 1971).

PATHOGENESIS

Mumps virus is usually spread by droplet infection (Gordon and Kilham 1949; Lerner 1970; Balraj and Miller 1995). There is an initial incubation period of 16–18 days, range 14–24 days, during which virus first replicates in the mucosa of the upper respiratory tract or eye. Infection then spreads to draining lymph nodes where further virus multiplication takes place, followed by a transient viremia, at which time virus dissemination occurs to other organs of the body (Kilham 1948; Lerner 1970; Carbone and Wolinsky 2001). Mumps virus can probably infect most organs of the body, but has a predilection for glandular tissue: most frequently affected are the salivary glands, testes, pancreas, and brain, and less frequently the heart, kidneys, ovaries, breasts, epididymis, prostate, joints, labyrinth, spinal cord, lung, liver, spleen, and thyroid. Mononuclear cell inflammation and edema occur in tissues during the incubation period and contribute to the tissue damage. Interferon is probably also important in pathogenesis, and can be detected in serum and saliva during the first 3 days of illness (Lerner 1970). The peripheral white blood cell count early in disease ranges between 2 400 and 30 000/mm^3 usually with a predominance of lymphocytes (Lerner 1970).

Infectious mumps virus is present in the blood for only a day or two at the onset of disease, but can be detected in the throat or saliva from 6 days before the onset of symptoms and may continue for up to 10 days after onset (Henle et al. 1948b; Kilham 1948; Brunell et al. 1968; Lerner 1970), cessation of excretion correlating with the local production of mumps-specific secretory IgA (Chiba et al. 1973). Mumps virus is also present in the urine for up to 14 days after the onset of illness (Utz et al. 1964; Lerner 1970). Kilham (1951) reported isolation of mumps virus from the breast milk of a woman who had parotitis 2 days before delivery, and Taparelli et al. (1988) isolated mumps virus from vaginal secretions. Mumps virus was recently isolated from semen during orchitis (Jin et al. 2004).

Mumps virus infects the ductal epithelium of the parotid gland producing intracytoplasmic inclusions, and the infected cells desquamate into the lumen of the duct. The duct is blocked by these cells and by leukocytes and other debris, causing dilatation above the blockage. There may also be an acute inflammatory infiltrate of periductal tissue involving lymphocytes and macrophages (Weller and Craig 1949; de Godoy et al. 1969). The lymphatics surrounding the gland become obstructed, with the production of edema that may spread down over the chest wall. Serum amylase levels usually rise coincident with the parotitis (Azimi et al. 1969; Lerner 1970).

Mumps virus infects the testes and much more rarely the ovaries. The seminiferous tubules are probably the site of virus multiplication leading to blockage of the tubules with epithelial cell debris and polymorphonuclear leukocytes, accompanied by local infiltration of lymphocytes and macrophages and interstitial edema. Partial atrophy of the testis may follow (Gall 1947; Carbone and Wolinsky 2001; Gnann 2002). The epididymis, spermatic cord, and prostate may also be affected by inflammation. Mumps virus has been isolated from testicular biopsies taken during orchitis (Hook et al. 1949; Bjorvatn 1973), and at postmortem from an 8-year-old boy with parotitis and meningoencephalitis, but no orchitis (Bistrian et al. 1972).

Involvement of the brain is common as shown by CSF pleocytosis in over half of mumps cases, although many do not have central nervous system (CNS) symptoms (Finkelstein 1938; Bang and Bang 1943; Lerner 1970). Usually the meninges are infected rather than the parenchyma. However, in mumps meningoencephalitis the basal leptomeninges, ependyma, and choroid plexus are infiltrated by lymphocytes and plasma cells. There is widespread edema, gliosis, perivascular cuffing, vascular dilatation, and engorgement, and degeneration of neurones (Taylor and Toreson 1963). Lesions may also be found in the spinal cord and mumps virus may be isolated from the brain postmortem (de Godoy et al. 1969). In secondary mumps postinfectious encephalomyelitis, the CNS lesions are caused by immunological destruction of the myelin sheaths. There is perivascular infiltration of mononuclear cells, edema, scattered foci of neuronophagia, microglial proliferation, swelling of astrocytes, and perivascular demyelination throughout the parenchyma (Donohue et al. 1955; de Godoy et al. 1969; Bistrian et al. 1972).

An acute interstitial inflammatory response may be present in the pancreas, with a mononuclear cell infiltrate, serous edema and swelling, and varying degrees of degeneration of exocrine epithelial cells. The islets of Langerhans may also be affected. The histology is similar to that in the parotid gland (Weller and Craig 1949; Craighead 1975).

The effect of mumps virus on the heart was described at postmortem in an 8-month-old girl (Brown and Richmond 1980). The heart was enlarged due to gross dilatation of all the chambers, there was pericardial effusion with mild pericarditis, and diffuse infiltration of the myocardium by lymphocytes, and occasional polymorphonuclear leukocytes. Mumps virus was isolated from the myocardium.

Transient subclinical renal dysfunction occurs in 100 percent of patients with mumps, with proteinuria in 20 percent and microscopic hematuria in 40 percent (Utz et al. 1964). Mumps virus replicates in renal tubular epithelial cells and the ureter (Weller and Craig 1949). A renal biopsy in a girl with persistent hematuria showed mild mesangial proliferative glomerulonephritis with deposition of IgA and IgM, C3, and mumps antigen in the glomerulus (Lin et al. 1990). A case of immunoglobulin A nephropathy in association with mumps infection was also reported by Fujieda et al. (2000). Kabacus et al. (1999) described an interstitial mononuclear cell infiltrate, edema, and focal tubular epithelial damage in the kidney at postmortem of a 14-year-old girl with nephritis.

Placental mumps infection may or may not lead to infection of the fetus. In one report there was a diffuse proliferative necrotizing villitis with areas of necrosis and mineralization in the fetal viscera. Intracytoplasmic inclusions were present in chorionic and fetal tissues (Garcia et al. 1980). Kurtz et al. (1982) reported mumps virus isolation from fetal tissues of a spontaneous first trimester abortion occurring on the 4th day of illness, and Takahashi et al. (1998) detected mumps virus RNA by reverse transcription polymerase chain reaction (RT-PCR) in cord blood cells of an infant with severe pulmonary symptoms whose mother was infected with mumps late in pregnancy.

CLINICAL FEATURES

Mumps is an acute infection mostly of children and young adults. Infection is subclinical overall in one quarter to one third of cases (Maris et al. 1946; Philip et al. 1959; Reed et al. 1967; Levitt et al. 1970; CDC 1989), but this depends on age. Between 10 and 14 years of age, symptoms are present in up to 90 percent of cases, whereas in children 2–3 years of age subclinical infection is frequent. Immunity following infection is usually lifelong, but re-infection can occur, sometimes symptomatically (Gut et al. 1995). The case fatality ratio is 1.6 to 3.8 per 10 000 (Carbone and Wolinsky 2001). The symptoms of mumps infection can be variable. There may be a prodromal phase of 1–7 days during which the temperature rises to 37.2–38.3°C, although it may reach above 40°C, and there may be headache, myalgia, anorexia, and malaise. The most common clinical presentation of mumps infection is swelling of the parotid gland which occurs in over 90 percent of symptomatic cases and is very often bilateral. In 75 percent of cases the contralateral gland swells 1–5 days after the first as symptoms in the first gland are subsiding. Initially there is pain or tenderness near the angle of the jaw and perhaps also earache. Maximum pain and swelling usually occurs within 48 h of onset, lasting for up to a week or more (Lerner 1970; Carbone and Wolinsky 2001), and is accompanied by dryness of the mouth. The skin over the gland is hot and flushed. Mumps infection in children under 5 years of age frequently presents as upper respiratory tract symptoms in the absence of parotitis (Cooney et al. 1975). The submaxillary and sublingual glands may also occasionally be involved.

Many other organs may be affected. The frequency of complications follows the frequency of infection, except for orchitis and oophoritis that occur much more often after puberty, and meningoencephalitis which is two to three times more common in males than in females. Mumps infection has not been reported to be more severe in immunocompromised children than in normal children, but the duration of symptoms and viral shedding may be prolonged (de Boer and de Vaan 1989; Tolpin 1991).

Orchitis occurs in about 20–38 percent of postpubertal male patients and much less frequently in prepubertal boys and infants (Werner 1950; Philip et al. 1959; Reed et al. 1967; Lerner 1970; Levy and Notkins 1971; CDC 1989). There may or may not have been preceeding parotitis 3 to 7 days earlier (Lerner 1970; Beard et al. 1977). Following experimental mumps infection, virus was isolated from saliva 10 days before the onset of orchitis (15 days postinfection) in a child who developed orchitis without parotitis (Henle et al. 1948b). Orchitis is usually unilateral, although bilateral involvement is seen in 17–40 percent of cases, and the second testicle may swell as the swelling in the first is subsiding (Werner 1950; Philip et al. 1959; Beard et al. 1977). There may be severe local pain, warmth, and tenderness, together with chills, sweating, swinging temperature, headaches, backache, nausea, and vomiting. The testicles may swell three- to four-fold within 5 days. There may also be associated epididymitis in 85 percent of cases (Lerner 1970). Testicular atrophy may result in one third to half the patients with orchitis. This is bilateral in 10 percent of those with atrophy, but mostly only one testicle is severely damaged (Werner 1950; Lerner 1970; Levy and Notkins 1971; Beard et al. 1977; CDC 1989). The sperm count may be normal, but transient or prolonged azoospermia may occur and anti-sperm antibodies may be produced (Jalal et al. 2004). Sterility is infrequent (CDC 1989).

Oophoritis, manifested by ovarian pain and pelvic tenderness, may occur in 0.5–7 percent of postpubertal females infected with mumps (Reed et al. 1967; Person et al. 1971; ASID 1974), but the symptoms are usually not as severe as orchitis in males. No association with infertility has been reported. Mastitis has been reported in 31 percent of postpubertal females in association with mumps infection, but the symptoms are mild and fleeting (Philip et al. 1959).

Symptoms reflecting central nervous system involvement may occur in up to 15 percent of mumps cases (Brown et al. 1948; CDC 1989), and are two to three times more frequent in males than in females (Azimi et al. 1969; Johnstone et al., 1972; ASID 1974; McDonald et al. 1989). A spectrum of disease is seen from mild CSF pleocytosis to severe encephalitis (Modlin et al. 1975). Most patients will have meningitis with fever, severe headache, vomiting, neck stiffness, and photophobia, but up to one quarter of these may also have symptoms of cerebral involvement, such as drowsiness, convulsions, slurred speech, twitching or rigidity of limbs, or altered sensory perception, denoting meningoencephalitis (Philip et al. 1959; Reed et al. 1967; Azimi et al. 1969; Lerner 1970; Johnstone et al. 1972; McDonald et al. 1989; Sosin et al. 1989). However, little change is usually seen in the EEG, even when clinical seizures are present (Gibbs et al. 1964).

Before mumps vaccination was introduced mumps was the most frequent cause of aseptic meningitis in the UK (Johnstone et al. 1972). Mumps meningitis may precede parotitis by a week or follow up to 3 weeks later, and in up to half of patients may occur in the absence of parotitis (Kilham 1949; Azimi et al. 1969; Wilfert 1969; Lerner 1970; Johnstone et al. 1972; Wolontis and Bjorvatn 1973). Mumps meningitis is usually mild and self-limiting, subsiding after 2–10 days without serious sequelae, but following mumps meningoencephalitis sequelae may persist for months to years. There may be difficulty in memory and learning, focal motor and sensory signs (Julkunen et al. 1985), ataxia, and behavioral disturbances along with electroencephalographic changes (Koskiniemi et al. 1983), as well as chronic encephalitis, seizures, and intellectual deterioration, polio-like paralysis or coma, and very rarely quadriplegia, single nerve palsy or weakness of the facial nerve, hydrocephalus, and psychomotor retardation (Bang and Bang 1943; Philip et al. 1959; Lerner 1970; Johnstone et al. 1972; Gonzalez-Gil et al. 2000; Carbone and Wolinsky 2001; Gnann 2002). The fatality rate following mumps encephalitis is between 0.5 and 2.3 percent (Modlin et al. 1975; CDC 1989).

Secondary postinfectious encephalitis involving demyelination may rarely occur 1–4 weeks after mumps infection with the sudden onset of fever, severe chills, paresis, convulsions, or coma, which may be accompanied by involuntary movements, cranial nerve lesions, ataxia, and upper motor neurone signs (Donohue et al. 1955; Taylor and Toreson 1963). Other very rare neurological complications of mumps include transverse myelitis, nystagmus, Ménière's disease, and bilateral neuroretinitis (Venketasubramanian 1997; Bansal et al. 1998; Khubchandani et al. 2002).

Deafness may occur secondary to endolymphatic labyrinthitis manifested by tinnitus, vertigo, and vomiting, in 0.02–0.3 percent of mumps patients. The deafness is usually unilateral and occurs with the same frequency in males and females (Bang and Bang 1943; Lerner 1970; Davis and Johnsson 1983). Mumps virus was grown at operation from inner ear perilymph (Balraj and Miller 1995). Deafness is usually transient (Vuori et al. 1962), but permanent sensorineural hearing loss may occur in up to one in 20 000 cases (ASID 1974; CDC 1989). Total bilateral deafness has been reported following asymptomatic mumps infection (Unal et al. 1998).

Pancreatitis characterized by upper epigastric pain, nausea, and vomiting, may occur following mumps infec-tion, with preceding parotitis being present in only two thirds of cases (Philip et al. 1959; Reed et al. 1967; Lerner 1970; Craighead 1975). Severe hemorrhagic pancreatitis associated with mumps has also been described (Feldstein et al. 1974). Despite many reports of a temporal association between mumps infection and the onset of diabetes mellitus, a causal relationship has not as yet been demonstrated (Craighead 1975; Notkins 1977; Carbone and Wolinsky 2001).

Electrocardiographic abnormalities may be seen in association with mumps infection, beginning 1–4 weeks after onset and lasting from 1 week to several months (Bengtsson and Örndahl 1954; Lansdown 1978). Cardiac symptoms are, however, rarely present although mild pericarditis and interstitial lymphocytic myocarditis have been reported (Lansdown 1978; Brown and Richmond 1980), and fatalities may occur following cardiac involvement (Lansdown 1978; Brown and Richmond 1980; Kabacus et al. 1999). A reported association between mumps infection and endocardial fibroelastosis is controversial (Hopps and Parkman 1979; Ni et al. 1997).

The joints may occasionally be affected by mumps virus infection, leading to mild or moderate migratory mono- or polyarthritis. This complication occurs mainly in young adults, with a male to female ratio of 5:1. Arthritis may appear up to 3 weeks before parotitis or follow up to 2–3 weeks later, usually lasting for 2 weeks or occasionally up to 6 months, but no residual joint damage results (Caranasos and Felker 1967; Gold et al. 1968; Lerner 1970; Gordon and Lauter 1984).

Transient renal dysfunction is frequent during mumps infection but rarely severe. However, a fatal case of interstitial nephritis and myocarditis was reported in a 14-year-old girl (Kabacus et al. 1999). Mumps infection has been temporally associated with subacute thyroiditis (Levy and Notkins 1971; Person et al. 1971; Bell et al. 1997), and mumps virus was grown from thyroid tissue in the acute stage of infection (Eylan et al. 1957; Lerner 1970). Transient abnormalities in liver function tests are occasionally seen in mumps infection, but clinical hepatitis is very rare (Lerner 1970; ASID 1974).

Fetal wastage may occur, usually within 2 weeks of clinical disease in the mother, in up to 27 percent of cases following mumps infection in the first trimester of pregnancy, rarely during the second trimester, and not in the third trimester or postnatally (Philip et al. 1959; Siegel et al. 1966; CDC 1989). Intrauterine mumps infection late in pregnancy may lead to severe pulmonary symptoms in the infant (Jones et al. 1980; Groenendaal et al. 1990; Takahashi et al. 1998), and perinatal infection in young infants may result in upper respiratory symptoms, thrombocytopenia, splenomegaly, and fever (Lacour et al. 1993). There is evidence that premature infants may be more susceptible than full-term infants to postnatal mumps infection (Glick et al. 1998). Clinical mumps is rare in infants during the first 2 years of life, but orchitis has been reported.

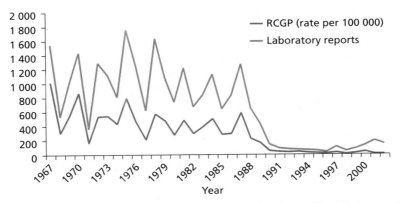

Figure 35.4 *Consultation rates and laboratory reports for mumps in England and Wales: 1967–2002. Source of data: Birmingham Research Unit, Royal College of General Practitioners (RCGP) and Health Protection Agency Communicable Disease Surveillance Centre*

THE IMMUNE RESPONSE FOLLOWING MUMPS VIRUS INFECTION OR VACCINATION

Both natural mumps infection and vaccination with live-attenuated vaccine induce cell-mediated immunity (CMI), humoral immunity (IgG, IgM, IgA) (Brown et al. 1970; Sarnesto et al. 1985), and long-term protection. Mumps-specific cytotoxic T cells and lymphoprolifera-tive responses are present in the blood, peaking 2 weeks after natural infection or a live vaccine booster dose and lasting for years (Ilonen 1979; McFarland et al. 1980; Chiba et al. 1982; Gans et al. 2001). Mumps-specific cytotoxic T cells and sensitized lymphocytes can also be detected in the CSF of patients with mumps meningitis (Fryden et al. 1978; Kreth et al. 1982; Fleischer and Kreth 1983).

During mumps infection a rise in serum antibody occurs, mumps-specific IgG being maximal during the third week of clinical disease (Ukkonen et al. 1981). Most IgG is of subclass 1, but IgG3 is also present (Sarnesto et al. 1985; Gut et al. 1995). A switch from low to high avidity IgG occurs about 180 days after infection (Narita et al. 1998). Mumps-neutralizing antibody is detectable 2 days after onset of parotitis in some patients, and peaks at 2–4 weeks (Brunell et al. 1968). Low, protective levels of antibody persist thereafter (Meyer et al. 1966; Lerner 1970), but may be boosted by natural re-infection. The level of mumps-neutralizing antibody detected after vaccinaton with live vaccine was found to be lower than after natural infection (Ennis et al. 1969). Immunity to clinical mumps is reported to correlate with a neutralizing antibody titer of >1 in 8, but the importance of protective cell mediated immunity is not known.

Mumps-specific IgM antibody is usually detectable in serum and saliva by 2–4 days after onset, and begins to wane in the first 2–6 months depending on the test used for detection (Brown et al. 1970; Chiba et al. 1973; Bjor-vatn 1974; Ukkonen et al. 1981; Gut et al. 1985; Sakata

et al. 1985). Anti-mumps IgM has also been reported in cases of secondary vaccine failure (Narita et al. 1998). Anti-mumps IgA antibody appears in serum and oral secretions during the first week of disease, and following vaccination, and persists for weeks to months (Chiba et al. 1973; Bjorvatn 1974; Friedman et al. 1983; Tanaka et al. 1992; Gut et al. 1995).

EPIDEMIOLOGY

Mumps infection occurs worldwide, man being the only natural host for the virus. Before the introduction of vaccination, mumps was a common endemic disease of children and young adults, most clinically apparent infections occurring between the ages of 4 and 14 years, with the peak at 5–9 years. Mumps is rare under 9 months of age (RCGP 1974; Modlin et al. 1975; Galbraith et al. 1984; CDC 1989), but in a study in England 63 percent of children had anti-mumps anti-body by 5 years of age and 87 percent were seropositive at 10 to 12 years (Morgan-Capner et al. 1988). This indi-cates that much infection occurs earlier than is apparent from the clinical data (Galbraith et al. 1984). Cooney et al. (1975) emphasized the role of young children in the spread of mumps infection via saliva due to the mild respiratory illness that occurs at this age. Urban commu-nities have a higher prevalence of mumps infection than rural communities. In England, the peak incidence of mumps infection occurred every 2–3 years in the prevac-cination era (Figure 35.4) (RCGP 1974; Galbraith et al. 1984; Anderson et al. 1987; Balraj and Miller 1995), but in less densely populated or remote areas outbreaks occur every 2–7 years. Mumps infection is seasonal in temperate climates in the northern hemisphere, with most cases occurring in late winter and spring (Lerner, 1970; RCGP 1974; Cooney et al. 1975; Modlin et al. 1975). However, seasonal variation has not been reported in tropical countries. Outbreaks of mumps have been reported in isolated communities (Philip et al. 1959; Reed et al. 1967), and are a particular problem in crowded environments, such as military establishments (Gordon and Kilham 1949), schools and colleges (London and Yorke, 1973; CDC 1989) and large social events involving young adults with close contact (Bell et al. 1997). There is only one serotype of mumps virus and immunity after natural infection is usually lifelong (Lerner 1970). However, reinfection has been reported in 1–2 percent of cases.

Since vaccination was introduced an at-risk cohort of older age groups has emerged (CDC 1989; Sosin et al. 1989; Bell et al. 1997; Visser et al. 1998) as predicted by Galbraith et al. (1984). The age group with the highest incidence of mumps infection changed from those under 15 years of age to those over 15 years of age 7 years after the introduction of MMR vaccination at 15 months of age in both England and Wales (Gay et al. 1997) and in Croatia (Bakasun 1997). An outbreak of mumps in 1996 in a secondary school in England was reported amongst 13–14 year olds who were too old to have been vaccinated with MMR, but too young to have natural immunity from previously circulating virus (Wehner et al. 2000).

TREATMENT

The treatment for mumps infection is symptomatic, i.e. rest and analgesics. Morphine may be needed for the relief of orchitis. Corticosteroids may be given for severe parotitis or orchitis. Gray (1973) reported that prednisolone reduced the pain of orchitis, but had no effect on the spread of infection from one testicle to the other, or on testicular atrophy. In another study of adult men with parotitis, intramuscular injection of 20 ml of gamma-globulin from human mumps convalescent serum significantly reduced the development of orchitis. There was no protective effect, however, from normal gamma-globulin (Gellis et al. 1945). Several recent studies reported a favorable outcome following experimental treatment of mumps orchitis with IFN-α-2B (Erpenbach 1991; Ruther et al. 1995; Ku et al. 1999), although in one study testicular atrophy was not prevented (Yeniyol et al. 2000).

PREVENTION

Isolation of patients is not effective in controlling the spread of mumps infection due to virus shedding by patients before symptoms are apparent and also by those who are infected subclinically (Henle et al. 1948b; Brunell et al. 1968; Lerner 1970). It was reported that the spread of mumps in a community outbreak was reduced by the early mass use of hyperimmune gamma-globulin (Copelovici et al. 1979). Normal or hyper-immune gammaglobulin given after exposure does not, however, protect from clinical mumps (Enders 1946; Reed et al. 1967; CDC 1989). Similarly vaccination with

inactivated or live vaccine late in the incubation period does not prevent clinical mumps (Meyer et al. 1966; Ennis et al. 1969), although the use of killed vaccine or MMR in susceptible groups of children or adults may contribute to the control of a mumps outbreak (Habel 1951; Ramsay et al. 1991).

Mumps infection has now been successfully controlled by vaccination in several countries. In the mid to late 1940s inactivated and live attenuated vaccines derived from monkey tissue or egg-passaged mumps virus, were tried in experimental animals and humans (Enders 1946; Enders et al. 1946; Henle et al. 1951a). A killed vaccine was introduced in 1950, but was discontinued in the USA in 1978 (Habel 1951; CDC 1989). Seroconversion was demonstrated after vaccination with the killed vaccine in 92 percent of recipients as determined by single radial hemolysis (SRH) or enzyme-linked immunosorbent assay (ELISA), but in only 58 percent of recipients by hemagglutination inhibition (HI) (Julkunen et al. 1984). In most cases, the antibody reacted with denatured HN or F protein. Killed vaccines give protection in about 80 percent of recipients, but it is only short-term protection and antibody subsequently wanes (Henle et al. 1951a; Lerner 1970). Anti-mumps IgM antibody is not detectable by radioimmunoassay (RIA) and cell mediated responses are delayed (Ilonen et al. 1981).

Live-attenuated mumps vaccines grown in cell culture were developed in the 1960s. Attenuation was achieved by serial passage of the virus in embryonated hens' eggs followed by chick embryo cell culture. The first safe and effective live-attenuated mumps vaccine was licensed in the USA in 1967 (Modlin et al. 1975; CDC 1989). Sero-conversion occurs in up to 97 percent of vaccinees within 4 weeks of vaccination with the live vaccine as detected by virus neutralization, in 75–94 percent by SRH or ELISA and in 38–67 percent by HI (Hilleman et al. 1968; Brunell et al. 1969; Ennis et al. 1969; Modlin et al. 1975; Julkunen et al. 1984; CDC 1989). Whilst 6-month-old infants were reported to have limited humoral immune responses to live mumps vaccine, probably due to the presence of maternal antibody, the cell-mediated response was equivalent to that of older infants (Gans et al. 2001). Protection lasts for at least 20 years (CDC 1989). This long-lasting protection post-vaccination may be due to boosting with naturally circulating wildtype virus in populations with only partial vaccination coverage (Modlin et al. 1975; Weibel et al. 1978). Even if mumps infection in a population is not prevented, fewer complications occur (Visser et al. 1998). Single mumps vaccine was later combined with measles and rubella in the live MMR vaccine. The serological response to mumps and long-term protection were reported to be the same following the combined vaccine as with the single live mumps vaccine (Hilleman et al. 1968; Modlin et al. 1975; Weibel et al. 1978). Vaccination with MMR produces mumps-specific gamma interferon in over 90 percent of vaccinees (Nakayama et al. 1990). In England and Wales, MMR was introduced in 1988, and was given at 12–15 months of age together with a catch-up program for preschool children (Gay et al. 1997). By 1998 childhood vaccination against mumps was being carried out with varying schedules in 82 countries (Galazka et al. 1999).

Since the introduction of mumps vaccination, the number of mumps cases have fallen dramatically in several countries (Galazka et al. 1999). In England and Wales the incidence of mumps was reduced by about 90 percent (Figure 35.4) (Balraj and Miller 1995; Gay et al. 1997), and by 98 percent over an 18-year period in the USA (CDC 1989). Mumps outbreaks have, however, recently been reported in vaccinated populations (Hersh et al. 1991; Briss et al. 1994; Cheek et al. 1995; Dias et al. 1996; Germann et al. 1996). These may be due to primary or secondary vaccine failure (Briss et al. 1994; Narita et al. 1998; Afzal and Minor 1999), and occurred mostly after only one dose of vaccine (Hersh et al. 1991). Gay et al. (1997) reported that 11 of 14 children aged 1–9 years confirmed with mumps after 1994 had previously been vaccinated. In the UK, 15–19 percent of those vaccinated at 12–18 months of age were found to be seronegative to mumps 4 years later by plaque reduction neutralization (PRN) (Miller et al. 1995) or ELISA (Pebody et al. 2002). Johnson et al. (1996) found that 11–13 year olds who had been vaccinated at 15 months of age had a lower mean titer of anti-mumps antibody than 4–6 year olds, although the prevalence of antibody was the same in each group. Therefore, although the incidence of mumps is reduced following one dose of vaccine, infection is not eliminated, and the risk of infection in older age groups leading to more complications is increased (Gay et al. 1997). A second dose of MMR at 4–6 years of age was recommended in the USA in 1989 (Galazka et al. 1999) and in the UK in 1996 (Pebody et al. 2002). In Sweden, it is given at 12 years of age (Broliden et al. 1998). A second MMR dose given at 11–13 years of age was reported to be as effective at boosting antibody levels as that given at 4–5 years of age (Johnson et al. 1996). In Finland, a two-dose MMR immunization program was introduced in 1982, and with very high childhood vaccination rates indigenous mumps had been eradicated by 1996. Between 1997 and 1999, only four cases of mumps occurred in Finland, all originating from outside the country, and no secondary cases occurred. Furthermore, infection did not spread from neighboring Russia where large mumps outbreaks were occurring in the unvaccinated population despite frequent travel between the two countries (Peltola et al. 2000).

Live mumps vaccine is contraindicated in immunosuppressed patients and pregnant women, in whom killed vaccine may be used. MMR vaccine may be given to asymptomatic HIV-infected children (CDC 1989; Dunn et al. 1998; Carbone and Wolinsky 2001; Gnann 2002).

The strain of mumps virus used in the original live vaccine was the Jeryl Lynn strain (Modlin et al. 1975). Subsequently the Urabe and Rubini strains have also been widely used in the vaccine following various attenuation protocols, as well as other strains including Leningrad-3, Hoshino, L-Zagreb, S-12, Torii, Miyahara, NK-M46, Sofia 6 (Brown and Wright 1998; Ito and Tsurudome 2002). Vaccination with the Jeryl Lynn strain has been associated with parotitis in vaccinees (Balraj and Miller 1995). Fever, rash, pruritis, and purpura may also be temporally related to vaccination (Modlin et al. 1975; CDC 1989). Mumps virus was not isolated from blood, urine, or saliva postvaccination with the Jeryl Lynn strain (Ennis et al. 1969), or from the throat after vaccination with the Miyahara or Hoshino strains, although mumps RNA was detected in the throat up to 26 days postvaccination with the latter two strains (Nagai and Nakayama 2001). However, in two of three seronegative pregnant women who were vaccinated 7–10 days prior to planned abortion, mumps virus was isolated from placental, but not fetal, tissues (Yamauchi et al. 1974). Mumps infection occurring in four army recruits who received MMR vaccine 16 days earlier, was shown to be caused by wild-type and not vaccine virus (Cohen et al. 1999). Several vaccines are now known to be mixtures of related strains (Boriskin et al. 1992; Afzal et al. 1993; Brown et al. 1996; Brown and Wright 1998). Recently a new vaccine, RIT/4385, derived from one of the two strains in Jeryl Lynn, has been evaluated in Europe (Usonis et al. 1999).

The live Urabe Am 9 strain mumps vaccine was developed in Japan (Yamanishi et al. 1973) and licensed in 1979. It was introduced in other countries in the 1980s to improve efficacy. High rates of seroconversion with the Urabe vaccine were subsequently reported in children from several countries including Brazil, South Africa, India, and China (Galazka et al. 1999), and significantly more children had mumps neutralizing antibody 4 years after receiving MMR vaccine containing the Urabe strain than vaccine containing the Jeryl Lynn strain (Miller et al. 1995). Mumps vaccine containing the Urabe strain of virus was found to be associated with parotitis in 0.7 percent of vaccinees (Balraj and Miller 1995), vaccinelike virus being isolated from the throat during parotitis (Forsey et al. 1990). Orchitis and transmission of virus to siblings was also reported (Sugiura and Yamada 1991; Sawada et al. 1993). More significantly, however, the Urabe strain was found to be associated with an unacceptable level of meningitis in vaccinees (Brown et al. 1991). Meningitis, found to occur within 2–4 weeks of vaccination, was first reported in Canada (McDonald et al. 1989) and subsequently in the UK, Belgium, France, Germany, and Japan (Balraj and Miller 1995). Vaccinelike virus was recovered from the CSF in between one in 1 000 and one in 11 000 vaccinees (Forsey et al. 1990; Brown et al. 1991; Sugiura and Yamada 1991; Miller et al. 1993). Meningitis was also a problem with two other mumps vaccines produced in Japan, from the Torii and Hoshino strains of virus (Ueda et al. 1995), with the Sofia-6 strain grown in guinea-pig cells and used in Bulgaria (Odisseev and Gacheva 1994), and with the Leningrad-3 and L-Zagreb strains in Slovenia and Croatia (Galazka et al. 1999). There was a predominance of meningitis in males, but the illness was mild with no sequelae (Sugiura and Yamada 1991; Balraj and Miller 1995). Urabe containing vaccines were subsequently withdrawn from many markets (Brown et al. 1991; Galazka et al. 1999). In the UK, Urabe containing MMR was replaced with vaccine containing the Jeryl Lynn strain in 1992, and no further cases of meningitis occurred postvaccination (Gay et al. 1997). Urabe Am9 vaccine is a mixture of strains, one of which has an A at nucleotide position 1081 of the HN gene leading to the amino acid Lys at position 335, which has been suggested by some authors (Brown et al. 1996) to be important in the causation of meningitis. It was suggested that this strain pre-existed in the vaccine virus rather than arising as a revertant (Brown and Wright 1998).

The Rubini strain of mumps virus was attenuated by passage in human diploid cells for use as a vaccine, and licensed in Switzerland in 1985 (Glück et al. 1986). It had a high apparent immunogenicity and a low incidence of side effects. However, recent mumps outbreaks in Switzerland and Singapore (Germann et al. 1996; Goh 1999), Portugal (Dias et al. 1996; Afzal et al. 1997b), Spain (Pons et al. 2000; Montes et al. 2002), and Italy amongst populations vaccinated with this strain suggest a low protective value (Germann et al. 1996; Chamot et al. 1998). Primary vaccine failure is probably occurring (Goh 1999), but secondary vaccine failure has also been suggested (Afzal and Minor 1999).

LABORATORY INVESTIGATIONS

Differential diagnosis

Parotid swelling may be due to a number of causes other than mumps virus infection, and laboratory confirmation of mumps is necessary in isolated cases. These causes include: other virus infections such as para-influenzaviruses 1 and 3, influenzavirus A, coxsackie virus, lymphocytic choriomeningitis virus (LCMV), echovirus, human immunodeficiency virus, Epstein–Barr virus, herpes simplex virus (HSV) and varicella-zoster virus; acute and chronic conditions such as tumors, Sjögren's syndrome, sarcoidosis, calculus, cirrhosis, diabetes mellitus, malnutrition, chronic renal failure, tuberculosis, amyloidosis, intraparotid hemorrhage, suppurative infections; and medications such as iodides, phenothiazines, phenylbutazone, didanosine, thiouracil (Tolpin 1991; Carbone and Wolinsky 2001; Gnann 2002). Similarly, orchitis or testicular enlargement may be due to enter-oviruses, mycoplasmas, gonococcal infection, tuberculosis, and non-infectious causes such as tumors, hernia, and torsion of a maldescended testicle (Gray 1973). Another complication of mumps infection, aseptic meningitis, may also be due to infection with other viruses including enteroviruses, LCMV, arboviruses, and HSV (Johnson 1982). In the absence of parotitis, laboratory confirmation of mumps infection is needed even during an epidemic.

Determination of immunity or susceptibility to mumps infection

The mumps skin test that was once widely used for determining immunity to mumps infection has been found to be unreliable, and results do not correlate with the presence of neutralizing antibody (Brunell et al. 1968; St Geme et al. 1975). Early serological tests used to detect antibody to mumps included CFT, HI, and virus neutralization (Henle et al. 1951b; Bashe et al. 1953; Buynak et al. 1967), although the HI test was not recommended for determining immune status because residual inhibitors in the serum can mask low titers of antibody (Kelen and McLeod 1977). There was variation in sensitivity between the tests with antibody remaining detectable by neutralization, but not by CFT or HI for months to years after infection (Ennis et al. 1968; Kelen and McLeod 1977). This, together with the specificity of the neutralization test, led to virus neutralization becoming the standard test for assessing past mumps infection (Meyer et al. 1966; Brunell et al. 1968; Kenny et al. 1970). Subsequently further tests were developed for the detection and quantification of anti-mumps antibody: indirect fluorescent antibody test (IFAT) (Brown et al. 1970), RIA (Daugharty et al. 1973; Forghani et al. 1976), hemolysis-in-gel (Grillner and Blomberg 1976; Väänänen et al. 1976), single radial immunodiffusion, hemolysis inhibition, and mixed hemadsorption (Norrby et al. 1977), enhanced virus neutralization (Sato et al. 1978), and ELISA (Leinikki et al. 1979; Popow-Kraupp 1981; Meurman et al. 1982). ELISA later became the assay of choice because of its sensitivity, specificity, speed, and low cost, and the large numbers of samples that can be tested simultaneously (Leinikki et al. 1979; Glikmann and Mordhorst 1986; Linde et al. 1987; Juto et al. 1989). Harmsen et al. (1992) reported a high level of correlation between mumps antibody as measured by indirect ELISA and that measured by a virus neutralization enzyme immunoassay, supporting an earlier suggestion that antibody detected by ELISA probably reflects immune status (Leinikki et al. 1979). This correlation was not, however, confirmed in a later study (Pipkin et al. 1999). Recently a quantitative immuno-PCR assay was developed in an attempt to increase the sensitivity and specificity of mumps antibody detection (McKie et al. 2002).

Diagnosis of recent mumps infection

SEROLOGICAL DIAGNOSIS

A serological diagnosis of mumps infection can be made by detection of seroconversion or a four-fold rise in mumps-specific IgG antibody in paired acute and convalescent sera, or the presence of mumps-specific IgM antibody in a single acute sample (Ukkonen et al. 1981; Meurman et al. 1982; Glikmann et al. 1986) or from a neonate (Takahashi et al. 1998). Two antigens were originally identified in the CFT, S antigen (soluble, nucleoprotein) and V antigen (surface glycoprotein, HN). Antibody to S antigen rises in the first 2 weeks of infection and then declines rapidly, becoming undetectable within a few months, whereas antibody to V antigen rises to high titer after the first week and persists for years (Henle et al. 1948a). Thus, a comparison of anti-S and anti-V titers could be used to identify recent mumps infection. An antibody rise may also be detected by neutralization, but it was reported that for maximal detection of antibody early after natural infection, and more especially after vaccination, a complement-mediated neutralization test was needed (Hishiyama et al. 1988).

Although mumps-specific IgM antibody can be detected in serum by several different assays, IFAT (Brown et al. 1970; Bjorvatn 1974), the hemadsorption immunosorbent test (Denoyel et al. 1982; van der Logt et al. 1982) and RIA (Daugharty et al. 1973), ELISA is now the most generally used assay (Meurman et al. 1982; Gut et al. 1985). An antibody capture format (MACRIA or MACELISA) gives rise to fewer false-positive and false-negative results than does the indirect test (Sakata et al. 1985). Recently a mumps MACELISA has been developed using recombinant nucleoprotein antigen (rNP) and an anti-rNP monoclonal antibody, which has equivalent sensitivity to the MACRIA (Samuel et al. 2002).

Saliva (i.e. oral fluid) samples are easier to collect than serum and the process is minimally invasive (Parry et al. 1987). Solid phase antibody capture immunoassays are particularly suited to the detection of low level antibody present in saliva, and thus saliva has been used as an alternative to serum for anti-mumps IgM detection in conjunction with both MACRIA (Perry et al. 1993; Jin et al. 2004) and MACELISA (Frankova and Sixtova 1987; Wehner et al. 2000). Mumps-specific IgA antibody is transiently present in saliva and may also detected by RIA (Friedman et al. 1983) or ELISA (Frankova and Sixtova 1987).

A problem encountered in the interpretation of mumps antibody tests is the presence of cross-reacting antibody to the parainfluenza viruses (Kelen and McLeod 1977; Hopps and Parkman 1979). This can be a particular problem with ELISA (Fedova et al. 1992; Harmsen et al. 1992), although less of a problem is found with IgM tests than with IgG (Brown et al. 1970; Meurman et al. 1982; Gut et al. 1985; Linde et al. 1987). Specificity in the mumps ELISA can be enhanced by the use of both an antibody capture format and a nucleoprotein antigen (Glikmann and Mordhorst 1986; Glikmann et al. 1986; Frankova et al. 1988). The effect of different antigens in the ELISA was also reported by Linde et al. (1987), who found that IgG antibody to mumps nucleoprotein rose earlier after infection than antibody to the glycoprotein, as had been reported respectively for the S and V antigens in the CFT (Henle et al. 1948a). Linde et al. (1987) and Gut et al. (1995) found that a high titer of anti-mumps IgG3 antibody to nucleoprotein antigen was diagnostic for recent mumps infection and could be used to distinguish mumps infection from infection with the parainfluenza viruses. Lehtonen and Meurman (1986) reported the use of an IgG avidity ELISA to distinguish early infection with mumps from parainfluenza virus infection.

DETECTION OF MUMPS VIRUS, ANTIGEN, AND RNA

In the acute stage of disease, mumps virus can be isolated from blood (Kilham 1948), saliva, throat washings, a swab of Stensen's duct orifice, or urine (Person et al. 1971). Mumps isolation from saliva is most successful during the first 4–5 days of symptoms (Chiba et al. 1973). Infectious mumps virus is present in urine for up to 2 weeks after onset, being isolated from 71 percent of samples taken during the first 5 days and from 58 percent taken between days 6 to 10 (Utz et al. 1964). The cell cultures susceptible to mumps virus are given above, but primary monkey kidney cells or human embryo kidney are probably the optimum cultures for primary isolation of virus (Utz et al. 1957; Person et al. 1971; Lennette et al. 1975; Kelen and McLeod 1977; Hopps and Parkman 1979). Characteristic CPE is not always present, but virus replication can be detected by hemadsorption using guinea-pig erythrocytes (see above). The isolate may be identified as mumps by IFAT, HI, hemadsorption inhibition, virus neutralization, ELISA, or more recently, by RT-PCR (Wolontis and Bjorvatn 1974; Lennette et al. 1975; Hopps and Parkman 1979; van Tiel et al. 1988; Boriskin et al. 1993). Rapid detection of virus may be achieved by an initial shell vial cell culture step followed by IFA, Vero, and LLC-MK2 being found to be the most sensitive cell lines followed by MDCK, MRC5, and HEp-2 (Germann et al. 1998; Reina et al. 2001). Alternatively when Vero cells were first inoculated and incubated overnight to amplify the virus followed by RT-PCR a sensitivity of detection of 1–20 units of infectious virus was reported (Boriskin et al. 1993). Mumps antigens can be detected by IFAT in nasopharyngeal cells or by EIA directly in saliva, and mumps RNA can be detected in saliva, throat swabs, urine, or umbilical cord blood by RT-PCR (Cusi et al. 1996; Afzal et al. 1997b; Takahashi et al. 1998; Jin et al.

2004). The timing of the samples is important, however, 69 percent of oral fluids being positive up to 7 days after onset. This falls to 20 percent between 8 and 14 days and 1.6 percent if taken later (Jin et al. 2002).

MUMPS MENINGITIS

CNS abnormalities can be detected in the majority of patients with symptoms of mumps infection (Bang and Bang 1943). There is frequently a CSF pleocytosis with, usually, <500 lymphocytes/mm^3 (Finkelstein 1938; Azimi et al. 1969; Johnstone et al. 1972), but >10 000 lymphocytes/mm^3 have been reported (Lerner 1970). The cell count peaks during the first week of illness, and wanes gradually over several weeks or months (Kilham 1949; Wilfert 1969; Wolontis and Bjorvatn 1973; Fryden et al. 1978; Vandvik et al. 1978; Link et al. 1981). The CSF glucose concentration is usually normal, but levels down to 17–41 percent of the serum level in 6–29 percent of all cases have been reported (Azimi et al. 1969; Wilfert 1969; Lerner 1970; Johnstone et al. 1972). Protein content is elevated in 39–70 percent of all cases, up to 100 mg/dl and occasionally exceeding 700 mg/dl (Kilham 1949; Azimi et al. 1969; Wilfert 1969; Fryden et al. 1978). Albumin indices are also elevated and may remain so for months (Link et al. 1981), reflecting damage to the blood–brain barrier.

Anti-mumps IgG, IgM, and IgA antibody can be detected in the CSF during mumps meningitis (Morishima et al. 1980; Vartdal and Vandvik 1983), and the nonspecific and specific antibody index for all three classes of antibody is also raised (Forsberg 1986). The IgG and IgM antibody are oligoclonal, whereas the IgA is polyclonal (Vartdal and Vandvik 1983). Between 30 and 43 percent of all patients with mumps meningitis have intrathecal synthesis of IgG and demonstrable oligoclonal immunoglobulins during the first 2 weeks of CNS symptoms, rising to 75 percent between 4 and 7 weeks, which may persist for more than 2 years even with apparently complete clinical recovery (Fryden et al. 1978; Vandvik et al. 1978; Link et al. 1981). In patients with clinical sequelae following mumps encephalitis intrathecal production of anti-mumps antibody may continue for up to 14 years (Julkunen et al. 1985). Using RIA, however, it was subsequently found that up to 91 percent of patients with acute meningitis showed mumps-specific IgG in the CSF (Reunanen et al. 1982), and using ELISA 66 percent had IgM (Forsberg 1986). Mumps-specific IgM antibody detected in the CSF by MACELISA showed no cross-reaction with the parainfluenza viruses (Glikmann et al. 1986).

In cases of mumps meningitis virus particles can be seen in the CSF by electron microscopy (Kelen and McLeod 1977). Mumps virus antigen can be detected in cells from the CSF by IF (Lerner 1970; Boyd and Vince-Ribarić 1973; Lindeman et al. 1974), or by a rapid capture ELISA (Chomel et al. 1997). It was reported

that mumps virus can be isolated from the CSF in at most half of those with meningitis (Utz et al. 1957; Azimi et al. 1969) within 8–9 days of the onset of neurological symptoms, 2–3 days being the optimum period for detection (Kilham 1949; Wolontis and Bjorvatn 1973). However, in a recent study, mumps was detected using nested RT-PCR in CSF from 96 percent of patients with clinical CNS disease and a diagnosis of mumps compared to only 39 percent detected by virus isolation (Poggio et al. 2000).

REFERENCES

Afzal, M.A. and Minor, P.D. 1999. Immune response and vaccine efficacy. *Vaccine*, **17**, 1813.

Afzal, M.A., Pickford, A.R., et al. 1993. The Jeryl Lynn vaccine strain of mumps virus is a mixture of two distinct isolates. *J Gen Virol*, **74**, 917–20.

Afzal, M.A., Buchanan, J., et al. 1997a. Clustering of mumps virus isolates by SH gene sequence only partially reflects geographical origin. *Arch Virol*, **142**, 227–38.

Afzal, M.A., Buchanan, J., et al. 1997b. RT-PCR based diagnosis and molecular characterisation of mumps viruses derived from clinical specimens collected during the 1996 mumps outbreak in Portugal. *J Med Virol*, **52**, 349–53.

Anderson, R.M., Crombie, J.A. and Grenfell, B.T. 1987. The epidemiology of mumps in the UK: a preliminary study of virus transmission, herd immunity and the potential impact of immunization. *Epidemiol Infect*, **99**, 65–84.

Association for the Study of Infectious Diseases, 1974. A retrospective survey of the complications of mumps. *J Roy Coll Gen Pract*, **24**, 552–56.

Azimi, P.H., Cramblett, H.G. and Haynes, R.E. 1969. Mumps meningoencephalitis in children. *JAMA*, **207**, 509–12.

Bakasun, V. 1997. Mumps in the region of Rijeka, Croatia. *Eur J Epidemiol*, **13**, 117–19.

Balraj, V. and Miller, E. 1995. Complications of mumps vaccines. *Rev Med Virol*, **5**, 219–27.

Bang, H.O. and Bang, J. 1943. Involvement of the central nervous system in mumps. *Acta Med Scand*, **113**, 487–505.

Bansal, R., Kalita, J., et al. 1998. Myelitis: a rare presentation of mumps. *Pediatr Neurosurg*, **28**, 204–6.

Bashe, W.J., Gotlieb, T., et al. 1953. Studies on the prevention of mumps. VI. The relationship of neutralizing antibodies to the determination of susceptibility and to the evaluation of immunization procedures. *J Immunol*, **71**, 76–85.

Beard, C.M., Benson, R.C., et al. 1977. The incidence and outcome of mumps orchitis in Rochester, Minnesota, 1935 to 1974. *Mayo Clin Proc*, **52**, 3–7.

Bell, A., Fyfe, M., et al. 1997. Outbreak of mumps among young adults – Vancouver, British Columbia. *Can Commun Dis Rep*, **23**, 169–72.

Bellini, W.J., Rota, P.A. and Anderson, L.J. 1998. Paramyxoviruses. In: Collier, L., Balows, A. and Sussman, M. (eds), *Topley and Wilson's microbiology and microbial infections*, Vol. 1. 9th edn. London: Arnold, 435–61.

Bengtsson, E. and Örndahl, G. 1954. Complications of mumps with special reference to the incidence of myocarditis. *Acta Med Scand*, **149**, 381–8.

Beveridge, W.I.B. and Lind, P.E. 1946. Mumps. 2. Virus haemagglutination and serological reactions. *Aust J Exp Biol Med Sc*, **24**, 127–32.

Beveridge, W.I.B., Lind, P.E. and Anderson, S.G. 1946. Mumps. I. Isolation and cultivation of the virus in the chick embryo. *Aust J Exp Biol Med Sc*, **24**, 15–19.

Bistrian, B., Phillips, C.A. and Kaye, I.S. 1972. Fatal mumps meningoencephalitis. Isolation of virus premortem and postmortem. *JAMA*, **222**, 478–9.

Bjorvatn, B. 1973. Mumps virus recovered from testicles by fine-needle aspiration biopsy in cases of mumps orchitis. *Scand J Infect Dis*, **5**, 3–5.

Bjorvatn, B. 1974. Incidence and persistence of mumps-specific IgM and IgA in the sera of mumps patients. *Scand J Infect Dis*, **6**, 125–9.

Boriskin, Y.S., Yamada, A., et al. 1992. Genetic evidence for variant selection in the course of dilute passaging of mumps vaccine virus. *Res Virol*, **143**, 279–383.

Boriskin, Yu.S., Booth, J.C. and Yamada, A. 1993. Rapid detection of mumps virus by the polymerase chain reaction. *J Virol Meth*, **42**, 23–32.

Boyd, J.F. and Vince-Ribarić, V. 1973. The examination of cerebrospinal fluid cells by fluorescent antibody staining to detect mumps antigen. *Scand J Infect Dis*, **5**, 7–15.

Briss, P.A., Fehrs, L.J., et al. 1994. Sustained transmission of mumps in a highly vaccinated population: assessment of primary vaccine failure and waning vaccine-induced immunity. *J Infect Dis*, **169**, 77–82.

Broliden, K., Abreu, E.R., et al. 1998. Immunity to mumps before and after MMR vaccination at 12 years of age in the first generation offered the two-dose immunization programme. *Vaccine*, **16**, 323–7.

Brown, E.G. and Wright, K.E. 1998. Genetic studies on a mumps vaccine strain associated with meningitis. *Rev Med Virol*, **8**, 129–42.

Brown, E.G., Furesz, J., et al. 1991. Nucleotide sequence analysis of Urabe mumps vaccine strain that caused meningitis in vaccine recipients. *Vaccine*, **9**, 840–2.

Brown, E.G., Dimock, K. and Wright, K.E. 1996. The Urabe AM9 mumps vaccine is a mixture of viruses differing at amino acid 335 of the hemagglutinin-neuraminidase gene with one form associated with disease. *J Infect Dis*, **174**, 619–22.

Brown, G.C., Baublis, J.V. and O'Leary, T.P. 1970. Development and duration of mumps fluorescent antibodies in various immunoglobulin fractions of human serum. *J Immunol*, **104**, 86–94.

Brown, J.W., Kirkland, H.B. and Hein, G.E. 1948. Central nervous system involvement during mumps. *Am J Med Sci*, **215**, 434–41.

Brown, N.J. and Richmond, S.J. 1980. Fatal mumps myocarditis in an 8-month-old child. *Br Med J*, **281**, 356–7.

Brunell, P.A., Brickman, A., et al. 1968. Ineffectiveness of isolation of patients as a method of preventing the spread of mumps. *N Engl J Med*, **279**, 1357–61.

Brunell, P.A., Brickman, A. and Steinberg, S. 1969. Evaluation of a live attenuated mumps vaccine (Jeryl Lynn). *Am J Dis Child*, **118**, 435–40.

Buynak, E.B., Whitman, J.E., et al. 1967. Comparison of neutralization and hemagglutination-inhibition techniques for measuring mumps antibody. *Proc Soc Exp Biol Med*, **125**, 1068–71.

Caranasos, G.J. and Felker, J.R. 1967. Mumps arthritis. *Arch Intern Med*, **199**, 394–8.

Carbone, K.M. and Wolinsky, J.S. 2001. Mumps virus. In: Knipe, D.M. and Howley, P.M. (eds), *Fields' Virology*, 4th edn. Philadelphia, PA: Lippincott Williams and Wilkins, 1381–400.

Centers for Disease Control. 1989. Mumps prevention. *Morb Mortal Wkly Rep*, **38**, 388–400.

Chamot, E., Toscani, L., et al. 1998. Estimation of the efficacy of three strains of mumps vaccines during an epidemic of mumps in the Geneva canton (Switzerland). *Rev Epidemiol San Pub*, **46**, 100–7.

Cheek, J.E., Baron, R., et al. 1995. Mumps outbreak in a highly vaccinated school population. Evidence for large-scale vaccination failure. *Arch Ped Adoles Med*, **149**, 774–8.

Chiba, Y., Horino, K., et al. 1973. Virus excretion and antibody responses in saliva in natural mumps. *Tohoku J Exp Med*, **111**, 229–38.

Chiba, Y., Tsutsumi, H., et al. 1982. Human leukocyte antigen-linked genetic controls for T cell-mediated cytotoxic response to mumps virus in humans. *Infect Immun*, **35**, 600–4.

Chomel, J.J., Robin, Y., et al. 1997. Rapid direct diagnosis of mumps meningitis by ELISA capture technique. *J Virol Meth*, **68**, 97–104.

Clarke, D.K., Sidhu, M.S., et al. 2000. Rescue of mumps virus from cDNA. *J Virol*, **74**, 4831–8.

Cohen, B.J., Jin, L., et al. 1999. Infection with wild-type mumps virus in army recruits temporally associated with MMR vaccine. *Epidemiol Infect*, **123**, 251–5.

Cooney, M.K., Fox, J.P. and Hall, C.E. 1975. The Seattle virus watch. VI. Observations on infections with and illness due to parainfluenza, mumps and respiratory syncytial viruses and *Mycoplasma pneumoniae*. *Am J Epidemiol*, **101**, 532–51.

Copelovici, Y., Strulovici, D., et al. 1979. Data on the efficiency of specific antimumps immunoglobulins in the prevention of mumps and of its complications. *Rev Rouman Med Virol*, **30**, 171–7.

Craighead, J.E. 1975. The role of viruses in the pathogenesis of pancreatic disease and diabetes mellitus. *Prog Med Virol*, **19**, 161–214.

Cusi, M.G., Bianchi, S., et al. 1996. Rapid detection and typing of circulating mumps virus by reverse transcription/polymerase chain reaction. *Res Virol*, **147**, 227–32.

Daugharty, H., Warfield, D.T., et al. 1973. Mumps class-specific immunoglobulins in radioimmunoassay and conventional serology. *Infect Immun*, **7**, 380–5.

Davis, L.E. and Johnsson, L.-G. 1983. Viral infections of the inner ear: clinical, virologic and pathologic studies in humans and animals. *Am J Otolaryngol*, **4**, 347–62.

de Boer, A.W. and de Vaan, G.A. 1989. Mild course of mumps in patients with acute lymphoblastic leukaemia. *Eur J Pediatr*, **148**, 618–19.

de Godoy, C.V.F., de Brito, T., et al. 1969. Fatal mumps meningoencephalitis. Isolation of virus from human brain (case report). *Rev Inst Med Trop São Paulo*, **11**, 436–41.

Denoyel, G.A., Gaspar, A. and Peyramond, D. 1982. A solid-phase reverse immunosorbent test (SPRIST) for the demonstration of specific-mumps virus IgM-class antibody. *Arch Virol*, **71**, 349–52.

Dias, J.A., Cordeiro, M., et al. 1996. Mumps epidemic in Portugal despite high vaccine coverage – preliminary report. *Eurosurveillance*, **1**, 25–8.

Domingo, E., Menendez-Arias, L. and Holland, J.J. 1997. RNA virus fitness. *Rev Med Virol*, **7**, 87–96.

Donohue, W.L., Playfair, F.D. and Whitaker, L. 1955. Mumps encephalitis. Pathology and pathogenesis. *J Pediatr*, **47**, 395–412.

Duc-Nguyen, H. 1968. Hemadsorption of mumps virus examined by light and electron microscopy. *J Virol*, **2**, 494–506.

Duc-Nguyen, H. and Henle, W. 1966. Replication of mumps virus in human leukocyte cultures. *J Bacteriol*, **92**, 258–65.

Dunn, D.T., Newell, M.L., et al. 1998. Routine vaccination and vaccine-preventable infections in children born to human immunodeficiency virus-infected mothers. European Collaborative Study. *Acta Paediatr*, **87**, 458–9.

Elango, N., Varsanyi, T.M., et al. 1988. Molecular cloning and characterization of six genes, determination of gene order and intergenic sequences and leader sequence of mumps virus. *J Gen Virol*, **69**, 2893–900.

Elango, N., Varsanyi, T.M., et al. 1989a. The mumps virus fusion protein mRNA sequence and homology among the *Paramyxoviridae* proteins. *J Gen Virol*, **70**, 801–7.

Elango, N., Kövamees, J., et al. 1989b. mRNA sequence and deduced amino acid sequence of the mumps virus small hydrophobic protein gene. *J Virol*, **63**, 1413–15.

Elliott, G.D., Yeo, R.P., et al. 1990. Strain-variable editing during transcription of the P gene of mumps virus may lead to the generation of non-structural proteins NS1 (V) and NS2. *J Gen Virol*, **71**, 1555–60.

Enders, J.F. 1946. Mumps: techniques of laboratory diagnosis, tests for susceptibility, and experiments on specific prophylaxis. *J Pediatr*, **29**, 129–42.

Enders, J.F., Levens, J.H., et al. 1946. Attenuation of virulence with retention of antigenicity of mumps virus after passage in the embryonated egg. *J Immunol*, **54**, 283–91.

Ennis, F.A., Douglas, R.D., et al. 1968. A plaque neutralization test for determining mumps antibodies. *Proc Soc Exp Biol Med*, **129**, 896–9.

Ennis, F.A., Douglas, R.D., et al. 1969. Clinical studies with virulent and attenuated mumps viruses. *Am J Epidemiol*, **89**, 176–83.

Erpenbach, K.H. 1991. Systemic treatment with interferon-alpha 2B: an effective method to prevent sterility after bilateral mumps orchitis. *J Urol*, **146**, 54–6.

Evans, S.A., Belsham, G.J. and Barrett, T. 1990. The role of the 5′ nontranslated regions of the fusion protein mRNAs of canine distemper virus and rinderpest virus. *Virology*, **177**, 317–23.

Eylan, E., Zmucky, R. and Sheba, C. 1957. Mumps virus and subacute thyroiditis. *Lancet*, **I**, 1062–3.

Fedova, D., Novotny, J. and Kubinova, I. 1992. Serological diagnosis of parainfluenza virus infections: verification of the sensitivity and specificity of the haemagglutination-inhibition (HI), complement-fixation (CF), immunofluorescence (IFA) tests and enzyme immunoassay (ELISA). *Acta Virol*, **36**, 304–12.

Feldstein, J.D., Johnson, F.R., et al. 1974. Acute hemorrhagic pancreatitis and pseudocyst due to mumps. *Ann Surg*, **180**, 85–8.

Finch, J.T. and Gibbs, A.J. 1970. Observations on the structure of the nucleocapsids of some paramyxoviruses. *J Gen Virol*, **6**, 141–50.

Finkelstein, H. 1938. Meningo-encephalitis in mumps. *JAMA*, **111**, 17–19.

Fleischer, B. and Kreth, H.W. 1983. Clonal analysis of HLA-restricted virus-specific cytotoxic T lymphocytes from cerebrospinal fluid in mumps meningitis. *J Immunol*, **130**, 2187–90.

Forghani, B., Schmidt, N.J. and Lennette, E.H. 1976. Sensitivity of a radioimmunoassay method for detection of certain viral antibodies in sera and cerebrospinal fluids. *J Clin Microbiol*, **4**, 470–8.

Forsberg, P. 1986. Studies on immunoglobulins and specific antibody in central nervous system infections. *Acta Neurol Scand*, **73**, Suppl 105, 1–76.

Forsey, T., Mawn, J.A., et al. 1990. Differentiation of vaccine and wild mumps viruses using the polymerase chain reaction and dideoxynucleotide sequencing. *J Gen Virol*, **71**, 987–90.

Frankova, V. and Sixtova, E. 1987. Specific IgM antibodies in the saliva of mumps patients. *Acta Virol*, **31**, 357–64.

Frankova, V., Holubova, J., et al. 1988. Contribution to laboratory diagnosis of mumps and parainfluenza. *Acta Virol*, **32**, 503–14.

Friedman, M., Hadari, I., et al. 1983. Virus-specific secretory IgA antibodies as a means of rapid diagnosis of measles and mumps infection. *Isr J Med Sci*, **19**, 881–4.

Fryden, A., Link, H. and Moller, E. 1978. Demonstration of cerebrospinal fluid lymphocytes sensitized against virus antigens in mumps meningitis. *Acta Neurol Scand*, **57**, 396–404.

Fujieda, M., Kinoshita, A., et al. 2000. Mumps associated with immunoglobulin A nephropathy. *Pediatr Infect Dis J*, **19**, 669–71.

Galazka, A.M., Robertson, S.E. and Kraigher, A. 1999. Mumps and mumps vaccine: a global review. *Bull World Health Organ*, **77**, 3–14.

Galbraith, N.S., Young, S.E.J., et al. 1984. Mumps surveillance in England and Wales 1962–81. *Lancet*, **1**, 91–4.

Galinski, M.S. and Wechsler, S.L. 1991. The molecular biology of the paramyxovirus genus. In: Kingsbury, D.W. (ed.), *The paramyxoviruses*. New York: Plenum Press, 41–82.

Gall, E.A. 1947. The histopathology of acute mumps orchitis. *Am J Pathol*, **23**, 637–51.

Gans, H., Yasukawa, L., et al. 2001. Immune responses to measles and mumps vaccination of infants at 6, 9, and 12 months. *J Infect Dis*, **184**, 817–26.

Garcia, A.G., Pereira, J.M., et al. 1980. Intrauterine infection with mumps virus. *Obstet Gynecol*, **56**, 756–9.

Gay, N., Miller, E., et al. 1997. Mumps surveillance in England and Wales supports introduction of two dose vaccination schedule. Communicable Disease Report. *CDR Rev*, **7**, R21–6.

Gellis, S.S., McGuiness, A.C. and Peters, M. 1945. A study of the prevention of mumps orchitis by gammaglobulin. *Am J Med Sci*, **210**, 661–4.

Germann, D., Ströhle, A., et al. 1996. An outbreak of mumps in a population partially vaccinated with the Rubini strain. *Scand J Infect Dis*, **28**, 235–8.

Germann, D., Gorgievski, M., et al. 1998. Detection of mumps virus in clinical specimens by rapid centrifugation culture and conventional tube cell culture. *J Virol Meth*, **73**, 59–64.

Gershon, A.A. 1995. Chickenpox, measles and mumps. In: Remington, J.S. and Klein, J.O. (eds), *Infectious diseases of the fetus and newborn infant*, 4th edn. Philadelphia: WB Saunders Company, 565–618, Chapter 13.

Gibbs, F., Gibbs, E., et al. 1964. Common types of childhood encephalitis: Electroencephalographic and clinical relationships. *Arch Neurol*, **10**, 111.

Glick, C., Feldman, S., et al. 1998. Measles, mumps, and rubella serology in premature infants weighing less than 1,000 grams. *South Med J*, **91**, 159–60.

Glikmann, G. and Mordhorst, C.H. 1986. Serological diagnosis of mumps and parainfluenza type-1 virus infections by enzyme immunoassay, with a comparison of two different approaches for detection of mumps IgG antibodies. *Acta Pathol Microbiol Immunol Scand Sect C Immunol*, **94**, 157–66.

Glikmann, G., Pedersen, M. and Mordhorst, C.H. 1986. Detection of specific immunoglobulin M to mumps virus in serum and cerebrospinal fluid samples from patients with acute mumps infection, using an antibody-capture enzyme immunoassay. *Acta Pathol Microbiol Immunol Scand Sect C Immunol*, **94**, 145–56.

Glück, R., Hoskins, J.M., et al. 1986. Rubini, a new live attenuated mumps vaccine virus strain for human diploid cells. *Dev Biol Stand*, **65**, 29–35.

Gnann, J.W. 2002. Mumps virus. In: Richman, D.D., Whitley, R.J. and Hayden, F.G. (eds), *Clinical virology*. Washington DC: ASM Press, 829–43.

Goh, K.T. 1999. Resurgence of mumps in Singapore caused by the Rubini mumps virus vaccine strain. *Lancet*, **354**, 1355–6.

Gold, H.E., Boxerbaum, B. and Leslie, H.J. 1968. Mumps arthritis. *Am J Dis Child*, **116**, 547–8.

Gonzalez-Gil, J., Zarrabeitia, M.T., et al. 2000. Hydrocephalus: a fatal late consequence of mumps encephalitis. *J Forensic Sci*, **45**, 204–7.

Gordon, J.E. and Kilham, L. 1949. Ten years in the epidemiology of mumps. *Am J Med Sci*, **218**, 338–59.

Gordon, S.C. and Lauter, C.B. 1984. Mumps arthritis: a review of the literature. *Rev Infect Dis*, **6**, 338–44.

Gray, J.A. 1973. Mumps. *Br Med J*, **1**, 338–40.

Gresser, I. and Enders, J.F. 1961. Cytopathogenicity of mumps virus in cultures of chick embryo and human amnion cells. *Proc Soc Exp Biol Med*, **107**, 804–7.

Grillner, L. and Blomberg, J. 1976. Hemolysis-in-gel and neutralization tests for determination of antibodies to mumps virus. *J Clin Microbiol*, **4**, 11–15.

Groenendaal, F., Rothbarth, P.H., et al. 1990. Congenital mumps pneumonia: a rare cause of neonatal respiratory distress. *Acta Paediatr Scand*, **79**, 1252–4.

Gut, J.P., Spiess, C., et al. 1985. Rapid diagnosis of acute mumps infection by a direct immunoglobulin M antibody capture enzyme immunoassay with labeled antigen. *J Clin Microbiol*, **21**, 346–52.

Gut, J.P., Lablache, C., et al. 1995. Symptomatic mumps virus reinfections. *J Med Virol*, **45**, 17–23.

Habel, K. 1945. Cultivation of mumps virus in the developing chick embryo and its application to studies of immunity to mumps in man. *Pub Health Rep*, **60**, 201–12.

Habel, K. 1951. Vaccination of human beings against mumps: vaccine administered at the start of an epidemic. II. Effect of vaccination upon the epidemic. *Am J Hyg*, **54**, 312–18.

Harmsen, T., Jongerius, M., et al. 1992. Comparison of a neutralization enzyme immunoassay and an enzyme-linked immunosorbent assay for evaluation of immune status of children vaccinated for mumps. *J Clin Microbiol*, **30**, 2139–44.

Harty, R.N. and Palese, P. 1995. Mutations within noncoding terminal sequences of model RNAs of Sendai virus: influence on reporter gene expression. *J Virol*, **69**, 5128–31.

Henle, G. and Deinhardt, F. 1955. Propagation and primary isolation of mumps virus in tissue culture. *Proc Soc Exp Biol Med*, **89**, 556–60.

Henle, G. and McDougall, C.L. 1947. Mumps meningo-encephalitis. Isolation in chick embryos of virus from spinal fluid of a patient. *Proc Soc Exp Biol Med*, **66**, 209–11.

Henle, G., Harris, S. and Henle, W. 1948a. The reactivity of various human sera with mumps complement fixation antigens. *J Exp Med*, **88**, 133–47.

Henle, G., Henle, W., et al. 1948b. Isolation of mumps virus from human beings with induced apparent or inapparent infections. *J Exp Med*, **88**, 223–32.

Henle, G., Bashe, W.J., et al. 1951a. Studies on the prevention of mumps. III. The effect of subcutaneous injection of inactivated mumps virus vaccines. *J Immunol*, **66**, 561–77.

Henle, G., Henle, W., et al. 1951b. Studies on the prevention of mumps. I. The determination of susceptibility. *J Immunol*, **66**, 535–49.

Hersh, B.S., Fine, P.E., et al. 1991. Mumps outbreak in a highly vaccinated population. *J Pediatr*, **119**, 187–93.

Hilleman, M.R., Buynak, E.B., et al. 1968. Live, attenuated mumps-virus vaccine. *N Engl J Med*, **278**, 227–32.

Hishiyama, M., Tsurudome, M., et al. 1988. Complement-mediated neutralization test for determination of mumps vaccine-induced antibody. *Vaccine*, **6**, 423–7.

Hook, E.W., Poole, S.A. and Friedewald, W.F. 1949. Virus isolation and serologic studies on patients with clinical mumps. *J Infect Dis*, **84**, 230–4.

Hopps, H.E. and Parkman, P.D. 1979. Mumps virus. In: Lennette, E.H. and Schmidt, N.J. (eds), *Diagnostic procedures for viral, rickettsial and chlamydial infections*, 5th edn. Washington DC: American Public Health Association., 633–53.

Horne, R.W., Waterson, A.P., et al. 1960. The structure and composition of the myxoviruses. I. Electron microscope studies of the structure of myxovirus particles by negative staining techniques. *Virology*, **11**, 79–98.

Huppertz, H.I. 1994. How could infectious agents hide in synovial cells? Possible mechanisms of persistent viral infection in a model for the etiopathogenesis of chronic arthritis. *Rheumatol Int*, **14**, 71–5.

Ilonen, J. 1979. Lymphocyte blast transformation response of seropositive and seronegative subjects to herpes simplex, rubella, mumps and measles virus antigens. *Acta Pathol Microbiol Scand Sect C Immunol*, **87C**, 151–7.

Ilonen, J., Salmi, A., et al. 1981. Lymphocyte blast transformation and antibody responses after vaccination with inactivated mumps virus vaccine. *Acta Pathol Microbiol Scand Sect C Immunol*, **89**, 303–9.

Ito, Y. and Tsurudome, M. 2002. Rubulavirus. In: Tidona, C.A. and Darai, G. (eds), *The Springer index of viruses*. Berlin: Springer-Verlag, 656–9.

Jalal, H., Bahadur, G., et al. 2004. Mumps epididymo-orchitis with prolonged detection of virus in semen and the development of anti-sperm antibodies. *J Med Virol*, **73**, 147–50.

Jin, L., Beard, S. and Brown, D.W. 1999. Genetic heterogeneity of mumps virus in the United Kingdom: identification of two new genotypes. *J Infect Dis*, **180**, 829–33.

Jin, L., Beard, S., et al. 2000. The genomic sequence of a contemporary wild-type mumps virus strain. *Virus Res*, **70**, 75–83.

Jin, L., Vyse, A. and Brown, D.W.G. 2002. The role of RT-PCR assay of oral fluid for diagnosis and surveillance of measles, mumps and rubella. *Bull World Health Organ*, **80**, 76–7.

Jin, L., Brown, D.W.G., et al. 2004. Genetic diversity of mumps virus in oral fluid specimens: application to mumps epidemiological study. *J Infect Dis*, **189**, 1001–8.

Johnson, C.D. and Goodpasture, E.W. 1934. An investigation of the etiology of mumps. *J Exp Med*, **59**, 1–19.

Johnson, C.E., Kumar, M.L., et al. 1996. Antibody persistence after primary measles-mumps-rubella vaccine and response to a second dose given at four to six vs. eleven to thirteen years. *Pediatr Infect Dis J*, **15**, 687–92.

Johnson, R.T. 1982. *Viral infections of the nervous system*. New York: Raven Press.

Johnstone, J.A., Ross, C.A.C. and Dunn, M. 1972. Meningitis and encephalitis associated with mumps infection. A 10-year survey. *Arch Dis Child*, **47**, 647–51.

Jones, J.F., Ray, C.G. and Fulginiti, V.A. 1980. Perinatal mumps infection. *J Pediatr*, **96**, 912–14.

Julkunen, I., Vaananen, P. and Penttinen, K. 1984. Antibody responses to mumps virus proteins in natural mumps infection and after vaccination with live and inactivated mumps virus vaccines. *J Med Virol*, **14**, 209–19.

Julkunen, I., Koskiniemi, M., et al. 1985. Chronic mumps virus encephalitis. Mumps antibody levels in cerebrospinal fluid. *J Neuroimmunol*, **8**, 167–75.

Juto, P., Settergren, B. and Mincheva-Nilsson, L. 1989. Serum IgG and IgM responses in mumps infection as measured by ELISA using a guinea pig capture antibody raised by intranasal immunization. *J Infect Dis*, **159**, 998–9.

Kabacus, N., Aydinoglu, H., et al. 1999. Fatal mumps nephritis and myocarditis. *J Trop Pediatr*, **45**, 358–60.

Kelen, A.E. and McLeod, D.A. 1977. Paramyxoviruses: comparative diagnosis of parainfluenza, mumps, measles, and respiratory syncytial virus infections. In: Kurstak, E. and Kurstak, C. (eds), *Comparative diagnosis of viral diseases. Human and related viruses, part A*, Vol. 1. New York: Academic Press, 503–607.

Kenny, M.T., Albright, K.L. and Sanderson, R.P. 1970. Microneutralization test for the determination of mumps antibody in Vero cells. *Appl Microbiol*, **20**, 371–3.

Khubchandani, R., Rane, T., et al. 2002. Bilateral neuroretinitis associated with mumps. *Arch Neurol*, **59**, 1633–6.

Kilham, L. 1948. Isolation of mumps virus from the blood of a patient. *Proc Soc Exp Biol Med*, **69**, 99–100.

Kilham, L. 1949. Mumps meningoencephalitis with and without parotitis. *Am J Dis Child*, **78**, 324–33.

Kilham, L. 1951. Mumps virus in human milk and in milk of infected monkey. *JAMA*, **146**, 1231–2.

Kim, S.H., Song, K.J., et al. 2000. Phylogenetic analysis of the small hydrophobic (SH) gene of mumps virus in Korea: identification of a new genotype. *Microbiol Immunol*, **44**, 173–7.

Knowles, W.A. and Cohen, B.J. 2001. Efficient isolation of mumps virus from a community outbreak using the marmoset lymphoblastoid cell line B95a. *J Virol Meth*, **96**, 93–6.

Koskiniemi, M., Donner, M. and Pettay, O. 1983. Clinical appearance and outcome in mumps encephalitis in children. *Acta Paediatr Scand*, **72**, 603–9.

Kreth, H.W., Kress, L., et al. 1982. Demonstration of primary cytotoxic T cells in venous blood and cerebrospinal fluid of children with mumps meningitis. *J Immunol*, **128**, 2411–15.

Ku, J.H., Kim, Y.H., et al. 1999. The preventive effect of systemic treatment with interferon-alpha 2B for infertility from mumps orchitis. *BJU Int*, **84**, 839–42.

Kurtz, J.B., Tomlinson, A.H. and Pearson, J. 1982. Mumps virus isolated from a fetus. *Br Med J*, **284**, 471.

Lacour, M., Maherzi, M., et al. 1993. Thrombocytopenia in a case of neonatal mumps infection: evidence for further clinical presentations. *Eur J Pediatr*, **152**, 739–41.

Lamb, R.A. 1993. Paramyxovirus fusion: a hypothesis for changes. *Virology*, **197**, 1–11.

Lansdown, A.B.G. 1978. Viral infections and diseases of the heart. *Prog Med Virol*, **24**, 70–113.

Lehtonen, O.-P.J. and Meurman, O.H. 1986. Avidity of IgG antibodies against mumps, parainfluenza 2 and Newcastle disease viruses after mumps infection. *J Virol Meth*, **14**, 1–7.

Leinikki, P.O., Shekarchi, I., et al. 1979. Evaluation of enzyme-linked immunosorbent assay (ELISA) for mumps virus antibodies. *Proc Soc Exp Biol Med*, **160**, 363–7.

Lennette, D.A., Emmons, R.W. and Lennette, E.H. 1975. Rapid diagnosis of mumps virus infections by immunofluorescence methods. *J Clin Microbiol*, **2**, 81–4.

Lerner, A.M. 1970. Guide to immunization against mumps. *J Infect Dis*, **122**, 116–21.

Levens, J.H. and Enders, J.F. 1945. The hemoagglutinative properties of amniotic fluid from embryonated eggs infected with mumps virus. *Science*, **102**, 117–20.

Levitt, L.P., Mahoney, D.H., et al. 1970. Mumps in a general population. A sero-epidemiologic study. *Am J Dis Child*, **120**, 134–8.

Levy, N.L. and Notkins, A.L. 1971. Viral infections and diseases of the endocrine system. *J Infect Dis*, **124**, 94–103.

Lin, C.Y., Chen, W.P. and Chiang, H. 1990. Mumps associated with nephritis. *Child Nephrol Urol*, **10**, 68–71.

Linde, G.A., Granstrom, M. and Orvell, C. 1987. Immunoglobulin class and immunoglobulin G subclass enzyme-linked immunosorbent assays compared with microneutralization assay for serodiagnosis of mumps infection and determination of immunity. *J Clin Microbiol*, **25**, 1653–8.

Lindeman, J., Muller, W.K., et al. 1974. Rapid diagnosis of meningoencephalitis, encephalitis. *Neurology (Minn)*, **24**, 143–8.

Link, H., Laurenzi, M.A. and Fryden, A. 1981. Viral antibodies in oligoclonal and polyclonal IgG synthesized within the central nervous system over the course of mumps meningitis. *J Neuroimmunol*, **1**, 287–98.

London, W.P. and Yorke, J.A. 1973. Recurrent outbreaks of measles, chickenpox and mumps. I. Seasonal variation in contact rates. *Am J Epidemiol*, **98**, 453–68.

Maris, E.P., Enders, J.F., et al. 1946. Immunity in mumps. IV. The correlation of the presence of complement-fixing antibody and resistance to mumps in human beings. *J Exp Med*, **84**, 323–39.

Matsumoto, T. 1982. Assembly of paramyxoviruses. *Microbiol Immunol*, **26**, 285–320.

McCarthy, M. and Lazzarini, R.A. 1982. Intracellular nucleocapsid RNA of mumps virus. *J Gen Virol*, **58**, 205–9.

McCarthy, M., Jubelt, B., et al. 1980. Comparative studies of five strains of mumps virus in vitro and in neonatal hamsters: evaluation of growth, cytopathogenicity, and neurovirulence. *J Med Virol*, **5**, 1–15.

McDonald, J.C., Moore, D.L. and Quennec, P. 1989. Clinical and epidemiologic features of mumps meningoencephalitis and possible vaccine-related disease. *Pediatr Infect Dis J*, **8**, 751–5.

McFarland, H.F., Pedone, C.A., et al. 1980. The response of human lymphocyte subpopulations to measles, mumps, and vaccinia viral antigens. *J Immunol*, **125**, 221–5.

McKie, A., Samuel, D., et al. 2002. Development of a quantitative immuno-PCR assay and its use to detect mumps-specific IgG in serum. *J Immunol Meth*, **261**, 167–75.

Meurman, O., Hanninen, P., et al. 1982. Determination of IgG- and IgM-class antibodies to mumps virus by solid-phase enzyme immunoassay. *J Virol Meth*, **4**, 249–56.

Meyer, M.B., Stifler, W.C. and Joseph, J.M. 1966. Evaluation of mumps vaccine given after exposure to mumps, with special reference to the exposed adult. *Pediatrics*, **37**, 304–15.

Miller, E., Goldacre, M., et al. 1993. Risk of aseptic meningitis after measles, mumps, and rubella vaccine in UK children. *Lancet*, **341**, 979–82.

Miller, E., Hill, A., et al. 1995. Antibodies to measles, mumps and rubella in UK children 4 years after vaccination with different MMR vaccines. *Vaccine*, **13**, 799–802.

Modlin, J.F., Orenstein, W.A. and Brandling-Bennett, A.D. 1975. Current status of mumps in the United States. *J Infect Dis*, **132**, 106–9.

Montes, M., Cilla, G., et al. 2002. Mumps outbreak in vaccinated children in Gipuzkoa (Basque Country), Spain. *Epidemiol Infect*, **129**, 551–6.

Morgan-Capner, P., Wright, J., et al. 1988. Surveillance of antibody to measles, mumps and rubella by age. *Br Med J*, **297**, 770–2.

Morishima, T., Miyazu, M., et al. 1980. Local immunity in mumps meningitis. *Am J Dis Child*, **134**, 1060–4.

Nagai, T. and Nakayama, T. 2001. Mumps vaccine virus genome is present in throat swabs obtained from uncomplicated healthy recipients. *Vaccine*, **19**, 1353–5.

Nakayama, T., Urano, T., et al. 1990. Evaluation of live trivalent vaccine of measles AIK-C strain, mumps Hoshino strain and rubella Takahashi strain, by virus-specific interferon-gamma production and antibody response. *Microbiol Immunol*, **34**, 497–508.

Narita, M., Matsuzono, Y., et al. 1998. Analysis of mumps vaccine failure by means of avidity testing for mumps virus-specific immunoglobulin G. *Clin Diagn Lab Immunol*, **5**, 799–803.

Ni, J., Bowles, N.E., et al. 1997. Viral infection of the myocardium in endocardial fibroelastosis. Molecular evidence for the role of mumps virus as an etiologic agent. *Circulation*, **95**, 133–9.

Norrby, E., Grandien, M. and Orvell, C. 1977. New tests for characterization of mumps virus antibodies: hemolysis inhibition, single radial immunodiffusion with immobilized virions, and mixed hemadsorption. *J Clin Microbiol*, **5**, 346–52.

Notkins, A.L. 1977. Virus-induced diabetes mellitus. *Arch Virol*, **54**, 1–17.

Odisseev, H. and Gacheva, N. 1994. Vaccinoprophylaxis of mumps using mumps vaccine, strain Sofia 6, in Bulgaria. *Vaccine*, **12**, 1251–4.

Okazaki, K., Tanabayashi, K., et al. 1992. Molecular cloning and sequence analysis of the mumps virus gene encoding the L protein and the trailer sequence. *Virology*, **188**, 926–30.

Orvell, C., Kalantari, M. and Johansson, B. 1997. Characterization of five conserved genotypes of the mumps virus small hydrophobic (SH) protein gene. *J Gen Virol*, **78**, 91–5.

Parry, J.V., Perry, K.R. and Mortimer, P.P. 1987. Sensitive assays for viral antibodies in saliva: an alternative to tests on serum. *Lancet*, **2**, 72–5.

Paterson, R.G. and Lamb, R.A. 1990. RNA editing by G-nucleotide insertion in mumps virus P-gene mRNA transcripts. *J Virol*, **64**, 4137–45.

Pebody, R.G., Gay, N.J., et al. 2002. Immunogenicity of second dose measles-mumps-rubella (MMR) vaccine and implication for serosurveillance. *Vaccine*, **20**, 1134–40.

Peltola, H., Davidkin, I., et al. 2000. Mumps and rubella eliminated from Finland. *JAMA*, **284**, 2643–7.

Perry, K.R., Brown, D.W., et al. 1993. The detection of measles, mumps and rubella antibodies in saliva using antibody capture radioimmunoassays. *J Med Virol*, **40**, 235–40.

Person, D.A., Smith, T.F. and Herrmann, E.C. 1971. Experiences in laboratory diagnosis of mumps virus infections in routine medical practice. *Mayo Clin Proc*, **46**, 544–8.

Philip, R.N., Reinhard, K.R. and Lackman, D.B. 1959. Observations on a mumps epidemic in a 'virgin' population. *Am J Hyg*, **69**, 91–111.

Pipkin, P.A., Afzal, M.A., et al. 1999. Assay of humoral immunity to mumps virus. *J Virol Meth*, **79**, 219–25.

Poggio, G.P., Rodriguez, C., et al. 2000. Nested PCR for rapid detection of mumps virus in cerebrospinal fluid from patients with neurological diseases. *J Clin Microbiol*, **38**, 274–8.

Pons, C., Pelayo, T., et al. 2000. Two outbreaks of mumps in children vaccinated with the Rubini strain in Spain indicate low vaccine efficacy. *Eurosurveillance*, **5**, 80–4.

Popow-Kraupp, T. 1981. Enzyme-linked immunosorbent assay (ELISA) for mumps virus antibodies. *J Med Virol*, **8**, 79–88.

Ramsay, M.E., Brown, D.W., et al. 1991. Saliva antibody testing and vaccination in a mumps outbreak. *CDR (Lond: Engl Rev)*, **1**, R96–8.

Reed, D., Brown, G., et al. 1967. A mumps epidemic on St. George Island, Alaska. *JAMA*, **199**, 967–71.

Reina, J., Ballesteros, F., et al. 2001. Evaluation of different continuous cell lines in the isolation of mumps virus by the shell vial method from clinical samples. *J Clin Pathol*, **54**, 924–6.

Reunanen, M., Salonen, R. and Salmi, A. 1982. Intrathecal immune responses in mumps meningitis patients. *Scand J Immunol*, **15**, 419–26.

Royal College of General Practitioners. 1974. The incidence and complications of mumps. *J Roy Coll Gen Pract*, **24**, 545–51.

Ruther, U., Stilz, S., et al. 1995. Successful interferon-alpha 2a therapy for a patient with acute mumps orchitis. *Eur Urol*, **27**, 174–6.

Sakata, H., Tsurudome, M., et al. 1985. Enzyme-linked immunosorbent assay for mumps IgM antibody: comparison of IgM capture and indirect IgM assay. *J Virol Meth*, **12**, 303–11.

Samuel, D., Sasnauskas, K., et al. 2002. High level expression of recombinant mumps nucleoprotein in *Saccharomyces cerevisiae* and its evaluation in mumps IgM serology. *J Med Virol*, **66**, 123–30.

Sarnesto, A., Julkunen, I. and Makela, O. 1985. Proportions of Ig classes and subclasses in mumps antibodies. *Scand J Immunol*, **22**, 345–50.

Sato, H., Albrecht, P., et al. 1978. Sensitive neutralization test for virus antibody. I. Mumps antibody. *Arch Virol*, **58**, 301–11.

Sawada, H., Yano, S., et al. 1993. Transmission of Urabe mumps vaccine between siblings. *Lancet*, **342**, 371.

Shelokov, A., Vogel, J.E. and Chi, L. 1958. Hemadsorption (adsorption-hemagglutination) test for viral agents in tissue culture with special reference to influenza. *Proc Soc Exp Biol Med*, **97**, 802–9.

Siegel, M., Fuerst, H.T. and Peress, N.S. 1966. Comparative fetal mortality in maternal virus diseases. A prospective study on rubella, measles, mumps, chicken pox and hepatitis. *N Engl J Med*, **274**, 768–71.

Sosin, D.M., Cochi, S.L., et al. 1989. Changing epidemiology of mumps and its impact on university campuses. *Pediatrics*, **84**, 779–84.

St Geme, J.W., Yamauchi, T., et al. 1975. Immunologic significance of the mumps virus skin test in infants, children and adults. *Am J Epidemiol*, **101**, 253–63.

Sugiura, A. and Yamada, A. 1991. Aseptic meningitis as a complication of mumps vaccination. *Pediatr Infect Dis J*, **10**, 209–13.

Takahashi, Y., Teranishi, A., et al. 1998. A case of congenital mumps infection complicated with persistent pulmonary hypertension. *Am J Perinatol*, **15**, 409–12.

Takeuchi, K., Tanabayashi, K., et al. 1996. The mumps virus SH protein is a membrane protein and not essential for virus growth. *Virology*, **225**, 156–62.

Tanabayashi, K., Takeuchi, K., et al. 1990a. Nucleotide sequence of the leader and nucleocapsid protein gene of mumps virus and epitope mapping with the in vitro expressed nucleocapsid protein. *Virology*, **177**, 124–30.

Tanabayashi, K., Takeuchi, K., et al. 1990b. Nucleotide sequence of the gene encoding the matrix protein of mumps virus (Miyahara strain). *Virus Genes*, **3**, 361–5.

Tanabayashi, K., Takeuchi, K., et al. 1992. Expression of mumps virus glycoproteins in mammalian cells from cloned cDNAs: both F and HN proteins are required for cell fusion. *Virology*, **187**, 801–4.

Tanabayashi, K., Takeuchi, K., et al. 1993. Identification of an amino acid that defines the fusogenicity of mumps virus. *J Virol*, **67**, 2928–31.

Tanaka, K., Baba, K., et al. 1992. Nasal antibody response to mumps virus after vaccination and natural infection. *Vaccine*, **10**, 824–7.

Taparelli, F., Squadrini, F., et al. 1988. Isolation of mumps virus from vaginal secretions in association with oophoritis. *J Infect*, **17**, 255–8.

Taylor, F.B. and Toreson, W.E. 1963. Primary mumps meningoencephalitis. *Arch Intern Med*, **112**, 216–21.

Tecle, T., Bottiger, B., et al. 2001. Characterization of two decades of temporal co-circulation of four mumps virus genotypes in Denmark: identification of a new genotype. *J Gen Virol*, **82**, 2675–80.

Tolpin, M.D. 1991. Mumps virus. In: Belshe, R.B. (ed.), *Textbook of human virology*, 2nd edn. St. Louis: Mosby-Year Book, 351–66.

Uchida, K., Shinohara, M., et al. 2001. Characterization of mumps virus isolated in Saitama Prefecture, Japan, by sequence analysis of the SH gene. *Microbiol Immunol*, **45**, 851–5.

Ueda, K., Miyazaki, C., et al. 1995. Aseptic meningitis caused by measles-mumps-rubella vaccine in Japan. *Lancet*, **346**, 701–2.

Ukkonen, P., Granström, M.-L. and Penttinen, K. 1981. Mumps-specific immunoglobulin M and G antibodies in natural mumps infection as measured by enzyme-linked immunosorbent assay. *J Med Virol*, **8**, 131–42.

Unal, M., Katircioglu, S., et al. 1998. Sudden total bilateral deafness due to asymptomatic mumps infection. *Int J Pediatr Otorhinol*, **45**, 167–9.

Usonis, V., Bakasenas, V., et al. 1999. Reactogenicity and immunogenicity of a new live attenuated combined measles, mumps and rubella vaccine in healthy children. *Pediatr Infect Dis J*, **18**, 42–8.

Utz, J.P., Kasel, J.A., et al. 1957. Clinical and laboratory studies of mumps. I. Laboratory diagnosis by tissue-culture technics. *N Engl J Med*, **257**, 497–502.

Utz, J.P., Houk, V.N. and Alling, D.W. 1964. Clinical and laboratory studies of mumps. IV. Viruria and abnormal renal function. *N Engl J Med*, **270**, 1283–6.

Väänänen, P., Hovi, T., et al. 1976. Determination of mumps and influenza antibodies by haemolysis-in-gel. *Arch Virol*, **52**, 91–9.

Valsamakis, A., Schneider, H., et al. 1998. Recombinant measles viruses with mutations in the C, V, or F gene have altered growth phenotypes in vivo. *J Virol*, **72**, 7754–61.

van der Logt, J.T., Heessen, F.W., et al. 1982. Hemadsorption immunosorbent technique for determination of mumps immunoglobulin M antibody. *J Clin Microbiol*, **15**, 82–6.

Vandvik, B., Norrby, E., et al. 1978. Mumps meningitis: prolonged pleocytosis and occurrence of mumps virus-specific oligoclonal IgG in the cerebrospinal fluid. *Eur Neurol*, **17**, 13–22.

van Regenmortel, M.H.V., Fauquet, C.M., et al. 2000. *Virus taxonomy. Classification and nomenclature of viruses. Seventh report of the International Committee on Taxonomy of Viruses.* San Diego: Academic Press.

van Tiel, F.H., Kraaijeveld, C.A., et al. 1988. Enzyme immunoassay of mumps virus in cell culture with peroxidase-labelled virus specific monoclonal antibodies and its application for determination of antibodies. *J Virol Meth*, **22**, 99–108.

Vartdal, F. and Vandvik, B. 1983. Characterization of classes of intrathecally synthesized antibodies by imprint immunofixation of electrophoretically separated sera and cerebrospinal fluids. *Acta Pathol Microbiol Immunol Scand Sect C Immunol*, **91**, 69–75.

Venketasubramanian, N. 1997. Transverse myelitis following mumps in an adult – a case report with MRI correlation. *Acta Neurol Scand*, **96**, 328–31.

Visser, L.E., González Perez, L.C., et al. 1998. An outbreak of mumps in the Province of Léon, Spain, 1995–1996. *Eurosurveillance*, **3**, 14–18.

Vuori, M., Lahikainen, E.A. and Peltonen, T. 1962. Perceptive deafness in connection with mumps: a study of 298 servicemen suffering from mumps. *Acta Otolaryngol*, **55**, 231–6.

Vuorinen, T., Nikolakaros, G., et al. 1992. Mumps and coxsackie B3 virus infection of human fetal pancreatic islet-like cell clusters. *Pancreas*, **7**, 460–4.

Waxham, M.N., Server, A.C., et al. 1987. Cloning and sequencing of the mumps virus fusion protein gene. *Virology*, **159**, 381–8.

Waxham, M.N., Aronowski, J., et al. 1988. Sequence determination of the mumps virus HN gene. *Virology*, **164**, 318–25.

Wehner, H., Morris, R., et al. 2000. A secondary school outbreak of mumps following the childhood immunization programme in England and Wales. *Epidemiol Infect*, **124**, 131–6.

Weibel, R.E., Buynak, E.B., et al. 1978. Persistence of antibody after administration of monovalent and combined live attenuated measles, mumps, and rubella virus vaccines. *Pediatrics*, **61**, 5–11.

Weller, T.H. and Craig, J.M. 1949. The isolation of mumps virus at autopsy. *Am J Pathol*, **25**, 1105–15.

Werner, C.A. 1950. Mumps orchitis and testicular atrophy. I. Occurrence. *Ann Intern Med*, **32**, 1066–74.

Wilfert, C.M. 1969. Mumps meningoencephalitis with low cerebrospinal-fluid glucose, prolonged pleocytosis and elevation of protein. *N Engl J Med*, **280**, 855–9.

Wollstein, M. 1916. An experimental study of parotitis (mumps). *J Exp Med*, **23**, 353–75.

Wolontis, S. and Bjorvatn, B. 1973. Mumps meningoencephalitis in Stockholm November 1964–July 1971. II. Isolation attempts from the cerebrospinal fluid in a hospitalized study group. *Scand J Infect Dis*, **5**, 261–71.

Wolontis, S. and Bjorvatn, B. 1974. Mumps meningoencephalitis in Stockholm. V. Virus isolations from samples of cerebrospinal fluid and urine – a comparison between some cell systems and typing techniques. *Scand J Infect Dis*, **6**, 117–23.

World Health Organization. 2001. Nomenclature for describing the genetic characteristics of wild-type measles viruses (update). *Wkly Epidemiol Rec*, **76**, 242–47.

Wu, L., Bai, Z., et al. 1998. Wild type mumps viruses circulating in China establish a new genotype. *Vaccine*, **16**, 281–5.

Yamanishi, K., Takahashi, M., et al. 1973. Studies on live mumps virus vaccine. V. Development of a new mumps vaccine 'AM9' by plaque cloning. *Biken J*, **16**, 161–6.

Yamauchi, T., Wilson, C. and St Geme, J.W. 1974. Transmission of live, attenuated mumps virus to the human placenta. *N Engl J Med*, **290**, 710–12.

Yates, P.J., Afzal, M.A. and Minor, P.D. 1996. Antigenic and genetic variation of the HN protein of mumps virus strains. *J Gen Virol*, **77**, 2491–7.

Yeniyol, C.O., Sorguc, S., et al. 2000. Role of interferon-alpha-2B in prevention of testicular atrophy with unilateral mumps orchitis. *Urology*, **55**, 931–3.

36

Respiroviruses: parainfluenza virus

RICHARD W. PELUSO AND ANNE MOSCONA

INTRODUCTION

Respiratory tract infections caused by respiroviruses, and specifically the human parainfluenza viruses, cause many of the most significant childhood diseases in both developed and underdeveloped areas of the world. This chapter is divided into two parts: the first part discusses properties of respiroviruses including human parainfluenza viruses types 1 and 3, and the second part discusses clinical and pathological aspects of infection with these pathogens.

PROPERTIES OF THE VIRUSES

Classification and structure

The respiroviruses comprise a genus within the *Paramyxoviridae* family whose members include the human pathogens parainfluenza virus types 1 and 3, bovine parainfluenza virus, *Sendai virus* (a mouse pathogen), and a number of other less-studied members, including murine parainfluenza virus type 1 and simian respirovirus 10. These viruses have features that distinguish them from other members of the *Paramyxovirinae*. They all possess both hemagglutinating and neuraminidase activities on their receptor-binding protein, and all have the ability to encode a nonstructural C protein. Like all other members of the *Paramyxovirinae*, these viruses, although pleimorphic, are roughly spherical in shape, are approximately 150-400 nm in diameter and possess a lipid envelope composed of host cell lipids and viral

glycoproteins that is derived from the plasma membrane of the host cell during budding. Figure 36.1 shows a schematic diagram of a representative respirovirus particle. All contain a negative-strand nonsegmented single-stranded RNA genome that is encapsidated by the viral nucleocapsid protein and forms a helical nucleocapsid (Choppin and Compans 1975). The viral RNA of each is approximately 15 500 nucleotides in length. Like all negative-strand RNA viruses, the respiroviruses encode and package an RNA-dependent RNA polymerase in the virion particles. The polymerase activity is only manifest on the RNA/NP helical nucleocapsid template and is attributed entirely to two viral proteins, L and P. There are approximately 50 P proteins and 300 L proteins per virion nucleocapsid (Lamb et al. 1976).

The negative-strand RNA genome of all respiroviruses contains six genes arranged in the order 3'-NP–P/V/C–M–F–HN–L-5'. The *NP* gene encodes the nucleocapsid protein that binds to the viral genome and antigenome during RNA synthesis, forming the characteristic helical nucleocapsids. The *P* gene of all respiroviruses encodes the phosphoprotein P (a subunit of the viral polymerase), another protein termed C, and for several members (Sendai and bovine parainfluenza type 3) also encodes a V protein via nontemplated nucleotide addition to the mRNA, a process referred to as RNA editing (see below). The *M* gene encodes a nonglycosylated membrane-associated protein, termed membrane or matrix protein. The M protein binds both to viral nucleocapsids and to viral glycoproteins that have been inserted into the host cell membrane, playing

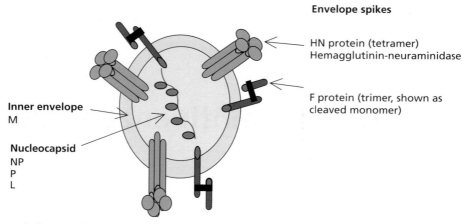

Figure 36.1 *Schematic diagram of a parainfluenza virus*

a role in virus assembly. The M protein also lends structure to the viral envelope, forming a protein layer between the lipid envelope and the helical nucleocapsid within. The F and HN genes encode the two integral membrane glycoproteins, the fusion (F) protein and the hemagglutinin-neuraminidase (HN). The F glycoprotein mediates fusion between the viral and host-cell membranes during infection, while the HN glycoprotein, possessing both receptor-binding and receptor-destroying activities (i.e. hemagglutinating and neuraminidase functions), is responsible for attachment of the virus particle to receptors on the cell, interaction with the F protein to mediate fusion between the viral and cell membranes, and release of progeny virus particles from infected cells. The *L* gene, comprising approximately 50 percent of the coding capacity of the virus, encodes the L protein, the catalytic subunit of the viral RNA polymerase.

Viral entry and membrane fusion: the roles of the surface glycoproteins

A characteristic feature of paramyxovirus infection in cell culture is the induction of cell fusion at neutral pH, resulting in the formation of syncytia. While several elements of the fusion process have been extensively studied, there remains much to learn about the precise role of each of the surface glycoproteins and the critical determinants of fusion. Several basic features of the glycoproteins are shown in Figure 36.2. Infection of cells by respiroviruses is initiated by attachment of the virus to the host cell through interaction of the HN glycoprotein with a neuraminic acid-containing molecule on the host cell surface. The fusion glycoprotein F is synthesized as a single polypeptide chain (F0) that forms a trimer before being cleaved by host-cell proteases to yield a membrane-distal (F2) and membrane-anchored subunit (F1). The new N-terminal region of the membrane-anchored subunit F1, termed the fusion

peptide, contains hydrophobic residues that insert into target membranes during fusion at neutral pH (reviewed in Hernandez et al. (1996)). Penetration and uncoating of the virus occur by fusion of the viral envelope with the plasma membrane of the cell, resulting in the release of the viral nucleocapsid into the cytoplasm. Infection also results in fusion between cells, which involves the interaction of F and HN proteins expressed on the surface of an infected cell with the membrane of an adjacent uninfected cell. The role of the receptor binding surface glycoprotein, HN, in this process has been the focus of much investigation in recent years, and is discussed in detail below.

THE HEMAGGLUTININ-NEURAMINIDASE

The HN proteins are type II transmembrane glycoproteins, oriented such that their NH_2 termini extend into the cytoplasm while the C termini are extracellular. The neuraminidase activity of HN is important for removing sialic acid residues from the viral and cellular surfaces to prevent self-aggregation and to allow for the release of newly formed virus. HN is present on the cell surface as a homotetramer composed of disulfide-linked homodimers (Markwell and Fox 1980; Thompson et al. 1988; Ng et al. 1989; Russell et al. 1994). The molecule contains a cytoplasmic domain, a membrane-spanning region, a stalk region, and a globular head. The membrane distal globular head region contains the sialic acid-binding site, which mediates attachment to sialic acid-containing receptor molecules on the cell surface to initiate infection. The recent publication of a suite of crystal structures of Newcastle disease virus (NDV) HN (Zaitsev et al. 2004) and parainfluenza virus type 3 HN (Lawrence et al. 2004) (shown in Figure 36.3 complexed with sialic acid) demonstrate the locations of the active site residue (T193 for parainfluenza virus type 3 HN) on the globular head of the molecule. These structures, when taken together with experimental data about the HN, promise to reveal much about the functions of HN and its interaction with F (see below).

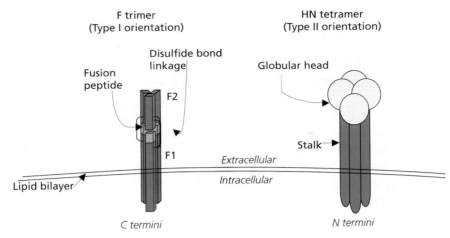

Figure 36.2 *F (fusion) and HN (receptor-binding) proteins*

RECEPTOR MOLECULES FOR PARAINFLUENZA VIRUSES

The receptors for parainfluenza viruses are known to be sialoglycoconjugates based upon their destruction by neuraminidases. Beyond this general classification, little is known. For human parainfluenza virus type 3 (HPIV-3) and other respiroviruses, the virus appears to be specific in its use of receptors (Moscona and Peluso 1996; Suzuki et al. 2001) in that it cannot make use of all potential sialic acid-containing surface molecules. For Sendai virus, specific gangliosides have been shown to be capable of functioning as receptors. Sendai virus binds to and fuses with liposomes containing gangliosides (Haywood 1974; Haywood and Boyer 1982), and three gangliosides belonging to the same family were shown to function as receptors for this virus in cultured cells (Markwell et al. 1981). It was shown that the minimal structure recognized by Sendai virus is NeuAcα2,3Gal. While glycolipids have been shown to function in initiating infection by Sendai virus, cell surface glycoproteins also contain the NeuAcα2,3Gal sequence as one possible type of carbohydrate modification. A number of studies have used

sialidases to destroy receptors, followed by sialyltransferases to resialylate the cell surface in order to determine the important sialic acid component of the receptor (Paulson et al. 1979; Markwell and Paulson 1980), but these experiments do not determine whether the biologically important glycoconjugate is a lipid or a protein since these enzymes can use either glycolipids or glycoproteins as substrates. In addition, although various studies with Sendai virus have assessed binding to erythrocytes or liposomes (Haywood 1974; Suzuki et al. 1985), it remains unclear which molecules are actually used on target cells. For example, Sendai virus was shown to bind to heparin, and this binding inhibited Sendai fusion with erythrocyte ghosts or liposomes (Ohki et al. 1992; Zschornig et al. 1993). Recently, it was suggested that HPIV-3 can utilize heparan sulfate (HS) during the cell entry process (Bose and Banerjee 2002). HPIV-3 interacted with HS-agarose in vitro, and cellular entry was reduced if HPIV-3 was preincubated with soluble HS or if target cells were treated with heparinase to remove cell surface HS. However, inhibition was incomplete, suggesting at least that additional cell surface molecules

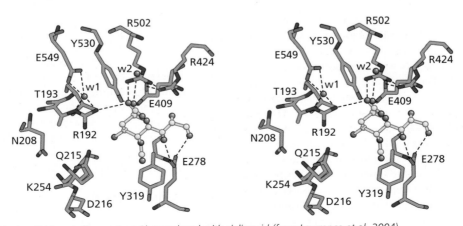

Figure 36.3 *HN active site (parainfluenza type 3) complexed with sialic acid (from Lawrence et al. 2004).*

are required. It is not known whether HS interacts with the HPIV-3 HN or F proteins. It is clear that HS is not used as the primary entry receptor, but it is possible that HS plays a secondary role and augments the efficiency of entry for HPIV-3, as well as Sendai viruses. While paramyxoviruses have many biological properties in common, several lines of investigation have now highlighted important differences between viruses of this family in regard to the viral entry and fusion processes, and it remains important to identify target receptors used by respiroviruses.

THE DUAL FUNCTION OF THE HN MOLECULES: A BALANCE OF ACTIVITIES

Unlike influenza viruses, in which separate surface glycoproteins are responsible for the neuraminidase and receptor-binding activities, the respirovirus HN is a dual function molecule. The existence of separate sites for the receptor binding and neuraminidase functions of the HN molecule has been debated extensively. Studies performed in various paramyxovirus family members with mutations in different HN residues have addressed this question by attempting to ascribe functional roles to these residues. The varied results failed to elucidate definitively whether the dual HN functions reside in the same or distinct sites. In studies of HPIV-3, both the neuraminidase and receptor binding activity of HN was inhibited by sialic acid analogues such as DANA (Levin Perlman et al. 1999) and 4-GU-DANA (Greengard et al. 2000). Passaging of HPIV-3 in the presence of 4-GU-DANA yielded an HN variant, ZM1, in which an alteration of residue 193 increased the receptor binding, as well as the neuraminidase activity, and conferred 4-GU-DANA resistance for both activities (Murrell et al. 2003). Analysis of this (4-GU-DANA-resistant) variant ZM1 supported the possibility of a single site capable of affecting both binding and enzymatic properties (Murrell et al. 2003) and the presence of a single, multifunctional site on HPIV-3 HN therefore appeared likely. A single site was also implicated in a study of bovine parainfluenza virus 3 (BPIV3) in which residue 193, the HPIV-3 193 correlate, affected both hemagglutinating and neuraminidase activities and thus suggested a single site (Shioda et al. 1988). Several studies employing monoclonal antibodies to select for Sendai virus escape variants postulated an HN with dual sites (Portner 1981; Portner et al. 1987; Thompson and Portner 1987; Gorman et al. 1990; Lyn et al. 1991). Initial crystallographic studies suggested that a single site on NDV HN was responsible for both activities (Crennell et al. 2000). However, a more recent study has identified an additional potential NDV HN receptor-binding site (Zaitsev et al. 2004). Recently, a third function of HN has become clear. Upon binding to receptor, parainfluenza HN plays a critical role in 'triggering' F to undergo its final conformational alteration that permits fusion (Porotto et al. 2003). This is discussed in detail below.

For influenza virus, the balance of NA and HA activities is important for the retention of in vivo viability. If virus binds receptor avidly, then entry will be efficient, while release will be hindered resulting in loss of viability. If receptor binding is reduced drastically, then entry of the virus is compromised resulting in a similar loss of viability. It is the balance of these two functions that determines the functional characteristics of influenza virus, including its ability to escape inhibition by a molecule like 4-GU-DANA. Balance of the dual functions of HN is also important for the functional characteristics of HPIV-3, even though the distinct biological activities of receptor binding and receptor destruction reside on a single molecule. For example, the fusogenic HPIV-3 variant C-0 incurred a single amino acid change that altered only its receptor binding affinity (Moscona and Peluso 1993). Another fusogenic HPIV-3 variant, C-28, possessed a single alteration that reduced the neuraminidase-specific activity while sparing its receptor binding affinity (Huberman et al. 1995). However, both variants exhibit similar highly fusogenic phenotypes distinct from wildtype HPIV-3. Thus, it is possible to affect HN functions separately, and, similar to influenza virus, the balance of binding and release influences the outcome of HPIV-3 infection. It is likely that the quantitative relationship between HN's receptor-binding and receptor-destroying functions determines the outcome of infection by parainfluenza viruses. It has been shown that virion release depends on this balance (Porotto et al. 2001). The ability of HN to trigger F to fuse (see below) is intimately related to HN's receptor bound state. Therefore, the balance between HN's two functions – binding and release from receptor – ultimately determines the third key HN function, the promotion of fusion, and thus viral entry (Porotto et al. 2001, 2003). Figure 36.4 presents a model of the several points of HN action in the cell during infection.

VIRAL INTERFERENCE

Viral interference is characterized by resistance of infected cells to infection by a challenge virus. This type of interference has been documented for several paramyxoviruses, including Sendai virus (Kimura et al. 1976) and NDV (Bratt and Rubin 1967a, b; Bratt and Rubin 1968) and was presumed to be due to the destruction of viral receptors by the viral neuraminidase. For HPIV-3, it was shown that interference is mediated by HN, and that the HN-mediated interference effect can be attributed to the presence of an active neuraminidase enzyme activity (Horga et al. 2000), indicating that the mechanism for attachment interference by a paramyxovirus is attributable to the viral neuraminidase.

THE FUSION PROTEIN

The fusion protein F, shown schematically in Figure 36.5, is important in the fusion process of all

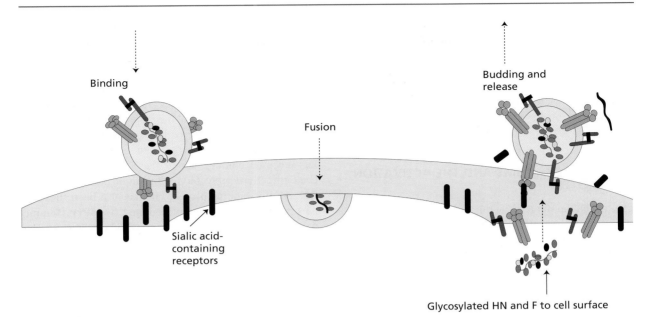

Binding

Budding and release

Fusion

Sialic acid-containing receptors

Glycosylated HN and F to cell surface

Figure 36.4 *Points of HN action*

paramyxoviruses (Lamb 1993; Plemper et al. 2003). The F proteins are type I integral membrane glycoproteins, synthesized as the inactive precursor F0, which trimerizes in the endoplasmic reticulum (Dutch et al. 2000). F0 is cleaved by a host cell protease during its transit to the cell surface to produce the active protein, which consists of two disulfide-linked subunits, F1 and F2 (Homma and Ouchi 1973; Scheid and Choppin 1974). After this cleavage, a new hydrophobic N-terminus is exposed. This is the fusion peptide, the region directly involved in mediating fusion of the viral envelope to the plasma membrane of the host cell. The

F protein cleavage sites contain multiple basic amino acids, and are cleaved in the trans-Golgi network by subtilisin-like endoproteases, furin and Kex2, with the sequence specificity of R–X–K/R–R. For several para-myxoviruses (e.g. Sendai, NDV) the efficiency of clea-vage has been shown to directly correlate with host range and tissue tropism of the virus, with greater 'cleavability' associated with virulence (Nagai et al. 1976, 1979; Nagai and Klenk 1977; Garten et al. 1980, 1992; Pritzer et al. 1990; Tashiro et al. 1990, 1992; Klenk and Garten 1994; Ortmann et al. 1994). It is also is likely that, by playing a role in determining the

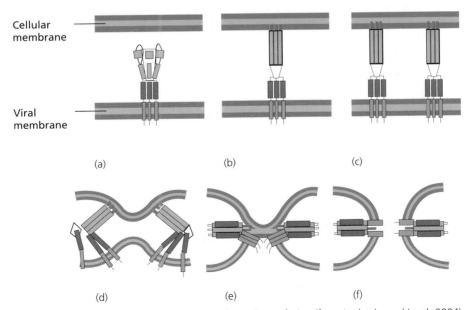

Cellular membrane

Viral membrane

(a)   (b)   (c)

(d)   (e)   (f)

Figure 36.5 *Schematic general model of fusion protein-mediated membrane fusion (from Jardetzky and Lamb 2004)*

budding efficiency from different cell types, the F protein affects cell and host tropism for the parainfluenza viruses (Okada et al. 1998). F proteins contain a hydrophobic domain (stop transfer signal) at the C terminus that anchors the protein in the membrane. It has been shown that the fusion activity of F is regulated in part by the cytoplasmic domain of the protein (Dutch and Lamb 2001; Tong et al. 2002; Seth et al. 2003).

FUSION MECHANISMS AND THE ACTIVATION OF F PROTEIN

The available data on viral fusion proteins of paramyxoviruses indicate that before initiating the fusion process, fusion proteins remain in a metastable state, which requires a trigger of some sort to induce the conformational change that leads to exposure of the fusion peptide (for a review, see Jardetzky and Lamb (2004)). A second 'activation' step is required for fusion readiness. For the parainfluenza viruses, this step requires interaction of the HN protein with its receptor. The triggering of the conformational change from a metastable fusion protein to a fusion-active state was initially elucidated for influenza HA (Carr and Kim 1993; Chen et al. 1998). The mechanism of this fusion activation in paramyxovirus F molecules is thought to have analogies to the influenza HA. The possibility of a common process is supported by the fact that the post-fusion conformation of HA, as well as several paramyxovirus F proteins, consist of a six-helix coiled-coil formed by three heterodimers of two heptad repeat (HR) regions (HRA and HRB). In this 'final' structure, the fusion peptide and the transmembrane domain are brought into proximity, allowing for membrane fusion (Skehel and Wiley 1998). For paramyxoviral F proteins, as well, the final F structure in which the fusion peptide is exposed requires formation of this stable six-helix structure leading to membrane merger (Baker et al. 1999). A schematic diagram of the process, from a recent review by Jardetsky and Lamb, is shown in Figure 36.5. Step (a) shows the metastable fusion protein; in (b) and (c) the fusion peptides are released and inserted into the target membrane. The proteins refold into a trimeric hairpin shape (d) and in (e) a helical coiled-coil rod forms next to the fusion peptide and refolding relocates the fusion peptides and transmembrane regions to the same end of this coiled coil, with the free energy that results from this step bringing the membranes closer together. With the completion of refolding, the most stable form of the protein is formed (f) and fusion is complete (Jardetzky and Lamb 2004).

The paramyxovirus F1 ectodomain contains two conserved heptad repeat (HR) regions, designated HRA and HRB, located near the fusion peptide and the transmembrane domains. Peptides derived from the HRA and HRB regions have been used to inhibit fusion

intermediates of F (Lamb and Kolakofsky 2001) and thereby to elucidate the mechanism whereby F mediates fusion. The HRA and HRB peptides are thought to inhibit fusion by preventing the F protein from forming the helical bundles required for fusion.

While for influenza virus the 'trigger' leading to conformational change of the fusion protein is the low pH of the endosome, for paramyxoviruses, which fuse at neutral pH at the cell surface, this trigger is likely to be HN-receptor binding. While the F protein is the molecule directly responsible for fusion of the lipid bilayers, the receptor-binding protein HN has also been shown to be essential for cell fusion mediated by HPIV. Interaction of HN with its receptor is required in order for F to promote membrane fusion during viral infection (Moscona and Peluso 1991; Horvath et al. 1992; Lamb 1993; Bagai and Lamb 1995). It has been proposed that upon binding sialic acid receptor, HN undergoes a receptor-induced conformational change, which in turn triggers a conformational change in F that allows fusion to occur (Lamb 1993; Porotto et al. 2003). Lamb recently showed that coexpression of HN with F of SV5 results in F protein susceptibility to HRA peptide inhibition, supporting the notion that HN binding to receptor induces a conformational change in F (Russell et al. 2001).

The triggering mechanism of paramyxovirus F at neutral pH is an area of active investigation. Lamb has shown that the free energy generated by the formation of the coiled-coil structure in F is the driving force for membrane fusion (Russell et al. 2001). There is evidence that the HN and F proteins interact (Tanabayashi and Compans 1996; Yao et al. 1997; Tong and Compans 1999). Recent work has supported the notion that HN interacts specifically with F protein to enable F to mediate fusion, and has generated models for this process. While, as above, co-expression of SV5 HN with F resulted in F protein susceptibility to HRA-region peptide inhibition, suggesting that HN binding to receptor induces a conformational change in F, the F protein fusion intermediate that was inhibited by the HRB peptide bound RBC independently of HN (or after HN had already exerted its action on F), and is likely to be the prehairpin stage of F immediately preceding membrane merger (Russell et al. 2001). The HRB peptide (corresponding to the region near the TM domain) binds F after the activation has already occurred, and F has been triggered to insert in the target membrane (and fusion at that point is independent of HN). The HN–receptor interaction is thus likely to be required for F protein function quite early in the triggering process. Many of the steps in the fusion and entry process remain to be understood. In particular, why is there a requirement for HN receptor binding, in order to initiate fusion promotion? What is the relationship between the 'docking' function of HN and its role in fusion promotion? A current model for paramyxovirus glycoprotein function proposes that HN attachment to receptor leads to interaction, which then triggers F (Russell et al. 2001). Alternatively an HN–F complex may form during trafficking to the surface, and HN attachment may lead to a conformational change in HN with a resulting release of F's fusion peptide (Russell et al. 2001). Models of possible mechanisms whereby binding of HN to receptor may contribute to activation of F are illustrated in Figure 36.6. The role of cell membrane constituents, including lipids and lipid rafts, in the organization of the glycoproteins for the fusion and entry process, and the potential role of cytoskeletal molecules in this process (Pastey et al. 1999; Pastey et al. 2000), remain to be clarified.

Primary transcription and replication

ROLES OF NONCODING SEQUENCES

As mentioned in Classification and structure, all respiroviruses contain six genes arranged in the order 3'-NP–P/V/C–M–F–HN–L-5'. In addition to the six mRNA-encoding portions of the genomic RNA, there are extragenic nucleotide sequences that control polymerase function. At the ends of the genome are short transcribed noncoding sequences that serve as polymerase-binding sites, as well as encapsidation signals. These sequences are called leader and antileader (or trailer) for the 3' and 5' ends, respectively. The leader RNA contains the signal to initiate binding of the NP protein to a nascent RNA product, and the promoter, or viral RNA polymerase binding site, on the negative-strand RNA template. The antileader (trailer) serves a similar dual function during the second stage of genome RNA replication, when full-length encapsidated plus-stranded RNA-containing nucleocapsids (antigenomes) are copied into progeny negative-strand RNA-containing nucleocapsids that are then packaged into progeny virions.

At the start of each gene, there are conserved sequences of ten nucleotides in length (3'-UCCRXXUUXC). Between each gene there is a trinucleotide sequence (3'-GYY) and at the end of each gene 11 conserved bases (3'-UXXUXXUUUUU), where R is a purine, Y is a pyrimidine, and X indicates no consensus (Kolakofsky et al. 1998). These sequences are believed to signal initiation of transcription and polyadenylation and termination of the mRNA. Except for the small number of intergenic nucleotides, all of the RNA of the viral genome is transcribed into either mRNA or leader RNAs, and most of the transcribed RNA is translated into viral proteins.

THE REPLICATION CYCLE

Replication of the virus occurs exclusively in the cytoplasm. Infecting virions fuse with the plasma membrane of the cell, releasing the viral nucleocapsid into the cytoplasm. The nucleocapsid contains the genome RNA in tight association with the viral NP protein, in the form an RNAse-resistant helical structure that is stable in

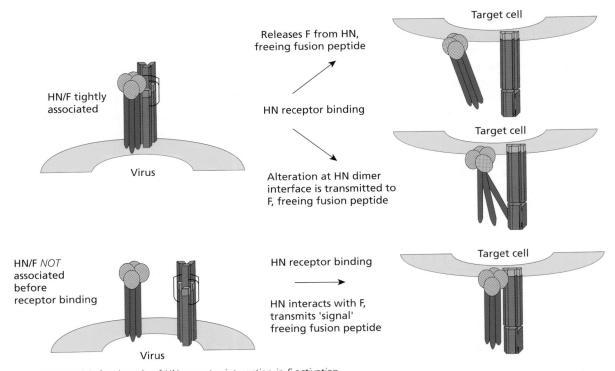

Figure 36.6 *Models for the role of HN–receptor interaction in F activation*

cesium chloride and readily visualized in the electron microscope. This RNA/protein complex is the template for both transcription and genome RNA replication, and there is no evidence that the structure uncoats further. Figure 36.7 represents this process, showing schematically that: (1) transcription and genome RNA replication both occur using the viral RNP nucleocapsid as a template; (2) during transcription multiple subgenomic mRNA molecules are made; (3) each subgenomic mRNA molecule is capped, methylated, and polyadenylated; and (4) during genome replication a full-length plus-stranded copy is made and encapsidated. This full-length positive-sense strand is the template for new progeny minus-sense nucleocapsids.

The virally encoded RNA polymerase is bound to the nucleocapsid as a complex of P and L proteins. Neither of these proteins bind to isolated viral RNA, indicating that protein–protein interactions are necessary in order for binding to occur. Thus, the infecting virion delivers an RNA–protein complex into the cell that is capable of transcribing and replicating the viral RNA genome. Purified virions can transcribe the viral RNA genome into multiple subgenomic capped and polyadenylated mRNAs if disrupted with a mild detergent and incubated in a simple salt mixture containing RNA precursors. However, genome RNA replication does not occur unless these in vitro systems are supplemented with cell extracts that are capable of supporting ongoing protein synthesis. These observations illustrate the fact that there are fundamental differences between the two processes of RNA synthesis that must occur during the growth of respiroviruses (transcription and genome RNA replication). One process, genome RNA replication, requires concurrent protein synthesis and perhaps multiple host-cell factors, while the other, transcription, occurs independently from host factors other than energy sources and nucleotide supply. Both processes are described in more detail below.

The first step in the viral growth process, termed primary transcription to denote transcription directly from the infecting nucleocapsid template, initiates at the exact 3' end of the genome in a primer-independent manner, first transcribing the short (approximately 50 nt) uncapped leader RNA. The synthesis of the leader RNA is followed sequentially by each of the other viral mRNAs in the order NP-P/V/C–M–F–HN–L. There is a polarity to the transcription process, so that genes located at the 3' end of the viral genome are transcribed more frequently than those at the 5' end. Each of the mRNAs is transcribed and present in infected cells as a function of its relative location on the negative sense viral genome. This polarity of transcription is a property of the viral coded RNA-dependent RNA polymerase complex.

The NP transcript is most abundant in infected cells and the L protein transcript is least abundant. The polymerase appears to pause at each intergenic junction and either reinitiates transcription at the next gene downstream or, alternatively, detaches from the nucleocapsid template and reinitiates upstream at the 3' leader region that contains the polymerase binding site or promoter. This 'decision' made by the polymerase at each gene junction, together with the fact that there is a single polymerase entry site at the 3' end of the genome, explains the sequential and polar nature of transcription. Transcription of each gene depends upon successful transcription and termination of the preceding upstream gene. Each mRNA is capped and methylated at its 5' end and polyadenylated at its 3' end, all carried out by the viral polymerase complex. Polyadenylation of the transcripts occurs through a polymerase chattering mechanism at a conserved stretch of U residues (U_5) at the end of each gene. The transcription of the P gene is more complex, and is discussed in more detail below.

THE 'RULE OF SIX'

The genomes of respiroviruses contain a total number of nucleotides that are evenly divisible by six. Taking advantage of the ability to generate recombinant infectious viruses from DNA clones ('reverse genetics'), it was observed that recombinant Sendai virus genomes that have a nucleotide number not divisible by six were

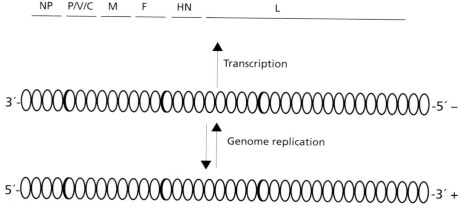

Figure 36.7 Transcription and genome RNA replication of respiroviruses

still assembled efficiently into nucleocapsids, but these genomes were very inefficiently transcribed or replicated (Pelet et al. 1996). This requirement for an optimal nucleotide number, or length evenly divisible by six, is referred to as the 'rule of six.' According to this model, the phasing of the nucleocapsid protein subunit on the viral genome is such that each protein subunit interacts with six nucleotides, and this phasing is important to maintain proper alignment of the 3' *cis*-nucleotide sequences that are recognized by the viral RNA polymerase complex during transcription and replication. Experimental evidence for this model has been obtained (Pelet et al. 1996; Kolakofsky et al. 1998; Vulliemoz and Roux 2001), and suggests that there is an optimal spacing for promoters on the viral genome relative to the NP proteins.

POLYCISTRONIC mRNAS AND ALTERNATE READING FRAMES

For five of the six genes, transcription generally leads to generation of a single mRNA species that encodes a single protein molecule. However, the *P* gene of respiroviruses encodes a number of proteins and, in several members of the family, more than one mRNA is synthesized. Each of the *P* genes of all of the members of this virus genus is transcribed directly into an mRNA that encodes the P protein. This mRNA also encodes a number of smaller protein products in an alternate reading frame from the P protein, and hence the P mRNA is bi-cistronic. The largest open reading frame encodes the P protein, of 568–603 amino acids in length. The second ORF, near the 5' end of the mRNA, is translated into a number of proteins called C, C', Y1, and Y2. These 'C' proteins, as they are commonly called, are a nested set of carboxy-coterminal proteins, with each protein encoded in the same reading frame, but differing by its start site on the mRNA. Not each member of the family encodes each protein. Sendai virus encodes all four, HPIV-1 encodes C' and C, while HPIV-3 and BPIV-3 encode just the C protein (Giorgi et al. 1983; Curran and Kolakofsky 1988). In Sendai virus the C, Y1, and Y2 proteins are synthesized by ribosomal choice at separate AUG codons, while C' is initiated using an ACG codon. All of these proteins are small (175–215 amino acids) and basic, with isoelectric points of over 10. The functions of the C proteins are incompletely understood. The C protein of HPIV-3 and the C proteins of Sendai virus are apparently required for virus growth in cultured cells since recombinant viruses that do not express these proteins replicate poorly (Kurotani et al. 1998; Latorre et al. 1998). In addition, as discussed below, these proteins may function in pathogenesis in the infected host.

NONTEMPLATED NUCLEOTIDE ADDITION

The *P* gene of most respiroviruses, in addition to encoding the P and 'C' proteins, also encodes at least one other protein using a second mRNA transcribed from the gene (HPIV-1 is the exception). The process by which this second mRNA is produced has been referred to as RNA editing, or nontemplated nucleotide addition. A sequence of nucleotides in the *P* gene is recognized by the viral polymerase as a signal for 'stuttering,' and the polymerase either ignores this stuttering signal and transcribes the P mRNA, or stutters and incorporates one or two nontemplated G residues at the precise editing site on the mRNA (Thomas et al. 1988; Vidal et al. 1990a, b; Hausmann et al. 1999a, b). The consequence of this nontemplated nucleotide addition is that the resultant mRNA allows access to a conserved short open reading frame called V. The V protein contains the N-terminus of the P protein fused to the V ORF. This V ORF is highly conserved among the viruses, is cysteine-rich and has been shown to bind zinc (Paterson et al. 1995). It is dispensable for viral growth in cell culture, and appears to function as a pathogenesis factor (see Interaction with the host cell). In several respiroviruses, addition of two nontemplated G residues allows access to a second ORF termed D (Galinski et al. 1992). Thus the *P* gene of most respiroviruses encodes a number of protein products through alternate codon usage and RNA editing.

THE SWITCH FROM TRANSCRIPTION TO REPLICATION

Replication of the viral genomic RNA is a process both linked to and distinct from transcription of the genomic RNA. Unlike transcription, replication of the viral RNA genome depends on ongoing protein synthesis, and therefore is linked to prior transcription of the viral genome. In addition, during the process of genome RNA replication, the nascent RNA molecule is assembled into the characteristic helical nucleocapsid structure. During replication all signals to the viral polymerase are ignored, including the transcriptional termination signals at the ends of each gene and the capping, methylation, polyadenylation, and RNA editing signals that are present on the template RNA. The viral genome and antigenome contain 3'U-OH and 5' pppA, respectively, rather than a cap and a poly(A) tail as in the mRNAs encoded by the genome.

Both transcription and genome RNA replication require the nucleocapsid template and the L and P proteins. The requirement for ongoing protein synthesis in order for RNA replication to occur is in part a consequence of the fact that the newly synthesized replication molecules are coassembled into nucleocapsids, and therefore NP protein is required in stoichiometric levels corresponding to the viral genome and antigenome RNAs (approximately 2 500 NP molecules per genome RNA). The NP protein that serves as the substrate for this assembly (NPo) is complexed with the P protein (Horikami et al. 1992). Binding of the P protein to free NPo is thought to prevent the self-assembly of free NP protein into higher order structures, and thus P protein acts as a molecular chaperone, delivering the NP to the assembling nucleocapsid while not, itself, becoming a part of the structure. The second stage of genome RNA replication occurs when the newly replicated and encapsidated full-length plus-stranded RNA (antigenome)-containing nucleocapsids are copied into negative-strand RNA-containing progeny nucleocapsids identical to the nucleocapsid that is packaged into progeny viral particles. These progeny viral nucleocapsids are templates for transcription and can greatly amplify the amount of viral mRNA and protein produced in an infected cell.

THE *NP* GENE

The nucleocapsid protein NP of respiroviruses is encoded by the 3′-proximal gene and is the most abundant viral protein in the infected cell. The protein in Sendai virus is 524 amino acids in length and is phosphorylated at its C-terminus (Hsu and Kingsbury 1982; Ryan et al. 1993). The protein's main function is to co-assemble with genomic and antigenomic RNAs to form the template for transcription and replication, the genome- and antigenome-containing nucleocapsid. When NP is expressed in the absence of other viral proteins it self-assembles into structures resembling viral nucleocapsids, suggesting that it can form higher order assemblies through protein–protein interactions. In infected cells, NPo is complexed with the P protein. Interaction with P protein prevents aggregation of free NPo, and it is the NPo–P protein complex that serves as the substrate for assembling NP/RNA nucleocapsid complexes. In addition to NP–NP and NPo–P interactions in nucleocapsid assembly, the NP protein on the nucleocapsid binds to the viral RNA and to the P subunit of the RNA polymerase of the virus. It has been demonstrated that the N-terminal 400 amino acids of the NP protein of Sendai virus are required for assembly into nucleocapsid templates (Buchholz et al. 1993; Curran et al. 1993). Further, these same 400 N-terminal amino acids of NP also retained the NPo–P interacting activity (Homann et al. 1991; Buchholz et al. 1994; Myers and Moyer 1997; Myers et al. 1997; Myers et al. 1999). The C-terminal portion of the protein appears to be necessary for binding of the P protein to the nucleocapsid (Ryan et al. 1993; Buchholz et al. 1994).

THE *L* GENE

The L proteins of all respiroviruses are greater than 2 000 amino acids in length and are encoded by approximately half of the viral genome. L is the least abundant protein in virus particles and in infected cells. It is likely that all of the enzymatic activities required for mRNA synthesis and genome RNA replication (polymerization, capping, methylation, polyadenylation) are encoded within this large multifunctional protein. However, a

detailed understanding of the structure/function of the L protein has yet to be obtained.

Sequence alignments have identified six conserved domains in the protein, (I–VI) (Poch et al. 1990; Sidhu et al. 1993). Several of the domains contain conserved sequence motifs that suggest possible functions. Domain II has a conserved charged RNA binding motif found in several other viruses (Smallwood et al. 1999). Domain III has a motif found in several other virus L proteins that has phosphodiester bond-forming activity (Smallwood et al. 2002). Domain VI contains a potential nucleotide binding motif. Domain III contains a motif found in the active site of several positive-stranded RNA virus polymerases and is believed to contain the polymerase active site (Jin and Elliott 1992; Sleat and Banerjee 1993; Schnell and Conzelmann 1995). Domains IV and V have no homology with any known polymerase-associated motifs.

The L protein, in order to be functional, must complex with the P protein and via this interaction bind to the nucleocapsid template. The P protein binding site has been localized to the N-terminal 350 amino acids of the L protein of Sendai virus (Holmes and Moyer 2002). A similar picture is emerging for the L protein of HPIV-3, where a short stretch of amino acids at the very N-terminus of the L protein interacts with the P protein of the virus (Malur et al. 2002). The L protein itself is an oligomer, and the oligomerization domain has been mapped to the N-terminal 174 amino acids (Cevik et al. 2003). However, L protein expressed alone is rapidly degraded, and its stability is increased by coexpression of the P protein (Horikami et al. 1997). It has been proposed that the L protein first oligomerizes, and then these oligomeric complexes interact with a complex of the P protein forming a stable and active RNA transcriptase/replicase complex (Cevik et al. 2003). The stoichiometry of the proteins in this polymerase complex have been suggested to be either L2–P4 or L2–P8. What is certain (see below) is that the P protein is a tetramer, while the state of the L protein is less certain at this time.

THE *P* GENE

The *P* gene of respiroviruses encodes a number of protein products, as described above. The P protein is the only one of these proteins that is essential for RNA synthesis. P is a phosphoprotein that acts as a molecular chaperone for the NPo protein in nucleocapsid assembly. However, the role that phosphorylation plays in modulating the function of the protein, if any, is uncertain (Hu et al. 1992, 1999). P is also an essential component of the viral RNA polymerase, forming a complex with the L protein both in solution and on the template, as well as serving to mediate binding of the polymerase complex to the nucleocapsid via P–NP interactions. Several facts have emerged concerning the structure/function of the P protein. Firstly, it oligo-merizes into a tetramer. A partially resolved molecular structure suggests the P protein complexes with itself via coiled-coil motifs (Tarboubiech et al. 2000a, b). Second, it complexes with the L protein to form the polymerase complex (Curran et al. 1994; Smallwood et al. 1994; De et al. 2000; Bousse et al. 2001). Third, it mediates binding of the polymerase to the nucleocapsid template; L does not bind to the nucleocapsid template alone (Horikami and Moyer 1995). Last, P acts as a molecular chaperone for NP during nucleocapsid assembly and prevents NP from self-assembling into higher order structures (Curran et al. 1995b; Horikami et al. 1996).

Several of the domains on the P protein that partici-pate in these varied activities have been mapped. The C terminus of the protein is capable of replacing the intact protein in supporting transcriptional activities (Curran et al. 1994). This fragment contains the domains/motifs required for oligomerization of the protein, for its inter-action with and stabilization of the L protein complex, and for its ability to bind to the nucleocapsid template (Ryan and Portner 1990; Curran et al. 1994, 1995a; Smallwood et al. 1994; Bowman et al. 1999; De et al. 2000; Bousse et al. 2001). The only domain or motif so far mapped to the N-terminus is that required for its chaperone function(Curran et al. 1995b).

Assembly and budding

Respiroviruses are formed by budding of newly repli-cated and assembled nucleocapsids containing the viral RNA genome along with the P and L proteins through modified areas of the plasma membrane that contain the F and HN transmembrane glycoproteins and the M protein. In polarized epithelial cells, the viruses bud from the apical surface of the cell. A detailed under-standing of the final assembly and budding process is lacking. However, it is likely that the nonglycosylated M protein binds to the nucleocapsid, condensing it, and preventing it from being transcribed or replicated. The M protein also likely interacts with the cytoplasmic tails of the HN and F proteins, and thereby mediates the alignment of the nucleocapsid and the areas of the plasma membrane containing viral glycoproteins in preparation for budding (Mottet et al. 1996, 1999; Coronel et al. 1999, 2001; Ali and Nayak 2000; Takimoto et al. 2001).

The M proteins of respiroviruses are small basic proteins and are a major component of virions. Their role in budding has been clearly shown by demon-strating the formation of virus-like particles in cells expressing just the M protein of HPIV-1 (Coronel et al. 1999, 2001). Interestingly, when NP was coexpressed, the budded particles contained structures closely resembling helical viral nucleocapsids. In similar systems, expression of the F protein alone led to the formation of virus-like

particles (Takimoto et al. 2001). These data indicate that there are inherent properties of more than one respir-ovirus protein that can lead to the formation of virus particles during the budding process, and there is specifi-city in protein–protein recognition during this budding process.

Interaction with the host cell

EVASION OF HOST DEFENSE MECHANISMS

Host cells have developed a variety of countermeasures in the face of viral infection. In some of these, an intra-cellular environment is created that is less hospitable for virus replication (the interferon (IFN)-induced antiviral state). Some cell types undergo apoptosis, which limits viral replication. Many viruses have been found to posess strategies for evading these host immune responses, particularly the innate immune response that plays a key role in controlling virus infection. Many viruses encode gene products that are capable of inhi-biting the host interferon response (Katze et al. 2002). For the paramyxoviruses, evasion of this response has been found to be mediated by the C and V proteins.

The Sendai virus C gene was one of the earliest exam-ples of an overlapping gene (Giorgi et al. 1983). The C gene open reading frame is found overlapping the amino-terminal end of the open reading frame for the P and V proteins (which are also expressed from the P gene mRNA via the mechanism of mRNA editing (Giorgi et al. 1983; Bellini et al. 1985), discussed in detail in Primary transcription and replication). C proteins carry a net positive charge and are expressed from the second ORF (+1 with respect to P). For Sendai virus, evasion of the interferon system is accomplished in several ways by the C protein (Garcin et al. 2003). Sendai virus C protein binds STAT1, preventing its acti-vation in response to IFN, and the carboxyl part of the C protein mediates this activity. A phenylalanine at position 170 of C is also critical for blocking STAT1 activation (Gotoh et al. 2001; Takeuchi et al. 2001; Garcin et al. 2002). In addition, Sendai C protein targets STAT1 for degradation, and the amino-terminal residues of the C proteins mediate this activity (Garcin et al. 2003).

The V proteins require the pseudotemplated addition of a single G residue to switch from the N terminal P to C terminal V ORF. V proteins of the parainfluenza viruses are fusion proteins containing a negatively charged and phosphorylated N terminus and a short, cysteine-rich zinc-binding domain at their C terminus (Paterson et al. 1995; Lamb and Kolakofsky 2001). The V proteins are involved in a wide range of mechanisms for evading the immune response. These have been found thus far to include prevention of apoptosis (He et al. 2002; Wansley and Parks 2002), cell-cycle alterations (Lin and Lamb 2000), inhibition of double-stranded RNA signaling (He et al. 2002; Poole et al. 2002), and prevention of IFN biosynthesis (He et al. 2002; Poole et al. 2002; Wansley and Parks 2002). V protein expression has been shown for several paramyxoviruses to inhibit IFN-responsive STAT proteins. The strategies whereby different V proteins inhibit STAT proteins have been found to be highly diverse. Most information about the function of these V proteins have been derived from study of closely related paramyxoviruses. For example, SV5 V proteins target STAT1 for degradation (Didcock et al. 1999; He et al. 2002), while HPIV type 2 V protein targets STAT2 (Parisien et al. 2001; Andrejeva et al. 2002). Mumps virus V protein can target both STAT1 (Nishio et al. 2002) and STAT3 (Ulane et al. 2003) and can also interact with cellular RACK1, potentially modifying IFN receptor activity (Kubota et al. 2002). Nipah virus V protein sequesters STAT1 and STAT2 in high-molecular-weight cytoplasmic complexes, thus preventing STAT protein nuclear accumulation (Rodriguez et al. 2002).

USE OF CELLULAR MACHINERY FOR VIRAL ENTRY AND/OR ASSEMBLY

After entering the target cell via fusion with the cell membrane, and release of the viral molecules into the cytoplasm, respiroviruses carry out their replicative cycle within the cytoplasm (as discussed in Primary transcription and replication) and then assemble and bud at the cell surface (discussed in Assembly and budding). The potential role of cytoskeletal molecules in the process of viral entry (Pastey et al. 1999, 2000), as well as the fascinating question of how the various viral constituents are directed during the parasitic phase of the life cycle to the correct cellular locations, remain to be clarified. It is possible that entry, fusion, and/or budding involve the participation of the cellular actin cytoskeleton, as well as microtubule function (Tashiro et al. 1993; Gupta et al. 1998; De and Banerjee 1999; Bose et al. 2001). In addition, host cellular proteins that are involved in cell mobility could be involved. For the related virus respiratory syncytial virus (RSV), it was shown that F binds RhoA, a small GTPase of the Ras superfamily, in yeast two-hybrid interaction studies (Pastey et al. 1999). RhoA controls cellular functions including actin reorganization, cell morphology, and motility. The interaction with RSV F was shown in vivo by mammalian two-hybrid assay and in RSV-infected HEp-2 cells by coimmunoprecipitation. Cells that overexpressed RhoA were used to show that RhoA correlated with fusogenicity by RSV, suggesting RhoA could play a role in RSV-induced syncytium formation. Subsequently, RhoA peptides were used to show that cell–cell fusion by HPIV-3 could be inhibited by a RhoA peptide corresponding to the region that binds RSV F (Pastey et al. 2000), suggesting a common component of the entry/

fusion mechanisms involving interaction between the F proteins and RhoA.

CLINICAL AND PATHOLOGICAL ASPECTS OF INFECTION WITH HUMAN PARAINFLUENZA VIRUSES

Croup (laryngotracheobronchitis)

ETIOLOGY

The parainfluenza viruses types 1, 2, and 3, taken together, are the most important cause of croup. HPIV-3 alone is responsible for approximately 11 percent of pediatric respiratory hospitalizations (Murphy 1988; Chanock 1990) and is a predominant cause of croup in young infants. HPIV 1 and 2 tend to infect older children and adolescents. Infection with HPIV in immunocompromised children (for example, transplant recipients) has been associated with a wide range of disease, from mild upper respiratory symptoms to severe disease requiring mechanical ventilation and leading to death, especially in young children, those whose infections occur soon after transplant, and those with the most intensive immunosuppression (Apalsch et al. 1995).

Other viral causes of croup include adenovirus, influenza A and B, rhinoviruses, RSV, measles and enteroviruses. Bacterial causes (such as *H. influenzae*, Group A hemolytic strep, *C. diphtheriae*, *S. pneumoniae*, *S. aureus* and *Mycoplasma pneumoniae*) are much less frequent. While RSV is the leading cause of acute lower respiratory tract infection in young children and causes a significant percentage of croup, it is more commonly seen as a cause of bronchiolitis. Influenza viruses (A and B) are also important causes of serious lower respiratory tract disease in children. Influenza A is an important cause of croup, as well as pneumonia and pharyngitis-bronchitis. Diphtheria caused by *Corynebacterium diphtheriae* is now a rare cause of croup. However, this organism may infect the larynx, trachea, and bronchi by extension from a pharyngeal infection or by primary infection, and result in a croupy cough with stridor.

EPIDEMIOLOGY

HPIV1 causes large seasonal outbreaks of illness, with rises in the number of croup cases every other year (odd-numbered years). HPIV-2 outbreaks generally follow those caused by HPIV-1. HPIV-3, in contrast, causes outbreaks each year, generally in the spring or summer (Hall 2001).

PATHOGENESIS IN THE HUMAN

Parainfluenza viruses replicate in the epithelium of the upper respiratory tract, and spread to the lower respiratory tract within 3 days. The pathogenesis in the lung has not yet been well studied as it has for RSV. Epithelial cells of the small airways become infected with resultant necrosis and imflammatory infiltrates. The interplay between virus-induced cell damage, beneficial immune responses and inflammatory responses that contribute to disease for HPIV-3 is still unknown, and this is an area of active investigation for parainfluenza virus research.

CLINICAL MANIFESTATIONS

Croup is the most common clinical manifestation of HPIV infection. Inflammatory obstruction of the airway produces the clinical picture in all forms of infectious croup, which include acute laryngitis, laryngotracheitis, and laryngotracheobronchitis. A mild upper respiratory syndrome usually precedes the clinical manifestations of croup. The clinical findings are produced by inflammatory obstruction of the airway in all forms of the illness. The severity and extent of the infectious process (and, likely, of the inflammatory response) determine the sites of obstruction in the laryngotracheobronchial tree. Milder cases are characterized by hoarseness and a barking ('croupy') cough. Low-grade fever, loss of appetite, and malaise may be the only constitutional signs, respiratory distress is absent or minimal, and the condition responds promptly to appropriate treatment and subsides in a few days. In patients with severe acute laryngitis the infection may descend rapidly to the trachea and bronchi, causing increased respiratory distress evidenced by nasal flaring and inspiratory retractions. In these cases, the site of obstruction is usually the subglottic area. Hoarseness is more marked, and breathing may become rapid and labored, with inspiratory stridor and retraction of the suprasternal notch, the supraclavicular spaces, the substernal region, and the intercostal spaces. Expiratory wheezes and various types of bronchitic rales are heard on auscultation of the chest. The illness can rapidly progress to respiratory failure with hypoxia, weakness, decreased air exchange, and death. Agitation, crying, and manipulation of the airway can aggravate the respiratory distress. The white blood cell count is frequently normal or mildly elevated, and radiographs classically show a 'steeple sign' indicative of subglottic edema.

In patients with infection limited to the laryngeal area, chest auscultation reveals inspiratory stridor and impaired aeration. The main site of obstruction lies below the vocal cords, where subglottic tissues bulge to meet in the midline. An exudate may add to the airway obstruction. In laryngotracheobronchitis, the most extensive type of croup, expiratory wheezes rales are heard on auscultation of the chest. Atelectasis resulting from plugging of a bronchus with exudate may result in localized areas of absent breath sounds, bronchial breathing, and dullness to percussion. If a main bronchus becomes plugged, cyanosis worsens, and the heart and mediastinum may be shifted to the affected side.

DIAGNOSIS

Diagnosis of HPIV infection in the clinical setting can be made by viral isolation, or by detection of antigen or nucleic acid. All three types of methods are currently available, and the use of reverse transcription polymerase chain reaction (RT-PCR) allows for the diagnosis of several respiratory viruses simultaneously. A multiplex RT-PCR assay for detecting HPIV 1, 2, and 3 was developed in 1995 (Fan and Henrickson 1996) and there is currently a highly sensitive and specific multiplex assay for detecting these viruses along with RSV and influenza viruses (Fan and Henrickson 1996; Fan et al. 1998; Kehl et al. 2001). These assay kits, as well as kits for antigen detection, allow for screening of children and are likely to be used more commonly in the future as more therapies for pediatric respiratory viruses become available.

TREATMENT

Novel antivirals for HPIV are under investigation, including molecules designed to inhibit viral fusion and entry, but no specific therapy is available as of November 2003. Most children with croup do not require hospitalization, and treatment is supportive, aimed at maintaining the airway and hydration. Avoiding agitation of the child is important, in order not to compromise the airway. If necessary, humidified supplemental oxygen may be administered by hood, mask, or nasal cannula. Steroids are beneficial in the treatment of croup (Kairys et al. 1989; Orlicek 1998; Wright et al. 2002) and nebulized steroids can be effective (Husby et al. 1993; Klassen et al. 1994, 1998; Johnson et al. 1998). Racemic epinephrine or L-epineprhine has been successfully used for the treatment of more severe cases of croup (Kuusela and Vesikari 1988; Waisman et al. 1992).

PREVENTION

The development of a vaccine for the parainfluenza viruses has been hampered by the need to induce an immune response in young infants whose immature immune systems and whose maternal antibody both interfere with the development of an adequate immune response. Experimental vaccines are under evaluation, with reasonable expectation that a vaccine for HPIV-3, and perhaps also HPIV1, will soon be feasible. Several strategies have been recently evaluated for HPIV-3 vaccines. Bovine parainfluenza type 3, attenuated in humans by nature of host range, has been shown to be infectious in seronegative recipients, with most vaccinees shedding virus or developing an immune response (Clements et al. 1996; Karron et al. 1996). Cold-adapted mutants of parainfluenza have been evaluated in both chimpanzees and in healthy infants. A cold-passaged mutant (cp45) was evaluated in seronegative chimpanzees and found to be attenuated in the upper and lower respiratory tracts. Immunized animals were resistant to wildtype PIV-3 challenge. The vaccine was also well tolerated when given intranasally to HPIV-3-seropositive and -seronegative children. One dose of vaccine induced a serum hemagglutination-inhibiting antibody response in 81 percent of vaccinees (Hall et al. 1993; Karron et al. 1995a, 1995b, 1995c). As for RSV, it is likely that with the recent increase in our understanding of the molecular contributions to attenuation, engineered live HPIV-3 vaccines can be designed to be ideally attenuated and immunogenic (Skiadopoulos et al. 1999a, b, c; Tao et al. 1999), and that this technology will enhance our ability to rapidly develop effective parainfluenza virus candidate vaccines suitable for children in the future.

Acute bronchiolitis

ETIOLOGY

While RSV is the leading cause of bronchiolitis in young children, accounting for 50–90 percent of all bronchiolitis hospitalizations, after RSV the human parainfluenza viruses type 3, and to a lesser extent type 1 and 2, are the most common causative agents of bronchiolitis (Collins et al. 1996).

PATHOGENESIS

Bronchiolitis is the result of a balance between cellular damage mediated by the viral pathogen and injury caused by the immune response of the host (Welliver 2000). Virus first replicates in the nasopharyngeal epithelium and spreads to the lower respiratory tract. Viral replication in the small airways causes inflammation, sloughing and necrosis of epithelium. Edema and increased mucous secretion cause plugging of the small airways, atelectasis, airway narrowing, and obstruction. Primary infection tends to be the most severe, and it is unclear whether this is due to immunopathologic mechanisms, immunologic immaturity or simply to the small size of the airways of the infected infants.

The immunology and immunopathogenesis of HPIV infection are complex and not fully understood, although it is clear that both humoral and cellular components of the immune system contribute to both pathogenesis and protection. Understanding of the interplay between virus-induced cell damage, beneficial immune responses and inflammatory responses will be key for the development of safe vaccine strategies and effective therapeutic interventions. This has been important, for example, in understanding mechanisms that may have contributed to enhanced disease observed after the administration of a formalin-inactivated RSV vaccine to infants (Scott et al. 1978; Connors et al. 1992; Waris et al. 1996; Prince et al. 1999, 2001; Openshaw et al. 2001). The pathologic changes that are present in children that have died with

parainfluenza infection suggest exaggerated inflammation (Aherne et al. 1970; Downham et al. 1975).

HPIV primary infection does not confer permanent immunity, and in fact repeated reinfection within a year of the previous infection is common in young children. Although reinfection with HPIV-3 can occur, immunity is usually sufficient to restrict virus replication from the lower respiratory tract and prevent severe disease. Mucosal IgA levels correlate with protection from replication of parainfluenza viruses in humans (Smith et al. 1966; Tremonti et al. 1968). Cell-mediated immunity is also an important contributor to prevention of disease: HPIV-3 infection of T cell-deficient infants can result in fatal giant-cell pneumonia (Smith et al. 1966; Tremonti et al. 1968) and HPF-induced pneumonia has a 30 percent mortality in bone marrow transplant recipients (Wendt et al. 1992). The desirablilty of a vaccine that would protect against HPIV-1, -2, and -3 is clear. An inactivated HPIV-1, -2, -3 vaccine used in infants in the late 1960s was immunogenic, but did not offer protection from infection (Chin et al. 1969; Fulginiti et al. 1969), and live attenuated viruses are now being considered as vaccine candidates (Clements et al. 1991; Karron et al. 1995a, 1995b). This underscores the importance of better defining the virus–host interactions that result in pathology versus immunity. The cotton rat (*Sigmodon hispidus*) is an excellent model for HPIV lower respiratory infection (Porter et al. 1991) and for testing potential therapies (Prince and Porter 1996), since experimental infection leads to bronchiolitis and interstitial pneumonia, mimicking human disease. When cotton rats were infected with wild-type HPIV-3 and with variant viruses containing single amino acid changes in the receptor-binding protein HN the pathology observed in lungs of infected animals was distinct: infection with viruses with variant HN resulted in far more severe alveolitis and interstitial pneumonitis even though there was little difference in magnitude and duration of virus replication (Prince et al. 2001). These findings are reminiscent of the cases of unexplained severe HPIV-3 disease in presumably normal children, and present a model to explore the role of HN–receptor interaction in immunopathogenesis that may translate into better understanding of HPIV-3 disease.

CLINICAL MANIFESTATIONS

Bronchiolitis usually begins as an ordinary upper respiratory tract infection with nasal discharge, cough, slight fever, fretfulness, and loss of appetite. The infant may rapidly worsen and develop rapid labored breathing, with retraction of the intercostal spaces, use of accessory respiratory muscles and cyanosis. Increasing obstruction leads to progressive hypoxemia, followed by exhaustion and death. Respirations are rapid, shallow, difficult, and often wheezy, with a rate of 60 to over 80 per minute. Inspiratory retraction is seen in the suprasternal notch and the intercostal and subcostal spaces. Cyanosis appears or is intensified during coughing or crying and can be continuous if the obstruction is severe.

Physical findings include overinflated lungs with hyperresonance to percussion. The diaphragm is depressed, and expiration is prolonged, and wheezing is prominent. Initial hypoxemia may be followed by respiratory acidosis and hypercapnia. Hyperinflation and diffuse interstitial pneumonitis are seen on chest X-ray in severe disease.

Risk factors predisposing to serious disease include underlying medical conditions such as prematurity, cardiopulmonary disease, immunodeficiency, metabolic disease, and some neuromuscular disorders. Assessment of the risk for progression to severe disease includes evaluation of underlying medical conditions, and the overall clinical status of the child. An oxygen saturation less than 95 percent by pulse oxymetry is a reliable objective predictor of progression to severe disease.

TREATMENT

The treatment of acute bronchiolitis should aim to relieve bronchiolar obstruction, correct hypoxemia and acidosis, control potential cardiac complications, provide supportive measures, and prevent or treat secondary bacterial infection.

Management of bronchiolitis is mainly supportive and symptomatic, aimed at providing adequate oxygenation and hydration. Close monitoring of the respiratory status is essential and cardiovascular support may be required in the presence of manifestations of developing heart failure. If the child has very severe bronchiolitis that progresses in spite of these measures, assisted ventilation may be needed.

The use of alpha- and beta-adrenergic agonists remains controversial. The individual response to these therapies is variable and their use must be assessed in each individual case. A trial of inhaled bronchodilators and evaluation of the response is recommended in most cases, particularly in patients with past history of reactive airway disease or asthma. If there is no significant improvement, the therapy may be discontinued.

Cellular damage caused by the immune system of the host is an important component in viral bronchiolitis. Because of this element of inflammation, corticosteroids have been considered and studied for the treatment of bronchiolitis, but to date these studies have failed to demonstrate significant efficacy. Other antiinflammatory agents, such as cromolyn sodium, budesonide, antileukotrienes, and antikinins, are currently being evaluated.

Pneumonia

ETIOLOGY

A variety of pathogens are etiologic agents of pneumonia in children in addition to the human parainfluenza viruses, including RSV and influenza virus and numerous bacterial agents. The incidence of viral pneumonia far outstrips that of bacterial and fungal pneumonia. The clinical manifestation of these various agents is dependent on the pathogen, the child's age and the immune status.

CLINICAL MANIFESTATIONS AND DIAGNOSIS

The clinical diagnosis of pneumonia is supported by the findings of fever, tachypnea, and crackles on lung examination. For many patients, this evaluation is sufficient and the need for pursuing further diagnostic evaluation, including complete blood count, chest radiograph, and blood culture, is based on the degree of toxicity and illness of the child. The most reliable indicator of a positive chest radiograph is the clinical finding of tachypnea. Approximately two out of three of patients with pneumonia present with this finding.

Clinical evidence may not be sufficient to differentiate between viral and bacterial etiologies. Conjunctivitis and otitis media are more often associated with bacterial than viral pneumonia (Ramsey et al. 1986), and wheezing is more commonly associated with viral etiologies (Turner et al. 1987; Forgie et al. 1991). The chest radiograph does not differentiate bacterial from viral pneumonia when radiographs are compared in a blinded fashion (McCarthy et al. 1981; Courtoy et al. 1989). Elevated CRP and absolute neutrophil are more reliable indicators of bacterial pneumonia than clinical and radiologic evidence (Korppi et al. 1997; McIntosh 2002).

REFERENCES

Aherne, W., Bird, T., et al. 1970. Pathological changes in virus infections of the lower respiratory tract in children. *J Clin Pathol*, **23**, 7–18.

Ali, A. and Nayak, D.P. 2000. Assembly of Sendai virus: M protein interacts with F and HN proteins and with the cytoplasmic tail and transmembrane domain of F protein. *Virology*, **276**, 289–303.

Andrejeva, J., Young, D.F., et al. 2002. Degradation of STAT1 and STAT2 by the V proteins of simian virus 5 and human parainfluenza virus type 2, respectively: consequences for virus replication in the presence of alpha/beta and gamma interferons. *J Virol*, **76**, 2159–67.

Apalsch, A.M., Green, M., et al. 1995. Parainfluenza and influenza virus infections in pediatric organ transplant recipients. *Clin Infect Dis*, **20**, 394–9.

Bagai, S. and Lamb, R.A. 1995. Quantitative measurement of paramyxovirus fusion: differences in requirements of glycoproteins between simian virus 5 and human parainfluenza virus 3 or Newcastle disease virus. *J Virol*, **69**, 6712–19.

Baker, K.A., Dutch, R.E., et al. 1999. Structural basis for paramyxovirus-mediated membrane fusion. *Mol Cell*, **3**, 309–19.

Bellini, W.J., Englund, G., et al. 1985. Measles virus P gene codes for two proteins. *J Virol*, **53**, 908–19.

Bose, S. and Banerjee, A.K. 2002. Role of heparan sulfate in human parainfluenza virus type 3 infection. *Virology*, **298**, 73–83.

Bose, S., Malur, A., et al. 2001. Polarity of human parainfluenza virus type 3 infection in polarized human lung epithelial A549 cells: role of microfilament and microtubule. *J Virol*, **75**, 1984–9.

Bousse, T., Takimoto, T., et al. 2001. Two regions of the P protein are required to be active with the L protein for human parainfluenza virus type 1 RNA polymerase activity. *Virology*, **283**, 306–14.

Bowman, M.C., Smallwood, S., et al. 1999. Dissection of individual functions of the Sendai virus phosphoprotein in transcription. *J Virol*, **73**, 6474–83.

Bratt, M. and Rubin, H. 1967a. Specific interference among strains of NDV. I. Demonstration and measurement of interference. *Virology*, **33**, 598–608.

Bratt, M. and Rubin, H. 1967b. Specific interference among strains of NDV. II. Comparison of interference of active and inactive virus. *Virology*, **35**, 381–94.

Bratt, M. and Rubin, H. 1968. Specific interference among strains of NDV. III. Mechanism of interference. *Virology*, **35**, 395–407.

Buchholz, C., Spehner, D., et al. 1993. The conserved N-terminal region of Sendai virus nucleocapsid protein NP is required for nucleocapsid assembly. *J Virol*, **67**, 5803–12.

Buchholz, C., Retzler, C., et al. 1994. The carboxy-terminal domain of Sendai virus nucleocapsid protein is involved in complex formation between phosphoprotein and nucleocapsid-like particles. *Virology*, **204**, 770–6.

Carr, C.M. and Kim, P.S. 1993. A spring-loaded mechanism for the conformational change of influenza hemagglutinin. *Cell*, **73**, 823–32.

Cevik, B., Smallwood, S., et al. 2003. The L-L oligomerization domain resides at the very N-terminus of the sendai virus L RNA polymerase protein. *Virology*, **313**, 525–36.

Chanock, R.M. 1990. Control of pediatric viral diseases: past successes and future prospects. *Pediatr Res*, **27**, Suppl. 6, S39–43.

Chen, J., Lee, K.H., et al. 1998. Structure of the hemagglutinin precursor cleavage site, a determinant of influenza pathogenicity and the origin of the labile conformation. *Cell*, **95**, 409–17.

Chin, J., Magoffin, R., et al. 1969. Field evaluation of a respiratory syncytial virus vaccine and a trivalent parainfluenza virus vaccine in a pediatric population. *Am J Epidemiol*, **89**, 449–63.

Choppin, P.W. and Compans, R. 1975. Reproduction of paramyxoviruses. In: Wagner, R.R. (ed.), *Comprehensive virology*. Vol. 4. New York: Plenum Press, 95–178.

Clements, M., Belshe, R., et al. 1991. Evaluation of bovine, cold-adapted human, and wild-type human parainfluenza type 3 viruses in adult volunteers and in chimpanzees. *J Clin Microbiol*, **29**, 1175–82.

Clements, M.L., Makhene, M.K., et al. 1996. Effective immunization with live attenuated influenza A virus can be achieved in early infancy. Pediatric Care Center. *J Infect Dis*, **173**, 44–51.

Collins, P., Chanock, R., et al. 1996. Parainfluenza viruses. In: Fields, B., Knipe, D.M. and Howley, P.M. (eds), *Fields virology*. Philadelphia: Lippincott-Raven Publishers.

Connors, M., Kulkarni, A.B., et al. 1992. Pulmonary histopathology induced by respiratory syncytial virus (RSV) challenge of formalin-inactivated RSV-immunized BALB/c mice is abrogated by depletion of CD4+ T cells. *J Virol*, **66**, 7444–51.

Coronel, E.C., Murti, K.G., et al. 1999. Human parainfluenza virus type 1 matrix and nucleoprotein genes transiently expressed in mammalian cells induce the release of virus-like particles containing nucleocapsid-like structures. *J Virol*, **73**, 7035–8.

Coronel, E.C., Takimoto, T., et al. 2001. Nucleocapsid incorporation into parainfluenza virus is regulated by specific interaction with matrix protein. *J Virol*, **75**, 1117–23.

Courtoy, I., Lande, A.E., et al. 1989. Accuracy of radiographic differentiation of bacterial from nonbacterial pneumonia. *Clin Pediatr (Phila)*, **28**, 261–4.

Crennell, S., Takimoto, T., et al. 2000. Crystal structure of the multifunctional paramyxovirus hemagglutinin-neuraminidase. *Nat Struct Biol*, **7**, 1068–74.

Curran, J. and Kolakofsky, D. 1988. Ribosomal initiation from an ACG codon in the Sendai virus P/C mRNA. *EMBO J*, **7**, 245–51.

Curran, J., Homann, H., et al. 1993. The hypervariable C-terminal tail of the Sendai paramyxovirus nucleocapsid protein is required for template function but not for RNA encapsidation. *J Virol*, **67**, 4358–64.

Curran, J., Pelet, T., et al. 1994. An acidic activation-like domain of the Sendai virus P protein is required for RNA synthesis and encapsidation. *Virology*, **202**, 875–84.

Curran, J., Boeck, R., et al. 1995a. Paramyxovirus phosphoproteins form homotrimers as determined by an epitope dilution assay, via predicted coiled coils. *Virology*, **214**, 139–49.

Curran, J., Marq, J.B., et al. 1995b. An N-terminal domain of the Sendai paramyxovirus P protein acts as a chaperone for the NP protein during the nascent chain assembly step of genome replication. *J Virol*, **69**, 849–55.

De, B.P. and Banerjee, A.K. 1999. Involvement of actin microfilaments in the transcription/replication of human parainfluenza virus type 3: possible role of actin in other viruses. *Microsc Res Tech*, **47**, 114–23.

De, B.P., Hoffman, M.A., et al. 2000. Role of NH(2)- and COOH-terminal domains of the P protein of human parainfluenza virus type 3 in transcription and replication. *J Virol*, **74**, 5886–95.

Didcock, L., Young, D.F., et al. 1999. The V protein of simian virus 5 inhibits interferon signalling by targeting STAT1 for proteasome-mediated degradation. *J Virol*, **73**, 9928–33.

Downham, M., Gardner, P., et al. 1975. Role of respiratory viruses in childhood mortality. *Br Med J*, **1**, 235–9.

Dutch, R.E. and Lamb, R.A. 2001. Deletion of the cytoplasmic tail of the fusion protein of the paramyxovirus simian virus 5 affects fusion pore enlargement. *J Virol*, **75**, 5363–9.

Dutch, R.E., Jardetzky, T.S., et al. 2000. Virus membrane fusion proteins: biological machines that undergo a metamorphosis. *Biosci Rep*, **20**, 597–612.

Fan, J. and Henrickson, K.J. 1996. Rapid diagnosis of human parainfluenza virus type 1 infection by quantitative reverse transcription-PCR-enzyme hybridization assay. *J Clin Microbiol*, **34**, 1914–17.

Fan, J., Henrickson, K.J., et al. 1998. Rapid simultaneous diagnosis of infections with respiratory syncytial viruses A and B, influenza viruses A and B, and human parainfluenza virus types 1, 2, and 3 by multiplex quantitative reverse transcription-polymerase chain reaction-enzyme hybridization assay (Hexaplex). *Clin Infect Dis*, **261**, 1397–402.

Forgie, I.M., O'Neill, K.P., et al. 1991. Etiology of acute lower respiratory tract infections in Gambian children: I. Acute lower respiratory tract infections in infants presenting at the hospital. *Pediatr Infect Dis J*, **10**, 33–41.

Fulginiti, V., Eller, J., et al. 1969. Respiratory virus immunization. I. A field trial of two inactivated respiratory virus vaccines; an aqueous trivalent parainfluenza virus vaccine and an alum-precipitated respiratory syncytial virus vaccine. *Am J Epidemiol*, **89**, 435–48.

Galinski, M.S., Troy, R.M., et al. 1992. RNA editing in the phosphoprotein gene of the human parainfluenza virus type 3. *Virology*, **186**, 543–50.

Garcin, D., Marq, J.B., et al. 2002. All four Sendai Virus C proteins bind Stat1, but only the larger forms also induce its mono-ubiquitination and degradation. *Virology*, **295**, 256–65.

Garcin, D., Marq, J.B., et al. 2003. The amino-terminal extensions of the longer Sendai virus C proteins modulate pY701-Stat1 and bulk Stat1 levels independently of interferon signaling. *J Virol*, **77**, 2321–9.

Garten, W., Berk, W., et al. 1980. Mutational changes of the protease susceptibility of glycoprotein F of Newcastle disease virus: effects on pathogenicity. *J Gen Virol*, **50**, 135–47.

Garten, W., Will, C., et al. 1992. Structure and assembly of hemagglutinin mutants of fowl plague virus with impaired surface transport. *J Virol*, **66**, 1495–505.

Giorgi, C., Blumberg, B.M., et al. 1983. Sendai virus contains overlapping genes expressed from a single mRNA. *Cell*, **35**, 829–36.

Gorman, W.L., Gill, D.S., et al. 1990. The hemagglutinin-neuraminidase glycoproteins of human parainfluenza virus type 1 and Sendai virus have high structure-function similarity with limited antigenic cross-reactivity. *Virology*, **175**, 211–21.

Gotoh, B., Komatsu, T., et al. 2001. Paramyxovirus accessory proteins as interferon antagonists. *Microbiol Immunol*, **45**, 787–800.

Greengard, O., Poltoratskaia, N., et al. 2000. The anti-influenza virus agent 4-GU-DANA (Zanamivir) inhibits cell fusion mediated by human parainfluenza virus and influenza virus HA. *J Virol*, **74**, 11108–14.

Gupta, S., De, B.P., et al. 1998. Involvement of actin microfilaments in the replication of human parainfluenza virus type 3. *J Virol*, **72**, 2655–62.

Hall, C.B. 2001. Respiratory syncytial virus and parainfluenza virus. *N Engl J Med*, **344**, 1917–28.

Hall, S.L., Sarris, C.M., et al. 1993. A cold-adapted mutant of parainfluenza virus type 3 is attenuated and protective in chimpanzees. *J Infect Dis*, **167**, 958–62.

Hausmann, S., Garcin, D., et al. 1999a. The versatility of paramyxovirus RNA polymerase stuttering. *J Virol*, **73**, 5568–76.

Hausmann, S., Garcin, D., et al. 1999b. Two nucleotides immediately upstream of the essential A6G3 slippery sequence modulate the pattern of G insertions during Sendai virus mRNA editing. *J Virol*, **73**, 343–51.

Haywood, A. 1974. Characteristics of Sendai virus receptors in a model membrane. *J Mol Biol*, **83**, 427–36.

Haywood, A. and Boyer, B. 1982. Sendai virus membrane fusion: Time course and effect of temperature, pH, calcium and receptor concentration. *Biochemistry*, **21**, 6041–6.

He, B., Paterson, R.G., et al. 2002. Recovery of paramyxovirus simian virus 5 with a V protein lacking the conserved cysteine-rich domain: the multifunctional V protein blocks both interferon-beta induction and interferon signaling. *Virology*, **303**, 15–32.

Hernandez, L.D., Hoffman, L.R., et al. 1996. Virus–cell and cell–cell fusion. *Annu Rev Cell Dev Biol*, **12**, 627–61.

Holmes, D.E. and Moyer, S.A. 2002. The phosphoprotein (P) binding site resides in the N terminus of the L polymerase subunit of sendai virus. *J Virol*, **76**, 3078–83.

Homann, H., Willenbrink, W., et al. 1991. Sendai virus protein-protein interactions studied by a protein-blotting protein-overlay technique: mapping of domains on NP protein required for binding to P protein. *J Virol*, **65**, 1304–9.

Homma, M. and Ouchi, M. 1973. Trypsin action on the growth of Sendai virus in tissue culture cells. Structural difference of Sendai viruses grown in eggs and tissue culture cells. *J Virol*, **12**, 1457–65.

Horga, M.A., Gusella, G.L., et al. 2000. Mechanism of interference mediated by human parainfluenza virus type 3 infection. *J Virol*, **74**, 11792–9.

Horikami, S.M., Curran, J., et al. 1992. Complexes of Sendai virus NP-P and P-L proteins are required for defective interfering particle genome replication in vitro. *J Virol*, **66**, 4901–8.

Horikami, S.M. and Moyer, S.A. 1995. Alternative amino acids at a single site in the Sendai virus L protein produce multiple defects in RNA synthesis in vitro. *Virology*, **211**, 577–82.

Horikami, S.M., Smallwood, S., et al. 1996. The Sendai virus V protein interacts with the NP protein to regulate viral genome RNA replication. *Virology*, **222**, 383–90.

Horikami, S.M., Hector, R.E., et al. 1997. The Sendai virus C protein binds the L polymerase protein to inhibit viral RNA synthesis. *Virology*, **235**, 261–70.

Horvath, C.M., Paterson, R.G., et al. 1992. Biological activity of paramyxovirus fusion proteins: factors influencing formation of syncytia. *J Virol*, **66**, 4564–9.

Hsu, C.H. and Kingsbury, D.W. 1982. Topography of phosphate residues in Sendai virus proteins. *Virology*, **120**, 225–34.

Hu, C.J., Kato, A., et al. 1999. Role of primary constitutive phosphorylation of Sendai virus P and V proteins in viral replication and pathogenesis. *Virology*, **263**, 195–208.

Hu, X.L., Ray, R., et al. 1992. Functional interactions between the fusion protein and hemagglutinin-neuraminidase of human parainfluenza viruses. *J Virol*, **66**, 1528–34.

Huberman, K., Peluso, R., et al. 1995. The hemagglutinin-neuraminidase of human parainfluenza virus type 3: Role of the neuraminidase in the viral life cycle. *Virology*, **214**, 294–300.

Husby, S., Agertoft, L., et al. 1993. Treatment of croup with nebulised steroid (budesonide): a double blind, placebo controlled study. *Arch Dis Child*, **68**, 352–5.

Jardetzky, T.S. and Lamb, R.A. 2004. Virology: a class act. *Nature*, **427**, 307–8.

Jin, H. and Elliott, R.M. 1992. Mutagenesis of the L protein encoded by Bunyamwera virus and production of monospecific antibodies. *J Gen Virol*, **73**, 2235–44.

Johnson, D.W., Jacobson, S., et al. 1998. A comparison of nebulized budesonide, intramuscular dexamethasone, and placebo for moderately severe croup. *N Engl J Med*, **339**, 498–503.

Kairys, S.W., Olmstead, E.M., et al. 1989. Steroid treatment of laryngotracheitis: a meta-analysis of the evidence from randomized trials. *Pediatrics*, **83**, 683–93.

Karron, R., Wright, P., et al. 1995a. A live attenuated bovine parainfluenza virus type 3 vaccine is safe, infectious, immunogenic, and phenotypically stable in infants and children. *J Infect Dis*, **171**, 1107–14.

Karron, R., Wright, P., et al. 1995b. A live human parainfluenza type 3 virus vaccine is attenuated and immunogenic in healthy infants and children. *J Infect Dis*, **172**, 1445–50.

Karron, R.A., Steinhoff, M.C., et al. 1995c. Safety and immunogenicity of a cold-adapted influenza A (H1N1) reassortant virus vaccine administered to infants less than six months of age. *Pediatr Infect Dis J*, **14**, 10–16.

Karron, R.A., Makhene, M., et al. 1996. Evaluation of a live attenuated bovine parainfluenza type 3 vaccine in two- to six-month-old infants. *Pediatr Infect Dis J*, **15**, 650–4.

Katze, M.G., He, Y., et al. 2002. Viruses and interferon: a fight for supremacy. *Nat Rev Immunol*, **2**, 675–87.

Kehl, S.C., Henrickson, K.J., et al. 2001. Evaluation of the Hexaplex assay for detection of respiratory viruses in children. *J Clin Microbiol*, **39**, 1696–701.

Kimura, Y., Norrby, E., et al. 1976. Homologous interference induced by a temperature sensitive mutant derived from an HJV carrier culture. *J Gen Virol*, **33**, 333–43.

Klassen, T.P., Feldman, M.E., et al. 1994. Nebulized budesonide for children with mild-to-moderate croup. *N Engl J Med*, **331**, 285–9.

Klassen, T.P., Craig, W.R., et al. 1998. Nebulized budesonide and oral dexamethasone for treatment of croup: a randomized controlled trial. *JAMA*, **279**, 1629–32.

Klenk, H.D. and Garten, W. 1994. Host cell proteases controlling virus pathogenicity. *Trends Microbiol*, **2**, 39–43.

Kolakofsky, D., Pelet, T., et al. 1998. Paramyxovirus RNA synthesis and the requirement for hexamer genome length: the rule of six revisited. *J Virol*, **72**, 891–9.

Korppi, M., Heiskanen-Kosma, T., et al. 1997. White blood cells, C-reactive protein and erythrocyte sedimentation rate in pneumococcal pneumonia in children. *Eur Respir J*, **10**, 1125–9.

Kubota, T., Yokosawa, N., et al. 2002. Association of mumps virus V protein with RACK1 results in dissociation of STAT-1 from the alpha interferon receptor complex. *J Virol*, **76**, 12676–82.

Kurotani, A., Kiyotani, K., et al. 1998. Sendai virus C proteins are categorically nonessential gene products but silencing their expression severely impairs viral replication and pathogenesis. *Genes Cells*, **3**, 111–24.

Kuusela, A.L. and Vesikari, T. 1988. A randomized double-blind, placebo-controlled trial of dexamethasone and racemic epinephrine in the treatment of croup. *Acta Paediatr Scand*, **77**, 99–104.

Lamb, R. 1993. Paramyxovirus fusion: A hypothesis for changes. *Virology*, **197**, 1–11.

Lamb, R. and Kolakofsky, D. 2001. Paramyxoviridae: the viruses and their replication. In: Fields, B., Knipe, D.M. and Howley, P.M. (eds), *Fields virology*. Philadelphia: Lippincott, Williams and Wilkins.

Lamb, R.A., Mahy, B.W.J., et al. 1976. The synthesis of Sendai virus polypeptides in infected cells. *Virology*, **69**, 116–31.

Latorre, P., Cadd, T., et al. 1998. The various Sendai virus C proteins are not functionally equivalent and exert both positive and negative effects on viral RNA accumulation during the course of infection. *J Virol*, **72**, 5984–93.

Lawrence, M.C., Borg, N.A., et al. 2004. Structure of the haemagglutinin-neuraminidase from human parainfluenza virus type III. *J Mol Biol*, **335**, 1343–57.

Levin Perlman, S., Jordan, M., et al. 1999. The use of a quantitative fusion assay to evaluate HN-receptor interaction for human parainfluenza virus type 3. *Virology*, **265**, 57–65.

Lin, G.Y. and Lamb, R.A. 2000. The paramyxovirus simian virus 5 V protein slows progression of the cell cycle. *J Virol*, **74**, 9152–66.

Lyn, D., Mazanec, M.B., et al. 1991. Location of amino acid residues important for the structure and biological function of the haemagglutinin-neuraminidase glycoprotein of Sendai virus by analysis of escape mutants. *J Gen Virol*, **72**, 817–24.

Malur, A.G., Choudhary, S.K., et al. 2002. Role of a highly conserved NH(2)-terminal domain of the human parainfluenza virus type 3 RNA polymerase. *J Virol*, **76**, 8101–9.

Markwell, M. and Fox, C. 1980. Protein–protein interactions within paramyxoviruses identified by native disulfide bonding or reversible chemical cross-linking. *J Virol*, **33**, 152–66.

Markwell, M. and Paulson, J. 1980. Sendai virus utilizes specific sialyloligosaccharides as host cell receptor determinants. *Proc Natl Acad Sci USA*, **77**, 5693–7.

Markwell, M., Svennerholm, L., et al. 1981. Specific gangliosides function as host cell receptors for Sendai virus. *Proc Natl Acad Sci USA*, **78**, 5406–10.

McCarthy, P.L., Spiesel, S.Z., et al. 1981. Radiographic findings and etiologic diagnosis in ambulatory childhood pneumonias. *Clin Pediatr (Phila)*, **20**, 686–91.

McIntosh, K. 2002. Community-acquired pneumonia in children. *N Engl J Med*, **346**, 429–37.

Moscona, A. and Peluso, R.W. 1991. Fusion properties of cells persistently infected with human parainfluenza virus type 3: Participation of hemagglutinin-neuraminidase in membrane fusion. *J Virol*, **65**, 2773–7.

Moscona, A. and Peluso, R.W. 1993. Relative affinity of the human parainfluenza virus 3 hemagglutinin-neuraminidase for sialic acid correlates with virus-induced fusion activity. *J Virol*, **67**, 6463–8.

Moscona, A. and Peluso, R.W. 1996. Analysis of human parainfluenza virus 3 receptor binding variants: evidence for the use of a specific sialic acid-containing receptor. *Microb Pathog*, **20**, 179–84.

Mottet, G., Muhlemann, A., et al. 1996. A Sendai virus vector leading to the efficient expression of mutant M proteins interfering with virus particle budding. *Virology*, **221**, 159–71.

Mottet, G., Muller, V., et al. 1999. Characterization of Sendai virus M protein mutants that can partially interfere with virus particle production. *J Gen Virol*, **80**, 2977–86.

Murphy, B.R. 1988. Current approaches to the development of vaccines effective against parainfluenza viruses. *Bull World Health Organ*, **66**, 391–7.

Murrell, M., Porotto, M., et al. 2003. Mutations in human parainfluenza virus type 3 HN causing increased receptor binding activity and resistance to the transition state sialic acid analog 4-GU-DANA (zanamivir). *J Virol*, **77**, 309–17.

Myers, T.M. and Moyer, S.A. 1997. An amino-terminal domain of the Sendai virus nucleocapsid protein is required for template function in viral RNA synthesis. *J Virol*, **71**, 918–24.

Myers, T.M., Pieters, A., et al. 1997. A highly conserved region of the Sendai virus nucleocapsid protein contributes to the NP-NP binding domain. *Virology*, **229**, 322–35.

Myers, T.M., Smallwood, S., et al. 1999. Identification of nucleocapsid protein residues required for Sendai virus nucleocapsid formation and genome replication. *J Gen Virol*, **80**, 1383–91.

Nagai, Y. and Klenk, H.D. 1977. Activation of precursors to both glycoproteins of Newcastle disease virus by proteolytic cleavage. *Virology*, **77**, 125–34.

Nagai, Y., Klenk, H.D., et al. 1976. Proteolytic cleavage of the viral glycoproteins and its significance for the virulence of Newcastle disease virus. *Virology*, **72**, 494–508.

Nagai, Y., Shimokata, K., et al. 1979. The spread of a pathogenic and an apathogenic strain of Newcastle disease virus in the chick embryo as depending on the protease sensitivity of the virus glycoproteins. *J Gen Virol*, **45**, 263–72.

Ng, D., Randall, R., et al. 1989. Intracellular maturation and transport of the SV percent type II glycoprotein HN: specific and transient association with GRP78-BiP in the ER and extensive internalization from the cell surface. *J Cell Biol*, **109**, 3273–89.

Nishio, M., Garcin, D., et al. 2002. The carboxyl segment of the mumps virus V protein associates with Stat proteins in vitro via a tryptophan-rich motif. *Virology*, **300**, 92–9.

Ohki, S., Arnold, K., et al. 1992. Effect of anionic polymers on fusion of Sendai virus with human erythrocyte ghosts. *Antiviral Res*, **18**, 163–77.

Okada, H., Seto, J.T., et al. 1998. Determinants of pantropism of the F1-R mutant of Sendai virus: specific mutations involved are in the F and M genes. *Arch Virol*, **143**, 2343–52.

Openshaw, P.J., Culley, F.J., et al. 2001. Immunopathogenesis of vaccine-enhanced RSV disease. *Vaccine*, **20**, Suppl. 1, S27–31.

Orlicek, S.L. 1998. Management of acute laryngotracheo-bronchitis. *Pediatr Infect Dis J*, **17**, 1164–5.

Ortmann, D., Ohuchi, M., et al. 1994. Proteolytic cleavage of wild type and mutants of the F protein of human parainfluenza virus type 3 by two subtilisin-like endoproteases, furin and Kex2. *J Virol*, **68**, 2772–6.

Parisien, J.P., Lau, J.F., et al. 2001. The V protein of human parainfluenza virus 2 antagonizes type I interferon responses by destabilizing signal transducer and activator of transcription 2. *Virology*, **283**, 230–9.

Pastey, M.K., Crowe, J.E., et al. 1999. RhoA interacts with the fusion glycoprotein of respiratory syncytial virus and facilitates virus-induced syncytium formation. *J Virol*, **73**, 7262–70.

Pastey, M.K., Gower, T.L., et al. 2000. A RhoA-derived peptide inhibits syncytium formation induced by respiratory syncytial virus and parainfluenza virus type 3. *Nat Med*, **6**, 35–40.

Paterson, R.G., Leser, G.P., et al. 1995. The paramyxovirus SV5 V protein binds two atoms of zinc and is a structural component of virions. *Virology*, **208**, 121–31.

Paulson, J., Sadler, J., et al. 1979. Restoration of specific myxovirus receptors to asialoerythrocytes by incorporation of sialic acid with pure sialyltransferases. *J Biol Chem*, **254**, 2120–4.

Pelet, T., Delenda, C., et al. 1996. Partial characterization of a Sendai virus replication promoter and the rule of six. *Virology*, **224**, 405–14.

Plemper, R.K., Lakdawala, A.S., et al. 2003. Structural features of paramyxovirus F protein required for fusion initiation. *Biochemistry*, **42**, 6645–55.

Poch, O., Blumberg, B., et al. 1990. Sequence comparison of five polymerases (L proteins) of unsegmented negative-strand RNA viruses: theoretical assignments of functional domains. *J Gen Virol*, **71**, 1153–62.

Poole, E., He, B., et al. 2002. The V proteins of simian virus 5 and other paramyxoviruses inhibit induction of interferon-beta. *Virology*, **303**, 33–46.

Porotto, M., Greengard, O., et al. 2001. Human parainfluenza virus type 3 HN-receptor interaction: the effect of 4-GU-DANA on a neuraminidase-deficient variant. *J Virol*, **76**, 7481–8.

Porotto, M., Murrell, M., et al. 2003. Triggering of human parainfluenza virus 3 fusion protein (F) by the hemagglutinin-neuraminidase (HN): an HN mutation diminishing the rate of F activation and fusion. *J Virol*, **77**, 3647–54.

Porter, D., Prince, G., et al. 1991. Pathogenesis of human parainfluenza virus 3 infection in two species of cotton rat: *Sigmodon hispidus* develops bronchiolitis, while *Sigmodon fulviventer* develops interstitial pneumonia. *J Virol*, **65**, 103–11.

Portner, A. 1981. The HN glycoprotein of Sendai virus: analysis of site(s) involved in hemagglutinating and neuraminidase activities. *Virology*, **115**, 375–84.

Portner, A., Scroggs, R.A., et al. 1987. Distinct functions of antigenic sites of the HN glycoprotein of Sendai virus. *Virology*, **158**, 61–8.

Prince, G. and Porter, D. 1996. Treatment of parainfluenza virus type 3 bronchiolitis and pneumonia in a cotton rat model using topical antibody and glucocorticosteroid. *J Infect Dis*, **173**, 598–608.

Prince, G., Prieels, J.P., et al. 1999. Pulmonary lesions in primary respiratory syncytial virus infection, reinfection and vaccine-enhanced disease in the cotton rat (*Sigmodon hispidus*). *Lab Invest*, **79**, 1385–92.

Prince, G.A., Curtis, S.J., et al. 2001. Vaccine-enhanced respiratory syncytial virus disease in cotton rats following immunization with Lot 100 or a newly prepared reference vaccine. *J Gen Virol*, **82**, 2881–8.

Prince, G.A., Ottolini, M.G., et al. 2001. Contribution of the human parainfluenza virus type 3 HN-receptor interaction to pathogenesis in vivo. *J Virol*, **75**, 12446–51.

Pritzer, E., Kuroda, K., et al. 1990. A host range mutant of Newcastle disease virus with an altered cleavage site for proteolytic activation of the F protein. *Virus Res*, **15**, 237–42.

Ramsey, B.W., Marcuse, E.K., et al. 1986. Use of bacterial antigen detection in the diagnosis of pediatric lower respiratory tract infections. *Pediatrics*, **78**, 1–9.

Rodriguez, J.J., Parisien, J.P., et al. 2002. Nipah virus V protein evades alpha and gamma interferons by preventing STAT1 and STAT2 activation and nuclear accumulation. *J Virol*, **76**, 11476–83.

Russell, C.J., Jardetzky, T.S., et al. 2001. Membrane fusion machines of paramyxoviruses: capture of intermediates of fusion. *EMBO J*, **20**, 4024–34.

Russell, R., Paterson, R., et al. 1994. Studies with cross-linking reagents on the oligomeric form of the paramyxovirus fusion protein. *Virology*, **199**, 160–8.

Ryan, K.W. and Portner, A. 1990. Separate domains of Sendai virus P protein are required for binding to viral nucleocapsids. *Virology*, **174**, 515–21.

Ryan, K.W., Portner, A., et al. 1993. Antibodies to Paramyxovirus nucleocapsid proteins define regions important for immunogenicity and nucleocapsid assembly. *Virology*, **193**, 376–3384.

Scheid, A. and Choppin, P. 1974. Identification of biological activities of paramyxovirus glycoproteins. Activation of cell fusion, hemolysis and infectivity by proteolytic cleavage of an inactive protein of Sendai virus. *Virology*, **57**, 470–90.

Schnell, M.J. and Conzelmann, K.K. 1995. Polymerase activity of in vitro mutated rabies virus L protein. *Virology*, **214**, 522–30.

Scott, R., Kaul, A., et al. 1978. Development of in vitro correlates of cell-mediated immunity to respiratory syncytial virus infection in humans. *J Infect Dis*, **137**, 810–17.

Seth, S., Vincent, A., et al. 2003. Mutations in the cytoplasmic domain of a paramyxovirus fusion glycoprotein rescue syncytium formation and eliminate the hemagglutinin-neuraminidase protein requirement for membrane fusion. *J Virol*, **77**, 167–78.

Shioda, T., Wakao, S., et al. 1988. Differences in bovine parainfluenza 3 virus variants studied by sequencing of the genes of viral envelope proteins. *Virology*, **162**, 388–96.

Sidhu, M.S., Menonna, J., et al. 1993. Canine distemper virus L protein gene: sequence and comparison with related viruses. *Virology*, **193**, 50–65.

Skehel, J.J. and Wiley, D.C. 1998. Coiled coils in both intracellular vesicle and viral membrane fusion. *Cell*, **95**, 871–4.

Skiadopoulos, M.H., Surman, S., et al. 1999a. Identification of mutations contributing to the temperature-sensitive, cold-adapted, and attenuation phenotypes of the live-attenuated cold-passage 45 (cp45) human parainfluenza virus 3 candidate vaccine. *J Virol*, **73**, 1374–81.

Skiadopoulos, M.H., Surman, S.R., et al. 1999b. Attenuation of the recombinant human parainfluenza virus type 3 cp45 candidate vaccine virus is augmented by importation of the respiratory syncytial virus cpts530 L polymerase mutation. *Virology*, **260**, 125–35.

Skiadopoulos, M.H., Tao, T., et al. 1999c. Generation of a parainfluenza virus type 1 vaccine candidate by replacing the HN and F glycoproteins of the live-attenuated PIV3 cp45 vaccine virus with their PIV1 counterparts. *Vaccine*, **18**, 503–10.

Sleat, D.E. and Banerjee, A.K. 1993. Transcriptional activity and mutational analysis of recombinant vesicular stomatitis virus RNA polymerase. *J Virol*, **67**, 1334–9.

Smallwood, S., Ryan, K.W., et al. 1994. Deletion analysis defines a carboxyl-proximal region of Sendai virus P protein that binds to the polymerase L protein. *Virology*, **202**, 154–63.

Smallwood, S., Easson, C.D., et al. 1999. Mutations in conserved domain II of the large (L) subunit of the Sendai virus RNA polymerase abolish RNA synthesis. *Virology*, **262**, 375–83.

Smallwood, S., Hovel, T., et al. 2002. Different substitutions at conserved amino acids in domains II and III in the Sendai L RNA polymerase protein inactivate viral RNA synthesis. *Virology*, **304**, 135–45.

Smith, C., Purcell, R., et al. 1966. Protective effect of antibody to parainfluenza type 1 virus. *N Eng J Med*, **275**, 1145–52.

Suzuki, Y., Suzuki, T., et al. 1985. Gangliosides as paramyxovirus receptor. Structural requirement of sialo-oligosaccharides in receptors for hemagglutinating virus of Japan (Sendai virus) and Newcastle disease virus. *J Biochem*, **97**, 1189–99.

Suzuki, T., Portner, A., et al. 2001. Receptor specificities of human respiroviruses. *J Virol*, **75**, 4604–13.

Takeuchi, K., Komatsu, T., et al. 2001. Sendai virus C protein physically associates with Stat1. *Genes Cells*, **6**, 545–57.

Takimoto, T., Murti, K.G., et al. 2001. Role of matrix and fusion proteins in budding of Sendai virus. *J Virol*, **75**, 11384–91.

Tanabayashi, K. and Compans, R.W. 1996. Functional interaction of paramyxovirus glycoproteins: identification of a domain in Sendai virus HN which promotes cell fusion. *J Virol*, **70**, 6112–18.

Tao, T., Skiadopoulos, M.H., et al. 1999. A live attenuated chimeric recombinant parainfluenza virus (PIV) encoding the internal proteins of PIV type 3 and the surface glycoproteins of PIV type 1 induces complete resistance to PIV1 challenge and partial resistance to PIV3 challenge. *Vaccine*, **17**, 1100–8.

Tarboubiech, N., Curran, J., et al. 2000a. On the domain structure and the polymerization state of the Sendai virus P protein. *Virology*, **266**, 99–109.

Tarboubiech, N., Curran, J., et al. 2000b. Tetrameric coiled coil domain of Sendai virus phosphoprotein. *Nat Struct Biol*, **7**, 777–81.

Tashiro, M., Yamakawa, M., et al. 1990. Organ tropism of Sendai virus in mice: proteolytic activation of the fusion glycoprotein in mouse organs and budding site at the bronchial epithelium. *J Virol*, **64**, 3627–34.

Tashiro, M., Seto, J.T., et al. 1992. Changes in specific cleavability of the Sendai virus fusion protein: implications for pathogenicity in mice. *J Gen Virol*, **73**, 1575–9.

Tashiro, M., Seto, J.T., et al. 1993. Possible involvement of microtubule disruption in bipolar budding of a Sendai virus mutant, F1-R, in epithelial MDCK cells. *J Virol*, **67**, 5902–10.

Thomas, S.M., Lamb, R.A., et al. 1988. Two mRNAs that differ by two nontemplated nucleotides encode the amino coterminal proteins P and V of the paramyxovirus SV5. *Cell*, **54**, 891–902.

Thompson, S.D. and Portner, A. 1987. Localization of functional sites on the hemagglutinin-neuraminidase glycoprotein of Sendai virus by sequence analysis of antigenic and temperature-sensitive mutants. *Virology*, **160**, 1–8.

Thompson, S., Laver, W., et al. 1988. Isolation of a biologically active soluble form of the hemagglutinin-neuraminidase protein of Sendai virus. *J Virol*, **62**, 4653–60.

Tong, S. and Compans, R.W. 1999. Alternative mechanisms of interaction between homotypic and heterotypic parainfluenza virus HN and F proteins. *J Gen Virol*, **80**, 107–15.

Tong, S., Li, M., et al. 2002. Regulation of fusion activity by the cytoplasmic domain of a paramyxovirus F protein. *Virology*, **301**, 322–33.

Tremonti, L., Lin, J., et al. 1968. Neutralizing activity in nasal secretions and serum in resistance of volunteers to parainfluenza virus type 2. *J Immunol*, **101**, 572–7.

Turner, R.B., Lande, A.E., et al. 1987. Pneumonia in pediatric outpatients: cause and clinical manifestations. *J Pediatr*, **111**, 194–200.

Ulane, C.M., Rodriguez, J.J., et al. 2003. STAT3 ubiquitylation and degradation by mumps virus suppress cytokine and oncogene signaling. *J Virol*, **77**, 6385–93.

Vidal, S., Curran, J., et al. 1990a. Editing of the Sendai virus P/C mRNA by G insertion occurs during mRNA synthesis via a virus-encoded activity. *J Virol*, **64**, 239–46.

Vidal, S., Curran, J., et al. 1990b. A stuttering model for paramyxovirus P mRNA editing. *EMBO J*, **9**, 2017–22.

Vulliemoz, D. and Roux, L. 2001. Rule of six: how does the Sendai virus RNA polymerase keep count? *J Virol*, **75**, 4506–18.

Waisman, Y., Klein, B.L., et al. 1992. Prospective randomized double-blind study comparing L-epinephrine and racemic epinephrine aerosols in the treatment of laryngotracheitis (croup). *Pediatrics*, **89**, 302–6.

Wansley, E.K. and Parks, G.D. 2002. Naturally occurring substitutions in the P/V gene convert the noncytopathic paramyxovirus simian virus 5 into a virus that induces alpha/beta interferon synthesis and cell death. *J Virol*, **76**, 10109–21.

Waris, M.E., Tsou, C., et al. 1996. Respiratory synctial virus infection in BALB/c mice previously immunized with formalin-inactivated virus induces enhanced pulmonary inflammatory response with a predominant Th2-like cytokine pattern. *J Virol*, **70**, 2852–60.

Welliver, R.C. 2000. Immunology of respiratory syncytial virus infection: eosinophils, cytokines, chemokines and asthma. *Pediatr Infect Dis J*, **19**, 780–3, discussion 784–85; 811–13.

Wendt, C., Weisdorf, D., et al. 1992. Parainfluenza virus respiratory infection after bone marrow transplantation. *N Engl J Med*, **326**, 921–6.

Wright, R.B., Pomerantz, W.J., et al. 2002. New approaches to respiratory infections in children. Bronchiolitis and croup. *Emerg Med Clin North Am*, **20**, 93–114.

Yao, Q., Hu, X., et al. 1997. Association of the parainfluenza virus fusion and hemagglutinin-neuraminidase glycoproteins on cell surfaces. *J Virol*, **71**, 650–6.

Zaitsev, V., von Itzstein, M., et al. 2004. Second sialic acid binding site in newcastle disease virus hemagglutinin-neuraminidase: implications for fusion. *J Virol*, **78**, 3733–41.

Zschornig, O., Arnold, K., et al. 1993. Effect of glycosaminoglycans and PEG on fusion of Sendai virus with phosphatidylserine vesicles. *Biochim Biophys Acta*, **1148**, 1–6.

37

Pneumovirus and Metapneumovirus: respiratory syncytial virus and human metapneumovirus

RALPH A. TRIPP

With the isolation of respiratory syncytial virus (RSV) in 1956, and its association with serious lower respiratory tract infection in young children, the significance of RSV as an important human pathogen was established. Recent discovery of human metapneumovirus (hMPV), a respiratory virus biologically and clinically related to RSV, has highlighted the importance of understanding the virus–host relationship between RSV and hMPV. The biology, replication, and virus and host factors that influence virus replication, immunity, and disease pathology are discussed.

HUMAN RESPIRATORY SYNCYTIAL VIRUS – THE TYPE SPECIES *PNEUMOVIRUS*

The *Paramyxoviridae* family includes numerous important human and avian respiratory tract pathogens. Human respiratory syncytial virus (HRSV) is a member of the *Pneumovirinae* subfamily and type species member of the *Pneumovirus* genus. RSV was first isolated in 1956 as the chimpanzee coryza agent (CCA) during an outbreak of respiratory illness in a chimpanzee colony (Morris et al. 1956). Shortly thereafter, RSV was isolated from an infant with bronchopneumonia, and from another infant with bronchitis (Chanock and Finberg 1957). It was named respiratory syncytial virus because of its characteristic ability to induce syncytia in cell lines. RSV is now recognized as a ubiquitous virus, and the most important cause of serious lower respiratory tract illness in infants and young children worldwide, as well as an important pathogen in the elderly, and those with compromised cardiac, pulmonary, or immune systems (Fixler 1996; Couch et al. 1997; Falsey 1998; Hall 1999; Simoes 1999; Falsey and Walsh 2000; Billings et al. 2001; CDC 2002; Staat 2002). RSV, followed by the parainfluenza viruses, is the primary cause of hospitalization for respiratory tract illness in young children. The infection rate in young children approaches 70 percent in the first year of life (Glezen and Denny 1973), and in the USA, lower respiratory tract disease develops in 20–30 percent of

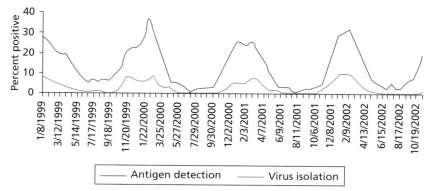

Figure 37.1 *The percent positive RSV tests in the USA from 1999 to 2002 by week of report to the National Respiratory and Enteric Virus Surveillance System. Weekly laboratory test result data are collected on a voluntary basis from reference laboratories in the USA. In the USA, RSV community outbreaks typically occur during late fall, winter, and early spring. There may be variation in the timing of outbreaks between regions and between communities in the same region.*

infected children requiring hospitalization (Shay et al. 1999). In immune compromised patients, or bone marrow or lung transplant recipients, RSV may cause respiratory failure leading to mortality rates of 70–100 percent (Hertz et al. 1989). RSV is a seasonal virus with peak rates of infection occurring annually during cold seasons in temperate climates, and in the rainy season in tropical climates. In the USA, most RSV infections occur during a period from October through March with peak activity usually in January or February (Figure 37.1). There are two major groups of RSV strains, A and B, and both strains circulate concurrently. The clinical severity of RSV infection has not been conclusively linked with infection by A or B strain. The significant public health burden mediated by RSV infection is exemplified by the dramatic infection rate in younger children, the percent of children hospitalized because of RSV-associated lower respiratory tract disease, and by the substantial mortality in the young and immune compromised. Despite four decades of efforts to unravel the complexities of RSV–host interactions, there is no effective vaccine to control RSV infection, and only limited prophylactic or therapeutic treatments. Although this work has led to a greater understanding of RSV immunobiology, significant efforts are still needed to understand the mechanisms of immunity and disease pathogenesis associated with infection, and their relationship to the newly discovered hMPV, in order to develop effective vaccines and treatments.

AVIAN PNEUMOVIRUS (APV) – THE TYPE SPECIES *METAPNEUMOVIRUS*

APV is a member of the *Pneumovirinae* subfamily, and type species member of the *Metapneumovirus* genus. In the USA, APV was first isolated in 1997 from turkeys with clinical signs of respiratory disease (Senne et al. 1997; Njenga et al. 2002). It is a ubiquitous virus that has

been isolated from fowl in Africa, Europe, and North America and South America (Njenga et al. 2002). The clinical signs of infection in turkeys include conjunctivitis, rhinitis, sinusitis, and tracheitis, which led to it initially being named *Turkey rhinotracheitis virus* (Collins and Gough 1988; Jirjis et al. 2002a). APV causes upper respiratory infection in both turkeys and chickens, and may rapidly spread through flocks via respiratory aspirate (Alkhalaf et al. 2002). Infection by APV infection is generally not associated with mortality, but is associated with high morbidity and exacerbated secondary infections, although it is possible to have infection without clinical signs (Seal 2000; Alkhalaf et al. 2002; Chary et al. 2002). Recovery usually takes place within 10–12 days. Morbidity may be 100 percent, and mortality, usually due to secondary bacterial infections, ranges from 0 to 90 percent (Alkhalaf et al. 2002; Jirjis et al. 2002a; Njenga et al. 2002). All ages of fowl are susceptible; however, APV disease is more severe in young birds. There are two strains of APV recognized, A and B, based on differences in the *G* glycoprotein of the virus (Njenga et al. 2002). Nucleotide sequence analysis of the *G* glycoprotein gene has indicated that isolates from the UK and France are similar and belong to strain A, and isolates from Spain, Italy, and Hungary are identical, and belong to strain B (Njenga et al. 2002).

CLASSIFICATION

RSV is a nonsegmented negative-strand RNA virus belonging to the family *Paramyxoviridae* (order *Mononegavirales*) which consists of two subfamilies and five genera. *Morbillivirus*, represented by *Measles virus*, *Rubulavirus*, represented by *Mumps virus* that includes parainfluenza virus 2 (PIV2), parainfluenza virus 4, *Newcastle disease virus* (NDV), and *Simian virus 5* (SV-5), *Respirovirus*, represented by *Sendai virus* that includes parainfluenza virus 1 and parainfluenza virus 3 form the subfamily *Paramyxovirinae* (Figure 37.2). The

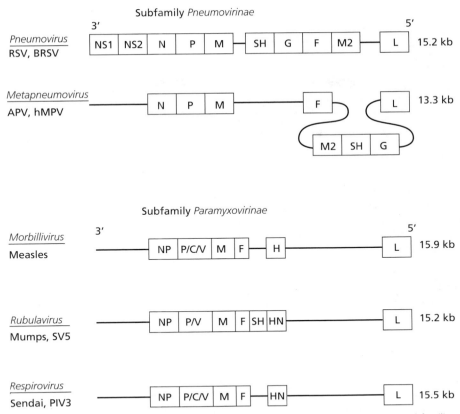

Figure 37.2 *Comparison of gene maps of members belonging to the* Pneumovirinae *and* Paramyxovirinae *subfamilies of nonsegmented negative-strand RNA viruses. The gene alignment is illustrated as genomic RNAs from 3' to 5'. Each box represents a separate encoded mRNA, and the acronyms for the encoded proteins. The box sizes and spacing are not to scale. Protein names: NS, nonstructural protein; N/NP, nucleocapsid protein; P, phosphoprotein; M, matrix protein; M2, second matrix protein; SH, small hydrophobic protein, G/HN/H, attachment protein; F, fusion protein; L, large polymerase protein; C, nonstructural protein; V, cysteine-rich protein. The* Rubulavirus *gene is indicated for mumps virus and SV-5 members; however, NDV, PIV2, and simian virus 41 do not have an SH gene.*

Pneumovirus genus, represented by RSV, includes bovine, ovine, and caprine RSV, and the *Metapneumovirus* genus is represented by APV (or *Turkey rhinotracheitis virus*) and tentatively includes hMPV, forming the subfamily *Pneumovirinae* (Figure 37.2). The *Morbillivirus*, *Rubulavirus*, and *Respirovirus* genera are highly interrelated, sharing significant amino acid homology for many proteins; however, the *Pneumovirus* genus is substantially different. The pneumoviruses have fusogenic activity (Zimmer et al. 2001), but do not hemagglutinate or have hemolytic activity (Richman et al. 1971), and neuraminidase activity is absent in both *Morbillivirus* and *Pneumovirus*. Pneumoviruses also differ from other paramyxoviruses in the diameter of the helical nucleocapsid that is 12–15 nm, rather than 18 nm (Bhella et al. 2002). In addition, pneumoviruses encode a larger number of mRNAs, but the lengths of genomic RNAs are similar to paramyxoviruses (Figure 37.2). *Pneumovirus* genome contains two nonstructural genes (*NS2, NS1*) followed by eight other genes namely, nucleocapsid (*N*), phosphoprotein (*P*), matrix (*M*), small hydrophobic (*SH*), surface attachment glycoprotein (*G*), surface fusion glycoprotein (*F*), second matrix (*M2*), and

RNA-dependent RNA polymerase (*L*) in the order 3'-*NS1–NS2–N–P–M–SH–G–F–M2–L*-5'. By contrast, the *Metapneumovirus* genome lack *NS* genes, and has a different gene order given by 3'-*N–P–M–F–M2–SH–G–L*-5'.

PNEUMOVIRUS PROTEINS

Electron microscopy (EM) and negative staining have shown that pneumovirus virions are pleomorphic, consisting of a nucleocapsid surrounded by a lipid envelope with a diameter ranging from 150 to 300 mm (Joncas et al. 1969; Norrby et al. 1970; Bachi and Howe 1973). A thin section EM of RSV particles budding from the plasma membrane of HEp-2 cells is shown in Figure 37.3. The lipid bilayer that surrounds the nucleocapsid is derived from the host-cell plasma membrane during the budding process, and contains three virally encoded surface transmembrane glycoproteins: G, F, and SH. The virion matrix proteins, M1 and M2, are non-glycosylated, and the N, P, and L proteins associate with genomic RNA to form the nucleocapsid. The NS1

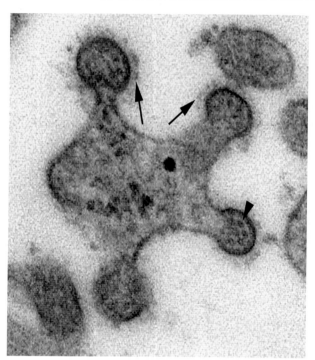

Figure 37.3 *RSV budding from the plasma membrane of HEp-2 cells. Cross-sections of the viral nucleocapsid (arrowhead) are enclosed within the viral envelope which has prominent surface projections (arrows). (Courtesy of C.S. Goldsmith, J. Hierholzer, and E.L. Palmer, Centers for Disease Control and Prevention, Atlanta, GA.)*

and NS2 proteins are not readily detectable in virions, but are found in RSV-infected cells.

The RSV genome consists of 15 222 nt that are transcribed into 11 major subgenomic mRNAs, each of which codes for a unique protein (Huang and Wertz 1982; Collins and Wertz 1983; Collins et al. 1984a, 1986; Dickens et al. 1984). The surface fusion glycoprotein (F), in combination with the surface attachment glycoprotein (G), is responsible for attachment, and the F glycoprotein is responsible for virus penetration and fusion of the viral envelope with host cell membranes and formation of syncytia. The F glycoprotein is structurally and functionally related to other paramyxoviruses (Collins et al. 1984b; Spriggs et al. 1986). It is a type I membrane glycoprotein of approximately 70 kDa that contains a cleaved N-terminal signal sequence anchored in the membrane by a C-terminal membrane anchor sequence allowing for >90 percent of the N-terminal molecule to be extracellular (Arumugham et al. 1989; Paradiso et al. 1989). The F glycoprotein is synthesized as precursor protein (F_0) in the endoplasmic reticulum consisting of a F_2 domain at amino acid positions 1–130, a cleavage site at amino acid positions 131–136, and an F_1 domain at amino acid positions 137–574. The F_0 protein precursor is cleaved by a trypsinlike protease into disulfide-linked F_1 and F_2 subunits in the trans-Golgi, constituting the biologically active form of the

molecule. The F_2 domain is modified by the addition of N-linked sugars, and the F glycoprotein is expressed as a trimer or tetramer (Collins et al. 1984b; Johnson and Collins 1988).

The G glycoprotein has a number of genetic, structural, and functional differences that are unique among the *Paramyxoviridae* viruses, and most virus attachment proteins in general (Satake et al. 1985; Wertz et al. 1985, 1989). The G glycoprotein forms from a polypeptide precursor (32 kDa) that ranges in amino acid length (292–299 amino acids) depending on the virus strain (Martinez et al. 1999; Sullender et al. 1991). The precursor is co-translationally modified by the addition of high mannose N-linked sugars to form an intermediate of 45 kDa, that is followed by addition of O-linked sugars in the trans-Golgi to achieve a mature form of approximately 90 kDa (Wertz et al. 1989; Collins and Mottet 1992). Most of the carbohydrate is of the O-linked variety, thus the G glycoprotein has high serine, threonine, and proline content (Collins 1990; Collins and Mottet 1992). The high proline content may reduce highly folded secondary structure contributing to an extended structure. The G glycoprotein is also palmitylated (Collins and Mottet 1992). The G glycoprotein is a type II glycoprotein with a single N-terminal hydrophobic region (amino acids 38–66) that serves as a signal peptide and membrane anchor (Wertz et al. 1985; Vijaya et al. 1988; Roberts et al. 1994; Lichtenstein et al. 1996). Proximal to the membrane anchor region is an extracellular ectodomain. In the middle of the ectodomain is a short protein segment and four cysteine residues (173, 176, 182, and 186) that are highly conserved in all RSV isolates (Sullender et al. 1991; Teng and Collins 2002). This region contains a CX3C chemokine motif (amino acids 182–186) that may facilitate virus attachment to cells expressing the CX3C chemokine receptor, CX3CR1 (Tripp et al. 2001). Flanking this region are two glycosylation sites that are highly divergent among all RSV isolates (Cane et al. 1991; Sullender et al. 1991). The G glycoprotein is expressed both membrane-bound and secreted by initiation of translation at an alternate in-frame AUG codon located in the middle of the hydrophobic transmembrane region (Roberts et al. 1994). Approximately 15 percent of the G glycoprotein synthesized in infected cells is secreted in a soluble form lacking the cytoplasmic domain and part of the signal-anchor sequence, but retaining the same characteristics as the membrane bound form, e.g. glycosylation and antibody reactivity (Hendricks et al. 1987, 1988).

The SH protein is a short (64 amino acids) minor surface glycoprotein with unknown function. Unpublished results from our laboratory suggest that SH expression may regulate apoptosis by inducing expression of the anti-apoptosis gene, *IEX-1L* (Domachowske et al. 2000) in RSV-infected human epithelial cells. The SH protein is membrane-anchored at a centrally located anchor sequence such that only a third of the molecule is extracellular. SH accumulates in the infected cell in different forms (Sho, SHg, SHp, SHt), but the SHo unglycosylated species is the most abundant form (Olmsted and Collins 1989; Collins et al. 1990a). All forms of SH, except for SHt, are transported to the cell surface, and only Sho and SHp are incorporated into the virion (Collins and Mottet 1993). The significance of the different forms is unknown, but conservation among human and bovine strains of RSV suggests that they may be involved in virus attachment, penetration, or viral uncoating (Collins et al. 1990a; Anderson et al. 1992), or may be important in regulating apoptosis.

RSV has three nucleocapsid-associated proteins, N, P, and L. The RNA binding protein, N, is a multifunctional protein of 391 amino acids that has a central role in transcription and replication of viral genomic RNA (Collins et al. 1984a, 1985). The phosphoprotein (P) is a key component of the viral RNA-dependent RNA polymerase complex, having two general functions as a transcription and replication factor, and as a chaperone for soluble L protein (Horikami et al. 1992). The P protein is smaller (241 amino acids) than most paramyxovirus P proteins (391–602 amino acids) and is dispensable for virus replication in vitro (Villanueva et al. 2000). However, phosphorylation of P protein is required for efficient virus replication in vitro and in vivo (Villanueva et al. 2000; Khattar et al. 2001). The large viral polymerase, L, is the least abundant of the structural proteins. The L protein is similar in length to other paramyxovirus counterparts (approximately 2 200 amino acids), but there is limited sequence homology within the paramyxoviruses (Stec et al. 1991). The N, P, and L proteins are the minimal *trans*-acting proteins required for RNA replication (Yu et al. 1995); however, RSV transcription and replication appears to lack the requirement that template length be an even multiple of an integer such as six, which is obligatory for nucleocapsid function of other paramyxoviruses, such as measles virus and Sendai virus (Samal and Collins 1996).

Unlike other negative-strand RNA viruses, pneumoviruses such as RSV have two matrix proteins, M and M2 (Collins et al. 1984a; Huang et al. 1985). The M protein is smaller (256 amino acids) than similar paramyxovirus counterparts (335–375 amino acids), and has limited sequence homology (Satake and Venkatesan 1984). The M2 protein (194 amino acids) is unique to pneumoviruses. M and M2 are nonglycosylated proteins that appear to be virion-associated. The M protein appears to functionally inactivate nucleocapsid transcription prior to packaging, and to mediate nucleocapsid association with the nascent envelope. The M2 protein appears to function as a transcription factor to increase polymerase processivity, and enhance readthrough of intergenic junctions during virus transcription (Hardy et al. 1999; Hardy and Wertz 2000). It has a Cys_3H_1 zinc-binding motif that is essential for its function, and

has been shown to interact with the N protein (Hardy and Wertz 2000).

Of the pneumovirus proteins, the function of NS1 and NS2 proteins are the least defined. NS1 and NS2 are considered nonstructural proteins as only trace amounts are detected in the virion (Huang et al. 1985; Collins et al. 1990a; Evans et al. 1996). Unique to pneumoviruses, the nonstructural proteins are encoded by separate mRNAs. NS1 and NS2 may act cooperatively to antagonize interferon (IFN)-α/β-induced antiviral responses, and NS2 protein appears to be rapidly processed and secreted (Schlender et al. 2000; Gotoh et al. 2001). Studies with recombinant RSVs with deletions in the *NS1* and *NS2* have shown that these genes are dispensable for virus replication in vitro; however, they provide auxiliary functions for efficient RSV replication in vitro and in vivo (Jin et al. 2000).

METAPNEUMOVIRUS PROTEINS

The *Metapneumovirus* genus has two members that cause respiratory disease, APV and the recently discovered hMPV (van den Hoogen et al. 2001; Stockton et al., 2002). Similar to the pneumoviruses, electron microscopy and negative staining have shown that metapneumovirus virions are pleomorphic, consisting of a nucleocapsid surrounded by a lipid envelope with a diameter ranging from 150 to 300 mm (Figure 37.4). APV has similar morphology and structural polypeptides compared with those of bovine, human, and murine pneumoviruses, but lacks the *NS* genes, making the genome shorter (13.3 kb). APV possesses a helical nucleocapsid 14 nm in diameter, and eight viral polypeptides with a gene order given by 3′-N–P–M–F–M2–SH–G–L-5′. hMPV has the same gene order.

The APV F glycoprotein consists of 538 amino acids, and the F1 and F2 subunits contain 102 residues (including the F1–F2 connecting peptide RRRR) and 436 residues, respectively. The F glycoprotein protein has approximately 40 percent amino acid identity with the F glycoprotein of RSV (*Pneumovirus* genus), but half that with members of the other two genera (*Respirovirus* and *Morbillivirus*) in the *Paramyxoviridae* family (Njenga et al. 2002). The putative hMPV F glycoprotein open reading frame encodes a 539 amino acid protein. Amino acid sequence analysis indicates 81 percent identity to group C APV, and only 10–20 percent homology with other paramyxovirus counterparts. The F1 and F2 subunits are similar to APV, and contain a conserved cleavage site (RQSR). Interestingly, a second cleavage site (RARR) occurring in RSV does not occur in metapneumoviruses. Similar to pneumoviruses, two heptad repeats (HRA and HRB) are located adjacent to the fusion peptide and transmembrane region, and are required for viral fusion.

The APV *G* gene is 1 193 nt in length and encodes a protein of 391 amino acids, which is larger than the RSV

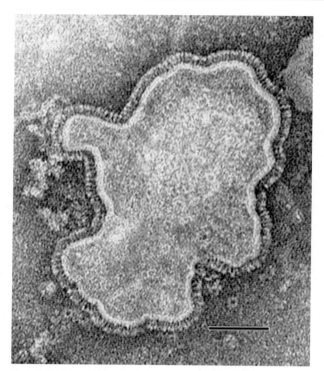

Figure 37.4 *A negative-stained electron micrograph of hMPV. This pleomorphic form of the virus is stain-penetrated, to permit visualization of portions of the virus envelope and nucleocapsid. A border composed of hMPV surface proteins occurs around the virus periphery. Bar marker represents 100 nm. (Courtesy of Charles Humphrey, Centers for Disease Control and Prevention, Atlanta, GA.)*

G glycoprotein (292–299 amino acids) (Ling et al. 1992). The APV *SH* gene is 589 nt in length, encoding a protein of 174 amino acids that is considerably larger than the RSV SH protein (64 amino acids) (Ling et al. 1992). Hydrophobicity profiles of APV SH and G glycoproteins show considerable similarity to those of the SH and G glycoproteins of RSV. The nucleotide sequences of the putative attachment protein (G glycoprotein) of APV isolates suggests that there are at least two distinct subgroups (A and B), similar to the grouping described for RSV (Juhasz and Easton 1994). Within the subgroups, there is nearly 100 percent amino acid identity; however, between the subgroups, there is considerable divergence. The hMPV *SH* gene encodes a 183 amino acid protein, which is the largest of all pneumovirus or metapneumovirus SH glycoproteins. The amino acid composition and hydrophobicity profile is similar to APV and pneumoviruses; however, hMPV SH glycoprotein contains 10 cysteine residues, compared to 16 for APV. The putative hMPV G glycoprotein open reading frame encodes a 236 amino acid protein. Several smaller open reading frames that lack start codons occur immediately following, or are in frame with, the G glycoprotein open reading frame, suggesting that additional coding sequences are expressed as separate proteins, or are expressed through RNA-editing events. The hMPV

G glycoprotein open reading frame is predicted to contain five N-linked glycosylation sites, similar to APV (Juhasz and Easton 1994; Njenga et al. 2002), but lower than RSV which has seven sites (Wertz et al. 1985). The predicted hydrophobicity profile of hMPV G glycoprotein is similar to the pneumoviruses, and the overall organization is consistent with an anchored type II transmembrane protein. However, the hMPV G glycoprotein lacks the cysteine secondary structure and CX3C chemokine motif in the G glycoprotein of pneumoviruses.

The APV nucleocapsid protein gene (*N*) comprises 1 197 nt, forming a single major open reading frame that potentially encodes a protein of 391 amino acid residues (Li et al. 1996). The predicted N protein is identical in length to human, bovine, and ovine RSV, and overall is approximately 41 percent similar, but has some regions of >90 percent identity (Njenga et al. 2002). The hMPV N protein is a 394 amino acid protein similar to APV. Amino acid sequence analysis indicates 88 percent overall identity to group C APV, but only 10 percent overall identity with other paramyxoviruses.

The APV phosphoprotein gene (*P*) comprises 855 nt containing one open reading frame encoding a protein of 278 amino acids (Ling et al. 1995). Comparison of the overall APV P protein sequence with that of the other pneumoviruses reveals amino acid identities ranging from 31 to 35 percent; however, there is much higher identity (approximately 70 percent) in a region of 57 residues that include a heptad repeat sequence. The putative hMPV P protein open reading frame encodes a 294 amino acid protein that shares 68 percent amino acid homology to group C APV. Similar to RSV and group C APV, the hMPV P protein open reading frame lacks cysteine residues.

The APV large viral polymerase gene (*L*) comprises 6 099 nt, and encodes a single major open reading frame of 2 004 amino acids (Randhawa et al. 1996). The APV L protein is the smallest described for any nonsegmented, negative-strand RNA virus. The protein contains six linear noncontiguous domains, a consensus ATP-binding site, and four polymerase motifs previously described for the L proteins of negative-strand RNA viruses. The *L* gene of hMPV encodes a 2 005 amino acid protein, and contains a consensus ATP-binding motif. Domain III in the hMPV L protein (amino acids 625–847) has 83 percent amino acid sequence identity with APV, and approximately 70 percent identity with RSV.

The APV M protein contains a hydrophobic domain common to pneumoviruses (Seal 1998). The M protein nucleotide sequence of group A strains is approximately 75 percent similar to group B strains (Seal 2000). The APV *M2* gene contains two overlapping open reading frames that encode the M2-1 protein of 184–186 and 71–73 amino acids that do not show any similarity to the equivalent RSV protein. The sequences of the intergenic regions of APV reveal the gene order to be 3′–*M*–*F*–*M2*–5′, compared to the 3′-*M–SH–G–F–M2*-5′ gene order of pneumoviruses. Determination of the nucleotide sequences in APV has established that *NS1* and *NS2* genes are absent in APV. The hMPV *M* gene, like APV, has two overlapping open reading frames, the first of which encodes a 187 amino acid M2-1 protein having 84 percent sequence identity to group C APV, the second of 71 amino acids. The hMPV M2-1 protein has three cysteine residues located within the first 30 amino acid residues conserved among all pneumoviruses, suggesting the possibility of a zinc-binding protein. Amino acid sequence comparison of the M2-2 open reading frame indicates approximately 60 percent identity to group C APV.

POLYMORPHISMS AMONG PNEUMOVIRUS AND METAPNEUMOVIRUS

The genomic organization of pneumoviruses and metapneumovirus are comparable, but there are distinct variations. Pneumovirus genomes (15.2 kb) contain two nonstructural genes (*NS1* and *NS2*), followed by the nucleocapsid (*N*), phosphoprotein (*P*), matrix (*M*), small hydrophobic (*SH*), surface glycoprotein (*G*), fusion (*F*), second matrix (*M2*), and large RNA-dependent, RNA polymerase (*L*) genes. By contrast, metapneumovirus genomes are smaller (13.4 kb), lack *NS1* and *NS2* genes, and the gene order is 3′-*N–P–MF–M2–SH–G–L*-5′. Genetic and antigenic polymorphisms are well documented for pneumoviruses such as RSV, where the *SH* and *G* genes have been shown to have the greatest diversity among strains (Sullender et al. 1990, 1991, 1998; Mlinaric-Galinovic et al. 1994; Zheng et al. 1999). For RSV A and B strains, there is approximately 25 percent antigenic relatedness overall, with F glycoproteins approximately 50 percent related and G glycoproteins approximately 1–10 percent related (Johnson et al. 1987a; Hendry et al. 1988). Divergence in the G glycoprotein is greatest in the ectodomain and related to poorly conserved *N*- and *O*-linked sugar acceptor sites (Johnson et al. 1987b; Sullender et al. 1991). A high percentage of nucleotide sequence differences occur in the G glycoprotein for A and B strains, for which nearly half encode amino acid substitutions (Cane et al. 1991; Sullender et al. 1991). It is possible that G glycoprotein diversity among RSV strains provides an advantage to the virus to evade previously induced immunity in the population. Sequence information indicates that multiple genotypes circulate simultaneously in the same community, and similar genotypes circulate in widely separated communities during different years (Peret et al. 1998, 2000). Immune pressure may contribute to diversity in the G glycoprotein, since it is one of the two major neutralizing antigens (the other the F glycoprotein), the ectodomain is extracellular, and sequence diversity is correlated with antigenic diversity.

Metapneumoviruses such as APV appear to have similar genetic and antigenic polymorphisms as the pneumoviruses. Comparison of the nucleotide and amino acid sequences of APV isolates indicate that the G glycoprotein is extremely variable between strains (38 percent nucleotide identity and 56 percent amino acid predicted sequence identity), but there is high nucleotide sequence identity (>99 percent) among strains (Bayon-Auboyer et al. 2000; Seal 2000; Njenga et al. 2002). APV strains also vary in patterns of neutralization by monoclonal antibodies reactive to the G glycoprotein (Njenga et al. 2002). Similar to RSV, the F glycoprotein and M protein of APV have extensive nucleotide and amino acid sequence identity within strains, but lower identity between strains (Naylor et al. 1998; Seal 2000; Seal et al. 2000). Sequence comparison between hMPV and APV shows high levels of nucleotide identity, and absence of *NS1* and *NS2* genes. Partial N, M, F, and L sequence comparison of hMPV isolates indicates that hMPV has two strains or clusters with 90–100 percent nucleotide identity within strains, and 80–90 percent identity between strains. Comparison of the four strains of APV to hMPV indicates 56–88 percent amino acid sequence identity within the nine open reading frames, and comparison of N, P, M, F, and M2 proteins indicated 80 percent overall amino acid identity. The APV *G* gene sequence is currently unavailable, but partial sequence information (personal communication) suggests that it has low sequence identity to hMPV.

VIRUS REPLICATION

Virions primarily attach to cells through the G glycoprotein. Attachment appears to be principally mediated by interaction of heparin-binding domains on the G glycoprotein with cell surface glycosaminoglycans (Krusat and Streckert 1997; Bourgeois et al. 1998; Feldman et al. 1999). However, recent evidence indicates that a CX3C chemokine motif located in the conserved region of the G glycoprotein (amino acids 182–186) may facilitate attachment through interaction with the CX3C chemokine receptor, CX3CR1 (Tripp et al. 2001), although this region is not required for attachment (Teng and Collins 2002). The G glycoprotein itself is not required for virion attachment to cells. Mutant RSV lacking *SH* and/or *G* genes have been shown to infect cells, likely through interaction with the F glycoprotein (Karron et al. 1997a; Teng et al. 2001; Techaarpornkul et al. 2002). Pneumoviruses penetrate cells by fusion with the plasma membrane, a process associated with the F glycoprotein (Bachi 1988). Penetration involves incorporation of the viral envelope into the cell membrane, and nucleocapsid release into the cytoplasm (Levine and Hamilton 1969; Hierholzer and Tannock 1986; Routledge et al. 1987; Arslanagic et al. 1996). The L protein initiates viral transcription and replication proceeds in the cytoplasm without nuclear involvement (Fearns and Collins 1999).

Transcription of pneumovirus mRNAs occurs in a 3′ to 5′ order from a single promoter near the 3′ end. Polymerase-mediated transcription results in a series of subgenomic mRNAs that are co-linear copies of the genes with no evidence of mRNA editing or splicing (Dickens et al. 1984; Huang et al. 1985; Kuo et al. 1996; Harmon et al. 2001; Krempl et al. 2002). Sequence and transcriptional mapping analysis of RSV mRNAs indicates that each transcript begins at the first nucleotide of the gene-start signal, is capped at the 5′ end, and polyadenylated at the 3′ end. Both mRNAs and proteins can be detected by 4 hours post-infection with peak mRNA synthesis and protein expression occurring 16–20 hours post-infection. The level of protein expressed is related to mRNA abundance (Dickens et al. 1984). In general, there is decreasing amounts of mRNAs with increasing gene distance from promoter sequence. RNA replication is dependent on active protein synthesis.

VIRUS ASSEMBLY

Virions assemble at the plasma membrane. Inclusion bodies containing viral ribonucleoprotein cores appear immediately below the plasma membrane. Nucleocapsids localize with cell membrane containing membrane viral glycoproteins. Virions mature in clusters at the apical surface in a filamentous form associated with caveolin-1, and extend from the plasma membrane (Brown et al. 2002). Experiments using human primary airway epithelial cell cultures have shown that ciliated epithelial cells are targeted by RSV, and that infection and shedding occurs via the apical membrane, and virus may be spread to neighboring ciliated cells by the motion of the cilia (Zhang et al. 2002).

INFECTION AND EXPERIMENTAL ANIMAL MODELS

Pneumoviruses and metapneumoviruses generally infect the superficial layers of the respiratory epithelium, but can grow in a wide variety of mammalian cells. There appear to be few differences in susceptibility to infection for most epithelial cell types, but significant differences in virus replication. For example, human nasal epithelial cell cultures, human bronchial epithelial cell cultures, and a human bronchoepithelial cell line (BEAS-2B) are equally susceptible to RSV infection; however, bronchial cells release less infectious virions than nasal cells (Becker et al. 1992), and RSV replicates better in ciliated epithelial cells compared to non-ciliated epithelial cells (Henderson et al. 1978; Zhang et al. 2002). In addition, a human epithelial cell line, HEp-2, and an African green monkey cell line, Vero, are commonly used to propagate pneumoviruses; however, only Vero cells effectively support metapneumovirus propagation (van den Hoogen et al. 2001). APV has been successfully isolated from infected turkeys using day-old chicken or turkey embryos, and chicken embryo fibroblasts and Vero cells support virus replication (Yachida et al. 1978; Goyal et al. 2000; Jirjis et al. 2002b; Patnayak et al. 2002).

Viral infection of susceptible cell lines results in a majority of cell-associated virions. A large fraction of the cell-associated virions are aggregated, and many virions released from the infected cell are defective and non-infectious (Levine and Hamilton 1969; Bachi 1988). Both pneumoviruses and metapneumoviruses are rather unstable, and rapidly lose infectivity during storage at −70°C, during handling, and during purification procedures. Freezing virus stocks in media containing 50 mM HEPES and 100 mM magnesium sulfate tends to stabilize the virions. Plaque assays can be used to readily quantify pneumoviruses; however, metapneumoviruses do not mediate quantifiable cytopathology or plaque formation (van den Hoogen et al. 2001). This limitation can be overcome by acetone fixation of infected cells and immunostaining to quantitate infected cells.

For pneumoviruses, a variety of experimental animals may be useful for experimental evaluation of infection or disease pathogenesis; however, there is great variation in permissiveness to infection. For RSV, the only experimental animal that approaches human permissiveness to infection and disease is the chimpanzee (Belshe et al. 1977; Collins et al. 1990b). Since this animal model is limited, the majority of RSV studies have focused on mice and cotton rats, which are semipermissive for RSV replication, but fail to fully emulate RSV disease associated in humans (Byrd and Prince 1997). BALB/c mice are the most commonly used experimental animal model for RSV infection, and much has been learned from its use; however, they appear less permissive to RSV infection than cotton rats (Prince et al. 1978, 1979, 1986). Histopathological studies of RSV disease in cotton rats has shown to better emulate the human condition than similar studies in mice. The choices for experimental animal models of metapneumovirus infection are less diverse. hMPV appears to be primarily a human pathogen; however, recent studies from our laboratory have shown that hMPV can infect and replicate in BALB/c mice, and there is strong preliminary evidence that cotton rats are also susceptible to infection (personal communication). APV is a pathogen of a variety of birds including turkeys, ducks, pheasants, and ostriches causing rhinotracheitis, and possibly a pathogen of chickens associated with swollen head syndrome (Cook 2000; Catelli et al. 2001; Shin et al. 2001).

DISEASE PATHOGENESIS

RSV is the leading cause of severe lower respiratory tract infection in infants and young children worldwide (Simoes 1999; Hall 2001; Krilov 2001; Law et al. 2002; McNamara and Smyth 2002; Weisman 2002), and may lead to a wide spectrum of respiratory illnesses. RSV infection is most common during infancy and early childhood (CDC 2000), but may also occur in adults, the immune compromised, and the elderly (Englund et al. 1991; Couch et al. 1997; Hall 1999; Han et al. 1999; Simoes 1999; Falsey and Walsh 2000). In infants, 25–40 percent of infections result in lower respiratory tract involvement, including pneumonia and bronchiolitis (Shay et al. 1999; Hall 2001). Viral replication initiates in the upper respiratory tract; however, it can spread to the lower airways by aspiration of secretions or via the respiratory epithelium involving the bronchi, bronchioles, and alveoli, and may continue to macrophages and monocytes (Domurat et al. 1985; Midulla et al. 1989; Becker et al. 1992). Infection is associated with necrosis of the bronchiolar epithelium, destruction of the ciliated epithelial cells, and a peribronchiolar infiltrate of lymphocytes and mononuclear cells (Price 1990; Lugo and Nahata 1993). Interalveolar thickening and filling of alveolar spaces with fluid released from edematous submucosal and advential tissues may lead to airways obstruction (Price 1990; Panitch et al. 1993). The characteristics of the immune response to RSV are not fully elucidated, and it is possible that damage of the epithelium and the bronchiolar ciliary cells may be associated with the host immune response, particularly RSV-specific $CD8^+$ cytotoxic T cells (CTL) (Garofalo et al. 1996).

RSV illness frequently begins with rhinorrhea and low-grade fever that is often accompanied by cough and wheezing (Price 1990; Lugo and Nahata 1993). At the beginning of illness, RSV replicates in the nasopharynx, reaching titers between 10^4 and 10^6 $TCID_{50}$/ml of nasal secretion in infants (Hall et al. 1975, 1976; Hall 1977). The titer deceases over time, and most patients recover within 1–2 weeks post-infection. Some infants continue to shed virus for 3 weeks after hospitalization, and disease severity may correlate with the duration of virus shedding (Hall et al. 1976). Approximately 60 percent of primary RSV infections are confined to the upper airways; however, during a period of 2–5 days, infection may progress to lower respiratory tract involvement. The mechanism for viral spread to the lower airways is not known, but may occur by epithelial ciliary action, or through aspirated secretions; however, RSV can spread cell to cell without emerging into the extracellular space. Severe disease generally involves lower respiratory tract infection, and physical examination may reveal otitis media, rales, and diffuse wheezing (Anderson 2000; Greenberg 2001; Panitch 2001; West 2002). The severity of the disease is directly related to the age of the patient. Infants under 6 months of age are the most severely affected, likely due to smaller, more easily obstructed airways and decreased ability to clear secretions. Illness may be particularly severe in premature infants, and in those with congenital cardiac or pulmonary disease (Krilov 2001; Shay et al. 2001; Aujard

and Fauroux 2002; Law et al. 2002). Apnea occurs in approximately 20 percent of infants hospitalized with RSV bronchiolitis (Bruhn et al. 1977; Church et al. 1984). The frequency of apnea increases significantly in premature infants, occurring early in the course of RSV disease. Apnea rarely lasts more than a few days, but about 10 percent of these patients require intubation and mechanical ventilation. The mechanisms that contribute to apnea are not well understood, but recent studies in mice suggest a link between RSV G glycoprotein binding to the CX3C chemokine receptor, CX3CR1, induction of the tachykinin, substance P, and subsequent depression of respiratory rates (Tripp et al. 2003).

In adults, the most common symptoms of RSV infection are those of the common cold which include rhinorrhea, sore throat, and cough. In the elderly, RSV may cause significant lower respiratory tract disease including pneumonia and some mortality (Han et al. 1999; Falsey and Walsh 2000). RSV is also a significant cause of morbidity and mortality in patients undergoing bone marrow or organ transplantation (Wendt 1997; Billings et al. 2002; Ison and Hayden 2002; Small et al. 2002). RSV reinfections occur frequently and are often associated with illness (Henderson et al. 1979); however, the cumulative effect of multiple re-infections appears to temper subsequent disease, an effect that is likely related to developing immunity. The severe disease observed in immune compromised or suppressed patients, and in experimental animal models, indicates that cell-mediated immunity is an important mechanism of host defense against RSV (Fishaut et al. 1980; Graham et al. 1991).

DIAGNOSIS

Parainfluenza viruses and bacteria that can cause respiratory tract illness complicate the diagnosis of RSV infection in infants less than 6 months of age. Presumptive diagnosis of RSV infection in young children can be made on the epidemiologic setting that includes seasonality and community outbreaks of diagnosed RSV infection. The specific diagnosis is established by isolation of RSV from respiratory secretions, including sputum, throat swabs, or nasopharyngeal washes. Infections in older children and adults cannot be differentiated with certainty from those caused by other respiratory viruses. Examining increases in titer of neutralizing serum antibodies may aid diagnosis of RSV infection in older children and adults; however, serological tests depend on fourfold or greater rises in complement-fixing or neutralizing antibody titers for useful diagnosis, and are less sensitive in children under 4 months of age (Richardson et al. 1978; Brandenburg et al. 1997). In addition, serological diagnosis requires comparison of acute and convalescent phase serum specimens, and is therefore not useful during acute illness. Virus obtained through sputum, throat swabs, or nasopharyngeal washes can be detected by tissue culture and immunostaining, by immunofluorescence, ELISA, or other techniques including detection of nucleic acid by reverse-transcriptase polymerase chain reaction (RT-PCR) (Paton et al. 1992; Falsey et al. 2002; Coiras et al. 2003).

MANAGEMENT AND TREATMENT

Infection with RSV is usually self-limiting, but may require supportive care including administration of oxygen, intravenous hydration, and intubation. Bronchodilators may be used if wheezing is part of the clinical presentation. Inhaled salbutamol may have some beneficial effects as a bronchodilator in moderate bronchiolitis (Kellner et al. 1996); however, racemic epinephrine appears to substantially improve airway resistance and clinical scores (Sanchez et al. 1993). Steroids, which are effective for alleviating wheezing in asthma, appear to have limited beneficial effect in RSV bronchiolitis (Roosevelt et al. 1996; De Boeck et al. 1997). The only specific antiviral drug licensed for RSV treatment is ribavirin. Ribavirin, a guanosine analogue, has antiviral activity in tissue culture and cotton rats (Hruska et al. 1982), but its effectiveness in decreasing the severity of clinical symptoms in young patients is questionable. When delivered as a continuous aerosol, ribavirin appears to have modest effects on the duration of virus shedding (Hall et al. 1983, 1985; Taber et al. 1983), but its use is now recommended only for immune compromised patients and those who are severely ill.

To prevent or reduce severe lower respiratory tract infection by RSV, prophylactic or therapeutic treatment with purified human intravenous immunoglobulin (Ig)G, RSV-IVIG (RespiGAM℠), or humanized anti-F glycoprotein monoclonal antibody, palivizumab (Synagis℠) has been investigated. RespiGAM℠, given parentally (2 g/kg/day) to infants and young children with RSV bronchiolitis or pneumonia was shown to reduce the amount of RSV shed; however, the mean duration of hospitalization was not affected by treatment (Hemming et al. 1987). However, RespiGAM℠ given monthly by intravenous infusion has been shown to reduce RSV-associated hospitalization by approximately 40 percent, and significantly reduced the severity of symptoms in high-risk patients who acquired RSV (Groothuis et al. 1993; Simoes et al. 1998). Synagis℠ exhibits neutralizing activity and, like RespiGAM℠, if administered monthly (15 mg/kg) has been shown to reduce RSV-associated hospitalization by approximately 55 percent (CDC 1998). Since monthly treatment with RespiGAM℠ or Synagis℠ appears necessary to reduce RSV-associated hospitalization, other agents that may be used in conjunction with these treatments to ameliorate RSV-associated disease are being investigated. Recent studies examining prophylactic or therapeutic treatment of RSV-infected BALB/c mice with neutralizing anti-F glycoprotein and anti-substance P monoclonal antibodies

have shown that prophylactic or therapeutic treatment with anti-substance P antibodies promptly reduces pulmonary inflammation, while anti-F antibody treatment reduces the virus load (Haynes et al. 2002), suggesting that combined antiviral and anti-inflammatory (substance P) antibody treatment may be effective in treating RSV disease in humans.

Small molecule inhibitors of RSV infection or replication have received some attention, particularly drugs that target the fusion process. Some peptide fusion inhibitors have been designed to interfere with heptad repeat domains in the F glycoprotein and disrupt their interaction, required during conformational rearrangement of the F glycoprotein that occurs in the later stages of the fusion process (Shigeta 2000; De Clercq 2002). A small-molecule inhibitor of RSV fusion is a peptide comprising amino acids 77–95 of RhoA (Pastey et al. 1999, 2000). RhoA is a small GTP-binding protein that has been shown to mediate virus-induced syncytium formation (Pastey et al. 1999, 2000; Gower et al. 2001). In studies of mice, in vivo administration of the RhoA peptide was shown to be effective in decreasing RSV titers if given at the time of infection; however, treatment at 4 days post-RSV infection was less effective at reducing viral titers, and did not alter the degree of pathogenesis when compared to mice treated with phosphate-buffered saline (PBS) alone. A similar picture has emerged for a variety of other small-molecule inhibitors that appear to be effective at inhibiting RSV infection in vitro, but their solubility, bioavailability, and effectiveness in vivo remains to be elucidated.

VACCINE DEVELOPMENT

RSV infection may cause severe lower respiratory tract infections early and late in life, and repeat infections with the same, or different strains of RSV are common. These indications suggest a lack of durable immunity. For an RSV vaccine to be effective, it must confer protection better than that associated with natural RSV infection, and for infants, must do so in the first weeks of life. These obstacles may require different vaccines and vaccination strategies. Early attempts to develop a safe and effective RSV vaccine failed. A formalin-inactivated, alum-precipitated RSV (FI-RSV) vaccine preparation that was administered intramuscularly to young children in an RSV vaccine trial in 1969 was not protective and when vaccinated children were subsequently exposed to natural RSV infection, they developed enhanced pulmonary disease with several fatalities (Kapikian et al. 1969; Kim et al. 1969). The enhanced pulmonary disease has been attributed to altered immunity to the FI-RSV vaccine; however, the exact mechanism is not completely understood. Recent studies from our laboratory examining FI-RSV-enhanced disease have shown that the absence of the G glycoprotein or G glycoprotein CX3C motif during FI-RSV vaccination or RSV challenge of FI-RSV-vaccinated mice, or treatment with anti-substance P or anti-CX3CR1 antibodies, reduces or eliminates enhanced pulmonary disease, modifies T-cell receptor (TCR) Vβ usage, and alters CC and CXC chemokine expression by pulmonary leukocytes (Haynes et al. 2003). These results suggest that the G glycoprotein, and in particular the G glycoprotein CX3C motif, may be key in the enhanced inflammatory response to FI-RSV vaccination, possibly through the induction of substance P.

The disastrous results associated with FI-RSV vaccination were unexpected since natural RSV infection induces a protective although incomplete immune response to infection. Thus, RSV vaccine efforts have been focused on development of attenuated vaccines. Development of temperature-sensitive or cold-passaged vaccine candidates and subsequent examination in adults indicated some effectiveness, but the attenuated vaccine candidates proved too unstable or virulent in children, and often reverted back to wild-type virus (Pringle et al. 1993; Karron et al. 1997b; Crowe et al. 1999; Gonzalez et al. 2000; Wright et al. 2000; Crowe 2001b; Krilov 2001). Clinical trials with candidate subunit vaccines have been explored. A series of trial studies examined the effectiveness of a full-length F glycoprotein vaccine (PFP) purified from RSV-infected cells (Paradiso et al. 1994; Tristram et al. 1994; Falsey and Walsh 1996; Dudas and Karron 1998; Groothuis et al. 1998; Gonzalez et al. 2000). An indication from the studies suggested that PFP was safe, but was only moderately immunogenic. A different series of clinical trials examined the effectiveness of a recombinant protein (BBG2Na) consisting of amino acids 13–230 of the RSV G glycoprotein fused to the C-terminal domain of streptococcal G protein (Libon et al. 1999; Kneyber et al. 2000; Goetsch et al. 2001; Power et al. 2001). These studies showed that BBG2Na was moderately immunogenic in adults, but did not offer significant protection. Investigation of other candidate subunit vaccines is proceeding, including development of DNA vaccines. Effective subunit vaccines may be useful in RSV seropositive groups at high risk, or immunizing pregnant women to enhance protection of their newborns (Crowe 2001b; Kneyber and Kimpen 2002).

Reverse genetics employing full-length RSV complementary DNA to produce transcripts of infectious RNA offers many advantages in RSV vaccine design. The entire RSV genome can be precisely manipulated to offer optimal immunogenicity and attenuation. Reverse genetics has been used to delete nonessential genes in the RSV genome with the hope of restricting replication in vivo, but not in vitro, thus permitting efficient vaccine production (Collins and Murphy 2002). Studies with recombinant RSV have shown that five RSV genes, *NS1*, *NS2*, *SH*, *G*, and *M1/M2* can be deleted or silenced individually, or in certain combinations, without dramatically altering viral replication in vitro (Collins and

Murphy 2002). Attenuation studies in chimpanzees have shown that recombinant RSV lacking the *SH* gene is least attenuated, whereas recombinant RSV lacking the *M2* gene is most attenuated (Teng et al. 2000). Attenuation of RSV vaccine candidates may also be achieved by taking advantage of the natural host restriction of RSV (Buchholz et al. 2000). Bovine RSV is over-attenuated and poorly immunogenic in seronegative chimpanzees (Buchholz et al. 2000); however, bovine RSV replication and immunogenicity can be improved by replacing the *F* and *G* genes with human RSV *F* and *G* genes (Schmidt et al. 2002). Strategies that focus on systemic replacement or deletion of RSV or bovine RSV genes in chimeric recombinant RSV are anticipated to yield useful vaccine candidates. Another advantage of recombinant RSV is the ability to alter or silence regions that may be associated with altered immunity or pathogenesis. For example, the RSV G glycoprotein has been shown to contain a CX3C chemokine motif (amino acids 182–186) that can bind to the CX3C chemokine receptor, CX3CR1, and mediate leukocyte chemotaxis in a fashion similar to fractalkine (Tripp et al. 2001). Recent studies from this laboratory suggest that the G glycoprotein, and in particular the G glycoprotein CX3C motif, is key in the enhanced inflammatory response to FI-RSV vaccination, possibly through the induction of substance P (Haynes et al. 2003). Therefore, ablation of this region may enhance the efficacy of recombinant RSV vaccine candidates.

IMMUNOLOGY AND HOST FACTORS

Innate immunity is the first line of defense providing early resistance to virus infection through a variety of host components. For respiratory viruses, innate immunity may be first mediated by mucus secreted by the membranes lining respiratory tract. Mucus acts as a protective barrier to block the adherence of respiratory viruses to epithelial cells, and ciliary movement, coughing, and sneezing removes virus particles trapped within mucus. In addition, a family of proteins called collectins has the ability to recognize foreign carbohydrate patterns, interact with phagocytic cells, and induce opsinization of the particles containing foreign carbohydrates (Lu et al. 2002; Shepherd 2002). The collectins, especially mannose-binding protein, and alveolar surfactant molecules SP-A and SP-D, are important agents in innate immunity (McCormack and Whitsett 2002), and SP-A is important in innate immunity to RSV infection (LeVine et al. 1999). SP-A binds to the RSV F glycoprotein, but not to the G glycoprotein, and neutralizes RSV infection in a calcium-dependent fashion (Ghildyal et al. 1999). If viruses penetrate to the respiratory epithelium, destructive soluble factors including enzymes and cytokines are released by the infected cells, or by resident phagocytic cells. Infected epithelial cells and alveolar macrophages release chemokines and pro-inflammatory cytokines that include tumor necrosis factor (TNF)-α, interleukin (IL)-1, IL-6, and CC and CXC chemokines (Becker et al. 1991; Arnold et al. 1995; Saito et al. 1997; Zhang et al. 2001). Expression of these soluble mediators of immunity contributes to airway inflammation, immune cell trafficking, bronchial hyperresponsiveness, and exacerbates mucus production. The CC chemokines, such as the macrophage inflammatory proteins (MIP), regulation on activation, normal T-cell expressed and secreted (RANTES), and eotaxin recruit a variety of granular cells to the site of infection or inflammation (Saito et al. 1997; Olszewska-Pazdrak et al. 1998). RANTES, eotaxin, and MIP-1α are potent chemokines for eosinophils and increased levels, or mRNA, in airway secretions or peripheral blood leukocytes have been found in infants with RSV bronchiolitis (Hornsleth et al. 2001; Noah et al. 2002; Smyth et al. 2002; Tripp et al. 2002). The CXC chemokine IL-8, a potent chemoattractant of neutrophils, has been found in secretions of RSV-infected children (Sheeran et al. 1999; Noah et al. 2002; Smyth et al. 2002), and experimentally infected adults (Noah and Becker 2000). Eosinophils are part of the nonspecific innate immune response and participate in inflammatory reactions. They contain cationic molecules that are useful for destroying infectious agents, especially helminths. Neutrophils are nondividing, short-lived cells containing primary azurophilic granules and secondary granules. The primary azurophilic granules contain myeloperoxidase together with other antimicrobial agents including defensins and cathepsin G. The secondary granules contain lactoferrin and other enzymes. Alveolar macrophages and dendritic cells are long-lived, tissue-resident cells that have an important role in phagocytosis and antigen presentation to the T-cell compartment. In this role they recognize and remove virally infected epithelial cells and debris, and present viral antigen to T cells, thereby initiating the adaptive immune response. Contact with virally infected cells, and the process of phagocytosis, activates macrophages and dendritic cells to secrete soluble mediators including interferons, lysozyme, and other factors that inhibit viral replication and upregulate the inflammatory response (Krilov et al. 1987; Lewis et al. 1989; Tsutsumi et al. 1996). Recognition of pathogens by phagocytic cells is achieved by pattern recognition receptors encoded in the germline (Hallman et al. 2001; Armant and Fenton 2002). The pattern recognition receptors (PRR) have broad specificity and recognize pathogen-associated molecular patterns (PAMP) that differ from pathogen to pathogen, but are not found in the host (Underhill and Ozinsky 2002). Thus, PAMPs are perceived as molecular signatures of infection by PRRs, resulting in activation of innate and adaptive immune responses (Barton and Medzhitov 2002; Sabroe et al. 2002). There are two major groups of PRRs – those that are secreted in the blood and lymph, and those on the surface of cells. Secreted PRRs include

components of the complement fixation pathway, e.g. C2, C3, and C4, and cell-surface PRRs include the Toll-like receptors (TLR) (Akira et al. 2001). There are 10 known TLRs, and three other candidate molecules, that specialize in recognition of different PAMPs. For example, TLR2 generally recognizes peptidoglycan of gram-positive bacteria, while TLR4 generally recognizes lipopolysaccharide in the outer membrane of gram-negative bacteria (Akira et al. 2001). Interestingly, the RSV F glycoprotein has been shown to stimulate innate immunity through activation of the shared components of CD14 and TLR4 (Kurt-Jones et al. 2000), and TLR4 appears to be important in the innate immune response to RSV infection (Haynes et al. 2001). TLR4-deficient mice challenged with RSV exhibit impaired natural killer (NK) cell and CD14$^+$-cell pulmonary trafficking, deficient NK-cell function, impaired IL-12 expression and impaired virus clearance. Activation of TLRs on phagocytic cells can trigger adaptive immune responses by up-regulation of T-cell co-stimulatory molecules and cytokines required for T-cell activation. In this role, phagocytic cells, particularly dendritic cells, have a key role in coupling innate and adaptive immune responses.

The adaptive immune response includes humoral and cell-mediated immunity. Antibodies located in the serum, lymphatics, and in secretory pathways mediate humoral immunity. There are five different classes of antibodies or immunoglobulins (Ig) known as IgD, IgA, IgM, IgE, and IgG, four subclasses of IgG, and two subclasses of IgA. Soluble antibodies and those on the surface of B cells recognize antigens in the native form. Resistance to respiratory virus infection in the upper airways is mediated by local, secretory IgA, and is transitory. More durable humoral resistance to infection seems to be associated with IgM, and especially IgG antibodies. In the newborn, passively acquired maternal IgG antibodies provide some protection from infection, a factor that may contribute to the reason why children under 8 weeks of age are rarely infected with RSV (Crowe 2001a). Maternal antibody levels diminish during the first 6 months of life (Brandenburg et al. 1997), leaving infants unprotected against RSV infection; however, serum and secretory antibodies appear within days of a primary RSV infection (McIntosh et al. 1978; Welliver et al. 1980). The serum and secretory antibody titers produced in infants are significantly lower than those of older subjects (Murphy et al. 1986a; de Sierra et al. 1993), and wane several months after primary infection of infants (Welliver et al. 1980). The diminished serum and neutralizing antibody response has been attributed to suppressive effects of maternally transferred antibodies (Crowe 2001a; Wright et al. 2002); however, immunological immaturity may also be important. Post-infection, serum antibody levels generally wane; however, higher levels are maintained over a longer period after repeated RSV infection (Murphy et al. 1986b; Wagner et al. 1989). As the infant matures, the presence of neutralizing IgA in respiratory secretions produced by local mucosal B cells may become more important. Studies of experimentally induced RSV disease in healthy adult volunteers indicate that the presence of nasal IgA neutralizing antibody correlates more closely with protection than does the presence of serum antibody (Mills et al. 1971). Complement is an important component of innate immunity and the humoral response to RSV infection. RSV-infected epithelial cells can activate complement by both the classical and alternative complement pathways (Edwards et al. 1986; Smith et al. 1981), and complement is important for enhanced antibody-mediated virus neutralization.

Cell-mediated immunity to respiratory virus infection involves $CD8^+$ CTLs, $CD4^+$ helper T cells, and innate immune cells, e.g. NK cells. The role of cell-mediated immunity in virus clearance is difficult to assess in humans; however, studies in patients with deficiencies in cellular immunity have shown that cellular immunity has a pivotal role in protection from severe RSV disease and limiting virus shedding (Fishaut et al. 1980; Chandwani et al. 1990). In vitro studies of human peripheral blood mononuclear cells (PBMC) have shown that NK cells and $CD4^+$ and $CD8^+$ T cells have potent antiviral responses. Exposure of adult PBMC to RSV immediately up-regulates NK activity, a feature dependent upon IL-15 induction (Fawaz et al. 1999). Infants hospitalized because of RSV infection have increased numbers of $CD16^+/CD56^+$ NK cells, and express T-helper-1 (Th1) and T-helper-2 (Th2) cytokines, and enhanced CC chemokine messenger RNA (Tripp et al. 2002). Antibody-dependent cellular cytotoxicity (ADCC), a feature associated with NK cells has been detected in human PBMC from RSV-infected individuals using serum antibodies and antibodies from nasopharyngeal secretions (Scott et al. 1977; Meguro et al. 1979; Cranage et al. 1981; Kaul et al. 1982). RSV-specific CTL responses in PBMC from infants with acute RSV infection can be detected rapidly after infection (Isaacs et al. 1987; Chiba et al. 1989). The response is age-dependent, as >65 percent of infants 6–24 months of age, and approximately 35 percent of infants under 5 months of age exhibit RSV-specific cellular cytotoxicity. Examination of the CTL repertoire of adults to RSV proteins showed that N, SH, F, M, M2 and NS2 proteins are targeted by CTLs with no predilection toward a particular major histocompatibility complex (MHC) phenotype (Bangham et al. 1986; Cherrie et al. 1992). Most data concerning RSV-specific $CD4^+$ or $CD8^+$ T-cell responses are derived from experimental animal studies, as it is difficult to assess responses in the lungs of infected patients, particularly infants and young children. Examining alterations of $CD4^+$ or $CD8^+$ T-cell responses in PBMC may be useful as a correlate of immune status; however, studies that examine bronchial lavage cells from infants infected with RSV may provide better information. For example, a study that examined bronchial lavage cells from infants infected with RSV identified large numbers of neutrophils in the upper airway (93 percent) and lower airway (76 percent), but few $CD4^+$ and $CD8^+$ T cells with median $CD4^+/CD8^+$ ratios being 22:1 in the upper airway, and 15:1 for the lower and upper airways (Everard et al. 1994). These results suggest that neutrophils probably have a major role in immunity and possibly RSV disease, and counter the hypothesis that excessive lymphocyte cytotoxicity is associated with RSV bronchiolitis.

The role of $CD4^+$ and $CD8^+$ T lymphocytes in terminating RSV infection, causing disease, and protecting from re-infection have been investigated using experimental animal models, particularly BALB/c mice. In BALB/c mice, the M2, F, and N proteins are the major targets for CTLs (Nicholas et al. 1990; Openshaw et al. 1990; Openshaw 1995b). Both $CD4^+$ and $CD8^+$ T-cell subsets have been shown to be involved in terminating RSV replication, as antibody depletion of both T-lymphocyte subsets markedly prolongs RSV replication (Graham et al. 1991). In addition, both $CD4^+$ and $CD8^+$ T cells have been shown to contribute to immunity and disease pathogenesis, although $CD8^+$ T cells appeared to have a dominant role in controlling RSV disease (Varga and Braciale 2002). Investigation of the RSV proteins associated with host resistance has shown that sensitization with F or G glycoproteins induces almost complete resistance to RSV challenge despite depletion of both $CD4^+$ and $CD8^+$ T cells prior to challenge, indicating that host resistance is mediated by the humoral response to F or G glycoproteins (Connors et al. 1992a). However, host resistance may also be mediated by sensitization with the M2 protein, and depletion of $CD8^+$ T cells abrogates M2-associated protection, while depletion of $CD4^+$ T cells has an intermediate effect (Connors et al. 1992a). Although both $CD4^+$ and $CD8^+$ T cells contribute to disease pathogenesis, passive transfer of RSV-specific $CD4^+$ T cells into RSV-immune mice mediates more severe immunopathology and pulmonary eosinophilia compared to transfer of $CD8^+$ T cells (Alwan et al. 1992). Distinct types of pulmonary disease are mediated by functionally different T-cell subsets reactive to different RSV proteins. Adoptive transfer of T-cell lines recognizing G glycoprotein into RSV-infected mice induces severe illness, characterized by pulmonary eosinophilia and hemorrhaging, compared to transfer of M2-specific, or F-glycoprotein-specific T-cell lines (Alwan et al. 1994). It is likely that Th2-type cytokine expression by the G-glycoprotein-specific T-cell lines contributed to the disease severity, since these cells were $CD4^+$ and expressed IL-4 and IL-5, whereas M2-specific or F-glycoprotein-specific T-cell lines were $CD4^+$ or $CD8^+$ and expressed Th1-type cytokines. The relationship of Th1- to Th2-type cytokine expression appears important in the outcome of RSV immunity or disease pathogenesis (Lemanske 1998; Welliver 2000;

Graham et al. 2002). Primary RSV infection induces a mixed Th1- and Th2-type cytokine response with limited disease pathogenesis (Openshaw et al. 2002), and from animal studies, it appears that early IFN-γ expression is key in controlling the Th1/Th2 cytokine balance (Spender et al. 1998; Boelen et al. 2002; Openshaw et al. 2002). Absence of IFN-γ early after primary infection or during subsequent RSV infections has been shown to result in a predominant Th2-type cytokine response and increased disease severity (Hussell et al. 1997; Boelen et al. 2002; Durbin et al. 2002). The relationship between phenotypes associated with cell activation and cytokine expression was investigated in RSV-infected BALB/c mice (Tripp et al. 2000c). In this study, CD54+ and CD102+ lymphocytes expressed higher levels of IL-2, IL-4, IL-5, and IFN-γ compared to CD44+, CD49d+ or CD62L^{lo} lymphocytes, and DNA analysis of lymphocytes expressing IL-2 or IFN-γ revealed higher G2/M levels compared to lymphocytes expressing IL-4 or IL-5, suggesting greater activation of Th1-type lymphocytes in the lungs in response to RSV infection.

IMMUNOPATHOLOGY AND THE RESPONSE TO RSV PROTEINS

Immune-mediated pathology was first indicated in clinical trials of FI-RSV vaccine parentally administered to infants who subsequently developed enhanced pulmonary disease upon natural RSV infection (Chin et al. 1969; Fulginiti et al. 1969; Kapikian et al. 1969; Kim et al. 1969). The vaccine failure is generally attributed to poor protection, and an unbalanced immune response to vaccination (Murphy et al. 1986c). The poor protection may be linked with a weak neutralizing secretory IgA response associated with parental vaccination, or an unbalanced humoral response to vaccination. FI-RSV vaccinees developed high titers of serum antibodies to the F glycoprotein, but these antibodies did not exhibit effective neutralizing activity (Murphy et al. 1986c). In addition, vaccinees had low levels of serum antibodies to the G glycoprotein, suggesting that G glycoprotein immunogenicity was altered by formalin-inactivation. Lung histopathology of FI-RSV vaccinees who died revealed extensive infiltration of neutrophils and eosinophils that is not associated with primary RSV infection in mice (Chin et al. 1969; Graham et al. 1993; Waris et al. 1996). Unfortunately, investigation of the CD4+ and CD8+ T-cell response was not available during this vaccine trial, thus cell-mediated responses to FI-RSV vaccination have been inferred from experimental animal studies.

FI-RSV vaccine studies in experimental animal models, particularly mice and cotton rats, suggest that enhanced pulmonary disease is primarily mediated by CD4+ T cells and Th2-type cytokines, as depletion of CD4+ T cells or IL-4 or IL-10 abrogates enhanced disease (Connors et al. 1992b, 1994). The RSV G glyco-

protein appears to sensitize for enhanced disease, skewed Th2-type cytokine and chemokine responses, and to enhance pulmonary expression of substance P, a neurogenic mediator of inflammation (Johnson et al. 1998; Johnson and Graham 1999; Graham et al. 2000; Tripp et al. 1999, 2000a, b, d). G glycoprotein sensitization for enhanced pulmonary disease has been shown to be associated with T-cell epitopes on the G glycoprotein comprising amino acids 185–193 (Srikiatkhachorn et al. 1999), 184–198 (Tebbey et al. 1998), or 193–202 (Sparer et al. 1998); however, the response mediated by the G glycoprotein may not be epitope-specific, since the form and site of administration of G glycoprotein available for antigen processing and presentation has been shown to be an important factor sensitizing for enhanced pulmonary disease (Bembridge et al. 1998). G-glycoprotein-associated Th2-type responses including high IL-4, IL-5, and IL-13 cytokine expression by infiltrating leukocytes, pulmonary eosinophilia, and extensive inflammation upon live RSV challenge (Openshaw 1995a; Graham et al. 2000; Openshaw et al. 2001). The T-cell repertoire is also altered by G-glycoprotein sensitization, characterized by constrained TCR Vβ14+ usage by CD4+ T cells responding to RSV challenge, and in vivo elimination of TCR Vβ14+ cells has been shown to abolish Th2-type pulmonary disease (Varga et al. 2001). A recent study from our laboratory indicates that FI-RSV-enhanced disease is associated with G-glycoprotein expression, and in particular the G-glycoprotein CX3C motif, and that pulmonary substance P expression contributes to the enhanced inflammatory response associated with FI-RSV vaccination (Haynes et al. 2003). Interestingly, G-glycoprotein-specific cytotoxic T-cell responses are not readily detected in humans or mice; however, mice sensitized to G glycoprotein generate Th1 and Th2 CD4+ T-cell responses (Hancock et al. 1996). By contrast, mice sensitized to RSV F glycoprotein induce potent cytotoxic T-cell responses, and Th1 CD4+ T-cell responses (Alwan and Openshaw 1993).

In addition to sensitizing for Th2-type CD4+ T-cell responses and altering the T-cell repertoire, the G glycoprotein has been associated with other immune modulatory features. BALB/c mice infected with wild-type RSV have markedly reduced pulmonary trafficking of neutrophils and NK cells, increased pulmonary substance P expression, and reduced CC and CXC chemokine mRNA expression by bronchoalveolar lavage (BAL) cells compared to mice infected with an RSV mutant lacking G and SH genes (Tripp et al. 1999, 2000a, 2000d). It is possible that skewed Th2-type CD4+ T-cell responses associated with G glycoprotein expression are affected by reduced CC and CXC chemokine expression. MIPs and inflammatory protein (IP)-10 are chemotactic for cells bearing the chemokine receptors CCR1, CCR5, and CXCR3 (Kabashima et al. 2001; Luther and Cyster 2001; Sauty et al. 2001). These chemokine receptors are preferentially expressed on

Th1 cells (Loetscher et al. 1998; Odum et al. 1999; Syrbe et al. 1999), thus decreased expression of MIP and IP-10 may impair recruitment of Th1-type cells favoring Th2-type cell recruitment. The G glycoprotein can also mimic the activities of the only known CX3C chemokine, fractalkine (Tripp et al. 2001). G glycoprotein contains a CX3C chemokine motif that interacts with the CX3C chemokine receptor, CX3CR1. The structural similarity between the G glycoprotein CX3C motif and the fractalkine CX3C motif is shown in Figure 37.5. G glycoprotein CX3C with CX3CR1 can compete with fractalkine for binding to CX3CR1, induce leukocyte chemotaxis in a fashion similar to fractalkine, and facilitate virus infection. The results suggest that G glycoprotein interaction with CX3CR1 may be important to the biology of RSV infection and possibly disease pathogenesis.

The form of the G glycoprotein appears to be important in immunity and disease pathogenesis. The secreted form of the G glycoprotein is more potent in inducing pulmonary eosinophilia than the membrane-anchored form (Johnson et al. 1998), and sensitization with the secreted form is associated with increased expression of IL-5, IL-13, and eotaxin (Johnson and Graham 1999). Pulmonary eosinophilia mediated by soluble G-glycoprotein sensitization does not require IL-4 expression, but does require IL-5, and if both IL-4 and IL-13 are inhibited at the time of immunization, the development of pulmonary eosinophilia upon RSV challenge is reduced (Johnson and Graham 1999). By contrast, presentation of RSV F in a soluble form does not sensitize for pulmonary eosinophilia, but does induce IL-4 and IL-5 (Bembridge et al. 1999). RSV-specific CD8[+] T cells and IL-12-activated NK cells appear to regulate development of G-glycoprotein-mediated enhanced disease. If RSV-specific CD8[+] T cells are present at the time of G-glycoprotein sensitization, the development of pulmonary eosinophilia and enhanced disease is reduced

(Alwan et al. 1994; Hussell et al. 1997). Similarly, IL-12-activated NK cells can reduce pulmonary eosinophilia mediated by G-glycoprotein sensitization, but do not enhance the severity of illness in the absence of CD8[+] T cells (Hussell and Openshaw 2000).

EPIDEMIOLOGY

Viral respiratory tract infections can be severe during infancy, and viral bronchiolitis is the most common cause of infant and young children hospitalization in the developed world (Leader and Kohlhase 2002; Staat 2002). RSV is the primary cause of lower respiratory tract infections among infants and young children, accounting for approximately 70 percent of all cases of viral bronchiolitis (Glezen et al. 1986). During a 17-year study period in the USA, an estimated 1.65 million hospitalizations for bronchiolitis occurred among children younger than 5 years, and 57 percent of these hospitalizations occurred among children <6 months of age (Shay et al. 1999). RSV activity in the USA monitored by the National Respiratory and Enteric Virus Surveillance System at the Centers for Disease Control and Prevention (CDC) has shown that RSV outbreaks occur between October and April (Figure 37.1). Examining the number of bronchiolitis hospitalizations in 1994–1996 from November through April in the USA, it is estimated that 51 240–81 985 annual bronchiolitis hospitalizations among children younger than 1 year were related to RSV infection (Shay et al. 1999). In the USA, the risk of primary RSV infection in infants <12 months of age ranges from 50 to 70 percent, and approximately 30–40 percent of children in this age group develop lower respiratory tract illness (Parrott et al. 1973; Glezen et al. 1986). By age 2, most children have experienced at least one RSV infection (CDC 2000), and the risk for lower respiratory tract illness remains high with re-infection, and through the first 5

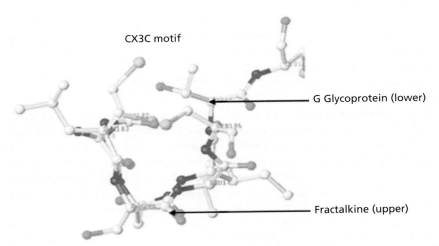

Figure 37.5 *Superimposed images of the CX3C motif of fractalkine and RSV G glycoprotein modeled using the molecular modeling program SYBYL. Forcefields were generated using SYBYL and charges calculated using the Gasteiger–Huckel and Kollman methods.*

years of life (Glezen et al. 1986; Wright et al. 1989). The risk of serious RSV infection is high in patients with underlying disorders of the cardiac, pulmonary, or immune system (Wendt 1997; Englund et al. 1999; Falsey and Walsh 2000; Whimbey and Ghosh 2000; Hall 2001; Aujard and Fauroux 2002; Greenberg 2002; Ison and Hayden 2002). Diagnostic studies using RT-PCR indicate that RSV may cause approximately 50 percent of all respiratory tract illness in adult patients. RSV is recognized as a major cause of serious disease in older adults and the elderly, and is associated with high morbidity and some mortality in older persons residing in nursing homes and in the community (Falsey 1998; Han et al. 1999). The relationship of serum antibody to RSV and risk of RSV infection suggests that older adults with low titers of serum neutralizing antibody may be at greater risk of developing symptomatic RSV infection than those who have high antibody titers (Falsey and Walsh 1998). Applying rates of RSV detection from prospective studies of lower respiratory tract illness in adults to national hospital discharge diagnosis and death certificate data, it is estimated that RSV causes 14 000–62 000 hospitalizations and 1 500–6 700 deaths each year in the USA in older adults and the elderly (Han et al. 1999). The impact of RSV strain variation on the epidemiology of RSV disease is not completely understood; however, RSV outbreaks appear to be community-based. The circulation patterns of RSV A and B strains appear genotypically distinct among communities with limited diversity between strains of the same genotype, but greater diversity in genotype in strains from different communities (Peret et al. 1998, 2000). Isolates of RSV strain A appear to be more common than strain B, and individual outbreaks of RSV infection may differ substantially in strain predominance; however, no substantial linkage has been made between strain variation, hospitalization, and disease severity. RSV is a major cause of nosocomial infections (Hall 1983), particularly for premature infants and the immune compromised (CDC 2002; Hall 2000; Jones et al. 2000; Heerens et al. 2002).

Nosocomial pneumonia is a common hospital-acquired infection in children, and is often fatal. Viruses, predominantly RSV, are the most common cause of pediatric nosocomial respiratory tract infections (Hall 1983; Mlinaric-Galinovic and Varda-Brkic 2000). Risk factors for nosocomial pneumonia include hospitalization during the RSV season, age, underlying chronic disease, admission to an intensive care unit, intubation, burns, surgery, immune suppression, and long hospitalization. The morbidity and cost associated with nosocomial RSV infection of infants is striking (Macartney et al. 2000). About 40 percent of nosocomial RSV infections are associated with lower respiratory tract disease in this young age group (Hall 1983). RSV appears to be nosocomially transmitted by fomites on the hands of hospital personnel (Hall et al. 1980). Medical staff infected with community-acquired or nosocomially acquired RSV are frequently unaware of RSV infection because infection may present as mild flulike illnesses. However, RSV infection may debilitate up to 40 percent of those infected, resulting in absence from work (Hall et al. 1978). The key to control of nosocomial transmission of RSV is compliance with guidelines for prevention and surveillance described by the CDC. Education of hospital personnel about the nature of RSV, active surveillance among patients, careful hand washing, and use of gloves and barriers are important in controlling infection (Snydman et al. 1988; Madge et al. 1992; Goldmann 2001); however, prevention through the use of masks and gowns has not been successful (Hall and Douglas 1981; Murphy et al. 1981).

The disease burden of hMPV is not well known. Recent identification of hMPV in the Netherlands was made from respiratory samples submitted for viral culture during the winter season associated with RSV infection (van den Hoogen et al. 2001). Approximately half the initial 28 samples were cultured from infants <1 year of age, and 96 percent were isolated from children <6 years of age. Seroprevalance studies of children aged 6–12 months indicated that approximately 25 percent had detectable antibodies to hMPV, and by age 5 all patients showed evidence of past exposure or infection. In Australia, three of 200 randomly chosen respiratory samples negative for known respiratory pathogens, were positive for hMPV on culture, RT-PCR, or both (Howe 2002). From Canada, 11 isolates from 10 patients aged 2 months to 87 years of age with acute respiratory tract illness during the winter season were identified as hMPV at the CDC (Peret et al. 2002). Two major groups or strains of hMPV were identified in Canadian isolates based upon sequence diversity. Similar to RSV, some of the hMPV isolates did not originate from a single outbreak, but were from unrelated cases of respiratory illness. The serological studies of hMPV infection in the Netherlands, and epidemiological features associated with studies at the CDC and in Australia, suggest that hMPV likely infects most children by age 5, co-circulates with RSV, and may cause repeated infections.

PERSPECTIVE

RSV disease remains a major public health problem, and limited prophylactic or therapeutic treatments are available. Significant progress is being made toward understanding the virus–host relationship related to immunity and disease pathogenesis, and these studies have led to several promising RSV vaccine candidates that are under clinical evaluation. The development of a safe and efficacious RSV vaccine remains a challenging task, as does preventing infection or controlling RSV infection in infants, the elderly, or immune-compromised patients. Success in these areas will likely require different vaccine and treatment strategies. Our limited understandings of durable immunity to RSV, immune-modulating activities of viral proteins, enhanced disease mechanisms associated with formalin-inactivated RSV vaccines and mechanisms that contribute to immunity or disease complicate vaccine development. Development of successful prophylactic or therapeutic treatments to reduce virus load and inhibit inflammation remains a priority. Progress towards these goals is occurring through experimental animal studies; however, more rapid translation of the findings to humans is required. The discovery of hMPV and its clinical relationship to RSV emphasizes the need for a better understanding of the disease burden associated with hMPV infection, the relationship between RSV and hMPV immunity, and the associated disease pathogenesis.

REFERENCES

Akira, S., Takeda, K. and Kaisho, T. 2001. Toll-like receptors: critical proteins linking innate and acquired immunity. *Nat Immunol*, **2**, 675–80.

Alkhalaf, A.N., Ward, L.A., et al. 2002. Pathogenicity, transmissibility, and tissue distribution of avian pneumovirus in turkey poults. *Avian Dis*, **46**, 650–9.

Alwan, W.H. and Openshaw, P.J. 1993. Distinct patterns of T- and B-cell immunity to respiratory syncytial virus induced by individual viral proteins. *Vaccine*, **11**, 431–7.

Alwan, W.H., Record, F.M. and Openshaw, P.J. 1992. CD4+ T cells clear virus but augment disease in mice infected with respiratory syncytial virus. Comparison with the effects of CD8+ T cells. *Clin Exp Immunol*, **88**, 527–36.

Alwan, W.H., Kozlowska, W.J. and Openshaw, P.J. 1994. Distinct types of lung disease caused by functional subsets of antiviral T cells. *J Exp Med*, **179**, 81–9.

Anderson, K., King, A.M., et al. 1992. Polylactosaminoglycan modification of the respiratory syncytial virus small hydrophobic (SH) protein: a conserved feature among human and bovine respiratory syncytial viruses. *Virology*, **191**, 417–30.

Anderson, L.J. 2000. Respiratory syncytial virus vaccines for otitis media. *Vaccine*, **19**, Suppl 1, S59–65.

Armant, M.A. and Fenton, M.J. 2002. Toll-like receptors: a family of pattern-recognition receptors in mammals. *Genome Biol*, **3**, REVIEWS3011.

Arnold, R., Konig, B., et al. 1995. Cytokine (IL-8, IL-6, TNF-alpha) and soluble TNF receptor-I release from human peripheral blood mononuclear cells after respiratory syncytial virus infection. *Immunology*, **85**, 364–72.

Arslanagic, E., Matsumoto, M., et al. 1996. Maturation of respiratory syncytial virus within HEp-2 cell cytoplasm. *Acta Virol*, **40**, 209–14.

Arumugham, R.G., Hildreth, S.W. and Paradiso, P.R. 1989. Evidence that the fusion protein of respiratory syncytial virus exists as a dimer in its native form. Brief report. *Arch Virol*, **106**, 327–34.

Aujard, Y. and Fauroux, B. 2002. Risk factors for severe respiratory syncytial virus infection in infants. *Respir Med*, **96**, Suppl B, S9–14.

Bachi, T. 1988. Direct observation of the budding and fusion of an enveloped virus by video microscopy of viable cells. *J Cell Biol*, **107**, 1689–95.

Bachi, T. and Howe, C. 1973. Morphogenesis and ultrastructure of respiratory syncytial virus. *J Virol*, **12**, 1173–80.

Bangham, C.R., Openshaw, P.J., et al. 1986. Human and murine cytotoxic T cells specific to respiratory syncytial virus recognize the viral nucleoprotein (N), but not the major glycoprotein (G), expressed by vaccinia virus recombinants. *J Immunol*, **137**, 3973–7.

Barton, G.M. and Medzhitov, R. 2002. Control of adaptive immune responses by Toll-like receptors. *Curr Opin Immunol*, **14**, 380–3.

Bayon-Auboyer, M.H., Arnauld, C., et al. 2000. Nucleotide sequences of the F, L and G protein genes of two non-A/non-B avian pneumoviruses (APV) reveal a novel APV subgroup. *J Gen Virol*, **81**, 2723–33.

Becker, S., Quay, J. and Soukup, J. 1991. Cytokine (tumor necrosis factor, IL-6 and IL-8) production by respiratory syncytial virus-infected human alveolar macrophages. *J Immunol*, **147**, 4307–12.

Becker, S., Soukup, J. and Yankaskas, J.R. 1992. Respiratory syncytial virus infection of human primary nasal and bronchial epithelial cell cultures and bronchoalveolar macrophages. *Am J Respir Cell Mol Biol*, **6**, 369–74.

Belshe, R.B., Richardson, L.S., et al. 1977. Experimental respiratory syncytial virus infection of four species of primates. *J Med Virol*, **1**, 157–62.

Bembridge, G.P., Garcia-Beato, R., et al. 1998. Subcellular site of expression and route of vaccination influence pulmonary eosinophilia following respiratory syncytial virus challenge in BALB/c mice sensitized to the attachment G protein. *J Immunol*, **161**, 2473–80.

Bembridge, G.P., Lopez, J.A., et al. 1999. Priming with a secreted form of the fusion protein of respiratory syncytial virus (RSV) promotes interleukin-4 (IL-4) and IL-5 production but not pulmonary eosinophilia following RSV challenge. *J Virol*, **73**, 10086–94.

Bhella, D., Ralph, A., et al. 2002. Significant differences in nucleocapsid morphology within the *Paramyxoviridae*. *J Gen Virol*, **83**, 1831–9.

Billings, J.L., Hertz, M.I. and Wendt, C.H. 2001. Community respiratory virus infections following lung transplantation. *Transpl Infect Dis*, **3**, 138–48.

Billings, J.L., Hertz, M.I., et al. 2002. Respiratory viruses and chronic rejection in lung transplant recipients. *J Heart Lung Transplant*, **21**, 559–66.

Boelen, A., Kwakkel, J., et al. 2002. Effect of lack of interleukin-4, interleukin-12, interleukin-18, or the interferon-gamma receptor on virus replication, cytokine response, and lung pathology during respiratory syncytial virus infection in mice. *J Med Virol*, **66**, 552–60.

Bourgeois, C., Bour, J.B., et al. 1998. Heparin-like structures on respiratory syncytial virus are involved in its infectivity in vitro. *J Virol*, **72**, 7221–7.

Brandenburg, A.H., Groen, J., et al. 1997. Respiratory syncytial virus specific serum antibodies in infants under six months of age: limited serological response upon infection. *J Med Virol*, **52**, 97–104.

Brown, G., Aitken, J., et al. 2002. Caveolin-1 is incorporated into mature respiratory syncytial virus particles during virus assembly on the surface of virus-infected cells. *J Gen Virol*, **83**, 611–21.

Bruhn, F.W., Mokrohisky, S.T. and McIntosh, K. 1977. Apnea associated with respiratory syncytial virus infection in young infants. *J Pediatr*, **90**, 382–6.

Buchholz, U.J., Granzow, H., et al. 2000. Chimeric bovine respiratory syncytial virus with glycoprotein gene substitutions from human respiratory syncytial virus (HRSV): effects on host range and evaluation as a live-attenuated HRSV vaccine. *J Virol*, **74**, 1187–99.

Byrd, L.G. and Prince, G.A. 1997. Animal models of respiratory syncytial virus infection. *Clin Infect Dis*, **25**, 1363–8.

Cane, P.A., Matthews, D.A. and Pringle, C.R. 1991. Identification of variable domains of the attachment (G) protein of subgroup A respiratory syncytial viruses. *J Gen Virol*, **72**, 2091–6.

Catelli, E., De Marco, M.A., et al. 2001. Serological evidence of avian pneumovirus infection in reared and free-living pheasants. *Vet Rec*, **149**, 56–8.

CDC. 1998. Palivizumab, a humanized respiratory syncytial virus monoclonal antibody, reduces hospitalization from respiratory syncytial virus infection in high-risk infants. The IMpact-RSV Study Group. *Pediatrics* **102**, 531–7.

CDC. 2000. Respiratory syncytial virus activity – United States, 1999–2000 season. *MMWR Morb Mortal Wkly Rep* **49**, 1091–3.

CDC. 2002. Respiratory syncytial virus activity – United States, 2000–01 season. *MMWR Morb Mortal Wkly Rep* **51**, 26–8.

Chandwani, S., Borkowsky, W., et al. 1990. Respiratory syncytial virus infection in human immunodeficiency virus-infected children. *J Pediatr*, **117**, 251–4.

Chanock, R.M. and Finberg, L. 1957. Recovery from infants with respiratory illness of a virus related to chimpanzee coryza agent CCA). II. Epidemiological aspects of infection in infants and young children. *Am J Hyg*, **66**, 291–54.

Chary, P., Rautenschlein, S., et al. 2002. Pathogenic and immunosuppressive effects of avian pneumovirus in turkeys. *Avian Dis*, **46**, 153–61.

Cherrie, A.H., Anderson, K., et al. 1992. Human cytotoxic T cells stimulated by antigen on dendritic cells recognize the N, SH, F, M, 22K, and 1b proteins of respiratory syncytial virus. *J Virol*, **66**, 2102–0.

Chiba, Y., Higashidate, Y., et al. 1989. Development of cell-mediated cytotoxic immunity to respiratory syncytial virus in human infants following naturally acquired infection. *J Med Virol*, **28**, 133–9.

Chin, J., Magoffin, R.L., et al. 1969. Field evaluation of a respiratory syncytial virus vaccine and a trivalent parainfluenza virus vaccine in a pediatric population. *Am J Epidemiol*, **89**, 449–63.

Church, N.R., Anas, N.G., et al. 1984. Respiratory syncytial virus-related apnea in infants. Demographics and outcome. *Am J Dis Child*, **138**, 247–50.

Coiras, M.T., Perez-Brena, P., et al. 2003. Simultaneous detection of influenza A, B and C viruses, respiratory syncytial virus, and adenoviruses in clinical samples by multiplex reverse transcription nested-PCR assay. *J Med Virol*, **69**, 132–44.

Collins, M.S. and Gough, R.E. 1988. Characterization of a virus associated with turkey rhinotracheitis. *J Gen Virol*, **69**, 909–16.

Collins, P.L. 1990. O glycosylation of glycoprotein G of human respiratory syncytial virus is specified within the divergent ectodomain. *J Virol*, **64**, 4007–12.

Collins, P.L. and Mottet, G. 1992. Oligomerization and post-translational processing of glycoprotein G of human respiratory syncytial virus: altered O-glycosylation in the presence of brefeldin A. *J Gen Virol*, **73**, 849–63.

Collins, P.L. and Mottet, G. 1993. Membrane orientation and oligomerization of the small hydrophobic protein of human respiratory syncytial virus. *J Gen Virol*, **74**, 1445–50.

Collins, P.L. and Murphy, B.R. 2002. Respiratory syncytial virus: reverse genetics and vaccine strategies. *Virology*, **296**, 204–11.

Collins, P.L. and Wertz, G.W. 1983. cDNA cloning and transcriptional mapping of nine polyadenylylated RNAs encoded by the genome of human respiratory syncytial virus. *Proc Natl Acad Sci U S A*, **80**, 3208–12.

Collins, P.L., Huang, Y.T. and Wertz, G.W. 1984a. Identification of a tenth mRNA of respiratory syncytial virus and assignment of polypeptides to the 10 viral genes. *J Virol*, **49**, 572–8.

Collins, P.L., Huang, Y.T. and Wertz, G.W. 1984b. Nucleotide sequence of the gene encoding the fusion (F) glycoprotein of human respiratory syncytial virus. *Proc Natl Acad Sci U S A*, **81**, 7683–7.

Collins, P.L., Anderson, K., et al. 1985. Correct sequence for the major nucleocapsid protein mRNA of respiratory syncytial virus. *Virology*, **146**, 69–77.

Collins, P.L., Dickens, L.E., et al. 1986. Nucleotide sequences for the gene junctions of human respiratory syncytial virus reveal distinctive features of intergenic structure and gene order. *Proc Natl Acad Sci U S A*, **83**, 4594–8.

Collins, P.L., Olmsted, R.A. and Johnson, P.R. 1990a. The small hydrophobic protein of human respiratory syncytial virus: comparison between antigenic subgroups A and B. *J Gen Virol*, **71**, 1571–6.

Collins, P.L., Purcell, R.H., et al. 1990b. Evaluation in chimpanzees of vaccinia virus recombinants that express the surface glycoproteins of human respiratory syncytial virus. *Vaccine*, **8**, 164–8.

Connors, M., Kulkarni, A.B., et al. 1992a. Resistance to respiratory syncytial virus (RSV) challenge induced by infection with a vaccinia virus recombinant expressing the RSV M2 protein (Vac-M2) is mediated by CD8+ T cells, while that induced by Vac-F or Vac-G recombinants is mediated by antibodies. *J Virol*, **66**, 1277–81.

Connors, M., Kulkarni, A.B., et al. 1992b. Pulmonary histopathology induced by respiratory syncytial virus (RSV) challenge of formalin-inactivated RSV-immunized BALB/c mice is abrogated by depletion of CD4+ T cells. *J Virol*, **66**, 7444–51.

Connors, M., Giese, N.A., et al. 1994. Enhanced pulmonary histopathology induced by respiratory syncytial virus (RSV) challenge of formalin-inactivated RSV-immunized BALB/c mice is abrogated by depletion of interleukin-4 (IL-4) and IL-10. *J Virol*, **68**, 5321–5.

Cook, J.K. 2000. Avian pneumovirus infections of turkeys and chickens. *Vet J*, **160**, 118–25.

Couch, R.B., Englund, J.A. and Whimbey, E. 1997. Respiratory viral infections in immunocompetent and immunocompromised persons. *Am J Med*, **102**, 2–9, discussion 25-26.

Cranage, M.P., Gardner, P.S. and McIntosh, K. 1981. In vitro cell-dependent lysis of respiratory syncytial virus-infected cells mediated by antibody from local respiratory secretions. *Clin Exp Immunol*, **43**, 28–35.

Crowe, J.E. Jr 2001a. Influence of maternal antibodies on neonatal immunization against respiratory viruses. *Clin Infect Dis*, **33**, 1720–7.

Crowe, J.E. Jr 2001b. Respiratory syncytial virus vaccine development. *Vaccine*, **20**, Suppl 1, S32–7.

Crowe, J.E. Jr, Randolph, V. and Murphy, B.R. 1999. The live attenuated subgroup B respiratory syncytial virus vaccine candidate RSV 2B33F is attenuated and immunogenic in chimpanzees, but exhibits partial loss of the ts phenotype following replication in vivo. *Virus Res*, **59**, 13–22.

De Boeck, K., Van der Aa, N., et al. 1997. Respiratory syncytial virus bronchiolitis: a double-blind dexamethasone efficacy study. *J Pediatr*, **131**, 919–21.

De Clercq, E. 2002. Highlights in the development of new antiviral agents. *Mini Rev Med Chem*, **2**, 163–75.

de Sierra, T.M., Kumar, M.L., et al. 1993. Respiratory syncytial virus-specific immunoglobulins in preterm infants. *J Pediatr*, **122**, 787–91.

Dickens, L.E., Collins, P.L. and Wertz, G.W. 1984. Transcriptional mapping of human respiratory syncytial virus. *J Virol*, **52**, 364–9.

Domachowske, J.B., Bonville, C.A., et al. 2000. Respiratory syncytial virus infection induces expression of the anti-apoptosis gene IEX-1L in human respiratory epithelial cells. *J Infect Dis*, **181**, 824–30.

Domurat, F., Roberts, N.J. Jr, et al. 1985. Respiratory syncytial virus infection of human mononuclear leukocytes in vitro and in vivo. *J Infect Dis*, **152**, 895–902.

Dudas, R.A. and Karron, R.A. 1998. Respiratory syncytial virus vaccines. *Clin Microbiol Rev*, **11**, 430–9.

Durbin, J.E., Johnson, T.R., et al. 2002. The role of IFN in respiratory syncytial virus pathogenesis. *J Immunol*, **168**, 2944–52.

Edwards, K.M., Snyder, P.N. and Wright, P.F. 1986. Complement activation by respiratory syncytial virus-infected cells. *Arch Virol*, **88**, 49–56.

Englund, J.A., Anderson, L.J. and Rhame, F.S. 1991. Nosocomial transmission of respiratory syncytial virus in immunocompromised adults. *J Clin Microbiol*, **29**, 115–19.

Englund, J.A., Whimbey, E. and Atmar, R.L. 1999. Diagnosis of respiratory viruses in cancer and transplant patients. *Curr Clin Top Infect Dis*, **19**, 30–59.

Evans, J.E., Cane, P.A. and Pringle, C.R. 1996. Expression and characterisation of the NS1 and NS2 proteins of respiratory syncytial virus. *Virus Res*, **43**, 155–61.

Everard, M.L., Swarbrick, A., et al. 1994. Analysis of cells obtained by bronchial lavage of infants with respiratory syncytial virus infection. *Arch Dis Child*, **71**, 428–32.

Falsey, A.R. 1998. Respiratory syncytial virus infection in older persons. *Vaccine*, **16**, 1775–8.

Falsey, A.R. and Walsh, E.E. 1996. Safety and immunogenicity of a respiratory syncytial virus subunit vaccine (PFP-2) in ambulatory adults over age 60. *Vaccine*, **14**, 1214–18.

Falsey, A.R. and Walsh, E.E. 1998. Relationship of serum antibody to risk of respiratory syncytial virus infection in elderly adults. *J Infect Dis*, **177**, 463–6.

Falsey, A.R. and Walsh, E.E. 2000. Respiratory syncytial virus infection in adults. *Clin Microbiol Rev*, **13**, 371–84.

Falsey, A.R., Formica, M.A. and Walsh, E.E. 2002. Diagnosis of respiratory syncytial virus infection: comparison of reverse transcription-PCR to viral culture and serology in adults with respiratory illness. *J Clin Microbiol*, **40**, 817–20.

Fawaz, L.M., Sharif-Askari, E. and Menezes, J. 1999. Up-regulation of NK cytotoxic activity via IL-15 induction by different viruses: a comparative study. *J Immunol*, **163**, 4473–80.

Fearns, R. and Collins, P.L. 1999. Model for polymerase access to the overlapped L gene of respiratory syncytial virus. *J Virol*, **73**, 388–97.

Feldman, S.A., Hendry, R.M. and Beeler, J.A. 1999. Identification of a linear heparin binding domain for human respiratory syncytial virus attachment glycoprotein G. *J Virol*, **73**, 6610–17.

Fishaut, M., Tubergen, D. and McIntosh, K. 1980. Cellular response to respiratory viruses with particular reference to children with disorders of cell-mediated immunity. *J Pediatr*, **96**, 179–86.

Fixler, D.E. 1996. Respiratory syncytial virus infection in children with congenital heart disease: a review. *Pediatr Cardiol*, **17**, 163–8.

Fulginiti, V.A., Eller, J.J., et al. 1969. Respiratory virus immunization. I. A field trial of two inactivated respiratory virus vaccines; an aqueous trivalent parainfluenza virus vaccine and an alum-precipitated respiratory syncytial virus vaccine. *Am J Epidemiol*, **89**, 435–48.

Garofalo, R., Mei, F., et al. 1996. Respiratory syncytial virus infection of human respiratory epithelial cells up-regulates class I MHC expression through the induction of IFN-beta and IL-1 alpha. *J Immunol*, **157**, 2506–13.

Ghildyal, R., Hartley, C., et al. 1999. Surfactant protein A binds to the fusion glycoprotein of respiratory syncytial virus and neutralizes virion infectivity. *J Infect Dis*, **180**, 2009–13.

Glezen, P. and Denny, F.W. 1973. Epidemiology of acute lower respiratory disease in children. *N Engl J Med*, **288**, 498–505.

Glezen, W.P., Taber, L.H., et al. 1986. Risk of primary infection and reinfection with respiratory syncytial virus. *Am J Dis Child*, **140**, 543–6.

Goetsch, L., Plotnicky-Gilquin, H., et al. 2001. BBG2Na an RSV subunit vaccine candidate intramuscularly injected to human confers protection against viral challenge after nasal immunization in mice. *Vaccine*, **19**, 4036–42.

Goldmann, D.A. 2001. Epidemiology and prevention of pediatric viral respiratory infections in health-care institutions. *Emerg Infect Dis*, **7**, 249–53.

Gonzalez, I.M., Karron, R.A., et al. 2000. Evaluation of the live attenuated cpts 248/404 RSV vaccine in combination with a subunit RSV vaccine (PFP-2) in healthy young and older adults. *Vaccine*, **18**, 1763–72.

Gotoh, B., Komatsu, T., et al. 2001. Paramyxovirus accessory proteins as interferon antagonists. *Microbiol Immunol*, **45**, 787–800.

Gower, T.L., Peeples, M.E., et al. 2001. RhoA is activated during respiratory syncytial virus infection. *Virology*, **283**, 188–96.

Goyal, S.M., Chiang, S.J., et al. 2000. Isolation of avian pneumovirus from an outbreak of respiratory illness in Minnesota turkeys. *J Vet Diagn Invest*, **12**, 166–8.

Graham, B.S., Bunton, L.A., et al. 1991. Role of T lymphocyte subsets in the pathogenesis of primary infection and rechallenge with respiratory syncytial virus in mice. *J Clin Invest*, **88**, 1026–33.

Graham, B.S., Henderson, G.S., et al. 1993. Priming immunization determines T helper cytokine mRNA expression patterns in lungs of mice challenged with respiratory syncytial virus. *J Immunol*, **151**, 2032–40.

Graham, B.S., Johnson, T.R. and Peebles, R.S. 2000. Immune-mediated disease pathogenesis in respiratory syncytial virus infection. *Immunopharmacology*, **48**, 237–47.

Graham, B.S., Rutigliano, J.A. and Johnson, T.R. 2002. Respiratory syncytial virus immunobiology and pathogenesis. *Virology*, **297**, 1–7.

Greenberg, D.P. 2001. Update on the development and use of viral and bacterial vaccines for the prevention of acute otitis media. *Allergy Asthma Proc*, **22**, 353–7.

Greenberg, S.B. 2002. Respiratory viral infections in adults. *Curr Opin Pulmon Med*, **8**, 201–8.

Groothuis, J.R., Simoes, E.A., et al. 1993. Prophylactic administration of respiratory syncytial virus immune globulin to high-risk infants and young children. The Respiratory Syncytial Virus Immune Globulin Study Group. *N Engl J Med*, **329**, 1524–30.

Groothuis, J.R., King, S.J., et al. 1998. Safety and immunogenicity of a purified F protein respiratory syncytial virus (PFP-2) vaccine in seropositive children with bronchopulmonary dysplasia. *J Infect Dis*, **177**, 467–9.

Hall, C.B. 1977. The shedding and spreading of respiratory syncytial virus. *Pediatr Res*, **11**, 236–9.

Hall, C.B. 1983. The nosocomial spread of respiratory syncytial viral infections. *Annu Rev Med*, **34**, 311–19.

Hall, C.B. 1999. Respiratory syncytial virus: A continuing culprit and conundrum. *J Pediatr*, **135**, 2–7.

Hall, C.B. 2000. Nosocomial respiratory syncytial virus infections: the 'Cold War' has not ended. *Clin Infect Dis*, **31**, 590–6.

Hall, C.B. 2001. Respiratory syncytial virus and parainfluenza virus. *N Engl J Med*, **344**, 1917–28.

Hall, C.B. and Douglas, R.G. Jr 1981. Nosocomial respiratory syncytial viral infections. Should gowns and masks be used? *Am J Dis Child*, **135**, 512–15.

Hall, C.B., Douglas, R.G. Jr. and Geiman, J.M. 1975. Quantitative shedding patterns of respiratory syncytial virus in infants. *J Infect Dis*, **132**, 151–6.

Hall, C.B., Douglas, R.G. Jr. and Geiman, J.M. 1976. Respiratory syncytial virus infections in infants: quantitation and duration of shedding. *J Pediatr*, **89**, 11–15.

Hall, C.B., Geiman, J.M., et al. 1978. Control of nosocomial respiratory syncytial viral infections. *Pediatrics*, **62**, 728–32.

Hall, C.B., Douglas, R.G. Jr. and Geiman, J.M. 1980. Possible transmission by fomites of respiratory syncytial virus. *J Infect Dis*, **141**, 98–102.

Hall, C.B., McBride, J.T., et al. 1983. Aerosolized ribavirin treatment of infants with respiratory syncytial viral infection. A randomized double-blind study. *N Engl J Med*, **308**, 1443–7.

Hall, C.B., McBride, J.T., et al. 1985. Ribavirin treatment of respiratory syncytial viral infection in infants with underlying cardiopulmonary disease. *JAMA*, **254**, 3047–51.

Hallman, M., Ramet, M. and Ezekowitz, R.A. 2001. Toll-like receptors as sensors of pathogens. *Pediatr Res*, **50**, 315–21.

Han, L.L., Alexander, J.P. and Anderson, L.J. 1999. Respiratory syncytial virus pneumonia among the elderly: an assessment of disease burden. *J Infect Dis*, **179**, 25–30.

Hancock, G.E., Speelman, D.J., et al. 1996. Generation of atypical pulmonary inflammatory responses in BALB/c mice after immunization with the native attachment (G) glycoprotein of respiratory syncytial virus. *J Virol*, **70**, 7783–91.

Hardy, R.W. and Wertz, G.W. 2000. The Cys_3-His_1 motif of the respiratory syncytial virus M2-1 protein is essential for protein function. *J Virol*, **74**, 5880–5.

Hardy, R.W., Harmon, S.B. and Wertz, G.W. 1999. Diverse gene junctions of respiratory syncytial virus modulate the efficiency of transcription termination and respond differently to M2-mediated antitermination. *J Virol*, **73**, 170–6.

Harmon, S.B., Megaw, A.G. and Wertz, G.W. 2001. RNA sequences involved in transcriptional termination of respiratory syncytial virus. *J Virol*, **75**, 36–44.

Haynes, L.M., Moore, D.D., et al. 2001. Involvement of Toll-like receptor 4 in innate immunity to respiratory syncytial virus. *J Virol*, **75**, 10730–7.

Haynes, L.M., Tonkin, J., et al. 2002. Neutralizing anti-F glycoprotein and anti-substance P antibody treatment effectively reduces infection and inflammation associated with respiratory syncytial virus infection. *J Virol*, **76**, 6873–81.

Haynes, L.M., Jones, L.P., et al. 2003. Enhanced disease and pulmonary eosinophilia associated with formalin-inactivated respiratory syncytial virus vaccination are linked to G glycoprotein CX3C-CX3CR1 interaction and expression of substance P. *J Virol*, **77**, 9831–44.

Heerens, A.T., Marshall, D.D. and Bose, C.L. 2002. Nosocomial respiratory syncytial virus: a threat in the modern neonatal intensive care unit. *J Perinatol*, **22**, 306–7.

Hemming, V.G., Rodriguez, W., et al. 1987. Intravenous immunoglobulin treatment of respiratory syncytial virus infections in infants and young children. *Antimicrob Agents Chemother*, **31**, 1882–6.

Henderson, F.W., Hu, S.C. and Collier, A.M. 1978. Pathogenesis of respiratory syncytial virus infection in ferret and fetal human tracheas in organ culture. *Am Rev Respir Dis*, **118**, 29–37.

Henderson, F.W., Collier, A.M., et al. 1979. Respiratory-syncytial-virus infections, reinfections and immunity. A prospective, longitudinal study in young children. *N Engl J Med*, **300**, 530–4.

Hendricks, D.A., Baradaran, K., et al. 1987. Appearance of a soluble form of the G protein of respiratory syncytial virus in fluids of infected cells. *J Gen Virol*, **68**, 1705–14.

Hendricks, D.A., McIntosh, K. and Patterson, J.L. 1988. Further characterization of the soluble form of the G glycoprotein of respiratory syncytial virus. *J Virol*, **62**, 2228–33.

Hendry, R.M., Burns, J.C., et al. 1988. Strain-specific serum antibody responses in infants undergoing primary infection with respiratory syncytial virus. *J Infect Dis*, **157**, 640–7.

Hertz, M.I., Englund, J.A., et al. 1989. Respiratory syncytial virus-induced acute lung injury in adult patients with bone marrow transplants: a clinical approach and review of the literature. *Medicine (Baltimore)*, **68**, 269–81.

Hierholzer, J.C. and Tannock, G.A. 1986. Respiratory syncytial virus: a review of the virus, its epidemiology, immune response and laboratory diagnosis. *Aust Paediatr J*, **22**, 77–82.

Horikami, S.M., Curran, J., et al. 1992. Complexes of Sendai virus NP-P and P-L proteins are required for defective interfering particle genome replication in vitro. *J Virol*, **66**, 4901–8.

Hornsleth, A., Loland, L. and Larsen, L.B. 2001. Cytokines and chemokines in respiratory secretion and severity of disease in infants with respiratory syncytial virus (RSV) infection. *J Clin Virol*, **21**, 163–70.

Howe, M. 2002. Australian find suggests worldwide reach for metapneumovirus. *Lancet Infect Dis*, **2**, 202.

Hruska, J.F., Morrow, P.E., et al. 1982. In vivo inhibition of respiratory syncytial virus by ribavirin. *Antimicrob Agents Chemother*, **21**, 125–30.

Huang, Y.T. and Wertz, G.W. 1982. The genome of respiratory syncytial virus is a negative-stranded RNA that codes for at least seven mRNA species. *J Virol*, **43**, 150–7.

Huang, Y.T., Collins, P.L. and Wertz, G.W. 1985. Characterization of the 10 proteins of human respiratory syncytial virus: identification of a fourth envelope-associated protein. *Virus Res*, **2**, 157–73.

Hussell, T. and Openshaw, P.J. 2000. IL-12-activated NK cells reduce lung eosinophilia to the attachment protein of respiratory syncytial virus but do not enhance the severity of illness in CD8 T cell-immunodeficient conditions. *J Immunol*, **165**, 7109–15.

Hussell, T., Baldwin, C.J., et al. 1997. CD8+ T cells control Th2-driven pathology during pulmonary respiratory syncytial virus infection. *Eur J Immunol*, **27**, 3341–9.

Isaacs, D., Bangham, C.R. and McMichael, A.J. 1987. Cell-mediated cytotoxic response to respiratory syncytial virus in infants with bronchiolitis. *Lancet*, **2**, 769–71.

Ison, M.G. and Hayden, F.G. 2002. Viral infections in immunocompromised patients: what's new with respiratory viruses? *Curr Opin Infect Dis*, **15**, 355–67.

Jin, H., Zhou, H., et al. 2000. Recombinant respiratory syncytial viruses with deletions in the *NS1, NS2, SH* and *M2-2* genes are attenuated in vitro and in vivo. *Virology*, **273**, 210–18.

Jirjis, F.F., Noll, S.L., et al. 2002a. Pathogenesis of avian pneumovirus infection in turkeys. *Vet Pathol*, **39**, 300–10.

Jirjis, F.F., Noll, S.L., et al. 2002b. Rapid detection of avian pneumovirus in tissue culture by microindirect immunofluorescence test. *J Vet Diagn Invest*, **14**, 172–5.

Johnson, P.R. and Collins, P.L. 1988. The fusion glycoproteins of human respiratory syncytial virus of subgroups A and B: sequence conservation provides a structural basis for antigenic relatedness. *J Gen Virol*, **69**, 2623–8.

Johnson, P.R. Jr, Olmsted, R.A., et al. 1987a. Antigenic relatedness between glycoproteins of human respiratory syncytial virus subgroups A and B: evaluation of the contributions of F and G glycoproteins to immunity. *J Virol*, **61**, 3163–6.

Johnson, P.R., Spriggs, M.K., et al. 1987b. The G glycoprotein of human respiratory syncytial viruses of subgroups A and B: extensive sequence divergence between antigenically related proteins. *Proc Natl Acad Sci U S A*, **84**, 5625–9.

Johnson, T.R. and Graham, B.S. 1999. Secreted respiratory syncytial virus G glycoprotein induces interleukin-5 (IL-5), IL-13, and eosinophilia by an IL-4-independent mechanism. *J Virol*, **73**, 8485–95.

Johnson, T.R., Johnson, J.E., et al. 1998. Priming with secreted glycoprotein G of respiratory syncytial virus (RSV) augments interleukin-5 production and tissue eosinophilia after RSV challenge. *J Virol*, **72**, 2871–80.

Joncas, J., Berthiaume, L. and Pavilanis, V. 1969. The structure of the respiratory syncytial virus. *Virology*, **38**, 493–6.

Jones, B.L., Clark, S., et al. 2000. Control of an outbreak of respiratory syncytial virus infection in immunocompromised adults. *J Hosp Infect*, **44**, 53–7.

Juhasz, K. and Easton, A.J. 1994. Extensive sequence variation in the attachment (G) protein gene of avian pneumovirus: evidence for two distinct subgroups. *J Gen Virol*, **75**, 2873–80.

Kabashima, H., Yoneda, M., et al. 2001. The presence of chemokine receptor (CCR5, CXCR3, CCR3)-positive cells and chemokine (MCP1, MIP-1alpha, MIP-1beta, IP-10)-positive cells in human periapical granulomas. *Cytokine*, **16**, 62–6.

Kapikian, A.Z., Mitchell, R.H., et al. 1969. An epidemiologic study of altered clinical reactivity to respiratory syncytial (RS) virus infection in children previously vaccinated with an inactivated RS virus vaccine. *Am J Epidemiol*, **89**, 405–21.

Karron, R.A., Buonagurio, D.A., et al. 1997a. Respiratory syncytial virus (RSV) SH and G proteins are not essential for viral replication in vitro: clinical evaluation and molecular characterization of a cold-passaged, attenuated RSV subgroup B mutant. *Proc Natl Acad Sci U S A*, **94**, 13961–6.

Karron, R.A., Wright, P.F., et al. 1997b. Evaluation of two live, cold-passaged, temperature-sensitive respiratory syncytial virus vaccines in chimpanzees and in human adults, infants, and children. *J Infect Dis*, **176**, 1428–36.

Kaul, T.N., Welliver, R.C. and Ogra, P.L. 1982. Development of antibody-dependent cell-mediated cytotoxicity in the respiratory tract after natural infection with respiratory syncytial virus. *Infect Immun*, **37**, 492–8.

Kellner, J.D., Ohlsson, A., et al. 1996. Efficacy of bronchodilator therapy in bronchiolitis. A meta-analysis. *Arch Pediatr Adolesc Med*, **150**, 1166–72.

Khattar, S.K., Yunus, A.S., et al. 2001. Deletion and substitution analysis defines regions and residues within the phosphoprotein of bovine respiratory syncytial virus that affect transcription, RNA replication, and interaction with the nucleoprotein. *Virology*, **285**, 253–69.

Kim, H.W., Canchola, J.G., et al. 1969. Respiratory syncytial virus disease in infants despite prior administration of antigenic inactivated vaccine. *Am J Epidemiol*, **89**, 422–34.

Kneyber, M.C. and Kimpen, J.L. 2002. Current concepts on active immunization against respiratory syncytial virus for infants and young children. *Pediatr Infect Dis J*, **21**, 685–96.

Kneyber, M.C., Moll, H.A. and de Groot, R. 2000. Treatment and prevention of respiratory syncytial virus infection. *Eur J Pediatr*, **159**, 399–411.

Krempl, C., Murphy, B.R. and Collins, P.L. 2002. Recombinant respiratory syncytial virus with the *G* and *F* genes shifted to the promoter-proximal positions. *J Virol*, **76**, 11931–42.

Krilov, L.R. 2001. Respiratory syncytial virus: update on infection, treatment and prevention. *Curr Infect Dis Rep*, **3**, 242–6.

Krilov, L.R., Hendry, R.M., et al. 1987. Respiratory virus infection of peripheral blood monocytes: correlation with ageing of cells and interferon production in vitro. *J Gen Virol*, **68**, 1749–53.

Krusat, T. and Streckert, H.J. 1997. Heparin-dependent attachment of respiratory syncytial virus (RSV) to host cells. *Arch Virol*, **142**, 1247–54.

Kuo, L., Grosfeld, H., et al. 1996. Effects of mutations in the gene-start and gene-end sequence motifs on transcription of monocistronic and dicistronic minigenomes of respiratory syncytial virus. *J Virol*, **70**, 6892–901.

Kurt-Jones, E.A., Popova, L., et al. 2000. Pattern recognition receptors TLR4 and CD14 mediate response to respiratory syncytial virus. *Nat Immunol*, **1**, 398–401.

Law, B.J., Carbonell-Estrany, X. and Simoes, E.A. 2002. An update on respiratory syncytial virus epidemiology: a developed country perspective. *Respir Med*, **96**, Suppl B, S1–7.

Leader, S. and Kohlhase, K. 2002. Respiratory syncytial virus-coded pediatric hospitalizations, 1997 to 1999. *Pediatr Infect Dis J*, **21**, 629–32.

Lemanske, R.F. Jr 1998. *Immunologic mechanisms in RSV-related allergy and asthma*. New York: American Thoracic Society.

LeVine, A.M., Gwozdz, J., et al. 1999. Surfactant protein-A enhances respiratory syncytial virus clearance in vivo. *J Clin Invest*, **103**, 1015–21.

Levine, S. and Hamilton, R. 1969. Kinetics of the respiratory syncytial virus growth cycle in HeLa cells. *Arch ges Virusforsch*, **28**, 122–32.

Lewis, C.E., McCarthy, S.P., et al. 1989. Heterogeneity among human mononuclear phagocytes in their secretion of lysozyme, interleukin 1 and type-beta transforming growth factor: a quantitative analysis at the single-cell level. *Eur J Immunol*, **19**, 2037–43.

Li, J., Ling, R., et al. 1996. Sequence of the nucleocapsid protein gene of subgroup A and B avian pneumoviruses. *Virus Res*, **41**, 185–91.

Libon, C., Corvaia, N., et al. 1999. The serum albumin-binding region of streptococcal protein G (BB) potentiates the immunogenicity of the G130-230 RSV-A protein. *Vaccine*, **17**, 406–14.

Lichtenstein, D.L., Roberts, S.R., et al. 1996. Definition and functional analysis of the signal/anchor domain of the human respiratory syncytial virus glycoprotein G. *J Gen Virol*, **77**, 109–18.

Ling, R., Easton, A.J. and Pringle, C.R. 1992. Sequence analysis of the 22K, SH and G genes of turkey rhinotracheitis virus and their intergenic regions reveals a gene order different from that of other pneumoviruses. *J Gen Virol*, **73**, 1709–15.

Ling, R., Davis, P.J., et al. 1995. Sequence and in vitro expression of the phosphoprotein gene of avian pneumovirus. *Virus Res*, **36**, 247–57.

Loetscher, P., Uguccioni, M., et al. 1998. CCR5 is characteristic of Th1 lymphocytes. *Nature*, **391**, 344–5.

Lu, J., Teh, C., et al. 2002. Collectins and ficolins: sugar pattern recognition molecules of the mammalian innate immune system. *Biochim Biophys Acta*, **1572**, 387–400.

Lugo, R.A. and Nahata, M.C. 1993. Pathogenesis and treatment of bronchiolitis. *Clin Pharm*, **12**, 95–116.

Luther, S.A. and Cyster, J.G. 2001. Chemokines as regulators of T cell differentiation. *Nat Immunol*, **2**, 102–7.

Macartney, K.K., Gorelick, M.H., et al. 2000. Nosocomial respiratory syncytial virus infections: the cost-effectiveness and cost–benefit of infection control. *Pediatrics*, **106**, 520–6.

Madge, P., Paton, J.Y., et al. 1992. Prospective controlled study of four infection-control procedures to prevent nosocomial infection with respiratory syncytial virus. *Lancet*, **340**, 1079–83.

Martinez, I., Valdes, O., et al. 1999. Evolutionary pattern of the G glycoprotein of human respiratory syncytial viruses from antigenic group B: the use of alternative termination codons and lineage diversification. *J Gen Virol*, **80**, 125–30.

McCormack, F.X. and Whitsett, J.A. 2002. The pulmonary collectins, SP-A and SP-D, orchestrate innate immunity in the lung. *J Clin Invest*, **109**, 707–12.

McIntosh, K., Masters, H.B., et al. 1978. The immunologic response to infection with respiratory syncytial virus in infants. *J Infect Dis*, **138**, 24–32.

McNamara, P.S. and Smyth, R.L. 2002. The pathogenesis of respiratory syncytial virus disease in childhood. *Br Med Bull*, **61**, 13–28.

Meguro, H., Kervina, M. and Wright, P.F. 1979. Antibody-dependent cell-mediated cytotoxicity against cells infected with respiratory syncytial virus: characterization of in vitro and in vivo properties. *J Immunol*, **122**, 2521–6.

Midulla, F., Huang, Y.T., et al. 1989. Respiratory syncytial virus infection of human cord and adult blood monocytes and alveolar macrophages. *Am Rev Respir Dis*, **140**, 771–7.

Mills, J.T., Kirk, J.E., et al. 1971. Experimental respiratory syncytial virus infection of adults. Possible mechanisms of resistance to infection and illness. *J Immunol*, **107**, 123–30.

Mlinaric-Galinovic, G. and Varda-Brkic, D. 2000. Nosocomial respiratory syncytial virus infections in children's wards. *Diagn Microbiol Infect Dis*, **37**, 237–46.

Mlinaric-Galinovic, G., Chonmaitree, T., et al. 1994. Antigenic diversity of respiratory syncytial virus subgroup B strains circulating during a community outbreak of infection. *J Med Virol*, **42**, 380–4.

Morris, J.A.J., Blount, R.E. and Savage, R.E. 1956. Recovery of cytopathogenic agent from chimpanzees with coryza. *Proc Soc Exp Biol Med*, **92**, 544–50.

Murphy, B.R., Alling, D.W., et al. 1986a. Effect of age and preexisting antibody on serum antibody response of infants and children to the F and G glycoproteins during respiratory syncytial virus infection. *J Clin Microbiol*, **24**, 894–8.

Murphy, B.R., Graham, B.S., et al. 1986b. Serum and nasal-wash immunoglobulin G and A antibody response of infants and children to respiratory syncytial virus F and G glycoproteins following primary infection. *J Clin Microbiol*, **23**, 1009–14.

Murphy, B.R., Prince, G.A., et al. 1986c. Dissociation between serum neutralizing and glycoprotein antibody responses of infants and children who received inactivated respiratory syncytial virus vaccine. *J Clin Microbiol*, **24**, 197–202.

Murphy, D., Todd, J.K., et al. 1981. The use of gowns and masks to control respiratory illness in pediatric hospital personnel. *J Pediatr*, **99**, 746–50.

Naylor, C.J., Britton, P. and Cavanagh, D. 1998. The ectodomains but not the transmembrane domains of the fusion proteins of subtypes A and B avian pneumovirus are conserved to a similar extent as those of human respiratory syncytial virus. *J Gen Virol*, **79**, 1393–8.

Nicholas, J.A., Rubino, K.L., et al. 1990. Cytolytic T-lymphocyte responses to respiratory syncytial virus: effector cell phenotype and target proteins. *J Virol*, **64**, 4232–41.

Njenga, M.K., Lwamba, H.M. and Seal, B.S. 2002. Metapneumoviruses in birds and humans. *Virus Res*, **83**, 119–29.

Noah, T.L. and Becker, S. 2000. Chemokines in nasal secretions of normal adults experimentally infected with respiratory syncytial virus. *Clin Immunol*, **97**, 43–9.

Noah, T.L., Ivins, S.S., et al. 2002. Chemokines and inflammation in the nasal passages of infants with respiratory syncytial virus bronchiolitis. *Clin Immunol*, **104**, 86–95.

Norrby, E., Marusyk, H. and Orvell, C. 1970. Ultrastructural studies of the multiplication of RS (respiratory syncytial) virus. *Acta Pathol Microbiol Scand [B] Microbiol Immunol*, **78**, 268.

Odum, N., Bregenholt, S., et al. 1999. The CC-chemokine receptor 5 (CCR5) is a marker of, but not essential for the development of human Th1 cells. *Tissue Antigens*, **54**, 572–7.

Olmsted, R.A. and Collins, P.L. 1989. The 1A protein of respiratory syncytial virus is an integral membrane protein present as multiple, structurally distinct species. *J Virol*, **63**, 2019–29.

Olszewska-Pazdrak, B., Casola, A., et al. 1998. Cell-specific expression of RANTES, MCP-1 and MIP-1alpha by lower airway epithelial cells and eosinophils infected with respiratory syncytial virus. *J Virol*, **72**, 4756–64.

Openshaw, P.J. 1995a. Immunity and immunopathology to respiratory syncytial virus. The mouse model. *Am J Respir Crit Care Med*, **152**, S59–62.

Openshaw, P.J. 1995b. Immunopathological mechanisms in respiratory syncytial virus disease. *Springer Semin Immunopathol*, **17**, 187–201.

Openshaw, P.J., Anderson, K., et al. 1990. The 22,000-kilodalton protein of respiratory syncytial virus is a major target for Kd-restricted cytotoxic T lymphocytes from mice primed by infection. *J Virol*, **64**, 1683–9.

Openshaw, P.J., Culley, F.J. and Olszewska, W. 2001. Immunopathogenesis of vaccine-enhanced RSV disease. *Vaccine*, **20**, Suppl 1, S27–31.

Openshaw, P.J.M., Matthews, S., et al. 2002. Immunopathogenesis of viral infections in children. In: Wardlaw, A.J. and Hamid, Q.A. (eds), *Textbook of respiratory cell and molecular biology*. London: Martin Dunitz, 283–98.

Panitch, H.B. 2001. Bronchiolitis in infants. *Curr Opin Pediatr*, **13**, 256–60.

Panitch, H.B., Callahan, C.W. Jr and Schidlow, D.V. 1993. Bronchiolitis in children. *Clin Chest Med*, **14**, 715–31.

Paradiso, P.R., Hu, B., et al. 1989. Antigenic structure of the fusion glycoprotein of respiratory syncytial virus. *Adv Exp Med Biol*, **251**, 273–8.

Paradiso, P.R., Hildreth, S.W., et al. 1994. Safety and immunogenicity of a subunit respiratory syncytial virus vaccine in children 24 to 48 months old. *Pediatr Infect Dis J*, **13**, 792–8.

Parrott, R.H., Kim, H.W., et al. 1973. Epidemiology of respiratory syncytial virus infection in Washington, D.C. II. Infection and disease with respect to age, immunologic status, race and sex. *Am J Epidemiol*, **98**, 289–300.

Pastey, M.K., Crowe, J.E. Jr and Graham, B.S. 1999. RhoA interacts with the fusion glycoprotein of respiratory syncytial virus and facilitates virus-induced syncytium formation. *J Virol*, **73**, 7262–70.

Pastey, M.K., Gower, T.L., et al. 2000. A RhoA-derived peptide inhibits syncytium formation induced by respiratory syncytial virus and parainfluenza virus type 3. *Nat Med*, **6**, 35–40.

Patnayak, D.P., Sheikh, A.M., et al. 2002. Experimental and field evaluation of a live vaccine against avian pneumovirus. *Avian Pathol*, **31**, 377–82.

Paton, A.W., Paton, J.C., et al. 1992. Rapid detection of respiratory syncytial virus in nasopharyngeal aspirates by reverse transcription and polymerase chain reaction amplification. *J Clin Microbiol*, **30**, 901–4.

Peret, T.C., Hall, C.B., et al. 1998. Circulation patterns of genetically distinct group A and B strains of human respiratory syncytial virus in a community. *J Gen Virol*, **79**, 2221–9.

Peret, T.C., Hall, C.B., et al. 2000. Circulation patterns of group A and B human respiratory syncytial virus genotypes in 5 communities in North America. *J Infect Dis*, **181**, 1891–6.

Peret, T.C., Boivin, G., et al. 2002. Characterization of human metapneumoviruses isolated from patients in North America. *J Infect Dis*, **185**, 1660–3.

Power, U.F., Nguyen, T.N., et al. 2001. Safety and immunogenicity of a novel recombinant subunit respiratory syncytial virus vaccine (BBG2Na) in healthy young adults. *J Infect Dis*, **184**, 1456–60.

Price, J.F. 1990. Acute and long-term effects of viral bronchiolitis in infancy. *Lung*, **168**, Suppl, 414–21.

Prince, G.A., Jenson, A.B., et al. 1978. The pathogenesis of respiratory syncytial virus infection in cotton rats. *Am J Pathol*, **93**, 771–91.

Prince, G.A., Horswood, R.L., et al. 1979. Respiratory syncytial virus infection in inbred mice. *Infect Immun*, **26**, 764–6.

Prince, G.A., Jenson, A.B., et al. 1986. Enhancement of respiratory syncytial virus pulmonary pathology in cotton rats by prior intramuscular inoculation of formalin-inactivated virus. *J Virol*, **57**, 721–8.

Pringle, C.R., Filipiuk, A.H., et al. 1993. Immunogenicity and pathogenicity of a triple temperature-sensitive modified respiratory syncytial virus in adult volunteers. *Vaccine*, **11**, 473–8.

Randhawa, J.S., Wilson, S.D., et al. 1996. Nucleotide sequence of the gene encoding the viral polymerase of avian pneumovirus. *J Gen Virol*, **77**, 3047–51.

Richardson, L.S., Yolken, R.H., et al. 1978. Enzyme-linked immunosorbent assay for measurement of serological response to respiratory syncytial virus infection. *Infect Immun*, **20**, 660–4.

Richman, A.V., Pedreira, F.A. and Tauraso, N.M. 1971. Attempts to demonstrate hemagglutination and hemadsorption by respiratory syncytial virus. *Appl Microbiol*, **21**, 1099–100.

Roberts, S.R., Lichtenstein, D., et al. 1994. The membrane-associated and secreted forms of the respiratory syncytial virus attachment glycoprotein G are synthesized from alternative initiation codons. *J Virol*, **68**, 4538–46.

Roosevelt, G., Sheehan, K., et al. 1996. Dexamethasone in bronchiolitis: a randomised controlled trial. *Lancet*, **348**, 292–5.

Routledge, E.G., Willcocks, M.M., et al. 1987. Expression of the respiratory syncytial virus 22K protein on the surface of infected HeLa cells. *J Gen Virol*, **68**, 1217–22.

Sabroe, I., Lloyd, C.M., et al. 2002. Chemokines, innate and adaptive immunity, and respiratory disease. *Eur Respir J*, **19**, 350–5.

Saito, T., Deskin, R.W., et al. 1997. Respiratory syncytial virus induces selective production of the chemokine RANTES by upper airway epithelial cells. *J Infect Dis*, **175**, 497–504.

Samal, S.K. and Collins, P.L. 1996. RNA replication by a respiratory syncytial virus RNA analog does not obey the rule of six and retains a nonviral trinucleotide extension at the leader end. *J Virol*, **70**, 5075–82.

Sanchez, I., De Koster, J., et al. 1993. Effect of racemic epinephrine and salbutamol on clinical score and pulmonary mechanics in infants with bronchiolitis. *J Pediatr*, **122**, 145–51.

Satake, M. and Venkatesan, S. 1984. Nucleotide sequence of the gene encoding respiratory syncytial virus matrix protein. *J Virol*, **50**, 92–9.

Satake, M., Coligan, J.E., et al. 1985. Respiratory syncytial virus envelope glycoprotein (G) has a novel structure. *Nucleic Acids Res*, **13**, 7795–812.

Sauty, A., Colvin, R.A., et al. 2001. CXCR3 internalization following T cell-endothelial cell contact: preferential role of IFN-inducible T cell alpha chemoattractant (CXCL11). *J Immunol*, **167**, 7084–93.

Schlender, J., Bossert, B., et al. 2000. Bovine respiratory syncytial virus nonstructural proteins NS1 and NS2 cooperatively antagonize alpha/beta interferon-induced antiviral response. *J Virol*, **74**, 8234–42.

Schmidt, A.C., Wenzke, D.R., et al. 2002. Mucosal immunization of rhesus monkeys against respiratory syncytial virus subgroups A and B and human parainfluenza virus type 3 by using a live cDNA-derived vaccine based on a host range-attenuated bovine parainfluenza virus type 3 vector backbone. *J Virol*, **76**, 1089–99.

Scott, R., de Landazuri, M.O., et al. 1977. Human antibody-dependent cell-mediated cytotoxicity against target cells infected with respiratory syncytial virus. *Clin Exp Immunol*, **28**, 19–26.

Seal, B.S. 1998. Matrix protein gene nucleotide and predicted amino acid sequence demonstrate that the first US avian pneumovirus isolate is distinct from European strains. *Virus Res*, **58**, 45–52.

Seal, B.S. 2000. Avian pneumoviruses and emergence of a new type in the United States of America. *Anim Health Res Rev*, **1**, 67–72.

Seal, B.S., Sellers, H.S. and Meinersmann, R.J. 2000. Fusion protein predicted amino acid sequence of the first US avian pneumovirus isolate and lack of heterogeneity among other US isolates. *Virus Res*, **66**, 139–47.

Senne, D.A., Edson, R.K., et al. 1997. Avian pneumovirus update. *Proceedings of American Veterinary Medical Association* 134th Annual Congress, Reno, NV, USA, 190.

Shay, D.K., Holman, R.C., et al. 1999. Bronchiolitis-associated hospitalizations among US children, 1980–1996. *JAMA*, **282**, 1440–6.

Shay, D.K., Holman, R.C., et al. 2001. Bronchiolitis-associated mortality and estimates of respiratory syncytial virus-associated deaths among US children, 1979–1997. *J Infect Dis*, **183**, 16–22.

Sheeran, P., Jafri, H., et al. 1999. Elevated cytokine concentrations in the nasopharyngeal and tracheal secretions of children with respiratory syncytial virus disease. *Pediatr Infect Dis J*, **18**, 115–22.

Shepherd, V.L. 2002. Distinct roles for lung collectins in pulmonary host defense. *Am J Respir Cell Mol Biol*, **26**, 257–60.

Shigeta, S. 2000. Recent progress in antiviral chemotherapy for respiratory syncytial virus infections. *Expert Opin Investig Drugs*, **9**, 221–35.

Shin, H.J., Njenga, M.K., et al. 2001. Susceptibility of ducks to avian pneumovirus of turkey origin. *Am J Vet Res*, **62**, 991–4.

Simoes, E.A. 1999. Respiratory syncytial virus infection. *Lancet*, **354**, 847–52.

Simoes, E.A., Sondheimer, H.M., et al. 1998. Respiratory syncytial virus immune globulin for prophylaxis against respiratory syncytial virus disease in infants and children with congenital heart disease. The Cardiac Study Group. *J Pediatr*, **133**, 492–9.

Small, T.N., Casson, A., et al. 2002. Respiratory syncytial virus infection following hematopoietic stem cell transplantation. *Bone Marrow Transplant*, **29**, 321–7.

Smith, T.F., McIntosh, K., et al. 1981. Activation of complement by cells infected with respiratory syncytial virus. *Infect Immun*, **33**, 43–8.

Smyth, R.L., Mobbs, K.J., et al. 2002. Respiratory syncytial virus bronchiolitis: disease severity, interleukin-8, and virus genotype. *Pediatr Pulmonol*, **33**, 339–46.

Snydman, D.R., Greer, C., et al. 1988. Prevention of nosocomial transmission of respiratory syncytial virus in a newborn nursery. *Infect Control Hosp Epidemiol*, **9**, 105–8.

Sparer, T.E., Matthews, S., et al. 1998. Eliminating a region of respiratory syncytial virus attachment protein allows induction of protective immunity without vaccine-enhanced lung eosinophilia. *J Exp Med*, **187**, 1921–6.

Spender, L.C., Hussell, T. and Openshaw, P.J. 1998. Abundant IFN-gamma production by local T cells in respiratory syncytial virus-induced eosinophilic lung disease. *J Gen Virol*, **79**, 1751–8.

Spriggs, M.K., Olmsted, R.A., et al. 1986. Fusion glycoprotein of human parainfluenza virus type 3: nucleotide sequence of the gene, direct identification of the cleavage-activation site, and comparison with other paramyxoviruses. *Virology*, **152**, 241–51.

Srikiatkhachorn, A., Chang, W. and Braciale, T.J. 1999. Induction of Th-1 and Th-2 responses by respiratory syncytial virus attachment glycoprotein is epitope and major histocompatibility complex independent. *J Virol*, **73**, 6590–7.

Staat, M.A. 2002. Respiratory syncytial virus infections in children. *Semin Respir Infect*, **17**, 15–20.

Stec, D.S., Hill, M.G. 3rd and Collins, P.L. 1991. Sequence analysis of the polymerase L gene of human respiratory syncytial virus and predicted phylogeny of nonsegmented negative-strand viruses. *Virology*, **183**, 273–87.

Stockton, J., Stephenson, I., et al. 2002. Human metapneumovirus as a cause of community-acquired respiratory illness. *Emerg Infect Dis*, **8**, 897–901.

Sullender, W.M., Anderson, K. and Wertz, G.W. 1990. The respiratory syncytial virus subgroup B attachment glycoprotein: analysis of sequence, expression from a recombinant vector, and evaluation as an immunogen against homologous and heterologous subgroup virus challenge. *Virology*, **178**, 195–203.

Sullender, W.M., Mufson, M.A., et al. 1991. Genetic diversity of the attachment protein of subgroup B respiratory syncytial viruses. *J Virol*, **65**, 5425–34.

Sullender, W.M., Mufson, M.A., et al. 1998. Antigenic and genetic diversity among the attachment proteins of group A respiratory syncytial viruses that have caused repeat infections in children. *J Infect Dis*, **178**, 925–32.

Syrbe, U., Siveke, J. and Hamann, A. 1999. Th1/Th2 subsets: distinct differences in homing and chemokine receptor expression? *Springer Semin Immunopathol*, **21**, 263–85.

Taber, L.H., Knight, V., et al. 1983. Ribavirin aerosol treatment of bronchiolitis associated with respiratory syncytial virus infection in infants. *Pediatrics*, **72**, 613–18.

Tebbey, P.W., Hagen, M. and Hancock, G.E. 1998. Atypical pulmonary eosinophilia is mediated by a specific amino acid sequence of the attachment (G) protein of respiratory syncytial virus. *J Exp Med*, **188**, 1967–72.

Techaarpornkul, S., Collins, P.L. and Peeples, M.E. 2002. Respiratory syncytial virus with the fusion protein as its only viral glycoprotein is less dependent on cellular glycosaminoglycans for attachment than complete virus. *Virology*, **294**, 296–304.

Teng, M.N. and Collins, P.L. 2002. The central conserved cystine noose of the attachment G protein of human respiratory syncytial virus is not required for efficient viral infection in vitro or in vivo. *J Virol*, **76**, 6164–71.

Teng, M.N., Whitehead, S.S., et al. 2000. Recombinant respiratory syncytial virus that does not express the NS1 or M2-2 protein is highly attenuated and immunogenic in chimpanzees. *J Virol*, **74**, 9317–21.

Teng, M.N., Whitehead, S.S. and Collins, P.L. 2001. Contribution of the respiratory syncytial virus G glycoprotein and its secreted and membrane-bound forms to virus replication in vitro and in vivo. *Virology*, **289**, 283–96.

Tripp, R.A., Moore, D., et al. 1999. Respiratory syncytial virus G and/or SH protein alters Th1 cytokines, natural killer cells, and neutrophils responding to pulmonary infection in BALB/c mice. *J Virol*, **73**, 7099–107.

Tripp, R.A., Jones, L. and Anderson, L.J. 2000a. Respiratory syncytial virus G and/or SH glycoproteins modify CC and CXC chemokine mRNA expression in the BALB/c mouse. *J Virol*, **74**, 6227–9.

Tripp, R.A., Jones, L., et al. 2000b. CD40 ligand (CD154) enhances the Th1 and antibody responses to respiratory syncytial virus in the BALB/c mouse. *J Immunol*, **164**, 5913–21.

Tripp, R.A., Moore, D. and Anderson, L.J. 2000c. TH(1)- and TH(2)-TYPE cytokine expression by activated T lymphocytes from the lung and spleen during the inflammatory response to respiratory syncytial virus. *Cytokine*, **12**, 801–7.

Tripp, R.A., Moore, D., et al. 2000d. Respiratory syncytial virus infection and G and/or SH protein expression contribute to substance P, which mediates inflammation and enhanced pulmonary disease in BALB/c mice. *J Virol*, **74**, 1614–22.

Tripp, R.A., Jones, L.P., et al. 2001. CX3C chemokine mimicry by respiratory syncytial virus G glycoprotein. *Nat Immunol*, **2**, 732–8.

Tripp, R.A., Moore, D., et al. 2002. Peripheral blood mononuclear cells from infants hospitalized because of respiratory syncytial virus infection express T helper-1 and T helper-2 cytokines and CC chemokine messenger RNA. *J Infect Dis*, **185**, 1388–94.

Tripp, R.A., Dakhama, A., et al. 2003. The G glycoprotein of respiratory syncytial virus depresses respiratory rates through the CX3C motif and substance P. *J Virol*, **77**, 6580–4.

Tristram, D.A., Welliver, R.C., et al. 1994. Second-year surveillance of recipients of a respiratory syncytial virus (RSV) F protein subunit vaccine, PFP-1: evaluation of antibody persistence and possible disease enhancement. *Vaccine*, **12**, 551–6.

Tsutsumi, H., Matsuda, K., et al. 1996. Respiratory syncytial virus-induced cytokine production by neonatal macrophages. *Clin Exp Immunol*, **106**, 442–6.

Underhill, D.M. and Ozinsky, A. 2002. Toll-like receptors: key mediators of microbe detection. *Curr Opin Immunol*, **14**, 103–10.

van den Hoogen, B.G., de Jong, J.C., et al. 2001. A newly discovered human pneumovirus isolated from young children with respiratory tract disease. *Nat Med*, **7**, 719–24.

Varga, S.M. and Braciale, T.J. 2002. RSV-induced immunopathology: dynamic interplay between the virus and host immune response. *Virology*, **295**, 203–7.

Varga, S.M., Wang, X., et al. 2001. Immunopathology in RSV infection is mediated by a discrete oligoclonal subset of antigen-specific CD4(+) T cells. *Immunity*, **15**, 637–46.

Vijaya, S., Elango, N., et al. 1988. Transport to the cell surface of a peptide sequence attached to the truncated C terminus of an N-terminally anchored integral membrane protein. *Mol Cell Biol*, **8**, 1709–14.

Villanueva, N., Hardy, R., et al. 2000. The bulk of the phosphorylation of human respiratory syncytial virus phosphoprotein is not essential but modulates viral RNA transcription and replication. *J Gen Virol*, **81**, 129–33.

Wagner, D.K., Muelenaer, P., et al. 1989. Serum immunoglobulin G antibody subclass response to respiratory syncytial virus F and G glycoproteins after first, second, and third infections. *J Clin Microbiol*, **27**, 589–92.

Waris, M.E., Tsou, C., et al. 1996. Respiratory synctial virus infection in BALB/c mice previously immunized with formalin-inactivated virus induces enhanced pulmonary inflammatory response with a predominant Th2-like cytokine pattern. *J Virol*, **70**, 2852–60.

Weisman, L.E. 2002. Current respiratory syncytial virus prevention strategies in high-risk infants. *Pediatr Int*, **44**, 475–80.

Welliver, R.C. 2000. Immunology of respiratory syncytial virus infection: eosinophils, cytokines, chemokines and asthma. *Pediatr Infect Dis J*, **19**, 780–3, discussion 784–5; 811–13.

Welliver, R.C., Kaul, T.N., et al. 1980. The antibody response to primary and secondary infection with respiratory syncytial virus: kinetics of class-specific responses. *J Pediatr*, **96**, 808–13.

Wendt, C.H. 1997. Community respiratory viruses: organ transplant recipients. *Am J Med*, **102**, 31–6, discussion 42–3.

Wertz, G.W., Collins, P.L., et al. 1985. Nucleotide sequence of the G protein gene of human respiratory syncytial virus reveals an unusual type of viral membrane protein. *Proc Natl Acad Sci U S A*, **82**, 4075–9.

Wertz, G.W., Krieger, M. and Ball, L.A. 1989. Structure and cell surface maturation of the attachment glycoprotein of human respiratory syncytial virus in a cell line deficient in O glycosylation. *J Virol*, **63**, 4767–76.

West, J.V. 2002. Acute upper airway infections. *Br Med Bull*, **61**, 215–30.

Whimbey, E. and Ghosh, S. 2000. Respiratory syncytial virus infections in immunocompromised adults. *Curr Clin Top Infect Dis*, **20**, 232–55.

Wright, A.L., Taussig, L.M., et al. 1989. The Tucson Children's Respiratory Study. II. Lower respiratory tract illness in the first year of life. *Am J Epidemiol*, **129**, 1232–46.

Wright, P.F., Karron, R.A., et al. 2000. Evaluation of a live, cold-passaged, temperature-sensitive, respiratory syncytial virus vaccine candidate in infancy. *J Infect Dis*, **182**, 1331–42.

Wright, P.F., Gruber, W.C., et al. 2002. Illness severity, viral shedding, and antibody responses in infants hospitalized with bronchiolitis caused by respiratory syncytial virus. *J Infect Dis*, **185**, 1011–18.

Yachida, S., Aoyama, S., et al. 1978. Plastic multiwell plates to assay avian infectious bronchitis virus in organ cultures of chicken embryo trachea. *J Clin Microbiol*, **8**, 380–7.

Yu, Q., Hardy, R.W. and Wertz, G.W. 1995. Functional cDNA clones of the human respiratory syncytial (RS) virus N, P and L proteins support replication of RS virus genomic RNA analogs and define minimal trans-acting requirements for RNA replication. *J Virol*, **69**, 2412–19.

Zhang, L., Peeples, M.E., et al. 2002. Respiratory syncytial virus infection of human airway epithelial cells is polarized, specific to ciliated cells, and without obvious cytopathology. *J Virol*, **76**, 5654–66.

Zhang, Y., Luxon, B.A., et al. 2001. Expression of respiratory syncytial virus-induced chemokine gene networks in lower airway epithelial cells revealed by cDNA microarrays. *J Virol*, **75**, 9044–58.

Zheng, H., Storch, G.A., et al. 1999. Genetic variability in envelope-associated protein genes of closely related group A strains of respiratory syncytial virus. *Virus Res*, **59**, 89–99.

Zimmer, G., Budz, L. and Herrler, G. 2001. Proteolytic activation of respiratory syncytial virus fusion protein. Cleavage at two furin consensus sequences. *J Biol Chem*, **276**, 31642–50.

38

Paramyxoviruses of animals

PAUL A. ROTA AND THOMAS BARRETT

This chapter describes the clinical and pathological aspects of infections caused by viruses of the family *Paramyxoviridae*, subfamily *Paramyxovirinae* that occur in birds and mammals (Figure 38.1). The emphasis is on viruses that are important veterinary pathogens, as well as those that also cause severe disease when transmitted to humans.

MORBILLIVIRUSES

Within the family *Paramyxoviridae*, members of an antigenically closely related group of viruses, the genus *Morbillivirus* (Figure 38.2) are responsible for some of the most devastating viral diseases in domestic and wild animal populations (Barrett 2001). Generally each virus species causes severe clinical signs in only one order of mammals, but the full host range in terms of infection is unknown. They share many clinical and pathological characteristics; in particular they are all highly immunosuppressive (Heaney et al. 2002). Despite this, animals which recover from an infection develop strong cellular and humoral immune responses, which give subsequent life-long protection, and can also give cross-protection against infection with other morbilliviruses.

Rinderpest

Rinderpest, also known as cattle plague, can infect a variety of cloven hoofed animals, for example cattle, buffalo, yak, and antelope, where it generally causes an acute febrile illness 3–15 days after infection. The term 'cattle plague' is now usually used to denote a severe outbreak of this disease in nonendemic areas, whereas 'rinderpest' is the term used most often in endemic regions. The last outbreak of classical cattle plague with very high mortality and economic losses occurred in Pakistan in 1994–1995 (Rossiter et al. 1998). In its most severe form it has been characterized as the disease of the three Ds: discharge, diarrhea, and death. Historically, rinderpest has been a major problem in Europe and Asia, but it was eliminated from Europe by the beginning of the twentieth century using zoosanitary control measures. Sporadic introductions, which were quickly contained, occurred in Europe, the Americas, and Australia in the early twentieth century. This led to the establishment of the Office International des Epizooties (OIE), an international veterinary organization which acts as a World Health Organization for animal diseases. As the disease was being eliminated from Europe it was introduced into Africa in about 1887 and caused a major pandemic on that continent killing over 90 percent of the cattle and buffalo, resulting in great social and economic hardship (Barrett and Rossiter 1999; Mack 1970).

CLINICAL AND PATHOLOGICAL MANIFESTATIONS

Virus enters by the respiratory route and replicates in the draining lymph nodes of the head and throat. White blood cells, lymphoblasts, and macrophages become infected and the virus spreads via the blood and lymph to other lymphatic tissues, and then to the lungs, mucous membranes, and gastrointestinal tract. Virus excretion begins 24–48 h before the onset of clinical signs and lasts for 7–10 days. Typically, the animal develops nasal and ocular congestion, which progresses to give profuse lacrimal and nasal discharges which can become mucopurulent. Necrotic lesions appear on all mucous

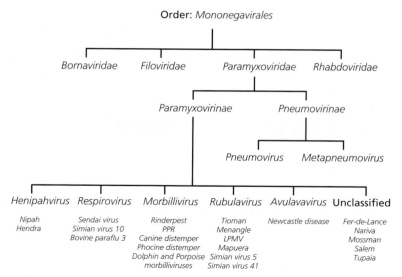

Figure 38.1 *Classification of the viruses within the order* Mononegavirales. *Family* Paramyxoviridae *is divided into two subfamilies, and there are five genera within the subfamily* Paramyxovirinae.

membranes, especially in the mouth where the lips, gums, buccal papillae, and tongue can be affected. Lesions on the mucous membranes and in the gastro-intestinal tract are responsible for the severe manifestations of the disease. The animals become depressed, anorexic, and emaciated because the mouth lesions make eating painful. The intestinal pain causes them to arch their backs and the hair becomes rough and soiled by the mucopurulent discharge and watery, often bloody, diarrhea. Severe diarrhea results in dehydration and the animals have sunken eyes and reduced skin turgor. Pregnant animals usually abort and recovery is prolonged in survivors, but results in life-long protection from disease. Pathological findings include severe

lymphodepletion, necrosis of the Peyer's patches and lesions in many parts of the digestive tract. The blood becomes concentrated and slow to circulate and the blood vessels in the longitudinal folds of the large intestine become distended and appear prominent, giving a marked striped appearance, the so-called zebra stripes. The lungs are generally minimally affected in rinderpest infections. Mortality can be as high as 70–90 percent in such severe cases, but there is considerable variation in the severity of symptoms, and even asymptomatic infections can occur, depending on the virulence of the virus strain involved and the host's innate resistance. Cattle of *Bos indicus* species are more resistant than *Bos taurus* species (Scott 1990). In endemic areas, mortalities of

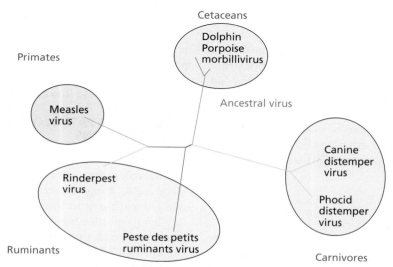

Figure 38.2 *Phylogenetic tree showing the relationships between the different morbilliviruses based on partial sequence of the P gene. A universal primer set was used to amplify a 429-base pair DNA fragment as described by Barrett et al. (1993). The tree was derived using the PHYLIP DNADIST and FITCH programmes (Felsenstein 1997). The branch lengths are proportional to the mutational differences between the viruses and the hypothetical common ancestor that existed at the nodes in the tree.*

30 percent, or less, are more normal. The pathogenesis of rinderpest infection has been extensively described (Brown and Torres 1994; Wamwayi et al. 1995; Wohlsein et al. 1993, 1995). The disease follows a similar course in wildlife species, except that skin lesions and corneal opacity are often seen, especially in buffalo and kudu, and this greatly increases the risk of predation (Kock et al. 1999).

EPIZOOTIOLOGY

The virus is present in all secretions and excretions from the infected animal but, since the virus is labile, it requires close contact for infection to occur, most often by infected air droplets. Contaminated fomites can also be a source of infection but nearly all outbreaks can be traced to the introduction of unvaccinated stock infected with the virus (Wamwayi et al. 1992; Rossiter 2001a; Rossiter et al. 1998). In endemic areas, rinderpest disease is most often seen in animals less than 2 years of age, as older animals are generally immune due to previous exposure. Maternal immunity protects the very young for up to 6 months. Until the mid-1990s, rinderpest was endemic in many parts of southern Asia, the Middle East, and Africa (Rweyemamu and Cheneau 1995); however, the intense vaccination campaigns carried out over the past decade have reduced the endemic region to a small area of eastern Africa on the borders of Somalia and Kenya. There are three distinct lineages of the virus, two African and a third found exclusively in Asia (Barrett et al., 1998) (Figure 38.3). The virus remaining in this last endemic focus is of African lineage 2 and appears to be maintained in cattle as a mild infection, but it becomes clinically apparent when it spreads, by means of trade and cattle movement, to areas where there are susceptible wildlife species such as buffalo, eland, and kudu (Kock et al. 1999). It has been suggested that rinderpest is the archetypal morbillivirus and it is likely that other morbilliviruses evolved form a ruminant virus of this type (Norrby et al. 1985).

CONTROL

All morbilliviruses are very sensitive to inactivation by heat, ultraviolet (UV) light, and chemicals, especially ones that disrupt the lipid envelope, so zoosanitary measures are very effective in controlling these infections. There is no effective treatment for rinderpest, but infection can easily be prevented by vaccination using a tissue culture attenuated vaccine developed by Plowright and Ferris (1962). There is only one serotype of rinderpest virus, as is the case for other morbillivirus species, and the attenuated vaccine is safe and gives life-long protection with a single shot. The main disadvantage of the vaccine is the inability to distinguish the vaccinated from naturally infected and recovered animals in serological assays. This would be a very useful characteristic to have at this final stage in the global eradication campaign and research is in progress to develop marker vaccines (Walsh et al. 2000).

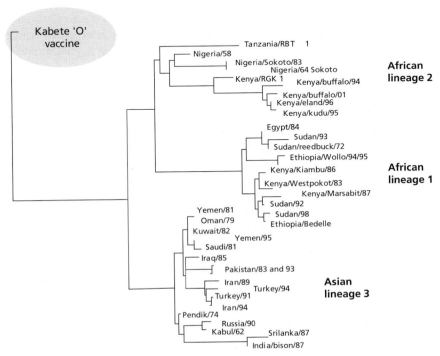

Figure 38.3 *The relationships between the different rinderpest viruses based on partial sequence data derived from the various fusion protein genes. A specific primer set was used to amplify a 372-base pair DNA fragment as described by Forsyth and Barrett (1995). The tree was derived as described in Figure 38.2.*

In nonendemic areas, a quarantine and slaughter policy has proved the most effective means of control. However, in endemic regions, or where cultural considerations prohibit slaughter, mass vaccination accompanied by restriction of animal movement and market closures are the control measures used. Because of the severe economic losses incurred as a result of rinderpest in Africa and Asia in the 1980s, a concerted international control and vaccination program was set up. This is now known as the Global Rinderpest Eradication Programme (GREP) with a target of eradication by 2010.

LABORATORY DIAGNOSIS

Rapid and accurate diagnosis of rinderpest has important implications for disease control programs as the clinical signs can be confused with those of other less serious diseases, such as bovine viral diarrhea and malignant catarrhal fever viruses. Classic cattle plague can be diagnosed clinically in nonendemic areas relatively easily but mild rinderpest, or disease in vaccinated populations, can only be diagnosed with certainty by laboratory testing. The virus can be detected by isolation in tissue culture cells (either primary bovine kidney cells or B95a cells), by antigen detection using various assays, for example agarose gel immunodiffusion, counterimmunoelectrophoresis, or preferably immunocapture enzyme-linked immunosorbent assay (ELISA) (Anderson et al. 1996; Libeau et al. 1994). A pen-side test, based on the use of virus-specific monoclonal antibodies, has been developed to detect virus antigen in samples taken in the field and this has greatly helped veterinarians investigating a potential outbreak to diagnose the disease and differentiate it from others with similar clinical manifestations (Wambura et al. 2000). Recently, reverse transcription polymerase chain reaction (RT-PCR) has been the method of choice for laboratory diagnosis as the resulting PCR product can be sequenced to give valuable information on the strain of virus involved (Forsyth and Barrett 1995; Barrett et al. 1998). Antibody responses can be detected in surviving animals, or following vaccination, by virus neutralization assays; however, for the large numbers of sera that are required to be tested for control programs a competitive ELISA has been developed which has proved highly robust and is routinely used in laboratories in countries where the virus remains a threat (Anderson and McKay 1994; Anderson et al. 1996). This assay is also being used for serosurveillance purposes to ensure that countries are free, and remain free, of disease.

Peste des petits ruminants virus

Peste des petits ruminants (PPR) is a disease mainly of sheep and goats, which is clinically very similar to rinderpest in large ruminants. Where it occurs it is considered to be one of the most economically important diseases in these species. Generally goats are more sensitive to PPR than sheep, but that can be strain-dependent. The disease was first seen in West Africa in the 1940s (Gargadennec and Lalanne 1942), but is now known to be widely distributed in sub-Saharan Africa. In the 1990s the Arabian peninsula, the Middle East, and most parts of the Indian subcontinent were swept by an epizootic of PPR where it has remained (Dhar et al. 2002; Ozkul et al. 2002).

CLINICAL AND PATHOLOGICAL MANIFESTATIONS

Like rinderpest, peste des petits ruminants virus (PPRV) infection is characterized by high fever, ocular and nasal discharges, necrosis in the mouth, and inflammation of the gastrointestinal tract leading to diarrhea and dehydration (Rossiter 2001b). However, unlike rinderpest in cattle, interstitial and suppurative pneumonia is commonly found in PPRV-infected animals and secondary bacterial infections (usually *Pasteurella* spp.) are often a complicating factor and so it can be easily confused with contagious caprine pleuropneumonia (CCPP). The pathological findings are very similar to those described for rinderpest infections, apart from the more marked lung involvement and severe bronchopneumonia. Giant cells are seen in the bronchioles and terminal alveoli, usually with intracytoplasmic and intranuclear inclusion bodies (Rossiter 2001b). Mortality rates in PPR epizootics can range from 10 to 90 percent and may vary with the host's innate resistance, body condition, age, complications resulting from secondary bacterial and parasitic infections, and perhaps, the virulence of the virus involved (Kitching 1988). However, little research has been carried out to establish these as facts.

EPIZOOTIOLOGY

The virus circulates in endemic areas in sheep and goats, but the full host range of this virus is unknown. There is no indirect transmission of the virus and no known wildlife reservoir; however, captive wildlife are known to be highly susceptible. Several species of wild antelope died as a result of infection in a zoo in the United Arab Emirates (Furley et al. 1987) and recently an epizootic killed many gazelle in a game park in Saudi Arabia (Abu Elzein et al. 2004). In West Africa, PPR is more prevalent in the more humid areas and shows a seasonal pattern. In the Middle East, the intensive trading of small ruminants for religious festivals spreads the virus. Due to the clinical and morphologic similarities of rinderpest and PPR, there was considerable confusion regarding which virus was circulating in large and small ruminants, especially in Asia, as these strains of rinderpest were known to infect sheep and goats and result in clinical disease. PPRV infection has been reported in buffalo in India and in cattle in West Africa (Anderson and McKay 1994; Govindarajan et al. 1997). This can interfere with the take of the rinderpest vaccine and cause confusion in serological surveillance; however, if the GREP is successful, this will no longer be an issue. PPRV isolates have been grouped into four distinct lineages on the basis of fusion (F) protein gene sequence similarities and they reflect the geographical distribution of virus strains (Shaila et al. 1996; Dhar et al. 2002) (Figure 38.4).

CONTROL

Zoosanitary measures, as applied to rinderpest control, are effective but often difficult to implement because of the large numbers of animals involved and the nomadic nature of many small ruminant pastoralists. These are often amongst the poorest members of society and depend very heavily on small ruminants for economic survival. Vaccination of herds is the most effective means of controlling PPR and at first, because of the close antigenic relatedness, the rinderpest vaccine was used to protect animals against PPR, but a homologous vaccine has now been developed and is widely used to control the disease (Couacy-Hymann et al. 1995). In endemic areas, captive wild animals should be kept well separated from local sheep and goat flocks, as the safety of the PPR vaccine in wild species has not yet been established.

LABORATORY DIAGNOSIS

The virus can be isolated most easily in primary sheep or goat kidney or skin cell cultures and it can also be grown after several blind passages in Vero cells. Laboratory techniques for detecting the virus have developed in parallel with those for rinderpest because of the need for differential diagnosis of the two infections and specific antibody, antigen and RNA detection tests are now available to distinguish the two viruses (Forsyth and Barrett 1995; Anderson et al. 1996; Libeau et al. 1994).

Canine distemper virus

Canine distemper virus infects a variety of carnivores, most notably the dog, mink, and ferret among domestic species. The epizootiology in wild carnivores is poorly understood but infections in these species have been more extensively studied in recent years.

CLINICAL AND PATHOLOGICAL MANIFESTATIONS

Disease is most often seen in young animals, but can also occur in older animals. Infection begins in the upper respiratory tract and, after an incubation period which can range from 1 to 6 weeks, spreads in a similar fashion to other morbilliviruses, that is from the local lymph nodes via the lymph and blood to other lymphatic

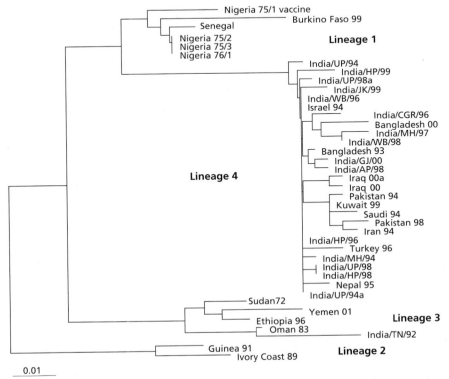

Figure 38.4 *The relationships between the different peste des petits ruminants viruses based on partial sequence data derived from the fusion protein gene. A specific primer set was used to amplify a 372-base pair DNA fragment as described by Forsyth and Barrett (1995). The tree was derived as described in Figure 38.2.*

tissues and then to the upper and lower respiratory tracts, gastrointestinal mucosa, and brain. Following an initial febrile response, infected animals suffer depression and develop mucopurulent nasal and ocular discharges, vomiting, diarrhea, and pneumonia, signs commonly seen in other morbillivirus infections. A dry cough may develop which progresses to a moist cough. However, the most striking difference between canine distemper and the ruminant morbilliviruses is the virus' ability to infect neurons and other cells of the nervous system, but the neurotropism of isolates can also vary considerably (Stettler et al. 1997). Brain infection results in a nonsuppurative encephalitis, meningoencephalitis, neuronal necrosis, and demyelination. Neurological signs such as seizures, tremors, disorientation, incoordination, coma, or behavioral changes are often present and can develop acutely weeks or months later. Another aspect of the disease that differs from that caused by rinderpest and PPR infections is a hyperkeratosis that commonly develops on the foot pads (so-called 'hard pad'). There can be considerable variation in the severity of disease and this is partly related to differences in the infecting strain, often referred to as a biotype, and the individual and species involved (Appel 1987). A strong humoral antibody response to the virus may result in mild or inapparent disease and the virus is cleared quickly but if a weak response is mounted, and the animal recovers from the inevitable disease, it can shed virus for 2 to 3 months. While early development of circulating antibody has been shown to be crucial for protection and recovery from canine distemper infections that is not the case for the ruminant morbilliviruses where a cell-mediated response appears to be more important for protection.

EPIZOOTIOLOGY

Canine distemper is found worldwide, with the exception of hot arid regions, and results in periodic disease outbreaks, mostly seen in domestic dogs, but a variety of wildlife species are highly susceptible. For example, disease has been observed in several species of large cat in American zoos, lions and hyenas in the Serengeti plains in Africa, javelinas in Arizona, ferrets, mink, raccoons, coyotes, badgers, foxes, bears, pandas, and seals (Appel 1987; Appel and Summers 1995; Haas et al. 1996; Harder et al. 1996; Roelke-Parker et al. 1996). A retrospective study of pathological specimens from large cats that died of unknown causes in a Swiss zoo indicated that canine distemper was not a new infection in these species (Myers et al. 1997). Ferrets are particularly susceptible to distemper infections and the virus has threatened the survival of the black-footed ferret, a highly endangered species in the USA (Carpenter et al. 1976). Virus is usually maintained in dog populations by transmission to susceptible young via respiratory, ocular, and nasal secretions, which contain the virus. Like all morbilliviruses, it is highly contagious but requires close contact for transmission. In enzootic areas, the density of the susceptible population is an important factor in maintenance and spread and disease is most often seen in young animals after the maternal antibody has waned. In isolated populations, as for other morbilliviruses, epizootics occur which can be severe and affect all age groups (Leighton et al. 1988).

CONTROL

Modified live virus vaccines, the Onderstepoort and Rockborn strains developed in the 1950s, have been very successful in controlling disease in domestic dogs and mink. Maternal antibody decreases the effectiveness of the vaccine, so vaccine should be given after maternal antibody begins to wane at 6–9 weeks of age (Chapuis 1995). Most vaccination protocols recommend giving a second dose at 12–15 weeks of age to ensure an effective vaccination. Live virus vaccines have also been used in nondomestic species, but this is risky and they should only be used if proven safe in that species. Vaccine-induced immunosuppression can be a problem in animals such as the panda (Bush et al. 1976; Deem et al. 2000). Threatened and endangered wild carnivores are best protected by ensuring good vaccination cover in domestic dogs living near wildlife reservations and minimizing contact. Domestic dogs were considered the most likely source of the virus that infected the lions, hyenas, and wild dogs in Africa (Roelke-Parker et al. 1996).

LABORATORY DIAGNOSIS

The virus can be isolated in cell culture or virus-specific antigens and RNA can be detected in infected secretions, blood, and affected tissues. Vero and dog kidney cells have been used for virus isolation, although not all strains grow well in these culture systems. Pulmonary alveolar macrophages and mitogen-stimulated canine or ferret blood lymphocytes are the most sensitive cell culture system for canine distemper virus (Appel et al. 1992). Viral antigens can be detected by immunofluorescence in conjunctival smears or by immunohistochemistry carried out on fixed tissues. Viral RNA can be detected by RT-PCR assays using specific primer sets (Forsyth and Barrett 1995; Kennedy et al. 2000). The most important differential diagnosis is for rabies virus because of the implications for human health.

Morbillivirus infections of aquatic mammals

Morbillivirus infections in marine mammals were unknown before 1987, but since then several newly recognized members of the genus *Morbillivirus* have been identified as the etiological agent of disease and mortality in the orders *Pinnipedia* (seals) and *Cetacea* (whales, porpoises, and dolphins). The first to be recognized was phocine (seal) distemper virus, which had severe ecological consequences for the European harbor seal (*Phoca vitulina*). Thousands of this species died along the coasts of northern Europe in 1988 (Osterhaus and Vedder 1988). The virus was also identified in European gray seals (*Halichoerus grypus*), but they have proved to be more resistant to the virus. Subsequently two other morbilliviruses were isolated from marine mammals, namely the dolphin and porpoise morbilliviruses (Barrett and Rima 2002; Kennedy et al. 1988; Domingo et al. 1990). The genetic similarity of the dolphin and porpoise viruses would indicate that they are variations of the same virus and they are collectively referred to as the cetacean morbillivirus (Barrett et al. 1993). Canine distemper virus has also been shown to infect and kill several species of seal (Kennedy et al. 2000; Grachev et al. 1989; Mamaev et al. 1995).

CLINICAL MANIFESTATIONS

Seals infected with either phocine distemper virus or canine distemper virus show a loss of body condition (reduced blubber thickness) along with the normal signs of a morbillivirus infection, fever, serous or mucopurulent oculonasal discharge, conjunctivitis, dyspnea, diarrhea, lethargy nervous signs, and abortion in pregnant females. Pneumonia was the main gross pathological finding in seals with the airways containing mucopurulent, blood-stained, or frothy exudates. Central nervous system (CNS) degeneration was also observed. Clinical data for infected cetaceans are less comprehensive as sick animals have not been observed under confined conditions and no experimental infections have been carried out. During the epizootic in the Mediterranean in 1990–1991, many striped dolphins (*Stenella coeruleoalba*) were found to be in poor body condition and loss of fat stores led to decreased buoyancy. Skin lesions and necrosis of the buccal mucosa, lymphodepletion, and hemoconcentration were commonly observed. Other clinical signs in striped dolphins included tachycardia, abnormal respiratory rates, lethargy, and reduced sound emissions. Bronchopneumonia was the most marked pathological feature in dolphins, along with CNS degeneration. The majority of the sick seals and dolphins had nonsuppurative encephalitis, some with signs of demyelination, which explained their behavioral changes (Domingo et al. 1992; Duignan et al. 1992).

EPIZOOTIOLOGY

Phocine distemper virus

The small size and scattered nature of European seal populations means it is unlikely that they could maintain this virus in circulation and indeed the virus disappeared from these populations following the epizootic in 1988. In 2002, another outbreak, following an almost identical course, occurred. Infection most probably results when interspecies transmission introduces or reintroduces the

virus to a susceptible population. The similarities in the course of the two European outbreaks may be explained by the migratory and breeding habits of the seals and there is a growing consensus among some seal biologists that gray seals may be key vectors in the transmission of phocine distemper between harbor seal colonies in European waters. This is especially so where large geographical jumps are made. Harbor seals usually return to the same haulout, whereas gray seals do not and move much greater distances between these sites. Another factor may be the relative resistance of this species to the virus enabling it to transmit without necessarily showing severe clinical disease. Since it is likely that most virus transmission occurs on land, their mixing at shared haulout sites most probably explains the timing in early summer to autumn. More than 20 000 seals died during each of the two European phocine distemper outbreaks. The original source of virus in the 1988 and 2002 outbreaks was probably Arctic harp seals (*Phoca groenlandica*), which came into contact with northern European gray seals (Dietz et al. 1989). Serological evidence suggests that the disease is endemic in many species of Arctic seals and has affected Atlantic walruses (*Odobenus rosmarus*), but the full host range and clinical disease induced in most species has not been fully determined (Duignan et al. 1997; Nielsen et al. 2000). Phocine distemper virus can also threaten terrestrial mammals and during the 1988 epizootic in Europe the virus clinically infected farmed mink in Denmark (Blixenkrone-Møller et al. 1990) and there is evidence for phocine distemper and dolphin distemper virus antibodies in Canadian terrestrial carnivores (Philippa et al. 2004).

As mentioned above, phocine distemper is not the only morbillivirus known to cause disease in seals and canine distemper virus infection can also result in significant mortality in these species. Immediately prior to the European seal epizootic, during the winter of 1987–1988, Lake Baikal seals (*Phoca sibirica*) suffered an unusual and severe mortality and there was no possible epidemiological connection between the two events (Grachev et al. 1989). Subsequently canine distemper virus, rather than phocine distemper virus, was shown to have been the etiological agent in the outbreak (Mamaev et al. 1995). Similarly, mass die-offs occurred in Caspian Sea seals (*Phoca caspica*) in 1997 and 2000, which were also attributed to canine distemper virus (Forsyth et al. 1998; Kennedy et al. 2000). Although not proven, the source of the virus is likely to have terrestrial carnivores, such as wolves, which prey on seal pups. Canine distemper virus has also been implicated in the deaths of thousands of crabeater seals (*Lobodon carcinophagus*) in the Antarctic in the 1950s. Since there are no terrestrial carnivores in the Antarctic, it is thought likely that sledge dogs used at that time were the source of the virus, or possibly the animals were infected by contact with carnivores in New Zealand or South America during migrations. A subsequent serological survey of Antarctic seals showed them to have a high prevalence of canine distemper-specific antibodies (Bengtson et al. 1991). All morbillivirus infections in seals are clinically similar and so differential diagnosis has to be made, which is most easily done by RT-PCR using universal morbillivirus primer sets and primer sets specific for each virus species (Mamaev et al. 1995; Kennedy et al. 2000).

Cetacean morbillivirus

Cetacean species in all the major oceans of the world have been reported to be seropositive for this virus (Duignan et al. 1996; Van Bressem et al. 2001). The pilot whale (*Globicephala* spp.) appears to be the reservoir and vector for transmission of the cetacean morbillivirus to other species. They move in large groups, known as pods, over great ocean distances and have a worldwide distribution. Over 90 percent of pilot whales involved in mass strandings between 1982 and 1993 were morbillivirus seropositive (Duignan et al. 1995a, b). Although the first report of a cetacean morbillivirus was in 1988 in a porpoise caught off the coast of Northern Ireland (Kennedy et al. 1988), subsequently it was shown that a mass die-off of Atlantic bottlenose dolphins (*Tursiops truncatus*) that occurred along the Atlantic coast of the USA in 1987–1988 was probably the result of morbillivirus infection since more than 50 percent of the animals were found to be morbillivirus positive (Lipscomb et al. 1994). Originally the mortality was thought to have been due to brevitoxins produced by red tides of dinoflagellates. Another epizootic occurred in the Gulf of Mexico in 1993–1994 (Lipscomb et al. 1994). There is also serological evidence of exposure of Florida manatees (order *Sirenia*) to morbillivirus infection but no reports of disease or unusual mortality in this species have been reported (Duignan et al. 1995c).

Some evidence also links the cetacean morbillivirus with seal mortality, although not on the same massive scale seen with phocine or canine distemper viruses. A minor outbreak of disease in seals occurred 1998 along the Belgian and northern French coasts and morbillivirus antigen and nucleic acid were detected in tissues from sick animals which were genetically closely related to either the cetacean morbillivirus or canine distemper virus (Jauniaux et al. 1998). The rare monk seal population of the eastern Mediterranean was not severely affected during an epizootic of this virus which killed thousands of striped dolphins in these waters in 1990–1991; however, the cetacean morbillivirus was found in carcasses of monk seals that died in large numbers off the coast of Mauritania in 1997 (Van de Bildt et al. 2000). At the time, an algal bloom was also considered to be an exacerbating or primary factor, which may have contributed to the very high mortality among adult seals at that time (Harwood 1998).

The long-term effects on marine mammal populations infected with morbilliviruses is not clear and will depend on whether the species concerned is already at dangerously low numbers, for example the Mediterranean monk seals and the Caspian Sea seals (Kennedy et al. 2000; Osterhaus et al. 1992). The catastrophic die-off in one of the few remaining colonies of monk seals off the Mauritanean coast in 1997 wiped out an estimated 70 percent of the population within the space of 1 month, a figure representing about one-third of the total world population, leaving only a few hundred remaining (Harwood 1998). However, in populations with healthier numbers, the situation is not so serious and following the 1988 epizootic the European seal populations recovered their normal levels within a few years.

CONTROL

Control of wildlife diseases is extremely difficult and vaccination poses great logistical problems. One exception has been the success in controlling rabies in wildlife using the vaccinia virus recombinant vaccine, but this required very long and careful development (Pastoret and Brochier 1996). Similar attempts at vaccinating seals with a vaccinia recombinant expressing the canine distemper virus fusion (F) protein failed as the virus did not replicate and elicit an immune response (Van Bressem et al. 1991). Vaccination of wildlife also raises ethical questions concerning the effects of the disturbance such an intervention would have on the population and whether there would be uncontrolled spread of the vaccine in the environment. Protection of vulnerable animals in marine wildlife parks and seal sanctuaries would be acceptable as the animals could be confined until the excretion of any vaccine virus had ceased. In any event, there is no currently licensed vaccine for use in these species. Because of the close antigenic relationship between morbilliviruses, strong cross-protection to infection is given by vaccines for other morbilliviruses. An experimental CDV-ISCOM vaccine has been shown to protect seals from PDV, but the duration of the immunity induced remains uncertain (Visser et al. 1992). Canine distemper vaccines have not been fully tested for safety in seals and these vaccines have been shown to cause death in other wildlife species (Bush et al. 1976; Carpenter et al. 1976; Sutherland-Smith et al. 1997); however, a small trial of live attenuated canine distemper vaccine in seals was successfully carried out in England during the 2002 phocine distemper outbreak. The consensus at present is that wildlife is best protected by vaccination to control diseases in domestic species, for example vaccination of cattle has proved an effective means of eliminating rinderpest from wildlife in Africa, but this is not an option for protecting marine mammals from morbillivirus infection since the marine morbilliviruses are rarely found in terrestrial mammals. Because of the threat posed by canine distemper to seals, it is recommended that unvaccinated dogs should not be allowed to mix with seals and sledge dogs are no longer used in the Antarctic.

AVULAVIRUSES (NEWCASTLE DISEASE VIRUS)

Newcastle disease virus (NDV) is responsible for outbreaks of severe disease among poultry throughout the world. Since outbreaks reported to the OIE result in severe trade limitations, this disease has serious economic consequences. NDV, also called fowl pest or avian paramyxovirus type 1 (APMV-1), is a member of the subfamily *Paramyxovirinae*. Recently, avian para-myxoviruses have been designated as a new genus, *Avulavirus* (Chang et al. 2001). The genomes of several rubulaviruses, except NDV, contain a small hydrophobic (SH) protein gene that is also not present among the respiroviruses (Lamb and Kolakofsky 2001). Interest-ingly, the avian paramyxovirus-6 (APMV6) genome was reported to contain a putative SH protein gene (Chang et al. 2001).

Clinical manifestations of infection

NDV causes epidemic disease in a wide range of domes-ticated and wild birds, most notably among poultry (Alexander 1995). It has been isolated from all orders of birds. The incubation period averages 5–6 days, with a range of 2–15 days. The type and severity of disease varies with the infecting virus strain, as well as the age and species of the infected bird. For example, younger chickens are subject to more severe disease than older chickens. Although there is a continuum of clinical presentations, isolates have been separated arbitrarily into four groups based on the presence of enteric or neural disease and the speed with which they kill embry-onating hens' eggs. All strains reduce egg production in chickens.

NDV strains are divided into three pathotypes based on disease severity (Alexander 1997). Lentogenic strains are associated with no, or mild, respiratory tract symp-toms and some have been developed into live virus vaccines. Young birds are most likely to develop illness when infected with these strains. The mesogenic form is associated with an acute respiratory illness of moderate severity that is sometimes associated with life-threatening nervous system complications. Neurotropic velogenic strains are associated with respiratory and neurological disease, such as paralysis of the legs. In outbreaks, death can occur in 5–10 percent or more of infected birds. Viscerotropic-velogenic strains cause an acute, often lethal, infection with hemorrhagic gastro-intestinal lesions. In outbreaks, mortality rates can be as high as 90 percent.

Virulence of NDV is dependent on the amino acid sequence of the cleavage site of the F protein (Glickman et al. 1988), which determines the ability of the F protein to be cleaved by cellular proteases (Gotoh et al. 1992). Mesogenic or velogenic strains have dibasic amino acids in the F protein cleavage sequence, while the F proteins of lentogenic NDV strains do not have this motif (Glickman et al. 1988).

Both wild-type and vaccine strains of NDV can infect humans (Chang 1981). After an incubation period of 1–4 days, the patient sometimes develops conjunctivitis, which is usually unilateral and, occasionally, systemic symptoms such as fever, myalgia, and malaise. Symp-toms usually resolve within a week.

Epizootiology

NDV can spread by inhalation or ingestion of infectious virus. Large amounts of infectious virus can be excreted in the feces, which is likely to be the source of infectious virus in most instances. NDV can be introduced into new populations through natural movement of infected birds (e.g. migration, shipping infected birds from one location to another) or by fomites such as contaminated food, equipment, or water. The virus can be transmitted quickly and efficiently in crowded populations, such as poultry houses. Humans presumably become infected by contamination of the hands and autoinoculation of the conjunctiva or by inhalation of aerosolized virus. Most human infections have occurred after exposure to wild-type virus in slaughterhouses or laboratories or while administering the vaccine.

Pathology, pathogenesis, and immune response

The virus infects via the respiratory or gastrointestinal tract or the conjunctivae. With virulent strains, the virus first causes a local lytic infection and then the bird becomes viremic and the virus spreads to infect multiple organs, including the brain, heart, kidneys, and reticulo-endothelial system. The speed and efficiency with which it infects different tissues seem to be key to its virulence and this, in turn, depends on the host species and strain of NDV. Efficient cleavage of the glycoproteins in a wide range of cell types is characteristic of highly viru-lent strains (Rott and Klenk 1988). The titer of the inoculum can also alter the course of the infection. A low-titer inoculum can ameliorate disease caused by a virulent strain.

Vaccination or naturally acquired infection confers resistance to further disease. Passively acquired antibody can also provide protection from disease. It has not yet been determined which components of the immune response are responsible for controlling and clearing established infection in the bird.

Laboratory diagnosis

Diagnosis of NDV is often important in the context of control measures that are to be undertaken, and requires isolation and the characterization of the virus as virulent, avirulent, or possibly vaccinelike. Respiratory, fecal, or cloacal specimens from live birds or tissue specimens from affected organs from dead birds can be used to isolate the virus. Cell culture systems or embryonic chicken (or other fowl) eggs from flocks known to be pathogen-free or NDV-free can be used to isolate the virus. The virus is then characterized by determining its virulence in embryonating hens' eggs, day-old chicks or 6-week-old chickens. Molecular methods to characterize strains and track transmission are being developed and may provide alternative ways to determine virulence (Seal et al. 1995; Alexander 1999).

Antibodies against NDV can be detected by a variety of tests, including neutralization, hemagglutination inhibition and enzyme immunoassays (EIA). Antibody tests have been used primarily to demonstrate past infection or a response to vaccination.

Control

Vaccination and transmission control programs have been used to prevent NDV infection. Live virus vaccines developed from B1 or Lasota lentogenic strains are most widely used. For poultry, the vaccines can be administered in a variety of ways: orally in water, by intranasal or intraocular inoculation, or by aerosols. Quarantine of imported birds and quarantine and slaughter of infected flocks have been an integral part of NDV control in a number of countries.

Other avian paramyxoviruses

Eight other serotypes of avian paramyxoviruses have been isolated from a variety of birds. Although NDV is the most important pathogen from an economic standpoint, other viruses in the group have sometimes been associated with serious disease.

HENIPAVIRUSES

Viruses belonging to the recently described genus *Henipavirus* within the family *Paramyxoviridae* emerged during the past decade. These viruses were initially identified as the etiologic agents responsible for outbreaks of febrile respiratory illnesses of veterinary livestock. When transmitted to humans from infected animals, these viruses were responsible for severe encephalitic or respiratory diseases that often had fatal outcomes (Murray et al. 1995a; Chua et al. 2000). The two viruses in this genus, Hendra virus and Nipah virus are different from most other paramyxoviruses because they have a broad host range both in vivo and in vitro. Fruit-eating bats appear to be a natural reservoir for the henipaviruses, although isolation of these viruses from this reservoir has been infrequent. Humans are infected via intermediate hosts such as horses or pigs, by exposure to infected fruit bats, or by direct human-to-human transmission.

Hendra virus is the type species of the genus *Henipavirus*, and both Hendra virus and Nipah virus have genetic characteristics and replication strategies that are similar to those of other members of the subfamily *Paramyxovirinae*. The henipaviruses also have several unique genetic features that distinguish them. The genomes of Hendra virus and Nipah virus are 18 234 and 18 246 nucleotides, respectively, making them the largest paramyxovirus genomes reported (Harcourt et al. 2001; Wang et al. 2000). The increased size is due to a longer open reading frame (ORF) encoding the phosphoprotein (P) and the unusually long nontranslated regions that flank each gene (Harcourt et al. 2000, 2001; Wang et al. 1998, 2000; Yu et al. 1998a,b). The *P* gene of these viruses encodes three nonstructural proteins (C, V, and W) in addition to P. The C protein is encoded by a second ORF that initiates 23 nucleotides downstream of the P ORF translational initiation site (Harcourt et al. 2000; Wang et al. 1998). In addition to the C ORF, HV has another ORF in the *P* gene that encodes a putative, arginine rich, small basic protein (SB) of 65 amino acids (Wang et al. 1998), which has not yet been detected in infected cells (Wang et al. 2001).

The *P* genes of both Hendra virus and Nipah virus contain an RNA editing site that it is identical to the editing site found in measles virus (MeV) (Harcourt et al. 2000; Wang et al. 1998). The addition of a single G allows expression of the V protein, while addition of two Gs allows expression of a protein analogous to the W protein of Sendai virus (Delenda et al. 1998; Harcourt et al. 2000; Vidal et al., 1990). The V and W proteins appear to be virulence factors since cells expressing both V and W of Nipah virus block activation of an IFN-inducible promoter in primate cells (Park et al. 2003). Expression of IFN-α and IFN-γ-driven reporter genes was inhibited by the expression of the V of Nipah virus or HV in the presence of IFN. The V of Nipah virus formed high molecular weight complexes of 300–500 kDa with STAT1 and STAT2, which prevented both the activation and nuclear transportation of STAT1 (Rodriguez et al. 2002, 2003).

The L proteins of the henipaviruses have the six linear domain structures found within the polymerase proteins of all viruses in the order *Mononegavirales*. A highly conserved GDNQ sequence within domain III is conserved in most of the *Mononegavirales* viruses but is changed to GDNE in the henipaviruses and tupaia virus (Poch et al. 1990; Tidona et al. 1999; Harcourt et al. 2000; Wang et al. 2001).

The cleavage site of the fusion (F) protein of the henipaviruses contains a single basic amino acid and thus does not contain the R–X–R/K–R consensus sequence for furin proteases that is seen in the morbilliviruses, rubulaviruses, and pneumoviruses (Lamb and Kolakofsky 2001). The cellular protease(s) that cleaves the F of henipaviruses is unidentified, though basic amino acids are not required for cleavage (Moll et al. 2004). The henipaviruses are unique in that they have a leucine residue at the amino terminus of F_1 instead of the phenylalanine found in most other members of the family *Paramyxoviridae* (Harcourt et al. 2000; Wang et al. 2001). The G proteins of the henipaviruses have no known hemagglutinin or neuraminidase activities (Harcourt et al. 2000; Yu et al. 1998a).

Epidemiology and transmission

Hendra virus has been associated with two human and 17 horse deaths in three separate incidents in Australia during 1994–1999 (Murray et al. 1995a, 1995b; Selvey et al. 1995). The last known incident of Hendra virus infection occurred during January 1999 in Australia and involved a fatality in a single, adult mare, but no human infections (Field et al. 2000; Hooper et al. 2000). Antibodies to Hendra virus were detected in several fruit bat species in Queensland and the virus isolated from a fruit bat was indistinguishable from that isolated from horses and humans (Young et al. 1996; Halpin et al. 1999, 2000) suggesting that these bats may be a natural reservoir for Hendra virus. Transmission to horses may have occurred through the ingestion of material recently contaminated by the urine or infected fetal tissue of fruit bats (Halpin et al. 1999; Field et al. 2000).

The first known human infections with Nipah virus occurred during an outbreak of severe febrile encephalitis in peninsular Malaysia and Singapore in 1998–1999. Direct contact with pigs was the primary source of human infection (CDC 1999a, b; Chua et al. 2000). This outbreak began in October 1998 near the city of Ipoh and then spread southward in conjunction with the movement of pigs, resulting in three other clusters of human disease near Kuala Lumpur. In Singapore, abattoir workers who slaughtered pigs imported from outbreak-affected areas in Malaysia were exclusively affected (Paton et al. 1999; Chew et al. 2000). A total of 265 patients (104 fatal) with viral encephalitis and 11 patients (one fatal) with laboratory-confirmed Nipah virus disease were reported in Malaysia and Singapore, respectively. Adult males who were primarily involved in pig farming or pork production activities accounted for the majority of cases. Although Nipah virus is excreted in respiratory secretions and urine of patients (Chua et al. 2001), a survey of healthcare workers in Malaysia demonstrated no evidence of human-to-human transmission (Mounts et al. 2001).

Because of the virologic similarities between Nipah virus and Hendra virus, surveillance for the natural reservoir for Nipah virus was focused on bats. Neutralizing antibodies to Nipah virus were found in four fruit-bat species and one insectivorous-bat species in peninsular Malaysia (Yob et al. 2001), and antibodies have been detected in Cambodian bats (Olson et al. 2002). Nipah virus has recently been isolated from the urine of Malaysian fruit bats roosting on Tioman Island (Chua et al. 2002).

Nipah virus has been established as the cause of fatal, febrile encephalitis in human patients in Bangladesh during the winters of 2001, 2003, and 2004. A Nipah virus-like virus was identified as the cause of the outbreaks in 2001 and 2003 based on results from serologic testing (Hsu et al. 2004); however, Nipah virus was isolated from patients with acute disease in 2004. Though antibodies to Nipah virus were detected in fruit bats from the affected areas in 2004, an intermediate animal host was not identified. It is likely that the virus was transmitted directly from bats to humans. Human-to-human transmission of Nipah virus was also documented during the outbreak in Bangladesh (ICDDRB 2004a,b; WHO 2004).

Clinical and pathological manifestations

Little is known concerning the clinical disease and associated pathology in the natural hosts of the henipaviruses, and studies are in progress to further address these questions. Natural or experimental Hendra virus infections of bats are asymptomatic though the bats seroconvert and viral antigen and some live virus can be detected (Williamson et al. 1998; Halpin et al. 2000; Field et al. 2001). Horses and cats naturally infected with Hendra virus show clinical signs that include depression, anorexia, profuse nasal discharge, and labored breathing with pulmonary edema and congestion. Pneumonic and hemorrhagic lesions are seen in the lungs and death occurs within 2 days of infection. Virus can be isolated from the urine of infected animals (Williamson et al. 1998; Field et al. 2001). Experimental infection of horses was less severe than natural disease. Nipah virus infection of golden hamsters results in fatal neurological disease, thus providing a small animal model for studying the pathogenesis of Nipah virus (Wong et al. 2003).

In the first reported cases of Hendra virus infection in humans, patients had abrupt onset of an influenza-like illness, characterized by myalgia, headaches, lethargy, and vertigo (Selvey et al. 1995). Based on the exposure history of the two people involved, the incubation period for the acute disease caused by Hendra virus is approximately 5–7 days. One patient remained lethargic for 6 weeks but recovered fully, while the other succumbed to infection. In the second reported Hendra virus incident, the single patient initially presented with features of meningitis, including headache, drowsiness, vomiting, and neck stiffness. Following complete recovery, this patient presented 13 months later with neurological disease and died shortly thereafter.

The onset of Nipah virus disease is abrupt, usually with the development of fever and severe encephalitis. Fever (97 percent), headache (65 percent), dizziness (36 percent), vomiting (27 percent), and reduced level of consciousness (21 percent) were the most common clinical features noted during the outbreaks in Malaysia and Singapore (Goh et al. 2000). In addition to the neurological symptoms described above, acute respiratory distress was also noted in many patients during the Nipah virus outbreak in Bangladesh in 2004 (ICDDRB 2004a, b). The exact incubation period of Nipah virus disease in humans is not known but ranged from several days to 2 months, and was 2 weeks or less in the majority of patients.

The pathogenesis of Hendra virus in humans showed a severe interstitial pneumonia (Selvey et al. 1995; Murray et al. 1995a) and leptomeningitis (O'Sullivan et al. 1997). In contrast, a multiorgan vasculitis associated with infection of endothelial cells was the main pathologic feature of Nipah virus infection (Parashar et al. 2000) with infection being most pronounced in the central nervous system with necrotic foci of neuronal degeneration. Evidence of endothelial infection and vasculitis was also seen in other organs, including the lung, heart, spleen, and kidney. Nipah virus has been isolated from cerebrospinal fluid, tracheal secretions, throat swab, nasal swab, and urine specimens of patients (Goh et al. 2000; Chua et al. 2001).

During the outbreak in Malaysia, direct contact with pigs was the primary source of human Nipah virus infection, with no evidence of human-to-human transmission (Parashar et al. 2000). Although pigs showed extensive infection of the upper and lower airways, with evidence of tracheitis, and bronchial and interstitial pneumonia, the mortality rate was less than 5 percent. A harsh, nonproductive cough (called the mile-long cough) was a prominent clinical feature, but other signs such as lethargy or aggressive behavior indicated some neurological involvement (Chua et al. 2000; Hooper and Williamson 2000; Hooper et al. 2000). Serologic studies demonstrated evidence of infection among other species of animals, including dogs and cats on and near farms with Nipah virus-infected pigs (Chua et al. 2000; Hooper et al. 2000), though it is unclear whether humans were at risk from exposure to infected animals other than pigs (Goh et al. 2000; Parashar et al. 2000).

Control

Since interruption of transmission of Hendra and Nipah viruses from their reservoirs to intermediate hosts or directly to humans is difficult, early identification of infected animals and humans and use of appropriate personal protective equipment in healthcare and agricultural settings are the keys to prevention. Since person-to-person transmission of Nipah virus has been documented, those in contact with patients, including healthcare workers, should use standard droplet precautions during contact with secretions, excretions, and body fluids of patients.

No vaccines or antiviral drugs are currently available for Hendra virus or Nipah virus. In vitro, ribavirin has a demonstrated antiviral effect against Hendra virus. During the Nipah virus outbreak in Malaysia, patients receiving ribavirin either orally or intravenously showed a lower mortality rate (Chong et al. 2001).

Laboratory diagnosis

Analysis of serum samples from outbreaks indicated that Nipah virus and Hendra virus infections generate a humoral immune response in humans. IgM was present in serum shortly after the onset of Nipah virus infection and nearly all patients were antibody-positive by the third day (Ramasundrum et al. 2000). IgG was detected 10–29 percent of Nipah virus-infected patients within the first 10 days of illness, and in 100 percent of patients after 17–18 days.

Because of their ability to cause severe disease in animals and humans, work with live Nipah virus and Hendra virus must be conducted at BSL-4. ELISA assays to detect IgG and IgM antibodies are routinely used to detect Hendra virus and Nipah virus infections. These assays often use inactivated or expressed antigens and, therefore, have the advantage that they do not need to be conducted at BSL-4. Also, IgG antibodies can be detected by using standard serum neutralization tests. Immunohistochemistry has proven extremely useful for detecting Nipah virus antigens in fixed tissue samples. Both Hendra virus and Nipah virus can be isolated on Vero-E6 cells from cerebrospinal fluid, nasal samples, and urine samples from infected individuals (Goh et al. 2000; Chua et al. 2001). Various RT-PCR assays have been used to detect RNA from Hendra virus and Nipah virus in a variety of clinical samples and tissues (Halpin et al. 2000; Daniels et al. 2001; Guillaume et al. 2004).

RUBULAVIRUSES

Several viruses in the genus *Rubulavirus* have been isolated from animals. During the search for the reservoir of Nipah virus in Malaysia, a previously undescribed rubulavirus, Tioman virus, was isolated from a small number of fruit bats. Tioman virus has not been associated with disease in bats or any other animal (Chua et al. 2002). Menangle virus is antigenically related to Tioman virus, and was originally isolated from stillborn piglets in a piggery in New South Wales Australia in 1997. Infections resulted in degeneration of the brain and spinal cord and an increase in the number of abortions and stillbirths associated with deformities. Fruit bats living near the affected piggeries were seropositive for antibodies to Menangle virus. Two of over 250 humans who worked in the piggery also had antibodies to Menangle virus and reported an influenza-like illness following exposure to the infected pigs (Chant et al. 1998; Philbey et al. 1998). No further outbreaks of Menangle virus have been reported. Another porcine paramyxovirus, La-Piedad Michoacan-Mexico virus (LPMV), was identified as the agent responsible for fatal disease in piglets and has been endemic in Mexico since 1980. Bats do not play a role in the tranmission of LPMV (Linne et al. 1992; Salas-Rojas et al. 2004). Another respirovirus, Mapuera virus, has also been detected in bats (Henderson et al. 1995).

UNASSIGNED PARAMYXOVIRUSES

A number of new paramyxoviruses have been isolated recently from various animal species, but have not yet been assigned to a genus. Sixteen paramyxovirus isolates from reptilian species (Ahne et al. 1999) have been described; the archetype is fer-de-lance virus, which causes highly pathogenic respiratory infections in snakes. This virus has been completely sequenced and has a novel gene located between the N and P genes, which has no counterpart in any of the other viruses of the family. Fer-de-lance virus has been proposed as the type species for a new genus, *Ferlavirus*, within the subfamily *Paramyxovirinae* (Kurath et al. 2004). A number of paramyxoviruses have been isolated from rodents, including Nariva virus and Mossman virus (Roos and Wollmann 1979; Miller et al. 2003). Tupaia virus was discovered in a cell line derived from tree shrews (Tidona et al. 1999) and Salem virus was isolated from the mononuclear cells of a horse during an outbreak of disease in the USA in 1992 (Renshaw et al. 2000). Mossman, Tupaia, and Salem viruses are unclassified members of the subfamily *Paramyxovirinae* that are most closely related to the morbilliviruses and henipaviruses (Miller et al. 2003). The natural distribution and pathogenic potential of these novel paramyxoviruses are mostly unexplored.

REFERENCES

Abu Elzein, E.M., Housawi, F., et al. 2004. Severe PPR infection in gazelles kept under semi-free range conditions in Saudi Arabia. *J Vet Microbiol*, **51**, 68–71.

Ahne, W., Batts, W.N., et al. 1999. Comparative sequence analyses of sixteen reptilian paramyxoviruses. *Virus Res*, **63**, 65–7.

Alexander, D.J. 1995. The epidemiology and control of avian influenza and Newcastle disease. *J Comp Pathol*, **112**, 105–26.

Alexander, D.J. 1997. Newcastle disease and other *Paramyxoviridae* infections. In: Calnek, B.W., Barnes, H.J., et al. (eds), *Diseases of poultry*, 10th edn. Ames, IA: Iowa State University Press, 541–69.

Alexander, D.J. 1999. Newcastle disease. In: Swayne, D.E., Glisson, J.R., et al. (eds), *A laboratory manual for the isolation and identification of avian pathogens*, 4th edn. Kennett Square, PA: American Association of Avian Pathologists, 156–63.

Anderson, J. and McKay, J.A. 1994. The detection of antibodies against peste des petits ruminants virus in cattle, sheep and goats and the possible implications to rinderpest control programmes. *Epi Infect*, **112**, 225–31.

Anderson, J., Barrett, T. and Scott, G.R. 1996. *Manual on the diagnosis of rinderpest*. Rome: FAO, 143 pp.

Appel, M.J.G. 1987. Canine distemper virus. In Appel, M.J.G. (ed.), *Virus infections of vertebrates*, Vol. 1. Virus infections of carnivores. Amsterdam: Elsevier, 133–59.

Appel, M.J.G. and Summers, B.A. 1995. Pathogenicity of morbilliviruses for terrestrial carnivores. *Vet Microbiol*, **44**, 187–91.

Appel, M.J.G., Pearce-Kelling, S. and Summers, B.A. 1992. Dog lymphocyte cultures facilitate the isolation and growth of virulent canine distemper virus. *J Vet Diag Invest*, **4**, 258–63.

Barrett, T. 2001. Morbilliviruses: dangers old and new. In: Smith, G.L., McCauley, J.W. and Rowlands, D.J. (eds), *New challenges to health: the threat of virus infection*. Cambridge: Cambridge University Press, 155–78, Society for General Microbiology Symposium 60.

Barrett, T. and Rima, B.K. 2002. Molecular biology of morbillivirus diseases of marine mammals. In: Pfeiffer, C.J. (ed.), *Molecular and cell biology of marine mammals*. Malabar, FL: Krieger Publishing, 161–72.

Barrett, T. and Rossiter, P.B. 1999. Rinderpest: the disease and its impact on humans and animals. *Adv Virus Res*, **53**, 89–110.

Barrett, T., Visser, I.L.G., et al. 1993. Dolphin and porpoise morbilliviruses are genetically distinct from phocine distemper virus. *Virology*, **193**, 1010–12.

Barrett, T., Forsyth, M., et al. 1998. Rediscovery of the second African lineage of rinderpest virus: its epidemiological significance. *Vet Rec*, **142**, 669–71.

Bengtson, J.L., Boveng, P., et al. 1991. Antibodies to canine distemper virus in Antarctic seals. *Marine Mamm Sci*, **71**, 85–7.

Blixenkrone-Møller, M., Svansson, V., et al. 1990. Phocid distemper virus: a threat to terrestrial mammals? *Vet Rec*, **127**, 263–4.

Brown, C.C. and Torres, A. 1994. Distribution of antigen in cattle infected with rinderpest virus. *Vet Path*, **31**, 194–200.

Bush, M., Montali, R.J., et al. 1976. Vaccine induced canine distemper in a lesser panda. *J Am Vet Med Assoc*, **169**, 959–60.

Carpenter, J.W., Appel, M.J., et al. 1976. Fatal vaccine-induced canine distemper virus infection in black-footed ferrets. *J Am Vet Med Assoc*, **169**, 961–4.

CDC. 1999a. Outbreak of Hendra-like virus – Malaysia and Singapore, 1998–1999. *Morbid Mortal Wkly Rep*, **48**, 265–9.

CDC. 1999b. Update: outbreak of Nipah virus – Malaysia and Singapore, 1999. *Morbid Mortal Wkly Rep*, **48**, 335–7.

Chang, P.W. 1981. Newcastle disease. In: Beran, G.W. (ed.), *CRC handbook series in zoonoses*. Boca Raton, FL: CRC Press, 261.

Chang, P.C., Hsieh, M.L., et al. 2001. Complete nucleotide sequence of avian paramyxovirus type 6 isolated from ducks. *J Gen Virol*, **82**, 2157–68.

Chant, K., Chan, R., NSW Expert Group, et al. 1998. Probable human infection with a newly described virus in the family *Paramyxoviridae*. *Emerging Infect Dis*, **4**, 273–5.

Chapuis, G. 1995. Control of canine distemper. *Vet Microbiol*, **44**, 351–8.

Chew, M.H., Arguin, P.M., et al. 2000. Risk factors for Nipah virus infection among abattoir workers in Singapore. *J Infect Dis*, **181**, 1760–3.

Chua, K.B., Bellini, W.J., et al. 2000. Nipah virus: a recently emergent deadly paramyxovirus. *Science*, **288**, 1432–5.

Chua, K.B., Lam, S.K., et al. 2001. The presence of Nipah virus in respiratory secretions and urine of patients during an outbreak of Nipah virus encephalitis in Malaysia. *J Infect*, **42**, 40–3.

Chua, K.B., Koh, C.L., et al. 2002. Isolation of Nipah virus from Malaysian Island flying-foxes. *Microbes Infect*, **4**, 145–51.

Chong, H.T., Kamarulzaman, A., et al. 2001. Treatment of acute Nipah encephalitis with ribavirin. *Ann Neurol*, **49**, 810–13.

Couacy-Hymann, E., Bidjeh, K., et al. 1995. Protection of goats against rinderpest by vaccination with attenuated peste des petits ruminants virus. *Res Vet Sci*, **59**, 106–9.

Daniels, P., Ksiazek, T. and Eaton, B.T. 2001. Laboratory diagnosis of Nipah and Hendra virus infections. *Microbes Infect*, **3**, 289–95.

Deem, S.L., Spelman, L.H., et al. 2000. Canine distemper in terrestrial carnivores: a review. *J Zoo Wildlife Med*, **31**, 441–51.

Delenda, C., Taylor, G., et al. 1998. Sendai viruses with altered P, V and W protein expression. *Virology*, **242**, 327–37.

Dhar, P., Barrett, T., et al. 2002. Recent epidemiology of peste des petits ruminants virus (PPRV). *Vet Microbiol*, **88**, 153–9.

Dietz, R., Ansen, C.T., et al. 1989. Clue to seal epizootic? *Nature*, **338**, 627.

Domingo, M., Ferrer, L., et al. 1990. Morbillivirus in dolphins. *Nature*, **348**, 21.

Domingo, M., Visa, J., et al. 1992. Pathologic and immunocytochemical studies of morbillivirus infection in striped dolphins (*Stenella coeruleoalba*). *Vet Pathol*, **29**, 1–10.

Duignan, P.J., Geraci, J., et al. 1992. Pathology of morbillivirus infection in striped dolphins (*Stenella coeruleoalba*) from Valencia and Murcia, Spain. *Can J Vet Res*, **56**, 242–8.

Duignan, P.J., House, C., et al. 1995a. Morbillivirus infection in two species of pilot whales (*Globicephala* sp.) from the western Atlantic. *Marine Mamm Sci*, **11**, 150–62.

Duignan, P.J., House, C., et al. 1995b. Morbillivirus infection in cetaceans of the Western Atlantic. *Vet Microbiol*, **44**, 241–9.

Duignan, P.J., House, C., et al. 1995c. Morbillivirus infections in manatees. *Marine Mamm Sci*, **11**, 51.

Duignan, P.J., House, C., et al. 1996. Morbillivirus infection in bottlenose dolphins: evidence for recurrent epizootics in the Western Atlantic and Gulf of Mexico. *Marine Mamm Sci*, **12**, 499–515.

Duignan, P.J., Nielsen, O., et al. 1997. Epizootiology of morbillivirus infection in harp, hooded and ringed seals from the Canadian Arctic and Western Atlantic. *J Wildlife Dis*, **33**, 7–19.

Felsenstein, J. 1997. An alternating least squares approach to inferring phylogenies from pairwise distances. *Syst Biol*, **46**, 101–11.

Field, H.E., Barratt, P.C., et al. 2000. A fatal case of Hendra virus infection in a horse in north Queensland: clinical and epidemiological features. *Aust Vet J*, **78**, 279–80.

Field, H.E., Young, P., et al. 2001. The natural history of Hendra and Nipah viruses. *Microbes Infect*, **3**, 307–14.

Forsyth, M. and Barrett, T. 1995. Evaluation of polymerase chain reaction for the detection of rinderpest and peste des petits ruminants viruses for epidemiological studies. *Virus Res*, **39**, 151–63.

Forsyth, M., Kennedy, S., et al. 1998. Canine distemper in a Caspian seal. *Vet Rec*, **143**, 662–4.

Furley, C.W., Taylor, W.P. and Obi, T.U. 1987. An outbreak of peste des petits ruminants in a zoological collection. *Vet Rec*, **121**, 443–7.

Gargadennec, L. and Lalanne, A. 1942. Peste des petits ruminants. *Bull Serv Zootech Epizoot Afr Occ Fran*, **5**, 16–21.

Glickman, R.L., Syddall, R.J., et al. 1988. Quantitative basic residue requirements in the cleavage-activation site of the fusion glycoprotein as a determinant of virulence for Newcastle disease virus. *J Virol*, **62**, 354–6.

Goh, K.J., Tan, C.T., et al. 2000. Clinical features of Nipah virus encephalitis among pig farmers in Malaysia. *N Engl J Med*, **342**, 1229–35.

Gotoh, B., Ohnishi, Y., et al. 1992. Mammalian subtilisin-related proteinases in cleavage activation of the paramyxovirus fusion glycoprotein: superiority of furin/PACE to PC2 or PC1/PC3. *J Virol*, **66**, 6391–7.

Govindarajan, R., Koteeswaran, A., et al. 1997. Isolation of pestes des petits ruminants virus from an outbreak in Indian buffalo (*Bubalus bubalis*). *Vet Rec*, **141**, 573–4.

Grachev, M.A., Kumarev, V.P., et al. 1989. Distemper virus in Baikal seals. *Nature*, **338**, 209.

Guillaume, V., Lefeuvre, A., et al. 2004. Specific detection of Nipah virus using real-time RT-PCR (TaqMan). *J Virol Meth*, **15**, 229–37.

Haas, L., Hofer, H., et al. 1996. Epizootic of canine distemper virus infection in Serengeti spotted hyaenas (*Crocuta crocuta*). *Vet Microbiol*, **49**, 147–52.

Halpin, K., Young, P.L., et al. 1999. Newly discovered viruses of flying foxes. *Vet Microbiol*, **68**, 83–7.

Halpin, K., Young, P.L., et al. 2000. Isolation of Hendra virus from pteropid bats: a natural reservoir of Hendra virus. *J Gen Virol*, **81**, 1927–32.

Harcourt, B.H., Tamin, A., et al. 2000. Molecular characterization of Nipah virus, a newly emergent paramyxovirus. *Virology*, **271**, 334–49.

Harcourt, B.H., Tamin, A., et al. 2001. Molecular characterization of the polymerase gene and genomic termini of Nipah virus. *Virology*, **287**, 192–201.

Harder, T.C., Kenter, M., et al. 1996. Morbilliviruses isolated from diseased captive large felids: pathogenicity for domestic cats and comparative molecular analysis. *J Gen Virol*, **77**, 397–405.

Harwood, J. 1998. What killed the monk seals? *Nature*, **393**, 17–18.

Heaney, J., Barrett, T. and Cosby, L. 2002. Inhibition of leucocyte proliferation by morbilliviruses. *J Virol*, **76**, 3579–84.

Henderson, G.W., Laird, C., et al. 1995. Characterization of Mapuera virus: structure, proteins and nucleotide sequence of the gene encoding the nucleocapsid protein. *J Gen Virol*, **76**, 2509–18.

Hooper, P.T. and Williamson, M.M. 2000. Hendra and Nipah virus infections. *Vet Clin N Am, Equine Pract*, **16**, 597–603.

Hooper, P.T., Gould, A.R., et al. 2000. Identification and molecular characterization of Hendra virus in a horse in Queensland. *Aus Vet J*, **78**, 281–2.

Hsu, V.P., Hussain, M.J., et al. 2004. Nipah virus encephalitis reemergence, Bangladesh. *Emerg Infect Dis*, **12**, 2082–7.

ICDDRB. 2004a. Nipah encephalitis outbreak over wide area of western Bangladesh, 2004. *Hlth Sci Bull*, **2**, 7–11.

ICDDRB. 2004b. Person-to-person transmission of Nipah virus during outbreak in Faridpur District. *Hlth Sci Bull*, **2**, 5–9.

Jauniaux, T., Charlier, G., et al. 1998. Lesions of morbillivirus infection in a fin whale (*Balaenoptera physalus*) stranded along the Belgian coast. *Vet Rec*, **143**, 423–4.

Kennedy, S., Smyth, J.A., et al. 1988. Viral distemper found in porpoises. *Nature*, **336**, 21.

Kennedy, S., Kuiken, T., et al. 2000. Canine distemper virus identified as cause of recent mass mortality in Caspian seals (*Phoca caspica*). *Emerg Infect Dis*, **6**, 637–9.

Kitching, R.P. 1988. The economic significance and control of small ruminant viruses in North Africa and West Asia. In Thompson, E.F., Thompson, F.S. (eds), *Increasing small ruminant productivity in semi-arid areas*. Proceedings of a Workshop held at the International Center for Agricultural Research in the Dry Areas, Aleppo, Syria, 1987. Dordrecht: Kluwer Academic, 225–36.

Kock, R.A., Wambua, J., et al. 1999. Rinderpest epidemic in wild ruminants in Kenya 1993–1997. *Vet Rec*, **145**, 275–83.

Kurath, G., Batts, W.N., et al. 2004. Complete genome sequence of Fer-de-Lance virus reveals a novel gene in reptilian paramyxoviruses. *J Virol*, **78**, 2045–56.

Lamb, R.A. and Kolakofsky, D. 2001. *Paramyxoviridae*: the viruses and their replication. In: Knipe, D.M., Howley, P.M., et al. (eds), *Fields' virology*. Philadelphia: Lippincott, Williams and Wilkins, 1305–41.

Leighton, T., Ferguson, M., et al. 1988. Canine distemper in sled dogs. *Can Vet J*, **29**, 299.

Libeau, G., Diallo, A., et al. 1994. Rapid differential diagnosis of rinderpest and peste des petits ruminants using an immunocapture ELISA. *Vet Rec*, **134**, 300–4.

Lipscomb, T.P., Schulman, F.Y., et al. 1994. Morbilliviral disease in Atlantic bottlenose dolphins (*Tursiops truncatus*) from the 1987–1988 epizootic. *J Wldl Dis*, **30**, 567–71.

Linne, T., Berg, M., et al. 1992. The molecular biology of the porcine paramyxovirus LPMV. *Vet Microbiol*, **33**, 263–73.

Mack, R. 1970. The great African cattle plague epidemic of the 1890s. *Trop Anim Hlth Prod*, **2**, 210–19.

Mamaev, L., Denikina, N.N., et al. 1995. Characterisation of morbilliviruses isolated from Lake Baikal seals (*Phoca sibirica*). *Vet Microbiol*, **44**, 251–9.

Miller, P.J., Boyle, D.B., et al. 2003. Full-length genome sequence of Mossman virus, a novel paramyxovirus isolated from rodents in Australia. *Virology*, **317**, 330–44.

Murray, K., Selleck, P., et al. 1995a. A morbillivirus that caused fatal disease in horses and humans. *Science*, **268**, 94–7.

Murray, K., Rogers, R., et al. 1995b. A novel morbillivirus pneumonia of horses and its transmission to humans. *Emerg Infect Dis*, **1**, 31–3.

Moll, M., Diederich, S., et al. 2004. Ubiquitous activation of the Nipah virus fusion protein does not require a basic amino acid at the cleavage site. *J Virol*, **78**, 9705–12.

Mounts, A.W., Kaur, H., Nipah Virus Nosocomial Study Group, et al. 2001. A cohort study of health care workers to assess nosocomial transmissibility of Nipah virus, Malaysia, 1999. *J Infect Dis*, **183**, 810–13.

Myers, D.L., Zurbriggen, A., et al. 1997. Distemper: not a new disease in lions and tigers. *Clin Diagnost Lab Immunol*, **4**, 180–4.

Nielsen, O., Stewart, R.E., et al. 2000. A morbillivirus antibody survey of Atlantic walrus, narwhal and beluga in Canada. *J Wildl Dis*, **36**, 508–17.

Norrby, E., Sheshberadaran, H., et al. 1985. Is rinderpest virus the archevirus of the *Morbillivirus* genus? *Intervirology*, **23**, 228–32.

Olson, J.G., Rupprecht, C., et al. 2002. Antibodies to Nipah-like virus in bats (*Pteropus lylei*) in Cambodia. *Emerg Infect Dis*, **8**, 987–8.

Osterhaus, A.D.M.E. and Vedder, E.J. 1988. Identification of virus causing recent seal deaths. *Nature*, **335**, 20.

Osterhaus, A.D.M.E., Visser, I.K.G., et al. 1992. Morbillivirus threat to Mediterranean monk seals? *Vet Rec*, **130**, 141–2.

Ozkul, A., Akca, Y., et al. 2002. Prevalence, distribution and host range of peste des petits ruminants virus in Turkey. *Emerg Infect Dis*, **8**, 708–12.

O'Sullivan, J.D., Allworth, A.M., et al. 1997. Fatal encephalitis due to novel paramyxovirus transmitted from horses. *Lancet*, **349**, 93–5.

Parashar, U.D., Sunn, L.M., et al. 2000. Case-control study of risk factors for human infection with a new zoonotic paramyxovirus, Nipah virus, during a 1998–1999 outbreak of severe encephalitis in Malaysia. *J Infect Dis*, **181**, 1755–9.

Park, M.S., Shaw, M.L., et al. 2003. Newcastle disease virus (NDV)-based assay demonstrates interferon-antagonist activity for the NDV V protein and the Nipah virus V, W and C proteins. *J Virol*, **77**, 1501–11.

Pastoret, P.P. and Brochier, B. 1996. The development and use of a vaccinia-rabies recombinant oral vaccine for the control of wildlife rabies: a link between Jenner and Pasteur. *Epi Infect*, **116**, 235–40.

Paton, N.I., Leo, Y.S., et al. 1999. Outbreak of Nipah-virus infection among abattoir workers in Singapore. *Lancet*, **354**, 1253–6.

Philbey, A.W., Kirkland, P.D., et al. 1998. An apparently new virus (family *Paramyxoviridae*) infectious for pigs, humans, and fruit bats. *Emerg Infect Dis*, **4**, 269–71.

Philippa, J.D., Leighton, F.A., et al. 2004. Antibodies to selected pathogens in free-ranging terrestrial carnivores and marine mammals in Canada. *Vet Rec*, **55**, 135–40.

Plowright, W. and Ferris, R.D. 1962. Studies with rinderpest virus in tissue culture. The use of attenuated culture virus as a vaccine for cattle. *Res Vet Sci*, **3**, 172–82.

Poch, O., Blumberg, B.M., et al. 1990. Sequence comparison of five polymerases (L proteins) of unsegmented negative-strand RNA viruses: theoretical assignment of functional domains. *J Gen Virol*, **71**, 1153–62.

Ramasundrum, V., Tan, C.T., et al. 2000. Kinetics of IgM and IgG seroconversion in Nipah virus infection. *Neurol J Southeast Asia*, **5**, 23–8.

Renshaw, R.W., Glaser, A.L., et al. 2000. Identification and phylogenetic comparison of Salem virus, a novel paramyxovirus of horses. *Virology*, **270**, 417–29.

Rodriguez, J.J., Parisien, J.P. and Horvath, C.M. 2002. Nipah virus V protein evades alpha and gamma interferons by preventing STAT1 and STAT2 activation and nuclear accumulation. *J Virol*, **76**, 11476–83.

Rodriguez, J.J., Wang, L.F. and Horvath, C.M. 2003. Hendra virus V protein inhibits interferon signaling by preventing STAT1 and STAT2 nuclear accumulation. *J Virol*, **77**, 11842–5.

Roelke-Parker, M.E., Munson, L., et al. 1996. A canine distemper virus epidemic in Serengeti lions (*Panthera leo*). *Nature*, **379**, 441–5.

Roos, R.P. and Wollmann, R. 1979. Non-productive paramyxovirus infection: Nariva virus infection in hamsters. *Arch Virol*, **62**, 229–40.

Rott, R. and Klenk, H.D. 1988. Molecular basis of infectivity and pathogenicity of Newcastle disease virus. In: Alexander, D.J. (ed.), *Developments in veterinary virology: Newcastle disease*. Boston, MA: Kluwer Academic, 98–112.

Rossiter, P.B. 2001a. Rinderpest. In: Williams, E.S. and Barker, I.K. (eds), *Infectious diseases of wild mammals*. London: Manson Publishing, 37–45.

Rossiter, P.B. 2001b. Peste des petits ruminants. In: Williams, E.S. and Barker, I.K. (eds), *Infectious diseases of wild mammals*. London: Manson Publishing, 45–50.

Rossiter, P.B., Hussain, M., et al. 1998. Cattle plague in Shangri-La: observations on a severe outbreak of rinderpest in northern Pakistan 1994–1995. *Vet Rec*, **143**, 39–42.

Rweyemamu, M.M. and Cheneau, Y. 1995. Strategy for the global rinderpest eradication programme. *Vet Microbiol*, **44**, 369–76.

Salas-Rojas, M., Sanchez-Hernandez, C., et al. 2004. Prevalence of rabies and LPM paramyxovirus antibody in non-hematophagous bats captured in the Central Pacific coast of Mexico. *Trans R Soc Trop Med Hyg*, **98**, 577–84.

Seal, B.S., King, D.J. and Bennett, J.D. 1995. Characterization of Newcastle disease virus isolates by reverse transcription PCR coupled to direct nucleotide sequencing and development of sequence database for pathotype prediction and molecular epidemiologic analysis. *J Clin Microbiol*, **33**, 2624–30.

Scott, G.R. 1990. Rinderpest virus. In: Dinter, Z. and Morein, B. (eds), *Virus infections of vertebrates*. Amsterdam: Elsevier, 341–54.

Selvey, L.A., Well, R.M., et al. 1995. Infection of humans and horses by a newly described morbillivirus. *Med J Austr*, **162**, 642–5.

Shaila, M.S., Shamaki, D., et al. 1996. Geographic distribution and epidemiology of peste des petits ruminants viruses. *Virus Res*, **43**, 149–53.

Stettler, M., Beck, K., et al. 1997. Determinants of persistence in canine distemper viruses. *Vet Microbiol*, **57**, 83–93.

Sutherland-Smith, M.R., Rideout, B.A., et al. 1997. Vaccine-induced canine distemper in European mink, *Mustela lutreola*. *J Zoo Wildl Med*, **28**, 312–18.

Tidona, C.A., Kurz, H.W., et al. 1999. Isolation and molecular characterization of a novel cytopathogenic paramyxovirus from tree shrews. *Virology*, **258**, 425–34.

Van Bressem, M.F., Meurichy, J., et al. 1991. Attempt to vaccinate orally harbour seals against phocid distemper. *Vet Rec*, **129**, 362.

Van Bressem, M.F., Van Waerebeek, K., et al. 2001. An insight into the epidemiology of dolphin morbillivirus worldwide. *Vet Microbiol*, **81**, 287–304.

Van de Bildt, M.W.G., Martina, B.E.E., et al. 2000. Identification of morbilliviruses of probable cetacean origin in carcasses of Mediterranean monk seals (*Monachus monachus*). *Vet Rec*, **146**, 691–4.

Vidal, S., Curran, J. and Kolakofsky, D. 1990. Editing of the Sendai virus P/C mRNA by G insertion occurs during mRNA synthesis via a virus-encoded activity. *J Virol*, **64**, 239–46.

Visser, I.K.G., Vedder, E.J., et al. 1992. Canine distemper virus ISCOMs induce protection in harbour seals against phocid distemper but still allow subsequent infection with phocid distemper virus-1. *Vaccine*, **10**, 435–8.

Walsh, E.P., Baron, M.D., et al. 2000. Recombinant rinderpest vaccines expressing membrane anchored proteins as genetic markers: evidence of exclusion of marker protein from the virus envelope. *J Virol*, **74**, 10165–75.

Wambura, P.N., Moshy, D.W., et al. 2000. Diagnosis of rinderpest in Tanzania by a rapid chromatographic strip-test. *Trop Anim Hlth Prod*, **32**, 141–5.

Wamwayi, H.M., Kariuki, D.P., et al. 1992. Observations on rinderpest in Kenya, 1986–1989. *Rev Sci Tech Off Int Epiz*, **11**, 769–84.

Wamwayi, H.M., Fleming, M. and Barrett, T. 1995. Characterisation of African isolates of rinderpest virus. *Vet Microbiol*, **44**, 151–63.

Wang, L.F., Michalski, W.P., et al. 1998. A novel P/V/C gene in a new member of the *Paramyxoviridae* family, which causes lethal infection in humans, horses, and other animals. *J Virol*, **72**, 1482–90.

Wang, L.F., Yu, M., et al. 2000. The exceptionally large genome of Hendra virus: support for creation of a new genus within the family *Paramyxoviridae*. *J Virol*, **74**, 9972–9.

Wang, L.F., Harcourt, B.H., et al. 2001. Molecular biology of Hendra and Nipah viruses. *Microbes Infect*, **3**, 279–87.

Williamson, M., Hooper, P., et al. 1998. Transmission studies of Hendra virus (equine morbillivirus) in fruit bats, horses, and cats. *Aust Vet J*, **76**, 813–18.

Wohlsein, P., Trautwein, G., et al. 1993. Viral antigen distribution in organs of cattle experimentally infected with rinderpest virus. *Vet Pathol*, **30**, 544–54.

Wohlsein, P., Wamwayi, H.M., et al. 1995. Pathomorphological and immunohistological findings in cattle experimentally infected with rinderpest virus isolates of different pathogenicity. *Vet Microbiol*, **44**, 141–7.

Wong, K.T., Grosjean, I., et al. 2003. A golden hamster model for human acute Nipah virus infection. *Am J Pathol*, **163**, 2127–37.

WHO. 2004. Nipah virus outbreak(s) in Bangladesh, January–April 2004. *Wkly Epidemiol Rec*, **17**, 168–71.

Yob, J.M., Field, H., et al. 2001. Nipah virus infection in bats (order *Chiroptera*) in peninsular Malaysia. *Emerg Infect Dis*, **7**, 439–41.

Young, P.L., Halpin, K., et al. 1996. Serologic evidence for the presence in Pteropus bats of a paramyxovirus related to equine morbillivirus. *Emerg Infect Dis*, **2**, 239–40.

Yu, M., Hansson, E., et al. 1998a. The attachment protein of Hendra virus has high structural similarity but limited primary sequence homology compared with viruses in the genus *Paramyxovirus*. *Virology*, **251**, 227–33.

Yu, M., Hansson, E., et al. 1998b. Sequence analysis of the Hendra virus nucleoprotein gene: comparison with other members of the subfamily *Paramyxovirinae*. *J Gen Virol*, **79**, 1775–80.

Coronaviruses, toroviruses, and arteriviruses

STUART G. SIDDELL, JOHN ZIEBUHR, AND ERIC J. SNIJDER

PROPERTIES OF THE VIRUSES

Introduction

Coronaviruses, toroviruses, and arteriviruses are enveloped, positive-strand RNA viruses that infect vertebrates and can cause disease in their natural hosts. The genome organization and replication strategy are similar in all three groups of viruses but the differences in morphology and in genome size of the arteriviruses clearly set them apart. Coronaviruses and toroviruses are usually associated with respiratory or enteric disorders, although other organs (for example, the central nervous system (CNS)) can also be involved. The outcome of arterivirus infection can range from an asymptomatic, persistent carrier-state to lethal hemorrhagic fever.

The combination of features that distinguishes coronaviruses, toroviruses, and arteriviruses from other positive-strand RNA viruses are primarily in the structure and function of the replicase gene:

- The replicase gene comprises two overlapping open reading frames (ORF), and expression of the downstream ORF is mediated by −1 ribosomal frameshifting.
- Sequence analysis has identified common coding regions, e.g. motifs characteristic of proteinase, polymerase, helicase, and endoribonuclease, that are located at specific positions within the replicase gene. The signature organization of these domains can be expressed as (M-3CL-M)–RdRp–(Zn-HEL)–NendoU,

where M-3CL-M represents a chymotrypsin-like proteinase (with a substrate specificity resembling that of picornavirus 3C proteinases) flanked by two hydrophobic transmembrane domains, RdRp is RNA-dependent RNA polymerase, (Zn-HEL) is a putative multinuclear Zn-finger-like domain associated with a superfamily 1 helicase domain and NendoU is a uridylate-specific endoribonuclease.

- In the infected cell, viral gene expression is mediated by a set of four or more 3′ co-terminal subgenomic mRNAs. Only the ORFs contained within the 5′ unique regions of each mRNA, i.e. the regions not found in the next smallest mRNA, are expressed as protein.

The features that distinguish coronaviruses, toroviruses, and arteriviruses from each other are two-fold:

1 There are significant differences in structure and function of the nucleocapsid protein gene. The molecular weights of the nucleocapsid protein are 50–60 kDa for coronaviruses, ca. 19 kDa for toroviruses and 12–14 kDa for arteriviruses. The nucleocapsid structure also has different morphologies: helical-spherical for coronaviruses, helical-tubular for toroviruses, and isometric for arteriviruses.

2 In addition to the common motifs listed above, coronaviruses and toroviruses have motifs indicative of additional replicase gene functions related to RNA processing. These include a putative exonuclease (ExoN), 2′-O-ribose methyl transferase (2-O-MT) and cyclic phophodiesterase (CPD).

A number of other features help to define and distinguish these three groups of viruses. They include the organization of the virus genome, genome size, evidence of discontinuous RNA synthesis during subgenomic mRNA production, the structure and function of the virus envelope (glyco)proteins and the intracellular budding of virus particles (de Vries et al. 1997; Gonzalez et al. 2003; Holmes 2001a; Lai and Holmes 2001; Snijder et al. 2003a; Snijder and Meulenberg 1998; van Vliet et al. 2002; Ziebuhr et al. 2000).

Classification

At the present time the coronaviruses and the toroviruses represent two genera of the family *Coronaviridae*. The arteriviruses are designated as a separate, monogeneric family, the *Arteriviridae* (they were previously assigned to the family *Togaviridae*). The families *Coronaviridae* and *Arteriviridae* are united in the order *Nidovirales* (Cavanagh 1997). The viruses that currently comprise the families *Coronaviridae* and

Arteriviridae are listed, with their abbreviations and natural hosts, in Table 39.1.

Twenty four viruses are now classified as species in the *Coronaviridae* (Spaan et al. 2005). The prototype of the genus *Coronavirus* is avian *Infectious bronchitis virus* (IBV). The name coronavirus is derived from the solar coronalike (Latin *corona*: crown) appearance of virus particles in negatively stained electron micrographs. The prototype of the genus *Torovirus* is *Equine torovirus* (previously Berne virus), the name torovirus being derived from the curved tubular (Latin *torus*: lowest convex molding in the base of a column) morphology of the nucleocapsid structure. In addition to the viruses listed in Table 39.1, a further coronavirus, rabbit coronavirus (RbCoV) is considered as a tentative species of the genus and there have been recent reports of a novel human coronavirus, HCoV-HKUI (Woo et al. 2005) and a bat coronavirus, BaCoV (Poon et al. 2005). Also, although *Feline infectious peritonitis virus* (FIPV), *Sialodacryoadenitis virus* (SDAV), *Human coronavirus NL63* (HCoV-NL63), and *Porcine respiratory coronavirus* (PRCoV) are now recognized as coronavirus species,

Table 39.1 *Coronaviruses, toroviruses, and arteriviruses*

Natural host	Virus	Abbreviation
Coronaviruses		
Chicken	*Infectious bronchitis virus*	IBV
Cattle	*Bovine coronavirus*	BCoV
Dog	*Canine enteric coronavirus*	CCoV
Cat	*Feline coronavirus*	FCoV
Cat	*Feline infectious peritonitis virus*	FIPV
Humans	*Human coronavirus 229E*	HCoV-229E
Humans	*Human coronavirus NL63*	HCoV-NL63
Humans	*Human coronavirus OC43*	HCoV-OC43
Humans	*SARS-coronavirus*	SARS-CoV
Humans	*Human enteric coronavirus*	HECoV
Mouse	*Murine hepatitis virus*	MHV
Rat	*Rat coronavirus*	RtCoV
Rat	*Sialodacryoadenitis virus*	SDAV
Pig	*Porcine epidemic diarrhoea virus*	PEDV
Pig	*Transmissible gastroenteritis virus*	TGEV
Pig	*Porcine hemagglutinating encephalomyelitis virus*	HEV
Pig	*Porcine respiratory coronavirus*	PRCoV
Turkey	*Turkey coronavirus*	TCoV
Pheasant	*Pheasant coronavirus*	PhCoV
Shearwater	*Puffinosis coronavirus*	PCoV
Toroviruses		
Horse	*Equine torovirus*	EToV
Cattle	*Bovine torovirus*	BToV
Humans	*Human torovirus*	HToV
Pig	*Porcine torovirus*	PToV
Arteriviruses		
Horse	*Equine arteritis virus*	EAV
Mouse	*Lactate dehydrogenase-elevating virus*	LDV
Monkey	*Simian haemorrhagic fever virus*	SHFV
Pig	*Porcine reproductive and respiratory syndrome virus*	PRRSV

limited sequence data suggests that they could also be considered as variants of *Feline coronavirus* (FCoV), RtCoV, *Human coronavirus 229E* (HCoV-229E), and *Transmissible gastroenteritis virus* (TGEV), respectively. The sequence relationships of coronaviruses and toroviruses have been analyzed in detail (Gonzalez et al. 2003) and a revision of the current taxonomy is expected.

Four viruses are classified as species in the *Arteriviridae* (Snijder et al. 2005). The prototype of the family is *Equine arteritis virus* (EAV). The name arterivirus is derived from arteritis (inflammation of an artery), a disease caused by EAV. Previously, *Porcine respiratory and reproductive syndrome virus* (PRRSV) was also referred to as swine infertility and respiratory syndrome virus (SIRSV) or Lelystad virus. The four arterivirus species are antigenically distinct and no detailed serological cross-reactions have been reported. Phylogenetic analysis of arterivirus replicase proteins indicates that the four arterivirus species each constitute a branch within the genus, with each species represented by a cluster of strains. *Lactate dehydrogenase-elevating virus* (LDV) and PRRSV are most closely related to each other.

Finally, it should be mentioned that sequence analysis of *Gill-associated virus* (GAV) and *Yellow head virus* (YHV), which infect prawns, indicates that they are related to coronaviruses, toroviruses, and arteriviruses (Cowley et al. 2000) and justifies placing them in a genus *Okavirus* in the family *Roniviridae* in the order *Nidovirales* (Chapter 20, Gonzalez et al. 2003). However, these viruses will not be discussed further in this chapter.

Morphology and structure

Coronaviruses are pleomorphic but roughly spherical enveloped particles, 120–160 nm in diameter with a characteristic 'fringe' of surface projections 20 nm long. An inner 'fringe' of short surface projections is sometimes seen on murine hepatitis virus (MHV), bovine coronavirus (BCoV), turkey coronavirus (TCoV), and human coronavirus OC43 (HCoV-OC43) particles. Toroviruses are also pleomorphic, enveloped particles, 120–140 nm in diameter; they are disk-, kidney- or rod-shaped and, like the coronaviruses, are decorated with 15–20 nm surface projections. The nucleocapsid of both coronaviruses and toroviruses is helical but differs in morphology. Coronavirus nucleocapsids are extended when the structure is relaxed but they may be organized into spherical, possibly icosahedral, superstructures in the virus particle (Escors et al. 2001; Risco et al. 1996; Salanueva et al. 1999). A gap separating the internal core from the envelope has been observed in coronaviruses using cryoelectron microscopy. The nucleocapsids of toroviruses are tubular. Arteriviruses are 45–60 nm in diameter and consist of an isometric nucleocapsid of 25–35 nm that is surrounded by a lipid envelope. No prominent surface projections are seen on the virion but a surface pattern of relatively small and indistinct projections has been observed. The morphological features and the assignment of structural proteins to the coronavirus, torovirus, and arterivirus virions are illustrated in Figure 39.1.

Coronaviruses have an estimated molecular mass of 400×10^6 kDa and a buoyant density in sucrose of 1.15–1.20 g/cm^3. The buoyant density in CsCl is 1.23–1.24 g/cm^3 and the sedimentation coefficient $S_{20,w}$ is 300–500. Coronaviruses are sensitive to heat, lipid solvents, non-ionic detergents, formaldehyde, oxidizing agents, and UV-irradiation. Some coronaviruses are resistant to acid pH and/or dessication. Toroviruses have a buoyant density of 1.14–1.18 g/cm^3 in sucrose and an estimated sedimentation coefficient ($S_{20,w}$) of 400–500. Virus infectivity is stable between pH 2.5 and 9.7 but rapidly inactivated by heat, organic solvents, and irradiation. Arteriviruses have a buoyant density in sucrose of 1.13–1.17 g/cm^3 and 1.17–1.20 g/cm^3 in CsCl. The sedimentation coefficient is 214S–230S. Temperature, pH, and lipid solvents affect virion stability and virions are highly unstable in solutions containing low concentrations of detergents.

Genome structure and function

The genome of coronaviruses and toroviruses is a positive-strand RNA molecule of ca. 27 000–31 500 nucleotides (nt). This estimate of size is based on the nucleotide sequence of nine complete coronavirus genomes and the nucleotide sequence of the equine torovirus (EToV) genome (see www.ncbi.nlm.nih.gov/entrez/) (van Vliet et al. 2002). The coronavirus and torovirus genomic RNAs have a 5′ cap structure, and are polyadenylated at their 3′ end. It is generally accepted that the genomic RNA of coronaviruses and toroviruses is infectious, a conclusion that is based on the initiation of infection in susceptible cells with RNA extracted from purified virions and the initiation of infection with transcripts from cDNA clones corresponding to full-length coronavirus genomic RNA (Almazan et al. 2000; Casais et al. 2001; Thiel et al. 2001a; Yount et al. 2000; Yount et al. 2003; Yount et al. 2002).

The positive-strand RNA genome of arteriviruses is significantly smaller than that of coronaviruses and toroviruses. Sequence analysis of the EAV, LDV, and PRRSV genomes indicates a size of ca. 12 700–15 700 nt (see www.ncbi.nlm.nih.gov/entrez/). The genomic RNA of arteriviruses is polyadenylated at the 3′ end. It has been reported that the genomic RNA of simian haemorrhagic fever virus (SHFV) has a 5′ cap structure (Sagripanti et al. 1986). Cap analogue was found to be an essential component of the in vitro transcription reactions used to generate infectious RNA from PRRSV and EAV full-length cDNA templates (Meulenberg et al. 1998; van Dinten et al. 1997).

REGULATORY ELEMENTS

The genomes of coronaviruses and toroviruses contain a 5′ non-translated region (NTR) of several hundred

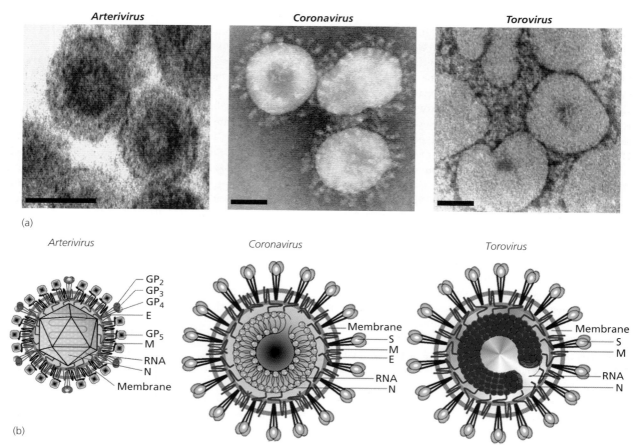

Figure 39.1 *Electron micrographs and schematic representations of coronavirus, torovirus, and arterivirus virion structure showing the locations of the structural proteins. The stoichiometry of the virion components is shown arbitrarily. E, envelope protein; GP$_5$, major glycoprotein; GP$_2$, GP$_3$, GP$_4$, minor glycoproteins; M, membrane protein; N, nucleoprotein; S, spike glycoprotein. The scale bar represents 50 nm.*

nucleotides. This region is almost devoid of AUG codons but a small ORF of 3–11 codons is conserved in the 5′ NTR of viruses examined to date. It has been speculated that this 'mini-ORF' may play a role in regulating translation from the genomic RNA (Senanayake and Brian 1999). The 5′ NTR of arteriviruses is relatively short, about 150–220 nt. Although small ORFs have been identified in this region for EAV, PRRSV, and SHFV (Snijder and Meulenberg 1998). The EAV intra-leader ORF was shown to be completely dispensable for EAV replication in cell culture (Molenkamp et al. 2000).

By analogy with other positive-strand RNA viruses, it can be expected that secondary (or tertiary) structures in the 5′ NTR of coronaviruses, toroviruses, and arteriviruses will have a role in the synthesis and packaging of virus RNA. Van den Born and colleagues (2004) have predicted and analyzed the secondary structure of the 5′ proximal region of the EAV genome. Their analysis suggests that secondary structures in this region play a role in the promotion of nidovirus plus-strand RNA synthesis from genomic and subgenomic templates. It remains to be shown exactly which of the predicted structural elements are involved and if, for example,

additional RNA–protein interactions are important. Similar secondary structures have also been predicted in the 5′ NTR of other arteriviruses, coronaviruses, and toroviruses (Chang et al. 1996; Shieh et al. 1987; Van den Born et al. 2004).

As is described in more detail in the section 'Transcription,' coronavirus and arterivirus gene expression is mediated by the production of a set of subgenomic mRNAs in the infected cell. An element that plays an important role in this process is the so-called transcription-regulating sequence (TRS). In coronaviruses and toroviruses, this motif is a species-specific AU-rich sequence of ca. 10 nt, located within the 5′ NTR and upstream of the ORFs that are destined to become 5′ proximal in the subgenomic mRNAs. In the arteriviruses, the motif is also an AU-rich, species-specific sequence of 6 nt. Secondary structure predictions of the 5′ NTR of many coronaviruses and arteriviruses (Van den Born et al. 2004) places the 5′ TRS (which is termed the leader TRS, see below) in a hairpin loop structure referred to as the 'leader TRS hairpin' or LTH. This structure is thought to be critical for the process of discontinuous RNA synthesis that takes place during the production of coronavirus and arterivirus virus minus-strand RNA.

As for many other viruses, the packaging of coronavirus and arterivirus genomes is a process that involves the interaction of virus structural proteins and elements in the genomic RNA. It has been shown for the coronaviruses MHV and BCoV that the packaging of genomic RNA is, at least partially, mediated by an RNA element located at the 3' end of the replicase gene (Cologna and Hogue 2000; Fosmire et al. 1992). In contrast, the packaging signal of TGEV has been located at the 5' end of the genome, specifically, within the first 640 nt (Escors et al. 2003). Also, it has been shown that DI-RNA sequences from the 5' and 3' NTR of IBV are required for minigenome incorporation into viral particles (Dalton et al. 2001). It is possible that for some coronaviruses, the packaging signal may be comprised of multiple elements but more data are needed to resolve this apparent discrepancy. The packaging signals of arteriviruses have not been mapped.

The 3' NTR of coronaviruses and arteriviruses comprises 60–150 nt (arteriviruses) or 200–500 nt (coronaviruses and toroviruses) following the last functional ORF and preceding the polyadenylate tract. It can be expected that secondary (or tertiary) structures in the 3' NTR will have important roles in virus replication. Indeed, at the very 3' end of the MHV 3' NTR an extensive complex structure containing multiple stem loops and bulges has been identified and shown to have a role in DI-RNA replication (Liu et al. 2001). This structure incorporates a common motif, $^G/_U$GGAAGAGC$^U/_C$, that is found 70–80 nt from the 3' end of all coronavirus 3' NTRs examined to date. Also, the 3' NTR of the MHV and BCoV genomes has been shown to include phylogenetically conserved structures, the 3' NTR bulged stem loop and the 3' NTR pseudoknot, that are postulated to represent a molecular switch that controls an, as yet unidentified, aspect of viral RNA synthesis (Goebel et al. 2004). There has been no detailed analysis of the arterivirus 3' NTR and the only significant nucleotide sequence conservation that has been found in the 3' NTR is located immediately upstream of the polyadenylate tract. However, it has become clear that RNA signals involved in arterivirus replication extend into the coding sequences in the 3'-proximal region of the genome (Molenkamp et al. 2000). In the case of PRRSV, a so-called 'kissing interaction' between the loop sequences of RNA hairpin structures in the 3' NTR and the nucleocapsid protein gene was recently found to be crucial for minus-strand RNA synthesis (Verheije et al. 2002b).

OPEN READING FRAMES

The available data suggest that coronavirus and arterivirus genomes contain between six and 14 functional ORFs. The easiest to define are those located toward the 3' end of the genome, encoding the structural proteins (Figure 39.2). For coronaviruses and toroviruses, these are the spike (S), membrane (M), and nucleocapsid protein (N) ORFs and for the arteriviruses these are ORFs encoding the major surface glycoprotein (GP$_5$), three minor glycoproteins (see the section on structural proteins) and the envelope (E), membrane (M), and nucleocapsid (N) proteins. The gene order, 5'-surface glycoprotein(s) ORF(s)/membrane protein ORF/nucleocapsid protein ORF-3', is conserved in the genome of all coronaviruses and arteriviruses studied to date.

The genomes of coronaviruses contain a fourth structural protein ORF, encoding the E (envelope) protein, located 5' proximal to the M protein ORF. The genomes of toroviruses and a subset of coronaviruses (e.g. HCoV-OC43, MHV, BCoV) also contain an additional structural protein gene, the hemagglutinin-esterase (HE) ORF. The location of this ORF in coronaviruses is 5' proximal to the S protein gene, and in toroviruses it lies between the M and N protein genes (Cornelissen et al. 1997; Snijder et al. 1991). It seems that the HE gene is not essential and may be converted to a pseudogene; for example, during prolonged passage of virus in tissue culture. Recently, it has been suggested that the SARS-coronavirus (SARS-CoV) genome encodes an additional structural protein (currently known as the 3a protein) that is associated with the spike glycoprotein (Zeng et al. 2004).

In the arteriviruses, the glycoprotein encoded by the PRRSV ORF2a, its homologues encoded by ORF2b in EAV and LDV, as well as the EAV and PRRSV ORF3 and ORF4 glycoproteins, were experimentally identified as minor virion components (de Vries et al. 1992; Faaberg and Plagemann 1995; Meulenberg and Petersen-den Besten 1996; Snijder et al. 1999; van Nieuwstadt et al. 1996; Wieringa et al. 2002). It should be noted that the PRRSV ORF3 glycoprotein was suggested to be a minor structural glycoprotein in a European PRRSV isolate (van Nieuwstadt et al. 1996) but a nonstructural protein in a Canadian isolate (Mardassi et al. 1998). Finally, a small, nonglycosylated envelope protein, encoded by ORF2a in EAV and ORF2b in PRRSV, was detected in virus particles and designated E (for envelope) protein (Snijder et al. 1999; Wu et al. 2001).

In the SHFV genome, the region corresponding to that between ORF 1b and ORF 5 in the other three arteriviruses contains three additional ORFs, covering about 1.6 kb (Smith et al. 1997). On the basis of limited sequence similarities, it was postulated that these SHFV ORFs (named ORFs 2a, 2b, and 3) have arisen from the duplication of the SHFV homologues of EAV/LDV/PRRSV ORFs 2–4 by an RNA recombination event (Godeny et al. 1998). Except for this putative triple gene duplication in SHFV, the genetic composition and gene order of all arteriviruses are identical.

With respect to ORFs that encode nonstructural proteins, the corona- and arterivirus genome is dominated by the replicase gene (also referred to as the RNA polymerase gene or RNA polymerase locus). The

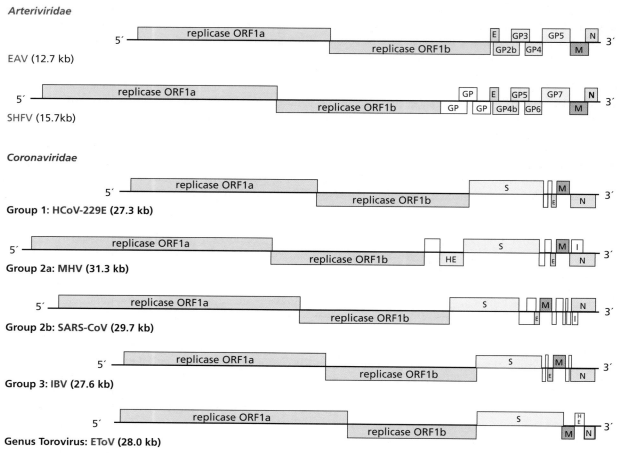

Figure 39.2 *Genomic structure of coronaviruses, toroviruses, and arteriviruses. The genomic ORFs of representative arteri- and coronaviruses are indicated and the names of the replicase protein and structural protein genes are given. References to the nomenclature of the accessory protein genes can be found in the text. Note that the HE protein gene of EToV is a pseudogene but that a functional HE protein is expressed from the BToV genome (Cornelissen et al. 1997). Note also that the arterivirus and coronavirus genomes are drawn to different scales.*

replicase gene consists of two large ORFs encompassing ca. 10 000 nt (arteriviruses) or 20 000 nt (coronaviruses and toroviruses) toward the 5′ end of the genome. These ORFs, ORF1a and ORF1b, overlap in the −1 reading frame. The extent of the overlap varies but invariably encompasses a specific sequence motif, UUUAAAC (or GUUAAAC in the case of EAV), which is referred to as the 'slippery' sequence. Immediately downstream of the slippery sequence is a characteristic RNA structure, the pseudoknot, which can be formed by base pairing. Together, these two elements mediate −1 ribosomal frameshifting during expression of the replicase gene (Brierley 1995). The translation products of the 1a and 1b ORFs are extensively processed by virus-encoded proteinases and, as described below in the section entitled Replicase, produce a large number of proteins that assemble to form a functional replication-transcription complex.

In contrast to the replicase gene, the pattern and arrangement of the remaining nonstructural protein ORFs in the genomes of nidoviruses depend on the virus genus. In the toroviruses and arteriviruses, there is no evidence for nonstructural genes other than the replicase gene. In the coronaviruses there is a diverse and complex pattern of nonstructural genes, even for viruses that are considered to be closely related. The reasons for this complexity are probably two-fold. First, many coronavirus genes seem to encode proteins with accessory functions. Thus, under certain conditions (for example, adaptation and propagation in cultured cells), mutations accumulate which lead to the inactivation and even deletion of these genes. Second, not only divergence from a common ancestor but also RNA recombination seems to have been a major driving force in the evolution of nidoviruses (see also Chapter 20, The order *Nidovirales*). It is particularly interesting to note that the SARS-CoV genome encodes a large number of nonstructural proteins that are probably not involved in RNA synthesis and that many of the ORFs encoding these proteins appear to have no counterparts in other coronaviruses.

Replication

A hallmark of the order *Nidovirales* is the production of a set of multiple, subgenomic, 3′ co-terminal mRNAs in the infected cell. The subgenomic mRNAs are synthesized in nonequimolar amounts but in relatively constant proportions throughout the replication cycle. The structural relationship of these subgenomic mRNAs to the genomic RNA is illustrated for MHV, EAV, and EToV in Figure 39.3. The replication of the coronavirus MHV and the arterivirus EAV have been studied most intensively and it is assumed that these viruses set a paradigm for other nidoviruses. However, it is also clear that the replication of coronaviruses, toroviruses, and arteriviruses differs, at least in some details. One particularly notable difference is the fact that, in contrast to the subgenomic mRNAs of coronaviruses and arteriviruses,

all but the largest of the subgenomic transcripts of toroviruses lack a 5′ leader sequence derived from the 5′-proximal region of the genome (see below).

TRANSCRIPTION

The process by which nidoviruses generate multiple subgenomic mRNAs in the infected cell is complex and not fully understood. A detailed description of the extensive and sometimes conflicting literature in this area is beyond the scope of this chapter and only a summary of the most important aspects is presented here. For more information, the reader is referred to the

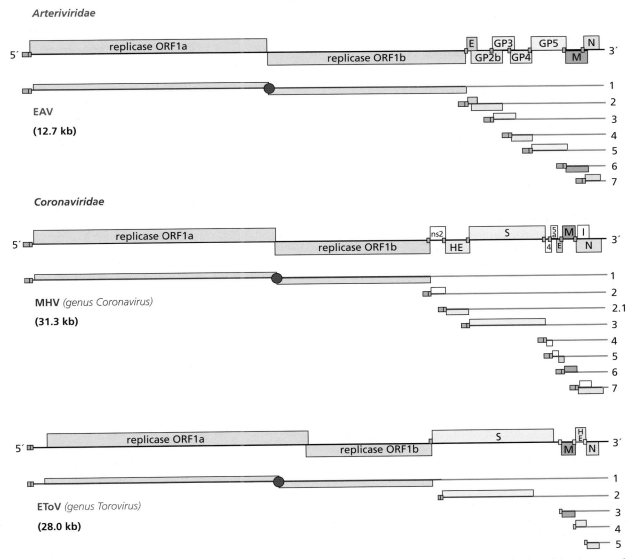

Figure 39.3 *The genome expression strategies of EAV, MHV, and EToV. The figure shows the genomic organization of the viruses and the structural relationships of the genome-length and subgenome-length mRNAs. The leader sequence and TRS sequences found at the 5′ end of EAV and MHV mRNAs, as well as the genome-length and subgenome-length mRNA2 of EToV are indicated as blue and orange boxes, respectively. The TRS-like element found at the 5′ end of EToV subgenome-length mRNAs 3, 4, and 5 is indicated as a yellow box. The ribosomal frameshifting element found in genome-length mRNA1 is indicated as a green circle and the translated region of each mRNA is indicated in green (the translationally silent regions are indicated in red). Only the translated ORFs are indicated for each mRNA.*

published literature and references therein (Alonso et al. 2002; Baric and Yount 2000; Curtis et al. 2004; Lai and Holmes 2001; Pasternak et al. 2001, 2004; Sawicki et al. 2001; Snijder and Meulenberg 2001; van der Most and Spaan 1995; van Vliet et al. 2002; Zuniga et al. 2004).

- The polycistronic genomic RNA of nidoviruses is infectious.
- Coronavirus and arterivirus subgenomic mRNAs are comprised of non-contiguous sequences. At their 5′ end they have a leader sequence of 65–100 nt (coronaviruses) or 150–210 nts (arteriviruses) that is derived from the 5′-proximal region of the genome. In toroviruses, only the largest subgenomic mRNA contains a short leader sequence derived from the 5′ end of the genome. All smaller torovirus subgenomic mRNAs do not contain this leader sequence.
- The site at which the leader and body of the mRNA are joined is defined by the position of a specific TRS, a conserved regulatory sequence preceding the mRNA body (body TRS). This sequence is also present at the 3′ end of the leader (leader TRS). The TRS is often referred to as the intergenic region or leader-body junction site in the older literature on coronaviruses and arteriviruses, respectively. In the case of all but the largest of the torovirus subgenomic mRNAs, the 5′ end of the mRNA is defined by a similar conserved regulatory sequence, apparently without the subsequent acquisition of the genomic 5′ leader sequence via a discontinuous RNA synthesis event as is found in coronaviruses and arteriviruses.
- The fusion of leader and body sequences of subgenomic mRNAs, as it occurs in coronaviruses and arteriviruses and the largest subgenomic mRNA of toroviruses, relies on a mechanism in which specific base-pairing interactions between RNA sequences and higher order RNA structures play an important role. This process appears to resemble sequence similarity-assisted RNA recombination, as it occurs in many positive strand RNA viruses (Nagy and Simon 1997).

In the coronaviruses:

- The bulk of the mRNA in the cell is produced from transcription intermediates that contain subgenome-length, negative-strand RNA. There is one transcription intermediate per mRNA species.
- The bulk of the subgenome-length negative-strand RNAs has an antileader sequence at their 3′ end.
- The subgenome-length RNAs (positive or negative strand) are not able to initiate a transcription complex.

It has also been shown that EAV-infected cells contain a set of subgenome-length transcription intermediates and that each intermediate contains a subgenome-length minus-strand RNA with an antileader sequence (den Boon et al. 1996).

These observations have been interpreted using two different models that essentially attempt to explain three basic questions. (1) How do subgenome-length templates arise? (2) How are the leader and body sequences of sg mRNAs joined? (3) What is the role of the conserved transcription-regulating sequences during subgenomic RNA synthesis?

The first model proposes that the genomic RNA enters the cell and is translated to produce RNA replicase that is used to synthesize a full-length negative-strand copy of the genome, the so-called antigenome. Transcription is initiated from the 3′ end of the antigenome and a leader transcript, identical to the 5′-proximal part of the genome, is synthesized. This leader RNA is then used to prime transcription of the different mRNA bodies, a process for which base pairing of the leader TRS (the TRS at the 3′ end of the leader RNA) with each of the body TRS complements in the antigenome would be a necessary interaction to synthesize a complete set of subgenomic mRNAs. The essential features of this model are that the discontinuous step takes place during positive-strand RNA synthesis and that the complement of each body TRS acts essentially as a promoter for subgenomic mRNA synthesis.

The second model has a different 'scenario.' Again, the genomic RNA enters the cell and is translated to produce RNA replicase. The RNA replicase is then used, however, to produce not only antigenome but also a set of subgenome-length negative-strand RNAs, the 3′ ends of which are defined by the body TRSs. These negative-strand RNAs then acquire an antileader sequence by a discontinuous 3′ terminal extension process that involves a crucial base pairing interaction between the body TRS complement at the 3′ end of the nascent minus strand and the leader TRS in the 5′ end of the genomic template (Pasternak et al. 2001; Zuniga et al. 2004). Subsequently, the subgenome-length negative-strand RNAs are completed by addition of the antileader sequence (the complement of the genomic leader sequence) and the subgenome-length minus-strand templates carry the RNA replicase into a transcription complex and act as templates for viral mRNA synthesis in the cell. In this model, discontinuous RNA synthesis takes place during the production of negative-strand RNA synthesis and the body TRSs act essentially as attenuators of RNA synthesis (Sawicki and Sawicki 1998).

Using the newly developed reverse genetics systems for arteriviruses (Meulenberg et al. 1998; van Dinten et al. 1997) and coronaviruses (Almazan et al. 2000; Thiel et al. 2001a; Yount et al. 2000), two important aspects of nidovirus discontinuous RNA synthesis were recently addressed (Pasternak et al. 2001; van Marle et al. 1999a; Zuniga et al. 2004). The first, which applies to both transcription models, is the base-pairing interaction between the leader TRS and the complement of the body TRS in the viral negative strand. By site-directed mutagenesis, it was shown that disruption of this base-pairing interaction can dramatically affect subgenomic mRNA synthesis, whereas the introduction of compensatory mutations could restore subgenomic mRNA synthesis. The second aspect is the origin of the TRS that forms the leader-body junction in the mRNA molecule. Whereas the first model predicts this sequence to be a copy of the leader TRS, the discontinuous minus strand extension model predicts exactly the opposite, i.e. the sequence in the mRNA should be a copy of the body intergenic region or TRS. Using EAV TRS mutants with partial transcriptional activity, it was demonstrated that, indeed, the body TRS determines the sequence at the mRNA leader-body junction. Together with biochemical data obtained for coronaviruses (Baric and Yount 2000; Sawicki et al. 2001), these results provide strong evidence for the discontinuous minus strand extension model.

The remarkable recent data on the structure of torovirus subgenomic mRNAs (van Vliet et al. 2002), and the reported absence of a common 5' leader sequence in roniviruses (see Chapter 20, The order *Nidovirales*), have made it clear that the production of subgenomic RNAs by discontinuous RNA synthesis is not a universal feature of nidoviruses. The largest subgenomic mRNA of toroviruses is most likely generated in a manner similar to that proposed above for coronaviruses and arteriviruses. Namely, a short piece of identical sequence, present both at the 3' end of the leader and the 5' end of the body segment, functions as the crossover site for an RNA recombination-like process during negative-strand RNA synthesis. This process may be enhanced by a predicted RNA hairpin located just upstream of the proposed attenuation site. However, for the remaining subgenomic RNAs of toroviruses, and for those of roniviruses, it was proposed that minus-strand synthesis is attenuated at the conserved ('TRS-like') sequence upstream of the body segment and that these attenuated minus-strand RNAs can function directly as templates for subgenomic mRNA synthesis. It is important that the minus-strands generated in cells infected with roniviruses and toroviruses are investigated in detail, to confirm that subgenome-length minus-strands indeed exist and result from attenuation of minus-strand RNA synthesis. However, if this is the case, it may be that the attenuation of minus strand RNA synthesis is, in fact, the common feature that unites the mechanisms used to produce subgenomic mRNAs in different nidoviruses. This conclusion would then provoke the question of the functions associated with the nidovirus leader sequence and, ultimately, the nature of the cis-acting signals needed for the promotion of nidovirus plus strand RNA synthesis. Finally, it should be noted that, in addition to the interactions described above, many other, as yet undiscovered, RNA–RNA, RNA–protein and protein–protein interactions are expected to play a role in nidovirus subgenomic mRNA synthesis

(Pasternak et al. 2000; Shi et al. 2000; Tijms et al. 2001; van Dinten et al. 2000; Yu and Leibowitz 1995; Zhang and Lai 1995).

TRANSLATION

The production of a 3' co-terminal set of subgenomic mRNAs in the infected cell allows for the expression of genes that are located internally on the nonsegmented genome. By and large, the viral mRNAs are thought to be functionally monocistronic although usually, with the exception of the smallest mRNA, they are structurally polycistronic. This conclusion is based mainly on the in vitro translation of coronavirus mRNAs and conforms to the conventional 'ribosome scanning' model of translational initiation. Thus, taking MHV as an example (Figure 39.3), the smallest mRNA, mRNA 7, encodes the nucleocapsid protein, mRNA 6 encodes the membrane protein, mRNA 3 encodes the spike protein, and so on. If the genomic sequence is known and the position of the functional body TRSs or intergenic regions has been determined by sequence analysis of mRNAs, a 'translational model' can be deduced for each of the viruses belonging to the order *Nidovirales*. It should be noted, however, that for arteriviruses, toroviruses, and even the majority of coronaviruses, this 'model' still needs to be confirmed by experiment.

The model outlined above describes the basic translational strategy of nidoviruses. However, Figure 39.3 indicates that there have to be exceptions. For example, MHV has no subgenomic mRNAs that could account for the expression of ORFs 1b, E, or I in this manner. It is now clear that nidoviruses also use a variety of alternative translation strategies to express some of their gene products.

In several coronaviruses (Brierley 1995; Brierley and Pennell 2001; Thiel et al. 2003), EToV (Snijder et al. 1990) and EAV (den Boon et al. 1991) the region of RNA that encompasses the overlap of ORFs 1a and 1b is able to mediate a high frequency of −1 ribosomal frameshifting. Thus, ORF1b is expressed as a fusion protein with the ORF1a gene product. As described above, ribosomal frameshifting is mediated by a 'shifty' sequence, the actual position at which frameshifting takes place, and an RNA pseudoknot which is believed to slow or halt the ribosome as it translates this sequence. The most likely mechanism of frameshifting is simultaneous slippage of two ribosome-bound tRNAs present in the aminoacyl and peptidyl sites of the ribosome during decoding of the 'shifty' sequence. The mechanistic aspects of nidovirus −1 ribosomal frameshifting have been analyzed in some detail (Brierley et al. 1997; Liphardt et al. 1999; Marczinke et al. 2000; Napthine et al. 1999).

The subgenomic mRNAs encoding the E proteins of MHV (mRNA 5) and IBV (mRNA 3) contain two and three ORFs, respectively, in their 5' unique regions. The

E ORF is 3'-proximal in both cases and the mRNAs are functionally bi- and tricistronic, respectively (Budzilowicz and Weiss 1987; Liu et al. 1991). Therefore, the expression of the E ORF has to involve the internal initiation of protein synthesis. The unique region of both mRNAs contains an element that is able to mediate the internal entry of ribosomes and initiate protein synthesis in a cap-independent manner (Jendrach et al. 1999; Liu and Inglis 1992). This element has not yet been characterized in detail. A similar element has also been recognized in the mRNA 3 of certain TGEV strains (O'Connor and Brian 2000). In the arterivirus group, mRNA 2 of EAV was proposed to be a functionally bicistronic mRNA from which both the GP$_{2b}$ glycoprotein and the newly discovered E protein are expressed (Snijder et al. 1999). Likewise, mRNA 2 of LDV and PRRSV and mRNA 4 of SHFV are probably used to express the corresponding genes of these other arteriviruses. Another mRNA of SHFV, mRNA 2, was proposed to be functionally bicistronic but, in this case, the expression of two ORFs (2a and 2b) from this mRNA remains to be demonstrated (Godeny et al. 1998).

Sequence analysis of the nucleocapsid protein gene of SARS-CoV, MHV, and related coronaviruses (Parker and Masters 1990; Snijder 2003a) has revealed an ORF, the internal or I ORF, which, in BCoV, is expressed in infected cells and encodes a 23-kDa, membrane-associated protein (Senanayake et al. 1992). The internal protein is translated from the same mRNA as the nucleocapsid protein, and it has been suggested, mainly on theoretical grounds, that the initiation of internal protein synthesis conforms to the 'leaky ribosomal scanning' model proposed by Kozak (Kozak 1999). Similar considerations apply to some of the small ORFs in the 3'-proximal region of the SARS-CoV genome (Snijder et al. 2003a).

Nonstructural polypeptides

REPLICASE

The replicase gene of viruses belonging to the order *Nidovirales* encodes two polyproteins of extraordinary size and complexity. The translation of ORF1a theoretically produces a polyprotein, pp1a, of 450–500 kDa (coronaviruses) or 190–260 kDa (arteriviruses). Alternatively, as described above, −1 ribosomal frameshifting is used to express an ORF1ab-encoded fusion protein, pp1ab, with a potential molecular weight of 750–800 kDa (coronaviruses) or 350–420 kDa (arteriviruses). Moreover, the polyproteins themselves are not the end products of replicase gene expression. Instead, they are co- and post-translationally cleaved by viral proteinases that are part of these polyproteins to produce a complex array of functional gene products.

Sequence analysis of the predicted nidovirus replicase polyproteins has revealed a number of putative functional domains that appear to have been conserved during evolution (Brown and Brierley 1995; de Vries et al. 1997; Gorbalenya 2001; Gorbalenya et al. 1989a; Snijder et al. 2003a; Snijder and Spaan 1995; Ziebuhr 2004a,b). These domains and their approximate positions are illustrated in Figure 39.4.

The ORF1a-encoded part of nidovirus pp1a and pp1ab polyproteins contains several proteinase domains, which are of two types. First, papainlike cysteine proteinase (PLpro) domains are located in the N-proximal half of the polyprotein. These may be single domains (SARS-CoV) or multiple domains (e.g. MHV and PRRSV). Nidovirus PLpro domains are generally linked with zinc-finger domains (Figure 39.4) (Snijder et al. 1995; Herold et al. 1999; Tijms et al. 2001) and have similar (sometimes overlapping) substrate specificities (Ziebuhr et al. 2001). At most PLpro cleavage sites, small aliphatic residues are conserved at the P1 and P1′ positions (Ziebuhr et al. 2000). Second, towards the C-terminal end of pp1a, a 3C-like proteinase domain (3CLpro) is found. In coronaviruses (and roniviruses), the active site nucleophile of this proteinase is a cysteine residue, whereas its arterivirus counterpart contains an active site serine (Hegyi et al. 2002; Liu and Brown 1995; Lu et al. 1995; Snijder et al. 1996; Ziebuhr et al. 1997, 2003). The 3CLpros of coronaviruses and arteriviruses are members of the large superfamily of chymotrypsin-like proteolytic enzymes that share a two-β-barrel fold (Gorbalenya et al. 1989b). There are significant structural differences between the coronavirus and arterivirus 3CLpros, for example, with respect to their sizes, subdomain organizations, and principal catalytic residues (Anand et al. 2002, 2003; Barrette-Ng et al. 2002). Despite these differences, the 3CLpros of coronaviruses and arteriviruses have similar substrate specificities (Hegyi and Ziebuhr 2002; Snijder et al. 1996; Thiel et al. 2003; Wassenaar et al. 1997; Ziebuhr et al. 1995, 2000). Thus, both enzymes cleave at sites that have a glutamine (coronaviruses) or glutamic acid (arteriviruses) at the P1 position and a small residue (usually glycine, alanine, or serine) at the P1′ position.

An important secondary function of pp1a appears to be the anchoring of the nidovirus replication complex to intracellular membranes (see below). Hydrophobic domains that flank the 3CLpro at either side are conserved in the pp1a proteins of all nidoviruses (Gorbalenya 2001; Snijder and Meulenberg 1998; Ziebuhr 2004a) (Figure 39.4). In the ORF1b-encoded product, which is expressed only as part of pp1ab, four domains have been conserved in all nidoviruses. The first is a RNA-dependent RNA polymerase module (RdRp) that is also found in a wide variety of putative RNA-dependent RNA polymerases. The alteration of the polymerase 'core' motif from glycine–aspartic acid–aspartic acid (GDD) to serine–aspartic acid–aspartic acid (SDD) is a feature that seems to be characteristic for the nidoviruses (Gorbalenya et al. 1989a). The second is a

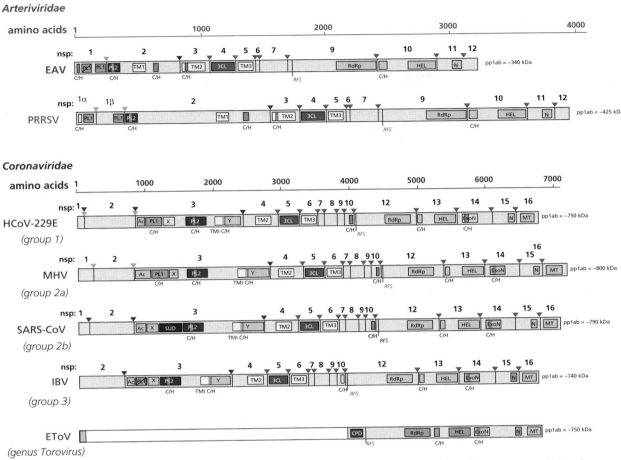

Figure 39.4 *The replicase gene organization of representative arteriviruses and coronaviruses. The replicase gene organization is depicted in the form of the polyprotein pp1ab. The delineation of amino acids encoded in ORF1a and ORF1b is indicated as RFS (ribosomal frameshift) and arrows represent sites in pp1ab that are cleaved by papainlike proteinases (orange and blue) or the main (3CL) proteinase (red). The proteolytic cleavage products are numbered and within the cleavage products, the location of domains that have been identified as structurally or functionally related are highlighted. These include domains with conserved Cys and His residues (C/H), putative transmembrane domains (TM), domains with conserved features (Ac, X, and Y), and domains that have been associated with proteolysis (PL1, PL2, and 3CL), RNA-dependent RNA synthesis (RdRp), helicase (HEL), exonuclease (ExoN), uridylate-specific endoribonuclease (N), and methyl transferase (MT) activities. Note that the arterivirus and coronavirus polyproteins are drawn to different scales.*

cysteine–histidine-rich motif that has been proposed to function as multinuclear zinc-finger (ZF) domain and was implicated in viral RNA synthesis (van Dinten et al. 1997, 2000). The third, and part of the same protein as the ZF domain, is a helicase domain. The location of the helicase domain downstream of the polymerase module in the polyprotein is unusual and characteristic of nidoviruses. And fourth is a conserved domain near the C-terminal end of pp1ab that was recently identified as a uridylate-specific endoribonuclease (NendoU) (Ivanov et al. 2004b; Snijder et al. 2003a). There are a number of (putative) additional RNA-processing activities (Snijder et al. 2003a) that appear to be differentially conserved among nidoviruses, indicating that the enzymology of viral RNA synthesis and/or some virus–host interactions may differ among the various nidovirus families and genera. Thus, for example, all nidoviruses (except for the arteriviruses)

have been predicted to encode 3′-to-5′ exoribonuclease and 2′-O-ribose methyltransferase functions in ORF1b (Figure 39.4). Coronaviruses (but not arteriviruses and roniviruses) also encode a putative ADP-ribose 1″-phosphatase activity that is conserved in only very few plus-strand RNA viruses (Gorbalenya et al. 1991; Snijder et al. 2003a). Finally, toroviruses and group 2 coronaviruses (excluding SARS-CoV) encode a putative cyclic phosphodiesterase that is located at the C-terminus of the torovirus ORF1a encoded polyprotein, whereas the coronavirus homologue is expressed from a sg RNA (rather than being part of the replicase polyprotein itself) (Snijder et al. 2003a). The activities of most of the nidovirus RNA-processing enzymes remain to be characterized.

Compared with other positive-strand RNA viruses, the biochemical analysis of functions encoded in the nidovirus replicase is still at an early stage (for a comprehensive review, see Ziebuhr (2004a)). There have been occasional reports of RNA-dependent RNA polymerase activity in subcellular fractions of coronavirus-infected cells or coronavirus-infected cells permeabilized with lysolecithin. However, there is no evidence that these systems can initiate RNA synthesis and their application has been very limited. Coronavirus RdRps and their nidovirus relatives have been classified as an outgroup of superfamiliy 1 RdRps (Koonin 1991). A molecular model for the coronavirus RdRp domain, which resides in the C-terminal two-thirds of nsp12 (Gorbalenya et al. 1989a) (Figure 39.4), has recently been reported (Xu et al. 2003). Furthermore, it has been proposed that the MHV nsp12 interacts through a protein segment located upstream of the C-terminal RdRp core domain with ORF1a-encoded proteins, such as nsp4 (3CL^{pro}), nsp8, and nsp9 (Brockway et al. 2003). Crystal structure analysis of SARS-CoV nsp9 and biochemical data have shown that nsp9 is a single-stranded RNA-binding protein (Egloff et al. 2004; Sutton et al. 2004) and genetic data obtained for MHV have implicated nsp10 in minus-strand synthesis (Siddell et al. 2001). Taken together, the data suggest that the small proteins encoded by the 3′-proximal region of ORF1a may have co-factor functions for the RdRp and be directly or indirectly involved in viral RNA synthesis.

In the replicase polyprotein, the RdRp domain is C-terminally flanked by a multidomain protein, called nsp10 in arteriviruses and nsp13 in coronaviruses, which contains N-terminal ZF and C-terminal helicase domains (Figure 39.4). Nidovirus helicases have been shown to have NTPase, RNA 5′-triphosphatase as well as RNA and DNA duplex-unwinding activities (Bautista et al. 2002; Heusipp et al. 1997; Ivanov et al. 2004a; Ivanov and Ziebuhr 2004; Seybert et al. 2000a, 2005; Tanner et al. 2003). Coronavirus and arterivirus helicases appear to act processively and unwind their substrates with 5′-to-3′ polarity (Ivanov et al. 2004a; Ivanov and Ziebuhr 2004; Seybert et al. 2000a, 2005). The N-terminal ZF was recently shown to be required for the enzymatic activities of nidovirus helicases (Seybert et al. 2005). Both the in vitro activities of nsp10/nsp13 and RNA replication of EAV in tissue culture were found to be extremely sensitive to substitutions of conserved Cys and His residues in the ZF domain (Seybert et al. 2005; van Dinten et al. 2000). Furthermore, point mutations that selectively inactivate EAV sg RNA synthesis (van Dinten et al. 1997, 2000; van Marle et al. 1999b) were identified and mapped to the region connecting the ZF and helicase domains of the protein. The flexibility of this spacer was postulated to be essential for the function of the protein in sg RNA synthesis. Furthermore, the most N-terminal cleavage product of the EAV replicase, nsp1, was implicated in the regulation of sg RNA synthesis. The protein was shown to be dispensable for genome replication, but absolutely required for sg RNA synthesis (Tijms et al. 2001).

Recently, manganese-dependent, uridylate-specific endoribonuclease activities (NendoU) were established for nsp15 of SARS-CoV and HCoV-229E (Ivanov et al. 2004b; Snijder et al. 2003a; Bhardwaj et al. 2004) (Figure 39.4). The nsp15 activity was shown to be critically involved in coronavirus RNA synthesis. Although nsp15 is capable of cleaving both single-stranded and double-stranded RNA in vitro, the biologically relevant substrate was proposed to be double-stranded RNA, which is cleaved more effectively and specifically at GU and GUU sequences (Ivanov et al. 2004b). 2′-O-ribose-methylated RNA substrates proved to be resistant to cleavage by nsp15, indicating that the putative 2′-O-ribose methyltransferase domain residing adjacent to NendoU in the coronavirus replicase polyprotein may control or modulate the ribonucleolytic activity of nsp15.

Also, there are an ever-increasing number of reports on the characterization of arterivirus and coronavirus proteinases and the proteolytic processing of the replicase gene products. A detailed review of these data is beyond the scope of this chapter (for recent reviews, see Ziebuhr 2004a; Ziebuhr et al. 2000). Briefly, the papain-like proteinases seem to be largely responsible for the processing in *cis* of N-terminal and N-proximal products from the ORF1a-encoded region of the replicase polyproteins, whilst the 3C-like proteinases are likely to function mainly in *trans* and are responsible for self-excision and processing of the pp1a and pp1ab polyproteins downstream of the proteinase domain itself (Figure 39.4). Because of their key role in polyprotein processing, nidovirus 3C-like proteinases are considered to be attractive targets for antiviral (in particular, anti-SARS) drug development (Anand et al. 2003; Davidson and Siddell 2003). Over the past years, significant progress has been made in the functional and structural characterization of these enzymes. Thus, for example, crystal structures of several coronavirus and arterivirus 3C-like proteinases have been reported and the binding modes of proteinase substrates have been elucidated by X-ray structure analysis of inhibitors bound to the active sites of TGEV and SARS-CoV 3CLpros, respectively (Anand et al. 2002, 2003; Barrette-Ng et al. 2002; Shi et al. 2004; Yang et al. 2003). The structural information provides an excellent basis for rational drug design and, because of the conserved substrate specificity of coronavirus 3CLpros, even the development of broad-spectrum proteinase inhibitors suitable for the therapy of human and animal coronavirus infections may be a tractable goal (Anand et al. 2003; Hegyi and Ziebuhr 2002; Thiel et al. 2003). Also, other nidovirus replicative proteins, such as the RNA-processing enzymes, RNA-binding proteins, RdRp, and the helicase, might be targets for selective antiviral therapies (Davidson and Siddell 2003), although their characterization is still at an early stage.

INTRACELLULAR LOCALIZATION OF THE REPLICASE

Over the past decade, the association of their replication complex with intracellular membranes (of different origin) has emerged as a common feature of positive-strand RNA viruses that replicate in eukaryotic cells (see, for example, Ahlquist et al. 2003; Mackenzie et al. 1999; Rust et al. 2001; Salonen et al. 2003) and references therein). The association of viral replicases with (modified) cellular membranes is thought to be an important advantage in creating a suitable (micro)-environment for viral RNA synthesis. Furthermore, the formation of membrane-bounded complexes may aid in shielding double-stranded RNA replication intermediates from double-stranded RNA activated host defense mechanisms such as RNA interference and interferon-induced pathways.

The subcellular localization of the replicase has only been studied in detail for the arterivirus EAV and for the coronavirus MHV. In the case of EAV, most replicase subunits (including RdRp and helicase) localize to virus-induced double-membrane structures that are likely derived from the endoplasmic reticulum (ER) (Pedersen et al. 1999; van der Meer et al. 1998). These paired membranes and double membrane vesicles (DMV) were shown previously to be induced by arterivirus infection. DMVs that strikingly resemble those seen in virus-infected cells could also be induced by expressing a part of the EAV pp1a protein (nsp2 and nsp3) (Pedersen et al. 1999; Snijder et al. 2001), indicating that their generation does not depend on viral replication or the presence of ORF1b-encoded protein functions. All cleavage products of the EAV pp1a and pp1ab polyproteins (with the exception of a fraction of nsp1; Tijms et al. 2002) and de novo synthesized RNA (as visualized by BrUTP labeling) colocalize to membranes in the perinuclear region of infected cells (Pedersen et al. 1999; van der Meer et al. 1998). Also, a substantial proportion of the EAV nucleocapsid protein was found in this region of the cell, but its involvement in genome replication or subgenomic (sg) RNA synthesis is highly unlikely, since nucleocapsid gene expression can be inactivated without a significant effect on either process (Molenkamp et al. 2000; Tijms et al. 2002).

For the only coronavirus studied in some detail thus far, MHV, the situation is less clear-cut, which may be partially due to the use of (i) a variety of cell lines, (ii) different cellular marker proteins, and (iii) antisera recognizing different MHV replicase subunits (compare, for example, Bost et al. 2001; Denison et al. 1999; Gosert et al. 2002; Shi et al. 1999, van der Meer et al. 1998). The majority of the MHV replicase subunits were found to be associated with intracellular membranes. During the peak of MHV RNA synthesis, key nonstructural proteins, like RdRp and helicase, de novo synthesized RNA, and also the viral nucleocapsid protein, were found to colocalize in punctate cytoplasmic foci (Denison et al. 1999; Shi et al. 1999; van der Meer et al. 1998). Ultra-structural studies of the replicase complex in MHV-infected cells have remained equivocal thus far. While the results of one study pointed mainly to membranes of (late) endosomal origin as the site of viral replication (van der Meer et al. 1998), a more recent study (Gosert et al. 2002) identified virus-induced double-membrane structures, resembling those implicated in the RNA synthesis of arteriviruses. Although all reports support the membrane association of MHV (and more recently also SARS-CoV) RNA synthesis, a variety of different cellular compartments (including ER, Golgi complex, endosomes, and autophagosomes) have been implicated in viral RNA synthesis (Ivanov et al. 2004a; Prentice et al. 2004a,b). Furthermore, the localization of, in particular, the MHV helicase protein, was reported to change later in infection (Bost et al. 2001).

Although further studies are necessary before definite conclusions can be reached, it does appear that major differences between arterivirus and coronavirus replication complexes may exist. In general, it is unclear how the nidovirus replicase associates with membranes. The most relevant questions are: (i) the mechanism of membrane insertion of the replicase subunits that anchor the complex, (ii) the coordination of proteolytic processing and membrane association, (iii) the role of protein–protein interaction (between viral proteins and possibly between viral and host proteins), and (iv) the interaction with host membranes, including the formation of double membranes and DMVs.

ACCESSORY PROTEINS

In the case of the arterivirus EAV, it has been shown that none of the ORFs downstream of the replicase gene are required for genome replication or subgenomic (sg) mRNA synthesis (Molenkamp et al. 2000). Each of these genes seems to encode a structural protein that is essential for the production of infectious progeny virus (Wieringa et al. 2003a). In the case of coronaviruses, there are a variety of proteins of unknown function encoded downstream of the replicase gene. Little more is known about them than their predicted molecular weights and putative structural features deduced from computer-assisted analyses (Brown and Brierley 1995) (see Figure 39.4). They do not appear to be essential for coronavirus sg RNA synthesis (Thiel et al. 2001b). The expression of some of the accessory proteins has been confirmed in coronavirus-infected tissue culture cells (reviewed in Brown and Brierley 1995) and evidence of post-translational modification (e.g. phosphorylation of the BCoV ORF2 protein) (Cox et al. 1991) has been obtained. Recently, the crystal structure of the SARSCoV ORF7a protein revealed an Ig-like fold for this intracellular membrane protein (Nelson et al. 2005). The picture, however, remains very incomplete. Despite this lack of information, two interesting observations have been made. First, for some coronaviruses, variants have been obtained that are defective for the expression of one or more of these proteins but are able, nevertheless, to replicate normally in tissue culture. Thus, for example, MHV variants defective for the expression of the ORF2, ORF4 or ORF5a gene products have normal properties in vitro (Schwarz et al. 1990; Yokomori and Lai 1991). Consistent with this idea, other studies show that deletion of the accessory genes from the MHV or FIPV genomes, result in replication-competent viruses that are, nevertheless, attenuated in mice and cats respectively, suggesting that these proteins provide a selective advantage in the natural host (de Haan et al. 2002b; Haijema et al. 2004). Second, it seems that the functions carried by some proteins of the *Coronaviridae* may be looked upon as 'genetic cassettes.' Thus, for example, the MHV CPDase domain is encoded by ORF2 whereas its EToV homologue is encoded at the 3' end of the ORF1a (Snijder et al. 1991). Another example of this concept is the proteins encoded by ORFs 4a and 4b of HCoV-229E, which seem to be equivalent to the single protein encoded by ORF3 of porcine epidemic diarrhoea virus (PEDV) (Duarte et al. 1994). In a similar vein, SARS-CoV has been predicted to encode as many as eight accessory proteins. Also in this case, it seems that (at least some of) these proteins are not essential in tissue culture. Thus, for example, a deletion in ORF7b was observed upon passage of the Frankfurt 1 strain of SARS-CoV in tissue culture (Thiel et al. 2003). Furthermore, SARS-CoV isolates obtained from SARS patients differed from SARS-CoV-like viruses isolated from Himalayan palm civets (and one human isolate, GZ01) by a 29-nucleotide deletion in ORF8 (Guan et al. 2003), generating two smaller ORFs, 8a and 8b. The biological

significance of the deletion (e.g. in terms of pathogenesis and/or adaptation to the human host) remains to be investigated. Thus far, only one of the SARS-CoV accessory proteins, the ORF3a protein, has been characterized in some detail (Yu et al. 2004; Zeng et al. 2004). Sequence comparison of diverse SARS-CoV isolates suggests a correlation of specific substitutions in the ORF3a and spike protein genes, suggesting that the biological function of the ORF3a protein is closely associated with spike protein functions (Zeng et al. 2004). The study suggests that the ORF3a protein associates with the SARS-CoV spike protein by intermolecular disulfide bridges and it is proposed that the ORF3a protein may be an additional structural protein.

Structural polypeptides

Whereas the RNA replicase provides clear evidence of an evolutionary link between viruses of the order *Nidovirales*, the structural proteins indicate a complex phylogeny, probably involving both recombination and evolution from a common ancestor. For example, the nucleoproteins of corona-, toro-, and arteriviruses show no sign of any relationship (apart from the features common to almost all nucleoproteins) whilst the envelope proteins of coronaviruses and toroviruses are clearly related both structurally and functionally. The structural proteins of coronaviruses, toroviruses, and arteriviruses are listed in Table 39.2.

NUCLEOCAPSID AND MEMBRANE POLYPEPTIDES

The nucleoprotein of corona-, toro-, and arteriviruses is a basic phosphoprotein that associates with the genomic RNA to form the nucleocapsid structure. However, the

Table 39.2 *Structural proteins of corona-, toro-, and arteriviruses*

Protein		Molecular weight (kDa)			Glycosylation	Abundance	Comments
		Corona	Toro-	Arteri-			
Nucleoprotein	N	50–69	19	12	No	Major	Basic, phosphorylated
Membrane	M	23–35	27	16	Only coronavirus	Major	Multi-membrane-spanning protein
Spike	S	180–220	200	...[a]	Yes	Major	Peplomer structure with coiled-coil elements
Envelope	E	9–12	...	7–9	No	Minor	Integral membrane protein
Hemagglutinin esterase	HE	65	65	...	Yes	Major	Subset of coronaviruses, disulfide-linked homodimer
Glycoprotein	GP_2	...	...	23–28	Yes	Minor	Part of $GP_2/Gp_3/GP_4$ heterotrimer
Glycoprotein	GP_3	...	...	18–29	Yes	Minor	Part of $GP_2/Gp_3/GP_4$ heterotrimer
Glycoprotein	GP_4	...	...	16–20	Yes	Minor	Part of $GP_2/Gp_3/GP_4$ heterotrimer
Glycoprotein	GP_5	...	...	30–45	Yes	Major	Disulfide-linked heterodimers with M

a) No such protein described.

nature of this association must be very different for the three groups of viruses. First, the sizes of the nucleocapsid proteins differ markedly and, secondly, the three groups of virus structures have very different morphologies. In a relaxed configuration, the coronaviruses and toroviruses have a helical nucleocapsid, which is unique among positive-strand RNA enveloped viruses, whilst the arteriviruses have an isometric (cubical) nucleocapsid. Recent data suggests that the coronavirus nucleocapsid protein binds to RNA with little sequence specificity (Narayanan et al. 2003a). Sequence comparisons and some partial structural information on coronavirus and arterivirus nucleocapsid proteins suggest a multidomain structure (Huang et al. 2004; Laude and Masters 1995), but the specific functions of the various domains remain to be elucidated. The partial crystal structure of the PRRSV N protein suggests that it may represent a new class of capsid-forming protein, with domains distinctly different from those of other known enveloped viruses (Doan and Dokland 2003). Both coronavirus and arterivirus nucleocapsid proteins assemble into higher order structures in virus-infected cells and when expressed as recombinant proteins (He et al. 2004; Narayanan et al. 2003b; Surjit et al. 2004; Wootton and Yoo 2003). Also, it has been noted that both the coronavirus and arterivirus nucleocapsid proteins have nucleo-nucleolar transport signals and a fraction of the protein synthesized in infected cells localizes to the nucleolus (Hiscox et al. 2001; Rowland et al. 2003; Tijms et al. 2002). However, it is not clear if this phenotype is linked, for example, to the viral modulation of nucleolar function, or simply a case of fortuitous molecular mimicry.

Coronaviruses and arteriviruses both have a multi-membrane-spanning protein, M. For most M proteins, it is thought that one of the hydrophobic transmembrane domains functions as an internal signal sequence, although for the M proteins of TGEV, FCoV, and CCoV an amino terminal signal sequence is present. Transient expression studies have revealed that the M protein also carries a signal for retention in the Golgi apparatus (coronavirus) or endoplasmic reticulum (torovirus and arterivirus) of the cell. Only when it is associated with other components of the virion does the M protein proceed beyond these compartments. Despite the striking similarities in structure of coronavirus and arterivirus M proteins, there are also significant differences. For example, only the M proteins of coronaviruses are glycosylated. In BCoV, MHV, and HCoV-OC43, O-glycosylation has been demonstrated; for the other coronaviruses, N-glycosylation is found (de Haan et al. 2002a; Rottier 1995).

Recent studies have shed some light on the role of the M protein in coronavirus budding. It appears that the coronavirus M protein may exist in two conformations. In TGEV, approximately two-thirds of the molecules are triple-membrane spanning and have a N_{exo}-C_{endo} configuration: the remaining molecules are quadruple-membrane spanning and have a N_{exo}-C_{exo} configuration. The molecules with an intravirion carboxyl-terminus are thought to interact with the nucleocapsid structure (Escors et al. 2001). Consistent with this conclusion, studies on MHV have suggested that the M protein interacts with the nucleocapsid structure, either by an M protein–N protein interaction (Kuo and Masters 2002) or by specifically binding to the packaging signal in the genomic RNA (Narayanan et al. 2003a). In any case, the M protein would link the incorporation of nucleocapsid structures to the virus budding process. Finally, de Haan and colleagues have shown that there are strong homotypic interactions between MHV M proteins and they suggest that these lateral interactions within the viral membrane generate the major driving force for envelope formation (de Haan et al. 1998, 2000). As discussed below, the coronavirus M protein is also believed to interact with the spike glycoprotein. Very little is known about the functional role(s) of the arterivirus M protein. It has been shown that the EAV and LDV M and GP_5 proteins are associated in virus particles as disulfide-linked heterodimers and that covalent linkage is essential for virus infectivity (Snijder et al. 2003b).

The coronavirus envelope protein, E, is predicted to have a hydrophobic region, located in the amino terminal half of the polypeptide, which is flanked by charged residues. Adjacent to this hydrophobic domain is a cysteine-rich region, followed by an abundance of charged residues in the carboxy half of the polypeptide (Siddell 1995). These features are indicative of an integral membrane protein, and a membrane location for the E proteins of IBV, TGEV, and MHV virions has been demonstrated. Recently, a cation-selective ion channel function has been demonstrated for the SARSCoV E protein (Wilson et al. 2004). The E protein, together with the M protein, has been shown to facilitate coronavirus particle formation (Bos et al. 1996; Fischer et al. 1998; Vennema et al. 1996) and recent data has shown that the E protein accumulates in and induces curvature into the pre-Golgi membranes where coronaviruses assemble by budding (Arbely et al. 2004; Raamsman et al. 2000). Although there is clear evidence for the importance of the E protein in the assembly of coronaviruses, it is not absolutely essential (Kuo and Masters 2003). The E protein is also reported to induce apoptosis (An et al. 1999). The identification of the E protein of arteriviruses has further extended the collection of structural proteins of this virus group (Snijder et al. 1999; Wu et al. 2001). The hydropathy profile of this small hydrophobic non-glycosylated protein suggests that it is an integral membrane protein with an uncleaved signal-anchor sequence in the central part of the molecule.

MAJOR GLYCOPROTEINS

The coronavirus and torovirus spike glycoproteins have a number of features in common: a large number (18–35) of potential N-glycosylation sites, an N-terminal signal sequence, a C-terminal transmembrane anchor domain, putative heptad repeat domains and, with the exception of some coronaviruses (e.g. TGEV, FCoV, SARSCoV, and HCoV-229E), a centrally located, arginine-rich cleavage site for a 'trypsinlike' proteinase. When post-translational cleavage takes place (which varies according to the virus and the cell) the quaternary structure of the protein is an oligomer (dimer or trimer), each monomer being comprised of two subunits, S1 (amino terminal) and S2 (carboxyl terminal) that are noncovalently linked. The S1 subunit is thought to be a globular protein that comprises the bulbous head of the peplomer. The heptad repeat domains, which are located in the S2 subunit, are thought to generate intrachain coiled-coil secondary structure (more precisely, antiparallel six helix bundles) and provide the stalk of the peplomer with its rigid, elongated structure (Cavanagh 1995). More detailed structural analysis of the coronavirus spike protein fusion core suggests that it shares significant similarity with both the low pH-induced conformation of influenza hemagglutinin and the fusion core of human immunodeficiency virus (HIV) gp41 (Bosch et al. 2003; Ingallinella et al. 2004; Tripet et al. 2004; Liu et al. 2004; Xu et al. 2004a, b). This suggests that the mechanisms for the viral fusion of coronaviruses might be quite similar to those of other class I virus fusion proteins. The MHV S protein is acylated, and it has been speculated that fatty acid chains are associated with a cluster of cysteine residues located in the C-terminal, hydrophilic tail of the protein. The same region has been implicated in spike protein-mediated membrane fusion (Chang et al. 2000; Ye et al. 2004). Finally, the assembly of the coronavirus spike protein into virions involves an interaction between the charge-rich carboxyl-terminal region of the endodomain, most probably with the membrane protein (de Haan et al. 1999).

The spike protein of coronaviruses has at least two major functions in virus replication. First, it binds to cellular receptors to initiate the infection process. The S protein–receptor interaction is complex and may involve the recognition of carbohydrates as well as protein. However, the major class of protein receptor for MHV has been identified as isoforms of the Bgp glycoprotein, a group of murine, carcinoembryonic antigen (CEA)-related glycoproteins in the biliary glycoprotein subgroup (Dveksler et al. 1993; Hemmila et al. 2004). Similarly, the metalloproteinase, aminopeptidase N (also called CD13 in humans) has been identified as the protein receptor for TGEV and HCoV-229E (Delmas et al. 1992; Yeager et al. 1992). Finally, angiotensin-converting enzyme 2 (ACE2) has been identified as a functional receptor for the SARS-CoV (Li et al. 2003; To and Lo 2004). It seems clear that the coronavirus spike protein is a major determinant of cell and species tropism (Casais et al. 2003; Haijema et al. 2003). The second major function of the S protein is to mediate membrane fusion. This activity is necessary for the fusion of viral and cellular membranes

at the cell surface during the initial stages of infection, and it may also occur later in infection by extensive formation of syncytia. In the coronaviruses, virus entry is thought to take place at the cell surface or within endosomes prior to their acidification. However, mutants of MHV that depend on low pH for fusion activity have been isolated (Gallagher et al. 1991) and SARS-CoV S-pseudotyped lentiviral vectors also display pH-dependent fusion (Yang et al. 2004a). Cleavage of the S protein seems to enhance its cell-to-cell fusion activity but is not required for virus infectivity (de Haan et al. 2004; Gombold et al. 1993). Bosch and colleagues have recently identified a putative fusion peptide in the S protein of a number of coronaviruses (Bosch et al. 2004).

The arterivirus major glycoprotein, GP_5 is sometimes considered as 'equivalent' to the coronavirus S protein but its structure is completely different and it appears to lack some of the important biological functions ascribed to the coronavirus spike glycoprotein. Recent analyses suggest that it is a polytopic class I protein; after removal of the signal peptide, the processed protein consists of an N terminal ectodomain (about 30 amino acids for LDV and PRRSV, 95 amino acids for EAV) which is N-glycosylated, an internal hydrophobic region that crosses the membrane three times and a C-terminal endodomain of 50–75 amino acids (Snijder et al. 2003b). The ectodomain of the EAV GP_5 protein carries one or two polylactosaminoglycans, a very unusual modification for a viral glycoprotein. The corresponding LDV protein was shown to carry 1–3 polylactoaminoglycans that strongly influence immunogenicity, sensitivity to antibody neutralization and neuropathogenicity (Li et al. 1998). At the present time, there is only limited information on the functions that are likely to be associated with this protein. The PRRSV GP_5–M protein hetrodimer has been implicated in attachment to a heparin-like receptor on the surface of porcine alveolar macrophages (Delputte et al. 2002) but studies with EAV chimeras make it clear that a factor other than the GP_5 ectodomain may determine the host specificity of arteriviruses (Dobbe et al. 2001). Likewise, the tropism of PRRSV M protein mutants carrying the ectodomain of other arteriviruses was unchanged, indicating that both ectodomains in the GP_5–M heterodimer can be replaced without a detectable effect on cell tropism (Verheije et al. 2002a). Recently, it has been shown that porcine sialoadhesin mediates the internalization of PRRSV into alveolar macrophages and that the presence of sialic acid on the virus is essential for attachment (Delputte and Nauwynck 2004; Vanderheijden et al. 2003).

The hemagglutinin-esterase glycoprotein is a structural protein that is restricted to a subset of the *Coronaviridae*. A strong hemagglutinating property and a second, shorter, fringe of peplomers on the virion surface characterize this subset, which includes HEV, BCoV, MHV, HCoV-OC43, and TCoV (Brian et al.

1995). Amongst the toroviruses, BToV has been shown to express a hemagglutinin-esterase protein (Cornelissen et al. 1997). It should be noted that some other coronaviruses (for example, TGEV and IBV) can also display strong hemagglutinating activity but this is a property of the surface glycoprotein S and is usually cryptic: treatment of the virus with, for example, neuraminidase is required to 'activate' hemagglutination. Finally, even for hemagglutinating coronaviruses, variants have been found that, for one reason or another, have lost the ability to express a functional HE protein. Thus, for example, the MHV strain A59 is defective in this respect. In the same way, it seems likely that the single isolate of EToV studied to date, which clearly carries the remnants of an HE protein gene but does not express an HE protein, is also a variant virus.

In the case of MHV, the HE protein is a disulfide-linked homodimer. The monomer polypeptide (65–75 kDa) has an N_{exo}–C_{endo} configuration and is N-glycosylated in the ectodomain. Transient expression of the MHV and BCoV HE proteins has shown that the protein has both hemagglutinin and esterase activities (Pfleiderer et al. 1991; Yoo et al. 1992). The acetylesterase activity of BCoV is specific for N-acetyl-9-O-neuraminic acid (Vlasak et al. 1988). Comparison of the coronavirus HE protein sequence and the sequence of the influenza C virus HEF protein reveals a remarkable degree of conservation, including, for example, many cysteine residues and the active site motif 'phenylalanine–glycine–aspartic acid–serine–arginine' (FGDSR) (Vlasak et al. 1988). It has been speculated that the *HE* gene of coronaviruses has been acquired by an RNA recombination event between ancestral nidoviruses and influenza C viruses (Luytjes et al. 1988; Snijder et al. 1991).

The importance of the coronavirus HE protein is not yet clear. On the one hand, there is evidence for a functional role: for example, monoclonal antibodies specific for the BCoV HE protein are able to neutralize virus infectivity. On the other hand, MHV A59, which does not have an HE protein, is able to replicate quite normally in tissue culture. Moreover, it has been shown that, even for coronaviruses that express high levels of HE, the HE–ligand interaction alone is not sufficient to mediate infection (Gagneten et al. 1995; Popova and Zhang 2002). One possibility is that the interaction of HE with N-acetyl-9-O-neuraminic acid serves to concentrate virus on the cell membrane and thereby facilitates the interaction of the coronavirus S protein with its specific protein receptor molecule. As the levels of cell surface N-acetyl-9-O-neuraminic acid can differ dramatically in vivo, this interaction may still be an important determinant of pathogenicity.

MINOR GLYCOPROTEINS

The minor arterivirus glycoprotein encoded by ORF2b (GP_{2b}; EAV/LDV) or ORF2a (GP_{2a}; PRRSV) is a conventional class I integral membrane protein with an N-terminal signal peptide, a C-terminal transmembrane segment, and 1–4 potential N-glycosylation sites. The protein is significantly under-represented in EAV particles (at least in relation to its intracellular abundance) (de Vries et al. 1992) and was shown to occur in EAV-infected cells in a variety of monomeric conformations and complexed with other minor glycoproteins (de Vries et al. 1995; Wieringa et al. 2003a). Complex formation is a prerequisite for GP_{2b} incorporation into virions, although the equivalent PRRSV protein was reported to be present in virions as a monomer (Meulenberg and Petersen-den Besten 1996). Recent mutagenesis studies using an EAV infectious cDNA clone revealed that cysteine residues in the GP_{2b} ectodomain form both intramolecular and intermolecular cysteine bridges, the latter involving a cysteine of the GP_4 ectodomain (Wieringa et al. 2003b).

The PRRSV and EAV GP_4 proteins were also identified as minor glycoprotein constituents of the virus particle (van Nieuwstadt et al. 1996; Wieringa et al. 2002). They contain an N-terminal signal sequence, a C-terminal membrane anchor and a small endodomain, which are typical properties of class I integral membrane proteins.

The EAV GP_3 protein is a heavily glycosylated integral membrane protein with an uncleaved N-terminal signal sequence and a hydrophobic C-terminal domain. The protein is inserted into the lipid bilayer by either or both of its hydrophobic termini and has no detectable endodomain (Hedges et al. 1999; Wieringa et al. 2002). Like GP_{2b} and GP_4, EAV GP_3 localizes to the endoplasmic reticulum, both in infected cells and in expression systems (Wieringa et al. 2002). There is no doubt about the presence of GP_3 in EAV particles (Wieringa et al. 2002), but conflicting data on the presence of PRRSV GP_3 in virions have been reported. Whereas GP_3 was detected in purified European PRRSV by using specific monoclonal antibodies (van Nieuwstadt et al. 1996), the protein could not be immunoprecipitated from a purified virus preparation of a North American isolate (Mardassi et al. 1998). However, small amounts of the latter protein were detected in a soluble form in the medium. Topological studies on the corresponding LDV protein also suggested it to be a secretory protein but, thus far, this protein could not be detected in cell lysates or the medium of infected cells (Faaberg and Plagemann 1997).

Recent studies on the GP_{2b}, GP_3, and GP_4 proteins of EAV have revealed various important properties of the arterivirus minor glycoproteins. By separately knocking out the expression of each of the EAV structural proteins in the context of a full-length EAV cDNA clone, it was shown that both major and minor structural proteins are required for the production of infectious progeny virus (Molenkamp et al. 2000). Subsequently, it was found that knock-out mutants for minor structural protein expression produce noninfectious subviral particles consisting of GP_5, M, N, and the viral RNA genome (Wieringa et al. 2004; Zevenhoven-Dobbe et al. 2004). These subviral particles did not differ from wild-type virus in terms of buoyant density, major structural protein composition, and appearance in electron microscopy. When one of the proteins GP_{2b}, GP_3, or GP_4 was missing, the incorporation of the other minor GPs was blocked and that of the E protein was greatly reduced (Wieringa et al. 2004). The absence of the E protein completely blocked the incorporation into virions of the three minor glycoproteins, which are present in equimolar amounts and form a heterotrimeric complex (Wieringa et al. 2003a). In infected cells, covalently linked GP_{2b}/GP_4 heterodimers associate with GP_3 to produce a $GP_{2b}/GP_3/GP_4$ complex that is required for incorporation of the three glycoproteins into virions. Following virus release, GP_3 becomes disulfide-linked to the GP_{2b}/GP_4 heterodimers, a postassembly maturation event that yields a complex of three covalently bound glycoproteins. Consequently, EAV particles contain both GP_{2b}/GP_4 heterodimers and $GP_{2b}/GP_3/GP_4$ heterotrimers (Wieringa et al. 2003a).

The above data indicate that EAV N, M, and GP_5 are the only structural proteins required for virus assembly, but that the disulfide-linked $GP_{2b}/GP_3/GP_4$ heterotrimer is required for virus infectivity, most likely because this complex is essential for attachment to the host cell surface. The higher order structure of the arterivirus E protein is unknown, but also this protein is essential for infectivity (Molenkamp et al. 2000) and may, in fact, be associated with the $GP_{2b}/GP_3/GP_4$ trimer (Wieringa et al. 2003b).

Immune responses

HUMORAL IMMUNITY

The surface glycoprotein, S (coronaviruses and toroviruses), and the major glycoprotein, GP_5 (arteriviruses), are the major inducers of neutralizing antibody during natural infection (Balasuriya et al. 2004a; Chirnside et al. 1995; Ostrowski et al. 2002; Spaan et al. 1988; Wissink et al. 2003). In the specific case of SARS-CoV, it also appears that the S protein is the only significant protective antigen among the structural proteins (Buchholz et al. 2004). The antigenic structure of the coronavirus S protein has been studied and the picture that emerges is complex (Cavanagh 1995). Essentially, the majority of virus neutralization (VN) epitopes seem to be located on the S1 subunit (or the amino terminal half of the S protein if it is not cleaved) and they are 'conformational' in the sense that they are comprised of amino acids that are brought into close proximity by the folding of the protein (Zhou et al. 2004). The VN epitopes are clustered into domains, one of which is usually immunodominant, although 2–3 domains may carry VN epitopes. Glycosylation seems to be an important component of VN epitope structure. Some studies have indicated that VN epitopes may be located on the S2 subunit (or carboxyl half of the protein) and that amino acids in the S2 subunit can modulate the recognition of VN epitopes located in the S1 subunit (Zhang et al. 2004a). It should be kept in mind that, although many VN epitopes have been defined, the mechanisms of virus neutralization remain essentially unknown.

Although the S and GP_5 proteins are the prime inducers of humoral immunity, antibody responses to other structural proteins may also have a role in protection. Some monoclonal antibodies specific for the MHV or TGEV M protein can neutralize virus infectivity in vitro (Fleming et al. 1989; Risco et al. 1995) and, as already mentioned, HE-specific antibodies are able to neutralize BCoV infection. It has been shown that E-specific antibodies are able to neutralize MHV infectivity in the presence of complement (Yu et al. 1994). The relevance of these observations to the situation in vivo is, however, unclear. The arterivirus, PRRSV, can be neutralized by monoclonal antibodies recognizing the ectodomain of the GP_4 protein (Meulenberg et al. 1997; van Nieuwstadt et al. 1996) and recombinant EAV N protein is able to induce neutralizing antibodies in mice (Tobiasch et al. 2001). Finally, immunization studies using alphavirus-based expression vectors have shown that the co-expression of EAV GP_5 and M is required for the induction of neutralizing antibodies in mice and horses (Balasuriya et al. 2000, 2002), although other reports indicate that the GP_5 ectodomain alone may suffice (Castillo-Olivares et al. 2001). A recombinant EAV lacking the immunodominant region of the GP_5 ectodomain was found to be viable and able to induce protective immunity in horses, indicating that immune effector mechanisms other than neutralizing antibodies binding to this region of GP_5 play an important role in protection against infection (Castillo-Olivares et al. 2003b).

CELL-MEDIATED IMMUNITY

As for most other viruses, the cell-mediated immune response to coronavirus and arterivirus infection is less well characterized than the humoral immune response. There is good evidence that the cell-mediated response is important in a variety of natural infections (Castillo-Olivares et al. 2003a; Loa et al. 2001; Paltrinieri et al. 1998) but, for technical reasons, most of the information we have relates to murine infections (MHV or LDV), often in an experimental setting. The coronavirus S, M, and N proteins, as well as the arterivirus N protein, are targets for cellular immune recognition (Plagemann 1996; Yang et al. 2004b). In a few cases, specific T-cell epitopes have been defined and helper or cytotoxic functions have been attributed to T-cell subpopulations. There is some preliminary evidence that nonstructural proteins may also represent T-cell immunogens (Stohlman et al. 1993).

In addition to MHC-restricted immune responses, coronavirus infections elicit lymphokine responses. Recent studies indicate that SARS-CoV infection elicits a response that is characterized by elevated levels of IL-6 cytokine, MCP-1, and IP-10 chemokines (Jones et al. 2004; Zhang et al. 2004b). Also, it is interesting to note that the SARS-CoV nucleocapsid protein has been shown to regulate cellular signaling (Subbarao et al. 2004). MHV infection of 129/Sv mice triggers a transient increase in the level of IL-12 (p40) mRNA present in pooled spleen cells (Coutelier et al. 1995). Also, the M protein of TGEV can induce, directly or indirectly, the production of interferon-α in lymphocytes (Baudoux et al. 1998, de Haan et al. 2003). The significance of these types of response for innate immunity has not yet been defined but there seems little doubt that they play an important role in particular situations.

CLINICAL AND PATHOLOGICAL ASPECTS

Introduction

The spectrum of disease caused by coronaviruses and arteriviruses is summarized in Table 39.3. As is the case with many viruses, the majority of infections are asymptomatic, perhaps reflecting the pathogenic equilibrium

reached during the co-evolution of host and pathogen. Many of the clinical diseases listed in Table 39.3 are, in fact, manifested only in immunodeficient animals (e.g. neonates or during pregnancy). In contrast, when a nonnatural host is infected, or when the natural host is infected by an unusual route or virus variant, fulminant disease can also ensue. In the following review, only natural infections of major importance are discussed. For a discussion of less common and experimental infections with coronaviruses and arteriviruses the reader is referred to other review articles (Dales and Anderson 1995; Foley and Leutenegger 2001; Garwes 1995; Haring and Perlman 2001; Holmes 2001b; Koopmans and Horzinek 1995; Paul et al. 2003; Plagemann et al. 1995).

Coronaviruses

HUMAN CORONAVIRUSES (INCLUDING SARS-COV)

Human coronaviruses (HCoV) are accepted as a major cause of respiratory tract illness in humans. HCoVs are

Table 39.3 Coronavirus and arterivirus infections in natural hosts

		Infection						
Virus	Host	Respiratory	Enteric	Reproductive	Neurologic	MPS	Other	Clinical disease
Coronaviruses								
IBV	Chicken	++	...	+	...	...	+[a]	Infectious bronchitis
BCoV	Cattle	...	++	...	...	...	...	Neonatal calf diarrhoea, winter dysentery
CCoV	Dog	...	++	...	...	...	...	Enteritis
FCoV	Cat	+	++	...	+	...	+[b]	Enteritis, infectious peritonitis
HCoV-229E	Human	++	...	...	...	...	...	Common cold
HCoV-OC43	Human	++	?	...	...	...	...	Common cold
SARS-CoV	Human	++	+					Severe acute respiratory syndrome
MHV	Mouse	+	++	...	+	...	+[c]	Enteritis, rhinitis, hepatitis
RtCoV	Rat	++	...	...	...	...	+[d]	Pneumonitis
PEDV	Pig	...	++	...	...	...	...	Epidemic diarrhoea
TGEV	Pig	+	++	...	...	...	...	Transmissible gastroenteritis
HEV	Pig	+	...	...	++	...	...	Vomiting and wasting disease
TCoV	Turkey	...	++	...	...	...	...	Transmissible enteritis
Toroviruses								
EToV	Horse	...	...	...	...	...	...	?
BToV	Cattle	+	++	...	...	...	...	Gastroenteritis
HToV		...	++	...	...	...	...	Gastroenteritis
PToV		...	++	...	...	...	...	Gastroenteritis
Arteriviruses								
EAV	Horse	+	...	+	...	++	+[e]	Rhinitis, abortion
LDV	Mouse	...	...	...	+	++	...	Generally asymptomatic
SHFV	Monkey	...	...	...	...	++	...	Generally asymptomatic
PRRSV	Pig	+	...	+	+	++	...	Pneumonia, abortion

MPS, mononuclear phagocyte system. ++, main target for infection; +, secondary target for infection. ?, circumstantial evidence of infection or disease. Other targets of infection are: [a]kidney; [b]serous membranes; [c]liver; [d]salivary, lacrimal glands; [e]arteries.

grouped into three major groups that are prototyped by HCoV-229E, HCoV-OC43, and SARS-CoV. HCoV-229E and HCoV-OC43 are mainly associated with common colds (Myint 1995). It has been estimated that up to 30 percent of clinical cases are due to infections with these two viruses. Typically, after an incubation period of about 3 days, patients develop general malaise, headache, nasal discharge, sneezing, and a mild sore throat (Tyrrell et al. 1993). About one-tenth of patients also have a fever and one-fifth will have a cough. Although most of these infections remain restricted to the upper respiratory tract there is evidence that HCoV-229E and HCoV-OC43 may also cause severe lower respiratory tract illness (El-Sahly et al. 2000; Falsey et al. 2002; Pene et al. 2003; Vabret et al. 2003; van Elden et al. 2004). Also, HCoV-NL63, a recently isolated HCoV that is closely related to HCoV-229E, was reported to be associated with lower respiratory tract infections, such as pneumonia and bronchiolitis, in young children (Fouchier et al. 2004, van der Hoek et al. 2004; Esper et al. 2005). Very recently, yet another human coronavirus, HCoV-HKU1, has been isolated from patients with pneumonia (Woo et al. 2005). HCoV-229E and HCoV-OC43 have also been associated with diseases outside the respiratory tract, for example with gastroenteritis (Zhang et al. 1994) and, possibly, neurological diseases (Arbour et al. 2000; Stewart et al. 1992). HCoV infections are thought to be transmitted by aerosols. The peak incidence of infection is in the winter and spring (Lina et al. 1996). Somewhere between 10 percent and 20 percent of individuals have serological responses indicative of HCoV-229E or HCoV-OC43 infection in any one year, although this figure may increase to 35 percent in some years (Monto and Lim 1974). A high percentage of infections occur despite pre-existing antibody, and the frequency of infection gradually diminishes with age (Callow et al. 1990). Little is known about the pathogenesis and immune response to HCoV-229E and HCoV-OC43 infection, mainly because there is no animal model available. Replication of the virus is optimal at 33–34°C and takes place in ciliated cells of the nasal epithelium (Afzelius 1994). Serum antibodies rise about 1 week after infection, peak at 2 weeks, and decline to low levels after about 12–18 months. The serum antibody response is mainly directed toward the surface protein although membrane- and nucleoprotein-specific immunoglobulins are also synthesized.

With very few exceptions, HCoVs are difficult to isolate and, even after adaptation to tissue culture, propagation in vitro is inefficient. Thus, the isolation of HCoVs in organ or tissue culture and the identification of HCoVs by electron microscopy or immunoelectron microscopy is possible only in specialized laboratories. Until a few years ago, the diagnosis of HCoV-229E and HCoV-OC43 infection relied mainly on serological methods, including, for example, enzyme-linked immunosorbent assay (ELISA), neutralization, immuno-

fluorescence, western-blotting, and complement fixation (Myint 1995). More recently, the detection of viral antigens and, in particular, RT-PCR methods have become the standard approach to the rapid diagnosis of 229E and OC43 infections (Hays and Myint 1998; Sizun et al. 1998; Stephensen et al. 1999; Vabret et al. 2001; Vallet et al. 2004; van Elden et al. 2004). Despite these advances, the detection of HCoV-229E and HCoV-OC43 infections is not generally done in routine diagnostic laboratories.

Another disease caused by a human coronavirus is the severe acute respiratory syndrome (SARS), a life-threatening and rapidly progressing form of pneumonia that first emerged in Guangdong province, China, in November 2002. Between February and July 2003 the virus infected more than 8 400 people worldwide and at the end of the epidemic more than 800 deaths had been recorded. SARS was shown to be caused by a previously unknown coronavirus, which was named SARS-CoV (Drosten et al. 2003; Ksiazek et al. 2003; Kuiken et al. 2003; Peiris et al. 2003a). The virus is generally believed to have evolved from an animal coronavirus that only recently crossed the species barrier to humans, although the natural reservoir of SARS-CoV remains to be identified (Guan et al. 2003). There is limited evidence that a very low number of people already had antibodies to SARS-CoV before the SARS outbreak, suggesting previous exposure to the same or a related coronavirus (Zheng et al. 2004). SARS-CoV is only distantly related to other animal and human coronaviruses (Marra et al. 2003; Rota et al. 2003) and has been classified (as the prototype of a new subgroup) in the coronavirus group 2, which also includes HCoV-OC43 (Gorbalenya et al. 2004; Snijder et al. 2003a). SARS-CoV is spread mainly by the respiratory and, possibly, fecal–oral routes (Ho et al. 2003b; Poutanen and McGeer 2004; Seto et al. 2003). Transmission requires close contact and, therefore, often occurs in hospital and health care settings from patients who are severely ill. It is generally believed that the virus is not transmitted from asymptomatic cases to contacts (Lee et al. 2003b). The clinical course of SARS is characterized by early nonspecific influenza-like symptoms, including persistent fever, chills, rigors, myalgia, and general malaise. After several days, respiratory symptoms (dry cough, rhinorrhea, shortness of breath) and gastrointestinal symptoms (nausea, vomiting, diarrhea) develop in most cases (Lee et al. 2003c; Loutfy et al. 2003; Ooi and Daqing 2003; Peiris et al. 2003a,b; Rainer 2004). About 8 days after the onset of fever, there is a rapid, often bilateral progression of ground glass opacies on chest radiographs. In a significant proportion of patients, multifocal and diffuse consolidation develops. The lung pathology may be associated with further complications, such as pneumomediastinum and pneumothorax, resulting in dramatically decreasing arterial oxygen saturation (Ooi and Daqing 2003; Peiris et al. 2003b). About 20 percent of the patients deteriorate with evidence of an acute respiratory distress syndrome (ARDS), requiring admission to an intensive care unit and mechanical ventilation. The overall case-fatality rate determined at the end of the outbreak in July 2003 was calculated to be about 11 percent. The fatality rate was extremely low in children (close to 0 percent), whereas in patients older than 65 years the mortality approached 50 percent. The laboratory diagnosis of SARS is based on RT-PCR and serology. RT-PCR is done from nasopharyngeal aspirate and swab samples and, if available, specimens from the lower respiratory tract (Emery et al. 2004). Viral RNA is also detectable in feces, serum, plasma, and urine. Viral load in respiratory samples and fecal samples peak at around 10–12 days and 15–17 days, respectively, after illness onset (Chan et al. 2004). To detect SARS-CoV infection as early as possible (i.e. in the first week of illness), multiple clinical samples should be collected and analyzed simultaneously. Positive RT-PCR results must be confirmed using primers specific for different parts of the SARS-CoV genome and tests should be done with multiple clinical samples. Seroconversion is a relatively delayed phenomenon and, consequently, not suitable as a rapid diagnostic test. Generally, SARS-CoV-specific IgG becomes detectable after 10–15 days of illness or even later. Serological assays, therefore, remain the gold standard for retrospective studies but are less suitable for rapid diagnosis. Anti-SARS-CoV IgG in the serum can be detected by immunofluorescence, enzyme-linked immunosorbent assays, and neutralization tests, which correlate very well with each other. The first serological assays to be developed and used during the SARS epidemic in 2003 were based on virus antigen produced from SARS-CoV-infected cells. This rapid development was possible because SARS-CoV, in contrast to most other HCoVs, grows to high titers in cell culture (for example, in Vero cells). Meanwhile, numerous diagnostic assays based on recombinant nucleocapsid (N), spike (S), and membrane (M) protein antigens are available, providing convenient tools that do not require biosafety level 3 laboratories. SARS-CoV antibodies show only very little cross-reactivity with antibodies specific for other human coronaviruses (Ksiazek et al. 2003). Negative SARS-CoV serology at 28 days after onset of symptoms is generally accepted to exclude the diagnosis of SARS-CoV infection.

To date, there have been no high-quality studies of any antiviral or immunosuppressive therapy. The few available studies indicate that therapies based on antiviral agents, such as ribavirin and oseltamivir, and immunosuppressive steroid therapy, may have severe side effects but there is only anecdotal evidence that these drugs significantly reduce the severity of the disease (Cyranoski 2003; Ho et al. 2003a; Loutfy et al. 2003; So et al. 2003; Tsang et al. 2003). However, SARS-CoV and other human coronaviruses proved to be sensitive to treatment with type I interferons, both in cell culture and animal models (Cinatl et al. 2003; Haagmans et al. 2004; Hensley et al. 2004; Hertzig et al. 2004), suggesting that type I interferons are promising drugs for SARS treatment protocols, which is consistent with pilot (mainly uncontrolled) clinical studies (Cinatl et al. 2004).

Thus far, the pathogenesis of SARS has been only poorly understood. The fact that, despite significantly reduced virus load, some patients deteriorate in the second week of illness suggests that the lung damage may be due to immunopathological mechanisms rather than virus replication. Animal models suitable to address this possibility and to investigate SARS-CoV pathogenesis in general are becoming increasingly available (Fouchier et al. 2003; Martina et al. 2003; Subbarao et al. 2004, ter Meulen et al. 2004; Wentworth et al. 2004; Yang et al. 2004b). The SARS outbreak has inspired many studies into virtually every aspect of SARS-CoV biology. The studies revealed promising therapeutic approaches, some of which might be used to develop drugs that are suitable to treat SARS-CoV infections. Candidate antivirals include fusion inhibitors (Bosch et al. 2004; Liu et al. 2004), inhibitors of the SARS-CoV main proteinase (Anand et al. 2003; Bacha et al. 2004; Hsu et al. 2004), recombinant antibodies (ter Meulen et al. 2004), and small compounds identified by screening of drug libraries (Wu et al. 2004). Finally, promising candidate vaccines have been developed that proved to be protective in SARS animal models (Bisht et al. 2004; Buchholz et al. 2004; Bukreyev et al. 2004; Yang et al. 2004b). The rapid progress in the improvement of diagnostic tests and the development of vaccines and antivirals should help to control future outbreaks of SARS more effectively.

AVIAN INFECTIOUS BRONCHITIS VIRUS

IBV is a pathogen of economic importance to the poultry industry worldwide. It causes a highly contagious disease affecting the respiratory, reproductive, neurological, and renal systems of chickens. IBV infection results in a drop in egg production in adult birds and damages the developing reproductive system in young birds. Infection of the respiratory tract, most probably by aerosols, is the most important route of transmission. Young chickens are most susceptible to infection and the clinical signs include nasal discharge, sneezing, coughing, and tracheal rales. IBV infection predisposes chickens to infection with secondary pathogens. Even young chickens will usually recover from an uncomplicated IBV infection, but the incidence of IBV-related nephritis, which can result in high mortality rates, seems to be increasing (Cavanagh and Naqi 2003; Cook and Mockett 1995; Ignjatovic and Sapats 2000; Lee et al. 2004).

Chickens respond to IBV infection by producing specific humoral antibodies of the IgM, IgG, and IgA subclasses. The major viral antigens are the S and M proteins, and the S protein is a major immunogen. High concentrations of VN antibodies are thought to prevent the spread of virus from its primary replication site to the reproductive and renal organs. Local immune responses, in particular IgA, play a significant role in controlling the respiratory infection. Finally, cell-mediated immune responses also develop after IBV infection. Cell-mediated immune responses to the S, N, and M proteins have been demonstrated (Ignjatovic and Galli 1993). At the moment, however, the relationship between cell-mediated immune responses and the degree of protective or long-term immunity has not been defined.

The diagnosis of IBV infection, in common with most other viruses, depends on three approaches: (1) isolation of the virus; (2) demonstration of a specific antibody response, usually by serological methods; and (3) demonstration of viral nucleic acid in clinical material.

IBV can be isolated in tracheal organ cultures and embryonated eggs and propagated in tissue cultures. Infected allantoic fluid and tracheal organ culture supernatant often contain enough virus particles to be visualized directly by electron microscopy. Alternatively, IBV isolates can be identified by immunofluorescence using polyclonal antisera or by antigen assays based on monoclonal antibodies. The existence of strain-specific monoclonal antibodies has also led to the development of serotype-specific ELISAs (Karaca and Naqi 1993).

A range of serological tests are available to detect IBV antibodies. They include immunofluorescence, hemagglutinin inhibition, ELISA, and virus neutralization. Probably the most sensitive tests are ELISAs using purified virus as antigen. In the future, it can be expected that these types of test will be significantly improved by the use of recombinant antigens (Chen et al. 2003; Guy et al. 2002; Wang et al. 2002). It is possible to detect IBV nucleic acids directly in clinical material. PCR is a rapid and sensitive method to amplify and identify IBV RNA (Jackwood et al. 2003; Liu et al. 2003). Combined with nucleotide sequencing (Lee et al. 2003a), PCR will probably also be the preferred method for distinguishing between IBV serotypes.

At the present time, the control of IBV relies almost exclusively on vaccination and management. Both live attenuated and inactivated vaccines are available. It is generally believed that both vaccines can be used, usually in combination, to induce high levels of humoral antibody and that immunity represents protection against reproductive and renal disease rather than protection against respiratory infection (Cook and Mockett 1995). There are also two major problems associated with the use of vaccine. First, there are many serotypes of IBV and, although it is not necessary to develop a different vaccine for each serotype, occasionally serotypes emerge against which existing vaccines are not fully effective. Secondly, although some serotypes probably emerge by antigenic drift, there is at least circumstantial evidence to suggest that they may also emerge by recombination, possibly involving the live vaccine virus itself (Cavanagh 2003; Lee and Jackwood 2000).

PORCINE TRANSMISSIBLE GASTROENTERITIS VIRUS

The severity of disease caused by porcine transmissible gastroenteritis virus TGEV is related to the age of the animal. Infection of the piglet during the first 2 weeks of life causes vomiting followed by profuse, watery diarrhea that eventually results in dehydration and frequently death within 2–5 days. In older pigs, similar clinical signs are manifested but the mortality rate drops as the body weight of the animal at the time of infection increases. Transmission of TGEV is primarily from the ingestion of contaminated material, usually feces or milk, and possibly via aerosols (Enjuanes and Van der Zeijst 1995; Garwes 1995). TGEV has been reported in a large number of countries, but with different incidence and prevalence of disease. In countries where pig breeding has not been intensified, transmissible gastroenteritis is essentially epizootic with an incidence of disease every 2–3 years. In this situation, new outbreaks of disease are probably due to the cyclic reintroduction of virus. In countries with intensive pig breeding, transmissible gastroenteritis infection has become essentially enzootic. In this situation, the virus probably establishes a persistent infection in adult animals, in the gut or respiratory tract.

The pathogenesis and immune response to TGEV infection, especially in newborn animals, are quite well understood. The virus primarily infects and replicates in the apical tubovascular system of villous absorptive cells in the jejunum and ileum. Clinical signs seem to result from an increase in osmotic pressure in the lumen of the small intestine, caused by a failure to absorb milk lactose combined with an abnormal level of sodium secretion into the lumen (Garwes 1995). Because immunity requires the secretion of antibodies into the lumen of the gut, the rapid progression of the disease in the newborn animal probably provides insufficient time for immunity to develop, irrespective of whether the animals have reached a state of immune competence. The main source of immune protection for neonates, therefore, has to be antibodies provided by the mother in colostrum and milk (de Diego et al. 1992). Surprisingly, it has been shown that colostrum from nonimmune sows can also provide some degree of protection (Enjuanes & Van der Zeijst 1995).

Several techniques are available for the rapid diagnosis of TGEV infection, including immunofluorescence, ELISA, nucleic acid hybridization, and RT-PCR (Enjuanes and Van der Zeijst 1995; Kim et al. 2000, 2001, Liu et al. 2001a; Paton and Lowings 1997). Most importantly, a panel of type-, group-, and interspecies-specific monoclonal antibodies have been developed to distinguish between viruses of the TGEV cluster, including PRCV (Sanchez et al. 1990). As described above, immune protection of piglets can be best achieved by natural lactogenic immunity provided by sows, by artificial lactogenic immunity using serum or protective monoclonal antibodies or, perhaps, by transgenic lactogenic immunity (Castilla et al. 1998). Virulent TGEV strains can be used to produce a solid immunity for both pregnant sows and their offspring (de Diego et al. 1992) but there is an obvious danger associated with this approach. Attenuated strains of TGEV and the PRCV variant have also been tested as vaccines but they have only limited efficacy (Saif and Wesley 1992). Efforts are being made to develop more effective vaccines. These may include noninfectious antigens that are targeted to the gut, and the use of live vectors with enteric tropism (Chen and Schifferli 2003, Lamphear et al. 2004; Liu et al. 2001b; Saif 1999; Sola et al. 2003).

FELINE CORONAVIRUS

Feline coronaviruses are a common cause of enteric disease in cats and, occasionally, they cause an immune-mediated disease known as feline infectious peritonitis (FIP). The enteric disease results in mild, transient diarrhoea that is self-limiting. FIP, however, is invariably lethal. Two distinct forms of FIP exist: the wet form, which is characterised by abdominal, and occasionally, pleural effusions, and the dry form, which is characterized by granuloma formation on the surface of tissues. In the dry form, the CNS is commonly involved but any organ may be affected. Feline coronavirus infection is enzootic in virtually all environments where large numbers of cats are kept and transmission is predominantly by the feco-oral route (de Groot and Horzinek 1995).

The patho-etiology of FIP is not well understood. It is known that purebred cats are predisposed to the development of FIP and the majority of cats develop FIP before 2 years of age (Foley et al. 1997; Poland et al. 1996). A widely held view is that FIP occurs when a cat is exposed to feline coronavirus variants that have mutated in the host and gained the ability to replicate in macrophages (Vennema et al. 1998). There is, however, no conclusive evidence to support this hypothesis. Also, it has been noted that, at least in experimental infections, seropositive cats develop an accelerated fulminating course of disease and this has been interpreted as evidence of 'antibody-dependent enhancement.' However, similar effects are seldom seen in natural infections (Hohdatsu et al. 1998). Finally, it has been postulated that a deregulated cytokine/chemokine response and the lack of an effective cell-mediated immune response plays a central role in the development of FIP (Paltrinieri et al. 2003). However, the available data is still preliminary.

With the exception of some laboratory-adapted strains, feline coronaviruses cannot be easily propagated in cell culture. Therefore infections are diagnosed by serological methods or, if the animals are shedding virus in the faeces, by using RT-PCR (Addie and Jarrett 2001; Addie et al. 2004; Addie et al. 2003). However, there is no specific diagnostic test for animals that are at increased risk of developing FIP or are in the earliest stages of the disease. Indeed, definitive diagnosis of FIP can only be made by histopathological examination of biopsy material or post-mortem material. As there is no effective treatment for FIP, environmental controls are currently the most powerful and widely used tools for the control of feline coronavirus infection. These include good hygiene, isolation, and early weaning. In the longer term, there is a clear need for an effective vaccine and/or the development of antiviral drugs that could be used to protect animals at greatest risk.

Toroviruses

BOVINE TOROVIRUS (PREVIOUSLY BREDA VIRUS)

There is clear evidence that torovirus infections are quite common in vertebrate species. Despite their potential veterinary and clinical relevance, the virus group has not been studied in great detail, in particular since propagation of toroviruses in cell culture has proven to be very difficult. Serological evidence of torovirus infection has been obtained in all ungulates that were tested using a bovine torovirus (BToV) neutralization assay (horses, cattle, sheep, goats, and pigs) and in rats, rabbits, and some species of feral mice (Weiss et al. 1984). Torovirus-like particles have also been observed and, in some cases, isolated from stool specimens from horses, cattle, pigs, humans, cats, and dogs (Koopmans and Horzinek 1995; Kroneman et al. 1998). Four torovirus genotypes were recently distinguished, exemplified by BToV (also known as bovine enteric torovirus), porcine torovirus (PToV), EToV, and human torovirus (HToV). In addition, sequence analysis revealed ample evidence for recurring intertypic recombination and predicts the existence of at least two additional, hitherto unknown, torovirus genotypes (Smits et al. 2003). It has been speculated that toroviruses may be associated with enteric disease in many species but, as yet, the only disease that can be definitely ascribed to a torovirus is BToV-related gastroenteritis in cattle.

Seroepidemiological studies in a number of countries show that the infection of cattle with BToV seems to be common throughout the world. In dairy cattle herds in the Netherlands, 85–95 percent of animals have antibodies to BToV by 1 year of age (Koopmans et al. 1989). Transmission probably takes place via the oral or the respiratory routes. BToV infections are usually limited to the gut, although there is some evidence for a possible respiratory involvement. The clinical signs of infection are watery diarrhea with dehydration, weakness, and depression. Predominantly affected are young animals 2–3 weeks of age; by the time they are 3–4 months old, they have only very mild or no diarrhea, in association with virus shedding. There is some preliminary evidence that persistent BToV infection can be established in a herd (Koopmans et al. 1990).

The pathogenesis of BToV infection centers on the destruction of crypt and villus epithelial cells, particularly in the small intestine. Although the epithelial cells are rapidly replaced, the new cells lack a mature brush border and thus present insufficient absorptive surface and digestive enzymes. This decrease in absorptive and digestive capacity causes an accumulation of lactose in the gut lumen, which in turn results in water and electrolytic retention leading to diarrhea. At least in young animals, the immune response following infection is probably of secondary importance, because protection depends mainly on maternal antibodies derived from colostrum and milk.

Attempts to isolate and propagate toroviruses have proved unsuccessful. In cell or tissue culture, BToV as well as HToV and PToV, have not been replicated to date. The isolation of EToV was a unique event that could be repeated only with the field sample of a single horse. The diagnosis of BToV infection has thus relied on immunological methods for the detection of BToV antigen or BToV-specific antibodies. However, there is evidence that BToV-infected animals shed ELISA-detectable amounts of virus for only 2–3 days (Woode et al. 1982), and the purification of BToV antigens from the feces of experimentally infected gnotobiotic calves is a laborious and expensive procedure. Nucleic acid hybridization, RT-PCR, and ELISA methods have been developed for the detection of BToV in clinical material (Hoet et al. 2003; Koopmans et al. 1991, 1993) and are used for diagnostic purposes and epidemiological studies. The control of torovirus-related disease currently depends on good management practices.

Arteriviruses

EQUINE ARTERITIS VIRUS

EAV was first isolated in 1953 from an aborted equine fetus. Serological evidence suggests that EAV is widespread in the horse population (Timoney and McCollum 1988) but infections are generally subclinical and usually lead only to a mild, often unrecognized, infection of the respiratory tract. If the virus does cause overt disease, the clinical symptoms are acute anorexia and fever, usually accompanied by palpebral edema, conjunctivitis, nasal catarrh, and edema of the legs, genitals, and abdomen (Plagemann and Moennig 1992). The clinical symptoms of EAV infection vary widely, probably reflecting, at least in part, differences in virulence among

EAV variants. Almost all naturally infected horses recover from EAV infection. Donkeys are the only other known host for the virus (Paweska 1994).

The primary mode of EAV transmission is assumed to be via the respiratory route by contact with aerosol secretions from acutely infected animals. The name 'equine arteritis virus' was derived from the characteristic necrosis of small muscular arteries following infection. Of greatest concern to the horse breeding industry, however, is the fact that the virus frequently causes abortion in pregnant mares (Golnik et al. 1986). Furthermore, a carrier state exists in seropositive stallions in which EAV is produced in the semen (Balasuriya et al. 2004b). These 'shedding stallions' may thus infect brood mares by the venereal route.

Studies of experimentally infected horses have indicated that, as with other arteriviruses, the initial replication of EAV takes place in lung macrophages. The virus infects the bronchial lymph nodes and then spreads throughout the body via the circulatory system. The cause of abortion in pregnant mares has not yet been elucidated. EAV-induced, macrophage-derived cytokines may contribute to the pathogenesis of EAV and the magnitude of the cytokine response may be linked to the virulence of the infecting virus strain (Moore et al. 2003). Neutralizing antibodies, mainly of the IgG class, are induced within a week of EAV infection, and this clears the virus from the circulation. Clearly, however, this does not always prevent the virus from establishing a persistent infection, particularly in stallions. Neutralizing antibodies generally persist for years, and protective immunity is presumed to be lifelong. Only one EAV serotype has been recognized, although European and North-American genotypes can be discriminated (Stadejek et al. 1999). As described above, the EAV GP_5 glycoprotein is the main inducer of neutralizing antibodies (Balasuriya et al. 2004a; Balasuriya et al. 2002; Castillo-Olivares et al. 2001; Chirnside et al. 1995).

Traditionally, the diagnosis of EAV infection has been based on the isolation and propagation of virus in tissue culture. The clinical materials most often used are nasopharyngeal, vaginal and rectal swabs or a buffy coat fraction from blood or semen. Rabbit kidney (RK-13), baby hamster kidney (BHK-21), and Vero cells are susceptible to infection and develop characteristic cytopathic effects.

Attempts to isolate virus from field cases have sometimes proved difficult. Several immunological assays for measuring EAV-specific antibodies in horse sera are available but the detection of neutralizing antibodies ($TCID_{50}$ and plaque reduction assays) are used most commonly. The determination of the nucleotide sequence of the EAV genome has also allowed the development of assays based on RT-PCR (Chirnside and Spaan 1990; Gilbert et al. 1997; St-Laurent et al. 1994). The control of EAV infection relies on a combination of vaccination and containment (Chirnside 1992;

Plagemann and Moennig 1992). At present, a live-attenuated and a killed virus vaccines are available. The live vaccine induces long-lasting protection against clinical disease but does not prevent reinfection with wild-type virus or temporary virus shedding (McCollum 1986). To avoid this problem, a formalin-inactivated vaccine (Fukunaga et al. 1984) has been developed. Increased knowledge of the antigenic properties of the EAV GP$_5$ protein may provide the basis for the development of an EAV subunit vaccine (Balasuriya et al. 2002; Castillo-Olivares et al. 2001; Chirnside et al. 1995; Giese et al. 2002). Furthermore, the development of reverse genetics systems for EAV (van Dinten et al. 1997) has opened the possibility of the development of vaccines based on the genetic engineering of the virus genome (Castillo-Olivares et al. 2003b; de Vries et al. 2001; Zevenhoven-Dobbe et al. 2004).

Porcine reproductive and respiratory syndrome virus

PRRSV is responsible for respiratory disease in pigs of all ages and for abortions and stillbirths in pregnant sows. The clinical signs of infection are transient fever, anorexia, and respiratory distress. Mortality is generally seen only in young piglets and is often associated with secondary infections (Meredith 1993; Plagemann 1996). Within the herd, PRRSV is thought to be transmitted mainly via aerosols but, as in the case of EAV, sexual transmission also occurs (Sur et al. 1997). The virus is present in nasal secretions and swine can be readily infected by intranasal inoculation. Fecal–oral transmission may, however, also take place and infection between herds may involve the movement of infected animals or fomites. In pregnant sows, PRRSV can be transmitted transplacentally, leading to reproductive failure in late gestation. The disease associated with PRRSV first appeared in the USA in the late 1980s. The first incidence of the disease in Europe was in northern Germany in 1991 and the virus is now common in the Netherlands and the UK. As with TGEV, the disease associated with PRRSV infection was originally epizootic, but more recently the incidence of acute disease has decreased and mild, even unapparent, infections are becoming more commonplace.

Lung macrophages are the primary site of PRRSV infection and replication. Their destruction is probably the cause of the increased susceptibility of infected pigs to secondary bacterial infections. The virus may also spread to other organs. In addition to interstitial pneumonia, lymphocytic encephalitis is a common lesion found in PRRSV-infected animals. The course of development of anti-PRRSV immunity is unconventional and many issues remain to be studied in detail (Murtaugh et al. 2002). The virus does not elicit the strong innate immune response seen in many other viral pathogens.

Humoral and cell-mediated immunity is induced and clears the virus from the circulation but not from lymphoid tissues, where the infection becomes persistent. As with other arteriviruses, the initial phase of PRRSV infection is characterized by transient suppression of the cellular immune response coupled with an enhanced response to T-cell-dependent and T-cell-independent antigens (Murtaugh et al. 1993). The weak cell-mediated immune response suggests that PRRSV suppresses T-cell recognition of infected macrophages (Xiao et al. 2004). PRRSV-specific humoral antibodies can be detected 1–2 weeks after infection and peak after 5–6 weeks. The neutralizing antibody component reaches a maximum after 4–6 weeks and, thereafter, virus is generally cleared from the circulation. There is evidence that virus may persist in swine herds for periods of 2 years or longer but it is not clear whether this represents persistence in the individual animal, reinfection of animals, or the infection of animals that have escaped earlier encounters with the virus.

The diagnosis and control of PRRSV infections still represents a significant problem. In tissue culture, PRRSV is most successfully isolated and propagated in primary pig lung macrophages. However, the costs involved preclude this as a routine diagnostic procedure. A number of continuous cell lines can be used for virus propagation but they do not seem to be equally susceptible to all isolates. Serologically, PRRSV infections can be detected by virus neutralization, immunofluorescence, and immunoperoxidase staining. However, it is clear that many isolates of PRRSV differ antigenically and it will be some time before the extent of this variation has been fully characterized (Drew et al. 1995). Finally, the detection of PRRSV RNA using RT-PCR is under development (Legeay et al. 1997; Suarez et al. 1994; Van-Woensel et al. 1994) and promises to be the method of choice for the detection of low levels of viral RNA in the tissues of infected pigs. Control measures essentially consist of the eradication of infected herds and restrictions on the movement of pigs from enzootic areas. Live-attenuated and killed vaccines are available to protect pigs. However, adverse effects of vaccination of Danish pig herds with a modified live PRRS vaccine have been described (Botner 1997), which were probably caused by reversion of the vaccine virus to virulence. Acute PRRS-like symptoms, including an increasing number of abortions and stillborn piglets, were experienced in vaccinated herds. Furthermore, vaccine virus was transmitted from vaccinated to nonvaccinated boars in several cases, resulting in viremia and shedding of vaccine virus into semen (Madsen et al. 1998). In this respect, the killed vaccines are safer but are less efficacious in the induction of protection. Promising results were obtained in DNA vaccination experiments with plasmids expressing the GP$_5$ protein of PRRSV (Pirzadeh and Dea 1998). Neutralizing antibodies and lymphocyte proliferation responses were detected in DNA-vaccinated pigs and the spread and clinical signs of challenge virus was reduced. As in the case of EAV, the immunogenic properties of the GP_5 ectodomain (Plagemann 2004; Wissink et al. 2003) suggest that the PRRSV major glycoprotein might be a good candidate for a DNA-based subunit vaccine. In addition, following the development of reverse genetics systems for PRRSV (Meulenberg et al. 1998; Nielsen et al. 2003; Truong et al. 2004), the first results from studies using vaccine viruses that have been attenuated by genetic engineering have recently been reported (Verheije et al. 2003).

REFERENCES

Addie, D.D. and Jarrett, O. 2001. Use of a reverse-transcriptase polymerase chain reaction for monitoring the shedding of feline coronavirus by healthy cats. *Vet Rec*, **148**, 649–53.

Addie, D.D., Schaap, I.A., et al. 2003. Persistence and transmission of natural type I feline coronavirus infection. *J Gen Virol*, **84**, 2735–44.

Addie, D.D., McLachlan, S.A., et al. 2004. Evaluation of an in-practice test for feline coronavirus antibodies. *J Feline Med Surg*, **6**, 63–7.

Afzelius, B.A. 1994. Ultrastructure of human nasal epithelium during an episode of coronavirus infection. *Virchows Arch*, **424**, 295–300.

Ahlquist, P., Noueiry, A.O., et al. 2003. Host factors in positive-strand RNA virus genome replication. *J Virol*, **77**, 8181–6.

Almazan, F., Gonzalez, J.M., et al. 2000. Engineering the largest RNA virus genome as an infectious bacterial artificial chromosome. *Proc Natl Acad Sci USA*, **97**, 5516–21.

Alonso, S., Izeta, A., et al. 2002. Transcription regulatory sequences and mRNA expression levels in the coronavirus transmissible gastroenteritis virus. *J Virol*, **76**, 1293–308.

An, S., Chen, C.J., et al. 1999. Induction of apoptosis in murine coronavirus-infected cultured cells and demonstration of E protein as an apoptosis inducer. *J Virol*, **73**, 7853–9.

Anand, K., Palm, G.J., et al. 2002. Structure of coronavirus main proteinase reveals combination of a chymotrypsin fold with an extra alpha-helical domain. *EMBO J*, **21**, 3213–24.

Anand, K., Ziebuhr, J., et al. 2003. Coronavirus main proteinase (3CLpro) structure: basis for design of anti-SARS drugs. *Science*, **300**, 1763–7.

Arbely, E., Khattari, Z., et al. 2004. A highly unusual palindromic transmembrane helical hairpin formed by SARS coronavirus E protein. *J Mol Biol*, **341**, 769–79.

Arbour, N., Day, R., et al. 2000. Neuroinvasion by human respiratory coronaviruses. *J Virol*, **74**, 8913–21.

Bacha, U., Barrila, J., et al. 2004. Identification of novel inhibitors of the SARS coronavirus main protease 3CLpro. *Biochemistry*, **43**, 4906–12.

Balasuriya, U.B., Heidner, H.W., et al. 2000. Expression of the two major envelope proteins of equine arteritis virus as a heterodimer is necessary for induction of neutralizing antibodies in mice immunized with recombinant Venezuelan equine encephalitis virus replicon particles. *J Virol*, **74**, 10623–30.

Balasuriya, U.B., Heidner, H.W., et al. 2002. Alphavirus replicon particles expressing the two major envelope proteins of equine arteritis virus induce high level protection against challenge with virulent virus in vaccinated horses. *Vaccine*, **20**, 1609–17.

Balasuriya, U.B., Dobbe, J.C., et al. 2004a. Characterization of the neutralization determinants of equine arteritis virus using recombinant chimeric viruses and site-specific mutagenesis of an infectious cDNA clone. *Virology*, **321**, 235–46.

Balasuriya, U.B., Hedges, J.F., et al. 2004b. Genetic characterization of equine arteritis virus during persistent infection of stallions. *J Gen Virol*, **85**, 379–90.

Baric, R.S. and Yount, B. 2000. Subgenomic negative-strand RNA function during mouse hepatitis virus infection. *J Virol*, **74**, 4039–46.

Barrette-Ng, I.H., Ng, K.K., et al. 2002. Structure of arterivirus nsp4. The smallest chymotrypsin-like proteinase with an alpha/beta C-terminal extension and alternate conformations of the oxyanion hole. *J Biol Chem*, **277**, 39960–6.

Baudoux, P., Carrat, C., et al. 1998. Coronavirus pseudoparticles formed with recombinant M and E proteins induce alpha interferon synthesis by leukocytes. *J Virol*, **72**, 8636–43.

Bautista, E.M., Faaberg, K.S., et al. 2002. Functional properties of the predicted helicase of porcine reproductive and respiratory syndrome virus. *Virology*, **298**, 258–70.

Bhardwaj, K., Guarino, L. and Kao, C.C. 2004. The severe acute respiratory syndrome coronavirus Nsp15 protein is an endoribonuclease that prefers manganese as a cofactor. *J Virol*, **78**, 12218–24.

Bisht, H., Roberts, A., et al. 2004. Severe acute respiratory syndrome coronavirus spike protein expressed by attenuated vaccinia virus protectively immunizes mice. *Proc Natl Acad Sci USA*, **101**, 6641–6.

Bos, E.C., Luytjes, W., et al. 1996. The production of recombinant infectious DI-particles of a murine coronavirus in the absence of helper virus. *Virology*, **218**, 52–60.

Bosch, B.J., van der Zee, R., et al. 2003. The coronavirus spike protein is a class I virus fusion protein: structural and functional characterization of the fusion core complex. *J Virol*, **77**, 8801–11.

Bosch, B.J., Martina, B.E., et al. 2004. Severe acute respiratory syndrome coronavirus (SARS-CoV) infection inhibition using spike protein heptad repeat-derived peptides. *Proc Natl Acad Sci USA*, **101**, 8455–60.

Bost, A.G., Prentice, E. and Denison, M.R. 2001. Mouse hepatitis virus replicase protein complexes are translocated to sites of M protein accumulation in the ERGIC at late times of infection. *Virology*, **285**, 21–9.

Botner, A. 1997. Diagnosis of PRRS. *Vet Microbiol*, **55**, 295–301.

Brian, D.A., Hogue, B.G. and Kienzle, T.E. 1995. The coronavirus haemagglutinin esterase protein. In: Siddell, S.G. (ed.), *The Coronaviridae*. New York: Plenum Press, 165–79.

Brierley, I. 1995. Ribosomal frameshifting viral RNAs. *J Gen Virol*, **76**, 1885–92.

Brierley, I. and Pennell, S. 2001. Structure and function of the stimulatory RNAs involved in programmed eukaryotic-1 ribosomal frameshifting. *Cold Spring Harb Symp Quant Biol*, **66**, 233–48.

Brierley, I., Meredith, M.R., et al. 1997. Expression of a coronavirus ribosomal frameshift signal in *Escherichia coli*: influence of tRNA anticodon modification on frameshifting. *J Mol Biol*, **270**, 360–73.

Brockway, S.M., Clay, C.T., et al. 2003. Characterization of the expression, intracellular localization, and replication complex association of the putative mouse hepatitis virus RNA-dependent RNA polymerase. *J Virol*, **77**, 10515–27.

Brown, T.D. and Brierley, I. 1995. The coronavirus nonstructural proteins. In: Siddell, S.G. (ed.), *The Coronaviridae*. New York: Plenum Press, 191–217.

Buchholz, U.J., Bukreyev, A., et al. 2004. Contributions of the structural proteins of severe acute respiratory syndrome coronavirus to protective immunity. *Proc Natl Acad Sci USA*, **101**, 9804–9.

Budzilowicz, C.J. and Weiss, S.R. 1987. In vitro synthesis of two polypeptides from a nonstructural gene of coronavirus mouse hepatitis virus strain A59. *Virology*, **157**, 509–15.

Bukreyev, A., Lamirande, E.W., et al. 2004. Mucosal immunisation of African green monkeys (*Cercopithecus aethiops*) with an attenuated parainfluenza virus expressing the SARS coronavirus spike protein for the prevention of SARS. *Lancet*, **363**, 2122–7.

Callow, K.A., Parry, H.F., et al. 1990. The time course of the immune response to experimental coronavirus infection of man. *Epidemiol Infect*, **105**, 435–46.

Casais, R., Thiel, V., et al. 2001. Reverse genetics system for the avian coronavirus infectious bronchitis virus. *J Virol*, **75**, 12359–69.

Casais, R., Dove, B., et al. 2003. Recombinant avian infectious bronchitis virus expressing a heterologous spike gene demonstrates that the spike protein is a determinant of cell tropism. *J Virol*, **77**, 9084–9.

Castilla, J., Pintado, B., et al. 1998. Engineering passive immunity in transgenic mice secreting virus-neutralizing antibodies in milk. *Nat Biotechnol*, **16**, 349–54.

Castillo-Olivares, J., de Vries, A.A., et al. 2001. Evaluation of a prototype sub-unit vaccine against equine arteritis virus comprising the entire ectodomain of the virus large envelope glycoprotein (G(L)): induction of virus-neutralizing antibody and assessment of protection in ponies. *J Gen Virol*, **82**, 2425–35.

Castillo-Olivares, J., Tearle, J.P., et al. 2003a. Detection of equine arteritis virus (EAV)-specific cytotoxic CD8+ T lymphocyte precursors from EAV-infected ponies. *J Gen Virol*, **84**, 2745–53.

Castillo-Olivares, J., Wieringa, R., et al. 2003b. Generation of a candidate live marker vaccine for equine arteritis virus by deletion of the major virus neutralization domain. *J Virol*, **77**, 8470–80.

Cavanagh, D. 1995. The coronavirus surface glycoprotein. In: Siddell, S.G. (ed.), *The Coronaviridae*. New York: Plenum Press, 73–113.

Cavanagh, D. 1997. Nidovirales: a new order comprising Coronaviridae and Arteriviridae. *Arch Virol*, **142**, 629–33.

Cavanagh, D. 2003. Severe acute respiratory syndrome vaccine development: experiences of vaccination against avian infectious bronchitis coronavirus. *Avian Pathol*, **32**, 567–82.

Cavanagh, D. and Naqi, S. 2003. Infectious bronchitis. In: Saif, Y.M., Barnes, H.J., et al. (eds), *Diseases of poultry*, 11th edn. Ames: Iowa State Press, 101–19.

Chan, K.H., Poon, L.L., et al. 2004. Detection of SARS coronavirus in patients with suspected SARS. *Emerg Infect Dis*, **10**, 294–9.

Chang, K.W., Sheng, Y. and Gombold, J.L. 2000. Coronavirus-induced membrane fusion requires the cysteine-rich domain in the spike protein. *Virology*, **269**, 212–24.

Chang, R.Y., Krishnan, R. and Brian, D.A. 1996. The UCUAAAC promoter motif is not required for high-frequency leader recombination in bovine coronavirus defective interfering RNA. *J Virol*, **70**, 2720–9.

Chen, H. and Schifferli, D.M. 2003. Construction, characterization, and immunogenicity of an attenuated Salmonella enterica serovar typhimurium pgtE vaccine expressing fimbriae with integrated viral epitopes from the spiC promoter. *Infect Immun*, **71**, 4664–73.

Chen, H., Coote, B., et al. 2003. Evaluation of a nucleoprotein-based enzyme-linked immunosorbent assay for the detection of antibodies against infectious bronchitis virus. *Avian Pathol*, **32**, 519–26.

Chirnside, E.D. 1992. Equine arteritis virus: an overview. *Br Vet J*, **148**, 181–97.

Chirnside, E.D. and Spaan, W.J. 1990. Reverse transcription and cDNA amplification by the polymerase chain reaction of equine arteritis virus (EAV). *J Virol Methods*, **30**, 133–40.

Chirnside, E.D., de Vries, A.A., et al. 1995. Equine arteritis virus-neutralizing antibody in the horse is induced by a determinant on the large envelope glycoprotein GL. *J Gen Virol*, **76**, 1989–98.

Cinatl, J., Morgenstern, B., et al. 2003. Treatment of SARS with human interferons. *Lancet*, **362**, 293–4.

Cinatl, J. Jr., Michaelis, M., et al. 2004. Role of interferons in the treatment of severe acute respiratory syndrome. *Expert Opin Biol Ther*, **4**, 827–36.

Cologna, R. and Hogue, B.G. 2000. Identification of a bovine coronavirus packaging signal. *J Virol*, **74**, 580–3.

Cook, J.K.A. and Mockett, A.P.A. 1995. Epidemiology of infectious bronchitis virus. In: Siddell, S.G. (ed.), *The Coronaviridae*. New York: Plenum Press, 317–35.

Cornelissen, L.A., Wierda, C.M., et al. 1997. Hemagglutinin-esterase, a novel structural protein of torovirus. *J Virol*, **71**, 5277–86.

Coutelier, J.P., Van-Broeck, J. and Wolf, S.F. 1995. Interleukin-12 gene expression after viral infection in the mouse. *J Virol*, **69**, 1955–8.

Cowley, J.A., Dimmock, C.M., et al. 2000. Gill-associated virus of Penaeus monodon prawns: an invertebrate virus with ORF1a and ORF1b genes related to arteri- and coronaviruses. *J Gen Virol*, **81**, 1473–84.

Cox, G.J., Parker, M.D. and Babiuk, L.A. 1991. Bovine coronavirus nonstructural protein ns2 is a phosphoprotein. *Virology*, **185**, 509–12.

Curtis, K.M., Yount, B., et al. 2004. Reverse genetic analysis of the transcription regulatory sequence of the coronavirus transmissible gastroenteritis virus. *J Virol*, **78**, 6061–6.

Cyranoski, D. 2003. Critics slam treatment for SARS as ineffective and perhaps dangerous. *Nature*, **423**, 4.

Dales, S. and Anderson, R. 1995. Pathogenesis and diseases of the central nervous system caused by murine coronaviruses. In: Siddell, S.G. (ed.), *The Coronaviridae*. New York: Plenum Press, 257–92.

Dalton, K., Casais, R., et al. 2001. cis-acting sequences required for coronavirus infectious bronchitis virus defective-RNA replication and packaging. *J Virol*, **75**, 125–33.

Davidson, A. and Siddell, S. 2003. Potential for antiviral treatment of severe acute respiratory syndrome. *Curr Opin Infect Dis*, **16**, 565–71.

de Diego, M., Laviada, M.D., et al. 1992. Epitope specificity of protective lactogenic immunity against swine transmissible gastroenteritis virus. *J Virol*, **66**, 6502–8.

de Groot, R.J. and Horzinek, M.C. 1995. Feline infectious peritonitis. In: Siddell, S.G. (ed.), *The Coronaviridae*. New York: Plenum Press, 293–315.

de Haan, C.A., Kuo, L., et al. 1998. Coronavirus particle assembly: primary structure requirements of the membrane protein. *J Virol*, **72**, 6838–50.

de Haan, C.A., Smeets, M., et al. 1999. Mapping of the coronavirus membrane protein domains involved in interaction with the spike protein. *J Virol*, **73**, 7441–52.

de Haan, C.A., Vennema, H. and Rottier, P.J. 2000. Assembly of the coronavirus envelope: homotypic interactions between the M proteins. *J Virol*, **74**, 4967–78.

de Haan, C.A., de Wit, M., et al. 2002a. O-glycosylation of the mouse hepatitis coronavirus membrane protein. *Virus Res*, **82**, 77–81.

de Haan, C.A., Masters, P.S., et al. 2002b. The group-specific murine coronavirus genes are not essential, but their deletion, by reverse genetics, is attenuating in the natural host. *Virology*, **296**, 177–89.

de Haan, C.A., de Wit, M., et al. 2003. The glycosylation status of the murine hepatitis coronavirus M protein affects the interferogenic capacity of the virus in vitro and its ability to replicate in the liver but not the brain. *Virology*, **312**, 395–406.

de Haan, C.A., Stadler, K., et al. 2004. Cleavage inhibition of the murine coronavirus spike protein by a furin-like enzyme affects cell–cell but not virus–cell fusion. *J Virol*, **78**, 6048–54.

de Vries, A.A., Chirnside, E.D., et al. 1992. Structural proteins of equine arteritis virus. *J Virol*, **66**, 6294–303.

de Vries, A.A., Raamsman, M.J., et al. 1995. The small envelope glycoprotein (GS) of equine arteritis virus folds into three distinct monomers and a disulfide-linked dimer. *J Virol*, **69**, 3441–8.

de Vries, A.A.F., Horzinek, M.C., et al. 1997. The genomic organization of the nidovirales: similarities and differences between arteri-, toro-, and coronaviruses. *Semin Virol*, **8**, 33–47.

de Vries, A.A., Glaser, A.L., et al. 2001. Recombinant equine arteritis virus as an expression vector. *Virology*, **284**, 259–76.

Delmas, B., Gelfi, J., et al. 1992. Aminopeptidase N is a major receptor for the entero-pathogenic coronavirus TGEV. *Nature*, **357**, 417–20.

Delputte, P.L. and Nauwynck, H.J. 2004. Porcine arterivirus infection of alveolar macrophages is mediated by sialic acid on the virus. *J Virol*, **78**, 8094–101.

Delputte, P.L., Vanderheijden, N., et al. 2002. Involvement of the matrix protein in attachment of porcine reproductive and respiratory syndrome virus to a heparinlike receptor on porcine alveolar macrophages. *J Virol*, **76**, 4312–20.

den Boon, J.A., Snijder, E.J., et al. 1991. Equine arteritis virus is not a togavirus but belongs to the coronaviruslike superfamily. *J Virol*, **65**, 2910–20.

den Boon, J.A., Kleijnen, M.F., et al. 1996. Equine arteritis virus subgenomic mRNA synthesis: analysis of leader-body junctions and replicative-form RNAs. *J Virol*, **70**, 4291–8.

Denison, M.R., Spaan, W.J., et al. 1999. The putative helicase of the coronavirus mouse hepatitis virus is processed from the replicase gene polyprotein and localizes in complexes that are active in viral RNA synthesis. *J Virol*, **73**, 6862–71.

Doan, D.N. and Dokland, T. 2003. Structure of the nucleocapsid protein of porcine reproductive and respiratory syndrome virus. *Structure (Camb)*, **11**, 1445–51.

Dobbe, J.C., van der Meer, Y., et al. 2001. Construction of chimeric arteriviruses reveals that the ectodomain of the major glycoprotein is not the main determinant of equine arteritis virus tropism in cell culture. *Virology*, **288**, 283–94.

Drew, T.W., Meulenberg, J.J., et al. 1995. Production, characterization and reactivity of monoclonal antibodies to porcine reproductive and respiratory syndrome virus. *J Gen Virol*, **76**, 1361–9.

Drosten, C., Gunther, S., et al. 2003. Identification of a novel coronavirus in patients with severe acute respiratory syndrome. *N Engl J Med*, **348**, 1967–76.

Duarte, M., Tobler, K., et al. 1994. Sequence analysis of the porcine epidemic diarrhea virus genome between the nucleocapsid and spike protein genes reveals a polymorphic ORF. *Virology*, **198**, 466–76.

Dveksler, G.S., Dieffenbach, C.W., et al. 1993. Several members of the mouse carcinoembryonic antigen-related glycoprotein family are functional receptors for the coronavirus mouse hepatitis virus-A59. *J Virol*, **67**, 1–8.

Egloff, M.P., Ferron, F., et al. 2004. The severe acute respiratory syndrome-coronavirus replicative protein nsp9 is a single-stranded RNA-binding subunit unique in the RNA virus world. *Proc Natl Acad Sci USA*, **101**, 3792–6.

El-Sahly, H.M., Atmar, R.L., et al. 2000. Spectrum of clinical illness in hospitalized patients with 'common cold' virus infections. *Clin Infect Dis*, **31**, 96–100.

Emery, S.L., Erdman, D.D., et al. 2004. Real-time reverse transcription-polymerase chain reaction assay for SARS-associated coronavirus. *Emerg Infect Dis*, **10**, 311–16.

Enjuanes, L. and Van der Zeijst, B.A.M. 1995. Molecular basis of transmissible gastroenteritis virus epidemiology. In: Siddell, S.G. (ed.), *The Coronaviridae*. New York: Plenum Press, 337–76.

Escors, D., Ortego, J., et al. 2001. The membrane M protein carboxy terminus binds to transmissible gastroenteritis coronavirus core and contributes to core stability. *J Virol*, **75**, 1312–24.

Escors, D., Izeta, A., et al. 2003. Transmissible gastroenteritis coronavirus packaging signal is located at the 5′ end of the virus genome. *J Virol*, **77**, 7890–902.

Esper, F., Weibel, C., et al. 2005. Evidence of a novel human coronavirus that is associated with respiratory tract disease in infants and young children. *J Infect Dis*, **191**, 492–8.

Faaberg, K.S. and Plagemann, P.G. 1995. The envelope proteins of lactate dehydrogenase-elevating virus and their membrane topography. *Virology*, **212**, 512–25.

Faaberg, K.S. and Plagemann, P.G. 1997. ORF 3 of lactate dehydrogenase-elevating virus encodes a soluble, nonstructural, highly glycosylated, and antigenic protein. *Virology*, **227**, 245–51.

Falsey, A.R., Walsh, E.E. and Hayden, F.G. 2002. Rhinovirus and coronavirus infection-associated hospitalizations among older adults. *J Infect Dis*, **185**, 1338–41.

Fischer, F., Stegen, C.F., et al. 1998. Analysis of constructed E gene mutants of mouse hepatitis virus confirms a pivotal role for E protein in coronavirus assembly. *J Virol*, **72**, 7885–94.

Fleming, J.O., Shubin, R.A., et al. 1989. Monoclonal antibodies to the matrix (E1) glycoprotein of mouse hepatitis virus protect mice from encephalitis. *Virology*, **168**, 162–7.

Foley, J.E. and Leutenegger, C. 2001. A review of coronavirus infection in the central nervous system of cats and mice. *J Vet Intern Med*, **15**, 438–44.

Foley, J.E., Poland, A., et al. 1997. Risk factors for feline infectious peritonitis among cats in multiple-cat environments with endemic feline enteric coronavirus. *J Am Vet Med Assoc*, **210**, 1313–18.

Fosmire, J.A., Hwang, K. and Makino, S. 1992. Identification and characterization of a coronavirus packaging signal. *J Virol*, **66**, 3522–30.

Fouchier, R.A., Kuiken, T., et al. 2003. Aetiology: Koch's postulates fulfilled for SARS virus. *Nature*, **423**, 240.

Fouchier, R.A., Hartwig, N.G., et al. 2004. A previously undescribed coronavirus associated with respiratory disease in humans. *Proc Natl Acad Sci USA*, **101**, 6212–16.

Fukunaga, Y., Wada, R. and Ka, M. 1984. Tentative preparation of an inactivated vaccine for equine viral arteritis. *Bull Eq Res Inst*, **21**, 56–64.

Gagneten, S., Gout, O., et al. 1995. Interaction of mouse hepatitis virus (MHV) spike glycoprotein with receptor glycoprotein MHVR is required for infection with an MHV strain that expresses the hemagglutinin-esterase glycoprotein. *J Virol*, **69**, 889–95.

Gallagher, T.M., Escarmis, C. and Buchmeier, M.J. 1991. Alteration of the pH dependence of coronavirus-induced cell fusion: effect of mutations in the spike glycoprotein. *J Virol*, **65**, 1916–28.

Garwes, D.J. 1995. Pathogenesis of the porcine coronaviruses. In: Siddell, S.G. (ed.), *The Coronaviridae*. New York: Plenum Press, 377–88.

Giese, M., Bahr, U., et al. 2002. Stable and long-lasting immune response in horses after DNA vaccination against equine arteritis virus. *Virus Genes*, **25**, 159–67.

Gilbert, S.A., Larochelle, R., et al. 1997. Typing of porcine reproductive and respiratory syndrome viruses by a multiplex PCR assay. *J Clin Microbiol*, **35**, 264–7.

Godeny, E.K., de Vries, A.A., et al. 1998. Identification of the leader-body junctions for the viral subgenomic mRNAs and organization of the simian hemorrhagic fever virus genome: evidence for gene duplication during arterivirus evolution. *J Virol*, **72**, 862–7.

Goebel, S.J., Hsue, B., et al. 2004. Characterization of the RNA components of a putative molecular switch in the 3′ untranslated region of the murine coronavirus genome. *J Virol*, **78**, 669–82.

Golnik, W., Moraillon, A. and Golnik, J. 1986. Identification and antigenic comparison of equine arteritis virus isolated from an outbreak of epidemic abortion of mares. *Zentralbl Veterinarmed B*, **33**, 413–17.

Gombold, J.L., Hingley, S.T. and Weiss, S.R. 1993. Fusion-defective mutants of mouse hepatitis virus A59 contain a mutation in the spike protein cleavage signal. *J Virol*, **67**, 4504–12.

Gonzalez, J.M., Gomez-Puertas, P., et al. 2003. A comparative sequence analysis to revise the current taxonomy of the family Coronaviridae. *Arch Virol*, **148**, 2207–35.

Gorbalenya, A.E. 2001. Big nidovirus genome. When count and order of domains matter. *Adv Exp Med Biol*, **494**, 1–17.

Gorbalenya, A.E., Donchenko, A.P., et al. 1989b. Cysteine proteases of positive strand RNA viruses and chymotrypsin-like serine proteases. A distinct protein superfamily with a common structural fold. *FEBS Lett*, **243**, 103–14.

Gorbalenya, A.E., Koonin, E.V., et al. 1989a. Coronavirus genome: prediction of putative functional domains in the non-structural polyprotein by comparative amino acid sequence analysis. *Nucleic Acids Res*, **17**, 4847–61.

Gorbalenya, A.E., Koonin, E.V. and Lai, M.M. 1991. Putative papain-related thiol proteases of positive-strand RNA viruses. Identification of rubi- and aphthovirus proteases and delineation of a novel conserved domain associated with proteases of rubi-, alpha- and coronaviruses. *FEBS Lett*, **288**, 201–5.

Gorbalenya, A.E., Snijder, E.J. and Spaan, W.J. 2004. Severe acute respiratory syndrome coronavirus phylogeny: toward consensus. *J Virol*, **78**, 7863–6.

Gosert, R., Kanjanahaluethai, A., et al. 2002. RNA replication of mouse hepatitis virus takes place at double-membrane vesicles. *J Virol*, **76**, 3697–708.

Guan, Y., Zheng, B.J., et al. 2003. Isolation and characterization of viruses related to the SARS coronavirus from animals in southern China. *Science*, **302**, 276–8.

Guy, J.S., Smith, L.G., et al. 2002. Development of a competitive enzyme-linked immunosorbent assay for detection of turkey coronavirus antibodies. *Avian Dis*, **46**, 334–41.

Haagmans, B.L., Kuiken, T., et al. 2004. Pegylated interferon-alpha protects type 1 pneumocytes against SARS coronavirus infection in macaques. *Nat Med*, **10**, 290–3.

Haijema, B.J., Volders, H. and Rottier, P.J. 2003. Switching species tropism: an effective way to manipulate the feline coronavirus genome. *J Virol*, **77**, 4528–38.

Haijema, B.J., Volders, H. and Rottier, P.J. 2004. Live, attenuated coronavirus vaccines through the directed deletion of group-specific genes provide protection against feline infectious peritonitis. *J Virol*, **78**, 3863–71.

Haring, J. and Perlman, S. 2001. Mouse hepatitis virus. *Curr Opin Microbiol*, **4**, 462–6.

Hays, J.P. and Myint, S.H. 1998. PCR sequencing of the spike genes of geographically and chronologically distinct human coronaviruses 229E. *J Virol Methods*, **75**, 179–93.

He, R., Dobie, F., et al. 2004. Analysis of multimerization of the SARS coronavirus nucleocapsid protein. *Biochem Biophys Res Commun*, **316**, 476–83.

Hedges, J.F., Balasuriya, U.B. and MacLachlan, N.J. 1999. The open reading frame 3 of equine arteritis virus encodes an immunogenic glycosylated, integral membrane protein. *Virology*, **264**, 92–8.

Hegyi, A. and Ziebuhr, J. 2002. Conservation of substrate specificities among coronavirus main proteases. *J Gen Virol*, **83**, 595–9.

Hegyi, A., Friebe, A., et al. 2002. Mutational analysis of the active centre of coronavirus 3C-like proteases. *J Gen Virol*, **83**, 581–93.

Hemmila, E., Turbide, C., et al. 2004. Ceacam1a-/- mice are completely resistant to infection by murine coronavirus mouse hepatitis virus A59. *J Virol*, **78**, 10156–65.

Hensley, L.E., Fritz, L.E., et al. 2004. Interferon-beta 1a and SARS coronavirus replication. *Emerg Infect Dis*, **10**, 317–19.

Herold, J., Siddell, S.G. and Gorbalenya, A.E. 1999. A human RNA viral cysteine proteinase that depends upon a unique Zn2+-binding finger connecting the two domains of a papain-like fold. *J Biol Chem*, **274**, 14918–25.

Hertzig, T., Scandella, E., et al. 2004. Rapid identification of coronavirus replicase inhibitors using a selectable replicon RNA. *J Gen Virol*, **85**, 1717–25.

Heusipp, G., Harms, U., et al. 1997. Identification of an ATPase activity associated with a 71-kilodalton polypeptide encoded in gene 1 of the human coronavirus 229E. *J Virol*, **71**, 5631–4.

Hiscox, J.A., Wurm, T., et al. 2001. The coronavirus infectious bronchitis virus nucleoprotein localizes to the nucleolus. *J Virol*, **75**, 506–12.

Ho, J.C., Ooi, G.C., et al. 2003a. High-dose pulse versus nonpulse corticosteroid regimens in severe acute respiratory syndrome. *Am J Respir Crit Care Med*, **168**, 1449–56.

Ho, P.L., Tang, X.P. and Seto, W.H. 2003b. SARS: hospital infection control and admission strategies. *Respirology*, **8**, Suppl, S41–5.

Hoet, A.E., Nielsen, P.R., et al. 2003. Detection of bovine torovirus and other enteric pathogens in feces from diarrhea cases in cattle. *J Vet Diagn Invest*, **15**, 205–12.

Hohdatsu, T., Yamada, M., et al. 1998. Antibody-dependent enhancement of feline infectious peritonitis virus infection in feline alveolar macrophages and human monocyte cell line U937 by serum of cats experimentally or naturally infected with feline coronavirus. *J Vet Med Sci*, **60**, 49–55.

Holmes, K.V. 2001a. Coronaviruses. In: Knipe, D.M. and Howley, P.M. (eds), *Fields virology*, 4th edn. Philadelphia, PA: Lippincott, Williams, Wilkins, 1187–203.

Holmes, K.V. 2001b. Enteric infections with coronaviruses and toroviruses. *Novartis Found Symp*, **238**, 258–69, discussion 269–75.

Hsu, J.T., Kuo, C.J., et al. 2004. Evaluation of metal-conjugated compounds as inhibitors of 3CL protease of SARS-CoV. *FEBS Lett*, **574**, 116–20.

Huang, Q., Yu, L., et al. 2004. Structure of the N-terminal RNA-binding domain of the SARS CoV nucleocapsid protein. *Biochemistry*, **43**, 6059–63.

Ignjatovic, J. and Galli, N. 1993. Immune responses to structural proteins of avian bronchitis virus. In: Coudert, F. (ed.), *Avian immunology in progress*. Paris: Institut National de Recherche Agronomique, 237–42.

Ignjatovic, J. and Sapats, S. 2000. Avian infectious bronchitis virus. *Rev Sci Tech*, **19**, 493–508.

Ingallinella, P., Bianchi, E., et al. 2004. Structural characterization of the fusion-active complex of severe acute respiratory syndrome (SARS) coronavirus. *Proc Natl Acad Sci USA*, **101**, 8709–14.

Ivanov, K.A. and Ziebuhr, J. 2004. Human coronavirus 229E nonstructural protein 13: characterization of duplex-unwinding, nucleoside triphosphatase and RNA 5′-triphosphatase activities. *J Virol*, **78**, 7833–8.

Ivanov, K.A., Thiel, V., et al. 2004a. Multiple enzymatic activities associated with severe acute respiratory syndrome coronavirus helicase. *J Virol*, **78**, 5619–32.

Ivanov, K.A., Hertzig, T., et al. 2004b. Major genetic marker of nidoviruses encodes a replicative endoribonuclease. *Proc Natl Acad Sci USA*, **101**, 12694–9.

Jackwood, M.W., Hilt, D.A. and Callison, S.A. 2003. Detection of infectious bronchitis virus by real-time reverse transcriptase-polymerase chain reaction and identification of a quasispecies in the Beaudette strain. *Avian Dis*, **47**, 718–24.

Jendrach, M., Thiel, V. and Siddell, S. 1999. Characterization of an internal ribosome entry site within mRNA 5 of murine hepatitis virus. *Arch Virol*, **144**, 921–33.

Jones, B.M., Ma, E.S., et al. 2004. Prolonged disturbances of in vitro cytokine production in patients with severe acute respiratory syndrome (SARS) treated with ribavirin and steroids. *Clin Exp Immunol*, **135**, 467–73.

Karaca, K. and Naqi, S. 1993. A monoclonal antibody blocking ELISA to detect serotype-specific infectious bronchitis virus antibodies. *Vet Microbiol*, **34**, 249–57.

Kim, O., Choi, C., et al. 2000. Detection and differentiation of porcine epidemic diarrhoea virus and transmissible gastroenteritis virus in clinical samples by multiplex RT-PCR. *Vet Rec*, **146**, 637–40.

Kim, S.Y., Song, D.S. and Park, B.K. 2001. Differential detection of transmissible gastroenteritis virus and porcine epidemic diarrhea virus by duplex RT-PCR. *J Vet Diagn Invest*, **13**, 516–20.

Koonin, E.V. 1991. The phylogeny of RNA-dependent RNA polymerases of positive-strand RNA viruses. *J Gen Virol*, **72**, 2197–206.

Koopmans, M. and Horzinek, M.C. 1995. The pathogenesis of torovirus infections in animals and humans. In: Siddell, S.G. (ed.), *The Coronaviridae*. New York: Plenum Press, 403–13.

Koopmans, M., van den Boom, U., et al. 1989. Seroepidemiology of Breda virus in cattle using ELISA. *Vet Microbiol*, **19**, 233–43.

Koopmans, M., Cremers, H., et al. 1990. Breda virus (Toroviridae) infection and systemic antibody response in sentinel calves. *Am J Vet Res*, **51**, 1443–8.

Koopmans, M., Snijder, E.J. and Horzinek, M.C. 1991. cDNA probes for the diagnosis of bovine torovirus (Breda virus) infection. *J Clin Microbiol*, **29**, 493–7.

Koopmans, M., Monroe, S.S., et al. 1993. Optimization of extraction and PCR amplification of RNA extracts from paraffin-embedded tissue in different fixatives. *J Virol Methods*, **43**, 189–204.

Kozak, M. 1999. Initiation of translation in prokaryotes and eukaryotes. *Gene*, **234**, 187–208.

Kroneman, A., Cornelissen, L.A., et al. 1998. Identification and characterization of a porcine torovirus. *J Virol*, **72**, 3507–11.

Ksiazek, T.G., Erdman, D., et al. 2003. A novel coronavirus associated with severe acute respiratory syndrome. *N Engl J Med*, **348**, 1953–66.

Kuiken, T., Fouchier, R.A., et al. 2003. Newly discovered coronavirus as the primary cause of severe acute respiratory syndrome. *Lancet*, **362**, 263–70.

Kuo, L. and Masters, P.S. 2002. Genetic evidence for a structural interaction between the carboxy termini of the membrane and nucleocapsid proteins of mouse hepatitis virus. *J Virol*, **76**, 4987–99.

Kuo, L. and Masters, P.S. 2003. The small envelope protein E is not essential for murine coronavirus replication. *J Virol*, **77**, 4597–608.

Lai, M.M.C. and Holmes, K.V. 2001. *Coronaviridae*: the viruses and their replication. In: Knipe, D.M., Howley, P.M., et al. (eds), *Fields virology*, 4th edn. Philadelphia, PA.: Lippincott, Williams, Wilkins, 1163–85.

Lamphear, B.J., Jilka, J.M., et al. 2004. A corn-based delivery system for animal vaccines: an oral transmissible gastroenteritis virus vaccine boosts lactogenic immunity in swine. *Vaccine*, **22**, 2420–4.

Laude, H. and Masters, P.S. 1995. The coronavirus nucleocapsid protein. In: Siddell, S.G. (ed.), *The Coronaviridae*. New York: Plenum Press, 141–63.

Lee, C.W. and Jackwood, M.W. 2000. Evidence of genetic diversity generated by recombination among avian coronavirus IBV. *Arch Virol*, **145**, 2135–48.

Lee, C.W., Hilt, D.A. and Jackwood, M.W. 2003a. Typing of field isolates of infectious bronchitis virus based on the sequence of the hypervariable region in the S1 gene. *J Vet Diagn Invest*, **15**, 344–8.

Lee, H.K., Tso, E.Y., et al. 2003b. Asymptomatic severe acute respiratory syndrome-associated coronavirus infection. *Emerg Infect Dis*, **9**, 1491–2.

Lee, N., Hui, D., et al. 2003c. A major outbreak of severe acute respiratory syndrome in Hong Kong. *N Engl J Med*, **348**, 1986–94.

Lee, C.W., Brown, C., et al. 2004. Nephropathogenesis of chickens experimentally infected with various strains of infectious bronchitis virus. *J Vet Med Sci*, **66**, 835–40.

Legeay, O., Bounaix, S., et al. 1997. Development of a RT-PCR test coupled with a microplate colorimetric assay for the detection of a swine Arterivirus (PRRSV) in boar semen. *J Virol Methods*, **68**, 65–80.

Li, K., Chen, Z. and Plagemann, P. 1998. The neutralization epitope of lactate dehydrogenase-elevating virus is located on the short ectodomain of the primary envelope glycoprotein. *Virology*, **242**, 239–45.

Li, W., Moore, M.J., et al. 2003. Angiotensin-converting enzyme 2 is a functional receptor for the SARS coronavirus. *Nature*, **426**, 450–4.

Lina, B., Valette, M., et al. 1996. Surveillance of community-acquired viral infections due to respiratory viruses in Rhone-Alpes (France) during winter 1994 to 1995. *J Clin Microbiol*, **34**, 3007–11.

Liphardt, J., Napthine, S., et al. 1999. Evidence for an RNA pseudoknot loop-helix interaction essential for efficient -1 ribosomal frameshifting. *J Mol Biol*, **288**, 321–35.

Liu, C., Kokuho, T., et al. 2001a. A serodiagnostic ELISA using recombinant antigen of swine transmissible gastroenteritis virus nucleoprotein. *J Vet Med Sci*, **63**, 1253–6.

Liu, C., Kokuho, T., et al. 2001b. DNA mediated immunization with encoding the nucleoprotein gene of porcine transmissible gastroenteritis virus. *Virus Res*, **80**, 75–82.

Liu, D.X. and Brown, T.D. 1995. Characterisation and mutational analysis of an ORF 1a-encoding proteinase domain responsible for proteolytic processing of the infectious bronchitis virus 1a/1b polyprotein. *Virology*, **209**, 420–7.

Liu, D.X. and Inglis, S.C. 1992. Internal entry of ribosomes on a tricistronic mRNA encoded by infectious bronchitis virus. *J Virol*, **66**, 6143–54.

Liu, D.X., Cavanagh, D., et al. 1991. A polycistronic mRNA specified by the coronavirus infectious bronchitis virus. *Virology*, **184**, 531–44.

Liu, H.J., Lee, L.H., et al. 2003. Detection of infectious bronchitis virus by multiplex polymerase chain reaction and sequence analysis. *J Virol Methods*, **109**, 31–7.

Liu, Q., Johnson, R.F. and Leibowitz, J.L. 2001. Secondary structural elements within the 3′ untranslated region of mouse hepatitis virus strain JHM genomic RNA. *J Virol*, **75**, 12105–13.

Liu, S., Xiao, G., et al. 2004. Interaction between heptad repeat 1 and 2 regions in spike protein of SARS-associated coronavirus: implications for virus fusogenic mechanism and identification of fusion inhibitors. *Lancet*, **363**, 938–47.

Loa, C.C., Lin, T.L., et al. 2001. Humoral and cellular immune responses in turkey poults infected with turkey coronavirus. *Poult Sci*, **80**, 1416–24.

Loutfy, M.R., Blatt, L.M., et al. 2003. Interferon alfacon-1 plus corticosteroids in severe acute respiratory syndrome: a preliminary study. *JAMA*, **290**, 3222–8.

Lu, Y., Lu, X. and Denison, M.R. 1995. Identification and characterization of a serine-like proteinase of the murine coronavirus MHV-A59. *J Virol*, **69**, 3554–9.

Luytjes, W., Bredenbeek, P.J., et al. 1988. Sequence of mouse hepatitis virus A59 mRNA 2: indications for RNA recombination between coronaviruses and influenza C virus. *Virology*, **166**, 415–22.

Mackenzie, J.M., Jones, M.K. and Westaway, E.G. 1999. Markers for trans-Golgi membranes and the intermediate compartment localize to induced membranes with distinct replication functions in flavivirus-infected cells. *J Virol*, **73**, 9555–67.

Madsen, K.G., Hansen, C.M., et al. 1998. Sequence analysis of porcine reproductive and respiratory syndrome virus of the American type collected from Danish swine herds. *Arch Virol*, **143**, 1683–700.

Marczinke, B., Hagervall, T. and Brierley, I. 2000. The Q-base of asparaginyl-tRNA is dispensable for efficient -1 ribosomal frameshifting in eukaryotes. *J Mol Biol*, **295**, 179–91.

Mardassi, H., Gonin, P., et al. 1998. A subset of porcine reproductive and respiratory syndrome virus GP3 glycoprotein is released into the culture medium of cells as a non-virion-associated and membrane-free (soluble) form. *J Virol*, **72**, 6298–306.

Marra, M.A., Jones, S.J., et al. 2003. The genome sequence of the SARS-associated coronavirus. *Science*, **300**, 1399–404.

Martina, B.E., Haagmans, B.L., et al. 2003. Virology: SARS virus infection of cats and ferrets. *Nature*, **425**, 915.

McCollum, W.H. 1986. Responses of horses vaccinated with avirulent modified-live equine arteritis virus propagated in the E. Derm (NBL-6) cell line to nasal inoculation with virulent virus. *Am J Vet Res*, **47**, 1931–4.

Meredith, M.J. 1993. *Porcine reproductive and respiratory syndrome*. Cambridge: University Press.

Meulenberg, J.J. and Petersen-den Besten, A. 1996. Identification and characterization of a sixth structural protein of Lelystad virus: the glycoprotein GP2 encoded by ORF2 is incorporated in virus particles. *Virology*, **225**, 44–51.

Meulenberg, J.J., van Nieuwstadt, A.P., et al. 1997. Posttranslational processing and identification of a neutralization domain of the GP4 protein encoded by ORF4 of Lelystad virus. *J Virol*, **71**, 6061–7.

Meulenberg, J.J., Bos-de Ruijter, J.N., et al. 1998. Infectious transcripts from cloned genome-length cDNA of porcine reproductive and respiratory syndrome virus. *J Virol*, **72**, 380–7.

Molenkamp, R., van Tol, H., et al. 2000. The arterivirus replicase is the only viral protein required for genome replication and subgenomic mRNA transcription. *J Gen Virol*, **81**, 2491–6.

Monto, A.S. and Lim, S.K. 1974. The Tecumseh study of respiratory illness: VI. Frequency of and relationship between outbreaks of coronavirus infection. *J Infect Dis*, **127**, 271–6.

Moore, B.D., Balasuriya, U.B., et al. 2003. Virulent and avirulent strains of equine arteritis virus induce different quantities of TNF-alpha and other proinflammatory cytokines in alveolar and blood-derived equine macrophages. *Virology*, **314**, 662–70.

Murtaugh, M., Collins, J.E. and Rossow, K.D. 1993. Porcine respiratory and reproductive syndrome. In: Lehman, A.D. (ed.), *Swine conference*. Minneapolis: University of Minnesota, 43–53.

Murtaugh, M.P., Xiao, Z. and Zuckermann, F. 2002. Immunological responses of swine to porcine reproductive and respiratory syndrome virus infection. *Viral Immunol*, **15**, 533–47.

Myint, S.H. 1995. Human coronavirus infections. In: Siddell, S.G. (ed.), *The Coronaviridae*. New York: Plenum Press, 389–401.

Nagy, P.D. and Simon, A.E. 1997. New insights into the mechanisms of RNA recombination. *Virology*, **235**, 1–9.

Napthine, S., Liphardt, J., et al. 1999. The role of RNA pseudoknot stem 1 length in the promotion of efficient -1 ribosomal frameshifting. *J Mol Biol*, **288**, 305–20.

Narayanan, K., Chen, C.J., et al. 2003a. Nucleocapsid-independent specific viral RNA packaging via viral envelope protein and viral RNA signal. *J Virol*, **77**, 2922–7.

Narayanan, K., Kim, K.H. and Makino, S. 2003b. Characterization of N protein self-association in coronavirus ribonucleoprotein complexes. *Virus Res*, **98**, 131–40.

Nelson, C.A., Pekosz, A., et al. 2005. Structure and intracellular targeting of the SARS-coronavirus Orf7a accessory protein. *Structure (Camb)*, **13**, 75–85.

Nielsen, H.S., Liu, G., et al. 2003. Generation of an infectious clone of VR-2332, a highly virulent North American-type isolate of porcine reproductive and respiratory syndrome virus. *J Virol*, **77**, 3702–11.

O'Connor, J.B. and Brian, D.A. 2000. Downstream ribosomal entry for translation of coronavirus TGEV gene 3b. *Virology*, **269**, 172–82.

Ooi, G.C. and Daqing, M. 2003. SARS: radiological features. *Respirology*, **8**, Suppl, S15–9.

Ostrowski, M., Galeota, J.A., et al. 2002. Identification of neutralizing and nonneutralizing epitopes in the porcine reproductive and respiratory syndrome virus GP5 ectodomain. *J Virol*, **76**, 4241–50.

Paltrinieri, S., Cammarata, M.P., et al. 1998. Some aspects of humoral and cellular immunity in naturally occuring feline infectious peritonitis. *Vet Immunol Immunopathol*, **65**, 205–20.

Paltrinieri, S., Ponti, W., et al. 2003. Shifts in circulating lymphocyte subsets in cats with feline infectious peritonitis (FIP): pathogenic role and diagnostic relevance. *Vet Immunol Immunopathol*, **96**, 141–8.

Parker, M.M. and Masters, P.S. 1990. Sequence comparison of the N genes of five strains of the coronavirus mouse hepatitis virus suggests a three domain structure for the nucleocapsid protein. *Virology*, **179**, 463–8.

Pasternak, A.O., Gultyaev, A.P., et al. 2000. Genetic manipulation of arterivirus alternative mRNA leader-body junction sites reveals tight regulation of structural protein expression. *J Virol*, **74**, 11642–53.

Pasternak, A.O., Van Den Born, E., et al. 2001. Sequence requirements for RNA strand transfer during nidovirus discontinuous subgenomic RNA synthesis. *EMBO J*, **20**, 7220–8.

Pasternak, A.O., Spaan, W.J. and Snijder, E.J. 2004. Regulation of relative abundance of arterivirus subgenomic mRNAs. *J Virol*, **78**, 8102–13.

Paton, D. and Lowings, P. 1997. Discrimination between transmissible gastroenteritis virus isolates. *Arch Virol*, **142**, 1703–11.

Paul, P.S., Halbur, P., et al. 2003. Exogenous porcine viruses. *Curr Top Microbiol Immunol*, **278**, 125–83.

Paweska, J.T. 1994. Equine viral arteritis in donkeys in South Africa [letter]. *J S Afr Vet Assoc*, **65**, 40.

Pedersen, K.W., van der Meer, Y., et al. 1999. Open reading frame 1a-encoded subunits of the arterivirus replicase induce endoplasmic reticulum-derived double-membrane vesicles which carry the viral replication complex. *J Virol*, **73**, 2016–26.

Peiris, J.S., Lai, S.T., et al. 2003a. Coronavirus as a possible cause of severe acute respiratory syndrome. *Lancet*, **361**, 1319–25.

Peiris, J.S., Chu, C.M., et al. 2003b. Clinical progression and viral load in a community outbreak of coronavirus-associated SARS pneumonia: a prospective study. *Lancet*, **361**, 1767–72.

Pene, F., Merlat, A., et al. 2003. Coronavirus 229E-related pneumonia in immunocompromised patients. *Clin Infect Dis*, **37**, 929–32.

Pfleiderer, M., Routledge, E., et al. 1991. High level transient expression of the murine coronavirus haemagglutinin-esterase. *J Gen Virol*, **72**, 1309–15.

Pirzadeh, B. and Dea, S. 1998. Immune response in pigs vaccinated with plasmid DNA encoding ORF5 of porcine reproductive and respiratory syndrome virus. *J Gen Virol*, **79**, 989–99.

Plagemann, P.G. 2004. GP5 ectodomain epitope of porcine reproductive and respiratory syndrome virus, strain Lelystad virus. *Virus Res*, **102**, 225–30.

Plagemann, P.G. and Moennig, V. 1992. Lactate dehydrogenase-elevating virus, equine arteritis virus, and simian hemorrhagic fever virus: a new group of positive-strand RNA viruses. *Adv Virus Res*, **41**, 99–192.

Plagemann, P.G.W. 1996. Lactate-dehydrogenase-elevating virus and related viruses. In: Knipe, D.M., Howley, P.M., et al. (eds), *Fields virology*, 3rd edn. Philidelphia, PA.: Lippincott, Williams & Wilkins. 1105–20.

Plagemann, P.G.W., Rowland, R.R., et al. 1995. Lactate dehydrogenase-elevating virus-an ideal persistent virus? *Semin Immunopathol*, **17**, 167–86.

Poland, A.M., Vennema, H., et al. 1996. Two related strains of feline infectious peritonitis virus isolated from immunocompromised cats infected with a feline enteric coronavirus. *J Clin Microbiol*, **34**, 3180–4.

Poon, L.L., Chu, D.K., et al. 2005. Identification of a novel coronavirus in bats. *J Virol*, **79**, 2001–9.

Popova, R. and Zhang, X. 2002. The spike but not the hemagglutinin/esterase protein of bovine coronavirus is necessary and sufficient for viral infection. *Virology*, **294**, 222–36.

Poutanen, S.M. and McGeer, A.J. 2004. Transmission and control of SARS. *Curr Infect Dis Rep*, **6**, 220–7.

Prentice, E., Jerome, W.G., et al. 2004a. Coronavirus replication complex formation utilizes components of cellular autophagy. *J Biol Chem*, **279**, 10136–41.

Prentice, E., McAuliffe, J., et al. 2004b. Identification and characterization of severe acute respiratory syndrome coronavirus replicase proteins. *J Virol*, **78**, 9977–86.

Raamsman, M.J., Locker, J.K., et al. 2000. Characterization of the coronavirus mouse hepatitis virus strain A59 small membrane protein E. *J Virol*, **74**, 2333–42.

Rainer, T.H. 2004. Severe acute respiratory syndrome: clinical features, diagnosis, and management. *Curr Opin Pulm Med*, **10**, 159–65.

Risco, C., Anton, I.M., et al. 1995. Membrane protein molecules of transmissible gastroenteritis coronavirus also expose the carboxy-terminal region on the external surface of the virion. *J Virol*, **69**, 5269–77.

Risco, C., Anton, I.M., et al. 1996. The transmissible gastroenteritis coronavirus contains a spherical core shell consisting of M and N proteins. *J Virol*, **70**, 4773–7.

Rota, P.A., Oberste, M.S., et al. 2003. Characterization of a novel coronavirus associated with severe acute respiratory syndrome. *Science*, **300**, 1394–9.

Rottier, P.J.M. 1995. The coronavirus membrane glycoprotein. In: Siddell, S.G. (ed.), *The Coronaviridae*. New York: Plenum Press, 115–39.

Rowland, R.R., Schneider, P., et al. 2003. Peptide domains involved in the localization of the porcine reproductive and respiratory syndrome virus nucleocapsid protein to the nucleolus. *Virology*, **316**, 135–45.

Rust, R.C., Landmann, L., et al. 2001. Cellular COPII proteins are involved in production of the vesicles that form the poliovirus replication complex. *J Virol*, **75**, 9808–18.

Sagripanti, J.L., Zandomeni, R.O. and Weinmann, R. 1986. The cap structure of simian hemorrhagic fever virion RNA. *Virology*, **151**, 146–50.

Saif, L.J. 1999. Enteric viral infections of pigs and strategies for induction of mucosal immunity. *Adv Vet Med*, **41**, 429–46.

Saif, L.J. and Wesley, R.D. 1992. Transmissible gastroenteritis. In: Leman, A.D. and Straw, B. (eds), *Diseases of swine*. Ames: Iowa State University Press, 362–86.

Salanueva, I.J., Carrascosa, J.L. and Risco, C. 1999. Structural maturation of the transmissible gastroenteritis coronavirus. *J Virol*, **73**, 7952–64.

Salonen, A., Vasiljeva, L., et al. 2003. Properly folded nonstructural polyprotein directs the Semliki Forest virus replication complex to the endosomal compartment. *J Virol*, **77**, 1691–702.

Sanchez, C.M., Jimenez, G., et al. 1990. Antigenic homology among coronaviruses related to transmissible gastroenteritis virus. *Virology*, **174**, 410–17.

Sawicki, S.G. and Sawicki, D.L. 1998. A new model for coronavirus transcription. *Adv Exp Med Biol*, **440**, 215–19.

Sawicki, D., Wang, T. and Sawicki, S. 2001. The RNA structures engaged in replication and transcription of the A59 strain of mouse hepatitis virus. *J Gen Virol*, **82**, 385–96.

Schwarz, B., Routledge, E. and Siddell, S.G. 1990. Murine coronavirus nonstructural protein ns2 is not essential for virus replication in transformed cells. *J Virol*, **64**, 4784–91.

Senanayake, S.D. and Brian, D.A. 1999. Translation from the 5′ untranslated region (UTR) of mRNA 1 is repressed, but that from the 5′ UTR of mRNA 7 is stimulated in coronavirus-infected cells. *J Virol*, **73**, 8003–9.

Senanayake, S.D., Hofmann, M.A., et al. 1992. The nucleocapsid protein gene of bovine coronavirus is bicistronic. *J Virol*, **66**, 5277–83.

Seto, W.H., Tsang, D., et al. 2003. Effectiveness of precautions against droplets and contact in prevention of nosocomial transmission of severe acute respiratory syndrome (SARS). *Lancet*, **361**, 1519–20.

Seybert, A., Hegyi, A., et al. 2000a. The human coronavirus 229E superfamily 1 helicase has RNA and DNA duplex-unwinding activities with 5′-to-3′ polarity. *RNA*, **6**, 1056–68.

Seybert, A., van Dinten, L.C., et al. 2000b. Biochemical characterization of the equine arteritis virus helicase suggests a close functional relationship between arterivirus and coronavirus helicases. *J Virol*, **74**, 9586–93.

Seybert, A., Posthuma, C.C., et al. 2005. A complex zinc finger controls the activities of nidovirus helicases. *J Virol*, **79**, 696–704.

Shi, J., Wei, Z. and Song, J. 2004. Dissection study on the severe acute respiratory syndrome 3C-like protease reveals the critical role of the extra domain in dimerization of the enzyme: defining the extra domain as a new target for design of highly specific protease inhibitors. *J Biol Chem*, **279**, 24765–73.

Shi, S.T., Schiller, J.J., et al. 1999. Colocalization and membrane association of murine hepatitis virus gene 1 products and de novo-synthesized viral RNA in infected cells. *J Virol*, **73**, 5957–69.

Shi, S.T., Huang, P., et al. 2000. Heterogeneous nuclear ribonucleoprotein A1 regulates RNA synthesis of a cytoplasmic virus. *EMBO J*, **19**, 4701–11.

Shieh, C.K., Soe, L.H., et al. 1987. The 5′-end sequence of the murine coronavirus genome: implications for multiple fusion sites in leader-primed transcription. *Virology*, **156**, 321–30.

Siddell, S.G. 1995. The small-membrane protein. In: Siddell, S.G. (ed.), *The Coronaviridae*. New York: Plenum Press, 181–9.

Siddell, S., Sawicki, D., et al. 2001. Identification of the mutations responsible for the phenotype of three MHV RNA-negative ts mutants. *Adv Exp Med Biol*, **494**, 453–8.

Sizun, J., Arbour, N. and Talbot, P.J. 1998. Comparison of immunofluorescence with monoclonal antibodies and RT-PCR for the detection of human coronaviruses 229E and OC43 in cell culture. *J Virol Methods*, **72**, 145–52.

Smith, S.L., Wang, X. and Godeny, E.K. 1997. Sequence of the 3′ end of the simian hemorrhagic fever virus genome. *Gene*, **191**, 205–10.

Smits, S.L., Lavazza, A., et al. 2003. Phylogenetic and evolutionary relationships among torovirus field variants: evidence for multiple intertypic recombination events. *J Virol*, **77**, 9567–77.

Snijder, E.J. and Meulenberg, J.J. 1998. The molecular biology of arteriviruses. *J Gen Virol*, **79**, 961–79.

Snijder, E.J. and Meulenberg, J.J.M. 2001. Arteriviruses. In: Knipe, D.M. and Howley, P.M. (eds), *Fields virology*. Philiadelphia, PA.: Lippincott, Williams, Wilkins, 1205–20.

Snijder, E.J. and Spaan, W. 1995. The coronaviruslike superfamily. In: Siddell, S.G. (ed.), *The Coronaviridae*. New York: Plenum Press, 239–55.

Snijder, E.J., den Boon, J.A., et al. 1990. The carboxyl-terminal part of the putative Berne virus polymerase is expressed by ribosomal frameshifting and contains sequence motifs which indicate that toro- and coronaviruses are evolutionarily related. *Nucleic Acids Res*, **18**, 4535–42.

Snijder, E.J., den Boon, J.A., et al. 1991. Comparison of the genome organization of toro- and coronaviruses: evidence for two nonhomologous RNA recombination events during Berne virus evolution. *Virology*, **180**, 448–52.

Snijder, E.J., Wassenaar, A.L., et al. 1995. The arterivirus Nsp2 protease. An unusual cysteine protease with primary structure similarities to both papain-like and chymotrypsin-like proteases. *J Biol Chem*, **270**, 16671–6.

Snijder, E.J., Wassenaar, A.L., et al. 1996. The arterivirus nsp4 protease is the prototype of a novel group of chymotrypsin-like enzymes, the 3C-like serine proteases. *J Biol Chem*, **271**, 4864–71.

Snijder, E.J., van Tol, H., et al. 1999. Identification of a novel structural protein of arteriviruses. *J Virol*, **73**, 6335–45.

Snijder, E.J., van Tol, H., et al. 2001. Non-structural proteins 2 and 3 interact to modify host cell membranes during the formation of the arterivirus replication complex. *J Gen Virol*, **82**, 985–94.

Snijder, E.J., Bredenbeek, P.J., et al. 2003a. Unique and conserved features of genome and proteome of SARS-coronavirus, an early split-off from the coronavirus group 2 lineage. *J Mol Biol*, **331**, 991–1004.

Snijder, E.J., Dobbe, J.C. and Spaan, W.J. 2003b. Heterodimerization of the two major envelope proteins is essential for arterivirus infectivity. *J Virol*, **77**, 97–104.

Snijder, E.J., Brinton, M.A., et al. 2005. Arteriviridae. In: Fauquet, C.M. and Mayo, M.A. (eds), *Virus taxonomy, VIIIth Report of the ICTV*. London: Elsevier-Academic Press, 963–72.

So, L.K., Lau, A.C., et al. 2003. Development of a standard treatment protocol for severe acute respiratory syndrome. *Lancet*, **361**, 1615–17.

Sola, I., Alonso, S., et al. 2003. Engineering the transmissible gastroenteritis virus genome as an expression vector inducing lactogenic immunity. *J Virol*, **77**, 4357–69.

Spaan, W., Cavanagh, D. and Horzinek, M.C. 1988. Coronaviruses: structure and genome expression. *J Gen Virol*, **69**, 2939–52.

Spaan, W.J.M., Cavanagh, D. 2005. Coronaviridae. In: Fauquet, C.M. and Mayo, M.A. (eds), *Virus taxonomy, VIIIth Report of the ICTV*. London: Elsevier-Academic Press, 945–62.

Stadejek, T., Bjorklund, H., et al. 1999. Genetic diversity of equine arteritis virus. *J Gen Virol*, **80**, 691–9.

Stephensen, C.B., Casebolt, D.B. and Gangopadhyay, N.N. 1999. Phylogenetic analysis of a highly conserved region of the polymerase gene from 11 coronaviruses and development of a consensus polymerase chain reaction assay. *Virus Res*, **60**, 181–9.

Stewart, J.N., Mounir, S. and Talbot, P.J. 1992. Human coronavirus gene expression in the brains of multiple sclerosis patients. *Virology*, **191**, 502–5.

St-Laurent, G., Morin, G. and Archambault, D. 1994. Detection of equine arteritis virus following amplification of structural and nonstructural viral genes by reverse transcription-PCR. *J Clin Microbiol*, **32**, 658–65.

Stohlman, S.A., Kyuwa, S., et al. 1993. Characterization of mouse hepatitis virus-specific cytotoxic T cells derived from the central nervous system of mice infected with the JHM strain. *J Virol*, **67**, 7050–9.

Suarez, P., Zardoya, R., et al. 1994. Direct detection of the porcine reproductive and respiratory syndrome (PRRS) virus by reverse polymerase chain reaction (RT-PCR). *Arch Virol*, **135**, 89–99.

Subbarao, K., McAuliffe, J., et al. 2004. Prior infection and passive transfer of neutralizing antibody prevent replication of severe acute respiratory syndrome coronavirus in the respiratory tract of mice. *J Virol*, **78**, 3572–7.

Sur, J.H., Doster, A.R., et al. 1997. Porcine reproductive and respiratory syndrome virus replicates in testicular germ cells, alters spermatogenesis, and induces germ cell death by apoptosis. *J Virol*, **71**, 9170–9.

Surjit, M., Liu, B., et al. 2004. The nucleocapsid protein of the SARS coronavirus is capable of self-association through a C-terminal 209 amino acid interaction domain. *Biochem Biophys Res Commun*, **317**, 1030–6.

Sutton, G., Fry, E., et al. 2004. The nsp9 replicase protein of SARS-coronavirus, structure and functional insights. *Structure (Camb)*, **12**, 341–53.

Tanner, J.A., Watt, R.M., et al. 2003. The severe acute respiratory syndrome (SARS) coronavirus NTPase/helicase belongs to a distinct class of 5′ to 3′ viral helicases. *J Biol Chem*, **278**, 39578–82.

ter Meulen, J., Bakker, A.B., et al. 2004. Human monoclonal antibody as prophylaxis for SARS coronavirus infection in ferrets. *Lancet*, **363**, 2139–41.

Thiel, V., Herold, J., et al. 2001a. Infectious RNA transcribed in vitro from a cDNA copy of the human coronavirus genome cloned in vaccinia virus. *J Gen Virol*, **82**, 1273–81.

Thiel, V., Herold, J., et al. 2001b. Viral replicase gene products suffice for coronavirus discontinuous transcription. *J Virol*, **75**, 6676–81.

Thiel, V., Ivanov, K.A., et al. 2003. Mechanisms and enzymes involved in SARS coronavirus genome expression. *J Gen Virol*, **84**, 2305–15.

Tijms, M.A., van Dinten, L.C., et al. 2001. A zinc finger-containing papain-like protease couples subgenomic mRNA synthesis to genome translation in a positive-stranded RNA virus. *Proc Natl Acad Sci USA*, **98**, 1889–94.

Tijms, M.A., van der Meer, Y. and Snijder, E.J. 2002. Nuclear localization of non-structural protein 1 and nucleocapsid protein of equine arteritis virus. *J Gen Virol*, **83**, 795–800.

Timoney, P.J. and McCollum, W.H. 1988. Equine viral arteritis, epidemiology and control. *Equine Vet Sci*, **8**, 54–9.

To, K.F. and Lo, A.W. 2004. Exploring the pathogenesis of severe acute respiratory syndrome (SARS): the tissue distribution of the coronavirus (SARS-CoV) and its putative receptor, angiotensin-converting enzyme 2 (ACE2). *J Pathol*, **203**, 740–3.

Tobiasch, E., Kehm, R., et al. 2001. Large envelope glycoprotein and nucleocapsid protein of equine arteritis virus (EAV) induce an immune response in Balb/c mice by DNA vaccination; strategy for developing a DNA-vaccine against EAV-infection. *Virus Genes*, **22**, 187–99.

Tripet, B., Howard, M.W., et al. 2004. Structural characterization of the SARS-coronavirus spike S fusion protein core. *J Biol Chem*, **279**, 20836–49.

Truong, H.M., Lu, Z., et al. 2004. A highly pathogenic porcine reproductive and respiratory syndrome virus generated from an infectious cDNA clone retains the in vivo virulence and transmissibility properties of the parental virus. *Virology*, **325**, 308–19.

Tsang, K.W., Ho, P.L., et al. 2003. A cluster of cases of severe acute respiratory syndrome in Hong Kong. *N Engl J Med*, **348**, 1977–85.

Tyrrell, D.A., Cohen, S. and Schlarb, J.E. 1993. Signs and symptoms in common colds. *Epidemiol Infect*, **111**, 143–56.

Vabret, A., Mouthon, F., et al. 2001. Direct diagnosis of human respiratory coronaviruses 229E and OC43 by the polymerase chain reaction. *J Virol Methods*, **97**, 59–66.

Vabret, A., Mourez, T., et al. 2003. An outbreak of coronavirus OC43 respiratory infection in Normandy, France. *Clin Infect Dis*, **36**, 985–9.

Vallet, S., Gagneur, A., et al. 2004. Detection of human Coronavirus 229E in nasal specimens in large scale studies using an RT-PCR hybridization assay. *Mol Cell Probes*, **18**, 75–80.

Van den Born, E., Gultyaev, A.P. and Snijder, E.J. 2004. Secondary structure and function of the 5′-proximal region of the equine arteritis virus RNA genome. *RNA*, **10**, 424–37.

van der Hoek, L., Pyrc, K., et al. 2004. Identification of a new human coronavirus. *Nat Med*, **10**, 368–73.

van der Meer, Y., van Tol, H., et al. 1998. ORF1a-encoded replicase subunits are involved in the membrane association of the arterivirus replication complex. *J Virol*, **72**, 6689–98.

van der Most, R.G. and Spaan, W.J.M. 1995. Coronavirus replication, transcription, and RNA recombination. In: Siddell, S.G. (ed.), *The Coronaviridae*. New York: Plenum Press, 11–31.

van Dinten, L.C., den Boon, J.A., et al. 1997. An infectious arterivirus cDNA clone: identification of a replicase point mutation that abolishes discontinuous mRNA transcription. *Proc Natl Acad Sci USA*, **94**, 991–6.

van Dinten, L.C., van Tol, H., et al. 2000. The predicted metal-binding region of the arterivirus helicase protein is involved in subgenomic mRNA synthesis, genome replication, and virion biogenesis. *J Virol*, **74**, 5213–23.

van Elden, L.J., van Loon, A.M., et al. 2004. Frequent detection of human coronaviruses in clinical specimens from patients with respiratory tract infection by use of a novel real-time reverse-transcriptase polymerase chain reaction. *J Infect Dis*, **189**, 652–7.

van Marle, G., Dobbe, J.C., et al. 1999a. Arterivirus discontinuous mRNA transcription is guided by base pairing between sense and antisense transcription-regulating sequences. *Proc Natl Acad Sci USA*, **96**, 12056–61.

van Marle, G., van Dinten, L.C., et al. 1999b. Characterization of an equine arteritis virus replicase mutant defective in subgenomic mRNA synthesis. *J Virol*, **73**, 5274–81.

van Nieuwstadt, A.P., Meulenberg, J.J., et al. 1996. Proteins encoded by open reading frames 3 and 4 of the genome of Lelystad virus (Arteriviridae) are structural proteins of the virion. *J Virol*, **70**, 4767–72.

van Vliet, A.L., Smits, S.L., et al. 2002. Discontinuous and non-discontinuous subgenomic RNA transcription in a nidovirus. *EMBO J*, **21**, 6571–80.

Vanderheijden, N., Delputte, P.L., et al. 2003. Involvement of sialoadhesin in entry of porcine reproductive and respiratory syndrome virus into porcine alveolar macrophages. *J Virol*, **77**, 8207–15.

Van-Woensel, P., Van-der-Wouw, J. and Visser, N. 1994. Detection of porcine reproductive respiratory syndrome virus by the polymerase chain reaction. *J Virol Methods*, **47**, 273–8.

Vennema, H., Godeke, G.J., et al. 1996. Nucleocapsid-independent assembly of coronavirus-like particles by co-expression of viral envelope protein genes. *EMBO J*, **15**, 2020–8.

Vennema, H., Poland, A., et al. 1998. Feline infectious peritonitis viruses arise by mutation from endemic feline enteric coronaviruses. *Virology*, **243**, 150–7.

Verheije, M.H., Welting, T.J., et al. 2002a. Chimeric arteriviruses generated by swapping of the M protein ectodomain rule out a role of this domain in viral targeting. *Virology*, **303**, 364–73.

Verheije, M.H., Olsthoorn, R.C., et al. 2002b. Kissing interaction between 3′ noncoding and coding sequences is essential for porcine arterivirus RNA replication. *J Virol*, **76**, 1521–6.

Verheije, M.H., Kroese, M.V., et al. 2003. Safety and protective efficacy of porcine reproductive and respiratory syndrome recombinant virus vaccines in young pigs. *Vaccine*, **21**, 2556–63.

Vlasak, R., Luytjes, W., et al. 1988. The E3 protein of bovine coronavirus is a receptor-destroying enzyme with acetylesterase activity. *J Virol*, **62**, 4686–90.

Wang, C.H., Hong, C.C. and Seak, J.C. 2002. An ELISA for antibodies against infectious bronchitis virus using an S1 spike polypeptide. *Vet Microbiol*, **85**, 333–42.

Wassenaar, A.L., Spaan, W.J., et al. 1997. Alternative proteolytic processing of the arterivirus replicase ORF1a polyprotein: evidence that NSP2 acts as a cofactor for the NSP4 serine protease. *J Virol*, **71**, 9313–22.

Weiss, M., Steck, F., et al. 1984. Antibodies to Berne virus in horses and other animals. *Vet Microbiol*, **9**, 523–31.

Wentworth, D.E., Gillim-Ross, L., et al. 2004. Mice susceptible to SARS coronavirus. *Emerg Infect Dis*, **10**, 1293–6.

Wieringa, R., de Vries, A.A., et al. 2002. Characterization of two new structural glycoproteins, GP(3) and GP(4), of equine arteritis virus. *J Virol*, **76**, 10829–40.

Wieringa, R., de Vries, A.A. and Rottier, P.J. 2003a. Formation of disulfide-linked complexes between the three minor envelope glycoproteins (GP2b, GP3, and GP4) of equine arteritis virus. *J Virol*, **77**, 6216–26.

Wieringa, R., de Vries, A.A., et al. 2003b. Intra- and intermolecular disulfide bonds of the GP2b glycoprotein of equine arteritis virus: relevance for virus assembly and infectivity. *J Virol*, **77**, 12996–3004.

Wieringa, R., de Vries, A.A.F., et al. 2004. Structural protein requirements in equine arteritis virus assembly. *J Virol*, **78**, 13019–27.

Wilson, L., McKinlay, C., et al. 2004. SARS coronavirus E protein forms cation-selective ion channels. *Virology*, **330**, 322–31.

Wissink, E.H., van Wijk, H.A., et al. 2003. The major envelope protein, GP5, of a European porcine reproductive and respiratory syndrome virus contains a neutralization epitope in its N-terminal ectodomain. *J Gen Virol*, **84**, 1535–43.

Woo, P.C., Lau, S.K., et al. 2005. Characterization and complete genome sequence of a novel coronavirus, coronavirus HKU1, from patients with pneumonia. *J Virol*, **79**, 884–95.

Woode, G.N., Reed, D.E., et al. 1982. Studies with an unclassified virus isolated from diarrheic calves. *Vet Microbiol*, **7**, 221–40.

Wootton, S.K. and Yoo, D. 2003. Homo-oligomerization of the porcine reproductive and respiratory syndrome virus nucleocapsid protein and the role of disulfide linkages. *J Virol*, **77**, 4546–57.

Wu, C.Y., Jan, J.T., et al. 2004. Small molecules targeting severe acute respiratory syndrome human coronavirus. *Proc Natl Acad Sci USA*, **101**, 10012–17.

Wu, W.H., Fang, Y., et al. 2001. A 10-kDa structural protein of porcine reproductive and respiratory syndrome virus encoded by ORF2b. *Virology*, **287**, 183–91.

Xiao, Z., Batista, L., et al. 2004. The level of virus-specific T-cell and macrophage recruitment in porcine reproductive and respiratory syndrome virus infection in pigs is independent of virus load. *J Virol*, **78**, 5923–33.

Xu, X., Liu, Y., et al. 2003. Molecular model of SARS coronavirus polymerase: implications for biochemical functions and drug design. *Nucleic Acids Res*, **31**, 7117–30.

Xu, Y., Liu, Y., et al. 2004a. Structural basis for coronavirus-mediated membrane fusion. Crystal structure of mouse hepatitis virus spike protein fusion core. *J Biol Chem*, **279**, 30514–22.

Xu, Y., Lou, Z., et al. 2004b. Crystal structure of severe acute respiratory syndrome coronavirus spike protein fusion core. *J Biol Chem*, **279**, 49414–19.

Yang, H., Yang, M., et al. 2003. The crystal structures of severe acute respiratory syndrome virus main protease and its complex with an inhibitor. *Proc Natl Acad Sci USA*, **100**, 13190–5.

Yang, Z.Y., Huang, Y., et al. 2004a. pH-dependent entry of severe acute respiratory syndrome coronavirus is mediated by the spike glycoprotein and enhanced by dendritic cell transfer through DC-SIGN. *J Virol*, **78**, 5642–50.

Yang, Z.Y., Kong, W.P., et al. 2004b. A DNA vaccine induces SARS coronavirus neutralization and protective immunity in mice. *Nature*, **428**, 561–4.

Ye, R., Montalto-Morrison, C. and Masters, P.S. 2004. Genetic analysis of determinants for spike glycoprotein assembly into murine coronavirus virions: distinct roles for charge-rich and cysteine-rich regions of the endodomain. *J Virol*, **78**, 9904–17.

Yeager, C.L., Ashmun, R.A., et al. 1992. Human aminopeptidase N is a receptor for human coronavirus 229E. *Nature*, **357**, 420–2.

Yokomori, K. and Lai, M.M. 1991. Mouse hepatitis virus S RNA sequence reveals that nonstructural proteins ns4 and ns5a are not essential for murine coronavirus replication. *J Virol*, **65**, 5605–8.

Yoo, D., Graham, F.L., et al. 1992. Synthesis and processing of the haemagglutinin-esterase glycoprotein of bovine coronavirus encoded in the E3 region of adenovirus. *J Gen Virol*, **73**, 2591–600.

Yount, B., Curtis, K.M. and Baric, R.S. 2000. Strategy for systematic assembly of large RNA and DNA genomes: transmissible gastroenteritis virus model. *J Virol*, **74**, 10600–11.

Yount, B., Denison, M.R., et al. 2002. Systematic assembly of a full-length infectious cDNA of mouse hepatitis virus strain A59. *J Virol*, **76**, 11065–78.

Yount, B., Curtis, K.M., et al. 2003. Reverse genetics with a full-length infectious cDNA of severe acute respiratory syndrome coronavirus. *Proc Natl Acad Sci USA*, **100**, 12995–3000.

Yu, C.J., Chen, Y.C., et al. 2004. Identification of a novel protein 3a from severe acute respiratory syndrome coronavirus. *FEBS Lett*, **565**, 111–16.

Yu, W. and Leibowitz, J.L. 1995. Specific binding of host cellular proteins to multiple sites within the 3′ end of mouse hepatitis virus genomic RNA. *J Virol*, **69**, 2016–23.

Yu, X., Bi, W., et al. 1994. Mouse hepatitis virus gene 5b protein is a new virion envelope protein. *Virology*, **202**, 1018–23.

Zeng, R., Yang, R.F., et al. 2004. Characterization of the 3a protein of SARS-associated coronavirus in infected vero E6 cells and SARS patients. *J Mol Biol*, **341**, 271–9.

Zevenhoven-Dobbe, J.C., Greve, S., et al. 2004. Rescue of disabled single cycle (DISC) equine arteritis virus using complementing cell lines that express minor structural proteins. *J Gen Virol*, **85**, 3709–14.

Zhang, H., Wang, G., et al. 2004a. Identification of an antigenic determinant on the S2 domain of the severe acute respiratory syndrome coronavirus spike glycoprotein capable of inducing neutralizing antibodies. *J Virol*, **78**, 6938–45.

Zhang, X. and Lai, M.M. 1995. Interactions between the cytoplasmic proteins and the intergenic (promoter) sequence of mouse hepatitis virus RNA: correlation with the amounts of subgenomic mRNA transcribed. *J Virol*, **69**, 1637–44.

Zhang, X.M., Herbst, W., et al. 1994. Biological and genetic characterization of a hemagglutinating coronavirus isolated from a diarrhoeic child. *J Med Virol*, **44**, 152–61.

Zhang, Y., Li, J., et al. 2004b. Analysis of serum cytokines in patients with severe acute respiratory syndrome. *Infect Immun*, **72**, 4410–15.

Zheng, B.J., Wong, K.H., et al. 2004. SARS-related virus predating SARS outbreak, Hong Kong. *Emerg Infect Dis*, **10**, 176–8.

Zhou, T., Wang, H., et al. 2004. An exposed domain in the severe acute respiratory syndrome coronavirus spike protein induces neutralizing antibodies. *J Virol*, **78**, 7217–26.

Ziebuhr, J. 2004a. The coronavirus replicase. *Curr Topics Microbiol Immunol*, **287**, 57–94.

Ziebuhr, J. 2004b. Molecular biology of severe acute respiratory syndrome coronavirus. *Curr Opin Microbiol*, **7**, 412–19.

Ziebuhr, J., Herold, J. and Siddell, S.G. 1995. Characterization of a human coronavirus (strain 229E) 3C-like proteinase activity. *J Virol*, **69**, 4331–8.

Ziebuhr, J., Heusipp, G. and Siddell, S.G. 1997. Biosynthesis, purification, and characterization of the human coronavirus 229E 3C-like proteinase. *J Virol*, **71**, 3992–7.

Ziebuhr, J., Snijder, E.J. and Gorbalenya, A.E. 2000. Virus-encoded proteinases and proteolytic processing in the Nidovirales. *J Gen Virol*, **81**, 853–79.

Ziebuhr, J., Thiel, V. and Gorbalenya, A.E. 2001. The autocatalytic release of a putative RNA virus transcription factor from its polyprotein precursor involves two paralogous papain-like proteases that cleave the same peptide bond. *J Biol Chem*, **276**, 33220–32.

Ziebuhr, J., Bayer, S., et al. 2003. The 3C-like proteinase of an invertebrate nidovirus links coronavirus and potyvirus homologs. *J Virol*, **77**, 1415–26.

Zuniga, S., Sola, I., et al. 2004. Sequence motifs involved in the regulation of discontinuous coronavirus subgenomic RNA synthesis. *J Virol*, **78**, 980–94.

Index

Notes

(Fig.) and (Tab.) refer to figures and tables respectively. *vs.* indicates a comparison or differential diagnosis.
To save space in the index, the following abbreviations have been used:
EBV - Epstein–Barr virus
HCMV - Human cytomegalovirus
HHV - human herpesvirus
HIV - human immunodeficiency virus
HPV - human papillomavirus
HSV - herpes simplex virus
HTLV - Human T-cell leukemia (lymphotrophic) virus
IL- interleukin
LCMV - Lymphocytic choriomeningitis virus
MHC - major histocompatibility complex
SV40 - Simian virus 40
VZV - varicella-zoster virus

Complete table of contents for *Topley & Wilson's Microbiology and Microbial Infections*

VIROLOGY, VOLUMES 1 AND 2

BACTERIOLOGY, VOLUMES 1 AND 2

MEDICAL MYCOLOGY

PARASITOLOGY

IMMUNOLOGY